W9-BPS-528

MENDELIAN INHERITANCE IN MAN

MENDELIAN INHERITANCE IN MAN

CATALOGS OF AUTOSOMAL DOMINANT, AUTOSOMAL RECESSIVE, AND X-LINKED PHENOTYPES

FOURTH EDITION

Victor A. McKusick, M.D.

The Johns Hopkins University Press

Baltimore and London

To my wife, Dr. Anne B. McKusick

Copyright © 1966, 1968, 1971, 1975 by The Johns Hopkins University Press
All rights reserved. No part of this book may be reproduced or transmitted
in any form or by any means, electronic or mechanical, including photocopying,
recording, xerography, or any information storage and retrieval system,
without permission in writing from the publisher.
Manufactured in the United States of America

The Johns Hopkins University Press, Baltimore, Maryland 21218
The Johns Hopkins University Press Ltd., London

Library of Congress Catalog Card Number 73-19636
ISBN 0-8018-1593-2

Originally published, 1966
Second edition, 1968
Third edition, 1971
Fourth edition, 1975

Library of Congress Cataloging in Publication data
will be found on the last printed page of this book.

CONTENTS

ON THE USE OF THE CATALOGS

In each of the three catalogs the entries are arranged alphabetically according to preferred designation. The entries in the dominant catalog are numbered consecutively beginning with number 10010. The numbers of entries in the recessive catalog begin with 20010. Those in the X-linkage catalog begin with 30010. Beginning with the third edition, a five-digit numbering system has been used. Numbers 1 through 9 for the terminal digit were left to accommodate future growth of the catalogs. Some geneticists expressed a desire to use the numbering system of these catalogs in diagnostic and bibliographic filing and were distressed by the change in numbering between the first and second editions. Having permanence in the numbering system has in several ways proved a boon to the maintenance of the catalogs.

In the subject index not only the preferred designation but also alternative designations and particularly conspicuous or distinctive phenotypic features are listed. The author index is provided as an aid in finding a condition whose position in the catalogs is uncertain; the searcher may, for example, recall that Dr. So-and-So described a particular unusual syndrome, but he may not know the designation under which it is entered.

The words "dominant," "recessive," and "X-linked," situated vertically at the margin of each page, are intended to serve as a quick guide for finding the desired section of the book.

An asterisk preceding an entry indicates that the particular mode of inheritance is considered quite certain. In the case of those without an asterisk, suggestions of the particular mode of inheritance are strong enough to warrant inclusion for heuristic purposes. Sometimes an asterisk has been omitted because of a strong suspicion that the entry represents a mutation allelic to another already asterisked. The aim is to provide one asterisked entry per locus. Thus, there are two reasons entries may be "in limbo": uncertainty about the particular mode of inheritance (or indeed, whether it is Mendelian) or uncertainty whether the given phenotype is nonallelic to another already asterisked. These are in the main mutually exclusive criteria.

Beginning with this fourth edition, upper case and lower case letters are being used. The computerization of the materials, however, places some limitations on the typography. (These limitations will, it is planned, be removed in future editions.) The oblique (/) is not available (but not often required). More serious deficiencies are the lack of special characters from foreign languages, such as the German umlaut and the French acute and grave accents. With this edition, ae, oe, and ue have been substituted for the German ä, ö, and ü, in most instances. Greek letters have been written out (for example, γ = gamma, δ = delta, and so on). Genetic notation (particularly superscripts) used in connection with blood groups and serum protein types also presented difficulty. As a rule, superscripts and subscripts have been placed in parentheses. For example, Xg^a = Xg(a) and Hb M_{Boston} = Hb M(Boston). Sometimes subscripts, especially when used to indicate isozymes, have been indicated by a hyphen, e.g., phosphoglucomutase-1. Italicization, often used, for example, in gene symbols in the genetic literature, is not available.

Q.v., an abbreviation used frequently in these catalogs, means *quod vide* "which see." In references, (NI) means "no initials given in the publication referenced."

The nosologic and other tables were a new feature of the third edition. They have been extended in this edition and should prove a useful guide to nosology in the areas covered. Also included is a table which purports to give an exhaustive listing of identified specific enzyme deficiencies. The information on the human chromosome map aims to keep abreast of this rapidly moving field. For other tables see HEMOGLOBIN in the dominant catalog.

FOREWORD

Background

These catalogs had their inception in 1960 when, in connection with an inquiry into the genetics of the X chromosome, it seemed desirable to examine the question "What genetic information is carried by the X chromosome of man?" The catalog of X-linked traits in man was first published in 1962 (McKusick, 1962). Two categories of traits were included: those for which X-linkage was considered proved and those for which the evidence was in various degrees suggestive but not conclusive. All traits, rare and common, were included.

In 1962 a study of genetic disorders in Old Order Amish communities was initiated. The question then arose, "What rare recessive disorders might one expect to encounter in inbred groups such as these?" Inbred populations afford an opportunity to detect "new" recessive phenotypes in man. A catalog of known recessive phenotypes would obviously be useful in recognizing these. The catalog was confined mainly to rare phenotypes, that is, those that in outbred populations have a homozygote frequency of 1 in 1,000 or less.

By 1963 the complexity of the catalog of recessives prompted adoption of computer methods for assembling, revising, and indexing.

In 1964 a catalog of dominant phenotypes was undertaken—with some hesitation because of the magnitude of the undertaking and the questionable status of a large number of traits for which "dominant inheritance with incomplete penetrance" had been suggested. Again, the catalog was confined mainly to uncommon traits. "Uncommon," however, was not precisely defined, so that some morphologic traits were included, as were anomalous hemoglobins, red cell antigenic types, leukocyte types, and serum protein types—co-dominant traits.

Organization

As in the original catalog of X-linked traits, two classes of entries have been made in each of the three catalogs. In the case of those marked with an asterisk, the particular mode of inheritance is, in the writer's opinion, quite certain, according to the criteria outlined below. In the case of the others, the evidence for the particular mode of inheritance is judged to be incomplete, yet sufficiently strong to warrant inclusion. It is considered important that these less certain items be included so that further families will be studied as they come to attention. Some of the instances with no asterisk are so classified, not because the mode of inheritance is not established, but because it is not clear that the given phenotype is distinct from that described in another entry or it is not certain that a locus distinct from one already asterisked is represented. An attempt has been made to give only one entry per locus.

Each entry consists of three parts: (1) a preferred designation (and sometimes frequently used synonyms); (2) a brief description of the phenotype, with a résumé of genetic information; and (3) key references. An attempt has been made to select references which are up to date and/or include particularly useful discussions of the genetics. The catalogs must be considered primarily a bibliographic guide. The discussion of each entry is necessarily brief. There are 10,197 references, mainly to the periodical literature, and 14,001 authors cited.

Two indices are provided. The author index is intended to help the reader find a particular entry. He may remember that Dr. So-and-so reported an unusual familial disorder about such-and-such a year but have no way of knowing under what title I have entered it. The author index will help him locate the appropriate title. The title index includes alternative designations and major symptoms or other features which do not appear in the title.

Included in the front material (pp. xxixff.) are nosologic and other tables, which, it is hoped, will enhance the usefulness of the catalogs.

Criteria

The definitions of *dominant* and *recessive* used in the preparation of these catalogs are those given by Mendel, who introduced the terms: "Those characters which are transmitted entire, or almost unchanged in the hybridization, and therefore in themselves constitute the characters of the hybrid, are termed the dominant, and those which become latent in the process recessive." Following Mendel, care has been taken always to use the terms *dominant* and *recessive* as attributes of a character—that is, a phenotype— and to have a specified phenotype in mind. The question, then, is whether the specific phenotype is observed in the heterozygote or only in the homozygote. Depending on the answer, the specifically defined trait is considered dominant or recessive, respectively.

Many of the phenotypes for which a particular mode of inheritance is indicated as proved might not meet criteria that experimental geneticists would be likely to lay down. A rare phenotype transmitted through several successive generations in a family without consanguinity, affecting both males and females and transmitted by both males and females, with male-to-male transmission, is considered autosomal dominant. When most of the cases are sporadic and few affected persons reproduce because of the gravity of the condition, the possibility that the nonfamilial cases represent the result of a new dominant mutation is supported by the finding of elevated mean paternal age (for example, Apert syndrome and fibrodysplasia ossificans progressiva).

In the case of a rare phenotype affecting brothers and sisters with normal parents but with instances of parental consanguinity, recessive inheritance has usually been considered very likely. In a "founder population" like the Amish, the ability to trace the ancestry of both parents in all cases back to a single common ancestral couple lends support to the recessive hypothesis. If the phenotype has been shown to result from an enzyme deficiency and especially if both parents show a partial deficiency, autosomal recessive inheritance is considered proved. In the case of oroticaciduria (25890), this judgment was made even when only one homozygote had been observed.

Pedigrees showing multiple affected males in two or more sibships connected through females were taken as evidence of X-linked recessive inheritance. When only males were affected by an enzyme deficiency and the mother (but not the father) showed an intermediate level of enzyme activity, X-linked recessive inheritance was considered highly probable. Pedigrees revealing a pattern in which all daughters but no sons among the offspring of affected males were affected were taken as evidence of X-linked dominant inheritance. X-linked dominant traits may be mistakenly labelled autosomal dominant, and in early stages, when only a few cases are known, X-linked recessive inheritance may suggest autosomal recessive inheritance. The difficulties of distinguishing X-linked inheritance from male-limited autosomal dominant inheritance (when affected males do not reproduce) are illustrated by disorders such as the testicular feminization syndrome (31370). This disorder also illustrates a method for proving X-linkage: the cloning of two populations of cells from fibroblast cultures derived from heterozygous females. One asterisked entry in the X-linkage catalog (31435) was made on the basis of studies of somatic cell hybrids. X-linkage of the seemingly homologous locus in another mammal was taken as supporting evidence of X-linkage in man, based on Ohno's Law of the Evolutionary Conservatism of the X chromosome (see p. lxxv). Thus, testicular feminization in man was considered X-linked when the homologous disorder in the mouse was shown to be X-linked.

Mendelism can be simulated by numerous mechanisms. Multifactorial inheritance is one (Edwards, 1960). Chromosomal aberrations undetectable by present methods are another. Many instances are now known in which, because a parent carries a "balanced" chromosomal rearrangement, two or more offspring suffer from a deficiency or excess of chromosomal material. Surely, some familial chromosomal rearrangements are beyond our present capacity for detection.

SC disease, as well as S-thal and E-thal diseases, is interesting because a characteristic phenotype is present which differs from that resulting from the homozygous state of either gene. In terms of the Mendelian definition of *dominant* and *recessive*, these phenotypes cannot be classified as either. There may be some conditions listed in the recessive catalog (because they occur in multiple sibs with normal parents) which, when the precise situation is known, will be found to be caused by two different mutant alleles (known as genetic compound or compound heterozygote, *not* double heterozygote). This form of disease should not show increased parental consanguinity (Haldane, 1938).

In dealing with recessives, especially when the parents are known to be related, the question sometimes arises whether two manifestations constitute a syndrome produced by the homozygous state of one mutant gene or, alternatively, whether homozygosity at two separate but perhaps linked loci, one for each manifestation, is involved. It is possible that some of the rare syndromes which appear as unasterisked entries in the recessive catalog represent the latter phenomenon.

Women with phenylketonuria may have several mentally retarded offspring apparently because of ill-effects of high phenylalanine concentrations on the fetal brain. This is a form of familial and genetic disease based on the genotype of the mother rather than on that of the affected individual. Breast-feeding hyperbilirubinemia (23790) is another human example, and "lethal milk" is an example in mice (Dickie *et al.*, 1969). It is to be recalled that, before its serologic basis was discovered, erythroblastosis fetalis was thought by some to be a Mendelizing disorder (Macklin, 1937). Congenital infection (for example, toxoplasmosis, listerellosis, rubella, cytomegalovirus disease, and of course, syphilis) can affect multiple sibs. The rubella virus acquired *in utero* is known to persist for several years after birth, and at least one instance is known of a rubella-damaged woman giving birth to a rubella-damaged infant (Menser *et al.*, 1968).

The phenotypic simulation of Mendelian disorders by fetal infections is an example of phenocopy. The converse also occurs. We (McKusick *et al.*, 1966) have observed a recessive syndrome of microcephaly and chorioretinopathy which rather precisely mimics toxoplasmosis. Goldberg and Hardy (1971) studied a family of X-linked cataract in which cytomegalovirus found in the lens of the proband seemed to be the cause of the cataract until a second affected male was born and the mother was found to have sutural cataracts typical of the carrier state. Usher syndrome (pigmentary retinal degeneration and congenital deafness, 27690) rather closely simulates rubella infection. In its cardiovascular aspects, the autosomal dominant type of stenotic arterial disease (18550), of which supravalvular aortic stenosis is a hallmark, closely matches both the hypercalcemia syndrome and rubella infection.

The distinction between genetic disease and slow-virus infection is not always clear-cut; see kuru (24530) and Creutzfeldt-Jakob disease (12340). Both are familial disorders in which a slow virus has been demonstrated by passage to laboratory primates.

Usefulness of the catalogs

For both applied and scientific reasons, I have considered it worthwhile to invest considerable effort in assembling and updating these catalogs. The reasons, in addition to those mentioned in the introduction, include the following:

1. Genetic counseling and the management of hereditary problems demand accurate diagnosis. Because genetic disorders are individually rare, so that most medical geneticists have a personal experience of only a few cases of a given disorder, familiarity with the experience reported in the literature is essential.

2. Genetic disorders give us insight into the normal. These catalogs of hereditary traits are like photographic negatives from which a positive picture of man's genetic constitution can be made. For example, the fact that agammaglobulinemia and classic hemophilia are X-linked disorders tells us that the X chromosome carries loci concerned with the synthesis of gamma globulin and clotting factor VIII. As complete knowledge as possible of the normal genetic constitution of man is bound to be useful in the long run. Physicians have a unique opportunity to contribute to the knowledge of what Richard Lewontin referred to as "man's mutational repertoire."

As mentioned earlier, these catalogs, despite the subtitle, purport to be listings of loci, not phenotypes. When multiple diverse phenotypes are produced by alleles, the locus is entered only once. Undoubtedly, some phenotypes resulting from alleles have been entered unwittingly as representing separate loci. For example, mutations at the beta hemoglobin locus can produce either cyanosis, polycythemia, or anemia (and the last can take any one of several different forms). If the biochemical nature of the mutations were unknown, these mutations might be listed separately in the catalogs. (Sickle cell anemia is listed in the dominant catalog simply because the beta locus is arbitrarily assigned to that catalog.)

The dominant catalog is swelled by arbitrary location there of loci which are definitely identified through chromosome assignment by cell hybridization. The first of these was thymidine kinase (18830). Subsequently, many others have been added to the list, as indicated in the tables on pages lvii ff. Also swelling the list of dominants are loci of structural genes for human polypeptides which have been completely sequenced (Dayhoff, 1972).

Table I presents information on the numerical status of genetic nosology in 1958 and through the successive editions of these catalogs.

TABLE I

Phenotype	Verschuer 1958	These Catalogs			
		1966	1968	1971	1975
Autosomal Dominant	285	269 (+568)	344 (+449)	415 (+528)	583 (+635)
Autosomal Recessive	89	237 (+294)	280 (+349)	365 (+418)	466 (+481)
X-linked	38	68 (+51)	68 (+55)	86 (+64)	93 (+78)
Total	412	574 (+913)	692 (+853)	866 (+1,010)	1,142 (+1,194)
		1,487	1,545	1,876	2,336

The numbers in parentheses relate to nonasterisked entries.

The numbers are of interest from several points of view. The ratio of "proved" autosomal dominants to "proved" autosomal recessives is of note: 583 dominants, 466 recessives. A few years ago the preponderance of dominants was even greater, but advances in biochemical genetics in the last few years have added many new items to the list of recessives, while fewer new dominants have been added. In experimental species, such as the mouse, recessives predominate.[1] This difference between man and mouse is largely the result of a difference in mating patterns. Most "visible" mutations—that is, those which cause phenotypic changes that are evident to the unaided senses—are recessive. In closely mating mice they are likely to become apparent promptly. In outbred man, however, a recessive mutation can occur and the gene be lost, either by chance or because of a disadvantage in the heterozygote, without ever "meeting up with itself" in a homozygote. Or if a homozygote occurs, it may, because of the small size of human families, be an isolated case and may not be recognized as representing a distinct genetic entity.

The catalog of X-linked traits represents the largest number of loci that have been identified on one chromosome in any metazoan, excepting *Drosophila.* Since 93 loci on the X chromosome have been identified, and since the X chromosome represents about 6 percent of the length of the haploid set of autosomes, one would expect that about 1,550 autosomal loci would be known. In fact, only about 1,050 are confidently known. The main deficiency is undoubtedly in the group of recessives. An X-linked recessive behaves as a dominant in the male. It is, for practical purposes, always expressed if the male has the gene. The number of X-linked dominants is close to what one would expect from the number of autosomal dominants and the length of the X chromosome relative to that of the autosomal complement.

The total number of loci[2] identified by these catalogs is a very small portion of the total number of genes. Estimates of the number of genes in man take at least three approaches (Vogel, 1964): (1) From the measured amount of DNA, and assuming a triplet code and 150 amino acids per polypeptide chain, one approach concludes that there is enough DNA to code for about ten million polypeptide chains. Redundancy, now known to be present in the mammalian genome (DNA-RNA hybridization techniques show that 30 percent or more of the DNA exists in multiple copies), greatly reduces this number. It is certain that much of the DNA must serve some function other than coding for the amino acid sequence of proteins. (2) From the relatively extensive information of *E. coli,* another approach concludes that several thousand genes would be required to code for all the proteins of its cell. Given the greater complexity of any multicellular organism—especially man—the number of genes may be one hundred times as great. The total number of genes in man probably is not less than 100,000. Thus the catalogs reveal perhaps only 1 percent of the whole. The number of entries in the catalogs reflects mainly the degree of genetic variability in man and, even more, man's ingenuity and persistence in detecting this variability. (3) From a review of various approaches in *Drosophila,* Bishop (1974) concluded that the organism may have 5,000-6,000 genes. Since man has 15 times as much DNA, one might expect about 100,000 genes in man.

An appreciable homology of genomal organization between man and some of his more closely related fellow animals is demonstrable (McKusick, 1962). The X chromosome has displayed particular stability in evolution, conserving certain loci which it carries in many species, probably because the sex-determining factors scattered through the X chromosome cannot be translocated to autosomes without disruptive effects on

1. Dr. Margaret C. Green (Bar Harbor, Maine, August, 1967) has estimated that in the house mouse the number of known autosomal dominant mutations is 99, autosomal recessives 207, and X-linked 12. In these enumerations the T locus was counted only once and loci for protein variants were counted singly, as dominants. Several recessive mutations known to be present at different loci, but having such closely similar phenotypes that they most likely would not be distinguished in man, were counted separately. Alleles producing phenotypes that were sufficiently different for allelism not to be suspected in the absence of genetic tests were also counted separately. The many histocompatibility loci were not counted.

2. It is likely that some of the phenotypes listed separately here—with the implication that they demonstrate the presence of separate loci—may be determined by mutant genes allelic to the genes for other phenotypes. The opposite error—listing as one locus a phenotype that can be caused by mutation at any one of several different loci—is at least equally likely, however.

reproduction. Attention should be directed constantly to the catalogs of X-linked traits in mice and other nonhuman mammals (see page lxxv), and although homologous linkage relationships in the autosomes are less likely, mouse linkages, such as albinism with the beta hemoglobin locus and transferrin with one malate dehydrogenase locus, should be kept in mind by students of human linkage. Linkage studies in subhuman primates might be particularly illuminating for human genetics.

3. Among the uses to which the catalogs may be put is "deletion-mapping" of the chromosomes. Observation of a specific autosomal recessive disorder in a patient with the *cri du chat* syndrome (deletion of the short arm of chromosome no. 5), for example, would provide evidence on the cartography of the particular genetic locus. Deletion-mapping in man has to date had relatively little success. The assignment of the acid phosphatase locus (17150) to the distal portion of the short arm of chromosome no. 2 by Ferguson-Smith *et al.* (1973) was the first definite example, and this is, of course, a protein polymorphism rather than a rare recessive trait.

4. The mode of inheritance can be a useful guide in the search for the basic defect in genetic disorders. Thanks to the margin of safety with which most enzyme systems are endowed, a gene-determined enzyme deficiency is likely to be reflected in the phenotype only in the homozygote. Contrariwise, when the mutation concerns a nonenzymic protein (for example, a structural protein such as collagen) it is plausible to presume that change in the amino acid sequence might alter the physical properties in such a way as to be reflected in the phenotype, even though only about half of the particular protein is of the mutant type. Almost all inborn errors of metabolism (defined in the strict Garrodian sense) are recessives. I believe one would be wasting his time to look for an enzyme defect in the Marfan syndrome, a dominant disorder. Obviously, there is much more to biochemical genetics than merely the determination of the amino acid sequence of proteins and the matter of whether these proteins are enzymes or not. Some genes determine enzymes that effect changes in the structure of nonenzymic proteins—for example, hydroxylate lysine in collagen. Mutation in such a gene results in a structural change in a nonenzymic protein and behaves as a recessive (cf. 22540). Speculation here about the existence in man of genetic control mechanisms of the Jacob-Monod type and about the genetic behavior to be expected of mutations therein would be useless. Nonetheless, the generalization stated above is probably true. In recessive disorders, an enzyme defect, or a defect in a peptide hormone such as growth hormone (see 26240), should be sought. In dominant disorders, abnormality in a nonenzymic protein is more likely. Theoretically, change in the specificity of an enzyme might be the result of mutation, so that it acts on a substrate it ordinarily would not touch. The enzymatic disorder resulting from such a mutation might behave as a dominant (Kirkman, 1970). For discussion of two dominant disorders whose biochemical bases are now known, see GOUT DUE TO INCREASED PRPP ACTIVITY (13984) and HYPERLIPOPROTEINEMIA, TYPE II (14440). In bacteria, "noninducible" mutations involve a change in a repressor such that its affinity for an inducer substance is lost and repression is maintained. Again, the enzymic deficiency would be expected to behave as a dominant.

In over 140 of the nearly 500 certain recessives, an enzyme deficiency has been demonstrated. This has been achieved since 1948 when the enzyme defect in methemoglobinemia (25080) was discovered and since 1952 when the Doctors Cori demonstrated deficiency of glucose-1-phosphatase in von Gierke disease (23220). The demonstration of enzyme deficiency has contributed to the list of confirmed recessives, since as mentioned earlier (pp. x ff.) complete deficiency in the offspring and intermediate levels in both parents is good evidence of recessive inheritance.

Heterogeneity and affinity ("splitting and lumping")

In the assembling of these three catalogs, consideration was necessarily constantly given to heterogeneity (Childs and Der Kaloustian, 1968), which is often discovered when a genetic disorder is examined closely; what at first is thought to be one entity is found to be several clinically similar (that is, phenotypically similar) but fundamentally (genotypically) distinct disorders (McKusick, 1969).

The principles of genetics force one to think of mutation as a *specific* etiologic mechanism which results in a *specific* disease entity. In 1930 Knut Faber, professor of medicine in Copenhagen, produced a monograph entitled *Nosography*, in which he traced the development of understanding of the classification of disease. To Gregor Mendel's principles he assigned a leading role in directing thought along lines of specific entities. The one other factor of comparable impact was the advent of the bacteriologic era with its focus on specific etiology and specific entities. One has but to recall that it was only a little more than a century ago that in many circles jaundice, dropsy, anemia, fever, and so on, were thought of as entities to realize the influence of bacteriologic and genetic discoveries on the conceptual base of medicine.

In medical genetics there is little place for expressions such as "spectrum of disease," "disease A is a mild form, or a variant, of disease B," and so on. Disease A and disease B are either the same disease, if they are based on the same mutation or different diseases. Phenotypic overlap is not necessarily grounds for considering them fundamentally the same or even closely related. For example, diagrams purporting to show the interrelationship of neurologic diseases (Myrianthopoulos *et al.*, 1964) are totally meaningless and also useless, except as an indication of phenotypic overlap.

What methods are available for demonstrating the heterogeneity of genetic disease in man? They can be outlined as follows:

I. Genetic Methods
   A. Mode of inheritance—for example, spastic paraplegia occurs in all three major modes (18260, 27080, 31290).
   B. Nonallelism of recessives—for example, parents with phenotypically identical recessive congenital deafness may have all normally hearing children.
   C. Linkage relationships—for example, one form of elliptocytosis is linked to the Rh blood group locus, but at least one other form is not.

II. Analysis of phenotype—for example, the mucopolysaccharidoses I and II are distinguishable by the presence or absence of corneal clouding.

III. Biochemical analysis—for example, hereditary nonspherocytic hemolytic anemia has many different forms each with a different enzyme defect.

IV. Physiological studies—for example, the X-linked hemophilias can be distinguished by mutual cross-correction of the clotting defect.

V. Studies of cells in culture.
   A. For example, the mucopolysaccharidoses are distinguishable by cell-mixing experiments.
   B. For example, cell hybridization studies permit recognition of distinct forms of xeroderma pigmentosum, depending on whether or not the defect in DNA repair disappears in the heterokaryon.

An experience in medical genetics much less frequent than discovery of heterogeneity is demonstration of *affinity*—that is, the discovery that phenotypes which appeared at first to represent separate entities are in fact the result of one and the same genotype. Wilson disease can be present in young patients as an essentially pure hepatic disorder and in older patients as a predominantly neurologic disorder. Familial Mediterranean fever may present the picture of primary amyloidosis without displaying at any time in its course the picture of episodic fever and polyserositis, and the converse may also occur. In man, final proof of genetic identity depends on demonstrating precisely the same chemical change at the molecular level. (See AMAUROSIS CONGENITA OF LEBER, TYPE 1 [20400], for a possible example of genetic affinity. Coffin syndrome and Lowry syndrome are disorders previously thought distinct but now convincingly shown to be one [30360].)

The laboratory, of course, has contributed heavily to the nosology of genetic disease. As mentioned earlier, studies of fibroblasts have confirmed the distinctness of several mucopolysaccharidoses which had been considered separate on other grounds; for example, co-cultivation of fibroblasts from patients with MPS I (Hurler syndrome) and MPS III (Sanfilippo syndrome) results in mutual correction of the metabolic defects. Although MPS I and MPS V (Scheie syndrome) are phenotypically very different, fibroblasts from patients with these two disorders, when grown in mixed culture, do not show cross-correction (Wiesmann and Neufeld, 1970). This may indicate that the responsible genes are alleles (McKusick *et al.*, 1972). The mutation may be in the same codon or in different codons of the particular cistron. The terms *euallele* and *heteroallele* can be used for these two situations, respectively, (Serra, 1965). Some of the patients with difficult-to-classify disturbances of mucopolysaccharide metabolism may be genetic compounds (compound heterozygotes, allozygotes, mixed heterozygotes) having, for example, the Hurler gene on one chromosome and the Scheie allele on the other. Other examples of phenotypic diversity resulting from allelic series and genetic compounds are given on pp. liiiff. (McKusick, 1973). If there is any place for use of the expression "variant of," etc., it is in relation to these allelic disorders.

Molecular genetics and the catalogs

A leading objective of medical genetics is to describe the defect in each disorder in as precise chemical terms as has been possible in many of the hemoglobinopathies. The catalogs provide a listing of all hemoglobin variants together with an indication of the amino acid substitution when known. As similarly detailed information becomes available on the variants of glucose-6-phosphate dehydrogenase, transferrins, and other polymorphic proteins, comprehensive cataloguing of these will probably be undertaken.

Genetics has been defined as the science of variation. Classically, without variation in a character, there could be no genetics. Molecular genetics and the development of new techniques in human genetics have to some extent removed the limitation. For example, interspecies cell hybridization permits study of the linkage relationships and chromosomal position of gene loci in man, even though no allelic variation at those loci is known. Assignment of the thymidine kinase locus to chromosome no. 17 was the first example, and there are now many more as outlined on p. lviiff. All loci positioned by study of somatic cell hybrids have been listed in the catalog even though no allelic variation in the locus is known in man. The one cistron–one polypeptide principle[3] leads to the conclusion that any well-characterized, unique polypeptide of man is governed by a specific gene. For that reason some polypeptides whose amino acid sequence is known in full are listed in the catalogs.

Other genetic variation

The Y chromosome is not represented in these catalogs. The only firm assignment to the Y chromosome is testis-determining factor(s) (see p. lxv). There may be one or more genes for histocompatibility on the Y chromosome of man (Wachtel *et al.*, 1974). Although Y-linkage may not be completely excluded, "hairy ears" (13950) seems more likely to be autosomal dominant with a strong male influence. There is no evidence, cytologic or genetic, for the existence in man of homologous segments of the X and Y chromosomes, between which crossing-over might occur and on which genes would give pedigree patterns referred to as partial sex linkage.

---

3. The special case of the immunoglobulins, in which more than one cistron appears to determine a single polypeptide (Edelman, 1970), is an exception that tests the rule.

These gene catalogs do not, furthermore, have any information on mitochondrial genes (Kroon and Saccone, 1974) in man, for the simple reason that nothing is known about them. In lower eukaryotes (especially yeasts) there is evidence that mitochondrial DNA codes for three components of cytochrome *c* oxidase, four components of the ATPase complex, one or two components of the cytochrome *b* complex, and a protein necessary for assembly of cytochrome *c*. Hutchison *et al.* (1974) presented evidence that in mammals, as in fungi and amphibia, mitochondrial DNA is derived solely from the mother.

Disorders and traits of multifactorial inheritance, for which empiric recurrence estimates are appropriate, are also not within the province of this book. Nor are the chromosomal aberrations of the relatively gross type demonstrable by means of existing methods, even the familial chromosomal variations that are essentially "Mendelizing." Chromosomal variation is being catalogued and computerized by Dr. D. S. Borgaonkar (1975), Department of Medicine, The Johns Hopkins University School of Medicine, using methods similar to those used in this catalog of Mendelian variation.

A caveat may be necessary for the genetically naive. The inclusion of an entry does not mean that the phenotype in question is always Mendelian. See, for example, VOLVULUS OF MIDGUT (19325); it would be absurd to conclude that wherever this phenotype occurs it is on the basis of autosomal recessive inheritance. To reduce this potential confusion somewhat, I have used "X-linked" in connection with the designation for the form of ichthyosis, mental retardation, cleft palate, hydrocephalus, etc., that has that mode of inheritance.

Some arbitrariness has been exercised as to which catalog carries a particular entry. Sickle cell anemia is recessive, but no entry for it appears in the recessive catalog inasmuch as an entry for the beta hemoglobin locus is in the dominant catalog. Alpha-1-antitrypsin deficiency does not appear in the recessive catalog because the alpha-1-antitrypsin locus is represented in the dominant catalog. There are several examples of enzymes which might be listed either in the dominant catalog because of polymorphism or in the recessive catalog because of deficiency.

Terminology

The terminology related to many genetic disorders presents difficulties, especially when the basic defect is unknown. The naming of syndromes is a rather helter-skelter, hit-or-miss process. Like all language, the naming of syndromes evolves; preferences are a matter of usage. Although personal bias has inevitably played a role in the choice of terms used here, I have attempted to use the most generally encountered term.

Optimally, the name for a genetic trait or disorder should have some relation to the basic defect, but, as I have said, this is often unknown. At least the name should be euphonious. It should be imaginative, in the sense that it should conjure up an *image* of the phenotype; that is, it should be mnemonic. It should also be appropriate for transmittal to patients. Tongue twisters and possibly embarrassing terms such as gargoylism are not acceptable. Some seven methods of naming have been used.

1) Eponyms are, improperly I think, maligned in some quarters. Admittedly, they should be used sparingly. Many, such as Ehlers-Danlos, Ellis-van Creveld, Marfan, Pelizaeus-Merzbacher, are too well established to be avoided, and in addition, no satisfactory noneponymic designation is available.

Most eponyms are physicians' names, but not all. I remind you of Hartnup and Byler diseases, which were named for patients. The virtue of eponyms is that they convey no preconceived notions as to the mechanism of the abnormality. The Hurler syndrome was, history showed (McKusick, 1972), a better designation than lipochondrodystrophy, which was long used by *Index Medicus*. As a rule, the possessive form of eponyms has *not* been used; for example, the Marfan syndrome, not Marfan's syndrome, will be found in the catalogs. The reason is that the eponym is merely a "handle"; often the man whose name is used was not the first to describe the condition or did not describe the full syndrome as it has subsequently become known. (Agreeing with Emerson that "consistency is the hobgoblin of little minds," I have retained in other writings of mine "Wilson's disease" and "Down's syndrome" and some other terms of which the nonpossessive form seems awkward to the tongue.) The nonpossessive form of eponyms is recommended by the latest edition (4th, 1971) of *Current Medical Information and Terminology.*

2) An unrecommended method of naming makes use of the first letter of the name of the family or families in which the disorder was first observed. Dr. John Opitz of Madison, Wisconsin, has been the main proponent of this system. His G syndrome (30700), BBB syndrome (31360), and SC syndrome (26900) are examples.

3) Another method is to pick out one striking feature, e.g., the whistling face syndrome (19370). Arachnodactyly was an early synonym for the Marfan syndrome but an unsatisfactory one because it is not an impressive feature of some bona fide cases and, in addition, occurs in many other conditions.

4) A fourth method constructs acronyms such as TAR syndrome (27400) and VATER association (19235) or combines the initials of features as in EMG syndrome (22560) and OFD syndrome (31120, 25210). These systems have mnemonic usefulness.

5) Geographic names for genetic disorders include familial Mediterranean fever (24910) and the Indiana (10490) and Portuguese (10480) varieties of amyloidosis. The Amsterdam type of malformation syndrome is now more commonly known as the Cornelia de Lange syndrome (21790). Thalassemia is essentially a geographic term. Geographic terms are inevitably ethnic as well—for example, the African type of G6PD deficiency.

6) A numbering system has been used in connection with the glycogenoses, the hyperlipoproteinemias, and the mucopolysaccharidoses. It has been particularly useful in connection with the last group of disorders. It is also used to differentiate the different forms of the orofaciodigital syndrome—OFD I (31120) and OFD II (25210).

7) In some cases the nature of the basic defect is used in the name, especially when it lends itself to easy typography and speaking. G6PD deficiency (glucose-6-phosphate dehydrogenase deficiency) is a successful example. Factor VIII deficiency is a synonym for hemophilia A.

There is little rhyme or reason to the use of *disorder, disease, syndrome,* and *anomaly. Disease* often has unhappy connotations to the layman; *disorder* or *syndrome* is more satisfactory.

Some inconsistency will be found in the use of designations such as valinemia or hypervalinemia, lysinemia or hyperlysinemia, methylmalonicaciduria or hypermethyl-malonicacidemia, and so on. It is hoped that the subject index is sufficiently exhaustive (with a full range of alternative designations indexed) for particular disorders to be found without difficulty, regardless of what designation I have used. Preferred designations have changed some with successive editions, even for conditions for which the defect remains obscure. Usage is the important consideration, as in all language. An example is cystic fibrosis of the pancreas, now generally known simply as *cystic fibrosis,* the designation used here. An attempt has been made in all instances to keep up with usage in nomenclature. The Noonan syndrome has become the preferred term for what was previously known as male Turner syndrome, female pseudo-Turner syndrome, Turner phenotype with normal karyotype, pterygium colli syndrome, Bonnevie-Ullrich syndrome, and so on. The naming of polymorphic enzymes has likewise evolved. For example, what was first called tetrazolium oxidase was termed indophenoloxidase by later workers and has now become most often known as superoxide dismutase.

To an increasing extent, the designation for an entry has been made the name of the enzyme or other gene product. For example, the entry entitled *LESCH-NYHAN*

SYNDROME in earlier editions has acquired the heading *HYPOXANTHINE GUANINE PHOSPHORIBOSYLTRANSFERASE*. Efforts have been made to conform to the recommendations of the Enzyme Commission (Florkin and Stotz, 1973). In future editions I expect to include the Enzyme Commission number for each enzyme; only a few have been included in this edition.

As mentioned earlier, a desideratum in nomenclature is terminology based on the nature of the fundamental defect. Mendelian disorders potentially lend themselves particularly well to precision in nomenclature. In the year 2084, for example, the "compleat" medical geneticist will probably be able to look at the phenotype and at the laboratory data and come up with a diagnostic label that is a statement of the specific abnormality in the genome. It might be something like 14-di-C164-17TA, meaning that on chromosome 14 both alleles of cistron no. 164 have adenine substituted for thymine as base no. 17 (paraphrased from Steinberg, 1971).

Concluding statements

It is difficult to master genetic nosology in every branch of medicine and difficult to maintain an overview of all medical literature. Aside from honest differences of opinion regarding the classification of some phenotypes and the interpretation of the evidence on modes of inheritance, errors may have crept in, and important omissions may exist. I have no illusions about either the infallibility or completeness of these catalogs. I would appreciate suggestions for increasing the usefulness of the catalogs and would like to have errors and omissions called to my attention.

The value of maintaining these catalogs on magnetic tape lies in the ease of revision and republication. I plan to keep them updated on a continuing basis and to republish whenever that is justified by the accumulation of new material. It is hoped that the catalogs will be *vade mecum* for the clinical geneticist—an inexpensive handbook that will make available the latest information on the nosology and genetics of hereditary diseases.

For the layman the large number of genetic disorders to which man is literally heir may come as an unhappy surprise. I am reminded of the following comment by Sir Thomas Browne in his *Religio Medici:*

> ... Men that look no further than their outsides, think health an appurtenance unto live, and quarrel with their constitutions for being sick; but I, that have examined the parts of man, and know upon what tender filaments that Fabrick hangs, do wonder that we are not always so; and considering the thousand doors that lead to death, do thank my God that we can die but once.

The Johns Hopkins Hospital   VICTOR A. McKUSICK, M.D.

REFERENCES

Bishop, J. O. The gene numbers game. Cell 2: 81-85, 1974.
Borgaonkar, D. S. *Chromosomal Variation in Man: A Catalog of Chromosomal Variants and Anomalies.* Baltimore: Johns Hopkins University Press, 1975.
Browne, T. *Religio Medici*, pt. 1, sec. 44. In G. Keynes, ed., *The Works of Sir Thomas Browne.* Vol. 1, p. 54. London: Faber & Gwyer, Ltd., 1928.
Childs, B., and Der Kaloustian, B. M. Genetic heterogeneity. New Eng. J. Med. 279: 1205-1212 and 1267-1274, 1968.

Dayhoff, M. O., ed. *Atlas of Protein Sequence and Structure 1972.* Vol. 5. Washington: National Biomedical Research Foundation, 1972.

Dickie, M. M.; Southard, J. L.; and Farnsworth, R. T. Two unusual mutations in the mouse. 40th Annual Report, The Jackson Laboratory, p. 77, 1969. See also Mouse Newsletter 41: 30, 1969.

Edelman, G. M. The structure and function of antibodies. Scientific American, August, 1970, pp. 34-42.

Edwards, J. H. The simulation of mendelism. Acta Genet. Statist. Med. 10: 63-70, 1960.

Ferguson-Smith, M. A.; Newman, B. F.; Ellis, P. M.; Thomson, D. M. G.; and Riley, I. D. Assignment by deletion of human red cell acid phosphatase gene locus to the short arm of chromosome 2. Nature N. B. 243: 271-273, 1973.

Florkin, M., and Stotz, E. H., eds. *Comprehensive Biochemistry.* Vol. 13: *Enzyme Nomenclature: Recommendations (1972) of the Commission on Nomenclature and Classification of Enzymes.* Amsterdam: Elsevier, 1973 (3rd ed.).

Garcia, A. G. P. Congenital toxoplasmosis in two successive sibs. Arch. Dis. Child. 43: 705-710, 1968.

Goldberg, M. F., and Hardy, J. M. B. X-linked cataract. In D. Bergsma, ed., *Clinical Delineation of Birth Defects.* Vol. 8: *The Eye.* Baltimore: Williams & Wilkins, 1971.

Haldane, J. B. S. A hitherto unexpected complication in the genetics of human recessives. Ann. Eugen. 8: 263-265, 1938.

Hutchison, C. A., III; Newbold, J. E.; Potter, S. S.; and Edgell, M. H. Maternal inheritance of mammalian mitochondrial DNA. Nature 251: 536-538, 1974.

Kirkman, H. N. Dominant mutations—biochemical basis for phenotype. In F. C. Fraser and V. A. McKusick, eds., *Congenital Malformations.* Amsterdam: Excerpta Medica, 1970.

Krech, U.; Konjajev, Z.; and Jung, M. Congenital cytomegalovirus infection in siblings from consecutive pregnancies. Helvet. Paed. Acta 26: 353-362, 1971.

Kroon, A. M., and Saccone, C., eds. *The Biogenesis of Mitochondria: Transcriptional, Translational, and Genetic Aspects.* New York: Academic Press, 1974.

Macklin, M. T. Erythroblastosis foetalis: a study of its mode of inheritance. Amer. J. Dis. Child. 53: 1245-1267, 1937.

McKusick, V. A. On the X chromosome of man. Quart. Rev. Biol. 37: 69-175, 1962.

McKusick, V. A.: On lumpers and splitters, or the nosology of genetic disease. Perspect. Biol. Med. 12: 298-312, 1969.

McKusick, V. A. *Heritable Disorders of Connective Tissue.* St. Louis: C. V. Mosby Co., 1972 (4th ed.).

McKusick, V. A. Phenotypic diversity of human diseases resulting from allelic series. Am. J. Human Genet. 25: 446-456, 1973.

McKusick, V. A.; Stauffer, M.; Knox, D. L.; and Clark, D. B. Chorioretinopathy with hereditary microcephaly. Arch. Ophthal. 75: 597-600, 1966.

McKusick, V. A.; Howell, R. R.; Hussels, I. E.; Neufeld, E. F.; and Stevenson, R. E. Allelism, nonallelism, and genetic compounds among the mucopolysaccharidoses. Lancet 1: 993-996, 1972.

Menser, M. A.; Slinn, R. F.; Dods, L.; Herzberg, R.; and Harley, J. D. Congenital rubella in a mother and son. Austral. Paed. J. 4: 200-202, 1968.

Myrianthopoulos, N. C.; Lane, M. H.; Silberberg, D. H.; and Vincent, B. L. Nerve conduction and other studies in families with Charcot-Marie-Tooth disease. Brain 87: 589-608, 1964.

O'Brien, S. J. On estimating functional gene number in eukaryotes. Nature N.B. 242: 52-54, 1973.

Ohno, S. *Sex Chromosomes and Sex-linked Genes.* Berlin: Springer-Verlag, 1967.

Rappaport, F.; Rabinovitz, M.; Toaff, R.; and Krochik, N. Genital listeriosis as a cause of repeated abortion. Lancet 1: 1273, 1960.

Saxbe, W. B., Jr. *Listeria monocytogenes* and Queen Anne. Pediat. 49: 97-101, 1972.

Serra, J. A. *Modern Genetics.* Vol. 1, pp. 397-398. London and New York: Academic Press, 1965.

Stagno, S.; Reynolds, D. W.; Lakeman, A.; Choramella, L. J.; and Alford, C. A. Congenital cytomegalovirus infection: consecutive occurrence due to viruses with similar antigenic composition. Pediat. 52: 788-794, 1973.

Steinberg, D. The metabolic basis of the Refsum syndrome. In D. Bergsma, ed., *Clinical Delineation of Birth Defects*. Vol. 6: *Nervous System*. Baltimore: Williams & Wilkins, 1971.

Verschuer, O. *Lehrbuch der Humangenetik*. Munich: Urban and Schwarzenberg, 1959.

Vogel, F. A. A preliminary estimate of the number of human genes. Nature 201: 847, 1964.

Wachtel, S. S.; Koo, G. C.; Zuckerman, E. E.; Hammerling, U.; Scheid, M. P.; and Boyse, E. A. Serological crossreactivity between H-Y (male) antigens of mouse and man. P.N.A.S. 71: 1215-1218, 1974.

Wiesmann, U., and Neufeld, E. F. Scheie and Hurler syndromes: apparent identity of the biochemical defect. Science 169: 72-74, 1970.

ACKNOWLEDGMENTS

I am indebted to a large number of colleagues in Baltimore and elsewhere for assistance over the years in assembling these catalogs. First, I would mention the research fellows and students who have worked with me since 1960 when the X-linked catalog was initiated. Second, I have been greatly assisted by the advice of many of my colleagues in The Johns Hopkins University. Colleagues elsewhere who have reviewed the catalogs at one stage or another include Alexander G. Bearn and O. J. Miller of New York City; Dick Hoefnagel of Hanover, N.H.; A Donald Merritt, W. DeMyer, and Wolfgang Zeman of Indianapolis; J. A. Fraser Roberts of London; Margery W. Shaw, formerly of Ann Arbor, now of Houston; John M. Opitz of Madison; George Fraser, formerly of London, Adelaide, Seattle, and Leiden, now of St. John's, Newfoundland; P. E. Becker of Göttingen; Arno G. Motulsky of Seattle; Herbert A. Lubs, Jr., formerly of New Haven, now of Denver; Mette Warburg of Copenhagen; David J. Weatherall, formerly of Liverpool, now of Oxford; Robert J. Gorlin of Minneapolis; Ernest Beutler and Akira Yoshida of Duarte, California; Jolin J. Mulvihill of Baltimore and Bethesda; Jürgen Spranger, formerly of Kiel, now of Mainz; and many others who will, I hope, forgive my failure to mention them by name. Collaboration with Drs. Margaret O. Dayhoff and Lois T. Hunt of the Biomedical Research Foundation, Silver Spring, Md., was helpful in cataloging the protein variants, particularly the hemoglobin variants. None of the errors in these catalogs can be attributed to any of the above, but without their help the catalogs would have been less accurate and less well organized.

Computerization was made possible by the sympathetic and ingenious assistance of Drs. Robert P. Rich and Richard H. Shepard of The Johns Hopkins Computing Center and was executed in the Division of Medical Genetics by David R. Bolling and his staff. Miss Sheila Manning, Mrs. Dixie Palma, Miss Rita Covington, and Miss Deborah Holifield deserve special mention for their work, both in computerization and in bibliographic verification. Particular thanks are due the staff of the William H. Welch Medical Library, without which this undertaking would have been, quite literally, impossible. I am also indebted to *Current Contents*, a weekly publication of the Institute for Scientific Information, Philadelphia. Regular scanning of the table of contents of journals covered by *Current Contents* has been a valuable first step in assembling nosologic information from the current literature. Finally, I am grateful to my patients; they have taught me much. The clinic and the library are the laboratories for research in genetic nosology.

Some aspects of the process of assembling the catalogs were supported by an NIH Genetics Training Grant (GM 00795), by an NIH Research Grant entitled "Mapping the Chromosomes of Man" (GM 10189), and most recently by an NIH Research Grant specifically for this work (GM 18676). The development of methods for computerization of the material and the processing of the catalogs took place in the Computing Center of The Johns Hopkins University School of Medicine.

GENERAL SOURCES

In assembling these catalogs, I have used several general sources, specialized monographs, and textbooks.

The older literature was reviewed in the following: R. R. Gates, *Human Heredity*, 2 vols. (New York: Macmillan, 1946); A. Sorsby, ed., *Clinical Genetics* (St. Louis: C. V. Mosby, 1953); and A. Touraine, *L'hérédité en médecine* (Paris; Masson, 1955).

The older literature is also usefully surveyed in *The Treasury of Human Inheritance* (1909–58), a series of reviews of the literature on a variety of genetic disorders; hemophilia, diabetes insipidus, dwarfism, angioneurotic edema, brachydactyly, polydactyly, osteogenesis imperfecta, Leber's optic atrophy, color blindness, retinitis pigmentosa, congenital stationary night blindness, multiple exostoses, cleidocranial dysostosis, Huntington's chorea, peroneal muscular atrophy, hereditary ataxias, spastic paraplegia, pseudohypertrophic muscular dystrophy, myotonic dystrophy, and Laurence-Moon syndrome. *The Treasury* was a publication of the Galton Laboratory, London (Cambridge University Press). Contributors include Julia Bell, Percy Stocks, William Bulloch, and Paul Fildes.

Comparable encyclopedic works of more recent publication include the following: P. E. Becker, ed., *Humangenetik: Ein kürzes Handbuch in fünf Bänden* (Stuttgart: G. Thieme, 1964); and L. Gedda, ed., *De Genetica Medica*, 6 vols. (Rome: G. Mendel Institute, 1961–62). The following also has bibliographic references and some unpublished observations: D. Bergsma, ed., *Birth Defects: Atlas and Compendium* (New York: National Foundation–March of Dimes, 1973).

The medical genetics literature for the six years 1958–63 inclusive was surveyed by my colleagues and myself in annual reviews published in the *Journal of Chronic Diseases* and collected in the following: V. A. McKusick *et al.*, *Medical Genetics 1958–1960* (St. Louis: C. V. Mosby, 1961); V. A. McKusick *et al.*, *Medical Genetics 1961–1963* (Oxford: Pergamon Press, 1966).

Useful in reviewing those forms of hereditary disease on which biochemical information is fullest were the following: H. G. Hers and F. Van Hoof, eds., *Lysosomes and Storage Disease* (New York: Academic Press, 1973); C. R. Scriver and L. E. Rosenberg, *Amino Acid Metabolism and Its Disorders* (Philadelphia: W. B. Saunders Co., 1973); J. B. Stanbury, J. B. Wyngaarden, and D. S. Fredrickson, eds., *The Metabolic Basis of Inherited Disease* (New York: Blakiston Division, McGraw-Hill, 1972) (3rd ed.).

The following journals were drawn on heavily: *Acta geneticae et gemellogiae*, *American Journal of Human Genetics*, *Annals of Human Genetics* (and its predecessor, *Annals of Eugenics*), *Clinical Genetics* (a newcomer), *Human Heredity* (and its predecessor, *Acta genetica et statistica medica*), *Journal de génétique humaine*, *Journal of Medical Genetics*, and *Social Biology* (and its predecessor, *Eugenics Quarterly*).

Beginning in 1968, annual conferences on the nosology of congenital and/or hereditary disorders, entitled "The Clinical Delineation of Birth Defects," have been held under the sponsorship of the National Foundation–March of Dimes, with publication by that organization. The published proceedings (edited by Dr. Daniel Bergsma) are a rich mine of information on genetic nosology. The 16 volumes on *Clinical Delineation of Birth Defects* have the following titles: I. Special lectures; II. Malformation syndromes; III. Limb malformations; IV. Skeletal dysplasias; V. Phenotypic aspects of chromosomal aberrations; VI. Nervous system; VII. Muscle; VIII. Eye; IX. Ear; X. Endocrine system; XI. Orofacial structures; XII. Skin, hair and nails; XIII. Gastrointestinal tract, liver, and pancreas; XIV. Blood; XV. Cardiovascular system; XVI. Urinary system and others.

Information concerning these publications can be obtained from Dr. Bergsma. Bibliographic referencing is somewhat confused by the fact that these proceedings are also part of the *Birth Defects: Original Article Series* published by the National Foundation–March of Dimes. The first five items listed above, each a separate volume, were part of Volume 5 of *Birth Defects: Original Article Series*, published in 1969.

The birth defects conferences that resulted in the 16 volumes listed above were held in Baltimore in five consecutive years, 1968 through 1972. Conferences have been held elsewhere since that time, namely, Boston in 1973 and Newport Beach, Calif., in 1974.

The proceedings are being published in D. Bergsma, ed., *Birth Defects: Original Article Series.*

Specialty monographs useful in assembling the catalogs included the following:

I. Eye

Deutman, A. F. *Hereditary Dystrophies of the Posterior Pole of the Eye.* Assen: Van Gorcum, 1971.

Duke-Elder, S. *System of Ophthalmology.* Vol. 3: *Normal and Abnormal Development,* pt. 2: Congenital Deformities. St. Louis: C. V. Mosby, 1963. Vol. 8: *Diseases of the Outer Eye,* pt. 1: Conjunctiva; pt. 2: Cornea. St. Louis: C. V. Mosby, 1965

Franceschetti, A.; François, J.; and Babel, J. *Les hérédo-dégénérescences chorio-rétiennes (dégénérescences tapéto-rétiennes).* 2 vols. Paris: Masson, 1963.

François, J. *Heredity in Ophthalmology.* St. Louis: C. V. Mosby, 1961.

François, J. *Congenital Cataracts.* Springfield, Ill.: Charles C Thomas, 1963.

Fraser, G. R., and Friedmann, A. I. *The Causes of Blindness in Childhood: A Study of 776 Children with Severe Visual Handicaps.* Baltimore: The Johns Hopkins Press, 1968.

Goldberg, M. F., ed. *Genetic and Metabolic Eye Disease.* Boston: Little, Brown & Co., 1974.

Waardenburg, P. J.; Franceschetti, A.; and Klein, D. *Genetics and Ophthalmology.* Springfield, Ill.: Charles C Thomas, 1961 (Vol. 1) and 1963 (Vol. 2).

Walsh, F. B., and Hoyt, W. F. *Clinical Neuro-Ophthalmology.* Baltimore: Williams & Wilkins, 1969 (3rd ed.).

II. Skin

Butterworth, R., and Strean, P. *Clinical Genodermatology.* Baltimore: Williams & Wilkins, 1962.

Cockayne, E. A. *Inherited Abnormalities of the Skin and Its Appendages.* London: Oxford University Press, 1933.

Gottron, H. A., and Schnyder, V. W. *Vererburg von Hautkrankheiten.* Berlin: Springer-Verlag, 1955. Vol. 7 of *Jadassohn Handbuch.*

III. Nervous System

Allen, N. Developmental and degenerative diseases of the brain. In T. W. Farmer, ed., *Pediatric Neurology.* New York: Hoeber Medical Division, Harper & Row, 1964.

Becker, P. E., ed. *Humangenetik: Ein kürzes Handbuch in fünf Bänden.* Vol. 5, pt. 1: *Krankheiten des Nervensystems.* Stuttgart: Georg Thieme Verlag, 1966.

Blackwood, W., *et al. Greenfield's Neuropathology.* Baltimore: Williams & Wilkins, 1963.

Ford, F. R. *Diseases of the Nervous System in Infancy, Childhood and Adolescence.* Springfield, Ill.: Charles C Thomas, 1966 (5th ed.).

Refsum, S. Genetic aspects of neurology. In A. B. Baker, ed., *Clinical Neurology.* New York: Hoeber Medical Division, Harper & Row, 1962 (2nd ed.).

IV. Muscle

Adams, R. D.; Denny-Brown, D.; and Pearson, C. M. *Diseases of Muscle.* New York: Harper & Row, 1962 (2nd ed.).

Walton, J. *Diseases of the Muscles.* Boston: Little Brown & Co., 1969 (2nd ed.).

Temtamy, S. *Genetic Factors in Hand Malformations.* Ph.D. dissertation, The Johns Hopkins University, 1966. Available through University Microfilms, Inc., Ann Arbor, Michigan.

Temtamy, S. A., and McKusick, V. A. *The Genetics of Hand Malformations.* New York: National Foundation–March of Dimes, 1975.

VI. Genetic Disorders of the Skeleton and of Connective Tissue in General

Kaufmann, H. J., ed. *Intrinsic Diseases of Bones.* Basel: S. Karger, 1973. Vol. 4 of *Progress in Pediatric Radiology.*

McKusick, V. A. *Heritable Disorders of Connective Tissue.* St. Louis: C. V. Mosby, 1972 (4th ed.).

Rubin, P. *The Dynamic Classification of Bone Dysplasias.* Chicago: Year Book Medical Publishers, 1963.

Spranger, J. W.; Langer, L. O., Jr.; and Weidemann, J. R. *Bone Dysplasias. An Atlas of Constitutional Disorders of Skeletal Development.* Stuttgart: Gustav Fischer Verlag, 1974.

VII. Endocrine System

Rimoin, D. L., and Schimke, R. N. *Genetic Disorders of the Endocrine Glands.* St. Louis: C. V. Mosby, 1971.

VIII. Immune System

Stiehm, E. R., and Fulginiti, V. A. *Immunologic Disorders in Infants and Children.* Philadelphia: W. B. Saunders, 1973.

IX. Mental Retardation

Holmes, L. B.; Moser, H. W.; Halldorsson, C. S.; Mack, C.; Pant, S. S.; and Matzilevich, B. *Mental Retardation: An Atlas of Diseases with Associated Physical Abnormalities.* New York: Macmillan, 1972.

X. Hematology

Weatherall, D. J., and Clegg, J. B. *The Thalassaemia Syndromes.* Oxford: Blackwell, 1972 (2nd ed.).

Williams, W. J.; Beutler, E.; Erslev, A. J.; and Rundles, R. W. *Hematology.* New York: McGraw-Hill, 1972.

Wintrobe, M. M.; Lee, G. R.; Boggs, D. R.; Bithell, T. C.; Athens, J. W.; and Foerster, J. *Clinical Hematology.* Philadelphia: Lea & Febiger, 1974 (7th ed.).

Most of the references (totalling 10,197, with 14,001 authors) are to articles in the periodical literature. Fields represented by more than 80 references each are listed in Table 1.

TABLE 1

Field of Journal	Number of References
Pediatrics	1,219
Human genetics and medical genetics	902

TABLE 1 (Continued)

Field of Journal	Number of References
Neurology, neuropathology, and mental deficiency	555
Ophthalmology	455
Hematology	329
Dermatology	299
Biochemistry	252
General genetics	204
Radiology	176
Orthopedics	126
Cardiology	84

Table 2 gives, in rank order, the specific journals which were referenced over 80 times.

TABLE 2

Journal	Number of References
New England Journal of Medicine	347
Lancet	329
Journal of Pediatrics	288
American Journal of Human Genetics	248
American Journal of Diseases of Children	213
Science	199
Nature (including *Nature New Biology*)	197
Pediatrics	187
Journal of Clinical Investigation	184
American Journal of Medicine	183
Archives of Disease in Children	177
Archives of Dermatology	157
Annals of Human Genetics (and *Annals of Eugenics*)	152
Journal of Medical Genetics	139
Journal of the American Medical Association	133
Archives of Neurology	132
Journal of Heredity	128
Blood	126
British Medical Journal	122
Neurology	113
Humangenetik	108
Annals of Internal Medicine	107
American Journal of Ophthalmology	102
Archives of Ophthalmology	102
Brain	95
Journal of Bone and Joint Surgery (U.S. and U.K.)	94
Proceedings of the National Academy of Sciences (U.S.)	80

A. NOSOLOGIC TABLES

B. OTHER TABLES

A. NOSOLOGIC TABLES

B. OTHER TABLES

DENTAL VARIATIONS AND ABNORMALITIES

The following is based on the classification of C. J. Witkop and S. Rao, Inherited defects in tooth structure, in D. Bergsma, ed., *Clinical Delineation of Birth Defects*, Vol. 11: *Orofacial Structures* (Baltimore: Williams and Wilkins, 1971), pp. 153-184. The Witkop-Rao classification also covered non-genetic causes of the given phenotype. This is essential for the genetic nosologists to keep phenocopies in mind. However, this part of the classification has been omitted here for economy of space. In December, 1974, Dr. Witkop kindly provided me with the latest revision of his classification. Drs. Ronald J. Jorgenson and L. Stefan Levin assisted in preparation of the following classification.

I. *Variants and anomalies of size, shape, and number*
- A. Primary (without associated extra-dental findings)
  1. Paramolar tubercle of Bolk (16820)
  2. Long upper central incisors (14730)
  3. Fused incisors (14725)
  4. Protuberant upper incisors (15430)
  5. "Shovel-shaped" incisors (14740)
  6. Carabelli anomaly (11470
  7. Odd-shaped teeth (18700)
  8. Microdontia (15680)
  9. Diastema (12590)
  10. Dens-in-dente (12530)
  11. Absent (or pegged) lateral incisors (15040)
  12. Absent central incisors (30240)
  13. Supernumerary teeth (18710)
  14. Hypodontia (partial anodontia) (10660, 31350)
- B. Secondary (part of generalized disorder)
  1. Hypodontia
     a. Tooth and nail syndrome (18950)
     b. Böök syndrome (11230)
     c. Anhidrotic ectodermal dysplasia (30510)
     d. Ellis-van Creveld syndrome (22550)
     e. Incontinentia pigmenti (30830)
     f. Hallermann-Streiff syndrome (13970)
     g. Focal dermal hypoplasia (30560)
     h. Lipoid proteinosis (24710)
     i. Rieger syndrome (18050)
     j. Otodental dysplasia (16675)
  2. Hyperdontia
     a. Cleidocranial dysplasia (11960)
     b. Gardner syndrome (17530)

II. *Defects in enamel*
- A. Primary (amelogenesis imperfecta)
  1. Hypoplastic forms
     a. Autosomal dominant hypoplastic-hypomaturation type with taurodontism (10445)—maybe TDO syndrome (13080)
     b. Autosomal dominant smooth, rough, pitted, and local hypoplastic forms (10453)
     c. X-linked rough hypoplastic form (30120)
  2. Hypocalcified form (10450)
  3. Hypomaturation forms
     a. X-linked hypomaturation form (30110)
     b. Autosomal recessive pigmented hypomaturation form (20470)
     c. Snow-capped teeth (18230)

B. Secondary to generalized disease
   1. Hypoplasia and/or hypocalcification
      a. Enamel hypoplasia with curly hair: tricho-donto-osseous syndrome (13080)
      b. Oculodentodigital dysplasia (16420)
      c. Epidermolysis bullosa dystrophica (22660)
      d. Focal dermal hypoplasia (30560)
      e. Morquio syndrome: mucopolysaccharidosis IV (25300)

III. *Defects in dentin*
  A. Primary
    1. Hereditary opalescent dentin (12550)
    2. Dentin dysplasia I (12540)
    3. Dentin dysplasia II (12542)
    4. Pulpal dysplasia (17845)
  B. Secondary (part of generalized disorder)
    1. Hereditary hypophosphatemia (30780)
    2. Osteogenesis imperfecta (16620)

IV. *Defects in both enamel and dentin*
  A. Primary
    1. Multiple odontomas (16435)
  B. Secondary (part of generalized disorder)
    1. Hypoplasia and/or hypocalcification
      a. Pseudohypoparathyroidism (30080)
      b. Hypoparathyroidism, Addison disease, moniliasis (24030)
    2. Pigmented and/or hypomaturation types
      a. Erythroblastosis fetalis
      b. Erythropoietic porphyria (26370)
    3. Odontoma-dysphagia syndrome (16433)

V. *Defects of cementum*
  A. Primary in cementogenesis
    1. Multiple cementomas
    2. Juvenile periodontosis (26095)
  B. Secondary to generalized disorder
    1. Cleidocranial dysplasia (11960)

VI. *Defects in both cementum and dentin*
  A. Primary (no genetic examples known)
  B. Secondary (part of generalized disorder)
    1. Hypophosphatasia (24150, 14630)

VII. *Miscellaneous abnormalities*
  A. Natal teeth as isolated abnormality (18705)
  B. Natal teeth accompanying systemic disorder
    1. Ellis-van Creveld syndrome (22550)
    2. Pachyonychia congenita (16720)
    3. Hallermann-Streiff syndrome (23410)
  C. Odontogenic keratocysts in basal cell nevus syndrome (10940)
  D. Periodontosis with Papillon-LeFèvre syndrome (24500)

TABLE A-II

EHLERS-DANLOS SYNDROMES

Number	Name	Clinical Features	Genetics	Biochemical Defect
E-D I	E-D, gravis type	Classic features, all severe	Autosomal dominant	Unknown
E-D II	E-D, mitis type	Classic features, all mild	Autosomal dominant	Unknown
E-D III	E-D, benign hypermobile type	Generalized marked joint hypermobility without skeletal deformity; skin features minimal	Autosomal dominant	Unknown
E-D IV	E-D, ecchymotic, arterial or Sack-Barabas type	Severe bruisability, very thin skin, rupture of bowel, rupture of large arteries, minimal joint laxity (e.g., limited to fingers)	Autosomal recessive	Deficient synthesis of type III collagen
E-D V	E-D, X-linked type	Stretchable skin striking, joint hypermobility minimal, skin fragility and bruisability variable	X-linked recessive	?Deficiency of lysyl oxidase
E-D VI	E-D, ocular type; lysyl hydroxylase deficiency; hydroxylysine-deficient collagen disease	Scoliosis, severe; skin features, moderate; blindness from retinal detachment or ocular rupture	Autosomal recessive	Deficiency of protocollagen lysyl hydroxylase
E-D VII	Arthrochalasis multiplex congenita; procollagen peptidase (or protease) deficiency	Short stature, severe joint laxity with congenital dislocations, moderate skin stretchability and bruisability	Autosomal recessive	Deficiency of procollagen protease (or peptidase)

xxxiii

HAND MALFORMATIONS

Temtamy's[1,2] system for classifying hand malformations has diagnostic usefulness. Three steps are involved:

1. According to the sole or predominant anomaly, the malformation is placed in one of ten main categories:

    I. Absence deformities
    II. Brachydactyly
    III. Syndactyly
    IV. Polydactyly
    V. Contracture deformities
    VI. Symphalangism
    VII. Carpal/tarsal synostosis
    VIII. Macrodactyly
    IX. Arachnodactyly
    X. Hand malformations with congenital ring constrictions

2. Each main category is divided into two subclasses according to whether or not malformation of other organs is associated.

3. By family studies the groupings achieved in the first two steps can often be extended. Even though categorization is unclear from study of the proband alone, the patterns of familial occurrence (or lack thereof) and, provided affected relatives are identified, the anatomy of malformation in these other affected persons may establish the diagnosis.

    I. Absence deformities
      A. Absence deformities as isolated malformations
        1. Terminal transverse defects
          a. Ectrodactyly: adactylia, acheiria (12980)
          b. Amelia and terminal transverse hemimelia (10440)
          c. Acheiropody (20050)
        2. Radial defects (17910)
        3. Ulnar defects
        4. Radioulnar defects
        5. Phocomelia
        6. Split-hand/split-foot deformity (18360)
      B. Absence deformities as a part of syndromes
        1. Terminal transverse defects as a part of syndromes
          a. Terminal transverse defects with orofacial malformations
            1) Ectrodactyly with orofacial malformations
            2) Aglossia-adactylia syndrome (10330)
            3) Ankyloglossum superius syndrome (10330)
            4) Hanhart syndrome (21630)
            5) Moebius syndrome (15790)
          b. Terminal transverse hemimelia with skull and scalp defects (10030)
          c. Terminal transverse hemimelia with ipsilateral dermatosis (24220)
        2. Radial defects as a part of syndromes
          a. Radial defects with orofacial malformations
            1) Nager acrofacial dysostosis (15440)

[1] S. Temtamy and V. A. McKusick, Synopsis of hand malformations with particular emphasis on genetic factors, in D. Bergsma, ed., *Clinical Delineation of Birth Defects*, Vol. 3: *Limb Malformations* (New York: National Foundation–March of Dimes, 1961), pp. 125–184.
[2] S. Temtamy and V. A. McKusick, *The Genetics of Hand Malformations* (New York: National Foundation–March of Dimes, in press).

MUCOPOLYSACCHARIDOSES

Catalog No.	Designation		Clinical Features
25280	MPS I H	Hurler syndrome	Early clouding of cornea, grave manifestations, death usually before age 10
	MPS I S	Scheie syndrome	Stiff joints, cloudy cornea, aortic regurgitation, normal intelligence, ?normal life-span
	MPS I H/S	Hurler-Scheie compound	Phenotype intermediate between Hurler and Scheie
30990	MPS II A	Hunter syndrome, severe	No clouding of cornea, milder course than in MPS IH, but death usually before age 15
	MPS II B	Hunter syndrome, mild	Survival to 30's to 50's, fair intelligence
25290	MPS III A	Sanfilippo syndrome A	Identical phenotype
25292	MPS III B	Sanfilippo syndrome B	Mild somatic, severe central nervous system effects
25300	MPS IV	Morquio syndrome (probably more than one allelic form)	Severe bone changes of distinctive type, cloudy cornea, aortic regurgitation
	MPS V	Vacant (now MPS I S)	
25320	MPS VI A	Maroteaux-Lamy syndrome, severe form	Severe osseous and corneal change, normal intellect
	MPS VI B	Maroteaux-Lamy syndrome, mild form	Mild osseous and corneal change, normal intellect
25322	MPS VII	β-glucuronidase deficiency (more than one allelic form?)	Hepatosplenomegaly, dysostosis multiplex, white cell inclusions, mental retardation

Genetics	Excessive Urinary MPS	Enzyme Deficient
Homozygous for MPS I H gene	Dermatan sulfate Heparan sulfate	α-L-iduronidase
Homozygosity for MPS I S gene	Dermatan sulfate Heparan sulfate	α-L-iduronidase
Genetic compound of MPS I H and I S genes	Dermatan sulfate Heparan sulfate	α-L-iduronidase
Hemizygous for X-linked gene	Dermatan sulfate Heparan sulfate	Sulfo-iduronide sulfatase
Hemizygous for X-linked allele for mild form	Dermatan sulfate Heparan sulfate	Sulfo-iduronide sulfatase
Homozygous for Sanfilippo A gene	Heparan sulfate	Heparan sulfate sulfatase
Homozygous for Sanfilippo B (at different locus)	Heparan sulfate	N-acetyl-α-D-glucosaminidase
Homozygous for Morquio gene	Keratan sulfate	?Chondroitin sulfate sulfatase
Homozygous for M-L gene	Dermatan sulfate	Arylsulfatase B
Homozygous for allele at M-L locus	Dermatan sulfate	Arylsulfatase B
Homozygous for mutant gene at beta-glucuronidase locus	Dermatan sulfate	β-glucuronidase

SEXUAL ABNORMALITIES

The following is based on the classification of J. L. Goldstein and J. D. Wilson, Hereditary disorders of sexual development in man, in A. G. Motulsky and W. Lenz, eds., *Birth Defects* (Amsterdam: Excerpta Medica, 1974), pp. 165–173.

I. Errors of genetic sex (No examples are known. The XO Turner syndrome is a chromosomal, i.e., non-Mendelian, example.)

II. Errors of gonadal sex
    A. Familial true hermaphroditism (23560)
    B. Sex reversal syndrome (15423)
    C. Pure gonadal dysgenesis, XX type (23330)
    D. Pure gonadal dysgenesis, XY type (30610)
    E. Familial anorchia (31065)

III. Errors of phenotypic sex
    A. Male pseudohermaphroditism
        1. Defect in androgen synthesis
            a. 20, 21-desmolase deficiency (20171)
            b. 3 β-hydroxysteroid dehydrogenase (20181)
            c. 17-hydroxylase deficiency (20211)
            d. Testicular 17, 20-desmolase deficiency (30915)
            e. Testicular 17-ketosteroid dehydrogenase deficiency (26430)
        2. Defect in androgen action ("androgen resistance")
            a. Complete testicular feminization syndrome (31370)
            b. Partial testicular feminization syndrome (31380)
            c. Incomplete male pseudohermaphroditism, type I (31210) (the following four "forms" may be all one or allelic)
                1) Lubs type (31380)
                2) Gilbert-Dreyfus type (30730)
                3) Reifenstein type (31230)
                4) Rosewater type (30650)
            d. Incomplete male pseudohermaphroditism, type II (pseudovaginal perineoscrotal hypospadias, 26460)
        3. Defective Müllerian duct regression: Hernia uteri inguinale (26155)
    B. Female pseudohermaphroditism
        1. Defect in corticosteroid synthesis
            a. 21-hydroxylase deficiency (20191)
            b. 11-hydroxylase deficiency (20201)
        2. Defect in Wolffian-Müllerian development (precise defect unknown)
            a. Rokitansky-Kuster-Hauser syndrome (27700)
            b. Cystic fibrosis (21970)

SKELETAL DYSPLASIAS: A CLINICAL CLASSIFICATION

The 1971 edition of *Mendelian Inheritance in Man* contained a modified draft of the classification of skeletal disorders devised by a small group which met in Paris in 1969—the so-called Paris Classification.

The following clinical classification is based, with their permission, on that given by Spranger and his colleagues: J. W. Spranger, L. O. Langer, Jr., and H. R. Wiedemann, *Bone Dysplasias: An Atlas of Constitutional Disorders of Skeletal Development* (Stuttgart: Gustav Fischer Verlag, 1974), pp. 359–365. Spranger and his colleagues intended their outline to permit the clinician rapidly to identify the diagnostic possibilities in a given case.

Conditions are divided into those presenting in the first year of life and those that first become evident in childhood and adolescence. (Some conditions appropriately appear in both categories.)

Each of the two categories is subdivided into short limb and normally proportioned types and the childhood-adolescence group into a third type, the short trunk type.

Those conditions which have diagnostic radiographic features in the newborn are indicated by an asterisk.

I. First year of life

    A. Short limbs

    Respiratory distress may be a problem in all of the short-limbed conditions since the ribs are also short.

       1. *Achondrogenesis, types IA and IB (20060, 20061)

        Head large in proportion to trunk; frequently stillborn, or neonatal respiratory distress with death in infancy. Two types which can be differentiated radiographically.

       2. *Achondroplasia (10080)

        Depressed nasal bridge, short fingers and toes.

       3. *Chondrodysplasia punctata, recessive (21510)

        Poor feeder, contractures, cataracts; frequently death in infancy.

       4. *Diastrophic dwarfism (22260)

        Proximally placed thumb, clubfeet, "blisters" on ears.

       5. Ellis–van Creveld syndrome (22250)

        Postaxial polydactyly of fingers, nail dysplasia; may be cardiac defects.

       6. Hypochondroplasia (14600)

        Rarely diagnosed in first year of life in absence of family history; may be short.

       7. *Hypophosphatasia, congenital lethal type (24150)

        Very soft calvarium, respiratory distress.

       8. *Kniest disease (15655)

        Prominent joints, frequently cleft palate; may be clubfeet.

       9. *Mesomelic dwarfism, Langer type (24970)

        Very short forearms and shanks with normal hands and feet.

10. *Mesomelic dwarfism, Nievergelt type (16340)

Very short shanks and, occasionally, forearms, frequently with bony protuberance at mid-shaft; restricted mobility of elbow joints; sometimes clubfeet.

11. Metaphyseal chondrodysplasia, McKusick type (25025)

Fine sparse hair, short body length present at birth. First radiographic change may be present near end of first year of life.

12. *Metaphyseal chondrodysplasia with thymolymphopenia (?)

No significant abnormalities other than short limbs in newborn, recurrent infections in first year of life.

13. *Metatropic dwarfism (25060)

Long, narrow thorax, frequently tail-like appendage over sacrum.

14. *Osteogenesis imperfecta, congenital recessive form or thick bone type (25940)

Soft calvaria, fractures.

15. *Short rib-polydactyly syndrome, Majewski type (26352)

Hydropic appearance; narrow thorax, preaxial and/or postaxial polydactyly; particular shortness of the tibia, multiple internal defects; early death.

16. *Short rib-polydactyly syndrome, Saldino-Noonan type (26353)

Hydropic appearance, narrow thorax, postaxial polydactyly; multiple internal defects; early death.

17. *Spondyloepiphyseal dysplasia congenita (18390)

May be cleft palate and clubfeet.

18. *Thanatophoric dwarfism (27365)

Depressed nasal bridge, very short fingers and toes, usually neonatal respiratory distress and death in infancy.

19. *Ulno-fibular dysplasia, Reinhardt-Pfeiffer type (19140)

Short forearms and shanks with normal hands and feet.

B. Normal body proportions

1. *Acrocephalosyndactylies (10120, 10130, 10140, 10160)

Syndactyly and other abnormalities of hands and feet, deformed cranium.

2. Arthro-ophthalmopathy (10830)

May be cleft palate, micrognathia, early severe myopia with high incidence of retinal detachment.

3. *Asphyxiating thoracic dysplasia (20850)

Frequently respiratory distress; may be postaxial polydactyly.

4. Caffey disease (11400)

Hyperirritability, fever, soft tissue swelling, bone pain.

5. *Chondrodysplasia punctata, dominant type (11865)

May be mongoloid facies, contractures, cataracts, foot deformity.

6. *Cleidocranial dysplasia (11960)

Large fontanels clavicles absent or hypoplastic to palpation.

7. Craniodiaphyseal dysplasia (21830)

Large head with broad nasal bridge with prominence of adjacent medial part of maxillary bones; may be cranial nerve palsies, blindness, or deafness.

8. Craniometaphyseal dysplasia (12300, 21840)

Large head with frontal bossing, broad nasal bridge with prominence of adjacent medial part of maxillary bones; may be cranial nerve palsies, blindness, or deafness.

9. Dysplasia epiphysealis hemimelica (12780)

May be asymmetric enlargement of knee and ankle regions; most cases not recognized in first year of life.

10. Enchondromatosis (16600)

May be leg-length discrepancy; most cases not recognized in first year of life.

11. G_M1 gangliosidosis, type I (23050)

Severe psychomotor retardation beginning at birth; occasionally, coarse facial features.

12. Hypercalcemia, idiopathic (23800)

Failure to thrive, irritability, anorexia, constipation, polyuria; may be elfin facies.

13. *Hypophosphatasia tarda, severe cases (24150)

Failure to thrive, may be bowlegs with pretibial skin dimples, clubfeet.

14. *Larsen syndrome (15025, 24560)

Flat nasal bridge, multiple joint dislocations, especially of knees and elbows, clubfeet; may be cleft palate.

15. *Metaphyseal chondrodysplasia, Jansen type (15640)

No significant clinical abnormalities in the newborn (characteristic radiographic findings are present in the newborn); may be symptoms of hypercalcemia.

16. Mucolipidosis II (25250)

Psychomotor retardation, Hurler-like clinical appearance beginning in early infancy.

17. Mucopolysaccharidosis I-H, Hurler disease (25280)

Progressive psychomotor retardation; usually no clinical dysmorphism in early infancy.

18. Nail-patella syndrome (16120)

Absence or hypoplasia of nails of thumbs and sometimes index fingers; may be absent patellae or palpable iliac horn.

19. Oculo-dento-osseous dysplasia (16420)

Syndactyly in hands, small eyes, medial epicanthal folds, hypoplastic thin nose with small nostrils.

20. *Osteodysplasty (16610)

May be neonatal respiratory distress; more commonly later in infancy and childhood with infection.

21. *Osteogenesis imperfecta, dominant form or thin bone type (16620)

Soft calvaria, fractures.

22. *Osteopetrosis with precocious manifestation (25970)

Enlargement of liver and spleen.

23. *Osteopetrosis with late manifestation (16660)

Rarely diagnosed in first year of life in absence of positive family history or of radiographs obtained for an unrelated indication. Radiographic abnormality may be present in the newborn.

24. Parastremmatic dwarfism (16840)

Stiffness, especially of spine; may be mild scoliosis and bowing of legs. (Stiffness may be present in the newborn.)

25. Pyknodysostosis (26580)

Large fontanels and wide skull sutures, small mandible.

26. *Tubular stenosis with periodic hypocalcemia (12700)

Short; may be tetany.

II. Childhood and adolescence

A. Short limbs

1. Achondroplasia (10080)

Dwarfed, depressed nasal bridge with typical nasal shape, usually large head, bowed legs, pelvic tilt, exaggerated lumbar lordosis.

Adult: Increased incidence of symptoms of spinal cord and/or rootlet compression with advancing age, usually in lumbar region, but also at the level of the foramen magnum and in the cervical region.

2. Asphyxiating thoracic dysplasia (20850)

Variably short limbs and small thorax, short fingers; may be postaxial polydactyly and renal disease.

3. Chondrodysplasia punctata, recessive type (21510)

Dwarfed, severe psychomotor retardation, cataracts, depressed nasal bridge, contractures; usually death in early childhood.

4. Dyschondrosteosis (12730)

Dwarfed or short in comparison with rest of family, mild shortening of shanks, shortening of forearms of variable degree which is frequently asymmetric, dorsal dislocation of distal ulna.

5. Ellis-van Creveld syndrome (22250)

Dwarfed, postaxial polydactyly of hands, short fingers, nail dysplasia, upper lip frenula, usually knock-knees; may be cardiac defects.

6. Hypochondroplasia (14600)

Dwarfed, normal facies, usually pelvic tilt and exaggerated lumbar lordosis; may be bowlegs.

7. Hypophosphatemic familial rickets (30780)

Mildly dwarfed or short in comparison with rest of family, relatively mild shortening of extremities, prominence of ends of long bones, deformity from rickets, usually bowing of lower extremities and genu varum; may be craniosynostoses.

Adult: Untreated individuals may develop extensive ligamentous calcification, thereby limiting motion, and may have progressive joint symptoms.

8. Mesomelic dwarfism, Langer type (24970)

Dwarfed, mild micrognathia, marked shortening of middle segments of upper and lower extremities, ulnar deviation of hands; hands and feet are normal.

9. Mesomelic dwarfism, Nievergelt type (16340)

Dwarfed with striking shortening of the shanks and, occasionally, of the forearms; restricted mobility of elbow joints.

10. Metaphyseal chondrodysplasia, Jansen type (15640)

Dwarfed, extreme shortening of lower extremities, with flexion of hips and knees, frequently hypercalcemia and mental retardation.

11. Metaphyseal chondrodysplasia, McKusick type (25025)

Usually dwarfed; thin hair and eyebrows, ligamentous laxity, flatfeet, usually short fingers and bowlegs.

12. Metaphyseal chondrodysplasia, Schmid type (15650)

Dwarfed or short in comparison with rest of family; may be fine hair; no other major clinical findings.

13. Multiple epiphyseal dysplasia (13240, 22690)

Dwarfed or short in comparison with rest of family; may be bowlegs or knock-knees, ligamentous laxity, abnormal gait.

Adult: Increased incidence of joint symptoms in lower extremities, especially hips and knees, with advancing age.

14. Pseudoachondroplasia (17715, 17717, 26415, 26416)

Dwarfed, normal facies, bowlegs or knock-knees, flatfeet, ligamentous laxity; may be scoliosis, which is usually mild.

Adult: Increased incidence of joint symptoms in lower extremities, especially hips and knees, with advancing age.

15. Pseudohypoparathyroidism, normocalcemic and hypocalcemic forms (30080)

Dwarfed or small, usually one or more short fingers or toes, knuckle sign on making fist, obese, may be mentally retarded, tetany, cataracts, subcutaneous calcification or ossification.

16. Ulno-fibular dysplasia, Reinhardt-Pfeiffer type (19140)

Short stature, short middle segments of upper and lower extremities, hands and feet are normal.

B. Short trunk

1. Diastrophic dwarfism (22260)

Dwarfed, usually short trunk secondary to progressive kyphoscoliosis, typical facies, deformity of cartilage of ears (cauliflower ears), resistant clubfeet, low-set hypermobile thumb, extension contractures of other fingers.

2. Dyggve-Melchior-Clausen disease (22380)

Dwarfed, usually mental retardation.

3. Kniest disease (15655)

Dwarfed with prominent joints and restricted joint mobility; round, flat face; frequently cleft palate, hearing deficit; occasionally myopia and retinal detachment.

4. Metatropic dwarfism (25060)

Dwarfed; usually progressive severe kyphoscoliosis, prominent joints.

5. Mucolipidosis I (25240)

Small stature, mild Hurler-like phenotype, clear corneae, sometimes progressive peripheral neuropathy specific storage cells in bone marrow, normal urinary mucopolysaccharides.

6. Mucolipidosis II (25250)

Dwarfed, severe Hurler-like phenotype, normal urinary mucopolysaccharides, particularly coarse fibroblast inclusions.

7. Mucolipidosis III (25260)

Dwarfed, coarse facial features, joint contractures, fine corneal opacities, normal urinary mucopolysaccharides.

8. Mucopolysaccharidosis I-H (25280)

Dwarfed, retarded, typical appearance, corneal clouding, increased mucopolysacchariduria.

9. Mucopolysaccharidosis I-S (25310)

Coarse facial features, joint contractures, corneal opacities, increased mucopolysacchariduria in childhood.

10. Mucopolysaccharidosis II (30990)

Hurler-like phenotype, small stature, clear corneae, impaired hearing, increased mucopolysacchariduria.

11. Mucopolysaccharidosis IV (Morquio) (25300)

Dwarfed, accentuated lower face, enamel hypoplasia, pigeon breast, fine corneal opacities, keratansulfaturia.

12. Mucopolysaccharidosis VI (25320)

Dwarfed, Hurler-like phenotype, corneal opacities, normal intelligence, increased mucopolysacchariduria.

13. Parastremmatic dwarfism (16840)

Dwarfed; usually kyphoscoliosis, so trunk is disproportionately short; flexion contractures, knobby knees, often with varus or valgus deformity.

14. Spondyloepiphyseal dysplasia congenita (18390)

Dwarfed, pelvic tilt and exaggerated lumbar lordosis, barrel chest, bowlegs or knock-knees, ligamentous laxity; frequently myopia and retinal detachment.

15. Spondyloepiphyseal dysplasia tarda (18410, 27160, 31340)

Dwarfed or short in comparison with rest of family, shorter than normal at 5 or 6 years of age; trunk becomes relatively shorter until growth ceases, barrel chest; may have back and/or hip pain in later childhood or adolescence.

Adult: Increased incidence of hip and back symptoms with increasing age.

16. Spondylometaphyseal dysplasia, Kozlowski type (27180)

Dwarfed or short; usually moderately severe kyphoscoliosis.

C. Normal proportions (or asymmetric limb length)

1. Arthro-ophthalmopathy (10830)

Usually thin, frequently early onset of myopia with high incidence of retinal detachment; may be cleft palate, kyphosis; joint symptoms are rare manifestations in childhood and adolescence.

Adult: Joint symptoms are more common in adults, retinal detachment.

2. Caffey disease (11400)

Residuals may be present in rare cases; synostosis between adjacent bones limiting normal function, bowing of bones in extremities, and length discrepancy in extremities.

Adult: Changes other than bony synostoses tend to have been corrected by normal bone growth by adulthood.

3. Chondrodysplasia punctata, dominant type (11865)

Usually small in comparison with rest of family, frequently asymmetric limb length; may be flat facies, scoliosis, partial alopecia, skin changes, cataracts.

4. Cleidocranial dysplasia (11960)

Dwarfed or small, relatively large head and small face, late eruption of permanent teeth, drooping shoulders, absent or hypoplastic clavicles.

5. Craniodiaphyseal dysplasia (21830)

Large head with frontal bossing, broad nasal bridge with prominence of adjacent medial part of maxillary bones which increases with age; mental retardation, cranial nerve palsies, blindness, or deafness.

6. Craniometaphyseal dysplasia (12300, 21840)

Large head with frontal bossing, broad nasal bridge with prominence of adjacent medial part of maxillary bones which increases with age; may be cranial nerve palsies, blindness, or deafness.

Adult: Symptoms due to neural foramina encroachment may increase with age, i.e., blindness, deafness, nerve palsies.

7. Diaphyseal dysplasia of Camurati and Engelmann (13130)

May be unusual gait when child starts to walk, pain and muscular weakness in extremities, usually thin habitus, rarely symptoms from encroachment in foramina in skull.

Adult: Muscular weakness and pain disappear to a large extent in adulthood.

8. Dysoteosclerosis (22430)

Short, increased bone fragility, dental anomalies; may be neurologic degeneration, macular skin atrophy.

9. Dysplasia epiphysealis hemimelica (?)

Usually lower extremity involved with overgrowth and hard masses at knee and ankle and varus or valgus deformity.

10. Enchondromatosis (16600)

Asymmetric limb length; may be hard tumors of hands and feet and in affected regions around joints.

11. Endosteal hyperostosis, recessive (?)

Prominent chin, facial nerve paralysis.

12. Fibrous dysplasia (17480)

Deformity of affected bones; may be fractures with minimal trauma. In McCune-Albright syndrome, brownish pigmented areas on skin and precocious puberty.

13. Frontometaphyseal dysplasia (22940)

Prominent bony supraorbital ridge, hirsutism; may be conductive deafness.

14. Hypophosphatasia tarda (14630, 24150)

No constant clinical features; may be small with deformity of lower extremities and craniosynostosis.

15. Hypothyroidism (e.g., 27440–27490)

Usually small, overweight, dry skin, coarse hair, constipation, and other clinical manifestations of defective thyroid function.

16. Idiopathic hypercalcemia (23800)

Short, mental retardation, broad mid-face and mouth, anteverted nose; may be supravalvular aortic stenosis and/or peripheral pulmonary artery stenosis.

17. Juvenile idiopathic osteoporosis (25975)

Bone pain especially in juxta-articular regions of lower extremities; may be disproportionately short trunk in severe cases and gross fractures of long bones. This is a self-limiting process which ends in late adolescence.

18. Larsen syndrome (15025, 24560)

Flat nasal bridge and mid-face, multiple dislocations of major joints usually with anterior dislocation of tibia on femur, clubfeet, short stature.

19. Melorheostosis

May be contractures, asymmetric limb shortening, swelling or atrophy of soft tissues, joint pain in affected area.

20. Metaphyseal chondrodysplasia, malabsorption, cyclic neutropenia (26040)

Short stature, intestinal malabsorption, recurrent infections.

21. Metaphyseal dysplasia of Pyle (26250)

Ends of long bones large to palpation; may be knock-knees.

22. Mucopolysaccharidosis III (25290, 25292)

Coarse facial features, mental retardation, heparansulfaturia.

23. Multiple cartilaginous exostoses (13370)

Hard masses most commonly near joints and of scapulae and ribs, often ulnar deviation of hand; may be limitation of motion of affected joint; rarely nerve compression.

24. Nail-patella syndrome (16120)

Absent or hypoplastic nails of thumbs and sometimes of index fingers, palpable iliac horns; may be absent or hypoplastic patellae, cubitus valgus, iris changes, renal disease.

Adult: The incidence of clinical renal disease increases with age.

25. Oculo-dento-osseous dysplasia (16420)

Syndactyly, camptodactyly, and ulnar clinodactyly of fingers, usually the fourth and fifth; small eyes (microcornea), medial epicanthal folds; hypoplastic thin nose with small nostrils; enamel hypoplasia.

26. Osteodysplasty (16610)

Small chest; distinctive facial appearance with prominent supraorbital ridges and eyes, and small jaw; may be kyphoscoliosis, respiratory and cardiac complications secondary to small thorax and/or spine changes.

27. Osteoectasia with hyperphosphatasia (23900)

Large head which becomes progressively larger throughout childhood, bowing of the extremities; may be fractures, optic atrophy, angioid retinal streaks.

28. Osteogenesis imperfecta, dominant form (16620)

Body proportions depend on deformity secondary to fractures; blue sclerae, tendency to fracture; may be deafness.

Adult: Fractures less common in adults; may be deafness from otosclerosis.

29. Osteolyses (16630, 25960, 27795, etc.)

Increased sensitivity; swelling, progressive deformities, and secondary contractures of affected segments, mostly of hands and/or feet; may be skin ulcerations and other findings according to type.

30. Osteopathia striata (16650)

No significant clinical findings, incidental finding on radiographs.

31. Osteopetrosis with late manifestation (16600)

Often incidental finding on radiographic study; may be fractures, anemia, symptoms from encroachment of neural foramina in skull; often short in comparison to rest of family.

32. Osteopetrosis with precocious manifestation (25970)

Dwarfed, hepatosplenomegaly, anemia, blindness; usually death in childhood.

33. Osteopoikilosis (16670)

Usually no significant clinical manifestations; may be connective tissue nevi of skin and, in females, precocious puberty with ultimate short stature.

34. Oto-palato-digital syndrome (31130)

Frontal bossing, ocular hypertelorism with antimongoloid slant of palpebral fissures, broad nasal root, small mouth with down-turned corners; may be cleft palate and deafness, thumbs and great toes spatulate and short.

35. Pachydermoperiostosis (16710)

    Seborrheic thickened skin of forehead, face, forearms,   and legs, clubbing of fingers.

36. Pyknodysostosis (26580)

    Dwarfed, open suture or sutures, most commonly the lambdoid; small jaw; may be fractures.

37. Sclerosteosis (26950)

    Peculiar face, cutaneous syndactyly of the fingers.

38. Tricho-rhino-phalangeal dysplasia, type I (19035, 27550)

    Fine, sparse hair, prominent philtrum; may be shortening of one or more fingers; frequently deviation at one or more interphalangeal joints; short or normal height.

39. Tricho-rhino-phalangeal dysplasia, type II (Langer-Giedion syndrome) (15023)

    Physical findings as in type I. Palpable bony masses as in multiple cartilaginous exostoses, mental retardation, short stature.

40. Tubular stenosis with periodic hypocalcemia (12700)

    Dwarfed, late closure of anterior fontanel; may be myopia, tetany from hypocalcemia, especially in stress situation (e.g., surgery).

ALLELIC SERIES AS THE BASIS OF PHENOTYPIC VARIATION

Disorders with Two or More Clinically Distinctive Forms Suspected of Being Allelic. (Enlarged from V. A. McKusick, Analytic review: Phenotypic diversity of human diseases resulting from allelic series, Am. J. Hum. Genet. 25: 446–456, 1973.)

I. Autosomal
   A. Enzyme (or other protein) deficiency known
      1. Acatalasia (20020)
      2. Acid phosphatase deficiency (20095)
      3. Adrenogenital syndrome due to 21-hydroxylase deficiency (20170)
      4. Afibrinogenemia (20240)
      *5. Alpha-1-antitrypsin deficiency (10740)
      6. Argininosuccinic-aciduria (20790)
      7. Cystathioninuria (cystathionase deficiency) (21950)
      8. Farber lipogranulomatosis (22800)
      9. Fucosidosis (α-L-fucosidase deficiency) (23000)
      10. Galactokinase deficiency (23020)
      *11. Galactosemia (galactose-1-phosphate uridyl transferase deficiency) (23040)
      *12. Gaucher disease (glucocerebrosidase deficiency) (23080, 23090, 23100)
      *13. Glucosephosphate isomerase deficiency (17240)
      14. Glycogen storage disease I (glucose-6-phosphatase deficiency) (23220)
      15. Glycogen storage disease II (alpha-1, 4-glucosidase deficiency) (23230)
      *16. Hemoglobin alpha variants (14180, 14185)
      *17. Hemoglobin beta variants (14190)
      18. Hemoglobin gamma variants (14220, 14225)
      19. Hemoglobin delta variants (14200)
      20. Histidinemia (23580)
      21. Homocystinuria (23620)
      22. Hyperlipoproteinemia II (14440)
      23. Hypophosphatasia (24150)
      24. Krabbe disease (24520)
      25. Maple syrup urine disease (keto acid decarboxylase deficiency) (24860)
      *26. Metachromatic leukodystrophy (cerebroside sulfatase deficiency) (25000, 25010, 25020)
      27. Methylenetetrahydrofolate reductase deficiency (23625)
      *28. MPS I (25240)
      *29. MPS IV (25300)
      30. MPS VI (25320)
      31. Neuronal ceroid-lipofuscinoses (20420, 20430, 20450)
      32. Niemann-Pick disease (sphingomyelinase deficiency) (25720)
      *33. Phenylketonuria (phenylalanine hydroxylase deficiency) (26160)
      34. Prothrombin deficiency or variation (12790, 24170)
      *35. Pseudocholinesterase deficiency (27240)
      *36. Pyruvate kinase deficiency hemolytic anemia (26620)
      37. Tay-Sachs disease (hexosaminidase A deficiency) (27280)
      38. Vitamin B12 metabolic defect (27740)
      39. Wolman disease; cholesterylester storage disease (27800, 21500)
      40. Xeroderma pigmentosum (27870, 27880)
   B. Enzymatic or other molecular basis not yet known
      *1. Achondroplasia-hypochondroplasia (10080, 14600)
      2. Amelogenesis imperfecta, hypoplastic type (10453)

Genetic compounds demonstrated or suspected with good reason are indicated by *. Compound heterozygotes are, of course, not likely to be observed in the case of rare X-linked traits.

3. Cataract, autosomal dominant forms (11570, 11580, 11590)
4. Cystic fibrosis (21970)
*5. Cystinosis (21980, 21990, 22000)
*6. Cystinuria (22010)
7. Diastrophic dwarfism (22260)
8. Ehlers-Danlos syndrome (13000)
*9. Epidermolysis bullosa (13170, 22650, 22660)
10. Fanconi renotubular syndrome (22770, 22780)
11. Iminoglycinuria (24260)
*12. Infantile cystic kidney (26320)
13. Keratosis palmaris et plantaris with esophageal cancer (14850)
14. Myotonic dystrophy (16090)
15. Renal glycosuria (23310)
16. Renal tubular acidosis with deafness (26730)
17. Spinal muscular atrophy (25330, 25340)
18. Spondyloepiphyseal dysplasia congenita (18390)
19. Von Recklinghausen neurofibromatosis (16220, 10100)

II. X-linked
 A. Enzyme (or other protein) deficiency known
  1. Fabry angiokeratoma (30150)
  2. Glucose-6-phosphate dehydrogenase deficiency (30590)
  3. Hemophilia A (30670)
  4. Hemophilia B (30690)
  5. Hypoxanthine-guanine phosphoribosyltransferase deficiency (30800)
  6. MPS II (30990)
  7. Testicular feminization syndrome (31370)
  8. Thyroid-binding globulin variants (31420)
 B. Molecular basis unknown
  1. Colorblindness, deutan (30380)
  2. Colorblindness, protan (30390)
  3. Ichthyosis (13810)
  4. Ocular albinism (30050, 30060)
  5. X-linked deafness (30440, 30450, 30460)
  6. X-linked muscular dystrophies (31000, 31010, 31020, 31030)

TABLE B-II

THE ETHNIC DISTRIBUTION OF DISEASE

Enlarged from A. Damon, Race, ethnic group and disease, Soc. Biol. 16: 69-80, 1969; V. A. McKusick, The ethnic distribution of disease in the United States, J. Chronic Dis. 20: 115-118, 1967; V. A. McKusick, Ethnic distribution of disease in non-Jews, Israel J. Med. Sci. 9: 1375-1382, 1973.

A. The ethnicity of disease: simply inherited disorders

Ethnic Group	Relatively High Frequency	Relatively Low Frequency
Ashkenazi Jews	Abetalipoproteinemia Bloom syndrome Dystonia musculorum deformans (recessive form) Familial dysautonomia Factor XI (PTA) deficiency Gaucher disease (adult form) Iminoglycinuria Niemann-Pick disease Pentosuria Spongy degeneration of brain Stub thumbs Tay-Sachs disease	Phenylketonuria
Mediterranean peoples (Italians, Greeks, Sephardic Jews)	Thalassemia (mainly β) G6PD deficiency, Mediterranean type Familial Mediterranean fever	Cystic fibrosis
Africans	Hemoglobinopathies, especially Hb S, Hb C, α- and β-thalassemia, persistent HbF G6PD deficiency, African type Adult lactase deficiency	Cystic fibrosis Hemophilia Phenylketonuria Wilson disease $E_1{}^a$ (pseudocholinesterase deficiency) Pi^z (α_1-antitrypsin deficiency)
Japanese (Koreans)	Acatalasia Oguchi disease Dyschromatosis universalis hereditaria	
Chinese	α-thalassemia G6PD deficiency, Chinese type Adult lactase deficiency	
Armenians	Familial Mediterranean fever	G6PD deficiency
Finns	Congenital nephrosis Lysinuric protein intolerance Aspartylglycosaminuria Neuronal ceroid lipofuscinosis, infantile type Cornea plana	Phenylketonuria Krabbe disease

Ethnic Group	Relatively High Frequency	Relatively Low Frequency
Norwegians	Cholestasis-lymphedema	
Eskimos	$E_1{}^S$ (pseudocholinesterase deficiency)	
French Canadians	Tyrosinemia	

B. The ethnicity of disease: disorders in which the genetics is complex or genetic factors are not proved

Ethnic Group	High Frequency	Low Frequency
Ashkenazi Jews	Hypercholesterolemia Diabetes mellitus Polycythemia vera Hyperuricemia Ulcerative colitis and regional enteritis Kaposi sarcoma Pemphigus vulgaris Buerger disease Leukemia Inguinal hernia	Cervical cancer Tuberculosis Alcoholism Pyloric stenosis

Irish	Major central nervous system
	  malformations (anencephaly,
	  encephalocele)	

Northern Europeans	Pernicious anemia	
Chinese	Nasopharyngeal cancer	
Japanese	Cleft lip-palate Cerebrovascular accidents Gastric carcinoma Gallbladder carcinoma (in females) Thrombosis of hepatic vein due to septum or membrane (in females) Pulseless disease (in females)	Otosclerosis Acne vulgaris Breast cancer Chronic lymphatic leukemia
Filipinos	Hyperuricemia (in U.S.)	
Polynesians (Hawaiians)	Clubfoot Coronary heart disease Diabetes mellitus	

Africans	Polydactyly
	Prehelical fissure
	Sarcoidosis
	Tuberculosis
	Hypertension
	Esophageal cancer
	Uterine fibroids
	Corneal arcus
		Major central nervous
		  system malformations
		  (anencephaly, encephalocele)
		Multiple sclerosis
		Skin cancer
		Osteoporosis and fracture
		  of hip and spine
		Pediculosis capitis

Ethnic Group	High Frequency	Low Frequency
	Cervical cancer	Polycythemia vera
	Ainhum	Pyloric stenosis
	Keloids	Gallstones
	Lupus erythematosus, systemic	Psoriasis
		Emphysema
		Chronic myeloid leukemia
		Legg-Perthes disease
		Parkinson disease
American Indians and Mexicans	Gallbladder disease	Duodenal ulcer
	Diabetes mellitus	
	Tuberculosis	
	Cleft lip-palate	
American Indians, Lapps, North Italians	Congenital dislocation of hip	
Icelanders	Glaucoma	
Eskimos	Salivary gland tumors	
	Otitis, deafness	

THE HUMAN GENE MAP

The following information is based, with minor revisions and additions, on the two International Workshops on Human Gene Mapping. The first was organized by Dr. Frank Ruddle and held in New Haven in June, 1973. The second was organized by Dr. Dirk Bootsma and held in The Netherlands in July, 1974. Both were sponsored by the National Foundation – March of Dimes, which published the proceedings of the first workshop as part of its *Birth Defects: Original Article Series* (Vol. X, part 3, 1974). The proceedings also appear in *Cytogenetics and Cell Genetics* 13: 1–216, 1974. The proceedings of the second workshop will be published similarly.

The following methods for mapping genes have been used:

1. F – study of traits in families; for example, linkage of ABO blood group and nail-patella syndrome. When anomalous chromosomes is one trait, Fc used; for example, Duffy blood group locus on chromosome No. 1.
2. S – study of traits and chromosomes in somatic cell hybrids.
3. A – *in situ* DNA-RNA annealing ("hybridization").
4. P – deductions from the amino acid sequence of proteins; for example, linkage of delta and beta hemoglobin loci from study of hemoglobin Lepore.
5. D – deletion mapping and gene dosage effects.
6. F-Fc, F-S, etc. – combination of F and Fc, F and S, etc.; for example, assignment of amylase loci to chromosome No. 1 by demonstration of linkage to Duffy (by family studies), which in turn is shown by family studies to be on chromosome No. 11.

The certainty with which assignment of genes to chromosomes has been made or the linkage between two loci established has been graded into the following classes:

C = confirmed = observed in at least two laboratories or in several families (not used in the following lists but can be assumed when one of the other symbols is not given).

P = provisional = based on evidence from one laboratory or one family.

I = inconsistent = results of different laboratories disagree.

The five digit numbers given here are entry numbers in McKusick's *Mendelian Inheritance in Man* (1971 and 1975 editions). Documentation on linkages and assignments is referenced in the entries indicated.

I. *Genetic map of the autosomes*

A total of over 1,100 loci on autosomes are known to exist, on the basis mainly of characteristic patterns of inheritance. As indicated by the following, some mapping information is available concerning at least 105 of these loci. About an equal number have been assigned by family study and by study of somatic cell hybrids.

A.   Chromosomal assignments (see Fig. 1, p. lx)

Chromosome No. 1 (see Fig. 2, p. lxii)

1p36		Phosphopyruvate hydratase (17245) S, F
1p32-1pter		6-phosphogluconate dehydrogenase (17220) F-S
1p31-1pter	(P)	Adenylate kinase-2 (10302) S
1p32-1pter		Rhesus blood group (11170) F-S, D
1p		Elliptocytosis-1 (13050) F
1p		Uridine monophosphate kinase (19173) F, S
1p32-1p33		Phosphoglucomutase-1 (17190) F-S
1p		Amylase, pancreatic (10465) F-F
1p		Amylase, salivary (10470) F-F
1p		Auriculo-osteodysplasia (10900) F
1p		Cataract, zonular pulverulent (11620) F
1p		Duffy blood group (11070) F
1q21-1q23	(P)	Uridyl diphosphate glucose pyrophosphorylase (19175) S

1q32	Peptidase C (17000) S
1q41-1q42	5S RNA gene(s) (18042) A
1q42	Fumarate hydratase (13927) S
1q44	Guanylate kinase (13927) S
1q43-1q44	Adenovirus 12-chromosome modification site-1 (10293) S

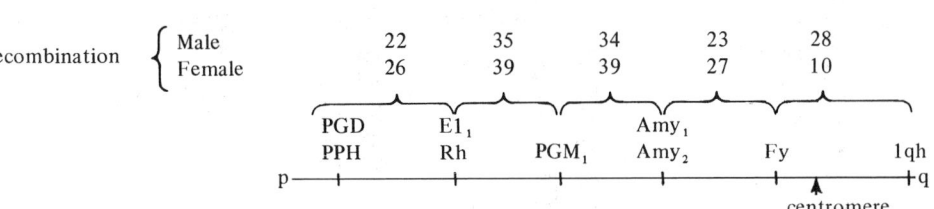

Recombination { Male   22   35   34   23   28
               Female   26   39   39   27   10

PGD   E1₁   Amy₁
PPH   Rh   PGM₁   Amy₂   Fy   1qh
p   centromere   q

Map of short arm of chromosome No. 1 based on family data (after Cook, Merritt, Rivas, Robson *et al.*, The Netherlands Conference, 1974).

Chromosome No. 2

(P)	2p23-2pter		Malate dehydrogenase-1 (15420) S
(P)	2p23		Acid phosphatase-1 (17150) D
	2p13-2q13	(I)	Galactose-1-phosphate uridyltransferase (23040) S
	2p11-2p22	(P)	Galactose + activator (13703) S
(P)	2q11, or 2q11-2q13		Isocitrate dehydrogenase-1 (14770) S
(I)	2q21-2q23	(P)	MNSs blood group (11130) Fc
	2q23		Hemoglobin alpha or beta (14180 or 14190) A
		(P)	Interferon-1 (14757) S
		(P)	Sclerotylosis (18160) F

Chromosome No. 3 (no confirmed assignment)

(I)   Galactose-1-phosphate uridyltransferase (23040) S

Chromosome No. 4

| | 4pter-4q26 | (P) | Phosphoglucomutase-2 (17200) S |
| | 4q23-4q27 | | Hemoglobin alpha or beta (14180 or 14190) A |

Chromosome No. 4 or 5

(P)   Adenine B, complement of auxotroph for (10255) S
(P)   Esterase activator (13325) S

Chromosome No. 5

Hexosaminidase B (14265) S
(P)   Interferon-2 (14758) S
(P)   Diphtheria toxin sensitivity (12615) S

Chromosome No. 6

(P) 6q22-6q23

HL-A histocompatibility region − S
    LA − first segregant series (14280) F
    FOUR − second segregant series (14283) F
    AJ − third segregant series (14284) F
    Mixed lymphocyte culture-1 and 2 (15785 15786) F
(P) Immune response (Ir) (14685) F
Glycine-rich β-glycoprotein (13847) F
Chido blood group (11043) F
Pepsinogen (16970) F
Malic enzyme-1 (15425) S
P blood group (11140) S,F
Phosphoglucomutase-3 (17210) S,F
Superoxide dismutase-2 (tetrameric or mitochondrial; indophenoloxidase B) (18547) S

[TABLE CONTINUES p. lxii]

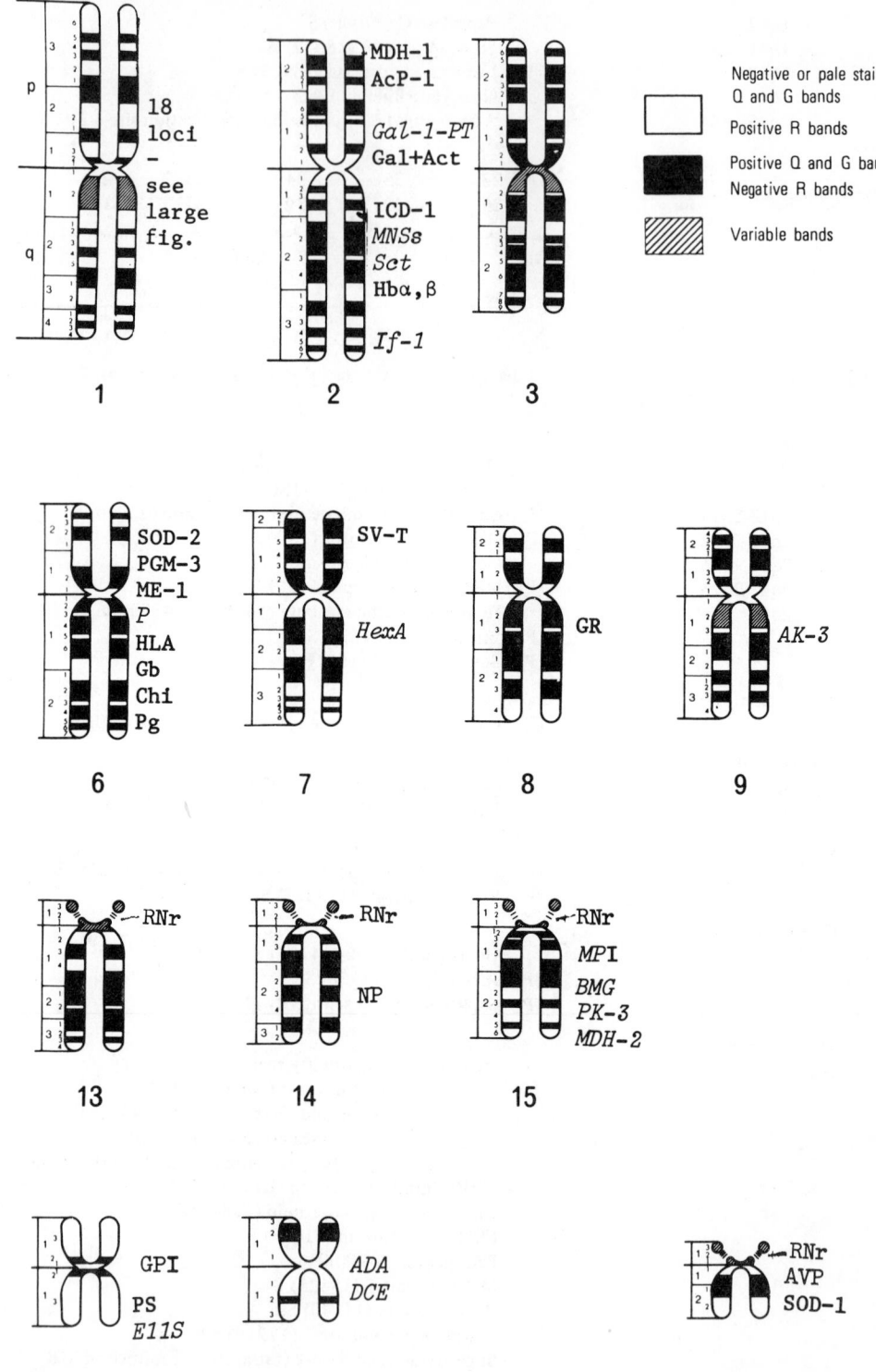

Fig. 1. A human gene map (Sept. 1, 1974). The banding pattern of the human chromosomes as indicated by special staining techniques is diagrammed (Paris Conference, 1971). To the left of

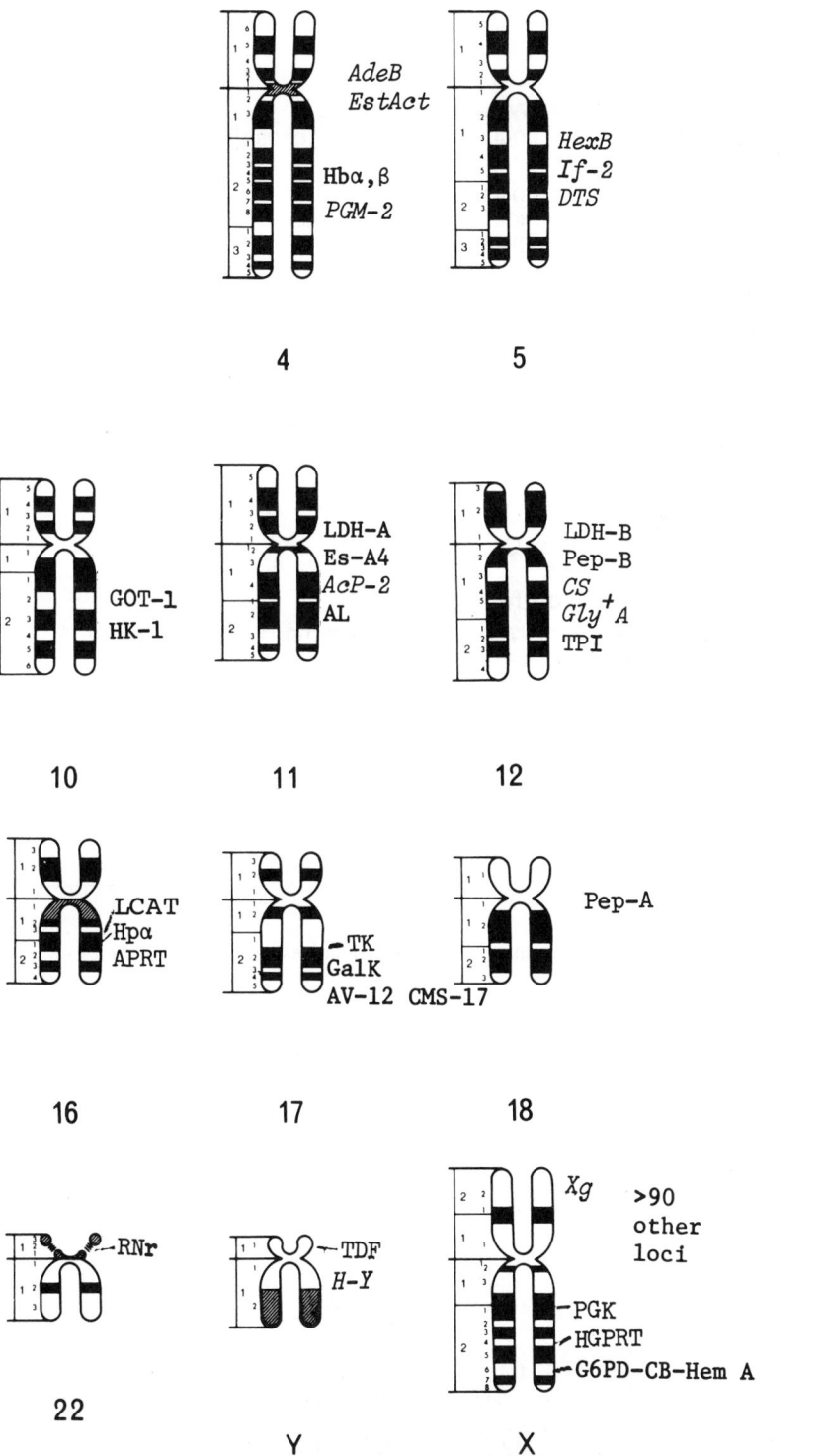

each chromosome, the symbols of genes which have been assigned to the given chromosome are given. When the assignment is inconclusive, the symbol is indicated in italics.

CHROMOSOME NO. 1

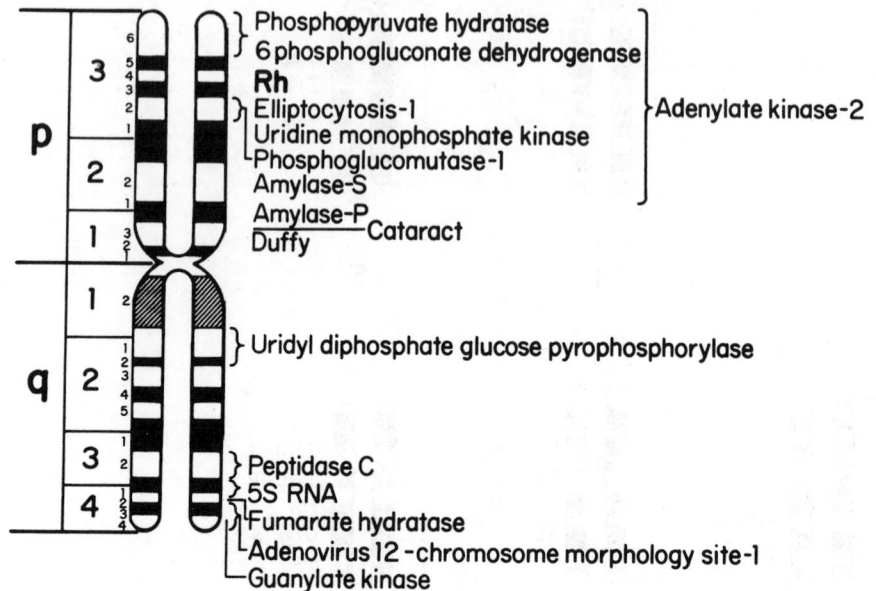

Fig. 2. A gene map of the human chromosome No. 1 (Sept. 1, 1974).

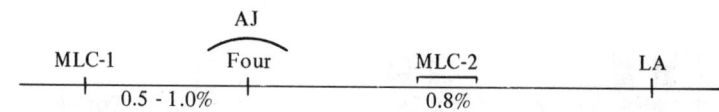

The major histocompatibility complex on chromosome 6 (after McDevitt and Bodmer, Lancet 1:1269-1274, 1974).

Chromosome No. 7

(P) SV40 T antigen (18680) S
Hexosaminidase A and/or C (27280) S

Chromosome No. 8

(P) Glutathione reductase (13820) S, D

Chromosome No. 9

(P) Adenylate kinase-3 (10303) S

Chromosome No. 10

Glutamate oxaloacetate transaminase-1 (13818) S
Hexokinase-1 (14260) S

Chromosome No. 11
(P) 11p

Lactate dehydrogenase A (15000) S
(P) Acid phosphatase-2 (20095) S
Esterase-A4 (13345) S
Killer antigen (14873) S

Chromosome No. 12
    12p   Lactate dehydrogenase B (15010) S
    12q14-12pter   Triosephosphate isomerase (19045) S
(P)   12q21   Peptidase B (16990) S

                           (P) Citrate synthase, mitochondrial (11895) S
                           (P) Serine hydroxymethylase (glycine A
                                      auxotroph complementing) (13845) S

Chromosome No. 13
    13p12   Ribosomal RNA (18045) A
                           (I)   Esterase D (13328) S

Chromosome No. 14
    14p12   Ribosomal RNA (18045) A
    14q   Nucleoside phosphorylase (16405) S

Chromosome No. 15
    15p12   Ribosomal RNA (18045) A
                           (P) β2-microglobulin (10970) S
                         (P) Malate dehydrogenase-2 (15410) S
                         (P) Mannosephosphate isomerase (15455) S
                         (P) Pyruvate kinase-3 (17905) S

Chromosome No. 16
    16q   Adenine phosphoribosyltransferase (10260) S
    16q   Haptoglobin, alpha (14010) Fc
    16q   Lecithin-cholesterol acyltransferase (24590) F
                         (I)   Esterase D (13328) S

Chromosome No. 17
    17q21-17q22   Thymidine kinase (18830) S
    17q21-17q22   Galactokinase (23020) S
    17q21-17q22   Adenovirus-12 chromosome modification site-17
                                   (10297) S

Chromosome No. 18
(P) 18q21-18qter   Peptidase A (16980) S, D

Chromosome No. 19

                            Phosphohexose isomerase (glucose-phosphate
                                 isomerase) (17240) S
(P) 19q   Polio sensitivity (17385) S
(P) 19q   (P) Echo 11 sensitivity (12915) S

Chromosome No. 20

                         (P) Adenosine deaminase (10270) S
                         (P) Desmosterol-to-cholesterol enzyme (12565) F

Chromosome No. 21
    21p12   Ribosomal RNA
                                Anti-viral protein (10745) S
(P) 21q21-21q22   Superoxide dismutase-1 (dimeric, or cytoplasmic;
                                 indophenoloxidase A) (18546) S

Chromosome No. 22
    22p12   Ribosomal RNA

B.   Syntenic autosomal loci for which assignment to a specific chromosome has not yet been achieved

     The tightness of the linkage is stated in general terms defined as follows:

very close – recombination less than 2%
close – recombination 2-6%
medium – recombination 6-22%
loose – recombination more than 22%

a. Lutheran (*Lu*) blood group locus (11120)
    secretor (*Se*) locus (18210)
    myotonic dystrophy locus (*Dm*) (16090)

    ] close (F)
    ] close (F)

b. ABO blood group locus (11030)
    nail-patella (*Np*) locus (16120)
    adenylate kinase-1 (*AK$_1$*) locus (10300)

    close (F)
    very close (F)
    (order unknown)

c. Hemoglobin beta locus (*HbB*) (14190)
    Hemoglobin delta locus (*HbD*) (14210)
    Hemoglobin gamma-A locus (*HbG-A*) (14220)
    Hemoglobin gamma-G locus (HbF-G) (14225)
(P) Hemoglobin epsilon locus (Hb Ep) (14210)

    all
    very
    close (F,P)

d. *Gm* immunoglobulin region

    γG$_4$] relative positions
    γG$_2$] unknown
    γG$_3$] linkage known
    ] from Lepore-like
    γG$_1$] myeloma protein

    Am$_2$ immunoglobulin locus (14700)

    α_1-antitrypsin (*Pi*) locus (10740)

    all
    very
    close
    (F,P)

    medium
    (F)

e. Transferrin (*Tf*) locus (19000)
    Pseudocholinesterase$_1$ (*E$_1$*) locus (17740)

    medium (F)

f. Albumin (*Alb*) locus (10360)
    Group-specific component (*Gc*) locus (13920)

    very close (F)

g. Pelger-Huët (*PH*) locus (16940)
    Unusual muscular dystrophy (*Mdu*) locus (15900)

    close (F)

h. Phenylthiocarbamide taste (*PTC*) locus (17120)
    Kell blood group (*K*) locus (11090)

    close (F)

i. Glutamate-pyruvate transaminase (*GPT*) locus (13820)
    Epidermolysis bullosa, Ogna type (*EBO*) locus (13195)

    close (F)

j. Lewis blood group (*Le*) locus (11110)
    Complement component-3 (*C3*) locus (12070)

    medium (F)

C. An "in limbo" group (autosomal syntenic groups or autosomal assignments suggested but not proved)

Dombrock blood group/MNSs
Lipoprotein-Ag (15200)/chromosome No. 21
ABO (11030)/chromosome No. 1
Spina bifida (18292)/HL-A (14280)
Chromosome 6/Gm (14710)
Chromosome 15/ABO (11030)
ABO (11030)/Xeroderma pigmentosum (27870)
Kidd blood group (11100)/chromosome 2 or 7
Cerebellar ataxia (16440)/HL-A (14280)
Hemoglobin alpha loci (14180, 14185)/Hemoglobin zeta locus (14228)

B. Mapping by family linkage studies (data assembled in Race and Sanger, *Blood Groups in Man*, 6th ed., in press)

1. *The colorblindness cluster*

Highly significant (lod > 3.0)

Nearly significant (lod approaching 3.0)

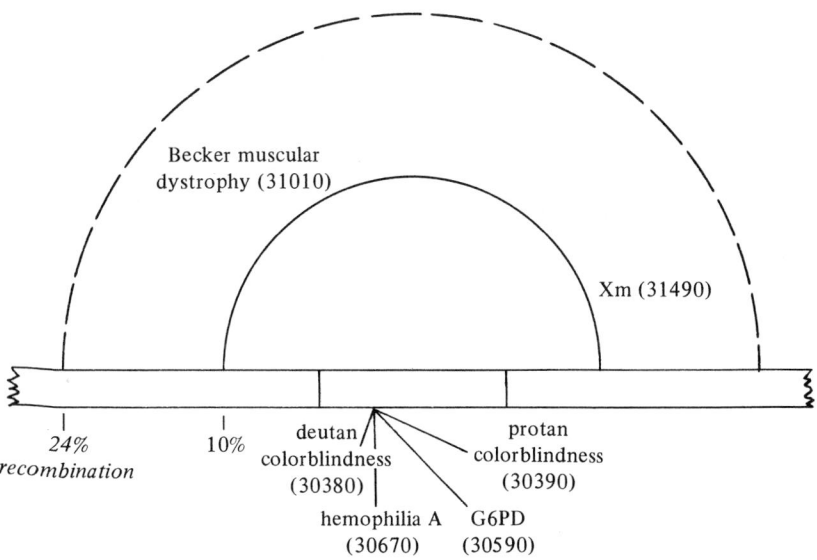

The order within the colorblindness cluster was suggested by the Rotterdam Workshop because recombination has been observed between the two forms of colorblindness but not among the loci within the cluster and those on the ends.

Xm and the Hunter locus (30990) may be linked. There is a suggestion also of linkage of muscular dystrophy with contractures (31030) and colorblindness.

2. *The Xg cluster*

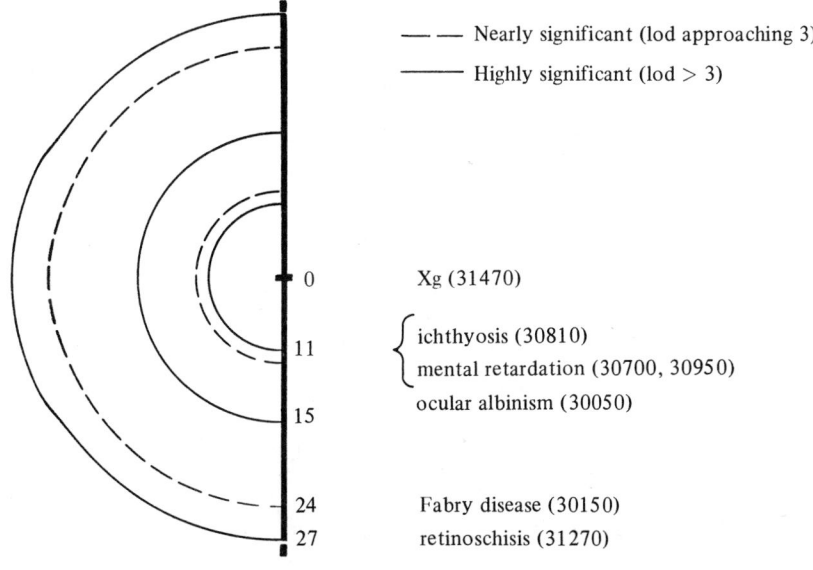

II. *Genetic map of the Y chromosome*

From the study of Y-chromosomal variants, factors which determine the differentiation of the indifferent gonads into testes are known to be located on the short arm of the Y chromosome. (Studies of sex anomalies suggest that a structural locus for testes is on the X chromosome and that the Y-borne locus, as well as one or more autosomal loci, serves a regulating function.) Histocompatibility antigens determined by the Y chromosome are known in the mouse (D. L. Gasser and W. K. Silvers, Genetics and immunology of sex-linked antigens, Adv. Immun. 15: 215–247, 1972) and may exist in man because mouse antisera react with human male lymphocytes but not with female lymphocytes (S. S. Wachtel; G. C. Koo; E. E. Zuckerman; U. Hammerling; M. P. Scheid; and E. A. Boyse. Serological crossreactivity between H-Y [male] antigens of mouse and man, Proc. Nat. Acad. Sci. 71: 1215–1218, 1974). That one or more genes concerned with stature are on the Y chromosome is suggested by the comparative heights of the XX, XY, and XYY genotypes. That the effect of the Y chromosome on stature is mediated through a mechanism other than androgen is suggested by the tall stature of persons with XY gonadal dysgenesis (30610).

III. *Genetic map of the X chromosome* (see Fig. 3 below)

From the characteristics of X-linked inheritance and in a unique instance from studies of somatic cell hybrids, at least 95 genetic loci have been assigned to the X chromosome. One (*TA*Tr, tyrosine aminotransferase regulator, 31435) was assigned by study of somatic cell hybrids. The others were assigned by pedigree pattern in the first instance at least; confirmation by other methods such as study of cell hybrids is available for some.

A. Regional assignments on the X chromosome by study of cell hybrids

Xp	Xg blood group (31470)
Centromere - Xq21	Phosphoglycerate kinase (PGK) (31180)
(P) Xq21 - Xq22	α-galactosidase (Fabry disease) (30150)
Xq22 - Xq25	Hypoxanthine-guanine phosphoribosyltransferase (HGPRT) (30800)
Xq25 - Xqter	Glucose-6-phosphate dehydrogenase (G6PD) (30590)
(P) Xq	Tyrosine aminotransferase regulator (31435)

[TABLE CONTINUES p. lxvi]

THE X CHROMOSOME

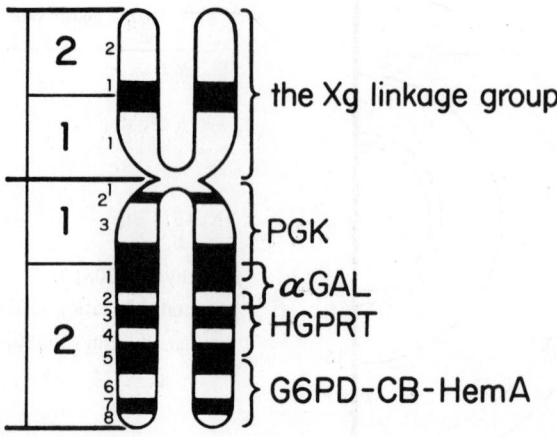

Fig. 3. A gene map of the human chromosome X (Sept. 1, 1974).

The linkage of Fabry disease with Xg might be inconsistent with the conclusions from hybrid cell studies that Xg is on the short arm and α-galactosidase is on the long arm.

Mental retardation is an indefinite phenotype. Hydrocephalus (30700) may present as mental retardation with little enlargement of the head. Linkage may be obscured by uncertainty as to which X-linked mental retardation syndrome is present in the particular family studied.

3. *Other data on Xg* (collected results of searches for linkage with *Xg* as of Spring, 1974)

Taken from a list in *Blood Groups in Man* 6th ed., in press. MRC Blood Group Unit, the Lister Institute, Chelsea Bridge Road, London SW1 W8RH.

Established	(sum of lods > 2 at some value of θ)
	ichthyosis (30810)
	ocular albinism (30050)
	retinoschisis (31270)
Probable	(sum of lods > 1 at some value of θ)
	Fabry disease (30150)
	mental retardation $\pm$ hydrocephalus (30700, 30950)
Possible	(sum of lods positive, but low, at $\theta = 0.3$)
	Lesch-Nyhan syndrome (30800)
	oligodontia (31350)
	congenital deafness (30450)
	thrombocytopenia (31390)
	nuclear cataract (30220)
	Xm (31490)
	testicular feminization (31370)
	mental retardation (30700, 30950)
	hypogammaglobulinemia (30030)
	Åland eye disease (30060)
	hypophosphatemia (30780)
	spondyloepiphyseal dysplasia tarda (31340)
Information Slight	keratosis follicularis (30880)
	colorblindness, blue-mono-cone-mono-chromatic (30370)
	macular dystrophy (30910)
	anophthalmos (30980)
	spastic paraplegia (31290)
	sideroblastic anemia (30130)
	dystrophy of the nose
	microphthalmia (30970)
	macular degeneration (30910)
	Ehlers-Danlos syndrome (30520)
	deafness, conductive (30440)
	obscure optic atrophy (30890)
	OFD syndrome (31120)
	pyridoxine responsive anemia (30130)
	cerebral sclerosis + Addison's disease (30010)
	chronic granulomatous disease (30640)
	congenital stationary night blindness (31050)
	choroido-retinal dystrophy (30320)
Unlikely	(sum of lods < -2 at $\theta = 0.1$, and between 0 and -2 at $\theta = 0.3$)
	retinitis pigmentosa (31260)
	Norrie disease (31060)
	choroideremia (30310)
	hydrocephalus (23660)
	renal diabetes insipidus (30480)
	Becker muscular dystrophy (31010)

low thyroxine binding globulin (31420)
increased thyroxine binding globulin (31420)
hypohidrotic ectodermal dysplasia (30510)

Excluded   (sum of lods < -2 at θ = 0.30)
G6PD (30590)
hemophilia A (VIII) (30670)
deutan colorblindness (30380)
protan colorblindness (30390)
Duchenne muscular dystrophy (31020)
Christmas disease (IX) (30690)

But, when the three-generation family evidence available for deutan, protan, G6PD, and hemophilia (VIII) is pooled, the score is 236 nonrecombinants and 193 recombinants: a recombination rate of 45% (expecting 50% recombination, X_1^2 = 4.3). So, is it just possible that this deutan cluster is not altogether out of reach of Xg, though time and expense would prevent the demonstration of direct linkage with Xg of any of the individual members of the cluster?

4.   *Other pairs of X-linked loci proven to be not closely linked*

colorblindness loci and retinitis pigmentosa (31260)
colorblindness loci and thyroxine-binding globulin (31420)
G6PD and thyroxine-binding globulin (31420)
hemophilia A (30670) and hypophosphatemia (30780)
HGPRT (30800) and G6PD (30590)
ichthyosis (30810) and colorblindness loci
ichthyosis and G6PD

PROTEIN DEFECTS IN INHERITED DISORDERS

A. *Enzymopathies: Disorders in Which Altered Activity (usually deficiency)*[1] *of a Specific Enzyme Has Been Demonstrated in Man*[2]

Condition	Enzyme with Deficient Activity	Catalog No.
1 Acatalasia	Catalase	20020
2 Acid phosphatase deficiency	Acid phosphatase	20095
3 Adrenal hyperplasia I	20, 21-desmolase*	20171
4 Adrenal hyperplasia II	3-β-hydroxysteroid dehydrogenase*	20180
5 Adrenal hyperplasia III	21-hydroxylase*	20191
6 Adrenal hyperplasia IV	11-β-hydroxylase*	20201
7 Adrenal hyperplasia V	17-hydroxylase*	20211
8 Albinism	Tyrosinase	20310
9 Aldosterone deficiency	18-OH-dehydrogenase	20340
10 Alkaptonuria	Homogentisic acid oxidase	20350
11 Angiokeratoma, diffuse (Fabry disease)	Ceramide trihexosidase	30150
12 Apnea, drug-induced	Pseudocholinesterase	27240
13 Argininemia	Arginase	20780
14 Argininosuccinic aciduria	Argininosuccinase	20790
15 Aspartylglycosaminuria	Specific hydrolase (AADG-ase)	20840
16 Ataxia, intermittent	Pyruvate decarboxylase	20880
17 Carnosinemia	Carnosinase	21220
18 Norum disease	Lecithin cholesterol acetyltransferase (LCAT)	24590
19 Citrullinemia	Arginosuccinic acid synthetase	21570
20 Crigler-Najjar syndrome	Glucuronyl transferase	21880
21 Cystathioninuria	Cystathionase	21950
22 Disaccharide intolerance I	Invertase	22290
23 Disaccharide intolerance II	Invertase, maltase	22300
24 Disaccharide intolerance III	Lactase	22310
25 Ehlers-Danlos syndrome, type V	Lysyl oxidase	30520
26 Ehlers-Danlos syndrome, type VI	Collagen lysyl hydroxylase	21655
27 Ehlers-Danlos syndrome, type VII	Procollagen peptidase	21656
28 Fanconi panmyelopathy	Exonuclease*	22790
29 Farber lipogranulomatosis	Ceramidase	22800
30 Formininotransferase deficiency	Formininotransferase*	22901
31 Fructose intolerance	Fructose-1-phosphate aldolase	22960
32 Fructosuria	Hepatic fructokinase	22980
33 Fucosidosis	α-L-fucosidase	23000
34 Galactokinase deficiency	Galactokinase	23020
35 Galactose epimerase deficiency	Galactose epimerase	23035
36 Galactosemia	Galactose-1-phosphate uridyl transferase	23040
37 Gangliosidosis, generalized, type I GM	β-galactosidase A, B, C	23050

[1] The form of gout due to increased activity of PPRP (13894) is the only disorder listed here with *increased* enzyme activity.

[2] The enzyme defect in many of these conditions is demonstrable in fibroblasts and in amniotic cells, so that antenatal diagnosis is possible.

In some conditions marked * (as well as some which are not listed) deficiency of a particular enzyme is suspected but has not been proved by direct study of enzyme activity.

	Condition	Enzyme with Deficient Activity	Catalog No.
38	Gangliosidosis, GM$_1$, type II or juvenile form	β-galactosidase B, C	23060
39	Gangliosidosis, GM(3)	Acetylgalactosaminyl transferase	23075
40	Gaucher disease	Glucocerebrosidase	23100
41	Glycogen storage disease I	Glucose-6-phosphatase	23220
42	Glycogen storage disease II	α-1-4-glucosidase	23230
43	Glycogen storage disease III	Amylo-1-6-glucosidase	23240
44	Glycogen storage disease IV	Amylo (1-4 to 1-6)-transglucosidase	23250
45	Glycogen storage disease V	Muscle phosphorylase	23260
46	Glycogen storage disease VI	Liver phosphorylase*	23270
47	Glycogen storage disease VII	Muscle phosphofructokinase	23280
48	Glycogen storage disease VIII	Liver phosphorylase kinase	30600
49	Gout	Hypoxanthine guanine phosphoribosyltransferase	30800
50	Gout	PPRP synthetase (increased)	13894
51	Granulomatous disease	NADPH oxidase	30640
52	Hemolytic anemia	Adenosine triphosphatase	10280
53	Hemolytic anemia	Adenylate kinase	20160
54	Hemolytic anemia	Aldolase A	20335
55	Hemolytic anemia	Diphosphoglycerate mutase	22280
56	Hemolytic anemia	γ-glutamylcysteine synthetase	23045
57	Hemolytic anemia	Glucose-6-phosphate dehydrogenase	30590
58	Hemolytic anemia	Glutathione peroxidase	23170
59	Hemolytic anemia	Glutathione synthetase	23190
60	Hemolytic anemia	Hexokinase	23570
61	Hemolytic anemia	Hexosephosphate isomerase	23575
62	Hemolytic anemia	Phosphoglycerate kinase	31180
63	Hemolytic anemia	Pyrimidine 5' nucleotidase	26612
64	Hemolytic anemia	Pyruvate kinase	26620
65	Hemolytic anemia	Triosephosphate isomerase	27580
66	Histidinemia	Histidase	23580
67	Homocystinuria I	Cystathionine synthetase	23620
68	Homocystinuria II	N (5, 10)-methylenetetrahydrofolate reductase	23625
69	β-hydroxyisovaleric-aciduria and methylcrotonylglysinuria	β-methylocrotonyl CoA carboxylase*	21020
70	Hydroxyprolinemia	Hydroxyproline oxidase	23700
71	Hyperammonemia I	Ornithine transcarbamylase	23720
72	Hyperammonemia II	Carbamyl phosphate synthetase	23730
73	Hyperglycinemia, ketotic form	Propionyl CoA carboxylase*	23200
74	Hyperglycinemia, nonketotic form	Glycine formininotransferase	23830
75	Hyperlipoproteinemia, type I	Lipoprotein lipase	23860
76	Hyperlysinemia	Lysine-ketoglutarate reductase	23870
77	Hyperprolinemia I	Proline oxidase	23950
78	Hyperprolinemia II	δ-1-pyrroline-5-carboxylate dehydrogenase*	23961
79	Hypoglycemia and acidosis	Fructose-1, 6-diphosphatase	22970
80	Hypophosphatasia	Alkaline phosphatase	14630
81	Immunodeficiency disease	Adenosine deaminase	24275
82	Immunodeficiency disease	Uridine monophosphate kinase	19173
83	Intestinal lactase deficiency (adult)	Lactase	22310
84	Isovalericacidemia	Isovaleric acid CoA dehydrogenase	24350
85	Ketoacidosis, infantile	Succinyl CoA: 3-ketoacid CoA-transferase	24505

	Condition	Enzyme with Deficient Activity	Catalog No.
86	Krabbe disease	A β-galactosidase	24520
87	Lactosyl ceramidosis	Lactosyl ceramidase	24550
88	Leigh necrotizing encephalomyelopathy	Pyruvate carboxylase	25600
89	Lipase deficiency, congenital	Lipase (pancreatic)	24660
90	Lysine intolerance	L-lysine: NAD-oxido-reductase	24790
91	Male pseudohermaphroditism	testicular 17, 20-desmolase	30915
92	Male pseudohermaphroditism	testicular 17-ketosteroid dehydrogenase*	26430
93	Male pseudohermaphroditism	α-reductase*	26460
94	Mannosidosis	α-mannosidase	24850
95	Maple sugar urine disease	Keto acid decarboxylase	24860
96	Metachromatic leukodystrophy	Arylsulfatase A (sulfatide sulfatase)	25010
97	Methemoglobinemia	NAD-methemoglobin reductase	25080
98	Methylmalonicaciduria I (B12-unresponsive)	Methylmalonic CoA mutase	25100
99	Methylmalonicaciduria II (B12-responsive)	Deoxyadenosyl transferase*	25110
100	Methylmalonicaciduria III	Methylmalonyl-CoA racemase	25112
101	Mucopolysaccharidosis I	α-L-iduronidase	25280
102	Mucopolysaccharidosis II	Sulfo-iduronide sulfatase	30990
103	Mucopolysaccharidosis IIIA	Heparan sulfate sulfatase	25290
104	Mucopolysaccharidosis IIIB	N-acetyl-α-D-glucosaminidase	25292
105	Mucopolysaccharidosis IV	6-sulfatase*	25300
106	Mucopolysaccharidosis VI	Arylsulfatase B	25320
107	Mucopolysaccharidosis VII	β-glucuronidase	25322
108	Myeloperoxidase deficiency with disseminated candidiasis	Myeloperoxidase (leukocyte)	25460
109	Niemann-Pick disease	Sphingomyelinase	25720
110	Ornithinemia	Ornithine ketoacid amino-transferase	25887
111	Oroticaciduria I	Orotidylic pyrophosphorylase and orotidylic decarboxylase	25890
112	Oroticaciduria II	Orotidylic decarboxylase	25892
113	Oxalosis I (Glycolic aciduria)	2-oxo-glutarate-glyoxylase carboligase	25990
114	Oxalosis II (Glyceric aciduria)	D-glycerate dehydrogenase	26000
115	Pentosuria	Xylitol dehydrogenase (L-xylulose reductase)	26080
116	Phenylketonuria	Phenylalanine hydroxylase	26160
117	Porphyria, acute intermittent	Uroporphyrinogen I synthetase	17600
118	Porphyria, congenital	Uroporphyrinogen III cosynthetase	26370
119	Pulmonary emphysema and/or cirrhosis	α-1-antitrypsin	20740
120	Pyridoxine-dependent infantile convulsions	Glutamic acid decarboxylase	26610
121	Pyridoxine-responsive anemia	Delta-aminolevulinic acid synthetase*	30130
122	Pyruvate carboxylase	Pyruvate carboxylase	26615
123	Refsum disease	Phytanic acid oxidase	26650
124	Renal tubular acidosis with deafness	Carbonic anhydrase B	26730
125	Richner-Hanhart syndrome	Tyrosine aminotransferase	24480
126	Rickets, vitamin-D-dependent	25-hydroxycholecalciferol*	26470
127	Sandhoff disease (GM$_2$ – gangliosidosis, type II)	Hexosaminidase A, B	26880
128	Sarcosinemia	Sarcosine dehydrogenase*	26890

	Condition	Enzyme with Deficient Activity	Catalog No.
129	Sulfite oxidase deficiency	Sulfite oxidase	27230
130	Tay-Sachs disease	Hexosaminidase A	27280
131	Thyroid hormonogenesis, defect in, II	Peroxidase*	27450
132	Thyroid hormonogenesis, defect in, IV	Iodotyrosine dehalogenase (deiodinase)	27480
133	Trypsinogen deficiency	Trypsinogen	27600
134	Tyrosinemia I	Para-hydroxyphenylpyruvate oxidase	27670
135	Tyrosinemia II	Tyrosine transaminase	27660
136	Valinemia	Valine transaminase	27710
137	Wolman disease	Acid lipase	27800
138	Xanthinuria	Xanthine oxidase	27830
139	Xanthurenic aciduria	Kynureninase	27860
140	Xeroderma pigmentosum	Ultraviolet specific endonuclease	27870
141	Xylosidase deficiency	Xylosidase	27890

B. *Other Diseases for Which a Molecular Defect Has Been Identified*

1. *Coagulopathies*
    a. Afibrinogenemia (Factor I deficiency) (20240)
    b. Hypoprothrombinemia (Factor II deficiency) (24170)
    c. Factor V deficiency (22740)
    d. Factor VII deficiency (22750)
    e. Hemophilia A (Factor VIII deficiency) (39670)
    f. Hemophilia B (Factor IX deficiency) (30690)
    g. Factor X deficiency (22760)
    h. Factor XI (PTA) deficiency (26490)
    i. Factor XII (Hageman factor) deficiency (23400)
    j. Factor XIII (fibrin-stabilizing factor) deficiency (30550)
    k. Antithrombin III deficiency (10730)
2. *Defects of the complement system*
    a. Angioneurotic edema (deficiency of Cl-esterase inhibitor) (10610)
    b. Complement component Clr, deficiency of (21695)
    c. Complement component-2, deficiency of (21700)
    d. Complement component-3, deficiency of (12070)
    e. Complement component-4, deficiency of (12080)
    f. Complement component-5, deficiency of (12090)
    g. Complement component-6, deficiency of (21708)
3. *Deficiencies of immunoglobulins* (e.g., 30030)
4. *Defects in transport proteins of blood, etc.*
    a. Abetalipoproteinemia (20010)
    b. Analbuminemia (20530)
    c. Analphalipoproteinemia (20540)
    d. Atransferrinemia (20930)
    e. Hemoglobinopathies (e.g., α, 14180; β, 14190)
    f. Macrocytic anemia due to deficiency of transcobalamin II (27535)
    g. Pernicious anemia due to deficiency of ileal factor (26110)
    h. Pernicious anemia due to deficiency of intrinsic factor (26100)
    i. Wilson disease (27790)
5. *Deficiencies of peptide hormones*
    a. Pituitary dwarfism I (26240)   Growth hormone deficiency
    b. ? some form of diabetes   Insulin deficiency
    c. Pituitary dwarfism II (26250)   Somatomedin deficiency

6. *Abnormalities in the collagens*
   a. Ehlers-Danlos type IV (13005)   ? Collagen III ("vascular collagen") defect
   b. Osteogenesis imperfecta   ? Collagen I ("collagen vulgaris") defect
      congenita (25940)
7. *Binding protein*
   a. Testicular feminization   Androgen-binding protein
      syndrome (31370)
   b. Hyperlipoproteinemia type II   Low density lipoprotein binding protein
      (14440)

VITAMIN-RESPONSIVE INBORN ERRORS OF METABOLISM

Based on S. H. Mudd, Vitamin-responsive genetic disease, J. Clin. Pathol., in press, 1974; C. R. Scriver, and L. E. Rosenberg, *Amino Acid Metabolism and Its Disorders* (Philadelphia: W. B. Saunders Co., 1973). (Many of the disorders discussed here occur in vitamin-responsive and vitamin-unresponsive forms, an illustration of genetic heterogeneity.)

A. *Biotin*
    1. Beta-methylcrotonylglycinuria due to beta-methylcrotonyl-CoA carboxylase deficiency (21020)
    2. Propionic acidemia due to propionyl-CoA carboxylase deficiency (23200)
B. *Folic acid*
    1. Congenital folate malabsorpsion (22905)
    2. Formiminotransferase deficiency (22910)
    3. Homocystinuria due to methylenetetrahydrofolate reductase deficiency (23625)
    4. Megaloblastic anemia due to dihydrofolate reductase deficiency (24930)
C. *Lipoic acid*
    1. Lactic acidosis due to pyruvate carboxylase deficiency (25600)
D. *Niacin*
    1. Hartnup disease (23450)
E. *Vitamin B1 (thiamine)*
    1. Lactic acidosis due to low Km pyruvate carboxylase deficiency (26615)
    2. Maple syrup urine disease due to branched-chain keto acid decarboxylase deficiency (24860)
    3. Megaloblastic anemia (24935)
    4. Pyruvate decarboxylase deficiency (20880)
F. *Vitamin B6 (pyridoxine)*
    1. Convulsions due to glutamic acid decarboxylase deficiency (26610)
    2. Cystathioninuria due to cystathionase deficiency (21950)
    3. Homocystinuria due to cystathionine synthase deficiency (23620)
    4. Oxalosis I due to deficiency of 2-oxo-glutarate-glyoxylate carboligase (25990)
    5. Sideroblastic anemia due to delta-aminolevulinic acid synthetase deficiency (30130)
    6. Xanthurenicaciduria due to kynureninase deficiency (27860)
G. *Vitamin B12*
    1. Megaloblastic anemia due to transcobalamin II deficiency (27535)
    2. Methylmalonic aciduria due to deficient adenosyl-B12 (25110)
    3. Methylmalonic aciduria and homocystinuria due to deficient adenosyl-B12 and methyl-B12 (27740)
    4. Pernicious anemia, congenital, due to deficiency of intrinsic factor (26100)
    5. Pernicious anemia, juvenile, due to defective ileal transport of vitamin B12 (26110)
    6. Transcobalamin I deficiency (21170)–no apparent pathologic consequences
H. *Vitamin C*
    1. Scurvy: the inborn error of metabolism from which all humans apparently suffer, the inability to synthesize ascorbic acid (24040)
    2. Ehlers-Danlos syndrome VI (22540)
I. *Vitamin D*
    1. Pseudo-vitamin-D-deficiency rickets (26470)
    2. Vitamin D resistant rickets, autosomal dominant (19310)
    3. X-linked hypophosphatemia (30780)

TABLE B-VI

X CHROMOSOME HOMOLOGIES IN MAMMALS

GENERAL REFERENCES

Green, E. L. *Biology of the Laboratory Mouse.* (2nd ed.). New York: McGraw-Hill, 1966.
McKusick, V. A. *On the X Chromosome of Man.* Washington, D.C.: A.I.B.S., 1964.
Ohno, S. *Sex Chromosomes and Sex-linked Genes.* Berlin: Springer-Verlag, 1967. Pp. 46–73.
Ohno, S. Evolution of sex chromosomes in mammals. Ann. Rev. Genet. 3: 495–524, 1969.
Ohno, S. *Evolution by Gene Duplication.* New York: Springer-Verlag, 1970.
Robinson, R. *Gene Mapping in Laboratory Mammals.* Part B. London, New York: Plenum Press, 1972.

A. *X-chromosomal homology in mammals: homology to man recognized or suspected* (Reference is given under entry number in catalog of X-linked traits.)

Catalog No.	Title	Other Species	References
30150	α-Galactosidase (Fabry angiokeratoma)	mouse	Ruddle, 1974
30510	Ectodermal dysplasia, anhidrotic	cattle, mouse (*Ta*, tabby)	Ohno, 1973
30590	Glucose-6-phosphate dehydrogenase	mouse, horse, donkey, brown hare, blue hare, kangaroo, Chinese hamster	Epstein, 1969; Ohno, 1967
30600	Glycogen storage disease VIII (phosphorylase kinase deficiency)	?mouse	Lyon *et al.*, 1967
30680	Hemophilia A	dog, ?horse	Brinkhous *et al.*, 1973
30690	Hemophilia B	dog	Brinkhous *et al.*, 1973
30780	Hypophosphatemia	mouse (*Hyp*)	Eicher, 1974
30800	Hypoxanthine guanine phosphoribosyl transferase	mouse, Chinese hamster	Epstein, 1972
30810	Ichthyosis	?mouse (scurfy, *sf*)	Eicher, 1974
30880	Keratosis follicularis spinulosa decalvans cum ophiasi	?mouse (sparse fur, *spf*)	Eicher, 1974
30940	Menkes syndrome	mouse (*Mo*, mottled allelic series), ?hamster	Rowe *et al.*, 1974 Yoon, 1974
31180	Phosphoglycerate kinase	mouse, kangaroo, Chinese hamster	Cooper *et al.*, 1971; Huijing *et al.*, 1973; Kozak *et al.*, 1974
31160	Pelizaeus-Merzbacher disease	?mouse (jimpy, *jp*)	Sidman *et al.*, 1964
31290	Spastic paraplegia	Syrian hamster	Nixon and Conneally, 1968

Catalog No.	Title	Other Species	References
31370	Testicular feminization	mouse (*Tfm*)	Goldstein, Wilson, 1972; Lyon, Hawkes, 1970; Ohno, Lyon, 1970
		cattle	Nes, 1966
		rat	Bullock, Bardin, 1972
31470	Xg blood group	gibbon	Ohno, 1967

B. *X-linked traits in mammals with no proved homology in man: selected examples* (Those X-linked loci in the mouse which have been mapped are given in the table above.)

1. *Antibody response to type III pneumococcal polysaccharide in the mouse*

In mice, Amsbaugh *et al.* (1972) showed that the ability to mount an IgM antibody response to type III pneumococcal polysaccharide is X-linked. The BALB/CAmN mouse was a higher responder, and CBA/HN a low responder. Other genes than the X-linked gene determine the level of response. In studies of normal volunteers given a polyvalent pneumococcal vaccine, Austrian (1974) found that a "fair number" failed to respond to one type of pneumococcal material, a few failed to respond to two types, and rare individuals failed to respond to three. There were also individual differences in type of immunoglobulin response, whether IgG or IgM.

Amsbaugh, D. F.; Hansen, C. T.; Prescott, B.; Stashak, P. W.; Barthold, D. R.; and Baker, P. J. Genetic control of the antibody response to type III pneumococcus polysaccharide in mice. I: Evidence that an X-linked gene plays a decisive role in determining responsiveness. J. Exp. Med. 136: 931–949, 1972.
Austrian, R. Personal communication, Sept. 4, 1974, Philadelphia.

2. *Carpal subluxation of the dog*

So much homology of X chromosome exists among mammals that the description of subluxation of the carpus as an X-linked trait in dogs is of great interest. The homologous condition in man is not known. The trait in dogs is very closely linked to the locus for hemophilia A. The two mutant genes were in repulsion and no recombination was observed in 49 opportunities (Pick *et al.*, 1967). The deformity is limited to the carporadial joints bilaterally. Pups appear normal at birth. Subluxation becomes evident at about 3 weeks of age when the pup begins to walk. No other effects of the gene are evident.

Pick, J. R.; Goyer, R. A.; Graham, J. B.; and Renwick, J. H. Subluxation of the carpus in dogs: An X chromosomal defect closely linked with the locus for hemophilia A. Lab. Invest. 17: 243–248, 1967.

3. *Cystinuria in the dog*

Cystine urinary calculi are well known in dogs (White, 1944). Brand (1940) and Hess (1942) observed that canine cystinuria is familial and concluded that it may be X-linked since all cases were in males. Treacher (1964) reported that the urine contains excessive lysine, arginine, and ornithine as in the human disease, but Holtzapple *et al.* (1971) noted an excess of only lysine and cystine. Furthermore, the latter group could not demonstrate in vitro any defect of transport in either gut or kidney.

Brand, E.; Cahill, G. F.; and Harris, M. M. Canine cystinuria. V: Family history of two cystinuric Irish terriers and cystine determination in dog urine. J. Biol. Chem. 133: 431–436, 1940.

Hess, W. C., and Sullivan, M. X. Canine cystinuria: the effect of feeding cystine, cysteine, and methionine at different protein levels. J. Biol. Chem. 143: 545–550, 1942.

Holtzapple, P. G.; Rea, C.; Bovee, K.; and Segal, S. Characteristics of cystine and lysine transport in renal and jejunal tissue from cystinuric dogs. Metabolism 20: 1016–1022, 1971.

Treacher, R. J. Quantitative studies on the excretion of the basic amino acids in canine cystinuria. Brit. Vet. J. 120: 178–185, 1964.

White, E. G. Urinary calculi in the dog with special reference to cystine stones. J. Comp. Path. 54: 16–25, 1944.

4. *Histocompatibility in the mouse*

Bailey (1963) demonstrated X-linked histocompatibility in the mouse.

Bailey, D. W. Histocompatibility associated with the X chromosome in mice. Transplantation 1: 70–74, 1963.

5. *Immune response to DNA*

In mice, Mozes and Fuchs (1974) found that the ability to respond to denatured DNA is regulated by a gene on the X chromosome. The interest for man arises from the homology of the X chromosomes of mammals, the familial nature of systemic lupus erythematosis in man (21695), the spontaneous occurrence of anti-nucleic acid antibodies in the serum of patients with this disease, and its occurrence more often in females than in males.

Mozes, E., and Fuchs, S. Linkage between immune response potential to DNA and X chromosome. Nature 249: 167–168, 1974.

6. *Irregular teeth in the mouse*

This character, symbolized *It*, is X-linked, lethal in males. In heterozygous females, one or both lower incisors are markedly reduced and sometimes absent. In extreme cases, upper incisors are absent also. Expression is variable with overlap of the normal. Heterozygotes are relatively inviable and reproduce poorly.

Phipps, E. L. Irregular teeth, *It*. Mouse Newsletter No. 40, p. 41, 1969.

7. *Mottled white in mouse and Syrian hamster*

This character occurs in both the mouse and the Syrian hamster (Ohno, 1970). The trait is observed only in females, thus demonstrating the same mode of inheritance as incontinentia pigmenti, OFD syndrome I, FDH, etc. Affected animals have a thinner than normal coat with normally colored fur intermingled with white. Some animals are almost entirely white, while others are only slightly grayer than normal. In litters from affected mothers, one-third of the offspring are normal males, one-third normal females, and one-third mottled-white females. Ohno (1974) maintains that *mottled white* is homologous to *mottled* in the mouse and therefore homologous to Menkes disease.

Magalhaes, H. Mottle-white, a sex-linked lethal mutation in the golden hamster, *Mesocricetus auratus*. (Abstract) Anat. Rec. 120: 752 only, 1954.

Ohno, S. *Evolution by Gene Duplication*. Berlin: Springer-Verlag, 1970.

Ohno, S. Personal communication, Oct. 3, 1974, Duarte, Calif.

8. *Myopathy in the dog*

In the dog, Wentink *et al.* (1972) described an X-linked myopathy manifested clinically by stiff gait, difficulty in swallowing, dirty cheeks from food particles, enlarged tongue, and atrophic muscles. Electromyography revealed high-frequency discharges suggestive of myotonia. Serum creatine phosphokinase and aldolase levels were very high. Abnormal mitochondria and unidentified electron-dense bodies were found on ultrastructural studies. See 30995, 31000, 31010, 31020, 31030, 31040, and 31045 for human X-linked myopathies, one of which may be homologous to this disorder in the dog.

Wentink, G. H.; Van der Linde-Sipman, J. S.; Meijer, A. E. F. H.; Kamphuizen, H. A. C.; Van Vorstenbosch, C. J. A. H. V.; Hartman, W.; and Hendriks, H. J. Myopathy with a possible recessive X-linked inheritance in a litter of Irish terriers. Vet. Pathol. 9: 328–349, 1972.

9. *Orange (tortoise-shell) in cat and Syrian hamster*

This character occurs in both the cat and the Syrian hamster (Ohno, 1970). The data in the cat is especially abundant (Doncaster, 1913; Bamber and Herdman, 1927, 1932). Soon after discovery of the XXY nature of the Klinefelter syndrome in man, several workers suggested that the tortoise-shell male is of XXY karyotype. This has several times been demonstrated to be the case (e.g., Loughman *et al.*, 1970), there usually being XY/XXY or other mosaicism. The gene is also known as yellow and is symbolized *To* (tortoise-shell). In both the cat and the hamster, both autosomal and X-linked yellow genes are known.

Ohno, S. *Evolution by Gene Duplication*. Berlin: Springer-Verlag, 1970.
Doncaster, L. On sex-limited inheritance in cats and its bearing on the sex-limited transmission of certain human abnormalities. J. Genet. 3: 11–23, 1913.
Bamber, R. C., and Herdman, E. C. The inheritance of black, yellow, and tortoiseshell coat colour in cats. J. Genet. 18: 87–97, 1927.
Loughman, W. D.; Frye, F. L.; and Condon, T. B. XY/XXY bone marrow mosaicism in three male tricolor cats. Am. J. Vet. Res. 31: 307–314, 1970.
Robinson, R. Sex-linked yellow in the Syrian hamster. Nature 212: 824–825, 1966.

10. *Striated in mice and streaked hairlessness in cattle*

Approximately perpendicular, irregularly narrow streaks of hide on various parts of the cow are affected. No males are affected. A deficiency of sons and an increased length of calving-interval in affected females support X-linked dominant inheritance with lethality in the male at an early embryonic stage.

Eldridge, F. E., and Atkeson, F. W. Streaked hairlessness in Holstein-Friesian cattle: a sex-linked lethal character. J. Hered. 44: 265–271, 1953.

C. *The map of the mouse X chromosome*

Unless otherwise indicated, information from M. C. Green, Mutant genes and linkages, in E. L. Green, ed., *Biology of the Laboratory Mouse* (New York: McGraw-Hill, 1966) (2nd ed.). References are provided there. See Fig. 4 opposite for a diagrammatic representation of the mouse X chromosome.

1. *sf* scurfy, X-linked recessive. Hemizygous males can first be recognized at about 11 days of age by reddening of the genital papilla. They develop scaliness, first of the tail and later of other parts of the body. The skin appears tight. The eyelids open late. Affected males usually die before or shortly after weaning. Survivors are small and sterile. Affected females have an XO karyotype. This mouse mutation may be homologous to X-linked ichthyosis (30810).

2. *spf*, sparse-fur, X-linked recessive. In affected hemizygous males and homozygous females, development of fur is late and patchy. By weaning the fur looks nearly normal. This mouse mutation may be homologous to human keratosis follicularis spinulosa decalvans cum ophiasi (30880).

3. *Hq*, harlequin, X-linked semidominant. Hemizygous males and homozygous females are completely bald but are fully viable and fertile. They are about one-third the weight of wild-type and heterozygous animals. Bald patches in heterozygotes give this mutation its name.

Barber, B. R. Mouse Newsletter, No. 45, pp. 34–35, July, 1971.
Isaacson, J. H.; Stewart, J.; and Falconer, D. S. Location of *Hq*. Mouse Newsletter, No. 50, p. 33, February, 1974.

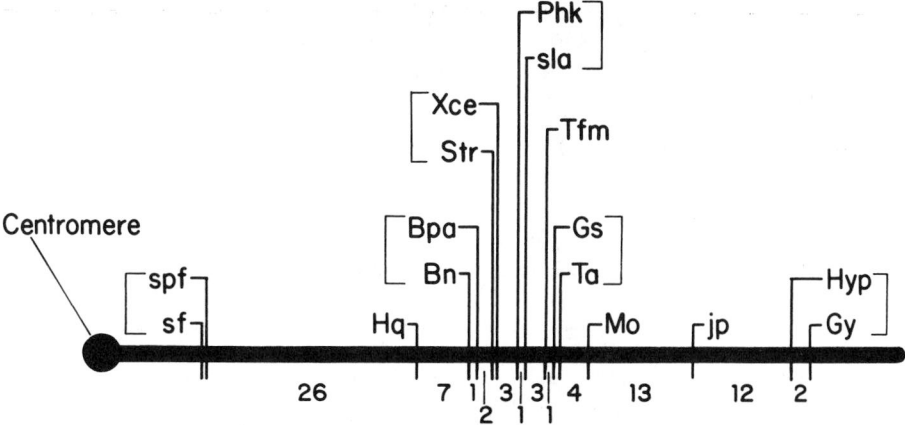

X CHROMOSOME OF MOUSE

Fig. 4.

---

4. *Bn*, bent-tail, X-linked semidominant. Tails of heterozygous females are more or less shortened, with one or several herds, and penetrance is incomplete. Tails of homozygous females
and hemizygous males are shorter and more kinked but not always clearly distinguishable
from the tails of heterozygotes. Homozygotes and hemizygotes may be less viable and fertile
than normals and heterozygotes.

5. *Bpa*, bare patches, X-linked dominant, lethal in the male. The mutant is first identifiable in
heterozygous females at 4–5 days of age by bare patches in the developing coat. The
patches later develop scabs. Males die at the small mole stage. Adult heterozygous females
resemble *Ta* or *Str*.

   Phillips, R. J. S.; Hawker, S. G.; and Moseley, H. J. Bare-patches, a new sex-linked gene in
   the mouse, associated with a high production of XO females. I: A preliminary report of
   breeding experiments. Genet. Res. 22: 91–99, 1973.

6. *Str*, striated, X-linked semidominant. Heterozygous females show transverse striping similar
to heterozygous "tabby" females. The dark stripes are due to shortening of the hairs and
not to a lack of zigzags as in tabby heterozygotes (*Ta/+*). Viability of heterozygotes appears
to be normal; they are underrepresented in segregating generations probably because of
misclassification ("reduced penetrance"). Hemizygous males die at 11–13 days of gestation.

7. *Xce*, X-chromosome controlling element. See 31467.

8. *Phk*, X-linked codominant electrophoretic polymorphism. See 30600.

9. *sla*, sex-linked anemia, X-linked recessive. In the mouse, an X-borne locus is apparently
concerned with transport of iron across the intestinal mucosa, specifically from the mucosal
cell into the blood, because an X-linked anemia of the mouse has a defect in this transport
(Pinkerton and Bannerman, 1967).

Edwards, J. A., and Bannerman, R. M. Hereditary defect of intestinal iron transport in mice with sex-linked anemia. J. Clin. Invest. 49: 1869–1871, 1970.

Pinkerton, P. H., and Bannerman, R. M. Hereditary defect of iron-absorption in mice. Nature 216: 482–483, 1967.

10. *Tfm*, testicular feminization, X-linked recessive. See 31370.

11. *Gs*, greasy, X-linked semidominant. Heterozygous females (*Gs*/+) resemble tabby heterozygotes (*Ta*/+). Homozygous females and hemizygous males have shiny fur like the corresponding tabby genotypes but lack the bare patches behind the ears, the dark middorsal stripe in agouti mice, and the characteristic sticky fell of the tail.

12. *Ta*, tabby, X-linked semidominant. Hemizygous males and homozygous females are characterized by absence of guard hairs in the coat, a bald patch behind each ear, bald tail with a few kinks near the tip, reduced aperture of the eyelids, a respiratory disorder, and a modified agouti pattern. Heterozygous females are most easily recognized if they are agouti, in which case they show transverse dark stripes. The dark stripes have no agouti bands on the hairs. Guard hairs are present in the bands, but zigzags are very deficient or absent. Tabby males breed satisfactorily but homozygous females are often sterile. Heterozygous females are normally fertile.

13. *Mo*, mottled, X-linked semidominant. The defect appears to concern copper transport across the intestinal mucosa and across cell membranes. Thus, it is homologous with Menkes disease (30940).

14. *jp*, jimpy, X-linked recessive. This mutation of the mouse may be homologous to Pelizaeus-Merzbacher disease (31160). It appears that *msd* is allelic.

Eicher, E. M., and Hoppe, P. C. Use of chimeras to transmit lethal genes in the mouse and to demonstrate allelism of the two X-linked male lethal genes *jp* and *msd*. J. Exp. Zool. 183: 181–184, 1973.

15. *Hyp*, hypophosphatemia, X-linked semidominant. This mutation seems to be homologous to human hereditary hypophosphatemia (30780). It was first described as osteopetrosis (*Op.*).

Eicher, E. M., and Southard, J. L. Mouse Newsletter No. 47, p. 46, July, 1972.

16. *Gy*, gyro, X-linked semidominant. Hemizygous males show circling behavior and abnormal development of the long bones and ribs. They are sterile. Heterozygous females show incomplete penetrance for circling behavior and no bony abnormalities. Lyon (1974) suggested that this disorder may be homologous to the oto-palato-digital syndrome (31130).

Lyon, M. F. Mechanisms and evolutionary origins of variable X-chromosome activity in mammals. Proc. Roy. Soc. Lond. B. 187: 243–268, 1974.

In addition to the 16 loci that have been mapped on the X chromosome in the mouse, three loci (G6PD, HGPRT, PGK) have been assigned to the mouse X chromosome by a comparison of enzyme levels in the XX and XO oocytes. The oocytes do not participate in lyonization. Furthermore, the XO mouse is fully fertile. Thus, any enzyme expressed in the oocyte should have a level in the XX oocytes twice as high as that in XO oocytes. Charles Epstein and colleagues (San Francisco) demonstrated the X chromosomal localization of G6PD and HGPRT; Leslie P. Kozak and associates (Bar Harbor), PGK. Furthermore, from study of somatic cell hybrids, α-galactosidase is known to be on the X chromosome in the mouse, just as it is in man.

Epstein, C. J. Mammalian oocytes: X-chromosome activity. Science 163: 1078–1079, 1969.

Epstein, C. J. Expression of the mammalian X chromosome before and after fertilization. Science 175: 1467–1468, 1972.

Kozak, L. P.; McLean, G. K.; and Eicher, E. M. X linkage of phosphoglycerate kinase in the mouse. Biochem. Genet. 11: 41–47, 1974.

In addition, histocompatibility and immune-response genes have been assigned to the mouse X chromosome as indicated elsewhere (B-V-B1, B-V-B4, B-V-B5).

AUTOSOMAL DOMINANT PHENOTYPES

BIOCHEMISTRY MINI-PRINT SERIES

'Prune belly' is a descriptive term for this syndrome, derived from the fact that the intestinal pattern is evident through the thin, lax, protruding abdominal wall in the infant. The full syndrome probably occurs only in males (Williams and Burkholder, 1967). Multiple cases (of the full syndrome) in families have rarely been reported (see below). If this is an X-linked recessive, multiple affected brothers should have been observed. If the disorder is due to fresh dominant mutation in each case, the male-limitation would be unexpected but not impossible. This malformation syndrome is one like Poland syndrome (q.v.) in being rather consistently reproduced in many cases but having no clearly demonstrable Mendelian basis. A possibly related syndrome was described in a single patient by Texter and Murphy (1968). The triad consisted of absence of the right testis, kidney and rectus abdominis muscle. A better prognosis than is usually thought to obtain was suggested by the series of 19 patients reported by Burke et al. (1969). In Lebanon where the rate of consanguinity is high, Afifi et al. (1972) described an affected offspring of first-cousin parents. Garlinger and Ott (1974) described two affected brothers in one family and two affected male cousins in a second. In the first family the parents were nonconsanguineous. In the second family the affected boys' mothers were half-sisters; they had different maternal grandmothers. The prune belly syndrome occurs with trisomy 18. Garlinger and Ott (1973) found 3 other reports of affected sibs, two of affected cousins, and one of concordant male twins. The majority of cases are, thus, sporadic.

Afifi, A. K., Rebeiz, J., Mire, J., Andonian, S. J. and Der Kaloustian, V. M.: The myopathology of the prune belly syndrome. J. Neurol. Sci. 15: 153-166, 1972.

Burke, E. C., Shin, M. H. and Kelalis, P. P.: Prune belly syndrome. Clinical findings and survival. Am. J. Dis. Child. 117: 668-671, 1969.

Garlinger, P. and Ott, J.: Prune belly syndrome: possible genetic implications. Birth Defects Orig. Art. Ser. 10 (8): 173-180, 1974.

Roberts, P.: Congenital absence of the abdominal muscles with associated abnormalities of the genito-urinary tract. Arch. Dis. Child. 31: 236-239, 1956.

Texter, J. H. and Murphy, G. P.: The right-sided syndrome: congenital absence of the right testis, kidney and rectus. Urologic diagnosis and treatment. Johns Hopkins Med. J. 122: 224-228, 1968.

Williams, D. I. and Burkholder, G. V.: The prune belly syndrome. J. Urol. 98: 244-251, 1967.

10020 ABDUCENS PALSY

Affected persons in two or more generations have been reported (Chavasse, 1938; Francois, 1961). Nuclear aplasia has been found in some cases (Phillips et al., 1932). This is a form of hereditary strabismus.

Chavasse, F. B.: The ocular palsies. Trans. Ophthalmol. Soc. U.K. 58: 493 and 497, 1938.

Francois, J.: Heredity in Ophthalmology. St. Louis: C. V. Mosby Co., 1961. P. 280.

Phillips, W. H., Dirion, J. K. and Graves, G. O.: Congenital bilateral palsy of abducens. Arch. Ophthalmol. 8: 355-364, 1932.

10030 ABSENCE DEFECT OF LIMBS, SCALP AND SKULL

The proband described by Adams and Oliver (1945) had (1) absence of the lower extremities below the mid-calf region and absence of all digits and some of the metacarpals of the right hand, (2) a denuded ulcerated area on the vertex of the scalp present at birth, and (3) a bony defect of the skull underlying the scalp defect. The proband had four unaffected brothers and a sister and brother with identical defects of limb, scalp and skull. The father was born with absence of toes II-V on the left foot, with short terminal phalanges of all fingers and with a scalp defect. The father was one of 10 children of whom three others had defects of the extremities. The father's father was said to have had short fingers. The proband's parents were not related. The skin and skull lesions are like those of aplasia cutis congenita (q.v.).

Adams, F. H. and Oliver, C. P.: Hereditary deformities in man due to arrested development. J. Hered. 36: 3-7, 1945.

10035 ACANTHOCYTOSIS WITH HYPO-BETA-LIPOPROTEINEMIA

Mars et al. (1969) described a family in which 14 persons in three generations had low serum levels of beta-lipoprotein, cholesterol and phospholipid. The proposita, a 37-year-old woman, had a demyelinating disorder of one year's duration. The family study was initiated because of the patient's low serum cholesterol. A dislike for dietary fat and unresponsiveness to local anesthetic agents used in dental surgery were found in many members of the family, but none of those examined had frank neurologic disease.

Mars, H., Lewis, L. A., Robertson, A. L., Jr., Butkus, A. and Williams, G. H., Jr.: Familial hypo-beta-lipoproteinemia. A genetic disorder of lipid metabolism with nervous system involvement. Am. J. Med. 46: 886-900, 1969.

*10050 ACANTHOCYTOSIS WITH NEUROLOGIC DISEASE

In addition to the form of acanthocytosis which accompanies abetalipoproteinemia (q.v.), Critchley, Clark and Wikler (1967) described an adult form of acanthocytosis associated with neurological abnormalities and apparently normal serum lipoproteins. The neurologic manifestations suggested those of the Gilles de la Tourette syndrome or Huntington chorea. Five of 10 sibs had neurologic manifestations. A niece had acanthocytes and a neurologic disorder suggesting Friedreich ataxia. The same disorder was probably reported by Levine (1964) and Estes et al. (1967) in a family in which 15 persons in 3 generations had some degree of neuronal impairment and 9 of these had acanthocytosis. Levine et al. (1968) concluded that the predominant neurologic involvement is neuronal. Critchley et al. (1970) reported a single case from England. Another family was reported by Aminoff (1972). Wasting of girdle and proximal limb muscles, absent tendon reflexes and disturbance of bladder function were other features.

Aminoff, M. J.: Acanthocytosis and neurological disease. Brain 95: 749-760, 1972.

Betts, J. J., Nicholson, J. T. and Critchley, E. M. R.: Acanthocytosis with normolipoproteinaemia: biophysical aspects. Postgrad. Med. J. 46: 702-707, 1970.

Critchley, E. M. R., Betts, J. J., Nicholson, J. T. and Weatherall, D. J.: Acanthocytosis, normolipo-proteinaemia and multiple tics. Postgrad. Med. J. 46: 698-701, 1970.

Critchley, E. M. R., Clark, D. B. and Wikler, A.: An adult form of acanthocytosis. Trans. Am. Neurol. Assoc. 92: 132-137, 1967.

Estes, J. W., Morley, T. J., Levine, I. M. and Emerson, C. P.: A new hereditary acanthocytosis syndrome. Am. J. Med. 42: 868-881, 1967.

Levine, I. M.: An hereditary neurologic disease with acanthocytosis. (Abstract) Neurology 14: 272 only, 1964.

Levine, I. M., Estes, J. W. and Looney, J. M.: Hereditary neurological disease with acanthocytosis. A new syndrome. Arch. Neurol. 19: 403-409, 1968.

*10060 ACANTHOSIS NIGRICANS

In all twenty-six patients with malignant acanthosis nigricans (secondary to visceral carcinoma) Curth and Aschner (1959) found no other affected persons in the family. On the other hand benign acanthosis nigricans is probably inherited as a Mendelian dominant. Jung et al. (1965) observed affected mother and daughter. The condition consists of thickening and hyperpigmentation of the skin of the entire body but especially in flexural areas. Lawrence et al. (1971) described a patient with acanthosis nigricans inherited from the father and telangiectasia (18730) inherited from the mother.

Curth, H. O. and Aschner, B. M.: Genetic studies on acanthosis nigricans. Arch. Dermatol. 79: 55-66, 1959.

Hermann, H.: Zur Erbpathologie der Acanthosis nigricans. Z. Menschl. Vererb. Konstitutionsl. 33: 193-202, 1955.

Jung, H. D., Bruns, W., Wulfert, P. and Mieler, W.: Ein Beitrag zum Krankheitsbild der Acanthosis nigricans benigna familiaris. Dtsch. Med. Wochenschr. 90: 1669-1673, 1965.

Lawrence, G., Thurston, C., Shultz, K. and Mengel, M.: Acanthosis nigricans, telangiectasia and diabetes mellitus. The Clinical Delineation of Birth Defects. XII. Skin, Hair and Nails. Baltimore: Williams and Wilkins, 1971. Pp. 322-323.

10070 ACHARD SYNDROME

Arachnodactyly, receding lower jaw and joint laxity limited to the hands and feet are features. Parish (1960) pictured a case. When Thursfield (1917-1918) reviewed the literature on Marfan syndrome, he remarked that the skeletal picture in the cases described by Achard (1902) differed from the others. The skull is broad and brachycephalic with small mandible. Although there is arachnodactyly the body proportions are not altered and the patient is not excessively tall.

Achard, C.: Arachnodactylie. Bull. Soc. Med. Hosp. Paris 19: 834-840, 1902.

Parish, J. G.: Heritable disorders of connective tissues with arachnodactyly. Proc. R. Soc. Med. 53: 515-518, 1960.

Parish, J. G.: Skeletal hand charts in inherited connective tissue disease. J. Med. Genet. 4: 227-238, 1967.

Thursfield, H.: Arachnodactyly. St. Bart's Hosp. Rep. 53: 35-40, 1917-18.

*10080 ACHONDROPLASIA

Although there are numerous simulating skeletal disorders, true achondroplasia is a well-delineated distinct entity which probably in all instances occurs as a new dominant mutation or by dominant inheritance. The chondrocranium is affected producing bulging skull, 'scooped out' bridge of the nose, and small foramen magnum. True megalencephaly occurs and appears to indicate effects of the gene other than those on the skeleton alone. Disproportion between the base of the skull and the brain results in internal hydrocephalus in some cases. In children caudad narrowing of the interpeduncular distance, rather than the normal caudad widening, and notch-like sacro-iliac groove are typical radiologic features. Also in children the epiphyseal ossification center shows a circumflex or chevron seat on the metaphysis. About seven-eighths of cases are the result of new mutation, there being a considerable reduction of effective reproductive fitness. Paternal age effect on mutation has been noted (Penrose, 1955). (It is of historic interest that Weinberg, of Hardy-Weinberg fame, noted (1912) in the data collected by Rischbieth and Barrington that sporadic cases were more often last born than first born.) The radiologic features of true achondroplasia and much concerning the natural history of the condition were presented by Langer et al. (1967) on the basis of a study of 101 cases. See THANATOPHORIC DWARFISM for a condition which is fatal in the first days of life and which simulates achondroplasia. Homozygosity for the achondroplasia gene results in a severe disorder of the skeleton with radiologic changes somewhat different from those of heterozygous achondroplasia and with early death as a result of respiratory embarrassment from the small thoracic cage and neurologic deficit from hydrocephalus (Hall et al., 1969). The confusion of true achondroplasia with other entities is illustrated by the two female sibs reported by Wallace et al. (1970) as examples of this condition. Both died in the neonatal period and showed, in addition to chondrodystrophy, central harelip, hypoplastic lungs and hydrocephalus. Without radiographic studies it is impossible to identify the nature of this condition but it is certainly not true achondroplasia. Jeune asphyxiating thoracic dystrophy, thanatophoric dwarfism and achondrogenesis are three possibilities. The report of Wallace et al. demonstrates why estimates of mutation rate have been falsely high. Hypochondroplasia (14600) may be caused by an allele at the achondroplasia locus.

Cohen, M. E., Rosenthal, A. D. and Matson, D. D.: Neurological abnormalities in achondroplastic children. J. Pediatr. 71: 367-376, 1967.

Dennis, J. P., Rosenberg, H. S. and Alvord, E. C., Jr.: Megalencephaly, internal hydrocephalus and other neurological aspects of achondroplasia. Brain 84: 427-445, 1961.

Hall, J. G., Dorst, J. P., Taybi, H., Scott, C. I., Langer, L. O., Jr. and McKusick, V. A.: Two probable cases of homozygosity for the achondroplasia gene. The Clinical Delineation of Birth Defects. IV. Skeletal Dysplasias. New York: National Foundation, 1969. Pp. 24-34.

Langer, L. O., Jr., Baumann, P. A. and Gorlin, R. J.: Achondroplasia. Am. J. Roentgenol. Radium Ther. Nuci. Med. 100: 12-26, 1967.

Maroteaux, P. and Lamy, P.: Achondroplasia in man and animals. Clin. Orthop. 33: 91-103, 1964.

Morch, E. T.: Chondrodystrophic dwarfs in Denmark. Op. Ex. Domo. Biol. Hered. Hum. U. Hafniensis 3: 1941.

Murdoch, J. L., Walker, B. A., Hall, J. G., Abbey, H., Smith, K. K. and McKusick, V. A.: Achondroplasia — a genetic and statistical survey. Ann. Hum. Genet. 33: 227-244, 1970.

Penrose, L. S.: Parental age and mutation. Lancet II: 312-313, 1955.

Penrose, L. S.: Parental age in achondroplasia and mongolism. Am. J. Hum. Genet. 9: 167-169, 1957.

Rimoin, D. L., Hughes, G. N., Kaufman, R. L., Rosenthal, R. E., McAlister, W. H. and Silberberg, R.: Endochondral ossification in achondroplastic dwarfism. N. Engl. J. Med. 283: 728-735, 1970.

Wallace, D. C., Exton, L. A., Pritchard, D. A., Leung, Y. and Cooke, R. A.: Severe achondroplasia. Demonstration of probable heterogeneity within this clinical syndrome. J. Med. Genet. 7: 22-26, 1970.

Weinberg, W.: Zur Vererbung des Zwergwuchses. Arch. Rass. u. Ges. Biol. 9: 710-717, 1912.

*10100 ACOUSTIC NEURINOMA, BILATERAL

Gardner and Frazier (1933) reported a family of five generations in which 38 members were affected with deafness. Of these, 15 later became blind. The average age of onset of deafness was 20 years. The average age at death of affected persons in the second generation was 72, in the third generation 63, in the fourth 42 and in the fifth 28. There was little or no evidence of von Recklinghausen disease (q.v.) in the family, suggesting that this is a separate mutation. A follow-up of the family was published in 1940. Although acoustic neuroma is sometimes a feature of neurofibromatosis (q.v.) bilateral acoustic neuroma is probably an isolated abnormality with dominant inheritance in some cases. The most convincing families are those of Gardner and Turner (1940) and of Feiling and Ward (1920). Moyes (1968) added a well-studied, extensively affected kindred with no evidence of von Recklinghausen disease. These cases represent in all probability a central nervous system form of multiple neurofibromatosis. Eldridge (1969) found no evidence of von Recklinghausen neurofibromatosis of the conventional type in the family of Gardner when he restudied it extensively. Two cases of the CNS form, one of them familial, were studied at autopsy by Perez Demoura et al. (1969), who incorrectly referred to the cases of Gardner and Frazier (1930) as representing von Recklinghausen disease. The case reported by Worster-Drought et al. (1937) were of the 'central' neurofibromatosis type. They pointed out that Wishart reported such a case in 1821.

Eldridge, R.: Bethesda, Md.: personal communication, 1969.

Feiling, A. and Ward, E.: A familial form of acoustic tumour. Br. Med. J. 1: 496-497, 1920.

Gardner, W. J. and Frazier, C. H.: Bilateral acoustic neurofibromas. A clinical study and survey of a family of five generations with bilateral deafness in 38 members. Arch. Neurol. Psychiat. 23: 266-302, 1930. (See also J. Hered. 22: 7-8, 1933.)

Gardner, W. J. and Turner, O.: Bilateral acoustic neurofibromas: further clinical and pathologic data on hereditary deafness and Recklinghausen's disease. Arch. Neurol. Psychiat. 44: 76-99, 1940.

Moyes, P. D.: Familial bilateral acoustic neuroma affecting 14 members from four generations. J. Neurosurg. 29: 78-82, 1968.

Perez Demoura, L. F., Hayden, R. C., Jr. and Conner, G. H.: Bilateral acoustic neurinoma and neurofibromatosis. Arch. Otolaryngnol. 90: 28-34, 1969.

Worster-Drought, C., Dickson, W. E. C. and McMenemey, W. H.: Multiple meningeal and perineural tumors with analogous changes in the glia and ependyma (neurofibroblastomatosis). Brain 60: 85-117, 1937.

Young, D. F., Eldridge, R. and Gardner, W. J.: Bilateral acoustic neuroma in a large kindred. J.A.M.A. 214: 347-353, 1970.

10110 ACROCEPHALOPOLYSYNDACTYLY TYPE I (ACPS I, OR NOACK SYNDROME)

Acrocephalopolysyndactyly differs from Apert syndrome (acrocephalosyndactyly) in the presence of polydactyly as an additional feature. Two types are recognized. Type I, or Noack syndrome, is dominant. Type II, or Carpenter syndrome, is recessive. Noack (1959) reported a 43-year-old man and his 11 month old daughter, both of whom exhibited acrocephaly and polysyndactyly. Enlarged thumbs and great toes with duplication of the latter (preaxial polydactyly) were described, as well as syndactyly. Intelligence was apparently normal. Follow-up of Noack's kindred by Pfeiffer appears to indicate that their disorder is the same as that referred to elsewhere as acrocephalosyndactyly type V (Pfeiffer type).

Gnamey, D, and Farriaux, J. P.: Syndrome dominant associant polysyndactylie, pouces en spatule, anomalies facials et retard mental (une forme particuliere de l'acrocephalo-polysyndactylie de type Noack). J. Genet. Hum. 19: 299-316, 1972.

Noack, M.: Ein Beitrag zum Krankheitsbild der Akrozephalosyndaktylie (Apert). Arch. Kinderheilk. 160: 168-171, 1959.

Pfeiffer, R. A.: Associated deformities of the head and hands. The Clinical Delineation of Birth Defects. III. Limb Malformations. New York: National Foundation, 1969. Pp. 18-34.

*10120 ACROCEPHALOSYNDACTYLY TYPE I (TYPICAL APERT SYNDROME)

Apert (1906) defined a syndrome characterized by skull malformation (acrocephaly of brachysphenocephalic type) and syndactyly of the hands and feet of a special type (complete distal fusion with a tendency to fusion also of the bony structures). The hand, when all the fingers are webbed, has been compared to a spoon and, when the thumb is free, to an obstetric hand. Blank (1960) in his review designated cases of ACS showing these malformations as typical Apert syndrome. Most cases of Apert syndrome are sporadic, but there are at least two reported instances of parent-to-child transmission. We (Roberts and Hall, 1971) have observed affected mother and daughter. Van den Bosch (quoted by Blank) observed the typical deformity in a mother and her son, and Weech (1927) reported Apert syndrome in a mother and her daughter. Blank (1960) assembled case material on 54 patients born in Great Britian. Two clinical categories were distinguished: (1) 'typical' acrocephalosyndactyly, to which Apert's name is appropriately applied; and (2) other forms lumped together as 'atypical' acrocephalosyndactyly. The feature distinguishing the two types is a mid-digital hand mass with a single nail common to digits II — IV, found in Apert syndrome and lacking in the others. 39 of the 54 were of Apert type. 6 of 12 autopsies showed visceral anomalies but in no two were these identical. A frequency of Apert syndrome of one in each 160,000 births was estimated. No patient married. Low frequency of consanguinity and failure to observe multiple sibs make recessive inheritance unlikely. No chromosomal abnormality is demonstrable. The evidence strongly suggests dominant inheritance, presumably autosomal in view of the equal sex ratio. Paternal age effect is demonstrable. Dodson et al. (1970) described deletion-translocation of the short arm of A chromosome 2 to the long arm of A chromosome 11 or 12 in a patient with Apert syndrome. They found reports of chromosomal abnormalities (all involving the A group) in three other cases of Apert syndrome. Schauerte and St-Aubin (1966) pointed out that progressive synostosis occurs in the feet, hands, carpus, tarsus, cervical vertebrae, and skull and proposed 'progressive synosteosis with syndactyly' as a more appropriate designation. Cohen (1973) provided a superb review of all the 'craniosynostosis syndromes.'

Apert, M. E.: De l'acrocephalosyndactylie. Bull. Soc. Med. Hosp. Paris 23: 1310-1330, 1906.

Blank, C. E.: Apert's syndrome (a type of acrocephalosyndactyly). Observations on a British series of thirty-nine cases. Ann. Hum. Genet. 24: 151-164, 1960.

Cohen, M. M., Jr.: An etiologic and nosologic overview of craniosynostosis syndromes. The Clinical Delineation of Birth Defects. XVII. Malformation Syndromes (cont.). Baltimore: Williams and Wilkins, 1973.

Dodson, W. E., Museles, M., Kennedy, J. L., Jr. and Al-Aish, M.: Acrocephalosyndactylia associated with a chromosomal translocation: 46,XX,t(2p-:Cq+). Am. J. Dis. Child. 120: 360-362, 1970.

Hoover, G. H., Flatt, A. E. and Weiss, M. W.: The hand and Apert's syndrome. J. Bone Joint Surg. 52A: 878-895, 1970.

Roberts, K. B. and Hall, J. G.: Apert's acrocephalosyndactyly in mother and daughter: cleft palate in the mother. The Clinical Delineation of Birth Defects. XI. Orofacial Structures. Baltimore: Williams and Wilkins, 1971. Pp. 262-264.

Schauerte, E. W. and St-Aubin, P. M.: Progressive synosteosis in Apert's syndrome (acrocephalosyndactyly): with a description of roentgenographic changes in the feet. Am. J. Roentgenol. Radium Ther. Nuci. Med. 97: 67-73, 1966.

Solomon, L. M., Fretzin, D. and Pruzansky, S.: Pilosebaceous abnormalities in Apert's syndrome. Arch. Dermatol. 102: 381-385, 1970.

Weech, A. A.: Combined acrocephaly and syndactylism occurring in mother and daughter. A case report. Bull. Hopkins Hosp. 40: 73-76, 1927.

10130 ACROCEPHALOSYNDACTYLY TYPE II (APERT-CROUZON DISEASE, OR VOGT CEPH-ALODACTYLY)

Vogt (1933) described cases presenting the hand and foot malformations characteristic of Apert disease, together with the facial characteristics of Crouzon disease, caused by an extremely hypoplastic maxilla. In the hands the syndactyly is less severe than in Apert disease and the thumbs and little fingers are usually free. Nager and de Reynier (1948) gave this deformity the name of Vogt cephalodactyly, while other authors called it Apert-Crouzon disease, indicating the similarity to both abnormalities. There are no reported instances of hereditary transmission; however, this could be due simply to low reproductive fitness. Many doubt seriously that Vogt cephalodactyly is a separate entity; they view it merely as Apert syndrome with unusually marked facial features (Temtamy and McKusick, 1975).

Nager, F. R. and De Reynier, J. P.: Das Gehoerorgan bei den angeborenen Kopfmissbildungen. Pract. Otorhinolaryngol. 10 (suppl. 2): 1-128, 1948.

Temtamy, S. A. and McKusick, V. A.: The Genetics of Hand Malformations. New York: National Foundation-March of Dimes, 1975 (to be published).

Vogt, A.: Dyskephalie (dysostosis craniofacialis, maladie De Crouzon 1912) und eine neuartige Kombination dieser Krankheit mit Syndaktylie der 4 Extremitaeten (Dyskephalodaktylie). Klin. Monatsbl. Augenheilkd. 90: 441-454, 1933.

*10140 ACROCEPHALOSYNDACTYLY TYPE III (CHOTZEN SYNDROME: ACROCEPHALY, SKULL ASYMMETRY AND MILD SYNDACTYLY)

In the family described by Saethre (1931), a mother, two daughters and probably other maternal relatives showed mild acrocephaly, asymmetry of the skull, and partial soft tissue syndactyly of fingers II and III and toes III and IV. Chotzen (1932) found identical malformations in a father and two sons. Bartsocas et al. (1970) described a Lithuanian kindred living in the United States in which 10 persons in 3 generations were affected, with several instances of male-to-male transmission. In 1961 Waardenburg reported the findings in 6 generations of a kindred. Asymmetry of the skull and orbits (plagiocephaly), strabismus and thin, long pointed nose were changes in the head. Some affected persons had bifid terminal phalanges of digits II and III and absence of the first metatarsal. Cleft palate, hydrophthalmos, cardiac malformation and contractures of elbows and knees were present in some. Aase and Smith (1970) described a syndrome in five members of three generations (with one instance of male-to-male transmission), comprising asymmetry of the face (hypoplasia of the left side), unusually shaped ear with prominent crus, and Simian crease. They pointed out similarities and differences from Waardenburg (1961) asymmetry of the face and skull with abnormalities of the digits. Gorlin (1971) is of the opinion that this is Chotzen syndrome.

Aase, J. M. and Smith, D. W.: Facial asymmetry and abnormalities of palms and ears: a dominantly inherited developmental syndrome. J. Pediatr. 76: 928-930, 1970.

Bartsocas, C. S., Weber, A. L. and Crawford, J. D.: Acrocephalosyndactyly type 3: Chotzen's syndrome. J. Pediatr. 77: 267-272, 1970.

Chotzen, F.: Eine eigenartige familiaere Entwicklungsstoerung (Akrocephalosyndaktylie, Dysostosis craniofacialis und Hypertelorismus). Monatschr. Kinderheilkd. 55: 97-122, 1932.

Gorlin, R. J.: Minneapolis, Minn.: personal communication, 1971.

Kreiborg, S., Pruzansky, S. and Pashayan, H.: The Saethre-Chotzen syndrome. Teratology 6: 287-294, 1972.

Saethre, M.: Ein Beitrag zum Turmschaedelproblem (Pathogenese, Erblichkeit und Symptomatologie). Deutsch. Z. Nervenheilk. 119: 533-555, 1931.

Waardenburg, P. J., Franceschetti, A. and Klein, D.: Genetics and Ophthalmology, vol. 1. Springfield, Ill.: Charles C Thomas, 1961. Pp. 301-354.

*10160 ACROCEPHALOSYNDACTYLY TYPE V (PFEIFFER TYPE)

Pfeiffer (1964) found 8 affected in 3 generations, with two instances of male-to-male transmission. The striking feature of the hand deformity was broad, short thumbs and big toes. The proximal phalanx of the thumb was either triangular or trapezoid (and occasionally fused with the distal phalanx) so that the thumb pointed outward (i.e., away from the other digits). Martsolf et al. (1971) described the case of an affected boy whose mother and maternal half-brother were said to be affected also. Another pedigree consistent with autosomal dominant inheritance was reported by Saldino et al. (1972). After restudying a family reported by Noack, Pfeiffer concluded that that family has the Pfeiffer syndrome rather than a distinct disorder (see 10110 for references).

Martsolf, J. T., Cracco, J. B., Carpenter, G. G. and O'Hara, A. E.: Pfeiffer syndrome: an unusual type of acrocephalosyndactyly with broad thumbs and great toes. Am. J. Dis. Child. 121: 257-262, 1971.

Pfeiffer, R. A.: Dominant erbliche Akrocephalosyndaktylie. Z. Kinderheilk. 90: 301-320, 1964.

Saldino, R. M., Steinbach, H. L. and Epstein, C. J.: Familial acropholosyndactyly (Pfeiffer syndrome). Am. J. Roentgenol. Radium Ther. Nuci. Med. 116: 609-622, 1972.

10170 ACROCYANOSIS

This may be the presenting complaint in the Ehlers-Danlos syndrome (q.v.) and this syndrome is, therefore, at least one basis for acrocyanosis that 'runs in a family.' (There is no evidence of a separate genetic basis for acrocyanosis.) For example, Gilbert and colleagues (1925) described a 22-year-old man who had had cyanosis of the hands, feet and ears from birth and showed other characteristic features of E-D. In his family several other persons had 'cyanosed limbs and ulcerated chilblains' in association with E-D.

Gilbert, A., Villaret, M. and Bosviel, G.: Sur un cas d'hyperelasticite congenitale des ligaments articulaires et de la peau. Bull. Soc. Med. Hosp. Paris 49: 303-307, 1925.

10180 ACRODYSOSTOSIS

Maroteaux and Malamut (1968) suggested that 'peripheral dysostosis' (q.v.) is a heterogeneous class. They described acrodysostosis as a condition in which peculiar facies (short nose, open mouth and prognathism) are associated with the small hands and feet. Mental deficiency is frequent. Inheritance or parental consanguinity is not yet known. Cone epiphyses occur in this condition. Robinow et al. (1971) reported nine cases and reviewed 11 from the literature. None was familial.

Arkless and Graham, C. B.: An unusual case of brachydactyly. Am. J. Roentgenol. Radium Ther. Nuci. Med. 99: 724-735, 1967.

Maroteaux, P. and Malamut, G.: L'acrodysostose. Presse Med. 76: 2189-2192, 1968.

Robinow, M., Pfeiffer, R. A., Gorlin, R. J., McKusick, V. A., Renuart, A. W., Johnson, G. F. and Summitt, R. L.: Acrodysostosis: a syndrome of peripheral dysostosis, nasal hypoplasia, and mental retardation. Am. J. Dis. Child. 121: 195-203, 1971.

*10185 ACROKERATOELASTOIDOSIS

This disorder was first described and named by Costa (1953). Jung (1973) studied an extensively affected family. The palms and soles are primarily affected. Involvement may extend to the dorsum of the hands and feet in severe cases. The lesions are nodulary and yellow with hyperkeratotic surfaces. The histology combines hyperkeratosis and disorganization of elastic fibers. No systemic manifestation has been detected.

Costa, O. G.: Akrokeratoelastoidosis: a hitherto undescribed skin disease. Dermatologica 107: 164-167, 1953.

Jung, E. G.: Acrokeratoelastoidosis. Humangenetik 17: 357-358, 1973.

*10190 ACROKERATOSIS VERRUCIFORMIS (HOPF)

The pedigree studied by Niedelman and McKusick (1962) contained instances of male-to-male transmission as well as unaffected daughters of affected males. Warty hyperkeratotic lesions are found on the dorsal aspect of the hands and feet and on the knees and elbows. Herndon and Wilson (1966) have emphasized the phenotypic overlap between this entity and Darier-White disease (q.v.) and have even proposed that they may not be separate entities. In the family they studied, 7 persons had typical acrokeratosis verruciformis, one or possibly two had Darier disease and three had minor disturbances of keratinization (white nails from subungual hyperkeratosis, or punctate keratoses of palms or soles).

Herndon, J. H., Jr. and Wilson, J. D.: Acrokeratosis verruciformis (HOPF) and Darier's disease. Genetic evidence for a unitary origin. Arch. Dermatol. 93: 305-310, 1966.

Niedelman, M. L. and McKusick, V. A.: Acrokeratosis verruciformis (HOPF). A follow-up study. Arch. Dermatol. 86: 779-782, 1962.

10200 ACROLEUKOPATHY, SYMMETRIC

Sugai, Saito and Hamada (1965) described mother and daughter with symmetric depigmentation of the great toes.

Sugai, T., Saito, T. and Hamada, T.: Symmetric acroleukopathy in mother and daughter. Arch. Dermatol. 92: 172-173, 1965.

*10210 ACROMEGALOID CHANGES, CUTIS VERTICIS GYRATA AND CORNEAL LEUKOMA

Rosenthal and Kloepfer (1962) described a 'new' syndrome with these three features in 13 persons of four generations of a Louisiana Negro family. Through the courtesy of Kloepfer, I saw affected members of this family in 1971. The corneal leukoma is an epithelial change. The hands, feet and chin are very large and the affected persons unusually tall. Although growth hormone assays had not been done, other endocrine studies and X-ray views of the sella turcica give no indication of pituitary dysfunction. One of the affected females examined had 9 living children. The skin of the hands is unusually soft and has an abnormal dermal ridge pattern, referred to as 'split ridges,' which permits identification of the disorder in children of preclinical age. A possible difference from the usual cutis verticis gyrata is a longitudinal orientation of the skin folds rather than transverse orientation. X-ray features were reported by Harbison and Nice (1971).

Harbison, J. B. and Nice, C. M., Jr.: Familial pachydermoperiostosis presenting as an acromegaly-like syndrome. Am. J. Roentgenol. Radium Ther. Nucl. Med. 112: 532-536, 1971.

Rosenthal, J. W. and Kloepfer, H. W.: An acromegaloid, cutis verticis gyrata, corneal leukoma syndrome. Arch. Ophthalmol. 68: 722-726, 1962.

10220 ACROMEGALY

Koch and Tiwisina (1959) reviewed 8 examples of affected persons in two successive generations including 4 instances of father and 1 or more sons affected. Some reported instances of familial acromegaly may in fact be pachydermoperiostosis, the acromegaloid-cutis gyrata-leukoma syndrome, or cerebral gigantism. Furthermore, familial acromegaly can be a partial expression of the multiple endocrine adenomatosis syndrome.

Koch, G. and Tiwisina, T.: Beitrag zur Erblichkeit der Akromegalie und der Hyperostosis generalisata mit Pachydermie. Aerztl. Forsch. 13: 489-504, 1959.

Koch, G.: Erbliche Hirngeschwuelste. Z. Menschl. Vererb. Konstitutionsl. 29: 400-423, 1949.

10230 ACROMELALGIA, HEREDITARY ('RESTLESS LEGS')

Because of paresthesia with first going to bed or sitting still for a time, the affected person cannot resist fidgeting with his feet. Huizinga (1957) described a family with affected persons in five generations. The condition involving the feet was relieved by cold and had its onset in adolescence. Bornstein (1961) and Ekbom (1960) also described familial aggregation.

Bornstein, B.: Restless legs. Psychiat. Neurol. 141: 165-201, 1961.

Ekbom, K. A.: Restless legs syndrome. Neurology 10: 868-873, 1960.

Huizinga, J.: Hereditary acromelalgia (or 'restless legs'). Acta Genet. Statist. Med. 7: 121-123, 1957.

9

D
O
M
I
N
A
N
T

10235 ACROMIAL DIMPLES

Dimples overlying the acromial process of the scapula, i.e., on the back of the shoulders, is a regular feature of the 18q- syndrome. Bianchine (1974) described acromial dimples in a four-year-old girl, her 30-year-old mother and her 65-year-old maternal grandmother. All three were generally healthy.

Bianchine, J. W.: Acromial dimples: a benign familial trait. Am. J. Hum. Genet. 26: 412-413, 1974.

10240 ACRO-OSTEOLYSIS

Lamy and Maroteaux (1961) described a dominant form in mother and son. Members of two earlier generations were also affected. No abnormality of sensation was present. Schinz (1951) described dominant inheritance of this disorder with onset between 8 and 22 years. Slowly progressive osteolysis of the phalanges in the hands and feet was associated with recurrent ulcers of the fingers and soles of the feet, elimination of bone sequestra and healing with loss of toes or fingers. Maroteaux (1970) found no basilar impression, or other changes in the skull or long bones to suggest that this was Cheney syndrome (q.v.). A phenocopy is produced in men working in the polymerization of vinyl chloride (Harris, Adams, 1967; Ross, 1970). Reed (1974) told me of other families.

Harms, I.: Ueber die familiaere Akro-osteolyse. Fortschr. Roentgenstr. 80: 727-733, 1954.

Harris, D. K. and Adams, W. G. F.: Acro-osteolysis occurring in men engaged in the polymerization of vinyl chloride. Br. Med. J. 3: 712-714, 1967.

Lamy, M. and Maroteaux, P.: Acro-osteolyse dominante. Arch. Fr. Pediatr. 18: 693-702, 1961.

Maroteaux, P.: Paris, France: personal communication, 1970.

Reed, W. B.: Burbank, Calif., personal communication.

Ross, J. A.: An unusual occupational bone change. In, Jelliffe, A. M. and Strickland, B. (eds.): Symposium Ossium. London: Livingstone, 1970.

Schinz, H. R., Baensch, W. E., Friedl, E. and Uehlinger, E. (eds.): Roentgen-diagnostics. Trans. in English by J. T. Case. New York: Grune and Stratton, vol. 1, 1951. Fig. 969 on P. 734.

*10250 ACRO-OSTEOLYSIS WITH OSTEOPOROSIS AND CHANGES IN SKULL AND MANDIBLE (CHENEY SYNDROME)

Cheney (1965) described a family living in the upper peninsula of Michigan in which the mother and four children had acro-osteolysis, multiple Wormian bones, hypoplasia of ramus of mandible. Different from pycnodysostosis, a recessive with osteosclerosis, the condition in Cheney's patients had osteoporosis with basilar impression as a feature. The mother was 57 and the affected children (4 of 6) were 35, 26, 21 and 13. Dorst and McKusick (1969) described a case. Herrmann et al. (1973) suggested the eponym of Hajdu-Cheney syndrome. They pointed out that the changes in the terminal phalanges in this condition as well as pycnodysostosis is 'pseudo-osteolysis,' that is a disorder development of bone rather than destruction of bone already found. Herrmann et al. (1973) exhaustively reviewed the previously reported cases and described one new case of this disorder. The authors suggest the name, arthro-dento-osteodysplasia (ADOD), for this disorder of connective tissue. They observed that acro-osteolysis, generalized osteoporosis and multiple fractures of the skull, spine and digits, short stature, persistent cranial sutures, multiple wormian bones, early loss of teeth and joint laxity were features associated in varying degrees with ADOD.

Cheney, W. D.: Acro-osteolysis. Am. J. Roentgenol. Radium Ther. Nuci. Med. 94: 595-607, 1965.

Dorst, J. P. and McKusick, V. A.: Acro-osteolysis (Cheney syndrome). The Clinical Delineation of Birth Defects. III. Limb Malformations. New York: National Foundation, 1969. Pp. 215-217.

Hajdu, N. and Kauntze, R.: Cranioskeletal dysplasia. Br. J. Radiol. 21: 42-48, 1948.

Herrmann, J., Zugibe, F. T., Gilbert, E. F. and Opitz, J. M.: Arthro-dento-osteo dysplasia (Hajdu-Cheney syndrome). Z. Kinderheilk 11: 1-18, 1973.

Herrmann, J., Zugibe, F. T., Gilbert, E. F. and Opitz, J. M.: Arthro-dento-osteo dysplasia (Hadju-Cheney syndrome). Review of a genetic 'acro-osteolysis' syndrome. Z. Kinderheilk. 114: 93-110, 1973.

10253 ACRORENAL SYNDROME

Dieker and Opitz (1969) described three patients with the association of major malformations of the kidneys and limbs, mainly absence deformities of digits. Curran and Curran (1972) described a case and pointed out that paternal age was sometimes increased (44 years in their case and 57 years in one of Dieker and Opitz).

Curran, A. S. and Curran, J. P.: Associated acral and renal malformations: a new syndrome? Pediatrics 49: 716-725, 1972.

Dieker, H. and Opitz, J. M.: Associated acral and renal malformations. The Clinical Delineation of Birth Defects. III. Limb Malformations. New York: National Foundation, 1969. Pp. 68-77.

*10255 ADENINE B+ AUXOTROPH, HUMAN COMPLEMENT FOR HAMSTER

Kao and Puck (1972) have shown that the locus is on either chromosome 4 or 5. The enzyme whose presence results in complementation is thought to be formylglycinamide ribotide amidotransferase.

Kao, F. D. and Puck, T. T.: Denver, Col.: personal communication through Dr. F. H. Ruddle, 1972.

Kao, F. T. and Puck, T. T.: Genetics of somatic mammalian cells: demonstration of a human esterase activator gene linked to the adeb gene. Proc. Natl. Acad. Sci. 69: 3273-3277, 1972.

*10260 ADENINE PHOSPHORIBOSYLTRANSFERASE

Mutant forms of APRT have been described by Kelley et al. (1968) and by Henderson et al. (1969) who found the inheritance to be autosomal. (The other purine phosphoribosyltransferase (HGPRT) is determined by an X-linked locus and is mutant in the Lesch-Nyhan syndrome (q.v.).) The heat-stable enzyme allele has a frequency of about 15 percent and the heat-labile enzyme allele of about 85 percent. This polymorphism might be a useful marker for linkage studies. No disease has been related to mutant forms of APRT. Kelly et al. (1968) found apparent heterozygosity in four persons in three generations of a family. The level of enzyme activity ranged from 21 to 37 percent, requiring some special explanation. That the enzyme is a dimer is one possibility. Fox et al. (1973) described a second family with partial deficiency of red cell APRT. By cell hybridization studies Tischfield and Ruddle (1974) concluded that the APRT locus is on chromosome no. 16. Mapping in relation to the haptoglobulin locus (14010) should be studied in families. Delbarre et al. (1974) found deficiency of APRT in persons with gout but recognized that purine overproduction was not necessarily caused by the APRT deficiency.

Delbarre, F., Aucher, C., Amor, B. De Gery, A., Cartier, P. and Hamet, M.: Gout with adenine phosphoribosyl transferase deficiency. Biomed. 21: 82-85, 1974.

Fox, I, H., Meade, J. C. and Kelley, W. N.: Adenine phosphoribosyltransferase deficiency in man. Report of a second family. Am. J. Med. 55: 614-619, 1973.

Henderson, J. F., Kelley, W. N., Rosenbloom, F. M. and Seegmiller, J. E.: Inheritance of purine phosphoribosyltransferases in man. Am. J. Hum. Genet. 21: 61-70, 1969.

Kelley, W. N., Levy, R. I., Rosenbloom, F. M., Henderson, J. F. and Seegmiller, J. E.: Adenine phosphoribosyltransferase deficiency: a previously undescribed genetic defect in man. J. Clin. Invest. 47: 2281-2289, 1968.

Tischfield, J. A. and Ruddle, F. H.: Assignment of the gene for adenine phosphoribosyltransferase to human chromosome 16 by mouse-human somatic cell hybridization. Proc. Natl. Acad. Sci. 71: 45-49, 1974.

*10270 ADENOSINE DEAMINASE

By means of a new and specific method, Spencer et al. (1968) demonstrated isozymes of adenosine deaminase and showed that there are 3 genetically determined phenotypes: ADA 1, ADA 2-1 and ADA 2. The frequency of the ADA(2) allele was estimated at 0.06 in Europeans, 0.04 in Negroes and 0.11 in Asiatic Indians. Giblett et al. (1973) found no measurable red cell ADA in two young unrelated girls with immune deficiency disease. The parents of the first case were related and the second case had, by history, a similarly affected sib. Furthermore, intermediate levels of ADA in the parents supported recessive inheritance. Since most of the ADA of lymphocytes is physicochemically identical to that in the red cell, it was suggested that the same locus as for red cell ADA polymorphism is involved. By study of mouse-man somatic cell hybrids, Creagan et al. (1973) showed that the locus for ADA can be assigned to chromosome no. 20.

Cook, P. J. L., Hopkinson, D. A. and Robson, E. B.: The linkage relationships of adenosine deaminase. Ann. Hum. Genet. 34: 187-188, 1970.

Creagan, R. P., Tischfield, J. A., Nichols, E. A. and Ruddle, F. H.: Autosomal assignment of the gene for the form of adenosine deaminase which is deficient in patients with combined immunodeficiency syndrome. (Letter) Lancet II: 1449 only, 1973.

Detter, J. C., Stamatoyannopoulos, G., Giblett, E. R. and Motulsky, A. G.: Adenosine deaminase: racial distribution and report of a new phenotype. J. Med. Genet. 7: 356-357, 1970.

Dissing, J. and Knudsen, J. B.: A new red cell adenosine deaminase phenotype in man. Hum. Hered. 19: 375-377, 1969.

Edwards, J. E., Allen, F. H., Glenn, K. P., Lamm, L. U. and Robson, E. B.: personal communication, 1972. (To be published in Histocompatibility Testing, 1972.)

Giblett, E. R., Anderson, J. E., Cohen, F., Pollara, B. and Meuwissen, H. J.: Adenosine-deaminase deficiency in two patients with severely impaired cellular immunity. Lancet II: 1067-1069, 1972.

Hopkinson, D. A., Cook, P. J. L. and Harris, H.: Further data on the adenosine deaminase (ADA) polymorphism and a report of a new phenotype. Ann. Hum. Genet. 32: 361-368, 1969.

Ritter, H., Wendt, G. G., Tariwerdian, G., Zelch, J., Rube, M. and Kirchberg, G.: Genetics and linkage analysis of adenosine deaminase. Humangenetik 14: 69-71, 1971.

Spencer, N., Hopkinson, D. A. and Harris, H.: Adenosine deaminase polymorphism in man. Ann. Hum. Genet. 32: 9-14, 1968.

Tariverdian, G. and Ritter, H.: Adenosine deaminase polymorphism (EC 3.5.4.4): Formal genetics and linkage relations. Humangenetik 7: 176-178, 1969.

Weitkamp, L. R.: Further data on the genetic linkage relations of the adenosine deaminase locus. Hum. Hered. 21: 351-356, 1971.

Weitkamp, L. R.: Genetic linkage relationships of the ADA and 6-PGD loci in 'Humangenetik.' (Letter) Humangenetik 15: 359-360, 1972.

*10280 ADENOSINE TRIPHOSPHATASE DEFICIENCY, ANEMIA DUE TO

In two kindreds Harvald et al. (1964) observed nonspherocytic hemolytic anemia due to deficiency of ATP-ase. At least two generations were affected in each family and father-son transmission was noted. Hanel et al. (1971) restudied the families and concluded that the trait is an irregular dominant. Only some of the heterozygotes, probably a minority, have hemolytic anemia.

Hanel, H. K., Cohn, J. and Harvald, B.: Adenosine-triphosphatase deficiency in a family with non-spherocytic haemolytic anaemia. Hum. Hered. 21: 313-319, 1971.

Harvald, B., Hanel, K. H., Squires, R. and Trap-Jensen, J.: Adenosine-triphosphatase deficiency in patients with non-spherocytic hemolytic anemia. Lancet II: 18-19, 1964.

Paglia, D. E., Valentine, W. N., Tartaglia, A. P. and Konrad, P. N.: Adenine nucleotide reductions associated with a dominantly transmitted form of nonspherocytic hemolytic anemia. (Abstract) Blood 36: 837 only, 1970.

*10290 ADENOSINE TRIPHOSPHATE, ELEVATED, OF ERYTHROCYTES

Brewer (1965) in this country and Zurcher et al. (1965) in Holland described high erythrocyte adenosine triphosphate as a dominantly inherited trait.

Brewer, G. J.: A new inherited abnormality of human erythrocyte-elevated erythrocyte adenosine triphosphate. Biochem. Biophys. Res. Commun. 18: 430-434, 1965.

Loos, J. A., Prins, H. K. and Zurcher, C.: Elevated ATP levels in human erythrocytes. In, Beutler, E. (ed.): Hereditary Disorders of Erythrocyte Metabolism. New York: Grune and Stratton, 1967.

Zurcher, C., Loos, J. A. and Prins, H. K.: Hereditary high ATP content of human erythrocytes. Folia Haematol. 83: 366-376, 1965.

*10293 ADENOVIRUS 12-CHROMOSOME MODIFICATION SITE-1

A site on the long arm of chromosome 1 is altered by exposure of cells in vitro to adenovirus 12 (2nd International Workshop on Human Gene Mapping, Rotterdam, July, 1974). See McDougall (1971).

McDougall, J. K.: Adenovirus induced chromosome aberrations in human cells. J. Gen. Virol. 12: 43-51, 1971.

*10297 ADENOVIRUS 12-CHROMOSOME MODIFICATION SITE-17

Adenovirus 12 produces an uncoiled segment in the long arm of chromosome 17. This is associated with elevated thymidine kinase (TK) activtiy. The TK locus (18830) is in the same region of 17q as that which shows the morphologic change.

*10300 ADENYLATE KINASE-1

Adenylate kinase, also known as myokinase, is a phosphotransferase which catalyzes the reversible conversion of 2 molecules of ADP to one of ATP plus one of AMP. The enzyme is present in red cells as well. Fildes and Harris (1966) found electrophoretic variation in red cells and defined 3 phenotypes, designated AK1, AK2-1 and AK2. All of the 141 children of two AK1 parents (62 such matings) were also AK1. Among the 136 children of AK1 by AK2-1 matings, 72 were AK1 and 64 AK2-1. AK1 and AK2 persons are thought to be homozygotes for a two-allele system and AK2-1 persons heterozygotes. The frequency of the rarer AK(2) allele is about 0.05 in the English and about 1 in 400 persons would be expected to be homozygous for this allele. Survey and family data are consistent. Rapley et al. (1967) concluded that the AK locus is linked to the ABO locus with a recombination value of about 0.20. Schleutermann et al. (1969) found that the nail-patella syndrome locus and the AK locus are very closely linked. No recombination was found in 53 opportunities. Bockelmann et al. (1968) concluded that adenylate kinase and pyruvate kinase are isozymes which share a polypeptide chain in common. Because of their similar functions a common evolutionary origin would be plausible. Singer and Brock (1971) identified a probably silent allele at the AK locus.

Bockelmann, W., Wolf, V. and Ritter, H.: Polymorphism of the phosphotransferases adenylate kinase and pyruvate kinase. Existence of a common subunit? Humangenetik 6: 78-83, 1968.

Bowman, J. E., Frischer, H., Ajmar, F., Carson, P. E. and Gower, M. K.: Population, family and biochemical investigation of human adenylate kinase polymorphism. Nature 214: 1156-1158, 1967.

Brock, D. J. H.: Evidence against a common subunit in adenylate kinase and pyruvate kinase. Humangenetik 10: 30-34, 1970.

Fildes, R. A. and Harris, H.: Genetically determined variation of adenylate kinase in man. Nature 209: 261-262, 1966.

Rapley, S., Robson, E. B., Harris, H. and Smith, S. M.: Data on the incidence, segregation and linkage relations of the adenylate kinase (AK) polymorphism. Ann. Hum. Genet. 31: 237-242, 1967.

Schleutermann, D. A., Bias, W. B., Murdoch, J. L. and McKusick, V. A.: Linkage of the loci for the nail-patella syndrome and adenylate kinase. Am. J. Hum. Genet. 21: 606-630, 1969.

Singer, J. D. and Brock, D. J.: Half-normal adenylate kinase activity in three generations. Ann. Hum. Genet. 35: 109-114, 1971.

Weitkamp, L. R., Sing, C. F., Shreffler, D. C. and Guttormsen, S. A.: The genetic linkage relations of adenylate kinase: further data on the ABO-AK linkage group. Am. J. Hum. Genet. 21: 600-605, 1969.

*10302 ADENYLATE KINASE-2

The existence of a second adenylate kinase locus linked to PGM-1 and peptidase C, i.e., on chromosome no. 1, was suggested by cell hybridization studies by Van Cong et al. (1972).

Van Cong, N., Billardon, C., Rebourcet, R., Kaouel, C. L-B., Picard, J. Y., Weil, D. and Frezal, J.: The existence of a second adenylate kinase locus linked to PGM-1 and peptidase-C. Ann. Genet. 15: 213-218, 1972.

*10303 ADENYLATE KINASE-3

The existence of a third adenylate kinase locus located on chromosome no. 9 is suggested by studies of somatic cell hybrids.

10310 ADIE SYNDROME

This is a stationary harmless disorder characterized by tonic, sluggishly reacting pupil and hypoactive or absent tendon reflexes. De Rudolf (1936) described it in mother and daughter, McKinney and Frocht (1940) in father and son, and affected sibs are reported (Mylius, 1938). The pupil (Laties and Scheie, 1965) is excessively sensitive to mecholyl (methacholine). In familial dysautonomia, a recessive (q.v.), the pupil is also mecholyl-sensitive and tendon reflexes are absent. It would be of interest to determine whether the reflexes return with parenteral administration of mecholyl as occurs in dysautonomia. An autopsied case was reported by Harriman and Garland (1968), who found neuronal degeneration in the ciliary ganglion. Selective degeneration of neurones in dorsal root ganglia may have been the basis for areflexia.

Adie, W. J.: Tonic pupils and absent tendon reflexes: a benign disorder sui generis: its complete and incomplete forms. Brain 55: 98-113, 1932.

De Rudolf, G.: Tonic pupils with absent tendon reflexes in mother and daughter. J. Neurol. Psychiat. 16: 367-368, 1936.

Harriman, D. G. F. and Garland, H.: The pathology of Adie's syndrome. Brain 91: 401-418, 1968.

Laties, A. M. and Scheie, H. G.: Adie's syndrome: duration of methacholine sensitivity. Arch. Ophthalmol. 74: 458-459, 1965.

McKinney, J. M. and Frocht, M.: Adie's syndrome: a non-luetic disease simulating tabes dorsalis. Am. J. Med. Sci. 199: 546-555, 1940.

Mylius, (NI): Ueber familiaeres Vorkommen der Pupillotonie. Klin. Monatsbl. Augenheilkd. 101: 598-599, 1938.

10320 ADIPOSIS DOLOROSA (DERCUM DISEASE)

Lynch and Harlan (1963) observed the disease in four members of three generations of one family and in two, possibly four, persons in two generations of a second family.

Cantu, J. M., Ruiz-Barquin, E., Jimenez, M., Castillo, L. and Ruiz-Macotela, E.: Autosomal dominant inheritance in adiposis dolorosa (Dercum's disease). Humangenetik 18: 89-91, 1973.

Lynch, H. T. and Harlan, W. L.: Hereditary factors in adiposis dolorosa (Dercum's disease). Am. J. Hum. Genet. 15: 184-190, 1963.

10325 ADRENOCORTICOTROPIN (ACTH)

ACTH, synthesized by the anterior pituitary gland, stimulates the adrenal cortex. Human ACTH has a molecular weight of 4,541 and contains 39 amino acids (Lee et al., 1961). It has structural similarities to melanotropin (MSH, see 15585).

Lee, T. H., Lerner, A. B. and Buettner-Janusch, V.: On the structure of human corticotropin (adrenocorticotropic hormone). J. Biol. Chem. 236: 2970-2974, 1961.

10330 AGLOSSIA-ADACTYLIA

The features are indicated by the name, although it is to be noted that both the aglossia and the adactylia may be only partial. No familial cases have been reported (Nevin et al., 1970).

Nevin, N. C., Dodge, J. A. and Kernohan, D. C.: Aglossia-adactylia syndrome. Oral Surg. 29: 443-446, 1970.

10340 AINHUM

A narrow strip of hardened skin, a constricting ring, forms on the little toe at the level of the digito-plantar fold and progresses to spontaneous amputation of the digit. Familial occurrence has been noted by Maass (1926) and by Da Silva Lima (1880).

Da Silva Lima, J. F.: On ainhum. Arch. Dermatol. Syph. 6: 367-376, 1880.

Horwitz, M. T. and Tunick, I.: Ainhum: report of six cases in New York. Arch. Dermatol. Syph. 36: 1058-1063, 1937.

Maass, E.: Beobachtungen ueber Ainhum. Arch. Schiffs- u. Tropenhygiene 30: 32-34, 1926.

10345 ALBINISM

Fitzpatrick et al. (1974) have observed a dominant form of albinism.

Fitzpatrick, T. B., Jimbow, K. and Donaldson, D. D.: Dominant oculo-cutaneous albinism. (Abstract) Br. J. Dermatol. 91: 23 only, 1974.

10350 ALBINISM-DEAFNESS

Tietz (1963) described 14 affected persons in 6 generations. The albinism was generalized but did not affect the eyes. The irides were blue. Nystagmus and other ocular abnormalities were absent. The medial canthi and nasal bridge were normal. Complete nerve deafness was present. The eyebrows were almost totally lacking. The albinism in this trait is hypopigmentation and not true albinism. The affected individuals tan, for example. Reed et al. (1967) thought this might have been merely a dominant type of deafness in unusually blond persons.

Reed, W. B., Stone, V. M., Boder, E. and Ziprkowski, L.: Pigmentary disorders in association with congenital deafness. Arch. Dermatol. 95: 176-186, 1967.

Tietz, W.: A syndrome of deaf-mutism associated with albinism showing dominant autosomal inheritance. Am. J. Hum. Genet. 15: 259-264, 1963.

*10360 ALBUMIN

Bisalbuminemia is an asymptomatic variation in serum albumin. Heterozygotes have two species of albumin, a normal type and one which migrates abnormally rapidly or slowly on electrophoresis. Acrocyanosis was present in two and probably three successive generations of the family reported by Williams and Martin (1960) but 4 other bisalbuminemic persons did not show acrocyanosis. Tarnoky and Lestas (1964) described a new type of bisalbuminemia in two sibs and the son of one of them. The usual type is demonstrable by filter paper electrophoresis. The new type was demonstrable by electrophoresis on cellulose acetate at pH 8.6, but not on filter paper or starch gel. A large number of albumin variants probably exist. 'Paralbuminemia' was suggested by Earle et al. (1959) as preferable to 'bisalbuminemia' which is perhaps appropriate for the heterozygous state only. Alloalbuminemia is the term suggested by Blumberg et al. (1968) for the variant albumins. In the family reported by Laurell and Nilehn (1966), a new type of paralbuminemia was associated with connective tissue disorders: systemic lupus erythematosus, ruptured knee meniscus, recurrent dislocation of shoulder, back pain. Weitkamp et al. (1966) concluded that the albumin locus indicated by bisalbuminemia is very closely linked with the locus for GC type. Using the Naskapi variant, Kaarsalo et al. (1967) found close linkage of the albumin and GC loci.

Melartin and Blumberg (1966) found an electrophoretic variant of albumin to be frequent in Naskapi Indians of Quebec and in lower frequency in other North American Indians. Homozygotes were found.

Wietkamp et al. (1967) compared the serum albumin variants of 19 unrelated families, using two electrophoretic systems. Five distinct classes were found. One class of variants was found only in North American Indians. The others were found only in persons of European descent.

Fraser, Harris and Robson (1959) found an anomalous plasma protein in 6 persons in two generations of a family, on two dimensional electrophoresis (paper first, followed by starch). The electrophoretic properties on paper were the same in the anomalous albumin and in normal albumin. This distinguishes the protein from that in bisalbuminemia as does also the fact that the amount of the anomalous protein is much less than that of the normal albumin in the presumably heterozygous persons. That the same locus as that which determines bisalbuminemia is involved here is suggested by the finding of Weitkamp et al. (1967) that the Fraser anomalous albumin is also linked to the GC locus. Relatively frequent different alloalbuminemias occur in various American Indians (Arends et al., 1969). The albumin variant first described by Fraser et al. (1959) in a Welch family has been characterized as a dimer by Jamieson and Ganguly (1969). The amino acid sequence has been determined in fragments of serum albumin of man (Dayhoff, 1972).

Adams, M. S.: Genetic diversity in serum albumin. J. Med. Genet. 3: 198-202, 1966.

Arends, T., Gallango, M. L., Layrisse, M., Wilbert, J. and Heinen, H. D.: Albumin Warao: new type of human alloalbuminemia. Blood 33: 414-420, 1969.

Blumberg, B. S., Martin, J. R. and Melartin, L.: Alloalbuminemia. Albumin Naskapi in Indians of the Ungava. J.A.M.A. 203: 180-185, 1968.

Darlington, G. J., Bernhard, H. P. and Ruddle, F. H.: Human serum albumin phenotype activation in mouse hepatoma-human leukocyte cell hybrids. Science 185: 859-862, 1974.

Dayhoff, M. O.: Serum albumin. Atlas of Protein Sequence and Structure 1972 (vol. 5). Washington: National Biomedical Research Foundation, 1972. P. D316.

Earle, D. P., Hutt, M. P., Schmid, K. and Gitlin, D.: Observations on double albumin: a genetically transmitted serum protein anomaly. J. Clin. Invest. 38: 1412-1420, 1959.

Efremov, G. and Braend, M.: Serum albumin: polymorphism in man. Science 146: 1679-1680, 1964.

Fraser, G. R., Harris, H. and Robson, E. B.: A new genetically determined plasma-protein in man. Lancet I: 1023-1024, 1959.

Jamieson, G. A. and Ganguly, P.: Studies on a genetically determined albumin dimer. Biochem. Genet. 3: 403-416, 1969.

Kaarsalo, E., Melartin, L. and Blumberg, B. S.: Autosomal linkage between the albumin and GC loci in humans. Science 158: 123-125, 1967.

Kueppers, F., Holland, P. V. and Weitkamp, L. R.: Albumin Santa Ana: a new inherited variant. Hum. Hered. 19: 378-384, 1969.

Lau, T. J., Sunderman, F. W., Jr., Weitkamp, L. R., Agarwall, S. S., Sutnick, A. I., Blumberg, B. S. and De Jimenez, R. B. C.: Albumin Cartago: a 'new' slow-moving alloalbumin. Am. J. Clin. Path. 57: 247-251, 1972.

Laurell, C. B. and Nilehn, J. E.: A new type of inherited serum albumin anomaly. J. Clin. Invest. 45: 1935-1945, 1966.

Melartin, L. and Blumberg, B. S.: Albumin Naskapi: a new variant of serum albumin. Science 153: 1664-1666, 1966.

Melartin, L.: Albumin polymorphism in man. Studies on albumin variants in North American native populations. Acta Path. Microbiol. Scand. 191 (suppl.): 1-50, 1967.

Melartin, L., Blumberg, B. S. and Lisker, R.: Albumin Mexico, a new variant of serum albumin. Nature 215: 1288-1289, 1967.

Sarcione, E. J. and Aungst, C. W.: Studies in bisalbuminemia: binding properties of the two albumins. Blood 20: 156-164, 1962.

Sarich, V. M.: Generation time and albumin evolution. Biochem. Genet. 7: 205-212, 1972.

Tarnoky, A. L. and Lestas, A. N.: A new type of bisalbuminaemia. Clin. Chim. Acta 9: 551-558, 1964.

Weitkamp, L. R. and Buck, A. A.: Phenotype frequencies for four serum proteins in Afghanistan: two 'new' albumin variants. Humangenetik 15: 335-340, 1972.

Weitkamp, L. R. and Chagnon, N. A.: Albumin maku: a new variant of human serum albumin. Nature 217: 759-760, 1968.

Weitkamp, L. R., Franglen, G., Rokala, D. A., Polesky, H. F., Simpson, N. E., Sunderman, F. W., Jr., Bell, H. E., Saave, J., Lisker, R. and Bohls, S. W.: An electrophoretic comparison of human serum albumin variants: eight distinguishable types. Hum. Hered. 19: 159-169, 1969.

Weitkamp, L. R., Renwick, J. H., Berger, J., Shreffler, D. C., Drachmann, O., Wuhrmann, F., Braend, M. and Frangle, G.: Additional data and summary for albumin-GC linkage in man. Hum. Hered. 20: 1-7, 1970.

Weitkamp, L. R., Robson, E. B., Shreffler, D. C. and Corney, G.: An unusual human serum albumin variant: further data on genetic linkage between loci for human serum albumin and group-specific component (GC). Am. J. Hum. Genet. 20: 392-397, 1968.

Weitkamp, L. R., Rucknagel, D. L. and Gershowitz, H.: Genetic linkage between structural loci for albumin and group specific component (GC). Am. J. Hum. Genet. 18: 559-571, 1966.

Weitkamp, L. R., Salzano, F. M., Neel, J. V., Porta, F., Geerdink, R. A. and Tarnoky, A. L.: Human serum albumin: twenty-three genetic variants and their population distribution. Ann. Hum. Genet. 36: 381-392, 1973.

Weitkamp, L. R., Shreffler, D. C., Robbins, J. L., Drachmann, O., Adner, P. L., Weime, R. J., Simon, N. M., Cooke, K. B., Sandor, G., Wuhrmann, F., Braend, M. and Tarnoky, A. L.: An electrophoretic comparison of serum albumin variants from nineteen unrelated families. Acta Genet. Statist. Med. 17: 399-405, 1967.

Wieme, R. J.: On the presence of two albumins in certain normal human sera and its genetic determination. Clin. Chim. Acta 5: 443-445, 1960.

Williams, D. I. and Martin, N. H.: Bisalbuminemia with curious acrocyanotic skin changes (two cases). Proc. R. Soc. Med. 53: 566-568, 1960.

*10370 ALCOHOL DEHYDROGENASE 1: ADH(1)

Polymorphism was investigated by Smith et al. (1971). They concluded that there are three ADH loci, responsible for three distinct polypeptide subunits, alpha, beta and gamma. At each of the ADH(2) and ADH(3) loci the evidence indicated that two different common alleles occur. The ADH isozymes are dimers. Any particular isozyme may be made up of two identical subunits coded by a specific allele at one of the loci, or of two non-identical subunits coded by alleles at two separate loci, or of two non-identical subunits coded by different alleles at the same locus. At least three autosomal gene loci may, they concluded, be concerned with determining the structure of alcohol dehydrogenase in man. ADH-1 is primarily active in the liver in early fetal life, becoming less active later in gestation and only weakly active during adult life. With the coenzyme NAD, this enzyme catalyzes the reversible conversion of organic alcohols to ketones or aldehydes. The physiologic function for alcohol dehydrogenase in the liver is the removal of ethanol formed by microorganisms in the intestinal tract. The enzyme from horse liver is a dimer with two very similar chains, called E for ethanol-active and S for steroid active. Sequence data are not available in man but the data on the horse liver enzyme are given in Dayhoff's atlas (1972). An atypical liver ADH was described by Von Wartburg and Schuerch (1968), in 2 of 50 English livers and in 12 of 59 Swiss livers. The difference studied concerned the ratio of activity at pH 10.8 and pH 8.8.

Dayhoff, M. O.: Dehydrogeneses. Atlas of Protein Sequence and Structure 1972 (vol. 5). Washington: National Biomedical Research Foundation, 1972. Pp. D141-D144.

Murray, R. F., Jr. and Price, P. H.: Ontogenetic, polymorphic, and interethnic variation in the isoenzymes of human alcohol dehydrogenase. Ann. N.Y. Acad. Sci. 197: 68-72, 1972.

Smith, M., Hopkinson, D. A. and Harris, H.: Alcohol dehydrogenase isozymes in adult human stomach and liver: evidence for activity of the ADH(3) locus. Ann. Hum. Genet. 35: 243-253, 1972.

Smith, M., Hopkinson, D. A. and Harris, H.: Developmental changes and polymorphism in human alcohol dehydrogenase. Ann. Hum. Genet. 34: 251-272, 1971.

Smith, M., Hopkinson, D. A. and Harris, H.: Studies on the properties of the human alcohol dehydrogenase isozymes determined by the different loci ADH(1), ADH(2) and ADH(3). Ann. Hum. Genet. 37: 49-67, 1973.

Smith, M., Hopkinson, D. A. and Harris, H.: Studies on the subunit structure and molecular size of the human dehydrogenase isozymes determined by the different loci, ADH(1), ADH(2), and ADH(3). Ann. Hum. Genet. 36: 401-414, 1973.

Von Wartburg, J. P. and Schuerch, P. M.: Atypical human liver alcohol dehydrogenase. Ann. N.Y. Acad. Sci. 151: 936-947, 1968.

*10372 ALCOHOL DEHYDROGENASE 2: ADH(2)

According to the conclusion of Smith et al. (see 10370), locus ADH-2 is expressed in the lung in early fetal life and remains active in this tissue throughout life. It is active also in liver after about the first trimester and gradually increases in activity so that in adults this locus is responsible for most of the liver ADH activity. It is active in the adult kidney. The 'atypical pH ratio' phenotype is probably determined by a variant allele at the ADH-2 locus.

*10373 ALCOHOL DEHYDROGENASE 3: ADH(3)

According to the conclusion of Smith et al. (see 10370), the ADH-3 locus is active in intestine and kidney in fetal and early postnatal life. Two alleles at the ADH-3 locus called 1 and 2 have a frequency of about 0.63 and 0.37, respectively.

10375 ALCOHOL SENSITIVITY

Wolff (1972) demonstrated that members of the Mongoloid race respond, after drinking amounts of alcohol that have no detectable effect on Caucasoids, with marked facial flushing and mild to moderate symptoms of intoxication. Group differences are present at birth, and are attributable in Wolff's view to differences in autonomic reactivity. The genetic basis is likely to be polygenic, but the operation of a single major gene might be worth seeking. The lower incidence of alcoholism in certain Mongoloid groups may have its basis in these observations. Fenna et al. (1971) concluded that ethanol is metabolized significantly faster in whites than in Eskimos or American Indians.

Fenna, D., Mix, L., Schaefer, O. and Gilbert, J. A. L.: Ethanol metabolism in various racial groups. Canad. Med. Assoc. J. 105: 472-475, 1971.

Wolff, P. H.: Ethnic differences in alcohol sensitivity. Science 175: 449-450, 1972.

Wolff, P. H.: Vasomotor sensitivity to alcohol in diverse mongoloid populations. Am. J. Hum. Genet. 25: 193-199, 1973.

*10380 ALDER ANOMALY

Azurophilic cytoplasmic inclusions of the polymorphonuclear leukocytes are inherited as an autosomal dominant. Francois, Barbier and de Rouck (1960) observed Alder anomaly and Fuchs atrophia gyrata chorioideae et retinae in the offspring of first-cousin parents both of whom had the Alder anomaly. They suggested that the eye disorder is the homozygous expression of the Alder anomaly gene. It is possible, of course, that the eye disorder was merely an unrelated recessive disorder and indeed later observations (see FUCHS ATROPHIA GYRATA in recessive catalog) supported this view. This change is probably morphologically indistinguishable from the Reilly granulations observed in mucopolysaccharidoses (Reilly, 1941). Alder (1939) originally described the change in a brother and sister who later at puberty developed changes in their hip joints. The brother was said to be in good health at age 28 (Davidson, 1961). Jordans (1947) reported a Dutch family showing a dominant inheritance pattern-9 affected persons in three generations with male-to-male transmission.

Alder, A.: Ueber konstitutionell bedingte Granulationsveraenderungen der Leukocyten. Deutsch. Arch. Klin. Med. 183: 372-378, 1939.

Davidson, W. M.: Inherited variations in leucocytes. Br. Med. Bull. 17: 190-195, 1961.

Francois, J., Barbier, F. and De Rouck, A.: Les conducteurs du gene de l'atrophia gyrata chorioideae et retinae de Fuchs (anomalie d'Alder). Acta Genet. Med. Gemellol. 9: 74-91, 1960.

Jordans, G. H. W.: Hereditary granulation anomaly of the leucocytes (Alder). Acta Med. Scand. 129: 348-351, 1947.

Reilly, W. A.: The granules in the leukocytes in gargoylism. Am. J. Dis. Child. 62: 489-491, 1941.

*10385 ALDOLASE-1

Electrophoretic variants were found by Charlesworth (1972). Harris (1974) concludes that three loci determine aldolase.

Charlesworth, D.: Starch-gel electrophoresis of four enzymes from human red blood cells: glyceraldehyde-3-phosphate dehydrogenase, fructoaldolase, glyoxalase II and sorbital dehydrogenase. Ann. Hum. Genet. 35: 477-484, 1972.

Harris, H.: London, personal communication, 1974.

10386 ALDOLASE-2

See ALDOLASE-1 (10385).

10387 ALDOLASE-3

See ALDOLASE-1 (10385).

10390 ALDOSTERONISM, SENSITIVE TO DEXAMETHASONE

Sutherland et al. (1966) and Salti et al. (1969) described a father and son with hypertension, low plasma renin activity and increased aldosterone secretion responsive to dexamethasone. Growth and sexual development were normal. At laparotomy the father was found to have multiple adrenocortical adenomas. This appears to be distinct from Conn syndrome (primary aldosteronism) which is not sensitive to dexamethasone.

Salti, I. S., Stiefel, M., Ruse, J. L. and Laidlaw, J. C.: Non-tumorous 'primary' aldosteronism. I. Type relieved by glucocorticoid (glucocorticoid-remediable aldosteronism). Canad. Med. Assoc. J. 101: 1-10, 1969.

Sutherland, D. J., Ruse, J. L. and Laidlaw, J. C.: Hypertension, increased aldosterone secretion and low plasma renin activity relieved by dexamethasone. Canad. Med. Assoc. J. 95: 1109-1119, 1966.

*10395 AL-M (ALPHA-2-MACROGLOBULIN)

This polymorphism has been demonstrated in Japanese persons. It is distinct from Gm, Am and haptoglobins. This factor is distinct from Xm (also a macroglobulin) as indicated by the autosomal inheritance and specific tests. Gene frequency of the allele whose product is demonstrated by the antiserum is about 0.16 in Japanese.

Leikola, J., Fudenberg, H. H., Kasukawa, R. and Milgrom, F.: A new genetic polymorphism of human serum: alpha(2) macroglobulin (AL-M). Am. J. Hum. Genet. 24: 134-144, 1972.

10400 ALOPECIA AREATA

Lubowe (1959) described a family with affected mother and affected daughter and son. Recent evidence suggests an autoimmune mechanism in this disorder. See AUTOIMMUNE DISEASES.

Lubowe, I. I.: The clinical aspects of alopecia areata, totalis, and universalis. Ann. N.Y. Acad. Sci. 83: 458-462, 1959.

10410 ALOPECIA CONGENITA WITH KERATOSIS PALMO-PLANTARIS

Stevanovic (1959) described a family with a dominant pattern of inheritance and hyperkeratosis of the palms and soles, and mild dystrophic changes of the fingernails.

Stevanovic, D. V.: Alopecia congenita. The incomplete dominant form of inheritance with varying expressivity. Acta Genet. Statist. Med. 9: 127-132, 1959.

*10420 ALPORT SYNDROME (HEREDITARY NEPHROPATHY AND DEAFNESS)

Partial sex linkage (location of the gene on the part of the X and Y chromosomes which is homologous) was suggested on the basis of the large Mormon kindred reported by Perkoff and his colleagues (1958). However, this possibility is excluded by other pedigrees (e.g., Cohen, Cassady, Hanna, 1961). Autosomal dominant inheritance with anomalous segregation (Shaw, Glover, 1961) seems more likely. Heterozygous mothers transmit the gene to more than 50 percent of daughters and probably also more than 50 percent of their sons. Walker (1966) has studied a family (N. P., 666088) with affected persons in four generations. Although the histology in two cases studied was consistent with Alport syndrome including the presence of foam cells, atypical features included absence of deafness in all affected persons, unusually long survival of affected males and death of one affected female in the early twenties. The kindred reported by Ohlsson (1963) differed from others reported in the fact that myopia was a conspicuous feature and the impairment of renal function in the affected males was relatively mild even in two over age 30 years. Ocular abnormalities have been observed in some patients (Arnott et al., 1966). A possibly distinct entity is hereditary nephritis without deafness reported by Dockhorn (1967) and by Reyersbach and Butler (1954). The case of Stanbury and Castleman (1968) had hypophosphatemia and nephrocalcinosis. At least 7 persons in 3 generations were affected. The proband had unilateral deafness and foam cells were demonstrated in the kidney. The family reported by Albert et al. (1969) may have suffered from a different disorder. Two sisters and a brother were affected. The females showed unusually severe abnormality for that sex. The major manifestation of renal disease in one sister was the nephrotic syndrome. None had deafness. The parents were normal and not related. Two otherwise unaffected brothers had congenital cataracts. See also NEPHRITIS, FAMILIAL, WITHOUT DEAFNESS OR OCULAR DEFECT. Immunofluorescent studies of Spear et al. (1970) were inconclusive as far as deciding on a possible immune basis of the nephropathy. Miller et al. (1970) showed that the vestibular neuroepithelium is involved as well as that of the cochlea. Pashayan et al. (1971) described a family with typical renal disease but almost no occurrence of deafness. Myers and Tyler (1972) reported the temporal bone histology on two cases. Both had severe deafness, but one had a histologically normal inner ear, whereas the other had a marked reduction in spinal ganglion cochlear neurons. This suggested to them that the Alport syndrome is either heterogeneous or has extraordinarily wide expression. Variability in histologic findings in the ear in the Alport syndrome led Myers and Tyler (1972) to conclude that it is a heterogeneous category. Teisberg et al. (1973) found that serum from patients with 'hereditary nephropathy' was able to break down the third component of complement in vitro. Furthermore, evidence of in vivo inactivation was described. They concluded that the underlying mechanism is an inherited defect in immunologic response. The family reported by Teisberg et al. (1973) may have had the disorder described as entry 16190.

Albert, M. S., Leeming, J. M. and Wigger, H. J.: Familial nephritis associated with the nephrotic syndrome. Am. J. Dis. Child. 117: 153-155, 1969.

Arnott, E. J., Crawfurd, M. D. A. and Toghill, P. J.: Anterior lenticonus and Alport's syndrome. Br. J. Ophthalmol. 50: 390-403, 1966.

Chazan, J. A., Zacks, J., Cohen, J. J. and Garella, S.: Hereditary nephritis. Clinical spectrum and mode of inheritance in five new kindreds. Am. J. Med. 50: 764-771, 1971.

Cohen, M. M., Cassady, G. and Hanna, B. L.: A genetic study of hereditary renal dysfunction with associated nerve deafness. Am. J. Hum. Genet. 13: 379-389, 1961.

Crawfurd, M. D. A. and Toghill, P. J.: Alport's syndrome of hereditary nephritis and deafness. Quart. J. Med. 37: 563-576, 1968.

Dockhorn, R. J.: Hereditary nephropathy without deafness. Am. J. Dis. Child. 114: 135-138, 1967.

Goyer, R. A., Reynolds, J., Jr., Burke, J. and Burkholder, P.: Hereditary renal disease with neurosensory hearing loss, prolinuria and ichthyosis. Am. J. Med. Sci. 256: 166-179, 1968.

Krickstein, H. I., Gloor, F. J. and Balogh, K.: Renal pathology in hereditary nephritis with nerve deafness. Arch. Pathol. 82: 506-517, 1966.

Marin, O. S. M. and Tyler, H. R.: Hereditary interstitial nephritis associated with polyneuropathy. Neurology 11: 999-1005, 1961.

Miller, G. W., Joseph, D. J., Cozad, R. L. and McCabe, B. F.: Alport's syndrome. Arch. Otolaryngol. 92: 419-432, 1970.

Mulrow, P. J., Aron, A. M., Gathman, G. E., Yesner, R. and Lubs, H. A.: Hereditary nephritis. Report of a kindred. Am. J. Med. 35: 737-748, 1963.

Myers, G. J. and Tyler, H. R.: The etiology of deafness in Alport's syndrome. Arch. Otolaryngol. 96: 333-340, 1972.

Ohlsson, L.: Congenital renal disease, deafness and myopia in one family. Acta Med. Scand. 174: 77-84, 1963.

Pashayan, H., Fraser, F. C. and Goldbloom, R. B.: A family showing hereditary nephropathy. Am. J. Hum. Genet. 23: 555-567, 1971.

Perkoff, G. T., Nugent, C. A., Jr., Dolowitz, D. A., Stephens, F. E., Carnes, W. H. and Tyler, F. H.: A follow-up study of hereditary chronic nephritis. Arch. Intern. Med. 102: 733-746, 1958.

Preus, M. and Fraser, F. C.: Genetics of hereditary nephropathy with deafness (Alport's disease). Clin. Genet. 2: 331-337, 1971.

Purriel, P., Drets, M., Pascale, E., Cestau, R. S., Borras, A., Ferreira, W. A., Delucca, A. and Fernandez, L.: Familial hereditary nephropathy (Alport's syndrome). Am. J. Med. 49: 753-773, 1970.

Reyersbach, G. C. and Butler, A. M.: Congenital hereditary hematuria. N. Engl. J. Med. 251: 377-380, 1954.

Schneider, R. G.: Congenital hereditary nephritis with nerve deafness. New York J. Med. 63: 2644-2648, 1963.

Shaw, R. F. and Glover, R. A.: Abnormal segregation in hereditary renal disease with deafness. Am. J. Hum. Genet. 13: 89-97, 1961.

Sherman, R. L., Churg, J. and Yudis, M.: Hereditary nephritis with a characteristic renal lesion. Am. J. Med. 56: 44-51, 1974.

Spear, G. S. and Slusser, R.: Alport's syndrome: emphasizing electron microscopic studies of the glomerulus. Am. J. Pathol. 69: 213-224, 1972.

Spear, G. S., Whitworth, J. M. and Konigsmark, B. W.: Hereditary nephritis with nerve deafness. Immunofluorescent studies on the kidney, with a consideration of discordant immunoglobulin-complement immunofluorescent reactions. Am. J. Med. 49: 52-63, 1970.

Stanbury, S. W. and Castleman, B.: Nephrocalcinosis and azotemia in a young man. N. Engl. J. Med. 278: 839-846, 1968.

Teisberg, P., Grottum, K. A., Myhre, E. and Flatmark, A.: In-vivo activation of complement in hereditary nephropathy. Lancet II: 356-358, 1973.

Turner, J. S., Jr.: Hereditary hearing loss with nephropathy (Alport's syndrome). Acta Otolaryngol. 271 (suppl.): 7-26, 1970.

Walker, W. G.: Baltimore, Md.: personal communication, 1966.

Westley, C. R.: Familial nephritis and associated deafness in a southwestern Apache Indian family. South. Med. J. 63: 1415-1419, 1970.

Whalen, R. E., Huang, S.-S., Peschel, E. and McIntosh, H. D.: Hereditary nephropathy, deafness and renal foam cells. Am. J. Med. 31: 171-186, 1961.

Williamson, D. A. J.: Alport's syndrome of hereditary nephritis with deafness. Lancet II: 1321-1323, 1961.

*10430 ALZHEIMER DISEASE OF BRAIN

Wheelan and Race (1959) studied a family in which the mother and five of ten children had Alzheimer disease. Possible linkage with the MNS locus was shown. Clinically, Alzheimer disease cannot be distinguished from Pick disease (q.v.). Schottky (1932) described presenile dementia in four generations. The diagnosis was confirmed at autopsy in a patient in the fourth generation. Lowenberg and Waggoner (1934) reported a family with unusually early onset. The father and four of five children were affected. Postmortem findings in one case were described. McMenemey and colleagues (1939) described four affected males in two generations with pathologic confirmation in one. From an extensive study in Sweden, Sjoegren, Sjoegren and Lindgren (1952) concluded that, although Pick disease may be dominant with important modifier genes, Alzheimer disease is probably multifactorial. Heston et al. (1966) described a family with 19 affected in 4 generations. Dementia was coupled with conspicuous Parkinsonism and long tract signs.

Heston, L. L., Lowther, D. L. W. and Leventhal, C. M.: Alzheimer's disease. A family study. Arch. Neurol. 15: 225-233, 1966.

Lowenberg, K. and Waggoner, R. W.: Familial organic psychosis (Alzheimer's type). Arch. Neurol. Psychiatry 31: 737-754, 1934.

McMenemey, W. H., Worster-Drought, C., Flind, J. and Williams, H. G.: Familial presenile dementia: report of a case with clinical and pathological features of Alzheimer's disease. J. Neurol. Psychopath. 2: 293-302, 1939.

Schottky, J.: Ueber praesenile Verblodungen. Zbl. Ges. Neurol. Psychiat. 140: 333-397, 1932.

Sjoegren, T., Sjoegren, H. and Lindgren, A. G. H.: Morbus Alzheimer and morbus Pick. A genetic, clinical and patho-anatomical study. Acta Psychiat. Neurol. Scand. 82 (suppl.): 1-152, 1952.

Wheelan, L. and Race, R. R.: Familial Alzheimer's disease; note on the linkage data. Ann. Hum. Genet. 23: 300-310, 1959.

Wolstenholme, G. E. W. and O'Connor, M.: Alzheimer's Disease and Related Conditions. (Ciba Foundation Symposium) London: J. and A. Churchill, 1970.

10440 AMELIA AND TERMINAL TRANSVERSE HEMIMELIA

Most cases are sporadic. Some families have affected relatives suggesting a complex genetic etiology.

Temtamy, S. A.: Genetic Factors in Hand Malformations. Ph. D. thesis, Johns Hopkins University, 1966.

*10445 AMELOGENESIS IMPERFECTA WITH TAURODONTISM

Winter et al. (1969) and Crawford (1970) have reported families. The amelogenesis imperfecta is of the hypoplastic-hypomaturation type. Taurodontism ('bull teeth') occurs as an isolated trait which is probably polygenic (see 27270). In the tricho-donto-osseous syndrome (13080), kinky hair and osteosclerosis are combined with the same dental defect.

Crawford, J. L.: Concomitant taurodontism and amelogenesis imperfecta in the American Caucasian. J. Dent. Child. 37: 171-175, 1970.

Winter, G. B., Lee, K. W. and Johnson, N. W.: Hereditary amelogenesis imperfecta. A rare autosomal dominant type. Br. Dent. J. 127: 157-164, 1969.

*10450 AMELOGENESIS IMPERFECTA, HYPOCALCIFICATION TYPE

The primary defect in amelogenesis imperfecta, hypocalcification type, is ectodermal although secondary changes occur in the exposed dentine. Chaudhry and colleagues (1959) reported five families with an autosomal dominant pattern of inheritance. There are two X-linked varieties. Clark and Clark (1933) studied two kindreds living in Maine and elsewhere in New England. Legend had it that the affected ancestor of one family came over on the Mayflower. Although presumed enamel defects 'running in families' were reported from a relatively early date, it is often difficult to be certain whether a dentine defect or an enamel defect was, in fact, involved in specific instances. Weinmann et al. (1945) made the useful division of enamel defects into two classes: (1) hereditary enamel hypoplasia, in which the enamel is deficient in quantity but hard in quality; and (2) hereditary enamel hypocalcification, in which the enamel is soft and undercalcified, although normal in quantity and histology. See AMELOGENESIS IMPERFECTA in the X-linkage catalog. This is the most frequent type of enamel dysplasia. Both the primary and the secondary dentitions are affected. The enamel is soft and friable. In older individuals the enamel may be completely worn away.

Chaudhry, A. P., Johnson, O. N., Mitchell, D. F., Gorlin, R. J. and Bartholdi, W. L.: Hereditary enamel dysplasia. J. Pediatr. 54: 776-785, 1959.

Clark, F. H. and Clark, C. S.: Absence of tooth enamel. A dominant hereditary anomaly in man. J. Hered. 24: 425-429, 1933.

Gardner, E. J.: A pedigree of brown teeth. The inheritance of brown, enamel-deficient teeth in a Utah family. J. Hered. 42: 289-290, 1951.

Rushton, M. A.: Hereditary enamel defects. Proc. R. Soc. Med. 57: 53-58, 1964.

Tsujii, T. and Obi, M.: A family of hereditary enamel hypoplasia. Jap. J. Hum. Genet. 6: 118-123, 1961.

Weinmann, J. P., Svoboda, J. F. and Woods, R. W.: Hereditary disturbances of enamel formation and calcification. J. Am. Dent. Assoc. 32: 397-418, 1945.

Witkop, C. J.: Genetics and dentistry. Eugen. Quart. 5: 15-21, 1958.

*10453 AMELOGENESIS IMPERFECTA, HYPOPLASTIC TYPE

There may be more than one distinct form of autosomal dominant hypoplastic amelogenesis imperfecta. For example, Witkop and Rao (1971) list smooth, rough and pitted forms, as well as a local form. These might be allelic disorders, comparable to the hemoglobin variants which have various changes in the beta chain. In the smooth hypoplastic type, many teeth fail to erupt and often have multiple calcifications of the pulp even in unerupted teeth. Numerous enameloid conglomerates are found histologically in areas of unerupted teeth.

Fischman, S. L. and Fischman, B. C.: Hypoplastic amelogenesis imperfecta: report of case. J. Am. Dent. Assoc. 75: 929-931, 1967.

Witkop, C. J. and Rao, S. R.: Inherited defects in tooth structure. The Clinical Delineation of Birth Defects. XI. Orofacial Structures. Baltimore: Williams and Wilkins, 1971. Pp. 153-184.

10460 AMENORRHEA-GALACTORRHEA SYNDROME

The association of secondary amenorrhea and galactorrhea is generally thought to occur in two distinct syndromes: the Forbes-Albright syndrome, where amenorrhea and galactorrhea are accompanied by a pituitary tumor, with or without prior pregnancy, and the Chiari-Frommel syndrome, where amenorrhea and galactorrhea commence after pregnancy, without associated pituitary tumor. This distinction may be artificial (Rimoin and Schimke, 1971), because the pituitary adenoma may be too small to identify clinically and progression from the benign to the neoplastic syndrome has been documented (Young et al., 1967). Linquette et al. (1967) described mother and daughter with amenorrhea-galactorrhea associated with pituitary adenoma. The mother first developed clinical signs after a pregnancy, whereas the daughter was never pregnant and amenorrhea followed emotional trauma. The sella turcica was enlarged in both and tumor was confirmed by craniotomy. The tumors resembled chromophobe adenomas, but there was fine eosinophilic granulation on tetrachrome staining, as seen in prolactin cells. Since the amenorrhea-galactorrhea syndrome has been described as a part of the multiple endocrine adenomatosis syndrome, it is not certain that the ailment in the mother and daughter reported by Linquette et al. (1967) represented a distinct entity.

Linquette, M., Herlant, M., Laine, E., Fossati, P. and Dupont-Lecompte, M.: Adenome prolactive chez une jeune fille dont la mere etait porteuse d'un adenome hypophysaire avec amenorrhee-galactorrhee. Ann. Endocrinol. 28: 773-780, 1967.

Rimoin, D. L. and Schimke, R. N.: Genetic Disorders of the Endocrine Glands. St. Louis: C. V. Mosby Co., 1971.

Young, R. L., Bradley, E. M., Goldzieher, J. W., Myers, P. W. and Lecocq, F. R.: Spectrum of nonpuerperal galactorrhea: report of two cases evolving through the various syndromes. J. Clin. Endocrinol. Metab. 27: 461-466, 1967.

*10465 AMYLASE, PANCREATIC (AMY-2)

Polymorphism is determined by agar gel electrophoresis. Kamaryt et al. (1971) assigned the locus to chromosome 1 by study of linkage with the 'uncoiled' variant used by Donohue et al. in assigning the Duffy blood group locus to chromosome 1. Hill et al. (1972) demonstrated probable linkage between the Amy-2 locus and the Duffy blood group locus.

Hill, C. J., Rowe, S. I. and Lovrien, E. W.: Probable genetic linkage between human serum amylase (Amy-2) and Duffy blood groups. Nature 235: 162-163, 1972.

Kamaryt, J., Adamek, R. and Vrba, M.: Possible linkage between uncoiler chromosome Un 1 and amylase polymorphism Amy 2 loci. Humangenetik 11: 213-220, 1971.

Merritt, D. A., Rivas, M. L., Bixler, D. and Newell, R.: Salivary and pancreatic amylase: electrophoretic characterizations and genetic studies. Am. J. Hum. Genet. 25: 510-522, 1973.

Merritt, D. A., Lovrein, E. W., Rivas, M. L. and Conneally, P. M.: Human amylase loci: genetic linkage with the Duffy blood group locus and assignment to linkage group I. Am. J. Hum. Genet. 25: 523-538, 1973.

*10470 AMYLASE, SALIVARY (AMY-1)

Kamaryt and Laxova (1965, 1966) found two amylase isoenzymes in serum, one produced by the salivary gland and the second by the pancreas. In 11 of 120 children a duplication of pancreatic enzyme band was found on starch gel electrophoresis and in each case one parent also showed the duplication. In the mouse the salivary and pancreatic amylases are determined by genes at closely linked loci (Sick and Nielsen, 1964). The separate loci have been designated Amy 1 (salivary) and Amy 2 (pancreatic). Polymorphism of both the salivary and the pancreatic serum amylases has been demonstrated in man. Ward et al. (1971) studied amylase in saliva and identified electrophoretic variants.

Kamaryt, J. and Laxova, R.: Amylase heterogeneity variants in man. Humangenetik 3: 41-45, 1966.

Kamaryt, J. and Laxova, R.: Amylase heterogeneity. Some genetic and clinical aspects. Humangenetik 1: 579-586, 1965.

McGeachin, R. L.: Multiple molecular forms of amylase. Ann. N.Y. Acad. Sci. 151: 208-212, 1968.

Sick, K. and Nielsen, J. T.: Genetics of amylase isozymes in the mouse. Hereditas 51: 291-296, 1964.

Ward, J. C., Merritt, A. D. and Bixler, D.: Human salivary amylase: genetics of electrophoretic variants. Am. J. Hum. Genet. 23: 403-409, 1971.

*10480 AMYLOIDOSIS I (ANDRADE OR PORTUGUESE TYPE)

Amyloidosis occurs with familial Mediterranean fever (a recessive), with cold hypersensitivity (a dominant) and in the syndrome of urticaria, deafness and amyloidosis (also a dominant). In addition three dominant types of systemic amyloidosis are recognized. In the Andrade type, observed in many patients in the northern coastal provinces of Portugal and in their Brazilian relatives, neuropathic manifestations begin and predominate in the legs, leading to the popular designation of 'foot disease.' Onset is between age 20 and 30 and death occurs 7-10 years later. The disease is milder in females. Vitreous opacities are frequent (Kaufman and Thomas, 1959). In both this and amyloidosis II the amyloid is peri-collagenous. In familial Mediterranean fever it is peri-reticular. The entire topic of amyloidosis was extensively reviewed by Cohen

(1967). Araki et al. (1968) reported a Japanese kindred with many members affected with the Portuguese type of amyloid neuropathy. Coimbra and Andrade (1971) reported the somewhat unexpected electron microscopic findings that demonstrate that the primary change is one of myelin degeneration, followed by axoplasmic degeneration and only subsequently by accumulation of amyloid deposits which do not cause nerve compression. This suggests that the amyloid accumulations are secondary to the peripheral nerve degeneration.

Andrade, C.: A peculiar form of peripheral neuropathy: familial atypical generalised amyloidosis with special involvement of peripheral nerves. Brain 75: 408-427, 1952.

Andrade, C., Canijo, M., Klein, D. and Kaelin, A.: The genetic aspects of the familial amyloidotic polyneuropathy. Portuguese type of paramyloidosis. Humangenetik 7: 163-175, 1969.

Araki, S., Mawatari, S., Ohta, M., Nakajima, A. and Kuroiwa, Y.: Polyneuritic amyloidosis in a Japanese family. Arch. Neurol. 18: 593-602, 1968.

Becker, P. E., Antunes, L., Rosario, M. and Barros, F.: Paramyloidose der peripheren Nerven in Portugal. Z. Menschl. Vererb. Konstitutionsl. 37: 329-364, 1963.

Cohen, A. S.: Amyloidosis. N. Engl. J. Med. 277: 522-530, 574-583 and 628-638, 1967.

Cohen, A. S.: The inherited systemic amyloidoses. In, Stanbury, J. B., Wyngaarden, J. B. and Fredrickson, D. S. (eds.): The Metabolic Basis of Inherited Disease. New York: McGraw-Hill, 1972 (3rd Ed.). Pp. 1273-1294.

Coimbra, A. and Andrade, C.: Familial amyloid polyneuropathy: an electron microscope study of the peripheral nerve in five cases. I. Interstitial changes. Brain 94: 199-206, 1971.

Coimbra, A. and Andrade, C.: Familial amyloid polyneuropathy: an electron microscope study of the peripheral nerve in five cases. II. Nerve fiber changes. Brain 94: 207-212, 1971.

Da Silva Horta, J., Filipe, I. and Duarte, S.: Portuguese polyneuritic familial type of amyloidosis. Pathol. Microbiol. 27: 809-825, 1964.

Heller, H., Sohar, E. and Gafni, J.: Classification of amyloidosis with special regard to the genetic types. Pathol. Microbiol. 27: 833-840, 1964.

Kaufman, H. E. and Thomas, L. B.: Vitreous opacities diagnostic of familial primary amyloidosis. N. Engl. J. Med. 261: 1267-1271, 1959.

*10490 AMYLOIDOSIS II (INDIANA OR RUKAVINA TYPE)

This type was observed by Rukavina et al. (1956) in many members of a religious sect of Swiss origin living in Indiana. We (Mahloudji et al., 1969) have observed it in an equally large number of persons of German extraction living in Frederick and Washington counties of Maryland. Neuropathic manifestations begin and predominate in the upper limbs. Carpal tunnel syndrome (pain, numbness and weakness referrable to the median nerve and atrophy of the abductor pollicis brevis muscle) is the characteristic feature and is relieved by decompression of the carpal tunnel. Onset is usually in the 40's and progression to generalized neuropathy is slow so that survival for 20 years or more after onset is the rule. The disease is milder in females. Vitreous opacities and visceral manifestations are less conspicuous than in amyloidosis I.

Mahloudji, M., Teasdall, R. D., Adamkiewicz, J. J., Hartmann, W. H., Lambird, P. A. and McKusick, V. A.: The genetic amyloidoses with particular reference to hereditary neuropathic amyloidosis, type II (Indiana or Rukavina type). Medicine 48: 1-37, 1969.

Rukavina, J. G., Block, W. D. and Curtis, A. C.: Familial primary systemic amyloidosis: an experimental, genetic and clinical study. J. Invest. Dermatol. 27: 111-131, 1956.

Rukavina, J. G., Block, W. D., Jackson, C. E., Falls, H. F., Carey, J. H. and Curtis, A. C.: Primary systemic amyloidosis: a review and an experimental, genetic and clinical study of 29 cases with particular emphasis on the familial form. Medicine 35: 239-334, 1956.

Schlesinger, A. S., Duggins, V. A. and Masucci, E. F.: Peripheral neuropathy in familial primary amyloidosis. Brain 85: 357-370, 1962.

10500 AMYLOIDOSIS III (CARDIAC FORM)

Frederiksen and colleagues (1962) in Denmark described a family in which 7 of 12 sibs had progressive heart failure due to cardiac amyloidosis. The onset of heart failure was at about age 40. The process progressed to death in 3 to 6 years. Cardiac catheterization showed constrictive-type right-ventricular pressure curves. The children and grandchildren of the affected persons were too young to show the condition. The father was living and well at age 74. The mother died in the influenza epidemic of 1918. She was said to have been always sickly and to have swollen legs — but did bear 12 offspring. Harrison and Derrick (1969) in a discussion of atrial standstill described Latin-American sibs with possible cardiac amyloidosis. Both parents and sister had died suddenly.

Allensworth, D. C., Rice, G. J. and Lowe, G. W.: Persistent atrial standstill in a family with myocardial disease. Am. J. Med. 775-784, 1969.

Frederiksen, T., Gotzsche, H., Harboe, N., Kiaer, W. and Mellemgaard, K.: Familial primary amyloidosis with severe amyloid heart disease. Am. J. Med. 33: 328-348, 1962.

Harrison, W. H., Jr. and Derrick, J. R.: Atrial standstill. A review, and presentation of two new cases of familial and unusual nature with reference to epicardial pacing in one. Angiology 20: 610-617, 1969.

*10510 AMYLOIDOSIS IV (IOWA OR VAN ALLEN TYPE)

In a family of English-Scottish-Irish extraction Van Allen et al. (1968) have been studying a form of amyloidosis apparently different from others listed here. Neuropathy dominates the clinical picture early in the course and nephropathy late in the course. Onset is at about 35 years, on the average, and average survival after onset is about 12 years with death ascribable in most cases to renal amyloidosis. Severe peptic ulcer disease occurred in some and hearing loss was also frequent. Cataracts were present in several but vitreous opacities were not observed. The pedigree was typical of autosomal dominant inheritance.

Van Allen, M. W., Frohlich, J. A. and Davis, J. R.: Inherited predisposition to generalized amyloidosis: clinical and pathological studies of a family with neuropathy, nephropathy and peptic ulcer. Neurology 19: 10-25, 1968.

*10512 AMYLOIDOSIS V (FINLAND OR MERETOJA TYPE)

The unique features of this variety of systemic amyloidosis are corneal lattice dystrophy and cranial neuropahty, manifesting, for example, by facial paresis. Meretoja (1973), in a massive investigatiom in Finland, identified 207 affected persons. Two cases, more severely affected than the others, were thought to represent homozygosity. Corneal lattice distriphy occurs as an isolated dominant and is due to local amyloid deposition (12220).

Meretoja, J.: Genetic aspects of familial amyloidosis with corneal lattice dystrophy and cranial neuropathy. Clin. Genet. 4: 173-185, 1973.

*10515 AMYLOIDOSIS, CEREBRAL ARTERIAL

In Iceland, Gudmundsson et al. (1972) studied a kindred in which 18 persons in 3 generations had cerebral hemorrhage, some of them at a young age. Cerebral arteries showed thickening of the walls with deposition of material with the characteristics of amyloid. Amyloid was not found in other arteries except in a case of long-standing tuberculosis.

Gudmundsson, G., Hallgrimsson, J., Jonasson, T. A. and Bjarnason, O.: Hereditary cerebral haemorrhage with amyloidosis. Brain 95: 387-404, 1972.

*10520 AMYLOIDOSIS, FAMILIAL VISCERAL

In 1932 and again in 1950, Ostertag wrote about a family with visceral amyloidosis. A woman, three of her children and one of her grandchildren were affected with chronic nephropathy, arterial hypertension and hepatosplenomegaly. Albuminuria, hematuria and pitting edema were early signs. The age of onset was variable. Death occurred about 10 years after onset. The visceral involvement by amyloid was found to be extensive. Maxwell and Kimbell (1936) described three brothers who died of visceral, especially renal, amyloidosis in their 40's. Chronic weakness, edema, proteinuria and hepatosplenomegaly were features. Although neither parent was known to be affected this may be the same disorder as that described by Ostertag (1932). I have followed up the family reported by Maxwell and Kimbell (1936). The father of the three affected brothers died at 72 after an automobile accident and their mother died suddenly at age 87 after being in apparent good health. A son of one of the brothers had frequent bouts of unexplained fever in childhood (as did his father and two uncles), accompanied at times by non-specific rash. At the age of 35, proteinuria was discovered and renal amyloidosis was diagnosed by renal biopsy. For two years thereafter he displayed the nephrotic syndrome followed in the next two years by uremia from which he died at age 39. Autopsy revealed amyloidosis most striking in the kidneys but also involving the adrenal glands and spleen. Some features of the family of Maxwell and Kimbell (1936) are similar to those of urticaria, deafness and amyloidosis (q.v.). No deafness was present in their family, however. Weiss and Page (1974) reported a family with two definite and four probable cases in three generations.

Maxwell, E. S. and Kimbell, I.: Familial amyloidosis with case reports. Med. Bull. Veterans Admin. 12: 365-369, 1936.

Ostertag, B.: Demonstration einer eigenartigen familiaeren Paramyloidose. Zbl. Path. 56: 253-254, 1932.

Ostertag, B.: Familiaere Amyloid-erkrankung. Z. Menschl. Vererb. Konstitutionsl. 30: 105-115, 1950.

Weiss, S. W. and Page, D. L.: Amyloid nephropathy of Ostertag: report of a kindred. In, Bergsma, D. (ed.): Clinical Delineation of Birth Defects. XVI. Urinary System and Others. Baltimore: Williams and Wilkins, 1974. Pp. 67-68.

*10525 AMYLOIDOSIS, PRIMARY CUTANEOUS (FAMILIAL LICHEN AMYLOIDOSIS)

Rajagopalan and Tay (1972) reported 19 persons in 4 successive generations of a Chinese family in Malaysia. Onset was around the age of puberty. The extent of cutaneous involvement increased with age but no systemic involvement occurred. Sagher and Shanon (1963) found 3 cases in 3 generations of a Russian-Jewish family. Tay (1971) reported affected mother and daughter. There are at least two reports of affected sibs. The disorder seems to be much more frequent in South America and Asia than in Europe or North America.

Rajagopalan, K. and Tay, C. H.: Familial lichen amyloidosis: report of 19 cases in 4 generations of a Chinese family in Malaysia. Br. J. Dermatol. 87: 123-129, 1972.

Shanon, J. and Sagher, F.: Interscapular cutaneous amyloidosis. Arch. Dermatol. 102: 195-198, 1970.

Tay, C. H.: Genodermatosis in Singapore. Asian J. Med. 7: 413, 1971.

*10530 AMYOTROPHIC DYSTONIC PARAPLEGIA

Gilman and Horenstein (1964) described dystonia, progressive amyotrophy, mental retardation, nystagmus, and incontinence of bowel and bladder in association with spastic paraplegia. Twelve members of 3 generations were involved to an extent varying from an asymptomatic condition to a severely disabling one beginning in late childhood.

Gilman, S. and Horenstein, S.: Familial amyotrophic dystonic paraplegia. Brain 87: 51-66, 1964.

*10540 AMYOTROPHIC LATERAL SCLEROSIS

Espinosa et al. (1962) concluded that the familial cases observed in the United States represent a different disorder from that in the cases on Guam and from that in many of the sporadic cases. Males and females are equally affected by the familial disease and the progression is less rapid than in the sporadic form which affects males twice as often as females.

Engel, Kurland and Klatzo (1959) described two affected American families. In one family of Pennsylvania Dutch stock at least eleven members of four generations were affected by what was locally and popularly termed 'Pecks' disease. Histopathologic studies revealed a consistent pattern of posterior column involvement. The reports to 1955 were reviewed by Kurland and Mulder (1955). In Germany Haberlandt (1961, 1963) concluded that amyotrophic lateral sclerosis (and its equivalent progressive bulbar palsy) is an irregular autosomal dominant in many instances. Progressive bulbar palsy of childhood (Fazio-Londe disease) is more likely to be recessive (q.v.).

Engel, W. K., Kurland, L. T. and Klatzo, I.: An inherited disease similar to amyotrophic lateral sclerosis with a pattern of posterior column involvement. An intermediate form? Brain 82: 203-220, 1959.

Espinosa, R. E., Okihiro, M. M., Mulder, D. W. and Sayre, G. P.: Hereditary amyotrophic lateral sclerosis: a clinical and pathologic report with comments on classification. Neurology 12: 1-7, 1962.

Green, J. B.: Familial amyotrophic lateral sclerosis occurring in 4 generations. Neurology 10: 960-962, 1960.

Haberlandt, W. F.: Aspects genetiques de la sclerose laterale amyotrophique. World Neurol. 2: 356-365, 1961.

Haberlandt, W. F.: Ergebnisse einer neurologisch-genetischen Studie im Nordwestdeutschen Raum. Proc. Sec. Intern. Cong. Hum. Genet. (Rome, Sept. 6-12, 1961) 3: 1645-1651, 1963.

Hirano, A., Kurland, L. T. and Sayre, G. P.: Familial amyotrophic lateral sclerosis. A subgroup characterized by posterior and spinocerebellar tract involvement and hyaline inclusions in the anterior horn cells. Arch. Neurol. 16: 232-243, 1967.

Kurland, L. T. and Mulder, D. W.: Epidemiologic investigations of amyotrophic lateral sclerosis. 2. Familial aggregations indicative of dominant inheritance. Neurology 5: 182 and 249, 1955.

Poser, C. M., Johnson, M. and Bunch, L. D.: Familial amyotrophic lateral sclerosis. Dis. Nerv. Syst. 26: 697-702, 1965.

Takahashi, K., Nakamura, H. and Okada, E.: Hereditary amyotrophic lateral sclerosis. Histochemical and electron microscopic study of hyaline inclusions in motor neurons. Arch. Neurol. 27: 292-299, 1972.

10550 AMYOTROPHIC LATERAL SCLEROSIS-PARKINSONISM DEMENTIA COMPLEX OF GUAM (ALS-PD)

Plato et al. (1969) found about the same level of inbreeding in affected sibships as in unaffected sibships and interpreted this as arguing against recessive inheritance. They found that affected sibships were more closely related to each other than to the 'general population' and interpreted this as suggesting dominant transmission, although a communicable factor could not be excluded. Segregation analysis adjusted for age was consistent with the conclusion that the disorder on Guam is an autosomal dominant completely penetrant in males but only about 50 percent penetrant in females.

Plato, C. C., Cruz, M. T. and Kurland, L. T.: Amyotrophic lateral sclerosis-Parkinsonism dementia complex of Guam: further genetic investigations. Am. J. Hum. Genet. 21: 133-141, 1969.

*10560 ANEMIA WITH MULTINUCLEATED ERYTHROBLASTS (DYSERYTHROPOIETIC ANEMIA, TYPE III)

Wolff and Von Hofe (1951) described in a mother and all three of her children mild anemia, macrocytosis in the peripheral blood, and giant multinuclear erythroblasts in the bone marrow. Two recessively inherited distinctive forms of congenital anemia with erythroblastic multinuclearity have been described (22410 and 22412).

Wolff, J. A. and Von Hofe, F. M.: Familial erythroid multinuclearity. Blood 6: 1274-1283, 1951.

10565 ANEMIA, CONGENITAL HYPOPLASTIC, OF BLACKFAN AND DIAMOND

Falter and Robinson (1972) described affected mother and daughter. Only the mother had aminoaciduria, suggesting that it was unrelated to the hematologic disorder. Forare (1963) described this disorder in two children with the same father and different mothers. Mott et al. (1969) reported a similar situation, namely, three affected children from two mothers and the same father.

Falter, M. L. and Robinson, M. G.: Autosomal dominant inheritance and amino aciduria in Blackfan-Diamond anemia. J. Med. Genet. 9: 64-66, 1972.

Forare, S. A.: Pure red cell anemia in step siblings. Acta Paediatr. 52: 159-160, 1963.

Mott, M. G., Apley, J. and Raper, A. B.: Congenital (erythroid) hypoplastic anaemia: modified expression in males. Arch. Dis. Child. 44: 757-760, 1969.

*10570 ANEMIA, NON-HEMOLYTIC NORMOCHROMIC

In northern Sweden, Bergstrom and Jacobsson (1962) discovered a new variety of non-hemolytic, normochromic anemia with low or normal reticulocyte count. They referred to it as hereditary benign erythroreticulosis. Fifteen members of four generations were affected. Bergstrom (1968) stated that no further families had been observed in Sweden but that new cases, to a total of about 20, had been detected in the reported family.

Bergstrom, I. and Jacobsson, L.: Hereditary benign erythroreticulosis. Blood 19: 296-303, 1962.

Bergstrom, I.: Ostersund, Sweden: personal communication, 1968.

*10580 ANEURYSM, INTRACRANIAL 'BERRY'

Ullrich and Sugar (1960) reported four families in each of which two members had cerebral aneurysms. We observed a 34-year-old man and his 13-year-old daughter, both of whom died of intracranial berry aneurysm. In some cases of polycystic kidneys (q.v.) berry aneurysm is an associated malformation (Jankowitz et al., 1971). Graf (1966) reported two pairs of affected sibs. 'Berry' aneurysm may have an increased frequency in persons with the Ehlers-Danlos syndrome and also occurs with coarctation of the aorta. Beumont (1968) described three affected sisters. Thierry et al. (1972) found 10 reports sufficiently detailed that autosomal dominant inheritance could be considered documented. Brisman and Abbassioun (1971) raised the question of prophylactic investigations in a family with a high frequency of mortality from ruptured aneurysms. Edelsohn et al. (1972) reported a family with affected father and three affected daughters and an affected son. Toglia and Samii (1972) reported two separate cases: two Negro sisters and two white brothers with intracranial aneurysms. One sister, age 38, developed six intracranial aneurysms, the largest at the left middle cerebral artery. Her sister suffered an aneurysm at the right anterior cerebral artery at age 43. In the second case, a 31-year-old male developed an aneurysm at the bifurcation of the basilar artery. His brother at age 34 developed an aneurysm at the same site as well as a smaller one at the left middle cerebral artery. Their father died of a subarachnoid hemorrhage at age 39. Toglia and Samii suggested that familial aneurysms may have favored locations and that multiple aneurysms may be more often familial than are single aneurysms. Berry aneurysm appears to have a genuinely lower frequency in Blacks than in whites in the U. S. and elsewhere.

Bannerman, R. M., Ingall, G. B. and Graf, C. J.: The familial occurrence of intracranial aneurysms. Neurology 20: 283-292, 1970.

Beumont, P. J.: The familial occurrence of berry aneurysm. J. Neurol. Neurosurg. Psychiatry 31: 399-402, 1968.

Brisman, R. and Abbassioun, K.: Familial intracranial aneurysms. J. Neurosurg. 34: 678-681, 1971.

Chakravorty, B. G. and Gleadhill, C. A.: Familial incidence of cerebral aneurysms. Br. Med. J. 1: 147-148, 1966.

Edelsohn, L., Caplan, L. and Rosenbaum, A. E.: Familial aneurysms and infundibular widening. Neurology 22: 1056-1060, 1972.

Graf, C. J.: Familial intracranial aneurysms. Report of four cases. J. Neurosurg. 25: 304-308, 1966.

Jankowitz, E., Banach, S. and Pikiel, L.: Intracranial familial aneurysms associated with polycystic kidneys. Neur. Neurochir. Pol., Pp. 263-265, 1971.

Kak, V. K., Gleadhill, C. A. and Bailey, I. C.: The familial incidence of intracranial aneurysms. J. Neurol. Neurosurg. Psychiatry 33: 29-33, 1970.

Thierry, A., Ballivet, J., Dumas, R. Et Al.: Les cas familiaux d'aneurysmes intra-craniens. Neuro-Chir. 18: 267-276, 1972.

Toglia, J. U. and Samii, A. R.: Familial intracranial aneurysms. Dis. Nerv. Syst. 33: 611-613, 1972.

Ullrich, D. P. and Sugar, O.: Familial cerebral aneurysms including one extracranial internal carotid aneurysm. Neurology 10: 288-294, 1960.

10590 ANGIOLIPOMAS, MULTIPLE

Klem (1949) described affected brother and sister whose deceased father was said to have been similarly affected. See description of histopathology and other features by Howard and Helwig (1960).

Howard, W. R. and Helwig, E. B.: Angiolipoma. Arch. Dermatol. 82: 924-931, 1960.

Klem, K. K.: Multiple lipoma-angiolipomas. Acta Chir. Scand. 97: 527-532, 1949.

10600 ANGIOMA RACEMOSUM VENOSUM

Segmentally related vascular anomalies of the spinal cord and skin are very rare. There is no evidence of a genetic basis.

Fine, R. D.: Angioma racemosum venosum of spinal cord with segmentally related angiomatous lesions of skin and forearm. J. Neurosurg. 18: 546-550, 1961.

*10610 ANGIONEUROTIC EDEMA

A considerable number of kindreds with angioneurotic edema transmitted in a typical autosomal dominant pattern have been described. In Trigg's family (1961) about twice as many males as females were affected. Two types are identifiable. One fails to synthesize the inhibitor of the first component of complement, whereas the other synthesizes an abnormal, nonfunctional protein. It is curious that this 'deficiency' is expressed in the heterozygote. All of the particular protein is either absent or abnormal, not approximately half as in heterozygotes for most disorders. See COLD HYPERSENSITIVITY for related condition. A family studied by Donaldson and Rosen (1964) had previously been reported by Heiner and Blitzer (1957). Cohen (1961) described a family with many cases in five generations. Although reported as giant urticaria, the same family was studied by Rosen and colleagues (1965) and shown to have a defect in a component of complement. Spaulding (1960) and Dennehy (1970) described apparently effective prophylaxis with testosterone. The latter also called attention to the fact that Nathaniel Hawthorne was apparently familiar with this disorder for in his 'House Of The Seven Gables' he described a family with members who gurgled in the throat and chest when excited and who would sometimes die this way, ever since a curse to choke on blood had been placed on one of their ancestors. Dennehy (1970) interpreted the following passage as an indication that Hawthorne recognized that a hereditary disease, not a curse, was responsible for the deaths: 'This mode of death has been an idiosyncrasy with his family, for generations past. . . . Old Maule's prophecy was probably founded on a knowledge of this physical predisposition in the Pyncheon race.' Three types of C1 esterase inhibitor in different families with angioneurotic edema were described by Rosen et al. (1971). Immunologically one had levels of inhibitor (an alpha-2 neuraminoglycoprotein) 17.5 percent of normal, a second group had levels 111 percent of normal and a third group represented by affected persons in a single kindred had more than 400 percent of normal. Although immunologically identical, the three types of inhibitor differed in electrophoretic and other characteristics from the normal and from each other. From immunofluorescence studies Johnson et al. (1971) concluded that deficient hepatic synthesis of the C1-inhibitor is the basis of the deficiency in plasma inhibitor. Epsilon aminocaproic acid is efficacious in treatment (Frank et al., 1972). Shokeir (1973) suggested that the mutation is in a repressor which fails to bind an inducer so that the operator site remains repressed. It was necessary to suggest that the repressor molecule has a very high affinity for the operator site so that the amount of unbound repressor present in the heterozygote suffices for repression of both operators. Shokeir (1973) encountered greater difficulty in explaining the 'genetic variant' form of angioedema. A possibility he suggested was that these persons are heterozygous for an enzyme which attaches an auxiliary group to the molecule (e.g. neuraminic acid) thereby altering its biologic but not is immunologic properties. If true, this hypothesis points to the existence of at least two loci at which mutation can lead to angioedema.

Austen, K. F. and Sheaffer, A. L.: Detection of hereditary angioneurotic edema by demonstration of a reduction in the second component of human complement. N. Engl. J. Med. 272: 649-656, 1965.

Cohen, J. D.: Chronic familial giant urticaria. Ann. Intern. Med. 54: 331-335, 1961.

De Marchi, M. J., Jacot-Guillarmod, H., Reesa, T. G. and Carbonara, A. O.: Hereditary angioedemia: report of a large kindred with a rare genetic variant of C'1-enterase inhibitor. Clin. Genet. 4: 229-235, 1973.

Dennehy, J. J.: Hereditary angioneurotic edema. Report of a large kindred with defect in C-Prime-1 esterase inhibitor and review of the literature. Ann. Intern. Med. 73: 55-59, 1970.

Donaldson, V. H. and Evans, R. R.: A biochemical abnormality in hereditary angioneurotic edema. Absence of serum inhibitor C'1-esterase. Am. J. Med. 35: 37-44, 1963.

Donaldson, V. H. and Rosen, F. S.: Action of complement in hereditary angioneurotic edema: the role of C-prime-1-esterase. J. Clin. Invest. 43: 2204-2213, 1964.

Frank, M. M., Sergent, J. S., Kane, M. A. and Alling, D. W.: Epsilon aminocaprotic acid therapy of hereditary angioneurotic edema. A double-blind study. N. Engl. J. Med. 286: 808-812, 1972.

Heiner, D. C. and Blitzer, J. R.: Familial paroxysmal dysfunction of the autonomic nervous system (a periodic disease), often precipitated by emotional stress. Pediatrics 20: 782-793, 1957.

Johnson, A. M., Alper, C. A., Rosen, F. S. and Craig, J. M.: C-prime-1 inhibitor: evidence for decreased hepatic synthesis in hereditary angioneurotic edema. Science 173: 553-554, 1971.

Landerman, N. S.: Hereditary angioneurotic edema. I. Case reports and a review of the literature. J. Allergy 33: 316-329, 1962.

Pickering, R. J., Kelly, J. R., Good, R. A. and Gewurz, H.: Replacement therapy in hereditary angioedema. Successful treatment of two patients with fresh frozen plasma. Lancet I: 326-330, 1969.

Rosen, F. S., Alper, C. A., Pensky, J., Klemperer, M. R. and Donaldson, V. H.: Genetically determined heterogeneity of the C-prime-1 esterase inhibitor in patients with hereditary angioneurotic edema. J. Clin. Invest. 50: 2143-2158, 1971.

Rosen, F. S., Charache, P., Pensky, J. and Donaldson, V. H.: Hereditary angioneurotic edema: two genetic variants. Science 148: 957-958, 1965.

Sheffer, A. L., Austen, K. F. and Rosen, F. S.: Tranexamic acid therapy in hereditary angioneurotic edema. N. Engl. J. Med. 287: 452-453, 1972.

Shokeir, M. H. K.: The genetics of hereditary angioedema: a hypothesis. Clin. Genet. 4: 494-499, 1973.

Spaulding, W. B.: Methyltestosterone therapy for hereditary episodic edema (hereditary angioneurotic edema). Ann. Intern. Med. 53: 739-745, 1960.

Trigg, J. W.: Hereditary angioneurotic edema: report of a case with gastrointestinal manifestations. N. Engl. J. Med. 264: 761-763, 1961.

10615 ANGIOTENSIN I

Human angiotensin I has a sequence identical to that of the horse. It has 14 amino acid residues. Angiotensin is formed from a precursor angiotensinogen which is produced by the liver and found in the alpha-globulin fraction of plasma. The lowering of blood pressure is a stimulus to secretion of renin by the kidney into the blood. Renin cleaves from angiotensinogen a terminal decapeptide angiotensin I. This is further altered by the enzymatic removal of a dipeptide to form angiotensin II.

Arakawa, K., Minohara, A., Yamada, J. and Nakamura, M.: Enzymatic degradation and electrophoresis of human angiotensin I. Biochim. Biophys. Acta 168: 106-112, 1968.

*10620 ANIRIDIA

Shaw, Falls and Neel (1960) ascertained 176 cases of aniridia in the lower Michigan peninsula. Forty isolated cases were considered mutants. The frequency in Michigan was about 1.8 x 10-5 and the mutation rate about 4 x 10-6 per gamete per generation. Affected persons may be visually handicapped because of nystagmus, cataract or glaucoma. The ratio of affected to normal among the offspring of an affected parent was 38 to 62, a significant difference from 50 to 50. Undoubtedly more than one 'cause' of aniridia exists. Aniridia is sometimes associated with Wilms tumor (q.v.) as a sporadic finding. Fraumeni (1972) is aware of only one patient with Wilms tumor and autosomal dominant aniridia. The patient was reported by Fraumeni and Glass (1968). In an economically depressed area of eastern Canada, Gove et al. (1961) identified 77 cases of aniridia descended from an affected woman born in 1824. The aniridias showed approximately a 20 percent elevation of reproductive activity as compared with the rest of the community, and this community was in turn nearly twice as fertile as the rest of Canada.

Fraumeni, J. F., Jr. and Glass, A. G.: Wilms' tumor and congenital aniridia. J.A.M.A. 206: 825-828, 1968.

Fraumeni, J. F., Jr.: Bethesda, Md.: personal communication, 1972.

Fraumeni, J. F., Jr.: The aniridia-Wilms' tumor syndrome. The Clinical Delineation of Birth Defects. II. Malformation Syndromes. New York: National Foundation, 1969. Pp. 198-201.

Gove, J. H., Shaw, M. W. and Bourque, G.: A family study of aniridia. Arch. Ophthalmol. 65: 81-94, 1961.

Neidhardt, M.: Wilms-tumor und Aniridie — ein genetisch fixiertes Syndrome? Klin. Paediatr. 184: 312-316, 1972.

Shaw, M. W., Falls, H. F. and Neel, J. V.: Congenital aniridia. Am. J. Hum. Genet. 12: 389-415, 1960.

10622 ANIRIDIA AND ABSENT PATELLA

Mirkinson and Mirkinson (1973) found this combination in a boy, his father, and his paternal grandmother. In the latter person bilateral cataracts and glaucoma complicated the aniridia. The patella was either hypoplastic or aplastic.

Mirkinson, A. E, and Mirkinson, N. K.: Manhasset, N.Y., personal communication, July 17, 1973.

10625 ANKYLOBLEPHARON FILIFORME ADNATUM AND CLEFT PALATE

Cleft palate or cleft lip or both, together with congenital filiform fusion of the eyelids, have been observed in families. Khanna (1957) described affected sisters, one of whom had cleft lip and palate. Other familial cases were reported by Ehlers and Jensen (1970) and by Lemtis and Neubauer (1959). Since clefts and ankyloblepharon occur together in the syndrome of cleft lip-palate, mucous pits of lower lip, popliteal pterygium, etc., it is not completely certain that this represents a separate mutation.

Ehlers, N. and Jensen, I. K.: Ankyloblepharon filiforme congenitum associated with harelip and cleft palate. Acta Ophthalmol. 48: 465-467, 1970.

Khanna, V. N.: Ankyloblepharon filiforme adnatum. Am. J. Ophthalmol. 43: 774-777, 1957.

Lemtis, H. and Neubauer, H.: Ankyloblepharon filiforme et membraniforme adnatum. Klin. Mbl. Augenheilk. 135: 510-516, 1959.

10630 ANKYLOSING SPONDYLITIS

Karten and colleagues (1962) demonstrated familial aggregation. Rheumatoid arthritis and positive tests for rheumatoid factor were found no more often in the relatives of spondylitics than in those of controls, suggesting that rheumatoid arthritis and ankylosing spondylitis are distinct entities. de Blecourt, Polman and De Blecourt-Meindersma (1961) found spondylitis 22.6 times more frequently in the relatives of spondylitic patients than in the relatives of controls. They suggested autosomal dominant inheritance with greater penetrance in males than in females. O'Connell (1959) arrived at the same conclusion. The familial incidence was higher when the proband was female. Kornstad and Kornstad (1960) described two families in which only females were affected. Emery and Lawrence (1967) presented data which they interpreted as indicating multifactorial inheritance. Linkage data were published by Kornstad and Kornstad (1960) and earlier by Riecker et al. (1950). Schlosstein et al. (1973) found HL-A specificity W27 in 35 of 40 cases of ankylosing spondylitis and in only 8 percent of normal controls.

Brewerton, D. A., Hart, F. D., Nicholls, A., Caffrey, M., James, D. C. O. and Sturrock, R. D.: Ankylosing spondylitis and HL-27. Lancet I: 904-907, 1973.

Caffrey, M. F. P. and James, D. C. O.: Human lymphocyte antigen association in ankylosing spondylitis. Nature 242: 121 only, 1973.

De Blecourt, J. J., Polman, A. and De Blecourt-Meindersma, T.: Hereditary factors in rheumatoid arthritis and ankylosing spondylitis. Ann. Rheum. Dis. 20: 215-220, 1961.

Emery, A. E. H. and Lawrence, J. S.: Genetics of ankylosing spondylitis. J. Med. Genet. 4: 239-244, 1967.

Karten, I., Ditata, D., McEwen, C. and Tanner, M.: A family study of rheumatoid (ankylosing) spondylitis. Arthritis Rheum. 5: 131-143: 1962.

Kornstad, A. M. G. and Kornstad, L.: Ankylosing spondylitis in two families showing involvement of female members only. With a search for linkage to genes determining blood group antigens. Acta Rheum. Scand. 6: 59-64, 1960.

O'Connell, D.: Heredity in ankylosing spondylitis. Ann. Intern. Med. 50: 1115-1121, 1959.

Riecker, H. H., Nell, J. V. and Test, A.: The inheritance of spondylitis rhizomelique (ankylosing spondylitis) in the K family. Ann. Intern. Med. 33: 1254-1273, 1950.

Schlosstein, L., Terasaki, P. I., Bluestone, R. and Pearson, C. M.: High association of an HL-A antigen, w27, with ankylosing spondylitis. N. Engl. J. Med. 288: 704-706, 1973.

10640 ANKYLOSING VERTEBRAL HYPEROSTOSIS WITH TYLOSIS

Beardwell (1969) described a family of Greek Cypriot extraction in which at least 8 persons in 4 sibships in two generations are known to have this combination. The tylosis was a punctate hyperkeratosis of the soles and palms. In addition, six persons had tylosis alone.

Beardwell, A.: Familial ankylosing vertebral hyperostosis with tylosis. Ann. Rheum. Dis. 28: 518-523, 1969.

10650 ANNULAR ERYTHEMA

Beare et al. (1966) described an Irish family in which four persons in three generations suffered from annular erythema.

Beare, J. M., Froggatt, P., Jones, J. H. and Neill, D. W.: Familial annular erythema, an apparently new dominant mutation. Br. J. Dermatol. 78: 59-68, 1966.

*10660 ANODONTIA, PARTIAL

Erwin and Cockern (1949) described absent second bicuspids and third molars in nine members of three generations.

Erwin, W. G. and Cockern, R. W.: A pedigree of partial anodontia. J. Hered. 40: 215-218, 1949.

10670 ANOMALOUS PULMONARY VENOUS RETURN

Neill and her colleagues (1960) described father and daughter with hypoplastic right lung with systemic arterial supply and venous drainage. They referred to the disorder as the 'scimitar syndrome' because of the radiographic appearance created by the anomalous vein draining the right lower lung and connecting with the inferior vena cava. The father was asymptomatic but had been rejected for military service because his heart was said to be on the right side. The daughter had severe pulmonary hypertension, frequent respiratory infections and marked hypoplasia of the right lung with dextroposition of the heart. Vinh et al. (1968) described a brother and sister, offspring of non-consanguineous parents, with total infra-diaphragmatic pulmonary venous return. In two brothers and a male paternal first cousin Paz and Castilla (1971) observed total anomalous pulmonary venous return. Kaufman et al. (1972) described total anomalous pulmonary venous return of the figure-of-eight type in two sisters and a daughter of their maternal uncle. Chelius et al. (1962) described partial anomalous pulmonary venous return in two brothers whose maternal grandmother died at age 42 of congenital heart disease.

Chelius, C. J., Rowe, G. C. and Grumpton, C. W.: Familial aspects of congenital heart disease. Am. J. Cardiol. 9: 508-514, 1962.

Kaufman, R. L., Boynton, R. C., Hartmann, A. F., Morgan, B. C. and McAlister, W. H.: Family studies in congenital heart disease III. Total anomalous venous connection in two sisters and their female maternal first cousin. Clinical Delineation of Birth Defects. XV. Cardiovascular System. Baltimore: Williams and Wilkins Co., 1972. Pp. 88-91.

Neill, C. A., Ferencz, C., Sabiston, D. C. and Sheldon, H.: The familial occurrence of hypoplastic right lung with systemic arterial supply and venous drainage: 'Scimitar syndrome.' Bull. Hopkins Hosp. 107: 1-21, 1960.

Paz, J. E. and Castilla, E. E.: Familial total anomalous pulmonary venous return. J. Med. Genet. 8: 312-314, 1971.

Vinh, L. T., Duc, T. V., Aicardi, J. and St. Thieffry, (NI): Retour veineux pulmonaire anormal total infra-diaphragmatique familiale. Arch. Fr. Pediatr. 25: 1141-1149, 1968.

*10690 ANONYCHIA-ECTRODACTYLY

Lees et al. (1957) described a condition of absence of some or all fingernails with variable absence of some phalanges and metacarpals. A suggestion of linkage with the Lutheran locus was presented.

Lees, D. H., Lawler, S. D., Renwick, J. H. and Thoday, J. M.: Anonychia with ectrodactyly: clinical and linkage data. Ann. Hum. Genet. 22: 69-79, 1957.

10700 ANONYCHIA-ONYCHODYSTROPHY

Timerman et al. (1969) described affected persons in at least four generations with male-to-male transmission. Some digits showed absent nails, others dystrophic nails. In some reported families absence of some or all nails apparently occurred without associated manifestations of the nail-patella syndrome (q.v.) and without absence of digits as in the anonychia-ectrodactyly syndrome (q.v.). Whether different from 'THUMBNAILS, ABSENCE OF' (q.v.) is not certain. Recessive anonychia has also been described.

Charteris, F.: A case of partial hereditary anonychia. Glasgow Med. J. 89: 207-209, 1918.

Hobbs, M. E.: Hereditary onychial dysplasia. Am. J. Med. Sci. 190: 200-206, 1935.

Timerman, I., Museteanu, C. and Simionescu, N. N.: Dominant anonychia and onychodystrophy. J. Med. Genet. 6: 105-106, 1969.

Vogel, F. and Dorn, H.: Anonychia congenita. In, Becker, P. E. (ed.): Humangenetik. Stuttgart: Georg Thieme Verlag, 1964. 4: 489-490.

10710 ANORECTAL ANOMALIES

Van Gelder and Kloepfer (1961) observed four sibs with anorectal stenosis or imperforate anus. Although the parents were unaffected the authors pointed out that failure of expression of a recent dominant mutation, carried by one parent, is a possibility. Kaijser and Malmstrom-Groth (1957) described imperforate anus with rectovaginal fistula in a mother and her two daughters. From the findings of Cozzi and Wilkinson (1968), anal stenosis seems particularly liable to familial occurrence, probably as an irregular dominant.

Cozzi, F. and Wilkinson, A. W.: Familial incidence of congenital anorectal anomalies. Surgery 64: 669-671, 1968.

Kaijser, K. and Malmstrom-Groth, A.: Anorectal abnormalities as a congenital familial incidence. Acta Paediatr. 46: 199-200, 1957.

Van Gelder, D. W. and Kloepfer, H. W.: Familial anorectal anomalies. Pediatrics 27: 334-336, 1961.

10720 ANOSMIA, CONGENITAL

Patterson and Lauder, (1948) described one family with onset of anosmia in middle age in mother and all three children. In each of two families, a single individual could not smell butyl mercaptan but could smell other odors and had normal parents. Admitting the meagerness of the material, they raised the question of recessive inheritance in this apparently congenital form of smell-blindness. In a Japanese kindred Yamamoto et al. (1966) found tremor and-or anosmia or hyposmia in 14 persons. They suggested that the two traits are independent dominants. Their findings may be equally consistent with the pleiotropic and variable effects of a single gene. In the Faroe Islands Lygonis (1969) found a large kindred in which 9 males and 19 females in 4 generations had anosmia with no other abnormality. Male-to-male transmission was observed several times. Singh et al. (1970) observed anosmia in 6 males in three generations. One male who transmitted the trait had only partial anosmia. Dominant inheritance was recorded by Mainland (1945) and Joyner (1963). Several instances of male-to-male transmission were observed. Singh et al. (1970) observed anosmia or hyposmia in 6 males in 3 consecutive generations. See KALLMANN SYNDROME. One of the patients of Hockaday (1966) with anosmia-hypogonadism had father and a brother with anosmia alone.

Hockaday, T. D. R.: Hypogonadism and life-long anosmia. Postgrad. Med. J. 42: 572-574, 1966.

Joyner, R. E.: Olfactory acuity in an industrial population. J. Occup. Med. 5: 37-42, 1963.

Lygonis, C. S.: Familiar absence of olfaction. Hereditas 61: 413-415, 1969.

Mainland, R. C.: Absence of olfactory sensation. J. Hered. 36: 143-144, 1945.

Patterson, P. M. and Lauder, B. A.: The incidence and probable inheritance of 'smell blindness' to normal butyl mercaptan. J. Hered. 39: 295-297, 1948.

Singh, N., Grewal, M. S. and Austin, J. H.: Familial anosmia. Arch. Neurol. 22: 40-44, 1970.

Wenzel, B. M.: Techniques in olfactometry: a critical review of the last one hundred years. Psychol. Bull. 45: 231, 1948.

Yamamoto, K., Ito, K. and Yamaguchi, M.: A family showing smell disturbance and tremor. Jap. J. Hum. Genet. 11: 36-38, 1966.

*10730 ANTITHROMBIN III DEFICIENCY

Egeberg (1965) described a pedigree in which persons in three generations had florid thrombophlebitis and other thrombotic disease associated with about half normal levels of antithrombin III. He suggested that antithrombin III may be the same as heparin cofactor. Antithrombin deficiency in individual patients with severe veno-occlusive disease and an impressive family history was also reported by Penick (1969) and by Nesje and Kordt (1970). See 13840 for a discussion of fibrinogen Oslo which is the basis of thrombophilia. Marciniak et al. (1974) described a large kindred from eastern Kentucky, with an extensive history of recurrent venous thrombosis and pulmonary embolism. Nine persons in three generations showed low antithrombin III levels (26 to 49 percent of normal). Five others were suspected of having the biochemical defect. Male-to-male transmission was noted. They concluded that antithrombin III is the sole blood component through which heparin exerts its anticoagulant effect.

Egeberg, O.: Inherited antithrombin deficiency causing thrombophilia. Thromb. Diath. Haemorrh. 13: 516-530, 1965.

Egeberg, O.: Thrombophilia caused by inheritable deficiency of blood antithrombin. Scand. J. Clin. Invest. 17: 92 only, 1965.

Marciniak, E., Farley, C. H. and DeSimone, P. A.: Familial thrombosis due to antithrombin III deficiency. Blood 43: 219-231, 1974.

Nesje, O. A. and Kordt, K. F.: Hypoantithrombinemi som arsak til mesenterialvenetrombose. Nord. Med. 83: 367-368, 1970.

Penick, G. D.: Blood states that predispose to thrombosis. In, Sherry, S., Brinkhous, K. M., Genton, E. and Stengle, J. M. (eds.): Thrombosis. Washington, D. C.: National Academy of Sciences, 1969.

*10740 ANTITRYPSIN, ELECTROPHORETIC VARIANT OF SERUM

Antitrypsin deficiency is discussed in the recessive catalog. In addition, electrophoretic variants of alpha(1)antitrypsin have been observed by Axelsson and Laurell (1965) who proposed that the gene for the electrophoretic variant is allelic with the deficiency gene. Kueppers and Bearn (1967) studied an Italian family with multiple members heterozygous for an electrophoretic variant which could not be distinguished from that which Axelsson and Laurell found in a Swedish family. The polymorphism of prealbumin described by Fagerhol and Braend (1965) was shown by Fagerhol and Laurell (1967) to be the same as the alpha(1)antitrypsin polymorphism. Fagerhol (1968) suggested that the system be called PI for protease inhibitor. A considerable number of codominant alleles have been described. The alleles have been given symbols according to the relative electrophoretic mobility of the allele product. The described phenotypes include FF, FM, FS, FZ, IM, MM, MS, MV, MX, MZ, SS, SZ, XZ and ZZ. The last phenotype ZZ is associated with lung disease. Aagenaes et al. (1972) described the clinical picture in children with the ZZ genotype as neonatal cholestasis. Five such cases were described.

Aagenaes, O., Matlary, A., Elgjo, K., Munthe, E. and Fagerhol, M.: Neonatal cholestasis in alpha-1-antitrypsin deficient children. Clinical, genetic, histological and immunohistochemical findings. Acta Paediatr. Scand. 61: 632-642, 1972.

Axelsson, U. and Laurell, C. B.: Hereditary variants of serum alpha-1-antitrypsin. Am. J. Hum. Genet. 17: 466-472, 1965.

Fagerhol, M. K. and Braend, M.: Serum prealbumin: polymorphism in man. Science 149: 986-987, 1965.

Fagerhol, M. K. and Gedde-Dahl, T., Jr.: Genetics of the PI serum types. Family studies of the inherited variants of serum alpha-1-antitrypsin. Hum. Hered. 19: 354-359, 1969.

Fagerhol, M. K. and Hauge, H. E.: The PI phenotype MP. Discovery of a ninth allele belonging to the system of inherited variants of serum alpha-1-antitrypsin. Vox Sang. 15: 396-400, 1968.

Fagerhol, M. K. and Laurell, C. B.: The PI system-inherited variants of serum alpha-1-antitrypsin. Prog. Med. Genet. 7: 96-111, 1970.

Fagerhol, M. K. and Laurell, C.-B.: The PI system — inherited variants of serum alpha(1)-antitrypsin. In, Steinberg, A. G. and Bearn, A. G. (eds.): Progress in Medical Genetics, New York: Grune and Stratton, chapter 6 vol. 7, 1970. Pp. 96-111.

Fagerhol, M. K. and Laurell, C. B.: The polymorphism of 'prealbumins' and alpha-1-antitrypsin in human sera. Clin. Chim. Acta 16: 199-203, 1967.

Fagerhol, M. K. and Tenfjord, O. W.: Serum PI types in some European, American, Asian and African populations. Acta Pathol. Microbiol. Scand. 72: 601-608, 1968.

Fagerhol, M. K.: The PI system. Genetic variants of serum alpha-1-antitrypsin. Series Hematol. 1: 153-161, 1968.

Gedde-Dahl, T., Jr., Fagerhol, M. K., Cook, P. J. L. and Noades, J.: Autosomal linkage between the GM and PI loci in man. Ann. Hum. Genet. 35: 393-400, 1972.

Kueppers, F. and Bearn, A. G.: An inherited alpha-1-antitrypsin variant. Humangenetik 4: 217-220, 1967.

Lieberman, J., Mittman, C. and Kent, J. R.: Screening for heterozygous alpha(1)-antitrypsin deficiency. III. A provocative test with diethylstilbestrol and effect of oral contraceptives. J.A.M.A. 217: 1198-1206, 1971.

*10745 ANTIVIRAL PROTEIN (AVP)

According to studies of mouse-man hybrid clones, the locus determining AVP is carried on chromosome no. 21 (Tan et al., 1973). AVP is a factor, presumably protein in nature, which mediates specific interferon inhibition of virus replication. AVP is higher in T21 cells than in normals or in T13 or T18 cells (Ruddle, 1974); thus there is dosage support of the AVP assignment to chromosome 21.

Ruddle, F.: New Haven, personal communication, 1974.

Tan, Y. H., Tischfield, J. and Ruddle, F. H.: The linkage of genes for the human interferon-induced antiviral protein and indophenoloxidase-B traits to chromosome G-21. J. Exp. Med. 37: 317-330, 1973.

10750 AORTIC ARCH ANOMALY WITH PECULIAR FACIES AND MENTAL RETARDATION

In a mother and three of her children, Strong (1968) found right aortic arch, mental subnormality and facial peculiarity difficult to describe. Three of the patients had esophageal indentation demonstrated by barium swallow, suggesting left ligamentum arteriosum or anomalous left subclavian artery. Two of the patients had microcephaly. A stillborn child had anencephaly and another died at 10 months with congenital heart disease and microcephaly.

Strong, W. B.: Familial syndrome of right-sided aortic arch, mental deficiency, and facial dysmorphism. J. Pediatr. 73: 882-888, 1968.

10755 AORTIC ARCH INTERRUPTION, FACIAL PALSY, AND RETINAL COLOBOMA

Levin et al. (1973) described monozygotic female twins with a syndrome of hypoplasia or interruption of the transverse aortic arch, facial weakness involving particularly the depressor anguli oris, and bilateral retinal coloboma. Marden and Ventres (1966) described macular coloboma and coarctation of the aorta in a single patient who also had the linear nevus sebaceous syndrome. Whether this is a genuine syndrome and whether it is Mendelian is not clear.

Levin, D. L., Muster, A. J., Newfeld, E. A., and Paul, M. H.: Concordant aortic arch anomalies in monozygotic twins. J. Pediatr. 83: 459-461, 1973.

Marden, P. M. and Ventres, P. M.: A new neurocutaneous syndrome. Am. J. Dis. Child. 112: 79-81, 1966.

*10760 APLASIA CUTIS CONGENITA

The mode of inheritance is not clear. Parent and child were affected in at least three families and sibs and cousins in others (Hodgman et al., 1965). A defect in the scalp and underlying calvaria characterizes this condition. Pap (1970) described a defect of the scalp and skull in four persons in three generations. Only the skin was involved in the affected persons in 3 generations of the family reported by Tisserand-Perrier (1953). Deeken and Caplan (1970) found aplasia cutis congenita of the midline occipital scalp in a father and two sons, who had two reportedly affected collateral relatives. Their series also contained two pairs of affected sibs. Cutlip et al. (1967) described mother and child.

Cutlip, B. D., Jr., Cryan, D. M. and Vineyard, W. R.: Congenital scalp defects in mother and child. Am. J. Dis. Child. 113: 597-599, 1967.

Hodgman, J. E., Mathies, A. W., Jr. and Levan, N. E.: Congenital scalp defects in twin sisters. Am. J. Dis. Child. 110: 293-295, 1965.

Johnsonbaugh, R. E., Light, I. J. and Sutherland, J. M.: Congenital scalp defects in father and son. Am. J. Dis. Child. 110: 297-298, 1965.

Lynch, P. J. and Kahn, E. A.: Congenital defects of the scalp. A surgical approach to aplasia cutis congenita. J. Neurosurg. 33: 198-202, 1970.

Pap, G. S.: Congenital defect of scalp and skull in three generations of one family: case report. Plast. Reconstr. Surg. 46: 194-196, 1970.

Tisserand-Perrier, M.: Transmission pendent plusieurs generations d'une aplasie cutanee circonscrite du vertex. Bull. Soc. Fr. Dermatol. Syph. 60: 77-78, 1953.

10770 APPENDICITIS, PRONENESS TO

Baker (1937) and others have reported families with numerous persons with appendicitis in a pattern consistent with dominant inheritance with irregular penetrance.

Baker, E. G. S.: A family pedigree for appendicitis. J. Hered. 28: 187-191, 1937.

10780 ARCUS CORNEAE (ARCUS SENILIS)

Although arcus may be a manifestation of a disorder of lipid metabolism, it is likely that this is by no means always the case. MacAraeg et al. (1968) showed that arcus corneae occurs in higher frequency in Negroes than in whites and develops at an earlier age. They could not relate it to diastolic hypertension, myocardial infarction or cerebrovascular accidents. Arcus corneae develops precociously in Tangier disease, Norum disease and in homozygotes for type II hyperlipoproteinemia.

Ahuja, Y. R.: L'heredite de l'arcus corneae. J. Genet. Hum. 8: 95-107, 1959.

MacAraeg, P. V. J., Jr., Lasagna, L. and Snyder, B.: Arcus not so senilis. Ann. Intern. Med. 68: 345-354, 1968.

10785 ARM FOLDING

If in folding his arms the right arm is on top, the person is classed R. Hand clasping (q.v.) is a comparable trait. Falk and Ayala (1971) concluded that although both traits are heritable to a significant extent, a simple Mendelian hypothesis is not tenable.

Falk, C. T. and Ayala, F. J.: Genetic aspects of arm folding and hand clasping. Jap. J. Hum. Genet. 15: 241-247, 1971.

10790 ARMS, MALFORMATION OF

Twelve cases of short, absent or partially fused radius and ulna and abnormalities of the digits were found in 3 generations by Stiles and Dougan (1940).

Stiles, K. A. and Dougan, P.: A pedigree of malformed upper extremities showing variable dominance. J. Hered. 31: 65-72, 1940.

10795 ARRHENOBLASTOMA — THYROID ADENOMA

Jensen et al. (1974) described ovarian tumors in a mother and two daughters. The tumor proved to be arrhenoblastoma in the two daughters. Thyroid adenomas occurred in several members of the family and was found frequently associated with ovarian arrhenoblastoma in young women surveyed separately. See 16695 and 16700.

Jensen, R. D., Norris, H. J. and Fraumeni, J. F., Jr.: Familial arrhenoblastoma and thyroid adenoma. Cancer 33: 218-223, 1974.

10800 ARTERIES, ANOMALIES OF

Gates (1946) cited a family in which the grandfather showed bilaterally a radial artery which passed over the supinator longus muscle 3-4 cm. above the wrist and ran over the radial extensors above the styloid process. All his children were said to have the same anomaly on the left side. Among his grandchildren the anomaly was found on both sides in 4, one side in 4 and neither side in seven. Barbosa Sueiro (1933-34) described the case of a man in whom the superficial cubital (ulnar) artery on the left arm ran along the medial border of the biceps, arising by precocious bifurcation of the branchial artery. There was also a superficial right interosseous artery. The latter condition was present also in the father and a brother and the former condition in the two brothers.

Barbosa Sueiro, M. B.: Observation de quelques arteres avec son trajet superficiel anormal chez quelques membres d'une famille. Arq. Anat. Anthrop. 16: 163-164, 1933-34.

Gates, R. R.: Human Genetics. New York: Macmillan, 1946. P. 1304.

10810 ARTHRITIS, SACRO-ILIAC

There is inadequate information provided in the report of Stauffer and Merrihew (1944) to be certain as to the nature of the ailment referred to by this designation. 22 persons in 4 generations were said to be affected.

Stauffer, J. and Merrihew, N. H.: A pedigree of sacro-iliac arthritis. J. Hered. 35: 112-118, 1944.

10815 ARTHROGRYPOSIS WITHOUT WEAKNESS

Daentl et al. (1974) described a father and his two daughters who had congenital contracture and deformity of the fingers, inguinal hernia, club foot, hip dislocation, small mandible, limiation of motion in the shoulders, elbows, wrist, knees and ankles, short neck, and elevated serum creatine phosphokinase. The authors gave an excellent review of familial forms of arthrogryposis and arthrogryposis-like disorders.

Daentl, D. L., Berg, B. O., Layzer, R. B. and Epstein, C. J.: A new familial arthrogryposis without weakness. Neurology 24: 55-60, 1974.

10820 ARTHROGRYPOSIS-LIKE HAND ANOMALY AND SENSORI-NEURAL DEAFNESS

Stewart and Bergstrom (1971) described a 'new' syndrome of arthrogryposis-like hand anomaly and sensori-neural deafness. Both features of the syndrome varied widely in severity. Two members of the most recent generation had only the hand anomaly.

Stewart, J. M. and Bergstrom, L.: Familial hand abnormality and sensori-neural deafness: a new syndrome. J. Pediatr. 78: 102-110, 1971.

*10830 ARTHRO-OPHTHALMOPATHY, HEREDITARY PROGRESSIVE (STICKLER SYNDROME)

Stickler et al. (1965) from a long experience at the Mayo Clinic with multiple members of a kindred described a new dominant entity consisting of progressive myopia beginning in the first decade of life and resulting in retinal detachment and blindness. Affected persons also exhibited premature degenerative changes in various joints with abnormal epiphyseal development and slight hypermobility in some. In a second paper Stickler and Pugh (1967) pointed out that the family reported by David (1953) probably had the same condition. Changes in vertebrae and hearing deficit were also noted. Opitz et al. (1972) suggested that the patients reported by Smith (1969), Walker (1971) and others may have had this syndrome. Wagner syndrome (14320) would seem more likely in these cases. Both- Stickler's patients and David's patient had dish face. A combination of retinal detachment, unusual facies and skeletal abnormalities occurs also in the Wagner syndrome (14320). Opitz (1972) pointed out that patients with this condition have the features of Pierre Robin syndrome. Hall (1974) described a family. One infant had died of Pierre Robin anomaly. The mother had spent the first 18 months of her life hospitalized for Pierre Robin syndrome. Later she developed progressive myopia, cataract and bilateral retinal detachments leading to bilateral enucleation in her teens. Young affected members had midface hypoplasia. None had joint hyperextensibility or Marfanoid habitus. Any deafness in the family was apparently explained by otitis media. Although examination or history gave no reason to suspect a skeletal abnormality, skeletal X-rays showed mild flattening of epiphyses and mild irregularity of the margins of the vertebral bodies (all changes suggesting a mild spondyloepiphyseal dysplasia).

Daniel, R., Kanski, J. J. and Glasspool, M. G.: Hyalo-retinopathy in the clefting syndrome. Br. J. Ophthalmol. 58: 96-102, 1974.

David, B.: Ueber einen dominanten Erbgang bei einer polytopen enchondralen Dysostose Typ Pfaundler-Hurler. Z. Orthop. 84: 657-660, 1953.

Hall, J.: Stickler syndrome presenting as a syndrome of cleft palate, myopia and blindness inherited as a dominant trait. Birth Defects Orig. Art. Ser. 10 (8): 157-171, 1974.

Opitz, J. M., France, T., Herrmann, J. and Spranger, J. W.: The Stickler syndrome. (Letter) N. Engl. J. Med. 286: 546-547, 1972.

Opitz, J. M.: Ocular anomalies in malformation syndromes. Trans. Am. Acad. Ophthalmol. Otolaryngol., P. 1193-1202, 1972.

Smith, W. K.: Pierre Robin syndrome in brothers. The Clinical Delineation of Birth Defects. II. Malformation Syndromes. New York: National Foundation, 1969. Pp. 220-221.

Spranger, J.: Hereditary arthro-ophthalmopathy. Ann. Radiol. 11: 359-364, 1968.

Stickler, G. B. and Pugh, D. G.: Hereditary progressive arthro-ophthalmopathy. II. Additional observations on vertebral abnormalities, a hearing defect, and a report of a similar case. Mayo Clin. Proc. 42: 495-500, 1967.

Stickler, G. B., Belau, P. G., Farrell, F. J., Jones, J. D., Pugh, D. G., Steinberg, A. G. and Ward, L. E.: Hereditary progressive arthro-ophthalmopathy. Mayo Clin. Proc. 40: 433-455, 1965.

Walker, B. A.: A syndrome of nerve deafness, eye anomalies and marfanoid habitus with autosomal dominant inheritance. The Clinical Delineation of Birth Defects. IX. The Ear. Baltimore: Williams and Wilkins, 1971. Pp. 137-139.

10833 ARTICHOKE, MODIFICATION OF TASTE BY

Eating the artichoke (Cynara scolymus) makes water taste sweet in some, but not all, subjects. Bartoshuk et al. (1972) encountered six males who failed to show the effect. They commented that whether the insensitivity to the effect has a genetic basis is unknown. The effect is induced by a temporary alteration in the tongue. Blakeslee (1935) reported that at the AAAS biologists' dinner in 1934, water tasted sweet to 60 percent of the nearly 250 persons present after eating artichokes as the salad course.

Bartoshuk, L. M., Lee, C.-H. and Scarpellino, R.: Sweet taste induced by artichoke (cynara scolymus). Science 178: 988-989, 1972.

Blakeslee, A. F.: A dinner demonstration of threshold differences in taste and smell. Science 81: 504-507, 1935.

*10834 ARYL HYDROCARBON HYDROXYLASE (AHH) INDUCIBILITY

Busbee et al. (1972) found three distinct groups in regard to inducibility of AHH measured in cultured lymphocytes 24 hours after introduction of 3-methylcholanthrene. AHH is one of the mixed function oxidases in the microsomal fraction. The three groups were designated low, intermediate and high. Family studies indicated diallelic determination at a single locus. Kellermann et al. (1973) found polymorphic inducibility of AHH in a study performed on lymphocytes. Since AHH is an enzyme involved in metabolism of carcinogens, the genetic difference might be relevant to the occurrence of cancer. Three-methylcholanthrene was used as the inducing agent. In a normal white U. S. population, Kellermann et al. (1973) found low, intermediate and high inducibility in the following proportions: 44.7 percent, 45.9 percent, 9.4 percent, respectively. Among 50 patients with bronchogenic cancer they found the following proportions: 4.0 percent, 66.0 percent and 30.0 percent, respectively.

Busbee, D. L., Shaw, C. R. and Cautrell, E. T.: Aryl hydrocarbon hydroxylase induction in human leucocytes. Science 178: 315-316, 1972.

Kellermann, G., Luyter-Kellermann, M. and Shaw, C. R.: Genetic variation of aryl hydrocarbon hydroxylase in human lymphocytes. Am. J. Hum. Genet. 25: 327-331, 1973.

Kellermann, G., Shaw, C. R. and Luyter-Kellermann, M.: Aryl hydrocarbon hydroxylase inducibility and bronchogenic carcinoma. N. Engl. J. Med. 289: 934-937, 1973.

10835 ARYLESTERASE, SERUM

Simpson (1971) found a unimodal distribution of arylesterase activity. From a study of twins heritability was estimated to be 74 percent. No discrete variants were detected. Variation is known in the rat (Augustinsson, Henricson, 1966).

Augustinsson, K.-B. and Henricson, B.: A genetically controlled esterase in rat plasma. Biochim. Biophys. Acta 124: 323-331, 1966.

Simpson, N. E.: Serum arylesterase levels of activity in twins and their parents. Am. J. Hum. Genet. 23: 375-382, 1971.

10840 ASPARAGUS, URINARY EXCRETION OF ODORIFEROUS COMPONENT OF

The odoriferous component seems to be methanethiol. Forty-six of 115 persons were excretors in the experience of Allison and McWhirter (1956). They suggested, furthermore, that 'excretor' is dominant to 'non-excretor.' I am told (Maas, 1972) that a non-excretor may become an excretor during pregnancy, the unborn child presumably being an excretor. This is yet to be tested.

Allison, A. C. and McWhirter, K. G.: Two unifactorial characters for which man is polymorphic. Nature 178: 748-749, 1956.

Maas, W, K.: New York City: personal communication, 1972.

10845 ATAXIA, LATE ONSET, WITH GLUCOSE INTOLERANCE (MACHADO DISEASE)

Nakano et al. (1972) described a form of dominantly inherited ataxia occurring in descendants of William Machado, a native of an island in the Portuguese Azores. The disorder began as ataxic gait after age 40. Six patients studied in detail showed abnormally large amounts of air in the posterior fossa on PEG, denervation atrophy of muscle and diabetes mellitus. The identity or distinctiveness from some other disorders previously included here is not clear.

Nakano, K. K., Dawson, D. M. and Spence, A.: Machado disease. A hereditary ataxia in Portuguese emigrants to Massachusettes. Neurology 22: 49-55, 1972.

*10850 ATAXIA, PERIODIC VESTIBULO-CEREBELLAR

In 16 members of a white, rural North Carolina family, Farmer and Mustian (1963) described recurrent attacks of vertigo, diplopia and ataxia beginning in early adulthood. Slowly progressive cerebellar ataxia occurred in some. Hill and Sherman (1968) described episodic cerebellar ataxia occurring particularly in children, with amelioration in later life and no permanent or progressive cerebellar abnormalities. A large kindred with autosomal dominant inheritance pattern was presented. The condition described by Farmer and Mustian (1963) was followed by progressive cerebellar degeneration and may be different. The same disorder may have been present in the families reported by Hill and Sherman (1968) and by White (1969).

Farmer, T. W. and Mustian, V. M.: Vestibulo-cerebellar ataxia. A newly defined hereditary syndrome with periodic manifestations. Arch. Neurol. 8: 471-480, 1963.

Hill, W. and Sherman, H.: Acute intermittent familial cerebellar ataxia. Arch. Neurol. 18: 350-357, 1968.

White, J. C.: Familial periodic nystagmus, vertigo and ataxia. Arch. Neurol. 20: 276-280, 1969.

*10860 ATAXIA, SPASTIC

In an Iranian family Mahloudji (1963) described a rare hereditary syndrome of spastic ataxia closely resembling disseminated sclerosis in 18 persons. The pedigree, covering five generations, strongly suggests transmission as an autosomal dominant. It appears to be the same disorder as was reported by Ferguson and Critchley (1929).

Ferguson, F. R. and Critchley, M.: A clinical study of an heredo-familial disease resembling disseminated sclerosis. Brain 52: 203-225, 1929.

Mahloudji, M.: Hereditary spastic ataxia simulating disseminated sclerosis. J. Neurol. Neurosurg. Psychiatry 26: 511-513, 1963.

10870 ATAXIA, WITH FASCICULATIONS

Singh and Sham (1964) described autosomal dominant inheritance of progressive ataxia associated with persistent fasciculations of the muscles of the limbs. Members of four sibships in three generations were affected.

Singh, H. and Sham, R.: Heredofamilial ataxia with muscle fasciculations (a report of two cases in brothers). Br. J. Clin. Pract. 18: 91-92, 1964.

10875 ATHROMBIA, ESSENTIAL

Essential athrombia is a qualitative platelet disorder characterized by a mild hemorrhagic diathesis and impaired platelet aggregation. Normal clot retraction and normal platelet factor 3 activity distinguish it from thrombasthenia (27380) and from thrombopathy (18780). The family reported by Goldman and Aledort (1972) was considered consistent with dominant inheritance, either autosomal or X-linked. There was a first-cousin mating in a critical part of the pedigree, and some critically informative members were concluded to be affected on clinical grounds only.

Goldman, B. A. and Aledort, L. A.: Essential athrombia: a family study. Ann. Intern. Med. 76: 269-273, 1972.

10877 ATRIAL CARDIOMYOPATHY WITH HEART BLOCK

In three of five sibs and in the son of one of the three sibs (a male), Williams et al. (1972) found first degree heart block and ectopic supraventricular rhythms progressing to persistent standstill with complete loss of response to direct atrial stimulation. Familial atrial standstill had been reported twice, but both were instances of amyloidosis (10500).

Williams, D. O., Jones, E. L., Nagle, B. and Smith, S.: Familial atrial cardiomyopathy with heart block. Quart. J. Med. 41: 491-508, 1972.

*10880 ATRIAL SEPTAL DEFECT

This congenital heart defect is one which is almost always sporadic. Yet occasional families in which multiple persons have isolated ASD suggest that a single 'major' gene may sometimes be responsible. The family reported by Zuckerman et al. (1962) suggests dominant inheritance. Zetterqvist (1960) reported a family with 8 proved and 5 probable cases of ASD of secundum type in 3 generations. Johansson and Sievers (1967) found 6 proved and 1 probable case of ASD in 3 generations. Furthermore, they were able to show that Zetterqvist's cases and theirs traced their ancestry to a common ancestral couple who lived in the 18th century. Zetterqvist et al. (1971) gave a full report on the family which they felt provided strong evidence for the existence of a single major gene as a determining factor. Sanchez-Cascos (1972) examined 109 cases of ASD, 84 of the ostium secundum type and 25 of the ostium primum type. Of these cases, 92 presented ASD as an isolated defect and 17 were associated with other malformations. Sanchez-Cascos concluded from the incidence of familial aggregation among first-degree relatives of affected cases, from the fact that the sex ratio deviated from 1 for his cases (0.64 males per 1 female) and from other findings that multifactorial inheritance is consistent with the demonstrated pattern of transmission. He also reported significant dermatoglyphic findings in these ASD cases-a high proportion of whorls and a parallel diminution in the number of ulnar loops.

Johansson, B. W. and Sievers, J.: Inheritance of atrial septal defect. (Letter) Lancet I: 1224-1225, 1967.

Sanchez-Cascos, A.: Genetics of atrial septal defect. Arch. Dis. Child. 47: 581-588, 1972.

Zetterqvist, P.: Multiple occurrence of atrial septal defect in a family. Acta Paediatr. 49: 741-747, 1960.

Zetterqvist, P., Turesson, I., Johansson, B. W., Laurell, S. and Ohlsson, N. M.: Dominant mode of inheritance in atrial septal defect. Clin. Genet. 2: 78-86, 1971.

Zuckerman, H. S., Zuckerman, G. H., Mammen, R. E. and Wassermil, M.: Atrial septal defect. Familial occurrence in four generations of one family. Am. J. Cardiol. 9: 515-520, 1962.

*10890 ATRIAL SEPTAL DEFECT WITH ATRIO-VENTRICULAR CONDUCTION DEFECTS

Amarasingham and Fleming (1967) and Kahler et al. (1966) reported a total of 3 families with this combination. Because of the rarity of conduction defects with atrial septal defects of the secundum type, this may be a specific Mendelizing form of atrial septal defect. Bizarro et al. (1970) referred to the form of atrial septal defect as fossa ovalis type (a synonym for secundum type). They demonstrated male-to-male transmission. The family of Weil and Allenstein (1961) probably represented an example of this syndrome.

Amarasingham, R. and Fleming, H. A.: Congenital heart disease with arrhythmia in a family. Br. Heart J. 29: 78-82, 1967.

Bizarro, R. O., Callahan, J. A., Feldt, R. H., Kurland, L. T., Gordon, H. and Brandenburg, R. O.: Familial atrial septal defect with prolonged atrioventricular conduction: a syndrome showing the autosomal dominant pattern of inheritance. Circulation 41: 677-684, 1970.

Kahler, R. L., Braunwald, E., Plauth, W. H., Jr. and Morrow, A. G.: Familial congenital heart disease. Familial occurrence of atrial septal defect with A-V conduction abnormalities, supravalvular aortic and pulmonic stenosis, and ventricular septal defect. Am. J. Med. 40: 384-399, 1966.

Weil, M. H. and Allenstein, B. J.: A report of congenital heart disease in five members of one family. N. Engl. J. Med. 265: 661-667, 1961.

*10900 AURICULO-OSTEODYSPLASIA

Beals (1967) gave this designation to a syndrome which he observed in many members of two families. Multiple osseous dysplasia, characteristic ear shape, and somewhat short stature were features. Dysplasia of the radiocapitellar joint, with or without radial-head dislocation, was a constant finding. Inheritance was unequivocally autosomal dominant. Kimberling (1972) reported possible linkage of auriculo-osteodysplasia to Rh and Duffy (which are now known to be on chromosome no. 1).

Beals, R. K.: Auriculo-osteodysplasia. A syndrome of multiple osseous dysplasia, ear anomaly, and short stature. J. Bone Joint Surg. 49A: 1541-1550, 1967.

Kimberling, W.: Computers and gene localization. In, Wright, S. W., Crandall, D. I. and Boyer, P. D. (eds.): Perspectives in Cytology. Springfield, Ill.: Charles C Thomas, 1972. p. 131.

10910 AUTOIMMUNE DISEASES

In many of the disorders in which autoimmunity has been incriminated, or at least accused, as a leading etiologic factor, familial aggregation is observed. The genetic significance of this is unclear. It is possible that if maternal antithyroid antibodies are responsible for athyreotic cretinism, then multiple sibs might be affected by this congenital anomaly without any genetic basis. Reports on the aggregation of possible antoimmune disorders include the following: Greenberg (1964) described two sisters with myasthenia gravis and thyrotoxicosis and a third sister with Hashimoto struma. See THYROID AUTOANTIBODIES. See ALOPECIA AREATA. See PERNICIOUS ANEMIA. See HYPOADRENOCORTICISM WITH HYPO-PARATHYROIDISM AND SUPERFICIAL MONILIASIS. See SCHMID SYNDROME. Pirofsky (1968) found that 20 percent of 44 patients with idiopathic autoimmune hemolytic anemia had close relatives with clinically detectable autoimmune disease.

Greenberg, J.: Myasthenia gravis and hyperthyroidism in two sisters. Arch. Neurol. 11: 219-222, 1964.

Pirofsky, B.: Hereditary aspects of autoimmune hemolytic anemia: a retrospective analysis. Vox Sang. 14: 334-347, 1968.

*10920 BALDNESS

Early baldness of the ordinary type has been thought to be autosomal dominant in males and to be autosomal recessive in females who transmit the trait if heterozygous but are bald only if homozygous (Osborn, 1916; Snyder and Yingling, 1935). The transmission through many successive generations as in the descendants of President John Adams suggests the operation of a single major gene.

Osborne, D.: Inheritance of baldness. Various patterns due to heredity and sometimes present at birth — a sex-limited character-dominant in man — women not bald unless they inherit tendancy from both parents. J. Hered. 7: 347-355, 1916.

Snyder, L. H. and Yingling, H. C.: The application of the gene-frequency method of analysis to sex-influenced factors, with special reference to baldness. Hum. Biol. 7: 608-615, 1935.

10930 BANKI SYNDROME

Banki (1965) described a Hungarian family in which members of 3 generations showed fusion of the lunate and cuneiform bones of the wrist, clinodactyly, clinometacarpy, brachymetacarpy and leptometacarpy (thin diaphysis). It appears to represent a unique dominant mutation.

Banki, Z.: Kombination erblicher Gelenk- und Knochenanomalien an der Hand. Zwei neue Roentgenzeichen. Fortschr. Roentgenstr. 103: 598-604, 1965.

*10940 BASAL CELL NEVUS SYNDROME (MULTIPLE BASAL CELL NEVI, ODONTOGENIC KERATOCYSTS AND SKELETAL ANOMALIES)

Gorlin and Goltz (1960) suggested autosomal dominant inheritance which now seems well established. (Meerkotter and Shear (1964) favored recessive inheritance. In the family they described both parents were normal but were related as second cousins. Of six children, one (the proband) was typically affected, one died at 6 weeks following an epileptic seizure and one died at two years of medulloblastoma.) Herzberg and Wiskemann (1963) described what they suggested may be considered the 'fifth phacomatosis,' basal cell nevus with medulloblastoma. A father and son had basal cell nevus. The son had medulloblastoma and congenital thoracic scoliosis. One of Cawson and Kerr's patients (1964) had astrocytoma with severe hydrocephalus. The palms and soles may show pits. Block and Clendenning (1963) described reduced responsiveness to parathormone. Other clinical features include mild mandibular prognathism, lateral displacement of the inner canthi, frontal and biparietal bossing, jaw cysts, kyphoscoliosis, fused ribs, imperfect segmentation of cervical vertebrae, characteristic lamellar calcification of the falx cerebri, ovarian fibromata and lymphomesenteric cysts which tend to calcify, short 4th and-or 5th metacarpal. The basal cell nevi occur in enormous numbers. Some may resemble seborrheic keratoses. Suicide is rather frequent in these unfortunate patients. Lip and-or palatal clefts probably occur with increased frequency. The basal cell nevus syndrome is one of the conditions which is accompanied by short fourth metacarpal. Lile et al. (1968) observed four cases in 3 generations. In two of these patients the terminal phalanx of the thumb was short. Bang (1970) described an 18 year old patient with keratocysts of the jaw, skeletal anomalies (bifid ribs, broad nasal root, spina bifida at T12, etc.), unresponsiveness to parathyroid hormone and possibly increased plasma calcitonin level. However, no basal cell carcinomas were present. The man and several relatives had ichthyosis. Ovarian carcinoma has been observed (Berlin et al., 1966).

Anderson, D. E. and Cook, W. A.: Jaw cysts and basal cell nevus syndrome. J. Oral Surg. 24: 15-26, 1966.

Anderson, D. E., Taylor, W. B., Falls, H. F. and Davidson, R. T.: The nevoid basal cell carcinoma syndrome. Am. J. Hum. Genet. 19: 12-22, 1967.

Bang, G.: Keratocysts, skeletal anomalies, ichthyosis, and defective response to parathyroid hormone in a patient without basal-cell carcinoma. Oral Surg. 29: 242-248, 1970.

Berlin, N. I., Van Scott, E. J., Clendenning, W. E., Archard, H. O., Block, J. B., Witkop, C. J. and Haynes, H. A.: Basal cell nevus syndrome. Ann. Intern. Med. 64: 403-421, 1966.

Block, J. B. and Clendenning, W. E.: Parathyroid hormone hyporesponsiveness in patients with basal-cell nevi and bone defects. N. Engl. J. Med. 268: 1157-1162, 1963.

Cawson, R. A. and Kerr, G. A.: The syndrome of jaw cysts, basal cell tumours and skeletal anomalies. Proc. Roy. Soc. Med. 57: 799-801, 1964.

Gorlin, R. J. and Goltz, R. W.: Multiple nevoid basal-cell epithelioma, jaw cysts and bifid rib: a syndrome. New Eng. J. Med. 262: 908-912, 1960.

Gorlin, R. J. and Pindborg, J. J.: Multiple basal nevi, odontogenic keratocysts and skeletal anomalies. Syndromes of the Head and Neck. New York: Blakiston Division, McGraw-Hill, 1964. Pp. 400-409.

Gorlin, R. J., Yunis, J. J. and Tuna, N.: Multiple nevoid basal cell carcinoma, odontogenic keratocysts and skeletal anomalies: a syndrome. Acta Dermatovener. 43: 39-55, 1963.

Herzberg, J. J. and Wiskemann, A.: Die fuenfte Phakomatose. Basalzellnaevus mit familaerer Belastung und Medulloblastom. Dermatologica 126: 106-123, 1963.

Howell, J. B. and Mehregan, A. H.: Pursuit of the pits in the nevoid basal cell carcinoma syndrome. Arch. Derm. 102: 586-597, 1970.

Lile, H. A., Rogers, J. F. and Gerald, B.: The basal cell nevus syndrome. Am. J. Roentgen. 103: 214-217, 1968.

Meerkotter, V. A. and Shear, M.: Multiple primordial cysts associated with bifid rib and ocular defects. Oral Surg. 18: 498-503, 1964.

Pollard, J. J. and New, P. F. J.: Hereditary cutaneomandibular polyoncosis: a syndrome of myriad basal-cell nevi of the skin, mandibular cysts, and inconstant skeletal anomalies. Radiology 82: 840-849, 1964.

Rater, C. J., Selke, A. C. and Van Epps, E. F.: Basal cell nevus syndrome. Am. J. Roentgen. 103: 589-594, 1968.

10950 BASILAR IMPRESSION, PRIMARY

Using a radiologic criterion Bull, Nixon and Pratt (1955) found primary basilar impression in 20 subjects. Of 39 available relatives 11 also showed basilar impression. Although first-cousin parents were found in one case, it was tentatively concluded that autosomal dominant inheritance is likely. Of the 20 probands, 10 were asymptomatic, 7 had a previous diagnosis of syringomyelia and 3 had symptoms and signs explicable by a local lesion at the level of the foramen magnum. Brocher (1955) described affected mother and daughter. Sax (1970) tells me of a family in which as many as 9 persons in four generations may have been affected, with one instance of male-to-male transmission. The proband, a 32-year-old man, presented with weakness mainly in the left arm and leg. He had a short neck, craniofacial asymmetry, left Horner syndrome, depressed reflexes in the arms, exaggerated reflexes in legs, Babinski sign, kyphoscoliosis. Cervical myelogram was thought to demonstrate hydromyelia.

Brocher, J. E. W.: Die Occipito-Cervical-Gegend. Stuttgart: Georg Thieme Verlag, 1955.

Bull, J. W. D., Nixon, W. L. B. and Pratt, R. T. C.: The radiological criteria and familial occurrence of primary basilar impression. Brain 78: 229-247, 1955.

Sax, D. S.: Boston, Mass.: personal communication, 1970.

10960 BEETURIA (BETACYANINURIA)

Beeturia is the urinary excretion of beet pigment (betacyanin) after oral ingestion of beets. Allison and McWhirter (1956) suggested that the trait is unifactorial and polymorphic. They concluded that 'non-excretor' is dominant to 'excretor.' Penrose (1957) challenged this idea. Watson, Luke and Inall (1963) found beeturia in 14 percent of persons. However, 80 percent of iron deficient subjects have beeturia. They suggested that iron and betacyanin may compete for an intestinal mucosal acceptor substance, perhaps apoferritin. Thus, iron deficiency interferes with the usefulness of beeturia as a genetic trait. Patients with iron deficiency have beeturia (Tunnessen et al., 1969).

Allison, A. C. and McWhirter, K. G.: Two unifactorial characters for which man is polymorphic. Nature 178: 748-749, 1956.

Penrose, L. S.: Two new human genes. (Letter) Br. Med. J. 1: 282 only, 1957.

Tunnessen, W. W., Smith, C. and Oski, F. A.: Beeturia. Am. J. Dis. Child. 117: 424-426, 1969.

Watson, W. C., Luke, R. G. and Inall, J. A.: Beeturia: its incidence and a clue to its mechanism. Br. Med. J. 2: 971-973, 1963.

*10970 BETA-2-MICROGLOBULIN

Beta-2-microglobulin is found in the serum of normal individuals and in the urine in elevated amounts in pateints with Wilson disease, cadmium poisoning and other conditions leading to renal tubular dysfunction. The protein is a single polypeptide chain of molecular weight 11,600. Its complete amino acid sequence was reported by Cunningham et al. (1973). Although the function of beta-2-microglobulin is not known, the close homolygy in sequence to immunoglobulins suggests a common evolutionary origin. Beta-2-microglobulin also has structural similarities to HL-A. By somatic cell hybridization Bodmer (1974) showed that a structural gene for this protein is on chromosome 15.

Bodmer, W.: Oxford, personal communication, 1974.

Cunningham, B. A., Wang, J. L., Berggard, I. and Peterson, P. A.: The complete amino acid sequence of beta-2-microglobulin. Biochemistry 12: 4811-4821, 1973.

Lindblom, J. B., Ostberg, I. and Peterson, P.: Beta-2-microglobulin on the cell surface. Relationship to HL-A antigens and the mixed lymphocyte culture reaction. Tissue Antigens 4: 186-196, 1974.

10980 BLADDER CANCER

Fraumeni and Thomas (1967) observed affected father and 3 sons. I have encountered two instances of affected father and son.

Fraumeni, J. F., Jr. and Thomas, L. B.: Malignant bladder tumors in a family. J.A.M.A. 201: 507-509, 1967.

*10990 BLEPHAROCHALASIS AND 'DOUBLE LIP' (ASCHER SYNDROME)

Franceschetti (1955) described it in father and daughter. Sagging eyelids and double upper lip are features. Nontoxic goiter is a variable feature.

Findlay, G. H.: Idiopathic enlargements of the lips: cheilitis granulomatosa, Ascher's syndrome and double lip. Br. J. Dermatol. 66: 129-138, 1954.

Franceschetti, A.: Cas observe: manifestation de blepharochalasis chez le pere, associe a des doubles levres apparaissant egalement chez sa filette agee d'un mois. J. Genet. Hum. 4: 181-182, 1955.

11000 BLEPHAROCHALASIS, SUPERIOR

The outer portion of the upper lid is loose-skinned and pendulous. Schulze (1965) traced the condition through 6 generations with 11 males and 3 females affected. Bismarck showed this condition. In minor form, this is sometimes called the Nordic type of eye fold. Panneton (1936) found the trait in 51 of 79 members of a French-Canadian family.

Panneton, P.: La blepharo-chalazis: a propos de 51 cas dans une meme famille. Arch. Ophtalmol. 53: 729-755, 1936.

Schulze, F.: Beitrag zur hereditaeren Blepharochalasis. Klin. Mbl. Augenheilk. 147: 863-877, 1965.

*11010 BLEPHAROPHIMOSIS, EPICANTHUS INVERSUS AND PTOSIS

Vignes (1889) probably first described this entity, a dysplasia of the eyelids. In addition to small palpebral fissures, epicanthus inversus, low nasal bridge, and ptosis of the eyelids are features (Sacrez et al., 1963; Johnson, 1964; Smith, 1970). The condition should be considered distinct from congenital ptosis. Smith (1970) described affected mother and daughter. Owens et al. (1960) updated the pedigree of a family which was first reported by Dimitry (1921) and which had affected members in 6 generations. The patients had the syndrome-triad consisting of blepharophimosis, ptosis and epicanthus inversus (fold curving in the mediolateral direction, inferior to the inner canthus). I got a first hand description of the disorder from a physician (Raviotta, 1971) who is an affected member (number 38) of the pedigree of Owens et al. (1960).

Dimitry, T. J.: Hereditary ptosis. Am. J. Ophthalmol. 4: 655-658, 1921.

Johnson, C. C.: Surgical repair of the syndrome of epicanthus inversus, blepharophimosis and ptosis. Arch. Ophthalmol. 71: 510-516, 1964.

Owens, N., Hadley, R. C. and Kloepfer, H. W.: Hereditary blepharophimosis, ptosis and epicanthus inversus. J. Intern. Coll. Surg. 33: 558-574, 1960.

Raviotta, J. J.: New Orleans, La.: personal communication, 1971.

Sacrez, R., Francfort, J., Juif, J. G. and De Grouchy, J.: Le blepharophimosis complique familial. Etude des membres de la famille Ble. Ann. Pediatr. 10: 493-501, 1963.

Smith, D. W.: Recognizable Patterns of Human Malformation. Genetic, Embryologic, and Clinical Aspects. Philadelphia: W. B. Sanders Co., 1970. Pp. 114-115.

Vignes, (NI): Epicanthus hereditaire. Rev. Gen. Opthalmol. 8: 438, 1889.

11020 BLOOD GROUP (RED CELL ANTIGEN TYPES)

The blood groups are inherited as co-dominant traits. Except for the Xg system, all are autosomal. (The serum protein types are also blood groups in the broad sense of the term but are discussed separately.) The standard reference on the blood groups is Race and Sanger (1968).

Ginsburg, V.: Enzymatic basis for blood groups in man. Adv. Enzymol. 36: 131-150, 1972.

Race, R. R. and Sanger, R.: Blood Groups in Man. Philadelphia: F. A. Davis Co., 1968 (5th ed).

The following are the major blood groups systems. At least 14 autosomal loci are identifiable. In addition, there is a considerable number of private systems (antigenic determinants of low frequency in the population) and public systems (antigenic determinants of high frequency in the population). Some of these are listed later. How many of them represent loci separate from the 14 others is not known. In addition to these, secretor factor (q.v.) might be considered an 'honorary blood group' and the Bombay phenotype (see recessive catalog) involves blood groups.

11025 BLOOD GROUP — ABO SUPPRESSOR

Rubinstein et al. (1973) found a healthy blood donor with no anti-A in his serum despite the fact that his red cells typed as O. A maternal half-brother, whose father was unrelated, lacked anti-B. The pedigree showed that the effect was due to dominant suppression of normal A1 and B genes. It is not certain that the suppressor is determined by a separate locus; as the authors indicated, there is precedence for mutation at the same locus (ABO) to be responsible. The authors favored a suppressor at the ABO locus. See 11115 for a Lutheran suppressor genetically independent of the Lutheran locus.

Rubinstein, P., Allen, F. H., Jr. and Rosenfield, R. E.: A dominant suppressor of A and B. Vox Sang. 25: 372-381, 1973.

*11030 BLOOD GROUP — ABO SYSTEM

This is the first blood group system discovered, by Landsteiner at the beginning of this century. The occurrence of natural antibody permitted identification of red cell types by agglutination of red cells when mixed with serum from some but not all other persons. At first the alternative genetic hypotheses were mainly (1) multiple alleles at a single locus and (2) two loci each with two alleles, one locus determining A and non-A and the other B and non-B. Application of the Hardy-Weinberg principle to population data by Bernstein and analysis of family data excluded the second alternative and established the former. Developments of the 1950's and 1960's include (1) demonstration of associations between particular disorders (peptic ulcer, gastric cancer, thromboembolic disease) and particular ABO phenotypes and (2) discovery of the biochemical basis of ABO specificity. It is known that the A and B alleles determine a specific glycosyl transferring enzyme. The specificity of the enzyme formed by the A allele is to add N-acetylgalactosaminosyl units to the ends of the oligosaccharide chains in the final stages of the synthesis of the ABO blood group macromolecule. The enzyme determined by the B allele may differ from that determined by the A allele by only a single amino acid, but its function is to add D-galactosyl units to the end. The O allele appears to be functionless. In studies of a familial 15p + chromosomal variant, Yoder et al. (1974) calculated a lod score of 1.428 at theta 0.32 for linkage between the p + region and the ABO blood group locus.

Yoder, F. E., Bias, W. B., Borgaonkar, D. S., Bahr, G. G., Yoder, I. I., Yoder, O. C. and Golomb, H. M.: Cytogenetics and linkage studies of a familial 15p+variant. Am. J. Hum. Genet. 26: 535-548, 1974.

*11035 BLOOD GROUP — AHONEN (AN)

Furuhjelm et al. (1972) described a rare 'new' blood type, An(a). It apparently is a blood group system distinct from ABO, MNS, P, Rh, secretor, Duffy, Kidd and Dombrock. Genetic independence from Lutheran, Kell, Yt, Diego and Colton has not been established.

Furuhjelm, U., Nevanlinna, H. R., Gavin, J. and Sanger, R.: A rare blood group antigen An(a) (Ahonen). J. Med. Genet. 9: 385-391, 1972.

*11040 BLOOD GROUP — AUBERGER SYSTEM

Although the alleles of the Auberger system have a frequency which would make it useful in linkage studies, the unavailability of antiserum excludes it from the list of linkage markers.

Salmon, C., Salmon, D., Liberge, G., Andre, R., Tippett, P. and Sanger, R.: Un nouvel antigene de groupe sanguin erythrocytaire present chez 80 percent des sujets de race blanche. Nouv. Rev. Fr. Hematol. 1: 649-661, 1961.

*11043 BLOOD GROUP — CHIDO SYSTEM

This was discovered by Harris et al. (1967). Robson (1974) informs me of evidence indicating close linkage to the HL-A locus. The frequency of Chido negativity is about 2 percent.

Harris, J. P., Tegoli, J., Swanson, J., Fisher, N., Gavin, J. and Noades, J.: A nebulos antibody responsible for cross-matching difficulties (Chido). Vox Sang. 12: 140-142, 1967.

Middleton, J., Crookston, M. C., Falk, J. A., Robson, E. B., Cook, P. J. L., Batchelor, J. R., Bodmer, J., Ferrara, G. B., Festenstein, H., Harris, H., Kissmeyer-Nielson, F., Lawler, S. D., Sachs, J. A. and Wolf, E.: Linkage of Chido and HLA. Tissue Antigens, in press, 1974.

Robson, E. B.: London, personal communication, March 21, 1974.

*11045 BLOOD GROUP — COLTON (CO)

Co(a) was described by Race and Sanger (1968) as 'well on the way to establishment as a separate system.' Its independence of Lutheran, Kell, Diego and Yt remained to be demonstrated.

Heisto, H., Van Der Hart, M., Madsen, G., Moes, M., Noades, J., Pickles, M. M., Race, R. R., Sanger, R. and Swanson, J.: Three examples of a new red cell antibody, anti-Co-(a). Vox Sang. 12: 18-24, 1967.

Race, R. R. and Sanger, R.: Blood Groups in Man. Philadelphia: F. A. Davis Co., 1968.

*11050 BLOOD GROUP — DIEGO SYSTEM

The Diego system shows polymorphism mainly in Mongolian peoples e.g., Chinese and American Indians.

*11060 BLOOD GROUP — DOMBROCK SYSTEM

Anti-Do(a) antibody was detected in a transfused patient, Mrs. Dombrock. About 64 per cent of northern Europeans are Do(a +), making the system a useful marker in linkage study (Swanson, Polesky, Tippett and Sanger, 1965). Tippett et al. (1972) found a hint of loose linkage between Do and MNS.

Molthan, L., Crawford, M. N. and Tippett, P.: Enlargement of the Dombrock blood group system: the finding of anti-Do(b). Vox Sang. 24: 382-384, 1973.

Polesky, H. F. and Swanson, J. L.: Studies on distribution of the blood group antigen Do(a) (Dombrock) and the characteristics of anti-Do(a). Transfusion 6: 268-270, 1966.

Swanson, J. L., Polesky, H. F., Tippett, P. and Sanger, R.: A 'new' blood group antigen, Do(a). Nature 206: 313 only, 1965.

Tippett, P.: Genetics of the Dombrock blood system. J. Med. Genet. 4: 7-11, 1967.

Tippett, P., Gavin, J. and Sanger, R.: The Dombrock system: linkage relations with other blood group loci. J. Med. Genet. 9: 392-395, 1972.

Williams, C. H. and Crawford, M. N.: The third example of anti-Do. Transfusion 6: 310 only, 1966.

*11070 BLOOD GROUP — DUFFY SYSTEM. SYMBOLIZED Fy(a) AND Fy(b)

The Duffy system enjoys the distinction of being one of the first whose genetic locus was assigned to a specific chromosome, i.e., no. 1 (Donahue et al., 1968). On the basis of families studied in Rochester, N.Y., Weitkamp (1972) could demonstrate no linkage of beta HB locus and Duffy, as had been suggested by Nance et al. (1970). An earlier suspicion of localization to chromosome 16 (Crawford et al., 1967) was apparently in error. Duffy and the locus for a form of hereditary cataract are closely linked (11680). From extensive family studies, Robson et al. (1973) arrived at a tentative map. From study of a family with a pericentric inversion of chromosome no. 1, Lee et al. (1974) suggested that the most probable location of the Fy locus is close to the centromere on the short arm (favored) or near the distal end of the centric heterochromatin on the long arm. Assuming that each arm of chromosome no. 1 is 140 male cM in length, Cook et al. (1974) concluded that, measured from the centromere, map positions are as follows: PGD 1p124; Rh 1p109; PGM-1 1p079; Fy 1p010; PEP-C 1q030.

Cook, P. J. L., Robson, E. B., Buckton, K. E., Jacobs, P. A. and Polani, P. E.: Segregation of genetic markers in families with chromosome polymorphisms and structural rearrangements involving chromosome no. 1. Ann. Hum. Genet. 37: 261-274, 1974.0574

Crawford, M. N., Punnett, H. H. and Carpenter, G. G.: Deletion of the long arm of chromosome 16 and an unexpected Duffy blood group phenotype reveal a possible autosomal linkage. Nature 215: 1075-1076, 1967.

Donahue, R. P., Bias, W. B., Renwick, J. H. and McKusick, V. A.: Probable assignment of the Duffy blood group locus to chromosome 1 in man. Proc. Natl. Acad. Sci. 61: 949-955, 1968.

Lee, C. S. N., Ying, K. L. and Bowen, P.: Position of the Duffy locus on chromosome 1 in relation to breakpoints for structural rearrangements. Am. J. Hum. Genet. 26: 93-102, 1974.

Nance, W. E., Conneally, M., Kang, K. W., Reed, T., Schroder, J. and Rose, S.: Genetic linkage analysis of human hemoglobin variants. Am. J. Hum. Genet. 22: 453-459, 1970.

Ritter, H.: Zur formalen Genetik des Duffy-systems. Untersuchung von 247 Familien. Humangenetik 4: 59-61, 1967.

Robson, E. B., Cook, P. J. L., Corney, G., Hopkinson, D. A., Noades, J. and Cleghorn, T. E.: Linkage data on Rh, PGM, PGD, peptidase C and Fy from family studies. Ann. Hum. Genet. 36: 393-399, 1973.

Weitkamp, L. R.: Rochester, N.Y.: personal communication, 1972.

11075 BLOOD GROUP — GERBICH (Ge)

Antibody demonstrating this antigen has been found in cases of feto-maternal incompatibility (Barnes and Lewis, 1961). Independence of ABO, MNS, P, Rh, Kell, Duffy, and Kidd systems has been demonstrated (Race and Sanger, 1968).

Barnes, R. and Lewis, T. L. T.: A rare antibody (anti-Ge) causing hemolytic disease of the newborn. Lancet II: 1285-1286, 1961.

Booth, P. B. and McLoughlin, : The Gerbich blood group system, especially in Melanesians. Vox Sang. 22: 73- , 1972.

Race, R. R. and Sanger, R.: Blood Groups in Man. Phila.: F. A. Davis Co., 1968. Pp. 385-389.

*11080 BLOOD GROUP — I SYSTEM

Tippett et al. (1960) described a Baltimore Negro family in which red cells were apparently of 'i' phenotype and their serum contained anti-'I.' This was the first direct evidence that the 'I' antigen is under genetic control. Anti-' I' had been first identified by Wiener et al. (1956). Anti-'i' was first recognized by Marsh and Jenkins (1960), leading to the 'reciprocal relationship hypothesis' of Marsh (1961). Bingham (1970) concluded, on the basis of the developmental pattern of the 'I' and 'i' antigens, that the corresponding antibodies may define two independent blood group systems. The matter cannot be considered resolved. Yamaguchi et al. (1972) presented evidence suggesting linkage of the Ii blood group locus and a recessive form of congenital cataract. In each of four Japanese families, two sibs were both homozygous for 'little eye' (no pun intended), and affected with a recessive form of cataract.

Bingham, C. P.: Anti-I and anti-i define two independent blood group systems. To be published, 1971.

Marsh, W. L. and Jenkins, W. J.: Anti-I: a new cold antibody. Nature 188: 753 only, 1960.

Marsh, W. L.: Anti-I: a cold antibody defining the Ii relationship in human red cells. Br. J. Haematol. 7: 200-209, 1961.

Tippett, P., Noades, J., Sanger, R., Race, R. R., Sausais, L., Holman, C. A. and Buttimer, R. J.: Further studies of the I antigen and antibody. Vox Sang. 5: 107-121, 1960.

Yamaguchi, H., Okubo, Y. and Tanaka, M.: A note on possible close linkage between the Ii blood locus and a congenital cataract locus. Proc. Japan Acad. 48: 625-628, 1972.

*11090 BLOOD GROUP — KELL-CELLANO SYSTEM

The Kell and Cellano blood groups are symbolized K and k, respectively. The Kell-Cellano system illustrates nicely the manner in which the understanding of several of the blood group systems have developed. The Kell type was first identified using an antibody developed by Mrs. Kell through the mechanism of materno-fetal incompatibility. Later when Mrs. Cellano was found to have an antibody developed by the same mechanism it was demonstrated that these antibodies were testing for antigens determined by allelic genes. Sutter is part of the Kell system. Close linkage of PTC tasting (17120) and Kell blood group have been demonstrated by several workers (e.g. Conneally et al., 1974).

Conneally, P. M., Nance, W. E. and Huntzinger, R. S.: Lingage analysis of Kell-Sutter and PTC loci. (Abstract) Am. J. Hum. Genet., in press, 1974.

Morton, N. E., Krieger, H., Steinberg, A. G. and Rosenfield, R. E.: Genetic evidence confirming the localization of Sutter in the Kell blood-group system. Vox Sang. 10: 608-613, 1965.

Stroup, M., MacIlroy, M., Walker, R. and Aydelotte, J. V.: Evidence that Sutter belongs to the Kell blood group system. Transfusion 5: 309-314, 1965.

*11100 BLOOD GROUP — KIDD SYSTEM.

On the basis of studies of a patient with deletion of part of the long arm of chromosome no. 7, Shokeir et al. (1973) proposed that the Kidd blood group is on the deleted segment. The parents were homozygous Jk(a) and Jk(b) and all nine sibs of the proband were heterozygous as one would expect. The proband herself was Jk(a). Hulten et al. (1968) previously suggested that the Kidd locus is on either chromosome no. 2 or a C group chromosome, but banding techniques were not then available.

Hulten, M., Lindsten, J., Pen-Ming, L. M., Fraccaro, M., Mannini, A., Trepolo, L., Robson, E. B., Heiken, A. and Tellingen, K. G.: Possible localization of the genes for the Kidd blood group on an autosome involved in a reciprocal translocation. Nature 211: 1067-1068, 1968.

Shokeir, M. H. K., Ying, K. L. and Pabello, P.: Deletion of the long arm of chromosome no. 7: tentative assignment of the Kidd (Jk) locus. Clin. Genet. 4: 360-368, 1973.

*11110 BLOOD GROUP — LEWIS SYSTEM

The Lewis system involves genetically variable antigens in the body fluids and only secondarily are the antigens absorbed to red cells. Grollman et al. (1969) showed that Lewis-negative women lack a specific fucosyltransferase which is present in the milk of Lewis-positive women. The enzyme is apparently required for synthesis of the structural determinants of both Lewis (a) and Lewis (b) specificity. The same enzyme is involved in the synthesis of milk oligosaccharides, because two oligosaccharides containing the relevant linkage were absent from the milk of Lewis-negative women. See 17150 for suggested linkage with acid phosphatase and chromosome no. 2. Weitkamp et al. (1973) presented evidence that the Lewis blood group locus and the C3 locus may be linked.

Grollman, E. F., Kobata, A. and Ginsburg, V.: An enzymatic basis for Lewis blood types in man. J. Clin. Invest. 48: 1489-1494, 1969.

Weitkamp, L. R., Johnston, E. and Gutlormsen, S. A.: Probable genetic linkage between the loci for the Lewis blood group and complement C3. Intern. Workshop on Human Gene Mapping, New Haven, Conn., June, 1973.

*11115 BLOOD GROUP — LUTHERAN SUPPRESSOR

Race and Sanger (1968) described a dominant independently segregating suppressor affecting the expression of Lutheran genes.

Race, R. R. and Sanger, R.: Blood Groups in Man. Philadelphia: F. A. Davis Co., 1968. Pp. 258-259.

*11120 BLOOD GROUP — LUTHERAN SYSTEM

Lutheran and secretor (q.v.) are linked (review by Cook, 1965).

Cook, P. J. L.: The Lutheran-secretor recombination fraction in man: a possible sex difference. Ann. Hum. Genet. 28: 393-401, 1965.

*11130 BLOOD GROUP — MNS SYSTEM

On the basis of studies in the family of a child with a translocation chromosome, German et al. (1968) suggested that the MN locus is either in the middle of chromosome no. 2 or near the distal end of the long arm of chromosome no. 4. Using 'banding techniques' German and Chaganti (1973) restudied the translocation they reported in 1968 and concluded that MN can be tentatively assigned to the area of band Q14 in the proximal portion of the long arm of chromosome no. 2. Hitherto deletion mapping had been surprisingly and disappointingly nonproductive. Weitkamp et al. (1972) have data suggesting that the MNS locus and the beta hemoglobin locus are linked. Linkage with the Alzheimer locus (10430) with the beta hemoglobin locus (14190) and with colonic polyposis (17510) has been suspected. Linkage between the MN

and beta hemoglobin loci has been suggested (Weitkamp et al., 1972). See 17150 for information on another
linkage with MNS.

German, J. and Chaganti, R. S. K.: Mapping human autosomes: assignment of the MN locus to a specific segment in the long arm of chromosone no. 2. Science 182: 1261-1262, 1973.

German, J., Walker, M. E., Stiefel, F. H. and Allen, F. H., Jr.: MN blood-group locus: data concerning the possible chromosomal location. Science 162: 1014-1015, 1968.

Weitkamp, L. R., Adams, M. S. and Rowley, P. T.: Linkage between the MN — and Hb beta-loci. Hum. Hered. 22: 566-572, 1972.

*11140 BLOOD GROUP — P SYSTEM

This locus is linked to ADA (10270), HL-A (14280) and PGM3 (17210) and the whole linkage group may be on chromosome no. 20. Cell hybrid studies suggest synteny of HL-A and P (Fellous et al., 1971). Family data are consistent, although only weakly supportive (Robson, 1974).

Fellous, M., Billardon, C., Dausset, J. and Frezal, J.: Linkage probable between locus HL-A and P. C. R. Acad. Sc. (Paris) 272: 3356-3359, 1971.

Robson, E. B.: London, personal communication, 1974.

11150 BLOOD GROUP — PRIVATE SYSTEMS (ANTIGENIC DETERMINANTS OF LOW FREQUENCY IN THE POPULATION)

Many of these have been found only in a single family. They include Levay, Jobbins, Becker, Ven, Cavaliere, Berrens, Wright, Batty, Romunde, Chr, Swann, Good, Bi, Tr, Webb (Wb). The relation, if any, of each to the major systems listed earlier is not known, mainly because the one or few families in which they have been found do not contribute enough information.

Yvart, J., Gerbal, A. and Salmon, C.: A new 'private' antigen: Hey. Vox Sang. 26: 41-44, 1974.

11160 BLOOD GROUP — PUBLIC SYSTEMS (ANTIGENIC DETERMINANTS OF HIGH FREQUENCY IN THE POPULATION)

These include Vel, Yt, Gerbich (Ge), Lan, Sm. The relation, if any, to each to the major systems listed earlier is not known. The I ('eye') blood group system may also be considered a public system. A listing of public systems, which may represent so-called monomorphic loci, is given by Nei and Roychoudhury (1974).

Nei, M. and Roychoudhury, A. K.: Genic variation within and between the three major races of man, Caucasoids, Negroids, and Mongoloids. Am. J. Hum. Genet. 26: 421-443, 1974.

*11165 BLOOD GROUP — RH BLOOD GROUPS, MODIFIER OF

Chown et al. (1972) described a genetic modifier for the Rh blood groups. Heterozygotes showed weakening of reaction of all Rh antigens. A homozygote also had a weak reaction with anti-U and anti-S, compensated hemolytic anemia and unconjugated hyperbilirubinemia. The modifier was clearly not linked with the Rh locus. The authors compared this 'modified' phenotype with the Rh-null phenotypes which have been described.

Chown, B., Lewis, M., Kaita, H. and Lowen, B.: An unlinked modifier of Rh blood groups: effects when heterozygous and when homozygous. Am. J. Hum. Genet. 24: 623-637, 1972.

*11170 BLOOD GROUP — RHESUS SYSTEM (Rh)

Rh, elliptocytosis, PGM(1) and 6PGD are all on the same chromosome. The first two loci appear to lie between the latter two (Renwick, 1971). Peptidase C is also a member of this linkage group which was thought carried by a C group chromosome (according to cell hybridization work of Nguyen et al., 1971). Newer information places it on chromosome no. 1. From cell hybridization studies, the Rh-elliptocytosis-PGM(1)-6PGD linkage group is known to be on chromosome no. 1. Jacobs et al. (1970) reported data suggesting a loose linkage between a translocation breakpoint near the end of the long arm of chromosome no. 1 and Rh. Lamm et al. (1970) published family data consistent with loose linkage of Duffy and PGM(1). Renwick (1971) suggested that PGM(1) is on the side of Rh remote from 6PGD and about 30 centimorgans from Rh. Cook et al. (1972) confirmed this interval. Although the Rh and Duffy loci are both on chromosome no. 1, they are too far apart to demonstrate linkage in family studies (Sanger et al., 1973). Marsh et al. (1974) found Rh-negative erythrocytes in an Rh-positive man suffering from myelofibrosis. Nucleated hemopoietic precursors were circulating in his blood, and these cells had an abnormal chromosome complement from which part of the short arm of chromosome no. 1 had been deleted. They concluded that the Rh locus probably lies on the distal segment of the short arm at some point between 1p32 and the end of the short arm. The conclusion is consistent with the finding of Douglas et al. (1973), that the PGM(1) locus, which is linked to Rh, is on the short arm of chromosome no. 1. Since the patient of Marsh et al. (1974) did not have deletion of the PGM(1) locus in the mutant clone, the Rh locus is probably distal to the PGM(1) locus.

Cook, P. J. L., Noades, J., Hopkinson, D. A., Robson, E. B., and Cleghorn, T. E.: Demonstration of a sex difference in recombination fraction in the loose linkage, Rh and PGM(1). Ann. Hum. Genet. 35: 239-242, 1972.

Douglas, G. R., McAlpine, P. J. and Harmerton, J. L.: Genetics 74: S65 only, 1973.

Jacobs, P. A., Brunton, M., Frackiewicz, A., Newton, M., Cook, P. J. L. and Robson, E. B.: Studies on a family with three cytogenetic markers. Ann. Hum. Genet. 33: 325-336, 1970.

Lamm, L. U., Kissmeyer-Nielsen, F. and Henningsen, K.: Linkage and association studies of two phosphoglucomutase loci (PGM-1 and PGM-3) to eighteen other markers. Hum. Hered. 20: 305-318, 1970.

Marsh, W. L., Chaganti, R. S. K., Gardner, F. H., Mayer, K., Nowell, P. C. and German, J.: Mapping human autosomes: evidence supporting assignment of Rhesus to the short arm of chromosome no. 1. Science 183: 966-968, 1974.

Nguyen, C., Billardon, C., Picard, J.-Y., Feingold, J. and Frezal, J.: Fourth World Congress of Human Genetics, Paris, 1971.

Renwick, J. H.: The Rhesus syntenic group in man. Nature 234: 475 only, 1971.

Sanger, R., Tippett, P., Gavin, J. and Race, R. R.: Failure to demonstrate linkage between the loci for the Rh and Duffy blood groups. Ann. Hum. Genet. (London) 38: 353-354, 1973.

*11173 BLOOD GROUP — Sd SYSTEM

Sd blood group substance is secreted into the saliva like ABO and Lewis substances.

MacVie, S. I., Morton, J. A. and Pickles, M. M.: The reactions and inheritance of a new blood group antigen, Sd(a). Vox Sang. 13: 485-492, 1967.

Renton, P. H., Howell, P., Ikin, E. W., Giles, C. M. and Goldsmith, K. L. G.: Anti-Sd(a), a new blood group antibody. Vox Sang. 13: 493-501, 1967.

*11175 BLOOD GROUP — SCIANNA SYSTEM

*11180 BLOOD GROUP — STOLTZFUS SYSTEM

An antibody which tests for an antigen in a seemingly 'new' blood group system was found in the Lancaster County Amish. It has been designated Stoltzfus, symbolized Sf.

Bias, W. B., Light-Orr, J. K., Krevans, J. R., Humphrey, R. L., Hamill, P. V. V., Cohen, B. H. and McKusick, V. A.: The Stoltzfus blood group, a new polymorphism in man. Am. J. Hum. Genet. 21: 552-558, 1969.

*11200 BLOOD GROUP — UL SYSTEM

In Finland Furuhjelm et al. (1968) found an antibody which tests for a previously unknown antigen called Ul(a). The antigen was present in 2.6 percent of Helsinki donors. Independence from Kell, Yt and Diego systems was not yet proved but it was independent of other systems. The Ul(a) locus may be within measurable distance of the ABO and adenylate kinase loci.

Furuhjelm, U., Nevanlinna, H. R., Nurkka, R., Gavin, J., Tippett, P., Gooch, A. and Sanger, R.: The blood group antigen Ul(a) (Karhula). Vox Sang. 15: 118-124, 1968.

11210 BLOOD GROUP — YT SYSTEM (CARTWRITGHT)

Eaton, B. R., Morton, J. A., Pickles, M. M. and White, K. E.: A new antibody anti-Yt(a), characterizing a blood group antigen of high incidence. Br. J. Haematol. 2: 333-341, 1956.

Giles, C. M., Metaxas-Buhler, M., Romanski, Y. and Metaxas, M. N.: Studies on the Yt blood group system. Vox Sang. 13: 171-180, 1967.

*11220 BLUE RUBBER BLEB NEVUS

This is a bladder-like variety of hemangioma found particularly on the trunk and upper arms. Nocturnal pain and regional hyperhidrosis are features. Bleeding hemangiomas of the gastrointestinal tract are an important complication. Berlyne and Berlyne (1960) demonstrated transmission through five generations. Other cases have been sporadic, perhaps new dominant mutations. Fretzin and Potter (1965) described a particularly dramatic case with involvement of the skin and gastrointestinal tract and angiomatous gigantism of the right arm requiring amputation in infancy. In a single case in a Japanese woman, Sakurane et al. (1967) described cavernous hemangiomas characteristic of blue rubber bleb nevi over the entire surface of the body and in the mucosa of the oropharynx, esophagus, distal ileum and anus. In addition the patient had multiple enchondromatosis. This, then, had many of the features of Maffucci syndrome (q.v.). Two families with affected persons in 3 and 5 successive generations, supporting autosomal dominant inheritance, were reported by Walshe et al. (1966).

Berlyne, G. M. and Berlyne, N.: Anaemia due to 'blue-rubber-bleb' naevus disease. Lancet II: 1275-1277, 1960.

Fine, R. M., Derbes, V. J. and Clark, W. H.: Blue rubber bleb nevus. Arch. Dermatol. 84: 802-805, 1961.

Fretzin, D. F. and Potter, B.: Blue rubber bleb nevus. Arch. Intern. Med. 116: 924-929, 1965.

Sakurane, H. F., Sugai, T. and Saito, T.: The association of blue rubber bleb nevus and Maffucci's syndrome. Arch. Derm. 95: 28-36, 1967.

Talbot, S. and Wyatt, E. H.: Blue rubber bleb naevi (report of a family in which only males were affected). Brit. J. Dermatol. 82: 37-39, 1970.

Walshe, M. M., Evans, C. D. and Warin, R. P.: Blue rubber bleb naevus. Br. Med. J. 2: 931-932, 1966.

11225 BONE DYSPLASIA WITH MEDULLARY FIBROSARCOMA

Arnold (1973) described several generations of a Vermont and New York kindred demonstrating multiple areas of necrosis in the diaphyses of the large tubular bones. The radiographic appearance of this skeletal condition resembled radiation osteitis, a highly premalignant condition. However, no source of radiation exposure was found in this family. Medullary fibrosarcoma, an uncommon bone tumor, was noted in 4 of the 12 affected members.

Arnold, W. H.: Hereditary bone dysplasia with sarcomatous degeneration. Ann. Intern. Med. 78: 902-906, 1973.

11227 BONE PAIN, PERIODIC

Reimann and Angelides, (1951) reported a kindred in which many members had episodic pain, they termed 'periodic arthralgia.' The kindred was studied further by Thompson and Merritt (1974), who concluded that the pain is located in the shafts of the long bones. It was reminiscent of the pain of sickle cell anemia. No instance of male-to-male transmission was noted. Thirty-three persons in 7 generations were considered affected.

Reimann, H. A. and Angelides, A. P.: Periodic arthralgia in twenty-three members of five generations of a family. J.A.M.A. 146: 713-716, 1951.

Thompson, B. H. and Merritt, A. D.: Dominantly inherited periodic bone pain. Birth Defects Orig. Art. Ser. 10: 245-248, 1974.

*11230 BOOK SYNDROME, OR PHC SYNDROME

In 1950 Book reported 25 affected persons in 4 generations of a Swedish family. The features are premolar aplasia (P), hyperhidrosis (H) and canities prematura (C). Inheritance is clearly autosomal dominant with high penetrance. No other family has been reported and there is no other report of this particular syndromal association.

Book, J. A.: Clinical and genetical studies of hypodontia. I. Premolar aplasia, hyperhidrosis, and canities prematura. A new hereditary syndrome in man. Am. J. Hum. Genet. 2: 240-263, 1950.

*11240 BRACHYCAMPTODACTYLY

Edwards and Gale (1970) described a family with 28 persons with a unique form of brachydactyly due to a combination of short metacarpals and metatarsals and short middle phalanges combined with camptodactyly. Urinary incontinence and longitudinal vaginal septum occurred in many affected persons. The marriage of affected cousins resulted in two presumably homozygous children with severe brachydactyly, polydactyly, syndactyly, deafness, mental retardation and, in the one of them who was female, vaginal septum.

Edwards, J. A. and Gale, R. P.: A kindred with an unusual congenital hand and foot anomaly: a new autosomal dominant trait with two probable homozygotes. (Abstract) Am. J. Hum. Genet. 22: 18A only, 1970.

*11241 BRACHYDACTYLY WITH HYPERTENSION

Bilginturan et al. (1973) described a 'new' form of brachydactyly manifested by shortening of both phalanges and metacarpals and associated, probably as a pleiotropic effect, with hypertension. An extensive pedigree was well documented.

Bilginturan, N., Zileli, S., Karacadag, S. and Pirnar, T.: Hereditary brachydactyly associated with hypertension. J. Med. Genet. 10: 253-259, 1973.

*11242 BRACHYDACTYLY WITH JOINT DYSPLASIA

Liebenberg (1973) reported a South African kindred with symmetrical, bilateral congenital anomalies of the elbows, wrists and hands occurring in 10 members through 5 generations. The elbows showed prominence of the radial head with an unusual olecranon process creating an appearance resembling anterior displacement of the joint. The wrists showed radial deviation and a flexion deformity of 20 degrees. X-rays showed abnormally shaped carpal bones with fusion of the triquetum and pisiform. Pronounced brachydactyly with club-shaped distal phalanges and small grooved fingernails were also seen. One affected child showed streblomicrodactyly of the little fingers. Liebenberg examined 5 of the 6 living affected members of this kindred.

Liebenberg, F.: A pedigree with unusual anomalies of the elbows, wrist and hands in five generations. S. Afr. Med. J. 47: 745-747, 1973.

11245 BRACHYDACTYLY, PREAXIAL, WITH HALLUX VARUS AND THUMB ABDUCTION

Christian et al. (1972) described short thumbs and first toes with abduction of these digits. The shortening involves the metacarpals, metatarsals and distal phalanges, while the proximal and middle phalanges are of normal length. Although no male-to-male transmission was observed, males and females were affected to a similar degree. Four successive generations and 6 sibships were affected.

Christian, J. C., Cho, K. S., Franken, E. A. and Thompson, B. H.: Dominant preaxial brachydactyly with hallux varus and thumb abduction. Am. J. Hum. Genet. 24: 694-701, 1972.

*11250 BRACHYDACTYLY, TYPE A1 (FARABEE TYPE)

In the classification of the brachydactylies, Bell's (1951) analysis has proved most useful. The type A brachydactylies have the shortening confined mainly to the middle phalanges. In the A1 type the middle phalanges of all the digits are rudimentary or fused with the terminal phalanges. The proximal phalanges of the thumbs and big toes are short. This trait has the distinction of being the first in man to be interpreted in Mendelian dominant terms (by Farabee in 1903). Haws and McKusick (1963) followed up on Farabee's family. The subjects are short of stature.

Bell, J.: On brachydactyly and symphalangism. In, Treasury of Human Inheritance. London: Cambridge Univ. Press, 5: 1-31, 1951.

Haws, D. V. and McKusick, V. A.: Farabee's brachydactylous kindred revisited. Bull. Hopkins Hosp. 113: 20-30, 1963.

*11260 BRACHYDACTYLY, TYPE A2 (BRACHYMESOPHALANGY II, MOHR-WRIEDT TYPE)

Shortening of the middle phalanges is confined to the index finger and the second toe, all other digits being more or less normal. Because of a rhomboid or triangular shape of the affected middle phalanx, the end of the second finger usually deviates radially. This rare form of brachydactyly has been described only 3 times in the literature. Temtamy (1966) added a fourth family, the first cases in Negroes. Mohr and Wriedt's family (1919) contained a possible homozygote.

Edelson, P. J.: Brachydactyly type A2 in an American Negro family. Clin. Genet. 3: 59 only, 1972.

Hanhart, E.: Die Entstehung und Ausbreitung von Mutationen beim Menschen. In, Handbuch der Erbbiologie des Menschen. 1: 288-370, 1940.

Mohr, O. L. and Wriedt, C.: A New Type of Hereditary Brachyphalangy I, Man. Washington: Carneg. Inst. (publ. 295) 1919. Pp. 5-64.

Temtamy, S. A.: Genetic Factors in Hand Malformations. Ph.D. thesis, Johns Hopkins University, 1966.

Ziegner, H.: Kasuistischer Beitrag zu den symmetrischen Missbildungen der Extremitaeten. Muenchen. Med. Wschr. 50: 1386-1387, 1903.

*11270 BRACHYDACTYLY, TYPE A3 (BRACHYMESOPHALANGY V, BRACHYDACTYLY-CLINO-DACTYLY)

Shortening is limited to the middle phalanx of the fifth finger. Because of rhomboid or triangular shape of the rudimentary middle phalanx, radial curvature (clinodactyly) of the fifth finger results. Dutta (1965) described 'simple radial deviation of the distal phalanx' without bony deformity of the middle or distal phalanx and with normal length of the digit. Whether this is a separate trait is uncertain. Type A3 brachydactyly is variable and may encompass the cases described by Dutta. (See also DYSTELEPHA-LANGY.) Bauer (1907) described the anomaly in four generations. Defining shortened fifth medial phalanges as those less than half the length of the fourth medial phalanx, Hertzog (1967) found the state much more frequent in Chinese than in Negroes. Population surveys suggest that the trait is more frequent in Mongoloids and American Indians than in whites or Negroes. The condition is more frequent in females. (Note that brachymesophalangy V and brachytelophalangy I are 'normal' forms of brachydactyly and that each has characteristic sex and population distributions.) X-ray changes consist of cone-shaped epiphyses with early union.

Bauer, B.: Eine bisher nicht beobachtete kongenitale, hereditaere Anomalie des Fingerskelettes. Deutsch. Z. Chir. 86: 252-259, 1907.

Dutta, P.: The inheritance of the radially curved little finger. Acta Genet. Statist. Med. 15: 70-76, 1965.

Hersh, A. H., Demarinis, F. and Stecher, R. M.: On the inheritance and development of clinodactyly. Am. J. Hum. Genet. 5: 257-268, 1953.

Hertzog, K. P.: Shortened fifth medial phalanges. Am. J. Phys. Anthrop. 27: 113-118, 1967.

*11280 BRACHYDACTYLY, TYPE A4 (BRACHYMESOPHALANGY II AND V, TEMTAMY TYPE)

Temtamy (1966) studied a pedigree with an unusual type of brachydactyly in four generations. The main features were brachymesophalangy affecting mainly the 2nd and 5th digits. The 4th digit when affected showed an abnormally shaped middle phalanx leading to radial deviation of the distal phalanx. The feet also showed absence of middle phalanges of the lateral four toes. The propositus had congenital talipes calcaneovalgus. A pedigree reported by Jeanselme (1923) had affected members in four generations and could represent the same type of brachydactyly. It was one of Bell's unclassified pedigrees. The affected members had brachydactyly of the 2nd and 5th fingers due to brachymesophalangy, and one affected member had club foot. Stiles and Schalck (1945) described a family in which many members of four generations had ulnar curvature of the second finger. Usually the fifth finger showed at least mild radial curvature and sometimes also the fourth finger. This is really a form of clinodactyly (q.v.).

Jeanselme, B. and Joannon, (NI): Brachydactylie symetrique familiale. Rev. Anthrop. 33: 1-23, 1923.

Stiles, K. A. and Schalck, J.: A pedigree of curved forefingers. J. Hered. 36: 211-216, 1945.

Temtamy, S. A.: Genetic Factors in Hand Malformations. Ph.D. Thesis, Johns Hopkins University, 1966.

*11290 BRACHYDACTYLY, TYPE A5 (ABSENT MIDDLE PHALANGES OF DIGITS II-V) WITH NAIL DYSPLASIA

In 13 persons in 4 generations, with male-to-male transmission, Bass (1968) found absence of the middle phalanges and nail dysplasia. The terminal phalanx of the thumb was duplicated.

Bass, H. N.: Familial absence of middle phalanges with nail dysplasia: a new syndrome. Pediatrics 42: 318-323, 1968.

*11300 BRACHYDACTYLY, TYPE B

In this form, as in the 4 types A, the middle phalanges are short but in addition the terminal phalanges are rudimentary or absent. Both fingers and toes are affected. The thumbs and big toes are usually deformed. This type of hand malformation presents the severest deformity in the brachydactyly group. Symphalangism is also a feature. There is also mild syndactyly between the digits leading some authors to describe this deformity as symbrachydactyly. In the feet there is syndactyly usually of the 2nd and 3rd toes. The first description of this hand deformity was in the pre-Mendelian era by MacKinder (1857) in six generations. MacArthur and McCullough (1932) described the same deformity in three generations and prefered the term 'apical dystrophy.' (see also COLOBOMA OF MACULA WITH TYPE B BRACHYDACTYLY.) Goeminne et al. (1970) observed affected persons in 5 generations.

Battle, H. I., Walker, N. F. and Thompson, M. W.: MacKinder's hereditary brachydactyly: phenotypic, radiological, dermatoglyphic and genetic observations in an Ontario family. Ann. Hum. Genet. 36: 415-424, 1973.

Goeminne, L., Agneessens, A. and Kunnen, M.: Perodactylie of apicale dystrofie: brachydactylie door hypofalangie II-V met bifide telefalangie I, in vijf generaties. Tijdschr. Geneeskunde. 9: 469-472, 1970.

MacArthur, J. W. and McCullough, E.: Apical dystrophy as inherited defect of hands and feet. Hum. Biol. 4: 179-207, 1932.

MacKinder, D.: Deficiency of fingers transmitted through six generations. Br. Med. J. 845-846, 1857.

*11310 BRACHYDACTYLY, TYPE C

Haws (1963) described an extensively affected Mormon kindred. The anomalies of the digits are of many types: brachydactyly of the middle phalanx of the index and middle fingers, triangulation of the fifth middle phalanx, brachymetapody, hyperphalangy (more than three phalanges per finger), symphalangism (q.v.), etc. About 600 family members were examined, of whom 86 were affected. The characteristic change should be considered a deformity of the middle and proximal phalanges of the second and third fingers, sometimes with hypersegmentation of the proximal phalanx. The ring finger may be essentially normal and project beyond the others. In a kindred with brachdactyly considered by the authors as type C, Robinson et al. (1968) found Legg-Perthes disease of the hip in 3 affected persons, 2 sisters and their maternal uncle.

Haws, D. V.: Inherited brachydactyly and hypoplasia of the bones of the extremities. Ann. Hum. Genet. 26: 201-212, 1963.

Pol, D.: 'Brachydactylie,' 'Klinodaktylie,' Hyperphalangie und ihre Grundlagen. Virchow. Arch. Path. Anat. 229: 388-530, 1921.

Robinson, G. C., Wood, B. J., Miller, J. R. and Baillie, J.: Hereditary brachydactyly and hip disease. Unusual radiological and dermatoglyphic findings in a kindred. J. Pediatr. 72: 539-543, 1968.

*11320 BRACHYDACTYLY, TYPE D ('STUB THUMB')

This type is characterized by short and broad terminal phalanges of the thumbs and big toes. Thomsen (1928) described this anomaly. In a unilateral case he pointed out that the epiphyseal line at the base of the anomalous phalanx was obliterated but was still demonstrable in the corresponding position on the normal thumb. Goodman and colleagues (1965) have also studied this 'normal' morphologic trait in detail. The trait has picturesque designations such as 'potter's thumb' and 'murderer's thumb.' It occurs as part of the heart-hand syndrome III (Tabatznik syndrome) and of Rubinstein syndrome (q.v.).

Breitenbecher, J. K.: Hereditary shortness of thumbs. J. Hered. 14: 15-21, 1923.

Goodman, R. M., Adam, A. and Sheba, C.: A genetic study of stub thumbs among various ethnic groups in Israel. J. Med. Genet. 2: 116-121, 1965.

Hefner, R. A.: Inherited abnormalities of the fingers. II. Short thumbs (brachymegalodactylism). J. Hered. 15: 433-440, 1924.

Sayles, L. P. and Jailer, J. W.: Four generations of short thumbs. J. Hered. 25: 377-378, 1934.

Thomsen, O.: Hereditary growth anomaly of the thumb. Hereditas 10: 261-273, 1928.

*11330 BRACHYDACTYLY, TYPE E

The brachydactyly is due mainly to shortening of the metacarpals and metatarsals. Wide variability in the number of digits affected occurs from person to person. The patients are moderately short of stature and have round facies but do not have ectopic calcification (or ossification), mental retardation or cataract as in pseudo-pseudohypoparathyroidism (q.v.) which is an otherwise similar entity. Male-to-male transmission of type E brachydactyly has been observed (McKusick and Milch, 1964), whereas the latter condition appears to be X-linked. This phenotype is a useful example of genetic heterogeneity, because in addition to the autosomal dominant isolated type and the X-linked Albright hereditary osteodystrophy, it also occurs with a chromosomal aberration, the XO Turner syndrome. Also see BRACHYDACTYLY-NYSTAGMUS-CEREBELLAR ATAXIA (Biemond syndrome I), a probable dominant trait. The obviously autosomal dominant pedigree reported by Goeminne (1965) also represented this entity and not Albright syndrome. Hertzog (1968) suggested that there are at least three subtypes: (E1) one in which shortening is limited to fourth metacarpals and-or metatarsals (Hortling, 1960); (E2) one in which variable combinations of metacarpals are involved, with shortening also of the first and third distal and the second and fifth middle phalanges (McKusick and Milch, 1964); and (E3) a dubious category which may have a variable combination of short metacarpals without phalangeal involvement. As peripheral dysostosis, Newcombe and Keats (1969) described an extensively affected kindred with a dominant pedigree pattern (their pedigree II). The description resembles that in the family of McKusick and Milch (1964) except for cone epiphyses. The authors felt that the presence of cone epiphyses in their family was a distinguishing feature. In a family reported by Gorlin and Sedano (1971), type E brachydactyly was associated with multiple impacted teeth. Gorlin and Sedano (1971) gave the designation 'cryptodontic metacarpalia' to type E brachydactyly associated with multiple impacted teeth. The clavicles were unusually straight and short. Whether this is a distinct entity is not clear.

Goeminne, L.: Albright's hereditary poly-osteochondrodystrophy (pseudo-pseudo hypoparathyroidism with diabetes, hypertension, arteritis and polyarthrosis). Acta Genet. Med. Gemellol. 14: 226-281, 1965.

Gorlin, R. J. and Sedano, H. O.: Cryptodontic brachymetacarpalia. The Clinical Delineation of Birth Defects. XI. Orofacial Structures. Baltimore: Williams and Wilkins, 1971. Pp. 200-203.

Hertzog, K. P.: Brachydactyly and pseudo-pseudohypoparathyroidism. Acta Genet. Med. Gemellol. 17: 428-437, 1968.

Hortling, H., Puupponen, E. and Koski, K.: Short metacarpal or metatarsal bones: pseudo-pseudohypo-parathyroidism. J. Clin. Endocrinol. Metab. 20: 466-472, 1960.

McKusick, V. A. and Milch, R. A.: The clinical behavior of genetic disease: selected aspects. Clin. Orthop. 33: 22-39, 1964.

Newcombe, D. S. and Keats, T. E.: Roentgenographic manifestations of hereditary peripheral dysostosis. Am. J. Roentgen. 106: 178-189, 1969.

11340 BRACHYDACTYLY-NYSTAGMUS-CEREBELLAR ATAXIA

Biemond (1934) described a syndrome consisting of brachydactyly (due to one short metacarpal and metatarsal), nystagmus and cerebellar ataxia in four generations of a family. Mental deficiency and strabismus were also present. Only a few members of the family had the full syndrome. Additional families are needed before this combination can be considered a single gene syndrome.

Biemond, A.: Brachydactylie, nystagmus en cerebellaire ataxie als familiair syndroom. Nederl. T. Geneesk. 78: 1423-1431, 1934.

11350 BRACHYRAPHIA

Brown (1933) described as Morquio disease the condition in a mother and two daughters. Lenz (1964) observed father and son with a very short spine and deformity of the anterior chest rather like that in Morquio disease. Except for marked changes in the femoral epiphyses, the extremities were normal. The vertebral bodies were small, irregular and radiolucent. Possibly this is the same condition as that referred to elsewhere as the dominant type of spondyloepiphyseal dysplasia tarda (q.v.). Perhaps the family of Lomus and Boyle (1959) in which 3 generations were affected had the same condition.

Brown, D. O. and MacDonald, C.: Three cases of familial osseous dystrophy. Aust. New Zeal. J. Surg. 3: 78-88, 1933.

Brown, D. O.: Morquio's disease. Med. J. Aust. 1: 598-600, 1933.

Lenz, W.: Anomalien des Wachstums und der Koerperform. In, Becker, P. E. (ed.): Ein kurzes Handbuch in fuenf Baenden. Stuttgart: Georg Thieme Verlag, 1964. 2: 88-89, fig. 30.

Lomas, J. J. P. and Boyle, A. C.: Osteo-chondrodystrophy (Morquio's disease) in three generations. Lancet II: 430-432, 1959.

11355 BRANCHIAL CLEFT ANOMALIES, CUP-SHAPED EARS, DEAFNESS

A mutation combining branchial cleft anomalies (11360) with 'cup ear' (12860) and deafness has been observed in an autosomal dominant pedigree pattern (Karmody and Feingold, 1974; Hoefnagel, 1973).

Hoefnagel, D.: Hanover, N. H., personal communication, June 4, 1973.

Karmody, C. and Feingold, M.: Autosomal dominant first and second brachial arch syndrome. A new inherited syndrome? Birth Defects Orig. Art. Ser. 10 (7): 31-40, 1974.

*11360 BRANCHIAL CLEFT ANOMALIES, INCLUDING BRANCHIAL CYSTS

The abnormality may be in the form of cysts, sinuses or fistulas, the last term being reserved for those instances in which there is communication between the skin and the pharynx. These are considered to be anomalies of the second brachial cleft. Although in at least one family, ear pits (q.v.) were also present, these are listed as separate mutations, because most families show either one or the other. Wheeler, Shaw and Cawley (1958) found branchial cysts and sinuses in four members of three generations of a family. Cysts, sinuses and skin tabs containing cartilage occurred in a line extending from a point anterior to the ear to the anterior border of the sternomastoid muscle at the level of the angle of the mandible and thence along the anterior border of this muscle to a point near its attachment to the sternum.

Muckle, T. J.: Hereditary branchial defects in a Hampshire family. Br. Med. J. 1: 1297-1299, 1961.

Wheeler, C. E., Shaw, R. F. and Cawley, E. P.: Branchial anomalies in three generations of one family. Arch. Dermatol. 77: 715-719, 1958.

11370 BREAST AND NIPPLES, ABSENCE OF

Pedigrees consistent with dominant inheritance have been reported. Fraser (1956) found absent breasts in 7 members of three generations. Goldenring and Crelin (1961) described it in mother and daughter. Recessive inheritance seemed more likely in the family of Kowlessar and Orti (1968) in which brother and sister were affected and the parents were first cousins. Hypoplasia or aplasia of the breasts and nipples occurs in anhidrotic ectodermal dysplasia. Trier (1965) observed affected mother and daughter. Wilson et al. (1972) described seven persons with absence or hypoplasia of the breasts in four generations. The observations do not permit distinction between autosomal and X-linked inheritance. Absence of the breast also occurs with Poland syndrome (17380).

Fraser, F. C.: Dominant inheritance of absent nipples and breasts. In, Novant' Anni Delle Leggi Mendeliane. Rome: Istituto Gregorio Mendel, 1956. P. 360.

Goldenring, H. and Crelin, E. S.: Mother and daughter with bilateral congenital amastia. Yale J. Biol. Med. 33: 466-467, 1961.

Kowlessar, M. and Orti, E.: Complete breast absence in siblings. Am. J. Dis. Child. 115: 91-92, 1968.

Trier, W. C.: Complete breast absence. Case report and review of the literature. Plast. Reconst. Surg. 36: 431-439, 1965.

Wilson, M. G., Hall, E. B. and Ebbin, A. J.: Dominant inheritance of absence of the breast. Humangenetik, in press, 1972.

*11380 BULLOUS ERYTHRODERMA ICHTHYOSIFORMIS CONGENITA (BROCQ)

Heimendinger and Schnyder (1962) described this disorder in a man and two of his three children, a son and a daughter. The condition is distinct from the non-bullous form inherited as a recessive. Gasser (1964) found, among 17 families with two or more affected persons, only sibs affected in 2, two successive generations affected in 12, and three generations affected in 3.

Barker, L. P. and Sachs, W.: Bullous congenital ichthyosiform erythrodermia. Arch. Dermatol. 67: 443-455, 1953.

Gasser, V.: Zur Klinik, Histologie und Genetik der 'Erythrodermie congenitale ichthyosiforme bulleuse (Brocq).' Arch. Klaus. Stift. Vererbungsforsch. 38: 23-59, 1964.

Heimendinger, J. and Schnyder, U. W.: Bullose 'Erythrodermie ichthyosiforme congenitale' in zwei Generationen. Helv. Paediatr. Acta 17: 47-55, 1962.

11390 BUNDLE BRANCH BLOCK

Combrink, Davis and Snyman (1962) described a family in which the mother had right bundle branch block and died at age 35 years in a Stokes-Adams attack. Of four children three had right bundle branch block. The mother's parents had both died suddenly in their 30's. One of her brothers was said to have a cardiac conduction disturbance and another had dextrocardia. Three other sibs were apparently normal. Segall (1961) described an instance of father, son and daughter (of French-Canadian and Negro intermixture) with right bundle branch block, and repeated Stokes-Adams attacks with various atrial arrhythmias and ventricular extrasystoles. The father died at 74 years, 14 years after the first fainting episode. Two asymptomatic brothers showed the electrocardiographic changes of Wolff-Parkinson-White. Deforest (1956) observed 'benign' left bundle branch block in 4 persons in two generations. Steenkamp described a family in which 6 of 17 members studied showed disturbance of rhythm or conduction.

Combrink, J. M., Davis, W. H. and Snyman, H. W.: Familial bundle branch block. Am. Heart J. 64: 397-400, 1962.

Deforest, R. E.: Four cases of 'benign' left bundle branch block in the same family. Am. Heart J. 51: 398-404, 1956.

Segall, H. N.: Congenital arrhythmias and conduction abnormalities in a father and four children. Canad. Med. Assoc. J. 84: 1283-1296, 1961.

Steenkamp, W. F. J.: Familial trifascicular block. Am. Heart J. 84: 758-760, 1972.

11400 CAFFEY DISEASE (INFANTILE CORTICAL HYPEROSTOSIS)

Autosomal dominant inheritance is suggested by the reports of Gerrard and colleagues (1961), Van Buskirk and colleagues (1961), Holman (1962) and others. Multiple sibs have been affected, suggesting autosomal recessive inheritance (e.g., Clemett and Williams, 1963). However, in at least two families (Van Buskirk, Tampas and Peterson, 1961; Gerrard, Holman, Gorman and Morrow, 1961) affected persons occurred in two generations. The condition has somewhat unusual features for a hereditary disorder. It rarely if ever appears after 5 months of age: it is sometimes present at birth and has been identified by X-ray in the fetus in utero. The acute manifestations are inflammatory in nature with fever and hot, tender swelling of involved bones (e.g., mandible, ribs). Despite striking radiologic changes in the acute stages, previously affected bones are often completely normal on restudy. Incontinentia pigmenti is another familial condition in which 'active' lesions at birth and early in life leave little or no residue. In this condition and in Caffey disease an infection could perhaps be the cause and not a mutant gene. Pickering and Cuddigan (1969) suggested that vascular occlusion secondary to thrombocytosis may be involved in the pathogenesis. Taj-Eldin and Al-Jawad (1971) describe a case followed since infancy with recurrences documented up to 19 years of age (1971). Male-to-male transmission was observed by Van Buskirk et al. (1961). Bull and Feingold (1974) reported two affected sisters, one of whom had affected son and daughter and the other had a normal daughter and affected son.

Bull, M. J. and Feingold, M.: Autosomal dominant inheritance of Caffey disease. In, Bergsma, D. (ed.): Skeletal Dysplasia. Miami, Fla.: Symposia Specialists, 1974. Pp. 139-146.

Clemett, A. R. and Williams, J. H.: The familial occurrence of infantile cortical hyperostosis. Radiology 80: 409-416, 1963.

Gerrard, J. W., Holman, G. H., Gorman, A. A. and Morrow, I. H.: Familial infantile cortical hyperostosis. J. Pediatr. 59: 543-548, 1961.

Holman, G. H.: Infantile cortical hyperostosis: a review. Quart. Rev. Pediat. 17: 24-31, 1962.

Pickering, D. and Cuddigan, B.: Infantile cortical hyperostosis associated with thrombocythaemia. Lancet II: 464-465, 1969.

Sherman, M. S. and Hellyer, D. T.: Infantile cortical hyperostosis. Review of the literature and report of 5 cases. Am. J. Roentgen. 63: 212-222, 1950.

Sidbury, J. B.: Infantile cortical hyperostosis. Postgrad. Med. 22: 211-215, 1957.

Taj-Eldin, S. and Al-Jawad, J.: Cortical hyperostosis. Infantile and juvenile manifestations in a boy. Arch. Dis. Child. 46: 565-566, 1971.

Van Buskirk, F. W., Tampas, J. P. and Peterson, O. S.: Infantile cortical hyperostosis: an inquiry into its familial aspects. Am. J. Roentgen. 85: 613-632, 1961.

11410 CALCIFICATION OF BASAL GANGLIA WITH OR WITHOUT HYPOCALCEMIA

Nichols, Holdsworth and Reinfrank (1961) reported a family in three generations of which members had a syndrome of calcification of the basal ganglia and hypocalcemia. It is not clear what relation these cases may have to pseudohypoparathyroidism. Roberts (1959) had reported a rather similar family with six affected persons in two generations including an instance of male-to-male transmission. Nigra (1970) restudied the family of Nichols et al. (1961) and found no evidence of parathormone unresponsiveness. Moskowitz et al. (1971) studied five cases in three sibships in two generations with male-to-male transmission. A greater than normal response of 3 prime, 5 prime-AMP to parathormone was observed. Moskowitz and Winickoff (1971) concluded that there are both autosomal dominant and autosomal recessive forms of idiopathic basal ganglion calcification. Male-to-male transmission was noted in some families, parental consanguinity in others. Significant neurologic abnormality related to basal ganglion dysfunction (choreoathetosis, Parkinsonism-like state, etc.) was observed. Hypocalcemia was not present, as it was in Nichol's family. Boller et al. (1973) described palilalia (compulsive repetition of a phrase or word) in mother and son with intracranial calcifications. Asymptomatic intracranial calcifications were present in other members of the family. An apparently recessive form of basal ganglion calcification was associated with steatorrhoea and mental retardation in four of 16 sibs in a family reported by Cockel et al. (1973). Autopsy showed normal parathyroid glands.

Boller, F., Boller, M., Denes, G., Timberlake, W. H., Zieper, I. and Albert, M.: Familial palilalia. Neurology 23: 1117-1125, 1973.

Cockel, R., Hill, E. E., Rushton, D. I., Smith, B. and Hawkins, C. F.: Familial steatorrhoea with calcification of the basal ganglia and mental retardation. Quart. J. Med. 42: 771-783, 1973.

Moskowitz, M. A., Winickoff, R. N. and Heinz, E. R.: Familial calcification of the basal ganglions: a metabolic and genetic study. N. Engl. J. Med. 285: 72-77, 1971.

Nichols, F. L., Holdsworth, D. E. and Reinfrank, R. F.: Familial hypocalcemia, latent tetany and calcification of the basal ganglia. Am. J. Med. 30: 518-528, 1961.

Nigra, T. P.: Bethesda, Md.: personal communication, 1970.

Roberts, P. D.: Familial calcification of the cerebral basal ganglia and its relation to hypoparathyroidism. Brain 82: 599-609, 1959.

11413 CALCITONIN

Calcitonin is a peptide hormone synthesized by the parafollicular cells of the thyroid. It causes reduction in serum calcium — an effect opposite to that of parathyroid hormone. Human calcitonin contains 32 amino acids and has a molecular weight of 3,421. See Dayhoff (1972) for sequence data.

Dayhoff, M. O.: Hormones, active peptides and toxins. Atlas of Protein Sequence and Structure 1972 (vol. 5). Washington: National Biomedical Research Foundation, 1972. P. D205.

Neher, R., Riniker, B., Rittel, W. and Zuber, H.: Thyrocalcitonin. II. Struktur von alpha-Thyrocalcitonin. Helv. Chim. Acta 51: 917-924, 1968.

*11415 CAMPTOBRACHYDACTYLY

In the large kindred reported by Edwards and Gale (1972) brachydactyly involved both the hands and the feet and congenital flexion contractures of the fingers. Syndactyly, polydactyly, septate vagina and urinary incontinence were present in some. Two severely affected children of affected first cousins were thought to be homozygotes.

Edwards, J. A. and Gale, R. P.: Camptobrachydactyly: a new autosomal dominant trait with two probable homozygotes. Am. J. Hum. Genet. 24: 464-474, 1972.

*11420 CAMPTODACTYLY

Camptodactyly is a hand malformation characterized by a contracture deformity of the proximal interphalangeal joints of the fingers. The little finger is the most frequently affected though any finger may be involved. This deformity is inherited as an autosomal dominant trait with variable penetrance. Hefner (1929, 1941) reported its occurrence in four generations. Camptodactyly, though often occurring as an isolated anomaly, is occasionally a feature of genetically distinct disorders (see CRANIOCARPOTARSAL DYSTROPHY). Symptoms include streblodactyly, congenital contracture of fingers, and congenital Dupuytren contracture. Parish, Horn and Thompson (1963) described flexion contractures of the fingers (streblodactyly: streblos = Gr. twisted, crooked) and aminoaciduria in 10 females of 3 generations of a family. In 2 females the hands were normal but the same aminoaciduria was present. 9 males were normal. Since all females in the direct line were affected by one or both of the traits mentioned, this is by definition hologynic. However, it is not, at least is not necessarily, a sex-linked dominant as the authors proposed. In most patients fingers II to V were affected. This entity may not be different from camptodactyly. Nevin, Hurwitz and Neill (1966) also found taurinuria in association with camptodactyly. The increased excretion of taurine seemed to be renal in origin. Taurine is not an amino acid but a sulfonated amine which arises as an end product of the metabolism of sulfur-containing amino acids. Several instances of male-to-male transmission were noted in the 4 families they studied. In a rural area of western North Carolina Murphy (1926) described camptodactyly in many members of 5 generations. Eleven of the affected persons also had knee-joint subluxation which was usually easily reduced.

Dutta, P.: The inheritance of the radially curved little finger. Acta Genet. Statist. Med. 15: 70-76, 1965.

Hefner, R. A.: Crooked little finger (minor streblomicrodactyly). J. Hered. 32: 37-38, 1941.

Hefner, R. A.: Inheritance of crooked little fingers (minor streblomicrodactyly). J. Hered. 20: 395-398, 1929.

Moore, W. G. and Messina, P.: Camptodactylism and its variable expression. J. Hered. 27: 27-30, 1936.

Murphy, D. P.: Familial finger contracture and associated familial knee-joint subluxation. J.A.M.A. 86: 395-397, 1926.

Nevin, N. C., Hurwitz, L. J. and Neill, D. W.: Familial camptodactyly with taurinuria. J. Med. Genet. 3: 265-268, 1966.

Parish, J. G., Horn, D. B. and Thompson, M.: Familial streblodactyly with amino-aciduria. Br. Med. J. 2: 1247-1250, 1963.

Welch, J. P. and Temtamy, S. A.: Hereditary contractures of the fingers (camptodactyly). J. Med. Genet. 3: 104-113, 1966.

11430 CAMPTODACTYLY, CLEFT PALATE, CLUB FOOT

Gordon et al. (1969) described affected persons in three generations. No similar family was found in the literature. A useful list of camptodactyly syndromes was provided.

Gordon, H., Davies, D. and Berman, M.: Camptodactyly, cleft palate and club foot. Syndrome showing the autosomal-dominant pattern of inheritance. J. Med. Genet. 6: 266-274, 1969.

11440 CANCER

Malignancy is observed with von Recklinghausen neurofibromatosis, tylosis, the several types of intestinal polyposis, von Hippel-Lindau syndrome, and basal cell nevus syndrome, all conditions listed in the dominant catalog. Xeroderma pigmentosum, a recessive, is complicated in all cases by skin malignancy. In addition, notable instances of 'cancer families' are on record. Whether these represent more than chance familial aggregation of common disorders is unclear. For example, Lynch et al. (1966) reported two large 'cancer families.' In one, nine of 11 sibs had histologically confirmed cancers, with four of these showing multiple primary tumors. In the second, seven of 13 sibs showed histologically proven cancers, with multiple primary malignant neoplasm in four. The two families contained 6 instances of the ordinarily rare combination of primary colonic and endometrial carcinoma. The 'cancer family' of Warthin is another notable example (Hauser and Weller, 1936). A virologic basis for familial aggregation, even transmission through successive generations, is possible. Lynch et al. (1966, 1967) suggest the existence of a syndrome which they call the cancer family syndrome and which is characterized by (1) increased occurrence of endometrial carcinoma and adenocarcinoma of the colon as well as multiple primary malignant neoplasms and (2) autosomal dominant inheritance. Lynch et al. (1973) suggested that among families with breast cancer some have an excess of ovarian cancer, others are prone to sarcoma, brain tumors and leukemia, whereas yet others have associated gastrointestinal cancer. Biochemical insight into familial susceptibility to cancer is beginning. Genetic differences in inducibility of aryl hydrocarbon hydroxylase (see 10834) may underlie susceptibility to lung cancer and colon cancer.

Brisman, R., Baker, R. R., Elkins, R. and Hartmann, W. H.: Carcinoma of lung in four siblings. Cancer 20: 2048-2053, 1967.

Dunstone, G. H. and Knaggs, T. W. L.: Familial cancer of the colon and rectum. J. Med. Genet. 9: 451-456, 1972.

Fielding, J. F.: Familial non-polypotic carcinoma of the colon. Br. Med. J. 1: 512-513, 1969.

Hauser, I. J. and Weller, C. V.: A further report on the cancer family of Warthin. Am. J. Cancer 27: 434-449, 1936.

Lynch, H. T. and Krush, A. J.: Cancer family 'G' revisited: 1895-1970. Cancer 27: 1505-1511, 1971.

Lynch, H. T. and Krush, A. J.: Heredity and adenocarcinoma of the colon. Gastroenterology 53: 517-527, 1967.

Lynch, H. T.: Hereditary Factors in Carcinoma. New York-Berlin: Springer, 1967.

Lynch, H. T., Krush, A. J. and Guirgis, H.: Genetic factors in families with combined gastrointestinal and breast cancer. Am. J. Gastroent. 59: 31-40, 1973.

Lynch, H. T., Shaw, M. W., Magnuson, C. W., Larsen, A. L. and Krush, A. J.: Hereditary factors in cancer: study of two large midwestern kindreds. Arch. Intern. Med. 117: 206-212, 1966.

11450 CANCER OF COLON

Cancer of the colon occurred in 7 members of 4 successive generations of the family reported by Kluge (1964), leading him to suggest a simple genetic basis for colonic cancer independent of polyposis. Morson (1973) studied a similar family.

Kluge, T.: Familial cancer of the colon. Acta Chir. Scand. 127: 392-398, 1964.

Mathis, V. M.: Familiares colon Karzinom. Ein Stammbaum aies den kanton Aargau. Schweiz. Med. Wchnschr. 92: 1673-1678, 1962.

Morson, B. C.: London, personal communication, 1973.

11455 CANCER, HEPATOCELLULAR

There are two reports of primary cancer of the liver in three brothers (Kaplan, Cole, 1965; Hagstrom, Baker, 1968). In these patients there was no recognized pre-existing liver disease. Denison et al. (1971) described two adult brothers who died of primary hepatocellular carcinoma. Both had micronodular cirrhosis with features of subacute progressive viral hepatitis. Australia antigen was demonstrated in the brother in whom it was sought. Their father had died much earlier of hepatocellular carcinoma.

Denison, E. K., Peters, R. L. and Reynolds, T. B.: Familial hepatoma with hepatitis-associated antigen. Ann. Intern. Med. 74: 391-394, 1971.

*11460 CANINE TEETH, ABSENCE OF UPPER PERMANENT

Dolamore (1925) described a case of persistent deciduous canines with absence of permanent successors in father and son. Gruneberg (1936) described the same in seven members of three generations of a German Jewish family.

Dolamore, W. H.: Absent canines. Br. Dent. J. 46: 5-8, 1925.

Gruneberg, H.: Two independent inherited tooth anomalies in one family. J. Hered. 27: 225-228, 1936.

11470 CARABELLI ANOMALY OF MAXILLARY MOLAR TEETH

Kraus (1951) was of the opinion that homozygosity of a gene is responsible for a pronounced tubercle, whereas the heterozygote shows slight grooves, pits, tubercles or bulge. He provided good pictures of the anomaly. Lee and Goose (1972) studied the inheritance of this and four other common dental traits, namely, shovel incisors (14740), maxillary molar cusp number, mandibular molar cusp number and fissure patterns. They concluded that all are probably multifactorial.

Dietz, V. H.: A common dental morphotropic factor: the Carabelli cusp. J. Am. Dent. Assoc. 31: 784-789, 1944.

Kraus, B. S.: Carabelli's anomaly of the maxillary molar teeth. Observations on Mexicans and Papago Indians and an interpretation of the inheritance. Am. J. Hum. Genet. 3: 348-355, 1951.

Lee, G. T. R. and Goose, D. H.: The inheritance of dental traits in a Chinese population in the United Kingdom. J. Med. Genet. 9: 336-339, 1972.

*11480 CARBONIC ANHYDRASE, ERYTHROCYTE, ELECTROPHORETIC VARIANTS OF (CA I)

By starch gel electrophoresis Tashian, Plato and Shows (1963) detected a genetically determined variant of erythrocyte carbonic anhydrase. Carbonic anhydrase has two isoenzymes with different amino acid sequences and specific activities. B and C are the designations for these two major forms. A is an earlier designation for a form which probably is a post-translationally, chemically modified B (Lindskog et al., 1971). Tashian (1969) reviewed the biochemical genetics of the two forms of red cell carbonic anhydrase, known as Ca I (or Ca B) and Ca II (or Ca C). These are under the control of separate autosomal loci. The amino acid change of several Ca I mutants has been determined (Carter et al., 1972). Moore et al. (1973) demonstrated the autosomal dominant inheritance of Ca I and Ca II variants. Shapira et al. (1974) found inactive mutant form of red cell carbonic anhydrase B in three persons with renal tubular acidosis and deafness (26730). The deficiency of Ca (B) function was considered etiologic. Ca I and Ca II are linked in the rodent genus Cavia (Carter, 1973). DeSimone et al. (1973) showed that they are closely linked in an Old World monkey Macaca nemestrina. Eicher (1974) finds that in the mouse the two carbonic anhydrase loci are tightly linked.

Carter, N. D.: Anhydrase II polymorphism in Africa. Hum. Hered. 22: 539-541, 1972.

Carter, N. D., Tashian, R. E., Huntsman, R. G. and Sacker, L.: Characterization of two new variants of red cell carbonic anhydrase in the British population: Ca ie Portsmouth and Ca ie Hull. Am. J. Hum. Genet. 24: 330-338, 1972.

Carter, N. D.: Carbonic anhydrase isozymes in Cavia porcellus, Cavia aperea and their hybrids. Comp. Biochem. Physiol. 43: 743-747, 1972.

DeSimone, J., Linde, M. and Tashian, R. E.: Evidence for linkage of carbonic anhydrase isozyme genes in the pig-tailed macaque, Macaca nemestrina. Nature N.B. 242: 55-56, 1973.

Eicher, E. M.: Bar Harbor, Maine, personal communication, 1974.

Lindskog, S., Henderson, L. E., Kannan, K. K., Liljas, A., Nyman, P. O. and Strandberg, B.: Carbonic anhydrase. In, Boyer, P. D. (ed.): The Enzymes. New York: Academic Press, 1971. Vol. 5, Pp. 587-665.

Marriq, C., Gulian, J. M. and Laurent, G.: Cleavage by cyanogen bromide of carbonic anhydrase from human erythrocyte B. Biochim. Biophys. Acta 221: 662-664, 1970.

Moore, M. J., Deutsch, H. F. and Ellis, F. R.: Human carbonic anhydrase. IX. Inheritance of variant erythrocyte forms. Am. J. Hum. Genet. 25: 29-35, 1973.

Shapira, E., Ben-Yoseph, Y., Eyal, G. and Russell, A.: Enzymatically inactive red cell carbonic anhydrase B in a family with renal tubular acidosis. J. Clin. Invest. 53: 59-63, 1974.

Tashian, R. E.: The esterases and carbonic anhydrases of human erythrocytes. In, Yunis, J. J. (ed.): Biochemical Methods in Red Cell Genetics. New York: Academic Press, 1969. Pp. 307-336.

Tashian, R. E., Goodman, M., Headings, V. E., Desimone, J. and Ward, R. H.: Genetic variation and evolution in the red cell carbonic anhydrase isozymes of Macaque monkeys. Biochem. Genet. 5: 183-200, 1971.

Tashian, R. E., Plato, C. C. and Shows, T. B., Jr.: Inherited variant of erythrocyte carbonic anhydrase in Micronesians from Guam and Saipan. Science 140: 53-54, 1963.

*11481 CARBONIC ANHYDRASE, ERYTHROCYTE, ELECTROPHORETIC VARIANTS OF (CA II)

See CARBONIC ANHYDRASE (Ca I). Electrophoretic variants of carbonic anhydrase C (Ca-C), otherwise known as Ca II, were described my Moore et al. (1971) in American Negroes. Tashian et al. (1968) found variants in monkeys.

Kuang-Tzu, D. and Deutsch, H. F.: Human carbonic anhydrases. XII. The complete primary structure of the C isozyme. J. Biol. Chem. 249: 2329-2337, 1974.

Lin, K.-T. and Deutsch, H. F.: Human carbonic anhydrases. XII. The complete primary structure of the C isozyme. J. Biol. Chem. 249: 2329-2337, 1974.

Moore, M. J., Funakoshi, S. and Deutsch, H. F.: Human carbonic anhydrase. VII. A new C type isozyme in erythrocytes of American Negroes. Biochem. Genet. 5: 497-504, 1971.

Tashian, R. E., Schreffler, D. C. and Shows, T. B.: Genetic and phylogenetic variation in the different molecular forms of mammalian erythrocyte carbonic anhydrases. Ann. N.Y. Acad. Sci. 151: 64-77, 1968.

11490 CARCINOID, INTESTINAL

Anderson (1966) observed appendiceal carcinoid in father and daughter. Eschback and Rinaldo (1962) reported fatal malignant carcinoid of the ileum in brother and sister. Duodenal carcinoid is described with multiple endocrine adenomatosis (q.v.).

Anderson, R. E.: A familial instance of appendiceal carcinoid. Am. J. Surg. 111: 738-740, 1966.

Eschbach, J. W. and Rinaldo, J. A., Jr.: Metastatic carcinoid: a familial occurrence. Ann. Intern. Med. 57: 647-650, 1962.

11500 CARDIAC ARRHYTHMIA (EXTRASYSTOLES)

Kuhn, Wolf and Stieler (1964) described two sisters with polymorphic and polytopic ventricular extrasystoles. One had syncopal attacks. A brother died suddenly at age 10 and the mother at age 40, under circumstances suggesting the presence of the same disorder.

Berg, K. J.: Multifocal ventricular extrasystoles with Adams-Stokes syndrome in siblings. Am. Heart J.: 60: 965-970, 1960.

Gault, J. H., Cantwell, J., Lev, M. and Braunwald, E.: Fatal familial cardiac arrhythmias. Am. J. Cardiol. 29: 548-553, 1972.

Kuhn, E., Wolf, D. and Stieler, M.: Familial polytopic and polymorphic extrasystoles. Jap. Heart J. 5: 81-84, 1964.

*11508 CARDIAC CONDUCTION DEFECT

Lynch et al. (1973) described a kindred in which many persons in several generations had a progressive atrioventricular conduction defect. Prolonged AV conduction had its onset usually in the 30's with loss of R waves in the right precordial leads. Arrythmia occurred only as a late manifestation. Syncopal attacks were the main symptom. Progression from first to third degree block was usually slow, but in a few persons a relatively fulminant course with death in two or three years was observed. Since the disorder appears to be limited to the concuction system, prognosis with artificial pacemaker should be excellent. The authors found several reports which may concern the same disorder.

Lynch, H. T., Mohiuddin, S., Sketch, M. H., Krush, A. J., Carter, S. and Runco, V.: Hereditary progressive atrioventricular conduction defect. A new syndrome? J.A.M.A. 225: 1465-1470, 1973.

Stephan, E.: Familial atrioventricular block. (Letter) J.A.M.A. 228: 697 only, 1974.

11510 CARDIAC CONDUCTION SYSTEM, DEFECT IN

Green et al. (1969) described a family in which sudden death occurred in at least 10 persons in 3 generations at an average age of 21 years (range 4-44). No clinical abnormalities were detectable in members of the family, including one who died suddenly. An abnormality of the conduction system was postulated but not definitely demonstrated.

Green, J. R., Jr., Krovetz, M. J., Shanklin, D. R., DeVito, J. J. and Taylor, W. J.: Sudden unexpected death in three generations. Arch. Intern. Med. 124: 359-363, 1969.

11520 CARDIOMYOPATHY, FAMILIAL IDIOPATHIC

Whitfield (1961) described a family in which 10 members were suffering, or had died, from cardiomyopathy and 6 others were probably affected. In this, as in all reported families, although both males and females are affected, transmission seemingly has occurred only through the female. Unaffected women have not borne affected children. Schrader and colleagues (1961) described two sisters with familial idiopathic cardiomegaly. Almost certainly the mother, who died at age 34, and probably one brother, who died at 16, had the same condition. In the family reported by Battersby and Glenner (1961) affected persons were limited to one sibship and deposits of a non-metachromatic, diastase-resistant, PAS-positive polysaccharide were described in the myocardium. One affected member had chronic pericardial effusion. Undoubtedly heterogeneity exists in the group of cardiomyopathies. Boyd et al. (1965) suggested that there may be three types: (1) form with predominantly fibrosis, (2) form with predominantly hypertrophy (see VENTRICULAR HYPERTRO- PHY, HEREDITARY) and (3) form with deposits described above. See AMYLOIDOSIS, CARDIAC FORM for another familial myocardopathy. Kariv and colleagues (1966) observed six affected persons in 3 generations. In two of these persons Adams-Stokes attacks required an artifical pacemaker. The affected males showed significant increase in the serum levels of multiple muscle-derived enzymes. Heterogeneity was suggested by the finding of normal serum enzyme levels in affected members of a second family. Rywlin et al. (1969) favored the view that obstructive and non-obstructive forms of familial cardiopathy are different expressions of a single entity. Machida et al. (1971) described a Japanese family with affected persons in two and perhaps three generations including male-to-male transmission. Classification into 'hypertrophic' and 'congestive' clinical types by Goodwin (1970) implies the same. Emanuel et al. (1971) suggested that both dominant and recessive forms may exist. Sommer et al. (1972) took an opposite view, that there is a separate non-obstructive familial cardiomyopathy. They described an Amish family with affected persons in three generations. Severity varied widely. The most severely affected pursued a rapidly fatal course whereas others manifested mainly conduction defects compatible with long survival.

Barry, M. and Hall, M.: Familial cardiomyopathy. Br. Heart J. 24: 613-624, 1962.

Battersby, E. J. and Glenner, G. G.: Familial cardiomyopathy. Am. J. Med. 30: 382-391, 1961.

Biorck, G. and Orinius, E.: Familial cardiomyopathies. Acta Med. Scand. 176: 407-424, 1964.

Bishop, J. M., Campbell, M. and Jones, E. W.: Cardiomyopathy in four members of a family. Br. Heart. J. 24: 715-725, 1962.

Boyd, D. L., Mishkin, M. E., Feigenbaum, H. and Genovese, P. D.: Three families with familial cardiomyopathy. Ann. Intern. Med. 63: 386-401, 1965.

Emanuel, R., Withers, R. and O'Brien, K.: Dominant and recessive modes of inheritance in idiopathic cardiomyopathy. Lancet II: 1065-1067, 1971.

Goodwin, J. F.: Congestive and hypertrophic cardiomyopathies. Lancet I: 731-739, 1970.

Kariv, I., Szeinberg, A., Fabian, I., Sherf, L., Kreisler, B. and Zelter, M.: A family with cardiomyopathy. Am. J. Med. 40: 140-148, 1966.

Machida, K., Iguchi, K., Yoshimi, S., Saito, Y., Sugishita, Y., Murayama, M., Mori, M., Yamaguchi, H., Ito, I. and Uede, H.: Familial cardiomyopathy. Immunological studies and review of literatures on autopsied cases in Japan. Jap. Heart J. 12: 40-49, 1971.

Rywlin, A. M., Barold, S. S., Linhart, J. W., Kramer, H. C., Meitus, M. L. and Samet, P.: Idiopathic familial cardiopathy. A study of two families. J. Genet. Hum. 17: 453-470, 1969.

Schrader, W. H., Pankey, G. A., Davis, R. B. and Theologides, A.: Familial idiopathic cardiomegaly. Circulation 24: 599-606, 1961.

Sommer, A., Sanz, G., Craenen, J. and Newton, W. A., Jr.: Familial cardiomyopathy. Clinical Delineation of Birth Defects. XV. Cardiovascular System. Baltimore: Williams and Wilkins Co., 1972.

Whitfield, A. G. W.: Familial cardiomyopathy. Quart. J. Med. 30: 119-134, 1961.

11530 CAROTENEMIA, FAMILIAL

Sharvill (1970) described very high levels of blood carotene in a woman, her mother, a sib and her son. Low levels of vitamin A were found at times. A defect in conversion of carotene to vitamin A was considered one possibility.

Sharvill, D. E.: Familial hypercarotinaemia and hypovitaminosis A. Proc. R. Soc. Med. 63: 605-606, 1970.

11540 CARPAL DISPLACEMENT (CARPAL BOSSING)

Ellsworth (1927) found displacement of the carpal bone group on the radius and ulna. The distal epiphyses of these bones were misshapen. Five females in four generations were affected in a pattern equally consistent with either autosomal or X-linked inheritance. Carpal bossing appears to be the same trait as Ellsworth described. A prominence is produced by a double beak between the third metacarpal and the capitate bone of the wrist. Photographs and X-rays were presented by Larson, Lazcano and Janes (1958), who estimated that it is present in about 26 percent of adults but only one of 50 children under 15 years of age. The genetics has not been worked out. Both genetic and environmental (e.g., occupational) factors may be involved.

Ellsworth, H. A.: Inheritance of carpal displacement. J. Hered. 18: 133 Only, 1927.

Larson, R. L., Lazcano, M. A. and Janes, J. M.: Carpal bossing, a common clinical entity. Mayo Clin. Proc. 33: 337-343, 1958.

*11545 CASEIN VARIANTS

Milk casein can be separated by urea starch electrophoresis into three regions, apparently alpha, beta and kappa casein. Alpha-variants and possibly beta-variants are present in the human population.

Voglino, G. F. and Ponzone, A.: Polymorphism in human casein. Nature N.B. 238: 149 only, 1972.

A chromosomal abnormality is known in this syndrome. However, because in many of the reported cases the abnormality is in only a portion of the patients' cells and because the mosaicism is sometimes transmitted through several generations, Mendelian factors may be important in its causation. The trivial name for the condition is derived from the vertical pupil which results from coloboma of the iris, one of the features of the syndrome. Other features include imperforate anus, preauricular tags or fistulas, heart malformations, urinary tract anomalies and mild to moderate mental retardation. The characteristic chromosomal change is the presence of a small extra acrocentric chromosome. It may be derived from an acrocentric chromosome by deletion — possibly from chromosome no. 14 (Pfeiffer et al., 1970).

Gerald, P. S., David, C., Say, B. and Wilkins, J.: Syndromal associations of imperforate anus: the cat eye syndrome. The Clinical Delineation of Birth Defects. XIII. G. I. Tract Including Liver and Pancreas. Baltimore: Williams and Wilkins, 1972. Pp. 79-84.

Pfeiffer, R. A., Heimann, K. and Hemiming, E.: Extra chromosome in 'cat eye' syndrome. (Letter) Lancet II: 97 only, 1970.

Schachenmann, G., Schmid, W., Fraccaro, M., Mannini, A., Tiepolo, L., Perona, G. P. and Sartori, E.: Chromosomes in coloboma and anal atresia. (Letter) Lancet II: 290 only, 1965.

*11550 CATALASE

Several rare electrophoretic variants of red cell catalase have been identified by Baur (1963). Nance et al. (1968) described electrophoretic variants of catalase and presented evidence suggesting linkage of the catalase locus with the haptoglobin locus. The relationship of the electrophoretic variants to acatalasia (q.v.) is unknown.

Baur, E. W.: Catalase abnormality in a Caucasian family in the United States. Science 140: 816-817, 1963.

Nance, W. E., Empson, J. E., Bennett, T. W. and Larson, L.: Haptoglobin and catalase loci in man: possible genetic linkage. Science 160: 1230-1231, 1968.

*11570 CATARACT, CRYSTALLINE ACULEIFORM OR FROSTED

Although recessive inheritance is suggested by some reports, dominant inheritance is clear from studies such as those of Romer (1926) and of Gifford and Puntenney (1937).

Gifford, S. R. and Puntenney, I.: Coralliform cataract and a new form of congenital cataract with crystals in the lens. Arch. Ophthalmol. 17: 885-892, 1937.

Romer, A.: Untersuchung ueber die Erblichkeit der Spiesskatarakt (Vogt). Arch. Klaus. Stift. Vererbungsforsch. 2: 207-220, 1926.

*11580 CATARACT, CRYSTALLINE CORALLIFORM

Both types of crystalline cataract (coralliform and aculeiform) are characterized by fine crystals in the axial region of the lens. Both are usually inherited as dominants, although in rare instances recessive inheritance is suspected. Dominant pedigrees of coralliform crystalline cataract were reported by Nettleship (1909), Riad (1938) and Jordan (1955).

Jordan, M.: Stammbaumuntersuchungen bei cataracta stellata coralliformis. Klin. Mbl. Augenheilk. 126: 469-475, 1955.

Nettleship, E.: Seven new pedigrees of hereditary cataract. Trans. Ophthal. Soc. U.K. 29: 188-211, 1909.

Riad, M.: Congenital familial cataract with cholesterin deposits. Brit. J. Ophthal. 22: 745-749, 1938.

*11590 CATARACT, FLORIFORM

Doggart (1957) recorded its transmission through 4 generations and Tosch (1958) through 5 generations.

Doggart, J. H.: Congenital cataract. Trans. Ophthal. Soc. U.K. 77: 31-37, 1957.

Tosch, C.: Beitrag zur Stammbaumforschung der Cataracta floriformis. Klin. Mbl. Augenheilk. 133: 60-66, 1958.

11610 CATARACT, MEMBRANOUS

Gruber (1945) described 6 cases in 4 generations. This should be considered a total cataract which has undergone regression or resorption.

Gruber, M.: Ueber primaere familiaere Linsendysplasie. Ophthalmologica 110: 60-73, 1945.

*11620 CATARACT, NUCLEAR (ALSO KNOWN AS COPPOCK CATARACT, DISCOID CATARACT AND PULVERULENT ZONULAR CATARACT)

Nettleship and Ogilvie (1906) described 18 cases in 4 generations. Harman (1909) reported 19 cases in 5 generations, Smith (1910) 26 in 4 generations, Lee and Benedict (1950) 63 in 6 generations, etc. Zonular pulverulent cataract was present in the family in which linkage with Duffy blood group was demonstrated by Renwick and Lawler (1963). The kindred had been earlier described by Nettleship (1909). In 1963 Renwick and Lawler referred to it as congenital zonular cataract. In 1970 Renwick referred to it as total nuclear cataract. In the latter publication the possibility that some other forms of dominant cataract might be linked with Duffy was discussed.

Harman, N. B.: Congenital cataract, a pedigree of five generations. Trans. Ophthalmol. Soc. U.K. 29: 101-108, 1909.

Lee, J. B. and Benedict, W. L.: Hereditary nuclear cataract. Arch. Ophthalmol. 44: 643-650, 1950.

Nettleship, E. and Ogilvie, F. M.: A peculiar form of hereditary congenital cataract. Trans. Ophthalmol. Soc. U.K. 26: 191-206, 1906.

Renwick, J. H. and Lawler, S. D.: Probable linkage between a congenital cataract locus and the Duffy blood group locus. Ann. Hum. Genet. 27: 67-84, 1963.

Renwick, J. H.: Eyes on chromosomes. J. Med. Genet. 7: 239-243, 1970.

Smith, P.: A pedigree of Doyne's discoid cataract. Trans. Ophthalmol. Soc. U.K. 30: 37-42, 1910.

*11630 CATARACT, NUCLEAR DIFFUSE NON-PROGRESSIVE

Opacity is limited to the fetal nucleus, resembles that of senile nuclear sclerosis, and is non-progressive. Vogt (1931) and Weber (1940) documented dominant inheritance.

Vogt, A.: Lehrbuch und Atlas der Spaltlampenmikroskopie des lebenden Auges. Linse und Zonula. Berlin: J. Springer, 1931.

Weber, E.: Weitere Untersuchungen ueber den kongenitalen, vererbten Kernstar (cataracta nuclearis diffusa congenita hereditaria Vogt). Schweiz. Med. Wschr. 70: 295-297, 1940.

*11640 CATARACT, NUCLEAR TOTAL

This is one of the most frequent types of severe congenital cataract which interferes seriously with vision. Dominant pedigrees were reported by Brown (1924), Parrow (1955) and others.

Brown, A. L.: Hereditary cataract. Am. J. Ophthalmol. 7: 36-38, 1924.

Parrow, R. D.: Hereditary cataract in two families. Acta Paediatr. 44: 460-464, 1955.

11650 CATARACT, OPACITY OF THE SUTURES (STELLATE, CORALLIFORM)

Jordan (1955) observed 24 affected persons in 3 generations.

Jordan, M.: Stammbaumuntersuchungen bei cataracta stellata coralliformis. Klin. Mbl. Augenheilk. 126: 469-475, 1955.

11660 CATARACT, POSTERIOR POLAR

Tulloh (1955) described 15 affected in 5 generations. Valk and Binkhorst (1956) described associated choroideremia and myopia in 2 generations. In Nettleship's family (1909, 1912) congenital posterior polar opacities were present and scattered cortical opacities appeared in childhood and progressed to total cataract.

Nettleship, E.: A pedigree of presenile or juvenile cataract. Trans. Ophthalmol. Soc. U.K. 32: 337-352, 1912.

Nettleship, E.: Seven new pedigrees of hereditary cataract. Trans. Ophthalmol. Soc. U.K. 29: 188-211, 1909.

Tulloh, C. G.: Heredity of posterior polar cataract with report of a pedigree. Br. J. Ophthalmol. 39: 374-379, 1955.

Valk, L. E. M. and Binkhorst, P. G.: A case of familial dwarfism, with choroideremia, myopia, posterior polar cataract and zonular cataract. Ophthalmologica 132: 299 only, 1956.

11670 CATARACT, TOTAL CONGENITAL

Meissner (1933) reported 22 cases in 6 generations of one family and 13 in five generations in a second. Three generations were affected in the family reported by Jahns (1938).

Jahns, H.: Angeborener Star in drei Generationen. Klin. Mbl. Augenheilk. 100: 481-482, 1938.

Meissner, M.: Augenaerztliches aus dem Blindeninstitut. Z. Augenheilk. 80: 48-58, 1933.

*11680 CATARACT, ZONULAR (PERINUCLEAR OR LAMELLAR)

Striking pedigrees were presented by Cridland (1918), Hilbert (1912), Jankiewicz and Freeberg (1956), Keizer (1952), Knapp (1926), and Marner (1949), among others. In Marner's family, 132 in 8 generations were affected, mainly by zonular cataract but some by nuclear, anterior polar, or stellate cataract. The opacities were progressive and 'anticipation' was suggested. In Harman's family (1910), malformation of the fingers was associated.

Cridland, A. B.: Three cases of hereditary cortical cataract, with a chart showing the pedigree of a family in which they occurred. Trans. Ophthalmol. Soc. U.K. 38: 375-376, 1918.

Harman, N. B.: Congenital cataract. In, Treasury of Human Inheritance. London: Cambridge Univ. Press, 1: (part 4) 126-169, 1910.

Hilbert, R.: Schichtstarbildung durch vier Generationen einer Familie. Muenchen. Med. Wschr. 59: 1272-1273, 1912.

Jankiewicz, H. and Freeberg, D. D.: A six generation pedigree of congenital zonular cataract. Am. J. Optom. 33: 555-557, 1956.

Keizer, D. P. R.: Congenitale cataract. Nederl. Tijdschr. Geneeskd. 96: 763-765, 1952.

Knapp, F. N.: Familial cataract: a study through five generations. Am. J. Ophthalmol. 9: 683-684, 1926.

Marner, E.: A family with eight generations of hereditary cataract. Acta Ophthalmol. 27: 537-551, 1949.

In this trait a forelock 4 to 6 inches long is present. The hair is usually finer than that of the rest of the head and may be more wavy than the rest. Stoddard (1939) described a family with affected persons in four generations. At least one skipped generation involved a male. Catatrichy is less evident in men than in women.

Stoddard, S. E.: Inheritance of 'natural bangs': catatrichy, new character dependent upon dominant autosomal gene. J. Hered. 30: 543-545, 1939.

11690 CELIAC SPRUE

McDonald, Dobbins and Rubin (1965) suggested that the mechanism of inheritance is autosomal dominant with incomplete penetrance. The matter was extensively reviewed by Frezal and Rey (1970) who concluded that Mendelism is unlikely. Familial aggregation is undoubted. Of three pairs of carefully studied identical twins only one was concordant. The authors thought this made a single-gene hypothesis unlikely, especially in view of the invariable anatomic relapse on re-exposure to gluten, even without clinical or biochemical signs. Falchuk et al. (1972) found that a particular HL-A type (HL-A 8) showed an abnormally high frequency in patients with this disorder. They interpreted this as indicating the presence of an abnormal 'immune response (IR) gene,' leading to the production of pathogenic antigluten antibody, or, alternatively a particular membrane configuration leading to binding of gluten to mucosal cells with subsequent tissue damage. Robinson et al. (1971) also concluded that celic disease is multifactorial, the genetic component in causation being polygenic and interacting with environmental factors. Dermatitis herpetiformis is frequently associated with duodeno-jejunal villous atrophy similar to that found in gluten-sensitive enteropathy (Brow et al., 1971). Both celiac disease and dermatitis herpetiformis have as a group a high frequency of a specific HL-A type, HL-A 8 (Falchuk et al., 1972; Katz et al., 1972).

Brow, J. R., Parker, F., Weinstein, W. M. and Rubin, C. E.: The small intestinal mucosa in dermatitis herpetiformis. I. Severity and distribution of the small intestinal lesion and associated malabsorption. Gastroenterology 60: 355-361, 1971.

Brow, J. R., Parker, F., Weinstein, W. M. and Rubin, C. E.: The small intestinal mucosa in dermatitis herpetiformis. II. Relationship of the small intestinal lesion to gluten. Gastroenterology 60: 362-369, 1971.

Falchuk, Z. M., Rogentine, G. N. and Strober, W.: Predominance of histocompatibility antigen HL-A 8 in patients with gluten-sensitive enteropathy. J. Clin. Invest. 51: 1602-1605, 1972.

Frezal, J. and Rey, J.: Genetics of disorders of intestinal digestion and absorption. In, Harris, H. and Hirschhorn, K. (eds.): Advances in Human Genetics 1: 275-336, 1970.

Gebhard, R. L., Falchuk, Z. M., Katz, S. I., Sessoms, C., Rogentine, G. N. and Strober, W.: Immunologic concomitants of small intestinal disease and relationship to histocompatiblity antigen HL-A8. J. Clin. Invest. 54: 98-103, 1974.

Katz, S. I., Falchuk, Z. M., Dahl, M. V., Rogentine, G. N. and Strober, W.: HL-A 8: a genetic link between dermatitis herpetiformis and gluten-sensitive enteropathy. J. Clin. Invest. 51: 2977-2980, 1972.

McDonald, W. C., Dobbins, W. O., III and Rubin, C. E.: Studies of the familial nature of celiac sprue using biopsy of the small intestine. N. Engl. J. Med. 272: 448-456, 1965.

Robinson, D. C., Watson, A. J., Wyatt, E. H., Marks, J. M. and Roberts, D. F.: Incidence of small-intestinal mucosal abnormalities and of clinical coeliac disease in the relatives of children with coeliac disease. Gut 12: 789-793, 1971.

*11700 CENTRAL CORE DISEASE OF MUSCLE

This disorder was first described in 1956 by Shy and Magee although the name was not given the entity until later. Five persons in five different sibships in three generations of the original family were affected. In the family studied by Engel et al. (1961) only the proband had clinical manifestations but his father had the same biochemical abnormality of muscle, namely, one involving the liberation of phosphate from glucose-6-phosphate. Central core disease is one of the conditions which produces the 'floppy infant' (amyotonia congenita of Oppenheim). Nemaline myopathy (q.v.) and central core disease have been described in the same family and indeed in the same patient (Afifi, Smith, Zellweger, 1965). It is possible that the 'central core' morphologic change is non-specific, i.e., may occur with other types of myopathy in addition to the specific entity to which the name can be applied. Bethlem et al. (1966) described a non-progressive myopathy in 3 females of three successive generations. The father of the earliest patient may have been affected. Histological findings of central core disease were found. Muscle cramps followed exercise and no hypotonia was present in infancy-features different from previously reported cases of central core disease. Creatine excretion in the urine was greatly increased. Creatine kinase and oxidative phosphorylation in the muscles were normal. Dubowitz and Roy (1970) described 4 cases in 3 generations. The disorders consisted of slowly progressive weakness since the age of 5 years resembling limb girdle muscular dystrophy. Only type 1 muscle fibers showed central cores.

Afifi, A. K., Smith, J. W. and Zellweger, H.: Congenital nonprogressive myopathy. Central core disease and nemaline myopathy in one family. Neurology 15: 371-381, 1965.

Bethlem, J., Van Gool, J., Hulsmann, W. C. and Meijer, A. E. F. H.: Familial non-progressive myopathy with muscle cramps after exercise. A new disease associated with cores in the muscle fibres. Brain 89: 569-588, 1966.

Dubowitz, V. and Roy, S.: Central core disease of muscle: clinical, histochemical and electron microscopic studies of an affected mother and child. Brain 93: 133-146, 1970.

Engel, W. K., Foster, J. B., Hughes, B. P., Huxley, H. E. and Mahler, R.: Central core disease — an investigation of a rare muscle cell abnormality. Brain 84: 167-185, 1961.

Shy, G. M. and Magee, K. R.: A new congenital non-progressive myopathy. Brain 79: 610-621, 1956.

Shy, G. M., Engel, W. K. and Wanko, T.: Central core disease: a myofibrillary and mitochondrial abnormality of muscle. Ann. Intern. Med. 56: 511-520, 1962.

*11710 CENTRALOPATHIC EPILEPSY

Metrakos and Metrakos (1961) concluded that the centrencephalic type of electroencephalogram (associated with 'centralopathic epilepsy') is an expression of an autosomal dominant gene, with the unusual characteristics of a very low penetrance at birth, a rapid rise to nearly complete penetrance for ages 4 and a half to 16 and a half years, and a gradual decline to almost no penetrance after the age of 40 and a half years. In this form of epilepsy seizures of varying clinical appearance are associated with paroxysmal, diffuse, bilateral synchronous spike-wave EEG abnormalities. From a family study Metrakos and Metrakos (1961) concluded that inheritance is autosomal dominant. Although their studies did not lead them to a definite dominant hypothesis, Bray and Wiser (1964, 1965) presented evidence for a genetic basis of one form of temporal lobe epilepsy.

Bray, P. F. and Wiser, W. C.: Evidence for a genetic etiology of temporal-central abnormalities in focal epilepsy. N. Engl. J. Med. 271: 926-933, 1964.

Bray, P. F. and Wiser, W. C.: Hereditary characteristics of familial temporal-central focal epilepsy. Pediatrics 36: 207-211, 1965.

Metrakos, K. and Metrakos, J. D.: Genetics of convulsive disorders. II. Genetic and electroencephalographic studies in centrencephalic epilepsy. Neurology 11: 474-483, 1961.

11720 CEREBELLAR ATAXIA

The spinocerebellar ataxias represent a nosologically confused category. Friedreich ataxia is clearly a recessive disorder. So-called Marie ataxia is characterized by late-onset and dominant inheritance. It probably is a heterogeneous category encompassing several of the conditions listed here as separate disorders under the general heading of either OLIVOPONTOCEREBELLAR ATROPHY (q.v.) or CEREBELLAR PAREN-CHYMAL DISORDER (q.v.). See also SPINO-PONTINE ATROPHY. Nosologic and genetic studies of the ataxias include those of Sjogren (1943). Nosologic studies based on pathologic findings were done by Greenfield (1954). The most extensive recent nosologic studies have been those of Konigsmark and his colleagues, who have insisted on histopathologic studies before they attempted to categorize a given family either reported or in their own experience. A form of cerebellar ataxia possibly distinct from the other forms discussed here was described by Becker et al. (1971). Pathologic findings included cerebellar cortical atrophy with Purkinje cell loss, pontine atrophy, spino-cerebellar fiber loss and vestibular neuronal loss.

Becker, P. E., Sabuncu, N. and Hopf, H. C.: Dominant erblicher Typ von 'cerebellarer Ataxie.' Z. Neurol. 199: 116-139, 1971.

Greenfield, J. G.: The Spino-cerebellar Degenerations. Oxford: Blackwell, 1954.

Sjogren, T.: Klinische und erbbiologische Untersuchungen ueber die Heredoataxien. Acta Psychiatry Neurol. Scand. 27 (suppl.): 1-200, 1943.

*11730 CEREBELLAR ATAXIA, ACUTE INTERMITTENT FAMILIAL

Hill and Sherman (1968) described acute self-limited intermittent cerebellar ataxia in at least 35 members in 5 generations of a Negro family. Presumably this is different from periodic vestibulo-cerebellar ataxia (q.v.) in which the attacks occur mainly in early adulthood rather than childhood and slowly progressive, irreversible symptoms develop in some patients.

Hill, W. and Sherman, H.: Acute intermittent familial cerebellar ataxia. Arch. Neurol. 18: 350-357, 1968.

*11740 CEREBELLO-PARENCHYMAL DISORDER I (CPD I; CEREBELLO-OLIVARY ATROPHY)

The disorders involving primarily the cerebellar parenchyma have been classed into six forms by Weiner and Konigsmark (1971). It is their classification which is followed here. CPA I is characterized by late onset (fifth or sixth decade), with unsteadiness of gait and speech difficulties and progressive dementia. Pathologically there is marked loss of Purkinje cells, especially in the superior cerebellum. Preservation of the pontine nuclei and fibers distinguish it from the olivopontocerebellar atrophies of which five types are described elsewhere. Affected families have been described by Hall et al. (1941), Richter (1950), Weber and Greenfield (1942) and others.

Hall, B., Noad, K. B. and Latham, O.: Familial cortical cerebellar atrophy. Brain 64: 178-194, 1941.

Hoffman, P. M., Stuart, W. H., Earle, K. M. and Brody, J. A.: Hereditary late-onset cerebellar degeneration. Neurology 21: 771-777, 1971.

Richter, R. B.: Late cortical cerebellar atrophy. A form of hereditary cerebellar ataxia. Am. J. Hum. Genet. 2: 1-29, 1950.

Weber, F. P. and Greenfield, J. G.: Cerebello-olivary degeneration: an example of heredo-familial incidence. Brain 65: 220-231, 1942.

Weiner, L. P. and Konigsmark, B. W.: Hereditary disease of the cerebellar parenchyma. The Clinical Delineation of Birth Defects. VI. The Nervous System. Baltimore: Williams and Wilkins, 1970. Pp. 192-196.

Mental dullness and in some cases signs of increased intracranial pressure are features. The latter is the result
of herniation of the cerebellar tonsils. First described by Lhermitte and Duclos (1920), a total of 35 cases
have been reported, according to Ambler et al. (1969), who described the disorder in mother and son.

Ambler, M., Pogacar, S. and Sidman, R.: Lhermitte-Duclos disease (granule cell hypertrophy of the
cerebellum): pathological analysis of the first familial cases. J. Neuropath. Exp. Neurol. 28: 622-647, 1969.

Lhermitte, J. and Duclos, P.: Sur un ganglioneurome diffus du cortex du cervelet. Bull. Assoc. Franc.
Cancer 9: 99-107, 1920.

*11770 CERULOPLASMIN

At least three variants determined by co-dominant alleles have been identified by starch gel electrophoresis
(Shreffler et al., 1967). Polymorphism has been found mainly in the American Negro. In Wilson disease
(27790) an abnormality of ceruloplasmin seems to be involved. However, because there is reason to think
a locus other than the polymorphic structural locus is involved, two separate asterisked entries are included
in the catalogs.

Kellermann, G. and Walter, H.: On the population genetics of the ceruloplasmin polymorphism.
Humangenetik 15: 84-86, 1972.

McCombs, M. L. and Bowman, B. H.: Demonstration of inherited ceruloplasmin variants in human
serum by acrylamide electrophoresis. Texas Rep. Biol. Med. 27: 769-772, 1969.

McCombs, M. L., Bowman, B. H. and Alperin, J. B.: A new ceruloplasmin variant, CP Galveston. Clin.
Genet. 1: 30-34, 1970.

Poulik, M. D.: Heterogeneity and structure of ceruloplasmin. Ann. N.Y. Acad. Sci. 151: 476-501, 1968.

Shokeir, M. H. and Shreffler, D. C.: Two new ceruloplasmin variants in Negroes — data on three
populations. Biochem. Genet. 4: 517-528, 1970.

Shokeir, M. H., Shreffler, D. C. and Gall, J. C., Jr.: Further electrophoretic variation in human
ceruloplasmin. Meeting, Am. Soc. Hum. Genet., Toronto, Dec. 1-3, 1967.

Shreffler, D. C., Brewer, G. J., Gall, J. C. and Honeyman, M. S.: Electrophoretic variation in human
serum ceruloplasmin: a new genetic polymorphism. Biochem. Genet. 1: 101-116, 1967.

*11780 CERUMEN, VARIATION IN

In Japanese Matsunaga (1962) described a dimorphism of ear wax, the two types being wet and dry. This
variation has been studied extensively in Japan since at least 1934. Less attention has been given to this
variation elsewhere, probably because Caucasians and Negroes have one type of cerumen, wet. In 80-85
percent of Japanese the cerumen is grey, dry and brittle. It is referred to as 'rice-bran ear wax' in Japanese.
In the other Japanese the cerumen is brown, sticky and wet. This is referred to as 'honey ear wax,' 'oily ear
wax' or 'cat ear wax.' In all except about 0.5 percent of Japanese classification is simple. Family studies
indicate monofactorial inheritance, with the rarer phenotype, wet wax, being dominant. Wet cerumen is often
associated with axillary odor, which in Japan because of its rarity is considered in the lay mind a pathologic
state requiring medical attention. Petrakis et al. (1967) found a high frequency of dry cerumen in
pure-blooded American Indians. No qualitative differences in chemical composition have been identified
(Kataura and Kataura, 1967). Petrakis, (1971) noted the positive correlation between wet ear wax and breast
cancer in several countries and suggested an association. This hypothesis seems reasonable because the
ceruminous gland and breast are both apocrine and share biochemical characteristics. Ing et al. (1973), in
a study of Chinese women in Hong Kong could not confirm the association.

Hyslop, N. E., Jr.: Ear wax and host defense. (Editorial) N. Engl. J. Med. 284: 1099-1100, 1971.

Ing, R., Petrakis, N. L. and Ho, H. C.: Evidence against association between wet cerumen and breast
cancer. Lancet I: 41 only, 1973.

Kataura, A. and Kataura, K.: The comparison of free and bound amino acids between dry and wet types
of cerumen. Tohoku J. Exp. Med. 91: 215-225, 1967.

Kataura, A. and Kataura, K.: The comparison of lipids between dry and wet types of cerumen. Tohoku
J. Exp. Med. 91: 227-237, 1967.

Martin, L. M. and Jackson, J. F.: Cerumen types in Choctaw Indians. Science 163: 677-678, 1969.

Matsunaga, E.: The dimorphism in human normal cerumen. Ann. Hum. Genet. 25: 273-286, 1962.

Petrakis, N. L.: Cerumen genetics and human breast cancer. Science 173: 347-349, 1971.

Petrakis, N. L., Molohan, K. T. and Tepper, D. J.: Cerumen in American Indians: genetic implications
of sticky and dry types. Science 158: 1192-1193, 1967.

11785 CERVICAL LIPODYSPLASIA, FAMILIAL

Green et al. (1970), Ozer et al. (1973) and Koebberling (1973) have described a condition of fat accumulation
around the neck, shoulders, buffalo hump area and genitalia associated with lean muscular limbs,
phlebectasia, insulin resistance, hyperglycemia, and type IV hyperlipoproteinemia. Affected members in the
family of Green et al. (1970) also had hyperuricemia. Only females had the full-blown disorder. Successive
generations were affected. Although no male-to-male transmission was observed, the disorder is probably
autosomal dominant.

Green, M. L., Gluck, C. J., Fujimoto, W. Y. and Seegmiller, J. E.: Benign symmetric lipomatosis (Launois-Bensaude adenolipomatosis) with gout and hyperlipoproteinemia. Am. J. Med. 48: 239-246, 1970.

Koebberling, J.: Ann Arbor, personal communication, 1973.

Ozer, F. L., Lichtenstein, J. R., Kwiterovich, P. O. and McKusick, V. A.: A 'new' genetic variety of lipodystrophy. (Abstract) Clin. Res. 21: 533 only, 1973.

11790 CERVICAL RIB

Weston (1956) found cervical ribs or enlarged transverse processes in 14 of 20 members of a family. The anomaly was particularly striking among the offspring of two affected parents, raising the question of homozygosity.

Weston, W. J.: Genetically determined cervical ribs: a family study. Br. J. Radiol. 29: 455-456, 1956.

11800 CERVICAL VERTEBRAL BRIDGE

The presence of a bony bridge on the first cervical vertebra, roofing the groove occupied by the vertebral artery, behaves as a dominant trait. The gene has a frequency of about 0.15.

Selby, S., Garn, S. M. and Kanareff, V.: The incidence and familial nature of a bony bridge on the first cervical vertebra. Am. J. Phys. Anthropol. 13: 129-141, 1955.

*11810 CERVICAL VERTEBRAL FUSION

C2-C3 fusion is the most common form of congenital fused cervical vertebrae and is probably dominant with variable expression. The best evidence for dominant inheritance was provided by Gunderson et al. (1967).

Gunderson, C. H. and Lubs, H. A.: Familial C2-3 fusion. (Abstract) Neurology 14: 272-273, 1964.

Gunderson, C. H., Greenspan, R. H., Glaser, G. H. and Lubs, H. A.: The Klippel-Feil syndrome: genetic and clinical reevaluation of cervical fusion. Medicine 46: 491-512, 1967.

11815 CHANDS (CURLY HAIR-ANKYLOBLEPHARON-NAIL DYSPLASIA SYNDROME)

Baughman (1971) described a seemingly distinctive 'new' syndrome, probably autosomal dominant. The hair was curly and nails hypoplastic. Ankyloblepharon was present at birth.

Baughman, F. A.: Chands: the curly hair-ankyloblepharon-nail dysplasia syndrome. The Clinical Delineation of Birth Defects. XII. Skin, Hair and Nails. Baltimore: Williams and Wilkins, 1971. Pp. 100-102.

*11820 CHARCOT-MARIE-TOOTH DISEASE

This is one of the entities which, like spastic paraplegia and retinitis pigmentosa, demonstrates autosomal dominant inheritance in some families, autosomal recessive inheritance in others and X-linked recessive inheritance in yet others. Norstrand and Margulies (1958) observed affected members in three generations. Gastrointestinal symptoms in the form of chronic diarrhea, nausea and vomiting were striking. Autopsy showed degeneration in the lateral horn area of the spinal cord. Stark (1958) described a large affected kindred. We have observed elevated cerebrospinal fluid protein, hyperhidrosis and penetrating foot ulcers in a case of the dominant form. This disorder begins with atrophy and weakness of the peroneal muscles and advances insidiously to involve other distal muscles of the leg and arm. Deep tendon reflexes are diminished or absent and pes cavus is commonly found. In the family reported first in the lay press by Verrill and followed up by England and Denny-Brown (1952) members had sensory and trophic changes in addition to classic peroneal muscular atrophy. Most have some sensory defect and this is not surprising in view of the fact that this is a neuropathy. Indeed, a case can be made for referring to the several forms of Charcot-Marie-Tooth disease as hereditary polyneuropathies. Charcot's description was reprinted by Brody and Wilkins (1967). The phenomenal case of a woman who was a patient in La Salpetriere, Paris, for 64 years was reported by Alajouanine et al. (1967). The diagnosis was made by Charcot in 1891. She died at age 80 years. Argyll-Robertson pupils and blindness from optic atrophy began 40-50 years after onset of other signs of disease. Whether this was a sporadic case of the recessive form (which the authors favored) or a new mutant for the dominant form was uncertain. Bradley and Aguayo (1969) described a family in which persons in 3 generations had chronic sensorineural polyneuropathy.

Alajouanine, T., Castaigne, P., Cambier, J. and Escourolle, R.: Maladie de Charcot-Marie. Etude anatomo-clinique d'une observation suivie pendant 65 ans. Presse Med. 75: 2745-2750, 1967.

Bradley, W. G. and Aguayo, A. J.: Hereditary chronic polyneuropathy. Electrophysiological and pathological studies in an affected family. J. Neurol. Sci. 9: 131-154, 1969.

Brody, I. A. and Wilkins, R. H.: Charcot-Marie-Tooth disease. Arch. Neurol. 17: 552-553, 1967.

Dawidenkow, S.: Charcot-Marie type. Z. Ges. Neurol. Psychiat. 108: 344-445, 1927.

Dawidenkow, S.: Neurotic muscular atrophy of Charcot-Marie type. Z. Ges. Neurol. Psychiatry 107: 259-320, 1927.

Dyck, P. J.: Histologic measurements and fine structure of biopsied sural nerve: normal, and in peroneal muscular atrophy, hypertrophic neuropathy, and congenital sensory neuropathy. Mayo Clin. Proc. 41: 742-774, 1966.

Dyck, P. J. and Lambert, E. H.: Lower motor primary sensory neuron diseases with peroneal muscular atrophy. I. Neurologic, genetic, and electrophysiologic findings in hereditary polymeuronpathies. Arch. Neurol. 18: 603-618, 1968.

Dyck, P. J. and Lambert, E. H.: Lower motor and primary sensory neuron disease with peroneal muscular atrophy. II. Neurologic, genetic, and electrophysiologic findings in various neuronal degenerations. Arch. Neurol. 18: 619-625, 1968.

Dyck, P. J., Lambert, E. H. and Mulder, D. W.: Charcot-Marie-Tooth disease: nerve conduction and clinical studies of a large kinship. Neurology 13: 1-11, 1963.

England, A. C. and Denny-Brown, D.: Sensory changes, and trophic disorder, in peroneal muscular atrophy (Charcot-Marie-Tooth type). Arch. Neurol. Psychiatry 67: 1-22, 1952.

Lucas, G. J. and Forster, F. M.: Charcot-Marie-Tooth disease with associated myopathy: a report of a family. Neurology 12: 629-636, 1962.

MacKlin, M. T. and Bowman, J. T.: Inheritance of peroneal atrophy. J.A.M.A. 86: 613-617, 1926.

Norstrand, I. F. and Margulies, M. E.: Peripheral neuronopathy (Charcot-Marie-Tooth disease) in association with gastrointestinal symptoms. New York J. Med. 58: 863-867, 1958.

Stark, P.: Etude clinique et genetique d'une famille atteinte d'atrophie musculaire progressive neurale (amyotrophie de Charcot-Marie). J. Genet. Hum. 7: 1-32, 1958.

11830 CHARCOT-MARIE-TOOTH DISEASE AND NEPHRITIS

Lemieux and Neemeh (1967) described two families each with multiple cases of C-M-T disease. In two of one family and one of the other chronic nephritis was also present. Foam cells were seen in the interstitium in one and two of the three had nerve deafness. A non-specific polyneuropathy, due possibly to chronic uremia, has been observed with Alport syndrome. The neurologic disorder in the cases of Lemieux and Neemeh (1967) was full-bloom C-M-T disease. Amyloidosis, a cause of nephritis and a condition mis-diagnosed as C-M-T disease, was apparently excluded.

Lemieux, G. and Neemeh, J. A.: Charcot-Marie-Tooth disease and nephritis. Canad. Med. Assoc. J. 97: 1193-1198, 1967.

*11840 CHERUBISM

Swelling of the lower face begins in the first years of life and progresses until the late teens. The enlargement is exaggerated by enlargement of submandibular lymph nodes. X-ray reveals multilocular cystic changes in the mandible and maxilla and often in the anterior ends of the ribs. The condition must be differentiated from Caffey disease (q.v.) in which the X-ray appearance is different and involvement of the skeleton, e.g., the tibia, is more widespread. It is, like Caffey disease, a benign self-limited condition treated by simple curettage. The condition has also been called familial benign giant-cell tumor of the jaw, familial multilocular cystic disease of the jaw, etc. Jones (1965) pointed out that lack of signs or history in either parent does not exclude the possibility of one being affected. In one of his cases (he was the first to describe the entity) the disorder would not have been discovered, or even suspected, were it not that X-rays were made in childhood in a deliberate search for the entity because of its occurrence in other members of the family. See FIBRO-OSSEOUS DYSPLASIA OF JAWS.

Anderson, D. E. and McClendon, J. L.: Cherubism-hereditary fibrous dysplasia of the jaws. I. Genetic considerations. Oral Surg. 15 (suppl. 2): 5-16, 1962.

Burland, J. G.: Cherubism: familial bilateral osseous dysplasia of the jaws. Oral Surg. 15 (suppl. 2): 43-68, 1962.

Jones, W. A.: Cherubism: a thumbnail sketch of its diagnosis and a conservative method of treatment. Oral Surg. 20: 648-653, 1965.

Khosla, V. M. and Korobkin, M.: Cherubism. Am. J. Dis. Child. 120: 458-461, 1970.

Salzano, F. M. and Ebling, H.: Cherubism in a Brazilian kindred. Acta Genet. Med. Gemellol. 15: 296-301, 1966.

Thompson, N.: Cherubism: familial fibrous dysplasia of the jaws. Br. J. Plast. Surg. 12: 89-103, 1959.

*11850 CHOLINESTERASE, VARIATION IN RED CELL

Genetic variations in serum cholinesterase ('pseudocholinesterase') are discussed elsewhere. In a man, his mother and his sister Johns (1962) found red cell cholinesterase reduced to about one-third the normal value. The patient was perfectly healthy. The 'defect' would not have been detected were it not for the fact that he worked in a plant manufacturing organophosphorous anticholinesterase compounds and was tested in connection with this employment. Coates and Simpson (1972) found electrophoretic variation in red cell acetylcholinesterase. Three phenotypes appeared to be determined by two co-dominant alleles. This was, to their knowledge, the first variation reported in a stromal enzyme. They proposed that with the method they developed for stabilizing human erythrocyte membranes other membrane-bound enzymes could be studied for genetic variation.

Coates, P. M. and Simpson, N. E.: Genetic variation in human erythrocyte acetylcholinesterase. Science 175: 1466-1467, 1972.

Johns, R. J.: Familial reduction in red cell cholinesterase. N. Engl. J. Med. 267: 1344-1348, 1962.

*11860 CHONDROCALCINOSIS ('CALCIUM GOUT')

This is a chronic articular disease characterized by acute intermittent attacks of arthritis, by the presence of calcium hypophosphate crystals in synovial fluid, cartilage and periarticular soft tissue and by X-ray evidence of calcium deposition in articular cartilage. The condition is sometimes a feature of hyperparathyroidism, hemochromatosis or diabetes mellitus. A genetic basis has been postulated in other cases. Also see

LIPOCALCIGRANULOMATOSIS. Under the designation of chondrocalcinosis articularis, Aschoff et al. (1966) described a family with four affected persons in two generations. The disorder was manifested clinically by episodic inflammatory involvement, acute or subacute, of one or more joints. Calcified hyaline and fibrous cartilages are demonstrable by X-ray, particularly in large joints. In articular cartilage a dense narrow band follows the contour of the epiphysis. Reginato et al. (1970) observed an unusually high frequency among natives of the Chiloe Island group. Twenty-eight patients were observed of whom 19 were aggregated in six kindreds. Parent-child involvement with no male-to-male transmission was observed in 3 of the families. In the other 3 families one or both parents were not screened. Since the Chilote group lives in an isolated area and is presumably inbred, recessive inheritance remains a possibility. In these cases involvement was polyarticular. Ankylosing of joints was a new feature observed in this study. Depressed activity of synovial pyrophosphohydrolase was suggested by the findings of Good and Starkweather (1969). The existence of at least one form of chondrocalcinosis inherited as an autosomal dominant is indicated by the large Dutch kindred studied by van der Korst et al. (1973). This has not been pursued further (Good, 1974). Male-to-male transmission and a dominant pedigree was observed in the Netherlands by van der Korst (1974). Autosomal dominant inheritance for a form of chondrocalcinosis is strongly supported by the pedigree reported by van der Korst et al. (1974). Father-to-son transmission was noted. Twenty-two cases in two generations were observed. Acute attacks occurred in only 14 of the 22 and 6 of the 14 had not yet sought medical care.

Aschoff, H., Boehm, P., Schoen, E. and Schurholz, K.: Hereditaere Chondrocalcinosis articularis. Untersuchung einer Familie. Humangenetik 3: 98-103, 1966.

Good, A. E. and Starkweather, W. H.: Synovial fluid pyrophosphate phosphohydrolase (PPPH) in pseudogout, gout and rheumatoid arthritis. (Abstract) Arthritis Rheum. 12: 298 only, 1969.

Good, A. E.: Madison, Wis., personal communication, 1974.

McCarty, D. J., Jr. and Haskin, M. E.: The roentgenographic aspects of pseudo-gout (articular chondrocalcinosis). An analysis of 20 cases. Am. J. Roentgen. 90: 1248-1257, 1963.

McCarty, D. J., Jr., Kohn, N. N. and Faires, J. S.: The significance of calcium phosphate crystals in the synovial fluid of arthritic patients. The 'pseudogout syndrome.' I. Clinical aspects. Ann. Intern. Med. 56: 711-737, 1962.

Moskowitz, R. and Katz, D.: Chondrocalcinosis (pseudogout syndrome). A family study. J.A.M.A. 188: 867-871, 1964.

Reginato, A., Valenzuela, F., Martinez, V., Passano, G. and Doza, S.: Polyarticular and familial chondrocalcinosis. Arthritis Rheum. 13: 197-213, 1970.

Twigg, H. L., Zvaifler, N. J. and Nelson, C. W.: Chondrocalcinosis. Radiology 82: 655-659, 1964.

Valsik, J., Zitnan, D. and Sitaj, S.: Articular chondrocalcinosis. II. Genetic study. Ann. Rheum. Dis. 22: 153-157, 1963.

Van der Korst, J. K., Geerards, J., and Driessens, F. C. M.: A hereditary type of idiopathic articular chondrocalcinosis. Survey of a pedigree. Am. J. Med. 56: 307-314, 1974.

*11865 CHONDRODYSPLASIA PUNCTATA (CHONDRODYSTROPHIA CALCIFICANS CONGENITA)

Spranger et al. (1971) concluded that the form of chondrodysplasia punctata to which the Conradi-Hunermann eponym is appropriately applied has predominantly epiphyseal, frequently asymmetric calcifications and dysplastic skeletal changes, a relatively good prognosis and autosomal dominant inheritance. They concluded that cataracts occur in only 17 percent of cases as compared with a frequency of 72 percent in the rhizomelic form which is a recessive and which is usually lethal in the first year of life. Skin changes occur in about 28 percent of cases of both forms. Conditions confused with chondrodysplasia punctata include Zellweger cerebrohepatorenal syndrome and multicentric epiphyseal ossification in multiple epiphyseal dysplasia. Bergstrom et al. (1972) described affected mother and child. The mother was born with short femora and humeri, the left leg shorter than the right, saddle nose, frontal bossing, flexion contractures at the hips and knees, left talipes equinovarus and hyperkeratosis with erythema of the left side of the body. The son lived only one hour.

Bergstrom, K., Gustavson, K. H. and Jorulf, H.: Chondrodystrophia calcificans congenita (Conradi's disease) in a mother and her child. Clin. Genet. 3: 158-161, 1972.

Spranger, J. W., Opitz, J. M. and Bidder, U.: Heterogeneity of chondrodysplasia punctata. Humangenetik 11: 190-212, 1971.

*11870 CHOREA, HEREDITARY BENIGN

Pincus and Chutorian (1967) and Haerer, Currier and Jackson (1967) described an early-onset, non-progressive form of chorea not associated with intellectual deterioration. The latter report concerned a Negro family. Because no male-to-male transmission was noted and because the condition was not manifested in two conductor females, X-linked dominant inheritance cannot be excluded. Possible dominant inheritance was demonstrated in two families by Chun et al. (1973).

Chun, R. W. M., Daly, R. F., Mansheim, B. J., Jr. and Wolcott, G. J.: Benign familial chorea with onset in childhood. J.A.M.A. 225: 1603-1607, 1973.

Haerer, A. F., Currier, R. D. and Jackson, J. F.: Hereditary nonprogressive chorea of early onset. N. Engl. J. Med. 276: 1220-1224, 1967.

Pincus, J. H. and Chutorian, A.: Familial benign chorea with intention tremor: a clinical entity. J. Pediatr. 70: 724-729, 1967.

Sadjadpour, K. and Amato, R. S.: Hereditary nonprogressive chorea of early onset. A new entity? Adv. Neurol. 1: 79-91, 1973.

*11880 CHOREOATHETOSIS, FAMILIAL PAROXYSMAL

Mount and Reback (1940) described a family with many members in five generations affected by paroxysmal choreoathetosis which was thought to be separate and distinct from Huntington chorea. The attacks lasted only a few minutes, occurred a few times a day and were not accompanied by unconsciousness. Alcohol, coffee, hunger, fatigue and tobacco were precipitating factors. Affected persons were said to be scattered thoughout the South from South Carolina to Oklahoma. Wagner, Mc Lees and Hatcher (1966) observed affected persons in 3 generations. Richards and Barnett (1968) suggested that it be called paroxysmal dystonic choreoathetosis to distinguish it from the more frequently reported movement induced (kinetogenic) familial (or nonfamilial) paroxysmal choreoathetosis with which it is often confused. They also suggested use of the eponym Mount-Reback for the dystonic form. See DYSTONIA, FAMILIAL PAROXYSMAL.

Hudgins, R. L. and Corbin, K. B.: An uncommon seizure disorder: familial paroxysmal choreoathetosis. Brain 89: 199-204, 1966.

Kato, M. and Araki, S.: Paroxysmal kinesigenic choreoathetosis. Arch. Neurol. 20: 508-513, 1969.

Mount, L. A. and Reback, S.: Familial paroxysmal choreoathetosis: preliminary report on a hitherto undescribed clinical syndrome. Arch. Neurol. Psychiat. 44: 841-847, 1940.

Richards, R. N. and Barnett, H. J.: Paroxysmal dystonic choreoathetosis. A family study and review of the literature. Neurology 18: 461-469, 1968.

Stevens, H.: Paroxysmal choreo-athetosis: a form of reflex epilepsy. Arch. Neurol. 14: 415-420, 1966.

Wagner, G. S., McLees, B. D. and Hatcher, M. A., Jr.: Familial paroxysmal choreo-athetosis. (Abstract) Neurology 16: 307 only, 1966.

Williams, J. and Stevens, H.: Familial paroxysmal chorea-athetosis. Pediatrics 31: 656-659, 1963.

11890 CIRRHOSIS, FAMILIAL

Joske and Laurence (1970) described a family in which the father and four of 10 children had chronic liver disease and raised immunoglobulin levels. A possible non-genetic basis is suggested by the example of hepatitis-associated antigen (HAA), or Australian antigen, in a mother and three children ascertained through one of the children who had neonatal giant cell hepatitis.

Bancroft, W. H., Warkel, R. L., Talbert, A. A. and Russell, P. K.: Family with hepatitis-associated antigen. Spectrum of liver pathology. J.A.M.A. 217: 1817-1820, 1971.

Joske, R. A. and Laurence, B. H.: Familial cirrhosis with autoimmune features and raised immunoglobulin levels. Gastroenterology 59: 546-552, 1970.

*11895 CITRATE SYNTHASE, MITOCHONDRIAL

The structural locus for this enzyme has been tentatively assigned to chromosome no. 12 by cell hybridization studies (van Heynigen et al., 1973).

Craig, I. W.: Procedure for the analysis of citrate synthase. Biochem. Genet., in press, 1973.

Van Heyningen, V., Craig, I. and Bodmer, W.: Genetic control of mitochondrial enzymes in human-mouse somatic cell hybrids. Nature 245: 509-512, 1973.

*11900 CLEFT CHIN

A bony peculiarity underlies the Y-shaped fissure of the chin. Guenther (1939) found 9 cases in 5 generations and Meirowsky (1924) 25 cases in 4 generations.

Guenther, H.: Anomalien und Anomaliekomplexe in der Gegend des ersten Schlundbogens. Z. Menschl. Vererb. Konstitutionsl. 23: 43-52, 1939.

Lebow, M. R. and Sawin, P. B.: Inheritance of human facial features: a pedigree study involving length of face, prominant ears and chin cleft. J. Hered. 32: 127-132, 1941.

Meirowsky, von: Kleine Beitraege zur Vererbungswissenschaft. Arch. Rass. u. Ges. Biol. 16: 439-443, 1924.

11910 CLEFT HAND AND ABSENT TIBIA

Roberts (1967) described a family in which persons in four generations had one cleft hand with a missing middle finger and flexed ring finger, whereas one other had in addition grossly deformed legs with missing tibias requiring amputation and a sib had only the severe leg deformity. Another member had absent forearms with the leg deformity.

Roberts, J. A. F.: Genetic Prognosis. An Introduction to Medical Genetics. London: Oxford U. Press, 1967. (4th Ed.) Pp. 253-280.

11920 CLEFT LIP AND-OR PALATE

Over 30 syndromes including a number which are either chromosomal or Mendelian in causation have cleft lip and-or palate as feature(s). As precise diagnosis as possible is necessary before falling back on empiric risk figures for genetic counseling. It is clear from family studies that cleft palate alone is genetically distinct from cleft lip with or without cleft palate.

*11930 CLEFT LIP AND-OR PALATE WITH MUCOUS CYSTS OF LOWER LIP

In 3 generations of a family Levy (1962) found malformations of the lower lip consisting of symmetrical lumps. Two sibs had cleft palate in addition to the lip anomaly. The literature for this syndrome has been analyzed by van der Woude (1954) where the autosomal dominant mode of inheritance was confirmed. It is possible that in some affected families, because of the variable expressivity of the gene, the syndrome is expressed only as pits. Baker (1964) reported such a pedigree with affected members in three generations showing pits as the only malformation. On the other hand, only harelip and-or cleft palate without pits could segregate in families as a dominant trait. Test and Falls (1947) described the condition transmitted through 5 generations. The rule that cleft palate alone and cleft lip with or without cleft palate behave differently does not hold in this disorder in which either type of cleft alone or the two in combination may occur.

Baker, B. R.: A family with bilateral congenital pits of the inferior lip. Oral Surg. 18: 494-497, 1964.

Bowers, D. G.: Congenital lower lip sinuses with cleft palate. Plast. Reconstr. Surg. 45: 151-154, 1970.

Cervenka, J., Gorlin, R. J. and Anderson, V. E.: The syndrome of pits of the lower lip and cleft lip and-or palate. Genetic considerations. Am. J. Hum. Genet. 19: 416-432, 1967.

Levy, J.: Zwillinge in einer Familie mit Unterlippenmissbildung. Acta Genet. Statist. Med. 12: 33-40, 1962.

Schneider, E. L.: Lip pits and congenital absence of second premolars: varied expression of the lip pits syndrome. J. Med. Genet. 10: 346-349, 1973.

Test, A. R. and Falls, H. F.: Dominant inheritance of cleft lip and palate in five generations. J. Oral Surg. 5: 292-297, 1947.

Van der Woude, A.: Fistula labii inferioris congenita and its association with cleft lip and palate. Am. J. Hum. Genet. 6: 244-256, 1954.

11940 CLEFT LIP-PALATE WITH SPLIT HAND AND FOOT

The three pedigrees described by Walker and Clodius (1963) suggest irregular autosomal dominant inheritance of the combination of split hand and-or foot and cleft lip-palate. Atresia of the lacrimal puncta or other deformity of the lacrimal duct was present in some. See EEC SYNDROME for the association of ectrodactyly, ectodermal dysplasia and cleft lip-palate (12990).

Cockayne, E. A.: Cleft palate-lip, hare lip, dacrocystitis, and cleft hand and foot. Biometrika 28: 60-63, 1936.

Walker, J. C. and Clodius, L.: The syndromes of cleft lip, cleft palate and lobster claw deformities of hands and feet. Plast. Reconstr. Surg. 32: 627-636, 1963.

*11950 CLEFT LIP-PALATE, MUCOUS CYSTS OF THE LOWER LIP, POPLITEAL PTERYGIUM, DIGITAL AND GENITAL ANOMALIES

Although Klein (1962) described a mother and a daughter with the features of this syndrome, suggesting dominant inheritance, Gorlin and Pindborg (1964) analyzing the literature favored an autosomal recessive mode of inheritance. Champion and Cregan's report of the syndrome in sibs supports the recessive hypothesis. Lewis (1948) described brother and sister with cleft palate and webbing of the lower limbs whose father had harelip and cleft palate. The webbing extended from the region of the ischial tuberosities to the heels. (Surgeons must be aware that the sciatic nerve can be situated in the web.) The girl was said to have 'bilateral incomplete harelip.' Hecht and Jarvinen (1967) observed affected mother and two sons in one family and affected mother and son and daughter in a second. The observation of affected father and son by Lewis (1948) excludes X-linked inheritance. Pterygium of the neck and arms does not occur in this syndrome. An intercrural pterygium causes distortion of the genitalia. Bifid scrotum and cryptorchidism are the rule in males and hypoplasia of the labia majora in females. Congenital ankyloblepharon filiforme occurs in some cases. The epithelial strands connecting the eyelids in ankyloblepharon filiforme have their counterpart in symmetrical epithelial strands running from the maxilla, as pictured by Rintala et al. (1970). Pfeiffer et al. (1970) described affected father and two sons with predominantly unilateral popliteal pterygium, anomalies of the skin around the nails, syndactyly, abnormality of the scrotum or cryptorchidism, cleft lip and palate, congenital fistulae of the lower lip, congenital bands of mucous membranes between jaws, and ankyloblepharon filiforme adnatum. Kind (1970) described affected mother and daughter. In addition to bilateral popliteal pterygium, aplasia of the labia majora, ankyloblepharon filiforme, filiform bands between the jaws, lip pits and cleft palate were present. See TURNER PHENOTYPE.

Bixler, D., Poland, C. and Nance, W. E.: Phenotypic variation in the popliteal pterygium syndrome. Clin. Genet. 4: 220-228, 1973.

Champion, R. and Cregan, J. C. F.: Congenital popliteal webbing in siblings. A report of two cases. J. Bone Joint Surg. 41B: 355-357, 1959.

Gorlin, R. J. and Pindborg, J. J.: Cleft lip-palate, popliteal pterygium digital and genital anomaly. Syndromes of the Head and Neck. New York: Blakiston Division, McGraw-Hill, 1964. Pp. 122-125.

Gorlin, R. J., Sedano, H. O. and Cervenka, J.: Popliteal pterygium syndrome: a syndrome comprising cleft lip-palate, popliteal and intercrural pterygia, digital and genital anomalies. Pediatrics 41: 503-509, 1968.

Hecht, F. and Jarvinen, J. M.: Heritable dysmorphic syndrome with normal intelligence. J. Pediatr. 70: 927-935, 1967.

Kind, H. P.: Popliteales pterygiumsyndrom. Helv. Paediatr. Acta 25: 508-516, 1970.

61

D
O
M
I
N
A
N
T

Klein, D.: Un curieux syndrome hereditaire: cheilo-palatoschizis avec fistules de la levre inferieure associe a une syndactylie, une onychodysplasie particuliere, un pterygion poplite unilateral et des pieds varus equins. J. Genet. Hum. 11: 65-71, 1962.

Lewis, E.: Congenital webbing of the lower limbs. Proc. Roy. Soc. Med. 41: 864 Only, 1948.

Pfeiffer, R. A., Tuente, W. and Reinken, M.: Das Kniepterygium-syndrom, ein autosomal-dominant vererbtes Missbildungssyndrom. Z. Kinderheilk. 108: 103-116, 1970.

Rintala, A. E., Laliti, A. Y. and Gylling, U. S.: Congenital sinuses of the lower lip in connection with cleft lip and palate. Cleft Palate J. 7: 336-346, 1970.

*11955 CLEFT PALATE LATERAL SYNECHIA SYNDROME (CPLS SYNDROME)

Fuhrmann et al. (1972) described a new syndrome of cleft palate combined with multiple cordlike adhesions between the free borders of the palate and lateral parts of the tongue and floor of the mouth. The full syndrome occurred in 5 persons, a sixth had cleft palate only and an unaffected male transmitted the disorder to two children with different mothers. The disorder is distinct from the ankyloglosson superius syndrome.

Fuhrmann, W., Koch, F. and Schweckendiek, W.: Autosomal dominante Vererbung von Gaumenspalte und Synechien zwischen Gaumen und Mundboden oder Zunge. Humangenetik 14: 196-203, 1972.

*11960 CLEIDOCRANIAL DYSPLASIA (FORMERLY CLEIDOCRANIAL DYSOSTOSIS)

Features include persistently open skull sutures with bulging calvarium, hypoplasia or aplasia of the clavicles permitting abnormal facility in apposing the shoulders, wide pubic symphysis, short middle phalanx of the fifth fingers, dental anomalies and often vertebral malformation. This disorder must be differentiated from pycnodysostosis (a recessive). Acro-osteolysis and bone sclerosis with tendency to fracture are differentiating features of pycnodysostosis. One of the most colorful families was described by Jackson (1951). The condition occurred in many descendants of a Chinese named Arnold who embraced the Mohammedan religion and 7 wives. Jackson was able to trace 356 descendants of whom 70 were affected by the 'Arnold head.' For translation of original description by Marie and Sainton (1898) see Bick (1968).

Bick, E. M.: The classic: on hereditary cleido-cranial dysostosis. Clin. Orthop. 58: 5-8, 1968.

Jackson, W. P. U.: Osteo-dental dysplasia (cleido-cranial dysostosis). The 'Arnold head.' Acta Med. Scand. 139: 292-307, 1951.

Kalliala, E. and Taskinen, P. J.: Cleidocranial dysostosis. Report of six typical cases and one atypical case. Oral Surg. 15: 808-822, 1962.

Lechelle, P., Thevenard, A. and Mignot, H.: Dysostose cleido-cranienne avec malformations vertebrales multiples et troubles nerveux. Caractere familial des malformations. Bull. Mem. Soc. Med. Hop. Paris 52: 1526-1530, 1936.

Levin, E. J. and Sonnenschein, H.: Cleidocranial dysostosis. New York J. Med. 63: 1562-1566, 1963.

Marie, P. and Sainton, P.: The classic: on hereditary cleido-cranial dysostosis. Clin. Orthop. 58: 5-8, 1968.

11970 CLINODACTYLY

Camptodactyly is flexure contracture of fingers, usually the fifth. Clinodactyly, which also involves the fifth finger, is a radial curvature. It is usually due to short, triangular middle phalanx. Clinodactyly also occurs in persons with the Marfan syndrome and in 'bird-headed dwarfs' (see recessive catalog), as well as in trisomy 21 (mongolism). See BRACHYDACTYLY TYPE A3 (11270).

11980 CLUB FOOT (TALIPES EQUINOVARUS)

Although genetic factors are clearly important, simple inheritance has not been established. Palmer (1964) suggested that two types may exist: (1) a group with normal sex ratio, normal maternal age curve, recurrence risk of about 10 percent and probable dominant inheritance with about 40 percent penetrance; and (2) a group born to younger mothers with preponderance of males and no clear pattern of inheritance. Book (1948) had estimated that the risk of recurrence in subsequently born children is between 3 and 8 percent if one child is affected and about 10 percent if one child and one parent are affected. Club foot is a feature of diastrophic dwarfism (q.v.).

Alberman, E. D.: The causes of congenital club foot. Arch. Dis. Child. 40: 548-554, 1965.

Book, J. A.: A contribution to the genetics of congenital clubfoot. Hereditas 34: 289-300, 1948.

Ching, G. H. S., Chung, C. S. and Nemechek, R. W.: Genetic and epidemiological studies of clubfoot in Hawaii: ascertainment and incidence. Am. J. Hum. Genet. 21: 566-580, 1969.

Palmer, R. M.: Hereditary clubfoot. Clin. Orthop. 33: 138-146, 1964.

Wynne-Davies, R.: Family studies and the cause of congenital club foot. Talipes equinovarus, talipes calcaneo-valgus and metatarsus varus. J. Bone Joint Surg. 46B: 445-476, 1964.

11990 CLUBBING OF DIGITS

Familial clubbing may be more frequent in Negroes than in whites. It is uncertain whether familial clubbing is distinct from pachydermoperiostosis (q.v.). Fischer, Singer and Feldman (1964) reported Negro families that showed strong sex influence, with males only or predominantly affected.

Curth, H. O., Firschein, I. L. and Alpert, M.: Familial clubbed fingers. Arch. Dermatol. 83: 828-836, 1961.

Fischer, D. S., Singer, D. H. and Feldman, S. M.: Clubbing, a review, with emphasis on hereditary acropachy. Medicine 43: 459-479, 1964.

12000 COARCTATION OF AORTA

Gough (1961) described the anomaly in father and son. He found 6 other reports of familial coarctation.

Gough, J. H.: Coarctation of the aorta in father and son. Br. J. Radiol. 34: 670-674, 1961.

*12010 COLD HYPERSENSITIVITY

After exposure to cold the patient develops urticarial wheals, pain and swelling of joints, chills and fever. Amyloidosis is also a feature of the syndrome of urticaria, deafness and amyloidosis (q.v.), a separate although somewhat similar entity. McKusick and Goodman (1962) noted that systemic amyloidosis is a complication of this condition and that amyloid nephropathy is a frequent cause of death. Doeglas (1973) examined 21 members of a kindred finding 10 affected. One of the 10 had leucocytosis during an attack. Derbes and Coleman (1972) reviewed the literature on familial cold urticaria and described several similar disorders to provide a basis for differential diagnosis.

Derbes, V. J. and Coleman, W. P.: Familial cold urticaria. Ann. Allergy 30: 335-341, 1972.

Doeglas, H. M. G.: Familial cold urticaria. Arch. Dermatol. 107: 136-137, 1973.

Doeglas, H. M. G., Bernini, L. F., Fraser, G. R., Van Loghem, E., Meera Khan, P., Nyenhuis, L. E. and Person, P. L.: A kindred with familial cold urticaria: linkage analysis. J. Med. Genet. 11: 31-34, 1974.

Kile, R. L. and Rusk, H. A.: A case of cold urticaria with unusual family history. J.A.M.A. 114: 1067-1068, 1940.

McKusick, V. A. and Goodman, R. M.: Pinnal calcification. Observations in systemic diseases not associated with disordered calcium metabolism. J.A.M.A. 179: 230-232, 1962.

Shepard, M. K.: Cold hypersensitivity. The Clinical Delineation of Birth Defects. XII. Skin, Hair and Nails. Baltimore: Williams and Wilkins, 1971. P. 352.

Tindall, J. P., Beeker, S. K. and Rosse, W. F.: Familial cold urticaria. A generalized reaction involving leukocytosis. Arch. Intern. Med. 124: 129-134, 1969.

Witherspoon, F. G., White, C. B., Bazemore, J. M. and Hailey, H.: Familial urticaria due to cold. Arch. Dermatol. Syph. 58: 52-55, 1948.

12013 COLLAGEN OF BASEMENT MEMBRANE

See COLLAGEN OF SKIN, TENDON AND BONE — ALPHA-1 POLYPEPTIDE (12015).

12014 COLLAGEN OF CARTILAGE — ALPHA-1 POLYPEPTIDE

See COLLAGEN OF SKIN, TENDON AND BONE — ALPHA-1 POLYPEPTIDE (12015).

12015 COLLAGEN OF SKIN, TENDON AND BONE — ALPHA-1 POLYPEPTIDE

Collagen has a triple-stranded ropelike coiled-coil structure. The major collagen of skin, tendon and bone is the same protein containing two alpha-1 polypeptide chains and one alpha-2 chain. Although these are long (the procollagen chain has a molecular weight of about 120,000, before the 'registration peptide' is cleaved off; see 22541), each messenger RNA is monocistronic (Lazarides and Lukens, 1971). Differences in the collagens from these three tissues are a function of the degree of hydroxylation of proline and lysine residues, aldehyde formation for cross-linking and glycosylation. The alpha-1 chain of the collagen of cartilage and that of the collagen of basement membrane are determined by different structural genes. The collagen of cartilage contains only one type of polypeptide chain, alpha-1, and this is determined by a distinct locus. The fetus contains a fetal collagen of distinctive structure.

Dayhoff, M. O.: Collagen alpha-1 chain. Atlas of Protein Sequence and Structure 1972 (vol. 5). Washington: National Biomedical Research Foundation, 1972. Pp. D297-D300.

Lazarides, E. and Lukens, L. N.: Collagen synthesis on polysomes in vivo and in vitro. Nature N.B. 232: 37-40, 1971.

12016 COLLAGEN OF SKIN, TENDON AND BONE — ALPHA-2 POLYPEPTIDE

See COLLAGEN OF SKIN, TENDON AND BONE — ALPHA-1 POLYPEPTIDE (12015).

12017 COLLAGEN, FETAL — ALPHA-1 POLYPEPTIDE

See COLLAGEN OF SKIN, TENDON AND BONE — ALPHA-1 POLYPEPTIDE (12015).

*12020 COLOBOMA OF IRIS

The defect is typically located in the lower part of the iris. Numerous pedigrees supporting dominant inheritance have been reported. Eldridge (1967) observed an affected family with dominant pedigree pattern. Snell (1908) observed 12 cases in 5 generations. This disorder is presumably distinct from aniridia (10620).

Eldridge, R.: Bethesda, Md., personal communication, 1967.

Francois, J.: Heredity in Ophthalmology. St. Louis: C. V. Mosby Co., 1961. Pp. 149-152.

Snell, S.: Carcinoma of orbit originating in a Meibomian gland. Trans. Ophthalmol. Soc. U.K. 28: 144-147, 1908.

*12030 COLOBOMA OF MACULA

Clausen (1921) described affected brother and sister who had, respectively, two affected sons and two affected daughters. Davenport (1927) described mother and son. Phillips (1970) gave a review.

Clausen, (N. I.): Typisches, beiderseitiges hereditaeres Makulakolobom. Klin. Mbl. Augenheilk. 67: 116 only, 1921.

Davenport, R. C.: Bilateral 'macular coloboma' in mother and son. Proc. R. Soc. Med. 21: 109-110, 1927.

Phillips, C. I.: Hereditary macular coloboma. J. Med. Genet. 7: 224-226, 1970.

12040 COLOBOMA OF MACULA WITH TYPE B BRACHYDACTYLY ('APICAL DYSTROPHY')

Sorsby (1935) described a mother and five children with bilateral pigmented macular coloboma and brachydactyly. One of the patients had unilateral absent kidney. Two other children and the father were unaffected. The skeletal defect was of the type described by MacArthur and McCullough (1932) as apical dystrophy and classified here as brachydactyly, type B (q.v.). Abnormalities are confined to the distal two phalanges. The distal phalanx may be completely absent. The distal phalanx of the thumb is usually broad or bifid. The brother and sister reported by Phillips and Griffiths (1969) in some ways resemble the patients of Sorsby.

MacArthur, J. W. and McCullough, E.: Apical dystrophy, an inherited defect of hands and feet. Hum. Biol. 4: 179-207, 1932.

Phillips, C. I. and Griffiths, D. L.: Macular coloboma and skeletal abnormality. Br. J. Ophthalmol. 53: 346-349, 1969.

Sorsby, A.: Congenital coloboma of the macula, together with an account of the familial occurrence of bilateral macular coloboma in association with apical dystrophy of hands and feet. Br. J. Ophthalmol. 19: 65-90, 1935.

12045 COMEDONES, FAMILIAL DYSKERATOTIC

Carneiro et al. (1972) described a family in which four members had disseminated comedo-like lesions which histologically showed distinctive dyskeratotic changes. Rodin et al. (1967) described widespread comedones in multiple family members. Dyskeratosis was not mentioned. No male-to-male transmission has been observed, it seems.

Carneiro, S. J., Dickson, J. E. and Knox, J. M.: Familial dyskeratotic comedones. Arch. Dermatol. 105: 249-251, 1972.

Rodin, H. H., Blankenship, M. L. and Bernstein, G.: Diffuse familial comedones. Arch. Dermatol. 95: 145-146, 1967.

12050 COMMISSURAL LIP PITS

These occur at the corners of the mouth. They are frequently of pencil-lead size, from 1 to 4 mm. deep and may be filled with cellular debris. Preauricular pits may be associated. Everett and Wescott (1961) found 2 cases among 1000 school children of Portland, Oregon. Witkop (1965) and these authors found evidence of dominant inheritance but could not distinguish between autosomal and X-linked dominance.

Everett, F. G. and Wescott, W. B.: Commissural lip pits. Oral Surg. 14: 202-209, 1961.

Witkop, C. J.: Genetic disease of the oral cavity. In, Tiecke, R. W. (ed.): Oral Pathology. New York: McGraw-Hill, 1965.

*12060 COMPLEMENT COMPONENT-2

Both heterozygotes and homozygotes for a deficiency state have been identified. No gene product is identifiable immunologically in the homozygote (Polley, 1968; Klemperer, 1969). A standardized nomenclature for variants of complement components was recommended by the World Health Organization (1968).

Klemperer, M. R.: Hereditary deficiency of the second component of complement in man: an immunochemical study. J. Immun. 102: 168-171, 1969.

Klemperer, M. R., Austen, K. F. and Rosen, F. S.: Hereditary deficiency of the second component of complement (C'2) in man: further observations on a second kindred. J. Immun. 98: 72-78, 1967.

Polley, M. J.: Inherited C-prime-2 deficiency in man: lack of immunochemically detectable C-prime-2 protein in serums from deficient individuals. Science 161: 1149-1151, 1968.

Ruddy, S. and Austen, K. F.: Inherited abnormalities of the complement system in man. Prog. Med. Genet. 7: 69-95, 1970.

World Health Organization: Bull. WHO 39: 935-938, 1968.

*12070 COMPLEMENT COMPONENT-3

In grandmother, mother, and two sons, Wieme and Demeulenaere (1967) found a double electrophoretic band corresponding apparently to complement component C-prime-3. By means of high voltage starch gel electrophoresis, Azen and Smithies (1968) also found electrophoretic polymorphism of the third component of complement. This component has many important functions in immune mechanisms. Alper and Propp (1968) independently found polymorphism of the third component of complement. Alper et al. (1972)

described a patient with striking susceptibility to pyogenic infection who was apparently homozygous for C3 deficiency. Her C3 levels were one-thousandth or less of normal. Many relatives, including both parents, had approximately half-normal levels. Weitkamp et al. (1973) presented evidence that the Lewis blood group locus and the C3 locus may be linked.

Alper, C. A., Colten, H. R., Rosen, F. S., Rabson, A. R. MacNab, G. and Gear, J. S. S.: Homozygous deficiency of C3 in a patient with repeated infections. Lancet II: 1179-1187, 1972.

Alper, C. A. and Propp, R. P.: Genetic polymorphism of the third component of human complement (C-prime-3). J. Clin. Invest. 47: 2181-2192, 1968.

Alper, C. A. and Rosen, F. S.: Studies of a hypomorphic variant of human C3. J. Clin. Invest. 50: 324-326, 1971.

Alper, C. A., Abramson, N., Johnston, R. B., Jr., Jandl, J. H. and Rosen, F. S.: Increased susceptibility to infection associated with abnormalities of complement-mediated functions and of the third component of complement (C3). N. Engl. J. Med. 282: 349-354, 1970.

Alper, C. A., Abramson, N., Johnston, R. B., Jr., Jandl, J. H. and Rosen, F. S.: Studies in vivo and in vitro on an abnormality in the metabolism of C3 in a patient with increased susceptibility to infection. J. Clin. Invest. 49: 1975-1985, 1970.

Alper, C. A., Colten, H. R., Rosen, S. F., Rabson, A. R., MacNab, G. M. and Gear, J. S. S.: Homozygous deficiency of C3 in a patient with repeated infections. Lancet II: 1179-1181, 1972.

Alper, C. A., Propp, R. P., Klemperer, M. R. and Rosen, F. S.: Inherited deficiency of the third component of human complement (C-prime-3). J. Clin. Invest. 48: 553-557, 1969.

Azen, E. A. and Smithies, O.: Genetic polymorphism of C-prime-3 (beta-1C-globulin) in human serum. Science 162: 905-907, 1968.

Goedde, H. W., Benkmann, H. G. and Hirth, L.: Genetic polymorphism of C'3(beta-1C-globulin) component of complement in a German and a Spanish population. Humangenetik 10: 231-234, 1970.

Muller-Eberhard, H. J.: Chemistry and reaction mechanisms of complement. Adv. Immunol. 8: 1-80, 1968.

Teisberg, P.: Another variant in the C3 system. Clin. Genet. 2: 298-302, 1971.

Teisberg, P.: New variants in the C3 system. Hum. Hered. 20: 631-637, 1970.

Weitkamp, L. R., Johnston, E. and Guttormsen, S. E.: Probable genetic linkage between the loci for the Lewis blood group and complement C3. Intern. Workshop on Human Gene Mapping. New Haven, Conn., June, 1973

Wieme, R. J. and Demeulenaere, L.: Genetically determined electrophoretic variant of the human complement component C-prime-3. Nature 214: 1042-1043, 1967.

*12080 COMPLEMENT COMPONENT-4

By the process of antigen-antibody crossed electrophoresis, Rosenfeld et al. (1969) demonstrated heterogeneity in the fourth component of complement. Subtypes A and A(1) seem to be inherited as co-dominant traits independent of subtype C. Partial deficiency of C4 was found in 3 persons during a screening of 42,000 healthy Japanese (Torisu et al., 1970). Ellman et al. (1970) found a deficiency of C4 in the guinea pig, where total deficiency was recessive.

Ellman, L., Green, I. and Frank, M.: Genetically controlled total deficiency of the fourth component of complement in the guinea pig. Science 170: 74-75, 1970.

Rosenfeld, S. I., Ruddy, S. and Austen, K. F.: Structural polymorphism of the fourth component of human complement. J. Clin. Invest. 48: 2283-2292, 1969.

Torisu, M., Sonozaki, H., Inai, S. and Arata, M.: Deficiency of the fourth component of complement in man. J. Immunol. 104: 728-737, 1970.

12090 COMPLEMENT COMPONENT-5, DEFICIENCY OF

Dysfunction of the fifth component of complement (C5) was found to be the basis for the deficiency in phagocytosis-enhancing activity of serum present in the proband, her mother and 15 other relatives (Miller and Nilsson, 1970). Genetic deficiency of C5 in mice was studied also. Jacobs and Miller (1972) reported a second family with deficiency of the fifth component of complement (C5). However, in this family two brothers were affected and the laboratory characteristics of the deficiency were different. The presence of low opsonic indices in relatives through each parent supported autosomal recessive inheritance. The clinical picture of affected children in both families was that described by Leiner in 1908. The four cardinal features are: (1) generalized seborrheic dermatitis, (2) intractable diarrhea, (3) recurrent local and systemic infections, usually of gram-negative etiology, and (4) marked wasting. The diagnostic test is for uptake of particles (baker's yeast) by leukocytes, since C5 is required for full opsonization. Immunochemical assays of C5 are normal. Recognition of this disorder is important because effective therapy is available. Fresh plasma contains opsonically active C5, which is absent in 5-day-old stored bank blood. The pedigree of the first family, as presented by Miller et al. (1968), is probably as consistent with recessive inheritance as dominant. The mode of inheritance cannot be considered established. Rosenfeld and Leddy (1974) found a kindred with C5 deficiency through studies of a Negro woman with systemic lupus erythematosus, frequent bacterial infections and absent serum hemolytic conplement activity. A healthy half-sister had almost no C5 and four relatives had about half normal levels. The ability of the proband's serum to promote phagocytosis of baker's yeast by normal or self neutrophiles was unimpaired — an apparent conflict with other studies cited above.

Jacobs, J. C. and Miller, M. E.: Fatal familial Leiner's disease: a deficiency of the opsonic activity of serum complement. Pediatrics 49: 225-232, 1972.

Miller, M. E. and Nilsson, U. R.: A familial deficiency of the phagocytosis-enhancing activity of serum related to a dysfunction of the fifth component of complement (C5). N. Engl. J. Med. 282: 354-358, 1970.

Miller, M. E., Seals, J., Kaye, R. and Levitsky, L. C.: A familial, plasma-associated defect of phagocytosis. A new cause of recurrent bacterial infections. Lancet II: 60-63, 1968.

Rosenfeld, S. I. and Leddy, J. P.: Hereditary deficiency of fifth component of complement (C5) in man. (Abstract) J. Clin. Invest. 53: 67A only, 1974.

12100 CONGENITAL HEART DISEASE

In the case of cardiovascular malformations as well as those of other systems, the occasional instances of parent-child involvement is to be expected. It is often uncertain whether this is more than one would expect on the basis of the modest familial aggregation which occurs with such malformations. When successively affected generations are observed in the case of a rare malformation such as supravalvar aortic stenosis or when three, four or more generations are affected, especially through several lines, simple autosomal dominant inheritance is quite likely. See the families reported by Kahler et al. (1966).

Carleton, R. A., Abelmann, W. H. and Hancock, E. W.: Familial occurrence of congenital heart disease: report of three families and review of the literature. N. Engl. J. Med. 259: 1237-1245, 1958.

Chelius, C. J., Rowe, G. G. and Crumpton, C. W.: Familial aspects of congenital heart disease. Am. J. Cardiol. 9: 508-514, 1962.

Kahler, R. L., Braunwald, E., Plauth, W. H., Jr. and Morrow, A. G.: Familial congenital heart disease. Familial occurrence of atrial septal defect with A-V conduction abnormalities, supravalvular aortic and pulmonic stenosis, and ventricular septal defect. Am. J. Med. 40: 384-399, 1966.

Nora, J. J., Dodd, P. F., McNamara, D. G., Hattwick, M. A. W., Leachman, R. D. and Cooley, D. A.: Risk to offspring of parents with congenital heart defects. J.A.M.A. 209: 2052-2053, 1969.

Pitt, D. B.: A family study of Fallot's tetrad. Aust. Ann. Med. 11: 179-183, 1962.

*12105 CONTRACTURAL ARACHNODACTYLY

Beals and Hecht (1971) described father and two sons affected in one kindred and father, daughter and son (by different mothers) affected in a second kindred. They proposed that the disorder be called 'contractural arachnodactyly' and further suggested that Marfan's patient (1896) did not have the Marfan syndrome as presently delineated but this disorder. They found several other reports, apparently of the same disorder, in the literature. Beyer et al. (1965) probably described the same condition in a mother and four children and some of the reports of combined Marfan syndrome and arthrogryposis multiplex congenita may be further examples (e.g., Reeve et al., 1960; Kingsley-Pillers, 1946). Epstein et al. (1968) described father and son with a connective tissue disorder with some features suggesting the Marfan syndrome and some suggesting osteogenesis imperfecta. Severe kyphoscoliosis, generalized osteopenia, flexion contractures of the fingers and abnormally shaped ears were among the characteristics. Abnormally shaped ('crumpled') ears have been emphasized by other students of this disorder.

Beals, R. K. and Hecht, F.: Congenital contractural arachnodactyly: a heritable disorder of connective tissue. J. Bone Joint Surg. 53A: 987-993, 1971.

Beyer, P., Klein, M. L. and Iszepy, E.: Maladie de Marfan avec raideurs articulaires importantes atteignant les quatre enfants de la meme fratrie et leur mere. Arch. Fr. Pediatr. 22: 210-216, 1965.

Epstein, C. J., Graham, C. B., Hodgkin, W. E., Hecht, F. and Motulsky, A. G.: Hereditary dysplasia of bone with kyphoscoliosis, contractures, and abnormally shaped ears. J. Pediatr. 73: 379-386, 1968.

Kingsley-Pillers, E. M.: Arachnodactyly with amyoplasia congenita. Proc. R. Soc. Med. 39: 696-697, 1946.

Lowry, R. B. and Guichon, V. C.: Congenital contractural arachnodactyly: a syndrome simulating Marfan's syndrome. Canad. Med. Assoc. J. 107: 531-533, 1972.

Marfan, M. A. B.: Un cas de deformation congenitale des quatre membres plus prononcee aux extremites, caracterisee par l'allongement des os avec un certain degre d'amincissement. Bull. Mem. Soc. Med. Hosp. Paris 13: 220-226, 1896.

Reeve, R., Silver, H. K. and Ferrier, P.: Marfan's syndrome (arachnodactyly) with arthrogryposis (amyoplasia congenita). Am. J. Dis. Child. 99: 101-106, 1960.

12110 CONTRACTURES WITH SCLERODERMA-LIKE CHANGES

Pichler (1968) described a father, daughter and son with flexion deformities of fingers and toes, limited motion of several other joints and the vertebral column, sclerodermatoid changes of the skin and generalized increase in the consistency of otherwise slightly underdeveloped muscles. Suspected myosclerosis could not be confirmed by biopsy. The appearance of the affected son rather suggests that of pseudo-Hurler polydystrophy (q.v.) but no corneal changes were described and autosomal dominant inheritance seems likely. This may be the same entity as that entered elsewhere as the stiff skin syndrome (18490).

Pichler, E.: Hereditaere Kontrakturen mit sklerodermieartigen Hautveraenderungen. Z. Kinderheilk. 104: 349-361, 1968.

*12120 CONVULSIONS, BENIGN FAMILIAL NEONATAL

Families have been reported in which multiple persons in an autosomal dominant pattern had neonatal convulsions which cleared spontaneously after a few weeks and were followed by normal psychomotor development (Bjerre and Corelius, 1968; Rett and Teubel, 1964). Pyridoxine dependency was excluded in all.

Bjerre, I. and Corelius, E.: Benign familial neonatal convulsions. Acta Paediat. Scand. 57: 557-561, 1968.

Rett, A. and Teubel, R.: Neugeborenenkraempfe im Rahmen einer epileptisch belasteten Familie. Wien. Klin. Wschr. 76: 609-613, 1964.

12125 CONVULSIVE DISORDER AND MENTAL RETARDATION

Juberg and Hellman (1971) reported a family in which 15 females, related either as sisters or first-cousins through their fathers, had a grand mal convulsive disorder of early onset associated with mental retardation. In the sibship of the fathers, 6 of 9 males had affected daughters. Their mother and her mother were said to have a convulsive disorder. Female-limited autosomal dominant inheritance was proposed.

Juberg, R. C. and Hellman, C. D.: A new familial form of convulsive disorder and mental retardation limited to females. J. Pediatr. 79: 726-732, 1971.

*12130 COPROPORPHYRIA

Many have commented that after the Swedish acute intermittent and South African variegate types of porphyria are excluded one is left with overlapping cases. Barnes and Whittaker (1965) described what may be a distinct entity. Four of 5 sibs were affected. The parents were not tested. Marked elevation of coproporphyria in the feces differentiated the condition from the Swedish type in which stool porphyrins are usually normal and from variegate porphyria, in which both coproporphyrin and protoporphyrin fractions are increased in the stool. The proband experienced typical acute porphyria. Constipation and abdominal colic were striking features in these patients. Goldberg et al. (1967) added 20 new cases. A massive excretion of coproporphyrin III in the urine and feces, predominantly the feces, was demonstrated. Attacks resembling those of acute intermittent porphyria were precipitated by drugs and during attacks porphobilinogen and delta-aminolevulinic acid were excreted in the urine in excess. Photosensitivity is occasionally present and the only manifestations may be psychiatric. About half of cases are asymptomatic. Dominant inheritance seems adequately established. This is a hepatic form of porphyria. Haeger-Aronson et al. (1968) reported familial cases. Cripps and Peters (1970) found that tranquilizers including meprobamate and chlorpromazine precipitated trouble. The first case, reported by Berger and Goldberg (1955), was the offspring of first-cousin parents, both of whom showed excessive excretion of coproporphyrin III. The authors suggested that the disorder is autosomal dominant and that their proband was homozygous. In the family of Haeger-Aronson et al. (1968) thirteen persons in 5 sibships of 2 generations showed latent coproporphyria, in addition to the symptomatic proband. Kaufman and Marver (1970) demonstrated increased ala synthetase activity in corproporphyria similar to that in acute intermittent porphyria. Increased hepatic delta-aminolevulinic acid synthetase has been demonstrated in three forms of hereditary porphyria: acute intermittent porphyria, porphyria variegata and coproporphyria (McIntyre, 1971).

Barnes, H. D. and Whittaker, N.: Hereditary coproporphyria with acute intermittent manifestations. Br. Med. J. 2: 1102-1104, 1965.

Berger, H. and Goldberg, A.: Hereditary coproporphyria. Br. Med. J. 2: 85-88, 1955.

Connon, J. J. and Turkington, V.: Hereditary coproporphyria. Lancet II: 263-264, 1964.

Cripps, D. J. and Peters, H. A.: Stool porphyrins in acute intermittent and hereditary coproporphyria. Adverse effects of tranquilizers. Arch. Neurol. 23: 80-84, 1970.

Goldberg, A., Rimington, C. and Lochhead, A. C.: Hereditary coproporphyria. Lancet I: 632-636, 1967.

Haeger-Aronson, B., Stathers, G. and Swahn, G.: Hereditary coproporphyria. Study of a Swedish family. Ann. Intern. Med. 69: 221-227, 1968.

Hunter, J. A. A., Khan, S. A., Hope, E., Beattie, A. D., Beveridge, G. W., Smith, A. W. M. and Goldberg, A.: Hereditary coproporphyria. Photosensitivity, jaundice and neuropsychiatric manifestations associated with pregnancy. Br. J. Dermatol. 84: 301-310, 1971.

Kaufman, L. and Marver, H. S.: Biochemical defects in two types of human hepatic porphyria. N. Engl. J. Med. 283: 954-958, 1970.

Lomholt, J. C. and With, T. K.: Hereditary coproporphyria. A family with unusually few and mild symptoms. Acta Med. Scand. 186: 83-85, 1969.

McIntyre, N., Pearson, A. J. G., Allan, D. J., Craske, S., West, G. M. L., Moore, M. R., Beattie, A. D., Paxton, J. and Goldberg, A.: Hepatic delta-aminolaevulinic acid synthetase in an attack of hereditary coproporphyria and during remission. Lancet I: 560-564, 1971.

*12140 CORNEA PLANA

Larsen and Eriksen (1949) described 13 patients in 3 generations of each of two families. Recessive inheritance (q.v.) seems well established in many other instances. Eriksson et al. (1973) described families.

Eriksson, A. W., Lehmann, W. and Forsius, H.: Congenital cornea plana in Finland. Clin. Genet. 4: 301-310, 1973.

Larsen, V. and Eriksen, A.: Cornea plana. Acta Ophthalmol. 27: 275-286, 1949.

Paufique and Bonnet (1966) described a family with affected members in three generations. Most of the affected persons also had strabismus. The cornea presented a 'dusty' opacity and a rough map-like surface with a peripheral condensation ring separated from the limbus by a narrow strip of normal cornea. The lesions are primarily in Bowman membrane with secondary involvement of the epithelium and superficial part of the stroma. Relapsing corneal erosions occur between ages 8 and 20 and again in more severe form at about 40 or 50 years. The ultrastructure was described by Rice et al. (1968) and Akiya and Brown (1971). Almost every epithelial cell, but especially the basal cells, showed degenerative changes, i.e., swollen mitochondria, large vacuoles, swelling and disruption of the endoplasmic reticulum. Bowman membrane was almost completely replaced by masses of disoriented collagen fibrils and smaller electron-dense fibrils whose composition and origin have not been determined.

D
O
M
I
N
A
N
T

Buecklers, M.: Ueber eine weitere familiaere Hornhautdystrophie (Reis). Klin. Mbl. Augenheilk. 114: 386-397, 1949.

Hall, P.: Reis-Bucklers dystrophy. Arch. Ophthalmol. 91: 170-173, 1974.

Malbran, E. S.: Corneal dystrophies: a clinical, pathological, and surgical approach. Am. J. Ophthalmol. 74: 771-809, 1972.

Paufique, L. and Bonnet, M.: La dystrophie corneenne heredo-familiale de Reis-Bucklers. Ann. Oculist. 199: 14-37, 1966.

Rice, N. S. C., Ashton, N., Jay, B. and Blach, R. K.: Reis-Bucklers' dystrophy: a clinico-pathological study. Br. J. Ophthalmol. 52: 577-603, 1968.

12160 CORNEAL DYSTROPHY, CONGENITAL

Maumenee (1960) observed 6 known afflicted persons in three generations of one family. The corneal dystrophies can, in the first instance, be classified according to the site of predominant involvement, the cornea having five layers, from outside inward, epithelium, Bowman membrane, stroma, Descemet membrane, and endothelium. Most cases are recessive. In an interesting twice-reported family (Turpin et al., 1939; Desvignes and Vigo, 1955) 13 were affected in 3 consecutive generations with five instances of male-to-male transmission.

Desvignes, P. and Vigo (NI): A case of corneal and parenchymal dystrophy of dominant type. Bull. Soc. Ophthalmol. Fr. 4: 220-225, 1955.

Feigin, R. D. and Caplan, D. B.: Corneal opacities in infancy and childhood. J. Pediatr. 69: 383-392, 1966.

Maumenee, A. E.: Congenital hereditary corneal dystrophy. Am. J. Ophthalmol. 50: 1114-1124, 1960.

Turpin, R., Tisserand, M. and Serane, J.: Opacites corneennes hereditaires et congenitales reparties sur trois generations et atteignant deux jumelles monozygotes. Arch. Ophtalmol. 3: 109-111, 1939.

12170 CORNEAL DYSTROPHY, CONGENITAL ENDOTHELIAL

Pearce et al. (1969) described a family with 39 affected members.

Pearce, W. G., Tripathi, R. C. and Morgan, G.: Congenital endothelial corneal dystrophy. Clinical, pathological, and genetic study. Brit. J. Ophthal. 53: 577-591, 1969.

*12180 CORNEAL DYSTROPHY, CRYSTALLINE, OF SCHNYDER

This disorder, beginning early in life, presents as an oval or annular clouding of the central part of the cornea with the periphery remaining clear. Involvement extends toward the limbus but usually leaves a clear peripheral area. Corneal sensitivity is normal. Slit-lamp examination shows in the opacified area many small iridescent needle-shaped shiny crystals of unknown composition. The opacity is located in the anterior portion of the stroma just posterior to Bowman membrane. The epithelium is normal. Gillespie and Covelli (1963) reported father-to-son transmission. The cornea has the appearance of crystalline dystrophy in cystinosis. Malbran et al. (1953) described a family. Luxenberg (1967) gave further information on members of a family reported by Fry and Pickett (1950). Clouding may be congenital but progresses little. The lesions are bilateral, centrally located and irregular in outline. Deposits occur in the anterior stroma near Bowman membrane and extend irregularly into deeper layers. Delleman and Winkelman (1968) described two families. In the first 21 persons in 6 generations were affected and genu valgum was rather constantly associated. By histochemistry and electron microscopy, the crystals were shown to be cholesterol (Garner and Tripathi, 1972).

Bron, A. J., Williams, H. P. and Carruthers, M. E.: Hereditary crystalline stromal dystrophy of Schnyder. I. Clinical features of family with hyperlipoproteinaemia. Br. J. Ophthalmol. 56: 383-399, 1972.

Delleman, J. W. and Winkelman, J. E.: Degeneratio corneae cristallinea hereditaria. A clinical, genetical and histological study. Ophthalmologica 155: 409-426, 1968.

Fry, W. E. and Pickett, W. E.: Crystalline dystrophy of cornea. Trans. Am. Ophthalmol. Soc. 48: 220-227, 1950.

Garner, A. and Tripathi, R. C.: Histopathology and ultrastructure. Br. J. Ophthalmol. 56: 400-408, 1972.

Gillespie, F. D. and Covelli, B.: Crystalline corneal dystrophy. Report of a case. Am. J. Ophthalmol. 56: 465-467, 1963.

Luxenberg, M.: Hereditary crystalline dystrophy of the cornea. Am. J. Ophthalmol. 63: 507-511, 1967.

Malbran, J. L., Paunessa, J. M. and Vidal, F.: Hereditary crystalline degeneration of cornea. Ophthalmologica 126: 369-378, 1953.

*12190 CORNEAL DYSTROPHY, GRANULAR TYPE (GROENOUW TYPE I)

In the macular, granular and lattice dystrophies the changes are in the corneal stroma rather than the epithelium. In this and the lattice type, the histologic findings are hyaline degeneration with absence of acid mucopolysaccharide deposition. See recessive catalog for MACULAR CORNEAL DYSTROPHY (GROENOUW TYPE II). The opacity in the granular type consists of grayish white granules with sharp borders mainly in a disc-shaped area in the center of the cornea. The peripheral cornea is usually clear and the cornea between granules is clear. Hyaline material separates the epithelium from Bowman membrane. Although this type can have its onset in the first 10 years, visual acuity during childhood is usually good.

Jones, S. T. and Zimmerman, L. E.: Histopathologic differentiation of granular, macular and lattice dystrophies of the cornea. Am. J. Ophthalmol. 51: 394-410, 1961.

*12200 CORNEAL DYSTROPHY, HEREDITARY POLYMORPHOUS POSTERIOR

Vacuoles are demonstrated in the posterior parts of the cornea by slit-lamp examination. Vision is not affected significantly in most cases. However, we have observed three affected persons in two generations of which one is legally blind. The affected persons in this family are obese with very similar facial features and widely spaced teeth. These characteristics may or may not be produced by the gene responsible for the corneal change. Schlichting (1941) noted depressions, vesicles and polymorphous opacities in Descemet membrane, with opacities in the deepest layers of the stroma, in father and 4-year-old daughter. Theodore (1939) reported 3 generations. Rubinstein and Silverman (1968) observed mother and two children affected. The mother and one child had rupture of Descemet membrane and the mother had glaucoma. McGee and Falls (1953) reported a family. The condition was first described by Koeppe (1916) under the name of keratitis bullosa interna, an appropriately descriptive designation. Pearce et al. (1969) reported a family in which 39 persons in five generations were affected with what they termed 'congenital endothelial corneal dystrophy.' A distortion of segregation ratio was noted in the offspring of affected females — an increased number of affected females and a deficiency of affected males. No biologic explanation could be found and it was concluded that the distorted sex ratio was a chance happening. The clouding of the cornea developed in the postnatal period and was usually well-established by early childhood. Changes in the posterior cornea, namely markedly reduced number of endothelial cells and thickening of Descemet membrane, was thought to be primary.

Bergman, G. D.: Posterior polymorphous degeneration of the cornea. Am. J. Ophthalmol. 58: 125-128, 1964.

Hogan, M. J. and Giambattista, B.: Hereditary deep dystrophy of the cornea (polymorphous). Am. J. Ophthalmol. 68: 777-788, 1969.

Koeppe, L.: Klinische Beobachtungen mit der Nernstspaltlampe und dem Hornhautmikroskop. Graefe Arch. Ophthalmol. 91: 363-379, 1916.

Kwedar, E. W.: Hereditary nonprogressive deep corneal dystrophy. Arch. Ophthalmol. 65: 127-129, 1961.

McGee, H. B. and Falls, H. F.: Hereditary polymorphous deep degeneration of the cornea. Arch. Ophthalmol. 50: 462-467, 1953.

Pearce, W. G., Tripathi, R. C. and Morgan, G.: Congenital endothelial corneal dystrophy. Clinical, pathological, and genetic study. Br. J. Ophthalmol. 53: 577-591, 1969.

Rubinstein, R. A. and Silverman, J. J.: Hereditary deep dystrophy of the cornea. Associated with glaucoma and ruptures in Descemet's membrane. Arch. Ophthalmol. 79: 123-126, 1968.

Schlichting, H.: Blasen- und dellenfoermige Endotheldystrophie der Hornhaut. Klin. Mbl. Augenheilk. 107: 425-435, 1941.

Theodore, F. H.: Congenital type of endothelial dystrophy. Arch. Ophthalmol. 21: 626-638, 1939.

*12210 CORNEAL DYSTROPHY, JUVENILE EPITHELIAL, OF MEESMANN

The condition usually appears in the first year or two of life, commencing with signs of irritation. The corneal changes, seen only with magnification, consist of myriads of fine punctate opacities in the epithelium and occasionally in Bowman membrane. Vision is only rarely impaired to a serious degree. Meesmann and Wilke (1939) studied three families with dominant inheritance and Stocker and Holt (1954, 1955) studied a family with affected members probably in 8 generations (4 generations were examined). Behnke and Thiel (1965) could demonstrate that all cases in Schleswig-Holstein were members of one kindred traced back to 1620. In the four living generations 120 cases were demonstrated. Progression does not occur. Alkemade and Van Balen (1966) observed 10 affected persons in one family. None had ocular complaints.

Alkemade, P. P. H. and Van Balen, A. T. M.: Hereditary epithelial dystrophy of the cornea. Br. J. Ophthalmol. 50: 603-605, 1966.

Behnke, H. and Thiel, H. J.: Uber die hereditaere Epitheldystrophie der Hornhaut (Typ Meesman-Wilke) in Schleswig-Holstein. Klin. Mbl. Augenheilk. 147: 662-672, 1965.

Meesmann, A. and Wilke, F.: Klinische und anatomische untersuchungen uber eine bisher unbekannte, dominant vererbte epitheldystrophieder hornhaut. Klin. Mbl. Augenheilk. 103: 361-391, 1939.

Snyder, W. B.: Hereditary epithelial corneal dystrophy. Am. J. Ophthalmol. 55: 56-61, 1963.

Stocker, F. W. and Holt, L. B.: A rare form of hereditary epithelial dystrophy of the cornea: a genetic, clinical, and pathologic study. Trans. Am. Ophthalmol. Soc. 52: 133-144, 1954.

69

D
O
M
I
N
A
N
T

Stocker, F. W. and Holt, L. B.: Rare form of hereditary epithelial dystrophy. Arch. Ophthalmol. 53: 536-541, 1955.

*12220 CORNEAL DYSTROPHY, LATTICE TYPE

Frayer and Blodi (1959) described a family. Grayish lines like cotton threads are mainly limited to a zone between the center of the cornea and the periphery, usually not extending to the limbus. Rounded dots with distinct borders are scattered everywhere. The cornea between opacities is relatively clear. Visual activity is usually normal in childhood. In this and the granular type, the histologic findings are hyaline degeneration and absence of acid mucopolysaccharide deposition. The changes involve particularly the central portion of the cornea, becoming first evident in adolescence and consisting of delicate, double-contoured, interdigitating, elongated deposits which form a reticular pattern in the corneal stroma. Recurrent corneal ulceration sometimes occurs. Progression to severe visual impairment by the fifth or sixth decade is the rule. No signs of systemic abnormality have been described. Klintworth (1967) presented evidence that corneal dystrophy of the lattice type is a local variety of amyloidosis. Lattice corneal dystrophy accompanied systemic amyloidosis of the Finnish type (10512).

Frayer, W. C. and Blodi, F. C.: The lattice type of familial corneal degeneration. A histopathologic study. Arch. Ophthalmol. 61: 712-719, 1959.

King, R. G., Jr. and Geeraets, W. J.: Lattice or Reis-Buecklers corneal dystrophy: a question of stromal pathology. Sth. Med. J. 62: 1163-1169, 1969.

Klintworth, G. K.: Lattice corneal dystrophy: an inherited variety of amyloidosis restricted to the cornea. Am. J. Pathol. 50: 371-399, 1967.

Meretoja, J.: Comparative histiopathological and clinical findings in eyes with lattice corneal dystrophy of two different types. Ophthalmologica 165: 15-37, 1972.

Ramsay, R. M.: Familial corneal dystrophy-lattice type. Trans. Canad. Ophthalmol. Soc. 23: 222-229, 1960.

Straatsma, B. R., Zeegen, P. D., Foos, R. Y., Feman, S. S. and Shabo, A. L.: Lattice degeneration of the retina. Am. J. Ophthalmol. 77: 619-649, 1974.

*12230 CORNEAL DYSTROPHY, PUNCTATE OR NODULAR

Onset is at about puberty. Bilateral nodular opacities of the cornea are characteristic. Groenouw (1933) demonstrated dominant inheritance.

Groenouw, A.: Knoetchenformige Hornhauttruebungen vererbt durch vier Generationen. Klin. Mbl. Augenheilk. 90: 577-580, 1933.

*12240 CORNEAL EROSIONS, RECURRING HEREDITARY

Franceschetti (1928) described a family in which six successive generations were affected. The disorder became manifest between 4 and 6 years. Recurring ulcerations are also seen in macular and lattice types of classical dystrophy. See also KERATITIS FUGAX HEREDITARIA. A follow-up in 1958 showed 40 affected members of the family (Franceschetti and Klein, 1961). Valle (1967) described a family with six affected persons in three sibships in two generations. The progenitor had Fuchs corneal dystrophy. Wales (1956) described affected persons in 3 generations.

Franceschetti, A. and Klein, D.: Chapter VIII — cornea. In, Waardenburg, P. J., Franceschetti, A. and Klein, D. (eds.): Genetics and Ophthalmology. Springfield, Ill.: Charles C Thomas, 1961. Pp. 447-543.

Franceschetti, A.: Hereditaere rezidivierende Erosion der Hornhaut. Z. Augenheilk. 66: 309-316, 1928.

Valle, O.: Hereditary recurring corneal erosions. A family study, with special reference to Fuch's dystrophy. Acta Ophthalmol. 45: 829-836, 1967.

Wales, H. J.: A family history of corneal erosions. Trans. Ophthalmol. Soc. New Zeal. 8: 77-78, 1956.

12250 CORTICOSTEROID-BINDING GLOBULIN (CBG), DECREASE IN

Doe et al. (1965) found decreased levels in 8 persons in three generations of a family. In no instance was there male-to-male transmission. The extent of the decrease was the same in males and females. CBG, otherwise known as transcortin, is an alpha-globulin. DeMoor et al. (1967) found a bimodal distribution of CBG levels in males but not in females, and the fathers of males with low levels showed normal levels. They felt that X-linked inheritance best accounts for the findings. Elevated CBG was found in a brother and sister by Lohrenz et al. (1968). Neither sib had children and the mother, the only surviving parent, had normal CBG levels.

DeMoor, P., Meulepas, E., Hendrikx, A., Heyns, W. and Vandenschrieck, H. G.: Cortisol-binding capacity of plasma transcortin: a sex-linked trait? J. Clin. Endocrinol. Metab. 27: 959-965, 1967.

Doe, R. P., Lohrenz, F. N. and Seal, U. S.: Familial decrease in corticosteroid-binding globulin. Metabolism 14: 940-943, 1965.

Lohrenz, F., Doe, R. P. and Seal, U. S.: Idiopathic or genetic elevation of corticosteroid-binding globulin? J. Clin. Endocrinol. Metab. 28: 1073-1075, 1968.

*12260 COSTOVERTEBRAL SEGMENTATION ANOMALIES

We (Rimoin et al., 1968) have seen a family in which father and son (1122178, 1222180) and probably two preceding generations were short of stature (less than five feet), the shortening being mainly in the trunk, and had multiple rib and vertebral anomalies. The number of ribs was reduced to 11 and several ribs were fused posteriorly. Hemivertebra and vertebral fusion were noted at multiple levels in the cervical and thoracic spine. No neurologic manifestations were present. Langer (1967) has shown us another family with multiple affected generations. The family reported as polydysspondyly by Rutt and Degenhardt (1959) had affected persons in 4 generations. Van de Sar (1952) found multiple hemivertebrae and rib anomalies in a mother and daughter. Multiple hemivertebrae also occur as a recessive. Polydysspondyly was described by Turpin et al. (1959) in association with a translocation involving group D and G chromosomes. De Grouchy et al. (1963) reported a similar condition in mother and daughter, both of whom carried a 14-15 translocation.

De Grouchy, J., Mlynarski, J. C., Maroteaux, P., Lamy, M., Deshaies, G., Benichou, C. and Salmon, C.: Syndrome polydysspondylique par translocation 14-15 et dyschondrosteose chez un meme sujet. Segregation familiale. Comp. Rend. Acad. Sci. 256: 1614-1616, 1963.

Langer, L. O., Jr.: Minneapolis, Minn.: personal communication, 1967.

Rimoin, D. L., Fletcher, B. D. and McKusick, V. A.: Spondylocostal dysplasia: a dominantly inherited form of short-trunked dwarfism. Am. J. Med. 45: 948-953, 1968.

Rutt, A. and Degenhardt, K.-H.: Beitrag zur Atiologie und Pathogenese von Wirbelsaulenmissbildungen. Arch. Orthop. Unfallchir. 57: 120, 1959. (see also, Ein kurzes Handbuch in funf Baenden. Becker, P. E. (ed.): Stuttgart: Georg Thieme Verlag, 2: 589 only, 1964.).

Turpin, R., Lejeune, J., Lafourcade, J. and Gautier, M.: Aberrations chromosomiques et maladies humaines. La polydysspondylie a 45 chromosomes. Comp. Rend. Acad. Sci. 248: 3636-3638, 1959.

Van de Sar, A.: Hereditary multiple hemivertebrae. Doc. De Med. Geograph. et Trop. 4: 23-28, 1952.

*12270 COUMARIN RESISTANCE

O'Reilly et al. (1964) described resistance to the hypoprothrombinemic effects of coumarin drugs, in 7 persons in three generations of a family with no male-to-male transmission. They postulated that an autosomal gene is responsible for the synthesis of a clotting factor dependent on vitamin K and that in this family affected persons have an abnormal factor with decreased affinity for the coumarin drug or increased affinity for vitamin K. Hereditary resistance to warfarin in rats, which may be a comparable condition, is inherited as an autosomal dominant (Greaves and Ayres, 1967). O'Reilly (1970) described a second kindred of which 18 members were shown to have relative resistance to oral anticoagulant drugs. Several instances of male-tomale transmission were observed. Of the various possible mechanisms for the relative resistance all could be excluded except mutation in the vitamin K-anticoagulant receptor site. Positive evidence favoring the latter included the correction of hypoprothrombinemia by small amounts of exogenous vitamin K and the fact that the anticoagulant dose-response curves for the probands of the two families studied by O'Reilly and normal subjects are parallel. Pool et al. (1968) concluded that the resistance to warfarin is due to a decreased affinity of the receptor sites in the liver to coumarin anticoagulant drugs.

Greaves, J. H. and Ayres, P.: Heritable resistance to warfarin in rats. Nature 215: 877-878, 1967.

O'Reilly, R. A.: The second reported kindred with hereditary resistance to oral anticoagulant drugs. N. Engl. J. Med. 282: 1448-1451, 1970.

O'Reilly, R. A., Aggeler, P. M., Hoag, M. S., Leong, L. S., and Kropatkin, M. L.: Hereditary transmission of exceptional resistance to coumarin anticoagulant drugs. The first reported kindred. N. Engl. J. Med. 271: 809-815, 1964.

Pool, J. G., O'Reilly, R. A., Schneiderman, L. J. and Alexander, M.: Warfarin resistance in the rat. Am. J. Physiol. 215: 627-631, 1968.

*12275 COXA VARA

Say et al. (1971) described coxa vara in three generations of a family and many other affected persons on Cyprus. Affected identical twins were reported by Martin (1942); and father, daughter and niece by Almond (1956).

Almond, H. G.: Familial infantile coxa vara. J. Bone Joint Surg. 38B: 539-544, 1956.

Martin, H.: Coxa vara congenita bei eineiigen Zwillingen. Arch. Orthop. Clin. 42: 230-240, 1942.

Say, B., Tuncbilek, E. and Pirnar, T.: Hereditary congenital coxa vara with dominant inheritance? Humangenetik 11: 266-268, 1971.

12277 COXA VARA, PATELLA APLASIA, TARSAL SYNOSTOSIS

Goeminne and Dujardin (1970) found the full syndrome in a mother, coxa vara and patella aplasia in one daughter and patella aplasia in a son.

Goeminne, L. and Dujardin, L.: Congenital coxa vara, patella aplasia and tarsal synostosis: a new inherited syndrome. Acta Genet. Med. Gemellol. 19: 534-545, 1970.

12280 CRANIAL DYSOSTOSIS WITH PRONOUNCED DIGITAL IMPRESSIONS (PSEUDO-CROU-ZON DISEASE)

In Crouzon disease and pseudo-Crouzon disease, the pronounced digital impressions, or convolutional markings, are identical. The essential difference is in the face. In pseudo-Crouzon disease there is no prognathism, the nose is not curved and divergent squint is usually lacking. Prominent forehead and some degree of exophthalmos are features. Franceschetti (1953) first delineated the condition. He (1968) pointed out that Walsh (1957) described a case as Crouzon disease. None of Franceschetti's cases were familial, but Dolivo and Gillieron (1955) described affected brother and sister. The mother, grandmother and great-grandmother were said to have oxycephaly.

Dolivo, G. and Gillieron, J.-D.: Une famille de pseudo-Crouzon. Confin. Neurol. 15: 114-118, 1955.

Franceschetti, A.: Cranial dysostosis with pronounced digital impressions (pseudo-Crouzon dysostosis). In, Congenital Anomalies of the Eye. St. Louis: C. V. Mosby Co., 1968. Pp. 81-84.

Franceschetti, A.: Dysostose cranienne avec calotte cerebriforme (pseudo-Crouzon). Confin. Neurol. 13: 161-166, 1953.

Walsh, F. B.: Clinical Neuro-ophthalmology. Baltimore: Williams and Wilkins Co., 1957 (2nd Ed.).

12285 CRANIO-ACRO-FASCIAL SYNDROME

Grosse (1974) described associated cardiac, craniofacial and hand anomalies in a father and daughter. The cardiac defect was combined ventricular septal defect and pulmonic stenosis. The craniofacial 'defect' consisted mainly of narrow head and face. Very minor abnormalities were present in the hands, e.g., Dupuytren contractures in the father.

Grosse, F. R.: The Rabenhorst-syndrome: a cardio-acral-fascial syndrome. Z. Kinderheilk. 117: 109-114, 1974.

12290 CRANIOFACIAL DYSOSTOSIS WITH DIAPHYSEAL HYPERPLASIA

Stanescu et al. (1963) described a curious syndrome in 9 members of a kindred with a pattern suggestive of autosomal dominant inheritance. The features included a peculiar form of cranio-facial dysostosis with small skull, thin cranial bone, depressions over the fronto-parietal and occipitoparietal sutures, poorly developed mandible, and exophthalmos. The limbs were short and by X-ray the cortices of the long bones were massively thickened.

Stanescu, V., Maximilian, C., Poenaru, S., Florea, I., Stanescu, R., Ionesco, V. and Ioanitiu, D.: Syndrome hereditaire dominant, reunissant une dysostose cranio-faciale de type particulier, une insuffisance de croissance d'aspect chondrodystrophique et un epaississement massif de la corticale des os longs. Rev. Franc. Endocr. Clin. 4: 219-231, 1963.

*12300 CRANIOMETAPHYSEAL DYSPLASIA

In the family described by Komins (1954) brother and sister were affected as well as the mother and a maternal uncle. Podlaha and Kratochvil (1963) and Lejeune et al. (1966) observed that craniometaphyseal dysplasia differs from Pyle disease (metaphyseal dysplasia) in the presence of conspicuous involvement of the craniofacial bones. Widening of the bridge of the nose develops and eventually leonine facies. Pressure on cranial nerves is responsible for a considerable part of the disability. It is likely that the cases in the family reported by Rimoin et al. (1969) and those reported by Spranger et al. (1965) should be considered dominant craniometaphyseal dysplasia reserving the term Pyle disease for the recessive disorder which is more nearly a 'pure' metaphyseal dysplasia with little or no craniofacial involvement. Spranger (1970) reviewed the skull X-ray of Pyle's original case and failed to find the intense increase in bone density characteristic of craniometaphyseal dysplasia. Furthermore the metaphyseal flare is notably abrupt in Pyle disease, producing the 'Erlenmeyer flask' deformity and is milder ('club-like') in craniometaphyseal dysplasia. Pyle disease is a recessive, whereas craniometaphyseal dysplasia is a dominant. The same family was reported by Rimoin et al. (1969) and by Gladney and Monteleone (1970). Stool and Caruso (1973) observed affected father and 15-month-old daughter. Both had peripheral facial palsy and the father was profoundly deaf.

Gladney, J. H. and Monteleone, P. L.: Metaphyseal dysplasia. Lancet II: 44-45, 1970.

Hassler, R.: Familiaere kranio-metaphysaere Dysplasie. Fortschr. Roentgenstr. 90: 704-713, 1959.

Holt, J. F.: The evolution of cranio-metaphyseal dysplasia. Ann. Radiol. 9: 209-214, 1966.

Komins, C.: Familial metaphyseal dysplasia (Pyle's disease). Br. J. Radiol. 27: 670-675, 1954.

Lejeune, E., Anjou, A., Bouvier, M., Robert, J., Vauzelle, J. L. and Jeanneret, J.: Dysplasie cranio-metaphysaire familiale. Rev. Rhum. 33: 714-726, 1966.

Mori, P. A. and Holt, J. F.: Cranial manifestations of familial metaphyseal dysplasia. Radiology 66: 335-343, 1956.

Podlaha, M. and Kratochvil, L.: Familial metaphysial dysplasia: Pyle's disease. Fortschr. Roentgenstr. 98: 158-162, 1963.

Rimoin, D. L., Woodruff, S. L. and Holman, B. L.: Craniometaphyseal dysplasia (Pyle's disease): autosomal dominant inheritance in a large kindred. The Clinical Delineation of Birth Defects. IV. Skeletal Dysplasias. New York: National Foundation, 1969. Pp. 96-104.

Spranger, J. W.: Familial metaphyseal dysplasia? (Letter) Lancet II: 475 only, 1970.

Spranger, J., Paulsen, K. and Lehmann, W.: Die kraniometaphysaere Dysplasie (Pyle). Z. Kinderheilk. 93: 64-79, 1965.

Stool, S. E. and Caruso, V. G.: Cranial metaphyseal dysplasia. Arch. Otolaryngol. 97: 410-412, 1973.

*12310 CRANIOSTENOSIS

Gordon (1959) found multiple cases in five of nine South.African families studied in detail. In four multiple sibs were involved. In the fifth the mother of an affected child was also affected. Under the designation 'scaphocephaly' Bell, Clare and Wentworth (1961) described the same condition in two families. In one family, 6 persons in three generations were said to be affected with male-to-male transmission and in another family two children of an unaffected woman, each by a different father, were affected. Murphy (1953) observed craniostenosis in father and son. Nance and Engel (1967) described a family in which the mother had marked dolichocephaly and two sons had severe craniostenosis with premature closure of sutures and a 'beaten metal' appearance of the calvarium by X-ray. The family was of unusual interest because the normal father and the two sons had a deletion of the short arm of one G chromosome which has been found as a normal variation in some families ('Christchurch chromosome') and was found by these workers in a patient with pycnodysostosis (q.v.) in which failure of closure of cranial sutures is a feature. Anderson and Geiger (1965) observed an infant with left coronal synostosis and father with sagittal synostosis. Bell, Clare and Wentworth (1961) observed 8 affected persons in 3 generations of one family and in 2 offspring of the same mother but different fathers. Sheldon (1931) reported five cases of oxycephaly in three generations. Intelligence was normal. The membrane bones of the skull showed a 'beaten copper' appearance by X-ray. In a large experience of 519 cases of craniostenosis, Shillito and Matson (1968) encountered 9 families in each of which two sibs were affected. In one the sibs were identical twins. Four pairs had synostosis of one or more coronal sutures. Familial involvement was highest in cases with coronal synostosis, particularly bilateral coronal involvement. Successive generations were especially often affected in cases of multiple or total synostosis.

Anderson, F. M. and Geiger, L.: Craniosynostosis. A survey of 204 cases. J. Neurosurg. 22: 229-240, 1965.

Bell, H. S., Clare, F. B. and Wentworth, A. F.: Case reports and technical notes of familial scaphocephaly. J. Neurosurg. 18: 239-241, 1961.

Freeman, J. M. and Berkowf, S.: Craniostenosis: review of the literature and report of thirty-four cases. Pediatrics 30: 57-70, 1962.

Gordon, H.: Craniostenosis. Br. Med. J. 2: 792-795, 1959.

Murphy, J. W.: Familial scaphocephaly in father and son. U.S. Armed Forces Med. J. 4: 1496-1499, 1953.

Nance, W. E. and Engel, E.: Autosomal deletion mapping in man. Science 155: 692-694, 1967.

Sheldon, W.: Hereditary and familial oxycephaly. Proc. R. Soc. Med. 24: 574-576, 1931.

Shillito, J., Jr. and Matson, D. D.: Craniosynostosis: a review of 519 surgical patients. Pediatrics 41: 829-853, 1968.

12320 CRANIUM BIFIDUM OCCULTUM

Terrafranca and Zellis (1953) described affected mother and two children. In one of the children a medial defect in the frontal bone was accompanied by symmetrical parietal lacunae like those described here as parietal foramina (q.v.), as well as cervical (C5-C7) and lumbosacral (L5-S1) spina bifida occulta. The other offspring had an identical frontal defect but less conspicuous parietal foramina and no spina bifida. The mother had a U-shaped frontal defect astride the metopic suture.

Terrafranca, R. J. and Zellis, A.: Congenital hereditary cranium bifidum occultum frontalis. Radiology 61: 60-66, 1953.

12330 CREATINE KINASE

Multiple forms (isozymes) are known. Creatine kinase exists as a dimer composed of two subunits. The muscle enzyme (MM) consists of two identical M subunits. The brain enzyme (BB) consists of two identical B subunits (Dawson et al., 1968). Other tissues show a third hybrid MB enzyme. Apparently polymorphism of creatine kinase has not been identified.

Dawson, D. M., Eppenberger, H. M. and Eppenberger, M. E.: Multiple molecular forms of creatine kinases. Ann. N.Y. Acad. Sci. 151: 616-626, 1968.

*12340 CREUTZFELDT-JAKOB DISEASE

Jacob et al. (1950) and his predecessors described the first reported family, the Becker kindred. Three generations may have been affected, with male-to-male transmission. Davidson and Rabiner (1940) described 3 affected sibs. Some question whether C-J disease should be considered a distinct entity. Friede and Dejong (1964) and later May et al. (1968) described affected father and 3 daughters. Onset was between 38 and 45 years. The illness lasted only 10 months to two years. The disorder began with forgetfulness and nervousness and progressed with jerky, trembling movements of the hands, loss of facial expression and unsteady gait. Pathologic findings included severe status spongiosus, diffuse nerve cell degeneration and some glial proliferation. Creutzfeldt-Jacob disease is undoubtedly a mixed category. Gibbs et al. (1968) reported a transmissible agent which reproduced the disease in a chimpanzee injected with brain material from a 59 year old English male. The familial disease appears to be no different from the sporadic one. Ferber et al. (1973) succeeded in transmitting the familial disease to the chimpanzee where the findings were the same as those from transmission of the sporadic disease. Among families studied by Gajdusek (1973) was one with 14 affected members from one of whom the disease was transmitted to the chimpanzee. The possibility that a 'slow virus' may be involved in Alzheimer disease (10430), Pick disease (17270) and Huntington chorea (14310) is under active study. Person-to-person transmission through a corneal transplant was suggested by the experience reported by Duffy et al. (1974). Kahana et al. (1974) described an aggregation of cases among Libyan Jews, a finding which supports either the viral or the genetic hypothesis or perhaps both. Zlotnik et al. (1974) transmitted the disease to the squirrel monkey.

Davidson, C. and Rabiner, A. M.: Spastic pseudosclerosis (disseminated encephalomyelopathy: corticopallidospinal degeneration). Arch. Neurol. Psychiatry 44: 578-598, 1940.

Duffy, P., Wolf, J., Collins, G., DeVoe, A. G., Streeten, B. and Cowen, D.: Possible person-to-person transmission of Creutzfeldt-Jakob disease. (Letter) N. Engl. J. Med. 290: 692-693, 1974.

Ferber, R. A., Wiesenfeld, S. L., Roos, R. P., Bobowick, A. R., Gibbs, C. J., Jr. and Gajdusek, D. C.: Familial Creutzfeldt-Jakob disease with a report on the transmission of the familial disease to the chimpanzee. Proc. Tenth Intern. Cong. Neurology, 1973.

Friede, R. L. and Dejong, R. N.: Neuronal enzymatic failure in Creutzfeldt-Jakob disease: a familial study. Arch. Neurol. 10: 181-195, 1964.

Gajdusek, D. C.: Bethesda, personal communication, 1973.

Gibbs, C. J., Jr., Gajdusek, D. C., Asher, D. M., Alpers, M. P., Beck, E., Daniel, P. M. and Matthews, W. B.: Creutzfeldt-Jakob disease (spongiform encephalopathy): transmission to the chimpanzee. Science 161: 388-389, 1968.

Jacob, H., Pyrkosch, W. and Strube, H.: Hereditary form of Creutzfeldt-Jakob disease (Backer family). Arch. Psychiatry 184: 653-674, 1950.

Kahana, E., Alter, M., Braham, J. and Sofer, D.: Creutzfeldt-Jakob disease: focus among Libyan Jews in Israel. Science 183: 90-91, 1974.

May, W. W., Itabashi, H. and Dejong, R. N.: Creutzfeldt-Jakob disease. II. Clinical, pathologic and genetic study of a family. Arch. Neurol. Psychiatry 19: 137-149, 1968.

Roos, R., Gajdusek, D. C. and Gibbs, C. J., Jr.: The clinical characteristics of transmissible Creutzfeldt-Jakob disease. Brain 96: 1-20, 1973.

Zlotnik, I., Grant, D. P., Dayan, A. D. and Earl, C. J.: Transmission of Creutzfeldt-Jakob disease from man to squirrel monkey. Lancet II: 435-438, 1974.

*12350 CROUZON CRANIOFACIAL DYSOSTOSIS

Crouzon disease is characterized by cranial synostosis, hypertelorism, exophthalmus and external strabismus, parrot-beaked nose, short upper lip, hypoplastic maxilla and a relative mandibular prognathism. The familial occurrence was noted by Crouzon in 1912 when he first described the syndrome. Subsequently, several investigators have demonstrated an autosomal dominant mode of inheritance. Shiller (1959) observed dominant transmission in four generations with 23 affected members. There was a marked variability in both cranial and facial manifestations of the syndrome. Andersen (1943) also traced the condition through 4 generations. Dodge et al. (1959) described five patients, three with typical Crouzon disease, two of these had a positive family history and one was sporadic. The other two cases, also sporadic, had syndactylism of both hands and feet, an association which has been designated as Vogt cephalodactyly (see ACROCEPHALO-SYNDACTYLY TYPES). Franceschetti (1953) described two unrelated cases which simulate Crouzon disease: however the patients do not have the facial manifestations. To differentiate these cases from Crouzon disease, Franceschetti coined the term 'pseudo-Crouzon syndrome.' Vulliamy and Normandale (1966) identified 14 cases of Crouzon disease in 4 generations of a family with several instances of male-to-male transmission. See PHOSPHATASE, PLACENTAL ALKALINE. See CRANIAL DYSOSTOSIS WITH PRONOUNCED DIGITAL IMPRESSIONS (PSEUDO-CROUZONS DISEASE). Three generations were affected in the family reported by Palacios and Schimke (1969). Flippen (1950) also traced the malformation through four generations, and Pinkerton and Pinkerton (1952) observed it in a mother and two of her three daughters. Juberg and Chambers (1973) suggested, on the basis of an affected brother and sister with unaffected non-consanguineous parents, that a recessive form of Crouzon disease exists. It seems more likely that they were dealing with a recessive form of craniostenosis (see 21850).

Andersen, P. F.: Craniofacial dysostosis (Crouzon's disease) as dominant hereditary disease. Nord. Med. 18: 993-996, 1943.

Crouzon, O.: Dysostose cranio-faciale hereditaire. Bull. Soc. Med. Hosp. Paris 33: 545-555, 1912.

Dodge, H. W., Wood, M. W. and Kennedy, R. L. J.: Craniofacial dysostosis.: Crouzon's disease. Pediatrics 23: 98-106, 1959.

Flippen, J. H., Jr.: Cranio-facial dysostosis of Crouzon. Report of a case in which the malformation occurred in four generations. Pediatrics 5: 90-96, 1950.

Franceschetti, A.: Dysostose cranienne avec calotte cerebriforme (pseudo-Crouzon). Confin. Neurol. 13: 161-166, 1953.

Juberg, R. C. and Chambers, S. R.: An autosomal recessive form of craniofacial dysostosis (the Crouzon syndrome). J. Med. Genet. 10: 89-93, 1973.

Palacios, E. and Schimke, R. N.: Craniosynostosis-syndactylism. Am. J. Roentgen. 106: 144-155, 1969.

Pinkerton, O. D. and Pinkerton, F. J.: Hereditary craniofacial dysplasia. Am. J. Ophthalmol. 35: 500-506, 1952.

Shiller, J. G.: Craniofacial dysostosis of Crouzon. A case report and pedigree with emphasis on heredity. Pediatrics 23: 107-112, 1959.

Vulliamy, D. G. and Normandale, P. A.: Cranio-facial dysostosis in a Dorset family. Arch. Dis. Child. 41: 375-382, 1966.

12360 CRYPTORCHIDISM, UNILATERAL

In 8 males in four generations, Perrett and O'Rourke (1969) described ipsilateral (right-sided) cryptorchidism. Corbus and O'Conor (1922) found several reports of families with multiple generations affected.

Corbus, B. C. and O'Conor, V. J.: The familial occurrence of undescended testes. Report of six brothers with testicular anomalies. Surg. Gynecol. Obstet. 34: 237-240, 1922.

Perrett, L. J. and O'Rourke, D. A.: Hereditary cryptorchidism. Med. J. Aust. 1: 1289-1290, 1969.

*12370 CUTIS LAXA

In some families the findings suggest that cutis laxa is inherited as a recessive (q.v.). However, Sestak (1962) reported affected father and daughter. See also the earlier report of dominant inheritance by Wiener (1925). (Beighton (1972) concluded that Wiener's family had the Ehlers-Danlos syndrome.) Goltz (1966) has a family with affected persons in successive generations. Balboni (1963) described a child with typical cutis laxa and multiple vascular anomalies including coarctation of the aorta. The father and a paternal uncle were thought to have the same condition. Beighton (1972) described two pedigrees with two or more generations affected. In each pedigree there was an instance of male-to-male transmission. In each case, however, the relevant males were not examined by the author. In the early report of Kopp (1888), the father had onset of cutis laxa at age 16 and in the son cutis laxa was present at birth. Other 'dominant' pedigrees were reported by Lewis (mother and daughter) (1948), Reidy (father and daughter) (1963) and Schreiber and Tilley (four generations) (1961). (Another of the families reported by Schreiber and Tilley (1961), vis. no. 1, had the acromegaloid syndrome (10210). As opposed to the recessive form of cutis laxa (21910), the dominant form is apparently free of pulmonary and other grave internal manifestations.

Balboni, F. A.: Cutis laxa and multiple vascular anomalies including multiple coarctation of the aorta. A case report. St. Francis Hosp. Bull. 19: 26-35, 1963.

Beighton, P. H.: The dominant and recessive forms of cutis laxa. J. Med. Genet. 9: 216-221, 1972.

Goltz, R. W.: Denver, Col.: personal communication, 1966.

Kopp, W.: Demonstration zweier Faelle von 'cutis laxa'. Muenchen. Med. Wschr. 35: 259, 1888.

Lewis, E.: Cutis laxa. Proc. R. Soc. Med. 41: 864, 1948.

Reidy, J. P.: Cutis hyperelastica (Ehlers-Danlos) and cutis laxa. Br. J. Plast. Surg. 16: 84-94, 1963.

Schreiber, M. M. and Tilley, J. C.: Cutis laxa. Arch. Dermatol. 84: 266-272, 1961.

Sestak, Z.: Ehlers-Danlos syndrome and cutis laxa: an account of families in the Oxford area. Ann. Hum. Genet. 25: 313-321, 1962.

Wiener, K.: Gummihaut (cutis laxa) mit dominanter Vererbung. Arch. Dermatol. Syph. 148: 599-601, 1925.

12380 CUTIS LAXA, CORNEAL CLOUDING, MENTAL RETARDATION

De Barsy et al. (1968) described a 22-month-old girl who had cutis laxa with defective development of elastic fibers in the skin. The corneas were cloudy due to degeneration in Bowman membrane. Psychomotor development was retarded and she was generally hypotonic. There was no known parental consanguinity, the father being Greek and the mother Flemish. This probably is a distinct syndrome. Hoefnagel et al. (1972) reported a male with a similar picture. The patient had congenital bilateral athetosis and the authors pointed out that the case of De Barsy et al. (1968) did also.

De Barsy, A. M., Moens, E. and Dierckx, L.: Dwarfism, oligophrenia and degeneration of the elastic tissue in skin and cornea. A new syndrome? Helv. Paediatr. Acta 23: 305-313, 1968.

Hoefnagel, D., Pomeroy, J., Wurster, D. and Saxon, A.: Congenital athetosis, mental deficiency, dwarfism and laxity of skin and ligaments. Helv. Paediatr. Acta 26: 397-402, 1971.

12385 CYLINDROMATOSIS

Almost certainly cylindroma is an entity distinct from benign cystic epithelioma (13270) and is probably inherited as an autosomal dominant, although a female preponderance raises questions of X-linked dominance (see 31310). Schuermann and Weber (1937) presented a pedigree with 9 persons affected in 4 generations. Six of the 9 were female. Although no male-to-male transmission was noted, two daughters of an affected male were unaffected. Reed (1972) is of the view that this is a quite distinct disorder from hereditary benign cystic epithelioma (13270). See the latter condition for a discussion of the view that they are the same. See Harper (1971) for a dramatic example of cylindromatosis.

Harper, P. S.: Turban tumors (cylindromatosis). The Clinical Delineation of Birth Defects. XII. Skin, Hair and Nails. Baltimore: Williams and Wilkins, 1971. Pp. 338-341.

Reed, W. B.: Burbank, Cal.: personal communication, 1972.

Schuermann, H. and Weber, K.: Beitrag zur Kenntnis der Spieglerschen Tumoren (Cylindrome) nebst einigen Bemerkungen zum Epithelioma adenoides cysticum. Arch. Dermatol. Syph. 175: 682-695, 1937.

12390 CYSTS OF THE JAW

Swift and Horowitz (1969) observed multiple jaw cysts and calcification of the falx cerebri in multiple members of 3 generations. There were none of the other features of basal cell nevus syndrome (q.v.) and Charcot-Marie-Tooth syndrome was segregating in the same family. Thus it is not certain that jaw cysts represented a distinct entity in this family.

Swift, M. R. and Horowitz, S. L.: Familial jaw cysts in Charcot-Marie-Tooth disease. J. Med. Genet. 6: 193-195, 1969.

*12395 CYTOCHROME B(5)

This protein is bound to the endoplasmic reticulum. Electrons are transferred to cytochrome B(5) from NADH by the action of cytochrome B(5) reductase, and can be transferred from cytochrome B(5) to molecular oxygen by another enzyme.

Dayhoff, M. O.: Cytochrome B group. Atlas of Protein Sequence and Structure 1972 (Vol. 5). Washington: National Biomedical Research Foundation, 1972. Pp. D29-D33.

*12397 CYTOCHROME C

This enzyme is located in the mitochondria of all aerobic cells. It is involved in the electron transport system which functions in oxidative phosphorylation. It accepts electrons from cytochrome B and transfers them to cytochrome oxidase. In the process the iron of the heme group (which is identical to that of hemoglobin and myoglobin) shifts from the ferrous to the ferric state. Human cytochrome C has 104 amino acid residues (Dayhoff, 1972) and a molecular weight of 11,458. Extensive comparative sequence data useful in study of the evolution of proteins are available.

Dayhoff, M. O.: Cytochrome C group. Atlas of Protein Sequence and Structure 1972 (vol. 5). Washington: National Biomedical Research Foundation, 1972. Pp. D7-D27.

12400 CYTOCHROME-RELATED DISEASE OF MUSCLE AND NERVOUS SYSTEM

Spiro et al. (1970) described a 46-year-old man and his 16-year-old son with progressive ataxia, predominantly proximal muscle weakness, areflexia, extensor plantar responses, dementia, concomitant nonspecific myopathia and neuropathic changes in muscle. Studies of muscle mitochondria showed very loose coupling of oxidative phosphorylation and marked reduction in cytochrome B content.

Spiro, A. J., Moore, C. L., Prineas, J. W., Strasberg, P. M. and Rapin, I.: A cytochrome-related inherited disorder of the nervous system and muscle. Arch. Neurol. 23: 103-112, 1970.

12410 DANUBIAN ENDEMIC FAMILIAL NEPHROPATHY (DEFN; BALKAN NEPHROPATHY)

The endemic nephropathy, commonly called 'Balkan' is more properly called Danubian. It occurs in a relatively restricted rural area of Roumania, Bulgaria and Yugoslavia near the Danubian Iron Gates. Clinical, epidemiologic and laboratory investigations are thought to have excluded selected forms (although not necessarily all forms) of infection, parasitism, intoxication, and radiation. 'No genetic factors are evident. Of paramount importance are household factors and living conditions' (Craciun and Rosculescu, 1970). On the other hand these authors state that 'the disease in a family may disappear within two or three generations.' The histologic end stage of the kidney lesion is thought to be a form of primary amyloidosis.

Craciun, E. C. and Rosculescu, I.: On Danubian endemic familial nephropathy (Balkan nephropathy). Some problems. Am. J. Med. 49: 774-779, 1970.

*12420 DARIER-WHITE DISEASE (KERATOSIS FOLLICULARIS)

Grossly this disorder is characterized by the formation of keratotic papules located especially in the 'seborrheic areas.' Histologically, one finds (1) mild non-specific perivascular infiltration in the dermis; (2) dermal villi protruding into the epidermis; (3) supra-basal detachment of the spinal layer leading to the formation of lacunae containing acantholytic cells; (4) in the more superficial epidermis, dyskeratotic round epidermal cells ('corps ronds'), the most distinctive feature; and (5) in the stratum corneum; 'grains' which resemble parakerotic cells embedded in a hyperkeratotic horny layer. A family with affected members in five generations was reported by Hitch, Callaway and Moseley (1941). See ACROKERATOSIS VERRUCI-FORMIS for discussion of phenotypic overlap with that condition. When bullous lesions are present, the condition is difficult to distinguish from benign familial pemphigus (q.v.). Niordson and Sylvest (1965) also suggested that Hailey and Hailey familial benign pemphigus is simply a bullous variant of Darier keratosis follicularis and that both may be variants of acrokeratosis verruciformis. They observed one patient with clinical and histopathologic features of all three entities. The father, brother, sister and son had acrokeratosis verruciformis.

Hitch, J. M., Callaway, J. L. and Moseley, V.: Familial Darier's disease (keratosis follicularis). Sth. Med. J. 34: 578-586, 1941.

Madden, J. F.: Darier's disease (mother and four daughters). Arch. Dermatol. Syph. 43: 735 only, 1941.

Niordson, A. M. and Sylvest, B.: Bullous dyskeratosis follicularis and acrokeratosis verruciformis. Arch. Dermatol. 92: 166-168, 1965.

Witkop, C. J. and Gorlin, R. J.: Four hereditary mucosal syndromes. Arch. Dermatol. 84: 762-771, 1961.

12430 DARWINIAN POINT (OF PINNA)

For pictures, see page 292 of Winchester (1958).

Winchester, A. M.: Genetics. A survey of the principles of heredity. Boston: Houghton Mifflin Co., 1958 (2nd Ed.).

12440 DARWINIAN TUBERCLE (OF PINNA)

Quelprud (1935) did an extensive twin and family study.

Quelprud, T.: Zur Erblichkeit des Darwinschen Hoockerchens. Z. Morph. Anthrop. 34: 343-363, 1934. Rev. Eugen. News 20: 3-4, 1935.

*12450 DEAFNESS, CONGENITAL, WITH KERATOPACHYDERMIA AND CONSTRICTIONS OF FINGERS AND TOES

Nockemann (1961) presented four generations of a family in which four members had hyperkeratosis, constrictions on the fingers and toes, and congenital deafness. The proband, a 20-year-old man, developed hyperkeratosis of the palms of his hands and soles of his feet beginning about two years of age, followed by involvement of his knees and elbows. Rubbing produced thickenings elsewhere. A few years later there developed ringshaped furrows of the skin in the region of the middle of the five fingers, followed by involvement of the toes. The proband had congenital deafness. The author presented three other family members in four generations with similar findings. They were all deaf and dumb. Drummond (1939) presented the case of a 19-year-old deaf-mute girl with constricting bands around three fingers of each hand. The bands were a quarter inch in width completely encircling each finger. Marked hyperkeratosis of the palms was also present, together with epidermal thickening over the knuckles and knees. Gibbs and Frank (1966) described affected father and daughter, but are surely mistaken in calling it a variant of mal de Meleda, a recessive. The presence of digital constrictions and the absence of leukonychia appear to distinguish this disorder from that listed under KNUCKLE PADS, LEUKONYCHIA AND SENSINEURAL DEAFNESS (q.v.). The hyperkeratosis and deafness reported by Morris et al. (1969) is probably a distinct entity, as they suggested. Their patient was an isolated case.

Drummond, M.: A case of unusual skin disease. Irish J. Med. Sci. 8: 85-86, 1939.

Gibbs, R. C. and Frank, S. B.: Keratoma hereditaria mutilans (Vohwinkel). Differentiating features of conditions with constriction of digits. Arch. Dermatol. 94: 619-625, 1966.

Hyde, J. N. and Montgomery, F. H.: A Practical Treatise of Diseases of the Skin. Philadelphia: Lea Brothers and Co., 1901. 6th Ed.

Morris, J., Ackerman, A. B. and Koblenzer, P. T.: Generalized spiny hyperkeratosis, universal alopecia, and deafness. A previously undescribed syndrome. Arch. Dermatol. 100: 692-698, 1969.

Nockemann, P. F.: Erbliche Hornhautverdickung mit Schnuerfurchen an Fingern und Zehen und Innenohrschwerhoerigkeit. Med. Welt. 2: 1894-1900, 1961.

12460 DEAFNESS, ECTODERMAL DYSPLASIA, POLYDACTYLISM AND SYNDACTYLISM

Robinson, Miller, and Bensimon (1962) presented the pedigree of 17 persons in three generations with five affected. The propositus was a 15-year-old girl with fissured small dystrophic nails, coniform teeth with partial anodontia, and syndactylism of the toes of the right foot with union of the first and second toes, and the third with the fourth toe. She had severe sensorineural hearing loss and had attended a school for the deaf. One brother was normal while another brother and a sister and their mother had similar nail and dental defects. All affected members had a high frequency hearing loss together with a 70 db low frequency loss in the propositus. The maternal grandmother of the propositus was thought to have a similar syndrome but was not available for study. The authors found elevation of electrolyte concentrations in sweat, suggesting this was a characteristic hidrotic form of ectodermal dysplasia with delayed primary and secondary dentition, misshapen and missing teeth, and dystrophic small nails. The pattern of inheritance was dominant. Feinmesser and Zelig (1961) described a family with onychodystrophy and neural deafness, but without abnormalities of the teeth or digits, and with probable recessive inheritance (q.v.), suggesting this is a separate disease. The hidrotic nature of the ectodermal dysplasia distinguishes this condition from that described under DEAFNESS WITH ECTODERMAL DYSPLASIA (q.v.).

Feinmesser, M. and Zelig, S.: Congenital deafness associated with onychodystrophy. Arch. Otolaryngol. 74: 507-508, 1961.

Robinson, G. C., Miller, J. R., and Bensimon, J. R.: Familial ectodermal dysplasia with sensori-neural deafness and other anomalies. Pediatrics 30: 797-802, 1962.

*12470 DEAFNESS, MID-TONE NEURAL

Onset is in childhood and the range affected is 500 to 4000 cps. Williams and Roblee (1962) described affected mother and 3 of her 6 children. This disorder was well delineated by Konigsmark et al. (1970) who emphasized that it can be progressive contrary to the conclusion of Williams and Roblee (1962). They observed four families, two of which were extensively affected. They pointed out that the family reported by Martensson (1960) may have had the same disorder.

Konigsmark, B. W., Salman, S., Haskins, H. and Mengel, M.: Dominant midfrequency hearing loss. Ann. Otolaryngol. 79: 1-12, 1970.

Martensson, B.: Dominant hereditary nerve deafness. Acta Otolaryngol. 53: 270-274, 1960.

Williams, F. and Roblee, L. A.: Hereditary nerve deafness. Arch. Otolaryngol. 75: 69-77, 1962.

*12480 DEAFNESS, PROGRESSIVE HIGH-TONE NEURAL

Several distinct types of dominantly inherited deafness are identifiable on the basis of associated manifestations, age of onset, tendency to progression, and tonal range involved. Studies of vestibular function might provide further differentiation. Dominant deafness without pigmentary anomaly as in Waardenburg syndrome (q.v.) almost certainly exists (see review by Fraser, 1964). 8-12 percent of profound deafness of childhood may be dominant (including fresh mutations). Dolowitz and Stephens (1961) described high tone neural deafness present at all ages but more severe in older members of four generations of a Mormon kindred. Slow progression of the hearing loss over a period of several decades was well demonstrated. Huizing et al. (1966) studied 5 generations of an extensive kindred in which 67 persons had non-congenital progressive perceptive deafness. Onset was in early childhood with impairment of high frequencies. The loss increased rapidly with gradual extension of the impairment to lower frequencies. Paparella et al. (1969) described the anatomic findings in two cases of dominant progressive sensorineural deafness.

Dolowitz, D. A. and Stephens, F. E.: Hereditary nerve deafness. Ann. Otol. 70: 851-859, 1961.

Fraser, G. R.: Review article: profound childhood deafness. J. Med. Genet. 1: 118-151, 1964.

Huizing, E. H., Van Bolhuis, A. H. and Odenthal, D. W.: Studies on progressive hereditary perceptive deafness in a family of 335 members. I. Genetical and general audiological results. Acta Otolaryng. 61: 35-41, 1966. II. Characteristic patterns of hearing deterioration. Ibid. 61: 161-167, 1966.

Paparella, M. M., Sugiura, S. and Hoshino, T.: Familial progressive sensorineural deafness. Arch. Otolaryngol. 90: 44-51, 1969.

*12490 DEAFNESS, PROGRESSIVE LOW-TONE

The Vanderbilt group (1968) described low-frequency deafness of sensorineural type in a large kindred. Speech development, intelligence, vestibular function and general physical condition were normal. Autosomal dominant inheritance was demonstrated. Above 2000 cycles per second hearing was normal or near normal. A localized abnormality of the cochlear apex was suggested. Konigsmark et al. (1971) studied 3 families.

Konigsmark, B. W., Mengel, M. C. and Berlin, C. I.: Dominant low-frequency hearing loss. Report of three families. Laryngoscope 81: 759-771, 1971.

Vanderbilt University Hereditary Deafness Study Group: Dominantly inherited low-frequency hearing loss. Arch. Otolaryngol. 88: 242-250, 1968.

12495 DEAFNESS, SENSORINEURAL, WITH PERIPHERAL NEUROPATHY AND ARTERIAL DISEASE

Stewart (1973) has informed me of a remarkable family in which a woman, a son and daughter, and the daughter of the daughter had a syndrome of early onset sensorineural deafness, skin rash, headache, peripheral arterial disease (leading to gangrene after a small dose of ergotamine), peripheral neuropathy, elevation of spinal fluid protein and cells, papilledema and contracted retinal arteries. Mild saddle nose was present. The family was reported by Campbell and Clifton (1950) as an example of familial toxoplasmosis, a diagnosis based on serologic findings and no longer considered tenable.

Campbell, A. M. G. and Clifton, F.: Adult toxoplasmosis in one family. Brain 73: 281-290, 1950.

Stewart, G.: Camperdown, N. S. W., personal communication, 1973.

12500 DEAFNESS, UNILATERAL

Smith (1939) described a sibship of eight children, four of whom had total deafness in one or the other ear. The tympanic membranes were normal. Labyrinthine testing was normal. There was no history of consanguinity, mumps, or syphilis. The mother, her father, and her sister also had unilateral deafness while another sister became deaf and dumb after measles. This latter sister married a deaf and dumb man. One of their three children, a girl, had unilateral deafness. She had two children, one of whom has unilateral deafness. Thus there were nine persons with total unilateral deafness in four generations. Four were deaf in the right ear and four in the left, while the side was unknown in one case. Everberg (1960) studied 122 children with total unilateral deafness in one ear and normal hearing in the other. More than one case of unilateral deafness in the same family was found in 12 of the 122 families of these children.

Everberg, G.: Unilateral anacusis. Clinical, radiological and genetic investigations. Acta Otolaryngol. 158 (suppl.): 366-374, 1960.

Smith, A. B.: Unilateral hereditary deafness. Lancet 237: 1172-1173, 1939.

*12510 DEAFNESS, WITH EAR PITS (PERHAPS TWO OR MORE TYPES)

Fourman and Fourman (1955) described a family of 108 in which 17 members had preauricular pits. Twelve were deaf and one was not. The others were too young for testing. Of those without pits three were deaf: one of these had a branchial pit. The deafness varied from mild to severe. In some it had been recognized from childhood, others who were certain they had been able to hear perfectly until they were about 20 years old, when their hearing began to deteriorate. Audiograms showed both high and low tone loss, usually high tones more than the low. Hearing testing was done on two of the three cases with deafness but without pits. This showed the same audiogram pattern. There was no evidence of vestibular disorder. The authors suggest earpits, deafness, and branchial fistulae are independent effects of a single dominant gene with incomplete penetrance.

Wildervanck (1962) reviews 16 members of a family 14 of whom had either deformed auricles, marginal pits, or preauricular appendages. Two members had a moderate conductive deafness. In one the deafness was bilateral and in the other it was unilateral. The mode of inheritance is dominant with full penetration. Wildervanck suggests this is a different syndrome from that of Fourman and Fourman. McLaurin et al. (1966) reported a kindred with abnormalities like those reported by Wildervanck (1962). Similar branchial cleft anomalies (q.v.), apparently without deafness, have been reported and may be genetically distinct.

Fourman, P. and Fourman, J.: Hereditary deafness in family with ear-pits (fistula auris congenita). Br. Med. J. 2: 1354-1356, 1955.

McLaurin, J. W., Kloepfer, H. W., Laguaite, J. K. and Stallcup, T. A.: Hereditary branchial anomalies and associated hearing impairment. Laryngoscope 76: 1277-1288, 1966.

Rowley, P. T.: Familial hearing loss associated with branchial fistulas. Pediatrics 44: 978-985, 1970.

Wildervanck, L. S.: Hereditary malformations of the ear in three generations. Acta Otolaryngol. 54: 553-560, 1962.

12520 DEAFNESS, WITH ECTODERMAL DYSPLASIA

Helweg-Larsen and Ludvigsen (1946) reported a kindred of 14 with anhidrotic ectodermal dysplasia, four of whom had defective hearing with onset between 35 and 45 years of age. Ellingson (1951) found hearing loss in two brothers with ectodermal dysplasia. See also ECTODERMAL DYSPLASIA, HIDROTIC, WITH NERVE DEAFNESS AND FINGER ANOMALIES.

Ellingson, R. J.: Major hereditary ectodermal dysplasia. J. Pediatr. 38: 191-198, 1951.

Helweg-Larsen, H. F. and Ludvigsen, K.: Congenital familial anhidrosis and neurolabyrinthitis. Acta Derm. Venerol. 26: 489-505, 1946.

12525 DEAFNESS — OPTIC ATROPHY SYNDROME

Konigsmark et al. (1974) described an association of congenital deafness with late onset, progressive optic atrophy. Six persons in four generations were affected. No male-to-male transmission was noted. However, males and females were equally severely affected and a daughter of an affected male was not affected.

Konigsmark, B. W., Knox, D. L., Hussels, I. E. and Moses, H.: Dominant congenital deafness and progressive optic nerve atrophy. Arch. Ophthalol. 91: 99-103, 1974.

12530 DENS IN DENTE AND PALATAL INVAGINATIONS

Dens in dente and deep palatal invaginations (lingual pits) of the secondary maxillary lateral incisors may be inherited as an autosomal dominant. Grahner et al. (1959) found in a study of 3000 Swedish children a frequency of about 3 per cent. In 58 families studied a similar defect was found in over one-third of parents. In the same family some had dens in dente and others had deep lingual pits. Lingual pits offer a favorable setting for development of caries.

Grahner, H., Lindahl, B. and Omnell, K. A.: Dens invaginatus. I. A clinical, roentgenological and genetical study of permanent upper lateral incisors. Odont. Rev. 10: 115-137, 1959.

12540 DENTINE DYSPLASIA ('ROOTLESS TEETH,' DENTINE HYPOPLASIA)

Both primary and secondary dentitions are affected. The color of the teeth is usually normal. Teeth are often malaligned in the arch and may exfoliate with minor trauma. By X-ray the dental roots are demonstrated to be markedly distorted and reduced in size. Rushton (1955) described the histologic characteristics. Finn (1962) expressed the view that this is a severe manifestation of dentinogenesis imperfecta and that transition between the two types is evident within families. Witkop (1965) states that he 'has personally examined over 1,000 cases of dentinogenesis imperfecta from 42 extensive kindreds and over 50 cases of dentin hypoplasia from 4 kindreds and has yet to find any case remotely resembling a transition from one disease to the other. The clinical, radiographic and histologic findings are distinctly different in the two conditions.' Absence of the lamina dura of the teeth, as detected by X-ray, suggests the diagnosis of hyperparathyroidism. However, Graham et al. (1965) found such in a father and two daughters with no evidence of deranged calcium or phosphorus metabolism. Dentin was abnormal making this a primary disorder of the teeth. Gorlin (1971) states that the disorder in this family was dentine dysplasia.

Finn, S. B.: Dentin and enamel anomalies. In, Witkop, C. J., Jr. (ed.): Genetics and Dental Health. New York: McGraw-Hill, 1962. Pp. 219-245.

Graham, W. L., Harley, J. B., Alberico, C. and Kelln, E. E.: Absent lamina dura associated with a developmental dentin abnormality. A family study. Arch. Intern. Med. 116: 837-841, 1965.

Logan, J., Becker, H., Silverman, S., Jr. and Pindborg, J. J.: Dentinal dysplasia. Oral. Surg. 15: 317-333, 1962.

Rushton, M. A.: Anomalies of human dentine. Ann. Roy. Coll. Surg. Eng. 16: 94-117, 1955.

Witkop, C. J.: Genetic disease of the oral cavity. In, Tiecke, R. W. (ed.): Oral Pathology. New York: McGraw-Hill, 1965.

*12542 DENTINE DYSPLASIA II (ANOMALOUS DYSPLASIA OF DENTINE)

Sheilds et al. (1973) described a 'new' heritable dental defect manifested as an amber, translucent discoloration and total pulpal obliteration in all primary teeth. Permanent teeth had a thistle-tube pulp configuration with ubiquitous pulp stones but normal coloration. They speculated that the abnormal dentine may have induced odontoblastic differentiation to give rise to the denticles. They proposed a classification of dentine defects into two major groups, dentine dysplasia and dentinogenesis imperfecta. They suggested that the condition in their family be called dentine dysplasia II.

Sheilds, E. D., Bixler, D. and El-Kafrawy, A. M.: A proposed classification for heritable human dentine defect with a description of a new entity. Arch. Oral Biol. 18: 543-553, 1973.

*12550 DENTINOGENESIS IMPERFECTA (CAPEDEPONT TEETH, OR OPALESCENT DENTINE)

The primary defect is mesodermal, involving dentine. An identical disorder occurs as part of the osteogenesis imperfecta syndrome. However, there is clearly a distinct entity inherited as a dominant and affecting only the teeth. Johnson (1959) described three families containing at least sixty-two affected persons. The teeth vary in color from opalescent blue to amber brown. The enamel splits from the dentine readily when subjected to occlusal stress. The frequency may be 1 in 6000 to 8000 children (Witkop, 1957). Study of a large affected kindred in a Maryland tri-racial isolate showed the variability in clinical picture (Hursey et al., 1956). This condition is also called hereditary brown teeth. Witkop and Rao (1971) prefer the term opalescent dentine for this condition as an isolated trait, reserving dentinogenesis imperfecta for the trait when it is combined with osteogenesis imperfecta. They gave an account of the genealogies of American kindreds. Shokeir (1972) described a probable homozygote. Sheilds et al. (1973) proposed that the variety of dentiogenesis imperfecta described the the Brandywine isolate by Hursey et al. (1956) was distinct from other reported dentinogenesis imperfecta. A significant number of the Brandywine cases had 'shell teeth' in which dentine formation ceased after the mantle layer was formed.

Hursey, R. J., Witkop, C. J., Jr., Miklashek, D. and Sackett, L. M.: Dentinogenesis imperfecta in a racial isolate with multiple hereditary defects. Oral Surg. 9: 641-658, 1956.

Ivancie, G. P.: Dentinogenesis imperfecta. Oral Surg. 7: 984-992, 1954.

Johnson, O. N., Chaudhry, A. P., Gorlin, R. J., Mitchell, D. F. and Bartholdi, W. L.: Hereditary dentinogenesis imperfecta. J. Pediatr. 54: 786-792, 1959.

Roberts, E. and Schour, I.: Hereditary opalescent dentine — dentinogenesis imperfecta. Am. J. Orthodont. 25: 267-276, 1939.

Sheilds, E. D., Bixler, D. and El-Kafrawy, A. M.: A proposed classification for heritable human dentine defect with a description of a new entity. Arch. Oral Biol. 18: 543-553, 1973.

Shokeir, M. H. K.: Dentinogenesis imperfecta: severe expression in a probable homozygote. Clin. Genet. 3: 442-447, 1972.

Wallace, J. R.: Hereditary dentinogenesis imperfecta. J. Pediatr. 65: 128-130, 1964.

Wilson, G. W. and Steinbecher, M.: Hereditary hypoplasia of the dentine. J. Am. Dent. Assoc. 16: 866-870, 1929.

Witkop, C. J. and Rao, S. R.: Inherited defects in tooth structure. The Clinical Delineation of Birth Defects. XI. Orofacial Structures. Baltimore: Williams and Wilkins, 1971. Pp. 153-184.

Witkop, C. J.: Hereditary defects in enamel and dentin. Acta Genet. Statist. Med. 7: 236-239, 1957.

Witkop, C. J., MacLean, C. J., Schmidt, P. J. and Henry, J. L.: Medical and dental findings in the Brandywine isolate. Ala. J. Med. Sci. 3: 382-403, 1966.

12553 DERMAL RIDGES, NELSON SYNDROME

David (1973) observed a single family in which inheritance was apparently autosomal dominant.

David, T. J.: Ridges-off-the-end syndrome in two families, and a third family with a new syndrome. Hum. Hered. 23: 32-41, 1973.

*12554 DERMAL RIDGES, PATTERNLESS

Disturbance of ridge formation resulting in scattered short ridges, or ridges simply comprising irregular dots, is a feature in patients with the Down syndrome and in some patients with limb malformations. It has also been observed as a familial disorder apparently transmitted as an autosomal dominant. Most earlier cases were reported from Japan (references in Holt, 1968) but it has also been reported in a Belgian pedigree by Dodinval (1971).

Dodinval, P., Lebanc, P., Delree, C. and Deslypere, P.: Dysplasie des cretes epidermiques a heredite dominante autosomique. Etude des dermatoglyphes d'une famille. Humangenetik 11: 230-236, 1971.

Holt, S. B.: The genetics of dermal ridges. Springfield, Ill.: Charles C Thomas, 1968.

David, T. J.: Ridges-off-the-end syndrome in two families, and a third family with a new syndrome. Hum. Hered. 23: 32-41, 1973.

*12555 DERMAL 'RIDGES-OFF-THE-END'

The cardinal characteristic is that the fingertip ridges, instead of running transversely, are vertical and run vertically off the end of the fingertips. Bilateral radial loops on the ring and little fingers (exceedingly rare in persons without this syndrome) are usual here. David (1971) concluded the trait is autosomal dominant. In his first family several other dominant traits were segregating independently. David (1973) described two further families and a third family, with the surname Nelson, in which a new dermatoglyphic syndrome occurred in mother and three children. Although the palmar features were the same as those in ROES, other features were clearly different.

David, T. J.: 'Ridges-off-the-end' — a dermatoglyphic syndrome. Hum. Hered. 21: 39-53, 1971.

David, T. J.: Ridges-off-the-end syndrome in two families, and a third family with a new syndrome. Hum. Hered. 23: 32-41, 1973.

12558 DERMATOGLYPHICS — FINGER RIDGE COUNT

Dermatoglyphics, as defined by finger ridge count, are considered a classic example of polygenic inheritance in man (Holt, 1968). Analysis of data by Spence et al. (1973) led to the suggestion that a single major autosomal locus with two additive alleles may account for over half the variation in absolute ridge count.

Holt, S. B.: The Genetics of Dermal Ridges. Springfield, Ill.: Charles C Thomas, 1968.

Spence, M. A., Elston, R. C., Namboodiri, K. K. and Pollitzer, W. S.: Evidence for a possible major gene effect in absolute finger ridge count. Hum. Hered. 23: 414-421, 1973.

12560 DERMATOSIS PAPULOSA NIGRA

Although nothing is clearly established about the genetics of this disorder, the occurrence predominantly in Negroes is consistent with a genetic basis. As many as 35 percent of adult Negroes may be affected. The disorder is somewhat more frequent in females. The papules occur most typically on the face below the eyes and on the cheeks. Castellani (1925) described and named this disorder, which he found to be very frequent among the Negroes of Jamaica and Central America. The lesions are black and dark-brown papules, sometimes cupoliform or at times flattened, situated on the face, principally on both malar regions, being rare or absent on the lower parts of the face and chin. Onset is usually about the time of puberty. Butterworth and Strean (1962) expressed the opinion that this condition is merely a variant of seborrheic keratoses that occurs predominantly in Negroes.

Butterworth, T. and Strean, L. P.: Clinical Genodermatology. Baltimore: Williams and Wilkins. 1962.

Castellani, A.: Observations on some diseases of Central America. J. Trop. Med. Hyg. 28: 1-14, 1925.

*12565 DESMOSTEROL-TO-CHOLESTEROL ENZYME

An enzyme which catalyzes conversion of desmosterol to cholesterol is determined by a locus on chromosome no. 20, according to cell hybrid studies (2nd International Workshop of Human Gene Mapping, Rotterdam, July, 1974). Desmosterol reductase is another name for the enzyme that converts desmosterol to cholesterol.

Croce, C. M.: Philadelphia, personal communication, 1974.

*12570 DIABETES INSIPIDUS, NEUROHYPOPHYSEAL TYPE

Normally the posterior pituitary hormones, antidiuretic hormone and oxytocin, are synthesized in the supraoptic and para-ventricular nuclei of the hypothalamus and transported within axons, possibly in a biologically inactive, bound form, to the posterior lobe of the pituitary where they are stored. One of the most dramatic examples of familial diabetes insipidus is that reported by Adolph Weil (1884) of Heidelberg and his son Alfred (1908). Seven generations were affected. Dolle (1950-52) reported a follow-up on this family. It contained numerous instances of male-to-male transmission. Braverman, Mancini and McGoldrick (1965) reported the postmortem findings in a case of pitressin-responsive diabetes insipidus. As in five previous reported cases, a striking decrease in the nerve cells of the supraoptic and paraventicular nuclei of the hypothalamus with associated mild gliosis was found. In this family the father and paternal grandmother were thought to have had diabetes insipidus. In the sibship of the proband, a male, two sisters had definite diabetes insipidus and a brother may have been affected. One child of each of three of the sibs was also thought to have the disorder. Dominant pedigrees of pitressin responsive diabetes insipidus were reported by Pender and Fraser (1953), Moehlig and Schultz (1955) and Martin (1959). One would scarcely expect a defect in synthesis of antidiuretic hormone to behave as a dominant. Isolated deficiencies of other pituitary hormones (e.g., sexual ateliosis) behave as recessives. An apparent defect in synthesis of vasopressin in the rat results in diabetes insipidus only in the homozygote, although the heterozygote shows reduced vasopressin. Oxytocin synthesis is not impaired (Valtin et al., 1965). Morphologic features suggest excessive activity of the hypothalamoneurohypophysial system which controls secretion of vasopressin (Sokol and Valtin 1965). Both autosomal dominant and X-linked inheritance of both renal and neurohypophyseal diabetes insipidus have been reported. Most often, however, the neurohypophyseal type is autosomal dominant and the renal type is X-linked. Autosomal dominant diabetes insipidus is associated with oligosyndactyly in the mouse (Falconer et al., 1964). The neurohypophyseal type is recessive in rats.

Braverman, L. E., Mancini, J. P. and McGoldrick, D. M.: Hereditary idiopathic diabetes insipidus. A case report with autopsy findings. Ann. Intern. Med. 63: 503-508, 1965.

Dolle, W.: Eine weitere Ergaenzung des Weilschen Diabetes-insipidus-Stammbaumes. Z. Menschl. Vererb. Konstitutionsl. 30: 372-374, 1950-52.

Falconer, D. S., Latsyzewski, M. and Isaacson, J. H.: Diabetes insipidus associated with oligosyndactyly in the mouse. Genet. Res. 5: 473-488, 1964.

Martin, F. I. R.: Familial diabetes insipidus. Quart. J. Med. 28: 573-582, 1959.

Moehlig, R. C. and Schultz, R. C.: Familial diabetes insipidus. Report of one of fourteen cases in four generations. J.A.M.A. 158: 725-727, 1955.

Pender, C. B. and Fraser, F. C.: Dominant inheritance of diabetes insipidus: a family study. Pediatrics 11: 246-254, 1953.

Sokol, H. W. and Valtin, H.: Morphology of the neurosecretory system in rats homogzygous and heterozygous for hypothalamic diabetes insipidus (Brattleboro strain). Endocrinology 77: 692-700, 1965.

Valtin, H.: Hereditary hypothalamic diabetes insipidus in rats (Brattleboro strain). Am. J. Med. 42: 814-827, 1967

Valtin, H., Sawyer, W. H. and Sokol, H. W.: Neurohypophysial principles in rats homozygous and heterozygous for hypothalamic diabetes insipidus (Brattleboro strain). Endocrinology 77: 701-706, 1965.

Weil, A.: Ueber die hereditaere Form des Diabetes insipidus. Deutsch. Arch. Klin. Med. 93: 180-290, 1908.

Weil, A.: Ueber die hereditaere Form des Diabetes insipidus. Virchow. Arch. Path. Anat. 95: 70-95, 1884.

12580 DIABETES INSIPIDUS, RENAL TYPE

Cannon (1955) traced a family back to 1813. The family contained 3 instances of male-to-male transmission. Assuming that the information was accurate and that consanguinity was not present, this excludes X-linked inheritance, which is more frequent. Cannon did note reduced penetrance in females with conductors not showing the disorder. This makes one suspicious that this was in fact the X-linked form of diabetes insipidus.

Cutler et al. (1955) proved the renal basis of the problem in this family. Bode and Crawford (1969) seem to have established the X-linked inheritance of the kindred reported by Cannon, by finding a suggestive tie-in with the very large, clearly X-linked pedigree descendant from persons who came to North America on the ship Hopewell. Ten Bensel and Peters (1970) restudied part of Cannon's pedigree and showed typical X-linked inheritance. Weller, Elliott and Gusman (1950), and Levinger and Escamilla (1955), described dominant pedigrees. One must distinguish renal and neurohypophyseal types in these reports, however.

Bode, H. H. and Crawford, J. D.: Nephrogenic diabetes insipidus in North America — the Hopewell hypothesis. N. Engl. J. Med. 280: 750-754, 1969.

Cannon, J. F.: Diabetes insipidus: clinical and experimental studies with consideration of genetic relationships. Arch. Intern. Med. 96: 215-272, 1955.

Cutler, R. E., Kleeman, C. R., Maxwell, M. H. and Dowling, J. T.: Physiologic studies in nephrogenic diabetes insipidus. J. Clin. Endocrinol. Metab. 22: 215-272, 1955.

Levinger, E. L. and Escamilla, R. F.: Hereditary diabetes insipidus: report of 20 cases in seven generations. J. Clin. Endocrinol. Metab. 15: 547-552, 1955.

Robinson, M. G., and Kaplan, S. A.: Inheritance of vasopressin-resistant ('nephrogenic') diabetes insipidus. Am. J. Dis. Child. 99: 164-174, 1960.

Weller, C. G., Elliott, W. and Gusman, A. R.: Hereditary diabetes insipidus: unusual urinary tract changes. J. Urol. 64: 716-721, 1950.

12585 DIABETES MELLITUS, AUTOSOMAL DOMINANT (MILD JUVENILE DIABETES MELLITUS)

Tattersall (1974) described three families with an autosomal dominant form of diabetes. This form had early onset, but mild and relatively uncomplicated course. For example, 7 out of 12 diabetics diagnosed under the age of 30 years had no retinopathy after an average duration of 37 years. In two of the families diabetes was associated with a low renal threshold for glucose. They noted transmission over at least 3 generations with 50 percent of affected children of an affected parent and an affected parent of almost all affected persons.

Tattersall, R. B.: Mild familial diabetes with dominant inheritance. Quart. J. Med. 43: 339-357. 1974.

*12590 DIASTEMA, DENTAL MEDIAL

A space between the superior central incisors is probably inherited as a dominant trait. Weninger (1933) studied 24 families, observing four generations affected in some. Persons with this trait have, in the past, been referred to as 'gat-toothed.'

Weninger, M.: Zur Vererbung des medianen Oberkiefertremas. Z. Morph. Anthrop. 32: 367-393, 1933.

12600 DIBASICAMINOACIDURIA I

Whelan and Scriver (1968) found excessive lysine, ornithine and arginine excretion in 13 members of a French-Canadian kindred. Plasma levels of these amino acids were normal. The endogenous renal clearance of the three amino acids was increased but that of cystine was normal. Intestinal absorption of L-lysine was impaired but that of L-cystine was normal. The relation to the disorder described in Finland and in Japan and called here dibasicaciduria II is unclear. Whelan and Scriver suggested that the two disorders may be allelic. The French-Canadian patients were asymptomatic except for mild intestinal malabsorption syndrome in the proband. The Finnish patients had severe protein intolerance. Kihara et al. (1973) described a presumed homozygote. The parents were first cousins of Italian extraction. Both parents and 9 other family members in four generations showed excretion patterns consistent with the heterozygous state. The homozygote was institutionalized because of mental retardation. She showed adverse reactions to three phenothiazines.

Kihara, H., Valente, M., Porter, M. T. and Fluharty, A. L.: Hyperdibasicaminociduria in a mentally retarded homozygote with a peculiar response to phenothiazines. Pediatrics 51: 223-229, 1973.

Whelan, D. T. and Scriver, C. R.: Hyperdibasicaminoaciduria: an inherited disorder of amino acid transport. Pediatr. Res. 2: 525-534, 1968.

12605 DIGITO-TALAR DYSMORPHISM

Sallis and Beighton (1972) described a new syndrome consisting of flexion deformity of the fingers and 'rocker-bottom' feet due to vertical talus. Fourteen persons in five generations were affected but no instance of male-to-male transmission was observed. Stevenson et al. (1974) described the same trait in a large American Negro family. They emphasized the ulnar deviation of the fingers. Their patients lacked vertical talus and short stature.

Sallis, J. G.: Dominantly inherited digito-talar dysmorphism. J. Bone Joint Surg. 54: 509-515, 1972.

Stevenson, R. E., Scott, C. I., Jr., and Epstein, M. J.: Dominantly inherited ulnar drift. To be published, 1974.

12607 DILUTION, PIGMENTARY

The term incomplete, or partial albinism or hypopigmentation would be appropriate. Fitzpatrick (1973) has observed a family with male-to-male transmission and knows of others. The iris transilluminates to an abnormal degree and the subjects have photophobia.

Fitzpatrick, T. B.: Boston, personal communication, 1973.

12610 DIMPLES, FACIAL

Cheek dimples may be inherited as an irregular dominant.

12620 DISSEMINATED SCLEROSIS (MULTIPLE SCLEROSIS)

Familial aggregation in this disease is not strong. However, Bas (1964) in a series of 91 cases found 3 instances of affected mother and daughter. From an extensive review, McAlpine (1965) concluded that the risk for a first degree relative of a patient with multiple sclerosis is at least 15 times that for a member of the general population but that no definite genetic pattern is discernible. See MULTIPLE SCLEROSIS-LIKE DISEASE. MacKay and Myrianthopoulos (1966) found that concordance is slightly higher in monozygotic than in dizygotic twins and that multiple sclerosis is about 20 times more frequent among relatives of probands than in the general population. The frequency declined as the relationship to the proband became more remote. They concluded that the family data consistent with autosomal recessive inheritance with reduced penetrance but that exogenous factors must be very strong. On the other hand, the concordance rate in monozygotic twins is so low that it is difficult to think that genetic factors are of great importance. There appear to be rare forms of multiple sclerosis or multiple sclerosis-like diseases which are genetic. Ekbom (1966) described a familial form of multiple sclerosis associated with narcolepsy. For example, in one family two brothers had MS, combined in one with narcolepsy. In another family three sisters had MS and of the three one had narcolepsy. See ATAXIA, SPASTIC.

Bas, H.: Sclerosis multiplex familiaris. Z. Aerztl. Fortbild. 58: 153-155, 1964.

Ekbom, K.: Familial multiple sclerosis associated with narcolepsy. Arch. Neurol. 15: 337-344, 1966.

MacKay, R. P. and Myrianthopoulos, N. C.: Multiple sclerosis in twins and their relatives. Final report. Arch. Neurol. 15: 449-462, 1966.

McAlpine, D.: Familial incidence and its significance. Multiple Sclerosis: a reappraisal. McAlpine, D., Lumsden, C. E. and Acheson, E. D. (eds.): Baltimore: Williams and Wilkins Co., 1965. Pp. 61-74.

*12630 DISTICHIASIS (TWO ROWS OF EYELASHES)

Fox (1962) reviewed the heredity of this anomaly. Dominant pedigrees were presented by Erdmann (1904) and by Cockayne (1933). Blatt (1924) traced double rows of eyelashes through three generations. See TRISTICHIASIS. The terms 'distichiasis' and 'tristichiasis' refer to two or three hairs per follicle. Much confusion exists, however, and 'distichiasis' and 'districhiasis' are often used interchangeably to mean 'two rows of eyelashes.' In three generations of a family Pico (1957) found 11 persons with congenital ectropion and of these 8 also had distichiasis. Two persons had distichiasis alone. Histologic study in two showed absence of Meibomian glands and replacement of the dense collagenous tissue of the tarsal plates by loose areolar tissue. Szily's observation (1923) suggested recessive inheritance. See LYMPHEDEMA WITH DISTICHIASIS.

Blatt, N.: Districhiasis congenita vera. Z. Augenheilk. 53: 325-338, 1924.

Cockayne, E. A.: Inherited Abnormalities of the Skin and its Appendages. London: Oxford U. Press, 1933.

Erdmann, P.: Ein Beitrag zur Kenntnis der Distichiasis congenita (hereditaria). Z. Augenheilk. 11: 427-444, 1904.

Fox, S. A.: Distichiasis. Am. J. Ophthal. 53: 14-18, 1962.

Pico, G.: Congenital ectropion and districhiasis. Etiologic and hereditary factors: a report of cases and review of the literature. Trans. Am. Ophthalmol. Soc. 55: 663-700, 1957.

Szily, A. von: Ueber Haarbildung in der Meibomschen Druese und ueber behaarte Meibomdruesen (sogenannte Districhiasis congenita vera). Klin. Mbl. Augenheilk. 70: 16-45, 1923.

12635 DOPAMINE BETA-HYDROXYLASE, PLASMA

Dopamine beta-hydroxylase (DBH; E.C.1.14.2.1), the enzyme that converts dopamine to norepinephrine, is present in the synaptic vesicles of postganglionic sympathetic neurons. Release of norepinephrine is accompanied by the simultaneous release of DBH. For this reason, it has been proposed that plasma DBH may serve as an index of sympathetic activity. Schanberg et al. (1974) found that subjects showed a wide range of values with a 'low' group and a 'high' group. The high group tended to show higher and less stable levels of blood pressure. Whether a major locus determines the plasma levels of DBH remains to be established. In a twin study Ross et al. (1973) found a high concordance for level of DBH activity in monozygotic twins than in dizygotic twins.

Ross, S. B., Wetterberg, L. and Myrhed, M.: Genetic control of plasma dopamine-beta-hydroxylase. Life Sciences 12: 529-532, 1973.

Schanberg, S. M., Stone, R. A., Kirshner, N., Gunnells, J. C. and Robinson, R. R.: Plasma dopamine beta-hydroxylase: a possible aid in the study and elevation of hypertension. Science 183: 523-525, 1974.

12640 DOUBLE ATHETOSIS (STATUS MARMORATUS, OR 'LITTLE'S DISEASE WITH INVOLUNTARY MOVEMENTS')

Patzig (1939) believed that the group of infantile cerebral palsies characterized by status marmoratus of the striatum (Vogt disease) is hereditary. He described the disorder in a girl, her father and his uncle. Eleven members of the father's family exhibited pronounced involuntary movements of a non-progressive athetoid nature.

Patzig, B.: Erbbiologie und Erbpathologie des Gehirns. In, Handbuch der Erbbiologie des Menschen. 5: (Part 1) 233-349, 1939.

Temtamy observed a mother and son with double nails on the little toes — one on top of the other. The woman's grandson (J. A., 988558) through an unaffected daughter had post-axial polydactyly (q.v.).

Temtamy, S. A.: Genetic Factors in Hand Malformations. Ph. D. Thesis, Johns Hopkins University, 1966.

*12660 DOYNE HONEYCOMB DEGENERATION OF RETINA

Characteristically small round white spots involving the posterior pole of the eye including the areas of the macula and optic disc appear in early adult life. Progression to form a mosaic pattern which Doyne (1899) aptly termed 'honeycomb' occurs thereafter. Doyne considered it to represent 'choroiditis.' However, Collins (1913) showed that the changes consist of swelling in the inner part of Bruch membrane. Failing vision usually developed considerably later than the ophthalmologic change. Doyne was an ophthalmologist in Oxford, England. Pearce (1967) did an extensive study of six kindreds living near Oxford. Some and possibly all may have been descendants from a common ancestor. Dominant inheritance with complete manifestation of the trait in persons surviving beyond early adult life was found. Families living elsewhere than England have been reported (see references given by Pearce, 1968).

Collins, E. T.: A pathological report upon a case of Doyne's choroiditis. Ophthalmoscope 11: 537-538, 1913.

Doyne, R. W.: A peculiar condition of choroiditis occurring in several members of the same family. Trans. Ophthalmol. Soc. U.K. 19: 71 Only, 1899.

Pearce, W. G.: Doyne's honeycomb retinal degeneration. Clinical and genetic features. Br. J. Ophthalmol. 52: 73-78, 1968.

Pearce, W. G.: Genetic aspects of Doyne's honeycomb degeneration of the retina. Ann. Hum. Genet. 31: 173-188, 1967.

12670 DRUSEN OF BRUCH MEMBRANE

Deutman and Jansen (1970) described a family in which 8 persons in 5 sibships had confirmed multiple drusen of Bruch membrane. There was no instance of male-to-male transmission but an affected male had two daughters who were negative by examination. They observed concordant monozygotic twins and affected boys 12 and 14 years old. They concluded that the family with 'crystalline retinal degeneration' reported by Evans (1950) had this condition. The authors also concluded that Doyne honeycomb choroiditis (q.v.) is the same condition.

Deutman, A. F. and Jansen, L. M. A. A.: Dominantly inherited drusen of Bruch's membrane. Br. J. Ophthalmol. 54: 373-382, 1970.

Evans, P. J.: Five cases of familial retinal abiotrophy. Trans. Ophthalmol. Soc. U.K. 70: 96 only, 1950.

*12680 DUANE SYNDROME (RETRACTION SYNDROME)

The features of the syndrome are congenital deficiency of ocular abduction, impairment of adduction, retraction and superior or inferior deviation of the globe on adduction and narrowing of the palpebral fissure on adduction. The condition is bilateral in twenty percent of cases. Transmission through 4 generations was reported by Cooper (1910) and through 3 generations by Waardenburg (1923), Laughlin (1937) and Zentmayer (1935). Heterogeneity almost certainly exists. Associated deformity of the upper extremity was reported by Gifford (1926), Crisp (1918) and Mennerich (1923). Ferrell, Jones and Lucas (1966) have described the association of a heart-hand syndrome (probably type II of Lewis, q.v.) in a dominant pattern of inheritance.

Cooper, H.: A series of cases of congenital ophthalmoplegia externa (nuclear paralysis) in the same family. Br. Med. J. 1: 917 only, 1910.

Crisp, W. H.: Congenital paralysis of the external rectus muscle. Am. J. Ophthalmol. 1: 172-176, 1918.

Ferrell, R. L., Jones, B. and Lucas, R. V., Jr.: Simultaneous occurrence of the Holt-Oram and the Duane syndromes. J. Pediatr. 69: 630-634, 1966.

Gifford, H.: Congenital defects of abduction and other ocular movements and their relation to birth injuries. Am. J. Ophthalmol. 9: 3-22, 1926.

Goldfarb, C. and Gannon, F. L.: Familial congenital lateral rectus palsy with retraction (Stilling-Duane-Turk syndrome). Dis. Nerv. Syst. 25: 17-21, 1964.

Laughlin, R. C.: Hereditary paralysis of the abducens nerve. Am. J. Ophthalmol. 20: 396-398, 1937.

Mennerich, P.: Ein Fall von Retraktionsbewegungen der Augen bei angeborenen Anomalien der aeusseren Augenmuskeln. Z. Augenheilk. 50: 173-180, 1923.

Waardenburg, P. J.: Congenital disturbances of motility. Am. J. Ophthalmol. 6: 44-45, 1923.

Zentmayer, W.: Mengel's bilateral deficiency of abduction. Arch. Ophthalmol. 13: 984 only, 1935.

12690 DUPUYTREN CONTRACTURE

Although this clearly runs in families and autosomal dominance with variable penetrance is likely, this mode of inheritance cannot be considered proven. There are certain fundamental similarities to Peyronie disease (q.v.) and the two are associated more frequently than chance alone would dictate. Knuckle pads (q.v.) are also associated frequently. Manson (1931) described affected father and three sons.

Hueston, J. T.: Dupuytren's contracture. Baltimore: Williams and Wilkins Co., 1963.

Kostia, J.: A Dupuytrens' contracture family. Ann. Chir. Gynaec. Fenn. 46: 351-358, 1957.

Lygonis, C. S.: Familial Dupuytren's contracture. Hereditas 56: 142-143, 1966.

Manson, J. S.: Heredity and Dupuytren's contracture. Br. Med. J. 2: 11 only, 1931.

Maza, R. K. and Goodman, R. M.: A family with Dupuytren's contracture. J. Hered. 59: 155-156, 1968.

Skoog, T.: Dupuytren's contraction with special reference to aetiology and improved surgical treatment: its occurrence in epileptics: note on knuckle-pads. Acta Chir. Scand. 138 (suppl.): 1-190, 1948.

12695 DWARFISM WITH TALL VERTEBRAE

In two sisters Fuhrmann et al. (1972) described a form of dwarfism with disproportionately tall vertebral bodies (i.e., reduced anteroposterior dimension). Other features were very slender, caudally directed lower ribs, coxa vara, and a cordate pelvis. Since the parents were not related and the mother showed minor changes (short stature and somewhat tall vertebrae), dominant inheritance with variable expressivity was suggested. Graff et al. (1972) described thanatophoric dwarfism in two male offspring of first-cousin Moroccan Jewish parents. In the second-born affected sib the diagnosis was made antenatally by X-ray.

Fuhrmann, W., Nagele, E., Gugler, R. and Adili, E.: Dwarfism with disproportionately high vertebral bodies. Humangenetik 16: 271-282, 1972.

Graff, G., Chemke, J. and Lancet, M.: Familial recurring thanatophoric dwarfism. Obstet. Gynec. 39: 515-520, 1972.

*12700 DWARFISM, CORTICAL THICKENING OF TUBULAR BONES, AND TRANSIENT HYPO-CALCEMIA

Kenny and Linarelli (1966) described mother and son who were markedly dwarfed with dense tubular bones and narrow marrow cavities. Both had self-limited bouts of hypocalcemia and hypophosphatemia documented at age 39 years in the mother and age 1 to 15 weeks in the son. Associated features were delayed closure of the fontanel, myopia and low birth weight. Mentation was normal. Radiologic features were presented in detail by Caffey (1967). The mother was 48 inches tall at age 39 years. An isolated case was reported by Wilson et al. (1973).

Caffey, J. P.: Congenital stenosis of medullary spaces in tubular bones and calvaria in two proportionate dwarfs, mother and son, coupled with transitory hypocalcemic tetany. Am. J. Roentgen. 100: 1-11, 1967.

Kenny, F. M. and Linarelli, L.: Dwarfism and cortical thickening of tubular bones. Transient hypocalcemia in a mother and son. Am. J. Dis. Child. 111: 201-207, 1966.

Wilson, M. G., Maronde, R. F., Mikity, V. G. and Shinno, N. W.: Dwarfism and congenital medullary stenosis (Kenny syndrome). The Clinical Delineation of Birth Defects. XIX. Skeletal Dysplasias (cont.). Baltimore: Williams and Wilkins, 1973.

12710 DWARFISM, LEVI OR 'SNUB-NOSED' TYPE

In 1910 Levi described two families with 'microsomie essentielle' displaying dominant inheritance. Body proportions were normal. Black (1961) referred to these as 'snub-nosed dwarfs,' a variety of low birth-weight dwarfism, and suggested that both dominant (illustrated by Levi cases) and recessive forms exist. The low birth weight is, perhaps, not well documented and this condition may in fact be sexual ateliosis, a recessive (q.v.). The phenotypes of the presumed dominant and recessive forms seem identical and possibly Levi's pedigree was an instance of quasi-dominance. On the other hand cases of primordial dwarfism in successive generations are cited by Warkany, Monroe and Sutherland (1961), notably the family studied by Selle (1920) in which 10 persons in 3 generations were affected.

Black, J.: Low birth weight dwarfism. Arch. Dis. Child. 36: 633-644, 1961.

Levi, E.: Contribution a la connaissance de la microsomie essentielle heredo-familiale: distinction de cette forme clinique d'avec les nanismes, les infantilismes et les formes mixtes de ces differentes dystrophies. N. Iconog. Salpet. 23: 552-570, 1910.

Selle, G.: Ueber Vererbung des echten Zwergwuchses. Inaug. Dissert., University Of Jena, 1920.

Warkany, J., Monroe, B. B. and Sutherland, B. S.: Intrauterine growth retardation. Am. J. Dis. Child. 102: 249-279, 1961.

*12720 DWARFISM, WITH STIFF-JOINTS AND OCULAR ABNORMALITIES

The features (Moore, Federman, 1965) are dwarfism with disproportionately short legs (height 54 to 57 inches), reduced joint mobility, and ocular abnormalities (hyperopia, glaucoma, cataract, retinal detachment). Seven members of three generations were affected in the one reported family, with male-to-male transmission. Although some features resemble those of Leri pleonosteosis, there is sufficient difference to indicate that this is a distinct entity. This may, however, be the same disorder as that described under the designation of arthro-ophthalmopathy.

Moore, W. T. and Federman, D. D.: Familial dwarfism and 'stiff joints.' Arch. Intern. Med. 115: 398-404, 1965.

*12730 DYSCHONDROSTEOSIS

The characteristics are typical deformity of the distal radius and ulna and proximal carpal bones and mesomelic dwarfism. The wrist deformity is often referred to as Madelung deformity. Langer (1965) reported

three families. A striking preponderance of affected females makes it important to observe male-to-male
transmission before autosomal transmission is completely accepted. It has been my impression that females
are more severely affected than males. Hence, the preponderance of affected females may be the result of bias
of ascertainment. The deformity of the forearm consists of bowing of the radius and dorsal dislocation of
the distal ulna. Motion is limited at the elbow and wrist. Lamy and Bienenfeld (1954) described affected
mother and son. The fibula was absent in both. Reviewing cases of Madelung deformity Felman and
Kirkpatrick (1969) concluded that patients taller than the 25th percentile for height probably do not have
dyschondrosteosis, that hereditary entity of Madelung deformity distinct from dyschondrosteosis exists, that
patients with the isolated Madelung deformity may be short, that marked shortening of the tibia relative to
the femur suggests dyschondrosteosis. Langer (1965) had taken the view that most or all Madelung deformity
is dyschondrosteosis. The most complete review of the subject of Madelung deformity is that by Anton et
al. (1938). Rullier et al. (1968) observed dyschondrosteosis in mother and two daughters. Nassif and
Harboyan (1970) described two brothers with Leri dyschondrosteosis, who also had middle ear deformities
and conductive hearing loss. Three sisters had the skeletal deformity with normal hearing. Lisker et al. (1972)
found a family informative for Rhesus and haptoglobin. No indication of close linkage was provided,
however. See 24970 for possible homozygosity.

Anton, J. I., Reitz, G. B. and Spiegel, M. B.: Madelung's deformity. Ann. Surg. 108: 411-439, 1938.

Felman, A. H. and Kirkpatrick, J. A., Jr.: Dyschondrosteose. Mesomelic dwarfism of Leri and Weill. Am. J. Dis. Child. 120: 329-331, 1970.

Felman, A. H. and Kirkpatrick, J. A., Jr.: Madelung's deformity: observations in 17 patients. Radiology 93: 1037-1042, 1969.

Herdman, R. C., Langer, L. O. and Good, R. A.: Dyschondrosteosis, the most common cause of Madelung's deformity. J. Pediatr. 68: 432-441, 1966.

Lamy, M. and Bienenfeld, C.: La dyschondrosteose. In, Gedda, L. (ed.): De Genetica Medica. Rome: Gregor Mendel Institute, 1954.

Langer, L. O., Jr.: Dyschondrosteosis, a hereditable bone dysplasia with characteristic roentgenographic features. Am. J. Roentgen. 95: 178-188, 1965.

Lisker, R., Gamboa, I. and Hernandez, J.: Dyschondrosteosis. A Mexican family with two affected males. Clin. Genet. 3: 154-157, 1972.

Nassif, R. and Harboyan, G.: Madelung's deformity with conductive hearing loss. Arch. Otolaryng. 91: 175-178, 1970.

Rullier, J., Labram, C., Lazarovici, A. M. and Rousselot, R.: Dyschondrosteose familiale. Etude de trois cas (mere et ses deux fils). Sem. Hosp. Paris 44: 2474-2479, 1968.

12740 DYSCHROMATOSIS SYMMETRICA HEREDITARIA

This disorder has, like dyschromatosis universalis hereditaria, been described only in Japanese. Relation of
the two conditions is not clear.

Komaya, G.: Symmetrische Pigmentanomalie der Extremitaeten. Arch. Dermatol. Syph. 147: 389-393, 1924.

12750 DYSCHROMATOSIS UNIVERSALIS HEREDITARIA

This anomaly has been described only in Japanese. It is characterized by pigmented flecks and spots over
much of the body. Suenaga's family could equally well or even better, be recessive and only quasi-dominant,
since a consanguineous marriage occurred in each of four successive generations. The apparent restriction
to Japanese is more consistent with this possibility.

Suenaga, M.: Genetical studies on skin diseases. VII. Dyschromatosis universalis hereditaria in five generations. Tohoku J. Exp. Med. 55: 373-376, 1952.

12755 DYSKERATOSIS CONGENITA, SCOGGINS TYPE

Scoggins et al. (1971) described a Negro family with a form of dyskeratosis congenita obviously inherited
as an autosomal dominant. Features included reticular hyperpigmentation of the skin (due to dermal
pigmentation, melanin having been released by melanocytes and taken up by dermal phagocytes), dystrophic
nails, osteoporosis, premalignant leukokeratosis of the mouth mucosa, absent finger prints, scant hair, poor
dentition, absent lacrimal puncta, palmar hyperkeratosis, anemia, endoreduplication on chromosome studies,
and a defect of the immune mechanism (probably in the afferent limb). The hematologic, immunologic and
chromosomal changes were rather like those of Fanconi panmyelopathy (22790). Three generations were
affected with male-to-male transmission. Dyskeratosis congenita is usually X-linked recessive (30500).

Scoggins, R. B., Prescott, K. J., Asher, G. H., Blaylock, W. K. and Bright, R. W.: Dyskeratosis congenita with Fanconi-type anemia: investigations of immunologic and other defects. (Abstract) Clin. Res. 19: 409 only, 1971.

*12760 DYSKERATOSIS, HEREDITARY BENIGN INTRAEPITHELIAL

Characteristic histologic changes of the prickle cell layer of the mucosa include numerous round,
waxy-appearing, eosinophilic cells which appear to be engulfed by normal cells giving a cell-within-cell
appearance. In a triracial isolate in North Carolina, Witkop and colleagues (1960) found this disorder in at
least 83 persons. The conjunctiva and oral mucous membranes are affected. The oral lesion, which grossly
resembles leukoplakia, is not precancerous. The eye lesions resemble pterygia (see PTERYGIUM). The only
symptoms are produced by involvement of the cornea with blindness. Histologically characteristic findings

are obtained in oral and eye scraping. Penetrance is about 97 per cent and there is little effect on reproductive fitness. Yanoff (1968) described the condition in mother and daughter. This was the only report of the condition in persons apparently unrelated to the North Carolinian tri-racial isolate, the 'Haliwa Indians,' studied by Witkop et al. (1961). However, Gorlin (1971) states that Yanoff's patients were in fact related to Witkop's.

Gorlin, R. J.: Minneapolis, Minn.: personal communication, 1971.

Von Sallmann, L. and Paton, D.: Hereditary benign intraepithelial dyskeratosis. I. Ocular manifestations. Arch. Ophthalmol. 63: 421-429, 1960.

Witkop, C. J., Jr. and Gorlin, R. J.: Four hereditary mucosal syndromes. Arch. Dermatol. 84: 762-771, 1961.

Witkop, C. J., Jr., Shankle, C. H., Graham, J. B., Murray, M. R., Rucknagel, D. L. and Byerly, B. H.: Hereditary benign intra-epithelial dyskeratosis. II. Oral manifestations and hereditary transmission. Arch. Pathol. 70: 696-711, 1960.

Yanoff, M.: Hereditary benign intra-epithelial dyskeratosis. Arch. Ophthalmol. 79: 291-293, 1968.

12770 DYSLEXIA, SPECIFIC ('CONGENITAL WORD-BLINDNESS')

Hallgren (1950) studied 116 families. Speech defects were associated in many instances, especially in males, and were probably determined by the same factor as dyslexia. Left-handedness and left-eyedness could not be shown to be associated. Genetic analysis suggested autosomal dominant inheritance. Zahalkova et al. (1972) concluded that dyslexia is inherited as an autosomal dominant with reduced penetrance in females.

Critchley, M.: The Dyslexic Child. London: William Heinemann, 1970.

Hallgren, B.: Specific dyslexia ('congenital word-blindness'). A clinical and genetic study. Acta Psychiatry Neurol. Scand. 65 (suppl.): 1-287, 1950.

Zahalkova, M., Vrzal, V. and Kloboukova, E.: Genetical investigations in dyslexia. J. Med. Genet. 9: 48-52, 1972.

12780 DYSPLASIA EPIPHYSEALIS HEMIMELICA

This condition is characterized by asymmetrical cartilaginous overgrowth of one or more epiphyses of a tarsal or carpal bone, and less often other bones. Males are affected about 3 times more often than females. The disorder appears to have no simple Mendelian basis. No familial case has been reported. Donalson (1953) described a patient whose monozygotic co-twin was not affected.

Donalson, J. S., Sankey, H. H., Girdany, B. R. and Donalson, W. F.: Osteochondroma of the distal femoral epiphysis. J. Pediatr. 43: 212-216, 1953.

Kettelkamp, D. B., Campbell, C. J. and Bonfiglio, M.: Dysplasia epiphysealis hemimelica. A report of fifteen cases and a review of the literature. J. Bone Joint Surg. 48A: 746-766, 1966.

Saxton, H. M. and Wilkinson, J. A.: Hemimelic skeletal dysplasia. J. Bone Joint Surg. 46B: 608-613, 1964.

Theodorou, S. and Lanitis, G.: Dysplasia epiphysialis hemimelica (epiphyseal osteochondromata). Report of two cases and review of the literature. Helv. Paediatr. Acta 23: 195-204, 1968.

*12790 DYSPROTHROMBINEMIA

In an extensive kindred, Shapiro et al. (1969) found 11 persons with half-normal plasma concentrations of biological prothrombin activity but normal immunoreactive prothrombin. They referred to the defective molecule as prothrombin Cardeza. The locus of the mutation may be the same as that for hypoprothrombinemia (q.v.) in which no cross-reacting material is identifiable. Three prothrombin variants are known — Barcelona, Cardega, San Juan (Shapiro et al., 1974). Shapiro et al. (1974) presented evidence that San Juan is in fact an example of a genetic compound, i.e., the parents were heterozygous for different prothrombin variants.

Shapiro, S. S., Martinez, J. and Holburn, R. R.: Congenital dysprothrombinemia: an inherited structural disorder of human prothrombin. J. Clin. Invest. 48: 2251-2259, 1969.

Shapiro, S. S., Maldonado, N. I., Fradera, J. and McCord, S.: Prothrombin San Juan: a complex new dysprothrombinemia. (Abstract) J. Clin. Invest. 53: 73A only, 1974.

*12800 DYSTELEPHALANGY (KIRNER DEFORMITY)

The tip of the fifth finger points toward the thenar eminence due to bowing of the distal phalanx. X-ray shows angulation of the metaphysis of the phalanx. The lesion is probably not manifest before the fifth year of age. A globular soft tissue mass at the tip of the fifth fingers without bone deformity is probably the minor manifestation. Autosomal dominant inheritance is supported by the findings of Blank and Girdany (1965), Brailsford (1953) and Wilson (1952). David and Burwood (1972) surveyed a selected population finding 18 cases of dystelephalangy in nine families. The incidence in the general population was 1 in 410. There were 12 affected females and 6 affected males: bilateral deformity was heavily favored in the females and unilateral deformity in the males. Pedigree studies favored dominant inheritance with incomplete penetrance. There was no association found between congenital heart disease and Kirner deformity.

Blank, E. and Girdany, B. R.: Symmetric bowing of the terminal phalanges of the fifth fingers in a family (Kirner's deformity). Am. J. Roentgen. 93: 367-373, 1965.

Brailsford, J. F.: Radiology of Bones and Joints. Baltimore: Williams and Wilkins, 1953 (5th Ed.). P. 64.

David, T. J. and Burwood, R. L.: The nature and inheritance of Kirner's deformity. J. Med. Genet. 9: 430-433, 2972.

Wilson, J. N.: Dystrophy of fifth finger: report of four cases. J. Bone Joint Surg. 34B: 236-239, 1952.

*12810 DYSTONIA MUSCULORUM DEFORMANS

Johnson, Schwartz and Barbeau (1962) described an extensively affected French-Canadian family. Minor manifestations interpreted as formes frustes were found in some family members. The neurologic picture in some cases of Wilson disease is very similar clinically. Zeman et al. (1959, 1960) traced the disorder through 4 generations and Larsson and Sjogren (1963) traced it through 5 generations. Rather than a hyperkinetic picture, some had a myostatic picture, such as was described by Wechsler and Brock (1922). A recessive form of the disease (22450) occurs with increased frequency among Jews. In the dominant form Wooten et al. (1973) found elevation of plasma dopamine-beta-hydroxylase. This is the enzyme which converts dopamine to nocephinephrine.

Eldridge, R.: The torsion dystonias: literature review and genetic and clinical studies. Neurology 20: 1-78, 1970.

Johnson, W., Schwartz, G. and Barbeau, A.: Studies on dystonia musculorum deformans. Arch. Neurol. 7: 301-313, 1962.

Larsson, T. and Sjogren, T.: Dystonia musculorum deformans. A clinical and genetic population study. Proc. Sec. Intern. Cong. Hum. Genet. (Rome, Sept. 6-12, 1961.) 3: 1659-1662, 1963.

Wechsler, I. S. and Brock, S.: Dystonia musculorum deformans with especial reference to a myostatic form and the occurrence of decerebrate rigidity phenomena. A study of six cases. Arch. Neurol. Psychiatr. 8: 538-552, 1922.

Wooten, F. G., Eldridge, R., Axelrod, J. and Stern, R. S.: Elevated plasma dopamine-beta-hydroxylase activity in autosomal dominant torsin dystonia. N. Engl. J. Med. 288: 284-287, 1973.

Zeman, W. and Dyken, P.: Dystonia musculorum deformans. Clinical, genetic and pathoanatomical studies. Psychiatry Neurol. Neurochir. 70: 77-121, 1967.

Zeman, W., Kaelbling, R. and Pasamanick, B.: Idiopathic dystonia musculorum deformans. Neurology 10: 1068-1075, 1960.

Zeman, W., Kaelbling, R. and Pasamanick, B.: Idiopathic dystonia musculorum deformans. I. The hereditary pattern. Am. J. Hum. Genet. 11: 188-202, 1959.

*12820 DYSTONIA, FAMILIAL PAROXYSMAL

Paroxysmal dystonia may occur in multiple sclerosis or hepatolenticular degeneration. It is characterized by assumption of unilateral dystonic postures without clonic movements or change in consciousness. It was reported as a 'pure entity,' in mother and 3 sons by Weber (1967). He claimed that only one family had previously been reported (Lance, 1963) and that this is distinct from familial paroxysmal choreoathetosis. (Possibly it is the same as the periodic dystonia reported by Smith and Heersema (1941), although they had multiple affected sibs with normal parents.) Kertesz (1967) called the condition paroxysmal kinesigenic choreoathetosis.

Kertesz, A.: Paroxysmal kinesigenic choreoathetosis. Neurology 17: 680-690, 1967.

Lance, J. W.: Sporadic and familial varieties of tonic seizures. J. Neurol. Neurosurg. Psychiatry 26: 51-59, 1963.

Smith, L. A. and Heersema, P. H.: Periodic dystonia. Proc. Mayo Clin. 16: 842-846, 1941.

Weber, M. B.: Familial paroxysmal dystonia. J. Nerv. Ment. Dis. 145: 221-226, 1967.

12830 EAR EXOSTOSES (EXOSTOSES OF EXTERNAL AUDITORY CANAL)

The trait is age and sex dependent being rare in young children and more frequent in males. Instances of involvement in multiple generations were reviewed by Hrdlicka (1935).

Hrdlicka, A.: Ear exostoses. Smithsonian Miscellaneous Collections 93: 1-100, 1935.

12840 EAR FLARE

'Near-head,' intermediate and 'flare' types can be recognized. The data of Kloepfer (1946) suggested complex genetics.

Kloepfer, H. W.: An investigation of 171 possible linkage relationships in man. Ann. Eugen. 13: 35-72, 1946.

12850 EAR FOLDING

Various unusual varieties of folding of the helix and other parts of the ear are described in families usually as an autosomal dominant 'with variable expressivity and reduced penetrance.'

Ahuja, Y. R. and Gupta, M.: Inheritance of an unusual ear type in man. Acta Genet. Med. Gemellol. 19: 454-456, 1970.

*12860 EAR MALFORMATION ('CUP EAR')

Potter (1937) described a bilateral congenital malformation of the pinna which is curled up like a cap or cup concealing the external auditory meatus when the subject is in lateral profile. Erich and Abu-Jamra (1965) observed transmission of the condition through four generations (in 17 cases in 8 sibships) and reviewed similar reports. Peterson and Schimke (1968) observed cup-shaped ears in members of 5 generations with at least 4 instances of male-to-male transmission. Their proband had Pierre Robin syndrome (q.v.). The embryology of the auricle and a large amount of clinical material on various anomalies of the auricle were presented by Rogers (1968).

Erich, J. B. and Abu-Jamra, F. N.: Congenital cup-shaped deformity of the ears transmitted through four generations. Mayo Clinic Proc. 40: 597-602, 1965.

Peterson, D. M. and Schimke, R. N.: Hereditary cup-shaped ears and the Pierre Robin syndrome. J. Med. Genet. 5: 52-55, 1968.

Potter, E. L.: A hereditary ear malformation transmitted through five generations. J. Hered. 28: 255-258, 1937.

Rogers, B. O.: Microtic, lop, cup and protruding ears: four directly inheritable deformities. Plast. Reconstr. Surg. 41: 208-231, 1968.

12870 EAR PITS

Although in at least one family (Muckle, 1961) both ear pits and lateral cervical sinuses opening at various levels on the anterior margin of the sternomastoid were present, sometimes in the same individual, most families have shown either ear pits only or branchial cleft anomalies (q.v.) only. Hence, ear pits are listed as a separate mutation. They occur in the upper anterior end of the helix. Ewing (1946) found them in 0.9 per cent of 3500 British service men. They occur more frequently in Negroes. Skin tags containing cartilage (Jenkins, 1928) occur in some affected persons (McKusick et al., 1964). These are considered abnormalities of the first branchial cleft. Muckle's family (1961) showed 'buck teeth' (projecting upper front teeth). Gualandri (1969) found 321 cases among 29,309 Milan school children. Pedigrees were prepared in 93 cases demonstrating autosomal dominant inheritance with about 85 percent penetrance. His use of the term fistula would be challenged by some who would call the lesion a sinus or simply a pit.

Cannon, F. E.: Inheritance of ear pits in six generations of a family. J. Hered. 32: 413-414, 1941.

Ewing, M. R.: Congenital sinuses of external ear. J. Laryng. 61: 18-23, 1946.

Gualandri, V.: Richerche genetiche sulla fistula auris congenita. Acta Genet. Med. Gemellol. 18: 51-68, 1969.

Jenkins, R.: The occurrence of a skin papillus through four human generations. J. Hered. 19: 174 only, 1928.

Martins, A. G.: Lateral cervical and preauricular sinuses: their transmission as dominant characters. Br. Med. J. 1: 255-256, 1961.

McKusick, V. A. and colleagues: Medical Genetics 1961-1963. Oxford: Pergamon Press, 1964. Fig. 12.

Muckle, T. J.: Hereditary branchial defects in a Hampshire family. Br. Med. J. 1: 1297-1299, 1961.

Quelprud, T.: Ear pit and its inheritance. Fistula auris congenita, described in 1864, still a genetical and embryological puzzle. J. Hered. 31: 379-384, 1940.

Simpkiss, M. and Lowe, A.: Congenital abnormalities in the African newborn. Arch. Dis. Child. 36: 404-406, 1961.

Stiles, K. A.: The inheritance of pitted ear. Genetics 26: 171 only, 1941. J. Hered. 36: 53-61, 1945.

Whitney, D. D.: Three generations of ear pits. J. Hered. 30: 323-324, 1939.

12880 EAR WITHOUT HELIX

We have observed mother and daughter (L.B., 1110726) with this peculiarity. The daughter had split-hand and split-foot deformity. MacCollum (1938) reported a large series but gave no genetic information.

MacCollum, D. W.: The lop ear. J.A.M.A. 110: 1427-1430, 1938.

12890 EARLOBE ATTACHMENT (ATTACHED VS. UNATTACHED)

Free earlobes are dominant in the view of some. Dutta and Ganguly (1965) suggested polygenic inheritance. There is a variety which is perhaps better classified as 'lobeless' than 'attached.' Lai and Walsh (1966) concluded that 'a simple Mendelian gene effect is unlikely to be responsible for the earlobe types.'

Dutta, P. and Ganguly, P.: Further observations on ear lobe attachment. Acta Genet. Statist. Med. 15: 77-86, 1965.

Lai, L. Y. C. and Walsh, R. J.: Observations on ear lobe types. Acta Genet. Statist. Med. 16: 250-257, 1966.

Mohanraju, C. and Mukherjee, D. P.: Ear lobe attachment in an Andhra village and other parts of India. Hum. Hered. 23: 288-297, 1973.

Powell, E. F. and Whitney, D. D.: Ear lobe inheritance. An unusual three-generation photographic pedigree-chart. J. Hered. 28: 185-186, 1937.

Suzuchi, A.: Genetic studies of the human earlappets. On the inheritance of the lobulus auriculae. Jap. J. Hum. Genet. 25: 157 only, 1950.

Wiener, A. S.: Complications in ear genetics. J. Hered. 28: 425-426, 1937.

12895 EARLOBE CREASE

Frank (1973) and Lichstein et al. (1974) suggested that a diagonal crease of the earlobe is an indication of increased risk of coronary heart disease. Whether the trait is Mendelian is not clear. The frequency of the trait seems to increase with the age of the cohort.

Frank, S. T.: Aural sign of coronary-artery disease. N. Engl. J. Med. 289: 327-328, 1973.

Lichstein, E., Chadda, K. D., Naik, D. and Gupta, P. K.: Diagonal earlobe crease: prevalence and implications as coronary risk factor. N. Engl. J. Med. 290: 615-616, 1974.

12910 EARS, ABILITY TO MOVE

Linder (1949) found a frequency of the trait among parents and sibs of probands leading to the idea that the ability is inherited as a somewhat irregular dominant. In 5 of 24 cases both parents lacked the trait.

Linder, L.: The ability to move the ears. Hereditas 35 (suppl.): 620-621, 1949.

12915 ECHO 11 SENSITIVITY

Gerald (1974) provisionally assigned a site determining cellular sensitivity to Echo 11 virus to chromosome no. 19. He concluded that the site is separate from that for polio sensitivity (17385).

Gerald, P. S.: Boston, personal communication, July 15, 1974.

*12920 ECTODERMAL DYSPLASIA, ABSENT DERMATOGLYPHIC PATTERN, CHANGES IN NAILS AND SIMIAN CREASE (BASAN SYNDROME)

Persons of both sexes in 3 generations were affected (Basan, 1965). Male-to-male transmission was noted. We have observed a five-and-one-half-year-old girl (M.B., 145 52 30) with this abnormality whose mother and grandmother are identically affected (Jorgenson, 1974).

Basan, M.: Ektodermale Dysplasie, fehlendes Papillarmuster. Nagelveraenderungen und Vierfingerfurche. Arch. Klin. Exp. Dermatol. 222: 546-557, 1965.

Jorgenson, R. J.: Ectodermal dysplasia with hypotrichosis, hypohidrosis, defective teeth, and unusual dermatoglyphics (Basan syndrome)? In, Bergsma, D. (ed.): Clinical Delineation of Birth Defects. XVI. Urinary System and Others. Baltimore: Williams and Wilkins, 1974. Pp. 323-325.

12930 ECTODERMAL DYSPLASIA, ANHIDROTIC

Richards and Kaplan (1969) described a girl infant with neonatal pyrexia due to anhidrotic ectodermal dysplasia. The mother had 'somewhat sparce hair and wrinkled appearance of the eyelids.' Two of the sisters and four of the brothers of the mother, as well as her mother had absence of upper canine teeth, as did also the son of a maternal uncle. The authors suggested autosomal dominant inheritance. Earlier Kerr et al. (1966) expressed the view that dominant inheritance had not been adequately documented. Certainly the family of Richards and Kaplan (1969) is consistent with X-linked inheritance with partial expression in heterozygous females.

Kerr, C. B., Wells, R. S. and Cooper, K. E.: Gene effect in carriers of anhidrotic ectodermal dysplasia. J. Med. Genet. 3: 169-176, 1966.

Richards, W. and Kaplan, M.: Anhidrotic ectodermal dysplasia. An unusual case of pyrexia in the newborn. Am. J. Dis. Child. 117: 597-598, 1969.

12940 ECTODERMAL DYSPLASIA, ANHIDROTIC, WITH CLEFT LIP AND CLEFT PALATE

Rapp and Hodgkin (1968) described mother, son and daughter with anhidrotic ectodermal dysplasia, cleft lip and cleft palate. The combination had not been previously recorded.

Rapp, R. S. and Hodgkin, W. E.: Anhidrotic ectodermal dysplasia: autosomal dominant inheritance with palate and lip anomalies. J. Med. Genet. 5: 269-272, 1968.

*12950 ECTODERMAL DYSPLASIA, HIDROTIC

Several reports have described an extensive kindred of French extraction which migrated to Canada, Scotland and northern United States (Clouston, 1929; 1939; Joachim, 1936; MacKay and Davidson, 1929; Wilkey and Stevenson, 1945). In contrast to the X-linked form, most of these patients have (1) normal sweat and sebaceous gland function, (2) total alopecia, (3) severe dystrophy of the nails, (4) hyperpigmentation of the skin, especially over the joints and (5) normal teeth. Strabismus, mental deficiency, clubbing of the fingers and palmar hyperkeratosis occur in some. Scriver et al. (1965) suggested a molecular abnormality of keratin. The hair was thin with reduced tensile strength, disorganized fibrillar structure by light microscopy, reduced birefringence in polarized light, and increased amount of reactive SH groups. The full report was provided by Gold and Scriver (1972).

Clouston, H. R.: A hereditary ectodermal dystrophy. Canad. Med. Assoc. J. 21: 18-31, 1929.

Clouston, H. R.: The major forms of hereditary ectodermal dysplasia. Canad. Med. Assoc. J. 40: 1-7, 1939.

Gold, R. J. M. and Scriver, C. R.: Properties of hair keratin in an autosomal dominant form of ectodermal dysplasia. Am. J. Hum. Genet. 24: 549-561, 1972.

Gold, R. J. M. and Scriver, C. R.: The characterization of hereditary abnormalities of keratin: Clouston's ectodermal dysplasia. The Clinical Delineation of Birth Defects. XII. Skin, Hair and Nails. Baltimore: Williams and Wilkins, 1971. Pp. 91-95.

Joachim, H.: Hereditary dystrophy of the hair and nails in six generations. Ann. Intern. Med. 10: 400-402, 1936.

MacKay, H. and Davidson, A. M.: Congenital ectodermal dysplasia. Br. J. Dermatol. 41: 1-5, 1929.

Scriver, C. R., Solomons, C. C., Davies, E., Williams, M. and Bolton, J.: A molecular abnormality of keratin in ectodermal dysplasia. (Abstract) J. Pediat. 67: 946 Only, 1965.

Wilkey, W. D. and Stevenson, G. H.: A family with inherited ectodermal dystrophy. Canad. Med. Assoc. J. 53: 226-230, 1945.

Williams, M. and Fraser, F. C.: Hidrotic ectodermal dysplasia — Clouston's family revisited. Canad. Med. Assoc. J. 96: 36-38, 1967.

*12960 ECTOPIA LENTIS

Usher (1924) reported seven affected persons in three successive generations. In these early reports one cannot be certain the Marfan syndrome (q.v.) was not present. Falls and Cotterman (1943) described a family with a large number of affected persons in five generations, and Chace (1945) observed three generations. I have restudied the family reported by McGavic (1966) as having Weill-Marchesani syndrome. They probably suffer from an autosomal dominant form of 'simple' ectopia lentis. Eleven members were affected. All members with or without ectopia lentis were short.

Chace, R. R.: Congenital bilateral subluxation of the lens. Arch. Ophthalmol. 34: 425-426, 1945.

Falls, H. F. and Cotterman, C. W.: Genetic studies on ectopia lentis. A pedigree of simple ectopia of the lens. Arch. Ophthalmol. 30: 610-620, 1943.

Harshman, J. P.: Glaucoma associated with subluxation of the lens in several members of family. Am. J. Ophthalmol. 31: 833-836, 1948.

McGavic, J. S.: Weill-Marchesani syndrome. Brachymorphism and ectopia lentis. Am. J. Ophthalmol. 62: 820-823, 1966.

Meyer, E. T.: Familial ectopia lentis and its complications. Br. J. Ophthalmol. 38: 163-172, 1954.

Usher, C. H.: A pedigree of congenital dislocation of lenses. Biometrika 16: 273-282, 1924.

12970 ECTOPIA LENTIS ET PUPILLAE

This condition is almost always recessive (q.v.). Walls and Heath (1959) described three affected sibs and an affected child of one of these. It seems most likely that this was the familiar recessive disorder, the normal parent of the affected member in the later generation being a heterozygote. For dominant inheritance to obtain, one must assume gonadal mosaicism or failure of expression in one of the parents of the affected sibs. These parents, it seems, were not examined.

Walls, G. L. and Heath, G. G.: Dominant ectopia lentis et pupillae. Am. J. Hum. Genet. 11: 166-168, 1959.

12980 ECTRODACTYLY

Ectrodactyly is derived from Greek ektroma (abortion) and daktylos (finger). The term is a non-specific one applied to a variety of malformations. It is probably best reserved for transverse terminal aphalangia, adactylia or acheiria. Cases defined in this way are usually sporadic. One hand is involved and the feet are not affected, as a rule. Congenital constriction rings ('amniotic bands') are sometimes associated. Many cases described as examples of autosomal dominant inheritance of ectrodactyly are in fact type B brachydactyly (q.v.). The family reported by Khosrovani (1959) may be such an instance. The anomaly called here split-hand deformity (q.v.) and sometimes called lobster-claw deformity is also called ectrodactyly, improperly I think.

Khosrovani, H.: Malformations of the hands and feet (ectrodactylia) through five successive generations of a large Vaudois family. J. Genet. Hum. 8: 1-59, 1959.

Temtamy, S. A.: Genetic Factors in Hand Malformations. Ph.D. Thesis, Johns Hopkins University, 1966.

12985 EDINBURGH MALFORMATION SYNDROME

Habel (1974) described an Edinburgh family in which five infant sibs in four sibships, four female and one male, were found to have consistently abnormal facial appearance, true or apparent hydrocephalus, retardation in motor and mental development, failure to thrive and death in the first months of life. Unexplained neonatal hyperbil: rubinemia and advanced bone age may be features. The affected infants were related as first-cousins or first-cousins once removed and there was no consanguinity in the family. A carp mouth and hairiness of the forehead suggested the Cornelia de Lange syndrome. A chromosomal abnormality was postulated but not demonstrated.

Habel, A.: 'Typus Edinburgensis?' Pediatrics 53: 425-430, 1974.

*12990 EEC SYNDROME (ECTRODACTYLY, ECTODERMAL DYSPLASIA, CLEFT LIP-PALATE)

Rudiger, Haase and Passarge (1970) suggested the designation EEC for the syndrome observed in a female child. The features were ectrodactyly of both hands and one foot, ectodermal dysplasia with severe keratitis and cleft lip-palate. This disorder is probably the same as that reported in one of the patients of Roselli and Guilienetti (1961) and probably different from the combination of ectrodactyly, anodontia and partial noncanalization of the lacrimal duct described in mother and son by Temtamy and McKusick (1969). See 11940, 12940, and 22500. Father-to-son transmission was described by Fraser (1971). Pashayan et al. (1974) described affected sisters (their cases 2 and 3).

Bixler, D., Spivack, J., Bennett, J. and Christian, J. C.: The ectrodactyly-ectodermal dysplasia-clefting (EEC) syndrome. Report of 2 cases and review of the literature. Clin. Genet. 3: 43-51, 1972.

Fraser, F. C.: Genetic counseling. Chapter 21 in McKusick, V. A. and Claiborne, R. (eds.) Medical Genetics. New York: Hospital Practice, 1973.

Levy, W. J.: Mesoectodermal dysplasia: a new combination of anomalies. Am. J. Ophthalmol. 63: 978-982, 1967.

Pashayan, H. M., Pruzansky, S. and Solomon, L.: The EEC syndrome. Report of six patients. Birth Defects Orig. Art. Ser. 10 (7): 105-120, 1974.

Pfeiffer, R. A.: Spalthald und Spaltfub, ektodermal dysplasie und Lippen-Kiefer-Gaumen-Spalte: ein autosomal dominant verebtes syndrome. Z. Kinderheilk. 115: 235-244, 1973.

Preus, M. and Fraser, F. C.: The lobster claw defect, cleft lip-palate, tear duct anomaly and renal anomalies. Clin. Genet. 4: 369-375, 1973.

Rosselli, D. and Gulienetti, R.: Ectodermal dysplasia. Br. J. Plast. Surg. 14: 190-204, 1961.

Rudiger, R. A., Haase, W. and Passarge, E.: Association of ectrodactyly, ectodermal dysplasia, and cleft lip-palate. Am. J. Dis. Child. 120: 160-163, 1970.

Swallow, J. N., Gray, O. P. and Harper, P. S.: Ectrodactyly, ectodermal dysplasia and cleft lip and plate (EEC syndrome). Br. J. Dermatol. 89: 54-56, 1973.

Temtamy, S. A. and McKusick, V. A.: Synopsis of hand malformations with particular emphasis on genetic factors. The Clinical Delineation of Birth Defects. III. Limb Malformations. New York: National Foundation, 1969. Pp. 125-184.

*13000 EHLERS-DANLOS SYNDROME (E-D TYPES I, II, III)

The main features are loose-jointedness and fragile and bruisable skin which heals with peculiar 'cigarette-paper' scars. Barabas (1966) concluded that most persons with this condition are born prematurely due to premature rupture of fetal membranes. In light of what is understood about the nature of this condition and the fact that the placenta is largely fetal in origin (and genotype), the conclusion is plausible. Graf (1965) reported brother and sister with Ehlers-Danlos syndrome who developed 'spontaneous' carotid-cavernous fistula. Internal complications include rupture of large vessels, hiatus hernia, spontaneous rupture of the bowel, diverticula of the bowel. Retinal detachment has been observed (Pemberton et al., 1966). Barabas (1967) suggested the existence of three distinct types of the Ehlers-Danlos syndrome. In the classical type the patients are born prematurely because of premature rupture of fetal membranes, and have severe skin and joint involvement but no varicose veins or arterial ruptures. A second (mild or 'varicose') group is not born prematurely and the skin and joint manifestations are not severe. However, varicose veins are severe. In a third ('arterial') group bruising is a paramount sign, including spontaneous ecchymoses during menstruation. Skin is soft and transparent but little extensible and joint hypermobility is limited to the hands. Severe and unexplained abdominal pain is a feature. Repeated arterial ruptures occur in these patients. Skin like that of E-D has been observed with a fibrinolytic defect (q.v.). Nordschow and Marsolais (1969) could demonstrate no abnormality of shrinkage temperature thermograms of tendon collagen from a hypermobile joint of an E-D patient. They supported the suggestion of Wechsler and Fisher (1964) that the defect concerns the amount of collagen produced. Varadi and Hall (1965) concluded that elastin is normal. Schofield et al. (1970) reported brother and sister in their 60's who suffered spontaneous rupture of the colon. They had joint laxity, and both bruised easily and sustained many lacerations from minor trauma. The father of the two sibs and the son of the brother may have also been affected. According to the classification which I currently (McKusick, 1972) follow, E-D I, or gravis type is the severe classic form; E-D II, or mitis type, is the mild classic form; E-D III is the benign hypermobility form. The last may be the same as the entry numbered 14790. E-D I, II and III are entered under one number because their genetic distinctness in terms of different loci being responsible is unknown. E-D IV is the arterial, ecchymotic or Sack type (13005). E-D V is the X-linked form (30520). E-D IV (22540) is the form due to deficiency of lysyl hydroxylase. E-D VII (22541) is the form due to deficiency of procollagen protease.

Barabas, A. P.: Ehlers-Danlos syndrome associated with prematurity and premature rupture of foetal membranes. Br. Med. J. 2: 682-684, 1966.

Barabas, A. P.: Heterogeneity of the Ehlers-Danlos syndrome: description of three clinical types and a hypothesis to explain the basic defect(s). Br. Med. J. 1: 612-613, 1967.

Beighton, P. H., Murdoch, J. L. and Votteler, T.: Gastrointestinal complications of the Ehlers-Danlos syndrome. Gut 10: 1004-1008, 1969.

Beighton, P. H., Price, A., Lord, J. and Dickson, E.: Variants of the Ehlers-Danlos syndrome. Clinical, biochemical, haematological, and chromosomal features of 100 patients. Ann. Rheum. Dis. 28: 228-245, 1969.

Bruno, M. S. and Narasimhan, P.: The Ehlers-Danlos syndrome: a report of four cases in two generations of a Negro family. N. Engl. J. Med. 264: 274-277, 1961.

Coventry, M. B.: Some skeletal changes in the Ehlers-Danlos syndrome. A report of two cases. J. Bone Joint Surg. 43A: 855-860, 1961.

Day, H. J. and Zarafonetis, C. J. D.: Coagulation studies in 4 patients with Ehlers-Danlos syndrome. Am. J. Med. Sci. 242: 565-573, 1961.

Goodman, R. M., Levitsky, J. M. and Friedman, I. A.: The Ehlers-Danlos syndrome and multiple neurofibromatosis in a kindred of mixed derivations, with special emphasis on hemostasis in the Ehlers-Danlos syndrome. Am. J. Med. 32: 976-983, 1962.

Graf, C. J.: Spontaneous carotid-cavernous fistula: Ehlers-Danlos syndrome and related conditions. Arch. Neurol. 13: 662-672, 1965.

Grahame, R. and Beighton, P.: Physical properties of the skin in the Ehlers-Danlos syndrome. Ann. Rheum. Dis. 28: 246-251, 1969.

Hegreberg, G. A., Padgett, G. A., Otto, R. L. and Henson, J. B.: A heritable connective tissue disease of dogs and mink resembling Ehlers-Danlos syndrome of man. I. Skin tensile strength properties. J. Invest. Dermatol. 54: 377-380, 1970.

Hines, C., Jr. and Davis, W. D.: Ehlers-Danlos syndrome with megaduodenum and malabsorption syndrome secondary to bacterial overgrowth: a report of the first case. Am. J. Med. 54: 539-543, 1972.

Imahori, S., Bannerman, R. M., Graf, C. J. and Brennan, J. C.: Ehlers-Danlos syndrome with multiple arterial lesions. Am. J. Med. 47: 967-977, 1969.

Lees, M. H., Menashe, V. D., Sunderland, C. O., Morgan, C. L. and Dawson, P. J.: Ehlers-Danlos syndrome associated with multiple pulmonary artery stenoses and tortuous systemic arteries. J. Pediat. 75: 1031-1036, 1969.

McKusick, V. A.: Heritable Disorders of Connective tissue. St. Louis: C. V. Mosby Co., 1972 (4th Ed.).

Nordschow, C. D. and Marsolais, E. B.: Ehlers-Danlos syndrome. Some recent biophysical observations. Arch. Pathol. 88: 65-68, 1969.

Pemberton, J. W., Freeman, H. M. and Schepens, C. L.: Familial retinal detachment and the Ehlers-Danlos syndrome. Arch. Ophthalmol. 76: 817-824, 1966.

Scarpelli, D. G. and Goodman, R. M.: Observations on the fine structure of the fibroblast from a case of Ehlers-Danlos syndrome with the Marfan syndrome. J. Invest. Dermatol. 50: 214-219, 1968.

Schofield, P. F., MacDonald, N. and Clegg, J. F.: Familial spontaneous rupture of the colon: report of two cases. Dis. Colon Rectum 13: 394-396, 1970.

Sestak, Z.: Ehlers-Danlos syndrome and cutis laxa: an account of families in the Oxford area. Ann. Hum. Genet. 25: 313-321, 1962.

Varadi, D. P. and Hall, D. A.: Cutaneous elastin in Ehlers-Danlos syndrome. Nature 208: 1224-1225, 1965.

Wechsler, H. L. and Fisher, E. R.: Ehlers-Danlos syndrome. Pathologic, histochemical and electron microscopic observations. Arch. Pathol. 77: 613-619, 1964.

13005 EHLERS-DANLOS SYNDROME — 'ARTERIAL,' 'ECCHYMOTIC,' OR SACK TYPE (E-D TYPE IV)

Within the Ehlers-Danlos syndrome as many as seven varieties can be identified (McKusick, 1972). These include two autosomal recessive forms: lysyl hydroxylase deficiency (22540) and procollagen protease deficiency (22541). These also include an X-linked form (30520). Severe ('gravis') and mild ('mitis') forms of classic E-D are recognized but may be allelic as may also the form called the simple hypermobility type of E-D. The seventh form is clinically distinctive and is clearly a dominant in its mode of inheritance, although whether X-linked or autosomal is not established to my satisfaction. The reported cases are few in number but the sex ratio is probably about 1.0, which speaks for autosomal inheritance. However, no father-to-son transmission is reported to my knowledge. The malignant form of E-D owes its bad reputation to a proneness to spontaneous rupture of bowel or large vessels. Paradoxically other manifestations are less dramatic than in some other forms of E-D. For example, joint hypermobility may be confined largely to the fingers and whereas the skin is strikingly thin and translucent, it is only mildly hyperextensible. Bruisability, however, is very striking. Barabas (1972) reported a family in which the mother and a 16-year-old brother died of aortic rupture and the proband had frequent hematomata and at least one intraperitoneal bleed. I have cared for a family in which the mother and sister died of aortic rupture and the proband (T. F., JHH 1432502) has survived aortic dissection (or rupture with false aneurysm formation).

Barabas, A. P.: Vascular complications in the Ehlers-Danlos syndrome, with, special reference to the 'arterial type' or Sack's syndrome. J. Cardiovas. Surg. 13: 160-167, 1972.

McKusick, V. A.: Heritable Disorders of Connective Tissue. St. Louis: C. V. Mosby Co., 1972 (4th Ed.).

Hole, B. V. and Wasserman, K.: Familial emphysema. Ann. Intern. Med. 63: 1009-1017, 1965.

Larson, R. K. and Barman, M. L.: The familial occurrence of chronic obstructive pulmonary disease. Ann. Intern. Med. 63: 1001-1008, 1965.

13010 ELASTOSIS PERFORANS SERPIGINOSA

Also known as hyperkeratosis follicularis et parafollicularis in cutem penetrans, elastoma intrapapillare perforans verruciformis, Kyrle disease, Miescher elastoma, etc., this condition occurs in the Marfan syndrome, the Ehlers-Danlos syndrome, osteogenesis imperfecta, pseudoxanthoma elasticum, and mongolism. In addition it probably occurs as an isolated genetic trait of which the inheritance may be dominant.

13020 ELECTROENCEPHALOGRAPHIC PECULIARITY: '14 AND 6 PER SEC. POSITIVE SPIKE' PHENOMENON

This peculiarity has been observed in identical twins (Vogel, 1965) and in parents and sibs of probands (Radin, 1964).

Radin, E. A.: Familial occurrence of the 14 and 6 per sec. Positive spike phenomenon. Electroenceph. Clin. Neurophysiol. 17: 566-570, 1964.

Vogel, F.: '14 and 6 per sec. positive spikes' in Schlaf-EEG von jugendlichen ein- und zweieiigen Zwillingen. Humangenetik 1: 390-391, 1965.

13030 ELECTROENCEPHALOGRAPHIC PECULIARITY: FRONTO-PRECENTRAL BETA WAVE GROUPS

Vogel (1966) suggested autosomal dominant inheritance of each of two types-(1) frontal beta-groups with high frequency (25-30 per sec.) and relatively low voltage, and (2) beta-groups with frequency of 20-25 per sec., higher voltage and precentral maximum.

Vogel, F.: Zur genetischen Grundlage fronto-parazentraler beta-Wellengruppen im EEG des Menschen. Humangenetik 2: 227-237, 1966.

13040 ELECTROENCEPHALOGRAPHIC PECULIARITY: OCCIPAL SLOW BETA WAVES

The alpha waves are replaced by 16-19 per second beta waves which show an occipital maximum and are blocked by opening of the eyes. From family data Vogel (1966) concluded the pattern is inherited as an autosomal dominant. The frequency was found to be about 0.6 percent among young males.

Berg, K. and Bearn, A. G.: Antibodies to inherited beta-lipoprotein antigens in the serum of multiply transfused patients. Clin. Genet. 1: 104-120, 1970.

Vogel, F.: Zur genetischen Grundlage occipitaler langsamer beta-Wellen im EEG des Menschen. Humangenetik 2: 238-245, 1966.

*13050 ELLIPTOCYTOSIS, RHESUS-LINKED TYPE

See below for description.

*13060 ELLIPTOCYTOSIS, RHESUS-UNLINKED TYPE

Two genetically distinct varieties of elliptocytosis are recognized by the fact that one is linked with the Rhesus locus and one is not. Phenotypic differences may be correlated with the differences in linkage relationships. Geerdink et al. (1967) found more hemolysis in the 'unlinked' type than in the 'linked' type. Peters et al. (1966) studying isolated red cell membranes demonstrated an abnormality in erythrocyte sodium transport. In a family in which both elliptocytosis and hereditary hemorrhagic telangiectasia were segregating, Roberts (1945) pointed out that even very small bodies of data are useful for excluding close linkage. The extensive study of elliptocytosis in Iceland reported by Jensson et al. (1967) shows how widely the manifestations may vary. All cases are plausibly considered to have the same gene. Additional evidence of heterogeneity in elliptocytosis may be provided by the effects of combination with beta-thalassemia. Aksoy and Erdem (1968) concluded that the combination sometimes results in mutual enhancement, whereas in other instances it does not. Nielsen and Strunk (1968) described a Dutch family in which, among the 7 offspring of related parents both with elliptocytosis, two died in infancy of severe anemia and a third had erythrocytes which showed more marked morphologic changes than in heterozygotes and had severe anemia which was compensated by splenectomy. All three were presumably homozygotes. Three other sibs were heterozygotes and one was stillborn. The elliptocytosis was of the Rh linked variety.

Aksoy, M. and Erdem, S.: Combination of hereditary elliptocytosis and heterozygous beta-thalassemia: a family study. J. Med. Genet. 5: 298-301, 1968.

Bannerman, R. M. and Renwick, J. H.: The hereditary elliptocytoses: clinical and linkage data. Ann. Hum. Genet. 26: 23-38, 1962.

Clarke, C. A., Donohoe, W. T. A., Finn, R., McConnell, R. B., Sheppard, P. M. and Nicol, D. S. H.: Data on linkage in man: ovalocytosis, sickling and the Rhesus blood group complex. Ann. Hum. Genet. 24: 283-287, 1960.

Geerdink, R. A., Nijenhuis, L. E. and Huizinga, J.: Hereditary elliptocytosis: linkage data in man. Ann. Hum. Genet. 30: 363-378, 1967.

Gomperts, E. D., Cayannis, F., Metz, J. and Zail, S. S.: Red cell membrane protein abnormality in hereditary elliptocytosis. Br. J. Haemat. 25: 415-420,1973.

Jensson, O., Jonasson, T. and Olafsson, O.: Hereditary elliptocytosis in Iceland. Br. J. Haematol. 13: 844-854, 1967.

Kuroda, S., Takeuchi, T. and Nagamori, H.: Data on the linkage between elliptocytosis and Rh blood type. Jap. J. Hum. Genet. 5: 112-118, 1960.

Morton, N. E.: The detection and estimation of linkage between the genes for elliptocytosis and the Rh blood type. Am. J. Hum. Genet. 8: 80-96, 1956.

Nielsen, J. A. and Strunk, K. W.: Homozygous hereditary elliptocytosis as the cause of haemolytic anemia in infancy. Scand. J. Haemat. 5: 486-496, 1968.

Peters, J. C., Rowland, M., Israels, L. G. and Zipursky, A.: Erythrocyte sodium transport in hereditary elliptocytosis. Canad. J. Physiol. Pharmacol. 44: 817-827, 1966.

Roberts, J. A. F.: Genetic linkage in man, with particular reference to the usefulness of very small bodies of data. Quart. J. Med. 14: 27-33, 1945.

13070 EMPHYSEMA

Larson and Barman (1965) described two kindreds, and Hole and Wasserman (1965) reported one, with multiple cases of chronic obstructive pulmonary disease (emphysema or chronic bronchitis or both). A correlation with smoking was suggested.

Hole, B. V. and Wasserman, K.: Familial emphysema. Ann. Intern. Med. 63: 1009-1017, 1965.

Larson, R. K. and Barman, M. L.: The familial occurrence of chronic obstructive pulmonary disease. Ann. Intern. Med. 63: 1001-1008, 1965.

*13080 ENAMEL HYPOPLASIA WITH CURLY HAIR (TRICHO-DENTO-OSSEOUS SYNDROME)

Robinson and Miller (1966) described autosomal dominant inheritance of enamel hypoplasia with associated strikingly curly hair. We (Lichtenstein et al., 1971) have traced the same condition through 6 generations of an Irish-American family. In affected members of this family, a feature not described by Robinson and Miller (1966) is mild increase in bone density, particularly in the skull. The dental defect has been observed alone (see AMELOGENESIS IMPERFECTA WITH TAURODONTISM). The finger nails showed either laminated splitting of the superficial layers or thick cornification. Apparently both keratin and enamel are defective.

Lichtenstein, J. R., Warson, R. W., Jorgenson, R. J. and McKusick, V. A.: The tricho-donto-osseous syndrome. Am. J. Hum. Genet. 24: 569-582, 1972.

Robinson, G. C., Miller, J. R. and Worth, H. M.: Hereditary enamel hypoplasia: its association with characteristic hair structure. Pediatrics 37: 498-502, 1966.

*13090 ENAMEL HYPOPLASIA, HEREDITARY LOCALIZED

The distribution is restricted mainly to the labial aspect of the anterior teeth and may affect the first dentition only. Pits and linear fissures oriented horizontally around the crown of the teeth are described. Witkop (1957, 1965) concluded that this is an autosomal dominant trait with incomplete penetrance and variable expressivity. He observed a kindred with many affected members.

Darling, A. I.: Some observations on amelogenesis imperfecta and calcification of the dental enamel. Proc. R. Soc. Med. 49: 759-766, 1956.

Witkop, C. J.: Genetic disease of the oral cavity. In, Tiecke, R. W. (ed.): Oral Pathology. New York: McGraw-Hill, 1965.

Witkop, C. J.: Hereditary defects in enamel and dentin. Acta Genet. Statist. Med. 7: 236-239, 1957.

*13110 ENDOCRINE ADENOMATOSIS, MULTIPLE

Underwood and Jacobs (1963) found father, son and daughter affected. Hypoglycemia was the presenting manifestation in all three. In addition to islet cell adenomas, the father had bronchial carcinoma and hyperparathyroidism from parathyroid adenomas. The son and daughter had been followed from childhood as cases of idiopathic epilepsy unresponsive to anticonvulsive therapy. The Zollinger-Ellison syndrome of intractable peptic ulcer with pancreatic islet adenoma is a facet of multiple endocrine adenomatosis. This disorder may present purely as hyperparathyroidism. Guida et al. (1966) described pituitary adenoma and duodenal carcinoid in patients with this condition. Bronchial carcinoid (Williams and Celestin, 1962) occurs as a feature of endocrine adenomatosis (q.v.). Wermer first reported 'his' syndrome in 1954 and Zollinger and Ellison 'theirs' in 1955. Recognition that they are one has subsequently occurred (Lulu et al., 1968). Kipnis et al. (1969) described a patient with MEA who succumbed to metastatic Schwannoma. One member of the family described as hereditary hyperparathyroidism by Cutler et al. (1964) was later reported to have a malignant Schwannoma, pituitary adenomas, multiple pancreatic islet cell adenomas and multiple adrenocortical adenomas. Snyder et al. (1972) reported 5 families and noted the previously described association of lipomas. Baylin et al. (1972), in a family with many affected members, demonstrated the usefulness of serum histaminidase in detecting metastases of medullary carcinoma of the thyroid as well as residual tumor after surgery. Serum calcitonin level was found reliable for early detection of localized medullary thyroid tumor. Vance et al. (1972), on the basis of studies of 8 affected members of a family, suggested that the primary genetic lesion in endocrine adenomatosis is one which leads to neoplasia and hyperfunction of the islets of Langerhans and that the other endocrine tumors arise as secondary effects of hypersecretion of islet hormones. There are families which have only hyperparathyroidism. Either of these represent a distinct entity or the theory of Vance et al. (1972) is not valid. A notable feature of this disease is intrafamilial uniformity. Some kindreds (e.g., Ballard et al., 1964; Wermer, 1954) have a high frequency of severe peptic ulcer disease with islet cell tumors, whereas other kindreds (e.g., Johnson et al., 1967) are devoid of peptic disease.

Aach, R. and Kissane, J.: Clinicopathologic conference: multiple endocrine adenomatosis. Am. J. Med. 47: 608-618, 1969.

Ballard, H. S., Frame, B. and Hartsock, R. J.: Familial multiple endocrine adenoma-peptic ulcer complex. Medicine 43: 481-516, 1964.

Baylin, S. B., Beaven, M. A., Keiser, H. R., Tashjian, A. H., Jr. and Melvin, K. E. W.: Serum histaminase and calcitonin levels in medullary carcinoma of the thyroid. Lancet I: 455-458, 1972.

Buchta, R. M. and Kaplan, J. M.: Zollinger-Ellison syndrome in a nine-year-old child: a case report and review of the entity in childhood. Pediatrics 47: 594-598, 1971.

Ellison, E. H. and Wilson, S. D.: The Zollinger-Ellison syndrome updated. Surg. Clin. N. Am. 47: 1115-1124, 1967.

Ellison, E. H. and Wilson, S. D.: The Zollinger-Ellison syndrome. Re-appraisal and evaluation of 260 registered cases. Ann. Surg. 160: 512-530, 1964.

Friesen, S. R., Schimke, R. N. and Pearse, A. G. E.: Genetic aspects of the Z-E syndrome: prospective studies in two kindred: antral gastrin cell hyperplasia. Ann. Surg. 176: 370-383, 1972.

Guida, P. M., Todd, J. E., Moore, S. W. and Beal, J. M.: Zollinger-Ellison syndrome with interesting variations. Report of twelve cases including one of carcinoid of the duodenum. Am. J. Surg. 112: 807-817, 1966.

Johnson, G. J., Summerskill, W. H. J., Anderson, V. E. and Keating, F. R.: Clinical and genetic investigation of a large kindred with multiple endocrine adenomatosis. N. Engl. J. Med. 277: 1379-1385, 1967.

Jones, B. S., O'Hagan, J. J., Phear, D. N. and Sheville, E.: A case of the Zollinger-Ellison syndrome associated with hyperplasia of salivary and Brunner's glands. Gut 11: 837-839, 1970.

Kipnis, D. and colleagues: Multiple endocrine adenomatosis. (Clinicopathologic conference) Am. J. Med. 47: 608-618, 1969.

Lulu, D. J., Corcoran, T. E. and Andre, M.: Familial endocrine adenomatosis with associated Zollinger-Ellison syndrome. Wermer's syndrome. Am. J. Surg. 115: 695-701, 1968.

Snyder, N., III, Scurry, M. T. and Deiss, W. P., Jr.: Five families with multiple endocrine adenomatosis. Ann. Intern. Med. 76: 53-58, 1972.

Snyder, N., Scurry, M. and Hughes, W.: Hypergastrinemia in familial multiple endocrine adenomatosis. Ann. Intern. Med. 80: 321-325, 1974.

Underwood, L. E. and Jacobs, N. M.: Familial endocrine adenomatosis. Am. J. Dis. Child. 106: 218-223, 1963.

Vance, J. E., Stoll, R. W., Kitabchi, A. E., Buchanan, K. D., Hollander, D. and Williams, R. H.: Familial nesidioblastosis as the predominant manifestation of multiple endocrine adenomatosis. Am. J. Med. 52: 211-227, 1972.

Vance, J. E., Stoll, R. W., Kitabchi, A. E., Williams, R. H. and Wood, F. C., Jr.: Nesidioblastosis in familial endocrine adenomatosis. J.A.M.A. 207: 1679-1682, 1969.

Way, L., Goldman, L. and Dunphy, J. E.: Zollinger-Ellison syndrome. An analysis of twenty-five cases. Am. J. Surg. 116: 293-304, 1968.

Wermer, P.: Genetic aspects of adenomatosis of endocrine glands. Am. J. Med. 16: 363-371, 1954.

Williams, E. D. and Celestin, L. R.: The association of bronchial carcinoid and pluriglandular adenomatosis. Thorax 17: 120-127, 1962.

Zollinger, R. M. and Ellison, E. H.: Primary pepticulcerations of the jejunum associated with islet cell tumors of the pancreas. Ann. Surg. 142: 709-728, 1955.

13120 ENDOMETRIOSIS

Endometriosis, often in the form of 'chocolate cysts' of the ovary, has been reported in sisters rather frequently and at least twice in mother and daughter(s).

Barnes, J.: Chocolate cysts of ovary (ovarian endometriosis) and pregnancy: report of two cases occurring in sisters. Proc. R. Soc. Med. 38: 324-325, 1945.

Frey, G. H.: The familial occurrence of endometriosis. Report of five instances and review of literature. Am. J. Obstet. Gynecol. 73: 418-421, 1957.

Gardner, G. H., Greene, R. R. and Ranney, B.: Histogenesis of endometriosis: recent contributions. Obstet. Gynecol. 1: 615-637, 1953.

Goodall, J. R.: A Study of Endometriosis, Endosalpingiosis, Endocervicosis, and Peritoneo-Ovarian Sclerosis: a Clinical and Pathologic Study. Philadelphia: J. B. Lippincott Co., 1943.

Velden, W. H.: Familiale endometricose een erfelijke aandoening? Nederl. Tijdschr. Geneeskd. 106: 1276-1281, 1962.

*13130 ENGELMANN DISEASE (PROGRESSIVE DIAPHYSEAL DYSPLASIA)

Lennon, Schechter and Hornabrook (1961) described a case of Engelmann disease and reviewed the literature. Characteristic is gross thickening of the cortex of bones, both on the periosteal surface and in the medullary canal. The process usually begins in the shaft of the femur or tibia but spreads to involve all bones. Onset is usually before 30 years, often before 10 years of age. All races and both sexes are affected. Nine examples of familial occurrence in one or two generations were mentioned. The sclerotic bone diseases are a confused group (see OSTEOPETROSIS). Several different and separate entities (including Van Buchem disease and Ribbing disease) were lumped together by Lennon et al. (1961). To confuse the matter further, Engelmann disease is called, by some, Camurati-Engelmann disease in recognition of the earlier description, but on review it seems likely that Camurati described a different entity. The skeletal disorder is often associated with muscular weakness, peculiar gait, pains in the legs, fatiguability and apparent undernutrition. The muscular weakness is not necessarily progressive and typical bone changes may be found in asymptomatic persons. Because of the associated features muscular dystrophy or poliomyelitis is sometimes diagnosed in these patients. Girdany (1959) described a family with 6 affected persons in 3 generations (no male-to-male transmission). A case reported by Singleton et al. (1956) had strikingly similar clinical features. Restudy indicates that three generations were affected in that family also. Father and two children (son and daughter) were affected in a family reported by Ramon and Buchner (1966). The father was much more severely affected than the offspring. Allen et al. (1970) reported improvement with corticosteroids. They presented a family in which 11 persons in three generations were known to have been affected. Sparkes and Graham (1972) reported a remarkable family with many affected persons in several successive generations. A particularly remarkable feature was lack of penetrance in persons who must have had the gene but, as adults at any rate, showed no abnormality by X-ray.

Allen, D. T., Saunders, A. M., Northway, W. H., Jr., Williams, G. F. and Schafer, I. A.: Corticosteroids in the treatment of Engelmann's disease: progressive diaphyseal dysplasia. Pediatrics 46: 523-531, 1970.

Clawson, D. K. and Loop, J. W.: Progressive diaphyseal dysplasia (Engelmann's disease). J. Bone Joint Surg. 46A: 143-150, 1964.

Girdany, B. R.: Engelmann's disease (progressive diaphyseal dysplasia) — a nonprogressive familial form of muscular dystrophy with characteristic bone changes. Clin. Orthop. 14: 102-109, 1959.

Lennon, E. A., Schechter, M. M. and Hornabrook, R. W.: Engelmann's disease. Report of a case with review of the literature. J. Bone Joint Surg. 43B: 273-284, 1961.

Ramon, Y. and Buchner, A.: Camurati-Engelmann's disease affecting the jaws. Oral. Surg. 22: 592-599, 1966.

Singleton, E. B., Thomas, J. R., Worthington, W. W. and Hild, J. R.: Progressive diaphyseal dysplasia (Engelmann's disease). Radiology 67: 233-240, 1956.

Sparkes, R. S. and Graham, C. B.: Camurati-Engelmann disease. Genetics and clinical manifestations with a review of the literature. J. Med. Genet. 9: 73-85, 1972.

Wilson, F. C. and Hundley, J. D.: Progressive diaphyseal dysplasia. Review of the literature and report of seven cases in one family. J. Bone Joint Surg. 55: 461-474, 1973.

*13140 EOSINOPHILIA, FAMILIAL

Naiman and colleagues (1964) observed eosinophilia in three generations of a family. No allergies were recorded. Zeni, Nardi and Frezza (1964) observed eosinophilia in 21 members of 3 generations of a kindred. Sparrevohn (1967) described an 18 month old girl with recurrent asthmatic bronchitis, recurrent pulmonary infiltrates, leukocytosis, persistent marked eosinophilia with 'shift to the left,' intermittent thrombocytopenia, eosinophilia of liver and bone marrow, cellular infiltration including mast cells and eosinophiles in skin and muscle, no signs of allergy by usual skin tests or of parasitism and a chronic but benign course. The mother and a brother had transient eosinophilia and similar changes in skin and muscle biopsy. Zuelzer and Apt (1949) described the above syndrome in young children. One of their patients had a sister with marked eosinophilia.

Naiman, J. L., Oski, F. A., Allen, F. H. and Diamond, L. K.: Hereditary eosinophilia. Report of a family and review of the literature. Am. J. Hum. Genet. 16: 195-203, 1964.

Sparrevohn, S.: Disseminated eosinophilic collagenosis and familial eosinophilia. Acta Paediatr. Scand. 56: 307-312, 1967.

Stewart, S. G.: Familial eosinophilia. Am. J. Med. Sci. 185: 21-29, 1933.

Zeni, G., Nardi, F. and Frezza, M.: In tema di ipereosinofilia constituzionale familiare idiopatica. Acta Med. Patav. 24: 589-602, 1964.

Zuelzer, W. W. and Apt, L.: Disseminated visceral lesions associated with extreme eosinophilia. Pathological and clinical observations on syndrome of young children. Am. J. Dis. Child. 78: 153-181, 1949.

*13150 EPICANTHUS

This is a normal finding in the fetus of all races. Dominant inheritance is quite clear in many pedigrees reviewed by Usher (1935). Epicanthus also occurs in association with hereditary ptosis (q.v.).

Usher, C. H.: Pedigrees of hereditary epicanthus. Biometrika 27: 5-25, 1935.

13160 EPIDERMOID CYSTS

Epidermoid cysts are keratinous cysts but may be impossible to distinguish clinically from sebaceous cysts (q.v.).

*13170 EPIDERMOLYSIS BULLOSA DYSTROPHICA

Scarring occurs with healing of lesions in the dystrophic form but not in the 'simplex' form. In the simplex type the blisters occur within the epidermis and are subcorneal, whereas the blisters are subepidermal in the dystrophic form. Davidson (1965) had six families with the dystrophic type of which four were dominant and two recessive.

Davison, B. C. C.: Epidermolysis bullosa. J. Med. Genet. 2: 233-242, 1965.

*13180 EPIDERMOLYSIS BULLOSA OF HANDS AND FEET (WEBER-COCKAYNE TYPE)

Readett (1961) described a family in which 14 members in 5 generations were known to have localized epidermolysis bullosa of the hands and feet. The pattern was that of an autosomal dominant. Adrenosteroid depressed bulla formation but recurrence occurred with stopping therapy. This disorder is sometimes called Weber-Cockayne syndrome. An enormous pedigree with many affected persons was reported from West Virginia by Cartledge and Myers (1943). The affected persons were descendants of one Zachariah Piles, born

in 1762. The blistering occurs only on the hands and feet and mainly in warm weather after unusual walking 97
or labor with hand tools.

D
O
M
I
N
A
N
T

Cartledge, J. L. and Myers, V. W.: Inherited foot blistering in an American family. J. Hered. 34: 24 only, 1943.

Cockayne, E. A.: Recurrent bullous eruption of the feet. Br. J. Dermatol. Syph. 50: 358-362, 1938.

Haldane, J. B. S. and Poole, R.: A new pedigree of recurrent bullous eruption of the feet. Four generations of foot blisters. J. Hered. 33: 17-18, 1942.

Readett, M. D.: Localized epidermolysis bullosa. Brit. Med. J. 1: 1510-1511, 1961.

*13190 EPIDERMOLYSIS BULLOSA SIMPLEX, KOEBNER TYPE

Davison (1965) limited the designation Cockayne type epidermolysis bullosa to the condition in which bullae are confined to the feet. The type with more extensive involvement was referred to as epidermolysis bullosa simplex. Nine families were of the simplex type and 4 of the Cockayne type. It appeared that in any one family all affected persons were of one type or the other. Passarge (1965) observed 21 affected persons in 4 generations of a family. On the basis of an extensive study in Norway and review of the literature, Gedde-Dahl (1971) arrived at the following classification of epidermolysis bullosa.

I. Epidermolysis bullosa simplex (autosomal dominant)

1. Koebner type. Gonadal mosaicism (germinal mosaicism, i.e., early germ cell mutation) occurred in one family.

2. Weber-Cockayne type. Blistering limited to the feet or feet and hands.

3. Ogna type (first delineated by Gedde-Dahl). Traumatic blistering associated with congenital generalized bruising tendency.

II. Epidermolysis bullosa dystrophica

1. Epidermolysis bullosa dystrophica albopapuloidea (Pasini). Autosomal dominant.

2. Epidermolysis bullosa dystrophica (Cockayne-Touraine). Autosomal dominant.

3. Epidermolysis bullosa dystrophica with autosomal recessive inheritance.

A. Congenital localized non-lethal type

B. Congenital generalized non-lethal type

C. Congenital generalized sub-lethal (mutilating) type

D. Lethal type

E. Congential generalized inverse type

F. Neurotrophic type (semitardive localized, non-lethal type with congenital deafness)

Gedde-Dahl presented evidence that some clinical variants of epidermolysis bullosa dystrophica are the result of the presence of two non-identical recessive alleles. Thus, the genes responsible for some or all of the several forms of recessive epidermolysis bullosa may be at the same locus.

Davison, B. C. C.: Epidermolysis bullosa. J. Med. Genet. 2: 233-242, 1965.

Gedde-Dahl, T., Jr.: Epidermolysis Bullosa. A clinical, genetic and epidermiological study. Baltimore: Johns Hopkins Press, 1971.

Passarge, E.: Epidermolysis bullosa hereditaria simplex. A Kindred affected in four generations. J. Pediatr. 67: 819-825, 1965.

*13195 EPIDERMOLYSIS BULLOSA SIMPLEX, OGNA TYPE

This disorder has thus far been identified only in one large Norwegian kindred (Gedde-Dahl, 1971). It was differentiated from the more generalized form of Koebner (13190) and the localized type of Weber and Cockayne (13180) by the occurrence of skin bruising in the Ogna type. Olaisen and Gedde-Dahl (1973) concluded that the locus for this disorder is closely linked (about 5 cM) to that for red cell soluble glutamate-pyruvate transaminase (13820).

Gedde-Dahl, T., Jr.: Epidermolysis bullosa. A clinical, genetic and epidermiological study. Baltimore: Johns Hopkins Press, 1971.

Olaisen, B. and Gedde-Dahl, T., Jr.: GPT-epidermolysis bullosa simplex (EBS Ogna) linkage in man. Hum. Hered. 23: 189-196, 1973.

*13200 EPIDERMOLYSIS BULLOSA WITH CONGENITAL LOCALIZED ABSENCE OF SKIN AND DEFORMITY OF NAILS

In the family reported by Bart et al. (1966), 26 persons were affected. Penetrance was complete. The syndrome consisted of congenital absence of skin on the lower extremities, blistering of skin and mucous membranes, and congenital absence or deformity of nails. The condition seems distinct from previously reported forms of local aplasia of skin and from various other types of epidermolysis bullosa. Congenital localized absence of skin is probably an occasional manifestation of epidermolysis bullosa, the result of in utero blistering (Bart, 1970). Father-son transmission was noted.

Bart, B. J.: Congenital localized absence of skin, blistering and nail abnormalities, a new syndrome. The Clinical Delineation of Birth Defects. XII. Skin, Hair and Nails. Baltimore: Williams and Wilkins, 1971. Pp. 118-120.

Bart, B. J.: Epidermolysis bullosa and congenital localized absence of skin. Arch. Dermatol. 101: 78-81, 1970.

Bart, B. J., Gorlin, R. J., Anderson, V. E. and Lynch, F. W.: Congenital localized absence of skin and associated abnormalities resembling epidermolysis bullosa. A new syndrome. Arch. Dermatol. 93: 296-304, 1966.

13210 EPILEPSY, PHOTOGENIC

Friedlander (1959) discussed an hereditary pattern of 'cerebral light sensitivity.' Davidson and Watson's data (1956) on 12 families is consistent with dominant inheritance with reduced penetrance. There was no instance of male-to-male transmission.

Davidson, S. and Watson, C. W.: Hereditary light sensitive epilepsy. Neurology 6: 231-261, 1956.

Friedlander, W. J.: Epilepsy. Am. J. Psychol. 1: 623-628, 1959.

Gerken, H., Doose, H., Volzke, E., Volz, C. and Hien-Volpel, K. F.: Genetics of childhood epilepsy with photic sensitivity. (Letter) Lancet I: 1377-1378, 1968.

13220 EPILEPSY, PRIMARY READING

Matthews and Wright (1967) reported the cases of mother and daughter with epilepsy and jaw-jerking provoked by reading.

Matthews, W. B. and Wright, F. K.: Hereditary primary reading epilepsy. Neurology 17: 919-921, 1967.

13230 EPILEPSY, READING

Rowan et al. (1970) described a girl who had major and minor seizures which were related to pattern and photosensitivity. The mother also had EEG discharges during reading. The daughter's attacks were precipitated by television-viewing. A younger sister had had one febrile convulsion. The father had had epilepsy between ages 5 and 8 years. No studies of him were reported.

Rowan, A. J., Heathfield, K. W. G. and Scott, D. F.: Is reading epilepsy inherited? J. Neurol. Neurosurg. Psychiatry 33: 476-478, 1970.

*13240 EPIPHYSEAL DYSPLASIA, MULTIPLE

Severe osteoarthritis of the hips develops in early adulthood. The diagnosis in the adult is aided by the changes in the distal tibia (Leeds, 1960). A deficiency in the lateral part of the distal tibial ossification center seen in children results in a sloping end of the tibia in adulthood. Short stature and brachydactyly are features. Considerable heterogeneity undoubtedly exists within this category. Chondrodystrophia calcificans congenita is a congenital form of multiple epiphyseal dysplasia (inherited as a recessive). Bachman and Norman (1967) described a 47 year old woman, height 61-and-one-half inches with marked hyperextensibility of fingers and precocious osteoarthritis of the hips. A son and a daughter had very flexible fingers and by hand X-ray delay in carpal ossification, proximal pseudo-epiphyses of metacarpals II-V, cone-cup epiphyses-metaphyses and widened joint spaces. Other joints showed extensive changes with widening of joint spaces and irregular epiphyses. The mother's mother, aunt, uncle and cousin had hyperextensibility of the fingers and premature osteoarthritis. These authors referred to the condition as peripheral dysostosis but it seems different from the peripheral dysostosis (q.v.) described by Singleton et al. (1960); the term 'peripheral' seems inappropriate, and the description suggests what others would call Fairbank multiple epiphyseal dysplasia. The condition described as enchondral dysostosis by Odman (1959) is probably the same condition as is also Elsbach (1959) microepiphyseal dysplasia. Almost certainly heterogeneity exists within the group of autosomal dominant multiple epiphyseal dysplasia. However, no one has succeeded in sorting out separate entities in a convincing manner. I suspect that the family with four affected persons in 3 generations reported by Cameron and Gardiner (1963) had multiple epiphyseal dysplasia, or perhaps a form of spondyloepiphyseal dysplasia, inasmuch as the spine was involved. Precocious osteoarthritis was a feature. Hulvey and Keats (1969) commented on the variability in the extent of spinal involvement and presented a family in which many members had severe peripheral involvement with no spinal involvement. The dividing line between multiple epiphyseal dysplasia and spondyloepiphyseal dysplasia tarda can be indistinct, witness the family reported by Diamond (1970).

Bachman, K. and Norman, A. P.: Hereditary peripheral dysostosis (3 cases). Proc. R. Soc. Med. 60: 21-22, 1967.

Berg, P. K.: Dysplasia epiphysialis multiplex: a case report and review of the literature. Am. J. Roentgen. 97: 31-38, 1966.

Cameron, J. M. and Gardiner, T. B.: Atypical familial osteochondrodystrophy. Br. J. Radiol. 36: 135-139, 1963.

Cowan, D. J.: Multiple epiphysial dysplasia. Br. Med. J. 2: 1629 only, 1963.

Diamond, L. S.: A family study of spondyloepiphyseal dysplasia. J. Bone Joint Surg. 52B: 1587-1594, 1970.

Elsbach, L.: Bilateral hereditary micro-epiphyseal dysplasia of the hips. J. Bone Joint Surg. 41B: 514-523, 1959.

Hoefnagel, D., Sycamore, L. K., Russell, S. W. and Bucknall, W. E.: Hereditary multiple epiphysial dysplasia. Ann. Hum. Genet. 30: 201-210, 1967.

Hulvey, J. T. and Keats, T. E.: Multiple epiphyseal dysplasia. A contribution to the problem of spinal involvement. Am. J. Roentgen. 106: 170-177, 1969.

Jacobs, P. A.: Dysplasia epiphysialis multiplex. Clin. Orthop. 58: 117-128, 1968.

Leeds, N. E.: Epiphysial dysplasia multiplex. Am. J. Roentgen. 84: 506-510, 1960.

Maudsley, R. H.: Dysplasia epiphysialis multiplex: a report of fourteen cases in three families. J. Bone Joint Surg. 37B: 228-240, 1955.

Murphy, M. C., Shine, I. B. and Stevens, D. B.: Multiple epiphyseal dysplasia. Report of a pedigree. J. Bone Joint Surg. 55A: 814-820, 1973.

Odman, P.: Hereditary enchondral dysostosis. Twelve cases in three generations mainly with peripheral location. Acta Radiol. 52: 97-113, 1959.

Singleton, E. B., Daeschner, C. W. and Teng, C. T.: Peripheral dysostosis. Am. J. Roentgen. 84: 499-505, 1960.

Watt, J. K.: Multiple epiphyseal dysplasia: report of four cases. Br. J. Surg. 39: 533-535, 1952.

13250 EPISTAXIS, HEREDITARY

Whether there are families with this condition transmitted as a simple dominant without telangiectasia is not clear. Fink (1940) described what was presumed to be such a family with transmission through six generations.

Fink, H. K.: Hereditary epistaxis in man. J. Hered. 31: 319-322, 1940.

13260 EPITHELIOMA CALCIFICANS OF MALHERBE

Kawamura and Sekimura (1939) observed affected brother and sister. Duperrat and Albert (1948) described five affected persons in two generations of a family. Geiser (1960) reported affected father and daughter. We (Harper, 1971) have observed two affected sisters who also had typical myotonic dystrophy a presumably unrelated trait. No information concerning their parents was available. Cantwell and Reed (1965) reported multiple calcifying epithelioma in association with myotonic dystrophy and Harper (1971) reported sibs with this combination and has seen at least 6 other confirmed instances of the association. Pilomatrixoma is the term for this tumor used by Jones and Campbell (1969). The lesions are firm, circumscribed tumors, usually in the head and neck area. They feel like buttons and are attached to the subcutaneous tissue and overlying skin.

Cantwell, A. R., Jr. and Reed, W. B.: Myotonia atrophica and multiple calcifying epithelioma of Malherbe. Acta Derm. Venerol. 45: 387-390, 1965.

Duperrat, B. and Albert (NI): Forme familiale de l'epithéliome de Malherbe. Bull. Soc. Fr. Dermatol. Syph. 55: 196, 1948.

Geiser, J. D.: Forme familiale d'epithelioma (calcifie) de Malherbe. Dermatologica 120: 361-365, 1960.

Harper, P. S.: Calcifying epithelioma of malherbe and myotonic dystrophy in sisters. The Clinical Delineation of Birth Defects. XII. Skin Hair and Nails. Baltimore: Williams and Wilkins, 1971. Pp. 343-345.

Jones, P. G. and Campbell, P. E.: Pilomatrixoma: a not uncommon hamartoma of infancy and childhood. Aust. Paediatr. J. 5: 162-166, 1969.

Kawamura, T. and Sekimura, T.: Zwei faelle von bei Bruder and Schwester vorkommendem verkalktem Epitheliom. Jap. J. Dermatol. Urol. 45: 41, 1939.

*13270 EPITHELIOMA, HEREDITARY MULTIPLE BENIGN CYSTIC (EPITHELIOMA ADENOIDES CYSTICUM OF BROOKE)

Fliegelman and Kruse (1948) described 10 cases in three generations. They indicated that despite some clinical similarities the disorder could be distinguished from syringocystadenoma, adenoma sebaceum and cylindroma. Some think that this and cylindroma are the same entity. Gartler and colleagues (1966), studying members of a family with affected members in four generations, found that females heterozygous for G6PD-deficiency had shown both G6PD-deficient and G6PD-normal cells in the same tumor, thus indicating multicellular origin. Ziprkowski and Schewach-Millet (1966) reported the dermatologic features in the same family. The skin tumors show differentiation in the direction of hair structures, hence the synonym trichoepithelioma. One affected person developed baso-squamous cell carcinoma. Welch, Wells and Kerr (1968) presented family data supporting the view that Ancell-Spiegler cylindromas and Brooke-Fordyce trichoepitheliomas are manifestations of a single entity. The term cylindroma was also applied by Billroth (1859) to a type of adenocarcinoma arising in salivary gland tissue (Evans et al., 1966).

Baden, H. P.: Cylindromatosis simulating neurofibromatosis. N. Engl. J. Med. 267: 296-297, 1962.

Billroth, T.: Beobachtungen ueber Geschwuelste der Speicheldruesen. Virchow. Arch. Path. Anat. 17: 357-375, 1859.

Evans, J. C., Efskind, J. and Roberts, T. W.: Cylindroma. Am. J. Roentgen. 96: 191-196, 1966.

Fliegelman, M. T. and Kruse, W. T.: Hereditary multiple benign cystic epithelioma. J. Invest. Derm. 11: 189-196, 1948.

Gartler, S. M., Ziprkowski, L., Krakowski, A., Ezra, R., Szeinberg, A. and Adam, A.: Glucose-6-phosphate dehydrogenase mosaicism as a tracer in the study of hereditary multiple trichoepithelioma. Am. J. Hum. Genet. 18: 282-287, 1966.

Welch, J. P., Wells, R. S. and Kerr, C. B.: Ancell-Spiegler cylindromas (turban tumours) and Brooke-Fordyce trichoepitheliomas. Evidence for a single genetic entity. J. Med. Genet. 5: 29-35, 1968.

Ziprkowski, L. and Schewach-Millet, M.: Multiple trichoepithelioma in a mother and two children. Dermatologica 132: 248-256, 1966.

*13280 EPITHELIOMA, SELF-HEALING SQUAMOUS (FERGUSON-SMITH TYPE)

This is considered to be a variety of multiple keratoacanthoma. It goes under many different names. Ereaux and Schopflocher (1965) observed affected brother and sister. Sommerville and Milne (1950) reported two cases in each of two successive generations. Affected father and son were referred to by Epstein, Biskind and Pollack (1957). Degos and colleagues (1964) described the condition in a woman and two daughters. Ferguson-Smith, geneticist son of the dermatologist who originally described this condition, and his colleagues (1971) assembled reliable information on 62 cases in the west of Scotland. It was considered possible that all the Scottish cases derived from a single mutation which occurred before 1790. The lesions were found more frequently on exposed areas of the skin and their distribution correspondingly differed between males and females.

Degos, R., Civatte, J., Touraine, B. and Guilaine, J.: Spontan heilende Epitheliome Ferguson-Smith und multiple familiaere Keratoacanthome. Hautarzt 15: 7-11, 1964.

Epstein, N. N., Biskind, G. R. and Pollack, R. S.: Multiple primary self-healing squamous-cell 'epitheliomas' of the skin: generalized keratoacanthoma. Arch. Dermatol. 75: 210-223, 1957.

Ereaux, L. P. and Schopflocher, P.: Familial primary self-healing squamous epithelioma of skin. Arch. Dermatol. 91: 589-594, 1965.

Ferguson-Smith, M. A., Wallace, D. C., James, Z. H. and Renwick, J. H.: Multiple self-healing squamous epithelioma. The Clinical Delineation of Birth Defects. XII. Skin, Hair and Nails. Baltimore: Williams and Wilkins, 1971. Pp. 157-163.

Sommerville, J. and Milne, J. A.: Self-healing squamous epithelioma of the skin. Br. J. Dermatol. 62: 485-490, 1950.

13290 ERDHEIM CYSTIC MEDIAL NECROSIS OF AORTA

Erdheim disease with dissecting aneurysm has been observed in brothers (Graham, Milne, 1952; von Meyenburg, 1939), in father and son (Fleming, Helwig, 1941) and in mother and daughter (Griffiths, Hayhurst, Whitehead, 1951) but clinical information in these reports is too scanty to permit exclusion of the Marfan syndrome (q.v.). Hanley and Jones (1967) reported dissecting aortic aneurysm in 2 sisters and the son of one of them. No stigmata of Marfan syndrome were present. Familial aortic rupture has been observed with the Sack variety of Ehlers-Danlos syndrome (13005). McKusick (1972) observed a father and son with congenital bicuspid aortic valve and medial necrosis of the aorta. Opitz (1973) studied a family with isolated Erdheim disease in a young woman, her father and her father's father.

Fleming, J. W. and Helwig, F. C.: Medionecrosis aortae idiopathica cystica with spontaneous rupture. Report of three cases with necropsies. J. Mo. Med. Assoc. 38: 86-88, 1941.

Graham, J. G. and Milne, J. A.: Dissecting aneurysm of the aorta: a review of 29 cases. Glasgow Med. J. 33: 320-330, 1952.

Griffiths, G. J., Hayhurst, A. P. and Whitehead, R.: Dissecting aneurysm of aorta in mother and child. Br. Heart J. 13: 364-368, 1951.

Hanley, W. B. and Jones, N. B.: Familial dissecting aortic aneurysm. A report of three cases within two generations. Br. Heart J. 29: 852-858, 1967.

McKusick, V. A.: Association of aortic valvular disease and cystic medial necrosis. (Letter) Lancet I: 1026-1027, 1972.

Opitz, J. M.: Madison, Wis., personal communication, Aug. 31, 1973.

Von Meyenburg, H.: Ueber spontane Aortenruptur bei zwei Bruedern. Schweiz. Med. Wschr. 20: 976-979, 1939.

*13300 ERYTHEMA PALMARE HEREDITARIUM

Symmetrical asymptomatic redness of the palms is similar to that seen with hepatic cirrhosis. Pregnancy may precipitate the appearance of hereditary erythema. I know of the trait in successive generations. Olivier (1956) described affected father and 4 (out of 9) affected children.

Lane, J. E.: Erythema palmare hereditarium. Arch. Dermatol. Syph. 20: 445-448, 1929.

Olivier, J.: Erythema palmo-plantaire hereditaire. Maladie de Lane. Arch. Belg. Dermatol. Syph. 12: 202-207, 1956.

13310 ERYTHROCYTOSIS, BENIGN FAMILIAL

This disorder is characterized by an increase in red blood cell mass with no increase in platelets and leukocytes, by a benign course and familial incidence. This is probably a condition distinct from polycythemia vera. The latter condition is more frequent in Jews than non-Jews in the United States (Modan, 1965) but shows no simple Mendelian pattern. A patient reported by Auerbach et al. (1958) was again reported by Cassileth and Hyman (1966) with family study. Engelking (1920) and Wieland (1932) separately reported a family in which 11 members of 3 generations were polycythemic. In some the abnormality was noted in childhood. Such families should be studied for a hemoglobinopathy. Polycythemia is a feature of several variant hemoglobins: Chesapeake, J (Capetown), Yakima, Kempsey, Rainier (Weatherall, 1969), Ypsilanti, Hiroshima. The heterozygotes show polycythemia, hence the phenotype is dominant. Alperin et al. (1967) reported finding elevated levels of erythropoietin in affected members of one family. Geary et al. (1967) observed polycythemia in 5 persons in three generations of a family and showed that the basis was thalassemia minor. The red cell count was elevated but total hemoglobin was normal, thus giving hypochromia. Hemoglobin A2 was elevated. More often thalassemia minor presents as refractory hypochromic anemia. Davey et al. (1968) found erythrocytosis in a brother and sister, offspring of a second-cousin marriage, and raised the question of recessive inheritance. The father had slight but persistent erythrocytosis. Apparently hemoglobin electrophoresis was not performed. Hemoglobin Olympia (q.v.) is an electrophoretically silent mutant form of hemoglobin which leads to erythrocytosis. Some instances of familial polycythemia with normal hemoglobin may represent a defect in the mechanisms for mantinining intra-erythrocytic pH (Charache, 1974).

Alperin, J. B., Levin, W. C., Alexanian, R. and Houston, E. W.: Familial erythrocytosis: a disorder due to increased erythropoietin production. To be published.

Auerbach, M. L., Wolff, J. A. and Mettier, S. R.: Benign familial polycythemia in childhood. Pediatrics 21: 54-58, 1958.

Cassileth, P. A. and Hyman, G. A.: Benign familial erythrocytosis: report of three cases and a review of the literature. Am. J. Med. Sci. 251: 692-697, 1966.

Charache, S.: Familial polycythemia. Mount Sinai J. Med. 37: 418-425, 1970.

Charache, S.: Baltimore, personal communication, Jan. 14, 1974.

Davey, M. G., Lawrence, J. R., Lander, H. and Robson, H. N.: Familial erythrocytosis. A report of two cases, and a review. Acta Haematol. 39: 65-74, 1968.

Engelking, E.: Ueber familiaere Polyzythaemie und die dabei beobachteten Augenveraenderungen. Klin. Mbl. Augenheilk. 64: 645-664, 1920.

Geary, C. G., Amos, H. E. and MacIver, J. E.: Benign familial polycythemia. J. Clin. Pathol. 20: 158-160, 1967.

Modan, B.: An epidemiological study of polycythemia vera. Blood 26: 657-667, 1965.

Spodaro, A. and Forkner, C. E.: Benign familial polycythemia. Arch. Intern. Med. 52: 593-602, 1933.

Stamatoyannopoulos, G., Nute, P. E., Adamson, J. W., Bellingham, A. J., Funk, D. and Hornung, S.: Hemoglobin olympia (beta 20 valine to methionine): an electrophoretically silent variant associated with high oxygen affinity and erythrocytosis. J. Clin. Invest. 52: 342-349, 1973.

Weatherall, D. J.: Polycythemia resulting from abnormal hemoglobins. New Eng. J. Med. 280: 604-606, 1969.

Wieland, W.: Weitere Untersuchungen ueber Polycythaemia vera im Kindesalter. Z. Kinderheilk. 53: 703-715, 1932.

*13320 ERYTHROKERATODERMIA VARIABILIS

Cowan (1962) presented cases of father and daughter with erythrokeratodermia. From early childhood the father had skin disease on the face, hands, forearms, legs and feet. Marked hyperkeratosis, hyperpigmentation and hypertrichosis were some of the features as well as erythema which varied from time to time and varied in site. The cardinal feature is the presence almost from birth of sharply outlined geographical areas of erythrokeratodermia. A particularly striking pedigree was assembled by Noordhoeck (1966). This was probably the condition present in the extensively affected kindred reported by Kelly and Kocsard (1970).

Brown, J. and Kierland, R. R.: Erythrokeratodermia variabilis. Report of three cases and review of the literature. Arch. Dermatol. 93: 194-201, 1966.

Cowan, M. A.: Erythrokeratodermia in father and daughter. Proc. Roy. Soc. Med. 55: 875-876, 1962.

Kelly, L. J. and Kocsard, E.: Congenital ichthyosis with erythema anulare centrifugum. A new form of ichthyosis affecting 12 members of a family of 31 in 5 generations. Dermatologica 140: 75-83, 1970.

Noordhoeck, F. J.: Over erythro- et keratodermia variabilis: on erythro- et keratodermia variabilis. Utrecht Thesis, 1950. (Cited by Schnyder, V. W. and Klunker, W.: Erbliche Verhornungsstoerungen der Haut. In, Gottron, H. A. and Schnyder, V. W. (eds.): Vererbung von Hautkrankheiten. Berlin: Springer-Verlag, 1966. P. 923.)

Schnyder, U. W. and Sommacal-Schopf, D.: Fourteen cases of erythro-keratodermia figurata variabilis within one family. Acta Genet. Statist. Med. 7: 204-206, 1957.

*13321 ESTERASE A

Using azo dye coupling techniques, and electrophoresis, Tashian (1969) defined several different esterases in human red cells. Three main groups, differing as to electrophoretic properties, substrate specificites and inhibition characteristics, were A, B and C esterases. Isozymes of carbonic anhydrase (11480, 11481) which also has esteratic activity, were demonstrated by similar techniques. Variants of esterase A were reported by Tashian and Shaw (1962) and Tashian (1965).

Tashian, R. E. and Shaw, M. W.: Inheritance of an erythrocyte acetylesterase variant of man. Am. J. Hum. Genet. 14: 295-300, 1962.

Tashian, R. E.: Genetic variation and evolution of the carboxylic esterases and carbonic anhydrases of primate erythrocytes. Am. J. Hum. Genet. 17: 257- , 1965.

*13322 ESTERASE A-4

By cell hybridization methods the structural locus for esterase A-4 has been localized to chromosone no. 11.

Shows, T. B.: Genetics of human-mouse cell hybrids linkage of human genes for lactate dehydrogenase-A and esterase-A-4. Proc. Natl. Acad. Sci. 69: 348-352, 1972.

*13325 ESTERASE ACTIVATOR

Kao and Puck (1972) found that hybrids formed from an adenine-requiring Chinese hamster cell and human fibroblasts uniformly display new esterase activity. Hybrids that grew in selective medium showed a single extra chromosome resembling a B-group human chromosome. They postulated a human activator gene linked to the ade B gene, located on a B-group chromosome, and capable of activating the mouse locus.

Kao, F. T. and Puck, T.T.: Genetics of somatic mammalian cells: demonstration of a human esterase activator gene linked to the Ade B gene. Proc. Natl. Acad. Sci. 69: 3273-3277, 1972.

13326 ESTERASE B

Esterase B of erythrocytes is primarily a butyryl esterase. No variants have been reported in population surveys to date. See ESTERASE A and ESTERASE D for bibliography.

13327 ESTERASE C

Esterase C is a rather weakly staining acetylesterase. No variant has been found. See ESTERASE A and ESTERASE D for bibliography.

*13328 ESTERASE D

Hopkinson et al. (1973) described another red cell esterase they called esterase D. Although studied in red cell hemolystates, esterase D was found in many different tissues in cloding cultured fibroblasts and lymphocytoid cells. Genetic polymorphism was discovered in European, Black and Indian populations.

Hopkinson, D. A., Mestriner, M. A., Cortner, J. and Harris, H.: Esterase D: a new human polymorphism. Ann. Hum. Genet. 37: 119-137, 1973.

*13330 ESTERASE ES-2, REGULATOR FOR

Klebe et al. (1970) using mouse-human hybrid somatic cells in culture, found that Es-2 esterase activity was depressed. Human chromosomes are selectively lost from the hybrid cells. Depression of esterase activity was present when human chromosome 10 was present and the activity returned to normal when chromosome 10 was lost. Thus, they concluded that the regulator 'element' is probably structurally linked to chromosome 10.

Klebe, R. J., Chen, T.-R. and Ruddle, F. H.: Mapping of a human genetic regulator element by somatic cell genetic analysis. Proc. Natl. Acad. Sci. 66: 1220-1227, 1970.

*13340 ESTERASE OF ERYTHROCYTES

Tashian and Shaw (1962) demonstrated co-dominant inheritance of an erythrocyte acetylesterase variant. These esterases catalyze the cleavage of carboxyl esters.

Tashian, R. E. and Shaw, M. W.: Inheritance of an erythrocyte acetylesterase variant of man. Am. J. Hum. Genet. 14: 295-300, 1962.

*13350 EXCHONDROSIS OF PINNA, POSTERIOR ('EAR BUMP')

A cartilaginous spur on the posterior aspect of the pinna rather close to its attachment to the side of the head is probably inherited as an irregular dominant (Quelprud: see Gates, 1947). The author and several members of his family in 3 generations show this trait. There are several instances of male-to-male transmission, a pair of concordantly affected monozygotic twins and no consanguinity.

Gates, R. R.: Human Heredity. New York: MacMillan, 1947. p. 249.

13360 EXOSTOSES OF HEEL

Gould (1942) described the condition in grandfather, father and son, i.e., males of three generations. X-rays were not described.

Gould, E. A.: Three generations of exostoses of the heel. Inherited from father to son. J. Hered. 33: 228 only, 1942.

*13370 EXOSTOSES, MULTIPLE

Krooth, Macklin and Hilbish (1961) reported on a study of the families of 6 persons with diaphyseal aclasis (multiple exostoses). The families were Chamorros, a Micronesian people who live in the Mariana Islands. The frequency of diaphyseal aclasis in the Chamorros of Guam was estimated at 1 in 1000. In published series the disease is more frequent in males than in females and more severe in affected males than in affected

Scholz and Murken (1963) did linkage studies with negative results. In a study of 56 patients Solomon (1963) found a sex ratio of 1 and reported that two-thirds of the patients had an affected parent. Solomon (1964) observed one family in which all 8 affected persons in four sibships of three generations showed exostoses on the bones of the hands and fingers with very few elsewhere. In no other patients of his study did the abnormality take this particular form. Other workers have found no correlation between members of the same family as to form and distribution of disease. For these reasons Solomon suggested that the particular family may suffer from a rare disorder due to a gene distinct from that causing most cases. Deformities of the forearms of the Madelung type occur in some cases. Two sibs who probably are cases of homozygosity (both parents were affected and came from exostosis families and the children showed unusually severe changes early) were observed by Giedion and colleagues (1972).

Giedion, A.: Zurich, Switzerland: personal communication, 1972.

Krooth, R. S., Macklin, M. T. and Hilbish, T. F.: Diaphysial aclasis (multiple exostoses) on Guam. Am. J. Hum. Genet. 13: 340-347, 1961.

Morgan, J. P., Carlson, W. D. and Adams, O. R.: Hereditary multiple exostosis in the horse. J. Am. Vet. Med. Assoc. 140: 1320-1322, 1962.

Scholz, W. and Murken, J. D.: Koppelungsuntersuchungen bei Familien mit multiplen cartilaeginaeren Exostosen. Z. Menschl. Vererb. Konstitutionsl. 37: 178-192, 1963.

Solomon, L.: Hereditary multiple exostosis. Am. J. Hum. Genet. 16: 351-363, 1964.

Solomon, L.: Hereditary multiple exostosis. J. Bone Joint Surg. 45B: 292-304, 1963.

Vinstein, A. L. and Franken, E. A., Jr.: Hereditary multiple exostoses: report of a case with spinal cord compression. Am. J. Roentgen. 112: 405-407, 1971.

13375 EXTRASYSTOLES, MULTIFORM VENTRICULAR WITH SHORT STATURE, HYPERPIGMENTATION AND MICROCEPHALY

Multiform ventricular extrasystoles as a dominant genetic trait is well known (see 11500). Char et al. (1974) described mother and son who had this disorder and in addition showed short stature, microcephaly, dull intelligence and cutaneous hyperpigmentation.

Char, F., Douglas, J. and Dungan, W. T.: Familial multiform ventricular extrasystoles with short stature, hyperpigmentation and microcephaly. To be published, 1974.

13380 EYEBROW, WHORL IN

Virchow (1912) found a whorl in the hair of the left eyebrow near the nose in 8 members of two generations. The progenitor in the next earlier generation may have shown it also.

Virchow, H.: Stellung der Haare im Brauenkopf. Z. F. Ethnol. 44: 402-403, 1912.

13400 FACIAL HYPERTRICHOSIS

Trotter and Danforth (1922) estimated a frequency of 27 percent in women. Obviously the frequency in man is not determinable. They found a correlation of about 0.8 between mother and daughter and suggested autosomal dominant inheritance.

Trotter, M. and Danforth, C. H.: The incidence and heredity of facial hypertrichosis in white women. Am. J. Phys. Anthropol. 5: 391-397, 1922.

13410 FACIAL PALSY, CONGENITAL UNILATERAL

Skyberg and Van der Hagen (1965) observed this in four generations with sixteen probably affected persons. No male-to-male transmission was identified but one affected male had an unaffected daughter. The stapedial reflex was absent suggesting involvement of the motor nucleus of the facial nerve. Carmena and Gomez Marcano (1943) reported four affected generations in a Spanish family. Autopsy in three cases showed partial agenesis of the facial motor nucleus. Wittig, Moreira and Freire-Maia (1967) observed congenital facial diplegia in three generations of a family. They suggested that the disorder in this family was the same as Moebius syndrome. Nuclear aplasia was present but different from Moebius syndrome (q.v.) which is an oculofacial palsy.

Carmena, M. and Gomez Marcano, E.: Paralysis facial hereditaria. Rev. Clin. Esp. 8: 266-268, 1943.

Skyberg, D. and Van der Hagen, C. B.: Congenital hereditary unilateral facial palsy in four generations. Acta Paediatr. Scand. 159 (suppl.): 77-79, 1965.

Wittig, E. O., Moreira, C. A. and Freire-Maia, N.: Familial congenital peripheral facial diplegia. (Letter) Lancet I: 282 only, 1967.

13420 FACIAL PARALYSIS

We have observed a man (1057218) who had onset of facial paralysis at the age of about 56. It began as inability to control the lower lip, which drooped. Progression occurred so that the lip became strikingly protruberant and everted with exposure of the lower gingival mucosa. Five years after onset he could not wrinkle his forehead. There was an intermittent twitch of the right side of the upper lip. The extraocular muscles were affected only very minimally and there was no ptosis. A striking feature was laxity of the skin raising the question of cutis laxa. Slit lamp examination showed a lattice type of corneal opacity bilaterally. The mother had the precisely identical disorder beginning at about the same stage of life and a son 20 years the proband's junior was said to be showing early signs. The disorder may represent a bilateral progressive hereditary facial nerve palsy. Electromyograms could not distinguish neural and muscular origin of the paralysis. Muscle biopsy was consistent with neurogenic atrophy. I suspect that the disorder in this family is, in fact, Melkersson syndrome (q.v.).

13430 FACIAL SPASM

Stocks (1922-23) made a distinction between facial tic (or habit spasm), which is a movement of a coordinated group of facial muscles not entirely beyond the control of the will and not occurring during sleep, and facial spasm, which is usually confined to the muscles supplied by the facial nerve or one branch thereof. The 18-year-old proband in Stocks' Polish family had rapid clonic spasm of the levator menti muscle between the chin and lower lip. The involvement was said to be limited to that muscle in other affected members of the family also. Cold and excitement aggravated the condition. Hellsing's family (1930) showed more extensive involvement and anisocoria and depressed tendon reflexes were noted. Considerable confusion exists between facial spasm and trembling chin (q.v.). It seems possible that the families of Stocks and of Goldsmith are ones of trembling chin and Hellsing's one of facial spasm.

Goldsmith, J. B.: The inheritance of 'facial spasm' and the effect of a modifying factor associated with high temper. J. Hered. 18: 185-187, 1927.

Hellsing, G.: Hereditaerer Facialiskrampf. Acta Med. Scand. 73: 526-537, 1930.

Stocks, P.: Facial spasm inherited through four generations. Biometrika 14: 311-315, 1922-23.

13440 FACTOR V (PROACCELERIN) EXCESS WITH SPONTANEOUS THROMBOSIS

Gaston (1966) reported a family in which a 6-year-old girl had iliofemoral thrombectomy, her father had bilateral leg amputations at age 34 for occlusive arterial disease, a father's cousin had recurrent thrombophlebitis beginning at age 18 and a son of the latter had recurrent leg and arm thrombophlebitis with pulmonary emboli. Plasma Factor V was found to be elevated in these persons.

Gaston, L. W.: Studies on a family with an elevated plasma level of Factor V (proaccelerin) and a tendency to thrombosis. J. Pediatr. 68: 367-373, 1966.

*13450 FACTOR VIII DEFICIENCY

Hensen, Mattern and Loeliger (1965) described a family in which 8 persons in four generations in an autosomal dominant pattern had Factor VIII deficiency. Normal bleeding times and lack of Factor VIII elevation after infusion of hemophilic plasma excluded Von Willebrand disease (q.v.). Veltkamp et al. (1968) confirmed these findings. No rise of Factor VIII occurred in a boy with hemophilia a when transfused with plasma from a girl in Hensen's family. Furthermore, the girl's plasma transfused into a woman with severe Von Willebrand disease had no effect on her Factor VIII level.

Hensen, A., Mattern, M. J. and Loeliger, E. A.: Haemophilia a with apparently autosomal dominant inheritance. Evidence for a second autosomal locus involved in Factor VIII production. Thromb. Diath. Haemorrh. 14: 341-345, 1965.

Veltkamp, J..J., Taconis, W. K. and Loeliger, E. A.: Autosomal Factor VIII deficiency. (Letter) Lancet II: 1303 only, 1968.

13455 FACTOR XII (HAGEMAN FACTOR) DEFICIENCY

Factor XII deficiency seemingly inherited as an autosomal dominant was reported by Bennett et al. (1972). The gene could be allelic with that responsible for the autosomal recessive form (23400).

Bennett, B., Ratnoff, O., Holt, J. B. and Roberts, H. R.: Hageman trait (Factor XII deficiency): a probable second genotype inherited as an autosomal dominant characteristic. Blood 40: 412-415, 1972.

13460 FANCONI RENOTUBULAR SYNDROME

In the kindred reported by Hunt et al. (1966) 8 persons in three generations may have been affected, although only a mother and son had the full-blown picture. Another presumably dominant pedigree is that of Ben-Ishay et al. (1961).

Ben-Ishay, D., Dreyfuss, F. and Ullmann, T. D.: Fanconi syndrome with hypouricemia in an adult. Family study. Am. J. Med. 31: 793-800, 1961.

Hunt, D. D., Stearns, G., McKinley, J. B., Froning, E., Hicks, P. and Bonfiglio, M.: Long-term study of a family with Fanconi syndrome without cystinosis (Detoni-Debre-Fanconi syndrome). Am. J. Med. 40: 492-510, 1966.

13470 FAVISM

Hemolytic anemia following ingestion of the bean of Vicia fava or exposure to its pollen is conditioned primarily by a deficiency of erythrocyte glucose-6-phosphate dehydrogenase, an X-linked genetic trait. Vicia fava apparently produces a substance which induces hemolysis of enzyme deficient red cells (Mager et al., 1965). In areas where the enzyme deficiency is frequent, favism shows familial aggregation probably not accounted for by the familial occurrence of the enzyme deficiency alone. Stamatoyannopoulos and colleagues (1966) interpreted studies in Greece as indicating the presence of an autosomal gene which in heterozygous state enhances the susceptibility to favism of G6PD-deficient persons. Beutler (1970) suggested that DOPA-quinone is the active hemolytic principle in fava beans. (Fava beans are the main commercial source of L-DOPA.) Differences in susceptibility to favism by G6PD-deficient persons may be related to differences in the enzymatic system which converts L-DOPA to DOPA-quinone. A genetic mechanism for susceptibility to favism on the part of G6PD-deficient persons is suggested by the findings of Bottini et al. (1971) that persons with favism are more often of a particular red-cell acid phosphatase type than would be expected on the basis of population frequencies.

Beutler, E.: L-DOPA and favism. (Editorial) Blood 36: 523-525, 1970.

Bottini, E., Lucarelli, P., Agostino, R., Palmarino, R., Businco, L. and Antognoni, G.: Favism: association with erythrocyte acid phosphatase phenotype. Science 171: 409-411, 1971.

Mager, J., Glaser, G., Razin, A., Izak, G., Bien, S. and Noam, M.: Metabolic effects of pyrimidines derived from fava bean glycosides on human erythrocytes deficient in glucose-6-phosphate dehydrogenase. Biochem. Biophys. Res. Commun. 20: 235-240, 1965.

Stamatoyannopoulos, G., Fraser, G. R., Motulsky, A. G., Fessas, P., Akrivakis, A. and Papayan-nopoulou, T.: On the familial predisposition to favism. Am. J. Hum. Genet. 18: 253-263, 1966.

*13480 FIBRINOGEN

In addition to afibrinogenemia (a recessive, 20240), fibrinogen may be functionally abnormal. Examples have been reported by Menache (1964), by Imperato and Dettori (1958) and by Jackson, Beck and Charache (1965). The last group (Beck et al., 1965), following the practice with hemoglobins, referred to the anomalous protein as fibrinogen (Baltimore). A mother and three daughters were affected in their family and a father and son in Menache's family. Beck, Charache and Jackson (1965) demonstrated an anomalous fibrinogen in a patient with increased tendency to thrombosis and paradoxically, a mild hemorrhagic diathesis. Three daughters by two different husbands were similarly affected. Menache (1964) described a different fibrinogen variant. In a family of Hungarian extraction, von Felten et al. (1966) found prolonged prothrombin time without hemorrhagic diathesis. Chemical studies suggested a molecular abnormality of fibrinogen. Von Felton, Duckert and Frick (1966) described a clotting disturbance, characterized by delayed aggregation of fibrin monomers, in father and son. Forman et al. (1968) described fibrinogen Cleveland which is immunoelectrophoretically distinct from fibrinogen Baltimore. Operative wounds showed dehiscence in two persons with the abnormal fibrinogen. The plasma in their 8 related persons of both sexes showed abnormally slow coagulation when thrombin was added. The fibrinogen described by Mammen et al. (1969) and called fibrinogen Detroit had characteristics different from fibrinogen Baltimore and fibrinogen Cleveland. Fibrinogen Oklahoma appears to have a structural defect such that cross-linkage is defective. Gralnick and Finlayson (1972) provided the tabulation of fibrinogen variants given below. Fibrinogen Detroit is the only one in which the specific amino acid substitution is known (Blomback et al., 1968). The distinctness of all the types is not proved. Most of the variants have been detected on coagulation tests in which plasma fibrinogen is converted to fibrin (thrombin time, reptilase test, prothrombin time). The times are prolonged or infinite (i.e., no clot is formed). Chemical or immunologic assays for fibrinogen are usually normal, however. Although the variants may be asymptomatic, abnormal bleeding, abnormal clotting, and wound dehiscence in isolation or in some combination have been observed. The defect in conversion of fibrinogen to fibrin is, in a few of the variants, at the first step, that of removal of fibrinopeptides A and B (catalyzed by thrombin) to form fibrin monomer. The majority, however, have the defect in the second stage, that of aggregation of fibrin monomer to form a fibrin gel. (The third step is covalent cross-linking of fibrin, catalyzed by activated Factor XIII, to form an insoluble clot.) Ratnoff and Bennett (1973) gave a table of fibrinogen variants. Martinez et al. (1974) described an abnormal fibrinogen associated with hypercatabolism. This so-called fibrinogen Philadelphia was noted in two sisters and the son of one of them. Only one was symptomatic, with excessive bleeding.

Beck, E. A., Charache, P. and Jackson, D. P.: A new inherited coagulation disorder caused by an abnormal fibrinogen ('fibrinogen Baltimore'). Nature 208: 143-145, 1965.

Beck, E. A., Shainoff, J. R., Vogel, A. and Jackson, D. P.: Functional evaluation of an inherited abnormal fibrinogen: fibrinogen 'Baltimore.' J. Clin. Invest. 50: 1874-1884, 1971.

Blomback, B. and Blomback, M.: Molecular defects and variants of fibrinogen. Nouv. Rev. Fr. Hematol. 10: 671-678, 1970.

Blomback, M., Blomback, B., Mammen, E. F. et al.: Fibrinogen Detroit a molecular defect in the N-terminal disulphide knot of human fibrinogen? Nature 218: 134-137, 1968.

Crum, E. D., Shainoff, J. R., Graham, R. C. and Ratnoff, O. D.: Fibrinogen Cleveland II. An abnormal fibrinogen with defective release of fibrinopeptide A. J. Clin. Invest. 53: 1308-1319, 1974.

Forman, W. B., Ratnoff, O. D. and Boyer, M. H.: An inherited qualitative abnormality in plasma fibrinogen: fibrinogen Cleveland. J. Lab. Clin. Med. 72: 455-472, 1968.

Funk, C. and Straub, P. W.: Hereditary abnormality of fibrin monomer aggregation ('fibrinogen Zurich II'). Europ. J. Clin. Invest. 1: 131, 1971.

Gralnick, H. R., Givelber, H. M., Shainoff, J. R. et al.: Fibrinogen Bethesda: a congenital dysfibrinogenemia with delayed fibrinopeptide release. J. Clin. Invest. 50: 1819-1830, 1971.

Gralnick, H. R., Givelber, H. and Finlayson, J. S.: Congenital dysfibrinogenemia: fibrinogen Bethesda II, in abstracts, International Society on Thrombosis and Haemostasis. Oslo, Norway: Villco Trykkeri, 1972.

Hampton, J. H. and Garrison, M. S.: Fibrinogen and fibrin-stabilizing factor. Med. Clin. N. Am. 56: 133-143, 1972.

Hampton, J. W., Morton, R. O., Bannerjee, D. and Kalmaz, E.: Defective fibrin cross-linkages: a genetic and biochemical study of three families. (Abstract) J. Clin. Invest. 50: 42A only, 1971.

Hasselback, R., Marion, R. B. and Thomas, J. W.: Congenital hypofibrinogenemia in five members of a family. Canad. Med. Assoc. J. 88: 19-22, 1963.

Imperato, C. and Dettori, A. G.: Ipofibrinogenemia congenita con fibrinoastenia. Helv. Paediatr. Acta 13: 380-399, 1958.

Jackson, D. P., Beck, E. A. and Charache, P.: Congenital disorders of fibrinogen. Fed. Proc. 24: 816-821, 1965.

Mammen, E. F., Prasad, A. S., Barnhart, M. I. and Au, C. C.: Congenital dysfibrinogenemia: fibrinogen Detroit. J. Clin. Invest. 48: 235-249, 1969.

Martinez, J., Holburn, R. R., Shapiro, S. and Erslen, A. J.: A hereditary hypodysfibrinogenemia characterized by fibrinogen hypercatabolism. J. Clin. Invest. 53: 600-611, 1974.

Menache, D.: Constitutional and familial abnormal fibrinogen. Thromb. Diath. Haemorrh. 10 (suppl. 13): 173-185, 1964.

Ratnoff, O. D. and Bennett, B.: The genetics of hereditary disorders of blood coagulation. Science, 179: 1291-1298, 1973.

Samama, M., Soria, C. et al.: Dysfibrinogenemie congenitale et familiale sans tendance hemorragique. Nouv. Rev. Fr. Haematol. 9: 817-832, 1969.

Soria, J., Samama, M., Soria, C. et al.: Two new cases of congenitale dysfibrinogenemia. Abstracts, International Society of Thrombosis and Haemostasis. Oslo, Norway: Villco Trykkeri, 1971, P. 58.

Streiff, F., Alexandre, P., Vigneron, C. et al.: Un nouveau cas d'anomalie constitutionelle et familiale du fibrinogene sans diathese hemorrhagique. Thromb. Diath. Haemorrh. 26: 565-576, 1971.

Verhaeghe, R., Verstraete, M., Vermylen, J. and Vermylen, C.: Fibrinogen 'Leuven', another genetic variant. Br. J. Haematol. 26: 421-434, 1974.

Verstraete, M.: Discussion. Thromb. Diath. Haemorrh. 39 (suppl): 334-337, 1970.

Von Felton, A., Duckert, F. and Frick, P. G.: Familial disturbance of fibrin monomer aggregation. Br. J. Haematol. 12: 667-677, 1966.

Winckelmann, G., Augustin, R. and Bandilla, K.: Congenital dysfibrinogenemia. Report of a new family (fibrinogen Wiesbaden). Abstracts, International Society on Thrombosis and Haemostasis. Oslo, Norway: Villco Trykkeri, 1971. P. 64.

Zietz, B. H. and Scott, J. L.: An inherited defect in fibrinogen polymerization: fibrinogen Los Angeles. (Abstract) Clin. Res. 18: 179, 1970.

13481 FIBRINOGEN CROSS-LINKAGE DEFECT, DUE TO DEFICIENCY OF TRANSGLUTAMI-NASE

An enzyme, plasma transglutaminase, which is activated by thrombin, catalyzes cross-linking of fibrinogen by covalent bonds involving the epsilon group of lysine and the gamma carboxylamide group of specific glutamines. Hampton et al. (1971) described deficiency of transglutaminase in a patient with bleeding.

Hampton, J. W., Morton, R. O., Bannerjee, D. and Kalmaz, E.: Defective fibrin cross-linkage: a genetic and biochemical study of three families. (Abstract) J. Clin. Invest. 50: 42A only, 1971.

13482 FIBRINOGEN — ALPHA POLYPEPTIDE CHAIN

Fibrinogen is a plasma glycoprotein synthesized in the liver. It is composed of three structurally different subunits, alpha, beta and delta. The subunit that carries the amino acid substitution is known for none of the fibrinogen variants (13480). Thrombin causes a limited proteolysis of the fibrinogen molecule during which fibrinopeptides A and B are released from the amino-terminal regions of the alpha and beta chains, respectively. The enzyme cleaves arginine-glycine linkages so that glycine is left as the amino-terminal amino acid on both chains. Thrombin also activates fibrin-stabilizing factor (see 22850, 30550) which in its activated form is a transpeptidase catalysing the formation of epsilon-(gamma-glutamyl)-lysine cross-links in fibrin. Fibrinopeptides, which have been sequenced in many species, may have a physiologic role as vasoconstrictors and may aid in local hemostasis during blood clotting. By amino acid sequencing, Doolittle et al. (1970) could find no variation of fibrinopeptides A and B from 125 persons.

Dayhoff, M. O.: Fibrinogen and fibrinopeptides. Atlas of Protein Sequence and Structure 1972 (vol. 5). Washington: National Biomedical Research Foundation, 1972. Pp. D87-D97.

Doolittle, R. F., Chen, R., Glasgow, C., Mross, B. and Weinstein, M.: The molecular constancy of fibrinopeptides A and B from 125 individual humans. Humangenetik 10: 15-29, 1970.

Doolittle, R. F., Takagi, T. and Cottrell, B. A.: Platelet and plasma fibrinogens are identical gene products. Science 185: 368-370, 1974.

13483 FIBRINOGEN — BETA POLYPEPTIDE CHAIN

See FIBRINOGEN — ALPHA POLYPEPTIDE CHAIN (13481).

13485 FIBRINOGEN — GAMMA POLYPEPTIDE CHAIN

See FIBRINOGEN — ALPHA POLYPEPTIDE CHAIN (13481).

13490 FIBRINOLYTIC DEFECT

Self and Matthews (1968) described a family in which multiple members in five generations showed hyper-extensible skin and a defect in fibrinolytic activity as indicated clinically by excessive bruising on minor trauma and spontaneous hematomas. Joints were not excessively mobile. The fibrinolytic defect was demonstrated by short euglobulin clot lysis time and decreased Factor XIII activity. Male-to-male transmission occurred.

Self, J. and Matthews, C.: Inherited fibrinolytic hyperactivity. Arch. Intern. Med. 122: 357-358, 1968.

*13500 FIBROCYSTIC PULMONARY DYSPLASIA

Koch (1965) observed a family with 3 definite and 5 probable cases. The features were progressive dyspnea and cyanosis, digital clubbing, pulmonary hypertension, polycythemia, diffuse pulmonary fibrosis by X-ray. The definite cases include an instance of father-son transmission. One patient developed bronchial carcinoma. The condition appears to be identical in all respects, including the development of carcinoma, to that described by McKusick and Fisher (1958). Rezek and Talbert (1962) reported affected father and daughter. Donohue and colleagues (1959) described a Canadian family with 8 cases of pulmonary fibrosis in four generations. Swaye et al. (1969) described 8 cases in 3 generations. In one, the diagnosis was made at age 3.5 years by lung biopsy. Two brothers had coexistent pulmonary fibrosis and bronchogenic cancer. It is by no means certain that the entity described here is distinct from pulmonary fibrosis, idiopathic (q.v.). Solliday et al. (1973) described father-to-son transmission.

Adelman, A. G., Chertkow, G. and Hayton, R. C.: Familial fibrocystic pulmonary dysplasia: a detailed family study. Canad. Med. Assoc. J. 95: 603-610, 1966.

Donohue, W. L., Laski, B., Uchida, I. and Munn, J. D.: Familial fibrocystic pulmonary dysplasia and its relation to the Hamman-Rich syndrome. Pediatrics 24: 786-813, 1959.

Koch, B.: Familial fibrocystic pulmonary dysplasia: observations in one family. Canad. Med. Assoc. J. 92: 801-808, 1965.

McKusick, V. A. and Fisher, A. M.: Congenital cystic disease of the lung with progressive pulmonary fibrosis and carcinomatosis. Ann. Intern. Med. 48: 774-790, 1958.

Rezek, P. R. and Talbert, W. R., Jr.: Kongenitale (familiaere) zystische Fibrose der Lunge. Wien. Klin. Wschr. 74: 869-873, 1962.

Solliday, N. H., Williams, J. A., Gaensler, E. A., Coutu, R. E. and Carrington, C. B.: Familial chronic interstitial pneumonia. Am. Rev. Resp. Dis. 108: 193-204, 1973.

Swaye, P., Van Ordstrand, H. S., McCormick, L. J. and Wolpaw, S. E.: Familial Hamman-Rich syndrome. Dis. Chest 55: 7-12, 1969.

Young, W. A.: Familial fibrocystic pulmonary dysplasia: a new case in a known affected family. Canad. Med. Assoc. J. 94: 1059-1061, 1966.

*13510 FIBRODYSPLASIA OSSIFICANS PROGRESSIVA

Most cases are sporadic. However, sufficient cases of affected twins and triplets are known to suggest a genetic basis. Furthermore, dominant inheritance is supported by observations of two or three successive generations affected and the finding of a paternal age effect in sporadic cases.

Becker, P. E. and Von Knorre, G. V.: Myositis ossificans progressiva. Ergeb. Inn. Med. Kinderheilk. 27: 1-31, 1968.

McKusick, V. A.: Heritable Disorders of Connective Tissue. St. Louis: C. V. Mosby Co., 1972 (4th Ed.).

Tuente, W., Becker, P. E. and Von Knorre, G. V.: Zur Genetik der Myositis ossificans progressiva. Humangenetik 4: 320-351, 1967.

Viparelli, V.: La miosite ossificante progressiva. Ann. Neuropsichiat. Psicoanal. 9: 297-324, 1962.

13520 FIBROMATOSIS, CONGENITAL GENERALIZED

This disorder was described by Stout (1954) who distinguished it from other forms of juvenile fibromatosis. The radiologic findings are similar to those of Ollier disease. Multiple cystic lesions involve the metaphyses. Multiple soft tissue nodules occur (Shnitka et al., 1958), as in multiple neurofibromatosis, but a cutaneous pigmentary anomaly is not a feature. Hower et al. (1971) described affected half-sisters with the same mother. Affected sibs have also been observed by McAdams (as cited by Stout et al., 1961). Bartlett et al. (1961) observed four cases among first cousins. The mother of affected brother and sister and the father of another affected brother-sister pair were sibs.

Bartlett, R. C., Otis, R. D. and Laakso, A. O.: Multiple congenital neoplasms of soft tissue. Cancer 14: 913-920, 1961.

Heiple, K. G., Perrin, E. and Aikawa, M.: Congenital generalized fibromatosis. A case limited to osseous lesions. J. Bone Joint Surg. 54A: 663-669, 1972.

Kauffman, S. L. and Stout, A. P.: Congenital mesenchymal tumors. Cancer 18: 460-476, 1965.

Shnitka, T. K., Asp, D. M. and Horner, R. H.: Congenital generalized fibromatosis. Cancer 11: 627-639, 1958.

Stout, A. P.: Juvenile fibromatoses. Cancer 7: 953-978, 1954.

Teng, P., Warden, M. J. and Cohn, W. L.: Congenital generalized fibromatosis (renal and skeletal) with complete spontaneous regression. J. Pediatr. 62: 748-753, 1963.

Touraine, A. and Ruel, H.: La polyfibromatose hereditaire. Ann. Derm. Syph. 29: 1-5, 1945.

13530 FIBROMATOSIS, GINGIVAL

It is not certain that a mutation 'gingival fibromatosis' exists separate from 'gingival fibromatosis with hypertrichosis.' The report of Zackin and Weisberger (1961) stated that there was 'slight hypertrichosis in all members of the family' which was of Italian ancestry. Whether persons without fibromatosis as well as those with it were hirsute was not clearly stated. Becker et al. (1967) described gingival fibromatosis without other features in mother, son and daughter. Ramon et al. (1967) described two brothers with features of gingival fibromatosis and of cherubism. The parents, Sephardic Jews, were first-cousins. They and six sibs were healthy. Witkop (1971) described an extensively affected kindred in which none of 13 examined persons with the gingival fibromatosis had hypertrichosis and none of many others with the gingival disorder had a history of hypertrichosis.

Becker, W., Collings, C. K., Zimmerman, E. R., De La Rosa, M. and Singdahlsen, D.: Hereditary gingival fibromatosis. A report on a family in which three members were affected with fibromatosis of the gingiva. Oral Surg. 24: 313-318, 1967.

Ramon, Y., Berman, W. and Bubis, J. J.: Gingival fibromatosis combined with cherubism. Oral Surg. 24: 435-448, 1967.

Witkop, C. J.: Heterogeneity in gingival fibromatosis. The Clinical Delineation of Birth Defects. XI. Orofacial Structures. Baltimore: Williams and Wilkins, 1971. Pp. 210-221.

Zackin, S. J. and Weisberger, D.: Hereditary gingival fibromatosis. Report of a family. Oral Surg. 14: 828-836, 1961.

*13540 FIBROMATOSIS, GINGIVAL, WITH HYPERTRICHOSIS

Extreme hirsutism with gingival fibromatosis follows a dominant pattern of inheritance (Weski, 1920; Garn and Hatch, 1950). I have seen a sporadic case of a severely retarded child who had muscular hypotonia in addition to hypertrichosis and gingival hyperplasia. The last two features are produced by dilantin — a phenocopy of the genetic disorder. There is no necessary relationship between the age of development of the gingival changes and the hypertrichosis. The latter may be present at birth but often appears at puberty (Anderson et al. 1969).

Anderson, J., Cunliffe, W. J., Roberts, D. F. and Close, H.: Hereditary gingival fibromatosis. Br. Med. J. 3: 218-219, 1969.

Foret, J., Dodinval, P. and Foret-Kestlicher, C.: Hyperplasie fibreuse idiopathique des gencives. J. Genet. Hum. 13: 337-350, 1964.

Garn, S. M. and Hatch, C. E.: Hereditary general gingival hyperplasia. J. Hered. 41: 41-42, 1950.

Weski, H.: Elephantiasis gingivae hereditaria. Deutsch. Mschr. Zahnheilk. 38: 557-584, 1920.

*13550 FIBROMATOSIS, GINGIVAL, WITH ABNORMAL FINGERS, FINGERNAILS, NOSE AND EARS AND SPLENOMEGALY

In two Asiatic Indian families (one living in the Caribbean and one in India) gingival fibromatosis occured in association with 'whittling' of the terminal phalanges and absence or dysplasia of the finger nails. The liver and spleen were enlarged. Gorlin (1967) called my attention to these reports. Laband et al. (1964) described this disorder in a 38-year-old Trinidad woman and 5 of her seven children. The family was of East-Indian origin. The mother showed large, soft ears, hypertension, hyperextensibility of metacarpophalangeal joints and splenomegaly. The five affected children had soft tissue enlargment of the nose and ears, splenomegaly, skeletal abnormalities, obscure or reduced size of toenails and thumbnails, short terminal phalanges and hypermobility of several joints. Alvandar (1965) observed 5 affected persons in three generations with one instance of male-to-male transmission. Associated features were thickening of the soft tissues of the nose and ear with softness of the cartilages, hyperextensible joints, and hepatomegaly.

Alvandar, G.: Elephantiasis gingivae. Report of an affected family with associated hepatomegaly, soft tissue and skeletal abnormalities. J. All India Dent. Assoc. 37: 349-353, 1965.

Gorlin, R. J.: Minneapolis, Minn.: personal communication, 1967.

Laband, P. F., Habib, G. and Humphreys, G. S.: Hereditary gingival fibromatosis. Report of an affected family with associated splenomegaly and skeletal and soft-tissue abnormalities. Oral Surg. 17: 339-351, 1964.

13560 FIBRO-OSSEOUS DYSPLASIA OF THE JAWS

Chatterjee and Mazumder (1967) described massive fibro-osseous dysplasia of the jaws in a man and his two sons. The tumorous involvement reached amazing proportions as shown in the published photographs. The father had progressive swelling of the upper jaw from childhood. Involvement of the lower jaw was later in onset.

Chatterjee, S. K. and Mazumder, J. K.: Massive fibro-osseous dysplasia of the jaws in two generations. Br. J. Surg. 54: 335-340, 1967.

13570 FIBROSIS OF EXTRAOCULAR MUSCLE

Hansen (1968) described a mother and a son and daughter with fibrosis of the extraocular muscles. The disorder is characterized clinically by anchoring of the eyes in downward gaze, ptosis and backward tilt of the head. Laughlin (1956) observed the condition in at least four generations of a family. It appears that no father-to-son transmission has been observed.

Hansen, E.: Congenital general fibrosis of the extraocular muscles. Acta Ophthalmol. 46: 469-476, 1968.

Laughlin, R. C.: Congenital fibrosis of the extraocular muscles: a report of six cases. Am. J. Ophthalmol. 41: 432-438, 1956.

Sandrow et al. (1970) described father and daughter with ulnar and fibular dimelia and peculiar facies. At birth the father was noted to have hand and foot anomalies described as syndactyly and polydactyly. Operations to correct digital webs and remove several supernumerary toes were performed. Bilateral clefts enlarged the inferior position margins of the nares. The daughter had identical nasal clefts and minor hands, with fusion of ten digits in rosebud fashion bilaterally. The fibula and ulna were duplicated bilaterally and the radius and tibia were missing. See 18874 and 18877.

Sandrow, R. E., Sullivan, P. D. and Steel, H. H.: Hereditary ulnar and fibular dimelia with peculiar facies. A case report. J. Bone Joint Surg. 52A: 367-370, 1970.

13580 FIBULA, RECURRENT DISLOCATION OF HEAD OF

Reeves (1967) reported two families, each with multiple affected persons in three generations. Generalized joint laxity was not present. Although Reeves favored X-linked dominant inheritance, one instance of male-to-male transmission was diagrammed.

Reeves, B.: Familial recurrent dislocation of the head of the fibula. Proc. R. Soc. Med. 60: 544-545, 1967.

13590 FIFTH DIGIT SYNDROME

Coffin and Siris (1970) described three unrelated girls with mental retardation and absent nail and terminal phalanx of the fifth finger. The nails and distal phalanges of the lateral toes were absent or hypoplastic. No similar cases were found in any of the three families. The same disorder was described by Senior (1971). In addition to short stature and very small toenails on the fifth digits, broad nose with prominent nares and mild mental retardation were features. No familial cases were seen by Senior (1971).

Coffin, G. S. and Siris, E.: Mental retardation with absent fifth fingernail and terminal phalanx. Am. J. Dis. Child. 119: 433-439, 1970.

Senior, B.: Impaired growth and onychodysplasia. Short children with tiny toenails. Am. J. Dis. Child. 122: 7-9, 1971.

*13600 FINGERPRINTS, ABSENCE OF

Baird (1964) reported a family in which 13 persons in 3 generations showed absent dermal ridges. The affected persons all showed transient congenital milia (small white papules, especially on the face, representing retention cysts). Some affected members also showed bilateral partial flexion contractures of the fingers and toes and webbing of the toes. See ECTODERMAL DYSPLASIA, ABSENT DERMATOGLYPHIC PATTERN, etc.

Baird, H. W.: Absence of fingerprints in four generations. Lancet II: 1250 only, 1968.

Baird, H. W., III: Kindred showing congenital absence of the dermal ridges (fingerprints) and associated anomalies. J. Pediatr. 64: 621-631, 1964.

David, T. J.: Congenital malformations of human dermatoglyphs. Arch. Dis. Child. 48: 191-198, 1973.

13610 FINGERS, RELATIVE LENGTH OF

The question is whether when the tip of the ring finger is placed on a line, the index finger reaches the line. Short index fingers is said to be dominant in men, recessive in women. Three phenotypes were noted-second longer than fourth, second equal to fourth and second shorter than fourth. Kloepfer (1946) studied the relative length of the index and middle fingers.

Blincoe, H.: Significant hand types in women according to relative lengths of fingers. Am. J. Phys. Anthrop. 20: 45-48, 1962.

Kloepfer, H. W.: An investigation of 171 possible linkage relationships in man. Ann. Eugen. 13: 35-71, 1946.

Philps, V. R.: Relative index finger length as a sex-influenced trait in man. Am. J. Hum. Genet. 4: 72-89, 1952.

13615 FLOOD FACTOR DEFICIENCY

Flood factor is defined as the agent in plasma which shortens the slightly long prothrombin time of several asymptomatic members of the Flood family studied by Quick and Hussey (1962). Its properties resemble those of Factor VII, from which it was distinguishable, however. Ten persons in 3 generations, with male-to-male transmission, were shown to be affected.

Quick, A. J. and Hussey, C. V.: Hereditary hypoprothrombinaemias. Lancet I: 173-177, 1962.

13620 FLUSHING OF EARS AND SOMNOLENCE

Kim (1969) noted a father and two sons, aged 7 and 11 years, with intermittent episodes of flushing of the ears associated with somnolence. It had its onset in all three at about the same time. The mother and another son were unaffected.

Kim, P. M.: Familial flushing and somnolence. (Letter) J.A.M.A. 210: 1289 only, 1969.

*13630 FLYNN-AIRD SYNDROME

In 10 members of five generations of a family, Flynn and Aird (1965) observed a neuroectodermal syndrome with some similarities to the syndromes of Werner, Refsum and Cockayne (all of which are, however, recessives). Male-to-male transmission occurred in three instances. Features included, in the eye: cataracts, atypical retinitis pigmentosa, myopia; in the ear: bilateral nerve deafness beginning as early as age 7; in the nervous system: ataxia, peripheral neuritis, epilepsy, elevation of cerebrospinal fluid protein and dementia; in the ectoderm: skin atrophy, chronic ulceration, baldness and striking dental caries; in the skeletal system: cystic changes of bone and joint stiffness.

Flynn, P. and Aird, R. B.: A neuroectodermal syndrome of dominant inheritance. J. Neurol. Sci. 2: 161-182, 1965.

13640 FOCAL EPITHELIAL HYPERPLASIA OF THE ORAL MUCOSA

Most cases of this rare lesion have been non-familial. However, Schock (1969) described the disorder in an Indian woman and three of her daughters. Most of the cases have been in American Indians, all the way from the Warm Springs Indians of Oregon to the Chavante Indians of Brazil. This disorder is thought to be viral, not genetic, although the proof is not yet complete.

Schock, R. K.: Familial focal epithelial hyperplasia. Report of a case. Oral Surg. 28: 598-602, 1969.

*13650 FOCAL FACIAL DERMAL DYSPLASIA (HEREDITARY SYMMETRICAL APLASTIC NEVI OF TEMPLES)

Brauer (1929) described 38 patients with this condition and traced it through 5 generations of a family in which 155 persons were said to have been affected. The affected progenitor was said to be one Johann Jokeb Van Bargen, who migrated to Germany from Holland in the 16th century. The resemblance to 'forceps marks' was noted. Unilateral occurrence was described in two. Affected persons in 4 generations were described by Church (1970). McGeoch and Reed (1971) studied an Australian family with many affected members of many generations. They called it focal facial dermal dysplasia. Although the main finding was a wrinkling or puckering of the skin at the temples, some patients showed guttate areas on the lateral aspects of the chin and midforehead. Father-to-son transmission has been observed in each of the three large kindreds (German, English, Australian). Histologically, the lesion is a mesodermal dysplasia with near absence of subcutaneous fat and with skeletal muscle almost contiguous with epidermis. The puckered skin is well accounted for by the hypoplasia of the corium and lack of fat.

Brauer, A.: Hereditaerer symmetrischer systematisierter Naevus aplasticus bei 38 Personen. Derm. Wschr. 89: 1163-1168, 1929.

Church, R. E.: Brit. Acad. Dermatology, Sheffield, July, 1970.

Jensen, N. E.: Congenital ectodermal dysplasia of the face. Br. J. Dermatol. 84: 410-416, 1971.

McGeoch, A. H. and Reed, W. B.: Familial focal facial dermal dysplasia. Arch. Dermatol. 107: 591-596, 1973.

McGeoch, A. H. and Reed, W. B.: Familial focal facial dermal dysplasia. The Clinical Delineation of Birth Defects. XII. Skin, Hair and Nails. Baltimore: Williams and Wilkins, 1971. Pp. 96-99.

13660 FRIEDREICH ATAXIA

It is likely that all cases which legitimately deserve this designation have recessive inheritance. However, Sylvester (1958) reported what he termed Friedreich ataxia in a father and six of his nine children. Optic atrophy and nerve deafness were associated features. Spillane (1940) described a family in which 21 persons (12 males and 9 females) in 6 generations had pes cavus and absent deep reflexes. This was probably Roussy-Levy hereditary areflexic dystasia (q.v.).

Spillane, J. D.: Familial pes cavus and absent tendon-jerks: its relationship with Friedreich's disease and peroneal muscular atrophy. Brain 63: 275-290, 1940.

Sylvester, P. E.: Some unusual findings in a family with Friedreich's ataxia. Arch. Dis. Child. 33: 217-221, 1958.

13670 FRONTODIGITAL SYNDROME

In 9 persons in 5 sibships of 3 generations, Marshall and Smith (1970) described cranial abnormalities, namely frontal bossing and a sagittal ridge. In six of the nine the thumbs and-or toes were broad. In two of the nine polydactyly and-or syndactyly were present. This is in fact polysyndactyly with peculiar skull shape q.v. (17570).

Marshall, R. E. and Smith, D. W.: Frontodigital syndrome: a dominantly inherited disorder with normal intelligence. J. Pediatr. 77: 129-133, 1970.

13674 FRONTOMETAPHYSEAL DYSPLASIA

Gorlin (1969) described a male patient with extraordinarily marked frontal hyperostosis giving great prominence to the supraciliary ridges, underdeveloped mandible, cryptorchidism, subluxated radial heads, and metaphyseal dysplasia resembling that in Pyle disease (metaphyseal dysplasia). This may be the disorder present in the case described by Walker (1969). Striking overgrowth of bone in the superciliary region was repaired by removal of excess bone. Danks et al. (1972) described progressive joint contractures especially in the hands, carpal osteolysis, and metachromatic granules in fibroblasts. Holt et al. (1972) reported two unrelated cases. Danks et al. 1972, 1973) have studied a third isolated case in which progressive contracture of the fingers and lysis and fusion of carpal bones are features. The patient had progressive ostosclerosis also. Fibroblasts showed metachromasia. All three patients were males. Nothing has been known of the genetics of this disorder until Weiss and Reynolds (1974) observed the disorder in a black male whose mother had the same disorder.

Danks, D. M. and Mayne, V.: Frontometaphyseal dysplasia: a progressive disease of bone and connective

Danks, D. M., Mayne, V., Hall, R. K. and McKinnon, M. C.: Frontometaphyseal dysplasia. A
progressive disease of bone and connective tissue. Am. J. Dis. Child. 123: 254-258, 1972.

Gorlin, R. J. and Cohen, M. M., Jr.: Frontometaphyseal dysplasia. A new syndrome. Am. J. Dis. Child.
118: 487-494, 1969.

Holt, J. F., Thompson, G. R..and Arenberg, I. K.: Frontometaphyseal dysplasia. Radiol. Clin. N. Am.
10: 225-243, 1972.

Stern, S. D., Arenberg, I. K., Ongal, R. M., Sandall, G. S. and Holt, J. F.: The ocular and cosmetic
problems in frontometaphyseal dysplasia. J. Pediatr. Ophthalmol. 9: 151-161, 1972.

Walker, B. A.: A craniodiaphyseal dysplasia or craniometaphyseal dysplasia? The Clinical Delineation
of Birth Defects. IV. Skeletal Dysplaisa. New York: National Foundation, 1969. Pp. 298-300.

Weiss, L. and Reynolds, W. A.: Familial frontometaphyseal dysplasia: evidence for dominant inheritance.
To be published, 1974.

13680 FUCHS EPITHELIAL AND ENDOTHELIAL DYSTROPHY OF THE CORNEA

Although evidence of a hereditary basis is scanty in the literature, Falls (1968) states that his experience
suggests autosomal dominant inheritance with greater expression in the female. Cross et al. (1971) presented
two new pedigrees and analyzed a previously reported one. They concluded that the disorder is probably
autosomal dominant. The female predilection was again noted. This disorder has an adult-onset, progressive
corneal degeneration characterized initially by central guttata and endothelial edema.

Cross, H. E., Maumenee, A. E. and Cantolino, S. J.: Inheritance of Fuchs' endothelial dystrophy. Arch.
Ophthalmol. 85: 268-272, 1971.

Falls, H. F.: Detection of the carrier state of genetically determined eye diseases. In, Congenital
Anomalies of the Eye. St. Louis: C. V. Mosby Co., 1968. Pp. 34-52.

*13685 FUMARATE HYDRATASE (FUMARASE)

This locus, symbolized FH, may be on chromosome no. 1 (van Someren, 1973). The work (van Someren et
al., 1974) was confirmed and study of anomalous chromosomes no. 1 suggested that the FH locus is in the
area 1q42.

Van Someren, H.: Intern. Workshop on Human Gene Mapping, New Haven, Conn., June, 1973.

Van Someren, H., Van Henegouwen, H. B. and De Wit, J.: Evidence for synteny between the human loci
for fumarate hydratase, UDG glucose pyrophosphorylase, 6-phosphogluconate dehydrogenase, phosphoglu-
comutase-1, and peptidase-C in man-Chinese hamster somatic cell hybrids. Cytogenet. Cell Genet. 13:
150-152, 1974.

13690 FUNDUS DYSTROPHY

Sorsby and Mason (1949) described five families with a fundus dystrophy which occurred in several
generations in a dominant pedigree pattern. It became manifest at about the age of 40 years, beginning as
a central (macular) lesion showing edema, hemorrhage and exudates. In the course of years atrophy with
pigmentation and extension peripherally occurred. The choroidal vessels became exposed and appeared
somewhat sclerotic. Within about 35 years after onset the entire fundus was involved. The choroidal vessels
disappeared by this stage and the terminal picture was one of extensive choroidal atrophy with pigmentation.
Night-blindness was not a feature at any stage. The authors considered the process to be primarily choroidal.
Sandvig (1955) described 13 cases of central choroidal degeneration in four generations of a family. Krill and
Archer (1971) described mother and three children with diffuse total choroidal vascular atrophy.

Krill, A. E. and Archer, D.: Classification of the choroidal atrophies. Am. J. Ophthalmol. 72: 562-585,
1971.

Sandvig, K.: Familial, central, areolar, choroidal atrophy of autosomal dominant inheritance. Acta
Ophthalmol. 33: 71-78, 1955.

Sorsby, A. and Mason, M. E. J.: A fundus dystrophy with unusual features (late onset and dominant
inheritance of a central retinal lesion showing oedema, haemorrhage and exudates developing into generalized
choroidal atrophy with massive pigment proliferation). Br. J. Ophthalmol. 33: 67-97, 1949.

13700 FUTCHER LINE

Futcher line is a linear discontinuity in intensity of pigmentation on the upper arm and deltoid area of
Negroes. It is located on the lateral aspect of the arm and marks the junction between the dorsal and ventral
parts of the extremity. Futcher (1938, 1940) found it bilaterally in 17.5 percent of Negroes regardless of age,
sex and intensity of over-all pigmentation. Another 2 percent had a line on one side only. Apparently no
family studies have been done.

Futcher, P. H.: A peculiarity of pigmentation of the upper arm of Negroes. Science 88: 570-571, 1938.

Futcher, P. H.: The distribution of pigmentation on the arm and thorax of man. Bull. Hopkins Hosp.
67: 372-373, 1940.

13703 GALACTOSE + ACTIVATOR

Chu (1974) presented evidence for a regular gene concerned with activation of a number of enzymes which have hexoses and hexosemonophosphates as substrates. The locus is thought (from study of cell hybrids) to be on the proximal portion of chromosome 2p.

Chu, E.: Ann Arbor, Mich., presentation at Second International Workshop on Human Gene Mapping, 1974.

13705 GAMMA-A-GLOBULIN, DEFECT IN ASSEMBLY OF

In a woman who had frequent respiratory infections, her mother and her son, Moroz et al. (1971) described absence of assembly of alpha-chains and light-chains to form IgA. Free alpha-chains were present in the serum and urine, and the urine also contained free light-chains. Studies in cultured tonsillar tissue showed synthesis and secretion of free alpha-chains and light-chains and normally assembled IgG and IgM.

Moroz, C., Amir, J. and De Vries, A.: A hereditary immunoglobulin A abnormality: absence of light-heavy-chain assembly. Study of immunoglobulin synthesis in tonsillar cells. J. Clin. Invest. 50: 2726-2733, 1971.

13710 GAMMA-A-GLOBULIN, SELECTIVE DEFICIENCY OF

In a Swiss kindred Stocker et al. (1968) described selective complete deficiency of gamma-A-globulin in two sisters, the son and daughter of one and the son of the other. Both parents of the two sisters had normal serum globulin. They suggested autosomal dominant inheritance but the evidence is meager. In fact Huntley and Stephenson (1968) favored autosomal recessive inheritance. The frequency of isolated IgA deficiency was 0.2 percent. Out of 24 deficient persons, 4 had rheumatoid arthritis and 2 had severe sinopulmonary disease. Hilman et al. (1969) found low IgA in a mother and two daughters. Nell et al. (1972) observed selective deficiency in 13 persons in 5 kindreds. Father and son and mother and daughter were affected in two of the families. In the other three recessive inheritance was suggested by the occurrence in double cousins and in multiple sibs. See 14687. Webb and Condemi (1974) found selective immunoglobulin A deficiency in a 43-year-old woman with far advanced chronic obstructive pulmonary disease. Her parents were uncle and niece. Other immunoglobulins and alpha-1-antitrypsin were normal. Among her relatives several had IgA deficiency, either definite or borderline. Her mother, aged 71 and two brothers, aged 48 and 44, had emphysema. Goldberg et al. (1968) reported a kindred in which inheritance seemed to be autosomal recessive.

Goldberg, L. S., Barnett, E. V. and Fudenberg, H. H.: Selective absence of IgA: a family study. J. Lab. Clin. Med. 72: 204-212, 1968.

Hilman, B. C., Mandel, I. D., Martinez-Tello, F. J. and Lieber, E.: Familial hypogammaglobulinemia-A. Ann. Allergy 27: 393-402, 1969.

Huntley, C. C. and Stephenson, R. L.: IgA deficiency: familial studies. N. Carolina Med. J. 29: 325-331, 1968.

Martin, G. I.: Inherited IgA deficiency. (Letter) Lancet II: 609 only, 1971.

Nell, P. A., Ammann, A. J., Hong, R. and Stiehm, E. R.: Familial selective IgA deficiency. Pediatrics 49: 71-79, 1972.

Stocker, F., Ammann, P. and Rossi, E.: Selective gamma-A-globulin deficiency, with dominant autosomal inheritance in a Swiss family. Arch. Dis. Child. 43: 585-588, 1968.

Tomkin, G. H., Mawhinney, M. and Nevin, N. C.: Isolated absence of IgA with autosomal dominant inheritance. Lancet II: 124-125, 1971.

Webb, D. R. and Condemi, J. J.: Selective immunoglobulin A deficiency and chronic obstructive lung disease. A family study. Ann. Intern. Med. 80: 681-621, 1974.

13720 GAMSTORP-WOHLFART SYNDROME (MYOKYMIA, MYOTONIA, MUSCLE WASTING, HYPERHIDROSIS)

Some of the features resembled Charcot-Marie-Tooth disease. However, myokymia and myotonia are not features of CMT and hyperhidrosis is said to be rare. Three unrelated patients were described. In one the inheritance was probably dominant. There is little to 'go on' in the reports of the other two. The myotonia may be what was called neuromyotonia by Mertens and Zschocke (1965) because there is continuous nerve activity. Stiffness is almost continual and anticonvulsants give relief. Grund (1938) reported affected brothers.

Gamstorp, I. and Wohlfart, G.: A syndrome characterized by myokymia, myotonia, muscular wasting and increased perspiration. Acta Psychiatry Scand. 34: 181-194, 1959.

Grund, G.: Ueber genetische Beziehungen zwischen Myotonie, Muskelkraempfen und Myokymie. (Zugleich Beitrag zur pathologie der neuralen Muskelatrophie). Deutsctieh. Z. Nervenheilk. 146: 3-14, 1938.

Mertens, H. G. and Zschocke, S.: Neuromyotonie. Klin. Wschr. 43: 917-925, 1965.

13722 GASTRIC JUICE PEPTIDES

Two peptides, one of 9 amino acids and one of 10 but otherwise identical, have been identified (Heathcote, Washington, 1970).

Heathcote, J. G. and Washington, R. J.: Peptides of normal human gastric juice. Int. J. Protein Res. 2: 117-126, 1970.

13725 GASTRIN

Human gastrin has a molecular weight of 2,117 and contains 17 amino acid residues. Gastrin I and gastrin II differ only in the presence of a sulfate ester group on tyrosine in the 12th position (Bentley et al., 1966). Both gastrin I and gastrin II (of normal sequence) are excreted in excess by pancreatic tumors in the

Zollinger-Ellison syndrome (Gregory et al., 1969). See 13110. Gastrin is normally formed by mucosal cells in the gastric antrum and by the D cells of the pancreatic islets. It is a hormone whose main function is to stimulate secretion of HCl by the gastrin mucosa. HCl inhibits gastrin formation.

Bentley, P. H., Kenner, G. W. and Sheppard, R. C.: Structure of human gastrins I and II. Nature 209: 583-585, 1966.

Gregory, R. A., Tracy, H. J., Agarwal, K. L. and Grossman, M. I.: Aminoacid constitution of two gastrins isolated from Zollinger-Ellison tumor tissue. Gut 10: 603-608, 1969.

13730 GAUCHER DISEASE

Hsia, Naylor and Bigler (1959) reported Gaucher disease in father and son. Although in the majority of instances Gaucher disease is autosomal recessive, a dominant form was suggested. The father in their case was German-Jewish and the mother Swedish-English. Even here, the mother may have been a carrier and this quasi-dominant mechanism is even more likely in reports of presumed dominant inheritance in Jewish groups where the frequency of the Gaucher gene may be relatively high.

Hsia, D. Y.-Y., Naylor, J. and Bigler, J. A.: Gaucher's disease: report of two cases in father and son and review of the literature. N. Engl. J. Med. 261: 164-169, 1959.

13740 GEOGRAPHIC TONGUE AND FISSURED TONGUE

Dawson and Pielou (1967) observed 18 persons with geographic tongue in 3 generations with probable autosomal dominant pattern. Some had fissured tongue also. Turpin and Caratzali (1936) concluded that one and the same gene is responsible for both geographic tongue and fissured tongue. Tobias (1945) reported dominant pedigrees.

Dawson, T. A. J. and Pielou, W. D.: Geographical tongue in three generations. Br. J. Dermatol. 79: 678-681, 1967.

Tobias, N.: Scrotal tongue and its inheritance. Arch. Dermatol. Syph. 52: 266 only, 1945.

Turpin, R. and Caratzali, A.: Contribution a l'etiologie de la glossite exfoliatrice marginee. Presse Med. 44: 1273-1274, 1936.

*13750 GIANT NEUTROPHILE LEUKOCYTES

Davidson, Milner and Lawler (1960) described giant neutrophile leukocytes in 7 members of 3 generations of a family. One to two percent of leukocytes showed the change.

Davidson, W. M., Milner, R. D. G. and Lawler, S. D.: Giant neutrophile leucocytes: an inherited anomaly. Br. J. Haematol. 6: 339-343, 1960.

13755 GIANT PIGMENTED HAIRY NEVUS

It has been thought that there is no genetic contribution to causation. However, Goodman et al. (1971) studied the families of three patients and found in each relatives with multiple small pigmented nevi. They suggested that at least some cases of GPHN may be determined by an autosomal dominant gene of variable expressivity.

Goodman, R. M., Caren, J., Ziprkowski, M., Padeh, B., Ziprkowski, L. and Cohen, B. E.: Genetic considerations in giant pigmented hairy naevus. Br. J. Dermatol. 85: 150-157, 1971.

*13760 GLAUCOMA

Using topical application of dexamethasone, Armaly (1966) concluded that subjects can be divided into three classes according to the response of intra-ocular pressure — high, intermediate and low. He interpreted these three phenotypes to correspond to the three genotypes of a two-allele system. Crombie and Cullen (1964) described juvenile open-angle glaucoma in 11 members of 5 generations. Harris (1965) observed 16 cases in 3 generations. The age of onset in 8 of these averaged 26 years. The angles of the anterior chambers were open in one patient on whom gonioscopy was performed early in the progress of the disease. In a Scottish family settled in Virginia, Courtney and Hill (1931) described 18 cases (10 males, 8 females) in five generations with two instances of failure of penetrance in the third generation. Onset was usually in the second or third generation and the course was rapid. Studies in families with and without cases of glaucoma led Armaly et al. (1968) to the conclusion that intraocular pressure and outflow facility are multifactorial in determination and that open-angle glaucoma is probably multifactorial also. Schwartz et al. (1972) found low concordance in a twin study of effect of corticosteroids on intraocular pressure and concluded that inheritance is multifactorial.

Armaly, M. F.: The heritable nature of dexamethasone induced ocular hypertension. Arch. Ophthalmol. 75: 32-35, 1966.

Armaly, M. F., Monstavicius, B. F. and Sayegh, R. E.: Ocular pressure and aqueous outflow facility in siblings. Arch. Ophthal. 80: 354-360, 1968.

Courtney, R. H. and Hill, E.: Hereditary juvenile glaucoma simplex. J.A.M.A. 97: 1602-1609, 1931.

Crombie, A. L. and Cullen, J. F.: Hereditary glaucoma. Occurrence in five generations of an Edinburgh family. Br. J. Ophthalmol. 48: 143-147, 1964.

Harris, D.: The inheritance of glaucoma. Am. J. Ophthalmol. 60: 91-95, 1965.

Schwartz, J. T., Reuling, F. H., Feinleib, M., Garrison, R. J. and Collie, D. J.: Twin heritability study of the effect of corticosteroids on intraocular pressure. J. Med. Genet. 9: 137-143, 1972.

In mother and daughter and probably in the mother's father, Minas and Podos (1968) observed open angle glucoma with elevated episcleral venous pressure, manifested by dilated episcleral veins.

Minas, T. F, and Podos, S. M.: Familial glucoma associated with elevated episceral venous pressure. Arch. Ophthalmol. 80: 202-208, 1968.

*13775 GLAUCOMA, HEREDITARY JUVENILE

Together Berg (1932) and Jerndal (1970) reported observations on 11 generations of a family with 25 out of 55 persons examined by an ophthalmologist were affected. All affected members showed dysgenesis of the iris and irido-corneal angle. Every member of the kindred with dysgenesis had developed glaucoma by age 8 years. Elevated intraocular pressure was found in two in the neonatal period. The goniodysgenesis had the same appearance as that in infantile congenital glaucoma, which is, however, clearly a distinct disorder in view of its recessive inheritance. Impressive 'dominant' pedigrees of juvenile glaucoma were reported by Courtney and Hill (1931), by Stokes (1940), by Allen and Ackerman (1942), and by others. The familial hypoplasia of the iris with glaucoma described by Weatherill and Hart (1969) may be the same but differs in the presence of greater variability in the goniodysgenesis.

Allen, T. D. and Ackerman, W. G.: Hereditary glaucoma in a pedigree of three generations. Arch. Ophthalmol. 27: 139-157, 1942.

Berg, F.: Erbliches jugendliches Glaukom. Acta Ophthalmol. 10: 568-587, 1932.

Courtney, R. H. and Hill, E.: Hereditary juvenile glaucoma simplex. J.A.M.A. 97: 1602-1609, 1931.

Jerndal, T.: Dominant goniodysgenesis with late congenital glaucoma. A re-examination of Berg's pedigree. Am. J. Ophthalmol. 74: 28-34, 1972.

Jerndal, T.: Goniodysgenesis and hereditary juvenile glaucoma. A clinical study of a Swedish pedigree. Acta Ophthalmol. (suppl. 107): 1-100, 1970.

Stokes, W. H.: Hereditary primary glaucoma. Arch. Ophthalmol. 24: 885-909, 1940.

Weatherill, J. R. and Hart, C. T.: Familial hypoplasia of the iris stroma associated with glaucoma. Br. J. Ophthalmol. 53: 433-438, 1969.

13780 GLIOMA OF BRAIN

King and Eisinger (1966) described glioma multiforme of the frontal lobes in father and daughter with development of symptoms at age 50 and 34 years, respectively. Others have reported multiple affected sibs or other relatives. Armstrong and Hanson (1969) described three sibs who died of brain glioma in adulthood.

Armstrong, R. M. and Hanson, C. W.: Familial gliomas. Neurology 19: 1061-1063, 1969.

King, A. B. and Eisinger, G.: May glioma multiforme be hereditary? Guthrie Clin. Bull. 35: 169-175, 1966.

Kjellin, K., Muller, R. and Astrom, K. E.: The occurrence of brain tumor in several members of a family. J. Neuropath. Exp. Neurol. 19: 528-537, 1960.

Parkinson, D. and Hall, C. W.: Oligodendrogliomas: simultaneous appearance in frontal lobes in siblings. J. Neurosurg. 19: 424-426, 1962.

Reese, W., Meredith, J. M. and Zfass, I. S.: Cerebral glioma in siblings. Sth. Med. J. 37: 424-428, 1944.

13790 GLOBULIN ANOMALY INVOLVING BETA (2A)-GLOBULIN

Wysocki and MacKiewicz (1965) described father and son with abnormal beta (2A)-globulin and a defect in coagulation and immunologic responses. A circulating anticoagulant directed against Factor VIII and various manifestations interpreted as autoimmune were described. In three other family members, beta (2A)-globulin was increased and in two was associated with a clotting defect. Another relative had the clotting defect without the protein abnormality. Except for the father and son these persons were all asymptomatic.

Wysocki, K. and MacKiewicz, S.: Familial anomalous beta (2A)-globulin accompanied by disorders of blood coagulation and pathologic immune phenomena. Arch. Intern. Med. 116: 351-356, 1965.

*13800 GLOMUS TUMORS, MULTIPLE

Gorlin, Fusaro and Benton (1960) reported five affected members of two generations of a family. The lesions tend to resemble cavernous hemangiomas. The distinctive feature is the presence of multiple layers of glomus cells lining the blood-filled cavities. The tumors are present at birth or appear in the first two decades. Isolated glomus tumor usually develops later (at about age 33 years on the average), is more frequently subungual than is the case with multiple tumors, and has no particular familial occurrence. Reed (1970) presented a pedigree of four persons with multiple glomus tumors in two generations.

Chasseuil, R. and Gautard, J.: Tumeurs glomiques familiales: 6 cas en 4 generations. Bull. Soc. Fr. Dermatol. Syph. 68: 635-636, 1961.

Gorlin, R. J., Fusaro, R. M. and Benton, J. W.: Multiple glomus tumor of the pseudocavernous hemangioma type. Arch. Dermatol. 82: 776-778, 1960.

Kaufman, L. R. and Clark, W. T.: Glomus tumors: report of 4 cases in same family. Ann. Surg. 114: 1102-1105, 1941.

Reed, W. B.: Genetische aspekte in der dermatologie. Hautarzt 21: 8-16, 1970.

115

Reinhard, M. and Luders, G.: Zur pathologie und klinik multipler familiarer glomustumoren. Arch. Klin. Exp. Dermatol. 237: 800-810, 1970.

13810 GLUCOGLYCINURIA

Renal glycosuria and hyperglycinuria without increased excretion of other amino acids were the features observed by Kaser, Cottier and Antener (1962). These workers found the combination in 14 persons in 7 sibships of three generations of one kindred with probable autosomal dominant inheritance.

Kaser, H., Cottier, P. and Antener, I.: Glucoglycinuria, a new familial syndrome. J. Pediatr. 61: 386-394, 1962.

*13815 GLUTAMATE OXALOACETATE TRANSAMINASE, MITOCHONDRIAL (GOT-2)

Davidson et al. (1970) demonstrated polymorphism of mitochondrial GOT. Soluble glutamic oxaloacetic transaminase of red cells, leukocytes and fibroblasts was not anomalous. In lower animals and plants, many mitochondrial enzymes show maternal inheritance, indicating that a separate mitochondrial genetic system is involved in their control. However, family studies showed that mitochondrial GOT is under the control of nuclear not mitochondrial DNA (Davidson et al., 1970).

Chen, S.-H. and Giblett, E. R.: Genetic variation of soluble glutamic-oxaloacetic transminase in man. Am. J. Hum. Genet. 23: 419-424, 1971.

Davidson, R. G., Cortner, J. A., Rattzaai, M. C., Ruddle, F. H. and Lubs, H. A.: Genetic polymorphisms of human mitochondrial glutamic oxaloacetic transaminase. Science 169: 391-392, 1970.

DeLorenzo, R. J. and Ruddle, F. H.: Glutamate transaminase (GOT) genetics in mus musculus: linkage, polymorphism, and phenotypes of the GOT-2 and GOT-1 loci. Biochem. Genet. 4: 259-273, 1970.

Lahav, M. and Szeinberg, A.: Red-cell glutamic-pyruvic transaminase polymorphism in several population groups in Israel. Hum. Hered. 22: 533-538, 1972.

*13818 GLUTAMATE OXALOACETATE TRANSAMINASE, SOLUBLE (GOT-1)

By analysis of mouse-human somatic cell hybrids, Creagan et al. (1973) concluded that the structural locus for cytoplasmic glutamate oxaloacetate transminase EC 2.6.1.1) is on chromosome 10.

Creagan, R., Tischfield, J., McMorris, F. A., Chen, S.-H., Hirschi, M., Chen, T.-T., Ricciuti, F. and Ruddle, F. H.: Assignment of the genes for human peptidase A to chromosome 18 and cytoplasmic glutamic oxaloacetate transaminase to chromosome 10 using somatic-cell hybrids. Cytogenet. Cell Genet. 12: 187-198, 1973.

*13820 GLUTAMATE-PYRUVATE TRANSAMINASE (GPT-1)

Chen and Giblett (1971) found polymorphism of this enzyme which is also known as alanine aminotransferase. It catalyzes the reversible conversion of L-alanine and alpha-ketoglutarate to L-glutamate and pyruvate. Like glutamic-oxaloacetic transaminase (GOT), malate dehydrogenase (MDH) and isocitrate dehydrogenase (ICD), it has two molecularly and presumably genetically distinct forms: one cytoplasmic (soluble) and one mitochondrial. Polymorphism of the soluble form was found in red cell hemolysates. Linkage of the GOT and GPT loci was suggested by very preliminary observations. Allele frequencies in the GPT system vary considerably in different populations but all those studied were in a range making GPT an efficient marker for study of linkage with other loci. Electrophoretic variants have also been studied by Kompf (1972). Olaisen and Gedde-Dahl (1973) found that the locus for soluble GPT and that for epidermolysis bullosa (13195) are linked.

Chen, S.-H. and Giblett, E. R.: Polymorphism of soluble glutamic-pyruvic transaminase: a new genetic marker in man. Science 173: 148-149, 1971.

Kompf, J.: Population genetics of soluble glutamic-pyruvic transminase (EC:2.6.1.2): gene frequencies in southwestern Germany. Humangenetik 14: 76-77, 1972.

Lahav, M. and Szeinberg, A.: A red-cell glutamic-pyruvic transaminase polymorphism in several population groups in Israel. Hum. Hered. 22: 533-538, 1972.

Olaisen, B. and Gedde-Dahl, T., Jr.: GPT-epidermolysis bullosa simplex (EBS Ogna) linkage in man. Hum. Hered. 23: 189-196, 1973.

13821 GLUTAMATE-PYRUVATE TRANSMINASE, MITOCHONDRIAL (GPT-2)

See 13820.

*13830 GLUTATHIONE REDUCTASE

Long (1967) found in a Negro a variant red cell glutathione reductase, characterized by greater electrophoretic mobility and enzyme activity per unit of hemoglobin than the normal. Inheritance was autosomal co-dominant. Three homozygotes were identified. The relation to gout is problematical. Also the relation of this locus to that responsible for glutathione reductase deficiency (q.v.) is unclear. By study of cell hybrids, Ruddle (1974) assigned the structural locus for glutathione reductase to chromosome no. 8. In cases of mosaic trisomy for chromosome no. 8, de la Chapelle (1974) found elevated glutathione reductase activity, with other enzymes normal.

De la Chapelle, A.: Helsinki, personal communication, 1974.

Long, W. K.: Glutathione reductase in red blood cells: variant associated with gout. Science 155: 712-713, 1967.

*13840 GLYCERALDEHYDE-3-PHOSPHATE DEHYDROGENASE

Variants have been found in a number of phyletically diverse organisms (Lebherz and Rutter, 1967). The combination of two different subunits (each determined by a separate gene) into tetramers was suggested by the existence of 5 isozymes as in lactic acid dehydrogenase. Variants were found in man by Charlesworth (1972). This enzyme catalyzes an important energy-yielding step in carbohydrate metabolism, the reversible oxidative phosphorylation of glyceraldehyde 3-phosphate in the presence of inorganic phosphate and nicotinamide adenine dinucleotide (NAD). The enzyme is thought to be a tetramer of identical chains. Sequence data were published in Dayhoff's atlas (1972). This enzyme catalyzes a critical energy-yielding step in carbohydrate metabolism, the reversible oxidative phosphorylation of glyceraldehyde 3-phosphate in the presence of inorganic phosphate and NAD. The enzyme is present in widely separated forms such as man, lobster and E. coli. Its rate of evolutionary change is one of the slowest known.

Charlesworth, D.: Starch-gel electrophoresis of four enzymes from human red blood cells: glyceraldehyde-3-phosphate dehydrogenase, fructoaldolase, glyoxalase II and sorbitol dehydrogenase. Ann. Hum. Genet. 35: 477-484, 1972.

Dayhoff, M. O.: Dehydrogenases. Atlas of Protein Sequence and Structure 1972 (vol. 5). Washington: National Biomedical Research Foundation, 1972. Pp. D141-D144.

Lebherz, H. G. and Rutter, W. J.: Glyceraldehyde-3-phosphate dehydrogenase variants in phyletically diverse organisms. Science 157: 1198-1199, 1967.

13841 GLYCEROL KINASE

This enzyme should be useful as a marker in cell hybridization studies of chromosome mapping.

Tischfield, J. A., Bernhard, H. P. and Ruddle, F. H.: A new electrophoretic-autoradiographic method for the visual detection of phosphotransferases. In press, 1973.

*13842 GLYCEROL-3-PHOSPHATE DEHYDROGENASE-1

Hopkinson et al. (1974) and others presented evidence that glycerol-3-phosphate dehydrogenase (EC no. 1.1.1.8) is a dimer of dissimilar subunits. Electrophoretic variants at each of two locus, designated GPD-1 and GPD-2, were described.

Hopkinson, D. A., Peters, J. and Harris, H.: Rare electrophoretic variants of glycerol-3-phosphate dehydrogenase: evidence for two structural gene loci (GPD-1 and GPD-2). Ann. Hum. Genet. 37: 477-484, 1974.

*13843 GLYCEROL-3-PHOSPHATE DEHYDROGENASE-2

See 13842.

*13845 GLYCINE AUXOTROPH A, HUMAN COMPLEMENT FOR HAMSTER (GLY A+)

By human-hamster hybrids Kao et al. (1969) have demonstrated that the human complement for hamster auxotroph A is located on chromosome no. 12. The enzyme, presence of which in human cells complements the deficiency in hamster cells, is thought to be serine hydroxymethylase.

Kao, F. T., Chasin, L. and Puck, T. T.: Genetics of somatic mammalian cells. X. Complementation analysis of glycine-requiring mutants. Proc. Natl. Acad. Sci. 64: 1284-1291, 1969.

*13847 GLYCINE-RICH BETA GLYCOPROTEIN

Alper et al. (1972) found evidence of extensive polymorphism in man of serum glycine-rich beta-glycoprotein. At least five components were demonstrated on electrophoresis. It was concluded that four alleles exist at a locus designated GB. GB(S) and GB(F) were found in all populations but in different proportions. Allen (1974) showed that GBG and HL-A are tightly linked. No recombinants were observed among 44 children from 12 informative families. The common alleles, Gb(S) and Gb(F), have a frequency of about .73 and .25, respectively. Alper et al. (1973) showed that GBG is the same as factor B in the properdin system (also known as C3 proaccelerator). Because of the tight linkage of GB and HL-A and the general characteristics of GB, homology is possible to the mouse S gene which determins a polymorphic serum protein and which lies in the midst of the HL-A region.

Allen, F. H., Jr.: Linkage of HL-A and GBG. Submitted to Vox Sang., 1974.

Alper, C. A., Boenisch, T. and Watson, L.: Genetic polymorphism-in human glycine-rich-beta glycoprotein. J. Exp. Med. 135: 68-80, 1972.

Alper, C. A., Goodkofsky, I. and Lepow, I. H.: The relationship of glycine-rich beta-glycoprotein to Factor B in the properdin system and to cobra-binding protein of human serum. J. Exp. Med. 137: 424-437, 1973.

13850 GLYCINURIA WITH OR WITHOUT OXALATE UROLITHIASIS

De Vries and colleagues (1957) found hyperglycinuria in a grandmother, her daughter and two granddaughters. The grandmother had had renal colic and renal oxalate stones were demonstrated in the two granddaughters of a Ashkenazic Jewish kindred. This family is apparently unique for the association of oxalate stones. It was plausibly suggested by Scriver (1968) that the glycinuria trait observed in these families was the heterozygous state of iminoglycinuria (q.v.), a disorder which has been described several times in Ashkenazic families. Greene et al. (1973) reported a family in which the father and two sons had hyperglycinuria. They were Ashkenazic. The proband was discovered when he was studied as a normal volunteer. The father had a history compatible with renal colic but had not been known to pass stones. One son had a life-long impairment of the sense of smell. Plasma glycine concentrations were normal. Intravenous proline infusion in one son showed a normal maximal transport rate for proline, but there was marked splay in the renal tubular titration curve for proline reabsorption, considered consistent with a 'Km' mutation affecting proline binding. They concluded that the mutation affecting glycine-proline-hydroxyproline renal transport in their family is different from that in previously described families. They suggested the designation iminoglycinuria type II. See 24260 for discussion of iminoglycinuria type I.

De Vries, A., Kochwa, S., Lazebnik, J., Frank, M. and Djaldetti, M.: Glycinuria, a hereditary disorder associated with nephrolithiasis. Am. J. Med. 23: 408-415, 1957.

Greene, M. L., Lietman, P. S., Rosenberg, L. E. and Seegmiller, J. E.: Familial hyperglycinuria. New defect in renal tubular transport of glycine and amino acids. Am. J. Med. 54: 265-271, 1973.

Scriver, C. R.: Renal tubular transport of proline, hydroxyproline, and glycine. III. Genetic basis for more than one mode of transport in human kidney. J. Clin. Invest. 47: 823-835, 1968.

*13860 GLYCOPROTEIN, ALPHA-1-ACID, OF SERUM

Variants of alpha-1-acid glycoprotein have been demonstrated in normal Caucasian and Japanese blood (Schmid et al., 1965). Family studies have not been reported. Johnson et al. (1969) presented twin and family data supporting the view that three phenotypes SS, FF and FS are determined by two codominant alleles.

Johnson, A. M., Schmid, K. and Alper, C. A.: Inheritance of human alpha(1)-acid glycoprotein (orosomucoid) variants. J. Clin. Invest. 48: 2293-2299, 1969.

Schmid, K., Tokita, K. and Yoshizaki, H.: The alpha-1-acid glycoprotein variants of normal Caucasian and Japanese individuals. J. Clin. Invest. 44: 1394-1401, 1965.

*13870 GLYCOPROTEIN, CONCENTRATION OF BETA-2-GLYCOPROTEIN I IN SERUM

Cleve and Rittner (1969) found 9 families out of 88 in which one parent and about half the children had intermediate concentrations of beta-2-glycoprotein I and were presumed to be heterozygous for a deficiency gene. Irregularities in other families limit the use of the trait in genetic studies. See 23300 for description of the probable homozygous state.

Cleve, H. and Rittner, C.: Further family studies on the genetic control of beta-2-glycoprotein I concentration in human serum. Humangenetik 7: 93-97, 1969.

Cleve, H.: Genetic studies on the deficiency of beta-2-glycoprotein I of human serum. Humangenetik 5: 294-304, 1968.

13880 GOITER, NON-TOXIC, WITH INTRATHYROIDAL CALCIFICATION

Murray et al. (1966) described a family in which members of five generations had non-toxic goiter appearing in the early teens. Calcification and firm, nodular consistency were unusual features. None of the known defects in thyroid hormonogenesis could be demonstrated. Radioactive iodine studies showed increased thyroid avidity and rapid turnover. No certain male-to-male transmission was observed.

Murray, I. P., Thomson, J. A., McGirr, E. M., MacDonald, E. M., Kennedy, J. S. and McLennan, I.: Unusual familial goiter associated with intrathyroidal calcification. J. Clin. Endocrinol. Metab. 26: 1039-1040, 1966.

13890 GOUT

Gout is a disorder in which, as in essential hypertension, diabetes mellitus and hypercholesterolemia, there is room for debate as to whether polygenic or monomeric inheritance is its genetic basis. Although numerous other factors, some genetic, some environmental, influence the level of serum uric acid and although the phenotype gout can probably be produced by non-genetic elevations of serum uric acid, classic familial gout may be a monomeric dominantly inherited disorder.

Evidence for both an increased rate of uric acid synthesis and an impaired net elimination of uric acid by the kidney has been advanced. In some reported families with both parents affected, children have been affected unusually early and severely and may represent homozygotes (Emmerson, 1960). The new view on the polygenic inheritance of gout is stated by Neel and colleagues (1965) and by Wyngaarden (1966). Hyperuricemia in Filipinos has been shown to result from interplay of environmental and genetic factors (Healey et al., 1967).

Emmerson, B. T.: Heredity in primary gout. Aust. Ann. Med. 9: 168-175, 1960.

Healey, L. A., Skeith, M. D., Decker, J. L. and Bayani-Sioson, P. S.: Hyperuricemia in Filipinos: interaction of heredity and environment. Am. J. Hum. Genet. 19: 81-85, 1967.

Neel, J. V., Rakic, M. T., Davidson, R. T., Valkenburg, H. A. and Mikkelson, W. M.: Studies on hyperuricemia. II. A reconsideration of the distribution of serum uric acid values in the families of Smyth, Cotterman, and Freyburg. Am. J. Hum. Genet. 17: 14-22, 1965.

Wyngaarden, J. B. and Kelley, W. N.: Gout. In, Stanbury, J. B., Wyngaarden, J. B. and Fredrickson, D. S. (eds.): The Metabolic Basis of Inherited Disease. New York: McGraw-Hill, 1972 (3rd Ed.). Pp. 889-968.

*13894 GOUT DUE TO INCREASED PHOSPHORIBOSYLPYROPHOSPHATE (PPRP OR PRPP) SYNTHETASE ACTIVITY

Becker et al. (1973) described two brothers with marked purine overproduction and clinical gout, who showed activity of PPRP synthetase in erythrocyte lysates 2.5 to 3 times greater than in normal persons or in other patients with gout. A daughter of one brother showed equally increased enzyme activity. Increased activity was thought to be a property of the mutant enzyme molecule. This is, perhaps, the first example of a dominant disorder due to increased enzyme activity. Sperling et al. (1972) likewise found increased PPRP synthetase activity in two brothers whose mother, although normouricemic with normal red cell PPRP, was a hyperexcretor of uric acid. The father was normal. They suggested X-linked recessive inheritance. Becker et al. (1973) concluded that the enzyme is structurally altered to result in increased activity per molecule. Decreased response of PRPP synthetase to feeback inhibition is another possible mechanism.

Becker, M. A., Meyer, L. J. and Seegmiller, J. E.: Gout with purine overproduction due to increased phosphoribosylphosphate synthetase activity. Am. J. Med. 55: 232-242, 1973.

Becker, M. A., Kostel, P. J., Meyer, L. J. and Seegmiller, J. E.: Human phosphoribyloprophosphate synthetase: increased enzyme specific activity in a family with gout and excessive purine synthesis. Proc. Natl. Acad. Sci. 70: 2749-2752, 1973.

De Vries, A. and Sperling, O.: Familial gouty malignant uric acid lithiasis due to mutant phosphoribosyl-pyrophosphatase synthetase. Der Urologe 12: 153-157, 1973.

Sperling, O., Eliam, G., Persky-Brosh, S. and de Vries, A.: Accelerated erythrocyte 5-phosphoribo-syl-1-pyrophosphate synthesis. A familial abnormality associated with excessive uric acid production and gout. Biochem. Med. 310-316, 1972.

*13895 GRANULOCYTE ANTIGEN

Although not as well studied genetically as the HL-A system, antigens characteristic of granulocytic leukocytes, not lymphocytes, have been demonstrated. The specificities labelled 5A and 5B by van Rood are now known to be granulocyte antigens. Granulocyte antigens are important to leukopenia of the newborn. They have been studied by Lalezari and others. N(a) and N(b) are granulocyte antigenic specificities.

Amos, B. L.: Durham, N. C.: personal communication, 1972.

Lalezari, L.: Montefiore Hosp., N. Y.: personal communication, 1972.

13900 GRANULOSIS RUBRA NASI

Binazzi (1958) described a kindred with 20 affected members in a clearly autosomal dominant pedigree pattern. Hellier (1937) described affected mother and daughter. This condition is characterized by redness and marked sweating confined to the nose and surrounding area of the face, with red papules and sometimes numerous small vesicles. It occurs most commonly in children, clearing up at puberty, but in rare instances persists into adulthood.

Binazzi, M.: Ulteriori relievi su di una osservazione di granulosis rubra nasi ereditaria. Rass. Dermatol. Sif. 11: 23-26, 1958.

Hellier, F. F.: Granulosa rubra nasi in mother and daughter. Brit. Med. J. 2: 1068 only, 1937.

13910 GRAYING OF HAIR, EARLY

This trait is likely to have many causes. It is a feature of both Book syndrome and of Waardenburg syndrome. Probably a simple form of premature graying is inherited as a dominant. Hare (1929) described 9 affected in five generations, with one instance of male-to-male transmission. The hair began to turn at 17 or 18 years and was white at 25 or 26 years. In some persons with premature graying black pigmentation of the eyebrow persists.

Hare, H. J. H.: Premature whitening of hair. J. Hered. 20: 31-32, 1929.

*13920 GROUP-SPECIFIC COMPONENT (Gc)

By immunoelectrophoresis Hirschfeld (1959) discovered polymorphism of the serum alpha-2-globulin called Gc for group-specific component. Gc1-1, Gc2-2, and Gc2-1 phenotypes can be distinguished also by starch or agar electrophoresis (Bearn et al., 1964). No evidence of linkage of Gc, transferrins, ABO, MN, Rh, and haptoglobins was found in a study in Finland (Seppala et al., 1967). See ALBUMIN VARIANTS for information on linkage. Gc appears to be the vitamin-D binding protein (Cavalli-Sporza, 1974).

Bearn, A. G., Bowman, B. H. and Kitchin, F. D.: Genetic and biochemical consideration of the serum group-specific component. Cold Spring Harbor Symposia Quant. Biol. 29: 435-442, 1964.

Cavalli-Sporza, L.: Stanford, personal communication, 1974.

Cleve, H., Kirk, R. L., Gajdusek, D. C. and Guiart, J.: On the distribution of the Gc variant Gc Aborigine in Melanesian populations: determination of Gc-types in sera from Tongariki Island, New Hebrides. Acta Genet. Statist. Med. 17: 511-517, 1967.

Hirschfeld, J.: Immune-electrophoretic demonstration of qualitative differences in human sera and their relation to the haptoglobins. Acta Pathol. Microbiol. Scand. 47: 160-168, 1959.

Rucknagel, D. L., Shreffler, D. C. and Halstead, S. B.: The Bangkok variant of the serum group-specific component (Gc) and the frequency of the Gc alleles in Thailand. Am. J. Hum. Genet. 20: 478-485, 1968.

Seppala, M., Ruoslahti, E. and Makela, O.: Inheritance and genetic linkage of Gc and TF groups. Acta Genet. Statist. Med. 17: 47-54, 1967.

13925 GROWTH HORMONE, PITUITARY

Growth hormone is synthesized by acidophilic cells of the anterior pituitary gland. Human growth hormone has a molecular weight of 22,005 and contains 190 amino acid residues (Niall et al., 1971). It is not known whether any of the growth hormone deficiency states (e.g., 26240) are a reflection of mutation of the structural locus for growth hormone.

Dayhoff, M. O.: Hormones, active peptides and toxins. Atlas of Protein Sequence and Structure 1972 (vol. 5). Washington: Biomedical Research Foundation, 1972. P. D202.

Niall, H. D., Hogan, M. L., Sauer, R., Rosenblum, I. Y. and Greenwood, F. C.: Sequence of pituitary and placental lactogenic and growth hormones: evolution from a primordial peptide by gene reduplication. Proc. Natl. Acad. Sci. 68: 866-869, 1971.

13926 GUANASE

Harris et al. (1970) found no genetic variants by electrophoretic means.

Harris, H., Hopkinson, D. A. and Robson, E. B.: The incidence of rare alleles determining electrophoretic variants: data on 43 enzyme loci in man. Ann. Hum. Genet. 37: 237-253, 1974.

*13927 GUANYLATE KINASE

From cell hybridization studies, Kahn (1973) concluded that this locus may be on chromosome no. 1.

Kahn, P. M.: Intern. Workshop on Human Gene Mapping, New Haven, Conn. June, 1973.

13930 GYNECOMASTIA, HEREDITARY

Male-limited autosomal dominant, autosomal recessive and X-linked modes of inheritance have been proposed. Wallach and Garcia (1962) reported a family in which two brothers, their father and their paternal uncle had bilateral gynecomastia beginning at puberty. The breasts were tender at the time of enlargement. The patients were well virilized and all endocrine assays yielded normal results. The authors postulated an inherited sensitivity of the breast to the normal hormonal milieu of the male.

Wallach, E. E. and Garcia, C.-R.: Familial gynecomastia without hypogonadism: a report of three cases in one family. J. Clin. Endocrinol. Metab. 22: 1201-1206, 1962.

*13935 HAIR ALPHA-PROTEIN

By electrophoresis Baden and Lee (1974) described polymorphism of one of the polypeptide chains of the alpha-fibrous proteins of human hair. A variant polypeptide was present in about 5 percent of Caucasians. Family studies showed co-dominant inheritance. No correlation with color, thickness or texture could be determined. Physical properties other than the electrophoretic ones were normal.

Baden, H. P. and Lee, L. D.: Polymorphism in hair alpha-proteins. (Abstract) Clin. Res. 22: 425A only, 1974.

13940 HAIR WHORL ('COW-LICK,' 'CROWN')

Whether the whorl in the scalp hair of the occipital area shows clockwise or counter-clockwise rotation is genetically determined. Bernstein (1946) suggested that clockwise direction is dominant to counter-clockwise direction. Brewster (1925) reported a family with double whorls or double crown; Lauterback (1927) described three crowns in one subject, one of them being a conspicuous one in the frontal area.

Bernstein, F.: Heredity of scalp whorls. S. B. Akad. Wiss. Wien. Phys.-Math. Kl., Pp. 61-62. Cited by Kloepfer, H. W.: An investigation of 171 possible linkage relationships in man. Ann. Eugen. 13: 35-71, 1946.

Brewster, E. T.: The inheritance of 'double crown.' J. Hered. 16: 345-346, 1925.

Lauterback, C. E. and Knight, J. B.: Variation in whorl of the head hair. J. Hered. 18: 107-115, 1927.

13950 HAIRY EARS (HYPERTRICHOSIS PINNAE AURIS)

The trait consists of long hairs growing from the helix of the pinna. Controversy has prevailed as to whether it is Y-linked or autosomal, or perhaps both (in different families). Rao (1970) proposed that hairy ears result from the interaction of two loci, one on the homologous segment of the X and Y and one on the non-homologous segment of the Y.

Dronamraju, K. R.: Y-linkage in man. Nature 201: 424-425, 1964.

Rao, D. C.: A contribution to the genetics of hypertrichosis of the ear rims. Hum. Hered. 20: 486-492, 1970.

Rao, D. C.: Hypertrichosis of the ear rims: two remarks on the two-gene hypothesis. Acta Genet. Med. Gemellol. 21: 216-220, 1972.

Rao, D. C.: Two-gene hypothesis for hairy pinnae of the ear. Acta Genet. Med. Gemellol. 19: 448-453, 1970.

Stern, C., Centerwall, W. R. and Sarkar, S. S.: New data on the problem of Y-linkage of hairy pinnae. Am. J. Hum. Genet. 16: 455-471, 1964.

13960 HAIRY ELBOWS

In an Amish kindred we have observed striking hypertrichosis limited mainly to the elbows (F. K., 1099001). The condition is probably dominant, although inbreeding makes recessive inheritance a possible explanation for the findings.

Beighton, P. H.: Familial hypertrichosis cubiti: hairy elbows syndrome. J. Med. Genet. 7: 158-160, 1970.

13975 HAND AND FOOT DEFORMITY WITH FLAT FACIES

Emery and Nelson (1970) reported a mother and daughter with the same disorder. The mother's condition was known by history only. Non-progressive deformities of the hands were first noted in childhood. The face was flat. Both were about 5 feet tall. The daughter was mentally retarded but the mother was considered unusually intelligent. The daughter was 'floppy' as a neonate. The first three metacarpophalangeal joints had flexion contractures and the thumbs showed contractures in extension at the interphalangeal joints. All the toes were clawed.

Emery, A. E. H. and Nelson, M. M.: A familial syndrome of short stature, deformities of the hands and feet, and an unusual facies. J. Med. Genet. 7: 379-382, 1970.

13980 HAND CLASPING PATTERN

From twin data, Freire-Maia (1961) concluded that hand clasping is genetic to an important degree. If in clasping the hands with entwining fingers those of the right hand are positioned above the corresponding fingers of the left hand, the individual is classified as R with the converse labelled L. The R frequency is higher in females than in males. Lai and Walsh (1965) doubted that genetic factors are significant in determining this trait. Falk and Ayala (1971) found significant parent-offspring correlations and suggested polygenic inheritance.

Falk, C. T. and Ayala, F. J.: Genetic aspects of arm folding and hand clasping. Jap. J. Hum. Genet. 15: 241-247, 1971.

Freire-Maia, A.: Twin data on hand clasping: a reanalysis. Acta Genet. Statist. Med. 10: 207-211, 1961.

Lai, L. Y. C. and Walsh, R. J.: The patterns of hand clasping in different ethnic groups. Hum. Biol. 37: 312-319, 1965.

Pons, J.: Hand clasping (Spanish data). Ann. Hum. Genet. 25: 141-144, 1961.

13990 HANDEDNESS

Annett (1964) postulated that right handedness is an incomplete dominant, or intermediate, i.e., that dominant homozygotes are always right handed with 'speech highly developed in the left hemisphere.' Recessive homozygotes are consistently left handed with speech in the right hemisphere. Heterozygotes may use either hand and develop speech in either hemisphere. From twin studies Rife (1940) concluded that handedness is a multifactorial trait.

Annett, M.: A model of the inheritance of handedness and cerebral dominance. Nature 204: 59-60, 1964.

Annett, M.: Handedness in families. Ann. Hum. Genet. 37: 93-105, 1973.

Rife, D. C.: Handedness with special reference to twins. Genetics 25: 178-186, 1940.

14000 HAND-FOOT-UTERUS (HFU) SYNDROME

The clinical features include small feet with unusually short great toes and abnormal thumbs. Females with the disorder have duplication of the genital tract (Stern et al., 1970). The radiographic changes were reviewed by Poznanski et al. (1970). These included short first metacarpal and metatarsal, short fifth fingers with clinodactyly, trapezuim-scaphoid fusion in the wrist, cuneiform-navicular fusion in the foot.

Poznanski, A. K., Stern, A. M. and Gall, J. C., Jr.: Radiographic findings in the hand-foot-uterus syndrome (HFUS). Radiology 95: 129-134, 1970.

Stern, A. M., Gall, J. C., Jr., Perry, B. L., Stimson, C. W., Weitkamp, L. R. and Poznanski, A. K.: The hand-foot-uterus syndrome. A new hereditary disorder characterized by hand and foot dysplasia, dermatoglyphic abnormalities, and partial duplication of the female genital tract. J. Pediat. 77: 109-116, 1970.

*14010 HAPTOGLOBIN, ALPHA LOCUS (Hp)

The haptoglobins, alpha-2-globulins whose name comes from their ability to bind protein, were found to be polymorphic when studied by Smithies using starch gel electrophoresis. Several haptoglobin variants have been identified in addition to the main types and evidence of genic evolution through duplication (by unequal crossing over) and subsequent independent mutation has been provided. Two loci are involved in haptoglobin synthesis, one for alpha and one for beta chains. Haptoglobin variants with change in electrophoretic mobility of the alpha polypeptide have been found (Giblett, Uchida and Brooks, 1966), whereas others, the 'Marburg' phenotypes, have alterations in the beta polypeptide chain (Cleve and Deicher, 1965). In man and some other mammals free heme is bound not by haptoglobin but by another plasma protein hemopexin. Polymorphism of this other protein has been shown in the pig (Lush, 1966). From study of cases of ring chromosome 13 and their families, Bloom, Gerald and Reisman (1967) conclude that the haptoglobin alpha locus may be located near one or the other end of chromosome 13. Black and Dixon (1968) reported the amino acid sequences of the alpha chains of haptoglobin. The findings confirmed the conclusion that the alpha(2) chain arose through partial gene duplication of the Hp(1) locus. Robson et al. (1969) presented evidence that the alpha haptoglobin locus is on the long arm of chromosome 16. In a family with 46t(2G-;16G +) and one with 46t(1-;16 +) haptoglobin type was linked with the translocation chromosome. The alpha (1F) and alpha (1S) chains differ by a single amino acid: at position 54, lysine and glutamic acid, respectively, are present (Black and Dixon, 1968). The primary structures of the alpha chain and of light chains of gamma globulins bear similarities and there are functional homologies since both form complexes with specific proteins. A common evolutionary origin is postulated. The fast and slow forms of alpha-1, so called from their electrophoretic mobilities differ in the amino acid at position 54, lysine (F) or glutamic acid (S). The alpha-2 chain (or rather the gene for it) originated through a chromosomal aberration (unequal crossing over) in a person who was heterozygous alpha-1F alpha-1S. The alpha-2 chain is nearly twice as long as the alpha-1 chain and consists of portions of alpha-1F and alpha-1S. Sequence data are summarized in Dayhoff's atlas (1972). The alpha-2 chain is not found in any species but man. Black and Dixon (1968) suggested that alpha-2 chains give a selective advantage because their increased size loss of the haptoglobulin complex by the kidney and at the same time hemoglobin binding is unimpaired and heme degradation enhanced. See 24590 for information on probable linkage of the alpha-haptoglobin locus and the LCAT locus.

Bias, W. B. and Migeon, B. R.: Haptoglobin: a locus on the D(1) chromosome? Am. J. Hum. Genet. 19: 393-398, 1967.

Black, J. A. and Dixon, G. H.: Amino-acid sequence of alpha chains of human haptoglobins. Nature 218: 736-741, 1968.

Bloom, G. E., Gerald, P. S. and Reisman, L. E.: Ring D chromosome: a second case associated with anomalous haptoglobin inheritance. Science 156: 1746-1748, 1967.

Cleve, H. and Deicher, H.: Haptoglobin 'Marburg': Untersuchungen ueber eine seltene erbliche Haptoglobin-variante mit zwei verschiedenen Phaenotypen inerhalb einer Familie. Humangenetik 1: 537-550, 1965.

Dayhoff, M. O.: Haptoglobulin. Atlas of Protein Sequence and Structure 1972 (vol. 5). Washington: National Biomedical Research Foundation, 1972. Pp. D309-D314.

Giblett, E. R., Hickman, G. C. and Smithies, O.: Variant haptoglobin phenotypes. Cold Spring Harbor Symposia Quant. Biol. 29: 321-326, 1964.

Giblett, E. R., Uchida, I. and Brooks, L. E.: Two rare haptoglobin phenotypes, 1-B and 2-B, containing a previously undescribed alpha polypeptide chain. Am. J. Hum. Genet. 18: 448-453, 1966.

Javid, J. and Yingling, W.: Immunogenetics of human haptoglobins. I. The antigenic structure of normal Hp phenotypes. J. Clin. Invest. 47: 2290-2296, 1968.

Kirk, R. L.: The haptoglobin groups in man. (Monographs in Human Genetics, vol. 4) Basel and New York: S. Karger, 1968.

Lush, I. E.: The Biochemical Genetics of Vertebrates Except Man. Philadelphia: W. B. Saunders, 1966.

Magenis, R. E., Hecht, F. and Lovrien, E. W.: Heritable fragile site on chromosome 16: probable localization of haptoglobin locus in man. Science 170: 85-87, 1970.

Robson, E. B., Polani, P. E., Dart, S. J., Jacobs, P. A. and Renwick, J. H.: Probable assignment of the alpha locus of haptoglobin to chromosome 16 in man. Nature 223: 1163-1165, 1969.

Smithies, O., Connell, G. E. and Dixon, G. H.: Chromosomal rearrangements and the evolution of haptoglobin genes. Nature 196: 232-236, 1962.

Smithies, O., Connell, G. E. and Dixon, G. H.: Inheritance of haptoglobin subtypes. Am. J. Hum. Genet. 14: 14-21, 1962.

Sutton, H. E.: The haptoglobins. In, Steinberg, A. G. and Bearn, A. G. (eds.): Progress in Medical Genetics. New York: Grune and Stratton, Chapter 6, vol. 7, 1970. Pp. 163-216.

*14020 HAPTOGLOBIN, BETA LOCUS (Bp)

Javid (1967) described a genetic variant of the haptoglobin beta polypeptide chain and suggested that the locus be called Bp ('binding peptide' since the beta chain binds hemoglobin), the longer known unlinked locus for the alpha chain being called Hp. Haptoglobin Marburg is also a beta chain variant. Cleve et al. (1969) concluded that haptoglobin Marburg is the result of a mutational event other than single base substitution. Haptoglobin P is another beta variant. Sequence data are summarized in Dayhoff's atlas (1972).

Cleve, H., Bowman, B. H. and Gordon, S.: Biochemical characterization of the beta-chain variant haptoglobin Marburg. Humangenetik 7: 337-343, 1969.

Dayhoff, M. O.: Miscellaneous proteins. Atlas of Protein Sequence and Structure 1972 (vol. 5). Washington: National Biomedical Research Foundation, 1972. P. D315.

Javid, J.: Haptoglobin 2-1 Bellevue, a haptoglobin beta-chain mutant. Proc. Natl. Acad. Sci. 57: 920-924, 1967.

Weerts, G., Nix, W. and Deicher, H.: Isolierung und nahere Charakterisierung eines neuen Haptoglobins: HP-Marburg. Blut 12: 65-77, 1965.

14030 HASHIMOTO STRUMA

In a family with several cases of Hashimoto struma, De Groot et al. (1962) demonstrated an abnormal small iodinated protein in the serum and suggested that a defect in thyroid basement membrane may account for the appearance of this protein in the blood. Three sibs, their father and their paternal aunt were affected. The paternal grandparents were dead. Hall et al. (1962) presented data which they felt supported autosomal dominant inheritance of the tendency to thyroid autoimmunity. Volpe et al. (1963) also found an impressive familial aggregation.

De Groot, L. J., Hall, R., McDermott, W. V., Jr. and Davis, A. M.: Hashimoto's thyroiditis: a genetically conditioned disease. N. Engl. J. Med. 267: 267-273, 1962.

Hall, R., Saxena, K. M. and Owen, S. G.: A study of the parents of patients with Hashimoto's disease. Lancet II: 1291-1292, 1962.

Volpe, R., Ezrin, C., Johnston, M. W. and Steiner, J. W.: Genetic factors in Hashimoto's struma. Canad. Med. Assoc. J. 88: 915-919, 1963.

Although most reports of congenital heart block have concerned affected sibs, two generations have in a few instances been affected (Fulton et al., 1910; Wallgren, Winblad, 1937; Wendkos, Study, 1947). In the family reported by Gazes et al. (1965), conduction disturbances occurred in three and probably a fourth generation. In most of the affected persons the heart block was of second degree with episodes of third degree (complete) atrioventricular dissociation, leading to Adams-Stokes seizures. The family of Wendkos and Study (1947) consisted of a father with the Wolff-Parkinson-White syndrome and two offspring with congenital complete heart block. In the family reported by Fulton et al. (1910) 3 to 1 block was thought to be present in the father, complete block in a 22-month-old son and 2 to 1 block in a 20-year-old daughter. Amatller-Trias et al. (1966) described father (age 43), son (age 19) and daughter (age 22) with first degree heart block (prolonged PR interval). Schaal et al. (1973) studied the family of a 69-year-old woman with right bundle branch block and left axis deviation, who later developed complete heart block. Six relatives had heart block and 26 had abnormal electrocardiograms. First degree heart block (prolonged PR interval) is a feature of a form of familial atrial septal defect and has been reported to precede more severe disturbances of AV conduction in cases of familial heart block (Paul et al., 1958). Gambetta et al. (1973) described a kindred in which 8 persons in 4 generations had prolonged PR interval. There was male-to-male transmission and two instances of skipped generation.

Amatller-Trias, A., Periz-Sague, A., Loran-Lleo, J. A., and Oses, H.: Bloqueo auriculo-ventricular de primer grado de tipo familiar. Med. Clin. 46: 27-34, 1966.

Fulton, Z. M. K., Judson, C. F. and Norris, G. W.: Congenital heart block occurring in a father and two children, one an infant. Am. J. Med. Sci. 140: 339-348, 1910.

Gambetta, M., Weese, J., Ginsburg, M. and Shapiro, D.: Sick sinus syndrome in a patient with familial PR prolongation. Chest 64: 520-523, 1973.

Gazes, P. C., Culler, R. M., Taber, E. and Kelly, T. E.: Congenital familial cardiac conduction defects. Circulation 32: 32-34, 1965.

Paul, M. H., Rudolph, A. M. and Nadas, A. S.: Congenital complete atrioventricular block: problems of clinical assessment. Circulation 18: 183- , 1958.

Schaal, S. F., Seidensticker, J., Goodman, R. and Wooley, C. F.: Familial right bundle-branch block, left axis deviation, multiple heart block, and early death. A heritable disorder of cardiac condition. Ann. Intern. Med. 79: 63-66, 1973.

Wallgren, A. and Winblad, S.: Congenital heart-block. Acta Paediatr. 20: 175-204, 1937.

Wendkos, M. H. and Study, R. S.: Familial congenital complete A-V heart blocks. Am. Heart J. 34: 138-142, 1947.

14050 HEART, MALFORMATION OF

Kojima et al. (1969) described hypoplastic left heart syndrome in sibs. Such familial aggregation is to be expected from a multifactorial causation. Nora et al. (1970) concluded that the frequency of congenital heart malformations in first degree relatives of probands is close to the square root of the population frequency, as was suggested by Edwards (1960) should be the case for a multifactorial disorder. Zetterqvist (1971) reported a family with many cases of various cardiac malformations.

Edwards, J. H.: Simulation of Mendelism. Acta Genet. Statist. Med. 10: 63-70, 1960.

Kojima, H., Ogimi, Y., Mizutani, K. and Nishimura, Y.: Hypoplastic-left-heart syndrome in siblings. (Letter) Lancet II: 701 only, 1969.

Nora, J. J., McGill, C. W. and McNamara, D. G.: Empiric recurrence risks in common and uncommon congenital heart lesions. Teratology 3: 325-330, 1970.

Zetterqvist, P.: Accumulation of different congenital heart defects in one pedigree. Clin. Genet. 2: 123-127, 1971.

14060 HEBERDEN NODES

These are bony excrescences of the phalanges of the distal interphalangeal joints of the fingers. They can be considered a variety of osteo-arthrosis, or degenerative arthritis. Stecher (1955) suggested that the disorder is sex-influenced so that it is dominant in women and recessive in males. It is also age-dependent, with penetrance complete after 70. In the general population Stecher estimated that 27 percent are heterozygotes and 3 percent homozygotes.

Stecher, R. M.: Heberden's nodes. A clinical description of osteo-arthritis of the finger joints. Ann. Rheum. Dis. 14: 1-10, 1955.

14070 HEINZ BODY ANEMIA

This is a form of non-spherocytic hemolytic anemia of Dacie type I (in vitro autohemolysis is not corrected by added glucose). After splenectomy, which has little benefit, basophilic inclusions called Heinz bodies are demonstrable in the erythrocytes. Before splenectomy diffuse or punctate basophilia may be evident. Most or all of these cases are probably instances of hemoglobinopathy. The hemoglobin demonstrates heat-lability and electrophoretic hemoglobin anomaly has been demonstrated in some, e.g. Hb Tacoma (q.v.).

Dacie, J. V., Grimes, A. J., Meisler, A., Steingold, L., Hemsted, E. H., Beaven, G. H. and White, J. C.: Hereditary Heinz-body anaemia. A report of studies on five patients with mild anaemia. Br. J. Haematol. 10: 388-402, 1964.

14080 HEMANGIOMAS

Norwood and Everett (1964) reported the remarkable case of a 21-year-old Negro female who during pregnancy developed large hemangiomas at many sites such as ear lobe and axilla and heart failure as a result. After delivery the hemangiomas rapidly subsided. The patient's mother and 6-year-old son had macular hemangiomas of the face and trunk and her brother had classical Klippel-Trenaunay-Weber syndrome of the right lower extremity. Beers and Clark (1942) described a family with cutaneous hemangiomas ranging in size from a millimeter to many centimeters in diameter, in 12 persons in 3 generations. Metatarsus atavicus (second toe longer than the first toe) was an independent dominant trait in this family. (See TOES, RELATIVE LENGTH OF 1ST AND 2ND.)

Beers, C. V. and Clark, L. A.: Tumors and short-toe — a dihybrid pedigree. A family history showing the inheritance of hemangioma and metatarsus atavicus. J. Hered. 33: 366-368, 1942.

Norwood, O. T. and Everett, M. A.: Cardiac failure due to endocrine dependent hemangiomas. Arch. Dermatol. 89: 759-760, 1964.

14090 HEMANGIOMAS OF SMALL INTESTINE

Bandler (1960) reported a family in three generations of which there were 3 proved and two possible instances of cavernous hemangioma involving almost the entire small intestine. One patient had mucocutaneous pigment spots precisely like those of the Peutz-Jeghers syndrome. See BLUE RUBBER NEVUS SYNDROME.

Bandler, M.: Hemangiomas of the small intestine associated with mucocutaneous pigmentation. Gastroenterology 38: 641-645, 1960.

14100 HEMANGIOMA-THROMBOCYTOPENIA SYNDROME (KASABACH-MERRITT SYNDROME)

With giant hemangiomas in small children, thrombocytopenia and red cell changes compatible with trauma ('microangiopathic hemolytic anemia') have been observed. The mechanism of the hematologic changes is obscure. No evidence of a simple genetic basis has been discovered.

Brizel, H. E. and Raccuglia, G.: Giant hemangioma with thrombocytopenia. Radioisotopic demonstration of platelet sequestration. Blood 26: 751-756, 1965.

Propp, R. P. and Scharfman, W. B.: Hemangioma-thrombocytopenia syndrome associated with microangiopathic hemolytic anemia. Blood 28: 623-633, 1966.

Rodriguez-Erdmann, F., Murray, J. E. and Moloney, W. C.: Consumption-coagulopathy in Kasabach-Merritt syndrome. Trans. Assoc. Am. Phys. 83: 168-175, 1970.

14110 HEMANGIOMATOSIS, DISSEMINATED

Burke et al. (1964) described two unrelated infants with a large number of small hemangiomata in many areas of the skin and also in the brain. Nothing is known of a possible genetic basis of these.

Burke, E. C., Winkelmann, R. K. and Strickland, M. K.: Disseminated hemangiomatosis. The newborn with central nervous system involvement. Am. J. Dis. Child. 108: 418-424, 1964.

*14120 HEMATURIA, BENIGN FAMILIAL

McConville, West and McAdams (1966) described dominant inheritance of benign familial hematuria. A chemical test for hematuria (paper strips impregnated at one end with orthotoluidine which in the presence of hemoglobin is oxidized to yield a blue color) was used. The disorder is a non-progressive condition not associated with other abnormalities such as deafness (see ALPORT SYNDROME). Earlier reports may have included some patients of this type (e.g., Livaditis and Ericsson, 1962; Ayoub and Vernier, 1965). Rogers et al. (1973) demonstrated thin glomerular capillary basement in affected persons.

Ayoub, E. M. and Vernier, R. L.: Benign recurrent hematuria. Am. J. Dis. Child. 109: 217-223, 1965.

Livaditis, A. and Ericsson, N. O.: Essential hematuria in children: prognostic aspects. Acta Paediatr. 51: 630-634, 1962.

McConville, J. M., West, C. D. and McAdams, A. J.: Familial and non-familial benign hematuria. J. Pediatr. 69: 207-214, 1966.

Rogers, P. W., Kurtzman, N. A., Bunn, S. M., Jr. and White, M. G.: Familial benign essential hematuria. Arch. Intern. Med. 131: 257-262, 1973.

14130 HEMIFACIAL ATROPHY, PROGRESSIVE (PARRY-ROMBERG SYNDROME)

This syndrome described in the last century by Parry (1825) and Romberg (1846) consists of slowly progressive atrophy of the soft tissues of essentially half the face accompanied usually by contralateral Jacksonian epilepsy, trigeminal neuralgia and changes in the eyes and hair (Walsh, 1939; Wartenberg, 1945). The number of familial cases is small but autosomal dominance with reduced penetrance is possible.

Franceschetti, A. and Koenig, H.: L'importance du facteur heredo-degeneratif dans l'hematrophie faciale progressive (Romberg). Etude des complications oculaires dans ce syndrome. J. Genet. Hum. 1: 27-64, 1952.

Klingmann, T.: Facial hemiatrophy. J.A.M.A. 49: 1888-1891, 1907.

Walsh, F. B.: Facial hemiatrophy: report of 2 cases. Am. J. Ophthalmol. 22: 1-10, 1939.

Wartenberg, R.: Progressive facial hemiatrophy. Arch. Neurol. Psychiatry 54: 75-96, 1945.

14135 HEMIFACIAL HYPERPLASIA WITH STRABISMUS

Facial hemihyperplasia (FH) involves abnormal growth of the facial skeleton and its soft tissue structure and viscera. The neuro-cranium and eyeball are unaffected. Facial asymmetry is a consequence of FH. Bencze et al. (1973) described three generations of a family demonstrating left side FH localized in the zygomatic and mandibular angle areas. The maternal grandmother of this kindred had facial asymmetry only, whereas one son and one daughter had the same facial asymmetry with the daughter also showing amblyopia of the eye on the affected side. This daughter had five affected offspring, all of whom also showed convergent strabismus of the eye on the affected side, one on the unaffected side and two showed alternating strabismus. Three of the sibs showed amblyopia on the affected side, but the two with alternating strabismus showed no amblyopia. Bencze et al. (1973) believe that the FH and ophthalmic problems in this family have a common genetic basis.

Bencze, J., Schnitzler, A. and Walawska, J.: Dominant inheritance of hemifacial hyperplasia associated with strabismus. Oral Med. 489-500, 1973.

Rowe, H. N.: Hemifacial hypertrophy. Oral Surg. 15: 572-587, 1962.

14140 HEMIFACIAL MICROSOMIA

The left side of the face is affected in a majority of cases (Gorlin and Pindborg, 1964).

Gellis, S. S. and Feingold, M.: Hemifacial microsomia (picture of the month). Am. J. Dis. Child. 122: 57-58, 1971.

Gorlin, R. J. and Pindborg, J. J.: Syndromes of the Head and Neck. New York: McGraw-Hill, 1964. P. 261 ff.

14150 HEMIPLEGIC MIGRAINE, FAMILIAL

Rosenbaum (1960) described a family. Vasoconstriction, followed by focal edema, is thought to be responsible for the neurologic manifestations. Ohta et al. (1967) described four cases in three generations and added a 'new' feature, persistent cerebellar manifestations. Young et al. (1970) commented on the occurrence of hemiplegic and ordinary migraine in the same family, suggesting that they are basically the same entity. See MIGRAINE.

Blau, J. N. and Whitty, C. W. M.: Familial hemiplegic migraine. Lancet II: 1115-1116, 1955.

Ohta, M., Araki, S. and Kuroiwa, Y.: Familial occurrence of migraine with a hemiplegic syndrome and cerebellar manifestations. Neurology 17: 813-817, 1967.

Rosenbaum, H. E.: Familial hemiplegic migraine. Neurology 10: 164-170, 1960.

Young, G. F., Leon-Barth, C. A. and Green, J.: Familial hemiplegic migraine, retinal degeneration, deafness, and nystagmus. Arch. Neurol. 23: 201-209, 1970.

*14160 HEMOCHROMATOSIS

Bothwell and colleagues (1959), Debre and colleagues (1958) and several others have concluded that one form of hemochromatosis is inherited as an autosomal dominant with incomplete penetrance in females because of loss of blood in menstruation and pregnancy. Features of the disease include cirrhosis of the liver, diabetes, hypermelanotic pigmentation of the skin and heart failure. Elevated serum iron is a diagnostically valuable finding which can be sought in relatives of full-blown cases. Prophylactic venesection is indicated.

Balcerzak, S. P., Westerman, M. P., Lee, R. E. and Doyle, A. P.: Idiopathic hemochromatosis. A study of three families. Am. J. Med. 40: 857-873, 1966.

Bothwell, T. H., Cohen, I., Abrahams, O. L. and Perold, S. M.: A familial study in idiopathic hemochromatosis. Am. J. Med. 27: 730-738, 1959.

Debre, R., Dreyfus, J.-C., Frezal, J., Labie, D., Lamy, M., Maroteaux, P., Schapira, F. and Schapira, G.: Genetics of haemochromatosis. Ann. Hum. Genet. 23: 16-30, 1958.

Johnson, G. B., Jr. and Frey, W. G., III: Familial aspects of idiopathic hemochromatosis. J.A.M.A. 179: 747-751, 1962.

Pollycove, M.: Hemochromatosis. In, Stanbury, J. B., Wyngaarden, J. B. and Fredrickson, D. S. (eds.): The Metabolic Basis of Inherited Disease. New York: McGraw-Hill, 1972 (3rd Ed.). Pp. 1051-1084.

Williams, R., Scheuer, P. J. and Sherlock, S.: The inheritance of idiopathic haemochromatosis. Quart. J. Med. 31: 249-265, 1962.

*14180 HEMOGLOBIN — ALPHA LOCUS — 1

The alpha and beta loci determine the structure of the two types of polypeptide chains in adult hemoglobin, Hb A, alpha 2-beta 2. The alpha locus also determines one polypeptide chain, the alpha chain, in fetal hemoglobin (alpha 2-gamma 2), in hemoglobin A2(alpha 2-delta 2), and in embryonic hemoglobin (alpha 2-epsilon 2). The following are mutations affecting the alpha chain, arranged according to location of the amino acid substitution. References are given later under the name of the particular hemoglobin variant, in alphabetic order. It is noteworthy that at least one mutant substitution is now known for 33 of the 141 amino acids of the alpha chain. Two different mutant substitutions for 7 of the 33 amino acids are known and in one other three substitutions.

POSITION	FROM	TO	HEMOGLOBIN
5	ALA	ASP	J (Toronto)
6	ASP	ALA	Sawara
12	ALA	ASP	J (Paris-1)
15	GLY	ARG	Ottawa
15	GLY	ASP	J (Oxford)
15	GLY	ASP	I (Interlaken)
16	LYS	GLU	I (Burlington)
16	LYS	GLU	I (Skamania)
21	ALA	ASP	J (Nyanza)
22	GLY	ASP	J (Medellin)
23	GLU	GLN	Memphis
23	GLU	LYS	Chad
23	GLU	VAL	G (Audhali)
27	GLU	GLY	G (Fort Worth)
30	GLU	GLN	G (Honolulu)
30	GLU	GLN	G (Singapore)
30	GLU	GLN	G (Hongkong)
30	GLU	LYS	O (Padua)
43	PHE	VAL	Torino
47	ASP	HIS	Sealy
47	ASP	HIS	Sinai
47	ASP	HIS	Hasharon
47	ASP	GLY	Umi
47	ASP	GLY	L (Ferrara)
47	ASP	GLY	Kokura
47	ASP	GLY	Tagawa II
48	LEU	ARG	Montgomery
50	HIS	ASP	J (Sardegna)
51	GLY	ARG	Russ
51	GLY	ASP	J (Abidjan)
53	ALA	ASP	J (Rovigo)
54	GLN	ARG	Shimonoseki
54	GLN	ARG	Hikoshima
54	GLN	GLU	Mexico
54	GLN	GLU	J (Paris-2)
54	GLN	GLU	Uppsala
57	GLY	ASP	Norfolk
57	GLY	ASP	G (Ibadan)
57	GLY	ASP	Nishiki I
57	GLY	ASP	Kagoshima
57	GLY	ARG	L (Persian Gulf)

58	HIS	TYR	M (Boston)
58	HIS	TYR	M (Osaka)
58	HIS	TYR	M (Gottenberg)
58	HIS	TYR	M (Leipzig-2)
60	LYS	ASN	Zambia
61	LYS	ASN	J (Budapest)
64	ASP	ASP	G (Waimanalo)
64	ASP	HIS	Q (India)
68	ASN	LYS	G (Bristol)
68	ASN	LYS	G (Philadelphia)
68	ASN	LYS	D (St. Louis)
68	ASN	LYS	Knoxville-1
68	ASN	LYS	Stanleyville-1
68	ASN	LYS	G (St-1)
68	ASN	LYS	X
71	ALA	GLU	J (Habana)
72	HIS	ARG	Daneshgah-Tehran
74	ASP	HIS	G (Taichung)
74	ASP	HIS	Q
74	ASP	ASN	G (Pest)
75	ASP	HIS	Q (Iran)
75	ASP	TYR	Winnipeg
78	ASN	LYS	Stanleyville-2
78	ASN	ASP	J (Singapore)
79	ALA	GLY	J (Singapore)
80	LEU	ARG	Ann Arbor
84	SER	ARG	Etobicoke
85	ASP	ASN	G (Norfolk)
85	ASP	TYR	Atago
85	ASP	VAL	Inkster
87	HIS	TYR	M (Kankakee)
87	HIS	TYR	M (Iwate)
90	LYS	THR	J (Rajappen)
90	LYS	ASN	J (Broussais)
90	LYS	ASN	Tagawa-I
92	ARG	LEU	Chesapeake
92	ARG	GLN	J (Capetown)
94	ASP	TYR	Setif
95	PRO	LEU	G (Georgia)
95	PRO	ALA	Denmark Hill
95	PRO	SER	Rampa
95	PRO	ARG	St. Lukes
102	SER	ARG	Manitoba

112	HIS	ASP	Hopkins-2	
112	HIS	GLN	Dakar	
114	PRO	ARG	Chiapas	
115	ALA	ASP	J(Tongariki)	
116	GLU	LYS	O(Indonesia)	
120	ALA	GLU	J(Meerut)	
120	ALA	GLU	J(Birmingham)	
136	LEU	PRO	Bibba	
141	ARG	PRO	Singapore	
141	ARG	NIL	Koelliker	

D
O
M
I
N
A
N
T

By dissociation-recombination experiments each of the following variant hemoglobins appears to have a substitution in the alpha chain but its nature has not been identified:

HEMOGLOBIN G(IBADAN)
HEMOGLOBIN J(INDIA)
HEMOGLOBIN J(MALAYA)
HEMOGLOBIN K(CALCUTTA)
HEMOGLOBIN K(MADRAS)
HEMOGLOBIN L(BOMBAY)
HEMOGLOBIN M(OLDENBURG)
HEMOGLOBIN Q(CHINESE)

*14185 HEMOGLOBIN — ALPHA LOCUS — (SECOND ALPHA LOCUS)

Two alpha loci are known to exist in some humans but not in all. Hemoglobins G(Pest) and J(Buda) show the existence of at least two alpha chains in the Hungarians studied, whereas hemoglobin J(Tongariki) indicates that in Melanesians only one alpha locus exists. The alpha locus is apparently double in Chinese (Kan, 1974) whereas in the American Negro chromosomes with single or double alpha loci are about equally frequent (Huisman, 1974).

Huisman, T. H. J.: Augusta, Ga., personal communication, 1974.

Kan, Y. W.: San Francisco, personal communication, 1974.

14186 HEMOGLOBIN — ALPHA LOCUS — (THIRD ALPHA LOCUS)

In apes Boyer et al. (1973) found evidence for a third alpha locus. No information is available in man.

Boyer, S. H., Noyes, A. N., Boyer, M. L. and Marr, K.: Hemoglobin 3-alpha chains in apes. J. Biol. Chem. 248: 992-1003, 1973.

*14190 HEMOGLOBIN — BETA LOCUS

The alpha and beta loci determine the structure of the two types of polypeptide chains in adult hemoglobin, Hb A. The following are mutations affecting the beta chain, arranged according to location of the amino acid substition. References are given later under the name of the particular hemoglobin variant, in alphabetic order. It is noteworthy that single substitution of 59 of the chain have been detected. For 9 of the 59 amino acids, two different mutant substitutions have been found and for two others three substitutions are known. By autoradiography using heavily labelled hemoglobin-specific messenger RNA, Price et al. (1972) found labelling of a chromosome no. 2 and a group B chromosome. They suggested that the beta-gamma-delta linkage group may be on the group B chromosome since the zone of labelling was longer on that chromosome than on the no. 2 (which by this reasoning is presumed to carry the alpha locus or loci). Study of a case of the Wolf-Hirschhorn syndrome (4p-) indicated that the B group chromosome involved is no. 4.

Hirschhorn, K.: New York, personal communication, 1974.

Price, P. M., Conover, J. H. and Hirschhorn, K.: Chromosomal localization of human hemoglobin structural genes. Nature 237: 340-342, 1972.

D
O
M
I
N
A
N
T

POSITION	FROM	TO	HEMOGLOBIN
2	HIS	TYR	Tokuchi
2	HIS	ARG	Deer Lodge
6	GLU	VAL	S
6	GLU	LYS	C
6	GLU	LYS	X
6	GLU	LYS	Arlington Park
6	GLU	ALA	G (Makassar)
6	GLU	VAL	C (Harlem)

(The above has a second change at beta 73, q.v.)

| 6 | GLU | VAL | C (Georgetown) |

(The above has a second change in the beta chain.)

7	GLU	GLY	G (San Jose)
6 OR 7	GLU	NIL	Leiden
7	GLU	LYS	Siriraj
7	GLU	LYS	G (Honan)
9	SER	CYS	Porto Alegre
10	ALA	ASP	Ankara
14	LEU	ARG	Sogn
16	GLY	ASP	J (Baltimore)
16	GLY	ASP	N (New Haven-2)
16	GLY	ASP	J (Trinidad)
16	GLY	ASP	J (Ireland)
16	GLY	ARG	D (Bushman)
17	LYS	GLU	Nagasaki
19	ASN	LYS	D (Ouled Rabeh)
20	VAL	MET	Olympia
22	GLU	LYS	E (Saskatoon)
22	GLU	ALA	G (Hsin-Chu)
22	GLU	ALA	G (Coushatta)
22	GLU	ALA	G (Saskatoon)
22	GLU	GLY	G (Taipei)
22	GLU	GLN	D (Iran)
23	VAL	NIL	Freiburg
24	GLY	ARG	Riverdale-Bronx
24	GLY	VAL	Savannah
25	GLY	ARG	G (Taiwan-Ami)
26	GLU	LYS	E
28	LEU	PRO	Genova
28	LEU	GLN	St. Louis
30	ARG	SER	Tacoma
32	LEU	PRO	Abraham Lincoln
32	LEU	PRO	Perth
35	TYR	PHE	Philly

37	TRP	SER	Hirose
39	GLN	LYS	Alabama
42	PHE	LEU	Bucuresti
42	PHE	LEU	Louisville
42	PHE	SER	Hammersmith
42-44or43-45		NIL	Niteroi
43	GLU	ALA	G (Galveston)
43	GLU	ALA	G (Texas)
43	GLU	ALA	G (Port Arthur)
46	GLY	GLU	K (Ibadan)
47	ASP	ASN	G (Copenhagen)
48	LEU	ARG	Okaloosa
50	THR	LYS	Edmonton
51	PRO	ARG	Willamette
52	ASP	ASN	Osu Christiansborg
52	ASP	ALA	Ocho Rios
56	GLY	ASP	J (Bangkok)
56	GLY	ASP	J (Meinung)
56	GLY	ASP	J (Korat)
56	GLY	ASP	J (Manado)
56-59		NIL	Tochigi
58	PRO	ARG	Dhofar
58	PRO	ARG	Yukuhashi
59	LYS	GLU	I (High Wycomb)
59	LYS	GLU	J (Kaoshiung)
59	LYS	THR	J (Honolulu)
61	LYS	ASN	Hikari
61	LYS	GLU	N (Seattle)
62	ALA	PRO	Duarte
63	HIS	TYR	M (Saskatoon)
63	HIS	TYR	M (Kurume)
63	HIS	TYR	M (Chicago)
63	HIS	TYR	M (Hamburg)
63	HIS	ARG	Zurich
66	LYS	GLU	I (Toulouse)
67	VAL	GLU	M (Milwaukee-1)
67	VAL	ASP	Bristol
67	VAL	ALA	Sydney
69	GLY	ASP	J (Rambam)
69	GLY	ASP	J (Cambridge)
70	ALA	ASP	Seattle
71	PHE	SER	Christchurch
73	ASP	ASN	C (Harlem)
73	ASP	ASN	Korle-Bu
74	GLY	ASP	Shepherds Bush
74,75	GLY,LEU	NIL	St. Antoine

77	HIS	ASP	J (Iran)
79	ASP	GLY	G (Hsi Tsou)
80	ASN	LYS	G (Szuhu)
83	GLY	ASP	Pyrgos
83	GLY	CYS	Ta-Li
85	PHE	SER	Buenos Aires
87	THR	LYS	D (Ibadan)
87	THR	NIL	Tours
88	LEU	PRO	Santa Ana
88	LEU	ARG	Boras
90	GLU	LYS	Agenogi
91	LEU	PRO	Sabine
91-95		NIL	Gun Hill
92	HIS	TYR	M (Hyde Park)
92	HIS	TYR	M (Akita)
92	HIS	GLN	St. Etienne
92	HIS	GLU	Istanbul
94	ASP	ASN	Oak Ridge
95	LYS	ASP	N
95	LYS	GLU	Arlington Park
95	LYS	GLU or GLN	N (Memphis)
95	LYS	GLU	N (Baltimore)
95	LYS	GLU	N (Jenkins)
95	LYS	GLU	Hopkins-1
97	HIS	GLN	Malmo
98	VAL	MET	Koln
98	VAL	GLY	Nottingham
99	ASP	HIS	Yakima
99	ASP	TYR	Ypsi
99	ASP	ASN	Kempsey
100	PRO	LEU	Brigham
101	GLU	GLN	Rush
102	ASN	THR	Kansas
102	ASN	LYS	Richmond
103	PHE	LEU	Heathrow
106	LEU	PRO	Southhampton
106	LEU	PRO	Casper
108	ASN	ASP	Yoshizuka
109	VAL	MET	San Diego
111	VAL	PHE	Peterborough
113	VAL	GLU	New York
117	HIS	ARG	P (Galveston)
120	LYS	GLU	Hijiyama

121	GLU	VAL	Beograd	
121	GLU	LYS	O (Arabia)	
121	GLU	GLN	D (Punjab)	
121	GLU	GLN	D (Los Angeles)	
121	GLU	GLN	D (Cyprus)	
121	GLU	GLN	D (Portugal)	
124	PRO	ARG	Khartoum	
126	VAL	GLU	Hofu	
129	ALA	ASP	J (Taichung)	
130	TYR	ASP	Wien	
131	GLN	GLU	Camden	
132	LYS	GLN	K (Woolwich)	
136	GLY	ASP	Hope	
141	LEU	ARG	Olmsted	
143	HIS	GLU	Little Rock	
143	HIS	ASP	Hiroshima	
143	HIS	ASP	Kenwood	
143	HIS	PRO	Syracuse	
143	HIS	ARG	Abruzzo	
144	LYS	ASN	Andrew-Minneapolis	
145	TYR	CYS	Rainier	
145	TYR	HIS	Bethesda	
146	HIS	ASP	Hiroshima	
146	PLUS 10		Tak	
	DELTA-BETA FUSION		Lepore	
	GAMMA-BETA FUSION		Kenya	
	BETA-DELTA FUSION		Miyada	
	BETA-DELTA FUSION		P (Congo)	

DOMINANT

By dissociation recombination experiments, each of the following variant hemoglobins appears to have a substitution in the beta chain but its nature has not been identified:

HEMOGLOBIN CASERTA
HEMOGLOBIN DURHAM-1
HEMOGLOBIN J(GEORGIA)
HEMOGLOBIN J(JAMAICA)
HEMOGLOBIN K
HEMOGLOBIN L
HEMOGLOBIN R(SAME AS DURHAM-1)
HEMOGLOBIN TSUKIJI

*14200 HEMOGLOBIN — DELTA LOCUS

The delta locus determines the delta, or non-alpha, chain of hemoglobin A2 (alpha 2-delta 2). The following are mutations affecting the delta chain arranged according to location of the amino acid substitution. References are given later under the name of the particular hemoglobin variant, in alphabetic order.

	POSITION		FROM		TO		HEMOGLOBIN	
D O M I N A N T	6		HIS		ARG		Sphakia	
	12		ASN		LYS		NYU	
	16		GLY		ARG		A(2)prime or B(2)	
	22		GLY		ASP		F(Kuala Lumur)	
	22		ALA		GLU		Flatbush	
	69		GLY		ARG		Indonesia	
	136		GLY		ASP		Babinga	

*14210 HEMOGLOBIN — EPSILON LOCUS

The epsilon locus determines the epsilon, or non-alpha, chain of embryonic hemoglobin (originally known as Gower-2). No mutations affecting the epsilon chain have yet been identified. Gower-1 is a tetramer of epsilon chains. The epsilon locus may be linked to the delta-beta complex. The amino acid sequence of the epsilon chain is similar to those of the delta and beta chains. Furthermore, the homologous chain, now called Y, in the mouse is linked to the beta locus (Gilman and Smithies, 1968).

Gilman, J. G. and Smithies, O.: Fetal hemoglobin variants in mice. Science 160: 885-886, 1968.

Huehns, E. R., Dance, N., Beaven, G. H., Hecht, F. and Motulsky, A. G.: Human embryonic hemoglobin. Nature 201: 1095-1097, 1964.

A. Tetramers of a single type of polypeptide chain
   Hemoglobin Augusta-1. Probably tetramer of S-beta chain.
   Hemoglobin Augusta-2. Probably tetramer of C-beta chain.
   Hemoglobin Barts. Tetramer of gamma chain.
   Hemoglobin Gower-1. Tetramer of epsilon chain.
   Hemoglobin H. Tetramer of beta chain.

B. Probable octomer
   Hemoglobin Porto-Alegre

C. Delta-beta fusion products
   Hemoglobin Lepore(Boston)
   Hemoglobin Pylos(same as last)
   Hemoglobin Lepore(Cyprus)
   Hemoglobin Lepore(Hollandia)
   Hemoglobin Lepore(The Bronx)

D. Beta-delta fusion products
   Hemoglobin Miyada
   Hemoglobin P(Congo)

E. Deletion of one or more amino acids
   Hemoglobin Freiburg
   Hemoglobin Gun Hill
   Hemoglobin Leiden
   Hemoglobin Tochigi
   Hemoglobin Niteroi
   Hemoglobin Lyon
   Hemoglobin St. Antoine
   Hemoglobin Tours

F. Two substitutions in beta chain
   Hemoglobin C(Georgetown)

G.   Substitution in both the alpha and the beta chain
     Hemoglobin X

H.   Interstital addition of amino acids
     Hemoglobin Grady

I.   Terminal addition of amino acids
     a. Through terminator mutation
     Hemoglobin Constant Spring
     b. Through frame-shift mutation
     Hemoglobin Wayne

*14220 HEMOGLOBIN — GAMMA LOCUS (136 ALANINE)

See 14225.

*14225 HEMOGLOBIN — GAMMA LOCUS (136 GLYCINE)

The gamma locus determines the gamma, or non-alpha, chain of fetal hemoglobin (alpha 2-gamma 2). Schroeder et al. (1968) have provided evidence for the existence of two types of gamma polypeptide chains, determined presumably by separate cistrons. Although not distinguishable by most of the physical methods used, sequencing has shown at least one amino acid difference: at position 136 one type has glycine (as indicated in the amino acid map shown on a previous page) and the second type has alanine. Presumably the two loci arose by gene duplication. The following are mutations affecting the gamma chain arranged according to location of the amino acid substitution. Each mutation occurs in only one of the gamma cistrons, e.g., the mutation of Hb F(Malta) is in the glycine 136 cistron. References are given later under the name of the particular hemoglobin variant, in alphabetic order. Huisman et al. (1972) concluded that there are four gamma structural loci. In the heterozygote gamma-G chain variants contribute either about one-fourth or one-eighth and the gamma-A chain variants either about one-eighth or one-sixteenth of the total Hb F. The four postulated gamma loci, two gamma-G loci termed M and L and two gamma-A loci likewise termed M and L, produce gamma chains in an approximate ratio of 4:2: 2:1. The following variant hemoglobin represent unusual genetic and biochemical changes.

Huisman, T. H. J., Schroeder, W. A., Bannister, W. H. and Grech, J. L.: Evidence for four nonallelic structural genes for the gamma chain of human fetal hemoglobin. Biochem. Genet. 7: 131-139, 1972.

Schroeder, W. A., Huisman, T. H. J., Shelton, J. R., Shelton, J. B., Kleihauer, E. F., Dozy, A. M. and Robberson, B.: Evidence for multiple structural genes for the gamma chain of human fetal hemoglobin. Proc. Nat. Acad. Sci. 60: 537-544, 1968.

AA AT 136	POSITION	FROM	TO	HEMOGLOBIN
GAMMA-GLY	1	GLY	CYS	F(Malaysia)
	5	GLU	LYS	F(Texas 1)
	6	GLU	LYS	F(Texas 2)
	12	THR	LYS	F(Alexandra)
	61	LYS	GLU	F(Jamaica)
	97	HIS	ARG	F(Dickinson)
	117	HIS	ARG	F(Malta)
	121	GLU	LYS	F(Hull)
GAMMA-GLY	125	GLU	ALA	F(Port Royal)

Other,variant fetal hemoglobins include the following:

HEMOGLOBIN AEGINA
HEMOGLOBIN BRISTOL-SINGAPORE
HEMOGLOBIN CYPRUS-1
HEMOGLOBIN F(ROMA)
HEMOGLOBIN FESSAS-PAPASPYROU

D O M I N A N T

*14228 HEMOGLOBIN — ZETA LOCUS

Zeta is an early embryonic chain which is substituted for the alpha chain in Hb Portla 1-1. Melderis et al. (1974) presented evidence for the zeta chain being homologous with the alpha chain. The zeta chain of mice, rabbits and man showed close similarities to each other and significant similarities to the alpha chain of these species.

Capp, G. L., Rigas, D. A. and Jones, R. T.: Evidence for a new hemoglobin chain (zeta chain). Nature 228: 278-280, 1970.

Melderis, H., Steinheider, G. and Osterlag, W.: Evidence for a unique kind of alpha-type globin chain in early mammalian embryos. Nature, in press, 1974.

The following is the amino acid sequence of the alpha, beta, gamma and delta chains of hemoglobin, starting with the -NH2 end of the chains. The alpha chain has 141 amino acid residues and the beta, gamma, and delta chains 146. The meaning of the three-letter designations of the amino acids is also given below. When a statement such as 'substitution of valine at beta 6' appears in the description of variant hemoglobins, the chart below will indicate what amino acid has been replaced.

```
THE ALPHA, BETA, GAMMA AND DELTA CHAINS OF NORMAL HUMAN HEMOGLOBINS

            1       2    3    4    5    6    7    8    9   10   11   12   13   14

ALPHA     VAL-    -LEU-SER-PRO-ALA-ASP-LYS-THR-ASN-VAL-LYS-ALA-ALA-TRP-

BETA      VAL-HIS-LEU-THR-PRO-GLU-GLU-LYS-SER-ALA-VAL-THR-ALA-LEU-TRP-
GAMMA     GLY-HIS-PHE-THR-GLU-GLU-ASP-LYS-ALA-THR-ILE-THR-SER-LEU-TRP-
DELTA     VAL-HIS-LEU-THR-PRO-GLU-GLU-LYS-THR-ALA-VAL-ASN-ALA-LEU-TRP-

            1    2    3    4    5    6    7    8    9   10   11   12   13   14   15


  15   16   17   18   19   20   21   22   23   24   25   26   27   28   29   30   31

GLY-LYS-VAL-GLY-ALA-HIS-ALA-GLY-GLU-TYR-GLY-ALA-GLU-ALA-LEU-GLU-ARG-

GLY-LYS-VAL-ASN-   -   -VAL-ASP-GLU-VAL-GLY-GLY-GLU-ALA-LEU-GLY-ARG-
GLY-LYS-VAL-ASN-   -   -VAL-GLU-ASP-ALA-GLY-GLY-GLU-THR-LEU-GLY-ARG-
GLY-LYS-VAL-ASN-   -   -VAL-ASP-ALA-VAL-GLY-GLY-GLU-ALA-LEU-GLY-ARG-

  16   17   18   19         20   21   22   23   24   25   26   27   28   29   30


  32   33   34   35   36   37   38   39   40   41   42   43   44   45   46        47

MET-PHE-LEU-SER-PHE-PRO-THR-THR-LYS-THR-TYR-PHE-PRO-HIS-PHE-   -ASP-

LEU-LEU-VAL-VAL-TYR-PRO-TRP-THR-GLN-ARG-PHE-PHE-GLU-SER-PHE-GLY-ASP-
LEU-LEU-VAL-VAL-TYR-PRO-TRP-THR-GLN-ARG-PHE-PHE-ASP-SER-PHE-GLY-ASN-
LEU-LEU-VAL-VAL-TYR-PRO-TRP-THR-GLN-ARG-PHE-PHE-GLU-SER-PHE-GLY-ASP-

  31   32   33   34   35   36   37   38   39   40   41   42   43   44   45   46   47


  48   49   50   51   52   53                       54   55   56   57   58   59

LEU-SER-HIS-GLY-SER-ALA-   -   -   -   -GLN-VAL-LYS-GLY-HIS-GLY-

LEU-SER-THR-PRO-ASP-ALA-VAL-MET-GLY-ASN-PRO-LYS-VAL-LYS-ALA-HIS-GLY-
LEU-SER-SER-ALA-SER-ALA-ILE-MET-GLY-ASN-PRO-LYS-VAL-LYS-ALA-HIS-GLY-
LEU-SER-SER-PRO-ASP-ALA-VAL-MET-GLY-ASN-PRO-LYS-VAL-LYS-ALA-HIS-GLY-

  48   49   50   51   52   53   54   55   56   57   58   59   60   61   62   63   64
```

| 60 | 61 | 62 | 63 | 64 | 65 | 66 | 67 | 68 | 69 | 70 | 71 | 72 | 73 | 74 | 75 | 76 |

LYS-LYS-VAL-ALA-ASP-ALA-LEU-THR-ASN-ALA-VAL-ALA-HIS-VAL-ASP-ASP-MET-

LYS-LYS-VAL-LEU-GLY-ALA-PHE-SER-ASP-GLY-LEU-ALA-HIS-LEU-ASP-ASN-LEU-
LYS-LYS-VAL-LEU-THR-SER-LEU-GLY-ASP-ALA-ILE-LYS-HIS-LEU-ASP-ASP-LEU-
LYS-LYS-VAL-LEU-GLY-ALA-PHE-SER-ASP-GLY-LEU-ALA-HIS-LEU-ASP-ASN-LEU-

| 65 | 66 | 67 | 68 | 69 | 70 | 71 | 72 | 73 | 74 | 75 | 76 | 77 | 78 | 79 | 80 | 81 |

| 77 | 78 | 79 | 80 | 81 | 82 | 83 | 84 | 85 | 86 | 87 | 88 | 89 | 90 | 91 | 92 | 93 |

PRO-ASN-ALA-LEU-SER-ALA-LEU-SER-ASP-LEU-HIS-ALA-HIS-LYS-LEU-ARG-VAL-

LYS-GLY-THR-PHE-ALA-THR-LEU-SER-GLU-LEU-HIS-CYS-ASP-LYS-LEU-HIS-VAL-
LYS-GLY-THR-PHE-ALA-GLN-LEU-SER-GLU-LEU-HIS-CYS-ASP-LYS-LEU-HIS-VAL-
LYS-GLY-THR-PHE-ALA-THR-LEU-SER-GLU-LEU-HIS-CYS-ASP-LYS-LEU-HIS-VAL-

| 82 | 83 | 84 | 85 | 86 | 87 | 88 | 89 | 90 | 91 | 92 | 93 | 94 | 95 | 96 | 97 | 98 |

| 94 | 95 | 96 | 97 | 98 | 99 | 100 | 101 | 102 | 103 | 104 | 105 | 106 | 107 | 108 | 109 | 110 |

ASP-PRO-VAL-ASN-PHE-LYS-LEU-LEU-SER-HIS-CYS-LEU-LEU-VAL-THR-LEU-ALA-

ASP-PRO-GLU-ASN-PHE-ARG-LEU-LEU-GLY-ASN-VAL-LEU-VAL-CYS-VAL-LEU-ALA-
ASP-PRO-GLU-ASN-PHE-LYS-LEU-LEU-GLY-ASN-VAL-LEU-VAL-THR-VAL-LEU-ALA-
ASP-PRO-GLU-ASN-PHE-ARG-LEU-LEU-GLY-ASN-VAL-LEU-VAL-CYS-VAL-LEU-ALA-

| 99 | 100 | 101 | 102 | 103 | 104 | 105 | 106 | 107 | 108 | 109 | 110 | 111 | 112 | 113 | 114 | 115 |

| 111 | 112 | 113 | 114 | 115 | 116 | 117 | 118 | 119 | 120 | 121 | 122 | 123 | 124 | 125 | 126 | 127 |

ALA-HIS-LEU-PRO-ALA-GLU-PHE-THR-PRO-ALA-VAL-HIS-ALA-SER-LEU-ASP-LYS-

HIS-HIS-PHE-GLY-LYS-GLU-PHE-THR-PRO-PRO-VAL-GLN-ALA-ALA-TYR-GLN-LYS-
ILE-HIS-PHE-GLY-LYS-GLU-PHE-THR-PRO-GLU-VAL-GLN-ALA-SER-TRP-GLN-LYS-
ARG-ASN-PHE-GLY-LYS-GLU-PHE-THR-PRO-GLN-MET-GLN-ALA-ALA-TYR-GLN-LYS-

| 116 | 117 | 118 | 119 | 121 | 122 | 123 | 124 | 125 | 126 | 127 | 128 | 129 | 130 | 131 | 132 |

| 128 | 129 | 130 | 131 | 132 | 133 | 134 | 135 | 136 | 137 | 138 | 139 | 140 | 141 |

PHE-LEU-ALA-SER-THR-VAL-LEU-THR-SER-LYS-TYR-ARG

VAL-VAL-ALA-GLY-VAL-ALA-ASN-ALA-LEU-ALA-HIS-LYS-TYR-HIS
MET-VAL-THR-GLY-VAL-ALA-SER-ALA-LEU-SER-SER-ARG-TYR-HIS
VAL-VAL-ALA-GLY-VAL-ALA-ASN-ALA-LEU-ALA-HIS-LYS-TRP-HIS

| 133 | 134 | 135 | 136 | 137 | 138 | 139 | 140 | 141 | 142 | 143 | 144 | 145 | 146 |

ALA - Alanine
ARG - Arginine
ASN - Asparagine
ASP - Aspartic Acid
CYS - Cysteine
GLN - Glutamine
GLU - Glutamic Acid
GLY - Glycine
HIS - Histidine
ILE - Isoleucine
LEU - Leucine

LYS - Lysine
MET - Methionine
NIL - Amino Acid Deleted
PHE - Phenylalanine
PRO - Proline
SER - Serine
THR - Threonine
TRP - Tryptophan
TYR - Tyrosine
VAL - Valine

D
O
M
I
N
A
N
T

HIS - Histidine
ILE - Isoleucine
LEU - Leucine
LYS - Lysine
MET - Methionine
NIL - Amino Acid Deleted
PHE - Phenylalanine
PRO - Proline
SER - Serine
THR - Threonine
TRP - Tryptophan
TYR - Tyrosine
VAL - Valine

The base sequences of the RNA genetic code (as presently understood) is given in the following table. From it the mutation responsible for each substitution can be deduced.

DOMINANT

	U	C	A	G
U	UUU · UUC · PHE UUA · UUG · LEU	UCU · UCC · UCA · UCG · SER	UAU · UAC · TYR UAA ---* UAG ---*	UGU · UGC · CYS UGA ---+ UGG · TRP
C	CUU · CUC · CUA · CUG · LEU	CCU · CCC · CCA · CCG · PRO	CAU · CAC · HIS CAA · CAG · GLN	CGU · CGC · CGA · CGG · ARG
A	AUU · AUC · ILE AUA --- AUG · MET	ACU · ACC · ACA · ACG · THR	AAU · AAC · ASN AAA · AAG · LYS	AGU · AGC · SER AGA · AGG · ARG
G	GUU · GUC · GUA · GUG · VAL	GCU · GCC · GCA · GCG · ALA	GAU · GAC · ASP GAA · GAG · GLU	GGU · GGC · GGA · GGG · GLY

* UAA and UAG are ochre and amber, respectively. They are both nonsense and may be termination punctuation. The code is reviewed by Crick, Scientific American, October, 1966.

+ Crick (Nature, Feb. 4, 1967) claims UGA is nonsense. It may be a 'spacer' between cistrons in a polycistronic message.

138 —HEMOGLOBIN A(2)INDONESIA.
Substitution of arginine for glycine at delta 69.

Eng, L. I.-L., Pribadi, W., Westendorf-Boerma, F., Efremov, G. D., Wilson, J. B., Reynolds, C. A. and Huisman, T. H. J.: Hemoglobin A(2)-Indonesia or alpha(2) beta(2) 69(E13)gly to arg. Biochem. Biophys. Acta 229: 335-342, 1971.

—HEMOGLOBIN A(2)PRIME, OR B(2).
Substitution of arginine for glycine at delta 16.

Ball, E. W., Meynell, M. J., Beale, D., Kynoch, P., Lehmann, H. and Strelton, A. O. W.: Haemoglobin alpha(2) prime: alpha 2 gamma 2 (16 glycine to arginine). Nature 209: 1217-1218, 1966.

Horton, B., Payne, R. A., Bridges, M. T. and Huisman, T. H. J.: Studies on an abnormal minor hemoglobin component Hb-beta(2). Clin. Chim. Acta 6: 246-253, 1961.

Vella, F. and Graham, B.: A variant of hemoglobin A(2) in Alberta Indianas. Clin. Biochem. 2: 455-460, 1969.

—HEMOGLOBIN ABRAHAM LINCOLN.
Substitution of proline for leucine at beta 32.

Honig, G. R., Green, D., Shamsuddin, M., Vida, L. N., Mason, R. G., Gnarra, D. J. and Maurer, H. S.: Hemoglobin Abraham Lincoln, beta 32 (beta 14) leucine to proline. An unstable variant producing severe hemolytic disease. J. Clin. Invest. 52: 1746-1755, 1973.

—HEMOGLOBIN ABRUZZO.
Substitution of arginine for histidine at beta 143.

Chiancone, E., Norne, J. E., Bonaventura, J., Bonaventura, C. and Forsen, S.: Nuclear magnetic resonance quadrupole relaxation study of chloride binding to hemoglobin Abruzzo (beta 143 his-to-arg). Biochim. Biophys. Acta 336: 403-406, 1974.

Tentori, L., Sorcini, M. C. and Buccella, C.: Hemoglobom Abruzzo: beta 143 (H 21) his to arg. Clin. Chim. acta 38: 258-262, 1972.

—HEMOGLOBIN AEGINA.
Possible abnormal gamma chain. Fast hemoglobin.

Fessas, P., Karaklis, A. and Gnafakis, N.: A further abnormality of foetal haemoglobin. Acta Haemat. 25: 62-70, 1961.

—HEMOGLOBIN AGENOGI.
Substitution of lysine for glutamic acid at beta 90.

Miyaji, T., Suzuki, H., Ohba, Y. and Shibata, S.: Hemoglobin Agenogi (alpha-2 beta-2 90 lys), a slow-moving hemoglobin of a Japanese family resembling hemoglobin E. Clin. Chim. Acta 14: 624-629, 1966.

—HEMOGLOBIN ALEXANDRA.
Abnormal gamma chain. See HEMOGLOBIN F(ALEXANDRA). Substitution of lysine for threonine at gamma 12.

Fessas, P., Mastrokalos, N. and Fostiropoulos, G.: New variant of human foetal haemoglobin. Nature 183: 30-31, 1959.

Loukopoulos, D., Kaltsoya, A. and Fessas, P.: On the chemical abnormality of Hb 'Alexandra,' a fetal hemoglobin variant. Blood 33: 114-118, 1969.

—HEMOGLOBIN ANKARA.
Substitution of aspartic acid for alanine at beta 10.

Arcasoy, A., Casey, R., Lehmann, H., Cavdar, A. O. and Berki, A.: A new hemoblobin J from Turkey-Hb Ankara (beta 10 ala-to-asp). FEBS Letters 42: 121-123, 1974.

—HEMOGLOBIN ANN ARBOR.
Substitution of arginine for leucine at alpha 80.

Adams, J. G., III, Winter, W. P., Rucknagel, D. L. and Spencer, H. H.: Biosynthesis of hemoglobin Ann Arbor: evidence for catabolic and feedback regulation. Science 176: 1427-1429, 1972.

—HEMOGLOBIN ARLINGTON PARK.
Substitution of lysine for glutamic acid at beta 6 and glutamic acid for lysine at beta 95. May have arisen either through a second mutation in a person with Hb C or Hb N(Baltimore), or through crossing-over in a person who was heterozygous for both mutant hemoglobins. See Hb C(HARLEM).

Adams, J. G., III and Heller P.: Hemoglobin Arlington Park (86 glu-to-lys, 95 lys-to-glu): a new hemoglobin with two amino acid substitutions in a single beta polypeptide chain. Am. J. Hum. Genet. 25: 10A, 1973.

—HEMOGLOBIN ATAGO.
Substitution of tyrosine for aspertic acid at alpha 85.

Fujiwara, N.: An amino acid substitution in Hb Atago, an abnormal human hemoglobin. J. Jap. Biochem. Soc. 42: 341-349, 1970.

—HEMOGLOBIN ATWATER ET AL.
Defect unknown. Fast hemoglobin.

Atwater, J., Baglioni, C. and Tocantins, L. M.: A variety of human hemoglobin with a 'fast' component, but unaltered tryptic digest 'fingerprint.' Proc. 9th Congr. Intern. Soc. Hematol., Mexico City, 1962. Pp. 115-119.

—HEMOGLOBIN AUGUSTA-1.
Possible tetramer of S-beta chain. Fast hemoglobin.

Huisman, T. H. J.: Properties and inheritance of the new fast hemoglobin type found in umbilical cord blood samples of Negro babies. Clin. Chim. Acta 5: 709-718, 1960.

Labie, D., Schroeder, W. A. and Huisman, T. H. J.: The amino acid sequence of the delta-beta chains of hemoglobin Lepore Augusta — Lepore Washington. Biochim. Biophys. Acta 127: 428-437, 1966.

—HEMOGLOBIN AUGUSTA-2.
Possible tetramer of C-beta chain. Fast hemoglobin.

Huisman, T. H. J.: Genetic aspects of two different minor haemoglobin components found in cord blood samples of Negro babies. Nature 188: 589-590, 1960.

—HEMOGLOBIN BABINGA.
Substitution of aspartic acid for glycine at delta 136.

De Jong, W. W. W. and Bernini, L. F.: Haemoglobin Babinga (delta 136 glycine-aspartic acid): a new delta chain variant. Nature 219: 1360-1362, 1968.

—HEMOGLOBIN BART'S.
Tetramer of gamma chain. Fast hemoglobin.

Ager, J. A. M. and Lehmann, H.: Observations on some 'fast' haemoglobins: K, J, N and Bart's. Brit. Med. J. 1: 929-931, 1958.

Hunt, J. A. and Lehmann, H.: Haemoglobin Bart's: a foetal haemoglobin without alpha chains. Nature 184: 872-873, 1959.

—HEMOGLOBIN BEILINSON.
May have substitution of glycine for aspartic acid at alpha 47. The change is in TP IV.

De Vries, A., Joshua, H., Lehmann, H., Hill, R. L. and Fellows, R. E.: The first observation of an abnormal hemoglobin in a Jewish family. Hemoglobin Beilinson. Brit. J. Haemat. 9: 484-486, 1963.

—HEMOGLOBIN BEOGRAD.
Substitution of valine for glutamic acid at beta 121.

Efremov, G. D., Duma, H., Ruvidic, R., Rolovic, Z., Wilson, J. B. and Huisman, T. H. J.: Hemoglobin Beograd or beta 121 glu-to-val (GH4). Biochim. Biophys. Acta 328: 81-83, 1973.

—HEMOGLOBIN BETHESDA.
Substitution of histidine for tyrosine at beta 145. See HB RAINIER.

Adamson, J. W., Hayashi, A., Stamatoyannopoulos, G. and Burger, W. F.: Erythrocyte function and marrow regulation in hemoglobin Bethesda (beta 145 histidine). J. Clin. Invest. 51: 2883-2888, 1972.

Bunn, H. F., Bradley, T. B., Davis, W. E., Drysdale, J. W., Burke, J. F., Beck, W. S. and Laver, M. B.: Structural and functional studies on hemoglobin Bethesda (alpha(2) beta(2) 145 his), a variant associated with compensatory erythrocytosis. J. Clin. Invest. 51: 2299-2309, 1972.

Hayashi, A., Stamatoyannopoulos, G., Yoshida, A. and Adamson, J.: Haemoglobin Rainier: beta-145 (HC2) tyr to cys and haemoglobin Bethesda: beta-145 (HC2) tyrosine to histidine. Nature 230: 264-267, 1971.

Hayashi, A., Stamatoyannopoulos, G., Yoshida, A. and Adamson, J.: Haemoglobin Rainier: beta-145 (HC2) tyr to cys and haemoglobin Bethesda: beta-145 (HC2) tyrosine to histidine. Nature 230: 264-267, 1971.

--HEMOGLOBIN BIBBA.
Substitution of proline for leucine at alpha 136.

Kleihauer, E. F., Reynolds, C. A., Dozy, A. M., Wilson, J. B., Moores, R. R., Berenson, M. P., Wright, C. S. and Huisman, T. H. J.: Hemoglobin Bibba or alpha(2)136 pro beta(2), an unstable alpha chain abnormal hemoglobin. Biochem. Biophys. Acta 154: 220-221, 1968.

—HEMOGLOBIN BIRMINGHAM (USA).
The designation of this hemoglobin was changed to Hb Montgomery when it was discovered that Hb Birmingham had already been used for an alpha variant hemoglobin from Birmingham, Eng. See Hemoglobin J (Birmingham).

Schneider, R. G.: Galveston, personal communication, March 5, 1974.

—HEMOGLOBIN BORAS.
Substitution of arginine for leucine at beta 88.

Hollender, A., Lorkin, P. A., Lehmann, H. and Svensson, B.: New unstable haemoglobin Boras: beta 88 (F4) leucine-arginine. Nature 222: 953-955, 1969.

—HEMOGLOBIN BRIGHAM.
Substitution of leucine for proline at beta 100. Cause of erythrocytosis.

Lokich, J. J., Moloney, W. C., Bunn, H. F., Bruckheimer, S. M. and Ranney, H. M.: Hemoglobin Brigham (beta 100 pro-to-leu). Hemoglobin variant associated with familial erythrocytosis. J. Clin. Invest. 52: 2060-2067, 1973.

—-HEMOGLOBIN BRISTOL.
Substitution of asparatic acid for valine at beta 67.

Steadman, J. H., Yates, A. and Huehns, E. R.: Idiopathic Heinz body anaemia: Hb Bristol (beta 67 (E 11) val-to-asp). Brit. J. Haemat. 18: 435-446, 1970.

—-HEMOGLOBIN BRISTOL-SINGAPORE.
Possibly abnormal gamma chain. Fast hemoglobin.

Raper, A. B., Ager, J. A. M. and Lehmann, H.: Haemoglobin 'Singapore-Bristol.' A 'fast' haemoglobin found in infants. Brit. Med. J. 1: 1537-1539, 1960.

—-HEMOGLOBIN BROUSSAIS.
Substitution of asparagine for lysine at alpha 90.

Traverse, P. M., Lehmann, H., Coquelet, M. L., Beale, D. and Isaacs, W. A.: Etude d'une hemoglobine J-alpha non encore decrite, dans une famille Francaise. C. R. Seanc. Soc. Biol. 160: 2270-2272, 1966.

Vella, F., Charlesworth, D., Lorkin, P. A. and Lehmann, H.: Hemoglobin Broussais: alpha 90 lys replaced by asn. Canad. J. Biochem. 48: 408-410, 1970.

—-HEMOGLOBIN BUCURESTI.
Substitution of leucine for phenylalanine at beta 42. The resulting Hb has a lower oxygen affinity than Hb A. The substitution leads to hemolytic anemia. Same as Hb Louisville.

Bratu, V., Lorkin, P. A., Lehmann, H. and Predescu, C.: Haemoglobin Bucuresti beta42 (CD1) phe to leu, a cause of unstable haemoglobin haemolytic anaemia. Biochim. Biophys. Acta 251: 1-6, 1971.

—-HEMOGLOBIN BUENOS AIRES.
Substitution of serine for phenylalanine at beta 85.

Lehmann, H.: Hamolyse aufgrund instabiler hamoglobine. In, Norwicki, L., Martin, H. and Schubert, J. C. F. (eds.): hamolyse-hamolytische Erkrankungen. Munich: J. F. Lehmanns Verlag, 1973.

Weinstein, B. I., White, J. M., Wiltshire, A. and Lehmann, H.: Hemoglobina Buenos Aires. Una nueva hemoglobina inestable. (Abstract) Medicina 32: 749 only, 1973.

—-HEMOGLOBIN BUSHWICK.
Substitution of valine for glycine at beta 74.

Rieder, R. F., Wolf, D. J., Clegg, J. B. and Lee, S. L.: Hemoglobin Bushwick, beta 74 (E18) gly-to-val: an unstable hemoglobin found in extremely small amounts. (Abstract) J. Clin. Invest. 65A only, 1974.

—-HEMOGLOBIN C.
Substitution of lysine for glutamic acid at beta 6.

Baglioni, C. and Ingram, V. M.: Four adult haemoglobin types in one person. Nature 189: 465-467, 1961.

Hunt, J. A. and Ingram, V. M.: A terminal peptide sequence of human haemoglobin? Nature 184: 640-641, 1959.

Itano, H. A. and Neel, J. V.: A new inherited abnormality of human hemoglobin. Proc. Nat. Acad. Sci. 36: 613-617, 1950.

—-HEMOGLOBIN C (GEORGETOWN).
Beta chain anomaly. Substitution of lysine for glutamic at beta 7. Second substitution also present but not identified. Sickles.

Pierce, L. E., Rath, C. E. and McCoy, K.: A new hemoglobin variant with sickling properties. New Eng. J. Med. 268: 862-866, 1963.

Lang, A., Lehmann, H., McCurdy, P. R. and Pierce, L.: Identification of haemoglobin C Georgetown (BBA 36186). Biochim. Biophys. Acta 278: 57-61, 1972.

—-HEMOGLOBIN C (HARLEM).
Double substitution in beta chain (valine for glutamic acid at beta 6 and asparagine for aspartic acid at beta 73). May be identical to C(Georgetown). See HEMOGLOBIN KORLE-BU. See HB ARLINGTON PARK for another doubly mutant beta hemoglobin chain.

Bookchin, R. M., Davis, R. P. and Ranney, H. M.: Clinical features of hemoglobin C(Harlem), a new sickling hemoglobin variant. Ann. Intern. Med. 68: 8-18, 1968.

Bookchin, R. M., Nagel, R. L. and Ranney, H. M.: The effect of beta 73 asn on the interactions of sickling hemoglobins. Biochim. Biophys. Acta 221: 373-375, 1970.

Bookchin, R. M., Nagel, R. L., Ranney, H. M. and Jacobs, A. S.: Hemoglobin C (Harlem): a sickling variant containing amino acid substitutions in two residues of the beta-polypeptide chain. Biochem. Biophys. Res. Comm. 23: 122-127, 1966.

—-HEMOGLOBIN CAMDEN.
Substitution of glutaminc acid for glutamine at beta 131.

Cohen, P. T. W., Yates, A., Bellingham, A. J., and Huehns, E. R.: Amino-acid substitution in the alpha-1-beta-1 intersubunit contact of haemoglobin Camden beta 131 (H9) gly to glu. Nature 243: 467-468, 1973.

Cotten, P., Yates, A. J., Bellingham, A. J. and Huehns, E. R.: (Beta 131 (H9) gln-to-glu). Amino acid substitution in the alpha-1 beta-1 intersubunit contact of Hb Camden. Nature 243: 467 only, 1973.

—HEMOGLOBIN CASERTA.
Beta chain anomaly.

Quattrin, N., Ventruto, V. and De Rosa, L.: Hemoglobinopathies in Campania with particular reference to the rare and new types. Blut 20: 292-295, 1970.

Ventruto, V., Baglioni, C., De Rosa, L., Bianchi, P., Colombo, B. and Quattrin, N.: Haemoglobin Caserta: an abnormal haemoglobin observed in a southern Italian family. Scand. J. Haemat. 2: 118-125, 1965.

—HEMOGLOBIN CASPER.
Substitution of proline for leucine at beta 106.

Jones, R. T., Koler, R. D., Duerst, M. and Stocklen, Z.: Hemoglobin Casper gamma 8 beta 106 leu-to-pro further evidence that hemoglobin mutations are not random. In Brewer, G. J. (ed.): Hemoglobin and Red Cell Structure and Function. Proc. 2nd Int. Conf. on Red Cell Metabolism and Functions. New York: Plenum Press, 1973.

Koler, R. D., Jones, R. T., Bigley, R. H., Litt, M., Lovrien, E., Brooks, R., Lahey, M. E. and Fowler, R.: Hemoglobin Casper: beta 106 (gamma 8) leu-to-pro. A contemporary mutation. Am. J. Med. 55: 549-558, 1973.

—HEMOGLOBIN CHAD.
Substitution of lysine for glutamic acid at alpha 23.

Boyer, S. H., IV, Crosby, E. F., Fuller, G. F., Ulenurm, L. and Buck, A. A.: A survey of hemoglobins in the Republic of Chad and characterization of hemoglobin Chad: alpha-2-23glu-lys beta-2. Am. J. Hum. Genet. 20: 570-578, 1968.

—HEMOGLOBIN CHESAPEAKE.
Polycythemia is a clinical feature. Leucine is substituted for arginine at alpha 92.

Charache, S., Weatherall, D. J. and Clegg, J. B.: Polycythemia associated with a hemoglobinopathy. J. Clin. Invest. 45: 813-822, 1966.

Clegg, J. B., Naughton, M. A. and Weatherall, D. J.: Abnormal human haemoglobins: separation and characterization of the alpha and beta chains by chromatography, and the determination of two new variants, Hb Chesapeake and Hb J (Bangkok). J. Molec. Biol. 19: 91-108, 1966.

—HEMOGLOBIN CHIAPAS.
Substitution of arginine for proline at alpha 114.

Jones, R. T., Brimhall, B. and Lisker, R.: Chemical characterization of hemoglobin Mexico and hemoglobin Chiapas. Biochem. Biophys. Acta 154: 488-495, 1968.

—HEMOGLOBIN CHRISTCHURCH.
Substitution of serine for phenylalanine at beta 71.

Carrell, R. W.: Christchurch, New Zealand: personal communication, 1970.

—HEMOGLOBIN CONSTANT SPRING.
Alpha chains have 172 amino acids rather than the normal 141. Clegg et al. (1971) suggested that this may reflect a chain termination mutation. Hb Constant Spring represents 1-2 percent of the hemoglobin of heterozygotes. When combined with the alpha-thalassemia gene, Hb H disease results. About 31 extra residues are attached to C-terminal end of the alpha chain, probably as a result of mutation in the terminating codon. Hemoglobin Tak (q.v.) is a termination defect of the beta chain. Hunt and Dayhoff (1972) searched 518 known protein sequences for a 31 amino acid sequence with the largest number of identities to that of the extra piece on hemoglobin Constant Spring. The sequence which had the greatest identity (9 amino acids) was the region 68-98 of the normal alpha chain. See hemoglobin Wayne for a further discussion.

Clegg, J. B., Weatherall, D. J. and Milner, P. F.: Haemoglobin Constant Spring--a chain termination mutant? Nature 234: 337-340, 1971.

Eng, L. I. L., Ganesan, J., Clegg, J. B. and Weatherall, D. J.: Homozygous state for Hb Constant Spring (slow-moving Hb X components). Blood 43: 251-260, 1974.

Hunt, L. T. and Dayhoff, M. O.: The origin of the genetic material in the abnormally long human hemoglobin alpha and beta chains. Biochem. Biophys. Res. Commun. 47: 699-704, 1972.

Milner, P. F., Clegg, J. B. and Weatherall, D. J.: Haemoglobin-H disease due to a unique haemoglobin variant with an elongated alpha-chain. Lancet I: 729-732, 1971.

—HEMOGLOBIN CYPRUS-1.
Possibly abnormal gamma chain.

Gillespie, J. E. O., White, C. J., Ellis, M. J., Beaven, G. H., Gratzer, W. B., Shooter, E. M. and Parkhouse, R. M. E.: Haemoglobin: a haemoglobin with unusual alkaline-denaturation properties in a Turkish-Cypriot woman. Nature 184: 18761877, 1959.

—HEMOGLOBIN D BETA-BUSHMAN.
Substitution of arginine for glycine at beta 16.

Wade, P. T., Jenkins, T. and Huehns, E. R.: Haemoglobin variant in a Bushman: haemoglobin D beta-Bushman (16 gly to arg). Nature 216: 688-690, 1967.

—-HEMOGLOBIN D (CYPRUS).
D (Cyprus) has a substitution in the beta chain.

Baglioni, C.: Abnormal human haemoglobins. VII. Chemical studies on haemoglobin D. Biochim. Biophys. Acta 59: 437-449, 1962.

Gammack, D. B., Huehns, E. R., Lehmann, H. and Shooter, E. M.: The abnormal polypeptide chains in a number of haemoglobin variants. Acta Genet. Statist. Med. 11: 1-16, 1961.

—-HEMOGLOBIN D (CYPRUS).
Substitution in alpha peptide 23.

Benzer, S., Ingram, V. M. and Lehmann, H.: Three varieties of human haemoglobin D. Nature 182: 852-854, 1958.

—-HEMOGLOBIN D (FRANKFURT).
Beta anomaly.

Gammack, D. B., Huehns, E. R., Lehmann, H. and Shooter, E. M.: The abnormal polypeptide chains in a number of haemoglobin variants. Acta Genet. Statist. Med. 11: 1-16, 1961.

Martin, H., Heupke, G., Pfleiderer, G. and Woerner, W.: Haemoglobin D in a Frankfurt family. Folia Haemat. 4: 233-241, 1960.

—-HEMOGLOBIN D (IBADAN).
Substitution of lysine for threonine at beta 87.

Watson-Williams, E. J., Beale, D., Irvine, D. and Lehmann, H.: A new haemoglobin, D Ibadan (beta-87 threonine to lysine), producing no sickle-cell haemoglobin D disease with haemoglobin S. Nature 205: 1273-1279, 1965.

—-HEMOGLOBIN D (IRAN).
Substitution of glutamine for glutamic acid at beta 22.

Rahbar, S.: Haemoglobin D Iran: beta 22 glutamic acid to glutamine (B4). Brit. J. Haemat. 24: 31-36, 1973.

Rohe, R. A., Sharma, V. S. and Ranney, H. M.: Double heterozygosity for beta thalassemia and hemoglobin D Iran (beta 22 glu to gln). (Abstract) Meeting Am. Soc. Hemat., Hollywood Fla., Dec. 3-6, 1972.

—-HEMOGLOBIN D (LOS ANGELES).
Same as hemoglobin D (Punjab).

Schneider, R. G., Ueda, S., Alperin, J. B., Levin, W. C., Jones, R. T. and Brimhall, B.: Hemoglobin D Los Angeles in two Caucasian families: hemoglobin SD disease and hemoglobin D thalassemia. Blood 32: 250-259, 1968.

—-HEMOGLOBIN D (MICHIGAN I).
Probably same as hemoglobin Kokura.

—-HEMOGLOBIN D (OULED RABAH).
Substitution of lysine for asparagine at beta 19.

Elion, J., Belkhodja, O., Wajcman, H. and Labie, D.: Two variants of hemoglobin D in the Algerian population: hemoglobin D (Ouled Rabah) beta 19 (B1) asn-to-lys and hemoglobin D Iran beta 22 (B4) glu-to-gln. Biochim. Biophys. Acta 310: 360-364, 1973.

—-HEMOGLOBIN D (PUNJAB).
Substitution glutamine for glutamic acid at beta 121.

Benzer, S., Ingram, V. M. and Lehmann, H.: Three varieties of human haemoglobin D. Nature 182: 852-854, 1958.

Bowman, R. and Ingram, V. M.: Abnormal human haemoglobin. VII. The comparison of normal human haemoglobin and haemoglobin D (Chicago). Biochim. Biophys. Acta 53: 569-573, 1961.

Ozsoylu, S.: Homozygous hemoglobin D Punjab. Acta Haemat. 43: 353-359, 1970.

Stout, C., Holland, C. K. and Bird, R. M.: Hemoglobin D in an Oklahoma family. Arch. Intern. Med. 114: 296-300, 1964.

—-HEMOGLOBIN D (ST. LOUIS).
Substitution of lysine for asparagine at alpha 68. Same as D (Washington), G (Philadelphia), G (Bristol), G (Azakuoli), Knoxville-1, and Stanleyville-1.

Schroeder, W. A. and Jones, R. T.: Some aspects of the chemistry and function of human and animal hemoglobins. Fortschr. Chem. Organ. Naturst. 23: 113-194, 1965.

—-HEMOGLOBIN DAKAR.
Substitution of glutamine for histidine at alpha 112.

Rosa, J., Maleknia, N., Vergoz, D. and Dunet, R.: Une nouvelle hemoglobine anormale: l'hemoglobine Ja-Paris 12 ala---asp. Nouv. Rev. Franc. Hemat. 6: 423-426, 1966.

—-HEMOGLOBIN DANESHGAH-TEHRAN.
Substitution of arginine for histidine at alpah 72.

Rahban, S., Nowzani, G. and Daneshmand, P.: Hemoglobin Daneshgah-Tehran alpha 72 (EF1) 143
histidine-to-arginine. Nature N. B. 245: 268-269, 1973.

D
O
M
I
N
A
N
T

—HEMOGLOBIN DEER LODGE.
Substitution of arginine for histidine at beta 2.

Labossiere, A., Vella, F., Hiebert, J. and Galbraith, P.: Hemoglobin Deer Lodge: alpha(2)beta(2)-his-to-arg. Clin. Biochem. 5: 46-50, 1972.

—HEMOGLOBIN DELTA CHAIN TETRAMER.
Not yet proven to be a tetramer.

Huehns, E. R.: A third haemoglobin abnormality in two individuals with Hb-H disease. In 'Haemoglobin-Colloquium.' H. Lehmann and K. Betke (eds.): Stuttgart: Georg Thieme Verlag, 1962. Pp. 76.

Huehns, E. R., Dance, N., Beaven, G. H. and Stevens, B. L.: Further investigations in haemoglobin H disease. Proc. 9th Congr. Intern. Soc. Hematol., Mexico City, 1962. Pp. 7-9.

—HEMOGLOBIN DENMARK HILL.
Substitution of alanine for proline at alpha 95.

Wiltshire, B. G., Clark, K. G. A., Lorkin, P. A. and Lehmann, H.: Haemoglobin Denmark Hill alpha — 95 (G2) pro-ala, a variant with unusual electrophoretic and oxygen-binding properties. Biochim. Biophys. Acta 278: 459-464, 1972.

—HEMOGLOBIN DHOFAR.
Substitution of arginine for proline at beta 58.

Marengo-Rowe, A. J., Lorkin, P. A., Gallo, E. and Lehmann, H.: Haemoglobin Dhofar-a new variant from southern Arabia. Biochem. Biophys. Acta 168: 58-63, 1968.

—HEMOGLOBIN DUARTE.
Substitution of proline for alanine at beta 62.

Beutler, E., Lang, A. and Lehmann, H.: Hemoglobin Duarte (beta 62 ala-to-pro): a new unstable hemoglobin with increased oxygen affinity. Blood 43: 527-536, 1974.

—HEMOGLOBIN DURHAM-I.
Beta chain anomaly.

Chernoff, A. I. and Pettit, N. M.: The amino acid composition of hemoglobin. III. A qualitative method for identifying abnormalities of the polypeptide chains of hemoglobin. Blood 24: 750-756, 1964.

—HEMOGLOBIN E.
Substitution of lysine for glutamic acid at beta 26.

Blackwell, R. Q., Yang, H. J., Liu, C. S. and Wang, C. C.: Structural identification of haemoglobin E in Filipinos. Trop. Geogr. Med. 22: 112-114, 1970.

Hunt, J. A. and Ingram, V. M.: Abnormal human haemoglobins. VI. The chemical difference between hemoglobin A and E. Biochim. Biophys. Acta 49: 520-536, 1961.

Shibata, S., Iuchi, I. and Hamilton, H. B.: The first instance of hemoglobin E in a Japanese family. Proc. Jap. Acad. 40: 846-851, 1962.

—HEMOGLOBIN E (SASKATOON).
Substitution of lysine for glutamic acid at beta 22.

Vella, F., Lorkin, P. A., Carrell, R. W.: A new hemoglobin variant resembling hemoglobin E. Hemoglobin E(Saskatoon): beta-22 glu replaced by lys. Canad. J. Biochem. 45: 1385-1391, 1967.

—HEMOGLOBIN EDMONTON.
Substitution of lysine for threonine at beta 50.

Labossiere, A., Hill, J. R. and Vella, F.: A new B-TP V hemoglobin variant: Hb Edmonton. Clin. Biochem. 4: 114-117, 1971.

—HEMOGLOBIN ETOBICOKE.
Substitution of arginine for serine at alpha 84.

Beale, D.: 1967, Cited by Dayhoff, M. O. and Eck, R. V., Loc. Cit.

Crookston, J. H., Farquharson, H. A., Beale, D. and Lehmann, H.: Hemoglobin Etobicoke: alpha 84(F5) serine replaced by arginine. Canad. J. Biochem. 47: 143-146, 1969.

—HEMOGLOBIN F.
Two forms of fetal hemoglobin are present in all persons: that in which the gamma chain has glycine at position 136 and that which has alanine at position 136. The finding is interpreted as indicating duplication of the gamma locus with mutation in one locus (Schroeder et al., 1968).

Schroeder, W. A., Huisman, T. H. J., Shelton, J. R., Shelton, J. B., Kleihauer, E. F., Dozy, A. M. and Robberson, B.: Evidence for multiple structural genes for the gamma chain of human fetal hemoglobin. Proc. Nat. Acad. Sci. 60: 537-544, 1968.

—HEMOGLOBIN F, HEREDITARY PERSISTENCE OF:
Not an abnormal hemoglobin. This state was first observed in Negroes (Conley et al., 1963) and thereafter in

Greeks and sporadically in other ethnic groups, e.g., Thais (see bibliography of Wasi et al., 1968). Two types of hereditary persistence of fetal hemoglobin have been found in Negroes. Some have only fetal hemoglobin with glycine at gamma 136 and others have both glycine 136 and alanine 136 forms of fetal hemoglobin. Greeks studied by Wasi et al. (1968) had only fetal hemoglobin of the alanine 136 type. These findings can be interpreted on the basis of various deletions involving a region containing several linked hemoglobin genes. Kazazian (1974) counted a minimum of seven different forms of hereditary persistence of fetal hemoblobins.

Conley, C. L., Weatherall, D. J., Richardson, S. N., Shephard, M. K. and Charache, S.: Hereditary persistence of fetal hemoglobin. A study of 79 affected persons in 15 Negro families in Baltimore. Blood 21: 261-281, 1963.67

Huisman, T. H. J., Schroeder, W. A., Adams, H. R., Shelton, J. R., Shelton, J. B. and Apell, G.: A possible subclass of the hereditary persistence of fetal hemoglobin. Blood 36: 1-9, 1970.

Huisman, T. H. J., Schroeder, W. A., Charache, S., Bethlenfalvay, N. C., Bouver, N., Shelton, R. J., Shelton, J. B. and Apell, G.: Hereditary persistence of fetal hemoglobin. Heterogeneity of fetal hemoglobin in homozygotes and in conjunction with beta-thalassemia. New Eng. J. Med. 285: 711-716, 1971.

Huisman, T. H. J., Schroeder, W. A., Stamatoyannopoulos, G., Bouver, N., Shelton, J. R., Shelton, J. B. and Apell, G.: Nature of fetal hemoglobin in the Greek type of hereditary persistence of fetal hemoglobin with and without concurrent beta-thalassemia. J. Clin. Invest. 49: 1035-1040, 1970.

Kazazian, H.: Baltimore, personal communication, 1974.

Siegel, W., Cox, R., Schroeder, W., Huisman, T. H. J., Penner, O. and Rowley, P. T.: An adult homozygous for persistent fetal hemoglobin. Ann. Intern. Med. 72: 533-536, 1970.

Wasi, P., Pootrakul, S. N. and Na-Nakorn, S.: Hereditary persistence of foetal haemoglobin in a Thai family: the first instance in the Mongol race and in association with haemoglobin E. Brit. J. Haemat. 14: 501-506, 1968.

Wheeler, J. T. and Krevans, J. R.: The homozygous state of persistent fetal hemoglobin and interaction of persistent fetal hemoglobin with thalassemia. Bull. Hopkins Hosp. 109: 217-233, 1961.

—HEMOGLOBIN F (ALEXANDRA).
Substitution of lysine for threonine at gamma 12.

Loukopoulos, D., Kaltsoya, A. and Fessas, P.: Brief report: on the chemical abnormality of Hb 'Alexandra,' a fetal hemoglobin variant. Blood 33: 114-118, 1969.

—HEMOGLOBIN F (DICKINSON).
Substitution of arginine for histidine at gamma 117.

Schneider, R. G., Brimhall, B. and Jones, R. T.: Galveston, Texas: Portland, Oregon, personal communication, 1970.

—HEMOGLOBIN F (FESSAS).

Fessas, P., Karaklis, A. and Gnafakis, N.: A further abnormality of foetal hemoglobin. Acta Haemat. 25: 62-70, 1961.

—HEMOGLOBIN F (HOUSTON).
A gamma chain defect. Probably substitution of alanine for glutamine. Similar or identical to hemoglobin F(Warren).

Schneider, R. G., Jones, R. T. and Suzuki, K.: Hemoglobin F-Houston: a fetal variant. Blood 27: 670-676, 1966.

—HEMOGLOBIN F (HULL).
Substitution of lysine for glutamic acid at gamma 121. The same substitution occurs at the homologous position in the alpha chain in hemoglobin O (Indonesia) and in the beta chain in hemoglobin O (Arab). Glutamine is substituted for glutamic acid at beta 121 in hemoglobin D (Punjab).

Sacker, L. S., Beale, D., Black, A. J., Huntsman, R. G., Lehmann, H. and Lorkin, P. A.: Haemoglobin F Hull (gamma 121 glutamic acid to lysine), homologous with Haemoglobins O Arab and O Indonesia. Brit. Med. J. 3: 531-533, 1967.

—HEMOGLOBIN F (JAMAICA).
Substitution of glutamic acid for lysine at position 61 of gamma 136 ala.

Ahern, E. J., Jones, R. T., Brimhall, B. and Gray, R. H.: Haemoglobin F Jamaica (gamma-A lys-to-ala). Brit. J. Haemat. 18: 369-375, 1970.

—HEMOGLOBIN F (KUALA LUMPUR).
Substitution of glycine and aspartic acid at position 22 of gamma 136 ala.

Eng, L. I. L., Wiltshire, B. B. and Lehmann, H.: Structural identification of Haemoglobin F (Kuala Lumpur): gamma 22 (B4) asp-to-gly; 136 ala. Biochim. Biophys. Acta 322: 224-230, 1973.

—HEMOGLOBIN F (MALAYSIA).
Substitution of cysteine for glycine at position 1 of gamma 136 glycine.

Eng, L. I. L., Kamuzora, H. and Lehmann, H.: Haemoglobin F (Malaysia gamma 1 (NA1) glycine-to-cysteine; 136 glycine. J. Med. Genet. 11: 25-30, 1974.

Substitution of arginine for histidine at position 117 in the glycine 136 gamma chain.

Cauchi, M. N., Clegg, J. B. and Weatherall, D. J.: Haemoglobin F (Malta): a new foetal haemoglobin variant with a high incidence in Maltese infants. Nature 223: 311-313, 1969.

—HEMOGLOBIN F (PORT ROYAL).
Substitution of alanine for glutamic acid at gamma-G 125.

Brimhall, B., Vedvick, T. S., Jones, R. T., Ahern, E., Palomino, E. and Ahern, V.: Haemoglobin F Port Royal (gamma-2 glu-to-ala). Brit. J. Haemat. 27: 313-318, 1974.

—HEMOGLOBIN F (ROMA).
Probable gamma chain defect.

Silvestroni, E. and Bianco, I.: A new variant of human fetal hemoglobin: Hb F-Roma. Blood 22: 545-553, 1963.

—HEMOGLOBIN F (TEXAS 1).
Substitution of lysine for glutamic acid at gamma 5.

Jenkins, G. C., Beale, D., Black, A. J., Huntsman, G. R. and Lehmann, H.: Haemoglobin F Texas 1(alpha-2, gamma-2-5 glu-lys): a variant of haemoglobin F. Brit. J. Haemat. 13: 252-255, 1967.

—HEMOGLOBIN F (TEXAS 2).
Substitution of lysine for glutamic acid at gamma 6.

Larkin, I. L., Baker, T., Lorkin, P. A., Lehmann, H., Black, A. J. and Huntsman, R. G.: Haemoglobin F Texas II (alpha-2 gamma-2 6 glu-lys), the second of the Haemoglobin F Texas variants. Brit. J. Haemat. 14: 233-238, 1968.

Schneider, R. G. and Jones, R. T.: Hemoglobin F Texas: gamma-chain variant. Science 148: 240-242, 1965.

—HEMOGLOBIN F (WARREN).
A gamma chain defect. Similar or identical to hemoglobin F (Houston).

Huisman, T. H. J., Dozy, A. M., Horton, B. E. and Wilson, J. B.: A fetal hemoglobin with abnormal gamma-polypeptide chains: Hemoglobin (Warren). Blood 26: 668-676, 1965.

—HEMOGLOBIN FESSAS-PAPASPYROU.
Same as Bart's.

Fessas, P. and Papaspyrou, A.: New 'fast' hemoglobin associated with thalassemia. Science 126: 1119 only, 1957.

Fessas, P.: Haemoglobin 'Bart's.' (Letter) Brit. Med. J. 2: 886 only, 1959.

—HEMOGLOBIN FLATBUSH.
Substitution of glutamic acid for alanine at delta 22.

Jones, R. T., Brimhall, B. and Huisman, T. H. J.: Structural characterization of two delta chain variants. Hemoglobin A-prime-2 (B2) and hemoglobin Flatbush. J. Biol. Chem. 242: 5141-5145, 1967.

—HEMOGLOBIN FLATBUSH (GEORGIA).
Delta chain anomaly.

Lee, R. C. and Huisman, T. H. J.: A variant of hemoglobin A-2 found in a Negro family. Blood 24: 495-501, 1964.

—HEMOGLOBIN FREIBURG.
Deletion of valyl residue no. 23 from otherwise normal beta chain probably occurred through triplet deletion resulting from unequal crossing-over between two normal beta loci in one parent of the proband. Two of three living children of the proband also had the abnormal hemoglobin whcih was accompanied by slight cyanosis in all three and by a hemolytic process in the proband.

Jones, R. T., Brimhall, B., Huisman, T. H. J., Kleihauer, E. and Betke, K.: Hemoglobin Freiburg: abnormal hemoglobin due to deletion of a single amino acid residue. Science 154: 1024-1027, 1966.

—HEMOGLOBIN G (ACCRA).
Substitution of asparagine for aspartic acid at beta 79. (No clinical or hematologic abnormality in the hemozygote.)

Edington, G. M., Lehmann, H. and Schneider, R. G.: Characterization and genetics of haemoglobin G. Nature 175: 850-851, 1955.

Gammack, D. B., Huehns, E. R., Lehmann, H. and Shooter, E. M.: The abnormal polypeptide chains in a number of haemoglobin variants. Acta Genet. Statist. Med. 11: 1-16, 1961.

Lehmann, H., Beale, D. and Boi-Doku, F. S.: Haemoglobin G (Accra). Nature 203: 363-365, 1964.

Milner, P. F.: High incidence of Hemoglobin G (Accra) in a rural district in Jamaica. J. Med. Genet. 4: 88-90, 1967.

—HEMOGLOBIN G (AUDHALI).
Substitution of valine for glutamic acid at alpha 23.

Marengo-Rowe, A. J., Beale, D. and Lehmann, H.: New human hemoglobin variant from southern

Arabia: G-Audhali (alpha-23(b4) glutamic acid-valine) and the variability of B4 in human haemoglobin. Nature 219: 1164-1166, 1968.

—HEMOGLOBIN G (BRISTOL).
Substitution of lysine at alpha 68.

Atwater, J., Schwartz, I. R. and Tocantins, L. M.: A variety of human hemoglobin with four distinct electrophoretic components. Blood 15: 901-908, 1960.

Baglioni, C. and Ingram, V. M.: Abnormal human hemoglobin. V. Chemical investigation of hemoglobins A, G, C, X from one individual. Biochim. Biophys. Acta 48: 253-265, 1961.

Dance, N., Huehns, E. R. and Shooter, E. M.: The chemical investigation of haemoglobins G Bristol and G Bristol-C. Biochim. Biophys. Acta 86: 144-148, 1964.

Gammack, D. B., Huehns, E. R., Lehmann, H. and Shooter, E. M.: The abnormal polypeptide chains in a number of haemoglobin variants. Acta Genet. Statist. Med. 11: 1-16, 1961.

Huehns, E. R. and Shooter, E. M.: The polypeptide chains of haemoglobin-A2 and haemoglobin-G2. J. Molec. Biol. 3: 257-262, 1961.

McCurdy, P. R., Pearson, H. and Gerald, P. S.: A new hemoglobinopathy of unusual genetic significance. J. Lab. Clin. Med. 58: 86-94, 1961.

Minnich, V., Cordonnier, J. K., Williams, W. J. and Moore, C. V.: Alpha, beta and gamma hemoglobin polypeptide chains during the neonatal period with description of a fetal form of hemoglobin D alpha-St. Louis. Blood 19: 137-167, 1962.

Raper, A. B., Gammack, D. B., Huehns, E. R. and Shooter, E. M.: Four haemoglobins in one individual: a study of the genetic interaction of Hb-G and Hb-C. Brit. Med. J. 2: 1257-1261, 1960.

Weatherall, D. J., Sigler, A. T. and Baglioni, C.: Four hemoglobins in each of three brothers. Genetic and biochemical significance. Bull. Hopkins Hosp. 111: 143-156, 1962.

—HEMOGLOBIN G (CHINESE).
The original G (Chinese) was found to have a beta chain substitution (Gammack et al., 1961). Several hemoglobins G in Chinese persons (Honolulu, Hong Kong, Singapore) were found by Swenson et al. (1962) to have substitution of glutamine for glutamic acid at alpha 30.

Gammack, D. B., Huehns, E. R., Lehmann, H. and Shooter, E. M.: The abnormal polypeptide chains in a number of haemoglobin variants. Acta Genet. Statist. Med. 11: 1-16, 1961.

Swenson, R. T., Hill, R. L., Lehmann, H. and Jim, R. T. S.: A chemical abnormality in hemoglobin G from Chinese individuals. J. Biol. Chem. 237: 1517-1520, 1962.

—HEMOGLOBIN G (COPENHAGEN).
Substitution of asparagine for aspartic acid at beta 47.

Sick, K., Beale, D., Irvine, D., Lehmann, H., Goodall, P. T. and MacDougall, S.: Hemoglobin G (Copenhagen) and hemoglobin J (Cambridge). Two new beta-chain variants of hemoglobin A. Biochim. Biophys. Acta 140: 231-242, 1967.

—HEMOGLOBIN G (COUSHATTA).
Substitution of alanine for glutamic at beta 22.

Bowman, B. H., Barnett, D. R. and Hite, R.: Hemoglobin G (Coushatta): a beta variant with a delta-like substitution. Biochem. Biophys. Res. Commun. 26: 466-470, 1967.

Schneider, R. G., Haggard, M. E., McNutt, C. W., Johnson, J. E., Bowman, B. H. and Barnett, D. R.: Hemoglobin G Coushatta: a new variant in an American Indian family. Science 143: 697-698, 1964.

—HEMOGLOBIN G (FORT WORTH).
Substitution of glycine for glutamic acid at alpha 27.

Schneider, R. G., Brimhall, B. and Jones, R. T.: Galveston, Texas and Portland, Oregon, personal communication, 1970.

—HEMOGLOBIN G (GALVESTON).
Substitution of alanine for glutamic at beta 43.

Bowman, B. H., Moreland, H. and Schneider, R. G.: A new haemoglobin variant (G-Galveston). Nature 193: 1298-1300, 1962.

Bowman, B. H., Oliver, C. P., Barnett, D. R., Cunningham, J. E. and Schneider, R. G.: Chemical characterization of three hemoglobins G. Blood 23: 193-199, 1964.

—HEMOGLOBIN G (GEORGIA).
Substitution of leucine for proline at alpha 95.

Huisman, T. H. J., Adams, H. R., Wilson, J. B., Efremov, G. D., Reynolds, C. A. and Wrightstone, R. N.: Hemoglobin G Georgia or alpha 95 leu (G-2) beta 2. Biochim. Biophys. Acta 200: 578-580, 1970.

—HEMOGLOBIN G (HONAN).
Substitution of lysine for glutamic acid at beta 7. Same as Hb Siriraj.

Blackwell, R. Q. and Liu, C. S.: Hemoglobin G Taichung: alpha 74 asp to his. Biochim. Biophys. Acta 200: 70-75, 1970.

—HEMOGLOBIN G (HONG KONG).
Same as Hemoglobin G(Honolulu).

—HEMOGLOBIN G (HONOLULU).
Same as G (HONG KONG) and G (SINGAPORE). Substitution of glutamine for glutamic acid at alpha 30.

Lehmann, H.: Haemoglobins and haemoglobinopathies. In, H. Lehmann and K. Betke (eds.): 'Haemoglobin-Colloquium.' Stuttgart: Georg Thieme Verlag, 1962. Pp. 1-14.

Swenson, R. T., Hill, R. L., Lehmann, H. and Jim, R. T. S.: A chemical abnormality in hemoglobin G from Chinese individuals. J. Biol. Chem. 237: 1517-1520, 1962.

—HEMOGLOBIN G (HSI-TSOU).
Substitution of glycine for aspartic acid at beta 79.

Blackwell, R. Q., Shih, T.-B., Wang, C.-L. and Liu, C.-S.: Biochim. Biophys. Acta 257: 49-53, 1972.

—HEMOGLOBIN G (HSIN-CHU).
Substitution of alanine for glutamic acid at beta 22. Same as Hb G (Coushatta) and Hb G (Saskatoon).

Blackwell, R. Q., Liu, C. S., Yang, H. J., Wang, C. C. and Huang, J. T. H.: Hemoglobin variant common to Chinese and North American Indians: alpha-2 beta-2 (22 glu-to-ala). Science 161: 381-382, 1968.

—HEMOGLOBIN G (IBADAN).
Alpha chain anomaly.

Gammack, D. B., Huehns, E. R., Lehmann, H. and Shooter, E. M.: The abnormal polypeptide chains in a number of haemoglobin variants. Acta Genet. Statist. Med. 11: 1-16, 1961.

Shooter, E. M., Skinner, E. R., Garlick, J. P. and Barnicot, N. A.: The electrophoretic characterization of haemoglobin G and a new minor haemoglobin G-2. Brit. J. Haemat. 6: 140-150, 1960.

—HEMOGLOBIN G (MAKASSAR).
Substitution of alanine for glutamic acid at beta 6.

Blackwell, R. Q., Oemijati, S., Pribadi, W., Weng, M. I. and Liu, C. S.: Hemoglobin G (Makassar): beta 6 glu to ala. Biochim. Biophys. Acta 214: 396-401, 1970.

—HEMOGLOBIN G (NORFOLK).
Substitution of asparagine for aspartic acid at alpha 85.

Huntsman, R. G., Lorkin, P. A. and Lehmann, H.: To be published.

—HEMOGLOBIN G (PARIS).
Alpha chain defect. Perhaps substitution of lysine for aspartic acid at 64, 74 or 85. The patient of Labie and Schapira (1966) had thrombocytopenic purpura.

Labie, D. and Schapira, G.: New variant of haemoglobin G: haemoglobin G (Paris). Nature 209: 1033-1034, 1966.

—HEMOGLOBIN G (PEST).
This and Hb J (Buda) occurred together in a Hungarian male with erythrocytosis. Both are alpha chain mutants and the occurrence of normal Hb A in this man shows the existence of at least two alpha loci. Substitution of asparagine for aspartic acid at alpha 74 or 75.

Brimhall, B., Hollan, S., Jones, R. T., Koler, R. D., Stocklen, Z. and Szelenyi, J. G.: Multiple alpha-chain loci for human hemoglobin. (Abstract) Clin. Res. 18: 184 only, 1970.

Brimhall, B., Duerst, M., Hollan, S. R., Stenzel, P., Szelenyi, J. and Jones, R. T.: Structural characterizations of hemoglobins J-Buda (alpha 61 (E10) lys-to-asn) and G-Pest (alpha 74 (EF3) asp-to-asn). Biochim. Biophys. Acta 336: 344-360, 1974.

Hollan, S. R., Szelenyi, J. G., Brimhall, B., Duerst, M., Jones, R. T., Koler, R. D. and Stocklen, Z.: Multiple alpha chain loci for human haemoglobins: Hb J (Buda) and Hb G (Pest). Nature 235: 47-50, 1972.

Jones, R. T.: Portland, Ore., personal communication, Jan. 30, 1973.

—HEMOGLOBIN G (PHILADELPHIA).
Same as D (Azakovli), D (Baltimore), D (St. Louis), Knoxville-1, and G (Azvakoli). Substitution of lysine for asparagine at alpha 68.

Baglioni, C. and Ingram, V. M.: Abnormal human hemoglobin. V. Chemical investigation of hemoglobins A, G, C, X from one individual. Biochim. Biophys. Acta 48: 253-265, 1961.

—HEMOGLOBIN G (PORT ARTHUR).
Same as Hb G (Galveston) and Hb G (Texas), q.v.

—HEMOGLOBIN G (SAN JOSE).
Substitution of glycine for glutamic acid at beta 7.

Hill, R. L. and Schwartz, H. C.: A chemical abnormality in haemoglobin G. Nature 184: 641-642, 1959.

Hill, R. L., Swenson, R. T. and Schwartz, H. C.: Characterization of a chemical abnormality in hemoglobin G. J. Biol. Chem. 235: 3182-3187, 1960.

Schwartz, H. C., Spaet, T. H., Zuelzer, W. W., Neel, J. V., Robinson, A. R. and Kaufman, S. F.: Combinations of hemoglobin G, hemoglobin S and thalassemia occurring in one family. Blood 12: 238-250, 1957.

—HEMOGLOBIN G (SASKATOON).
Substitution of lysine for glutamic acid at beta 22. Same as hemoglobin G (Coushatta) and hemoglobin G (Hsin-Chu).

> Vella, F., Isaacs, W. A. and Lehmann, H.: Hemoglobin G (Saskatoon): beta-22-glu-ala. Canad. J. Biochem. 45: 351-353, 1967.

—HEMOGLOBIN G (SINGAPORE).
Same as hemoglobin G (Honolulu).

—HEMOGLOBIN G (ST-1).
Substitution of lysine for asparagine at alpha 68.

> Bowman, B. H., Barnett, D. R., Hodgkinson, K. T. and Schneider, R. G.: Chemical characterization of haemoglobin G(St-1). Nature 211: 1305-1306, 1966.

—HEMOGLOBIN G (SZUHU).
Substitution of lysine for asparagine at beta 80.

> Blackwell, R. Q., Yang, H. J. and Wang, C. C.: Hemoglobin G (Szuhu): beta 80 asn replaced by lys. Biochim. Biophys. Acta 188: 59-64, 1969.

—HEMOGLOBIN G (TAEGN).
Same as G (Coushatta), G (Saskatoon) and G (Hsin-Chu).

> Blackwell, R. Q., Ro, I. H., Liu, C. S., Yang, H. J., Wang, C. C. and Huang, J. T. S.: Hemoglobin variant found in Koreans, Chinese, and North American Indians: alpha(2) beta(2) (22-glu-to-ala). Am. J. Phys. Anthrop. 30: 389-391, 1969.

—HEMOGLOBIN G (TAEGU).
Beta chain defect (probably in segment 18-30).

> Blackwell, R. Q., Huang, J. T. H. and Ro, I. H.: Hemoglobin variants in Koreans: hemoglobin G (Taegu). Science 158: 1056-1057, 1967.

> Blackwell, R. Q., Ro, I. H., Liu, C. S., Yang, H. J., Wang, C. C. and Huang, J. T. H.: Hemoglobin variant found in Koreans, Chinese, and North American Indians: alpha-2 beta-2 (22 glu-to-ala). Am. J. Phys. Anthrop. 30: 389-391, 1969.

—HEMOGLOBIN G (TAIPEI).
Substitution of glycine for glutamic acid at beta 22.

> Blackwell, R. Q., Yang, H. J. and Wang, C. C.: Hemoglobin G-Taipei: alpha-2-beta-2-22 glu replaced by gly. Biochim. Biophys. Acta 175: 237-241, 1969.

—HEMOGLOBIN G (TAIWAN-AMI).
Substitution of arginine for glycine at beta 25.

> Blackwell, R. Q. and Liu, C. S.: Hemoglobin G Taiwan-Ami: alpha(2)beta(2)25glu-to-arg. Biochem. Biophys. Res. Commun. 30: 690-696, 1968.

—HEMOGLOBIN G (TEXAS).
Substitution of alanine for glutamic acid at beta 43. Same as Hb G (Galveston) and Hb G (Port Arthur).

> Bowman, B. H., Oliver, C. P., Barnett, D. R., Cunningham, J. E. and Schneider, R. G.: Chemical characterization of three hemoglobins G. Blood 23: 193-199, 1964.

—HEMOGLOBIN G (WAIMANALO).
Substitution of asparagine for aspartic acid at alpha 64.

> Blackwell, R. Q., Jim, R. T. S., Tan, T. G. H., Weng, M. I., Liu, C. S. and Wang, C. L.: Hemoglobin G Waimanalo: alpha 64 asp-to-asn.

—HEMOGLOBIN GALLIERA GENOVA.
Defect unknown.

> Sansone, G. and Pick, C.: Familial haemolytic anaemia with erythrocyte inclusion bodies, bilifuscinuria and abnormal haemoglobin (haemoglobin Galliera Genova). Brit. J. Haemat. 11: 511-517, 1965.

—HEMOGLOBIN GENOVA.
Substitution of proline for leucine at beta 28. Unstable hemoglobin.

> Labie, D., Bernadou, A., Wajcman, H. and Bilski-Pasquier, G.: A familial observation of hemoglobin Genova beta 28(B10) leu-to-pro. A hematological, genetic and biochemical clinical study of a French family. Nouv. Rev. Franc. Hemat. 12: 502-505, 1972.

> Sansone, G., Carrell, R. W. and Lehmann, H.: Haemoglobin Genova: beta 28 (B10) leucine to proline. Nature 214: 877-879, 1967.

—HEMOGLOBIN GOWER-1.
Tetramer of epsilon chain.

—HEMOGLOBIN GOWER-2.
Alpha-2-epsilon-2.

> Huehns, E. R., Flynn, F. V., Butler, E. A. and Beaven, G. H.: Two new hemoglobin variants in a very young human embryo. Nature 189: 496-497, 1961.

—HEMOGLOBIN GRADY.

This hemoglobin is now seemingly unique in having an apparent insertion of threonine-glutamic acid-phenylalanine between AA no. 117 and 118 of the alpha chain. Eight hemoglobins with deletions are known (Leiden, Lyon, Freiburg, Niteroi, Tochigi, St. Antoine, Tours and Gun Hill).

Huisman, T. H. J., Wilson, J. B., Gravely, M. and Hubbard, M.: Hemoglobin Grady: a variant resulting from crossing over between hemoglobin-alpha loci on mispaired homologous chromosomes. (Abstract) Clin. Res. 22: 374A only, 1974.

—HEMOGLOBIN GUN HILL.

Deletion of amino acid residues 93-97 inclusive of beta chain probably through unequal crossing over. This unstable hemoglobin also has absence of half of the normal complement of heme. Other unstable hemoglobins include Hb Zurich, Hb Koln, Hb Geneva, Hb Sydbet, Hb Hammersmith and Hb Sinai.

Bradley, T. B., Jr., Wohl, R. C. and Rieder, R. F.: Hemoglobin Gun Hill: deletion of five amino acid residues and impaired heme-globin binding. Science 157: 1581-1583, 1967.

Rieder, R. F. and Bradley, T. B., Jr.: Hemoglobin Gun Hill: an unstable protein associated with chronic hemolysis. Blood 32: 355-369, 1968.

—HEMOGLOBIN H.

Tetramer of beta chains. Fast hemoglobin. Necheles et al. (1966) provided further evidence that Hb H disease results from mating of a parent with alpha thalassemia and a parent with a silent H gene, that double heterozygosity is necessary for Hb H disease. The findings of Na-Nakorn et al. (1969) leads to roughly the same conclusion. Among the newborn offspring of persons with Hb H, they found some with 1-2 percent Hb Bart's and others with 5-6 percent. They suggested that these two types of children are heterozygous for two different alpha-thal genes one of which is not detectable in the adult heterozygote.

Eng, L. I. L., Lopez, C. G. and Lopes, M.: Inheritance of haemoglobin H disease: a new aspect. Acta Haemat. 46: 106-120, 1971.

Jones, R. T., Schroeder, W. A., Balog, J. E. and Vinograd, J. R.: Gross structure of hemoglobin H. J. Am. Chem. Soc. 81: 3161 only, 1959.

Kattamis, C. and Lehmann, H.: The genetical interpretation of haemoglobin H disease. Hum. Hered. 20: 156-164, 1970.

Koler, R. D., Jones, R. T., Wasi, P. and Pootrukul, S. N.: Genetics of haemoglobin H and alpha-thalassaemia. Ann. Hum. Genet. 34: 371-377, 1971.

Na-Nakorn, S., Wasi, P., Pornpatkul, M. and Pootrakul, S. N.: Further evidence for a genetic basis of haemoglobin H disease from newborn offspring of patients. Nature 223: 59-60, 1969.

Necheles, T. F., Cates, M., Sheehan, R. G. and Meyer, H. J.: Hemoglobin H disease. A family study. Blood 28: 501-512, 1966.

Rigas, D. A., Koler, R. D. and Osgood, E. E.: New hemoglobin possessing a higher electrophoretic mobility than normal adult hemoglobin. Science 121: 372 only, 1955.

—HEMOGLOBIN HAMMERSMITH.

Substitution of serine for phenylalanine at beta 42. The normal phenylalanine at this site apparently 'stabilizes' the heme with which it is in contact. The substitution of serine leads to severe Heinz body hemolytic anemia.

Dacie, J. V., Shinton, N. K., Gaffney, P. J., Jr., Carrell, R. W. and Lehmann, H.: Haemoglobin Hammersmith (beta 42 (CD 1) phe to ser). Nature 216: 663-665, 1967.

—HEMOGLOBIN HASHARON.

Substitution of histidine for aspartic acid at alpha 47. Same as hemoglobin Sinai.

Charache, S., Mondzac, A. M. and Gessner, U.: Hemoglobin Hasharon (alpha-2 47 his(CD5)beta-2): a hemoglobin found in low concentration. J. Clin. Invest. 48: 834-847, 1969.

Halbrecht, I., Isaacs, W. A., Lehmann, H. and Ben-Porat, F.: Hemoglobin Hasharon (alpha 47 aspartic acid to histidine). Israel J. Med. Sci. 3: 827-831, 1967.

Ostertag, W. and Smith, E. W.: Hb Sinai, a new alpha chain mutant alpha his 47. Humangenetik 6: 377-379, 1968.

—HEMOGLOBIN HEATHROW.

Substitution of leucine for phenylalanine at beta 103.

White, J. M., Szur, L., Gillies, I. D. S., Lorkin, P. A. and Lehmann, H.: Familial polycythaemia caused by a new haemoglobin variant: Hb Heathrow, beta 103 (G5) phenylalanine to leucine. Brit. Med. J. 3: 665-667, 1973.

—HEMOGLOBIN HIJIYAMA.

Substitution of glutamic acid for lysine at beta 120.

Miyaji, T., Oba, Y., Yamamoto, K., Shibata, S., Iuchi, I. and Hamilton, H. B.: Hemoglobin Hijiyama: a new fast-moving hemoglobin in a Japanese family. Science 159: 204-206, 1968.

—HEMOGLOBIN HIKARI.

Substitution of asparagine for lysine at beta 61. Heterozygotes have about 60 per cent hemoglobin Hikari.

Shibata, S. and Iuchi, I.: Hemoglobin-Hikari (alpha-2-beta-2, T-7). A fast-moving hemoglobin demonstrated in two families of Japanese people, with a brief note on the abnormal hemoglobins of Japan which are likely to be confused with it. Proc. 9th Congr. Intern. Soc. Hematol., Mexico City, 1962. Pp. 65-70.

Shibata, S., Miyaji, T., Iuchi, I., Ueda, S. and Takeda, I.: Hemoglobin Hikari (alpha(2) A-B(2) 61 asp NH(2): a fast-moving hemoglobin found in two unrelated Japanese families. Clin. Chim. Acta 10: 101-105, 1964.

—-HEMOGLOBIN HIROSE.
Substitution of serine for tryptophan at beta 37.

Yanase, T., Hanada, M., Seita, M., Ohya, I., Ohta, Y., Imamura, T., Fujimura, T., Kawasaki, K. and Yamaoka, K.: Molecular basis of morbidity from a series of studies of hemoglobinopathies in western Japan. Jap. J. Hum. Genet. 13: 40-53, 1968.

—-HEMOGLOBIN HIROSHIMA.
Substitution of aspartic acid for histidine at beta 146 (formerly thought to be 143). Associated with increased oxygen affinity, decreased Bohr effect and erythremia.

Hamilton, H. B., Iuchi, I., Miyaji, T. and Shibata, S.: Hemoglobin Hiroshima (beta 143 histidine to aspartic acid): a newly identified fast moving beta chain variant associated with increased oxygen affinity and compensatory erythremia. J. Clin. Invest. 48: 525-535, 1969.

Perutz, M. F., Pulsinelli, P., Eyck, L. T., Kilmartin, J. V., Shibata, S., Miyaji, Y., Iuchi, I. and Hamilton, H. B.: Haemoglobin Hiroshima and the mechanism of the alkaline Bohr effect. Nature 232: 147-149, 1971.

—-HEMOGLOBIN HOFU.
Substitution of glutamic acid for valine at beta 126.

Miyaji, T., Ohba, Y., Yamamoto, K., Shibata, S., Iuchi, I. and Takenaka, M.: Japanese haemoglobin variant. Nature 217: 89-90, 1968.

—-HEMOGLOBIN HONOLULU.
Defect unknown.

Schneider, R. G. and Jim, R. T. S.: Haemoglobin: a new hemoglobin variant (the 'Honolulu type') in a Chinese. Nature 190: 454-455, 1961.

—-HEMOGLOBIN HOPE.
Substitution of aspartic for glycine at beta 136.

Minnich, V., Hill, R. J., Khuri, P. D. and Anderson, M. E.: Hemoglobin Hope: a beta chain variant. Blood 25: 830-838, 1965.

—-HEMOGLOBIN HOPKINS-1.
Substitution of glutamic acid for lysine at beta 95. Same as hemoglobin N (Baltimore).

Gottlieb, A. J., Robinson, E. A. and Itano, H. A.: Primary structure of Hopkins-1 haemoglobin-A. Nature 214: 189-190, 1967.

—-HEMOGLOBIN HOPKINS-2.
Substitution of aspartic acid for histidine at alpha 112. Fast hemoglobin.

Bradley, T. B., Jr., Boyer, S. H. and Allen, F. H., Jr.: Hopkins-2 hemoglobin: a revised pedigree with data on blood and serum groups. Bull. Hopkins Hosp. 108: 75-79, 1961.

Itano, H. A. and Robinson, E. A.: Genetic control of the alpha- and beta-chains of hemoglobin. Proc. Nat. Acad. Sci. 46: 1492-1501, 1960.

Ostertag, W.: Baltimore, Md.: personal communication, 1967.

Ostertag, W., Von Ehrenstein, G. and Charache, S.: Duplicated alpha-chain genes in Hopkins-2 haemoglobin of man and evidence for unequal crossing over between them. Nature 237: 90-94, 1972.

Smith, E. W. and Torbert, J. V.: Study of two abnormal hemoglobins with evidence for a new genetic locus for hemoglobin formation. Bull. Hopkins Hosp. 102: 38-45, 1958.

—-HEMOGLOBIN I.
Fast hemoglobin. Substitution of aspartic acid for lysine at alpha 16 was first reported by Murayama (1962). However, Crick pointed out that this substitution could not be accomplished by change in one base. Restudy by Beale and Lehmann (1965) and by Schneider et al. (1966) showed substitution of glutamic acid for lysine. Hemoglobin I was thought to show sickling but this has been shown to be due to faulty technique (Schneider et al., 1967).

Beale, D. and Lehmann, H.: Abnormal haemoglobins and the genetic code. Nature 207: 259-261, 1965.

Itano, H. A. and Robinson, E. A.: Formation of normal and double abnormal haemoglobins by recombination of haemoglobin I with S and C. Nature 183: 1799-1800, 1959.

Itano, H. A. and Robinson, E. A.: Genetic control of the alpha- and beta-chains of hemoglobin. Proc. Nat. Acad. Sci. 46: 1492-1501, 1960.

Labossiere, A. and Vella, F.: Hemoglobin I in a white family in Saskatoon. Clin. Biochem. 4: 104-113, 1971.

Murayama, M.: Chemical difference between normal human haemoglobin and haemoglobin-I. Nature 196: 276-277, 1962.

Rucknagel, D. L., Page, E. B. and Jensen, W. N.: Hemoglobin I: an inherited hemoglobin anomaly. Blood 10: 999-1009, 1955.

Schneider, R. G., Alperin, J. B. and Lehmann, H.: Sickling tests. Pitfalls in performance and interpretation. J.A.M.A. 202: 419-421, 1967.

Schneider, R. G., Alperin, J. B., Beale, D. and Lehmann, H.: Hemoglobin I in an American Negro family: structural and hematologic studies. J. Lab. Clin. Med. 68: 940-946, 1966.

Schwartz, I. R., Atwater, J., Repplinger, E. and Tocantins, L. M.: Sickling of erythrocytes with I-A electrophoretic haemoglobin pattern. Fed. Proc. 16: 115 only, 1957.

Thompson, R. B., Rau, P. J., Odom, J. and Bell, W. N.: The sickling phenomenon in a white male without Hb-S. Acta Haemat. 34: 347-353, 1965.

—HEMOGLOBIN I (BURLINGTON).
Alpha chain defect. Same as hemoglobin I.

O'Brien, C., Grey, M. J. and Jacobs, A. S.: A survey of cord bloods for abnormal hemoglobin, with further observations on hemoglobin I (Burlington). Am. J. Obstet. Gynec. 88: 816-822, 1964.

Ranney, H. M., O'Brien, C. and Jacobs, A. S.: An abnormal human foetal haemoglobin with an abnormal alpha-polypeptide chain. Nature 194: 743-745, 1962.

—HEMOGLOBIN I (HIGH WYCOMBE).
Substitution of glutamic acid for lysine at beta 59.

Boulton, F. E., Huntsman, R. G., Lehmann, H., Lorkin, P. and Romero-Herrera, A. E.: Myoglobin variants. (Abstract) Biochem. J. 118: 39P only, 1970.

—HEMOGLOBIN I (INTERLAKEN).
Substitution aspartic acid for glycine at alpha 15. Same as hemoglobin J (OXFORD).

Marti, H. R., Pik, C. and Mosimann, P.: Eine neue Haemoglobin I-Variante: Hb I (Interlaken). Acta Haemat. 32: 9-16, 1964.

—HEMOGLOBIN I (SKAMANIA).
Substitution of glutamic acid for lysine at alpha 16. Same as Hb I (Texas), etc.

Baur, E. W.: Hb alpha 2 glu beta 2(Hb I) in a Caucasian family: independent mutation or common origin? Humangenetik 6: 368-372, 1968.

—HEMOGLOBIN I (TEXAS).
Substitution of glutamic acid for lysine at alpha 16.

Bowman, B. H. and Barnett, D. R.: Amino-acid substitution in haemoglobin I (Texas variant). Nature 214: 499 only, 1967.

—HEMOGLOBIN I (TOULOUSE).
Substitution of glutamic acid for lysine at beta 66.

Rosa, J., Labie, D., Wajcman, H., Boigne, J. M., Cabannes, R., Bierme, R., Ruffie, J.: Hemoglobin I Toulouse: beta 66 (E10) lys to glu: a new abnormal hemoglobin with a mutation localized on the E10 porphyrin surrounding zone. Nature 223: 190-191, 1969.

—HEMOGLOBIN INDONESIA.
Substitution for aspartic acid for glycine at delta 136.

Eng, L. I., Pribadi, W., Westendorp-Boerma, F., Efremov, G. D., Wilson, J. B., Reynolds, C. A. and Huisman, T. H. J.: Hemoglobin A(2)-Indonesia or alpha(2) delta(2) 69(E13) gly-to-arg. Biochim. Biophys. Acta 229: 335-342, 1971.

—HEMOGLOBIN INKSTER.
Substitution of valine for aspartic acid at alpha 85.

Reed, R. E., Winter, W. P. and Rucknagel, D. L.: Haemoglobin Inkster (alpha 85 aspartic acid to valine) coexisting with beta-thalassaemia in a Caucasian family. Brit. J. Haemat. 26: 475-484, 1974.

—HEMOGLOBIN ISTANBUL.
Substitution of glutamine for histidine at beta 92. The patient was an apparent new mutation. The father was 41 years old, the mother 36, at his birth.

Aksoy, M., Erdem, S., Efremov, G. D., Wilson, J. B., Huisman, T. H. J., Schroeder, W. A., Shelton, J. R., Shelton, J. B., Ulitin, O. N. and Muftuoglu, A.: Hemoglobin Istanbul: substitution of glutamine for histidine in a proximal histidine (F8(92)beta). J. Clin. Invest. 51: 2380-2387, 1972.

—HEMOGLOBIN J (ABIDJAN).
Substitution of aspartic acid for glycine at alpha 51.

Cabannes, R., Renaud, R., Mauran, A., Pennors, H., Charlesworth, D., Price, B. G. and Lehmann, H.: Two fast haemoglobins in Ivory-Coast: Hb K Woolwich and a new haemoglobin Hb J Abidjan (alpha 51 gly to asp). Nouv. Rev. Franc. Hemat. 12: 289-300, 1972.

—HEMOGLOBIN J (BALTIMORE).
Substitution of aspartic acid for glycine at beta 16. Fast hemoglobin.

Weatherall, D. J.: Hemoglobin J (Baltimore) coexisting in a family with hemoglobin S-I. Bull Hopkins Hosp. 114: 1-12, 1964.

Wilkinson, T., Kronenberg, H., Isaacs, W. A. and Lehmann, H.: Haemoglobin J Baltimore interacting with beta-thalassaemia in an Australian family. Med. J. Aust. 1: 907-910, 1967.

—HEMOGLOBIN J (BANGKOK).
Substitution of aspartic acid for glycine at beta 56.

Clegg, J. B., Naughton, M. A. and Weatherall, D. J.: Abnormal human haemoglobins. Separation and characterization of the alpha and beta chains by chromatography, and the determination of two new variants, Hb Chesapeake and Hb J(Bangkok). J. Molec. Biol. 19: 91-108, 1966.

Pootrakul, S. N., Wasi, P. and Nakorn, S.: Haemoglobin J-Bangkok: a clinical, haematological and genetical study. Brit. J. Haemat. 13: 303-309, 1967.

—HEMOGLOBIN J(BIRMINGHAM).
Substitution of glutamic acid for alanine at alpha 120.

Kamuzora, H. and Lehmann, H.: A new hemoglobin variant. Hemoglobin J (Birmingham) alpha 120 (H3) ala-to-glu. Ann. Clin. Biochem. 11: 53-55, 1974.

—HEMOGLOBIN J (BROUSSAIS).
Substitution of asparagine for lysine at alpha 90.

Detraverse, P. M., Lehmann, H., Coquelet, M. L., Beale, D. and Isaacs, W. A.: Etude d'une hemoglobine J(alpha) non encore decrite, dans une famille Francaise. C. R. Soc. Biol. 160: 2270-2272, 1966.

—HEMOGLOBIN J (BUDA).
This and Hb G (Pest) occurred together in a Hungarian male with erythrocytosis. Both are alpha chain mutants and the occurrence of normal HB A in this man shows the existence of at least two alpha loci. Substitution of asparagine for lysine at alpha 61.

Brimhall, B., Duerst, M., Hollan, S. R., Stenzel, P., Szelenyi, J. and Jones, R. T.: Structural characterization of hemoglobins J-Buda (alpha 16 (E10) lys-to-asn) and G-Pest (alpha 74 (EF3) asp-to-asn). Biochim. Biophys. Acta 336: 344-360, 1974.

Hollan, S. R., Szelenyi, J. G., Brimhall, B., Duerst, M., Jones, R. T., Koler, R. D. and Stocklen, Z.: Multiple alpha chain loci for human haemoglobins: Hb J-Buda and Hb G-Pest. Nature 235: 47-50, 1972.

—HEMOGLOBIN J (CAMBRIDGE).
Substitution of aspartic acid for glycine at beta 69.

Sick, K., Beale, D., Irvine, D., Lehmann, H., Goodall, P. T. and MacDougall, S.: Hemoglobin G (Copenhagen) and hemoglobin J (Cambridge). Two new beta-chain variants of hemoglobin A. Biochim. Biophys. Acta 140: 231-242, 1967.

—HEMOGLOBIN J (CAPE TOWN).
Glutamine substitutes for arginine at alpha 92.

Botha, M. C., Beale, D., Issacs, W. A. and Lehmann, H.: Hemoglobin J Cape Town. Nature 212: 792-794, 1966.

—HEMOGLOBIN J (GEORGIA).
Beta chain anomaly. Fast hemoglobin.

Huisman, T. H. J. and Sydenstricker, V. P.: Haematology: difference in gross structure of two electrophoretically identical 'minor' hemoglobin components. Nature 193: 489-491, 1962.0767

Sydenstricker, V. P., Horton, B., Payne, R. A. and Huisman, T. H. J.: Studies on a fast hemoglobin variant found in a Negro family in association with thalassemia. Clin. Chim. Acta 6: 677-685, 1961.

—HEMOGLOBIN J(HABANA).
Substitution of glutamic acid for alanine at alpha 71.

Colombo, B., Vidal, H., Kamuzora, H. and Lehmann, H.: A new haemoglobin J-Habana-alpha 71 (E20) alanine-to-glutamic acid. Biochim. Biophys. Acta 351: 1-6, 1974.

—HEMOGLOBIN J (HONOLULU).
Substitution of threonine for lysine at beta 59. Same as hemoglobin J (Kaohsiung).

Blackwell, R. Q., Jim, R. T. S., Liu, C.-S., Weng, M.-I., Wang, C.-L. and Shih, T.-B.: Vox Sang. 22: 469-473, 1972.

—HEMOGLOBIN J (INDIA).
Alpha chain anomaly.

Lehmann, H.: Haemoglobins and haemoglobinopathies. In, H. Lehmann and K. Betke (eds.): 'Haemoglobin-Colloquium.' Stuttgart: Georg Thieme Verlag, 1962. Pp. 1-14.7

Raper, A. B.: Unusual haemoglobin variant in a Gujerati Indian. Brit. Med. J. 1: 1285-1286, 1957.

—HEMOGLOBIN J (IRAN).
Substitution of aspartic acid for histidine at beta 77.

Gammack, D. B., Huehns, E. R., Lehmann, H. and Shooter, E. M.: The abnormal polypeptide chains in a number of haemoglobin variants. Acta Genet. Statist. Med. 11: 1-16, 1961.

Rahbar, S., Beale, D., Isaacs, W. A. and Lehmann, H.: Abnormal haemoglobins in Iran. Observations of a new variant--haemoglobin J Iran (alpha 2 beta 2 his to asp). Brit. Med. J. 1: 674-677, 1967.

—HEMOGLOBIN J (IRELAND).
Same as hemoglobin J (Baltimore).

Went, L. N. and MacIver, J. E.: Sickle-cell haemoglobin-J disease. Brit. Med. J. 2: 138-139, 1959.

—HEMOGLOBIN J (JAMAICA).
Beta chain anomaly.

Gammack, D. B., Huehns, E. R., Lehmann, H. and Shooter, E. M.: The abnormal polypeptide chains in a number of haemoglobin variants. Acta Genet. Statist. Med. 11: 1-16, 1961.

—HEMOGLOBIN J (KAOHSIUNG).
Substitution of threonine for lysine at beta 59.

Blackwell, R. Q., Liu, C. S. and Shih, T. B.: Hemoglobin J Kaohsiung: beta 59 lys to thr. Biochim. Biophys. Acta 229: 343-348, 1971.

—HEMOGLOBIN J (KORAT).
Substitution of aspartic acid for glycine at beta 56.

Blackwell, R. Q. and Liu, C. S.: The identical structural anomalies of hemoglobin J(Meinung) and J(Korat). Biochem. Biophys. Res. Commun. 24: 732-738, 1966.

—HEMOGLOBIN J (MALAYA).
Alpha chain anomaly.

Lehmann, H.: Haemoglobins and haemoglobinopathies. In, H. Lehmann and K. Betke (eds.): 'Haemoglobin-Colloquium.' Stuttgart: Georg Thieme Verlag, 1962. Pp. 1-14.

—HEMOGLOBIN J (MANADO).
Substitution of aspartic acid for glycine at beta 56. Same as hemoglobin J (Meinung), Hemoglobin J (Korat) and Hb J (Bangkok).

Blackwell, R. Q., Liu, C. S., Eng, L. I. L. and Pribadi, W.: Fast hemoglobin variant in Minahassan people of Sulawesi, Chinese and Thais: alpha(2)beta(2) 56 gly-to-asp. Am. J. Phys. Anthrop. 32: 147-150, 1970.

—HEMOGLOBIN J (MEDELLIN).
Substitution of aspartic acid for glycine at alpha 22.

Gottlieb, A. J., Restrepo, A. and Itano, H. A.: Hb J (Medellin). Chemical and genetic study. Fed. Proc. 23: 172 only, 1964.

—HEMOGLOBIN J (MEERUT).
Substitution of glutamic acid for alanine at alpha 120.

Blackwell, R. Q., Wong, H. B., Wang, C.-L., Weng, M.-I. and Liu, C.-S.: Hemoglobin J-Meerut: alpha 120 ala-to-glu. Biochim. Biophys. Acta 351: 7-12, 1974.

—HEMOGLOBIN J (MEINUNG).
Substitution of aspartic acid for glycine at beta 56.

Blackwell, R. Q. and Liu, C. S.: The identical structural anomalies of hemoglobin J (Meinung) and J (Korat). Biochem. Biophys. Res. Commun. 24: 732-738, 1966.

—HEMOGLOBIN J (NYANZA).
Substitution of aspartic acid for alanine at beta 21.

Kendall, A. G., Barr, R. D., Lang, A. and Lehmann, H.: Biochim. Biophys. Acta 310: 357-359, 1973.

—HEMOGLOBIN J (OXFORD).
Substitution of aspartic acid for glycine at alpha 15. Same as hemoglobin I (Interlaken).

Liddell, J., Brown, D., Beale, D., Lehmann, H. and Huntsman, R. G.: A new haemoglobin J(alpha)-Oxford, found during a survey of an English population. Nature 204: 269-270, 1964.

—HEMOGLOBIN J (PARIS-1).
Substitution of aspartic acid for alanine at alpha 12.

Rosa, J., Maleknia, N., Vergos, D. and Dunet, R.: Une nouvelle hemoglobine anormale: l'hemoglobine J(alpha-Paris) 12 ala a asp. Nouv. Rev. Franc. Hemat. 6: 423-426, 1966.

Trincao, C., Demelo, J. M., Lorkin, P. A. and Lehmann, H.: Haemoglobin J Paris in the south of Portugal (Algarve). Acta Haemat. 39: 291-298, 1968.

—HEMOGLOBIN J (PARIS-2).
Substitution of glutamic acid for glutamine at alpah 54. Identical to hemoglobin Mexico.

Labie, D. and Rosa, J.: Sur une nouvelle hemoglobine anormale: l'hemoglobine J (alpha-54 glutamine a glutamique). Nouv. Rev. Franc. Hemat. 6: 426-430, 1966.

—HEMOGLOBIN J (RAMBAM).
Substitution of aspartic acid for glycine at beta 69.

Salomon, H., Tatarski, I., Dance, N., Huehns, E. R. and Shooter, E. M.: A new hemoglobin variant found in a Bedouin tribe: hemoglobin 'Rambam.' Israel J. Med. Sci. 1: 836-840, 1965.

—HEMOGLOBIN J (ROVIGO).
Substitution of aspartic acid for alanine at alpha 53.

Alberti, R., Mariuzzi, G. M., Artibani, L., Bruni, E. and Tentori, L.: A new haemoglobin variant: J-Rovigo alpha 53 (E-2) alanine to aspartic acid. Biochim. Biophys. Acta 342: 1-4, 2974.

—HEMOGLOBIN J (SARDEGNA).
Substitution of aspartic acid for histidine at alpha 50.

Tangheroni, W., Zorcolo, G., Gallo, E. and Lehmann, H.: Haemoglobin J (Sardegna): alpha 50(CD8) histidine--aspartic acid. Nature 218: 470-471, 1968.

—HEMOGLOBIN J (SINGAPORE).
Substitution of asparatic acid for asparagine at alpha 78 and glycine for alanine at alpha 79. Since no simple frame shift mechanism could be imagined, the possibliity of two separate mutations was favored by Blackwell et al. (1972), who suggested that two separate hemoglobins appropriately called Hb J (Singa) and Hb J (Pore) will be discovered eventually. Double mutation on the same chromosome would seem more likely than crossing-over in a compound heterozygote since the two codons involved are contiguous.

Blackwell, R. Q., Boon, W. H., Liu, C. S. and Weng, M. T.: Hemoglobin J Singapore: alpha - 78 asn to asp; alpha - 79 ala to gly. Biochim. Biophys. Acta 278: 482-490, 1972.

—HEMOGLOBIN J (TONGARIKI).
Substitution of aspartic acid for alanine at alpha 115. A homozygous individual had only anomalous hemoglobin suggesting the existence of only one alpha locus in Melanesians.

Abramson, R. K., Rucknagel, D. L., Shreffler, D. C. and Saave, J. J.: Homozygous Hb J Tongariki: evidence for only one alpha chain structural locus in Melanesians. Science 169: 194-196, 1970.

Beaven, G. H., Hornabrook, R. W., Fox, R. H. and Huehns, E. R.: Occurrence of heterozygotes and homozygotes for the alpha-chain haemoglobin variant Hb-J (Tongariki) in New Guinea. Nature 235: 46-47, 1972.

Gajdusek, D. C., Guiart, J., Kirk, R. L., Carrell, R. W., Irvine, D., Kynoch, P. A. M. and Lehmann, H.: Haemoglobin J Tongariki (alpha 115 alanine to aspartic acid): the first new haemoglobin variant found in a Pacific (Melanesian) population. J. Med. Genet. 4: 1-6, 1967.

—HEMOGLOBIN J (TORONTO).
Substitution of aspartic acid for alanine at alpha 5.

Crookston, J. H., Beale, D., Irvine, D. and Lehmann, H.: A new haemoglobin, J Toronto (alpha-5 alanine to aspartic acid). Nature 208: 1059-1060, 1965.

—HEMOGLOBIN J (TRINIDAD).
Substitution of glycine for aspartic acid at beta 16. Same as hemoglobin J (Baltimore).

Gammack, D. B., Huehns, E. R., Lehmann, H. and Shooter, E. M.: The abnormal polypeptide chains in a number of haemoglobin variants. Acta Genet. Statist. Med. 11: 1-16, 1961.

—HEMOGLOBIN K.
Beta chain anomaly.

O'Gorman, P., Lehmann, H., Allsopp, K. M. and Sukumaran, P. K.: Sickle cell haemoglobin K disease. Brit. Med. J. 2: 1381-1382, 1963.

—HEMOGLOBIN K (CALCUTTA).
Alpha chain anomaly. Fast hemoglobin.

Lehmann, H.: Haemoglobins and haemoglobinopathies. In, H. Lehmann and K. Betke (eds.): 'Haemoglobin-Colloquium.' Stuttgart: Georg Thieme Verlag, 1962. Pp. 1-14.67

—HEMOGLOBIN K (IBADAN).
Substitution of glutamic acid for glycine at beta 46. For reference see HEMOGLOBIN K (WOOLWICH).

—HEMOGLOBIN K (MADRAS).
Alpha chain anomaly.

Ager, J. A. M. and Lehmann, H.: Haemoglobin K in an East Indian and his family. Brit. Med. J. 1: 1449-1450, 1957.

—HEMOGLOBIN K (WOOLWICH).
Substitution of glutamine for lysine at beta 132.

Allan, N., Beale, D., Irvine, D. and Lehmann, H.: Three haemoglobins K: Woolwich, an abnormal, Cameroon and Ibadan, two unusual variants of human haemoglobin A. Nature 208: 658-661, 1965.

Ringelhann, B., Konotey-Ahulu, F. I. D., Talapatra, N. C., Nkrumah, F. K., Wiltshire, B. G. and Lehmann, H.: Haemoglobin K Woolwich (alpha 2 beta 2 132 lysine to glutamine) in Ghana. Acta Haemat. 45: 250-258, 1971.

—HEMOGLOBIN KAGOSHIMA.
Same as hemoglobin Norfolk.

Imamura, T.: Hemoglobin Kagoshima: an example of hemoglobin Norfolk in a Japanese family. Am. J. Hum. Genet. 18: 584-593, 1966.

Also known as hemoglobin Reissmann (q.v.). Substitution of threonine for aspartic acid at beta 102.

> Bonaventura, J. and Riggs, A.: Hemoglobin Kansas, a human hemoglobin with a neutral amino acid substitution and an abnormal oxygen equilibrium. J. Biol. Chem. 243: 980-991, 1968.

—HEMOGLOBIN KARAMOJO.
Alpha chain variant.

> Allbrook, D., Barnicot, N. A., Dance, N., Lawler, S. D., Marshall, R. and Mungai, J.: Blood groups, haemoglobin and serum factors of the Karamojo. Hum. Biol. 37: 217-237, 1965.

—HEMOGLOBIN KEMPSEY.
Substitution of asparagine for aspartic acid at beta 99.

> Reed, C. S., Hampson, R., Gordon, S., Jones, R. T., Novy, M. J., Brimhall, B., Edwards, M. J. and Koler, R. D.: Erythrocytosis secondary to increased oxygen affinity of a mutant hemoglobin, hemoglobin Kempsey. Blood 31: 623-632, 1968.

—HEMOGLOBIN KENWOOD.
Substitution of glutamic acid for lysine at beta 95. Identical to Hb N (Baltimore). This was previously reported incorrectly as having either aspartic acid or glutamic acid at beta 143. See personal communication from Heller in Hamilton et al. (1969).

—HEMOGLOBIN KENYA.
Huisman (1972) described a new hemoglobin in a healthy Kenyan male. The man was thought to have Hb S in combination with hereditary persistance of fetal hemoglobin. The abnormal hemoglobin was found to have a non-alpha chain with characteristics of the gamma chain at the NH2 end and of beta chain at the COOH end. The normal Hb F contained only gamma-G chains. From further studies of the family, Kendall et al. (1973) concluded that the order of linked genes is gamma-G-gamma-A, delta, and beta. Crossing-over occurred between residues 81 and 86 of the gamma and beta chains.

> Huisman, T. H. J., Schroeder, W. A. and Kendall, A. G.,: Hemoglobin Kenya, the product of nonhomologous crossing over of gamma and beta genes. (Abstract) Am. Soc. Hemat., Hollywood, Fla., Dec. 3-6, 1972.

> Kendall, A. G., Ojwang, P. J., Schroeder, W. A. and Huisman, T. H. J.: Hemoglobin Kenya, the product of a gamma-beta fusion gene: studies of the family. Am. J. Hum. Genet. 25: 548-563, 1973.

—HEMOGLOBIN KHARTOUM.
Substitution of arginine for proline at beta 124.

> Clegg, J. B., Weatherall, D. J., Boon, W. H. and Mustafa, D.: Two new haemoglobin variants involving proline substitutions. Nature 222: 379-380, 1969.

—HEMOGLOBIN KINGS COUNTY.
Probably beta chain defect. Observed in an American Negro family. Affected persons had nonspherocytic hemolytic Heinz body anemia.

> Sathiapalan, R. and Robinson, M. G.: Hereditary haemolytic anaemia due to an abnormal haemoglobin (haemoglobin Kings County). Brit. J. Haemat. 15: 579-587, 1968.

—HEMOGLOBIN KNOXVILLE-1.
Same as G (Philadelphia).

—HEMOGLOBIN KOELLIKER.
Not a genetic change. The C-terminal amino acid, no. 141, of the alpha chain (arginine) is missing, probably from the action of a carboxypeptidase present in normal palsma. This unusual fast hemoglobin is observed in persons with hemolysis.

> Marti, H. R., Beale, D. and Lehmann, H.: Haemoglobin Koelliker: a new acquired haemoglobin appearing after severe haemolysis: alpha-2 (minus 141 arg) beta-2. Acta Haemat. 37: 174-180, 1967.

—HEMOGLOBIN KOKURA.
Substitution of glycine for aspartic acid at alpha 47.

> Ooya, I., Kawamura, K., Seita, M., Hanada, M. and Hitsumoto, A.: Hemoglobin Kokura which was discovered in Kokura. 23rd Gen. Meeting Japan. Soc. Hematol. Kyoto, 1961.

> Yamaoka, K., Kawamura, K., Hanada, M., Seita, M., Hitsumoto, S. and Ooya, I.: Studies on abnormal haemoglobins. Jap. J. Hum. Genet. 5: 99-111, 1960.

—HEMOGLOBIN KOLN.
Substitution of methionine for valine at beta 98.

> Carrell, R. W., Lehmann, H. and Hutchison, H. E.: Haemoglobin Koln (beta-98 valine to methionine): an unstable protein causing inclusion body anaemia. Nature 210: 915-917, 1966.

> Eng, L. I.-L., Lopez, C. G., Eapen, J. S., Eravelly, J., Wiltshire, B. G. and Lehmann, H.: Unstable haemoglobin Koln disease in members of a Malay family. J. Med. Genet. 9: 340-343, 1972.

> Hutchison, H. E., Pinkerton, P. H., Waters, P., Douglas, A. S., Lehmann, H. and Beale, D.: Hereditary Heinz-body anaemia, thrombocytopenia, and haemoglobinopathy (Hb Koln) in a Glasgow family. Brit. Med. J. 2: 1099-1103, 1964.

Jackson, J. M., Way, B. J. and Woodliff, H. J.: A west Australian family with a haemolytic disorder associated with haemoglobin Koln. Brit. J. Haemat. 13: 474-481, 1967.

Jones, R. V., Grimes, A. J., Carrell, R. W. and Lehmann, H.: Koln haemoglobinopathy: further data and a comparison with other hereditary Heinz body anaemias. Brit. J. Haemat. 13: 394-408, 1967.

Miller, D. R., Weed, R. I., Stamatoyannopoulos, G. and Yoshida, A.: Hemoglobin Koln disease occurring as a fresh mutation: erythrocyte metabolism and survival. Blood 38: 715-729, 1971.

Pribilla, W.: Thalassemie-aehnliche Erkrankung mit neuem minor-Hb (Hb Koln). In, H. Lehmann and K. Betke (eds.): 'Haemoglobin-Colloquium.' Stuttgart: Georg Thieme Verlag, 1962. Pp. 1-14.

Pribilla, W., Klesse, P., Betke, K., Lehmann, H. and Beale, D.: Haemoglobin Koln disease: familial hypochromic hemolytic anemia with hemoglobin anomaly. Klin. Wschr. 43: 1049-1053, 1965.

—-HEMOGLOBIN KORLE-BU.
Substitution of asparagine for aspartic acid at beta 73. Since this same substitution is present, with the sickle hemoglobin change, as one of the two defects in hemoglobin C(Harlem), Konotey-Ahulu et al. (1968) suggested that the latter hemoglobin may have arisen by intracistronic crossing over in an individual with the Korly-Bu gene on one chromosome and the sickle gene on the other.

Konotey-Ahulu, F. I. D., Gallo, E., Lehmann, H. and Ringelhann, B.: Haemoglobin Korle-Bu (beta 73 aspartic acid to asparagine) showing one of the two amino acid substitutions of haemoglobin C Harlem. J. Med. Genet. 5: 107-111, 1968.

—-HEMOGLOBIN KOYA DORA.
Excessive length of alpha-like chain (with 155 or 156 amino acids rather than 141).

De Jong, W. W. W.: Leiden, personal communication, 1970.

—-HEMOGLOBIN L.
Beta chain anomaly.

Ager, J. A. M. and Lehmann, H.: Haemoglobin L: a new haemoglobin found in a Punjabi Hindu. Brit. Med. J. 2: 142-143, 1957.

Gammack, D. B., Huehns, E. R., Lehmann, H. and Shooter, E. M.: The abnormal polypeptide chains in a number of haemoglobin variants. Acta Genet. Statist. Med. 11: 1-16, 1961.

—-HEMOGLOBIN L (BOMBAY).
Alpha chain anomaly.

Sukumaran, P. K. and Pik, C.: Some observations on haemoglobin L(Bombay). Biochim. Biophys. Acta 104: 290-292, 1965.

—-HEMOGLOBIN L (FERRARA).
Substitution of glycine for aspartic acid at alpha 47. Same as hemoglobin Kokura. Same as hemoglobin Beilinson.

Nagel, R. L., Ranney, H. M., Bradley, T. B., Jacobs, A. and Udem, L.: Hemoglobin L Ferrara in a Jewish family associated with a hemolytic state in the propositus. Blood 34: 157-165, 1969.

Silvestroni, E., Bianco, I., Lucci, R. and Soffritti, E.: Presence of hemoglobin 'L' in natives of Ferrara and of hemoglobin 'D' in natives of Bologna. Acta Genet. Med. Gem. 9: 472-496, 1960.

Silvestroni, E., Bianco, I., Lucci, R. and Soffritti, E.: The hematological picture in carriers of Hb L, living in Ferrara. Associations and relations to microcythenia. Progr. Med. 16: 553-561, 1960.

—-HEMOGLOBIN L (PERSIAN GULF).
Substitution of arginine for glycine at alpha 57.

Rahbar, S., Kinderlerer, J. L. and Lehmann, H.: Haemoglobin L Persian Gulf: alpha 57 (E6) glycine leads to arginine. Acta Haemat. 42: 169-175, 1969.

—-HEMOGLOBIN LEIDEN.
Deletion of glutamic acid 6 or 7 in the beta chain.

De Jong, W. W. W., Went, L. N. and Bernini, L. F.: Abnormal haemoglobin — chemical characterization of hemoglobin Leiden. Nature 220: 788-789, 1968.

—-HEMOGLOBIN LEPORE.
Beta-delta fusion.

Baglioni, C. and Ventruto, V.: Human abnormal hemoglobins. II. A chemical study of hemoglobin Lepore from a homozygote individual. Europ. J. Biochem. 5: 29-32, 1968.

Gerald, P. S. and Diamond, L. K.: A new hereditary hemoglobinopathy (the Lepore trait) and its interaction with thalassemia trait. Blood 12: 835-844, 1958.

Huisman, T. H. J. and Sydenstricker, V. P.: Haemoglobin: difference in gross structure of two electrophoretically identical minor haemoglobin components. Nature 193: 489-491, 1962.

—-HEMOGLOBIN LEPORE (AUGUSTA).
Same as hemoglobin Lepore (Washington).

Labie, D., Schroeder, W. A. and Huisman, T. H. J.: The amino acid sequence of the delta-beta chains of hemoglobin Lepore (Augusta) — hemoglobin Lepore (Washington). Biochim. Biophys. Acta 127: 428-437, 1966.

—HEMOGLOBIN LEPORE (BALTIMORE). 157
Beta-delta fusion.

Ostertag, W. and Smith, E. W.: Hemoglobin-Lepore-Baltimore, a third type of a delta, beta crossover (delta 50, beta 86). Europ. J. Biochem. 10: 371-376, 1969.

—HEMOGLOBIN LEPORE (BOSTON).
Beta-delta fusion. Same as hemoglobin Pylos.

Baglioni, C.: The fusion of two peptide chains in hemoglobin Lepore and its interpretation as a genetic deletion. Proc. Nat. Acad. Sci. 48: 1880-1886, 1962.

—HEMOGLOBIN LEPORE (CYPRUS).
Beta-delta fusion.

Beaven, G. H., Gratzer, W. B., Stevens, B. L., Shooter, E. M., Ellis, M. J., White, J. C. and Gillespie, J. E. O.: An abnormal haemoglobin (Lepore-Cyprus) resembling haemoglobin Lepore and its interaction with thalassaemia. Brit. J. Haemat. 10: 159-170, 1964.

—HEMOGLOBIN LEPORE (HOLLANDIA).
Beta-delta fusion. Several hemoglobins Lepore have been shown to differ in the position of the cross-over between the delta and beta chains (Curtain, 1964).

Baglioni, C.: The fusion of two peptide chains in hemoglobin Lepore and its interpretation as a genetic deletion. Proc. Nat. Acad. Sci. 48: 1880-1886, 1962.

Barnabas, J. and Muller, C. J.: Haemoglobin Lepore (Hollandia). Nature 194: 931-932, 1962.

Barnabas, J. and Muller, C. J.: Haemoglobin Lepore (Hollandia). Nature 194: 931-932, 1962.6 Curtain, C. C.: A structural study of abnormal haemoglobins occurring in New Guinea. Aust. J. Exp. Biol. 42: 89-97, 1964.

Neeb, H., Beiboer, J. L., Jonxis, J. H., Kaars-Sijpesteijn, J. A. and Muller, C. J.: Homozygous Lepore haemoglobin disease appearing as thalassaemia major in two Papuan siblings. Trop. Geograph. Med. 13: 207-215, 1961.

Sijpesteijn, J. A. K. and Muller, C. J.: Homozygous Lepore haemoglobin disease appearing as thalassaemia major in two Papuan siblings. Trop. Geograph. Med. 13: 207, 1961.

—HEMOGLOBIN LEPORE (THE BRONX).
Beta-delta fusion.

Ranney, H. M. and Jacobs, A. S.: Simultaneous occurrence of haemoglobins C and Lepore in an Afro-American. Nature 204: 163-166, 1964.

—HEMOGLOBIN LEPORE (WASHINGTON).
Beta-delta fusion. Different hemoglobins Lepore show evidence that the cross-over occurred at different sites: e.g., Hb Lepore (Washington) has the shift-over somewhere between amino acids at 87 and 116 (Labie et al., 1966). (It is impossible to position it more precisely because the delta and beta chains are identical between these residues. Hb Lepore (Hollandia) has the shift-over between positions 22 and 50 (Curtain, 1964).

Ahern, E. J., Ahern, V. N., Aarons, G. H., Jones, R. T. and Brimhall, B.: Hemoglobin Lepore Washington in two Jamaican families: interaction with beta chain variants. Blood 40: 246-256, 1972.

Curtain, C. C.: A structural study of abnormal haemoglobins occurring in New Guinea. Aust. J. Exp. Biol. Med. Sci. 42: 89-97, 1964.

Labie, D., Schroeder, W. A., and Huisman, T. H. J.: The amino acid sequence of the delta-beta chains of haemoglobin Lepore Augusta = Lepore Washington. Biochim. Biophys. Acta 127: 428-437, 1966.

—HEMOGLOBIN LITTLE ROCK.
Substitution of glutamine for histidine at beta 143. Heterozygotes have marked erythrocytosis as in the case of Hb Chesapeake, J (Capetown), Malmo, Rainier, Bethesda, Yakima, Kempsey, and Hiroshima.

Bromberg, P. A., Alben, J. O., Bare, G. H., Balcerzak, S. P., Jones, R. T., Brimhall, B. and Padilla, F.: High oxygen affinity variant of haemoglobin Little Rock with unique properties. Nature N. B. 243: 177-179, 1973.

—HEMOGLOBIN LOUISVILLE.
Substitution of leucine for phenylalanine at beta 42. This hemoglobin shows decreased stability on warming to 65 degrees C. and an increased tendency to dissociate in the presence of sulfhydryl group-blocking agents. Clinically it results in mild hemolytic anemia.

Keeling, M. M., Ogden, L. L., Wrightstone, R. N., Wilson, J. B., Reynolds, C. A., Kitchens, J. L. and Huisman, T. H. J.: Hemoglobin Louisville (beta 42(CD1)phe to leu): an unstable variant causing mild hemolytic anemia. J. Clin. Invest. 50: 2395-2402, 1971.

—HEMOGLOBIN M.
As outlined below, several aberrant hemoglobins associated with methemoglobinemia have been identified. All are referred to as hemoglobin M. Some have alpha chain substitutions and some have beta chain substitutions. In all, the substitution is at a position critical to the globin-heme interrelationship. All move more slowly than hemoglobin A in alkaline electrophoresis.

—HEMOGLOBIN M (AKITA).
Substitution of tyrosine for histidine at beta 92.

Shibata, S., Miyaji, T., Iuchi, I., Ohba, Y. and Yamamoto, K.: Amino acid substitution in hemoglobin M (Akita). J. Biochem. 63: 193-198, 1968.

—HEMOGLOBIN M (BOSTON).
Same as M (Gothenburg), M (Osaka) and perhaps M (Leipzig-2). Substitution of tyrosine for histidine at alpha 58. Most the hemoglobins M have substitutions of the histidine at alpha 53, alpha 87, beta 63 or beta 92. These four amino acids are critical to the binding of the heme group. The exception is hemoglobin M (Milwaukee-1).

Betke, K.: Haemoglobin-M: Typen und ihre Differenzierung (Uebersicht). In, H. Lehmann and K. Betke (eds.): 'Haemoglobin-Colloquium.' Stuttgart: Georg Thieme Verlag, 1962. Pp. 39-47.

Gerald, P. S. and Efron, M. L.: Chemical studies of several varieties of Hb M. Proc. Nat. Acad. Sci. 47: 1758-1767, 1961.

Gerald, P. S., Cook, C. D. and Diamond, L. K.: Hemoglobin M. Science 126: 300-301, 1957.

Hansen, H. A., Jagenburg, O. R. and Johansson, B. G.: Studies on an abnormal hemoglobin causing hereditary congenital cyanosis. Acta Paediat. 49: 503-511, 1960.

Pulsinelli, P. D., Perutz, M. F. and Nagel, R. L.: Structure of hemoglobin M (Boston), a variant with a five-coordinated ferric heme. Proc. Nat. Acad. Sci. 70: 3870-3874, 1973.

—HEMOGLOBIN M (CHICAGO).
Same as hemoglobin M (Saskatoon).

Heller, P.: Hemoglobin M (Chicago) and M (Kankakee). In, H. Lehmann and K. Betke (eds.): 'Haemoglobin-Colloquium.' Stuttgart: Georg Thieme Verlag, 1962. Pp. 47-49.

Josephson, A. M., Weinstein, H. G., Yakulis, V. J., Singer, L. and Heller, P.: A new variant of hemoglobin M disease. Hemoglobin M (Chicago). J. Lab. Clin. Med. 59: 918-925, 1962.

—HEMOGLOBIN M (FREIBURG).
See HEMOGLOBIN FREIBURG.

—HEMOGLOBIN M (HAMBURG).
Same as M (Saskatoon).

Betke, K., Kleihauer, E., Gehring-Muller, R., Braunitzer, G., Jacobi, J. and Schmidt, D.: Hb M Hamburg, eine beta-Ketten-Anomalie: alpha-2 beta-2 (63 tyr). Klin. Wschr. 44: 961-966, 1966.

—HEMOGLOBIN M (HITA).
Same as hemoglobin M (Saskatoon).

Hanada et al.,: For reference see HEMOGLOBIN TAGAWA II.

—HEMOGLOBIN M (HYDE PARK).
Substitution of tyrosine for histidine at beta 92. Same as hemoglobin M (Milwaukee-2).

Heller, P., Coleman, R. D. and Yakulis, V.: Hemoglobin M: a new variant of abnormal methemoglobin in a Negro. (Abstract) Proc. Third Intern. Cong. Hum. Genet. (Chicago, Sept. 5-10), 1966. (Also J. Clin. Invest. 45: 1021 only, 1966.)

—HEMOGLOBIN M (IWATE).
Substitution of tyrosine for histidine at alpha 87.

Gerald, P. S. and Efron, M. L.: Chemical studies of several varieties of Hb M. Proc. Nat. Acad. Sci. 47: 1758-1767, 1961.

Meyering, C. A., Israels, A. L., Sebens, T. and Huisman, T. H.: Studies on the heterogeneity of hemoglobin. II. The heterogeneity of different human hemoglobin types in carboxymethylcellulose and in amberlite irc-50 chromatography. Quantitative aspects. Clin. Chim. Acta 5: 208-222, 1960.

Miyaji, T., Ueda, S., Shibata, S., Tamura, A. and Sasaki, H.: Further studies on the fingerprint of Hb M (Iwate). Acta Haemat. Jap. 25: 169-175, 1962.

Shibata, S.: Hereditary nigremia (geneticobiochemical aspects). Jap. J. Hum. Genet. 9: 193-206, 1964.

Shibata, S., Iuchi, I., Miyaji, T. and Ueda, S.: Spectroscopic characterization of hemoglobin M (Iwate) and hemoglobin M (Kurume), the two variants of hemoglobin M found in Japan. Acta Haemat. Jap. 24: 477-485 and 486-494, 1961.

Shibata, S., Tamura, A., Iuchi, I. and Takahashi, H.: Hemoglobin M-1. Demonstration of a new abnormal hemoglobin in hereditary nigremia. Acta Haemat. Jap. 23: 96-104, 1960.

Shimizu, A., Tsugita, A., Hayashi, A. and Yamamura, Y.: The primary structure of hemoglobin M (Iwate). Biochim. Biophys. Acta 107: 270-277, 1965.

Tamura, A.: Black blood disease. Jap. J. Hum. Genet. 9: 183-192, 1964.

—HEMOGLOBIN M (KANKAKEE).
Same as hemoglobin M (Iwate).

Heller, P.: Hemoglobin M (Chicago) and M (Kankakee). In, H. Lehmann and K. Betke (eds.): 'Haemoglobin-Colloquium.' Stuttgart: Georg Thieme Verlag, 1962. Pp. 47-49.R

Heller, P., Weinstein, H. G., Yakulis, V. J. and Rosenthal, I. M.: Hemoglobin M (Kankakee), a new variant of hemoglobin M. Blood 20: 287-301, 1962.

Substitution of threonine for asparagine at beta 102.

Reissman, K. R., Ruth, W. E. and Nomura, T.: A human hemoglobin with lowered oxygen affinity and impaired heme-heme interactions. J. Clin. Invest. 40: 1826-1833, 1961.

—HEMOGLOBIN M (LEIPZIG-1).
Chain anomaly unknown.

Betke, K., Groschner, E. and Bock, K.: Properties of a further variant of hemoglobin M. Nature 188: 864-865, 1960.

—HEMOGLOBIN M (MILWAUKEE-1).
Substitution of glutamic acid for valine at beta 67. This is now usually called simply Hb M (Milwaukee) since Hb M (Milwaukee-2) has been shown to be the same as Hb M (Hyde Park).

Gerald, P. S. and Efron, M. L.: Chemical studies of several varieties of Hb M. Proc. Nat. Acad. Sci. 47: 1758-1767, 1961.

Hayashi, A., Suzuki, T., Imai, K., Morimoto, H. and Watari, H.: Properties of hemoglobin M, Milwaukee-1 variant and its unique characteristic. Biochim. Biophys. Acta 194: 6-15, 1969.

Perutz, M. F., Pulsinelli, P. D. and Ranney, H. M.: Structure and subunit interaction of haemoglobin M Milwaukee. Nature N. B. 237: 259-263, 1972.

Pisciotta, A. V., Ebre, S. N. and Hinz, J. E.: Clinical and laboratory features of two variants of methemoglobin-M disease. J. Lab. Clin. Med. 54: 73-87, 1959.

—HEMOGLOBIN M (MILWAUKEE-2).
Same as hemoglobin M (Hyde Park).

Pisciotta, A. V., Ebre, S. N. and Hinz, J. E.: Clinical and laboratory features of two variants of methemoglobin-M disease. J. Lab. Clin. Med. 54: 73-87, 1959.

—HEMOGLOBIN M (OLDENBURG).
Probably substitution of histidine by tyrosine at alpha 87 and thus same as hemoglobin M (Iwate) and hemoglobin M (Kankakee).

Pik, C. and Tonz, O.: Nature of haemoglobin M (Oldenburg). Nature 210: 1182 only, 1966.

Tonz, O., Simon, H. A. and Hasselfeld, W.: Untersuchung einer grossen Haemoglobin-M-Sippe. Entdeckung eines neuen Blutfarbstoffes: Hb M-Oldenburg. Schweiz. Med. Wschr. 92: 1311-1313, 1962.

—HEMOGLOBIN M (OSAKA).
Substitution of tyrosine for histidine at alpha 58.

Hayashi, A., Yamamura, Y., Ogita, S. and Kikkawa, H.: Hemoglobin M (Osaka), a new variant of hemoglobin M. Jap. J. Hum. Genet. 9: 87-94, 1964.

Shimizu, A., Hayashi, A., Yamamura, Y., Tsugita, A. and Kitayama, K.: The structural study on a new hemoglobin variant, Hb M (Osaka). Biochim. Biophys. Acta 97: 472-482, 1965.

Suzuki, T., Hayashi, A., Yamamura, Y., Enoki, Y. and Tyuma, I.: Functional abnormality of hemoglobin M (Osaka). Biochem. Biophys. Res. Commun. 19: 691-695, 1965.

—HEMOGLOBIN M (RADOM).
Same as hemoglobin M (Saskatoon).

Murawski, K., Carta, S., Sorcini, M., Tentori, L., Vivaldi, G., Antonine, E., Brunori, M., Wyman, J., Bucci, E. and Rossi-Fanelli, A.: Observations on the structure and behavior of hemoglobin M (Radom). Arch. Biochem. 111: 197-201, 1965.

—HEMOGLOBIN M (RESERVE).
An alpha chain substitution. Reduced oxygen affinity and decreased reversible oxygen-binding capacity.

Overly, W. L., Rosenberg, A. and Harris, J. W.: Hemoglobin M (Reserve): studies on identification and characterization. J. Lab. Clin. Med. 69: 62-87, 1967.

—HEMOGLOBIN M (SASKATOON).
Same as M (Emory), M (Radom) and possibly M (Kurume) and M (H-W). Substitution of tyrosine for histidine at beta 63.

Gerald, P. S. and Efron, M. L.: Chemical studies of several varieties of Hb M. Proc. Nat. Acad. Sci. 47: 1758-1767, 1961.

Gerald, P. S. and George, P.: Second spectroscopically abnormal methemoglobin associated with hereditary cyanosis. Science 129: 393-394, 1959.

Heck, W. and Wolf, H.: Angeborener Herzfehler mit Cyanose durch pathologischen Blutfarbstoff (Hb-M). Ann. Paediat. 190: 135-146, 1958.

Horlein, H. and Weber, G.: Ueber chronische familiaere Methaemoglobine. Deutsch. Med. Wschr. 73: 476-478, 1948.

Shibata, S., Iuchi, I. and Miyaji, T.: Hemoglobin M disease in Japan. Israel J. Med. Sci. 1: 766-768, 1965.

Shibata, S., Iuchi, I., Miyaji, T. and Ueda, S.: Spectroscopic characterization of hemoglobin M (Iwate) and hemoglobin M (Kurume), the two variants of hemoglobin M found in Japan. Acta Haemat. Jap. 24: 477-485, 1961.

Shibata, S., Miyaji, T., Iuchi, I. and Ueda, S.: A comparative study of hemoglobin M (Iwate) and hemoglobin M (Kurume) by means of electrophoresis, chromatography and analysis of peptide chains. Acta Haemat. Jap. 24: 486-494, 1961.

—HEMOGLOBIN MAHIDOL.
Substitution of histidine for aspartic acid at alpha 76.

Pootrakul, S. and Dixon, G. H.: Hemoglobin Mahidol: a new hemoglobin alpha-chain mutant. Canad. J. Biochem. 48: 1066-1078, 1970.

—HEMOGLOBIN MALMO.
Substitution of glutamine for histidine at beta 97.

Berglund, S.: Erythrocytosis associated with haemoglobin Malmo, accompanied by pulmonary changes, occurring in the same family. Scand. J. Haemat. 9: 1-15, 1972.

Berglund, S. and Linell, F.: Fibrosis and carcinoma of the lung in a family with haemoglobin Malmo — anatomic findings. Scand. J. Haemat. 9: 424-432, 1972.

Boyer, S. H., Charache, S., Fairbanks, V. F., Maldonado, J. E., Noyes, A. and Gayle, E. E.: Hemoglobin Malmo beta-97 (FG-4) histidine to glutamine: a cause of polycythemia. J. Clin. Invest. 51: 666-676, 1972.

Fairbanks, V. F., Maldonado, J. E., Charache, S. and Boyer, S. H. Iv: Familial erythrocytosis due to electrophoretically undetectable hemoglobin with impaired oxygen dissociation (hemoglobin Malmo, alpha(2)beta(2) 97 gln). Mayo Clin. Proc. 46: 721-727, 1971.

Lorkin, P. A. and Lehmann, H.: Two new pathological haemoglobins: Olmsted beta 141 (H19) leu to arg and Malmo beta 97 (FG4) his to glu. Biochem. J. 118: 38P only, 1970.

—HEMOGLOBIN MANITOBA.
Substitution of arginine for serine at alpha 102.

Crookston, J. H., Farquharson, H. A., Kinderlerer, J. L. and Lehmann, H.: Hemoglobin Manitoba: alpha 102(G9)serine replaced by arginine. Canad. J. Biochem. 48: 911-914, 1970.

—HEMOGLOBIN MEMPHIS.
Substitution of glutamine for glutamic acid at alpha 23. A Hb S homozygote who also carries this abnormal hemoglobin has a mild form of sickle cell anemia.

Cooper, M. R., Kraus, A. P., Felts, J. H., Myers, R. and Kraus, L. M.: A third case of hemoglobin Memphis: sickle cell disease. Am. J. Med. 55: 535-541, 1973.

Kraus, A. P., Miyaji, T., Iuchi, I. and Kraus, L. M.: Hemoglobin Memphis, a new variant of sickle cell anemia. Trans. Ass. Am. Physicians 80: 297-304, 1968.

Kraus, A. P., Miyaji, T., Iuchi, I. and Kraus, L. M.: Hemoglobin Memphis, an alpha chain mutation — alpha 23 glutamine. (Abstract) Proc. Third Intern. Cong. Hum. Genet. (Chicago, Sept. 5-10), 1966.

—HEMOGLOBIN MEXICO.
Substitution of glutamic acid for glutamine at alpha 54. Fast hemoglobin.

Jones, R. T., Brimhall, B. and Lisker, R.: Chemical characterization of hemoglobin-Mexico and hemoglobin-Chiapas. Biochim. Biophys. Acta 154: 488-495, 1968.

Jones, R. T., Koler, R. D. and Lisker, R.: The chemical structure of hemoglobin Mexico determined by automatic peptide chromatography and subunit hybridization. Clin. Res. 11: 105 only, 1963.

Quattrin, N. and Ventruto, V.: Hemoglobin Mexico in a Sardinian woman. Helv. Med. Acta 33: 388-394, 1967.

—HEMOGLOBIN MIYADA.
A beta-delta fusion variant, i.e., the complement of hemoglobin Lepore. For explanation see HEMOGLOBIN P (CONGO).

Ohta, Y., Yamaoka, K., Sumida, I. and Yanase, T.: Haemoglobin Miyada, a beta-delta fusion peptide (anti-Lepore) type discovered in a Japanese family. Nature N.B. 234: 218-220, 1971.

Yanase, T., Hanada, M., Seita, M., Ohya, I., Ohta, Y., Imamura, T., Fujimura, T., Kawasaki, K. and Yamaoka, K.: Molecular basis of morbidity, from a series of studies of hemoglobinopathies in western Japan. Jap. J. Hum. Genet. 13: 40-53, 1968.

—HEMOGLOBIN MONTGOMERY.
See Hemoglobin Birmingham.

—HEMOGLOBIN N.
Alpha chain anomaly.

Silvestroni, E., Bianco, I. and Brancati, C.: Haemoglobins N and P in Italian families. Nature 200: 658-659, 1963.

—HEMOGLOBIN N.
Fast hemoglobin. Substitution of aspartic acid for lysine at beta 95.

Chernoff, A. I. and Weichselbaum, T. E.: A microhemolyzing technic for preparing solutions of hemoglobin for paper electrophoretic analysis. J. Clin. Path. 30: 120-125, 1958.

Gammack, D. B., Huehns, E. R., Lehmann, H. and Shooter, E. M.: The abnormal polypeptide chains in a number of haemoglobin variants. Acta Genet. Statist. Med. 11: 1-16, 1961.

—HEMOGLOBIN N (BALTIMORE).
Glutamic acid substitution for lysine at beta 95.

Clegg, J. B., Naughton, M. A. and Weatherall, D. J.: An improved method for the characterization of human haemoglobin mutants: identification of alpha-2, beta-2 (95 glu), haemoglobin N (Baltimore). Nature 207: 945-947, 1965.

—HEMOGLOBIN N (JENKINS).
Substitution of glutamic acid for lysine at beta 95. Same as hemoglobin N (Baltimore).

Dobbs, N. B., Jr., Simmons, J. W., Wilson, J. B. and Huisman, T. H. J.: Hemoglobin Jenkins or hemoglobin-N-Baltimore or alpha-2 beta-2(glu) 95. Biochim. Biophys. Acta 117: 492-494, 1966.

—HEMOGLOBIN N (MEMPHIS).
Substitution of either glutamic acid or glutamine for lysine at beta 95.

Schroeder, W. A. and Jones, R. T.: Some aspects of the chemistry and function of human and animal hemoglobins. Fortschr. Chem. Organ. Naturst. 23: 113-194, 1965.

—HEMOGLOBIN N (NEW HAVEN-2).
Same as hemoglobin J (Baltimore). Substitution of aspartic acid glycine at beta 16.

Chernoff, A. I. and Perillie, P. E.: The amino acid composition of hemoglobin B New Haven-2 or HgB N (New Haven). Biochem. Biophys. Res. Commun. 16: 368-372, 1964.

—HEMOGLOBIN N (SARDINIA).

Silvestroni, E. and Bianco, I.: Association of haemoglobin N and microcythaemia in a Sardinian family. Nature 191: 1208-1209, 1961.

—HEMOGLOBIN N (SEATTLE).
Substitution of glutamic acid for lysine at beta 61.

Jones, R. T., Brimhall, B., Huehns, E. R. and Motulsky, A. G.: Structural characterization of hemoglobin N (Seattle): alpha(2)beta(2)61 lys-to-glu. Biochim. Biophys. Acta 154: 278-283, 1968.

—HEMOGLOBIN NAGASAKI.
Substitution of lysine for glutamic acid at beta 17.

Maekawa, M., Maekawa, T., Fujiwara, N., Tabara, K. and Matsuda, G.: Hemoglobin Nagasaki (beta 17 glu): a new abnormal human hemoglobin found in one family in Nagasaki. Int. J. Protein Res. 2: 147-156, 1970.

—HEMOGLOBIN NEW YORK.
Substitution of glutamic acid for valine at beta 113. Found in Chinese-American family.

Ranney, H. M., Jacobs, A. S. and Nagel, R. L.: Haemoglobin New York. Nature 213: 876-878, 1967.

—HEMOGLOBIN NICOSIA.
Alpha chain substitution.

Fessas, C., Karaklis, A., Loukopoulos, D., Stamatoyannopoulos, G. and Fessas, P.: Hemoglobin Nicosia: an alpha-chain variant and its combination with beta-thalassaemia. Brit. J. Haemat. 11: 323-330, 1965.

—HEMOGLOBIN Nishiki I.
Same as hemoglobin Norfolk.

Hanada et al.: For reference see HEMOGLOBIN TAGAWA II.

—HEMOGLOBIN NORFOLK.
Substitution of aspartic acid for glycine at alpha 57. Fast hemoglobin.

Ager, J. A. M., Lehmann, H. and Vella, F.: Haemoglobin 'Norfolk': a new haemoglobin found in an English family. Brit. Med. J. 2: 539-541, 1958.

Baglioni, C.: A chemical study of hemoglobin-Norfolk. J. Biol. Chem. 237: 69-74, 1962.

Huntsman, R. G., Hall, M., Lehmann, H. and Sukumaran, P. K.: A second and a third abnormal haemoglobin in Norfolk. Hb G-Norfolk and Hb D-Norfolk. Brit. Med. J. 1: 720-722, 1963.

Lehmann, H. and Carrell, R. W.: Variations in the structure of human haemoglobins: with particular reference to the unstable haemoglobins. Brit. Med. Bull. 25: 14-23, 1969.

Imamura, T.: Hemoglobin Kagoshima: an example of hemoglobin Norfolk in a Japanese family. Am. J. Hum. Genet. 18: 584-593, 1966.

—HEMOGLOBIN NOTTINGHAM.
Substitution of glycine for valine at beta 98.

Gordon-Smith, E. C., Dacie, J. V., Blecker, T. E., French, E. A., Wiltshire, B. G. and Lehmann, H.:

Haemoglobin Nottingham, beta FG 5(98) val to gly: a new unstable haemoglobin producing severe hemoglysis. Proc. Roy. Soc. Med. 66: 539-540, 1973.

—HEMOGLOBIN NYU.

Substitution of lysine for asparagine at delta 12.

Ranney, H. M., Jacobs, A. S., Ramot, B. and Bradley, T. B., Jr.: Hemoglobin NYU, a delta chain variant, alpha 2 delta 2(12 lys). J. Clin. Invest. 48: 2057-2062, 1969.

—HEMOGLOBIN O (ARABIA).

Substitution of lysine for glutamic acid at beta 121. This hemoglobin has been found in the American Negroes and in Bulgarians as well as Arabs (Kamel et al., 1967).

Kamel, K. A., Hoerman, K. and Awny, A. Y.: Ethnological significance of hemoglobin alpha 2 beta 2 (121 lys). Am. J. Phys. Anthrop. 26: 107-108, 1967.

Kamel, K. A., Hoerman, K. and Awny, A. Y.: Hemoglobin alpha(2) beta(2) 121 lys: chemical identification in an Egyptian family. Science 156: 397-398, 1966.

Milner, P. F., Miller, C., Grey, R., Seakins, M., Dejong, W. W. and Went, L. N.: Hemoglobin O Arab: interaction with hemoglobin S and hemoglobin C. New Eng. J. Med. 283: 1417-1424, 1970.

Ramot, B., Fisher, S., Remez, D., Schneerson, R., Kahane, D., Ager, J. A. M. and Lehmann, H.: Haemoglobin O in an Arab family: sickle-cell haemoglobin O trait. Brit. Med. J. 2: 1262-1264, 1960.

Vella, F., Beale, D. and Lehmann, H.: Haemoglobin O Arab in Sudanese. Nature 209: 308-309, 1966.

—HEMOGLOBIN O (INDONESIA).

Substitution of lysine for glutamic acid at alpha 116.

Baglioni, C. and Lehmann, H.: Chemical heterogeneity of haemoglobin O. Nature 196: 229-231, 1962.

Eng, L. I. L. and Sadono, (NI): Haemoglobin O (Buginese X) in Sulawesi. Brit. Med. J. 1: 1461-1462, 1958.

Sansone, G., Centa, A., Sciarratta, V., Gallo, E. and Lehmann, H.: Haemoglobin O Indonesia (alpha 116 glu leads to lys) in an Italian family. Acta Haemat. 43: 40-47, 1970.

—HEMOGLOBIN OAK RIDGE.

Substitution of asparagine for aspartic acid at beta 94.

Imamura, T. and Riggs, A.: Identification of hemoglobin Oak Ridge with hemoglobin D Punjab (Los Angeles). Biochem. Genet. 7: 127-130, 1972.

Lehmann, H. and Carrell, R. W.: Variations in the structure of human haemoglobins: with particular reference to the unstable haemoglobins. Brit. Med. Bull. 25: 14-23, 1969.

—HEMOGLOBIN OCHO RIOS.

Substitution of alanine for aspartic acid at beta 52.

Beresford, C. H., Clegg, J. B. and Weatherall, D. J.: Haemoglobin Ocho Rios (beta 52 (D3) aspartic acid to alanine): a new beta chain variant of haemoglobin A found in combination with haemoglobin S. J. Med. Genet. 9: 151-153, 1972.

—HEMOGLOBIN OKALOOSA.

Substitution of arginine for leucine at beta 48.

Charache, S., Brimhall, B., Milner, P. and Cobb, L.: Hemoglobin Okaloosa (beta 48 (CD7) leucine to arginine) an unstable variant with low oxygen affinity. J. Clin. Invest. 52: 2858-2864, 1973.

—HEMOGLOBIN OLMSTED.

Substitution of arginine for leucine at beta 141.

Fairbanks, V. F., Opfell, R. W. and Burgert, E. O., Jr.: Three families with unstable hemoglobinopathies (Koln, Olmsted and Santa Ana) causing hemolytic anemia with inclusion bodies and pigmenturia. Am. J. Med. 46: 344-359, 1969.

Lorkin, P. A. and Lehmann, H.: Two new pathological haemoglobins: Olmsted beta 141 (H19) leu to arg and Malmo beta 97 (FG4) his to glu. Biochem. J. 118: 38P only, 1970.

—HEMOGLOBIN OLYMPIA.

Substitution of methionine for valine at beta 20. Since GUG to AUG is the only sinele base change which can result in this substitution, the codon for beta 20 can be uniquely identified as GUG.

Nute, P. E., Stamatoyannopoulos, G. and Funk, D.: Hemoglobin Olympia (beta 20 val to met): an electrophoretically silent variant associated with high oxygen affinity and erythrocytosis. (Abstract) J. Clin. Invest. 51: 70A only, 1972.

—HEMOGLOBIN OSU CHRISTIANSBORG.

Substitution of asparagine for aspartic acid at beta 52.

Konotey-Ahulu, F. I., Kinderlerer, J. L., Lehmann, H. and Ringelhann, B.: To be published, 1970.

—HEMOGLOBIN OTTAWA.

Substitution of arginine for glycine at alpha 15.

Vella, F., Casey, R., Lehmann, H., Labossiere, A. and Jones, T. G.: Haemoglobin Ottawa: alpha 15 gly-to-arg. Biochim. Biophys. Acta 336: 25-29, 1974.

Substitution of arginine for histidine at beta 117.

Schneider, R. G., Alperin, J. B., Brimhall, B. and Jones, R. T.: Hemoglobin P (alpha-2 beta-2 117 arg): structure and properties. J. Lab. Clin. Med. 73: 616-622, 1969.

Silvestroni, E., Bianco, I. and Brancati, C.: Haemoglobin P in a family of southern Italian extraction. Nature 191: 292-294, 1961, and Nature 200: 658-659, 1963.

—HEMOGLOBIN P (CONGO).
This is a beta-delta fusion variant, the complement of hemoglobin Lepore. Unlike the delta-beta fusion product of Lepore hemoglobin, the non-alpha chain resembles beta at the NH2-end. Furthermore, Hb A2 is present in normal concentrations and both Hb A and Hb S (or other beta variant) can be present in the patient heterozygous for hemoglobin P (Congo). The explanation for the origin of hemoglobin Lepore and hembolobin P (Congo) (nonhomologous pairing and unequal crossing-over) is diagrammed in fig. 2.20 (P. 41) of McKusick (1969).

Dherte, P., Lehmann, H. and Vandepitte, J.: Haemoglobin P in a family in the Belgian Congo. Nature 184: 1133-1135, 1959.

Gammack, D. B., Huehns, E. R., Lehmann, H. and Shooter, E. M.: The abnormal polypeptide chains in a number of haemoglobin variants. Acta Genet. Statist. Med. 11: 1-16, 1961.

Lambotte-Legrand, J., Lambotte-Legrand, C., Ager, J. A. and Lehmann, H.: L'hemoglobinose P. A propos d'un cas d'association des hemoglobines P et S. Rev. Hemat. 15: 10-18, 1960.

Lehmann, H. and Charlesworth, D.: Observations on haemoglobin P (Congo type). Biochem. J. 118: 12-13P, 1970.

Lehmann, H., Vandepitte, J. and Dherte, P.: Haemoglobin P in a family in the Belgian Congo. Nature 184: 1133-1135, 1959.

McKusick, V. A.: Human genetics. Englewood Cliffs, N. J.: Prentice-Hall, 1969.

—HEMOGLOBIN P (GALVESTON).
Substitution of arginine for histidine at beta 117.

Schneider, R. G., Alperin, J. B., Brimhall, B. and Jones, R. T.: Hemoglobin P (alpha 2 beta 2 117 arg): structure and properties. J. Lab. Clin. Med. 73: 616-622, 1969.

—HEMOGLOBIN PERTH.
Substitution of proline for leucine at beta 32. This is an unstable hemoglobin resulting in hemolytic anemia.

Jackson, J. M., Yates, A. and Huehns, E. R.: Haemoglobin Perth: beta 32 (B14) leu-to-pro, an unstable haemoglobin causing haemolysis. Brit. J. Haemat. 25: 607-610, 1973.

Jackson, J. M., Yates, A. and Huehns, E. R.: Haemoglobin Perth: beta 32 (B14) leu-to-pro, an unstable haemoglobin causing haemolysis. Brit. J. Haemat. 25: 607-610, 1973.3918 --HEMOGLOBIN PETERBOROUGH.
Substitution of phenylalanine for valine at beta 111.

King, M. A. R., Wiltshire, B. G., Lehmann, H. and Morimoto, H.: An unstable haemoglobin with reduced oxygen affinity: haemoglobin Peterborough, beta 111 (G13) valine to phenylalanine, its interaction with normal haemoglobin and with haemoglobin Lepore. Brit. J. Haemat. 22: 125-134, 1972.

—HEMOGLOBIN PHILLY.
Substitution of phenylalanine for tyrosine at beta 35. An unstable hemoglobin leading to hemolytic anemia. No electrophoretic abnormality.

Rieder, R. F., Oski, F. A. and Clegg, J. B.: Hemoglobin Philly (beta 35 tyrosine to phenylalanine): studies in the molecular pathology of hemoglobin. J. Clin. Invest. 48: 1627-1642, 1969.

—HEMOGLOBIN PIERCE ET AL.
Defect unknown.

Pierce, L. E., McCoy, K. and Rath, C. E.: A new hemoglobin variant with sickling properties. New Eng. J. Med. 268: 862-866, 1963.

Pierce, L. E., McCoy, K. and Rath, C. E.: A new hemoglobin variant with sickling properties. New Eng. J. Med. 268: 862-866, 1963.24 --HEMOGLOBIN PORTLAND-1.
This unique hemoglobin was found in a newborn infant with multiple congenital anomalies and complex autosomal chromosomal mosaicism. Its composition is gamma(2) X(2). The X-chain may be the epsilon chain whose synthesis persists until after birth because of the chromosomal anomaly. On the other hand, the X polypeptide chain may be under the control of a separate locus. Recent work indicates that the X-chain is indeed different from epsilon and therefore it is now called zeta.

Capp, G. I., Rigas, D. A. and Jones, R. T.: Hemoglobin Portland 1: a new human hemoglobin unique in structure. Science 157: 65-66, 1967.

Hecht, F., Jones, R. T. and Koler, R. D.: Newborn infants with Hb Portland 1, an indicator of alpha-chain deficiency. Ann. Hum. Genet. 31: 215-218, 1968.

—HEMOGLOBIN PORTO ALEGRE.
Substitution of cysteine for serine at beta 9.

Bonaventura, J. and Riggs, A.: Polymerization of hemoglobins of mouse and man: structural basis. Science 158: 800-802, 1967.

Seid-Akhavan, M., Ayres, M., Salzano, F. M., Winter, W. P. and Rucknagel, D. L.: Two more examples of Hb Porto Alegre, alpha-2-beta-2 9 ser-to-cys in Belem, Brazil. Hum. Hered. 23: 175-181, 1973.

Tondo, C. V., Salzano, F. M. and Rucknagel, D. L.: Hemoglobin Porto Alegre, a possible polymer of normal hemoglobin in a Caucasian Brazilian family. Am. J. Hum. Genet. 15: 265-279, 1963.

—HEMOGLOBIN PYLOS.
Beta-delta chain anomaly. See LEPORE (BOSTON).

Fessas, P., Stamatoyannopoulos, G. and Karaklis, A.: Hemoglobin 'Pylos': study of a hemoglobinopathy resembling thalassemia in the heteroxygous homozygous and double heterozygous state. Blood 19: 1-22, 1962.

—HEMOGLOBIN PYRGOS.
Substitution of aspartic acid for glycine at beta 83.

Tatsis, B., Sofroniadou, K. and Stergiopoulos, K.: Hemoglobin Pyrgos (alpha 2 beta 2 83 gly to asp): a new hemoglobin variant. (Abstract) Meeting Am. Soc. Hemat., Hollywood, Fla., Dec. 3-6, 1972.

—HEMOGLOBIN Q.
Two forms exist, one with substitution of histidine for aspartic acid at alpha 74 and one with the same change at alpha 75. The latter may be called Q (Iran).

Lorkin, P. A., Charlesworth, D., Lehmann, H., Rahbar, S., Tuchinda, S. and Eng, L. I. L.: Two haemoglobins Q, alpha 74 (EF3) and alpha 75 (EF4) aspartic acid to histidine. Brit. J. Haemat. 19: 117-125, 1970.

—HEMOGLOBIN Q (CHINESE).
Alpha chain anomaly.

Eng, L. I. L., Pillay, R. P. and Thuraisingham, V.: Further cases of haemoglobin Q-H disease (Hb Q-alpha thalassemia). Blood 28: 830-839, 1966.

Gammack, D. B., Huehns, E. R., Lehmann, H. and Shooter, E. M.: The abnormal polypeptide chains in a number of haemoglobin variants. Acta Genet. Statist. Med. 11: 1-16, 1961.

Vella, F., Wells, R. H. C., Ager, J. A. M. and Lehmann, H.: A haemoglobinopathy involving haemoglobin H and a new (Q) haemoglobin. Brit. Med. J. 1: 752-755, 1958.

—HEMOGLOBIN Q (INDIA).
Substitution of histidine for aspartic acid at alpha 64.

Sukumaran, P. K., Merchant, S. M., Desai, M. P., Wiltshire, B. G. and Lehmann, H.: Haemoglobin Q India (alpha-64 (E13) aspartic acid to histidine). Associated with beta-thalassemia observed in three Sindhi families. J. Med. Genet. 9: 436-442, 1971.

—HEMOGLOBIN R.
Same as hemoglobin Durham-I.

Chernoff, A. I. and Weichselbaum, T. E.: A microhemolyzing technic for preparing solutions of hemoglobin for paper electrophoretic analysis. Am. J. Clin. Path. 30: 120-125, 1958.

—HEMOGLOBIN RAINIER.
Causes erythrocytosis and is only adult hemoglobin that is alkali-resistant. Substitution of tyrosine by cysteine at beta 145. See HEMOGLOBIN BETHESDA with which Rainier was confused earlier.

Adamson, J. W., Parer, J. T. and Stamatoyannopoulos, G.: Erythrocytosis associated with hemoglobin Rainier: oxygen equilibria and marrow regulation. J. Clin. Invest. 48: 1376-1386, 1969.

Greer, J. and Perutz, M. F.: Three dimensional structure of haemoglobin Rainier. Nature 230: 261-264, 1971.

Hayashi, A., Stamatoyannopoulos, G., Yoshida, A. and Adamson, J.: Haemoglobin Rainier: beta 145 (HC2) tyrosine to cysteine and haemoglobin Bethesda: beta 145 (HC2) tyrosine to histidine. Nature 230: 264-267, 1971.

Salhany, J. M.: The deoxygenation kinetics of hemoglobin Rainier (alpha(2)beta(2) 145 tyr to cys). Biochim. Biophys. Res. Commun. 47: 784-789, 1972.

Stamatoyannopoulos, G. and Yoshida, A.: Single chain alkali resistance in hemoglobin Rainier: beta 145 tyrosine to histidine. Science 166: 1005-1006, 1969.

Stamatoyannopoulos, G., Yoshida, A., Adamson, J. and Heinenberg, S.: Hemoglobin Rainier (beta 145 tyrosine to histidine): alkali-resistant hemoglobin with increased oxygen affinity. Science 159: 741-743, 1968.

—HEMOGLOBIN RAJAPPEN.
Substitution of threonine for lysine at alpha 90.

Hyde, R. D., Kinderlerer, J. L., Lehmann, H. and Hall, M.: Hb Rajappen. To be published, 1970.

Substitution of serine for proline at alpha 95.

DeJong, W. W. W.: Leiden, Holland: personal communication, 1970.

DeJong, W. W. W., Bernini, L. F. and Kahn, P. M.: Haemoglobin Rampa: alpha 95 pro to ser (BBA 35815). Biochim. Biophys. Acta 236: 197-200, 1971.

—HEMOGLOBIN REISSMANN ET AL.
Same as hemoglobin Kansas. Hemoglobin with low affinity for oxygen.

Reissmann, K. R., Ruth, W. E. and Normura, T.: A human hemoglobin with lowered oxygen affinity and impaired heme-heme interactions. J. Clin. Invest. 40: 1826-1833, 1961.

—HEMOGLOBIN RICHMOND.
Substitution of lysine for asparagine at beta 102.

Efremov, G. D., Huisman, T. H. J., Smith, L. L., Wilson, J. B., Kitchens, J. L., Wrightstone, R. N. and Adams, H. R.: Hemoglobin Richmond, a human hemoglobin which forms asymmetric hybrids with other hemoglobins. J. Biol. Chem. 244: 61056116, 1969.

—HEMOGLOBIN RIVERDALE-BRONX.
Substitution of arginine for glycine at beta 24.

Ranney, H. M., Jacobs, A. S., Udem, L. and Zalusky, R.: Hemoglobin Riverdale-Bronx: an unstable hemoglobin resulting from the substitution of arginine for glycine at helical residue B6 of the beta polypeptide chain. Biochem. Biophys. Res. Commun. 33: 1004-1011, 1968.

—HEMOGLOBIN RUSH.
Substitution of glutamine for leucine acid at beta 101.

Adams, J. G., Winter, W. P., Tausk, K. and Heller, P.: Hemoglobin Rush (beta 101 (G-3) glu-to-gln): a new unstable hemoglobin causing mild hemolytic anemia. Blood 43: 261-270, 1974.

—HEMOGLOBIN RUSS.
Substitution of arginine for glycine at alpha 51.

Huisman, T. H. J. and Sydenstricker, V. P.: Difference in gross structure of two electrophoretically identical 'minor' hemoglobin components. Nature 193: 489-491, 1962.

Reynolds, C. A. and Huisman, T. H. J.: Hemoglobin Russ or alpha-2 (51 arg) beta-2. Biochim. Biophys. Acta 130: 541-543, 1966.

—HEMOGLOBIN S.
Substitution of valine for glutamic acid at beta 6. Hemoglobin C (Georgetown) also sickles.

Ingram, V. M.: Abnormal human haemoglobin. III. The chemical difference between normal and sickle cell haemoglobins. Biochim. Biophys. Acta 36: 402-411, 1959.

Pauling, L., Itano, H. A., Singer, S. J. and Wells, I. C.: Sickle cell anemia, a molecular disease. Science 110: 543-548, 1949.

—HEMOGLOBIN SABINE.
Substitution of proline for leucine at beta 91. The hemoglobin is unstable causing hemolytic anemia in the heterozygote.

Schneider, R. G., Ueda, S., Alperin, J. B., Brimhall, B. and Jones, R. T.: Hemoglobin Sabine at beta 91 (E7) leu-to-pro: an unstable variant causing severe anemia with inclusion bodies. New Eng. J. Med. 280: 739-745, 1969.

—HEMOGLOBIN SAINT ETIENNE.
Substitution of glutamine for histidine at beta 92. Same as hemoglobin Instanbul.

Beizard, Y., Courvalin, J. C., Solal, M. C., Garel, M. C., Rosa, J., Brizard, C. P. and Gibaud, A.: Febs Letters 27: 76-80, 1972.

—HEMOGLOBIN SAN DIEGO.
Substitution of methionine for valine at beta 109.

Anderson, N. L.: Hemoglobin San Diego (beta 109 (G11) val-to-met). Crystal structure of the deoxy form. J. Clin. Invest. 53: 329-333, 1974.

Nute, P. E., Stamatoyannopoulos, G., Hermodson, M. A. and Roth, D.: Hemoglobinopathic erythrocytosis due to a new electrophoretically silent variant, hemoglobin San Diego (beta 109 (G11) val-to-met). J. Clin. Invest. 53: 320-328, 1974.

—HEMOGLOBIN SANTA ANA.
Substitution of proline for leucine at beta 88.

Opfell, R. W., Lorkin, P. A. and Lehmann, H.: Hereditary non-spherocytic haemolytic anaemia with post-splenectomy inclusion bodies and pigmenturia caused by an unstable haemoglobin Santa Ana — beta 88 (F4) leucine-proline. J. Med. Genet. 5: 292-297, 1968.

—HEMOGLOBIN SAVANNAH.
Substitution of valine for glycine at beta 24.

Huisman, T. H. J., Brown, A. K., Efremov, G. D., Wilson, J. B., Reynolds, C. A., Uy, R. and Smith,

L. L.: Hemoglobin Savannah (beta 6 (24) beta-glycine to valine): an unstable variant causing anemia with inclusion bodies. J. Clin. Invest. 50: 650-659, 1971.

—HEMOGLOBIN SAWARA.
Substitution of alanine for aspartic acid at alpha 6. No pathologic effects were observed.

Sumida, I., Ohta, Y., Imammura, T. and Yanase, T.: Hemoglobin Sawara: alpha 6 (A4) aspartic acid to alanine. Biochim. Biophys. Acta 322: 23-26, 1973.

—HEMOGLOBIN SCOTT ET AL.
Defect unknown.

Scott, J. L., Haut, A., Cartwright, G. E. and Wintrobe, M. M.: Congenital hemolytic disease associated with red cell inclusion bodies, abnormal pigment metabolism and an electrophoretic hemoglobin abnormality. Blood 16: 1239-1252, 1960.

—HEMOGLOBIN SEALY.
Substitution of histidine for aspartic acid at alpha 47. (Of interest is the fact that the family in which this was found was Ashkenazic. Hemoglobin Beilinson was also found in an Ashkenazic Jewish family and has a substitution of glycine for aspartic acid at alpha 47.)

Schneider, R. G., Ueda, S., Alperin, J. B., Brimhall, B. and Jones, R. T.: Hemoglobin Sealy (alpha-47 his-2 beta-2): a new variant in a Jewish family. Am. J. Hum. Genet. 20: 151-156, 1968.

—HEMOGLOBIN SEATTLE.
Substitution of glutamic acid for alanine at beta 76.

Huehns, E. R., Hecht, F., Yoshida, A., Stammatoyannopoulos, G., Hartman, J. and Motulsky, A. G.: Hemoglobin-Seattle (alpha-2-beta-2-76 glu): an unstable hemoglobin causing chronic hemolytic anemia. Blood 36: 209-218, 1970.

Stamatoyannopoulos, G., Parer, J. T. and Finch, C. A.: Physiologic implications of a hemoglobin with decreased oxygen affinity (hemoglobin Seattle). New Eng. J. Med. 281: 915-919, 1969.

—HEMOGLOBIN SETIF.
Substitution of tyrosine for aspartic acid at alpha 94.

Wajcman, H., Beklhodja, O. and Labie, D.: Hb Setif: G1 (94) alpha — asp-tyr. A new chain hemoglobin variant with substitution of the residue involved in a hydrogen bond between unlike subunits. Fed. Europ. Biochem. Soc. 27: 298-300, 1972.

—HEMOGLOBIN SHEPHERDS BUSH.
Substitution of aspartic acid for glycine at beta 74.

White, J. M., Brain, M. C., Lorkin, P. A., Lehmann, H. and Smith, M.: Mild 'unstable haemoglobin haemolytic anaemia' caused by haemoglobin Shepherds Bush (beta 74 (E18) gly to asp). Nature 225: 939-941, 1970.

—HEMOGLOBIN SHIMONOSEKI.
Substitution of arginine for glutamine at alpha 54.

Hanada, M. and Rucknagel, D. L.: The characterization of hemoglobin Shimonoseki. Blood 24: 624-635, 1964.

Yamaoka, K., Kawamura, K., Hanada, M., Seita, M., Hitsumoto, S. and Ooya, I.: Studies on abnormal haemoglobins. Jap. J. Hum. Genet. 5: 99-111, 1960.

—HEMOGLOBIN SINAI.
Substitution of histidine for aspartic acid at alpha 47. Same as hemoglobin Hasharon.

Charache, S.: Baltimore, Md.: personal communication, 1967.

Ostertag, W. and Smith, E. W.: Hb Sinai, a new alpha chain mutant alpha his 47. Humangenetik 6: 377-379, 1968.

—HEMOGLOBIN SINGAPORE.
Substitution of proline for arginine at alpha 141.

Clegg, J. B., Weatherall, D. J., Boon, W. H. and Mustafa, D.: Two new haemoglobin variants involving proline substitutions. Nature 222: 379-380, 1969.

—HEMOGLOBIN SIRIRAJ.
Substitution of lysine for glutamic acid at beta 7.

Blackwell, R. Q., Liu, C. S. and Wang, C. L.: Hemoglobin Siriraj, beta — 7 (A4) glu-lys, in a Chinese subject in Taiwan. Vox Sang. 23: 433-438, 1972.

Tuchinda, S., Beale, D. and Lehmann, H.: A new haemoglobin in a Thai family. A case of haemoglobin Siriraj-beta thalassaemia. Brit. Med. J. 1: 1583-1585, 1965.

—HEMOGLOBIN SOGN.
Substitution of arginine for leucine at beta 14.

Monn, E., Gaffney, P. J. and Lehmann, H.: Haemoglobin Sogn (beta 14 arginine)--a new hemoglobin variant. Scand. J. Haemat. 5: 353-360, 1968.

—HEMOGLOBIN SOUTHAMPTON.
Substitution of proline for leucine at beta 106.

Hyde, R. D., Hall, M. D., Wiltshire, B. G. and Lehmann, H.: Haemoglobin Southampton, beta 106 (G8) leu to pro: an unstable variant producing severe haemolysis. Lancet II: 1170-1172, 1972.

—HEMOGLOBIN SPHAKIA.
Substitution of arginine for histidine at delta 2.

Jones, R. T., Brimhall, B., Huehns, E. R. and Barnicot, N. A.: Hemoglobin Sphakia: a delta-chain variant of hemoglobin A2 from Crete. Science 151: 1406-1408, 1966.

—HEMOGLOBIN ST. ANTOINE.
Two amino acids, glycine and leucine, are deleted from beta 74 and 75.

Wajcman, H., Labie, D. and Schapira, G.: Hemoglobin Tours: thr beta-87(F3) deleted and hemoglobin St. Antoine: gly-to-leu beta-74-75(E18-19) deleted. Consequences for oxygen affinity and protein stability. Biochim. Biophys. acta 295: 495-504, 1973.

—HEMOGLOBIN ST. LUKE'S.
Substitution of arginine for proline at alpha 95.

Bannister, W. H., Grech, J. L., Plese, C. F., Smith, L. L., Barton, B. P., Wilson, J. B., Reynolds, C. A. and Huisman, T. H. J.: Europ. J. Biochem. 29: 301-307, 1972.

—HEMOGLOBIN ST. MARY'S.
A possible 'core' hemoglobin variant.

Buchanan, A., Barkhan, P., Crome, P. E., Morrison, P. L. and Huehns, E. R.: 1965, unpublished.

—HEMOGLOBIN STANLEYVILLE-1.
Same as G (Philadelphia). Change from asparagine to lysine at alpha 68.

Dherte, P., Vandepitte, J., Ager, J. A. M. and Lehmann, H.: Stanleyville I and II. Two new variants of adult hemoglobin. Brit. Med. J. 2: 282-284, 1959.

—HEMOGLOBIN STANLEYVILLE-2.
Substitution of lysine for asparagine at alpha 78.

Van Ros, G., Beale, D. and Lehmann, H.: Hemoglobin Stanleyville-II (alpha 78 asparagine to lysine). Brit. Med. J. 4: 92-93, 1968.

—HEMOGLOBIN SUD-VIETNAM.
Defect unknown.

Albahary, C., Dreyfus, J. C., Labie, D., Schapira, G. and Tram, L.: Hemoglobines anormales au Sud-Vietnam. Hemoglobinose C homozygote. Trait E. hemoglobine nouvelle. Rev. Hemat. 13: 163-170, 1960.

—HEMOGLOBIN SYDNEY.
Substitution of alanine for valine at beta 67. Like hemoglobins Koln and Genova, this hemoglobin has no electrophoretic abnormality but is unstable, forming intracellular precipitates.

Carrell, R. W., Lehmann, H., Lorkin, P. A., Raik, E. and Hunter, E.: Haemoglobin Sydney: beta 67 (E 11) valine to alanine: an emerging pattern of unstable haemoglobins. Nature 215: 626-628, 1967.

—HEMOGLOBIN SYRACUSE.
Substitution of proline for histidine at beta 143.

Jensen, M., Bunn, H. F., Nathan, D. G. and Oski, F. A.: Hemoglobin Syracuse (beta 143 his-to-pro), a new variant with high oxygen affinity and interesting electrophoretic properties. Blood, in press, 1974.

—HEMOGLOBIN TA-LI.
Substitution of cysteine for glycine at beta 83.

Blackwell, R. Q., Liu, C.-S. and Wang, C.-L.: Biochim. Biophys. Acta 243: 467-474, 1971.

—HEMOGLOBIN TACOMA.
Substitution of serine for arginine at beta 30.

Baur, E. W. and Motulsky, A. G.: Hemoglobin Tacoma, a beta-chain variant associated with increased Hb A(2). Humangenetik 1: 621-634, 1965.

Brimhall, B., Jones, R. T., Baur, E. W. and Motulsky, A. G.: Structural characterization of hemoglobin Tacoma. Biochemistry 8: 2125-2129, 1969.

—HEMOGLOBIN TAGAWA 1.
Substitution of asparagine for lysine at alpha 90. Same as Hb J (Broussais).

Yanase, T., Hanada, M., Seita, M., Ohya, I., Ohta, Y., Imamura, T., Fujimura, T., Kawasaki, K. and Yamaoka, K.: Molecular basis of morbidity from a series of studies of hemoglobinopathies in western Japan. Jap. J. Hum. Genet. 13: 40-53, 1968.

—HEMOGLOBIN TAGAWA II.
Probably same as hemoglobin Kokura.

Hanada, M., Ohta, Y., Imamura, T., Fejimura, T., Kawasaki, K., Kosaka, K., Yamaoka, K. and Seita, M.: Studies of abnormal hemoglobins in western Japan. (Abstract) Jap. J. Hum. Genet. 9: 253-254, 1964.

The usual terminal dipeptide 145-146 of the beta chain is lacking and is replaced by 10 residues attached to the C-terminal end. Hemoglobin Constant Spring is a termination defect of the alpha chain. These two anomalous hemoglobins may shed light on normal chain termination and the nature of 'intergenic' DNA, i.e., in this case, that between the end of the beta-chain gene and the beginning of the next gene along the chromosome.

D
O
M
I
N
A
N
T

Flatz, G., Kinderlerer, J. L., Kilmartin, J. V. and Lehmann, H.: Haemoglobin Tak: a variant with additional residues at the end of the beta-chains. Lancet I: 732-733, 1971.

—HEMOGLOBIN TOCHIGI.
Deletion of residues 56-59 of the beta chain.

Shibata, S., Miyaji, T., Ueda, S., Matsvoka, M., Iuchi, I., Yamada, K. and Shinkai, N.: Hemoglobin Tochigi (beta 56-59 deleted). A new unstable hemoglobin discovered in a Japanese family. Proc. Jap. Acad. 46: 440-445, 1970.

—HEMOGLOBIN TOKUCHI.
Substitution of tyrosine for histidine at beta 2.

Shibata, S., Iuchi, I., Mazagi, T. and Takeda, I.: Hemoglobinopathy in Japan. Bull. Yamaguchi Med. Sch. 10: 1-9, 1963.

—HEMOGLOBIN TOKYO.
Defect unknown.

Fukutake, K. and Kato, K.: Hemolytic anemia due to a new abnormal hemoglobin. Proc. 8th Congr. Intern. Soc. Hemat., Tokyo, 1960. 2: 1220-1223, 1961.

—HEMOGLOBIN TORINO.
Substitution of valine for phenylalanine at alpha 43.

Beretta, A., Prato, V., Gallo, E. and Lehmann, H.: Haemoglobin Torino — alpha 43 (CD 1) phenylalanine replaced by valine. Nature 217: 1016-1018, 1968.

Prato, V., Gallo, E., Ricco, G., Mazza, U., Bianco, G. and Lehmann, H.: Haemolytic anaemia due to haemoglobin Torino. Brit. J. Haemat. 19: 105-115, 1970.

—HEMOGLOBIN TOULOUSE.
Substitution of glutamic acid for lysine at beta 66.

Labie, D., Rosa, J., Belkhodja, O. and Bierme, R.: Hemoglobin Toulouse alpha(2)beta(2)66(E10)lys to glu. Structure and consequences in molecular pathology. Biochim. Biophys. Acta 236: 201-207, 1971.

—HEMOGLOBIN TOURS.
Threonine is deleted at beta 87. See HB FREIBURG, LEIDEN, GUN HILL, TOCHIGI and ST. ANTOINE for other examples of deletion.

Wajacman, H., Labie, D. and Schapira, G.: Hemoglobin Tours: thr beta-87 (F3) deleted and hemoglobin St. Antoine: gly-to-leu beta-74-75 (E18-19) deleted. Consequences for oxygen affinity and protein stability. Biochim. Biophys. Acta 295: 495-504, 1973.

—HEMOGLOBIN TSUKIJI.
Beta chain anomaly.

Shibata, S. and Iuchi, I.: Hemoglobin-Hikari (alpha-2-beta-2,T-7). A fast-moving hemoglobin demonstrated in two families of Japanese people, with a brief note on the abnormal hemoglobins of Japan which are liable to be confused with it. Proc. 9th Congr. Intern. Soc. Hemat., Mexico City, 1962. Pp. 65-70.

—HEMOGLOBIN UBE-I.
Substitution of methionine for valine at beta 98. Identical to Hb Koln.

Ohba, Y., Miyaji, T. and Shibata, S.: Identical substitution in Hb Ube-1 and Hb Koln. Nature N. B. 243: 205-207, 1973.

Shibata, S., Iuchi, I., Miyaji, T., Ueda, S., Yamashita, K. and Suzuno, R.: A case of hemolytic disease associated with the production of Heinz bodies and of an abnormal hemoglobin (Hb Ube-1). Med. Biol. 59: 79-84, 1961.

—HEMOGLOBIN UBE-II.
Substitution of aspartic acid for asparagine at alpha 68.

Miyaji, T., Iuchi, I., Yamamoto, K., Ohba, Y. and Shibata, S.: Amino acid substitution of hemoglobin Ube 2(alpha 2 68 asp beta 2): an example of successful application of partial hydrolysis of peptide with 5 percent acetic acid. Clin. Chim. Acta 16: 347-352, 1967.

Shibata, S. and Iuchi, I.: Hemoglobin-Hikari (alpha-2 A-beta-2,T-7). A fast-moving hemoglobin demonstrated in two families of Japanese people with a brief note on the abnormal hemoglobins of Japan which are liable to be confused with it. Proc. 9th Congr. Intern. Soc. Hemat., Mexico City, 1962. Pp. 65-70.

—HEMOGLOBIN UMI.
Probably same as hemoglobin Kokura.

Janada, et al.: For reference see HEMOGLOBIN TAGAWA II.

Substitution of glutamic acid for glutamine at alpha 54.

Beckman, L., Christodoulou, C., Fessas, P., Loukopoulos, D., Kaltsoya, A. and Nilsson, L.-O.: A Swedish haemoglobin variant. Acta Genet. Statist. Med. 16: 362-370, 1966.

Fessas, P., Kaltsoya, A., Loukopoulos, D. and Nilsson, L.-O.: On the chemical structure of haemoglobin Uppsala. Hum. Hered. 19: 152-158, 1969.

—-HEMOGLOBIN WARREN.
Gamma chain anomaly.

Huisman, T. H. J., Dozy, A. M., Horton, B. E. and Wilson, J. B.: A fetal hemoglobin with abnormal gamma-polypeptide chains: hemoglobin Warren. Blood 26: 668-676, 1965.

—-HEMOGLOBIN WAYNE.
Two hemoglobins, Hb W1 and Hb W2, with anomalous alpha chains were observed in several members of a family. The alpha T-14 peptide was replaced by a new peptide which was different in the two. The sequence in Hb A which was missing was thr-ser-lys-tyr-arg - COOH. In W1 it was replaced by thr-ser-asn-thr-val-lys-leu-glu-pro-arg-COOH. Hb W2 had the same peptide except that aspartic acid had been substituted for asparagine in the third position. This was believed to represent the result of enzymatic deamidation of Hb W1. This is the first reported frameshift mutation in man. Deletion of a single nucleotide yields the sequence observed in Hb W1. If the usual nucleotide sequence in the alpha chain gene is ACX.UCX.AAA(G).UAC.CGU.UAA signifying thr-ser-lys-tyr-arg-terminator, then hemoglobin Wayne has had a deletion of the third nucleotide of codon 139 resulting in frame-shift to ACX.UCX.AAU.ACC-.GUU.AAG.CUG.GAG. which reads thr-ser-asn-thr-val-lys-leu-glu-etc. This interpretation agrees with that for hemoglobin Constant Spring (q.v.), which appears to be a change in the first nucleotide of the terminator codon so that the above sequence becomes ACX.UCX.AAA.UAC.CGU.CAA.GCU.GGA etc., which is read as thr-ser-lys-tyr-arg-gln-ala-gly-etc.

Seid-Akhavan, M., Winter, W. P., Abramson, R. K. and Rucknagel, D. L.: Hemoglobin Wayne: a frameshift variant occurring in two distinct forms. (Abstract) Blood 40: 927 only, 1972.

—-HEMOGLOBIN WIEN.
Substitution of aspartic acid for tyrosine at beta 130.

Perutz, M. F. and Lehmann, H.: Molecular pathology of human hemoglobin. Nature 219: 902-909, 1968.

—-HEMOGLOBIN WINNEPEG.
Substitution of tyrosine for aspartic acid at alpha 75.

Vella, F., Wiltshire, B., Lehmann, H. and Galbraith, P.: Hemoglobin Winnepeg. Clin. Biochem. 6: 66-70, 1973.

—-HEMOGLOBIN X.
Substitutions in both alpha and beta. At alpha 68, change of asparagine to lysine as in hemoglobin G (Philadelphia). At beta 6, change of glutamic acid to lysine as in hemoglobin C.

Baglioni, C. and Ingram, V. M.: Four adult haemoglobin types in one person. Nature 189: 465-467, 1961.

—-HEMOGLOBIN YAKIMA.
Substitution of histidine for aspartic acid at beta 99. Polycythemia occurs with this hemoglobinopathy as with hemoglobin Chesapeake.

Jones, R. T., Osgood, E. E., Brimhall, B. and Koler, R. D.: Hemoglobin Yakina. I. Clinical and biochemical studies. J. Clin. Invest. 46: 1840-1847, 1967.

Novy, M. J., Edwards, M. J. and Metcalfe, J.: Hemoglobin Yakima. II. High blood oxygen affinity associated with compensatory erythrocytosis and normal hemodynamics. J. Clin. Invest. 46: 1848-1854, 1967.

Novy, M. J., Edwards, M. J., Peterson, E. N. and Metcalfe, J.: Hemoglobin Yakima: oxygen hemoglobin equilibrium and cardiodynamic effects. (Abstract) Clin. Res. 15: 133 only, 1967.

Osgood, E. E., Jones, R. T., Brimhall, B. and Koler, R. D.: Hemoglobin Yakima: clinical and biochemical studies. (Abstract) Clin. Res. 15: 134 only, 1967.

—-HEMOGLOBIN YOSHIZUKA.
Substitution of aspartic acid for asparagine at beta 108. Reduced oxygen affinity like hemoglobin Kansas.

Imamura, T., Fujita, S., Ohta, Y., Hanada, M. and Yanase, T.: Hemoglobin Yoshizuka (G10(108) beta asparagine to aspartic acid): a new variant with a reduced oxygen affinity from a Japanese family. J. Clin. Invest. 48: 2341-2348, 1969.

—-HEMOGLOBIN YPSI.
Substitution in beta chain results in increased oxygen affinity leading to erythremia and abnormal polymerization manifested in heterozygotes by hybrid hemoglobin molecules containing both the Ypsi beta chain and the normal beta chain. Substitution of tyrosine for aspartic acid at beta 99.

Glynn, K. P., Penner, J. A. and Smith, J. R.: Familial erythrocytosis: a description of three families, one with hemoglobin Ypsilanti. Ann. Intern. Med. 69: 769-776, 1968.

Rucknagel, D. L.: Personal communication cited by Stamatoyannopoulos, G., Billingham, A. J., Lenfant, C. and Finch, C. A.: Ann. Rev. Med. 22: 221-234, 1971.

—-HEMOGLOBIN YUKUHASHI.
Substitution of arginine for proline at beta 58.

Yanase, T., Hanada, M., Seita, M., Ohya, I., Ohta, Y., Imamura, T., Fujimura, T., Kawasaki, K. and Yamaoka, K.: Molecular basis of morbidity from a series of studies of hemoglobinopathies in western Japan. Jap. J. Hum. Genet. 13: 40-53, 1968.

—-HEMOGLOBIN ZAMBIA.
Substitution of asparagine for lysine at alpha 60.

Barclay, G. P. T., Charlesworth, D. and Lehmann, H.: Abnormal haemoglobins in Zambia. A new hemoglobin Zambia alpha 60 (E9) lysine to asparagine. Brit. Med. J. 2: 595-596, 1969.

—-HEMOGLOBIN ZURICH.
Substitution of arginine for histidine at beta 63. Drug induced hemolysis.

Dickerman, J. D., Holtzman, N. A. and Zinkham, W. H.: Hemoglobin Zurich. A third family presenting hemolytic reactions to sulfonamides. Am. J. Med. 55: 638-642, 1973.

Frick, P. G., Hitzig, W. H. and Betke, K.: Hemoglobin Zurich. I. A new hemoglobin anomaly associated with acute hemolytic episodes with inclusion bodies after sulfonamide therapy. Blood 20: 261-271, 1962.R

Huisman, T. H. J., Horton, B., Bridges, M. T., Betke, K. and Hitzig, W. H.: A new abnormal human hemoglobin: hemoglobin-Zurich. Clin. Chem. Acta 6: 347-355, 1960.

Muller, C. J. and Kingma, S.: Haemoglobin Zurich beta 63 arg. Biochim. Biophys. Acta 50: 595 only, 1961.

Rieder, R. F., Zinkham, W. H. and Holtzman, N. A.: Hemoglobin Zurich. Clinical, chemical and kinetic studies. Am. J. Med. 39: 4-20, 1965.

14229 HEMOPEXIN

Hemopexin, a globulin synthesized by liver, accounts for about 1.4 percent of total serum protein. Like albumin, it binds with heme to form a brown-colored complex in vitro. Hemopexin is low in patients with hemolysis. It has been found in the serum of all mammals studied and it is polymorphic in rabbits and swine. Stewart and Lovrein (1971) sought electrophoretic polymorphism in man and found none.

Stewart, R. E. and Lovrein, E. W.: Haemopexin in human serum: a search for genetic polymorphism. Ann. Hum. Genet. 35: 19-24, 1971.

14230 HERNIA, DOUBLE INGUINAL

Weimer (1949) described a family in which at least one male in four successive generations had bilateral inguinal hernia. Autosomal dominance with sex influence was suggested. Familial hernia was reported also by Edwards (1974) and by Simpson et al. (1974).

Edwards, R. H.: Familial hernia. In, Bergsma, D. (ed.): Clinical Delineation of Birth Defects. XVI. Urinary System and Others. Baltimore: Williams and Wilkins, 1974. Pp. 329-331.

Simpson, J. L., Morillo-Cucci, G. and German, J.: Familial inguinal hernia affecting females. In, Bergsma, D. (ed.): Clinical Delineation of Birth Defects. XVI. Urinary System and Others. Baltimore: Williams and Wilkins, 1974. P. 332 only.

Weimer, B. R.: Congenital inheritance of inguinal hernia. J. Hered. 40: 219-220, 1949.

14240 HERNIA, HIATUS

Goodman et al. (1969) observed six affected persons in two generations. Five of the six were female. This disorder is sometimes called congenital short esophagus (Myles, 1959) or partial thoracic stomach. Carre and Froggatt (1970) described 8 definite cases in 3 successive generations of a family. Others were equivocally affected. Sidd et al. (1966) observed affected twins.

Carre, I. J. and Froggatt, P.: Oesophageal hiatus hernia in three generations of one family. Gut 11: 51-54, 1970.

Goodman, R. M., Wooley, C. F., Ruppert, R. D. and Freimanis, A. K.: A possible genetic role in esophageal hiatus hernia. J. Hered. 60: 71-74, 1969.

Myles, R. B.: Familial short oesophagus. Brit. J. Radiol. 12: 645-647, 1939.

Sidd, J. J., Gilliam, J. I. and Bushueff, D. P.: Sliding hiatus hernia in identical twins. Brit. J. Radiol. 39: 703-704, 1966.

14250 HETEROCHROMIA IRIDIS

Asymmetry in the pigmentation of the irides probably occurs as an isolated phenomenon inherited as a dominant (Calhoun, 1919). We have observed it in at least three cases of the Marfan syndrome. Damage to the cervical sympathetics, as in birth injury, may result in this trait, which represents in such instances a phenocopy. Whether hereditary heterochromia iridis ever exists independent of Horner syndrome (q.v.), Waardenburg syndrome (q.v.), or the piebald trait (q.v.) is not clear. The melanocytes of the uveal trait constitute a branching pseudo-syncytium richly innervated by sympathetic nerves. Pigmentation of the iris does not occur in the absence of this innervation. Sympathetic fibers leave the lateral horn of the gray matter of the first and second thoracic segments, pass out in the anterior roots and join the lateral sympathetic chain via the white rami communicantes. They then proceed to the superior cervical ganglion and along the distribution of the carotid artery to the head. Congenital Horner syndrome with associated heterochromia iridis can be produced by birth injury to the lower roots of the brachial plexus (Klumpke palsy). Heterochromia iridis is the designation which the purist reserves for different pigmentation in sectors of one iris, whereas heterochromia iridum is the term used when the two irides are of different color.

Calhoun, F. P.: Causes of heterochromia iridis with special reference to paralysis of the cervical sympathetics. Am. J. Ophthal. 2: 255-269, 1919.

Gladstone, R. M.: Development and significance of heterochromia of the iris. Arch. Neurol. 21: 184-192, 1969.

*14260 HEXOKINASE-1

Schimke and Grossbard (1968) reviewed studies of hexokinase isozymes. Shows (1973) presented evidence that hexokinase and cytoplasmic glutamate oxaloacetic transaminase are linked and are on chromosome no. 10.

Altay, C., Alpers, C. A. and Nathan, D. G.: Normal and variant isoenzymes of human blood cell hexokinase and the isoenzyme pattern in hemolytic anemia. Blood 36: 219-227, 1970.

Schimke, R. T. and Grossbard, L.: Studies on isozymes of hexokinase in animal tissues. Ann. N.Y. Acad. Sci. 151: 332-350, 1968.

Shows, T. B.: Genetic linkage of hexokinase and cytoplasmic glutamate oxaloacetic transaminase in man-mouse cell hybrids. Intern. Workshop, New Haven, Conn. June, 1973.

*14263 HEXOKINASE, WHITE CELL

Harris and Hopkinson (1972) made reference to unpublished data of the M. R. C. Human Biochemical Genetics Unit, Galton Laboratory, indicating polymorphism with frequency of heterozygosity of about 5 percent in Europeans.

Harris, H. and Hopkinson, D. A.: Average heterozygosity per locus in man: an estimate based on the incidence of enzyme polymorphisms. Ann. Hum. Genet. 36: 9-20, 1972.

*14265 HEXOSAMINIDASE B

The nature of the mutation in Tay-Sachs disease (27280), which shows deficiency of hexosaminidase A, is not known. Furthermore, the relationship between the A and B forms of hexosaminidase is not known. However, at least one structural locus is, presumably, concerned with hexosaminidase B. By study of somatic cell hybrids, Gilbert et al. (1974) showed; that a locus determining hexosaminidase B is on chromosome No. 5. See 27280 for similar information concerning hexosaminidase A.

Gilbert, F., Kucherlapati, R., Creagan, R. P., Murnane, M. J., Darlington, G. J. and Ruddle, F. H.: Tay-Sachs' disease: the assignment of genes for hexosaminidase A and B to chromosomes 7 and 5 in man. Proc. Natl. Acad. Sci., in press, 1974.

Lalley, P. A., Rattazzi, M. C. and Shows, T. B.: Human beta-D-N-Acetylhexosaminidase A and B: expression and linkage relationships in somatic hybrids. Proc. Natl. Acad. Sci. 71: 1569-1573, 1974.

Swallow, D. M., Stokes, D. C., Corney, G. and Harris, H.: Differences between the N-acetyl hexosaminidase isozymes in serum and tissues. Ann. Hum. Genet. 37: 287-302, 1974.

14270 HIP, DISLOCATION OF, CONGENITAL

The genetics is considered complex. Joint laxity, normally greater in females than in males, probably accounts for the preponderance of affected females over males. Persistent laxity (q.v.), often of familial nature, is probably a factor especially in males. Hip dysplasia with dislocation occurs in high frequency in the German shepherd dog. Autosomal dominant inheritance is favored by Bornfors, Palsson and Skude (1964). Dislocation of the hip is an occasional feature of conditions with simple inheritance, e.g., Marfan syndrome and Ehlers-Danlos syndrome. Record and Edwards (1958) estimated the risk of recurrence in subsequently born sibs to be about 5 percent.

Bornfors, S., Palsson, K. and Skude, G.: Hereditary aspects of hip dysplasia in german shepherd dogs. J. Am. Vet. Med. Assoc. 145: 15-20, 1964.

Carter, C. O. and Wilkinson, J. A.: Genetic and environmental factors in the etiology of congenital dislocation of the hip. Clin. Orthop. 33: 119-128, 1964.

Carter, C. O. and Wilkinson, J. A.: Persistent joint laxity and congenital dislocation of the hip. J. Bone Joint Surg. 46B: 40-45, 1964.

Record, R. G. and Edwards, J. H.: Environmental influences related to the etiology of congenital dislocation of the hip. Brit. J. Prev. Soc. Med. 12: 8-22, 1958.

*14273 HISTIOCYTIC DERMATOARTHRITIS

Four members of a family, father, daughter and two sons, presented with papulo-nodular eruptions, symmetric arthritis and ocular lesions. Zayid and Farraj (1973) described this condition as resembling, but distinct from multicentric reticulohistiocytosis. The four affected family members showed multiple benign cutaneous histiocytic nodules on the face and limbs (no xanthelasmas or mucosal lesions were noted) and symmetric destructive seronegative rheumatoid-like polyarthritis. The father and two sons showed ocular lesions including glaucoma, uveitis and cataracts. This condition had an onset early in childhood for the sibs and in adolescence for the father.

Zayid,,I. and Farraj, S.: Familial histiocytic dermatoarthritis. A new syndrome. Am. J. Med. 54: 793-800, 1973.

*14274 HISTOCOMPATABILITY ANTIGEN — 5(Ke) SYSTEM

The 5 (or Ke) system involves antigens shared by leukocytes and other tissues, except red cells. In this it is like HL-A (14280). It is not linked to HL-A and has weak histocompatibility properties. The Ke antibody was discovered in a multiparous woman (Lalezari and Bernard, 1965).

Lalezari, P. and Bernard, G. E.: Identification of a specific leukocyte antigen: another presumed example of 5(b). Transfusion 5: 135-142, 1965.

14275 HISTONE IV

In its 110 amino acids histone IV of cattle and garden peas differ by only two (Delange and Smith, 1971).

Delange, R. J. and Smith, E. L.: Histones: structure and function. Ann. Rev. Biochem. 40: 279-314, 1971.

*14280 HL-A HISTOCOMPATIBILITY TYPE, LA OR FIRST SEGREGANT SERIES

Bach and Amos (1967) concluded that a single locus with 15 or more alleles controls reactivity in mixed leukocyte culture tests, and that genes at this locus also control most of the specificities measured by cytotoxic antiserums to leukocytes. This may be the major histocompatibility locus in man. Bernard (1967) called discovery of the Hu-1 (now called HL-A) system as important an event in biology as discovery of the ABO and Rh systems, perhaps more important. HL-A in the new nomenclature means 'human leukocyte' and A refers to the fact that this is the first locus designated. The usefulness of HL-A typing for selection of kidney donors was demonstrated by Patel et al. (1968). By gel filtration Mann et al. (1969) separated soluble preparations of HL-A alloantigens into components having either 'LA' specificity or '4' specificity. This may indicate that the HL-A 'locus' is a region with several different cistrons. Furthermore, family data indicates the existence of two 'segregant series.' Antigens 1, 2, 3, 9, 10 and 11 are mutually exclusive members of one allelic series whereas a different array of antigens constitute a second series (Bach and Bach, 1970). The relation of the isoantigenic variants identified in human fibroblast cultures to the HL-A system is not known. Both the HL-A system in man and the H-2 system in mice seem to have haploid expression in sperm. Recombination has been observed within the HL-A system (Bodmer et al., 1970). The LA and 4 loci are very closely linked (Kissmeyer-Nielsen and Thorsby, 1970). The ratio of female to male recombination fractions is 1.6 (Lamm et al., 1971). The HL-A loci are linked to the PGM(3) locus, the distance being about 0.15 morgans in females (Lamm et al., 1971). Linkage with the alpha haptoglobin locus is suspected (Bias, 1970) but not proved. Lamm et al. (1972) reviewed the evidence that the 4 and LA loci are about 1 centimorgan apart and presented evidence that the PGM-3 locus is on the 4 side of the HL-A region. Kissmeyer-Nielsen et al. (1972) reviewed the genetics of HL-A, including the close linkage of 'LA' and '4' and the linkage of HL-A. An immune response locus (14685) is thought to be closely linked to the HL-A locus or part of the HL-A region. Studies of HL-A antigens solubilized from cell membranes indicate that the products of the two loci reside on different molecules,- and no firm linkage between the two molecular products exists in the cell membrane. Solheim et al. (1973) presented evidence for a third segregant HL-A series, the 'AJ' series. AJ appears to be between LA and FOUR but closer to FOUR. Weitkamp et al. (1974) showed that recombination between the LA and FOUR loci was 50 percent greater in females than in males but age had no effect. The chimpanzee has two main allelic series of leukocyte antigens (Balner et al., 1974) and the Rhesus monkey has histocompatibility-linked immune-response genes (Dorf et al., 1974).

Adman, R. and Pious, D. A.: Isoantigenic variants: isolation from human diploid cells in culture. Science 168: 370-372, 1970.

Bach, F. H. and Amos, D. B.: Hu-1 major histocompatibility locus in man. Science 156: 1506-1508, 1967.

Bach, M. L. and Bach, F. H.: The genetics of histocompatibility. Hosp. Practice 5 (no. 8): 33-44, 1970.

Balner, H., D'Amaro, J. and Visser, T. P.: Tissue typing of chimpanzees: I. Evidence for two allelic series of leukocyte antigens. Transplant. Proc. 6: 141-149, 1974.

Bernard, J.: La decouverte du systeme principal d'histocompatibilite de l'homme. (Editorial) Presse Med. 75: 2369 only, 1967.

Bias, W. B.: Baltimore, Md.: personal communication, 1970.

Bodmer, W. F.: Evolutionary significance of the HL-A system. Nature, 237: 139-145, 1972.

Bodmer, W. F., Bodmer, J. G. and Tripp, M.: Recombination between the LA and 4 loci of the HL-A system. In, Histocompatibility Testing. Copenhagen: Munksgaard, 1970. Pp. 187-191.

Bodmer, W. F., Bodmer, J. G., Adler, S., Payne, R. and Bialek, J.: Genetics of '4' and 'LA' human leukocyte groups. Ann. N.Y. Acad. Sci. 129: 473-489, 1966.

Ceppellini, R. and Van Rood, J. J.: The HL-A system. I. Genetics and molecular biology. Seminars in Hemat. 11: 233-252, 1974.

Dausset, J.: Similarities between the HL-A system and other immunogenetic systems. (Editorial) Vox Sang. 23: 153-164, 1972.

Dausset, J., Ivanyi, P., Colombani, J., Feingold, N. and Legrand, L.: Le systeme Hu-1. Etudes genetiques de population et de familles. Nouv. Rev. Fr. Hematol. 7: 897-899, 1967.

Dorf, M. E., Balner, H., De Groot, M. L. and Benaceraff, B.: Histocompatibility-linked immune-response genes in the Rhesus monkey. Transplant. Proc. 6: 119-124, 1974.

Edwards, J. H., Allen, F. H., Glenn, K. P., Lamm, L. U., and Robson, E. B.: The linkage relationships of HL-A. Histocompatibility Workshop 1972.

Engelfriet, C. P. and Britten, A.: The cytotoxic test for leucocyte antibodies. A simple and reliable technique. Vox. Sang. 10: 660-674, 1965.

Fellous, M. and Dausset, J.: Probable haploid expression of HL-A antigens on human spermatozoon. Nature 225: 191-193, 1970.

Kissmeyer-Nielsen, F. and Thorsby, E.: Human transplantation antigens. Transplant. Rev. 4: 1-176, 1970.

Kissmeyer-Nielsen, F., Jorgensen, F. and Lamm, L. U.: The HL-A system in clinical medicine. Johns Hopkins Med. J., in press, 1972.

Kissmeyer-Nielsen, F., Svejgaard, A. and Hauge, M.: Genetics of the human HL-A transplantation system. Nature 219: 1116-1119, 1968.

Kissmeyer-Nielsen, F., Svejgaard, A., Ahrons, S. and Nielsen, L. S.: Crossing-over within the HL-A system. Nature 224: 75-76, 1969.

Lamm, L. U., Svejgaard, A. and Kissmeyer-Nielsen, F.: Further evidence for PGM(3): HL-A is another linkage in man. Nature 231: 109-110, 1971.

Lamm, L. U., Kissmeyer-Nielsen, F., Svejgaard, A., Petersen, G. B., Thorsby, E., Mayr, W. and Hogman, C.: On the orientation of the HL-A region and the PGM(3) locus in the chromosome. Tissue Antigens 2: 205-214, 1972.

Mann, D. L., Rogentine, G. N., Jr., Fahey, J. L. and Nathenson, S. G.: Molecular heterogeneity of human lymphoid (HL-A) alloantigens. Science 163: 1460-1462, 1969.

Patel, R., Mickey, M. R. and Terasaki, P. I.: Serotyping for homotransplantation of kidneys from unrelated donors. N. Engl. J. Med. 279: 501-506, 1968.

Payne, R., Tripp, M., Weigle, J., Bodmer, W. F. and Bodmer, J. G.: A new leukocyte isoantigen system in man. Cold Spring Harbor Symposia Quant. Biol. 29: 285-295, 1964.

Solheim, B. G., Bratlie, A., Sandberg, L., Staub-Nielsen, L. and Thorsby, E.: Further evidence of a third HL-A locus. Tissue Antigens 3: 439-453, 1973.

Thorsby, E., Sandberg, L., Lindholm, A. and Kissmeyer-Nielsen, F.: The HL-A system. Evidence of a third sub-locus. Scand. J. Haematol. 7: 195-200, 1970.

Van Leeuwen, A., Eernisse, J. G. and Van Rood, J. J.: A new leucocyte group with two alleles: leucocyte group five. Vox Sang. 9: 431-446, 1964.

Van Rood, J. J. and Van Leeuwen, A.: Leukocyte grouping. A method and its application. J. Clin. Invest. 42: 1382-1390, 1963.

Van Rood, J. J.: Leucocyte grouping and organ transplantation. Br. J. Haematol. 16: 211-220, 1969.

Van Rood, J. J.: Tissue typing and organ transplantation. Lancet I: 1142-1146, 1969.

Van Someren, H., Westerveld, A., Hagemeijer, A., Mees, J. R., Meera Khan, P. and Zaalberg, O. B.: Human antigen and enzyme markers in man-Chinese hamster somatic cell hybrids: evidence for synteny between the HL-A, PGM-3, ME-1, and IPO-B loci. Proc. Natl. Acad. Sci. 71: 962-965, 1974.

Walford, R. L., Finkelstein, S., Hanna, C. and Collins, Z.: Third sublocus in the HL-A human transplantation system. Nature 224: 74-75, 1969.

Weitkamp, L. R., Van Rood, J. J., Thorsby, E., Bias, W., Fotino, M., Lawler, S. D., Dausset, J., Mayr, W. R., Bodmer, J., Ward, F. S., Seignalet, J., Payne, R., Kissmeyer-Nielsen, F., Gatti, R. A., Sachs, J. A. and Lamm, L. U.: The relation of parental sex and age to recombination in the HL-A system. Hum. Hered. 23: 197-205, 1973.

*14283 HL-A HISTOCOMPATIBILITY TYPE, FOUR OR SECOND SEGREGANT SERIES

See 14280.

*14284 HL-A HISTOCOMPATIBILITY TYPE, A-J OR THIRD SEGREGANT SERIES

See 14280.

14285 HL-A MODIFIER

Bias et al. (1973) presented evidence for the existence of an unlinked gene which modifies HL-A antigen expression. In a sibship of seven, three of four individuals who inherited the haplotype W29-W10 showed modified expression of W10.

Bias, W. B., Hopkins, K. A., Hutchinson, J. R. and Hsu, S. H.: Evidence for an unlinked gene which modifies HL-A antigen expression. Tissue Antigens 4: 36-41, 1974.

*14290 HOLT-ORAM SYNDROME (HEART AND HAND SYNDROME)

Although the abnormality of the upper extremities is more extensive in some cases, the characteristic finding is thumb anomaly with atrial septal defect. The thumb may be absent or may be a triphalangeal, non-opposable, finger-like digit. The thumb metacarpal has both a proximal and a distal epiphyseal ossification center. McKusick (1961) reported mother and daughter with atrial septal defect and absent or triphalangeal, finger-like thumb. In 1966 the daughter gave birth to a male infant with upper extremity phocomelia and ventricular septal defect. The involvement of the arm was more extensive and the cardiovascular involvement more varied in the families described by Lewis et al. (1965) and Harris et al. (1966) than in that of Holt and Oram (1960). However it is not certain that these represent a separate mutation. Poznanski et al. (1970) pointed out that carpal abnormalities, e.g. extra carpal bones, are more specific for the Holt-Oram syndrome than changes in the thumb. Posteriorly and laterally protruberant medial epicondyles of the humerus were seen in several patients. Rybak et al. (1971) described many cases in four generations of a Polish family and concluded that partial deletion of the long arm of a B-group chromosome was related to the abnormality. They suggested that the single case of Ockey et al. (1967) had the Holt-Oram syndrome: a similar deletion of the long arm of a group B chromosome was present.

Emerit, I., De Grouchy, J., Laval-Jeantet, M., Corone, P. and Vernant, P.: Malformations complexes des membres superieurs associees a une cardiopathie congenitale. A propos de six observations. Acta Genet. Med. Gemellol. 14: 132-163, 1965.

Gall, J. C., Jr., Stern, A. M., Cohen, M. M., Adams, M. S. and Davidson, R. T.: Holt-Oram syndrome: clinical and genetic study of a large family. Am. J. Hum. Genet. 18: 187-200, 1966.

Harris, L. C. and Osborne, W. P.: Congenital absence or hypoplasia of the radius with ventricular septal defect: ventriculo-radial dysplasia. J. Pediatr. 68: 265-272, 1966.

Holt, M. and Oram, S.: Familial heart disease with skeletal malformations. Br. Heart J. 22: 236-242, 1960.

Lewis, K. B., Bruce, R. A., Baum, D. and Motulsky, A. G.: The upper limb-cardiovascular syndrome. An autosomal dominant genetic effect on embryogenesis. J.A.M.A. 193: 1080-1086, 1965.

McKusick, V. A. and colleagues: Medical genetics 1960. J. Chronic Dis. 14: 1-198, 1961 (fig. 45).

Ockey, C. H., Feldman, G. V., MacAulay, M. E. and Delaney, M. J.: A large deletion of the long arm of chromosome no. 4 in a child with limb abnormalities. Arch. Dis. Child. 42: 428-434, 1967.

Poznanski, A. K., Gall, J. C., Jr. and Stern, A. M.: Skeletal manifestations of the Holt-Oram syndrome. Radiology 94: 45-54, 1970.

Rybak, M., Kozlowski, K., Kleczkowska, A., Lewandowska, J., Sokolowski, J. and Soltysik-Wilk, E.: Holt-Oram syndrome associated with ectromelia and chromosomal aberrations. Am. J. Dis. Child. 121: 490-495, 1971.

*14300 HORNER SYNDROME

Durham (1958) described congenital Horner syndrome in a boy and his father, paternal aunt and uncle and a first cousin. The boy showed ptosis and pupillary changes on the left. The right iris was brown, the left blue. These findings like those of Calhoun (1919) illustrate the role of normal sympathetic innervation of the iris in its pigmentation.

Calhoun, F. P.: Causes of heterochromia iridis with special reference to paralysis of cervical sympathetic. Am. J. Ophthalmol. 2: 256-269, 1919.

Durham, D. G.: Congenital hereditary Horner's syndrome. Arch. Ophthalmol. 60: 939-940, 1958.

*14310 HUNTINGTON CHOREA

Choreic movements and dementia are the leading features. The age at onset is highly variable: some show signs in the first decade and some not until over 60 years of age. The mode is between 30 and 40 years (Chandler and colleagues, 1960). Reed and Neel (1959), in a study of 196 kindreds, found only eight in which both parents of a single patient with Huntington chorea were 60 years of age or older and normal. Reed and Chandler (1958) estimated the frequency of recognized Huntington chorea in the Michigan lower peninsula to be about 4.12 x 10 (to the minus 5), and the total frequency of heterozygotes to be about 1.01 x 10 (to the minus 4). Vessie (1932) traced the ancestry of the families studied by Huntington. About 1000 cases in twelve generations descendant from two brothers in Suffolk, England, could be identified. The intrafamilial variability is illustrated by the report by Campbell et al. (1961) of the juvenile rigid form in two brothers in a kindred in which for three preceding generations disease of more classic type had occurred. Barbeau (1970) pointed out that patients with the juvenile form of Huntington chorea seem more often to have inherited their disorder from the father than from the mother. Brackenridge (1972) showed a relationship between age of onset of symptoms in parent and child. Wallace and Hall (1972) suggested that in Queensland, Australia, two possibly allelic forms may exist, one with early onset and one with late onset.

Barbeau, A.: Parental ascent in the juvenile form of Huntington's chorea. (Letter) Lancet II: 937 only, 1970.

Bird, E. D., Caro, A. J. and Pilling, J. B.: A sex related factor in the inheritance of Huntington's chorea. Ann. Hum. Genet. 37: 255-260, 1974.

Brackenridge, C. J.: Familial correlations for age at onset and age at death in Huntington's disease. J. Med. Genet. 9: 23-32, 1972.

Brackenridge, C. J.: The relation of type of initial symptoms and line of transmission to ages at onset and death in Huntington's disease. Clin. Genet. 2: 287-297, 1971.

Brackenridge, C. J.: Relationship of parental age of ridigity in Huntington's disease. J. Med. Genet. 11: 136-140, 1974.

Byers, R. K. and Dodge, J. A.: Huntington's chorea in children: report of four cases. Neurology 17: 587-596, 1967.

Campbell, A. M. G., Corner, B. D., Norman, R. M. and Urich, H.: The rigid form of Huntington's disease. J. Neurol. Neurosurg. Psychiatry 24: 71-77, 1961.

Chandler, J. H., Reed, T. E. and Dejong, R. N.: Huntington's chorea in Michigan. Neurology 10: 148-153, 1960.

Klawans, H. L., Jr., Paulson, G. W., Ringel, S. P. and Barbeau, A.: L-dopa in the detection of presymptomatic Huntington's chorea. N. Engl. J. Med. 286: 1332-1334, 1972.

Lyon, R. L.: Huntington's chorea in the Moray Firth area. Br. Med. J. 1: 1301-1306, 1962.

Myrianthopoulos, N. C.: Huntington's chorea. J. Med. Genet. 3: 298-314, 1966.

Perry, T. L., Hansen, S. and Kloster, M.: Huntington's chorea, deficiency of gamma-amniobutyric acid in brain. N. Engl. J. Med. 7: 337-342, 1974.

Reed, T. E. and Chandler, J. H.: Huntington's chorea in Michigan. I. Demography and genetics. Am. J. Hum. Genet. 10: 201-225, 1958.

Reed, T. E. and Neel, J. V.: Huntington's chorea in Michigan. II. Selection and mutation. Am. J. Hum. Genet. 11: 107-136, 1959.

Vessie, P. R.: Original article on the transmission of Huntington's chorea for 300 years — the Bures family group. J. Nerv. Ment. Dis. 76: 553-573, 1932.

Wallace, D. C. and Hall, A. C.: Evidence of genetic heterogeneity in Huntington's chorea. J. Neurol. Neurosurg. Psychiatry 35: 789-800, 1972.

*14320 HYALOIDEO-RETINAL DEGENERATION OF WAGNER

Wagner (1938) described 13 members of a Canton Zurich family with a peculiar lesion of the vitreous and retina. Ten additional affected members were observed by Boehringer, Dieterle and Landolt (1960) and 5 more by Ricci (1961). In Holland Jansen (1962) described two families with a total of 39 affected persons. Alexander and Shea (1965) reported a family. In the last report, characteristic facies (epicanthus, broad sunken nasal bridge, receeding chin) was noted. Genu valgum was present in all. In addition to typical changes in the vitreous, retinal detachment occurs in some and cataract is another complication. See

AUTOSOMAL RECESSIVE HYALOIDEO-TAPETORETINAL DEGENERATION OF FAVRE. Irregular autosomal dominant inheritance was suggested by van Balen and Falger (1970) on the basis of three large pedigrees and the syndromal association of cleft palate was emphasized. This disorder is, of course, a 'cause' of familial retinal detachment (Edmund, 1961). Marshall (1958) reported four generations of a family in which seven members had (1) nasal defect and facies characteristic of anhidrotic ectodermal dysplasia; (2) congenital and juvenile cataracts; (3) myopia and fluid vitreous; (4) spontaneous, sudden maturation and absorption of congenital cataract; (5) luxation of cataract; (6) congenital hearing loss. Deficiency in sweating was minimal. The transmission was dominant. Ruppert et al. (1970) described father and daughter with features like those in Marshall's family, namely, saddle nose, myopia, and deafness and in the father cataracts. Cohen et al. (1971) described a father and two sons and two daughters with myopia, hyaloideo-retinal degeneration, retinal detachment, flat face from maxillary hypoplasia, and in the father and two of his children submucous cleft palate. Families which the authors felt had the same disorder also included those reported by Delaney et al. (1963) and Frandsen (1966). Retinal detachment with complicating cataract and cleft palate occurred in multiple members of a family reported by Delaney et al. (1963). Two brothers reported as Pierre Robin syndrome with eye complications by Smith and Stowe (1961) and by Smith (1969) probably had this condition (see 26180). Differentiation of the Wagner syndrome and the Stickler syndrome (10830) are difficult. Zellweger et al. (1974) considered Marshall syndrome a separate and distinct entity. They provided a report of the third recorded family, the others being those of Marshall (1958) and Ruppert et al. (1970).

Alexander, R. L. and Shea, M.: Wagner's disease. Arch. Ophthalmol. 74: 310-318, 1965.

Boehringer, H. R., Dieterle, P. and Landolt, E.: Zur Klinik und Pathologie der degeneratio hyaloideo-retinalis hereditaria (Wagner). Ophthalmologica 139: 330-338, 1960.

Bundey, S. E. and Leffler, A. T.: Retinal degeneration and midline submucous cleft of the palate (Wagner-Cervenka syndrome). In, Bergsma, D. (ed.): Clinical Delineation of Birth Defects. XVI. Urinary System and Others. Baltimore: Williams and Wilkins, 1974. Pp. 342-343.

Cohen, M. M., Jr., Knobloch, W. H. and Gorlin, R. J.: A dominantly inherited syndrome of hyaloideo-retinal degeneration, cleft palate, and maxillary hypoplasia (Cervenka's syndrome). The Clinical Delineation of Birth Defects. XI. Orofacial Structures. Baltimore: Williams and Wilkins, 1971.

Delaney, W. V., Podedeuorny, W. and Havener, W. H.: Inherited retinal detachment. Arch. Ophthalmol. 69: 44-50, 1963.

Edmund, J.: Familial retinal detachment. Acta Ophthalmol. 39: 644-654, 1961.

Frandsen, E.: Hereditary hyaloideo-retinal degeneration (Wagner) in a Danish family. Acta Ophthalmol. 44: 223-232, 1966.

Jansen, L. M. A. A.: Degeneratio hyaloideo-retinalis hereditaria. Ophthalmologica 144: 458-464, 1962.

Marshall, D.: Ectodermal dysplasia: report of kindred with ocular abnormalities and hearing defect. Am. J. Ophthalmol. 45: 143-156, 1958.

Ricci, A.: Clinique et transmission hereditaire des degenerescences vitreo-retiniennes. Bull. Soc. Ophthalmol. Fr. 61: 618-662, 1961.

Ruppert, E. S., Buerk, E. and Pfordresher, M. F.: Hereditary hearing loss with saddle-nose and myopia. Arch. Otolaryngol. 92: 95-98, 1970.

Smith, J. L. and Stowe, F. R.: The Pierre Robin syndrome (glossoptosis, micrognathia, cleft palate). A review of 39 cases with emphasis on associated ocular lesions. Pediatrics 27: 128-133, 1961.

Smith, W. K.: Pierre Robin syndrome in brothers. The Clinical Delineation of Birth Defects. II. Malformation Syndromes. New York: National Foundation, 1969. Pp. 220-221.

Van Balen, A. T. M. and Falger, E. L. F.: Hereditary hyaloideo-retinal degeneration and palatoschisis. Arch. Ophthalmol. 83: 152-162, 1970.

Wagner, H.: Ein bisher unbekanntes Erbleiden des Auges (degeneratio hyaloideo-retinalis hereditaria), beobachtet im Kanton Zuerich. Klin. Mbl. Augenheilk. 100: 840-858, 1938.

Zellweger, H., Smith, J. K. and Grutzner, P.: The Marshall syndrome: report of a new family. J. Pediatr. 84: 868-871, 1974.

14340 HYDRONEPHROSIS

Cannon (1954) described a curious family in which five males in three successive generations had unilateral hydronephrosis. MacKay (1945) observed congenital megalo-ureters with hydronephrosis in 3 sibs (bilateral in 2). Two other sibs were said to have died of congenital sarcoma of the kidney. The paternal grandfather died of pyonephrosis. The father died of cerebral hemorrhage at 56. Jewell and Buchert (1962) observed four cases in three generations. Aaron and Robbins (1948) found hydronephrosis without hydroureters and aberrant renal vessels possibly responsible for obstruction at the uretero-pelvic junction in sibs. Simpson and German (1970) described seven families with multiple cases of urinary trait anomalies, most of them a form of obstructive uropathy and reviewed the literature on cases in sibs, twins and other relatives.

Aaron, G. and Robbins, M. A.: Hydronephrosis due to aberrant vessels: remarkable familial incidence with report of cases. J. Urol. 60: 702-705, 1948.

Cannon, J. F.: Hereditary unilateral hydronephrosis. Ann. Intern. Med. 41: 1054-1060, 1954.

Grosse, F. R., Kaveggia, L. and Opitz, J. M.: Familial hydronephrosis. Z. Kinderheilk. 114: 313-322, 1973.

Jewell, J. H. and Buchert, W. I.: Unilateral hereditary hydronephrosis: a report of four cases in three consecutive generations. J. Urol. 88: 129-136, 1962.

MacKay, H.: Congenital bilateral megalo-ureters with hydronephrosis. A remarkable family history. Proc. R. Soc. Med. 38: 567-568, 1945.

Simpson, J. L. and German, J.: Familial urinary tract anomalies. (Letter) J.A.M.A. 212: 2264 only, 1970.

*14350 HYPERBILIRUBINEMIA I (GILBERT DISEASE)

In a series of 58 patients, Foulk and colleagues (1959) found a family history of jaundice in 8 and in 5 of these jaundice had been present in successive generations. Billing, Williams and Richards (1964) presented indirect evidence of a defect of uptake of bilirubin into the liver cell. This disorder is difficult to distinguish from prolonged post-hepatitic hyperbilirubinemia. The characteristics are normal liver function tests of the usual type, normal liver histology, no evidence of hemolysis and delayed clearance of bilirubin from the blood (Nixon and Monahan, 1967). Powell et al. (1967) observed affected persons in successive generations. Black and Billing (1969) found hepatic bilirubin UDP-transferase to be about 25 percent of normal in 11 patients with Gilbert syndrome.

Berk, P. D., Bloomer, J. R., Howe, R. B. and Berlin, N. I.: Constitutional hepatic dysfunction (Gilbert's syndrome). A new definition based on kinetic studies with unconjugated radiobilirubin. Am. J. Med. 49: 296-305, 1970.

Billing, B. H., Williams, R. and Richards, T. G.: Defects in hepatic transport of bilirubin in congenital hyperbilirubinaemia: an analysis of plasma bilirubin disappearance curves. Clin. Sci. 27: 245-257, 1964.

Black, M. and Billing, B. H.: Hepatic bilirubin UDP-glucoronyl transferase activity in liver disease and Gilbert's syndrome. N. Engl. J. Med. 280: 1266-1271, 1969.

Black, M. and Sherlock, S.: Treatment of Gilbert's syndrome with phenobarbitone. Lancet I: 1359-1361, 1970.

Foulk, W. T., Butt, H. R., Owen, C. A., Jr. Whitcomb, F. F., Jr. and Mason, H. L.: Constitutional hepatic dysfunction (Gilbert's disease): its natural history and related syndromes. Medicine 38: 25-46, 1959.

Nixon, J. C. and Monahan, G. J.: Gilbert's disease and the bilirubin tolerance test. Canad. Med. Assoc. J. 96: 370-373, 1967.

Powell, L. W., Hemingway, E., Billing, B. H. and Sherlock, S.: Idiopathic unconjugated hyperbilirubinemia (Gilbert's syndrome). A study of 42 families. N. Engl. J. Med. 277: 1108-1112, 1967.

Schmid, R.: Hyperbilirubinemia. In, Stanbury, J. B., Wyngaarden, J. B. and Fredrickson, D. S. (eds.): The Metabolic Basis of Inherited Disease. New York: McGraw-Hill, 1972 (3rd Ed.). Pp. 1141-1178.

14370 HYPERBILIRUBINEMIA III (ROTOR DISEASE)

Like the Dubin-Johnson syndrome this is a form of conjugated hyperbilirubinemia. The two disorders are not clearly distinguished. Three sibs from a first-cousin marriage were affected in the family reported by Pereira Lima, Utz and Roisenberg (1966), suggesting recessive inheritance. Dollinger et al. (1967) observed father and 3 of 5 children with what they considered to be the Rotor syndrome. However, occult hemolysis was also present.

Dollinger, M. R., Brandborg, L. L., Sartor, V. E. and Bernstein, J. M.: Chronic familial hyperbilirubinemia. Hepatic defects associated with occult hemolysis. Gastroenterology 52: 875-881, 1967.

Pereira Lima, J. E., Utz, E. and Roisenberg, I.: Hereditary nonhemolytic conjugated hyperbilirubinemia without abnormal liver cell pigmentation. A family study. Am. J. Med. 40: 628-633, 1966.

Schiff, L., Billing, B. H. and Oikawa, Y.: Familial nonhemolytic jaundice with conjugated bilirubin in the serum: a case study. N. Engl. J. Med. 260: 1315-1318, 1959.

*14380 HYPERBILIRUBINEMIA, ARIAS TYPE

Arias (1962) demonstrated glucuronyl transferase deficiency in eight patients with chronic nonhemolytic jaundice and serum unconjugated bilirubin levels of 6.2 to 18.8 mg. percent. Arias et al. (1969) concluded that this is a disorder distinct from Crigler-Najjar syndrome, which also has deficiency of hepatic glucuronyl transferase activity. In the Crigler-Najjar type hyperbilirubinemia is severe and frequently accompanied by kernicterus. The bile is almost colorless and contains traces of unconjugated bilirubin only. Transmission is autosomal recessive and phenobarbital does not influence the hyperbilirubinemia. In the Arias type bilirubinemia is less severe without kernicterus. The bile is pigmented and contains bilirubin glucuronide. The transmission is autosomal dominant. Phenobarbital administration causes prompt disappearance of jaundice. Since patients with the Arias type have a disorder almost only of cosmetic significance, long-term phenobarbital treatment is useful. The response to phenobarbital, which may represent induction, and the dominant inheritance lead me to suspect that the defect in the Arias type is in a controller gene and not in the structural gene for glucuronyl transferase. Sleisenger et al. (1967) described an Irish kindred in which persons with life-long jaundice occurred in 4 generations, in a dominant pedigree pattern with male-to-male transmission. Hepatic glucuronyl transferase activity was low in affected individuals, by direct or indirect test. The condition differs from the Crigler-Najjar syndrome (which has deficiency of the same enzyme) in mode of inheritance, lack of brain damage and favorable prognosis. It is probably the the same condition as that reported by Arias (1962).

Arias, I. M.: Chronic unconjugated hyperbilirubinemia without overt signs of hemolysis in adolescents and adults. J. Clin. Invest. 41: 2233-2245, 1962.

Arias, I. M., Gartner, L. M., Cohen, M., Ben-Ezzer, J. and Levi, A. J.: Chronic nonhemolytic unconjugated hyperbilirubinemia with glucuronyl transferase deficiency: clinical, biochemical, pharmacologic and genetic evidence for heterogeneity. Am. J. Med. 47: 395-409, 1969.

Sleisenger, M. H., Kahn, I., Barniville, H., Rubin, W., Ben Ezzer, J. and Arias, I. M.: Nonhemolytic unconjugated hyperbilirubinemia with hepatic glucuronyl transferase deficiency: a genetic study in four generations. Trans. Assoc. Am. Physicians 80: 259-266, 1967.

*14385 HYPERBRADYKININISM

This familial disorder is characterized by orthostatic light-headedness of syncope, facial erythema, excessive orthostatic fall in pulse pressure and rise in pulse rate, ecchymoses and purple discoloration of the legs after standing (Streeten et al., 1972). Plasma concentrations of bradykinin were elevated. Impaired destruction of circulating bradykinin was suggested, because of low concentrations of bradykininase-I. Clinical improvement occurred with administration of propranolol, fluorocortisone or cyproheptadine ('Periactin'). The families described were three in number: a woman and her daughter, a 23-year-old female student and her 50-year-old father and 16-year-old brother, another woman and her daughter.

Streeten, D. H. P., Kerr, L. P., Kerr, C., Prior, J. C. and Dalakos, T. G.: Hyperbradykininism: a new orthostatic syndrome. Lancet II: 1048-1053, 1972.

14400 HYPERHEPARINEMIA

Congenital hemorrhagic diathesis due to an excess of a clotting inhibitor has not been fully established. Quick (1957) diagnosed congenital hyperheparinemia in a woman with abnormal bleeding from age 3. Heni and Krauss (1956) described a similar condition in a father and daughter. In both instances the in vitro clotting defect was repaired by protamine sulphate and by toluidine blue, and Quick achieved correction of the defect in vivo as well.

Heni, F. and Krauss, I.: Angeborene familiaere Gerinnungsstoerung durch heparinartigen Hemmkoerper. Klin. Wschr. 34: 747-749, 1956.

Quick, A. J.: Hemorrhagic Diseases. Philadelphia: Lea and Febiger, 1957.

14410 HYPERHIDROSIS, GUSTATORY

Mailander (1967) described excessive sweating of the face with eating in five persons of three generations. There was no male-to-male transmission and one instance of 'skipped generation' was known.

Mailander, J. C.: Hereditary gustatory sweating. J.A.M.A. 201: 203-204, 1967.

14415 HYPERKERATOSIS LENTICULARIS PERSTANS

Beveridge and Langlands (1973) described 2 generations of a kindred manifesting hyperkeratosis lenticularis perstans (HLP). The mother and four children showed the typical hyperkeratotic lesions on the lower leg and dorsum of the foot, however, involvment of the trunk, thigh, arms and dorsum of the hand may occur. The pink or reddish-brown scaly papules from one to five mm. in size developed in the third or fourth decade of life. Interestingly, this family had a high incidence of skin tumors, including squamous and basal cell cancers, in areas other than those affected by the hyperkeratotic lesions. The authors suggest that there may be an inherited tendency to epithelial neoplasia in this family.

Bean (1969) first reported the familial occurrence of HLP without skin tumors. In 1970 he reported finding HLP in 3 generations of his previously documented family. HLP is sometimes called Flegel disease after the man who first described the condition.

Bean, S. F.: Hyperkeratosis lenticularis perstans. A clinical, histopathological and genetic study. Arch. Derm. 99: 705-709, 1969.

Bean, S. F.: The genetics of hyperkeratosis lenticularis perstans. Arch. Derm. 106: 72 Only, 1972.

Beveridge, G. W. and Langlands, A. O.: Familial hyperkeratosis lenticular perstans associated with tumors of the skin. Brit. J. Derm. 88: 453-458, 1973.

Flegel, H.: Hyperkeratosis lenticularis perstans. Hautarzt. 9: 362-364, 1958.

*14420 HYPERKERATOSIS, LOCALIZED EPIDERMOLYTIC

Usually this condition has not been distinguished from keratosis palmaris et plantaris. The distinguishing feature is the presence of histologic and kinetic findings of epidermolysis, despite the same clinical picture. Klaus et al. (1970) demonstrated dominant inheritance and male-to-male transmission.

Klaus, S., Weinstein, G. D. and Frost, P.: Localized epidermolytic hyperkeratosis. A form of keratoderma of the palms and soles. Arch. Dermatol. 101: 272-275, 1970.

*14425 HYPERLIPIDEMIA, COMBINED

Goldstein et al. (1973) gave the designation 'familial combined hyperlipidemia' to the most common genetic form of hyperlipidemia identified in a study of survivors of coronary occlusions. Affected persons characteristically showed elevation of both cholesterol and triglycerides in the blood. The combined disorder was shown to be distinct from familial hypercholesterolemia (Fredrickson type II 14440) and from familial hypertriglyceridemia (14575) for the following reasons: (1) lipid distributions in relatives were unique; (2) unlike familial hypercholesterolemia, children of affected persons did not express hypercholesterolemia; and

(3) informative matings suggest that variable expression of a single gene rather than segregation for two separate genes was responsible.

Goldstein, J. L., Schrott, H. G., Hazzard, W. R., Bierman, E. L. and Motulsky, A. G.: Hyperlipidemia in coronary heart disease. Genetic analysis of lipid levels in 176 families and delineation of a new inherited disorder, combined hyperlipidemia. J. Clin. Invest. 52: 1544-1568, 1973.

14430 HYPERLIPOPROTEINEMIA (TYPE II) AND DEAFNESS

Raphael and Hyde (1970) described the association of congenital deafness with type II hyperlipoproteinemia in mother and daughter.

Raphael, S. S. and Hyde, T. A.: Deaf-mutism and type-II hyperlipoproteinaemia. (Letter) Lancet I: 892 only, 1970.

*14440 HYPERLIPOPROTEINEMIA II (HYPERBETALIPOPROTEINEMIA, HYPER-LOW-DENSI-TY-LIPOPROTEINEMIA, ESSENTIAL FAMILIAL HYPERCHOLESTEROLEMIA, FAMILIAL HYPERCHOLESTEROLEMIC XANTHOMATOSIS, XANTHOMA TUBEROSUM MULTIPLEX, FAMILIAL XANTHOMA)

On a normal diet, the blood shows an increase in beta-lipoproteins. Reflecting the composition of these lipoproteins, cholesterol is increased whereas phospholipids and triglycerides remain within normal limits. This is the most frequent type of hyperlipidemia. Features are xanthoma tuberosum and tendinosum, corneal arcus, and atheromatosis. This is probably dominant with a wide range of variability of severity as is commonplace with dominants. Terminology and nosology of the hyperlipoproteinemias are confused largely because understanding is imperfect. Fredrickson and Lees (1966) make particular use of paper electrophoresis in identification of lipoprotein factors in the plasma and changes therein. In a French-Canadian kindred, Hould et al. (1969) observed hypercholesterolemia with severe xanthomatosis in three sibs and one of their second cousins. Both parents were apparently heterozygotes. Both had hypercholesterolemia and mild xanthomata, as did some relatives of each of them. Thus hyperbetalipoproteinemia might be listed in either the dominant or the recessive catalog. This phenotype may be genetically heterogeneous. For a suggested classification of the hyperlipoproteinemias, see Beaumont et al. (1970). Schrott et al. (1972) presented studies on a large Aleutian kindred supporting autosomal dominant inheritance as opposed to a polygenic basis which is considered most likely by some. The cholesterol of plasma low-density lipoprotein was elevated without change in the level of plasma triglyceride and early xanthomas and coronary atherosclerosis were associated. Goldstein and Brown (1973) studied cultured skin fibroblasts from 3 unrelated persons homozygous for the familial hypercholesterolemia gene and found a 40-60 fold higher level of activity of 3-hydroxy-3-methylglutaryl coenzyme A reductase (HMG CoA reductase), the rate-controlling enzyme in cholesterol biosynthesis. The enhanced enzyme activity resulted from complete absence of normal feedback suppression by low density lipoproteins. The HMG CoA reductase of mutant cells had apparently normal kinetics. This, coupled with the evidence that this enzyme is normally regulated not by allosteric effectors but by alterations in enzyme synthesis and degradation, suggests that the primary genetic abnormality does not involve the structural gene for the enzyme itself but rather a hitherto unidentified gene whose product is necessary for the mediation of feedback control by lipoproteins. The fibroblasts of heterozygotes showed a pattern of enzyme regulation intermediate between those of controls and homozygotes. Goldstein and Brown (1973) demonstrated that the defect involves the regulation of 3-hydroxy-3-methylglutaryl coenzyme A reductase. The hypothesis of Goldstein and Brown (1974) is that a cell-surface receptor for LDL (low density lipoprotein) is defective or missing so that both degradation of LDL and inhibition of HMG CoA reductase are impaired. Kwiterovich et al. (1974) studied the children of 90 matings in which one parent had hyperlipoproteinemia, type II, and one did not. They concluded that the data fitted a monogenic model and not a polygenic model. Goldstein (1974) observed a possible genetic compound for the type II hypercholesterolemia locus.

Beaumont, J. L., Carlson, L. A., Cooper, G. R. and Fredrickson, D. S.: Classification of hyperlipidaemias and hyperlipoproteinemias. Bull. WHO 43: 891-915, 1970.

Brown, M. S. and Goldstein, J. L.: Familial hypercholesterolemia: defective binding of lipoproteins to cultured fibroblasts associated with impaired regulation of 3-hydroxy-3-methylglutaryl coenzyme A reductase activity. Proc. Natl. Acad. Sci. 71: 788-792, 1974.

Epstein, F. H., Block, W. D., Hand, E. A. and Francis, T., Jr.: Familial hypercholesterolemia, xanthomatosis and coronary heart disease. Am. J. Med. 26: 39-53, 1959.

Fredrickson, D. S. and Levy, R. I.: Familial hyperlipoproteinemia. In, Stanbury, J. B., Wyngaarden, J. B. and Fredrickson, D. S. (eds.): The Metabolic Basis of Inherited Diseases. New York: McGraw-Hill, 1972 (3rd Ed.). Pp. 545-614.

Fredrickson, D. S.: Plasma lipoproteins: micellar models and mutants. Trans. Assoc. Am. Phys. 82: 68-86, 1969.

Fredrickson, D. S., Levy, R. I. and Lees, R. S.: Fat transport in lipoproteins-an integrated approach to mechanisms and disorders. N. Engl. J. Med. 276: 215-225, 1967.

Goldstein, J. L. and Brown, M. S.: Familial hypercholesterolemia: identification of a defect in the regulation of 3-hydroxy-3-methylglutaryl coenzyme A reductase activity associated with overproduction of cholesterol. Proc. Natl. Acad. Sci. 70: 2804-2808, 1973.

Goldstein, J. L. and Brown, M. S.: Expression of the familial hypercholesterolemia gene in heterozygotes: model for a dominant disorder in man. (Abstract) Clin. Res. 22: 559A only, 1974.

Goldstein, J. L.: Dallas, personal communication, 1974.

Harlan, W. R., Jr., Graham, J. B. and Estes, E. H.: Familial hypercholesterolemia: a genetic and metabolic study. Medicine 45: 77-110, 1966.

Hould, F., Leclerc, R. and Marcoux, J.: Essential familial hypercholesterolemia with xanthomatosis. Pediatrics 43: 455-459, 1969.

Khachadurian, A. K.: The inheritance of essential familial hypercholesterolemia. Am. J. Med. 37: 402-407, 1964.

Kwiterovich, P. O., Jr., Fredrickson, D. S. and Levy, R. I.: Familial hypercholesterolemia (one form of familial type II hyperlipoproteinemia): a study of its biochemical, genetic, and clinical presentation in childhood. J. Clin. Invest. 53: 1237-1249, 1974.

Nevin, N. C. and Slack, J.: Hyperlipidaemic xanthomatosis. II. Mode of inheritance in 55 families with essential hyperlipidaemia and xanthomatosis. J. Med. Genet. 5: 9-28, 1968.

Ott, J., Schrott, H. G., Goldstein, J. L., Hazzard, W. R., Allen, F. H., Jr., Falk, C. T. and Motulsky, A. G.: Linkage studies in a large kindred with familial hypercholesterolemia. Am. J. Hum. Genet. 26: 598-603, 1973.

Schrott, H. G., Goldstein, J. L., Hazzard, W. R., McGoodwin, M. M. and Motulsky, A. G.: Familial hypercholesterolemia in a large kindred. Evidence for a monogenic mechanism. Ann. Intern. Med. 76: 711-720, 1972.

Slack, J. and Nevin, N. C.: Hyperlipidaemic xanthomatosis. I. Increased risk of death from ischaemic heart disease in first degree relatives of 53 patients with essential hyperlipidaemia and xanthomatosis. J. Med. Genet. 5: 4-8, 1968.

Wheeler, E. O.: The genetic aspects of atherosclerosis. Am. J. Med. 23: 653-660, 1957.

14450 HYPERLIPOPROTEINEMIA III (FAMILIAL HYPERBETA AND PREBETALIPO-PROTEINEMIA, FAMILIAL HYPERCHOLESTEROLEMIA WITH HYPERLIPEMIA, HYPERLIPEMIA WITH FAMILIAL HYPERCHOLESTEROLEMIC XANTHOMATOSIS, CARBOHYDRATE-INDUCED HYPERLIPEMIA)

On a normal diet, the patient shows increased amounts of both beta- and pre-beta-lipoproteins. Plasma cholesterol and phospholipids are elevated and glycerides may be elevated. Carbohydrate induces or exacerbates the hyperlipidemia. Often tuberous and planar and sometimes tendon xanthomas occur as well as precocious atherosclerosis and abnormal glucose tolerance. The relation between types II (the pure beta-lipoprotein disorder) and III is uncertain. Furthermore, Matthews (1968) concluded that types III and IV are consequences of the same mutant gene(s).

Fredrickson, D. S., Levy, R. I. and Lees, R. S.: Fat transport in lipoproteins — an integrated approach to mechanisms and disorders. N. Engl. J. Med. 276: 215-225, 1967.

Matthews, R. J.: Type III and IV familial hyperlipoproteinemia. Evidence that these two syndromes are different phenotypic expressions of the same mutant gene(s). Am. J. Med. 44: 188-199, 1968.

Roberts, W. C., Levy, R. I. and Fredrickson, D. S.: Hyperlipoproteinemia: a review of the five types with first report of necropsy findings in type 3. Arch. Pathol. 90: 46-56, 1970.

14460 HYPERLIPOPROTEINEMIA IV (CARBOHYDRATE INDUCED HYPERLIPEMIA)

On a regular diet the patient demonstrates increased pre-beta-lipoprotein. Plasma glycerides are persistently increased. Plasma cholesterol and phospholipids are usually within normal limits. Precocious sclerosis, abnormal glucose tolerance and atheroeruptive xanthoma may occur. The disorder is probably a dominant but experience is thus far limited. Indeed, Fredrickson and Levy (1972) have only recently suggested this category. In an old American family living in New England, Schreibman et al. (1969) described hyperpre-beta-lipoproteinemia behaving as an autosomal dominant with reduced penetrance. Although triglyceride levels as high as 2000 mg. per 100 ml. were observed in some children of this family, precocious atherosclerosis was not observed. The absence of obesity and glucose intolerance may account for the favorable prognosis. Heterogeneity of type IV hyperlipoproteinemia is suggested by these observations. Goldman et al. (1972) emphasized the association of rheumatic manifestations.

Blankenhorn, D. H., Chin, H. P. and Lau, F. Y. K.: Ischemic heart disease in young adults. Ann. Intern. Med. 69: 21-34, 1968.

Fredrickson, D. S. and Levy, R. I.: Familial hyperlipoproteinemia. In, Stanbury, J. B., Wyngaarden, J. B. and Fredrickson, D. S. (eds.): The Metabolic Basis of Inherited Diseases. New York: McGraw-Hill, 1972 (3rd Ed.). Pp. 545-614.

Goldman, J. A., Glueck, C. J., Abrams, N. R., Steiner, P. and Herman, J. H.: Musculoskeletal disorders associated with type-IV hyperlipoproteinaemia. Lancet II: 449-452, 1972.

Schreibman, P. H., Wilson, D. E. and Arky, R. A.: Familial type IV hyperlipoproteinemia. N. Engl. J. Med. 281: 981-985, 1969.

14470 HYPERNEPHROMA (ADENOCARCINOMA OF KIDNEY)

Rusche (1953) observed hypernephroma in two brothers. Both had distant metastasis as the first manifestation and both were in their early 30's at the time of diagnosis. Brinton (1960) described a family in which two brothers and a sister had hypernephroma. The father had died of kidney tumor and the mother of cancer, site unstated. One of the patients had polycythemia, a known accompaniment of hypernephroma on occasion. It should be noted that hypernephroma and cerebellar hemangioblastoma which histologically resembles hypernephroma are features of von Hippel-Lindau disease. Polycythemia also occurs with cerebellar hemangioblastoma.

Brinton, L. F.: Hypernephroma — familial occurrence in one family. J.A.M.A. 173: 888-890, 1960.

Rusche, C.: Silent adenocarcinoma of the kidneys with solitary metastases occurring in brothers. J. Urol. 70: 146-151, 1953.

*14475 HYPEROSTOSIS CORTICALIS GENERALISATA, BENIGN FORM OF WORTH, WITH TORUS PALATINUS

Maroteaux et al. (1971) described a benign form of osteosclerosis associated with torus palatinus. Worth and Wollin (1966) first described the condition. The entity has usually been labeled osteopetrosis incorrectly. The form of the bones is not altered. The cortex of the shafts of the long bones is thickened. This is a benign and usually asymptomatic disorder.

Maroteaux, P., Fontaine, G., Scharfman, W. and Farriaux, J. P.: L'hyperostose corticale generalisee a transmission dominante (type Worth). Arch. Fr. Pediatr. 28: 685-698, 1971.

Worth, H. M. and Wollin, D. G.: Hyperostosis corticalis generalisata congenita. J. Canad. Assoc. 17: 67-74, 1966.

14480 HYPEROSTOSIS FRONTALIS INTERNA (MORGAGNI-STEWART-MOREL SYNDROME)

In addition to thickening of the inner table of the frontal bone, obesity and hypertrichosis may be present. This condition affects mainly females. Knies and Le Fever (1941) reported mother and three children affected. Thus, the disorder may be dominant, but whether autosomal or X-linked is not known. Lieberman (1967) has observed 5 affected females in three generations. No case of male-to-male transmission is known. Rosatti (1972) described a family with 12 affected members (10 of them females) in 4 successive generations. Gegick et al. (1973) found elevated serum alkaline phosphatase levels in about half of patients.

Gegick, C. G., Danowski, T. S., Khurana, R. C., Vidalon, C., Nolan, S., Stephan, T., Chae, S. and Wingard, L.: Hyperostosis frontalis interna and hyperphosphatasemia. Ann. Intern. Med. 79: 71-75, 1973.

Knies, P. T. and Le Fever, H. E.: Metabolic craniopathy: hyperostosis frontalis interna. Ann. Intern. Med. 14: 1858-1892, 1941.

Lieberman, B.: Oakland, Calif.: personal communication, 1967.

Moore, S.: Hyperostosis Cranii (Stewart-Morel Syndrome, Metabolic Craniopathy, Morgagni's Syndrome, Stewart-Morel-Moore Syndrome (Ritvo), le Syndrome de Morgagni-Morel). Springfield, Ill.: Charles C Thomas, 1955.

Rosatti, P.: Une famille atteinte d'hyperostose frontale interne (syndrome de Morgagni-Morel) a travers quatre generations successives. J. Genet. Hum. 20: 207-252, 1972.

14490 HYPEROXALURIA

Oxalosis seems to be a recessive in most instances. A few observations suggest dominant inheritance. Shepard et al. (1960) reported a family with hyperoxaluria in two and perhaps three successive generations. Oxalate urinary stones occur commonly throughout the world. Most patients with oxalate stones have normal urinary oxalate excretion. Gram (1932) described an extensive pedigree of oxalate urolithiasis in five generations. Urinary oxalate concentrations were not reported. Several presumed carrier females did not have calculi. Fifteen males (and no females) in 10 sibships were affected. The systematic genetic study of calcium oxalate renal calculi done by Resnick et al. (1968) lead to the conclusion that although familial aggregation is undoubted, monogenic inheritance can be excluded and the findings are compatible with the hypothesis that the tendency to form calcium oxalate renal stones is regulated by a polygenic system, with less risk for females than males. Hyperoxaluria occurs with various forms of intestinal disease as an abnormality in absorption of dietary oxalate (Smith and Hofmann, 1974).

Gram, H. C.: The heredity of oxalic urinary calculi. Acta Med. Scand. 78: 268-281, 1932.

Resnick, M., Pridgen, D. B. and Goodman, H. O.: Genetic predisposition to calcium oxalate renal calculi. N. Engl. J. Med. 278: 1313-1318, 1968.

Shepard, T. H., Jr., Lee, L. W. and Krebs, E. G.: Primary hyperoxaluria. II. Genetic studies in a family. Pediatrics 25: 869-871, 1960.

Smith, L. H. and Hofmann, A. F.: Acquired hyperoxaluria, urolithiasis, and intestinal disease: a new digestive disorder? (Editorial) Gastroenterology 66: 1257-1268, 1974.

14500 HYPERPARATHYROIDISM

Familial hyperparathyroidism is usually part of endocrine adenomatosis (q.v.). Primary chief-cell hyperplasia is the usual histologic change in the hyperparathyroidism of that condition and also in the type which occurs in families without evidence of other endocrine disease. This suggests that discovery of this histologic change should prompt study for other endocrine disease in the patient and for other cases in the family. Cases of apparently isolated familial hyperparathyroidism have been reported by Cameron et al. (1966), Cutler et al. (1964), and Peters et al. (1966), among others. The pedigrees have usually been consistent with autosomal dominant inheritance. Families with multiple cases of parathyroid adenoma have been described by Cassidy and Anderson (1960), Jackson, Talbert and Taylor (1960) and others. Such families may have multiple endocrine adenomatosis, although the possibility of a separate and distinct dominantly inherited entity cannot be excluded (Cutler, Reiss and Ackerman, 1964). Cutler et al. (1964) among others have emphasized that chief cell hyperplasia rather than adenoma may be the characteristic histologic change in the familial cases of hyperparathyroidism. The two types of changes are often distinguished with difficulty. Jackson and Boonstra (1967) studied 8 families each with multiple cases (55 in all) of parathyroid adenoma. In at least three kindreds some individuals had other endocrine adenomata.

Cameron, K. M., Ogg, C. S. and Harrison, A. R.: Familial hyperparathyroidism. Lancet II: 1006-1007, 1966.

Cassidy, C. E. and Anderson, A. S.: A familial occurrence of hyperparathyroidism caused by multiple parathyroid adenomas. Metabolism 9: 1152-1158, 1960.

Cutler, R. E., Reiss, E. and Ackerman, L. V.: Familial hyperparathyroidism: a kindred involving eleven cases, with a discussion of primary chief-cell hyperplasia. N. Engl. J. Med. 270: 859-865, 1964.

Graber, A. L. and Jacobs, K.: Familial hyperparathyroidism. Medical and surgical considerations. J.A.M.A. 204: 542-544, 1968.

Grevsten, S., Grimelius, L. and Thoren, L.: Familial hyperparathyroidism. Upsala J. Med. Sci. 79: 109-115, 1974.

Jackson, C. E. and Boonstra, C. E.: The relationship of hereditary hyperparathyroidism to endocrine adenomatosis. Am. J. Med. 43: 727-734, 1967.

Jackson, C. E., Talbert, P. C. and Taylor, H. D.: Hereditary hyperparathyroidism. J. Indiana Med. Assoc. 53: 1313-1316, 1960.

Peters, N., Chalmers, T. M., Rack, J. H., Truscott, B. M., and Adams, P. H.: Familial hyperparathyroidism. Postgrad. Med. J. 42: 228-233, 1966.

*14510 HYPERPIGMENTATION OF EYELIDS

Hunziker (1962) described a family in which 10 persons in three generations (in an autosomal dominant pattern) showed hyperpigmentation of the eyelids. Peters (1918) traced this trait through five generations. Goodman and Belcher (1969) described two kindreds with many affected members.

Goodman, R. M. and Belcher, R. W.: Periorbital hyperpigmentation. An overlooked genetic disorder of pigmentation. Arch. Dermatol. 100: 169-174, 1969.

Hunziker, N.: A propos de l'hyperpigmentation familiale des paupieres. J. Genet. Hum. 11: 16-21, 1962.

Peters, R.: Auffallende Dunkelfaerbung der unteren Lider als erhebliche Anomalie. Centrbl. Prakt. Augenheilk. 42: 8-11, 1918.

14520 HYPERPIGMENTATION OF FULDAUER AND KUIJPERS

Fuldauer and Kuijpers (1964) described a pigmentary anomaly in many members of a Dutch family. Although the paper was entitled 'Incontinentia Pigmenti,' the distribution of the hyperpigmentation was quite different, being located on the wrists, hands, and neck and less consistently on the axillary folds, dorsa of the feet and lines of the hands. Futhermore incontinentia pigmenti is probably an X-linked dominant lethal in males. Many males were affected in this family.

Fuldauer, M. L. and Kuijpers, P. B.: An inherited pigmentary anomaly (incontinentia pigmenti)? Nederl. T. Geneesk. 108: 1613-1623, 1964.

14525 HYPERPIGMENTATION, FAMILIAL PROGRESSIVE

Familial progressive hyperpigmentation (FPH) was observed by Chernosky et al. (1971) in four individuals in two generations of a Negro family. It was characterized by patches of cutaneous hyperpigmentation which were present at birth and increased in size and number with age. Eventually large areas of skin became hyperpigmented. A mother had two affected children by different husbands.

Chernosky, M. E., Anderson, D. E., Chang, J. P., Shaw, M. W. and Romsdahl, M. M.: Familial progressive hyperpigmentation. Arch. Dermatol. 103: 581-591, 1971.

*14540 HYPERTELORISM (GREIG SYNDROME)

Although hypertelorism means an excessive distance between any paired organs (e.g., the nipples), the use of the word has come to be confined to ocular hypertelorism. Pseudohypertelorism occurs in Waardenburg syndrome (q.v.) in which lateral displacement of the inner canthus gives a mistaken impression of excessive distance between the eyes. Bojlen and Brems (1938) traced the anomaly through five generations. Friede (1954) described mother and daughter. Hypertelorism is thought to be the consequence of arrest in development of the greater wings of the sphenoid, making them smaller than the lesser wings and thus fixing the orbits in the widely separated fetal position.

Abernethy, D. A.: Hypertelorism in several generations. Arch. Dis. Child. 2: 361-365, 1927.

Bojlen, K. and Brems, T.: Hypertelorism (Greig). Acta Pathol. Microbiol. Scand. 15: 217-258, 1938.

Friede, R.: Ueber physiologische Euryopie und pathologischen Hypertelorismus ocularis. Graefe Arch. Ophthalmol. 155: 359-385, 1954.

14550 HYPERTENSION, ESSENTIAL

The Pickering school holds that blood pressure has a continuous distribution, that multiple genes and multiple environmental factors determine the level of one's blood pressure just as the determination of stature and intelligence is multifactorial, and that 'essential hypertension' is merely the upper end of the distribution. In this view the person with essential hypertension is one who happens to inherit an aggregate of genes determining hypertension (and also is exposed to exogenous factors which favor hypertension). The Platt school takes the view that essential hypertension is a simple Mendelian dominant trait. See McKusick (1960) for review. I find the Pickering point of view more consistent with the observations. McDonough and colleagues (1964) defended the monogenic idea.

Acheson, R. M. and Fowler, G. B.: On the inheritance of stature and blood pressure. J. Chronic Dis. 20: 731-746, 1967.

McDonough, J. R., Garrison, G. E. and Hames, C. G.: Blood pressure and hypertensive disease among Negroes and whites. A study in Evans County, Georgia. Ann. Intern. Med. 61: 208-228, 1964.

McKusick, V. A.: Genetics and the nature of essential hypertension. (Editorial) Circulation 22: 857-863, 1960.

*14560 HYPERTHERMIA OF ANESTHESIA

Denborough et al. (1962) observed a family in which 11 of 38 persons who had general anesthesia died. The 11 included father-daughter and mother-son and daughter combinations. Explosive hyperthermia seems to occur in these cases. Wilson et al. (1967) suggested that 'uncoupling of oxidative phosphorylation' is the defect. Thus, this condition may be a pharmacogenetic disorder. Hypertonicity of voluntary muscles is often associated with malignant hyperpyrexia. Elevation of creatine phosphokinase, phosphate and potassium in the blood indicated severe muscle damage (Denborough et al. 1970). High levels of CPK were found in a patient who had survived malignant pyrexia and in his father, paternal aunt and sister. Two of the relatives showed mild myopathy affecting mainly the legs. Kalow (1970) pointed out rigidity as a feature of the syndrome and raised the possibility of two disorders one with and one without rigidity. Mortality is higher in the cases with rigidity. In some cases rigidity may occur in the absence of fever. Kalow (1970) stated that his most extensively involved kindred fits dominant inheritance and referred to 11 other instances of familial occurrence in his series. He concluded that 'there is no doubt that the condition can be inherited as an autosomal dominant.' The malignant hyperthermia which occurs on the basis of a genetic defect in Landrace pigs is not only clinically identical with the human syndrome, but also identical in many of the biochemical features (Britt and Kalow, 1970). Kalow et al. (1970) suggested that malignant hyperthermia with and without rigidity are distinct entities. Elevated levels of serum creatine phosphokinase and clinical examination indicate the presence of a dominantly inherited myopathy in patients with malignant hyperpyrexia (King et al., 1972). King et al. (1972) referred to it as Evans myopathy, presumably for the family name. Myotonia congenita is also accompanied by susceptibility to hyperpyrexia. There are both dominant and recessive forms of myotonia congenita (q.v.). King et al. (1972) found hyperpyrexia in a case of the dominant form. A third group of patients with myopathy and malignant hyperpyrexia are all males with physical abnormalities including short stature, cryptorchidism, pectus carinatum, lumbar lordosis, thoracic kyphosis, and unusual facies.

Aldrete, J. A., Padfield, A., Solomon, C. C. and Rubright, M. W.: Possible predicative tests for malignant hyperthermia during anesthesia. J.A.M.A. 125: 1465-1469, 1971.

Britt, B. A. and Kalow, W.: Malignant hyperthermia: aetiology unknown. Canad. Anaesth. Soc. J. 17: 316-330, 1970.

Denborough, M. A., Ebeling, P., King, J. O. and Zapf, P. W.: Myopathy and malignant hyperpyrexia. Lancet I: 1138-1140, 1970.

Denborough, M. A., Forster, J. F. A., Hudson, M. C., Carter, N. G. and Zapf, P. W.: Biochemical changes in malignant hyperpyrexia. Lancet I: 1137-1138, 1970.

Denborough, M. A., Forster, J. F. A., Lovell, R. R. H., Maplestone, P. A. and Villiers, J. D.: Anaesthetic death in a family. Br. J. Anaesth. 34: 395-396, 1962.

Denborough, M. A. and Moulds, R. F. W.: Identification of susceptibility to malignant hyperpyrexia. Br. Med. J. 2: 245-246, 1974.

Isaacs, H. and Barlow, M. B.: The genetic background to malignant hyperpyrexia revealed by serum creatine phosphokinase estimations in asymptomatic relatives. Br. J. Anaesth. 42: 1077-1084, 1970.

Kalow, W.: Rigidity and malignant hyperthermia associated with anaesthesia. Humangenetik 9: 237-239, 1970.

Kalow, W., Britt, B. A., Terreau, M. E. and Haist, C.: Metabolic error of muscle metabolism after recovery from malignant hyperthermia. Lancet II: 895-898, 1970.

King, J. O., Denborough, M. A. and Zapf, P. W.: Inheritance of malignant hyperpyrexia. Lancet I: 365-370, 1972.

Moulds, R. F. W. and Denborough, M. A.: Biochemical basis of malignant hyperpyrexia. Br. Med. J. 2: 241-244, 1974.

Nelson, T. E., Jones, E. W., Henrickson, R. L., Falk, S. M. and Kerr, D. D.: Procine malignant hyperthermia: observations on the occurrence of pale, soft, exudative musculature among susceptible pigs. Am. J. Vet. Res. 35: 347-350, 1974.

Stephens, C. R.: Fulminant hyperthermia during anesthesia and surgery. J.A.M.A. 202: 178-182, 1967.

Wilson, R. D., Dent, T. E., Traber, D. L., McCoy, N. R. and Allen, C. R.: Malignant hyperpyrexia with anesthesia. J.A.M.A. 202: 183-186, 1967.

*14570 HYPERTRICHOSIS, UNIVERSALIS

We have observed a 6-year0old boy (JHH, 1251544) with extreme generalized hypertrichosis (Beighton,

1970). He was born with double eyebrows. The father, grandfather and great-grandfather had excessive hair over the entire body until about age 4. Other males in each generation escaped the excessive hairiness and it may have been transmitted through an unaffected female. There was no gingival fibromatosis (q.v.) in this family. Felgenhauer (1969) described affected mother, son and daughter and reviewed the literature exhaustively. Dominant inheritance was demonstrated by the family of Peter Gonzales who was born in the Canary Islands in 1556 and later lived in the court of King Henry II of France. He, three of his children and some in the next generation were affected (Ravin and Hodge, 1969). Affected mother and son are described by Durand and Durand (1957).

Beighton, P. H.: Congenital hypertrichosis lanuginosa. Arch. Dermatol. 101: 669-672, 1970.

Durand, J. and Durand, A.: Pictorial History of the American Circus. New York: A. S. Barnes, 1957. p. 104.

Felgenhauer, W. R.: Hypertrichosis lanuginosa universalis. J. Genet. Hum. 17: 1-44, 1969.

Ravin, J. G. and Hodge, G. P.: Hypertrichosis portrayed in art. J.A.M.A. 207: 533-535, 1969.

*14575 HYPERTRIGLYCERIDEMIA

Relatives of affected persons (ascertained in a study of survivors of coronary occlusion) were found to have normal cholesterol distribution and bimodal triglyceride distribution (Goldstein et al., 1973). Hypertriglyceridemia is not completely expressed in affected children.

Fredrickson, D. S. and Levy, R. I.: Familial hyperlipoproteinemias. In, Stanbury, J. B., Wyngaarden, J. B. and Fredrickson, D. S., (eds.): The Metabolic Basis of Inherited Disease. New York: McGraw-Hill Book Co., 1972 (3rd Ed.).

Goldstein, J. L., Schrott, H. G., Hazzard, W. R., Bierman, E. L. and Motulsky, A. G.: Hyperlipidemia in coronary heart disease. Genetic analysis of lipid levels in 176 families and delineation of a new inherited disorder, combined hyperlipidemia. J. Clin. Invest. 52: 1544-1568, 1973.

*14580 HYPERTROPHIA MUSCULORUM VERA

This condition must be distinguished from myotonia congenita and from the Debre-Semelaigne syndrome of congenital hypothyroidism. Poch et al. (1971) described a well documented family with male-to-male transmission. Striking hypertrophy of the calf muscles and less constantly of the masseter muscles were found.

Poch, G. F., Sica, E. P., Taratuto, A. and Weinstein, I. H.: Hypertrophia musculorum vera. Study of a family. J. Neurol. Sci. 12: 53-61, 1971.

*14590 HYPERTROPHIC NEUROPATHY OF DEJERINE-SOTTAS

Andermann and colleagues (1962) described Dejerine-Sottas hypertrophic neuropathy in grandfather, father and 4-year-old daughter. Features were nystagmus, distal muscular weakness, distal sensory change, pes cavus and exacerbations and remissions. Isaacs (1960) described a family in which paralysis of the extremities was precipitated by cold weather. No sensory changes occurred in the family of Russell and Garland (1930), restudied by Croft and Wadia (1957) with tracing of the disorder through five generations. On the other hand Andermann et al. (1962) described sensory changes. They also demonstrated advanced involvement of cranial and spinal nerves. Spinal nerve root enlargement was demonstrable by myelography. An abnormality of pyruvate tolerance deserves further study. Elevated spinal fluid protein is often found in this condition and in Refsum syndrome, a recessive (q.v.). Bedford and James (1956) also observed a family with affected members in five generations. The onset is usually with weakness and deformity of the feet and lower limbs. 'Onion bulb' formation makes the histologic diagnosis. Despite the apparent dominant inheritance as outlined above, the cases described by Dejerine and Sottas (1893) were sibs with presumably unaffected parents. Onset was in infancy in Fanny Roy and at age 14 in Henri Roy. The patients showed clubfoot, kyphoscoliosis, generalized weakness and muscular atrophy with fasciculations beginning first in the leg muscles, decreased reactivity to electric stimulation, areflexia, marked distal sensory loss in all four extremities, incoordination in the arms, Romberg sign, miosis, decreased pupillary reaction to light, nystagmus. Fanny died at 45. Autopsy showed the peripheral nerves to be increased in size, firm and gelatinous. Only rare nerve fibers contained myelin. Dyck et al. (1970) found changes in nerves and liver suggesting a systemic defect in the metabolism of ceramide hexosides and ceramide hexoside sulfates. Thomas et al. (1972) studied 9 kindreds. Two types were suggested. In one onset was in childhood with leg weakness and foot deformity and only mild sensory changes. In a second type sensory loss was severe and often associated with chronic ulceration of the feet.

Andermann, F., Lloyd-Smith, D. L., Mavor, H. and Mathieson, G.: Observations on hypertrophic neuropathy of Dejerine and Sottas. Neurology 12: 712-724, 1962.

Austin, J. H.: Observations on the syndrome of hypertrophic neuritis (the hypertrophic interstitial radiculo-neuropathies). Medicine 35: 187-237, 1956.

Bedford, P. D. and James, F. E.: A family with the progressive hypertrophic polyneuritis of Dejerine and Sottas. J. Neurol. Neurosurg. Psychiatry 19: 46-51, 1956.

Croft, P. B. and Wadia, N. H.: Familial hypertrophic polyneuritis: review of a previously reported family. Neurology 7: 356-366, 1957.

Dejerine, J. and Sottas, J.: Sur la nevrite interstitielle hypertrophique et progressive de l'enfance. C. R. Soc. Biol. 45: 63-96, 1893.

Deleon, G. A.: Progressive ventral sensory loss in sensory radicular neuropathy and hypertrophic neuritis. Johns Hopkins Med. J. 125: 53-61, 1969.

Dyck, P. J., Ellefson, R. D., Lais, A. C., Smith, R. C., Taylor, W. F. and Van Dyke, R. A.: Histologic and lipid studies of sural nerves in inherited hypertrophic neuropathy: preliminary report of a lipid abnormality in nerve and liver in Dejerine-Sottas disease. Mayo Clin. Proc. 45: 286-327, 1970.

Isaacs, H.: Familial chronic hypertrophic polyneuropathy with paralysis of the extremities in cold weather. S. Afr. Med. J. 34: 758-761, 1960.

Russell, W. R. and Garland, H. G.: Progressive hypertrophic polyneuritis, with case reports. Brain 53: 376-384, 1930.

Thomas, P. K., Calne, D. B. and King, R. H. M.: Autosomal dominant forms of hereditary hypertrophic neuropathy. Proc. 3rd Intern. Cong. Neuro-Genetics and Neuro-Ophthalmology, Brussels, 1970. Monographs Hum. Genet. 6: 210 only, 1972.

14595 HYPOBETALIPOPROTEINEMIA

As a clinical entity, familial hypobetalipoproteinemia is ill defined. The consistent laboratory findings of reduced serum cholesterol and betalipoprotein define it as a distinct syndrome. Brown et al. (1974) found four reported kindreds and added a fifth. Only two of the patients in the reported families had symptoms. Mars et al. (1969) observed a family in which one of the hypobetalipoproteinemic persons had signs and symptoms of progressive demyelination of the central nervous system, lack of responsiveness to local anesthesia, and dislike for animal fats and milk. The family reported by Brown et al. (1974) contained child psychomotor retardation. Although the peripheral blood smear showed no acanthocytes, the red cells on symptomatic and asymptomatic persons became acanthocytotic when placed in tissue culture medium with 10 percent autologous serum. An asterisk has been omitted because of uncertainty of relationship to abetalipoproteinemia (20010).

Brown, B. J., Lewis, L. A. and Mercer, R. D.: Familial hypobetalipoproteinemia: report of a case with psychomotor retardation. Pediatrics 54: 111-113, 1974.

Mars, H., Lewis, L. A., Robertson, A. L., Jr., Butkus, A. and Williams, G. H., Jr.: Familial hypobetalipoproteinemia: a genetic disorder of lipid metabolism with nervous system involvement. Am. J. Med. 46: 886-900, 1969.

14600 HYPOCHONDROPLASIA

This condition resembling true achondroplasia is probably not rare. It probably is a dominant. The head is not affected. The spinal canal narrows in its caudad portion as in true achondroplasia. The fingers are short but the hand is not of the trident type. The term is Lamy and Maroteaux' (1961). Beals (1969) described five kindreds with clear evidence of autosomal dominant inheritance. This chondrodystrophy which resembles achondroplasia can be distinguished on clinical and radiographic grounds. The pelvis is normal. The neurological complications of achondroplasia are not a constant feature. This form of short limb dwarfism does not show tibial bowing and the proximal fibula is not extended. Father-to-daughter and mother-to-daughter transmission have been reported. No asterisk is assigned this entry because hypochondroplasia probably is caused by an allele of achondroplasia (10080). The evidence comes from observation of the presumed genetic compound in an offspring of an achondroplastic father and a hypochondroplastic mother (McKusick et al., 1973).

Beals, R. K.: Hypochondroplasia. A report of five kindreds. J. Bone Joint Surg. 51A: 728-736, 1969.

Lamy, M. and Maroteaux, P.: Les Chondrodystrophies Genotypiques. Paris: L'Expansion Scientifique Francaise, 1961. P. 26.

McKusick, V. A., Kelly, T. E. and Dorst, J. P.: Observations suggesting allelism of the achondroplasia and hypochondroplasia genes. J. Med. Genet. 10: 11-16, 1973.

Walker, B. A., Murdoch, J. L., McKusick, V. A., Langer, L. O. and Beals, R. K.: Hypochondroplasia. Am. J. Dis. Child. 122: 95-104, 1971.

14610 HYPOFIBRINOGENEMIA

Families seem to exist in which hypofibrinogenemia is segregating in a dominant pattern and in which the disorder on the one hand cannot be related to liver disease and on the other hand is probably not the heterozygous state of congenital afibrinogenemia (Imperato, Dettori, 1958; Revol, 1962). Some of these may be the same entity as discussed under FIBRINOGEN VARIANTS (q.v.).

Imperato, C. and Dettori, A. G.: Ipofibrinogenemia congenita con fibrinoastenia. Helv. Paediatr. Acta 13: 380-399, 1958.

Revol, L.: Les grandes hypofibrinemies constitutionelles hemorrhagiques. Hemostase 2: 243-254, 1962.

*14615 HYPOMELANOSIS OF ITO ('INCONTINENTIA PIGMENTI ACHROMIANS')

Although some features are similar to those of classic incontinentia pigmenti the differences are sufficient to establish it as a separate disorder. Abnormalities of the eyes and the musculoskeletal and central nervous systems occur in some (Jelinek et al., 1973). Parent-child affection was reported by Grosshans et al. (1971) and by Rubin (1972). Father-son involvement was described in the latter report.

Grosshans, E. M., Stoebner, P., Bergoend, H. and Stoll, C.: Incontinentia pigmenti achromians (ITO). Dermatologica 142: 65-78, 1971.

Jelinek, J. E., Bart, R. S. and Schiff, G. M.: Hypomelanous of ITO (incontinentia pigmenti achromians'). Report of three cases and review of the literature. Arch: Dermatol. 107: 596-601, 1973.

Rubin, M. B.: Incontinentia pigmenti achromians. Arch. Dermatol. 105: 424-425, 1972.

Aceto et al. (1966) reported fetal and infantile hyperparathyroidism due to maternal hypoparathyroidism. The second and third offspring, a girl and a boy of the affected mother had hypoparathyroidism. The fathers of at least two of the offspring were different. Benson and Parsons (1964) described hypoparathyroidism in a mother and two of her children. They found no circulating antibodies to parathyroid hormone. Barr et al. (1971) reported hypoparathyroidism in two generations of two unrelated kindreds. In one kindred there was father-son transmission.

Aceto, T., Jr., Batt, R. E., Bruck, E., Schultz, R. B. and Perez, Y. R.: Intrauterine hyperparathyroidism: a complication of untreated maternal hypoparathyroidism. J. Clin. Endocrinol. Metab. 26: 487-492, 1966.

Barr, D. G. D., Prader, A., Esper, U., Rampini, S., Marrian, V. J. and Forfar, J. O.: Chronic hypoparathyroidism in two generations. Helv. Paediatr. Acta 26: 507-521, 1971.

Benson, P. F. and Parsons, V.: Hereditary hypoparathyroidism presenting with oedema in the neonatal period. Quart. J. Med. 33: 197-208, 1964.

*14630 HYPOPHOSPHATASIA

In the family reported by Silverman (1962) a father and 2 sons had hypophosphatasia. The paternal grandmother may have been affected. No evidence of heterozygosity was obtained in the propositus' wife and two unaffected children. Clinical features were early loss of teeth, bowed legs diagnosed as rickets and requiring osteotomy, and beaten-copper appearance of skull X-ray. The propositus had served in the U.S. Air Force. Danovitch et al. (1968) also suggested dominant inheritance as the mechanism in the family they studied. Three female cousins, the daughters of three sisters, and their mothers had low serum alkaline phosphatase and elevated urinary phosphoethanolamine. Two of the cousins had premature loss of primary teeth. Intestinal alkaline phosphatase was normal. Jardon et al. (1970) described a woman who was asymptomatic until age 50 years. She showed pseudofracture of the proximal femur and calcification of paraspinous ligaments like those in adults with hypophosphatemic rickets (q.v.).

Danovitch, S. H., Baer, P. N. and Laster, L.: Intestinal alkaline phosphatase activity in familial hypophosphatasia. N. Engl. J. Med. 278: 1253-1260, 1968.

Jardon, O. M., Burney, D. W. and Fink, R. L.: Hypophosphatasia in an adult. J. Bone Joint Surg. 52: 1477-1484, 1970.

Silverman, J. L.: Apparent dominant inheritance of hypophosphatasia. Ann. Intern. Med. 110: 191-198, 1962.

14640 HYPOPLASIA OF TEETH

Brown (1944) described a 19-year-old boy with underdeveloped dental roots and early exfoliation of the teeth. The father and a paternal uncle were edentulous.

Brown, H. C.: Hypoplasia of the dentition. Am. J. Orth. Oral Surg. 30: 102-103, 1944.

14650 HYPOTENSION, ORTHOSTATIC (SHY-DRAGER SYNDROME)

Lewis (1964) described a family in which several members had a neurologic disorder manifested by orthostatic hypotension, amyotrophy, ataxia, rigidity, tremor and sphincter disturbance. Six persons in three generations with two instances of possible male-to-male transmission were observed. Onset was in middle life and the disease progressed slowly without impairment of intellect. Vanderhaeghen et al. (1970) suggested that two forms of idiopathic orthostatic hypotension exist, on the basis of clinico-pathologic correlations. Walton (1969) has observed male-to-male transmission.

Lewis, P.: Familial orthostatic hypotension. Brain 87: 719-728, 1964.

Shy, G. M. and Drager, G. A.: A neurological syndrome associated with orthostatic hypotension: a clinical-pathologic study. Arch. Neurol. 2: 511-527, 1960.

Vanderhaeghen, J. J., Perier, O. and Sternon, J. E.: Pathological findings in idiopathic orthostatic hypotension. Arch. Neurol. 22: 207-214, 1970.

Walton, J. N.: Newcastle-Upon-Tyne, England: personal communication, 1969.

*14653 HYPOTRICHOSIS WITH LIGHT-COLORED HAIR AND FACIAL MILIA

Parrish et al. (1972) described this syndrome in 11 members of 3 generations with no male-to-male transmission but one normal daughter of an affected male making X-linked dominance unlikely. A markedly reduced density of scalp hair was the only abnormality identified. Sparcity of hair was less marked in adults than in children. A defect in the induction phase of hair development during fetal life was postulated. 'Melanization' of the hair shaft is reduced.

Goldsmith, L. A. and Baden, H. P.: The analysis of genetically determined hair defects. The Clinical Delineation of Birth Defects. XII. Skin, Hair and Nails. Baltimore: Williams and Wilkins, 1971. Pp. 86-90.

Parrish, J. A., Baden, H. P., Goldsmith, L. A. and Matz, M. H.: Studies of the density and the properties of the hair in a new inherited syndrome of hypotrichosis. Ann. Hum. Genet. 35: 349-356, 1972.

*14655 HYPOTRICHOSIS, HEREDITARY (MARIE UNNA TYPE)

Peachey and Wells (1971) reported three kindreds, each with several members with hereditary hypotrichosis of the type reported by Marie Unna in 1925. Affected persons were born with little or no eyebrows, eyelashes or body hair. Characteristically coarse, wiry, twisted hair developed in early childhood and was followed by the development of alopecia.

Peachey, R. D. and Wells, R. S.: Hereditary hypotrichosis (Marie Unna type). Trans. St. John's Hosp. Dermatol. Soc. 57: 157-166, 1971.

*14660 ICHTHYOSIS HYSTRIX GRAVIOR (LAMBERT TYPE ICHTHYOSIS, 'PORCUPINE MAN')

Y-linkage was suggested on the basis of the famous Lambert pedigree. Penrose and Stern (1958) disproved this, however, and concluded that autosomal dominant inheritance is likely.

Penrose, L. S. and Stern, C.: Reconsideration of the Lambert pedigree (ichthyosis hystrix gravior). Ann. Hum. Genet. 22: 258-283, 1958.

*14670 ICHTHYOSIS VULGARIS (ICHTHYOSIS SIMPLEX)

Wells and Kerr (1965) suggested that dominant ichthyosis vulgaris is distinguishable clinically from the X-linked variety. In the dominant form, the first skin involvement is usually noted after the first three months of life and less of the body surface is affected. Lesions are rarely observed in the axillae or anticubital and popliteal fossae but the palms and soles often show increased markings. There are some histologic differences also. A considerable proportion of patients with dominant ichthyosis have asthma, eczema or hayfever. This may not be a separate entity, however. For a useful classification and discussion of the various forms of ichthyosis, see Schnyder (1970).

Anton-Lamprecht, I. and Hofbauer, M.: Ultrastructural distinction of autosomal dominant ichthyosis vulgaris and X-linked recessive ichthyosis. Humangenetik 15: 261-264, 1972.

Kuokkanen, K.: Ichthyosis vulgaris. A clinical and histopathological study of patients and their close relatives in the autosomal dominant and sex-linked forms of the disease. Acta Derm. Venerol. 49 (suppl. 62): 1-72, 1969.

Schnyder, U. W.: Inherited ichthyoses. Arch. Dermatol. 102: 240-252, 1970.

Wells, R. S. and Kerr, C. B.: Genetic classification of ichthyosis. Arch. Dermatol. 92: 1-6, 1965.

14680 ICHTHYOSIS, BULLOUS TYPE

Schnyder (1970) concluded that this represents a separate entity.

Schnyder, U. W.: Inherited ichthyoses. Arch. Dermatol. 102: 240-252, 1970.

Siemens, H. W.: Dichtung und Wahrheit ueber die Ichthyosis bullosa, mit Bemerkungen zur Systematik der Epidermolysen. Arch. Dermatol. Syph. 175: 590-608, 1937.

*14685 IMMUNE RESPONSE (Ir)

Levine et al. (1972) found that clinical ragweed pollenosis (hay fever) and IgE antibody production specific for antigen E (the major purified protein antigen from ragweed pollen extract) correlated closely with HL-A haplotypes in successive generations of seven families. The correlation was thought to be based on the existence of an Ir locus closely linked to the HL-A locus (14280). Blumenthal et al. (1974) extensively studied a kindred spanning three generations, for skin sensitivity to antigen E of ragweed and for HL-A type (14280). They concluded that a locus controlling sensitivity to angigen E (IrE) is linked to the HL-A complex and that the order is first locus (LA), second locus (FOUR), IrE. They used the designation of the complex as HL-1.

Blumenthal, M. N., Amos, D. B., Noreen, H., Mendell, N. R. and Yunis, E. J.: Genetic mapping or Ir locus in man: linkage to second locus of HL-A.. Science 184: 1301-1303, 1974.

Levine, B. B. and Stember, R. H. and Fotino, M.: Ragweed hay fever: genetic control and linkage to HL-A haplotypes. Science 178: 1201-1203, 1972.

McDevitt, H. O. and Bodmer, W. F.: HL-A, immune-response genes, and disease. Lancet I: 1269-1275, 1974.

14686 IMMUNE RESPONSE ASSOCIATED ANTIGENS (Ia)

In the mouse and presumably in man, there are lymphocyte alloantigens, designated as Ia (immune response associated) antigens, found mainly on B lymphocytes. The MLC genes (15785, 15786), the Ir genes (14685) and the Ia antigens map in the same region in the mouse. It is not clear whether the three are different effects of the same gene or separate genes mapping in the same region. The existence of immune response associated antigens in man is highly probable, because of the close homolyogy of the H-2 and HL-A regions in mouse and man. See McDevitt and Bodmer (1974) for disscussion and references.

McDevitt, H. O and Bodmer, W. F.: HL-A, immune-response genes, and disease. Lancet I: 1269-1275, 1974.

14687 IMMUNOGLOBULIN A, LEVEL OF

The low levels of immunoglobulin A in the 18-long-arm deletion syndrome may indicate the localization on the long arm of one or more genes concerned with the synthesis of immunoglobulin (Hecht, 1969). Grundbacher (1972) concluded that selective immunoglobin A deficiency is probably multifactorial. Descreased IgA occurs also in some cases of the 21q-syndrome or anti-mongolism (Kelch et al. 1971), further weakening any claims of structural gene for IgA on chromosome 18. See 13710.

Grundbacher, F. J.: Genetic aspects of selective immunoglobulin A deficiency. J. Med. Genet. 9: 344-347, 1972.

Hecht, F.: IgA and partial deletions of chromosome 18. Lancet I: 100, 1969.

Kelch, R. P., Franklin, M. and Schmickel, R. D.: Group D deletion syndrome. J. Med. Genet. 8: 341-345, 1971.

*14690 IMMUNOGLOBULIN Am(1)

The Gm and Inv types are variants of IgG, immunoglobulin G. Vyas and Fudenberg (1970) described allotype of IgA, using isoantibodies from a patient who displayed an anaphylactoid transfusion reaction.

Vyas, G. N. and Fudenberg, H. H.: Immunobiology of human anti-IgA: a serologic and immunogenetic study of immunization to IgA in transfusion and pregnancy. Clin. Genet. 1: 45-64, 1970.

*14700 IMMUNOGLOBULIN Am(2) (IgA HEAVY CHAIN LOCUS)

Kunkel et al. (1969) defined a system they called Am(2). The Am(2) and Gm systems, involving IgA and IgG, respectively, appear to be closely linked in man. Gamma A and gamma G markers are closely linked in the mouse. The system of Vyas and Fudenberg (1969) is not linked to Gm. Van Loghem et al. (1970) showed that the Gm and Am(2) loci are closely linked but Gm and Inv unlinked. No asterisk precedes this entry because information now available indicates that Am(2) is identical to Am(1). Both are markers of IgA(2). See Curtain et al. (1972).

Curtain, C. C., Van Loghem, E., Fudenberg, H. H., Tindale, N. B., Simmons, R. T., Doherty, R. L. and Vos, G.: Distribution of the immunoglobulin markers at the IgG1, IgG2, IgG3, IgA(2), and kappa-chain loci in Australian Aborigines: comparison with New Guinea populations. Am. J. Hum. Genet. 24: 145-155, 1972.

Kunkel, H. G., Smith, W. K., Joslin, F. G., Natvig, J. B. and Litwin, S. D.: Genetic marker of the gamma A2 subgroup of gamma A immunoglobulins. Nature 223: 1247-1248, 1969.

Van Loghem, E., Natvig, J. B. and Matsumoto, H.: Genetic markers of immunoglobulins in Japanese families. Inheritance of associated markers belonging to one IgA and three IgG subclasses. Ann. Hum. Genet. 33: 351-359, 1970.

Vyas, G. N. and Fudenberg, H. H.: Immunogenetic study of Am(1), the first allotype of human IgA. Clin. Res. 17: 469 only, 1969.

14705 IMMUNOGLOBULIN E (IgE), BASIC LEVEL OF, IN SERUM

From determinations of IgE levels in 29 families, Bias et al. (1973) suggested the existence of 'an autosomal dominant gene coding for a substance which represses the biosynthesis or controls the metabolism of IgE'.

Bias, W. B., Marsh, D. G. and Ishigaka, K.: Genetic control of the immune response in man. Am. J. Hum. Genet. 25: 16A, 1973.

*14710 IMMUNOGLOBULIN Gm-1 (IgG HEAVY CHAIN LOCUS)

At least two separate autosomal loci determining serologic type of gamma globulin have been identified. One is referred to as the Gm locus and the other as the Inv locus. The genetics of the gamma globulins promises to be as revealing of general principles as has been that of the hemoglobins. The Gm system is associated with the heavy chains of the IgG molecules and the Inv system with the light chains. (See Nature 209: 653, 1966, recommended notation for Gm and Inv types.) Hood and Ein (1968) presented evidence that antibody light chains are an exception to the rule of 'one gene, one polypeptide chain.' Two separate loci (a specific region locus and a common region locus) appear to code for a single, continuous polypeptide chain. Absence of certain immunoglobulins in patients with deleted chromosome 18 suggests the localization of structural and-or controller genes to that chromosome (Finley et al., 1968). Three closely linked loci (IgG1, IgG2 and IgG3) are thought to be responsible for the Gm specificities. Lovrien et al. (1972) found suggestive evidence of linkage of the Gm locus with the alpha-haptoglobin locus which is known to be on the long arm of chromosome no. 16. Van Loghem et al. (1970) presented evidence on the linkage relationship of immunoglobulin markers (gamma 1, 2, 3, Am). That the gamma-G3 and gamma-G1 loci are closely linked is indicated by the findings in a Lepore-type myeloma protein (Kunkel et al. 1969). A fourth IgG locus (gamma-G4) is identifiable in the cluster, but its position relative to the other loci is unknown. Weitkamp et al. (1974) presented evidence that Pi (10740) and AcP(1) (17150) are linked. If true, the Gm-Am(2) cluster is situated on the short arm of chromosone no. 2.

Borgaonkar, D. S., Bias, W. B., Chase, G. A., Sadasivan, G., Herr, H. M., Golomb, H. M., Bahr, G. F. and Kunkel, L. M.: Identification of a C6-G21 translocation chromosome by Q-M and Giemsa banding techniques in a patient with Down's syndrome, with possible assignment of Gm locus. Clin. Genet. 4: 53-57, 1973.

Ceppellini, R., Dray, S., Fabey, J. L., Franklin, E. C., Fudenberg, H., Gell, P. G. H., Goodman, H. C., Grubb, R., Harboe, M., Kirk, R. L., Oudin, J., Ropartz, C., Smithies, O., Steinberg, A. G. and Trnka, Z.: Notation for genetic factors in human immunoglobulins. Genetics 53: 235-241, 1966.

Fahey, J. L.: Antibodies and immunoglobulins. Structure and function. J.A.M.A. 194: 71-74, 1965.

Finley, S. C., Finley, W. H., Noto, T. A., Uchida, I. A. and Roddam, R. F.: IgA absence associated with a ring-18 chromosome. (Letter) Lancet I: 1095-1096, 1968.

Gedde-Dahl, T., Jr., Fagerhol, M. K., Cook, P. J. L. and Noades, J.: Autosomal linkage between the Gm and Pi loci in man. Ann. Hum. Genet. 35: 393-400, 1972.

Grubb, R.: The Genetic Markers of Human Immunoglobins. New York: Springer, 1970.

Hill, R. L., Delaney, R., Fellows, R. E., Jr. and Lebovitz, H. E.: The evolutionary origins of the immunoglobulins. Proc. Natl. Acad. Sci. 56: 1762-1769, 1966.

Hood, L. and Ein, D.: Immunoglobulin lambda chain structure: two genes, one polypeptide chain. Nature 220: 764-767, 1968.

Kunkel, H. G., Natvig, J. B. and Joslin, F. G.: A 'Lepore' type of hybrid gamma globulin. Proc. Natl. Acad. Sci. 62: 144-149, 1969.

Lennox, E. S. and Cohn, M.: Immunoglobulins. Ann. Rev. Biochem. 36: 365-402, 1967.

Lovrien, E. W., Magenis, R. E., Rowe, S. I. and Hazard, S.: Possible genetic linkage between Hp(alpha) and Gm. Proc. Am. Soc. Hum. Genet. p. 40A, 1972.

Natvig, J. B. and Kunkel, H. G.: Human immunoglobulins: classes, subclasses, genetic variants, and idiotypes. Adv. Immunol. 16: 1-59, 1973.

Oudin, J.: Genetic regulation of immunoglobulin synthesis. J. Cell. Physiol. 67 (suppl. 1): 77-108, 1966.

Steinberg, A. G. and Bearn, A. G.: Progress in Medical Genetics. New York: Grune and Stratton, 3: 1964.

Steinberg, A. G.: Gammaglobulin polymorphisms in man. Ann. Rev. Genet. 3: 25-32, 1969.

Van Loghem, E., Natvig, J. B. and Matsumoto, H.: Genetic markers of immunoglobulins in Japanese famiIes. Inheritance of associated markers belonging to one IgA subclass and three IgG subclasses. Ann. Hum. Genet. 33: 351-360, 1970.

Weitkamp, L. R., Johnston, E. and Guttormsen, S. A.: Genetic linkage of Pi and AcP(1). (Abstract) Am. J. Hum. Genet. 26: 92A only, 1974.

*14711 IMMUNOGLOBULIN Gm-2

See 14710.

*14712 IMMUNOGLOBULIN Gm-3

See 14710.

*14713 IMMUNOGLOBULIN Gm-4

See 14710.

14717 IMMUNOGLOBULIN: HEAVY DELTA CHAIN LOCUS

This locus determins the heavy chain of IgD. No idiotypic variation is known. See 14722.

14718 IMMUNOGLOBULIN: HEAVY EPSILON CHAIN LOCUS

This locus determines the heavy chain of IgE. No idiotypic variation is known. See 14722.

14719 IMMUNOGLOBULIN: HEAVY Mu CHAIN LOCUS

This locus determines the heavy chain unique to IgM. No idiotypic variation is known. See 14722.

*14720 IMMUNOGLOBULIN: INV LOCUS (KAPPA LIGHT CHAIN LOCUS)

Inv(-1,3) homozygotes have valine at position 191 of the kappa-type light polypeptide chains whereas Inv(1,3) heterozygotes have some chains with leucine and some with valine at this position (Terry et al., 1969).

Terry, W. D., Hood, L. E. and Steinberg, A. G.: Genetics of immunoglobulin kappa chains: chemical analysis of normal human light chains of differing Inv types. Proc. Natl. Acad. Sci. 63: 71-77, 1969.

14722 IMMUNOGLOBULIN: LAMBDA LIGHT CHAIN LOCUS

Although no idiotypic variation of lambda light chains has been found (comparable to Inv and Gm variants of kappa light chains and gamma heavy chains), the existence of at least one locus for lambda light chains can be inferred from the amino acid sequence of immunoglobulins. The same type of evidence indicates the existence of mu, delta, and epsilon heavy chain loci which determine the structure of heavy chains in IgM, IgD and IgE, respectively. Each immunoglobulin molecule is composed of two heavy chains and two light chains. Since there are five types of heavy chains and two types of light chains, a minimum of 10 classes of immunoglobulins result. Actually, as indicated elsewhere (14710), since there are at least four subtypes of gamma heavy chains, there are at least 32 types of immunoglobulins.

14725 INCISORS, FUSED

Passarge and Bosman (1971) observed the trait in father and son, and Schulze (1964) in sibs. Moody and Montgomery (1934) found fused incisors in females of three generations.

Moody, E. and Montgomery, L. B.: Hereditary tendencies in tooth formation. J. Am. Dent. Assoc. 21: 1774-1776, 1934.

Passarge, E. and Bosman, H.: Fusion of lateral incisors as autosomal dominant trait. The Clinical Delineation of Birth Defects. XI. Orofacial Structures. Baltimore: Williams and Wilkins, 1971. Pp. 194-195.

Schulze, C.: Anomalien, Missbildungen und Krankheiten der Zaehne, des Mundes und der Kiefer. In, Becker, P. E. (ed.): Handbuch der Humangenetik. Stuttgart: Georg Thieme Verlag, 1964. vol. II, p. 364.

14730 INCISORS, LONG UPPER CENTRAL

Although a single major gene may be involved and this trait behaves as a simple dominant, data actually proving this are apparently not available.

Hrdlicka, A.: Normal variation of teeth and jaws and orthodonty. Int. J. Orthod. Dent. Child. 21: 1099-1114, 1935.

Hyde, W.: Heredity in relation to size of the teeth. J. Am. Dent. Assoc. 25: 1762-1767, 1938.

14740 INCISORS, 'SHOVEL-SHAPED'

The incisors are hollowed out on their lingual surface, creating a resemblance to a shovel or a sugar scoop. The lateral incisors are more often or more markedly affected than the middle incisors. The trait is particularly frequent in the Mongoloid race. Family studies have, apparently, not been performed.

Koski, K. and Hautala, E.: On the frequency of shovel-shaped incisors in the Finns. Am. J. Phys. Anthropol. 10: 127-132, 1952.

Portin, P. and Alvesala, L.: The inheritance of shovel shape in maxillary central incisors. Am. J. Phys. Anthropol. 41: 59-62, 1974.

Riesenfeld, A.: Shovel-shaped incisors and a few other dental features among the native people of the Pacific. Am. J. Phys. Anthropol. 14: 505-521, 1956.

*14745 INDOPHENOLOXIDASE A (IPO-A)

When starch gels are stained by the phenazine-tetrazolum technique, in addition to the appearance of blue bands marking the site of isozymes under investigation, light or achromatic areas appear. The bands are the effects of an oxidase which oxidizes tetrazolium dyes in the presence of phenazine and light. Brewer (1967) observed an electrophoretic variant of the three generations of a family with presumed male-to-male transmission. Indophenoloxidase is otherwise known as tetrazolium oxidase. Brewer (1967) demonstrated tetrazolium oxidase in several human tissues and classified the enzyme as an indophenol oxidase. The physiologic function of the enzyme is not known. In the dog there is a genetic polymorphism of red cell tetrazolium oxidase (Baur and Schorr, 1969). In man genetic variation is rare. Baur (cited by Baur and Schorr, 1969) has observed an electrophoretic variant of tetrazolium oxidase in a Caucasian mother and one of two children. Ruddle et al. (1972), by mouse-man cell hybridization, could demonstrate that indophenoloxidase A is determined by a locus on chromosome no. 21. IPO-A is a dimer and IPO-B, a tetramer. Welch and Mears (1972) found an unusually high frequency of a variant in one of the Orkney Islands. IPO-B is determined by a locus thought to be on chromosome no. 6. Beckman (1973) referred to this enzyme as superoxide dismutase (symbolized SOD) and reported on the frequency of the 'Morenci' phenotype in a population of northern Sweden. Beckman et al. (1973) found two isozymes of superoxide dismutase, A and B, in extracts of human tissues. Isozyme A is a soluble form, whereas B is mitochondrial. Isozyme A is lacking from polymorphonucleas leukocytes and isozyme B from erythrocytes. The presence of hybrid molecules in heterozygotes indicates that SOD-A is a dimer of two identical subunits. Berg (1974) showed me pedigrees which makes kinkage with Ag unlikely even thought both loci have been tentatively assigned to chromosome no. 21.

Baur, E. W. and Schorr, R. T.: Genetic polymorphism of tetrazolium oxidase in dogs. Science 166: 1524-1525, 1969.

Beckman, G.: Population studies in northern Sweden. Polymorphism of superoxide dismutase. Hereditas 73: 305-310, 1973.

Beckman, G., Lundgren, E. and Tarnvik, A.: Superoxide dismutase isozymes in different human tissues, their genetic control and intracellular localization. Hum. Hered. 23: 338-345, 1973.

Berg, K.: Oslo, personal communication, 1974.

Brewer, G. J.: Achromatic regions of tetrazolium stained starch gels: inherited electrophoretic variation. Am. J. Hum. Genet. 19: 674-680, 1967.

Ritter, H. and Wendt, G. G.: Indophenol oxidase variability. Humangenetik 14: 72 only, 1971.

Ruddle, F. H.: New Haven, Conn.: personal communication, 1972.

Welch, S. G. and Mears, G. W.: Genetic variants of human indophenol oxidase in the Westray Island of the Orkneys. Hum. Hered. 22: 38-41, 1972.

*14746 INDOPHENOLOXIDASE B (IPO-B)

According to the results of studies of mouse-man hybrid clones, the locus is carried by chromosome no. 6 (Ruddle et al. 1972). This indophenoloxidase is probably a tetramer whereas IPO-A is a dimer. The locus for mitochondrial has been assigned to chromosome no. 6 by study of somatic cell hybrids (Creagan et al., 1973). It is syntenic with cytoplasmic malic enzyme (E.C.1.1.1.40) (15425). It is tetrameric. See 23370 for a discussion of significance of superoxide.

Creagan, R., Tischfield, J., Ricciuti, F. and Ruddle, F. H.: Chromosome assignments of genes in man using mouse-human somatic cell hybrids: mitochondrial superoxide dismutase (indophenol oxidase-B, tetrameric) to chromosome 6. Humangenetik 20: 203-209, 1973.

Ruddle, F. H.: New Haven, Conn.: personal communication, 1972.

*14750 INHIBITOR OF PROTHROMBIN CONSUMPTION, HEMORRHAGIC DISORDER DUE TO

In 4 generations of a family (with one instance of male-to-male transmission), Robinson et al. (1967) described a mild bleeding disorder associated with increased concentrations of a natural inhibitor of prothrombin consumption in the serum. The inhibitor was directed specifically toward activated Stuart factor and resembled that commonly observed in systemic lupus erythematosus. A similar agent was found in normal plasma but in much smaller amounts.

Robinson, A. J., Aggeler, P. M., McNicol, G. P. and Douglas, A. S.: An atypical genetic haemorrhagic

disease with increased concentration of a natural inhibitor of prothrombin consumption. Br. J. Haematol.
13: 510-527, 1967.

14753 INOSINE TRIPHOSPHATASE

Harris et al. (1974) found no genetic variants by electrophoretic means.

Harris, H., Hopkinson, D. A. and Robson, E. B.: The incidence of rare alleles determining electrophoretic variants: data on 43 enzyme loci in man. Ann. Hum. Genet. 37: 237-253, 1974.

14755 INSECT STINGS, HYPERSENSITIVITY TO

Hecht (1971) described a family, presumably his own, in which a male and two sons of his brother had exquisite sensitivity to insect stings. This is a situation of possible genetic sensitivity to an environmental insult, comparable to familial farmer's lung (q.v.) and pulmonary edema of mountaineers (17840), as well as less esoteric and more clearly established examples such as favism, suxamethonium sensitivity and malignant hyperpyrexia of anesthesia.

Hecht, F.: Familial hypersensitivity to insect stings. (Letter) Lancet II: 469 only, 1971.

*14757 INTERFERON-1

This locus may be on chromosome no. 2, according to cell hybridization studies (Tan et al., 1973). An interferon-2 locus (14758) is on chromosome 5. Tan et al. (1974) considered several possible explanations for two loci being necessary for production of interferon. First, one of two chromosomes may contain a gene that codes for a specific receptor site necessary for processing of interferon inducers into a signal that activates the structural gene for interferon; the other chromosome may carry the structural gene. Second, both chromosomes may carry a gene that codes for an interferon subunit. Third, one chromosome may have a gene for a pre-interferon and the other a gene involved in processing the active form. In the African green monkey, Cassingena et al. (1971) assigned the structural gene for interferon to a small subtelocentric chromosome, probably A8 or A9. According to Stock and Hsu (1973), these chromosomes are homologous to human chromosome 5.

Cassingena, R., Chany, C., Vignal, M., Suarex, H., Estrade, S. and Lazar, P.: Use of monkey-mouse hybrid cells for the study of the cellular regulation of interferon production and action. Proc. Natl. Acad. Sci. 68: 580-584, 1971.

Stock, A. D. and Hsu, T. C.: Evolutionary conservatism in arrangement of genetic material. A comparative analysis of chromosome banding between the Rhesus macaque (2n=42, 84 arms) and the African green monkey (2n=60, 120 arms). Chromosoma 43: 211-224, 1973.

Tan, Y. H., Armstrong, J. A. and Ho, M.: The regulation of cellular interferon production: enhancement by antimetabolites. Proc. Natl. Acad. Sci. 67: 464-471, 1970.

Tan, Y. H., Creagan, R. P. and Ruddle, F. H.: Assignment of the genes of the human interferon system to chromosomes 2 and 5. Cytogenet. Cell Genet. 13: 115-157, 1974.

*14758 INTERFERON-2

See 14757.

*14760 IRIS HYPOPLASIA WITH GLAUCOMA

Berg (1932) described 22 affected in 6 generations. McCulloch (1950) described 18 affected in 5 generations. Weatherill and Hart (1969) observed it in many members of 5 generations. Not only is the stroma of the iris hypoplastic but the iris is also light in color, a feature that antedates development of glaucoma and permits recognition of affected persons at birth. See RIEGER SYNDROME which has somewhat similar ocular features.

Berg, F.: Erbliches jugendliches Glaukom. Acta Ophthalmol. 10: 568-587, 1932.

McCulloch, J. C.: Iridoschisis as a cause of glaucoma. Am. J. Ophthalmol. 33: 1398-1400, 1950.

Weatherill, J. R. and Hart, C. T.: Familial hypoplasia of the iris stroma associated with glaucoma. Br. J. Ophthalmol. 53: 433-438, 1969.

*14765 ISOCITRIC DEHYDROGENASE, MITOCHONDRIAL

See ISOCITRIC DEHYDROGENASE, SOLUBLE.

*14770 ISOCITRIC DEHYDROGENASE, SOLUBLE

Henderson (1965) described electrophoretic polymorphism of this enzyme in mice. However, using the cell-hybrid method which relies on interspecies variation rather than polymorphism, Boone et al. (1972) could show that the IDH locus is on chromosome 20. NADP-dependent ICD occurs in two structurally distinct forms: mitochondrial and soluble (also called supernatant or cytoplasmic). Chen et al. (1972) found rare variants of the soluble form and concluded that the structural gene is probably autosomal and that it is distinct from the locus governing the mitochondrial form. Shows (1971) presented cell hybridization data suggesting that soluble malate dehydrogenase and isocitrate dehydrogenase are syntenic. The assignment of soluble IDH and soluble MDH (15420) to chromosome 20 was withdrawn (Ruddle, 1973). Creagan et al. (1974) presented evidence that these two syntenic loci are on chromosome 2.

Boone, C., Chen, T. and Ruddle, F. H.: Assignment of three human genes to chromosomes (LDH-A to 11, TK to 17 and IDH to 20) and evidence for translocation between human and mouse chromosomes in somatic cell hybrids. Proc. Natl. Acad. Sci. 68: 510-514, 1972.

Chen, S.-H., Fossum, B. L. G. and Giblett, E. R.: Genetic variation of the soluble form of NADP-dependent isocitric dehydrogenase in man. Am. J. Hum. Genet. 24: 325-329, 1972.

Creagan, R. P., Carritt, B., Chen, S., Kucherlapati, R., McMorris, F. A., Ricciuti, F., Tan, Y. H., Tischfield, J. A. and Ruddle, F. H.: Chromosome assignments of genes in man using mouse-human somatic cell hybrids: cytoplasmic isocitrate dehydrogenase (IDH 1) and malate dehydrogenase (MDH 1) to chromosme 2. Am. J. Hum. Genet. 26: 604-613, 1974.

Henderson, N. S.: Isozymes of isocitrate dehydrogenase: subunit structure and intracellular location. J. Exp. Zool. 158: 263-273, 1965.

Henderson, N. S.: Intracellular location and genetic control of isozymes of NADP-dependent isocitrate dehydrogenase and malate dehydrogenase. Ann. N.Y. Acad. Sci. 151: 429-440, 1968.

Ruddle, F. H.: Linkage analysis in man by somatic cell genetics. Nature 242: 165-169, 1973.

Shows, T. B.: (Abstract) IV Internat. Congr. Human Genetics, Paris, 1971. P. 165.

Shows, T. B.: Genetics of human-mouse somatic cell hybrids: linkage of human genes for isocitrate dehydrogenase and malate dehydrogenase. Biochem. Genet. 7: 193-204, 1972.

Turner, B. M., Fisher, R. A., Garthwaite, E., Whale, R. J. and Harris, H.: An account of two new ICD-S variants not detectable in red blood cells. Ann. Hum. Genet. 37: 469-476, 1974.

14780 JOINT CONTRACTURES WITH OTHER ABNORMALITIES

Aase and Smith (1968) described a syndrome in father and two children. The infants one stillborn and one who survived only two months had virtually identical findings: hydrocephalus, cleft palate and severe joint contractures. The father had joint contractures from birth, deformed ears and bilateral ptosis. One of the infants was male. One had congenital neuroblastoma and the other had multiple ventricular septal defects and a single sternal ossification center. The same condition may have been present in the infant reported by Potter and Parrish (1942). See PSEUDO-ARTHROGRYPOSIS.

Aase, J. M. and Smith, D. W.: Dysmorphogenesis of joints, brain and palate: a new dominantly inherited syndrome. J. Pediatr. 73: 606-609, 1968.

Potter, E. L. and Parrish, J. M.: Neuroblastoma, ganglioneuroma and fibroneuroma in a stillborn fetus. Am. J. Pathol. 18: 141-152, 1942.

*14790 JOINT LAXITY, FAMILIAL

Carter and Sweetnam (1960) noted dominant inheritance in several families that suffered from recurrent dislocation of joints, particularly the shoulder. Recurrent dislocation of the patella (q.v.) may be an independent dominant trait in some families. Other dominant pedigrees are referred to by McKusick (1972).

Beighton, P. H. and Horan, F. T.: Dominant inheritance in familial generalized articular hypermobility. J. Bone Joint Surg. 52B: 145-147, 1970.

Carter, C. and Sweetnam, R.: Recurrent dislocation of the patella and of the shoulder. Their association with familial joint laxity. J. Bone Joint Surg. 42B: 721-727, 1960.

Kirk, J. A., Ansell, B. M. and Bywaters, E. G. L.: The hypermobility syndrome. Ann. Rheum. Dis. 26: 419-425, 1967.

McKusick, V. A.: Heritable Disorders of Connective Tissue. St. Louis: C. V. Mosby Co., 1972 (4th Ed.).

14800 KAPOSI SARCOMA

Zeligman (1960) observed the disorder in father and son. Although a characteristic ethnic occurrence (Italian and Jewish) has been noted, this was perhaps only the second instance of familial incidence.

Zeligman, I.: Kaposi's sarcoma in a father and son. Bull. Hopkins Hosp. 107: 208-212, 1960.

14810 KELOIDS

Over-growth of connective tissue of the skin occurs after trauma. Bloom (1956) described cases in five generations. Bohrod (1937) speculated that sexual selection favored the genotype of keloids formation. He presented evidence that cicatrization was practiced as a pubertal rite by Africans and that 'good' scar formers may have been on the average more fertile. Cosman et al. (1961) found a familial incidence of 3 percent. I (1966) have seen a transverse keloid over the upper sternum in father and son who recalled no trauma preceding the development of the keloid.

Bloom, D.: Heredity of keloids: review of the literature and report of a family with multiple keloids in five generations. New York J. Med. 56: 511-519, 1956.

Bohrod, M. G.: Keloids and sexual selection: a study in the racial distribution of disease. Arch. Dermatol. Syph. 36: 19-25, 1937.

Cosman, B., Crikelair, G. F., Ju, D. M., Gaulin, J. C. and Lattes, R.: The surgical treatment of keloids. Plast. Reconstr. Surg. 27: 335-358, 1961.

McKusick, V. A.: Heritable Disorders of Connective Tissue. St. Louis: C. V. Mosby Co., 1972 (4th Ed.). Fig. 10-11, P. 430.

*14820 KERATITIS FUGAX HEREDITARIA

Valle (1964) described this as a new entity in 10 members of 4 generations. The disease begins between the ages of 4 and 12 years and is characterized by acute attacks of keratitis occurring 2 to 8 times a year. No permanent corneal opacities result. Attacks become milder and less frequent after age 50. Also see CORNEAL EROSIONS, RECURRING HEREDITARY which may be the same disorder.

Valle, O.: Keratitis fugax hereditaria. Duodecim 80: 659-664, 1964.

14830 KERATOCONUS

Irregular autosomal dominant inheritance was suggested by Falls and Allen (1969), who observed affected aunt and niece. The mother who presumably transmitted the trait had astigmatism and other features they interpreted as forme fruste of keratoconus. They cited several instances of multigeneration involvement including the family of Stahli (1925) with transmission through 3 generations. Keratoconus is frequent in cases of amaurosis congenita of Leber (20400).

Falls, H. F. and Allen, A. W.: Dominantly inherited keratoconus. Report of a family. J. Genet. Hum. 17: 317-324, 1969.

Staehli, J.: Weitere Mitteilungen ueber die Vererbung des Keratoconus. Klin. Mbl. Augenheilk. 75: 465-466, 1925.

*14840 KERATOSIS PALMARIS ET PLANTARIS FAMILIARIS (TYLOSIS)

This condition is characterized by diffuse hyperkeratosis of the palms and soles. The condition usually becomes first evident between the ages of 3 and 12 months. Low serum vitamin A has been found in some cases. The family of Anderson and Klintworth (1961) also had clinodactyly, probably as an independent trait. In addition to the diffuse type referred to here a punctate type (see KERATOSIS PALMO-PLANTARIS PAPULOSA) and a linear or striate form (see KERATOSIS PALMO-PLANTARIS STRIATA) are recognized on morphologic grounds. It is quite possible that these are genetically distinct from the diffuse type but such cannot be considered proved. See HYPERKERATOSIS, LOCALIZED EPIDERMOLYTIC, for description of a condition grossly indistinguishable but histologically different. This disorder is sometimes referred to as keratosis of Greither (1952).

Anderson, I. F. and Klintworth, G. K.: Hypovitaminosis-A in a family with tylosis and clinodactyly. Br. Med. J. 1: 1293-1297, 1961.

Chung, H.-L.: Keratoma palmare et plantare hereditarium, with special reference to its mode of inheritance as traced in six and seven generations, respectively, in two Chinese families. Arch. Derm. Syph. 36: 303-313, 1937.

Greither, A.: Keratosis extremitatum hereditaria progrediens mit dominantem Erbgang. Hautarzt 3: 198-203, 1952.

Klintworth, G. K. and Anderson, I. F.: Tylosis palmaris et plantaris familiaris associated with clinodactyly. S. Afr. Med. J. 35: 170-175, 1961.

*14850 KERATOSIS PALMARIS ET PLANTARIS WITH ESOPHAGEAL CANCER

The same disorder as that described above was associated with esophageal cancer in the two kindreds (which perhaps are related) studied in Liverpool by Howel-Evans and colleagues (1958). The disorder is apparently distinct. Whether allelic with the other form is unknown. From Oxford, Shine and Allison (1966) described another family in which multiple members showed the association. Affected members showed congenital sliding hiatal hernia and lower esophagus lined by gastric mucosa. Harper et al. (1970) gave further information on the Liverpool families and added two further families each with one case of esophageal cancer with tylosis. Age of onset of the tylosis appears to be a feature distinguishing the cancer-prone from the nonprone form. Tylosis is late in onset in the form with esophageal cancer. Shine and Allison (1966) suggested that 'probably a different allele in this pedigree' is involved than in the pedigrees of Howel-Evans et al. (1958). Esophageal cancer was later in onset (average 61 years as compared with average 45 in the Howel-Evans families) and a sliding hiatal hernia was present.

Harper, P. S., Harper, R. M. J. and Howel-Evans, A. W.: Carcinoma of the oesophagus with tylosis. Quart. J. Med. 39: 317-333, 1970.

Howel-Evans, W., McConnell, R. B., Clarke, C. A. and Sheppard, P. M.: Carcinoma of the oesophagus with keratosis palmaris et plantaris (tylosis): a study of two families. Quart. J. Med. 27: 413-429, 1958.

Shine, I. and Allison, P. R.: Carcinoma of the esophagus with tylosis. Lancet I: 951-953, 1966.

14860 KERATOSIS PALMO-PLANTARIS PAPULOSA

Late onset complicates genetic study. In 14 families reported by Schirren and Dinger (1965) direct transmission was observed. Females are less severely involved.

Schirren, V. and Dinger, R.: Untersuchungen bei Keratosis palmo-plantaris papulosa. Arch. Klin. Exp. Derm. 221: 481-495, 1965.

14870 KERATOSIS PALMO-PLANTARIS STRIATA

The lesions of the hands consist of a streak of hyperkeratosis running the length of each finger and onto the palm. Bologna (1966) reported a case in which involvement of males predominated in a striking manner.

Bologna, E. I.: Dominant verebliche Durch vier Generationen geschlechtsgebundene Keratosis palmaris striata (linearia). Dermatol. Wschr. 152: 446-457, 1966.

*14873 KILLER ANTIGEN OF PUCK

Puck et al. (1972) demonstrated a cell surface antigen which from evidence provided by hamster-man hybrids is determined by a locus on chromosome no. 11. Bodmer (1974) referred to KA as SA 1 species antigen 1.

Bodmer, W.: Oxford, personal communication, 1974.

Puck, T. T., Wuthier, P., Jones, C. and Kao, F. T.: Genetics of somatic mammalian cells: lethal antigens as genetic markers for study of human linkage groups. Proc. Natl. Acad. Sci. 68: 3102-3106, 1971.

14880 KLEEBLATTSCHAEDEL (CLOVERLEAF SKULL) SYNDROME

Only a few dozen cases have been described, all sporadic. The head has a flattened, trilobular configuration, caused by hydrocephalus in combination with congenital synostosis of the coronal and lambdoidal sutures. In the most severe form there is grotesque exophthalmos with corneal ulcerations. Bony deformities and ankylosis at the elbows occur in some cases. Nothing is known of a possible genetic basis. Paternal age effect should be sought. See THANATOPHORIC DWARFISM in the recessive catalog. Cohen (1973) points out that Kleeblattschaedel is a component of many syndromes, e.g. it is found in some cases of Crouzon syndrome (12350), Pfeiffer syndrome (10160) and Carpenter syndrome (20100).

Angel, C. R., McIntrye, M. S. and Moore, R. C.: Cloverleaf skull: Kleeblatts-Chaedel-deformity syndrome. Am. J. Dis. Child. 114: 198-202, 1967.

Cohen, M. M., Jr.: An etiologic and nosologic overview of craniosynostosis syndromes. The Clinical Delineation of Birth Defects. XVII. Malformation Syndromes (cont.). Baltimore: Williams and Wilkins, 1973.

Gruber, G. B.: Ueber einen akrocephalen Reliefschaedel. Ein Beitrag zur Frage der partiellen Chondrodystrophie. Beitr. Pathol. Anat. 97: 9-21, 1936.

Holtermueller, K. and Wiedemann, H. R.: The clover-leaf skull syndrome. Med. Wschr. 14: 439-446, 1960.

Welter, H.: Zur Frage des Hydrocephalus chondrodystrophicus congenitus. Beitr. Pathol. Anat. 97: 1-8, 1936.

14886 KLIPPEL-FEIL DEFORMITY, CONDUCTIVE DEAFNESS, ABSENT VAGINA

Park et al. (1971) described two unrelated females with a syndrome which previously has, it seems, not been recognized. Both had absent vagina, Klippel-Feil deformity of the cervical spine, short stature (about 5 feet) and conductive deafness from malformation of the temporal bones and ossicles. Secondary sexual characteristics were normal. One of the patients had absent left kidney and ectopic right kidney. Nothing is known of the genetics. Baird and Lowry (1974) described two unrelated patients who had absent vagina and Klippel-Feil syndrome, but no deafness. The abnormality in sexual development in this syndrome may be the same as that in the Rokitansky-Kuster-Hauser syndrome (27700) which is thought to be autosomal recessive.

Baird, P. A. and Lowry, R. B.: Absent vagina and Klippel-Feil anomaly. Am. J. Obstet. Gynecol. 118: 290-291, 1974.

Park, I. J., Jones, H. W., Jr., Nager, G. T., Chen, S. C. A. and Hussels, I. E.: A new syndrome in two unrelated females: Klippel-Feil deformity, conductive deafness and absent vagina. The Clinical Delineation of Birth Defects. X. Endocrine System. Baltimore: Williams and Wilkins, 1971. Pp. 311-317.

14890 KLIPPEL-FEIL SYNDROME

Dominant inheritance with reduced penetrance and variable expression is suggested by several reports including those of Bauman (1932), Bizarro (1938), Clemmesen (1936), Erskine (1946) and Jarcho and Levin (1938). There are clearly several genetic entities in this general category. One or more may be recessive and some may have no simple genetic basis (Lubs, personal communication). Klippel and Feil recognized three morphologic types of cervical vertebral fusion: I. Massive fusion of many cervical and upper thoracic vertebrae into bony blocks. II. Fusion at only one or two interspaces, although hemivertebrae, occipito-atlantal fusion, and other anomalies might be associated. III. Both cervical fusion and lower thoracic or lumbar fusion. Gunderson, Greenspan, Glaser and Lubs (1967) did family studies. C2-3 fusion, a subtype of category II, may be a simple dominant. The ear and spine changes are probably identical to those of the Wildervanck syndrome (31460).

Bauman, G. I.: Absence of the cervical spine. Klippel-Feil syndrome. J.A.M.A. 98: 129-132, 1932.

Bizarro, A. H.: Brevicollis. Lancet II: 828-829, 1938.

Clemmesen, V.: Congenital cervical synostosis (Klippel-Feil's syndrome): four cases. Acta Radiol. 17: 480-490, 1936.

Erskine, C. A.: An analysis of the Klippel-Feil syndrome. Arch. Pathol. 41: 269-281, 1946.

Jarcho, S. and Levin, P. M.: Hereditary malformation of the vertebral bodies. Bull. Hopkins Hosp. 62: 216-226, 1938.

14900 KLIPPEL-TRENAUNAY-WEBER SYNDROME

The features are large cutaneous hemangiomata with hypertrophy of the related bones and soft tissues. It resembles, clinically and in its lack of definite genetic basis, Sturge-Weber syndrome (18530) and indeed the two have been associated in some cases (Harper, 1971). Suggestions of a genetic 'cause' are meager (Waardenburg, 1963). See HEMANGIOMAS. I have seen a case of presumed K-T-W syndrome in which the affected parts were cool not warm.

Brooksaler, F.: The angioosteohypertrophy syndrome (Klippel-Trenaunay-Weber syndrome). Am. J. Dis. Child. 112: 161-164, 1966.

with nevus of Ota and Oto. Arch. Dermatol. 102: 640-645, 1970.

Harper, P. S.: Sturge-Weber syndrome with Klippel-Trenaunay-Weber syndrome. The Clinical Delineation of Birth Defects. XII. Skin, Hair and Nails. Baltimore: Williams and Wilkins, 1971. Pp. 314-317.

Koch, G.: Zur Klinik, Symptomatologie, Pathogenese und Erbpathologie des Klippel-Trenaunay-Weberschen syndroms. Acta Genet. Med. Gemellol. 5: 326-370, 1956.

Waardenburg, P. J.: Hypertrophic haemangiectasia (Klippel-Trenaunay-Weber's syndrome). In, Genetics and Ophthalmology. Springfield, Ill.: Charles C Thomas, 2: 1381-1386, 1963.

14910 KNUCKLE PADS

These are sometimes associated with Dupuytren contractures (q.v.) and it is not completely certain that a different gene is involved. Camptodactyly (q.v.) also has an uncertain relationship.

Allison, J. R., Jr. and Allison, J. R., Sr.: Knuckle pads. Arch. Dermatol. 93: 311-316, 1966.

Garrod, A. E.: Concerning pads upon the finger joints and their clinical relationship. Br. Med. J. 2: 8 only, 1904.

Weber, F. P.: A note on Dupuytren's contraction, camptodactylia and knuckle-pads. Br. J. Dermatol. Syph. 50: 26-31, 1938.

White, W. H.: On pads on the finger joints. Quart. J. Med. 1: 479-480, 1908.

*14920 KNUCKLE PADS, LEUKONYCHIA AND SENSINEURAL DEAFNESS

Bart et al. (1967) described a kindred in which many members had knuckle pads, leukonychia and deafness due to a lesion of the cochlea. Keratosis palmaris et plantaris was present in some. Male-to-male transmission was thought to have occurred in two instances. The condition described by Schwann (1963) was probably the same. The presence of leukonychia and the absence of digital constrictions appear to distinguish this disorder from the one listed as 'deafness, congenital, with keratopachydermia and constrictions of fingers and toes' (q.v.).

Bart, R. S. and Pumphrey, R. E.: Knuckle pads, leukonychia and deafness — a dominantly inherited syndrome. N. Engl. J. Med. 276: 202-207, 1967.

Schwann, J.: Keratosis palmaris et plantaris cum surditate congenita et leuconychia totali unguium. Dermatologica 126: 335-353, 1963.

*14930 KOILONYCHIA, HEREDITARY

Heidensleben (1960) observed koilonychia in father and child. The child also had cataract. Bergeson and Stone (1967) reported 12 affected persons in 4 generations with several instances of male-to-male transmission. Hellier (1950) reported 16 affected in 5 generations. Schleutermann et al. (1970) described eight affected persons in 5 generations with no male-to-male transmission and no clear evidence of close linkage. Linkage with the ABO locus was excluded. Char (1971) described 8 cases in four generations of a family. An extensively affected kindred was reported by Handa et al. (1960).

Bergeson, J. R. and Stone, O. J.: Koilonychia. A report of familial spoon nails. Arch. Dermatol. 95: 351-353, 1967.

Char, F.: Hereditary koilonychia. The Clinical Delineation of Birth Defects. XII. Skin, Hair and Nails. Baltimore: Williams and Wilkins, 1971. P. 274.

Graciansky, P. and Bovhulle, S.: Association de koilonychie et de leukonychie transmises en dominance. Bull. Soc. Fr. Dermatol. Syph. 68: 15-17, 1961.

Handa, Y., Handa, K., Kosaka, S. and Mitani, K.: A note in the genetics of koilonychia. Wakeyama Med. Rep. 5: 143-150, 1960.

Heidensleben, E.: Hereditary congenital koilonychia accompanied by syndermatotic cataract. Acta Ophthalmol. 38: 1-4, 1960.

Hellier, F. F.: Hereditary koilonychia. Br. J. Dermatol. 62: 213-214, 1950.

Schleutermann, D. A., Bias, W. B. and McKusick, V. A.: A kindred of koilonychia: linkage data. Am. J. Hum. Genet. 22: 390-395, 1970.

*14940 KOK DISEASE

Kok and Bruyn (1962) described a 'new' hereditary disease, inherited as an autosomal dominant and characterized by onset at birth with hypertonia in flexion which disappears in sleep, exaggerated startle response, strong brain-stem reflexes (especially head-retraction reflex) and, in some, epilepsy. There were 29 affected persons in six generations. Hypertonia diminished during the course of the first year of life. The startle reflex was sometimes accompanied by acute generalized hypertonia causing the patient to fall like a log to the ground. The description is somewhat reminiscent of the 'Jumping Frenchmen of Maine' (Stevens, 1966). Suhren et al. (1966) described a family in which 25 persons in 5 generations with numerous instances of male-to-male transmission were afflicted with transient congenital hypertonia and hypokinesia in the waking state, later in life greatly exaggerated startle reaction sometimes associated with falling, markedly hyperactive brain-stem reflexes (e.g., head retraction, palmo-mental and snout reflexes) and a momentary generalized jerking on falling asleep. The findings were interpreted as indicating uninhibited nonciceptive reflex pattern as a result of a defect in maturation. Improvement accompanied barbiturate medication. (I question the etymologic and orthographic propriety of 'hypereflexia.') (As kindly pointed out to me by Went (1974), Kok and Suhren are one person.)

Kok, O. and Bruyn, G. W.: An unidentified hereditary disease. (Letter) Lancet I: 1359 only, 1962.

Stevens, H.: Jumping Frenchmen of Maine. Arch. Neurol. 12: 311-314, 1966.

Suhren, O., Bruyn, G. W. and Tuynman, J. A.: Hyperflexia. A hereditary startle syndrome. J. Neurol. Sci. 3: 577-605, 1966.

Went, L. N.: Leyden, personal communication, 1974.

14950 KYRLE DISEASE

Kyrle disease is a follicular keratosis. The horny papules may be situated anywhere except the palms, soles and mucous membranes. They eventually acquire a central keratotic plug that upon removal leaves a crater that matches the shape of the plug (Kyrle signe). The lesions come in crops, last several weeks, and eventually disappear with minimal or no scarring. The histologic appearance is responsible for the Latin name 'hyperkeratosis follicularis et parafollicularis in cutem penetrans.' The perforating character of the lesions is reminiscent of elastosis perforans . Tessler et al. (1973) described a family with dominant inheritance but no instance of male-to-male transmission. Posterior subcapsular cataracts were present in 3 young adults with the skin disease.

Tessler, H. H., Apple, D. J. and Goldberg, M. F.: Ocular findings in a kindred with Kyrle disease. Arch. Ophthal. 90: 278-280, 1973.

14960 LABIA MINORA, INCOMPLETE ADHESION OF

Barbosa Sueiro and Piloto (1964) reported 5 cases occurring in 4 generations of a family.

Barbosa Sueiro, M. B. and Piloto, R.: Aderencia incompleta dos pequenos labios com caracter familiar. Arqu. Anat. Antrop. 32: 187-192, 1964.

*14970 LACRIMAL DUCT DEFECT

Schnyder (1920) described a defect of the tear ducts in members of three generations of a family. Imperforate naso-lacrimal ducts with or without absence of puncta and canaliculi has been described in a dominant pedigree pattern by Bischler (1957), Lumbroso (1960), Town (1943) and others. See also ORBITAL MARGIN, HYPOPLASIA OF. See also CLEFT LIP-PALATE WITH SPLIT HAND AND FOOT.

Bischler, V.: Le facteur hereditaire dans obstructions des voies lacrymales et plus particulierement dans l'atresie des points et canalicules lacrymaux. Mod. Prob. Ophthal. 1: 584-590, 1957.

Lumbroso, B. D.: On a case of congenital atresia of the lacrimal ducts with familial characteristics. Acta Genet. Med. Gemellol. 9: 290-295, 1960.

Schnyder, W. F.: Uber familiaeres Vorkommen resp. die Vererbung von Erkrankungen der Traenenwege. Z. Augenheilk. 44: 257-261, 1920.

Town, A. E.: Congenital absence of lacrimal puncta in three members of a family. Arch. Ophthalmol. 29: 767-771, 1943.

*14973 LACRIMO-AURICULO-DENTO-DIGITAL SYNDROME (LADD)

Hollister et al. (1973) described a Mexican man who had a combination of manifestations to which they gave this name. Five of eight children (four girls and one boy) had the same syndrome. The lacrimal feature was aplasia or hypoplasia of the puncta with obstruction of the nasal lacrimal ducts. The auricular features were cup-shaped pinnas with mixed hearing deficit. The dental features included small and peg-shaped lateral maxillary incisors and mild enamel dysplasia. The digital features were variable but included fifth finger clinodactyly, duplication of the distal phalanx of the thumb, triphalangeal thumb, syndactyly. All of the features of this syndrome have been reported as isolated traits inherited as autosomal dominants (see 14970, 12860, 19070, 15040, etc.) but the syndromal association has, it seems, not been reported before. In a Mexican man and 5 of his 8 children (including one son) Hollister et al. (1973) observed a syndrome of obstruction of nasolacrimal ducts, hypoplasia or aplasia of the lacrimal puncta, cup-shaped ears, hearing loss, and dental and digital abnormalities. Levy (1967) described a sporadic case of this association. Temtamy (1974) suggested that a better acronym for this syndrome is LARD (lacrimo-auriculo-radio-dental).

Hollister, D. W., Klein, S. H., Dejager, H. J., Lachman, R. S. and Rimoin, D. L.: Lacrimo-auriculo-dento-digital (LADD) syndrome. The Clinical Delineation of Birth Defects. XXII. Malformation Syndromes (cont.). Baltimore: Williams, and Wilkins, 1972.

Hollister, D. W., Klein, S. H., Dejager, H. J., Lachman, R. S. and Rimoin, D. L.: The lacrimo-auriculo-dento-digital syndrome. J. Pediatr. 83: 438-444, 1973.

Levy, W. J.: Mesoectodermal dysplasia: a new combination of anomalies. Am. J. Ophthalmol. 63: 978-982, 1967.

Temtamy, S. A.: Baltimore, personal communication, 1974.

14975 LACTALBUMIN

Lactalbumin is one of the principle proteins of milk. Its structural similarity to lysozyme (see 15345) indicates an evolutionary kinship to that enzyme which is closer than that between hemoglobin chains and myoglobin. By itself lactalbumin has no known enzymatic activity. However, it represents the B chain of lactose synthetase, an enzyme found only in lactating mammary gland. The A chain of lactose synthetase is N-acetyllactosamine synthetase, an enzyme bound to the membranes of the Golgi system in many tissues, not only breast. In other tissues, without lactalbumin, the B chain functions in the synthesis of the carbohydrate part of glycoproteins. Hormonal regulation of the synthesis of lactalbumin by mammary tissue controls the synthesis of lactose. Thus, in evolution lactalbumin lost its lysozyme-type activity and acquired a new function, that of modifying the action of another enzyme so that it functions in the synthesis of lactose. Human lactalbumin has a molecular weight of 14,076 and contains 123 amino acid residues. The estimated difference in structure between lactalbumins and lysozymes is 59 percent.

Dayhoff, M. O.: Lactalbumin and lysozymes. Atlas of Protein Sequence and Structure 1972 (vol. 5). Washington: National Biomedical Research Foundation, 1972. Pp. D133-D140.

*15000 LACTATE DEHYDROGENASE, LOCUS A

Boyer, Fainer and Watson-Williams (1963) detected an electrophoretic variant of the B subunit of LDH. Family studies could not be done. The pattern was consistent with the hypothesis that LDH isozymes are tetramers of two different subunits. In the heterozygote LDH-1, -2, -3, -4 and -5 occur in proportions 1 : 4 : 6 : 4 : 1, as in Markert's dissociation-reassociation experiments.

Nance, Claflin and Smithies (1963) observed a genetically determined variant LDH in the red cells of four members of two generations of a Brazilian family. The mutation involves the A subunit. Close linkage with MNS, haptoglobin and Gm loci was excluded. This is the first instance in which practical considerations permitted demonstration of the variant in multiple relatives. Unlike the findings of Shaw and Barto (1963) in Peromyscus and of Boyer, Fainer and Watson-Williams in man, the findings in the Brazilian family did not suggest random association between the products of the mutant and wild type alleles. In trout the loci coding for subunits A and B are linked (Morrison and Wright, 1966). Studies using human-mouse somatic cell hybrids indicate that the LDH-A and LDH-B loci are not linked (Nabholz et al., 1969). LDH variants, involving either the A or the B subunit, seem to be unusually frequent in India (Das et al., 1970).

Blake, N. M., Kirk, R. L., Pryke, E. and Sinnett, P.: Lactate dehydrogenase electrophoretic variant in a New Guinea highland population. Science 163: 701-702, 1969.

Boyer, S. H., IV, Fainer, D. C. and Watson-Williams, E. J.: Lactate dehydrogenase variant from human blood: evidence for molecular subunits. Science 141: 642-643, 1963.

Das, S. R., Mukherjee, B. N., Das, S. K., Ananthakrishnan, R., Blake, N. M. and Kirk, R. L.: LDH variants in India. Humangenetik 9: 107-109, 1970.

Davidson, R. G., Fildes, R. A., Glen-Bott, A. M., Harris, H., Robson, E. B. and Cleghorn, T. E.: Genetical studies on a variant of human lactate dehydrogenase (subunit A). Ann. Hum. Genet. 29: 5-17, 1965.

Morrison, W. J. and Wright, J. E.: Genetic analysis of three lactate dehydrogenase isozyme systems in trout: evidence for linkage of genes coding subunits A and B. J. Exp. Zool. 163: 259-270, 1966.

Nabholz, M., Miggiano, V. and Bodmer, W. F.: Genetic analysis with human-mouse somatic cell hybrids. Nature 223: 358-363, 1969.

Nance, W. E., Claflin, A. and Smithies, O.: Lactic dehydrogenase: genetic control in man. Science 142: 1075-1077, 1963.

Shaw, C. R. and Barto, E.: Genetic evidence for the subunit structure of lactate dehydrogenase isozymes. Proc. Natl. Acad. Sci. 50: 211-214, 1963.

Shows, T. B.: Genetics of human-mouse somatic cell hybrids: linkage of human genes for lactate dehydrogenase-A and esterase-A4. Proc. Natl. Acad. Sci. 69: 348-352, 1972.

Van Someren, H., Kah., Westerveld, A. and Bootsma, D.: Human genetics- two new linkage groups carrying different loci for LDH and glutamic-pyruvic transaminase found. Nature 240: 221-222, 1972.

Vesell, E. S.: Genetic control of isozyme patterns in human tissue. In, Steinberg, A. G. and Bearn, A. G. (eds.): Progress in Medical Genetics. New York: Grune and Stratton, 4: 1965.

*15010 LACTATE DEHYDROGENASE, LOCUS B

See above. LDH-B and peptidase B (16990) are linked (Silvana Santachiara, et al., 1970) and both loci are on chromosome no. 12 (Chen et al., 1973). Kitamura et al. (1971) reported the first case of a complete deficiency of lactate dehydrogenase subunit H(B) in serum, saliva and erythrocytes of a 64-year-old male with mild diabetes. Study made on family members revealed low LDH activity in their serum also linked with decreased relative activity of the H4(B4) fraction. Based on the comparison of the calculated ratio of H to M subunits in normal and affected family members, it was hypothesized that the proband is homozygous while the abnormal family members are heterozygous, assuming a single gene is involved. In a case of deletion of the short arm of chromosome no. 12, Weiss et al. (1973) found evidence that LDH-B is located there.

Chen, T. R., McMorris, F. A., Creagan, R., Ricciuti, F., Tischfield, J. and Ruddle, F.: Assignment of the genes for malate oxidoreductase decarboxylating to chromosome 6 and peptidase B and lactate dehydrogenase B to chromosome 12 in man. Am. J. Hum. Genet. 25: 200-207, 1973.

Kitamura, M., Iijima, N., Hashimoto, F. and Hiratsuka, A.: Hereditary deficiency of subunit H of lactate dehydrogenase. Clin. Chim. Acta 34: 419-423, 1971.

Mayeda, K., Weiss, L., Lindahl, R. and Dully, M.: Localization of the human lactate dehydrogenase B gene on the short arm of chromosome 12. Am.·J. Hum. Genet. 26: 59-64, 1974.

Silvana Santachiara, A., Nabholz, M., Miggiano, V., Darlington, A. J. and Bodmer, W. F.: Linkage between human lactate dehydrogenase B and peptidase B genes. Nature 227: 248-251, 1970.

Van Someren, H., Kah., Westerveld, A. and Bootsma, D.: Human genetics-two new linkage groups carrying different loci for LDH and glutamic-pyruvic transaminase found. Nature 240: 221-222, 1972.

Weiss, L., Mayeda, K., Lindahl, R. and Dully, M.: Localization of human LDH-B gene of the short arm of chromosome 12. (Abstract) Am. J. Hum. Genet. 25: 85A only, 1973.

*15015 LACTATE DEHYDROGENASE, LOCUS C (TESTICULAR VARIANT X)

Zinkham et al. (1964) have found a distinctive LDH isozyme in mature testis of many species including man. It is polymorphic in the pigeon where one can infer that a locus separate from the A and B loci control it. The same is almost certainly true in the human also. This is a gene which functions only in one sex and only in one tissue. The locus determining the testicular variant X is called LDH(C). Zinkham et al. (1969) found that the B and C loci are closely linked, possibly contiguous. Since LDH B and C have remained closely linked for a long evolutionary period, they are probably closely linked in man. This would mean that LDH(C) is on chromosome no. 12.

Blanco, A., Zinkham, W. H. and Kupchyk, L.: Genetic control and ontogeny of lactate dehydrogenase in pigeon testes. J. Exp. Zool. 156: 137-152. 1964.

Zinkham, W. H. and Isensee, H.: Genetic control of lactate dehydrogenase synthesis in the somatic and genetic tissues of pigeons. Johns Hopkins Med. J. 139: 11-25, 1972.

Zinkham, W. H.: A unique form of lactate dehydrogenase in human sperm: biological and clinical significance. Johns Hopkins Med. J. 130: 1-10, 1972.

Zinkham, W. H., Blanco, A. and Clowry, L. J., Jr.: An unusual isozyme of lactic dehydrogenase in mature testes: localization, ontogeny, and kinetic properties. Ann. N.Y. Acad. Sci. 121: 571-588, 1964.

Zinkham, W. H., Blanco, A. and Kupchyk, L.: Lactate dehydrogenase in pigeon testes: gentetic control of three loci. Science 144: 1353-1354, 1964.

Zinkham, W. H., Isensee, H. and Renwick, J. H.: Linkage of lactate dehydrogenase B and C loci in pigeons. Science 164: 185-187, 1969.

15017 LACTIC ACIDOSIS, CHRONIC ADULT FORM

Sussman et al. (1970) described a 28-year-old woman with chronically elevated lactic acid, pyruvic acid and increased lactate-to-pyruvate ratio. Alcohol ingestion and moderate exercise increased lactate levels. Hyperuricemia was present as in glycogen storage disease and as in that condition uric acid clearance was apparently depressed. The mother and three of the mother's sibs also showed abnormal lactate response to the combination of alcohol ingestion and exercise.

Sussman, K. E., Alfrey, A., Kirsch, W. M., Zweig, P., Felig, P. and Messner, F.: Chronic lactic acidosis in an adult. A new syndrome associated with an altered redox state of certain NAD-NADH coupled reactions. Am. J. Med. 48: 104-112, 1970.

15020 LACTOGEN, PLACENTAL

Also called chorionic somato-mammotropin or HCS, this peptide hormone is structurally, immunologically, and functionally similar to pituitary growth hormone (13925). It is synthesized by the placental syncytiotrophoblast and therefore its genetic determination is a function of the fetal genome. Human lactogen has 190 amino acid residues and a molecular weight of 22,125.

Dayhoff, M. O.: Hormones, active peptides and toxins. Atlas of Protein Sequence and Structure 1972 (vol. 5). Washington: National Biomedical Research Foundation, 1972. P. D201.

15023 LANGER-GIEDION SYNDROME

This disorder has similarities to the tricho-rhino-phalangeal syndrome, particularly with regard to facies and cone-shaped epiphysis. Distinguishing features are mental retardation, microcephaly, multiple exostoses and redundant skin. Less consistent features include hyperextensible joints, recurrent upper respiratory tract infections and delayed speech development. All cases have been sporadic and a majority have been males.

Giedion, A.: Die periphere Dysostose (pD) — ein Sammelbegriff. Fortschr. Roentgenstr. 110: 507-534, 1969.

Hall, B. D., Langer, L. O., Giedion, A., Smith, D. W., Cohen, M. M. Jr., Beals, R. K. and Brandner, M.: Langer-Giedion syndrome. Clinical Delineation of Birth Defects, in press, 1974.

Langer, L. O.: The thoracic-pelvic-phalangeal dystrophy. Clinical Delineation of Birth Defects. IV. Skeletal System. New York National Foundation-March of Dimes, 1969. Pp. 55-64.

*15025 LARSEN SYNDROME

Harris and Cullen (1971) described affected mother and daughter. Bilateral dislocation of the knees, pes cavus, cylindrically shaped fingers and characteristic facies (wide-spaced eyes, flattened nasal bridge and prominent forehead) were present in both. The maternal grandfather is said to have had similar facies. One of the original cases of Larsen et al. (1950), age 23 years in 1972, has an affected child. Features in addition to knee dislocations included flat face, accessory carpal bones and short terminal phalanges creating pseudoclubbing. Both recessive (see 24560) and dominant forms seem to exist. Multiple congenital dislocations with osseous anomalies and unusual facies are characteristic. Anterior dislocation of the tibia on the femur is usual. A juxtacalcaneal accessory ossification center and abnormality of vertebrae are observed. Although usually this condition is recessive, dominant inheritance seems certain from the reports of Latta et al. (1971) and of McFarlane (1929). Phenotypic differences of the dominant and recessive types have not been delineated.

Harris, R. and Cullen, C. H.: Autosomal dominant inheritance in Larsen's syndrome. Clin. Genet. 2: 87-90, 1971.

Larsen, L. J., Schottstaedt, E. R. and Bost, F. C.: Multiple congenital dislocations associated with characteristic facial abnormality. J. Pediatr. 37: 574-581, 1950.

Latta, R. J., Grahm, C. B., Aase, J., Scham, S. M. and Smith, D. W.: Larsen's syndrome: a skeletal dysplasia with multiple joint dislocations and unusual facies. J. Pediatr. 78: 291-298, 1971.

McFarlane, A. L.: A report on four cases of congenital genu recurvatum occurring in one family. Br. J. Surg. 34: 388-391, 1947.

15030 LARYNX, CONGENITAL PARTIAL ATRESIA OF

Baker and Savetsky (1966) described affected mother and 2 children.

Baker, D. C., Jr. and Savetsky, L.: Congenital partial atresia of the larynx. Laryngoscope 76: 616-620, 1966.

*15040 LATERAL INCISORS, ABSENCE OF

The upper lateral incisors are absent or hypoplastic. A pointed tooth is a partial expression of the gene. The trait was present in one-third of a Swiss group studied by Joehr (1934). Furthermore, all affected members of the isolate were descendants of one man, born in the 18th century. Schultz (1934) found the condition in one gorilla and one gibbon. Woolf (1971) found that in 71 of 103 families of probands with missing maxillary lateral incisors one or more first-, second-, or third-degree relatives had a missing or peg-shaped maxillary incisor. He concluded that at least part of the genetic component is autosomal dominant with reduced penetrance and variable expressivity. Recessive or polygenetic inheritance in some families was also considered plausible. Families showed a high degree of intrafamilial concordance for type of minor anomaly, especially if the proband had bilaterally absent lateral incisors.

Grahnen, H.: Hypodontia in the permanent dentition. Odont. Rev. 7 (suppl. 3): 419-421, 1965.

Joehr, A. C.: Reduktionserscheinungen an den oberen Seitlichen schneidezaehnen. Arch. Klaus. Stift. Vererbungsforsch. 9: 73-133, 1934.

Keeler, C. E. and Short, R.: Hereditary absence of upper lateral incisors. J. Hered. 25: 391-392, 1934.

Mandeville, L. C.: Congenital absence of permanent maxillary lateral incisor teeth. A preliminary investigation. Ann. Eugen. 15: 1-10, 1950.

Montagu, M. F. A.: The significance of the variability of the upper lateral incisor teeth in man. Hum. Biol. 12: 323-358, 1940.

Rantanen, A. V.: On the frequency of the missing and peg-shaped maxillary lateral incisor among Finnish students. Am. J. Phys. Anthrop. 14: 491-496, 1956.

Schultz, A. H.: Inherited reductions in the dentition of man. Hum. Biol. 6: 627-631, 1934.

Schultz, A. H.: The hereditary tendency to eliminate the upper lateral incisors. Hum. Biol. 4: 34-40, 1932.

Witkop, C. J.: Studies of intrinsic disease in isolates with observations on penetrance and expressivity of certain anatomical traits. In, Pruzansky, S. (ed.): Congenital Anomalies of the Face and Associated Structures. Springfield, Ill.: Charles C Thomas, 1961.

Woolf, C. M.: Missing maxillary lateral incisors: a genetic study. Am. J. Hum. Genet. 23: 289-296, 1971.

15050 LATTICE DEGENERATION OF RETINA LEADING TO RETINAL DETACHMENT

Lattice degeneration of the retina with later development of retinal detachment in many non-myopic persons was observed by Everett (1968). The familial occurrence of lattice degeneration in non-myopes was earlier reported by Gartner (1960).

Everett, W. G.: Study of a family with lattice degeneration and retinal detachment. Am. J. Ophthalmol. 65: 229-232, 1968.

Gartner, J.: Erbbedingte aequatoriale Degenerationen Nichtmyoper: Solitaerformen und oraparallele Baender. Klin. Mbl. Augenheilk. 136: 523-539, 1960.

15060 LEGG-CALVE-PERTHES DISEASE

Wamosher and Farhi (1963) described a Jewish family in which 8 members of 3 generations were affected. Boys predominate heavily in all reports of sporadic cases of the disease. In the families with multiple cases the sex ratio has been closer to 1. A similar phenomenon has been observed in ankylosing spondylitis (q.v.) and in congenital dislocation of the hip. When familial the disorder may be more likely to show bilateral involvement. McNutt (1962) suggested that a peculiarity in vascular supply of the femoral head and neck may be inherited as the factor predisposing to this disorder. I have seen affected father and two sons. Stephens and Kerby (1946) observed many affected persons in five generations. Caffey (1968) is of the view that coxa plana, as he terms this condition, really represents at least in its initiation a stress fracture and not avascular necrosis. Gray et al. (1972) found evidence suggesting polygenic inheritance.

Caffey, J. P.: The early roentgenographic changes in essential coxa plana: their significance in pathogenesis. Am. J. Roentgen. 103: 620-634, 1968.

Goff, C. W.: Legg-Calve-Perthes syndrome (LCPS). An up-to-date critical review. Clin. Orthop. 22: 93-107, 1962.

Gray, I. M., Lowry, R. B. and Renwick, D. H. G.: Incidence and genetics of Legg-Perthes disease (osteochondritis deformans) in British Columbia: evidence of polygenic determination. J. Med. Genet. 9: 197-202, 1972.

McNutt, W.: Inherited vascular pattern of the femoral head and neck as a predisposing factor to Legg-Calve-Perthes disease. Texas Rep. Biol. Med. 20: 525-531, 1962.

Stephens, F. E. and Kerby, J. P.: Hereditary Legg-Calve-Perthes disease. J. Hered. 37: 153-160, 1946.

Wamoscher, Z. and Farhi, A.: Hereditary Legg-Calve-Perthes disease. Am. J. Dis. Child. 106: 97-100, 1963.

15070 LEIOMYOMA OF VULVA AND ESOPHAGUS

Wahlen and Astedt (1965) described this combination in mother and daughter. The esophageal tumor was an obstructing lesion in the lower portion. In both women the presenting complaint with reference to the vulval lesions was enlargement of the clitoris due to growth of the tumor at its base. Chromosome and endocrinologic studies showed nothing abnormal. The authors emphasized that leiomyoma of the vulva should prompt X-ray studies of the esophagus and leiomyoma of the esophagus should prompt search for vulval leiomyoma.

Wahlen, T. and Astedt, B.: Familial occurrence of coexisting leiomyoma of vulva and oesophagus. Acta Obstet. Gynecol. Scand. 44: 197-203, 1965.

*15080 LEIOMYOMATA, HEREDITARY MULTIPLE, OF SKIN

Multiple small tumors composed of smooth muscle fibers develop in the skin. Malignant transformation is rare. The tumors are thought to arise from the erector pilorum muscles. The pedigree as reported by Kloepfer et al. (1958) was more suggestive of recessive inheritance (q.v.) than of dominant inheritance as they suggested. However, several critical members of the pedigree were not available for examination. Dominant inheritance with incomplete penetrance is supported by the pedigree of Mezzadra (1965), who described cutaneous leiomyomata in 3 generations. Uterine myomata were associated. This and Kloepfer's family were Italian. Weilbaecher (1967) observed a Swedish family with five affected in three generations and male-to-male transmission. Rudner et al. (1972) described identical twins both with multiple cutaneous leiomyoma and both with a history of hysterectomy for uterine leiomyoma. Reed et al. (1973) also emphasized the association of uterine myomata.

Berendes, U., Kuhner, A. and Schnyder, U. W.: Segmentary and disseminated lesions in multiple hereditary cutaneous leiomyoma. Humangenetik 13: 81-82, 1971.

Kloepfer, H. W., Krafchuk, J., Derbes, V. and Burks, J.: Hereditary multiple leiomyoma of the skin. Am. J. Hum. Genet. 10: 48-52, 1958.

Mezzadra, G.: Leiomioma cutaneo multiplo ereditario. Studio di un caso sistematizzato in soggetto maschile appartenente a famiglia portatrice di leiomiomatosi cutanea E fibromiomatosi uterina. Minerva Dermatol. 40: 388-393, 1965.

Reed, W. B., Walker, R. and Horowitz, R.: Cutaneous leimyomata with uterine leiomyomata. Acta Derm. Venerol. 53: 1-8, 1973.

Rudner, E. J., Schwartz, O. D. and Greekin, J. N.: Multiple cutaneous leiomyoma in identical twins. Arch. Dermatol. 104: 81-82, 1972.

Weilbaecher, R. G.: New Orleans, La.: personal communication, 1967.

15090 LENTIGINES

Pipkin and Pipkin (1950) observed eight cases in three generations of a Maltese-Lebanese family. Six of the affected had nystagmus.

Pipkin, A. C. and Pipkin, S. B.: A pedigree of generalized lentigo. J. Hered. 41: 79-82, 1950.

15100 LENTIGINOSIS, CENTROFACIAL NEURO-DYSRAPHIC

Touraine (1955), who first described this condition (1941), stated that in 17 families in which he examined multiple members a total of 32 cases were discovered. In 9 of the families a parent and one or more children were affected. In 5 families with a total of 15 cases only two or more sibs were affected. He quoted an instance of affected mother and four children. Mental retardation is frequently associated.

Touraine, A.: L'Heredite en Medecine. Paris: Masson, 1955.

Touraine, A.: Une nouvelle neuro-ectodermose congenitale: la lentiginose centro-faciale et ses dysplasies associees. Ann. Dermatol. Syph. 8: 453-473, 1941.

*15110 LEOPARD SYNDROME

Walther et al. (1967) found asymptomatic cardiac changes in a mother and her son and daughter, associated with generalized lentigo. The electrocardiogram in the son suggested myocardial infarction. The mother was shown by cardiac catheterization to have mild pulmonary stenosis. Watson (1967) reported three families in which two generations contained persons with generalized lentigines. Many of these had valvular pulmonary stenosis. In all, 14 persons were affected. We have observed mother and daughter with striking generalized lentigines (694841, 693586). Both were deaf and both have a striking heart murmur. The nature of the cardiac malformation has not been elucidated. Similar generalized lentigines were described by Moynahan (1962) in three unrelated patients (2 females, 1 male). Growth was stunted. In one girl, one ovary was absent and the other hypoplastic. The boy had hypospadias and undescended testes. Endocardial and myocardial fibroelastosis may have been present. Intelligence was normal but behavior childish. Matthews (1968) reported mother and two half-sib children with generalized lentigines, electrocardiographic changes and murmurs. A history of male-to-male transmission was recorded. Lentigines were also present in the cardiac syndrome reported by Forney et al. (see MITRAL REGURGITATION, CONDUCTIVE DEAFNESS, etc.). Gorlin et al. (1969) presented evidence for dominant inheritance. Polani and Moynahan (1972) gave a full report of 8 patients and their families. They were impressed with the occurrence of left-sided obstructive cardiomyopathy and none of their patients were deaf. 'Progressive cardiomyopathic lentiginosis' was the term they proposed. It would seem that there must be more than one form of this disease.

Capute, A. J., Rimoin, D. L., Konigsmark, B. W., Esterly, N. B. and Richardson, F.: Congenital deafness and multiple lentigines. A report of cases in a mother and daughter. Arch. Dermatol. 100: 207-213, 1969.

Gorlin, R. J., Anderson, R. C. and Blaw, M.: Multiple lentigines syndrome. Complex comprising multiple lentigenes, electrocardiographic conduction abnormalities, ocular hypertelorism, pulmonary stenosis, abnormalities of genitalia, retardation of growth, senorineural deafness, and autosomal dominant hereditary pattern. Am. J. Dis. Child. 117: 652-662, 1969.

Matthews, N. L.: Lentigo and electrocardiographic changes. N. Engl. J. Med. 278: 780-781, 1968.

Moynahan, E. J.: Multiple symmetrical moles, with psychic and somatic infantilism and genital hypoplasia: first male case of a new syndrome. Proc. R. Soc. Med. 55: 959-960, 1962.

Pickering, D., Laski, B., MacMillan, D. C. and Rose, V.: 'Little leopard' syndrome. Arch. Dis. Child. 46: 85-90, 1971.

Polani, P. E. and Moynahan, E. J.: Progressive cardiomyopathic lentiginosis. Quart. J. Med. 41: 205-225, 1972.

Selmanowitz, V. J., Orentreich, N. and Felsenstein, J. M.: Lentiginosis profusa syndrome. (Multiple lentigines syndrome). Arch. Dermatol. 104: 393-401, 1971.

Sommer, A., Contras, S. B., Craenen, J. M. and Hosier, D. M.: A family study of the leopard syndrome. Am. J. Dis. Child. 121: 520-523, 1971.

Swanson, S. L., Santen, R. J. and Smith, D. W.: Multiple lentigines syndrome: new findings of hypogonadotrophism, hyposmia, and unilateral renal agenesis. J. Pediatr. 78: 1037-1039, 1971.

Walther, R. J., Polansky, B. and Grots, I. A.: Electrocardiographic abnormalities in a family with generalized lentigo. Meeting, Am. College of Cardiol., Washington, D. C., Feb. 17, 1967.

Watson, G. H.: Pulmonary stenosis, cafe-au-lait spots, and dull intelligence. Arch. Dis. Child. 42: 303-307, 1967.

*15120 LERI PLEONOSTEOSIS

Rukavina and associates (1959) reported the disorder in four generations of a family. The features were short stature, mongoloid facies, short spade-like hands, broad thumbs in valgus position, genu recurvatum and generalized limitation of joint mobility, thickening of the palmar and forearm fasciae, enlargement of the posterior neural arches of the cervical vertebrae and shuffling short-stepped gait.

Rukavina, J. G., Falls, H. F., Holt, J. F. and Block, W. D.: Leri's pleonosteosis: a study of a family with a review of the literature. J. Bone Joint Surg. 41A: 397-408, 1959.

15130 LEUCINE AMINOPEPTIDASE OF PLACENTA

Beckman et al. (1966) found 3 placental lap types. (Lap enzymes in the serum of pregnant women probably are not derived from placenta) genetic studies remain to be done. Beckman et al. (1969) in a later publication stated a preference for the designation amino acid naphthylamidase.

Beckman, L., Beckman, G., Mi, M. P. and De Simone, J.: The human placental amino acid naphthylamidases: their molecular interrelations and correlations with perinatal factors. Hum. Hered. 19: 249-257, 1969.

Beckman, L., Bjorling, G. and Christodoulou, C.: Pregnancy enzymes and placental polymorphism. II. Leucine aminopeptidase. Acta Genet. Statist. Med. 16: 122-131, 1966.

Scandalios, J. G.: Human serum leucine aminopeptidase. Variation in pregnancy and in disease states. J. Hered. 58: 153-156, 1967.

15140 LEUKEMIA, CHRONIC LYMPHATIC

Chronic lymphatic leukemia seems especially prone to familial occurrence. Furbetta and Solinas (1963) reported affected grandfather, son, and grandson.

Furbetta, D. and Solinas, P.: Hereditary chronic lymphatic leukemia. Proc. Sec. Intern. Cong. Hum. Genet. (Rome, Sept. 6-12, 1961.) 2: 1078-1079, 1963.

McPhedran, P., Heath, C. W., Jr. and Lee, J.: Patterns of familial leukemia. Ten cases of leukemia in two interrelated families. Cancer 24: 403-407, 1969.

Wisniewski, D. and Weinreich, J.: Lymphatische Leukaemie bei Vater und Sohn. Blut 12: 241-244, 1966.

15143 LEUKEMOID REACTION

Smith and Herring (1971) described hereditary leukemoid reaction in mother and two children. The mother had been suspected of leukemia at an early age and had been treated with methane for a time.

Smith, L. G. and Herring, W. B.: Hereditary leukemoid reaction. (Abstract) Clin. Res. 19: 432 only, 1971.

15150 LEUKOCYTE NUCLEAR APPENDAGES, HEREDITARY PREVALENCE OF

Seaman (1959) described a family with nuclear projections of the nuclei of neutrophilic leukocytes simulating the drumsticks but not sex-specific. Such were present in 76 percent of the neutrophiles of the male proband and in 25-56 percent of those of his father, uncle, two sons and a daughter but in neither of his wives.

Seaman, G.: Sur une anomalie constitutionnelle hereditaire du noyau des polynucleaires neutrophiles. Rev. Hematol. 14: 409-412, 1959.

*15160 LEUKONYCHIA TOTALIS

Medansky and Fox (1960) described white nails in fourteen members of five generations of a family. Kruse et al. (1951) observed father-son transmission.

Harrington, J. F.: White fingernails. Arch. Intern. Med. 114: 301-306, 1964.

Juhlin, L.: Hereditary leukonychia. Acta Derm. Venerol. 43: 136-141, 1963.

Kruse, W. T., Cawley, E. P. and Cotterman, C. W.: Hereditary leukonychia totalis. J. Invest. Derm. 17: 135-140, 1951.

Medansky, R. S. and Fox, J. M.: Hereditary leukonychia totalis. Arch. Derm. 82: 412-414, 1960.

15165 LIPOATROPHIC DIABETES

Dunnigan et al. (1974) described a dominantly inherited disorder in 6 females in 4 generations. Three of the 6 were personally examined by the authors. Features were symmetric lipoatrophy of the trunk and limbs with rounded, full face, tubero-eruptive xanthomata, acanthosis nigricans, insulin-resistant hyperinsulinism. In a second family from the same region of northern Scotland and therefore probably related to the first, 6 females in 3 generations were affected. X-linked dominant inheritance is as plausible as autosomal dominant inheritance. No comment was made on abortions, which if excessive might suggest a mode of inheritance like that of incontinentia pigmenti (30830) and the OFD syndrome (31120). This syndrome is distinct from congenital lipodystrophy (26970), a recessive; from progressive partial lipodystrophy, a seemingly non-Mendelian disorder that occurs predominantly in females who exhibit loss of fat from the face and trunk with normal or excessive fat deposition on the pelvic girdle and lower limbs; and from the acquired lipoatrophic diabetes that was described by Lawrence (1946). The last condition begins in adolescence or early adult life and shares with some other members of this group hepatosplenomegaly (leading to frank cirrhosis in some cases), acanthosis nigricans, hyperlipemia, and insulin-resistant diabetes.

Dunnigan, M. G., Cochrane, M. A., Kelly, A. and Scott, J. W.: Familial lipoatrophic diabetes with dominant transmission. A new syndrome. Quart. J. Med. 43: 33-48, 1974.

Lawrence, R. D.: Lipodystrophy and hepatomegaly with diabetes, lipaemia, and other metabolic disturbances: a case throwing light on the action of insulin. Lancet I: 724-731, 773-775, 1946.

15170 LIPOMA OF THE CONJUNCTIVA

Saebo (1948) described 3 persons in three successive generations: grandfather, mother and daughter. The tumor is distinctive from the dermo-lipoma of the Goldenhar syndrome.

Saebo, J.: Lipoma conjunctivae in three generations. Acta Ophthalmol. 26: 447-450, 1948.

15180 LIPOMATOSIS, FAMILIAL BENIGN CERVICAL

We observed three brothers with a collar of fat around the neck in the submandibular area and involving the nape of the neck. The age of onset was said to be 45, 39 and 29 years in the three patients. The mother was said to be definitely unaffected, having died at age 61, but two sisters and a maternal aunt were also affected. In advanced stages the process extended into the upper mediastinum. In the three brothers lipomata of conventional type were present in the epitrochlear area, back, axillae, internal aspect of forearm, etc. Brodie (1846) is said to have first described diffuse symmetrical lipomatosis with predilection for the neck. It was called 'fat neck' (Fetthals) by Madelung (1888). In cretinism we have seen not only the supraclavicular fossa but also the axillae filled with fat. When the cretinism is familial this may raise a suspicion of a separate recessively inherited supraclavicular lipomatosis. Cervical lipomatosis was associated with gout and hyperlipoproteinemia type IV in the sisters reported by Greene et al. (1970). Oligomenorrhea, muscle cramps, pes cavus and extensor plantar reflexes were also described. Lyon (1910) reported a striking case which was familial. Michon and Rose (1935) observed familial cases. Taylor et al. (1961) described surgical procedures adopted in a case similar to those reported by McKusick et al. (1962). It is entirely likely that most of these cases, as well as the familial cases noted above, represent an unusual localization of multiple lipomatosis (15290). See CERVICAL LIPODYSPLASIA, FAMILIAL (11785) for a distinct disorder.

Brodie, B. C.: Clinical Lectures on Surgery, Delivered at St. George's Hospital. Philadelphia: Lea and Blanchard, 1846. Pp. 201-202.

Greene, M. L., Glueck, C. J., Fujimoto, W. Y. and Seegmiller, J. E.: Benign symmetric lipomatosis (Launois-Bensaude adenolipomatosis) with gout and hyperlipoproteinemia. Am. J. Med. 48: 239-246, 1970.

Lyon, I. P.: Adiposis and lipomatosis: considered in reference to their constitutional relations and symptomatology. Arch. Intern. Med. 6: 28-120, 1910.

Madelung, (NI): Ueber den Fetthals (diffuses Lipom des Halses). Arch. Klin. Chir. 37: 106-130, 1888.

McKusick, V. A. and colleagues: Medical Genetics 1961. J. Chronic Dis. 15: 417-572, 1962 (fig. 24).

Michon, P. and Rose, F.: Adenolipomatose symetrique familiale. Bull. Soc. Frc. Dermatol. Syph. 42: 1005-1007, 1935.

Taylor, L. M., Beahrs, O. H. and Fontana, R. S.: Benign symmetric lipomatosis. Proc. staff meet. Mayo Clinic 36: 96-100, 1961.

*15190 LIPOMATOSIS, MULTIPLE

Stephens and Isaacson (1959) observed seventeen cases in three generations. Usually the condition did not become evident until the age of about 35 years, although in one lipomas were present at age 9. The gastrointestinal tract may be involved (Lang et al., 1959).

Humphrey, A. A. and Kingsley, P. C.: Familial multiple lipomas: report of a family. Arch. Dermatol. Syph. 37: 30-34, 1938.

Krabble, K. H. and Bartels, E. D.: La lipomatose circonscripte multiple. Copenhagen: Munksgaard, 1944.

Kurzweg, F. T. and Spencer, R.: Familial multiple lipomatosis. Am. J. Surg. 82: 762-765, 1951.

Lang, C. S., Leagus, C. and Stahlgren, L. H.: Intestinal lipomatosis. Surgery 46: 1054-1059, 1959.

Shanks, J. A., Paranchych, W. and Tuba, J.: Familial multiple lipomatosis. Canad. Med. Assoc. J. 77: 881-884, 1957.

Stephens, F. E. and Isaacson, A.: Hereditary multiple lipomatosis. J. Hered. 50: 51-53, 1959.

*15200 LIPOPROTEIN TYPES — Ag SYSTEM

Blumberg et al. (1963) described a polymorphic system including serum beta lipoprotein distinct from that discovered by Berg. They detected this by the study of patients who had received multiple transfusions. The first type was called Ag-a; the second was called Ag-b. Blumberg and colleagues (1964) proposed the symbol LP for lipoprotein. Lower case letters are used for designating different loci (i.e., LPa, LPb, LPc, etc.) and superscript numbers for alleles at the locus (i.e., LPa-1, LPa2, etc.). Gene symbols are underlined in manuscript or typescript and italicized in print. Retention of the Ag designation may be advisable to avoid confusion with the Berg type. Jackson (1974) observed a family in which variation of a chromosome no. 21 appeared to be linked with Ag type. The peak lod score was 2.1 at a recombination fraction of 0.0. Berg (1974), on the other hand, found considerable recombination with IPO-A (14745), in family studies IPO-A is known to be on chromosome 21 from hybrid cell studies.

Allison, A. C. and Blumberg, B. S.: Serum lipoprotein allotypes in man. Progress in Medical Genetics. Steinberg, A. G. and Bearn, A. G. (eds.): New York: Grune and Stratton, 4: 176-201, 1965.

Blumberg, B. S., Alter, H. J. and Riddell, N. M.: Inherited antigenic differences in human serum beta lipoproteins. A second antiserum. J. Clin. Invest. 42: 867-875, 1963.

Blumberg, B. S., Alter, H. J., Riddell, N. M. and Erlandson, M.: Multiple antigenic specificities of serum lipoproteins detected with sera of transfused patients. Vox Sang. 9: 128-145, 1964.

Butler, R. and Brunner, E.: On the genetics of the low density lipoprotein factors Ag(c) and Ag(e). Hum. Hered. 19: 174-179, 1969.

Butler, R., Brunner, E., Morganti, G., Vierucci, A., Scaloumbacas, N. and Politis, E.: A new factor in the Ag-system: Ag(g). Vox Sang. 18: 85-89, 1970.

Jackson, L. G.: Philadelphia, personal communication, 1973.

Jackson, L., Falk, C. T., Allen, F. H., Jr. and Barr, M.: A possible gene assignment to chromosome 21. Intern. Workshop on Human Gene Mapping, New Haven, Conn., June, 1973. Cytogenet. Cell Genet. 13: 100-102, 1974.

Morganti, G., Beolchini, P. E., Butler, R., Brunner, E. and Vierucci, A.: Contribution to the genetics of serum beta-lipoproteins in man. IV. Evidence for the existence of the Ag(A1-D) and Ag(C-G) loci, closely linked to the Ag(X-Y) locus. Humangenetik 10: 244-253, 1970.

*15210 LIPOPROTEIN TYPES — Ld SYSTEM

In the serum of a multiply transfused boy, Berg (1965) found an isoprecipitin against a factor in the serum low-density lipoprotein of about 42 percent of healthy persons. He named the factor Ld for 'low-density.'

Berg, K.: A new serum type system in man — the Ld system. Vox Sang. 10: 513-527, 1965.

*15220 LIPOPROTEIN TYPES — Lp SYSTEM

Berg and Mohr (1963) discovered a new serum protein system called Lp (for lipoprotein) by the intravenous injection of rabbits with isolated human serum beta-lipoprotein from one individual. The resulting antibody distinguishes two distinct types of human beta-lipoprotein. Berg and Mohr (1963) demonstrate regular dominant inheritance. The Lp-a allele has a frequency of 0.19 in Norwegians. The authors concluded that this system is independent of the Ag system of Blumberg. Berg and Bearn (1967) suggested that at least four lipoprotein systems exist: Ag, Lp, Ld and Lt. Schultz and Shreffler (1972) espoused a polygenic determination of Lp antigen, whereas Berg (1972) maintained his monodocus hypothesis.

Berg, K.: The Lp system — interpretations and views. In, deGrouchy et al. (Eds.): Human Genetics (IVth Int. Congress of Human Genetics, 1971). Amsterdam: Excerpta Medica, 1972. Pp. 352-362.

Berg, K. and Mohr, J.: Genetics of Lp system. Acta Genet. Statist. Med. 13: 349-360, 1963.

Berg, K.: Lack of linkage between the Lp and Ag serum systems. Vox Sang. 12: 71-74, 1967.

Butler, R.: Polymorphism of the human low-density lipoproteins. Vox Sang. 12: 2-17, 1967.

Schultz, J. S. and Shreffler, D. C.: Genetics and immunochemistry of the Lp antigen of human serum, in, de Grouchy et al. (eds.): Human Genetics (IVth Int. Congress of Human Genetics, 1971). Amsterdam: Excerpta Medica, 1972. Pp. 345-351.

15230 LIPOPROTEIN TYPES — Lt SYSTEM

For references, see 15200.

15240 LIPOPROTEIN, VARIANT OF BETA ('DOUBLE BETA-LIPOPROTEIN')

Seegers, Hirschhorn, Burnett, Robson and Harris (1965) have observed double beta-lipoprotein in 6 families. The relation of the locus revealed by this mutant form to those studied by the lipoprotein types of Berg and Blumberg is unknown.

Seegers, W., Hirschhorn, K., Burnett, L., Robson, E. and Harris, H.: Double beta-lipoprotein: a new genetic variation in man. Science 149: 303-304, 1965.

15250 LUDER-SHELDON SYNDROME

Luder and Sheldon (1955) and Sheldon et al. (1961) described cases of generalized aminoaciduria with loss of glucose and phosphate as well. Mild rickets with late onset or no bone disease occurred. Three generations were affected. Dominant inheritance is unusual for a defect of this type. The affected persons were female twins, their father and his father.

Luder, J. and Sheldon, W.: A familial tubular absorption defect of glucose and amino-acids. Arch. Dis. Child. 30: 160-164, 1955.

Sheldon, W., Luder, J. and Webb, B.: A familial tubular absorption defect of glucose and amino acids. Arch. Dis. Child. 36: 90-95, 1961.

15260 LUNULAE OF FINGERNAILS

Size of the lunulae and indeed their presence or absence is a variable matter presumably under genetic control, although no systemic investigation of the genetics has been performed. The lunulae are usually largest on the thumbnail and if present at all are most likely to be found on the thumb. Azure lunulae occur in Wilson disease.

15270 LUPUS ERYTHEMATOSUS, SYSTEMIC (SLE)

Although familial aggregation of clinical SLE, of related disorders such as dermatomyositis, and of protein abnormalities is rather frequently observed, a simple Mendelian mechanism is not established. Lappat and Cawein (1968) suggested that drug-induced, specifically procainamide-induced, systemic lupus erythematosus is an expression of a pharmacogenetic polymorphism. Among close relatives of a procainamide SLE proband, they found three with antinuclear antibody in the serum and in all five 'significant' history or laboratory findings suggesting an immunologic disorder. Three had a coagulation abnormality. The finding of complement deficiency (see 12090) in cases of lupus as well as associated with particular HL-A types points to genetic factors responsible for familial aggregation of this disease. On the other hand the evidence for viral etiology suggests non-genetic explanations.

First, M. R.: Familial systemic lupus erythematosus. S. Afr. J. 47: 742-744, 1973.

Kohler, P. F., Perry, J., Campion, W. M. and Smyth, C. J.: Hereditary angioedema and 'familial lupus' erythematosus in identical twin boys. Am. J. Med. 56: 406-411, 1974.

Lappat, E. J. and Cawein, M. J.: A familial study of procainamide-induced systemic lupus erythematosus. A question of pharmacogenetic polymorphism. Am. J. Med. 45: 846-852, 1968.

Larsen, R. A.: Family studies in systemic lupus erythematosus (SLE). I. A proband material from central Norway. Acta. Med. Scand. suppl. 543: 11-20, 1972.

Larsen, R. A. and Godal, T.: Family studies in systemic lupus erythematosus (SLE)-IX. Thyroid diseases and antibodies. J. Chron. Dis. 25: 225-234, 1972.

Leonhardt, T.: Family studies in systemic lupus erythematosus. Acta Med. Scand. 176 (suppl. 416): 1-156, 1964.

Lewis, R., Tannenberg, W., Smith C. and Schwartz, R.: Human systemic lupus erythematosus and C-type RNA viruses. (Abstract) Clin. Res. 22: 422A only, 1974.

Pollak, V. E.: Antinuclear antibodies in families of patients with systemic lupus erythematosus. N. Engl. J. Med. 271: 165-171, 1964.

Siegel, M., Lee, S. L., Widelock, D., Gwon, N. V. and Kravitz, H.: A comparative family study of rheumatoid arthritis and systemic lupus erythematosus. N. Engl. J. Med. 273: 893-897, 1965.

15280 LYMPHANGIECTASIA, INTESTINAL

Under the designation 'familial idiopathic dysproteinemia' Homburger and Petermann (1949) described a disorder characterized by edema of the legs, with ulcers in the males and 'functional vascular changes' in the females, by dysproteinemia of variable type and sometimes discernable only by electrophoresis, by a number of congenital malformations and by a high incidence of stillbirths. Persons in three generations were affected and male-to-male transmission occurred. Subsequently these patients have been found to have intestinal loss of protein presumably because of lymphangiectasia (Waldmann et al., 1961; Waldmann and

Schwab, 1965). Murphy (1972) gave clinical follow-up. Lymphopenia due to exaggerated intestinal loss is also a feature. Double vortex pilorum ('hair whorl') and usually prominent 'floating ribs' (ribs 11 and 12) were present. Parfitt (1966) described three sibs (2 females, one male) affected out of 5. All had neonatal edema. The small bowel showed dilated lymphatic spaces and partial villous atrophy. Cottom, London and Wilson (1961) reported neonatal hypoproteinemia in two sibs and other probable cases are known. See also LYMPHEDEMA, HEREDITARY I (15310) and ENTEROPATHY, PTOTEIN-LOSING (22630). Patients with intestinal lymphangiectasia have hypogammaglobulinemia, lymphocytopenia, skin anergy and impaired allograft rejection. Peripheral blood lymphocytes show impaired in vitro blastic transformation (Weiden et al., 1972). This is attributable to depletion of lymphocytes necessary for transformation. The situation is comparable to experimental thoracic duct drainage.

Cottom, D. G., London, D. R. and Wilson, B. D. R.: Neonatal oedema due to exudative enteropathy. Lancet II: 1009-1012, 1961.

Homburger, F. and Petermann, M. L.: Studies on hypoproteinemia. II. Familial idiopathic dysproteinemia. Blood 4: 1085-1108, 1949.

Murphy, E. A.: Familial lymphatic dysplasia with intestinal lymphangiectasia. The Clinical Delineation of Birth Defects. XIII. G. I. Tract Including Liver and Pancreas. Baltimore: Williams and Wilkins, 1972. Pp. 180-181.

Parfitt, A. M.: Familial neonatal hypoproteinaemia with exudative enteropathy and intestinal lymphangiectasis. Arch. Dis. Child. 41: 54-62, 1966.

Waldmann, T. A. and Schwab, P. J.: IgG(7s gamma globulin) metabolism in hypogammaglobulinemia: studies in patients with defective gamma globulin synthesis, gastrointestinal protein loss, or both. J. Clin. Invest. 44: 1523-1533, 1965.

Waldmann, T. A., Steinfeld, J. L., Dutcher, T. F., Davidson, J. D. and Gordon, R. S., Jr.: The role of the gastrointestinal system in 'idiopathic hypoproteinemia.' Gastroenterology 41: 197-207, 1961.

Weiden, P. L., Blaese, R. M., Strober, W., Block, J. B. and Waldmann, T. A.: Impaired lymphocyte transformation in intestinal lymphangiectasia: evidence for at least two functionally distinct lymphocyte populations in man. J. Clin. Invest. 51: 1319-1325, 1972.

15290 LYMPHEDEMA AND CEREBRAL ARTERIOVENOUS ANOMALY

Avasthey and Roy (1968) reported a woman with lymphedema of the feet beginning in her teens and a cerebrovascular anomaly indicated by a loud systolic bruit over the temples and transmitted down the carotids. A son, aged 20 years, likewise had foot lymphedema and a cranial bruit and by angiogram a large extracranial arteriovenous malformation over the parietal region. Two other sons had lymphedema, cerebrovascular malformation and primary pulmonary hypertension. One son was normal and the only daughter had lymphedema of both feet and bilateral temporo-parietal bruit.

Avasthey, P. and Roy, S. B.: Primary pulmonary hypertension, cerebrovascular malformation, and lymphoedema feet in a family. Br. Heart J. 30: 769-775, 1968.

15300 LYMPHEDEMA AND PTOSIS

In a family reported by Bloom (1941), lymphedema of the legs occurred in five generations and six affected persons in 3 consecutive generations also had ptosis. Falls and Kertesz (1964) made brief reference to a family in which the male proband had ptosis and lymphedema and the father ptosis.

Bloom, D.: Hereditary lymphedema (Nonne-Milroy-Meige). Report of a family with hereditary lymphedema associated with ptosis of the eyelids in several generations. New York J. Med. 41: 856-863, 1941.

*15310 LYMPHEDEMA, HEREDITARY I (NONNE-MILROY, OR EARLY-ONSET TYPE)

Edema is present from birth. Rosen (1962) observed congenital chylous ascites in an affected infant. Marked loss of albumin into the intestinal tract with consequent hypoproteinemia was demonstrated. The father had recurrent swelling of the scrotum beginning at the age of 20 years. Hurwitz and Pinals (1964) observed persistent bilateral pleural effusion in two such patients. The protein content of the pleural fluid was high. Milroy (1928), a physician in Omaha, Nebraska, described the disorder in a family in which many of the affected persons were prominent in public and professional life.

Esterly, J. R.: Congenital hereditary lymphoedema. J. Med. Genet. 2: 93-98, 1965.

Hurwitz, P. A. and Pinals, D. J.: Pleural effusion in chronic hereditary lymphedema (Nonne, Milroy, Meige's disease). Report of two cases. Radiology 82: 246-248, 1964.

Milroy, W. F.: Chronic hereditary edema: Milroy's disease. J.A.M.A. 91: 1172-1175, 1928.

Rosen, F. S., Smith, D. H., Earle, R., Jr., Janeway, C. A. and Gitlin, D.: The etiology of hypoproteinemia in a patient with congenital chylous ascites. Pediatrics 30: 696-706, 1962.

15320 LYMPHEDEMA, HEREDITARY II (MEIGE, OR LATE-ONSET TYPE)

Edema develops about the time of puberty (Goodman, 1962). Meige (1898) described 8 cases in four generations. No male-to-male transmission was observed. Goodman (1962) reported the condition in two sisters and a brother with presumed normal parents who were not known to be related.

Goodman, R. M.: Familial lymphedema of the Meige's type. Am. J. Med. 32: 651-656, 1962.

Juchems, R.: Das hereditaere Lymphoedem, Typ Meige. Klin. Wschr. 41: 328-332, 1963.

Meige, H.: Dystrophie oedemateuse hereditaire. Presse Med. 6: 341-343, 1898.

Osterland, G.: Beobachtungen zum Nonne-Milroy-Meige-Syndrom. Z. Menschl. Vererb. Konstitutionsl. 36: 108-117, 1961.

15330 LYMPHEDEMA, WITH ADULT ONSET AND YELLOW NAILS

Wells (1966) described a family with 8 cases in 4 sibships of two generations. In the proband the onset was in the legs at the age of 51. At times edema also affected the genitalia, hands, face, and even the vocal cords. Lymphangiograms were interpreted as showing primary hypoplasia of lymphatics. The proband had yellow nails and grew poorly. The nail changes were noted before lymphedema. Zerfas and Wallace (1966) described a sporadic case with onset of lymphedema at age 10. Recurrent pleural effusion occurs in some cases.

Samman, P. D. and White, W. F.: The 'yellow nail' syndrome. Br. J. Dermatol. 76: 153-157, 1964.

Wells, G. C.: Yellow nail syndrome with familial primary hypoplasia of lymphatics, manifest late in life. Proc. R. Soc. Med. 59: 447 Only, 1966.

Zerfas, A. J. and Wallace, H. J.: Yellow nail syndrome with bilateral bronchiectasis. Proc. Roy. Soc. Med. 59: 448 only, 1966.

*15340 LYMPHEDEMA, WITH DISTICHIASIS

Robinow et al. (1970) described the syndrome in a father and a daughter and son. The lymphedema was always of late onset. Spinal changes were asymptomatic. Chynn (1967) saw these in combination with spinal extradural cyst (q.v.) in two and perhaps three Negro sibs. Falls and Kertesz (1964) described (see also Neel and Schull, 1954) a family with distichiasis and lymphedema. Of a sibship of 5, four had bilateral lymphedema of the legs and distichiasis, one was normal. One of the four had striking webbed neck whereas two of the others were thought to have mild webbing. The lymphedema was of the type which has onset at puberty. Several of the affected persons complained of photophobia and had partial ectropion of the lateral third of the lower lids, giving them a wide-eyed appearance. The father and one of his brothers reportedly had lymphedema, distichiasis and webbed neck. The paternal grandmother had lymphedema. An affected paternal uncle died of metastatic fibrosarcoma originating in an edematous leg. See PTERYGIUM COLLI SYNDROME. Hoover (1971) has studied a family with the lymphedema-distichiasis syndrome in three generations. Irritation of the cornea, with corneal ulceration in some cases, brings the patients to the attention of ophthalmologists.

Chynn, K.-Y.: Congenital spinal extradural cyst in two siblings. Am. J. Roentgen. 101: 204-215, 1967.

Falls, H. F. and Kertesz, E. D.: A new syndrome combining pterygium colli with developmental anomalies of the eyelids and lymphatics of the lower extremities. Trans. Am. Ophthalmol. Soc. 62: 248-275, 1964.

Hoover, R. E.: Baltimore, Md.: personal communication, 1971.

Neel, J. V. and Schull, W. J.: Human Heredity. U. of Chicago Press, 1954. Pp. 50-51.

Robinow, M., Johnson, G. F. and Verhagen, A. D.: Distichiasis-lymphedema. A hereditary syndrome of multiple congenital defects. Am. J. Dis. Child. 119: 343-347, 1970.

15345 LYSOZYME

Lysozyme catalyzes the hydrolysis of certain mucopolysaccharides of bacterial cell walls. It is found in spleen, lung, kidney, white blood cells, plasma, saliva, milk and tears. As was pointed out by Flemming (1921), who first discovered this enzyme, it is particularly abundant in cartilage. In structure it resembles lactalbumin (14975). Human lysozyme has a molecular weight of 14,602 and contains 129 amino acid residues.

Dayhoff, M. O.: Lactalbumin and lysozyme. Atlas of Protein Sequence and Structure 1972 (vol. 5). Washington: National Biomedical Research Foundation, 1972. Pp. D133-D140.

15350 MACROCEPHALY, PSEUDOPAPILLEDEMA AND MULTIPLE HEMANGIOMATA

Riley and Smith (1960) described mother and two children of seven who had macrocephaly, pseudopapilledema and multiple hemangiomata. Two other sibs had macrocephaly and pseudopapilledema. Intellect and vision were unimpaired.

Riley, H. D., Jr. and Smith, W. R.: Macrocephaly, pseudopapilledema and multiple hemangiomata: a previously undescribed heredofamilial syndrome. Pediatrics 26: 293-300, 1960.

15360 MACROGLOBULINEMIA, WALDENSTROM

Vannotti (1963) observed this in mother and son; and Seligman, Danon and Fine (1963) had an instance of mother and two sons affected. Brown et al. (1967) found an abnormal chromosome in some lymphocytes of 5 members of one family. Three of the 5 had protein abnormalities. See also Elves and Brown (1968).

Brown, A. K., Elves, M. W., Gunson, H. H. and Pell-Ilderton, R.: Waldenstrom's macroglobulinaemia. A family study. Acta Haematol. 38: 184-192, 1967.

Elves, M. W. and Brown, A. K.: Cytogenetic studies in a family with Waldenstrom's macroglobulinaemia. J. Med. Genet. 5: 118-122, 1968.

Massari, R., Fine, J. M. and Metais, R.: Waldenstrom's macroglobulinaemia observed in two brothers. Nature 196: 176-178, 1962.

Seligman, M., Danon, F. and Fine, J. M.: Immunological studies in familial beta-2-macroglobulinaemias. Proc. Soc. Exp. Biol. Med. 114: 482-486, 1963.

Vannotti, A.: Etude clinique d'un cas de macroglobulinemie de Waldenstrom a caractere familial, associe a des troubles endocriniens. Schweiz. Med. Wschr. 93: 1744-1746, 1963.

15365 MACROTHROMBOCYTOPATHIA, NEPHRITIS AND DEAFNESS

Epstein et al. (1972) described two unrelated families each with two members with this combination. In one family, a third member, a young child, had the platelet disorder and a mild hearing loss. Except for the greater severity in females, the renal disease was indistinguishable from that of Alport syndrome (10420). Likewise, the high frequency sensorineural hearing loss was similar to that of the Alport syndrome. Thrombocytopenia was present with giant platelets showing abnormal ultrastructure and defective adherence to glass. Bleeding time was prolonged. Aggregation of platelets in response to collagen and epinephrine and release of factor 3 were impaired. The release of nucleotide after exposure to collagen was abnormally low. Inheritance was clearly dominant but no male-to-male transmission was noted to corroborate autosomal inheritance. The fact that females were as severely affected as males makes X-linked dominance unlikely, however.

Epstein, C. J., Sahud, M. A., Piel, C. F., Goodman, J. R., Bernfield, M. R., Kushner, J. H. and Ablin, A. R.: Hereditary macrothrombocytopathia, nephritis and deafness. Am. J. Med. 52: 299-310, 1972.

*15370 MACULAR DEGENERATION, POLYMORPHIC VITELLINE FORM

As will be seen from the title of papers referenced below, many different designations have been employed. More than one entity may well be represented. Yet the evidence is not adequate for delineating more than one. Davis and Hollenhorst (1955) described a kindred containing at least 24 affected persons in five generations. The age of onset of manifest visual disability varied from very early childhood to adolescence. Cystoid macular degeneration was described in a dominant pedigree pattern by Falls (1949) and Sorsby et al. (1956). Vail and Shock (1965) followed up on an extensively affected kindred and reported histologic findings in a patient who died at 78 years of age. Best disease is sometimes called vitelline macular dystrophy. Eight persons were affected in the family reported by Best (1905) and follow-up (Vossius, 1921; Jung, 1936) increased the number to 22. Characteristically funduscopic changes are in advance of visual impairment. A yellow mass like the yolk of an egg (hence the name) in the macular area later becomes deeply and irregularly pigmented and a process called 'scrambling the egg' by Braley (1966) takes place. The egg-like lesion is probably present at birth. Examination of relatives is essential to diagnosis in advanced cases. Friedenwald and Maumenee (1951) observed affected mother and daughter.

Best, F.: Ueber eine hereditaere Maculaaffektion. Z. Augenheilk. 13: 199-212, 1905.

Braley, A. E. and Spivey, B. E.: Hereditary vitelline macular degeneration. A clinical and functional evaluation of a new pedigree with variable expressivity and dominant inheritance. Arch. Ophthalmol. 72: 743-762, 1964.

Braley, A. E.: Dystrophy of the macula. Am. J. Ophthalmol. 61: 1-24, 1966.

Davis, C. T. and Hollenhorst, R. W.: Hereditary degeneration of the macula: occurring in five generations. Am. J. Ophthalmol. 39: 637-643, 1955.

Deutman, A. F.: Electro-oculography in families with vitelliform dystrophy of the fovea. Detection of the carrier state. Arch. Ophthalmol. 81: 305-316, 1969.

Falls, H. F.: Hereditary congenital macular degeneration. Am. J. Hum. Genet. 1: 96-104, 1949.

Francois, J.: Vitelliform degeneration of the macula. Bull. N.Y. Acad. Med. 44: 18-27, 1968.

Friedenwald, J. S. and Maumenee, A. E.: Peculiar macular lesions with unaccountably good vision. Arch. Ophthal. 45: 567-570, 1951.

Jung, E. E.: Ueber eine Sippe mit angeborener Maculadegeneration. Giessen: Seibert, 1936.

Krill, A. E., Morse, P. A., Potts, A. M. and Klien, B. A.: Hereditary vitelliruptive macular degeneration. Am. J. Ophthalmol. 61: 1405-1415, 1966.

Sorsby, A., Savory, M., Daney, J. B. and Fraser, R. J. L.: Macular cysts: a dominantly inherited affection with a progressive course. Br. J. Ophthalmol. 40: 144-158, 1956.

Vail, D. and Shock, D.: Hereditary degeneration of the macula. II. Follow-up report and histopathologic study. Trans. Am. Ophthalmol. Soc. 63: 51-63, 1965.

Vossius, A.: Ueber die Bestsche familiaere Maculadegeneration. Arch. Ophtalmol. 105: 1050-1059, 1921.

15380 MACULAR DEGENERATION, SENILE

Streiff and Babel (1963) described senile macular changes in an 80-year-old mother and her 50-year-old daughter. Because of the late onset of the abnormality dominant inheritance is more likely. Furthermore because of the late onset affected members of successive generations are not likely to be observed. Braley (1966) stated that senile macular degeneration runs in families. 'Nearly every patient I have seen has had other members of the family similarly affected.' Visual disturbance without ophthalmoscopic findings may be present by age 50 and fundus changes become apparent only after age 70.

Braley, A. E.: Dystrophy of the macula. Am. J. Ophthalmol. 61: 1-24, 1966.

Streiff, E. B. and Babel, J.: La senescence de la retine. Prog. Ophthalmol. 13: 1-75, 1963.

15385 MACULAR DYSTROPHY WITH AMINOACIDURIA

Lefler et al. (1971) described a family in which members of four generations were affected. Onset was late in the first decade of life. Color vision remained intact thus distinguishing the disorder, in the opinion of the authors, from Stargardt disease. A random urine of 11 of 17 affected family members showed generalized aminoaciduria and two showed increased glycine. It was not made clear whether members without macular dystrophy had aminoaciduria. The authors thought the abnormality was different from other reported forms of macular dystrophy.

Lefler, W. H., Wadsworth, J. A. C. and Sidbury, J. B., Jr.: Hereditary macular dystrophy and amino-aciduria. Am. J. Ophthalmol. 71 (suppl.): 224-230, 1971.

*15410 MALATE DEHYDROGENASE, MITOCHONDRIAL (MDH-2, OR MOR-2)

In leukocytes and placentas Davidson and Cortner (1967) found polymorphism of the malate dehydrogenase that is bound to mitochondria, so-called M-MDH. The fact that mitochondrial malate dehydrogenase was indistinguishable from normal in persons with variation in the supernatant MDH indicates that a separate locus is involved in its genetic determination. Mendelian segregation rather than maternal inheritance of M-MDH suggests that not all mitochondrial proteins are coded by mitochondrial DNA. Mitochondrial glutamic oxaloacetic transaminase (q.v) is also determined by nuclear genes. (The form of MDH studied by Davidson and Cortner (1967) was NAD-dependent.) From study of hybrid cells the locus for MDH-2 is known to be on chromosome no. 7 (2nd International Workshop on Human Gene Mapping, Rotterdam, July, 1974).

Davidson, R. G. and Cortner, J. A.: Mitochondrial malate dehydrogenase: a new genetic polymorphism in man. Science 157: 1569-1571, 1967.

Shows, T. B.: Genetics of human-mouse somatic cell hybrids: linkage of human genes for isocitrate dehydrogenase and malate dehydrogenase. Biochem. Genet. 7: 193-204, 1972.

*15420 MALATE DEHYDROGENASE, CYTOPLASMIC (NAD-DEPENDENT MDH; MDH-1, OR MOR-1)

Malate dehydrogenase (EC 1.1.1.37) catalyzes a reversible reaction in the citric acid cycle: L-malate plus NAD to form oxaloacetate plus NADH. This enzyme is therefore called the NAD-dependent form of malate dehydrogenase. The designation MOR comes from the oxidoreductase function of the enzyme. MDH is syntenic with isocitrate dehydrogenase (14770) but chromosomal assignment has not been achieved (Shows, 1972). Davidson and Cortner (1967) observed an inherited variant of supernatant malate dehydrogenase of erythrocytes. The variant was found in a Negro woman and her two sons, uncovered in a survey of 1470 Negroes and 1440 whites. The electrophoretic nature of the variant suggested that the molecule is a dimer with mutation in the gene controlling one of the elements and that this gene is autosomal.

Blake, N. M., Kirk, R. L., Simons, M. J. and Alpers, M. P.: Genetic variants of soluble malate dehydrogenase in New Guinea populations. Humangenetik 11: 72-74, 1970.

Davidson, R. G. and Cortner, J. A.: Genetic variant of human erythrocyte malate dehydrogenase. Nature 215: 761-762, 1967.

Leakey, T. E. B., Coward, A, R., Warlow, A. and Mourant, A. E.: The distribution in human populations of electrophoretic variants of cytoplasmic malate dehydrogenase. Hum. Hered. 22: 542-551, 1972.

Ruddle, F. H.: New Haven, Conn.: personal communication, 1972.

Shows, T. B.: Genetics of human-mouse somatic cell hybrids: linkage of human genes for isocitrate dehydrogenase and malate dehydrogenase. Biochem. Genet. 7: 193-204, 1972.

15423 MALE-DETERMINING FACTOR

Kasdan et al. (1973) described a family in which a paternally transmitted, non-Y, male-determining autosomal gene was postulated as the only plausible explanation. Sex reversal mutations have been observed in the goat (Hamerton et al., 1969) and mouse (Cattanach et al., 1971). In the goat, the disorder is recessive, whereas it is dominant in the mouse. The autosomal gene, in these cases, apparently causes the indifferent gonad of genetic females to differentiate partially or completely into a testis. Over 40 men with a 46XX karyotype have been reported (de la Chapelle, 1972). The phenotype resembles that of the Klinefelter syndrome. Translocation of Y-chromosome material to an autosome cannot be excluded as the cause in at least some cases.

Cattanach, B. M., Pollard, C. E. and Hawkes, S. G.: Sex-reversed mice: XX and XO males. Cytogenetics 10: 318-337, 1971.

De la Chapelle, A.: Nature and origin of males with XX sex chromosomes. Am. J. Hum. Genet. 24: 71-105, 1972.

Hamerton, J. L., Dickson, J. M., Pollard, C. E., Grieves, S. A. and Short, R. V.: Genetic intersexuality in goats. J. Reprod. Fertil., Suppl. 7: 25-51, 1969.

Kasdan, R., Nankin, H. R., Troen, P., Wald, N., Pan, S. and Yanaihara, T.: Paternal transmission of maleness in XX human beings. N. Engl. J. Med. 288: 539-545, 1973.

*15425 MALIC ENZYME (NADP-DEPENDENT MALATE DEHYDROGENASE), CYTOPLASMIC (ME-1; MOD-1)

This enzyme (EC 1.1.1.40) catalyzes the reversible oxidative decarboxylation of malate and is a link between the glycolytic pathway and the citric acid cycle. The reaction is L-malate plus NADP to form pyruvate, CO_2 and NADPH. The enzyme is also called NADP-dependent malate dehydrogenase. Each of the malate dehydrogenases has a soluble and a mitochondrial form. Electrophoretic variants of mitochondrial malic enzyme have been demonstrated in the mouse (Shows et al., 1970) and in man (Cohen and Omenn 1972). It has not been possible to map the mitochondrial enzymes by mouse-man hybridization methods because the enzymes in the two species have identical electrophoretic mobilities. Ruddle (1972) has evidence that the soluble form of malic enzyme is determined by a locus on chromosome no. 6.

Chen, T. R., McMorris, F. A., Creagan, R., Ricciuti, F., Tischfield, J. and Ruddle, F.: Assignment of the genes for malate oxidoreductase decarboxylating to chromosome 6 and peptidase B and lactate dehydrogenase B to chromosome 12 in man. Am. J. Hum. Genet. 25: 200-207, 1973.

Cohen, P. T. W. and Omenn, G. S.: Genetic variation of the cytoplasmic and mitochondrial malic enzymes in the monkey: Macaca nemestrina. Biochem. Genet. 7: 289-301, 1972.

Cohen, P. T. W. and Omenn, G. S.: Human malic enzyme high-frequency polymorphism in the mitochondrial form. Biochem. Genet. 7: 303-311, 1972.

Ruddle, F. H.: New Haven, Conn.: personal communication, 1972.

Shows, T. B., Chapman, V. M. and Ruddle, F. H.: Mitochondrial malate dehydrogenase and malic enzyme: mendelian inherited electrophoretic variants in the mouse. Biochem. Genet. 4: 707-718, 1970.

*15427 MALIC ENZYME, MITOCHONDRIAL (ME-2; MOD-2)

See 15425. This is a third example of a mitochondrial enzyme determined by nuclear genes, the others being MDH (15420) and GOT (13820).

*15455 MANNOSEPHOSPHATE ISOMERASE

By study of mouse-man hybrids Ruddle et al. (1972) have demonstrated that mannose phosphate isomerase is determined by a locus on chromosome no. 7. By human-mouse cell hybridization Shows (1972) demonstrated that pyruvate kinase (EC 2.7.1.40) and mannosephosphate isomerase (EC 5.3.1.8) are syntenic. The kinase is PK-3 or leukocyte PK, which is distinct from erythrocyte PK, deficiency of which leads to hemolytic anemia (26620). The PK-3 and MPI loci may be on chromosome no. 7.

McMorris, F. A., Chen, T. R., Ricciuti, F., Tischfield, J., Creagan, R. and Ruddle, F.: Chromosome assignments in man of the genes for two hexosphosphate isomerase. Science 179: 1129-1131, 1973.

Ruddle, F. H.: New Haven, Conn.: personal communication, 1972.

Shows, T. B.: Linkage of loci for human pyruvate kinase and mannosephosphate isomerase in somatic cell hybrids. Am. Soc. Hum. Genet., Phila., Oct., 1972.

Shows, T. B.: Somatic cell genetics of enzyme markers associated with three human linkage groups. In, Davidson, R. L. (ed.): Proc. Conf. Somatic Cell Hybridization, Orlando, Fla., 1973.

15460 MARCUS GUNN PHENOMENON ('JAW-WINKING,' OR MAXILLO-PALPEBRAL SYNKINESIS)

Although it usually persists into adult life, this phenomenon is seen in its most marked forms in infancy when the rapid spasmodic movements of the lid are apparent during sucking and thus are noted soon after birth. It is typically unilateral and is associated with ptosis. The phenomenon has been observed in sucessive generations on several occasions. Kirkham (1969) described brother and sister with unilateral Marcus Gunn phenomenon.

Cooper, E. L.: The jaw-winking phenomenon. Report of a case. Arch. Ophthalmol. 18: 198-203, 1937.

Falls, H. F., Kruse, W. T. and Cotterman, C. W.: Three cases of Marcus Gunn phenomenon in 2 generations. Am. J. Ophthalmol. 32: 53-59, 1949.

Grant, F. C.: The Marcus Gunn phenomenon: report of a case with suggestions as to relief. Arch. Neurol. Psychiatry 35: 487-500, 1936.

Kirkham, T. H.: Familial Marcus Gunn phenomenon. Br. J. Ophthalmol. 53: 282-283, 1969.

Leri, A. and Weill, J.: Phenomene de Marcus Gunn (synergie palpebro-maxillaire) congenital et hereditaire. Bull. Soc. Med. Hosp. Paris 53: 875-880, 1929.

*15470 MARFAN SYNDROME

Cardinal features occur in three areas- in the eye, especially subluxation of the lenses; in the skeletal system, especially excessive length of the extremities; and in the cardiovascular system, especially dissecting and-or diffuse aneurysm of the ascending aorta. Homocystinuria, a recessive, also produces ectopia lentis and vascular lesions. Furthermore ectopia lentis is a feature of sulfo-cysteinuria and of Weill-Marchesani syndrome. Metachromasia of fibroblasts was reported by Matalon and Dorfman (1968).

Massumi, R. A., Lowe, E. W., Misanik, L. F., Just, H. and Tawakkoi, A.: Multiple aortic aneurysms (thoracic and abdominal) in twins with Marfan's syndrome: fatal rupture during pregnancy. J. Thorac. Cardiovasc. Surg. 53: 223-230, 1967.

Matalon, R. and Dorfman, A.: The accumulation of hyaluronic acid in cultured fibroblasts of the Marfan syndrome. Biochem. Biophys. Res. Commun. 32: 150-154, 1968.

McKusick, V. A.: Heritable Disorders of Connective Tissue. St. Louis: C. V. Mosby Co., 1972 (4th Ed.).

15475 MARFANOID HYPERMOBILITY SYNDROME

Walker et al. (1968) described a 27-year-old man with a Marfanoid habitus, pectus excavatum, and camptodactyly V, but no evidence of aortic or eye involvement, although a systolic click was heard over the heart and mesodermal anomalies were found in the angle of the anterior chamber. Very marked joint hypermobility and excessive stretchability of the skin suggested Ehlers-Danlos syndrome but no other features of that condition were present. The patient reported by Goodman et al. (1965, 1969) as having both E-D and Marfan syndromes probably had this disorder and other examples are perhaps the cases of Roederer (1951) and Coventry (1961). Little information of the genetics is available. Relatives of Goodman's patient were said to be similarly affected. In 1974 I re-studied the patient of Walker et al. (1968) and found that he had aortic regurgitation. Valvular heart disease occurred also in Goodman's family.

Coventry, M. B.: Some skeletal changes in the Ehlers-Danlos syndrome. A report of two cases. J. Bone Joint Surg. 43A: 855-860, 1961.

Goodman, R. M., Baba, N. and Wooley, C. F.: Observations on the heart in a case of combined Ehlers-Danlos and Marfan syndromes. Am. J. Cardiol. 24: 734-742, 1969.

Goodman, R. M., Wooley, C. F., Frazier, R. L. and Covault, L.: Ehlers-Danlos syndrome occurring together with the Marfan syndrome. Report of a case with other family members affected. N. Engl. J. Med. 273: 514-519, 1965.

Roederer, C.: Syndrome d'Ehlers-Danlos syndrome atypique coincidant avec une dolichostenomelie. Arch. Fr. Pediatr. 8: 192-195, 1961.

Walker, B. A., Beighton, P. H. and Murdoch, J. L.: The marfanoid hypermobility syndrome. Ann. Intern. Med. 71: 349-352, 1969.

15480 MAST CELL DISEASE

The cutaneous manifestation is termed urticaria pigmentosa. Generalized involvement, which may be fatal, is sometimes observed. Burgoon et al. (1968) observed the disorder in father and daughter. Selmanowitz et al. (1970) described cutaneous mastocytosis in 8 females in three generations with a male carrier representing a 'skipped generation.' They also reviewed experience in twins. Selmanowitz and Orentreich (1970) stated that about 40 familial cases and six concordant pairs of monozytotic twins are known. Both dominant and recessive inheritance has been postulated (Shaw, 1968).

Burgoon, C. F., Jr., Graham, J. H. and McCaffree, D. L.: Mast cell disease. A cutaneous variant with multisystem involvement. Arch. Dermatol. 98: 590-605, 1968.

Selmanowitz, V. J., Orentreich, N., Tiangco, C. C. and Demis, D. J.: Uniovulvar twins discordant for cutaneous mastocytosis. Arch. Dermatol. 102: 34-41, 1970.

Selmanowitz, V. J. and Orentreich, N.: Mastocytosis: a clinical genetic evaluation. J. Hered. 61: 91-94, 1970.

Shaw, J. M.: Genetic aspects of urticaria pigmentosa. Arch. Dermatol. 97: 137-138, 1968.

15500 MAXILLOFACIAL DYSOSTOSIS

Peters and Hovels (1960) described the familial nature of the syndrome.

Peters, A. and Hovels, O.: Die Dysostosis maxillo-facialis, eine erbliche, typische Fehlbildung des 1. Visceralbogens. Z. Menschl. Vererb. Konstitutionsl. 35: 434-444, 1960.

*15510 MAY-HEGGLIN ANOMALY

The May-Hegglin anomaly consists of cytoplasmic RNA-containing inclusions of the leukocytes in association with giant platelets. The inclusions are the so-called Dohle bodies which are also seen, though only transiently, with acute infections. Oski and colleagues (1962) observed the anomaly in a mother and her two children. Of 24 reported cases 9 had thrombocytopenia. On the basis of electron microscopic studies, Jenis et al. (1971) suggested that the inclusions represented paracrystalline arrays of depolymerized ribosomes. See DOHLE BODIES AND LEUKEMIA (22335).

Godwin, H. A. and Ginsburg, A. D.: May-Hegglin anomaly: a defect in megakarocyte. Br. J. Haematol. 26: 117-128, 1974.

Jenis, E. H., Takeuchi, A., Dillon, D. E., Ruymann, F. B. and Rivkin, S.: The May-Hegglin anomaly: ultrastructure of the granulocyte inclusion. Am. J. Clin. Pathol. 55: 187-196, 1971.

Jordan, S. W. and Larsen, W. E.: Ultrastructural studies of the May-Hegglin anomaly. Blood 25: 921-932, 1965.

Oski, F. A., Naiman, J. L., Allen, D. M. and Diamond, L. K.: Leukocytic inclusions — Dohle bodies — associated with platelet abnormality (the May-Hegglin anomaly). Report of a family and review of the literature. Blood 20: 657-667, 1962.

15520 MEDIOSTERNAL DEPIGMENTATION LINE

Kisch and Nasuhoglu (1953) described a mediosternal, longitudinally directed streak of hypopigmentation in five Negroes. I have observed this, but no systematic family studies have been done. See FUTCHER LINE and RAINDROP DEPIGMENTATION for other pigment peculiarities in Negroes.

Kisch, B. and Nasuhoglu, A.: Mediosternal depigmentation line in Negroes. Exp. Med. Surg. 11: 265-267, 1953.

*15530 MEGADUODENUM AND-OR MEGACYSTIS

Law and Ten Eyck (1962) reported the association of megaduodenum and megacystis in 9 members of a family of Italian extraction. Male-to-male transmission was observed. Weiss (1938) reported megaduodenum alone in 6 persons in 3 generations of a German family. Newton (1968) treated two Negro males with megaduodenum. One of them also had magacystis and the father probably had megaduodenum. Marfanoid habitus was noted. Oberhelman, in discussing Newton's paper, referred to a family with multiple cases of megaduodenum. Tobenkin (1964) described megacystis with nonobstructive vesicoureteral reflux in a mother and her three daughters. The history of unilateral nephrectomy in the maternal grandmother suggested that three generations may have been affected. No comment on associated megaduodenum was made.

Law, D. H. and Ten Eyck, E. A.: Familial megaduodenum and megacystis. Am. J. Med. 33: 911-922, 1962.

Newton, W. T.: Radical enterectomy for hereditary megaduodenum. Arch. Surg. 96: 549-553, 1968.

Tobenkin, M. I.: Hereditary vesicoureteral reflux. Sth. Med. J. 57: 139-147, 1964.

Weiss, W.: Zur Aetiologie des Megaduodenums. Deutsch. Z. Chir. 251: 317-330, 1938.

*15535 MEGALENCEPHALY

DeMyer (1972) reported instances of apparently autosomal dominant megalencephaly. Male-to-male transmission occurred in some instances. In a family with three generations affected the proband also had mediastinal ganglioneuroblastoma. In the group of megalencephalics as a whole, males predominated. It is of interest, therefore, that X-linked megalencephaly has been suggested (see 24800). Most persons with megalencephaly are mentally retarded. DeMyer (1972) told me of information he had received on other families showing autosomal dominant inheritance of megalencephaly. Hall (1974) also told me of such families.

DeMyer, W. E.: Indianopolis, personal communication, Dec., 1972.

DeMyer, W. E.: Megalencephaly in children. Clinical syndromes, genetic patterns, and differential diagnosis from other causes of megalocephaly. Neurology 22: 634-643, 1972.

Hall, J. G.: Seattle, personal communication, 1974.

15550 MEGALODACTYLY

One or two fingers are grotesquely enlarged. Barsky (1967) and others have found no report of familial occurrence.

Barsky, A. J.: Macrodactyly. J. Bone Joint Surg. 49A: 1255-1266, 1967.

Rechnagel, K.: Megalodactylism. Report of 7 cases. Acta Orthop. Scand. 38: 57-66, 1967.

15560 MELANOMA, MALIGNANT

Katzenellenbogen and Sandbank (1967) described dizygotic twins each with malignant melanoma. Cawley (1952) observed this malignancy in father, son and daughter. Several writers (e.g. Moschella, 1961; Schoch, 1963; Salomon et al., 1963) commented on the usual fair complexion, blue eyes and multiple ephelides in these patients. Smith, Henly, Knox and Lane (1966) described affected mother and son. Anderson et al. (1967) described malignant melanoma in at least 15 members of three generations of a single kindred. Early age of onset and a tendency for multiple primary lesions were features they noted. Andrews (1968) reported brother and sister. Lynch and Krush (1968) described two families with malignant melanoma in two generations in one and three generations in another. Anderson (1971) reported 36 pedigrees totaling 106 members each having cutaneous melanoma. He noted, in addition to earlier age at onset and increased frequency of multiple primary lesions when compared to non-familial cases, a higher survival rate. A comparison of monozygotic and dizygotic twins for melanoma might be of importance because of cases of melanoma in non-blood-related members of the same household (Robinson and Manheimer, 1972).

Anderson, D. E.: Clinical characteristics of the genetic variety of cutaneous melanoma in man. Cancer 28: 721-725, 1971.

Anderson, D. E., Smith, J. L., Jr. and McBride, C. M.: Hereditary aspects of malignant melanoma. J.A.M.A. 200: 741-746, 1967.

Andrews, J. C.: Malignant melanoma in siblings. Arch. Dermatol. 98: 282-283, 1968.

Cawley, E. P.: Genetic aspects of malignant melanoma. Arch. Derm. Syph. 65: 440-450, 1952.

Katzenellenbogen, I. and Sandbank, M.: Malignant melanoma in twins. Arch. Dermatol. 94: 331-332, 1967.

Lynch, H. T. and Krush, A. J.: Heredity and malignant melanoma: implications for early cancer detection. Canad. Med. Assoc. J. 99: 17-21, 1968.

Moschella, S. L.: A report of malignant melanoma of the skin in sisters. Arch. Dermatol. 84: 1024-1025, 1961.

Robinson, M. J. and Manheimer, L.: Familial melanomas. (Letter) J.A.M.A. 220: 277 only, 1972.

Salomon, T., Schnyder, I. W. and Storck, H.: A contribution to the question of heredity in malignant melanomas. Dermatologica 126: 65-75, 1963.

Schoch, E. P., Jr.: Familial malignant melanoma. A pedigree and cytogenetic study. Arch. Dermatol. 88: 445-455, 1963.

Smith, F. E., Henly, W. S., Knox, J. M. and Lane, M.: Familial melanoma. Arch. Intern. Med. 117: 820-823, 1966.

Turkington, R. W.: Familial factor in malignant malanoma. J.A.M.A. 192: 77-82, 1965.

Wallace, D. D., Beardmore, G. L. and Exton, L. A.: Familial malignant melanoma. Ann. Surg. 177: 15 only, 1973.

Wallace, D. C., Exton, L. A. and McLeod, G. R.: Genetic factor in malignant melanoma. Cancer 27: 1262-1266, 1971.

15570 MELANOMA, MALIGNANT INTRAOCULAR

Bowen, Brady and Jones (1964) reported malignant intraocular melanoma in a 45-year-old white female and in her 26-year-old daughter. Davenport (1927) reported this malignancy in three successive generations.

Bowen, S. F., Brady, H. and Jones, V. L.: Malignant melanoma of eye occurring in two successive generations. Arch. Ophthal. 71: 805-806, 1964.

Cawley, E. P.: Genetic aspects of malignant melanoma. Arch. Dermatol. Syph. 65: 440-450, 1952.

Davenport, R. C.: Familial history of choroidal sarcoma. Br. J. Ophthalmol. 11: 443-445, 1927.

*15580 MELANOSIS, UNIVERSAL

Scheidt (1926) described 14 affected in 4 successive generations. Orth (1929) described 2 families, each with four affected generations. Pegum (1955) and Wende and Bauckus (1919) described generalized hyperpigmentation beginning in infancy in a pair of sibs. Tvaroh and Kares (1968) described 5 affected in 3 generations.

Leber, R.: Ueber eine Familie mit erblichem universellem Melanismus. Z. Kinderheilk. 58: 142-147, 1936.

Orth, H.: Ueber zwei Falle von erblichem Melanismus. Arch. Dermatol. Syph. 158: 95-97, 1929.

Pegum, J. S.: Diffuse pigmentation in brothers. Proc. R. Soc. Med. 48: 179-180, 1955.

Scheidt, W.: Einige Ergebnisse biologischer Familienerhebungen. Arch. Rass. u. Ges. Biol. 17: 135-139, 1926.

Tvaroh, F. and Kares, B.: Familial occurrence of diffuse melanosis. Plzen. Lek. Sborn. 22 (suppl.): 35-38, 1968.

Wende, G. W. and Bauckus, H. H.: A hitherto undescribed generalized pigmentation of the skin appearing in infancy in brother and sister. J. Cutan. Dis. 37: 685-701, 1919.

15585 MELANOTROPIN, BETA (MELANOCYTE STIMULATING HORMONE, MSH)

Human beta melanotropin has 22 amino acid residues and a molecular weight of 2,661 (Harris, 1959).

Harris, J. I.: Structure of a melanocyte-stimulating hormone from the human pituitary gland. Nature 184: 167-169, 1959.

*15590 MELKERSSON SYNDROME

The features are chronic swelling of the face, peripheral facial palsy which may be bilateral and tends to relapse, and in some cases lingua plicata. The disease often begins in childhood or youth. The swelling is localized especially to the lips. Kunstadter (1965) described a case with onset at 5 and one-half years. The maternal grandmother developed unilateral Bell palsy without facial edema at age 68. A maternal aunt at 10 years of age developed unilateral Bell palsy with questionable edema and recovered completely. Carr (1966) found at least four other reported families in which two generations were affected and one instance of three generations affected.

Carr, R. D.: Is the Melkersson-Rosenthal syndrome hereditary? Arch. Dermatol. 93: 426-427, 1966.

Kunstadter, R. H.: Melkersson's syndrome. A case report of multiple recurrences of Bell's palsy and episodic facial edema. Am. J. Dis. Child. 110: 559-561, 1965.

15600 MENIERE DISEASE

Although genetic factors probably are involved to a significant extent, it is unusual to find more than one case of episodic vertigo and hearing loss in the same family. Bernstein (1965) reported seven such families. In one family identical female twins and the daughter of one of the twins were affected. Three families had migraine also in certain members. (Also see ATASIS, PERIODIC VESTIBULO-CEREBELLAR.)

Bernstein, J. M.: Occurrence of episodic vertigo and hearing loss in families. Ann. Otol. 74: 1011-1021, 1965.

15610 MENINGIOMA

Although the mode of inheritance is not clear, a few reports have indicated familial occurrence of meningioma.

Gaist, G. and Piazza, G.: Meningiomas in two members of the same family (with no evidence of neurofibromatosis). J. Neurosurg. 16: 110-113, 1959.

Joynt, R. J. and Perret, G. E.: Meningiomas in a mother and daughter. Cases without evidence of neurofibromatosis. Neurology 11: 164-165, 1961.

Sahar, A.: Familial occurrence of meningiomas.: Case report. J. Neurosurg. 23: 444-445, 1965.

15620 MENTAL RETARDATION

In two families with undifferentiated mental retardation occurring in members of multiple generations, Dekaban and Klein (1968) concluded that dominant transmission (i.e., a single major gene) could be responsible.

Dekaban, A. S. and Klein, D.: Familial mental retardation. Acta Genet. Statist. Med. 18: 206-228, 1968.   213

15625 METACHONDROMATOSIS

Maroteaux (1971) described two families with skeletal radiologic features of both multiple exostoses (13370) and Ollier disease (16600). He suggested that inheritance is autosomal dominant and gave it the name metachondromatosis. Lachman et al. (1974) reported a case.

Lachman, R. S., Cohen, A., Hollister, D. and Rimoin, D. L.: Metachondromatosis. Birth Defects Orig. Art. Ser. 10: 171-178, 1974.

Maroteaux, P.: La metachondromatose. Z. Kinderheilk. 109: 246-261, 1971.

15630 METACHROMASIA OF FIBROBLASTS

Danes et al. (1970) have described six families in which metachromasia can be traced through normal individuals in at least three generations. The basis for the metachromasia is not known. Increased concentrations of mucopolysaccharides is not the explanation. Possibly this cellular characteristic is an expression of the heterozygous state of some recessive disorders.

Danes, B. S., Scott, J. E. and Bearn, A. G.: Further studies on metachromasia in cultured human fibroblasts. Staining of glycosaminoglycans (mucopolysaccharides) by alcian blue in salt solutions. J. Exp. Med. 132: 765-774, 1970.

*15640 METAPHYSEAL CHONDRODYSPLASIA, MURK JANSEN TYPE

This disorder was formerly known as metaphyseal dysostosis. Stoeckenius (1966) described affected mother and child. The mother's condition may have been the result of new dominant mutation. Her father was 40-years-old at her birth. Lenz (1967) saw the same family. The mother was only 102 cm. tall. The extreme disorganization of the metaphyses of the long bones and of the metacarpal and metatarsal bones is in sharp contrast with the almost normal appearance of the epiphyseal centers, which on X-ray appear widely separated from the long bones. The chin is receding. The fingers, especially the distal phalanges, are very short. The spine, pelvis and lower legs are distorted. De Haas et al. (1969) gave a follow-up of the original case of Murk Jansen. The striking feature at age 44 was the development of nearly normal bone structure with, however, marked deformity and dwarfing. Sclerosis in the cranial bones, including the petrous bone leading to deafness, was demonstrated. Hypercalcemia has been noted in cases in childhood (Lenz, 1969; Holt and Dent in discussion of Lenz, 1969). See the follow-up by Lenz (1969).

De Haas, W. H. D., De Boer, W. and Griffioen, F.: Metaphyseal dysostosis. A late follow-up of the first reported case. J. Bone Joint Surg. 51B: 290-299, 1969.

Lenz, W.: Diagnosis in medical genetics. In, Crow, J. F. and Neel, J. V. (eds.): Proc. 3rd. Intern. Cong. Hum. Genet., Sept., 1966. Baltimore: Johns Hopkins Press, 1967. Pp. 29-36.

Lenz, W.: Discussion. The Clinical Delineation of Birth Defects. IV. Skeletal Dysplasias. New York: National Foundation, 1969. Pp. 71-72.

Ozonoff, M. B.: Metaphyseal dysostosis of Jansen. Radiology 93: 1047-1050, 1969.

Stoeckenius, N.I.: Cited by Lenz, W.: Symposion uber generalisierte Anomalien des Skeletes. Mschr. Kinderheilk. 114: 157-158, 1966.

*15650 METAPHYSEAL CHONDRODYSPLASIA, SCHMIDT TYPE

This disorder was formerly known as metaphyseal dysostosis. This is not a true dysostosis (since it is not primarily a disorder of bone formation), nor is the primary defect in the metaphyses. Irregularities of the metaphyseal ends of bones of the extremities are demonstrated radiologically. Bowlegs and coxa vara result. There is a recessive type of metaphyseal dysostosis (Spahr type). Rosenbloom and Smith (1965) described 24 affected persons in one kindred. In 1943 Stephens reported on a Morman kindred in which over 40 members of four generations were affected with what he considered to be achondroplasia. The X-ray findings as demonstrated in his figures and as reviewed by Caffey (1963) are, however, those of metaphyseal dysostosis. In a 3-year-old child the inter-peduncular distances and greater sciatic groove were quite normal and the typical metaphyseal changes were demonstrated. Affected women went through vaginal deliveries successfully and were usually accompanied only by a midwife. Stephens (1943) suggested that the original mutation could be identified. The first affected ancestor, born in 1833, was said to have normal parents and 11 unaffected sibs. In a girl with metaphyseal chondrodysplasia said to be intermediate in phenotype between the Jansen and Schmidt types, Cooper et al. (1973) demonstrated distintion of the rough surfaced endoplasmic reticulum cisternae of chondrocytes due to accumulation of what appeared to be a protein. Cooper and Ponsetti (1973) studied an affected girl. Electron microscopy of her chondrocytes from the iliac crest area and ulnar epiphyseal plate revealed dilated rough endoplasmic reticulum (RER) cisternal containing a granular material. Cartilage matrix collagen and osteoid appeared to be normal. Osteoblasts and osteocytes showed a slight degree of RER dilatation.

Caffey, J. P.: Quoted by Dr. William R. Christensen, Salt Lake City, 1963.

Cooper, R. R., Pedrini-Mille, A. and Ponseti, I. V.: Metaphyseal dysostosis: a rough surfaced endoplasmic reticulum storage defect. Lab. Invest. 28: 119-125, 1973.

Cooper, R. R. and Ponsetti, I. V.: Metaphyseal dysostosis: description of an ultrastructural defect in the epiphyseal plate chondrocytes. Case report. J. Bone Joint Surg. 55A: 485-495, 1973.

Daeschner, C. W., Singleton, E. B., Hill, L. L. and Dodge, W. F.: Metaphyseal dysostosis. J. Pediatr. 57: 844-854, 1960.

David, J. E. A. and Palmer, P. E. S.: Familial metaphysial dysplasia. J. Bone Joint Surg. 40B: 86-93, 1958.

Dent, C. E. and Normand, I. C. S.: Metaphyseal dysostosis, type Schmid. Arch. Dis. Child. 39: 444-454, 1964.

Miller, S. M. and Paul, L. W.: Roentgen observations in familial metaphyseal dysostosis. Radiology 83: 665-673, 1964.

Peterson, J. C.: Metaphyseal dysostosis: questionably a form of vitamin D-resistant rickets. J. Pediatr. 60: 656-663, 1962.

Rosenbloom, A. L. and Smith, D. W.: The natural history of metaphyseal dysostosis. J. Pediatr. 66: 857-868, 1965.

Stephens, F. E.: An achondroplastic mutation and the nature of its inheritance. J. Hered. 34: 229-235, 1943.

Stickler, G. B., Maher, F. T., Hunt, J. C., Burke, E. C. and Rosevear, J. W.: Familial bone disease resembling rickets (hereditary metaphyseal dysostosis). Pediatrics 29: 996-1004, 1962.

*15652 METATARSUS VARUS, TYPE I

Juberg and Touchstone (1974) described type 1 metatarsus varus in 9 persons in 4 generations with male-to-male transmission. Metatarsus varus is a malformation of the anterior foot that results in inward angulation. Type 1, the most common form, shows adduction of the anterior foot, high longitudial arch, concavity of the medial border and convexity of the lateral border of the foot, and neutral position of the heel. Type 2 is a deformity residual after correction of the more severe forms of clubfoot. The third form, the rarest, usually has a fixed valgus deformity of the heel and is often associated with other anomalies. The first and third types have been noted to 'run in families' as multifactorial traits. A Mendelian form is indicated by the kindred of Juberg and Touchstone (1974).

Juberg, R. C. and Touchstone, W. J.: Congenital metatarsus varus in four generations. Clin. Genet. 5: 127-132, 1974.

*15655 METATROPIC DWARFISM, TYPE II (KNIEST DISEASE)

This disorder resembles classic metatropic dwarfism in many respects but is probably an autosomal dominant. Cartilage obtained by biopsy feels soft. Histology shows lacunae in the cartilage giving it a Swiss-cheese appearance. Electron microscopy shows abnormality of the collagen of cartilage. The patients have inability to make a tight fist, seemingly because of thin joint spaces, and have a violaceous line of the palms. The face is rather characteristically flat. Siggers et al. (1974) reported eight patients. Two were identical twins; the others were sporadic. Cleft palate was present in 5, deafness in 6, retinal detachment in 3. They cited cases in mother and daughter known to Dr. J. Spranger of Kiel. The mean paternal age of the eight cases was 28.5.

Kniest, W.: Zur Abgrenzung der Dysostosis enchondralis von der Chondrodystrophie. Z. Kinderheilk. 43: 633-640, 1952.

Rimoin, D. L.: Torrance, Calif.: personal communication, 1971.

Siggers, D. C., Rimoin, D. L., Dorst, J. P., Doty, S. B., Williams, B. R., Hollister, D. W., Silberberg, R., Granley, R. E., Kaufman, R. L. and McKusick, V. A.: The Kniest syndrome. In, Bergsma, D. (ed.): Skeletal Dysplasias. Miami, Fla.: Symposia Specialists, 1974. Pp. 193-208.

15660 MICROCORIA, CONGENITAL

Ardouin et al. (1964) described a family in which 25 persons had small pupils due apparently to hypoplasia of the dilator muscle of the iris. Myopia was present in all.

Ardouin, M., Urvoy, M. and Lefranc, J.: Microcorie congenitale. Bull. Soc. Fr. Ophthalmol. 64: 356-363, 1964.

15670 MICROCORNEA, GLAUCOMA AND ABSENT FRONTAL SINUSES

Grandmother, mother, son and daughter showed this combination in the family reported by Holmes and Walton (1969).

Holmes, L. B. and Walton, D. S.: Hereditary microcornea, glaucoma, and absent frontal sinuses: a family study. J. Pediatr. 74: 968-972, 1969.

15680 MICRODONTIA, GENERALIZED

In the family reported by Steinberg, Warren and Warren (1961) either autosomal dominant or sex-linked dominant inheritance is possible.

Steinberg, A. G., Warren, J. F. and Warren, L. M.: Hereditary generalized microdontia. J. Dent. Res. 40: 58-62, 1961.

*15685 MICROPHTHALMIA-CATARACT

Capella et al. (1963) reported a family in which 12 persons in 4 generations had microphthalmia and congenital cataract. No instance of male-to-male transmission was noted. Harman (1909) observed a family with 9 cases in 5 generations, showing anterior polar cataracts, microphthalmia, nystagmus and strabismus.

Capella, J. A., Kaufman, H. E., Lill, F. J. and Cooper, G.: Hereditary cataracts and microphthalmia. Am. J. Ophthalmol. 56: 454-458, 1963.

Harman, N. B.: Congenital cataract, a pedigree of five generations. Trans. Ophthalmol. Soc. U.K. 29: 101-108, 1909.

15690 MICROPHTHALMOS WITH MYOPIA AND CORECTOPIA

Usher (1921) described a family with eleven cases in 4 generations including three instances of male-to-male transmission. Myopia and displaced pupil were associated with microphthalmos.

Usher, C. H.: A pedigree of microphtalmia with myopia and corectopia. Br. J. Ophthalmol. 5: 289-299, 1921.

15700 MICROPHTHALMOS, ANTERIOR (MICROCORNEA)

Friedman and Wright (1952) reported a pedigree with 8 cases in 5 generations.

Friedman, M. W. and Wright, E. S.: Hereditary microcornea and cataract in five generations. Am. J. Ophthalmol. 35: 1017-1021, 1952.

15710 MICROPHTHALMOS, PIGMENTARY RETINOPATHY, GLAUCOMA

Hermann (1958) reported a family with microphthalmos in 13 members of 4 generations. Some also had pigmentary retinopathy and some had glaucoma.

Hermann, P.: Le syndrome: microphtalmie-retinite pigmentaire-glaucome. Arch. Ophthalmol. 18: 17-24, 1958.

15715 MICROSPHEROPHAKIA WITH HERNIA

Johnson et al. (1971) described a family in which 11 persons in four generations had microspherophakia with upward dislocation of the lens, myopia, retinal detachment and inguinal hernias in various combinations. No other stigmata of either the Marfan or the Marchesani syndrome were detected. They suggested that this is a distinctive connective tissue disorder. No male-to-male transmission occurred in their family. As an isolated trait microspherophakia has been thought to be recessive (q.v.).

Johnson, V. P., Grayson, M. and Christian, J. C.: Dominant microspherophakia. Arch. Ophthalmol. 85: 534-537, 1971.

*15720 MIDPHALANGEAL (MID-DIGITAL) HAIR

The genetic determination of presence or absence of hair on the dorsal aspect of the middle phalanx was first suggested by Danforth (1921). The presence of hair is dominant.

Beckman, L. and Book, J. A.: Distribution and inheritance of mid-digital hair in Sweden. Hereditas 45: 215-220, 1959.

Bernstein, M. E.: The middigital hair genes. Their inheritance and distribution among the white race. J. Hered. 40: 127-131, 1949.

Bernstein, M. M. and Burke, B. S.: The incidence and Mendelian transmission of mid-digital hair in man. J. Hered. 33: 45-53, 1942.

Danforth, C. H.: Distribution of hair on the digits in man. Am. J. Phys. Anthropol. 4: 189-204, 1921.

Saldanha, P. H. and Guinsburg, S.: Distribution and inheritance of middle phalangeal hair in a white population of Sao Paulo, Brazil. Hum. Biol. 33: 237-249, 1961.

15730 MIGRAINE

Familial aggregation for migraine is undoubted. Allan (1928) favored dominant inheritance. Among 500 patients, at least one parent was affected in 91 percent. Among offspring of affected by affected matings, 83.3 percent were affected; affected by unaffected, 61 percent; and unaffected by unaffected, 3.7 percent. Goodell et al. (1953) found values of 69 percent, 44 percent and 29 percent in the three types of matings and favored recessive inheritance with about 70 percent penetrance. Refsum (1968) gave an extensive review.

Allan, W.: Inheritance of migraine. Arch. Intern. Med. 42: 590-599, 1928.

Goodell, H., Lewontin, R. and Wolff, H. G.: The familial occurrence of migraine headache: a study of heredity. Arch. Neurol. Psychiatry 72: 325-334, 1954.

Refsum, S.: Genetic aspects of migraine. In, Vinken, P. J. and Bruyn, G. W. (eds.): Handbook of Clinical Neurology. Amsterdam: North-Holland Publishing Co. 1968, vol. 5, chapter 25. Pp. 258-269.

*15740 MILIA, MULTIPLE ERUPTIVE

Thies and Schwarz (1961) described this condition. Heard et al. (1971) described a seemingly identical situation in a man who had onset of the abnormality in childhood and whose father had the same condition. (The father died at age 72 of carcinoma of the colon.) The case of Thies and Schwarz was not familial and was late in onset.

Heard, M. G., Horton, W. A. and Hambrick, G. W., Jr.: Multiple eruptive milia. The Clinical Delineation of Birth Defects. XII. Skin, Hair and Nails. Baltimore: Williams and Wilkins, 1971. Pp. 333-337.

Thies, W. and Schwarz, E.: Multiple eruptive milia — an organoid follicle hamartoma. Arch. Klin. Exp. Dermatol. 214: 21-34, 1961.

15745 MILIA-HYPOTRICHOSIS SYNDROME

Goldsmith and Baden (1971) described a family in which persons in three generations had milia (confined to the face) and sparse, hypopigmented scalp hair. Since there was no male-to-male transmission, differentiation from X-linked dominant inheritance is impossible.

Goldsmith, L. A. and Baden, H. P.: The analysis of genetically determined hair defects. The Clinical Delineation of Birth Defects. XII. Skin, Hair and Nails. Baltimore: Williams and Wilkins, 1971. Pp. 86-90.

15750 MILK PROTEINS, VARIANTS OF

Polymorphism is known in the proteins of milk (as well as in those of seminal fluid) of cattle. Such should be sought in man.

Bell, K., Hopper, K. E., McKenzie, H. A., Murphy, W. H. and Shaw, D. C.: A comparison of bovine alpha-lactalbumin A and B of Droughtmaster. Biochim. Biophys. Acta 214: 437-444, 1970.

Bell, K., McKenzie, H. A., Murphy, W. H. and Shaw, D. C.: Beta-lactoglobulin (Droughtmaster): a unique protein variant. Biochim. Biophys. Acta 214: 427-436, 1970.

15760 MIRROR MOVEMENTS, HEREDITARY

Mirror movements predominantly of the hand, not associated with other neurologic abnormality and with no abnormality of the cervical vertebrae, are inherited as a dominant with incomplete penetrance.

Regli, F., Filippa, G. and Wiesendanger, M.: Hereditary mirror movements. Arch. Neurol. 16: 620-623, 1967.

15765 MITOCHONDRIAL MYOPATHY, LIPID TYPE

Worsfield et al. (1974) reported biochemical findings in affected members of a kindred in which persons in four generations showed a myopathy whose expression ranged from sub-clinical to moderately severe weakness and wasting clinically resembling fascioscapulohumeral dystrophy, but which on ultrastructural grounds had been designated a 'mitochondrial myopathy' (Hudgson et al., 1972; Johnson et al., 1973). In vitro oxidative phosphorylation by mitochondria showed reduced or absent respiratory control. Greatly increased muscle lipid, in the form of triglyceride, was demonstrated.

Hudgson, P., Bradley, W. G. and Jenkinson, M.: Familial 'mitochondrial' myopathy. A myopathy associated with disordered oxidative metabolism in muscle fibres. Part I. (Clinical, electrophysiological and pathological findings). J. Neurol. Sci. 16: 343-370, 1972.

Johnson, M. A., Fulthorpe, J. J. and Hudgson, P.: Lipid storage myopathy. A clinicopathiologically recognizable entity? Acta Neuropathol. 24: 97-106, 1973.

Worsfield, M., Park, D. C. and Pennington, R. J.: Familial 'mitochondrial' myopathy. A myopathy associated with disordered oxidative metabilism in muscle fibres. Part II. Biochemical findngs. J. Neurol. Sci. 19: 261-274, 1973.

*15770 MITRAL REGURGITATION

Hunt and Sloman (1969) described a family in which multiple members of two generations had a systolic click followed by a late systolic murmur or a late systolic murmur alone. In one member the systolic murmur became loud and pansystolic during a few years observation. Systolic click and late systolic murmur have been related to flail mitral valve or floppy mitral valve. Incompetence of the posterior or mural leaflet is the usual finding of cineangiocardiography in such cases. This anomaly of the mitral valve is frequently found in the Marfan syndrome but certainly occurs as an isolated finding and might be familial. Shell et al. (1969) studied the families of four patients with this syndrome and in all four found a number of relatives with mid-late systolic clicks, late systolic murmurs, pansystolic murmurs, abnormal electrocardiograms and unexplained premature sudden death. Successive generations were affected and male-to-male transmission occurred. Stannard et al. (1967) observed familial incidence in 3 families.

Hunt, D. and Sloman, G.: Prolapse of the posterior leaflet of the mitral valve occurring in eleven members of a family. Am. Heart J. 78: 149-153, 1969.

Shappell, S. D., Marshall, C. E., Brown, R. E. and Bruce, T. A.: Sudden death and the familial occurrence of mid-systolic click, late systolic murmur syndrome. Circulation 48: 1128-1134, 1973.

Shell, W. E., Walton, J. A., Clifford, M. E. and Willis, P. W., III: The familial occurrence of the syndrome of mid-late systolic click and late systolic murmur. Circulation 39: 327-337, 1969.

Sreenivasan, V. V., Liebman, J., Linton, D. S. and Downs, T. D.: Posterior mitral regurgitation in girls possibly due to posterior papillary muscle dysfunction. Pediatrics 42: 276-290, 1968.

Stannard, M. and Rigo, S. J.: Prolapse of the posterior leaflet of the mitral valve: chromosome studies in three sisters. Am. Heart J. 75: 282-283, 1968.

Stannard, M., Sloman, J. G., Hare, W. S. C. and Goble, A. J.: Prolapse of the posterior leaflet of the mitral valve. A clinical, familial, and cineangiographic study. Br. Med. J. 3: 71-74, 1967.

15780 MITRAL REGURGITATION, CONDUCTIVE DEAFNESS, AND FUSION OF CERVICAL VERTEBRAE AND OF CARPAL AND TARSAL BONES

In a mother and two daughters, Forney, Robinson and Pascoe (1966) observed congenital mitral regurgitation, congenital perceptive deafness due to stapes footplate fixation, fusion of cervical vertebrae and of carpal and tarsal bones, striking freckling of the face and iris, and short stature (mother less than 5 feet). The maternal grandfather was short of stature and his father was both short and deaf. Thus, the condition may have passed through four generations.

Forney, W. R., Robinson, S. J. and Pascoe, D. J.: Congenital heart disease, deafness, and skeletal malformations: a new syndrome? J. Pediatr. 68: 14-26, 1966.

*15785 MIXED LYMPHOCYTE CULTURE (MLC) LOCUS

There is evidence that response in mixed lymphocyte culture is determined by a locus closely linked to the HL-A region. The genetic control of stimulation in the mixed lymphocyte culture reaction is determined by a separate gene (MLR-S) closely linded to the FOUR locus of the HL-A chromosomal region. Dupont et al. (1974) present three additional examples of sibs with recombination between the FOUR locus and the MLR-S locus. The occurrence of four recombinant children in one family, with four other children representing all possible HL-A haplotype combinations, strongly supported mapping of the MLR-S determinants outside the HL-A chromosomal region. An additional locus within the HL-A region appears to be involved in weak mixed lymphocyte reactions.

Dupont, B., Good, R. A., Hansen, G. S., Jensild, C., Nielsen, L. S., Park, B. H., Svejgaard, A., Thomsen, M. and Yunis, E.: Two separate genes controlling stimulation in mixed lymphocyte. Proc, Natl. Acad. Sci. 71: 52-56, 1974.

15786 MIXED LYMPHOCYTE CULTURE (MLC) LOCUS II

See 15785.

*15790 MOEBIUS SYNDROME (CONGENITAL FACIAL DIPLEGIA)

Van der Wiel (1957) described the disorder in 46 persons in 6 generations and Fortanier and Speijer (1935) found 15 cases in 3 generations. Congenital paralysis of the sixth and seventh cranial nerves was observed in multiple members of families by Wilbrand and Saenger (1921). Affected members of the family of Krueger and Friedrich (1963) occurred in three generations. See FACIAL PALSY, CONGENITAL UNILAT-ERAL. Hanissian et al. (1970) reported the Moebius syndrome in both of presumably monozygotic, Negro, male twins. The facial nerves were small or absent at autopsy in both cases. Sprofkin and Hillman (1956) described a patient with arthrogryposis and Moebius syndrome who had a sib with arthrogryposis only.

Fortanier, A. H. and Speijer, N.: Eine Erblichkeitsforschung bei einer Familie mit angeborenen Beweglichkeitsstoreungen der Hirnnerven (infantiler Kernschwund von Moebius). Genetica 17: 471-486, 1935.

Hanissian, A. S., Fuste, F., Hayes, W. T. and Duncan, J. M.: Mobius syndrome in twins. Am. J. Dis. Child. 120: 472-475, 1970.

Krueger, K. E. and Friedrich, D.: Familiaere kongenitale Motilitaetsstoerungen der Augen. Klin. Mbl. Augenheilk. 142: 101-117, 1963.

Sprofkin, B. E. and Hillman, J. W.: Moebius's syndrome — congenital oculofacial paralysis. Neurology 6: 50-54, 1956.

Van der Wiel, H. J.: Hereditary congenital facial paralysis. Acta Genet. Statist. Med. 7: 348 only, 1957.

Wilbrand, H. and Saenger, A.: Die Neurologie des Auges. Muenchen und Wiesbaden 8: 179 only, 1921.

*15795 MOLAR I REINCLUSION

Nijenhuis and Bosker (1974) have observed several families with a dental anomaly consisting of recession ('reinclusion') of the first molars into the bone. Linkage with blood group P was suggested (lod score + 2.14 at theta 0.00).

Nijenhuis, L. E.: Amsterdam, personal communication concerning work with H. Bosker of Groningen, 1974.

*15800 MONILETHRIX

Alopecia may be the presenting manifestation. The degree of alopecia is variable from patient to patient and from time to time in the same individual. Perifollicular hyperkeratosis is a consistent feature. Microscopically the hair is beaded.

Baker, H.: An investigation of monilethrix. Br. J. Dermatol. 74: 24-30, 1962.

Salamon, T. and Schnyder, U. W.: Ueber die Monilethrix. Arch. Klin. Exp. Dermatol. 215: 105-136, 1962.

Solomon, I. L. and Green, O. C.: Monilethrix: its occurrence in seven generations, with one case that responded to endocrine therapy. New Eng. J. Med. 269: 1279-1282, 1963.

15810 MONOPHALANGY OF GREAT TOE

Monophalangy of the great toes as an isolated hereditary defect was described by Frankel (1871).

Frankel, B.: Ueber einen Fall von erblicher Difformitaet. Klin. Wschr. 8: 418-419, 1871.

15825 MOSAICISM, CHROMOSOMAL

Chromosomal mosaicism based on a Mendelizing tendency to non-disjunction (25730) or satellite association (18110) is discussed elsewhere. A curious example of familial mosaicism is that for the Philadelphia chromosome, as reported by Hirschhorn (1968) and Weiner (1965). The proband, a 65-year-old man, had classic chronic myeloid leukemia (CML) with Ph(1) chromosome in all bone marrow and peripheral blood cells examined without phytohemagglutinin (PHA). His father died of leukemia of undetermined type and a brother and sister died of well documented CML without chromosome studies. The sister's son died of thymoma at 32. The proband's daughter age 29 and two of his sons ages 7 and 5 showed Ph(1) chromosome in some cells of the peripheral blood cultured without PHA. Lymphocytes stimulated with PHA showed normal karyotypes.

Hirschhorn, K.: Cytogenetic alterations in leukemia. Perspectives in Leukemia. New York: Grune and Stratton, 1968. Pp. 113-122.

Weiner, L.: A family with high incidence of leukemia and unique Ph(1) chromosome findings. Eighth Annual Meeting, Am. Soc. Hematology. Philadelphia, 1965.

*15830 MOUTH, INABILITY TO OPEN COMPLETELY, AND SHORT FINGER-FLEXOR TENDONS

Hecht and Beals (1969) described father and four children (2 sons, 2 daughters) with inability to open the mouth completely with resulting problems in mastication, short finger-flexor tendons such that dorsiflexion of the wrist resulted in camptodactyly and short leg muscles resulting in foot deformity. The father's mother was probably also affected. Wilson et al. (1969) described the same syndrome in 9 persons in 4 generations. They ascribed the finger peculiarity to shortening of the flexor profundus muscle-tendon unit. DeJong (1971) described a Dutch family with many affected members.

DeJong, J. G. Y.: A family showing strongly reduced ability to open the mouth and limitation of some movements of the extremities. Humangenetik 13: 210-217, 1971.

Hecht, F. and Beals, R. K.: Inability to open the mouth fully: an autosomal dominant phenotype with facultative campylodactyly and short stature. The Clinical Delineation of Birth Defects. III. Limb Malformations. New York: National Foundation, 1969. Pp. 96-98.

Wilson, R. V., Gaines, D. L., Brooks, A., Carter, T. S. and Nance, W. E.: Autosomal dominant inheritance of shortening of the flexor profundus muscle-tendon unit with limitation of jaw excursion. The Clinical Delineation of Birth Defects. III. Limb Malformations. New York: National Foundation, 1969. Pp. 99-102.

*15835 MULTIPLE HAMARTOMA SYNDROME

Only one case had been reported prior to the report of Weary et al. (1972). This was the report of the Cowden family for whom Lloyd and Dennis (1963) named the disorder. Multiple hamartomatous lesions especially of the skin, mucous membranes, breast and thyroid are encountered. Hamartomatous polyps of the colon and other intestines occur also. Affected brother and sister were observed by Gentry et al. (1974). Gentry et al. (1974) observed affected persons in 4 generations, with father-to-son transmission.

Gentry, W. C., Jr., Reed, W. B., Burnett, J. W., Siegel, J. M. and Colton, G. J.: Cowden disease. Report of 4 cases and a review of the English literature. In press, 1974.

Gentry, W. C., Jr., Eskritt, N. R. and Gorlin, R. J.: Multiple hamartoma syndrome (Cowden disease). Arch. Dermatol. 109:521-525, 1974.

Lloyd, K. M. and Dennis, M.: Cowden's disease: a possible new symptom complex with multiple system involvement. Ann. Intern. Med. 58: 136-142, 1963.

Weary, P. E., Gorlin, R. J., Gentry, W. C., Jr., Comer, J. E. and Greer, K. E.: Multiple hamartoma syndrome (Cowden's disease). Arch. Dermatol. 106: 682-690, 1972.

15840 MULTIPLE SCLEROSIS-LIKE DISEASE (SEE ATAXIA, SPASTIC)

Gayle and Williams (1933) described 17 cases in 4 generations of a disorder beginning in the sixth decade with stiffness in the leg muscles, followed by stumbling, dysarthria, and loss of memory. Although progression to severe spastic paraplegia occurred, the disorder did not shorten life. These patients lived in Accomac and Northampton counties on the eastern shore of Virginia.

Gayle, R. F., Jr. and Williams, J. P.: A familial disease of the central nervous system resembling multiple sclerosis. Sth. Med. J. 26: 242-246, 1933.

*15850 MUSCULAR ATROPHY, ATAXIA, RETINITIS PIGMENTOSA, DIABETES INSIPIDUS

In 10 persons in 4 generations, Furukawa et al. (1968) found muscular atrophy, ataxia, retinitis pigmentosa and diabetes insipidus. No reported case seemed to be identical.

Furukawa, T., Takagi, A., Nakao, K., Sugita, H., Tsukagoshi, H. and Tsubaki, T.: Hereditary muscular atrophy with ataxia, retinitis pigmentosa, and diabetes mellitus. A clinical report of a family. Neurology 18: 942-947, 1968.

*15860 MUSCULAR ATROPHY, JUVENILE (KUGELBERG-WELANDER SYNDROME)

A dominant form of this disorder, which is usually inherited as a recessive, was suggested by Tsukagoshi et al. (1966) and by others. Quasi-dominance due to consanguinity is possible, especially in the Japanese kindred. In three generations and 8 sibships of a Negro family, Armstrong, Fogelson and Silberberg (1966) reported a proximal muscular atrophy like Kugelberg-Welander disease but the inheritance was clearly dominant. See SCAPULOPERONEAL AMYOTROPHY in this catalog. Fenichel et al. (1967), Garvie and Woolf (1966) and Magee and DeGong (1960), among others, have reported dominant pedigrees. Several reports beginning with Timme (1917) have described a family with a dominant variety of proximal 'muscular dystrophy' with onset at age 3 or 4 but little if any effect on longevity and useful life. Gowers sign (climbing up the legs to rise from the floor) is noted early and the difficulty in getting up from the floor increases with age. Achilles tendon lengthening is required. Young (1971) gave the most recent information on the family, which has 13 affected persons in four generations. The fact that the disorder did not prevent productive life is indicated by the biography of one of the affected persons (Young, 1967), William Stewart Young, co-founder of Occidental College and the subject of an autopsy report by Butt et al. (1939), who wrongly labeled the disorder as dystrophia myotonica. There has been no cataract, myotonia, diabetes, or mental retardation in the family (Young, 1972). (Myotonic dystrophy is a distal myopathy.) One of the affected members of the family, son of William Stewart Young, gave a useful description of mechanical aids for patients with muscular disability (Young, 1949). The clinical picture is most consistent with an autosomal dominant spinal muscular atrophy.

Armstrong, R. M., Fogelson, M. H. and Silberberg, D. H.: Familial proximal spinal muscular atrophy. Arch. Neurol. 14: 208-212, 1966.

Butt, E. M., Hall, E. M. and Courville, C. B.: Progressive muscular dystrophy (dystrophia myotonica). Bull. Los Angeles Neurol. Soc. 4: 58-68, 1939.

Fenichel, G. M., Emery, E. S. and Hunt, P.: Neurogenic atrophy simulating facioscapulohumeral dystrophy. Arch. Neurol. 17: 257-260, 1967.

Garvie, J. M. and Woolf, A. L.: Kugelberg-Welander syndrome (hereditary proximal spinal muscular atrophy). Br. Med. J. 1: 1458-1461, 1966.

Magee, K. R. and DeJong, R. N.: Neurogenic muscular atrophy simulating muscular dystrophy. Arch. Neurol. 2: 677-682, 1960.

Timme, W.: Progressive muscular dystrophy as an endocrine disease. Arch. Intern. Med. 19: 79-104, 1917.

Tsukagoshi, H., Sugita, H., Furukawa, T., Tsubaki, T. and Ono, E.: Kugelberg-Welander syndrome with dominant inheritance. Arch. Neurol. 14: 378-381, 1966.

Young, N. M.: William Stewart Young, Builder of California Institutions. Glendale, Calif.: Arthur H. Clark Co., 1967.

Young, P. T.: Claremont, Calif.: personal communication, 1972.

Young, P. T.: Mechanical aids for patients with muscular disability. J. Bone Joint Surg. 31A: 428-430, 1949.

Zellweger, H., Simpson, J., McCormick, W, F. and Ionasescu, V.: Spinal muscular atrophy with autosomal dominant inheritance: report of a new kindred. Neurology 22: 957-963, 1972.

15865 MUSCULAR ATROPHY, MALIGNANT NEUROGENIC

Zatz et al. (1971) described a Brazilian kindred of Italian origin in which 7 members had neurogenic muscular atrophy with an unusually malignant and rapid course. Onset varied from ages 28 to 62 years and death from respiratory paralysis occurred within one year. Male-to-male transmission was observed.

Zatz, M., Penha-Serrano, C., Frota-Pessoa, O. and Klein, D.: A malignant form of neurogenic muscular atrophy in adults, with dominant inheritance. J. Genet. Hum. 19: 337-354, 1971.

15870 MUSCULAR ATROPHY, PROGRESSIVE

Brown (1951, 1960) described two New England families, Wetherbee and Farr by name, in which progressive degeneration of the anterior horn cells of the spinal cord and bulbar palsy as a cause of death behaved as a dominant trait.

Brown, M. R.: 'Wetherbee ail.' The inheritance of progressive muscular atrophy as a dominant trait in two New England families. N. Engl. J. Med. 245: 645-647, 1951.

Brown, M. R.: The inheritance of progressive muscular atrophy as a dominant trait in two New England families. N. Engl. J. Med. 262: 1280-1282, 1960.

15880 MUSCULAR DYSTROPHY, BARNES TYPE

Barnes (1932) described a family with muscular dystrophy of a type which may be distinct from any of the others presented in these catalogs. The disease had affected many persons in 6 generations of a family, with many instances of male-to-male transmission. The myopathy was exceedingly protean with predominantly pseudo-hypertrophic or distal character in some patients. In others it could be confused with peroneal atrophy. At least one showed myotonia of some thigh muscles.

Barnes, S.: Myopathic family, with hypertrophic, pseudohypertrophic, atrophic and terminal (distal in upper extremities) stages. Brain 55: 1-46, 1932.

*15890 MUSCULAR DYSTROPHY, FACIO-SCAPULO-HUMERAL

Justin-Besancon and colleagues (1964) gave autopsy findings in one of Landouzy's original patients who died at age of 86 years. Three affected generations were added to the four described by Landouzy. Some cases show congenital absence of part or all of certain muscles such as a pectoral. The relationship of the congenital defect of muscle to the dystrophy is unclear. Tyler and Stephens (1950, 1953) reported 17 families. In one kindred 150 members were affected over six generations. A girl, whose face alone was affected at age 9 when examined by Landouzy and Dejerine (whose names are attached eponymously to this condition), did not develop weakness of the arms until 60 and of the legs until 70 and survived to age 85 years. In her family affected members were distributed in 8 generations. Morton and Chung (1959) estimated the frequency to be about 2 per million living persons with a frequency in each million births, of about 4 persons destined to develop the trait. Fertility is little reduced and the mutation rate is not more than 5 per 10 million gametes.

Justin-Besancon, L., Pequignot, H., Contamin, F., Delavierre, P. and Rolland, P.: Myopathie du type Landouzy-Dejerine. Rapport d'une observation historique. Sem. Hosp. Paris 40: 2990-2999, 1964.

Morton, N. E. and Chung, C. S.: Formal genetics of muscular dystrophy. Am. J. Hum. Genet. 11: 360-379, 1959.

Tyler, F. H. and Stevens, F. E.: Studies in disorders of muscle. II. Clinical manifestations and inheritance of facioscapulohumeral dystrophy in a large family. Ann. Intern. Med. 32: 640-660, 1950.

Tyler, F. H.: The inheritance of neuromuscular disorders. Res. Publ. Assoc. Res. Nerv. Ment. Dis. 33: 283-292, 1953.

*15900 MUSCULAR DYSTROPHY, PROXIMAL

Schneiderman (1969) described a family with muscular dystrophy of gradual onset and slow progression, affecting mainly the proximal limb muscles and sparing the face. Linkage with the Pelger-Huet anomaly was demonstrated. The recombination fraction was about 0.25. This form of muscular dystrophy, which has the characteristics of a limb-girdle type, may be the same as that reported by Bacon and Smith (1971).

Bacon, P. A. and Smith, B.: Familial muscular dystrophy of late onset. J. Neurol. Neurosurg. Psychiatry 34: 93-97, 1971.

Schneiderman, L. J., Sampson, W. I., Schoene, W. C. and Haydon, G. B.: Genetic studies of a family with two unusual autosomal dominant conditions: muscular dystrophy and Pelger-Huet anomaly. Clinical, pathologic and linkage considerations. Am. J. Med. 46: 380-393, 1969.

15910 MUSCULAR HYPOPLASIA, CONGENITAL UNIVERSAL, OF KRABBE

The muscular hypoplasia is congenital and generalized and no or little progression of muscular weakness occurs. This condition was called muscular infantilism by Gibson (1921) who observed affected members of four generations. Schreier and Huperz (1956) described cases. Ford (1961) described affected mother and daughter who have subsequently been shown to have nemaline myopathy (q.v.). This suggests that a number of separate conditions will be found to answer to the above description. Thurmon (1971) has shown me a father and daughter with universal muscular hypoplasia in whom no specific myopathy such as nemaline myopathy could be identified by special studies.

Ford, F. R.: Diseases of the Nervous System in Infancy, Childhood and Adolescence. Springfield, Ill.: Charles C Thomas, 1961 (4th Ed.). P. 1259.

Gibson, A.: Muscular infantilism. Arch. Intern. Med. 27: 338 only, 1921.

Schreier, K. and Huperz, R.: Ueber die Hypoplasia musculorum generalisata congenita. Ann. Paediatr. 186: 241-248, 1956.

Thurmon, T. F.: New Orleans, La.: personal communication, 1971.

15920 MUSCULAR SHORTENING AND DYSTROPHY

In three generations of a French-Canadian family, Hauptmann and Thannhauser (1941) observed a disorder manifested by inability to flex the neck and slight webbing due to shortened muscle as well as limitation on spinal flexion and elbow extension from the same cause. The limb-girdle muscles were underdeveloped and weak. The condition apparently was not progressive.

Hauptmann, A. and Thannhauser, S. J.: Muscular shortening and dystrophy. A heredofamilial disease. Arch. Neurol. Psychiat. 46: 654-664, 1941.

15930 MYASTHENIA GRAVIS

Noyes (1930) noted myasthenia gravis in a father and two daughters. Herrmann (1966) reported affected father and son. The familial aggregation, although definite and impressive, does not conform to a simple Mendelian pattern. In a sample of 70 patients with myasthenia gravis, Jacob et al. (1968) found no instance of familial occurrence. They provided a comprehensive survey of the reported familial cases and pointed out differences from their own series, particularly earlier onset in the familial cases. Namba et al. (1971) pointed out, on the basis of 85 families with multiple cases (excluding transient neonatal myasthenia in offspring of myasthenic mothers), that the familial aggregation most often involves sibs and that affected persons in more than two generations have never been reported.

Herrmann, C., Jr.: Myasthenia gravis occurring in families. Neurology 16: 75-85, 1966.

Jacob, A., Clack, E. R. and Emery, A. E. H.: Genetic study of sample of 70 patients with myasthenia gravis. J. Med. Genet. 5: 257-261, 1968.

Namba, T., Brunner, N. G., Brown, S. B., Muguruma, M. and Grob, D.: Familial myasthenia gravis. Report of 27 patients in 12 families and review of 164 patients in 73 families. Arch. Neurol. 25: 49-60, 1971.

Noyes, A. P.: A case of myasthenia gravis with certain unusual features. Rhode Island Med. J. 13: 52-59, 1930.

15940 MYASTHENIA, FAMILIAL LIMB-GIRDLE

McQuillen (1966) described limb-girdle myasthenia in 3 of 3 sibs and in their father. Two of the children also had dystrophic changes in the weak muscles. The atrophy was not marked, however, and no oculobulbar involvement was present. Response to anti-cholinesterase therapy was striking and sustained. Electromyography suggested a defect of both muscle and the neuromyal junction.

McQuillen, M. P.: Familial limb-girdle myasthenia. Brain 89: 121-132, 1966.

15943 MYELIN (A1) PROTEIN, BASIC

This protein has been fully sequenced (Eylar et al., 1971). Sheremata et al. (1974) found a temporal relationship between clinical attacks of illness in multiple sclerosis and cellular hypersensitivity to basic myelin protein.

Eylar, E. H., Brostoff, S., Hashim, G. and Westall, F. C.: Basic A1 protein of the myelin membrane: the complete amino acid sequence. J. Biol. Chem. 246: 5770-5784, 1971.

Sheremata, W., Cosgrove, J. B. R., Hylar, E. H.: Cellular hypersensitivity to basic myelin (A1) protein and clinical multiple sclerosis. N. Engl. J. Med. 291: 14-17, 1974.

15945 MYELIN MEMBRANE ENCEPHALITOGENIC PROTEIN

This protein has been isolated from the myelin of the central nervous system of several mammals including man and represents up to 30 percent of total myelin protein. Its molecular weight is about 18,000, with 170 amino acids. Antibodies against this protein 'raised' in an animal of another species causes allergic encephalomyelitis with demyelination when reinjected into an animal of the species from which the myelin membrane protein was derived.

Chao, L.-P. and Einstein, E. R.: Localization of the active site through chemical modification of the encephalitogenic protein. J. Biol. Chem. 245: 6397-6403, 1970.

Dayhoff, M. O.: Myelin membrane encephalitogenic protein. Atlas of Protein Sequence and Structure 1972 (vol. 5). Washington: National Biomedical Research Foundation, 1972. P. D324.

15950 MYELINATED OPTIC NERVE FIBERS

Normally the optic nerve fibers are myelinated only after their passage through the lamina cribosa. Sometimes, however, the myelin sheath begins sooner producing a white area near the disk. Pseudopapilledema (q.v.) is a distinct condition. Francois (1961) cited a family with 10 cases in two generations and a few other instances suggesting dominant inheritance. In a few descriptions the anomaly was limited to one sibship.

Francois, J.: Heredity in Ophthalmology. St. Louis: C. V. Mosby Co., 1961. P. 495.

*15960 MYOCLONIC EPILEPSY, HARTUNG TYPE

This form appears to be distinct from the two types which are inherited as autosomal recessives (q.v.). Furthermore, unlike those forms no Lafora bodies were found at autopsy and only diffuse atrophy was present.

Hartung, E.: Zwei Faelle von Paramyoclonus multiplex mit Epilepsie. Zentbl. Ges. Neurol. Psychiat. 56: 150-153, 1920.

Vogel, F., Hafner, H. and Diebold, K.: Zur Genetik der progressiven Myoklonusepilepsien (Unverricht-Lundborg). Humangenetik 1: 437-475, 1965.

15970 MYOCLONUS AND ATAXIA

In 1921 Ramsay Hunt described the association of generalized myoclonus and signs of cerebellar dysfunction, especially intention tremor, under the designation of dyssynergia cerebellaris myoclonica. Autopsy in one case confirmed his impression of a lesion in the dentate nucleus of the cerebellum. His cases were non-familial. Gilbert, McEntee and Glaser (1963) described two females and two males in three sibships of a family with the combination of myoclonus and ataxia. Cerebrospinal fluid uric acid was elevated in two. Autosomal dominant inheritance with reduced penetrance was suggested.

Gilbert, G. J., McEntee, W. J., III and Glaser, G. H.: Familial myoclonus and ataxia. Pathophysiologic implications. Neurology 13: 365-372, 1963.

Hunt, J. R.: Dyssynergia cerebellaris myoclonica-primary atrophy of the dentate system: a contribution to the pathology and symptomatology of the cerebellum. Brain 44: 490-538, 1921.

15980 MYOCLONUS, CEREBELLAR ATAXIA AND DEAFNESS

May and White (1968) described a new syndrome of familial myoclonus, cerebellar ataxia and deafness and concluded that it is autosomal dominant. Evidence is meager, however a mother and son had the full syndrome. Hearing loss was noted in childhood or early adulthood. Myoclonic jerks and cerebellar symptoms began at age 14 in the son. See DEAF-MUTISM AND FAMILIAL MYOCLONUS EPILEPSY.

May, D. L. and White, H. H.: Familial myoclonus, cerebellar ataxia, and deafness: specific genetically-determined disease. Arch. Neurol. 19: 331-338, 1968.

*15990 MYOCLONUS, HEREDITARY ESSENTIAL

This disorder consists of sudden, brief muscular contractions affecting mainly the proximal muscles of the extremities. The twitchings are aggravated by excitement and disappear during sleep. Epilepsy and intellectual deterioration do not occur. We know of affected mother and son (P7063). In another family, of French-Canadian background, a father and 5 of his 9 children show onset of myoclonus in the first or second decade and benign course, without seizures, dementia or neurologic signs other than myoclonus (Mahloudji and Pikielny, 1966). Because of the uncertainty of the nature of the case on the basis of which Friedreich in 1881 introduced the term paramyoclonus multiplex, these cases might best be called hereditary essential myoclonus. Daube and Peters (1966) reported two families in which affected members occurred in at least four generations of each with male-to-male transmission in each but some skipped generations. Symonds (1953) described nocturnal myoclonus in a man and five of his six children.

Biemond, A.: Paramyoclonus multiplex (Friedreich). Clinical and genetic aspects. Psychiat. Neurol. Neurochir. 66: 270-276, 1963.

Daube, J. R. and Peters, H. A.: Hereditary essential myoclonus. Arch. Neurol. 15: 587-594, 1966.

Korten, J. J., Notermans, S. L. H., Frenken, C. W. G. M., Gabreels, F. J. M. and Joosten, E. M. G.: Familial essential myoclonus. Brain 97: 131-138, 1974.

Lindermulder, F. G.: Familial myoclonia occurring in three successive generations. J. Nerv. Ment. Dis. 77: 489-491, 1933.

Littlejohn, W. S.: Familial myoclonus: report of four cases with electroencephalograms. Sth. Med. J. 42: 404-410, 1949.

Mahloudji, M. and Pikielny, R. T.: Hereditary essential myoclonus. Brain 90: 669-674, 1967.

Symonds, C. P.: Nocturnal myoclonus. J. Neurol. Neurosurg. Psychiatry 16: 166-171, 1953.

*16000 MYOGLOBIN

Two structural variants of myoglobin were described by Boyer, Fainer and Naughton (1963). Boulton et al. (1969) studied muscle obtained post mortem from 2500 persons. Two myoglobin variants were found and in one of these substitution of lysine for glutamic acid as the 53rd residue was demonstrated. Human myoglobin has 152 residues. Later Boulton et al. (1970) described a variant myoglobin with substitution of glutamine for arginine as residue 138.

Boulton, F. E. and Huntsman, R. G.: Abnormal human myoglobin: 53(D4) glutamic acid lysine. Nature 223: 832-833, 1969.

Boulton, F. E., Huntsman, R. G., Lehmann, H., Lorkin, P. A. and Romero-Herrera, A. E.: Myoglobin variants. (Abstract) Biochem. J. 118: 39P only, 1970.

Boulton, F. E., Huntsman, R. G., Yawson, G. I., Romero-Herrera, A. E. and Lorkin, P. A.: The second variant of human myoglobin: 138(H16) arginine to glutamine. Br. J. Haematol. 20: 69-74, 1971A.

Boyer, S. H., IV, Fainer, D. C. and Naughton, M. A.: Myoglobin inherited structural variation in man. Science 140: 1228-1231, 1963.

Romero-Herrera, A. E. and Lehmann, H.: The amino acid sequence of human myoglobin and its minor fractions. Proc. R. Soc. London 186B: 249-279, 1974.

*16010 MYOKYMIA

Spontaneous muscle twitches occur in many persons and have no grave significance. They may be confused with fasciculations which occur with amyotrophic lateral sclerosis. I know of a family with multiple affected members in a dominant inheritance pattern. The family derived from a tri-racial (Caucasoid, Negro, Indian) group in Robson Co., N. C. (H. O., JHH917242). Sheaff (1952) described affected father and two sons. Wieczorek and Greger (1962) described a dominant pedigree. Sheaff (1952) observed myokymia in a man and his four sons. In a portion of muscle removed for biopsy fasciculations persisted for 8 minutes. Affected persons probably have an increased frequency of muscle cramps ('night cramps').

Sheaff, H. M.: Hereditary myokymia. Syndrome or disease entity associated with hypoglycemia and disturbed thyroid function. Arch. Neurol. Psychiatry 68: 236-247, 1952.

Wieczorek, V. and Greger, J.: Ueber ein familiaer gehaeuftes Vorkommen von Myokymie. Psychiat. Neurol. Med. Psychol. 14: 452-455, 1962.

*16015 MYOPATHY, CENTRONUCLEAR

Centronuclear myopathy is an example of genetic heterogeneity. Recessive (25520) and X-linked (31040) forms have been suspected and the family reported by McLeod et al. (1972) makes autosomal dominant inheritance quite certain. Muscle weakness had its onset between the first and third decades, was slowly progressive and was primarily proximal in distribution but sometimes involved the facial musculature. External ophthalmoplegia and pharyngeal weakness were not features. Sixteen members of the family were affected. Karpati et al. (1970) reported affected mother and daughter. Pathologically there was atrophy predominantly of type I muscle fibers, with central nuclei and pale central zones with variably staining granules. These changes are indistinguishable from those in the other genetic varieties.

Karpati, G., Carpenter, S. and Nelson, R. F.: Type I muscle fibre atrophy and central nuclei: a rare familial neuromuscular disease. J. Neurol. Sci. 10: 489-500, 1970.

McLeod, J. G., Baker, W. C., Lethlean, A. K. and Shorey, C. D.: Centronuclear myopathy with autosomal dominant inheritance. J. Neurol. Sci. 15: 375-388, 1972.

16020 MYOPATHY, CONGENITAL, WITH CRYSTALLINE INTRANUCLEAR INCLUSIONS

Jenis et al. (1969) described a white female from unrelated parents who showed extreme muscular weakness and hypotonia from birth and died of respiratory insufficiency at 2 months of age. Intranuclear and sarcoplasmic inclusions were found in muscle cells. There were no sibs. Hence, the genetics is completely obscure.

Jenis, E. H., Lindquist, R. R. and Lister, R. C.: New congenital myopathy with crystalline intranuclear inclusions. Arch. Neurol. 20: 281-287, 1969.

*16030 MYOPATHY, DISTAL, WITH ONSET IN INFANCY

Foot drop and finger weakness are leading features. Although onset is in infancy, the ailment is not incapacitating and progression after adolescence does not occur. Autosomal dominant inheritance seems quite certain.

Magee, K. R. and Dejong, R. N.: Hereditary distal myopathy with onset in infancy. Arch. Neurol. 13: 223
387-390, 1965.

Willebois, A. E. M., Bethlem, J., Meyer, A. E. F. H. and Simons, A. J. R.: Distal myopathy with onset
in early infancy. Neurology 18: 383-390, 1968.

16040 MYOPATHY, DUE TO GLYCOLYTIC ABNORMALITY

Satoyoshi and Kowa (1967) described myopathy studied in detail in two brothers but also present by history
in a sister, their mother and a son of one sister. Onset was about age 35 years with delayed muscle pain and
stiffness on exertion but absence of contracture or weakness on ischemic exercise. Phosphofructokinase
activity was about 40 percent of normal in skeletal muscle. Oral ingestion of fructose relieved the symptoms.
The possible role of an inhibitor in the process was proposed. Glycogen storage disease VII (q.v.), a recessive,
has deficiency of muscle phosphofructokinase.

Satoyoshi, E. and Kowa, H.: A myopathy due to glycolytic abnormality. Arch. Neurol. 17: 248-256, 1967.

*16050 MYOPATHY, LATE DISTAL HEREDITARY

On the basis of 78 probands and 171 secondary cases, Welander (1951) delineated distal myopathy as a
distinct entity with dominant inheritance. The 249 affected persons were distributed in 72 kindreds. The mean
age at onset was 47 years (range 20-77). Weakness and wasting of the small muscles of hands was the first
manifestation in 89 percent. Fasciculations, myotonia and sensory changes were notably absent. About 70
percent of the probands were aware of their hereditary predisposition at the time of first examination. The
disorder was very slowly progressive and apparently did not shorten life. The first description of this type
is attributed to Gowers. The relationship to the four with onset in childhood described by Dahlgaard (1960)
and that with onset in infancy described by Magee and DeJong (1965) is uncertain. Welander (1957)
described the homozygous state. Both parents were affected, 7 of 16 children had distal myopathy and 2 of
these were unusually severe with early proximal involvement. Sumner et al. (1971) described an English
family with 5 of 6 sibs affected. The father may have been affected. They considered this a distinct entity
from Welander's Swedish cases because of the earlier onset (age 15-20). The clinical course, however, does
not appear appreciably different. Markesbery et al. (1974) reported autopsy findings and the occurrence of
cardiomyopathy.

Dahlgaard, E.: Myopathia distalis tarda hereditaria. Acta Psychiat. Neurol. Scand. 35: 440-447, 1960.

Magee, K. R. and DeJong, R. N.: Hereditary distal myopathy with onset in infancy. Arch. Neurol. 13:
387-390, 1965.

Markesbery, W. R.,,Griggs, R. C., Leach, R. P. and Lapham, L. W.: Late onset hereditary distal
myopathy. Neurology, 24: 127-134, 1974.

Sumner, D., Crawford, M. A. and Harriman, D. G. F.: Distal muscle dystrophy in an English family.
Brain 94: 51-60, 1971.

Wallis, K., Deutsch, V. and Azizi, E.: Hypertension in a case of Von Recklinghausen's neurofibromatosis.
Helvet. Paediatr. Acta 25: 147-153, 1970.

Welander, L.: Homozygous appearance of distal myopathy. Acta Genet. Statist. Med. 7: 321-325, 1957.

Welander, L.: Myopathia distalis tarda hereditaria. Acta Med. Scand. 141 (suppl. 265): 1-124, 1951.

16060 MYOPATHY, LIMITED TO FEMALES

Henson et al. (1967) described a slowly progressive limb-girdle type of muscular dystrophy in 8 females in
4 sibships in 2 generations of a family. Female-limited autosomal dominant inheritance was favored. This
may be an X-linked dominant, lethal in the hemizygous male. See 30995.

Henson, T. E., Muller, J. and DeMyer, W. E.: Hereditary myopathy limited to females. Arch. Neurol.
17: 238-247, 1967.

*16070 MYOPIA

Myopia of severe degree was transmitted through 4 generations in the family reported by Francois (1961).
Franceschetti (1953) observed a family with 10 cases in 4 generations. Four suffered detachment of the retina.
Myopia in a sense is a metric character. Variation in many components of the eye contributes to its refractive
capacity (Sorsby et al., 1962). Some myopia, perhaps most, is multifactorial in causation. Some environmental
causes of myopia are identifiable.

Franceschetti, A.: Haute myopie avec decollement retinien hereditaire. J. Genet. Hum. 2: 283-284, 1953.

Francois, J.: Heredity in Ophthalmology. St. Louis: C. V. Mosby Co., 1961.

Sorsby, A., Sheridan, M. and Leary, G. A.: Refraction and its components in twins. Medical research
council: special reprint series. London: (no. 303), 1962.

*16080 MYOTONIA CONGENITA (ALSO SEE PARAMYOTONIA CONGENITA)

This is the disorder described by Thomsen (1875) in his own family. Isaacs (1959) studied the disorder in
a mother and her son and daughter. Quinine, local procain, procain amide, insulin, injections of 50 percent
magnesium sulfate, curarization, sodium loading and sodium depletion had no effect on the mother's
myotonia. However, marked improvement occurred when potassium depletion was achieved with cortisone
and chlorothiazide. The daughter was treated with chlorothiazide only and improved. Pasternack and
Lindqvist (1962) described 6 cases in 3 generations, and personally examined four. With the follow-up by
Thomasen (1948), Thomsen's family showed 64 affected persons in 7 generations without skips. The pedigree

of Birt (1908), who like Thomsen was himself affected showed skipped generations. Possible homozygotes were reported by Te Kamp (1907). Somatic mutation is a possible explanation in the case of monomelic myotonia congenita reported by Celesia et al. (1967).

Birt, A.: A study of Thomsen's disease (congenital myotonia) by a sufferer from it. Montreal Med. 37: 771-784, 1908.

Celesia, G. G., Andermann, F., Wiglesworth, F. W. and Robb, J. P.: Monomelic myopathy. Congenital hypertrophic myotonic myopathy limited to one extremity. Arch. Neurol. 17: 69-77, 1967.

Isaacs, H.: The treatment of myotonia congenita. S. Afr. Med. J. 33: 984-986, 1959.

Katzenstein-Sutro, E., Bosch-Gwalter, T. and Rosenmund, H.: Myotonie congenitale de Thomsen et ses criteres differentiels avec les autres maladies musculaires: etude d'une famille presentant un groupement special de symptomes, en tenant specialement compte de l'elimination de ribose dans l'urine. J. Genet. Hum. 9: 1-64, 1960.

Pasternack, A. and Lindqvist, C.: Thomsen's disease. Observations on strength-duration curves in myotonia. Ann. Paediat. Fenn. 8: 284-291, 1962.

Te Kamp, (NI): Ein Beitrag zur Kenntnis der Myotonia congenita sog. Thomsenschen Krankheit. Deutsch. Med. Wschr. 33: 1005 only, 1907.

Thomasen, E.: Myotonia, Thomsen's disease. Paramyotonia, and dystrophia myotonica. Op. Ex. Domo Biol. Hered. Hum. U. Hafniensis 17: 11-251, 1948.

Thomsen, J.: Tonische Kramepfe in willkuerlich beweglichen Muskeln in Folge von ererbter psychischer Disposition. Ataxia Musularis? Arch. Psychiatry Nervenkr. 76: 706, 1875.

*16090 MYOTONIC DYSTROPHY (STEINERT DISEASE)

The features are myotonia, muscle wasting (e.g., in the temporal muscles and those of the neck), cataract, hypogonadism, frontal balding, EKG changes. Anticipation-earlier onset in more recent generations- is described but is probably an artifact of ascertainment (Penrose, 1948). Bosma and Brodie (1969) demonstrated both myotonia and weakness in patients with swallowing and speech disability. In the cytoplasm of cultured skin fibroblasts Swift and Finegold (1969) found an abnormally large amount of material with the staining properties of acid mucopolysaccharides. Schwindt et al. (1969) claimed that 25 to 50 percent of patients have abdominal symptoms due to cholelithiasis. Bundey et al. (1970) found that the most useful method for identifying subclinical cases is slit-lamp examination (for lens changes), followed by electromyography (for myotonic discharges), and in third position as to level of success, by measurement of immunoglobulins. They estimated that about a quarter of index cases are the result of new mutation. In selected families it may be feasible to perform amniocentesis for determination of secretor status of the fetus and thereby predict inheritance of the allele for myotonic dystrophy based upon the Dm-Se linkage. The affected spouse must be heterozygous at the secretor locus and the coupling between Dm and Se or Se must be established; the unaffected spouse must not be homozygous secretor-positive. It is best if that spouse be secretor-negative, but useful information for counseling can be obtained if he is heterozygous for secretor. In some cases the secretor phenotype of the fetus may establish the genotype in the parents. Finally, recombination between Dm and Se introduces a degree of uncertainty into the counseling (Schrott et al., 1973).

Bosma, J. F. and Brodie, D. R.: Cineradiographic demonstration of pharyngeal area myotonia in myotonic dystrophy patients. Radiology 92: 104-109, 1969.

Bundey, S. and Carter, C. O.: Genetic heterogeneity for dystrophia myotonica. J. Med. Genet. 9: 311-315, 1972.

Bundey, S., Carter, C. O. and Soothill, J. F.: Early recognition of heterozygote for the gene for dystrophia myotonica. J. Neurol. Neurosurg. Psychiatry 33: 279-293, 1970.

Caughey, J. E. and Myrianthopoulos, N. C.: Dystrophia Myotonica and Related Disorders. Springfield, Ill.: Charles C Thomas, 1963.

Dumaine, L. and Lozeron, P.: Contribution a l'etude clinique et genetique de la dystrophie myotonique (Steinert) et de la myotonie congenitale (Thomsen). J. Genet. Hum. 10: 221-296, 1961.

Harper, P. S., Rivas, M. L., Bias, W. B., Hutchinson, J. R., Dyken, P. R. and McKusick, V. A.: Genetic linkage confirmed between the locus for myotonic dystrophy and the ABH-secretion and Lutheran blood group loci. Am. J. Hum. Genet. 24: 310-316, 1972.

Klein, D.: La Dystrophie Myotonique (Steinert) et la Myotonie Congenitale (Thomsen) en Suisse. Geneve: Edition Medicine et Hygiene, 1957.

Lynas, M. A.: Dystrophia myotonica with special reference to Northern Ireland. Ann. Hum. Genet. 21: 318-351, 1957.

Penrose, L. S.: The problems of anticipation in pedigrees of dystrophia myotonica. Ann. Eugen. 14: 125-132, 1948.

Pruzanski, W.: Variants of myotonic dystrophy in pre-adolescent life (the syndrome of myotonic dysembryoplasia). Brain 89: 563-568, 1966.

Renwick, J. H., Bundey, S. E., Ferguson-Smith, M. A. and Izatt, M. M.: Confirmation of linkage of the loci for myotonic dystrophy and ABH secretion. J. Med. Genet. 8: 407-416, 1971.

Schrott, H. G., Karp, L. and Omenn, G. S.: Prenatal prediction in myotonic dystrophy: guidelines for genetic counseling. Clin. Genet. 4: 38-45, 1973.

Schwindt, W. D., Bernhardt, L. C. and Peters, H. A.: Cholelithiasis and associated complications of myotonia dystrophica. Postgrad. Med. 46: 80-83, 1969.

Swift, M. R. and Finegold, M. J.: Myotonic muscular dystrophy: abnormalities in fibroblast culture. Science 165: 294-296, 1969.

*16100 NAEGELI SYNDROME

This disorder was earlier confused with incontinentia pigmenti (see X-linked catalog). Naegeli (1927) described the syndrome in a father and two daughters. Franceschetti and Jadassohn (1954) documented dominant inheritance. Differences from incontinentia pigmenti include (1) equal frequency in males and females, (2) plantar and palmar hypohidrosis and hyperkeratosis, and (3) uncommon blistering and inflammatory phenomena. Franceschetti and Jadassohn (1954) maintained that this disorder is distinct from incontinentia pigmenti (an X-linked trait). The cardinal features are reticular cutaneous pigmentation, discomfort provoked by heat with diminished sweat gland function, poor teeth and moderate hyperkeratosis of the palms and soles. Males and females are equally affected.

Berlin, C.: Congenital generalized melanoleucoderma associated with hypodontia, hypotrichosis, stunted growth and mental retardation occurring in two brothers and two sisters. Dermatologica. 123: 227-243, 1961.

Franceschetti, A. and Jadassohn, W.: A propos de l'incontinentia pigmenti, delimitation de deux syndromes differents figurant sous le meme terme. Dermatologica 108: 1-28, 1954.

Kitamura, K. and Hirako, T.: Ueber zwei Japanische Falle einer eigenartigen retikulaeren Pigmentierung: zur Frage der dermatose pigmentaire reticulee (Franceschetti-Jadassohn). Dermatologica 110: 97-107, 1955.

Naegeli, B.: Familiaerer Chromatophorennaevus. Schweiz. Med. Wschr. 57: 48 only, 1927.

Vilanova, X. and Aguade, J. P.: Incontinentia pigmenti. Troubles sudoripares fonctionnels dysplastiques et pigmentaires chez les ascendants. Ann. Dermeratol. Syph. 86: 247-258, 1959.

16110 NAILBEDS, PIGMENTATION OF

Pigmented nailbeds occur in a certain proportion of Negroes. The pigmentation may be confused with cyanosis or may make evaluation of cyanosis difficult. Dark pigmentation of the nailbeds was correlated with pigmentation of fungiform papillae of the tongue (27525) in a Negro family studied by Norum (1974). The teen-age brother and sister also had black cerumen and an unexplained history of black staining of diapers as infants. Apocrine chromidrosis (Shelley and Hurley, 1954) has no known familial basis. It is not certain that aprocine chromidrosis was present in sibs reported by Norum (1974).

Norum, R. A.: Association of pigmented nails, pigmented fungiform papillae of tongue, and apocrine chromidrosis. In, Bergsma, D. (ed.): Clinical Delineation of Birth Defects. XVI. Urinary System and Others. Baltimore: Williams and Wilkins, 1974. Pp. 351-352.

Shelly, W. B. and Hurley, H. H., Jr.: Localization chromidrosis. Arch. Dermatol. Syph. 69: 449-471, 1954.

*16120 NAIL-PATELLA SYNDROME

Dysplasia of the nails and absent or hypoplastic patellae are the cardinal features but others are iliac horns, abnormality of the elbows interfering with pronation and supination, and in some cases nephropathy. The nail-patella locus and the ABO blood group locus are linked. The recombination fraction is about 10 percent but is higher in females than in males. Nephropathy was an associated abnormality in the family of Hawkins and Smith (1950). The renal change resembles glomerulonephritis. It is relatively benign although fatality at a young age from this complication has been described (Leahy, 1966). This condition is sometimes called Turner syndrome, but this leads to confusion with the XO syndrome. The renal disorder in the case of Simila et al. (1970) took the appearance of congenital nephrosis. In the family eight had nail-patella syndrome of whom five also had renal disease. The seeming familial aggregation of the renal complications suggests two separate genes, one for a nephropathic form and one for a non-nephropathic form. They might be allelic since no heterogeneity has been detected in the linkage with the ABO locus. As demonstrated by electron microscopy by Morita et al. (1973), among others, many collagen fibrils are present in the thickened basement membranes and in mesangial matrix of otherwise normal glomeruli. Abnormalities of collagen at this site have been demonstrated also in Alport syndrome (10420). Both of these conditions may be special forms of heritable disorders of connective tissue.

Bennett, W. M., Musgrave, J. E., Campbell, R. A., Elliot, D., Cox, R., Brooks, R. E., Lovrien, E. W., Beals, R. K. and Porter, G. A.: The nephropathy of the nail-patella syndrome: clinicopathologic analysis of 11 kindreds. Am. J. Med. 54: 304-319, 1973.

Cottereill, C. P. and Jacobs, P.: Hereditary arthro-osteo-onychodysplasia associated with iliac horns. Brit. J. Clin. Pract. 15: 933-941, 1961.

Darlington, D. and Hawkins, C. F.: Nail patella syndrome with iliac horns and hereditary nephropathy. Necropsy report and anatomical dissection. J. Bone Joint Surg. 49B: 164-174, 1967.

Eisenberg, K. S., Potter, D. E. and Bovill, E. G., Jr.: Osteo-onychodystrophy with nephropathy and renal osteodystrophy. A case report. J. Bone Joint Surg. 54: 1301-1305, 1972.

Hawkins, C. F. and Smith, O. E.: Renal dysplasia in a family with multiple hereditary abnormalities including iliac horns. Lancet I: 803-808, 1950.

Leahy, M. S.: The hereditary nephropathy of osteo-onychodysplasia (nail patella syndrome). Am. J. Dis. Child. 112: 237-241, 1966.

Morita, T., Laughlin, O., Kawano, K. and Kimmelstiel, P.: Nail-patella syndrome. Arch. Intern. Med. 131: 271-277, 1973.

Pillay, V. K.: Onycho-osteodysplasia (nail-patella syndrome). Study of a Chinese family with this condition. Ann. Hum. Genet. 28: 301-307, 1965.

Renwick, J. H. and Lawler, S. D.: Genetical linkage between the ABO and nail-patella loci. Ann. Hum. Genet. 19: 312-331, 1955.

Renwick, J. H. and Schulze, J.: Male and female recombination fractions for the nail patella: ABO linkage in man. Ann. Hum. Genet. 28: 379-392, 1965.

Schroeder, G.: Osteo-onycho-dysplasia hereditaria. Z. Menschl. Vererb. Konstitutionsl. 36: 42-73, 1961.

Simila, S., Vesa, L. and Wasz-Hockert, O.: Hereditary onycho-osteodysplasia (the nail-patella syndrome) with nephrosis-like renal disease in a newborn boy. Pediatrics 46: 61-65, 1970.

Vernier, R. L., Hoyer, J. R. and Michael, A. F.: The nail-patella syndrome — pathogenesis of the kidney lesion. In, Bergsma, D. (ed.): Clinical Delineation of Birth Defects. XVI. Baltimore: Williams and Wilkins, 1974. Pp. 57-59.

Von Knorre, G.: Ueber die hereditaere arthro-osteo-onycho-dysplasie (Turner-Kieser-syndrom). Z. Menschl. Vererb. Konstitutionsl. 36: 118-129, 1961.

Zimmerman, C.: Iliac horns: a pathognomonic roentgen sign of familial onycho-osteodysplasia. Am. J. Roentgen. 86: 478-483, 1961.

16140 NARCOLEPSY

In three generations of a family Daly and Yoss (1959) found 12 definite and 3 possible cases. Whereas about two-thirds of all cases of narcolepsy (sleeping attacks) are associated with cataplexy (paroxysmal attacks of weakness or frank paralysis, associated especially with strong emotion), only one-third of the affected persons in this family displayed cataplexy. Furthermore, in these the weakness was mild. Narcolepsy is as difficult to document and to study genetically as is schizophrenia. Therefore, a simple inherited form cannot be considered fully established. Three of the 12 affected persons in the family of Daly and Yoss (1959) had cataplectic attacks. Gelardi and Brown (1967) reported on a family in which 11 persons in 4 generations had cataplexy. Three may have had narcolepsy. No instance of male-to-male transmission occurred in the pedigree. In a later publication, Yoss (1970) reported studies with infrared pupillography in narcolepsy families, leading to the conclusion that narcolepsy is polygenic, i.e., that the affected persons are at one end of a spectrum. When a person is awake and alert in total darkness his pupils are large. During sleep the pupils are small. The pupils are intermediate in size when the subject is between these two extremes. This is the basis of infrared pupillography as a guage of wakefulness. The author suggested that it would be very unusual for two persons with philagrypnia (ability to stay alert with little sleep) to have an offspring with narcolepsy.

Daly, D. D. and Yoss, R. E.: A family with narcolepsy. Mayo Clin. Proc. 34: 313-320, 1959.

Gelardi, J. A. M. and Brown, J. W.: Hereditary cataplexy. J. Neurol. Neurosurg. Psychiatry 30: 455-457, 1967.

Yoss, R. E.: The inheritance of diurnal sleepiness as measured by pupillography. Mayo Clin. Proc. 45: 426-437, 1970.

*16150 NASAL GROOVE, FAMILIAL TRANSVERSE

This is a red furrow which extends across the nose just proximal to the alae nasi. It is usually noticed early in childhood and at that stage may have a rose color. Anderson observed two rather extensively affected families. An instance of male-to-male-transmission occurred in one.

Anderson, P. C.: Familial transverse nasal groove. Arch. Dermatol. 84: 316-317, 1961.

16160 NAVICULAR BONE, ACCESSORY

This is present in about 5 percent of persons. It causes an undue prominence on the medial side of the foot. It is sometimes referred to as an accessory or secondary medial malleolus. Sometimes it is fused with the navicular to form an abnormally large tuberosity on the latter bone.

Moseley, H. F.: Static disorders of the ankle and foot. Ciba Clinical Symposia 9: 83-110, 1957.

16170 NECROBIOSIS LIPOIDICA AND PERIODONTOSIS

In one family (A. K., 1136340) I have observed a skin lesion resembling necrobiosis lipoidica diabeticorum in association with periodontal disease leading to early loss of teeth. The skin lesions consisted of symmetrical patches on the front of the shins, about five inches long, covered by parchment skin and discolored by blood pigments. The appearance resembled that in the Ehlers-Danlos syndrome. The knees showed small 'cigarette-paper scars' and easy bruisability of the skin was noted. Loosejointedness and general bruisability and cutaneous fragility were not present. Furthermore, although the histology of the lesions of the skin suggested necrobiosis lipoidica diabeticorum no evidence of diabetes was uncovered in any member of the family.

*16180 NEMALINE MYOPATHY

The mother and daughter described by Ford (1961) as cases of congenital universal muscular hypoplasia of Krabbe were shown by Hopkins et al. (1966) to have this disorder. The rod-like inclusions in muscle may be precipitated myosin. The relation to central core disease (q.v.) awaits clarification. The two have been reported in the same family. Spiro and Kennedy (1965) also observed affected mother and daughter. X-linked dominant inheritance is, of course, also possible. The pathologic fibrillar material is similar to and continuous with the substance which constitutes the Z-bands (Price et al., 1965) and may be tropomyosin B. Conventional histopathological preparations may be normal or nearly normal. The condition described by Gibson (1921) was present in three generations and may be this disorder. The dominant inheritance and the anomalous material of Z-band origin suggest that a simple amino acid substitution may be demonstrated eventually in this disorder. This is a non-progressive form of congenital myopathy with abnormal threadlike structures in muscle cells on histologic examination. In the family of Shy et al. (1963) both parents of two affected sibs showed minor abnormalities which might be interpreted as heterozygous effects. The clinical picture is that of the 'floppy infant' (see MYOTONIA CONGENITA). An older case studied by Engel et al. (1964) suggested slow progression of the disease through late childhood. Pearson et al. (1967) described 3 affected sibs out of 8. The mother, although clinically normal, had minor histologic alterations of skeletal muscle. Narrow, highly arched palate is a feature of all these cases, as it sometimes is in myotonic dystrophy with childhood onset of manifestations. In each of three brothers with this condition, Danowski et al. (1973) found a distinct beta globulin peak upon serum protein electrophoresis. This sharp beta peak was caused by an increase in the C3 component of serum complement. Both parents were normal. The report of Gonatas et al. (1966) concerned two brothers who had normal parents but were related to the cases of Spiro and Kennedy (1965), their father being a brother to the mother of the Spiro-Kennedy report. This disorder is probably autosomal dominant with rather wide variability in severity. Price et al. (1965) studied two Negro sisters.

Danowski, T. S., Fisher, E. R., Wald, N., Wester, J. W. and Zawadzki, Z. A.: Rod myopathy: beta globulin peak and increased complement. Metabolism 22: 597-604, 1973.

Engel, W. K., Wanko, T. and Fenichel, G. M.: Nemaline myopathy. A second case. Arch. Neurol. 11: 22-39, 1964.

Ford, F. R.: Diseases of the Nervous System in Infancy, Childhood and Adolescence. Springfield, Ill.: Charles C Thomas, 1961. (4th Ed.) Pp. 1259-1260.

Gibson, A.: Muscular infantilism. Arch. Intern. Med. 27: 338 only, 1921.

Gonatas, N. K., Shy, G. M. and Godfrey, E. H.: Nemaline myopathy. The origin of nemaline structures. New Eng. J. Med. 274: 535-539, 1966.

Hopkins, I. J., Lindsey, J. R. and Ford, F. R.: Nemaline myopathy. A long-term clinicopathologic study of affected mother and daughter. Brain 89: 299-310, 1966.

Pearson, C. M., Coleman, R. F., Fowler, W. M., Jr., Mommaerts, W. F. H. M., Munsat, T. L. and Peter, J. B.: Skeletal muscle. Basic And Clinical Aspects And Illustrative New Diseases. Ann. Intern. Med. 67: 614-650, 1967.

Price, H. M., Gordon, G. B., Pearson, C. M., Munsat, T. L. and Blumberg, J. M.: New evidence for excessive accumulation of Z-band material in nemaline myopathy. Proc. Natl. Acad. Sci. 54: 1398-1406, 1965.

Shy, G. M.: Central core disease and nemaline myopathy. In, Stanbury, J. B., Wyngaarden, J. B. and Fredrickson, D. S. (eds.): The Metabolic Basis of Inherited Disease. New York: McGraw-Hill, 1966 (2nd Ed.) Pp. 952-962.

Shy, G. M., Engel, W. K., Somers, J. E. and Wanko, T.: Nemaline myopathy. A new congenital myopathy. Brain 86: 793-810, 1963.

Spiro, A. J. and Kennedy, C.: Hereditary occurrence of nemaline myopathy. Arch. Neurol. 13: 155-159, 1965.

16190 NEPHRITIS, FAMILIAL, WITHOUT DEAFNESS OR OCULAR DEFECT

Ben-Ishay, Biran and Ullman (1967) described a Jewish-Kurdish family with many cases of nephritis in four generations. Differences from Alport syndrome included rarity of gross hematuria, proteinuria being the presenting manifestation, and absence of deafness. The family of Goldman and Haberfelde (1959) may be of the same type. Perkoff (1967) gave a general review of hereditary renal disease. Walker (1974) tells me of families which may represent the same disorder. The same disorder may have been present in the family of Teisberg et al. (1973). Serum from their patients was able to break down the third component of complement in vitro. Furthermore, evidence of in vivo inactivation was described. The authors concluded that the underlying mechanism is an inherited defect in immunologic response. A dominant nephritis without associated features has been observed in unrelated females by Walker (1974) and by Spector (1974).

Ben-Ishay, D., Biran, S. and Ullmann, T. D.: Familial nephritis. Israel J. Med. Sci. 3: 106-112, 1967.

Goldman, R. and Haberfelde, G. C.: Hereditary nephritis: report of a kindred. N. Engl. J. Med. 261: 734-738, 1959.

Perkoff, G. T.: The hereditary renal diseases. N. Engl. J. Med. 277: 79-85, and 129-138, 1967.

Spector, D. A.: Baltimore, personal communication, 1974.

Teisberg, P., Grottum, K. A., Myhre, E. and Flatmark, A.: In-vivo activation of complement in hereditary nephropathy. Lancet II: 356-358, 1973.

Walker, W. G.: Baltimore, Md., personal communication, 1974.

16200 NEPHROPATHY, FAMILIAL, WITH GOUT

Rosenbloom et al. (1967) described a family in which multiple males in three generations died from renal failure at a relatively early age. All had hyperuricemia early in the course and gout. No distinctive histologic findings were yielded by renal biopsy. Transmission from father to son excluded X-linked inheritance. See McKusick (1974) for pedigree of the family of Rosenbloom et al. (1967). A family observed by Leumann (1972) may have the same disorder (in a mother and two daughters). The urine was entirely normal but the uric acid was elevated, the mother had onset of gout at age 18 years, glomerular filtration rate was reduced and biopsy showed interstitial nephropathy. The erythrocyte-sedimentation rate was elevated in all three.

Leumann, E.: Zurich, Switzerland: personal communication, 1972.

McKusick, V. A.: Familial nephropathy with gout. In, Bergsma, D. (ed.): Clinical Delineation of Birth Defects. XVI. Urinary System and Others. Baltimore: Williams and Wilkins, 1974. Pp. 178-179.

Rosenbloom, F. M., Kelley, W. N., Carr, A. A. and Seegmiller, J. E.: Familial nephropathy and gout in a kindred. (Abstract) Clin. Res. 15: 270 only, 1967.

*16210 NEURITIS WITH BRACHIAL PREDILECTION

The disorder described by Jacob, Andermann and Robb (1961) is manifested by recurring brachial neuritis or mononeuritis multiplex. The legs are involved only in instances of severe arm involvement. They observed 14 similar episodes in 7 patients in two unrelated families. Attacks were featured by incapacitating pain, weakness, wasting, depression of reflexes, and sensory loss. Narrow face with close-set eyes was a feature. Taylor (1960) studied a family in which five generations were affected by single or recurrent attacks of mononeuritis with a particular predilection for proximal brachial localization. The trait behaved as an autosomal dominant one with high penetrance. Clinically, the picture closely resembled serum neuritis, suggesting that the fundamental defect might be- a genetic susceptibility to 'hyperergic reactions.'

Geiger, L. R., Mancall, E. L., Penn, A. S. and Tucker, S. H.: Familial neuralgic amyotrophy. Report of three families with review of the literature. Brain 97: 87-102, 1974.

Jacob, J. C., Andermann, F. and Robb, J. P.: Heredofamilial neuritis with brachial predilection. Neurology 11: 1025-1033, 1961.

Smith, B. H., Ramakrishna, T. and Schlagenhauff, R. R.: Familial branchial neuropathy: two case reports with discussion. Neurology 21: 941-945, 1971.

Taylor, R. A.: Heredofamilial mononeuritis multiplex with brachial predilection. Brain 83: 113-137, 1960.

*16220 NEUROFIBROMATOSIS

The only consistent features are cafe-au-lait spots and fibromatous skin tumors. Tumors of nerve trunks are likely to be palpable. Other occasional features included pendulous tumors, scoliosis, pseudoarthrosis of the tibia, pheochromocytoma, meningioma, glioma, acoustic neuroma, optic neuroma, mental retardation, hypertension, hypoglycemia. Hayes and colleagues (1961) reported hypoglycemia associated with massive intraperitoneal tumor of mesodermal origin in a patient with typical cutaneous lesions. Gastrointestinal bleeding is another manifestation. Fibromas may occur in the iris and glaucoma occurs in rare instances (Grant and Walton, 1968). Unusual clinical manifestations were described by Diekmann et al. (1967); hypertension due to renal artery stenosis, hypertrophy of the clitoris. Benedict et al. (1968) studied the pigmentary anomaly of neurofibromatosis in relation to that of Albright polyostotic fibrous dysplasia. Gross appearance of the pigmented areas was not always reliable. However special microscopic studies showed giant pigment granules in Malpighian cells or melanocyte of normal skin and of neurofibromatosis spots but rarely in Albright syndrome. Nicolls (1969) described two cases of sectorial neurofibromatosis which he plausibly interpreted as representing somatic mutation. One had a mediastinal neurofibroma and in the skin area corresponding segmentally to the site of the internal lesion five small neurofibromas. Involvement of the heart in neurofibromatosis was described and reviewed by Rosenquist et al. (1970) who also reviewed involvement of renal and other arteries, abdominal aorta and carotid artery. Crowe et al. (1956) suggested that the presence of six spots each more than 1.5 cm. in diameter is necessary for the diagnosis. Crowe (1964) suggested axillary freckling as an especially useful diagnostic clue. See ACOUSTIC NEUROMA for a discussion of 'central neurofibromatosis,' a probably separate entity. The patients described by Hashemian (1953) apparently had Recklinghausen neurofibromatosis, although the skin changes were not as striking as in some patients. We have observed very similar intestinal tumors in a patient (G. R., 368525) with striking skin changes of neurofibromatosis. Johnson and Charneco (1970) suggested that the cafe-au-lait spot of neurofibromatosis can be distinguished from the innocent spot which occurs in normal persons and from the pigmented areas of Albright disease by the presence of a large number of DOPA-positive melanocytes which have giant pigment granules in the cytoplasm. Fialkow et al. (1971) concluded from analysis of neurofibromas from G6PD A-B heterozygotes with von Recklinghausen disease that each tumor must originate in many cells, perhaps at least 150. Neurofibromatosis is associated with a tendency to malignant degeneration of the neurofibromas in an estimated 3% to 15% of cases. Knight et al. (1973), reviewed 69 patients with single and 45 patients with multiple neurofibromas were reviewed. Five patients in the group were found to have a total of 11 secondary malignant lesions including 3 fibrosarcomas, 3 squamous cell carcinomas and one neurofibrosarcoma among other forms. Some earlier studies have reported mainly sarcomas associated with neurofibromatosis. D'Agostino et al. (1963) discovered 21 cases of secondary neoplasms in his study of 678 cases of neurofibromatosis. Crowe et al. (1956) discovered 6 secondary malignant lesions in 168 patients with neurofibromatosis. Schenkein et al. (1974) reported increased nerve growth stimulating activity in the serum of patients with von Recklinghausen disease.

Benedict, P. H., Szabo, G., Fitzpatrick, T. B. and Sinesi, S. J.: Melanotic macules in Albright's syndrome and in neurofibromatosis. J.A.M.A. 205: 618-626, 1968.

Boudin, G., Pepin, B. and Vernant, C.: Les tumeurs multiples du systeme nerveux au cours de la maladie

Buntin, P. T. and Fitzgerald, J. F.: Gastrointestinal neurofibromatosis: a rare cause of chronic anemia. Am. J. Dis. Child. 119: 521-523, 1970.

Charron, J. W. and Gariepy, G.: Neurofibromatosis of bladder: case report and review of the literature. Canad. J. Surg. 13: 303-306, 1970.

Crowe, F. W., Schull, W. J. and Neel, J. V.: A Clinical, Pathological and Genetic Study of Multiple Neurofibromatosis. Springfield, Ill.: Charles C Thomas, 1956.

Crowe, F. W.: Axillary freckling as a diagnostic aid in neurofibromatosis. Ann. Intern. Med. 61: 1142-1143, 1964.

D'Agostino, A. N., Soule, E. H. and Miller, R. H.: Sarcomas of the peripheral nerves and somatic soft tissue associated with multiple neurofibromatosis. Cancer 16: 1015-1027, 1963.

Diekmann, L., Huther, W. and Pfeiffer, R. A.: Ungewoehnliche Erscheinungsformen der Neurofibromatose (von Recklinghausensche Krankheit) im Kindesalter. Z. Kinderheilk. 101: 191-222, 1967.

Fialkow, P. J., Sagebiel, R. W., Gartler, S. M. and Rimoin, D. L.: Multiple cell origin of hereditary neurofibromas. New Eng. J. Med. 284: 298-300, 1971.

Fienman, N. L. and Yakovac, W. C.: Neurofibromatosis in childhood. J. Pediatr. 76: 339-346, 1970.

Grant, W. M. and Walton, D. S.: Distinctive gonioscopic findings in glaucoma due to neurofibromatosis. Arch. Ophthalmol. 79: 127-134, 1968.

Hashemian, H.: Familial fibromatosis of small intestine. Br. J. Surg. 40: 346-350, 1953.

Hayes, D. M., Spurr, C. L., Felts, J. H. and Miller, E. C., Jr.: Von Recklinghausen's disease with massive intra-abdominal tumor and spontaneous hypoglycemia: metabolic studies before and after perfusion of abdominal cavity with nitrogen mustard. Metabolism 10: 183-199, 1961.

Izumi, A. K., Rosato, F. E. and Wood, M. G.: Von Recklinghausen's disease associated with multiple neurolemomas. Arch. Dermatol. 104: 172-176, 1971.

Johnson, B. L. and Charneco, D. R.: Cafe-au-lait spot in neurofibromatosis and in normal individuals. Arch. Dermatol. 102: 442-446, 1970.

Knight, W. A., Murphy, W. K. and Gottlieb, J. A.: Neurofibromatosis associated with malignant neurofibromas. Arch. Dermatol. 107: 747-750, 1973.

Miles, J., Pennybacker, J. and Sheldon, P.: Intrathoracic meningocele. Its development and association with neurofibromatosis. J. Neurol. Neurosurg. Psychiatry 32: 99-110, 1969.

Nager, G. T.: Association of bilateral VIIIth nerve tumors with meningiomas in von Recklinghausen's disease. Laryngoscope 74: 1220-1261, 1964.

Newman, A. and So, S. K.: Bilateral neurofibroma of the intrathoracic vagus associated with von Recklinghausen's disease. Am. J. Roentgen. 112: 389-392, 1971.

Nicolls, E. M.: Somatic variation and multiple neurofibromatosis. Hum. Hered. 19: 473-479, 1969.

Philippart, M.: Neurofibromatose hereditaire a large spectre phenotypique (famille SN). J. Genet. Hum. 10: 338-346, 1961.

Rosenquist, G. C., Krovetz, L. J., Haller, J. A., Jr., Simon, A. L. and Bannayan, G. A.: Acquired right ventricular outflow obstruction in a child with neurofibromatosis. Am. Heart J. 79: 103-108, 1970.

Schenkein, I., Bueker, E. D., Helson, L., Axelrod, F. and Dancis, J.: Increased nerve-growth stimulating activity in disseminated neurofibromatosis. N. Engl. J. Med. 290: 613-614, 1974.

Smith, C. J., Hatch, F. E., Johnson, J. G. and Kelly, B. J.: Renal artery dysplasia as a cause of hypertension in neurofibromatosis. Arch. Intern. Med. 125: 1022-1026, 1970.

Taylor, P. E.: Encapsulated glioma of the sylvian fissure associated with neurofibromatosis. Report of a case with histopathological comparison of surgical lesion and autopsy specimen following recurrence. J. Neuropath. Exp. Neurol. 21: 566-578, 1962.

*16230 NEUROMATA, MUCOSAL, WITH ENDOCRINE TUMORS

Williams and Pollock (1966) described two unrelated patients with multiple true neuromas, pheochromocytoma and thyroid carcinoma. The thyroid cancer was of the medullary type as in the PTC syndrome (q.v.). Indeed the relationship of these is unclear. Although the association of pheochromocytoma with neurofibromatosis is well known, the nervous tumor is a true neuroma, i.e., consists mainly of nerve cells, in this condition. They are not associated with cafe-au-lait spots. They occur as pedunculated nodules on the eyelid margins, lips and tongue. The lips are diffusely hypertrophied with a 'Negroid' appearance. Neuromas occur also in the tongue. The father of one of Williams and Pollock's cases had very thick lips and eyelid and tongue lesions like his daughters. He had a medullary thyroid cancer and had died at age 38 after an abdominal operation, having had symptoms suggestive of pheochromocytoma. Schimke et al. (1968) reported cases also. Cunliffe et al. (1968) demonstrated calcitonin-secretion in a medullary carcinoma of the thyroid. The patient was a 19-year-old girl with acne, features of Marfan syndrome, neuromas of tongue and eyelid, prominent lips, nodular goiter, pigmentation of hands, feet and circumoral area, proximal myopathy, loose motions, and flushing attacks. (The first patient with this syndrome I saw was referred to me as possible Marfan syndrome.) The features suggesting Marfan syndrome were high arched palate, pectus excavatum, bilateral pes cavus, high patella and scoliosis. Marfanoid habitus and pes cavus are striking features in most. Megacolon or colonic diverticula also occur. Mucosal neuromas involve the lips, anterior tongue, conjunctiva and nasal and laryngeal mucosa. Medullated nerve fibers traverse the cornea. Bartlett et al. (1968) described affected persons in 6 generations. Prophylactic thyroidectomy has been performed in some persons at risks (Wolfe et al., 1973). In addition to histaminase, DOPA decarboxylase is high in medullary carcinoma of the thyroid (Atkins et al., 1973). The latter enzyme is found in pheochromocytomas also.

Atkins, F. L., Beaven, M. A. and Keiser, H. R.: DOPA decarboxylase in medullary carcinoma of the thyroid. N. Engl. J. Med. 289: 545-548, 1973.

Bartlett, R. C., Bean, L. R. and Mandelstam, P.: Hereditary study of neuroendocrine dysplasia in six generations. Int. Assoc. Dent. Res. (San Francisco, March 21-24), 1968. P. 36.

Baum, J. L. and Adler, M. E.: Pheochromocytoma, medullary thyroid carcinoma, multiple mucosal neuroma. A variant of the syndrome. Arch. Ophthalmol. 87: 574-584, 1972.

Baylin, S. B., Beaven, M. A., Engelman, K. and Sjoersdma, A.: Elevated histaminase activity in medullary carcinoma of the thyroid gland. N. Engl. J. Med. 283: 1239-1244, 1970.

Braley, A. E.: Medullated corneal nerves and plexiform neuroma associated with pheochromocytoma. Trans. Am. Ophthal. Soc. 52: 189-197, 1954.

Cunliffe, W. J., Black, M. M., Hall, R., Johnston, I. D. A., Hudgson, P., Shuster, S., Gudmundsson, T. V., Joplin, G. F., Williams, E. D., Woodhouse, N. J. Y., Galante, L. and MacIntyre, I.: A calcitonin-secreting thyroid carcinoma. Lancet II: 63-66, 1968.

Gorlin, R. J. and Mirkin, B. L.: Multiple mucosal neuromas, pheochromocytoma, medullary carcinoma of the thyroid and marfanoid body build with muscle wasting. Syndrome of hyperplasia and neoplasia of neural crest derivatives. A unitarian concept. Z. Kinderheilk. 113: 313-321, 1972.

Gorlin, R. J., Sedano, H. O., Vickers, R. A. and Cervenka, J.: Multiple mucosal neuromas, pheochromocytoma and medullary carcinoma of the thyroid — a syndrome. Cancer 22: 293-299, 1968.

Schimke, R. N., Hartmann, W. H., Prout, T. E. and Rimoin, D. L.: Pheochromocytoma, medullary thyroid carcinoma and multiple neuromas. N. Engl. J. Med. 279: 1-7, 1968.

Williams, E. D. and Pollock, D. J.: Multiple mucosal neuromata with endocrine tumours: a syndrome allied to von Recklinghausen's disease. J. Pathol. Bact. 91: 71-80, 1966.

Wolfe, H. J., Melvin, K. E. W., Cervi-Skinner, S. J., Al-Saadi, A. A., Juliar, J. F., Jackson, C. E. and Tashjian, A. H., Jr.: C-cell hyperplasia preceding medullary thyroid carcinoma. N. Engl. J. Med. 289: 437-441, 1973.

*16235 NEURONAL CEROID-LIPOFUSCINOSIS, DOMINANT OR PARRY TYPE

The strikingly consistent clinical picture has onset about 31 years and presents as a cerebellar syndrome. Major fits, myoclonic jerks, and progressive dementia are other features. The affected persons have hypertension. Boehme et al. (1971) reported 11 cases in 4 generations of a family named Parry from the southern part of New Jersey. Zeman and Dyken (1969) abandoned the age-dependent classification of 'amaurotic familial idiocies' and divided them into the gangliosidoses and the neuronal ceroid-lipofuscinoses. The latter group, of which the biochemical lesions remain obscure, includes amaurotic idiocy, late infantile type (20450), amaurotic idiocy, juvenile type (20420) and amaurotic idiocy, adult type (20430). All of these are recessive. The disorder in the Parry kindred was clearly dominant. Several similar reported families were found but none which could be confidently said to be identical.

Boehme, D. H., Cottrell, J. C., Leonberg, S. C. and Zeman, W.: A dominant form of neuronal ceroid-lipofuscinosis. Brain 94: 745-760, 1971.

Zeman, W. and Dyken, P.: Neuronal ceriod-lipofuscinosis (Batten's disease). Relationship to amaurotic familial idiocy? Pediatrics 44: 570-583, 1969.

*16237 NEUROPATHY, CONGENITAL, WITH ARTHROGRYPOSIS MULTIPLEX

Yuill and Lynch (1974) described this disorder in three males of successive generations and the sister of the youngest male. The syndrome was present at birth and showed little progression. Three of the patients had arthrogryposis multiplex. This disorder could be confused with a congenital myopathy.

Yuill, G. M. and Lynch, P. G.: Congenital non-progressive peripheral neuropathy with arthrogryposis multiplex. J. Neurol. Neurosurg. Psychiatry 37: 316-323, 1974.

*16240 NEUROPATHY, HEREDITARY SENSORY RADICULAR

Mandell and Smith (1960) described a case. The manifestations were Charcot-type arthropathy, recurrent ulceration of the lower extremities and signs of radicular sensory deficiency in both the upper and the lower extremities, without any motor dysfunction.

Hicks (1922) described a family in which ten members suffered from perforating ulcers of the feet and shooting pains about the body, and deafness. The first symptoms appeared between 15 to 36 years of age. First to appear was a corn on a big toe, followed by a painless ulcer with bony debris. Other toes then became involved. Shooting pains then appeared, similar to the lightning pains of tabes dorsalis. At about the same time the patient begins to suffer from bilateral deafness, progressing to total deafness over several years. Neurological examination shows disappearance of ankle, then knee jerks. Cranial nerves are normal with the exception of the auditory nerve. An extensor plantar response is never obtained, the pupils react normally, and there is no nystagmus. Sensation of the arms is normal. There is loss of pain, touch, heat and cold over the feet. The pathology is completely unknown. Though others have reported hereditary perforating ulcers of the feet (q.v.) there is no mention of deafness or shooting pains.

Denny-Brown (1951) reported the clinical and autopsy findings of a 53-year-old woman, a member of the family reported by Hicks (1922). At the age of 22 an ulcer formed on her right great toe requiring a year to heal. Since then she suffered from recurrent ulceration, each lasting six to nine months, sometimes extending to bone. In her early twenties she first noticed shooting pains in her legs, sometimes in her arms. Deafness began at the age of 40 years and progressed to almost total deafness by 53 years of age. Neurological examination 53 years of age showed loss of all sensation in the lower legs with loss of pain and temperature sensation in the thighs and hands. Autopsy showed a small brain. The most severe changes were a marked loss of ganglion cells in the sacral and lumbar dorsal root ganglia. There were less severe changes in C-8 and T-1 ganglia. The remaining ganglion cells showed great proliferation of subcapsular dendrites. Clear hyalin bodies were seen in the involved ganglia representing possibly an amyloid mass around capillaries. No mention was made of the temporal bones.

Heller and Robb (1955) described a French-Canadian family in which five had full-blown disease and three had an incomplete form. Although dominant inheritance was proposed for this family also, recessive inheritance seems equally or more likely. No amyloid was found on dorsal root ganglion biopsy. These authors suggested that Morvan disease was the same as this. Most of Morvan's cases (1883-1889) came from Brittany. Many of the features suggest acro-osteolysis (recessive catalog). Mandell and Smith (1960) observed sensory radicular neuropathy in grandfather, father and male proband.

Dyck, Kennel, Magal and Kraybill (1965) described a family in which the presence of peroneal muscular atrophy and pes cavus suggested Charcot-Marie-Tooth disease. Biopsy of the skin from the pad of the great toe of affected persons using the cholinesterase technique showed normal numbers of Meissner corpuscles in a 14-year-old boy with early signs suggestive of the disorder but no corpuscles in a 37-year-old man and a 28-year-old woman with well-developed disease. The authors commented on the similarities between four entities — this one and those which carry the eponyms Charcot-Marie-Tooth, Roussy-Levy and Dejerine-Sottas.

Campbell and Hoffman (1964) reported two families. DeLeon (1969) described a case which like theirs had amyotrophy. This may, therefore, be a separate entity. Congenital sensory neuropathy resulting in insensitivity to pain seemed to be dominant in the family reported by Ervin and Sternbach (1960) and that of Silverman and Gilden (1959). Wallace (1968) studied an extensively affected Australian kindred.

Campbell, A. M. G. and Hoffman, H. L.: Sensory radicular neuropathy associated with muscle wasting in two cases. Brain 87: 67-74, 1964.

Clarke, J. M. and Groves, E. W. H.: Remarks on syringomyelia (sacro-lumbar type) occurring in a brother and sister. Br. Med. J. 2: 737-740, 1909.

DeLeon, G. A.: Progressive ventral sensory loss in sensory radicular neuropathy and hypertrophic neuritis. Johns Hopkins Med. J. 125: 53-61, 1969.

Denny-Brown, D.: Hereditary sensory radicular neuropathy. J. Neurol. Neurosurg. Psychiatry 14: 237-252, 1951.

Dyck, P. J., Kennel, A. J., Magal, I. V. and Kraybill, E. N.: A Virginia kinship with hereditary sensory neuropathy: peroneal muscular atrophy and pes cavus. Mayo Clin. Proc. 40: 685-694, 1965.

Ervin, F. R. and Sternbach, R. A.: Hereditary insensitivity to pain. Trans. Am. Neurol. Assoc. 86: 70-74, 1960.

Heller, I. H. and Robb, P.: Hereditary sensory neuropathy. Neurology 5: 15-29, 1955.

Hicks, E. P. and Camp, M. B.: Hereditary perforating ulcer of the foot. Lancet I: 319-321, 1922.

Mandell, A. J. and Smith, C. K.: Hereditary sensory radicular neuropathy. Neurology 10: 627-630, 1960.

Ogryzlo, M. A.: A familial peripheral neuropathy of unknown etiology resembling Morvan's disease. Canad. Med. Assoc. J. 54: 547-553, 1946.

Schultze, F.: Familiaer auftretendes malum perforans der Fuesse (familiaere lumbale Syringomyelie). Deutsch. Med. Wschr. 43: 545-547, 1917.

Silverman, F. N. and Gilden, J. J.: Congenital insensitivity to pain, a neurologic syndrome with bizarre skeletal lesions. Radiology 72: 176-190, 1959.

Smith, E. M.: Familial neurotrophic osseous atrophy. A familial neurotrophic condition of the feet with anesthesia and loss of bone. J.A.M.A. 102: 593-595, 1934.

Tocantins, L. M., and Reimann, H. A.: Perforating ulcers of feet, with osseous atrophy in family with other evidences of dysgenesis (hare lip, cleft palate): an instance of probable myelodysplasia. J.A.M.A. 112: 2251-2255, 1939.

Wallace, D. C.: A Study of an Hereditary Neuropathy. U. of Sydney M.D. Thesis, 1968.

*16250 NEUROPATHY, HEREDITARY, WITH LIABILITY TO PRESSURE PALSIES

This disorder seems to be distinct from neuritis with brachial predilection (q.v.). Families were reported by Davies (1954) and by Earl and colleagues (1964). The latter group found that motor nerve conduction velocity was reduced in some clinically normal family members. Staal, De Weerdt, and Went (1965) studied a family in which members in 4 generations showed transient unilateral peroneal palsies. The neuropathy manifested itself especially after prolonged work in a kneeling position. The family, living in Holland, knew the disease as 'bulb diggers' palsy. Other nerve palsies, such as ulna, occur as well (Davies, 1954). Females are less severely affected. The relationship to neuritis with brachial predilection is unclear. Guillozet and Mercer (1973) described 4 cases of recurrent brachial neuropathy in 3 generations of a family. These patients showed recurrent attacks of pain, weakness and sometimes muscle-wasting in the arms and hands. These attacks generally were known to gradually remit, sometimes leaving residual weakness or muscular atrophy. The brachial plexus is primarily involved in this condition. However the lower cranial nerves and the sympathetic nervous system may also be affected.

Behse, F., Buchthal, F., Carlsen, F. and Knapplis, G. G.: Hereditary neuropathy with liability to pressure palsies: electrophysiological and histopathological aspects. Brain 95: 777-794, 1972.

Davies, D. M.: Recurrent peripheral-nerve palsies in a family. Lancet II: 266-268, 1954.

Earl, C. J., Fullerton, P. M., Wakefield, G. S. and Schretta, H. S.: Hereditary neuropathy, with liability to pressure palsies: a clinical and electrophysiological study of four families. Quart. J. Med. 33: 481-498, 1964.

Guillozet, N. and Mercer, R. D.: Hereditary recurrent brachial neuropahty. Am. J. Dis. Child. 125: 884-887, 1973.

Staal, A., De Weerdt, C. J. and Went, L. N.: Hereditary compression syndrome of peripheral nerves. Neurology 15: 1008-1017, 1965.

16260 NEUROPATHY, WITH PARAPROTEIN IN SERUM, CEREBROSPINAL FLUID AND URINE

Gibberd and Gavrilescu (1966) described a family in which four persons in three generations had a progressive hypertrophic polyneuritis associated with an abnormal protein in serum, cerebrospinal fluid and urine. Motor and sensory changes began at about age 50 years. Nerve conduction velocity was delayed. Sural nerve on biopsy showed marked demyelination with Schwann cell proliferation. The total spinal fluid protein was only slightly increased.

Gibberd, F. B. and Gavrilescu, K.: A familial neuropathy associated with a paraprotein in the serum, cerebrospinal fluid and urine. Neurology 16: 130-134, 1966.

*16270 NEUTROPENIA, CHRONIC FAMILIAL

Levine (1959) described an affected 14 and one-half-year-old-boy who also showed hyperplastic gingivitis. The father and two sibs also had chronic neutropenia. Clubbing of the fingers and hyperglobulinemia were other features. Although recessive forms of congenital neutropenia have been more frequently described, the family described by Hitzig (1959) suggests dominant inheritance of one form. The father, age 36, a son age 8 and a daughter age 4 were affected. The blood and marrow findings were similar to those in the recessive form described by Kostermann. However, severe infections were not a feature. Cutting and Lang (1964) observed 9 cases of benign chronic neutropenia in 3 generations of a family. The neutropenia was constant.

Cutting, H. O. and Lang, J. E., Jr.: Familial benign chronic neutropenia. Ann. Intern. Med. 61: 876-887, 1964.

Hitzig, W. H.: Familiaere Neutropenie mit dominantem Erbgang und Hypergammaglobulinamie. Helv. Med. Acta 26: 779-784, 1959.

Levine, S.: Chronic familial neutropenia, with marked periodontal lesions. Report of a case. Oral Surg. 12: 310-314, 1959.

16280 NEUTROPENIA, CYCLIC

Hahneman and Alt (1958) described a 29-year-old man who from an early age had neutropenia recurring every 21 days and accompanied by infection. Complete remission occurred at age 18 years. The man's daughter was seen at the age of 2 years with similar periodic disease recurring each 14 days. Torrioli-Riggio (1958) also reported cases. Morley et al. (1967) described 20 cases in 5 families. Clinical manifestations usually began in childhood and improved thereafter. The commonest are fever, oral ulcerations and skin infections. Neutropenia occurs at intervals of 15-35 days. It is often accompanied by monocytosis and sometimes by anemia, eosinophilia or thrombocytopenia. Male-to-male transmission occurred. Cyclic neutropenia in the collie dog is accompanied by gray fur, leads to early death from pyogenic infections and is an autosomal recessive (Dale et al., 1970). Weiden et al. (1974) showed by transplantation of grey collie bone marrow into normal dogs which had been irradiated that the basic defect is in the stem cell. There are sufficient similarities between the canine and human disease (Guerry et al., 1972) to suggest that the same may be true in man. Weiden et al. (1974) showed by transplantation of grey collie bone marrow into normal dogs which had been irradiated that the basic defect is in the stem cell. There are sufficient similarities between the canine and human disease (Guerry et al., 1972) to suggest that the same may be true in man.

Dale, D. C., Alling, D. W. and Wolff, S. M.: Cyclic hematopoiesis: the mechanism of cyclic neutropenia in grey collie dogs. J. Clin. Invest. 51: 2197-2204, 1972.

Dale, D. C., Ward, S. B., Kimball, H. R. and Wolff, S. M.: Studies of neutrophil production and turnover in grey collie dogs with cyclic neutropenia. J. Clin. Invest. 51: 2190-2196, 1972.

Dale, D. C., Kimball, H. R. and Wolff, S. M.: Studies of cyclic neutropenia in gray collie dogs. (Abstract) Clin. Res. 18: 402 only, 1970.

Guerry, D. D., Dale, D. C., Omine, M., Perry, S. and Wolff, S. M.: Studies on the mechanism of human cyclic neutropenia. (Abstract) Br. J. Haematol. 40: 951 only, 1972.

Meuret, G. and Fliedner, T. M.: Zellkinetik der Granulopoiese und des Neutrophilensystems bei einem Fall von zyklischer Neutropenie. Acta Haematol. 43: 48-63, 1970.

Morley, A. A., Carew, J. P. and Baikie, A. G.: Familial cyclical neutropenia. Br. J. Haematol. 13: 719-738, 1967.

Page, A. R. and Good, R. A.: Studies on cyclic neutropenia. A clinical and experimental investigation. Am. J. Dis. Child. 94: 623-661, 1957.

Torrioli-Riggio, G.: Considerazioni su una famiglia di granulopenici. Acta Genet. Med. Gemellol. 7: 237-248, 1958.

Weiden, P. L., Robinett, B., Graham, T. C., Adamson, J. and Storb, R.: Canine cyclic neutropenia. A stem cell defect. J. Clin. Invest. 53: 950-953, 1974.

16282 NEUTROPHIL CHEMOTACTIC DEFECT

In three children with congenital ichthyosis and recurrent infections with Trichophyton rubrum, Miller et al. (1973) identified an abnormality of neutrophil movement. Numbers, morphology, and phagocytic and bacteriocidal activities were normal. Although random mobility was normal, chemotaxis of leukocytes from the patients and their fathers was deficient. (In the 'lazy leukcoyte syndrome' (24585) random movement is also defective.) A girl in one family and a brother and sister in a second were affected. In each family the father showed the same defect of neutrophil movement. The father of the two affected sibs had been plagued by recurrent Trichophyton rubrum infections but did not have ichthyosis.

Miller, M. E., Norman, M. E., Koblenzer, P. J. and Schonauer, T.: A new familial defect of neutrophil movement. J. Lab. Clin. Med. 82: 1-8, 1973.

16283 NEUTROPHILIA, HEREDITARY

Herring et al. (1974) described an apparently autosomal dominant form of lifelong persistent neutrophilia in a mother and three of her four children. The neutrophiles were morphologically and functionally normal. Associated findings were hepatosplenomegaly, histiocytes of Gaucher type, and thickened calcavia due to widened diploe. Leukocyte alkaline phosphatase, serum vitamin B12 levels and heat-labile serum alkaline phosphatase were elevated. The course was benign. No previous report was found. This disorder differs from the familial myeloproliferative syndrome (25470) by the mode of inheritance and benign course. It is also distinct from hereditary eosinophilia (13140).

Herring, W. B., Smith, L. G., Walker, R. I. and Herion, J. C.: Neutrophilia. Am. J. Med. 56: 729-734, 1974.

*16285 NEUTROPHIL-SPECIFIC ANTIGEN: NA LOCUS

Neutrophil antigens have been identified in the course of study of isoimmune neonatal neutropenia due to feto-maternal incompatibility. (Since it occurs in multiple sibs, neonatal neutropenia might simulate a recessive disorder.) Two loci, termed NA and NB, have been identified (Lalezari and Radel, 1974). Two alleles at each locus are known. These are known as NA1 and NA2, NB1 and NB2.

Lalezari, P. and Radel, E.: Neutrophil-specific antigens immunology and clinical significance. Seminars Hematol. 11: 281-290, 1974.

*16286 NEUTROPHIL-SPECIFIC ANTIGEN: NB LOCUS

See 16285.

*16290 NEVI (PIGMENTED MOLES)

Although it is a common observation that nevi occur in families, probably with dominant transmission, the study by Denaro (1944) is one of the few which has examined the matter specifically. Multiple pigmented moles are a feature of one chromosomal aberration, the Turner syndrome, as pointed out by Sharpey-Schafer (1941). Estabrook (1928) reported affected persons in 5 generations of a family. (His term nevus spilus comes from the Greek 'spilos' for 'spot.'). Goodman et al. (1971) described three unrelated cases of giant pigmented hairy nevi in which other members of pedigrees exhibited multiple small pigmented nevi. They considered the presence of six such small nevi as indication of the presence of a mutant gene.

Denaro, S. J.: The inheritance of nevi. J. Hered. 35: 215-218, 1944.

Estabrook, A. H.: A family with birthmarks (nevus spilus) for five generations. (Abstract) Eugen. News 13: 90-92, 1928.

Goodman, R. M., Caren, J., Ziprkowski, M., Padeh, B., Ziprkowski, L. and Cohen, B. E.: Genetic considerations in giant pigmented hairy naevus. Br. J. Dermatol. 85: 150-157, 1971.

Meirowski, E.: Moles and malformations of the skin in their relationship to inheritance and phylogenesis (new and old investigations). Br. J. Dermatol. 54: 99-121, 1942.

Sharpey-Schafer, E. P.: Case of pterygo-nuchal infantilism (Turner's syndrome), with post-mortem findings. Lancet II: 559-560, 1941.

*16300 NEVI FLAMMEI, FAMILIAL MULTIPLE

Shelley and Livingood (1949) described 12 cases in 7 sibships in 4 generations of a family, with five instances of male-to-male transmission. Two generations were skipped in one branch of the family. Referred to as birthmarks, these consist of dark red, nonelevated, sharply circumscribed patches which blanch on pressure with a glass, leaving a residual brown hyperpigmentation.

Shelley, W. B. and Livingood, C. S.: Familial multiple nevi flammei. Arch. Dermatol. Syph. 59: 343-345, 1949.

*16310 NEVUS FLAMMEUS OF THE NAPE OF THE NECK

Nevus flammeus nuchae occurs in about 5 percent of persons. Sometimes called port wine stains, these consist of a faint non-elevated red area of variable size and irregular outline on the nape of the neck. An exceedingly extensive pedigree demonstrating dominant inheritance was published by Zumkeller (1957). Sklarz (1955) questioned the significance of genetic factors. However, Shafar and Doig (1955), like Zumkeller (1957) and others, insisted on a genetic basis.

Corson, E. F.: Nevus flammeus nuchae, its occurrence and abnormalities. Am. J. Med. Sci. 187: 121-124, 1934.

Oster, J. and Nielsen, A.: Nuchal naevi and interscapular telangiectases. Incidence in Danish school children. Acta Paediatr. Scand. 59: 416-423, 1970.

Shafar, J. and Doig, A.: The 'nape naevus.' Br. Med. J. 1: 913 only, 1955.

Sklarz, E.: Telangiectatic ('nape') naevi. Br. Med. J. 1: 1221 only, 1955.

Zumkeller, R.: A propos de la frequence et de l'heredite du naevus vasculosus nuchae (unna). Incidence and heredity of nevus vasculosus nuchae unna. J. Genet. Hum. 6: 1-12, 1957.

16320 NEVUS SEBACEUS OF JADASSOHN

Convulsive disorders and multiple developmental abnormalities as well as mental retardation are often associated. Mehregan and Pinkus (1965) pointed out characteristics of the natural history. In the first stage there is alopecia with absent or primitive hair follicles and numerous small hypoplastic sebaceous glands. At puberty the lesions become verrucous with hyperplastic sebaceous glands. In late stages benign or malignant tumors develop. Apparently no familial cases have been observed. The syndrome is included here for heuristic purposes only.

Lantis, S., Leyden, J., Thew, M. and Heaton, C.: Nevus sebaceus of Jadassohn. Arch. Dermatol. 98: 117-123, 1968.

Mehregan, A. H. and Pinkus, H.: Life history of organoid nevi. Arch. Dermatol. 91: 574-588, 1965.

16330 NEVUS SEBACEUS, LINEAR, WITH CONVULSIONS AND MENTAL RETARDATION

Feuerstein and Mims (1962) described 2 unrelated patients with linear nevus sebaceus of the midline of the face associated with epilepsy, focal EEG abnormalities and mental retardation. Nothing is known about a possible genetic basis.

Feuerstein, R. C. and Mims, L. C.: Linear nevus sebaceus with convulsions and mental retardation. Am. J. Dis. Child. 104: 675-679, 1962.

*16340 NIEVERGELT SYNDROME

This disorder is characterized by specific deformities of the radius, ulna, tibia and fibula. Radio-ulnar synostosis and a typical rhomboid shape of the tibia and fibula are observed. Nievergelt (1944) reported an affected man who transmitted the syndrome to three sons, each by a different wife. In a second family 9 persons (2 males and 7 females) in 3 generations were affected. (This may, however, have been a different disorder.) A characteristic rhomboidal shape of the tibia and fibula help differentiate this condition from achondrogenesis (q.v.) and from recessive micromelic dwarfism (q.v.). The X-ray changes, completely specific, are well demonstrated in the sporadic cases reported by Solonen and Sulamaa (1958). The cases called Nievergelt syndrome by Blockey and Lawrie (1963) were in fact instances of mesomelic dwarfism, a recessive (q.v.).

Dubois, H. J.: Nievergelt-Pearlman syndrome: synostosis in feet and hands with dysplasia of elbows. Report of a case. J. Bone Joint Surg. 52B: 325-329, 1970.

Nievergelt, K.: Positiver Vaterschaftsnachweis auf grund erblicher Missbildungen der Extremitaten. Arch. Klaus. Stift. Vererbungsforsch. 19: 157 only, 1944.

Solonen, K. A. and Sulamaa, M.: Nievergelt syndrome and its treatment. A case report. Ann. Chir. Gynaec. Fenn. 47: 142-147, 1958.

*16350 NIGHT BLINDNESS, CONGENITAL STATIONARY (HEMERALOPIA)

The most famous affected family is that descendant for some 11 generations from Jean Nougaret, a butcher from Provence who settled in a small village near Montpellier in the south of France. Florent Cunier, the Belgian ophthalmologist who founded Annales d'oculistique, heard of the family, examined some affected members and stimulated M. Chauvet, a local antiquarian, to assemble the family genealogy. It was Chauvet who showed that Nougaret was the common ancestor of all persons in the district with night blindness. His genealogy listed 629 persons of whom 86 were night blind. Cunier published the findings in 1838. Nettleship followed up on the family in 1907. By this time 135 night-blind persons were known. Vision was unimpaired in daylight, the fundi were normal and general health was excellent. The excess of normal over affected observed in this family among offspring of affected persons may be a matter of incomplete penetrance or incomplete recording of mild cases — a view subscribed to by the geneticist William Bateson who discussed the paper. Attempts at further follow up in 1949 by Dejean et al. indicated that the village inhabited by Nougaret's descendants was no longer an isolate. Francois, Verriest and De Rouck (1965) observed a family with at least four affected in three generations. All were females. See editorial (1970) for an interesting biography of Nettleship.

Carroll, F. and Haig, C.: Congenital stationary night blindness without ophthalmoscopic or other abnormalities. Arch. Ophthalmol. 50: 35-44, 1953.

Cunier, F.: Ann. Ocul. 1: 32, 1838.

Cunier, F.: Annales de la societe de medicin de Gand 4: 385-395, 1838.

Dejean, C. and Gassenc, R.: Note sur la genealogie de la famille Nougaret, de Vendemian. Bull. Soc. Ophthalmol. Fr. 96: 96-100, 1949.

Editorial: Edward Nettleship (1845-1913): Veterinarian-dermatologist-ophthalmologist-geneticist. J.A.M.A. 214: 751-752, 1970.

Francois, J., Verriest, G. and De Rouck, A.: A new pedigree of idiopathic congenital night-blindness: transmitted as a dominant hereditary trait. Am. J. Ophthal. 59: 621-625, 1965.

Nettleship, E.: A history of congenital stationary night-blindness in nine consecutive generations. Trans. Ophthalmol. Soc. U.K. 27: 269-293, 1907.

Snyder, C.: Jean Nougaret, the butcher from Provence, and his family. Arch. Ophthalmol. 69: 676-678, 1963.

*16360 NIPPLES INVERTED (MAMMILLAE INVERTITA)

Romanus (1948) described 7 cases in 5 sibships in 4 generations.

Romanus, T.: A pedigree showing the incidence of malformation of the nipples. Acta Genet. Statist. Med. 1: 168-173, 1948.

16370 NIPPLES, SUPERNUMERARY

Rather extensive literature supporting dominant inheritance was reviewed by Gates (1947). In the guinea pig this trait behaves as an autosomal dominant. Klinkerfuss (1924) found polymastia in 5 females in 4 generations. The extra breast consisted of a mass in one or both axillae which enlarged in pregnancy and lactation. In some but not all a nipple was associated with the adventitious breast tissue. It may have communicated with the main breast tissue because it swelled before nursing and shrunk with nursing. Pierre Marie (1893) also observed supernumerary breasts in four generations and noted an association with twinning.

Fernet, C.: Bull. Soc. Med. Hosp. Paris 10: 457-484, 1893.

Gates, R. R.: Human Genetics. New York: MacMillan, 1947. 2: 843 ff.

Goertzen, B. L. and Ibsen, H. L.: Supernumerary mammae in guinea pigs. J. Hered. 42: 307-311, 1951.

Klinkerfuss, G. H.: Four generations of polymastia. J.A.M.A. 82: 1247-1248, 1924.

*16380 NODAL RHYTHM

Bacos, Eagan and Orgain (1960) presented a family in which 9 members of 3 generations exhibited nodal rhythm with bradycardia and tended to develop paroxysms of atrial fibrillation in the fourth decade of life.

Bacos, J. M., Eagan, J. T. and Orgain, E. S.: Congenital familial nodal rhythm. Circulation 22: 887-895, 1960.

16390 NON-HEME PROTEIN OF ERYTHROCYTE

Hewitt (1963) found in the red cells of Cynomolgus and Rhesus monkeys a non-heme protein which migrates toward the cathode on electrophoresis in starch gel at pH 8.5. Two variant forms, Y and Z, existed, with YY, YZ and ZZ animals in proportions consistent with simple inheritance. Polymorphism of the protein has not been recognized in man.

Hewitt, L. F.: Proteins in the erythrocyte of monkeys. Proc. R. Soc. Biol. 159: 536-543, 1963.

*16395 NOONAN SYNDROME

Baird and De Jong (1972) described seven cases in three generations. One affected woman had five affected children (out of 6) with two different husbands. Seizures and anomalous upper lateral incisors may have been coincidental. Among 95 male patients with pulmonary stenosis, Celermajer et al. (1968) found the Turner phenotype in 8. In 5 of these, karyotyping was performed. In 4 the chromosomes were normal. In one an extra acrocentric chromosome was present. Noonan (1968) reported 19 cases of whom 17 had pulmonary stenosis and 2 had patent ductus arteriosus. Twelve were males and 7 were females. Deformity of the sternum with precocious closures of sutures was a frequent feature. Kaplan et al. (1968) described two brothers with elevated alkaline phosphatase levels and in one of them malignant Schwannoma of the forearm. In 3 families Nora and Sinha (1968) observed mother-to-offspring transmission, through 3 generations in one family. They suggested X-linked dominant inheritance either of a single mutant gene or a submicroscopic deletion. See PTERYGIUM COLLI SYNDROME. Abdel-Salem and Temtamy (1969) reported two affected sibs from a first-cousin marriage. A deceased female sib may have been affected also. They suggested autosomal recessive inheritance. Krieger and Espiritu (1972) described the Turner phenotype in a brother and sister who showed contractures of the hands referred to as arthrogryposis multiplex congenita (which would seem an unnecessarily confusing designation best reserved for cases with evidence of defective joint development or either a neuropathic or a myopathic basis). The parents were apparently normal. Diekmann et al. (1967) described two brothers and a sister, with normal and unrelated parents, who had somatic characteristics of the Noonan syndrome, particularly pterygium colli and deformed sternum, and had myocardopathy leading to death at ages 12 and 10 in two of them. A particularly convincing pedigree for autosomal dominant inheritance was reported by Bolton et al. (1974), who found the condition in a man and 4 sons (in a sibship of 10). Four of the five affected persons had pulmonic stenosis. Father-to-son transmission was reported by Qazi et al. (1974).

Abdel-Salem, E. and Temtamy, S. A.: Familial Turner phenotype. J. Pediatr. 74: 67-72, 1969.

Baird, P. A. and De Jong, B. P.: Noonan's syndrome (XX and XY Turner phenotype) in three generations of a family. J. Pediatr. 80: 110-114, 1972.

Bolton, M. R., Pugh, D. M., Mattioli, L. F., Dunn, M. I. and Schimke, N.: The Noonan syndrome: a family study. Ann. Intern. Med. 80: 626-629, 1974.

Celermajer, J. M., Bowdler, J. D. and Cohen, D. H.: Pulmonary stenosis in patients with the Turner phenotype in the male. Am. J. Dis. Child. 116: 351-358, 1968.

Diekmann, L., Pfeiffer, R. A., Hilgenberg, F., Bender, F. and Reploh, H. D.: Familiare kardiomypathie mit pterygium colli. Munic. Med. Wschr. 109: 2638-2645, 1967.

Kaplan, M. S., Opitz, J. M. and Gosset, F. R.: Noonan's syndrome. A case with elevated serum alkaline phosphatase levels and malignant Schwannoma of the left forearm. Am. J. Dis. Child. 116: 359-366, 1968.

Krieger, I. and Espiritu, C. E.: Arthrogryposis multiplex congenita and the Turner phenotype. Am. J. Dis. Child. 123: 141-144, 1972.

Levy, E. P., Pashayan, H., Fraser, F. C. and Pinsky, L.: XX and XY Turner phenotypes in a family. Am. J. Dis. Child. 120: 36-43, 1970.

Noonan, J. A.: Hypertelorism with Turner phenotype. A new syndrome with assoiciated congenital heart disease. Am. J. Dis. Child. 116: 373-380, 1968.

Nora, J. J. and Sinha, A. K.: Direct familial transmission of the Turner phenotype. Am. J. Dis. Child. 116: 343-350, 1968.

Qazi, Q. H., Arnon, R. G., Paydar, M. H. and Mapa, H. C.: Familial occurrence of Noonan syndrome. Am. J. Dis. Child. 127: 696-698, 1974.

16400 NOSE, ANOMALOUS SHAPE OF ('POTATO NOSE')

Benjamins and Stibbe (1926) described a Dutch family in which 6 males and 8 females in two generations showed a 'potato nose.'

Benjamins, C. E. and Stibbe, F. H.: Een merkwaardig geval van aangeboren afwijking van den uitwendigen neus. (Bigdrage tot de kennis der erfelijkheid van dergelijde afivijkingen). Nederl. T. Geneesk. 70: 2543-2549, 1926.

*16405 NUCLEOSIDE PHOSPHORYLASE

Edwards et al. (1971) described electrophoretic variants of nucleoside phosphorylase, the enzyme which catalyzes the phosphorolytic cleavage of inosine to hypoxanthine. The enzyme appears to be a trimer. Family studies indicated autosomal co-dominant inheritance of the variants. This enzyme is known to be determined by a structural locus on chromosome 14 (Ruddle, 1972), from the findings in cell hybridization studies. See Ricciuti and Ruddle, 1973.

Edwards, Y. H., Hopkinson, D. A. and Harris, H.: Inherited variants of human nucleoside phosphorylase. Ann. Hum. Genet. 34: 395-408, 1971.

Ricciuti, F. and Ruddle, F. H.: Assignment of nucleoside phosphorylase to D-14 and localization of X-linked loci in man by somatic cell genetics. Nature N.B. 241: 180-182, 1973.

Ricciuti, F. and Ruddle, F. H.: Assignment of three gene loci (PGK, HGPRT, G6PD) to the long arm of the human X-chromosome by somatic cell genetics. Genetics 74: 661-678, 1973.

Ruddle, F. H.: New Haven, Conn.: personal communication, 1972.

*16410 NYSTAGMUS, CONGENITAL

Allen (1942) described a family with many affected members. We have observed this as a probably dominant trait among the Old Order Amish of Holmes Co., Ohio.

Allen, M.: Three pedigrees of eye defects: primary hereditary nystagmus. Case study with genealogy. J. Hered. 33: 454-456, 1942.

Dichgans, J. and Kornhuber, H. H.: Eine seltene Art des hereditaeren Nystagmus mit autosomal-dominantem Erbgang und besonderem Erscheinungsbild: vertikale Nystagmuskomponente und Stoerung des vertikalen und horizontalen optokinetischen Nystagmus. Acta Genet. Statist. Med. 14: 240-250, 1964.

Jayalakshmi, P., Scott, T. F. M., Rucker, S. H. and Schaffer, D. B.: Infantile nystagmus: a prospective study of spasmus nutans, congenital nystagmus, and unclassified nystagmus of infancy. J. Pediatr. 77: 177-187, 1970.

*16415 NYSTAGMUS, HEREDITARY VERTICAL

Marmor (1973) reported three families in two of which the mother and one or more children were affected. Forsythe (1955) and Dichgans and Kornhuber (1964) described families in which male-to-male transmission was observed. Vertical nystagmus most often signifies acquired disease. The familial disorder is a motor-type vertical (and horizontal) nystagmus with associated mild ataxia. Most of the affected persons had absent optokinetic nystagmus and a hyperactive vestibulo-ocular response.

Dichgans, J. and Kornhuber, H. H.: Eine seltene Art des hereditaren Nystagmus mit autosomal-dominantem Erbgang und besonderem Erscheinungsbild: vertikale Nystagmuskomponente und Stoerung des vertikalen und horizontalen optokinetischen Nystagmus. Acta Genet. 14: 240-250, 1964.

Forsythe, W. I.: Congenital hereditary vertical nystagmus. J. Neurol. Neurosurg. Psychiatry 18: 196-198, 1955.

Marmor, M. F.: Hereditary vertical nystagmus. Arch. Ophthalmol. 90: 107-111, 1973.

16417 NYSTAGMUS, VOLUNTARY

This is a rare nonpathologic finding. The subjects can voluntarily initiate and maintain rapid to-and-fro synchronous movements of the eyes. The trait has been described in sibs (Goldberg and Jampel, 1962) and in mother and three children (Keyes, 1973).

Goldberg, R. and Jampel, R.: Voluntary nystagmus in a family. Arch. Ophthalmol. 68: 32-35, 1962.

Keyes, M. J.: Voluntary nystagmus in two generations. Arch. Neurol. 29: 63-64, 1973.

*16420 OCULODENTODIGITAL DYSPLASIA (ODD SYNDROME): OCULO-DENTO-OSSEOUS SYNDROME

Gillespie (1964) described brother and sister with bilateral microphthalmos, abnormally small nose, hypotrichosis, dental anomalies, fifth finger camptodactyly, syndactyly of the fourth and fifth fingers and missing toe phalanges. The condition reported as acrocephalosyndactyly by Mohr (1939) and characterized by bilateral syndactyly of the 4th and 5th fingers is probably the same condition. The father and five of his children (including three sons) presented craniofacial deformity and complete syndactyly of the 4th and 5th fingers of the hand. This type of syndactyly, designated as type III syndactyly (q.v.), also occurs as an isolated malformation. In two unpublished pedigrees Renwick (1967) found that a constant and characteristic feature of the syndrome is the absence of the middle phalanx of those toes (2nd through 5th) that normally have three phalanges. Lightwood and Lewis (1963) reported father and son. Eidelman et al. (1967) observed affected brother and sister. Rajic and De Veber (1966) reported a family with many affected members in 3 generations but no male-to-male transmission. Eye features include microphthalmos, microcornea and glaucoma. The teeth were small with what was termed enamelogenesis imperfecta. The phalanges and metacarpals were widened and syndactyly of fingers 4 and 5 was present. These authors used the designation 'oculodentoosseous dysplasia.' O'Rourk and Bravos (1969) have observed the sporadic case of a boy with an oculodentodigital dysplasia probably distinct from that described above and therefore tentatively desibnated ODD syndrome II. Rather than syndactyly of fingers 4 and 5 the patient showed unilateral pre-axial polydactyly of the hand, laterally curved fifth finger on the right, fifth finger camptocdactyly on the left, and absent terminal phalanges of right fingers II and V.

Eidelman, E., Chosack, A. and Wagner, M. L.: Orodigitofacial dysostosis and oculodentodigital dysplasia. Oral Surg. 23: 311-319, 1967.

Gillespie, F. D.: A hereditary syndrome: 'dysplasia oculodentodigitalis.' Arch. Ophthalmol. 71: 187-192, 1964.

Gorlin, R. J., Meskin, L. H. and Geme, J. W.: Oculodentodigital dysplasia. J. Pediatr. 63: 69-75, 1963.

Lightwood, J. M. and Lewis, G. M.: The Holmes-Adie syndrome in a boy with acute juvenile rheumatism and bilateral syndactyly. Arch. Dis. Child. 38: 86-88, 1963.

Mohr, O. L.: Dominant acrocephalosyndactyly. Hereditas 25: 193-203, 1939.

O'Rourk, T. R., Jr. and Bravos, A.: An oculo-dento-digital dysplasia. The Clinical Delineation of Birth Defects. II. Malformation Syndromes. New York: Williams and Wilkins, 1969. Pp. 226-227.

Rajic, D. S. and De Veber, L. L.: Hereditary oculodentoosseous dysplasia. Ann. Radiol. 9: 224-231, 1966.

Renwick, J. H.: Glasgow, Scotland: personal communication, 1967.

Sugar, H. S., Thompson, J. P. and Davis, J. D.: The oculo-dento-digital dysplasia syndrome. Am. J. Ophthalmol. 61: 1448-1451, 1966.

*16430 OCULOPHARYNGEAL MUSCULAR DYSTROPHY

Victor, Hayes and Adams (1962) described a family with oculopharyngeal muscular dystrophy, an autosomal dominant disorder coming on in late life and characterized by dysphagia and progressive ptosis of the eyelids. Nine members of three generations were known to be affected. One affected member also had total external ophthalmoplegia and weakness of the limb-girdle muscles. The combination of ptosis and pharyngeal palsy was first noted in 1915 by Taylor who also commented on the familial nature of the syndrome. Hayes and colleagues (1963) succeeded in locating Taylor's original family and found that members of two subsequent generations had developed the disorder. In a family with this disorder observed in The Johns Hopkins Hospital the anal and vesical sphincters were also involved (Teasdall, Schuster, Walsh, 1964). Many cases have been of French-Canadian descent. The family reported by Schotland and Rowland (1964) may have had this disorder. Ten members had ptosis, ophthalmoparesis, dysphagia, and weakness and wasting of face, neck and distal limb muscles. Barbeau (1966) showed that all of the numerous reported French-Canadian cases could be traced back to a single ancestor who emigrated from France in the 1600's. Morgan-Hughes and Mair (1973) studied 4 patients with oculoskeletal myopathy. All complained of generalized muscle weakness and fatigability. All showed bilateral ptosis with external ophthalmoplegia, facial and sternocleidomastoid weakness and diffuse wasting in the limbs. Two patients were dysphagic and one had pigmentary retinal degeneration. Triceps biopsies revealed certain isolated or clustered muscle fibers to contain accumulations of sarcoplasmic matter. The number of abnormal fibers ranged from 18% to 8% with no relation between the number of affected fibers and the severity or duration of the symptoms.

Electron microscopy showed degenerative muscle fiber changes in all biopsy samples as well as striking abnormalities of muscle cell mitochondria. The mitochondria were seen to have laminated crystalline inclusions within the cristae. Some mitochondria were large with expanded area between the cristae. Sometimes the intercristal spaces were wide and electron dense. The authors stated that similar types of mitochondrial abnormalities have been described in other forms of myopathy. See Olson et al. (1972) for another study of this condition.

Barbeau, A.: The syndrome of hereditary late onset ptosis and dysphagia in French-Canada. In Kuhn, E. (ed.): Symposium ueber progressive Muskeldystrophie, Myotonie, Myasthenie. Berlin: Springer-Verlag, 1966. Pp. 102-109.

Bray, G. M., Kaarsoo, M. and Ross, R. T.: Ocular myopathy with dysphagia. Neurology 15: 678-684, 1965.

Hayes, R., London, W., Seidman, J. and Embree, L.: Oculopharyngeal muscular dystrophy. (Letter) N. Engl. J. Med. 268: 163 only, 1963.

Morgan-Hughes, J. A. and Mair, W. G. P.: Atypical muscle mitochondria in oculoskeletal myopathy. Brain 96: 215-224, 1973.

Murphy, S. F. and Drachman, D. B.: The oculopharyngeal syndrome. J.A.M.A. 203: 1003-1008, 1968.

Olson, W., Engel, W. K., Walsh, G. O. and Einaugler, R.: Oculocraniosomatic neuromuscular disease with 'ragged-red' fibers. Arch. Neurol. 26: 193-211, 1972.

Schotland, D. L. and Rowland, L. P.: Muscular dystrophy. Features ocular myopathy, distal myopathy, and myotonic dystrophy. Arch. Neurol. 10: 433-445, 1964.

Taylor, E. W.: Progressive vagus-glossopharyngeal paralysis with ptosis. Contribution to group of family diseases. J. Nerv. Ment. Dis. 42: 129-139, 1915.

Teasdall, R. D., Schuster, M. M. and Walsh, F. B.: Sphincter involvement in ocular myopathy. Arch. Neurol. 10: 446-448, 1964.

Victor, M., Hayes, R. and Adams, R. D.: Oculopharyngeal muscular dystrophy. A familial disease of late life characterized by dysphagia and progressive ptosis of the eyelids. N. Engl. J. Med. 267: 1267-1272, 1962.

16433 ODONTOMA-DYSPHAGIA SYNDROME

Schonberger (1974) described severe dysphagia in father and son with multiple odontomas. A case previously reported in the literature had the same combination. Hypertrophy of the smooth muscles of the esophagus was thought to be the cause of the dysphagia.

Schonberger, W.: Angeborene multiple Odontome und Dysphagie bie Vater und Sohn — eine syndromhafte Verknuepfung? Z. Kinderheilk. 117: 101-108, 1974.

16435 ODONTOMAS, MULTIPLE

Schmidseder and Hausamen (1973) described multiple odontomas in a father and his two sons.

Schmidseder, R. and Hausamen, J. E.: Familiaeres Auftreten angeborener, multipler Odontome. Dtsch. Zahnaerztl. Zschr. 28: 628-632, 1973.

*16440 OLIVOPONTOCEREBELLAR ATROPHY I (OPCA I; MENZEL TYPE)

Symptoms usually begin in the third or fourth decades of life, usually about 30. In addition to cerebellar signs, there are upper motor neurone signs and extensor plantar responses. Involuntary choreiform movements may occur. Characteristic families were reported by Menzel (1890) and by Waggoner et al. (1938) and Destunis (1944). The nosology of the olivopontocerebellar atrophies followed here is that of Konigsmark and Weiner (1970) who identify five types. In addition some reported families defy precise classification into one of the five types. See also CEREBELLO-PARENCHYMAL DISORDER, of which six types are recognized. Yakura et al. (1974) suggested that Marie cerebellar ataxia is linked to HL-A (14280). As noted elsewhere (11720), Marie ataxis is probably heterogeneous.

Critchley, M. and Greenfield, J. G.: Olivo-ponto-cerebellar atrophy. Brain 71: 343-364, 1948.

Destunis, G.: Die olivo-ponto-cerebellaere Heredoataxie. Zbl. Ges. Neurol. Psychiat. 177: 683, 1944.

Geary, J. R., Jr., Earle, K. M. and Rose, A. S.: Case report: olivoponto-cerebellar atrophy. Neurology 6: 218-224, 1956.

Konigsmark, B. W. and Weiner, L. P.: The olivo-ponto-cerebellar atrophies: a review. Medicine 49: 227-242, 1970.

Menzel, P.: Beitrag zur Kenntniss der hereditaeren Ataxie und Kleinhirnatrophie. Arch. Psychiatr. Nervenkr. 22: 160-190, 1890.

Waggoner, R. W., Lowenberg, K. and Speicher, K. G.: Hereditary cerebellar ataxia. Report of a case and genetic study. Arch. Neurol. Psychiatr. 39: 570-586, 1938.

Yakura, H., Wakisaka, A., Fujimoto, S. and Itakura, K.: Hereditary ataxia and HL-A genotypes. (Letter) 239
N. Engl. J. Med. 291, 154-155, 1974.

*16450 OLIVOPONTOCEREBELLAR ATROPHY III (OPCA III; WITH RETINAL DEGENERATION)

Weiner et al. (1967) found 27 affected persons in 5 generations. They suggested that the families of Woodworth et al. (1959) and of Carpenter and Schumacher (1966) may have suffered from the same entity. Froment, Bonnet and Colrat (1937) described four affected persons in three successive generations. They referred to the neurologic lesion as spinocerebellar degeneration. The character of the retinopathy was variable being peripheral in the first generation, macular in the second and macular and circumpapillary in the third. Retinal degeneration with cerebellar ataxia in a dominant pedigree pattern was also reported by Bjork, Lindblom and Wadensten (1956) and others. Havener (1951) described macular degeneration with cerebellar ataxia in a 28-year-old Negro. Cerebellar involvement was much less severe than in a daughter who died at 3 years with profound involvement. Foster and Ingram (1962) described a family with at least 7 affected members of 3 generations. Severity varied widely with infant death in at least one case and survival to middle age in other affected persons. Halsey et al. (1967) found degenerative changes in the retina and cerebellum of 11 persons in three generations of a North Carolina Negro family. Blindness and ataxia were the clinical features. Fundus changes were mainly macular. Onset was usually in middle age although 3 had onset in adolescence. Consanguinity and skipped generations suggest recessive inheritance. However, a high illegitimacy rate in this population could account for the pedigree pattern by accounting for apparently 'skipped' generations with a dominant trait. Jampel, Okazaki and Bernstein (1961) reported spinocerebellar ataxia with external ophthalmoplegia and retinal degeneration in 8 members of a Negro family (in 4 sibships of 3 generations). Ophthalmoplegia was progressive and appeared to have a supranuclear basis. Ptosis never occurred. Retinal degeneration began in the macular area and progressed to the periphery. Reports of the same syndrome were found in the literature, e.g., Alfano and Berger (1957). In other reports only external ophthalmoplegia or only retinal degeneration was associated with ataxia.

Alfano, J. E. and Berger, J. P.: Retinitis pigmentosa, ophthalmoplegia, and spastic quadriplegia. Am. J. Ophthalmol. 43: 231-240, 1957.

Bjork, A., Lindblom, U. and Wadensten, L.: Retinal degeneration in hereditary ataxia. J. Neurol. Neurosurg. Psychiatry 19: 186-193, 1956.

Carpenter, S. and Schumacher, G. A.: Familial infantile cerebellar atrophy associated with retinal degeneration. Arch. Neurol. 14: 82-94, 1966.

Foster, J. B. and Ingram, T. T. S.: Familial cerebro-macular degeneration and ataxia. J. Neurol. Neurosurg. Psychiatry 25: 63-68, 1962.

Froment, J., Bonnet, P. and Colrat, A.: Heredo-degenerations retinienne et spino cerebelleuse. Variantes ophtalmoscopiques et neurologiques presentees par trois generations successives. J. Med. Lyon, no vol: 153-163, 1937.

Halsey, J. H., Jr., Scott, T. R. and Farmer, T. W.: Adult hereditary cerebelloretinal degeneration. Neurology 17: 87-90, 1967.

Havener, W. H.: Cerebellar-macular abiotrophy. Arch. Ophthalmol. 45: 40-43, 1951.

Jampel, R. S., Okazaki, H. and Bernstein, H.: Ophthalmoplegia and retinal degeneration associated with spinocerebellar ataxia. Arch. Ophthal. 66: 247-259, 1961.

Weiner, L. P., Konigsmark, B. W., Stoll, J., Jr. and Magladery, J. W.: Hereditary olivopontocerebellar atrophy with retinal degeneration. Report of a family through six generations. Arch. Neurol. 16: 364-376, 1967.

Woodworth, J. A., Beckett, R. S. and Netsky, M. G.: A composite of hereditary ataxias. A familial disorder with features of olivopontocerebellar atrophy, Leber's optic atrophy and Friedreich's ataxia. Arch. Intern. Med. 104: 594-606, 1959.

*16460 OLIVOPONTOCEREBELLAR ATROPHY IV (OPCA IV; SCHUT-HAYMAKER TYPE)

Both the clinical and the pathologic pictures in the disorder described in a large kindred by Schut (1950) and by Schut and Haymaker (1951) were variable. Symptoms varied from those of spinocerebellar ataxia to spastic paraplegia. Identification as a form of OPCA is based on the presence of the major pathology in the inferior olivary nucleus and cerebellum with variable positive involvement. The spinal cord showed variable loss of anterior motor horn cells and changes in the spinocerebellar tracts and posterior funiculus. Involvement of cranial nerves IX, X and XII was another distinguishing feature. Currier et al. (1972) reported on a family as extensively affected as the Vandenberg family of Schut.

Currier, R. D., Glover, G., Jackson, J. F. and Tipton, A. C.: Spinocerebellar ataxia: study of a large kindred. I. General information and genetics. Neurol. 22: 1040-1043, 1972.

Schut, J. W. and Haymaker, W.: Hereditary ataxia: pathologic study of 5 cases of common ancestry. J. Neuropath. Clin. Neurol. 1: 183-213, 1951.

Schut, J. W.: Hereditary ataxia: clinical study through six generations. Arch. Neurol. Psychiat. 63: 535-568, 1950.

*16470 OLIVOPONTOCEREBELLAR ATROPHY V (OPCA V; WITH DEMENTIA AND EXTRAPYRA-MIDAL SIGNS)

Affected kindreds were reported by Carter and Sukavajana (1956), Konigsmark and Lipton (1970) and Chandler and Bebin (1956). In addition to cerebellar signs, rigidity and mental deterioration were consistent features. Neuronal loss was observed in the basal ganglia in all cases. Cortical changes correlated with dementia. Carter and Sukavajana (1956) described a father and five sons and a daughter (out of a sibship of 19) with a familial form of cerebello-olivary degeneration with late development of rigidity and dementia. Post-mortem showed profound cerebellar atrophy with degeneration in the olivary nuclei and substantia nigra.

Carter, H. R. and Sukavajana, C.: Familial cerebello-olivary degeneration with late development of rigidity and dementia. Neurology 6: 876-884, 1956.

Chandler, J. H. and Bebin, J.: Hereditary cerebellar ataxia: olivopontocerebellar type. Neurology 6: 187-195, 1956.

Konigsmark, B. W. and Lipton, H. L.: Dominant olivopontocerebellar atrophy with dementia and extrapyramidal signs. Report of a family through three generations. The Clinical Delineation of Birth Defects. VI. The Nervous System. Baltimore: Williams and Wilkins, 1970. Pp. 178-191.

Konigsmark, B. W. and Weiner, L. P.: The olivopontocerebellar atrophies: a review. Medicine 49: 227-242, 1970.

16480 ONYCHOLYSIS, PARTIAL, WITH SCLERONYCHIA

Schulze (1966) described mother and two children with onycholysis of the distal part of the fingernails, which were thickened. The disease was thought to have occurred in five generations.

Schulze, H. D.: Hereditaere Onycholysis partialis mit Skleronychie. Derm. Wschr. 152: 766-775, 1966.

*16490 OPHTHALMO-MANDIBULO-MELIC DYSPLASIA

The above designation was given by Pillay (1964) to a syndrome he observed in a father and two sons. Changes were found in the eye (corneal clouding), in the mandible (temporo-mandibular fusion, absent coronoid process, obtuse mandibular angle) and limbs (radio-humeral and radio-ulnar dislocations, aplasia of the lateral humeral condyle, radial head and distal ulna, etc.). Chromosome studies were negative.

Pillay, V. K.: Ophthalmo-mandibulo-melic dysplasia, an hereditary syndrome. J. Bone Joint Surg. 46A: 858-862, 1964.

*16500 OPHTHALMOPLEGIA, FAMILIAL STATIC

Lees (1960) described congenital static familial ophthalmoplegia. Ptosis, almost completely fixed eyes, nystagmoid movements and unequal pupils were features. Males in three successive generations and 7 persons in all were affected. Lees thought the lesion to be in the posterior longitudinal bundle and its connections with the oculomotor nuclei. Transmission through several generations with male-to-male transmission has been noted by Bradburne (1912) and many others. The palsy is thought to be of nuclear origin. Ptosis, immobility of the eyeball and paralysis of the pupil to accommodation are features. Holmes (1956) described 9 affected in four generations of a family, with congenital onset.

Bradburne, A. A.: Hereditary ophthalmoplegia in five generations. Trans. Ophthalmol. Soc. U.K. 32: 142-153, 1912.

Holmes, W. J.: Hereditary congenital ophthalmoplegia. Am. J. Ophthalmol. 41: 615-618, 1956.

Lees, F.: Congenital static familial ophthalmoplegia. J. Neurol. Neurosurg. Psychiatry 23: 46-51, 1960.

16510 OPHTHALMOPLEGIA, PIGMENTARY DEGENERATION OF RETINA AND CARDIOMYOPATHY

Kearns (1965) reported 9 unrelated patients with ophthalmoplegia, pigmentary degeneration of the retina and cardiomyopathy as leading features. Less consistent features were weakness of facial, pharyngeal, trunk and extremity muscles, deafness, small stature, electroencephalographic changes and markedly increased cerebrospinal fluid protein. In none of the 9 was a positive family history present. Refsum disease (q.v.) should be considered.

Kearns, T. P.: External ophthalmoplegia, pigmentary degeneration of the retina, and cardiomyopathy: a newly recognized syndrome. Trans. Ophthalmol. Soc. U.K. 63: 559-625, 1965.

16520 OPTIC ATROPHY WITH DEMYELINATING DISEASE OF CNS

Lees, MacDonald and Turner (1964) described a kindred in 5 generations of which 12 males and 3 females were affected with optic neuritis accompanied in some by neurologic manifestations resembling disseminated sclerosis. One had ataxia, right leg weakness and dysarthria. Another developed left hemiparesis during a two-week period and then recovered partially. Went (1974) is of the view that this kindred is an example of Leber optic atrophy and not a separate entity.

Lees, F., MacDonald, A. M. E. and Turner, J. W. A.: Leber's disease with symptoms resembling disseminated sclerosis. J. Neurol. Neurosurg. Psychiatry 27: 415-421, 1964.

Went, L. N.: Leyden, personal communication, 1974.

16530 OPTIC ATROPHY, CATARACT AND NEUROLOGIC DISORDER

Garcin et al. (1961) described optic atrophy, cataract, and neurologic disorder in 14 persons in 7 sibships of four generations with several instances of male-to-male transmission. Considerable variability was observed. Cataract was usually recognized in the first decade. The authors discussed the relation of this disorder to syndromes of Behr, of Marinesco and Sjogren and of Friedreich. Since all of these three are recessives, there can be no doubt that the entity they reported was distinct.

Garcin, R., Raverdy, P., Delthil, S., Man, H. X. and Chimenes, H.: Sur une affection heredo-familiale associant cataracte, atrophie optique, signes extra-pyramidaux et certains stigmates de la maladie de Friedreich. (Sa position nosologique par rapport au syndrome de Behr, au syndrome de Marinesco-Sjogren et a la maladie de Friedreich avec signes oculaires). Rev. Neurol. 104: 373-379, 1961.

*16540 OPTIC ATROPHY, CONGENITAL

Iverson (1958) reported congenital optic atrophy in three generations. The clear autosomal dominant pattern of inheritance and congenital nature distinguish it from Leber optic atrophy. See 19090.

Iverson, H. A.: Hereditary optic atrophy. Arch. Ophthalmol. 59: 850-853, 1958.

Kjer, P.: Infantile optic atrophy with dominant mode of inheritance. Op. ex Domo Biol. Hered. Hum. U. Hafniensis 42: 146 only, 1959.

*16550 OPTIC ATROPHY, JUVENILE

Caldwell et al. (1971) described two families with insidious onset of optic atrophy in childhood. There were no neurologic, congenital or developmental abnormalities. They classified the familial optic atrophies into six groups: congenital dominant, congenital recessive, juvenile dominant, juvenile recessive, Leber (perhaps X-linked), and Behr (recessive). The features of the six were usefully compared.

Caldwell, J. B. H., Howard, R. O. and Riggs, L. A.: Dominant juvenile optic atrophy. A study of two families and review of hereditary disease in childhood. Arch. Ophthalmol. 85: 133-147, 1971.

16560 ORBITAL MARGIN, HYPOPLASIA OF

Urrets-Zavalia (1955) observed two families with a syndrome consisting of agenesis of the orbital margin, hypoplasia of the palpebral skin and tarsal plates and variable defects of the lacrimal passages including ectopia and elongation of the lower punctum, shortening or absence of the inferior canaliculi, supernumerary canaliculi, or atresia of the naso-lacrimal duct. In some a small coloboma of the inner part of the lower lids and congenital anomalies of the extra-ocular muscles were present.

Urrets-Zavalia, A., Jr.: Familial primary hypoplasia of the orbital margin. Trans. Am. Acad. Ophthalmol. Otolaryngol. 59: 42-59, 1955.

16565 OROSOMUCOID

This is an alpha-1 acid glycoprotein found in the blood plasma. It is a monomer about 210 amino acid residues in length. Its amino acid sequence has been determined through 192 amino acids.

Dayhoff, M. O.: Orosomucoid. Atlas of Protein Sequence and Structure 1972 (vol. 5). Washington: National Biomedical Research Foundation, 1972. Pp. D-310 and D-316.

16567 OSSIFIED EAR CARTILAGES

Kirsch (1953) described ossification of the external ears in grandfather, father and son. Ossification occurs with calcification of the ear cartilages in hereditary conditions such as diastrophic dwarfism (22260), cold sensitivity (12010) and Keutel syndrome (24515).

Kirsch, R.: Vererbbare Verknoecherung der Ohrmuschel. Z. Laryng. Rhinol. 32: 729-734, 1953.

*16570 OSTEOARTHROPATHY OF FINGERS, FAMILIAL

Allison and Blumberg (1958) described the type of avascular necrosis of the phalangeal epiphyses to which the name of Thiemann is sometimes attached. Painless deformity at the proximal interphalangeal joints began in childhood or adolescence. A consanguineous mating of two affected persons resulted in particularly severe deformity in two of six offspring. These two may have been homozygotes.

Allison, A. C. and Blumberg, B. S.: Familial osteoarthropathy of the fingers. J. Bone Joint Surg. 40B: 538-545, 1958.

16580 OSTEOCHONDRITIS DISSECANS (ASEPTIC NECROSIS)

Each of the large number of possible localizations has an eponym, e.g., of phalangeal epiphyses (Thiemann, q.v.), of tibial tubercle (Osgood-Schlatter), of head of femur (Legg-Calve-Perthes), of spine (Scheuermann), of tarsal scaphoid (Kohler), of semilunar bone of the wrist (Kienbock), of the head of the second metatarsal (Frieberg), of the capitellum of the humerus (Panner), of the patella (Larsen-Johanssen). Dominant inheritance has been suggested in relation to several of these. Gardiner (1955) reported osteochondritis dissecans of the knees in a sister and two brothers. The term 'dissecans' comes from 'dis' meaning 'from' and 'secare' meaning 'cut off,' and is not to be confused with 'desiccans' derived from 'desiccare' meaning to 'dry up.' Dissecans refers to the appearance of part of the bone having been cut away.

Gardiner, T. B.: Osteochondritis dissecans in three members of one family. J. Bone Joint Surg. 37B: 139-141, 1955.

Harbin, M. and Zollinger, R.: Osteochondritis of growth centers. Surg. Gynecol. Obstet. 51: 145-161, 1930.

Smith, A. D.: Osteochondritis of the knee joint: a report of three cases in one family and a discussion of the etiology and treatment. J. Bone Joint Surg. 42A: 289-294, 1960.

16590 OSTEOCHONDRITIS DISSECANS OF MULTIPLE SITES

Stougaard (1961) observed osteochondritis dissecans of the knees and-or elbows in 9 persons in three generations. A pair of twins thought to be identical were affected. We have observed osteochondritis dissecans in the femur at the knee and in the capitellum of the humerus in two brothers who also show hypertelorism, finger contractures, peculiarly shaped ears, sternal deformity and cryptorchidism. This may be a syndrome. (It is also listed in the recessive catalog because of the uncertainty in the mode of inheritance.) Both parents seem normal. Zellweger and Ebnother (1951) reported a family in which the four affected members were also dwarfed. In the family reported by Pick (1955) the affected mother and 3 affected daughters were short. On the other hand some authors have commented on a tall, slender habitus. Tobin (1957) described father and 2 sons with the combination of osteochondritis dissecans and tibia vara (q.v.). A daughter had only osteochondritis dissecans.

Hanley, W. B., McKusick, V. A. and Barranco, F. T.: Osteochondritis dissecans and associated malformations in brothers. A review of familial aspects. J. Bone Joint Surg. 49A: 925-937, 1967.

Mueller, W. and Hetzar, W.: Familiaere generalisierte Osteochondritis dissecans zahlreicher Gelenke und der Eirbelsaeule. Deutsch. Z. Chir. 241: 795-804, 1933.

Pick, M. P.: Familial osteochondritis dissecans. J. Bone Joint Surg. 37B: 142-145, 1955.

Stougaard, J.: The hereditary factor in osteochondritis dissecans. J. Bone Joint Surg. 43B: 256-258, 1961.

Tobin, W. J.: Familial osteochondritis dissecans with associated tibia vara. J. Bone Joint Surg. 39A: 1091-1105, 1957.

Zellweger, H. and Ebnother, M.: Ueber eine familiaere Skelettstoerung mit multilocularen, aseptischen Knochennekrosen, insbesondere mit Osteochondritis dissecans. Helv. Paediatr. Acta 6: 95-111, 1951.

16600 OSTEOCHONDROMATOSIS (ENCHONDROMATOSIS, DYSCHONDROPLASIA)

Ollier disease is the eponymous designation. When hemangiomata are associated, the condition is known as Maffucci syndrome. Neither condition seems to be genetically determined in a simple Mendelian manner. There are a few instances of familial occurrence of Ollier disease, however. Steudel (1891-2) described two affected brothers and Rossberg (1959) reported affected brother and sister whose paternal grandfather was also affected. Lamy et al. (1954) observed 3 affected sibs and Carbonell and Vineta (1962) reported affected brother and sister. Dominant inheritance with reduced penetrance is possible.

Anderson, I. F.: Maffucci's syndrome: report of a case with a review of the literature. S. Afr. Med. J. 39: 1066-1070, 1965.

Andren, L., Dymling, J. F., Elner, A. and Hogeman, K. E.: Maffucci's syndrome: report of four cases. Acta Chir. Scand. 126: 397-405, 1963.

Carbonell Juanico, M. and Vineta Teixido, J.: Otro caso de discondroteosis generalizada congenita, tipo Ollier. Rev. Esp. Pediatr. 18: 91-99, 1962.

Cauble, W. G. and Bowman, H. S.: Dyschondroplasia and hemangiomas (Maffucci's syndrome): presentation of a case. Arch. Surg. 97: 678-681, 1968.

Lamy, M., Aussannaire, M., Jammet, M. L. and Nezelof, C.: Trois cas de maladie d'Ollier dans une fratrie. Bull. Soc. Med. Hosp. Paris 70: 62-70, 1954.

Rossberg, A.: Zur Erblichkeit der Knochenchondromatose. Fortschr. Roentgenstr. 90(1): 138-139, 1959.

Steudel, (NI): Multiple Enchondrome der Knochen in Verbindung mit venoesen Angiomen der Weichteile. Bruns Beir. Klin. Chir. 8: 503-521, 1891-2.

*16610 OSTEODYSPLASTY OF MELNICK AND NEEDLES

Melnick and Needles (1966) described families which contained multiple cases in multiple generations of a severe congenital bone disorder characterized by typical facies (exophthalmos, full cheeks, micrognathia and malalignment of teeth), flaring of the metaphyses of long bones, s-like curvature of bones of legs, irregular constrictions in the ribs, sclerosis of base of skull. Male-to-male transmission was noted in one case. 'Osteodysplasty' was the term suggested by Coste et al. (1968) who described an affected 58-year-old woman. Bone disease was recognized in infancy when she began to walk. Normal childbirth was impossible because of contracted pelvis. Osteoarthritis of the lumbar spine and hips gave much pain. Her height was normal. Striking facies comprised exophthalmos, high forehead, full red cheeks and receding chin. X-rays showed curved long bones, tortuous ribboned ribs and deformed clavicles, scapula and pelvis.

Coste, F., Maroteaux, P. and Chouraki, L.: Osteodysplasty (Melnick and Needles' syndrome). Report of a case. Ann. Rheum. Dis. 27: 360-366, 1968.

Maroteaux, P., Chouraki, L. and Coste, F.: L'osteodysplastie (syndrome de Melnick et de Needles). Presse Med. 76: 715-718, 1968.

Melnick, J. C. and Needles, C. F.: An undiagnosed bone dysplasia. A two family study of 4 generations and 3 generations. Am. J. Roentgen. 97: 39-48, 1966.

*16620 OSTEOGENESIS IMPERFECTA

Although it now seems clear that some cases of osteogenesis imperfecta congenita are recessive, osteogenesis imperfecta is usually dominant. In addition to frequent fractures, loose jointedness, blue sclerae and progressive deafness are features. Aortic regurgitation has been reported in OI, e.g., by Jornod et al. (1968). Solomons and Styner (1969) reported that bone collagen of OI inhibits calcification in vitro. Treatment of the collagen with pyrophosphatase in the presence of magnesium ion removed the inhibition. Elevated serum and urinary pyrophosphate in patients declined with administration of magnesium sulfate. Francis et al. (1974) suggested that cases of osteogenesis imperfecta fall into two groups: those with mild bone disease and blue sclerae and those with severe bone disease and white sclerae. According to them, furthermore, patients with blue sclerae tend to have a reduced amount of collagen which has normal stability. Whereas those with white sclerae have a normal amount of collagen with reduced stability. 'Stability' was measured by resistance to depolymerization by pronase, heat, or cold alkali. These workers suggested that a defect in cross-linking of collagen is present in the severe form of the disease.

Francis, M. J. O., Smith, R. and Bauze, R. J.: Instability of polymeric skin collagen in osteogenesis imperfecta. Br. Med. J. 1: 421-424, 1974.

Freda, V. J., Vosburgh, G. J. and Di Liberti, C.: Osteogenesis imperfecta congenita: a presentation of 16 cases and review of the literature. Obstet. Gynecol. 18: 535-547, 1961.

Heckman, B. A. and Steinberg, I.: Congenital heart disease (mitral regurgitation) in osteogenesis imperfecta. Am. J. Roentgen. 103: 601-607, 1968.

Jornod, J., Rothlin, M. and Uehlinger, E.: Anomalies cardiovasculaires de la maladie de Lobstein. Schweiz. Med. Wschr. 98: 795-798, 1968.

McKusick, V. A.: Heritable Disorders of Connective Tissue. St. Louis: C. V. Mosby Co., 1972 (4th Ed).

Scott, P. P., McKusick, V. A. and McKusick, A. B.: The nature of osteogenesis imperfecta in cats. Evidence that the disorder is primarily nutritional, not genetic, and therefore not analogous to the disease in man. J. Bone Joint Surg. 45A: 125-134, 1963.

Smars, G.: Osteogenesis Imperfecta in Sweden: Clinical Genetic, Epidemiological and Socio-Medical Aspects. Stockholm: Svenska Bokforlaget, 1961.

Smars, G., Beckman, L. and Book, J. A.: Osteogenesis imperfecta and blood groups. Acta Genet. Statist. Med. 11: 133-136, 1961.

Solomons, C. C. and Styner, J.: Osteogenesis imperfecta: effect of magnesium administration on pyrophosphate metabolism. Calc. Tiss. Res. 3: 318-326, 1969.

*16630 OSTEOLYSIS, HEREDITARY, OF CARPAL BONES WITH NEPHROPATHY

Shurtleff and colleagues (1964) observed a family with 11 affected persons in three generations. Osteolysis of the carpal bones leads to disappearance of these in older cases. Deformity of the hands suggesting arthritis also occurred in severe cases. Hypertension and renal failure were internal complications. Arteriolar thickening was the basis of these changes. Caffey (1961) described father and son. The father died of uremia (personal observation). Torg et al. (1969) suggested that sporadic cases such as that of Lagier and Rutishauer (1965) and that of Torg and Steel (1968) represent a separate disorder. It seems that they are indistinguishable (except quantitatively in terms of severity of renal disease) from the inherited cases and probably represent new dominant mutations. Gluck and Miller (1972) reported a family with males affected in 3 successive generations. Nephropathy and hypertension were not present and the authors cited a personal communication from Dr. J. Schaller indicating that 'this association has not been substantiated with time' in the family reported by Shurtleff et al. (1964). Kohler et al. (1973) described a father and 3 sibs with hereditary osteolysis. The osteolysis was most severe in the carpal and tarsal bones. The osteolysis was also present and spreading in adjacent areas. All the affected showed arthritic symptoms in childhood, painless deformities of the wrists and feet and a Marfan-like appearance. Mild deterioration of the elbow was present in the children. No hypertension or renal involvement was seen. These patients demonstrated an elevated alkaline phosphatase reflecting the process of bone destruction.

Caffey, J. P.: Idiopathic familial multiple carpal necrosis. Pediatric X-ray Diagnosis. Chicago: Yearbook Medical Publishers, (4th Ed.) 1961. P. 984.

Gluck, J. and Miller, J. J., III: Familial osteolysis of the carpal and tarsal bones. J. Pediatr. 81: 506-510, 1972.

Kohler, E., Babbitt, D., Huizenga, B. and Good, T. A.: Hereditary osteolysis. A clinical, radiological and chemical study. Radiology 108: 99-106, 1973.

Lagier, R. and Rutishauer, E.: Osteoarticular changes in a case of essential osteolysis. J. Bone Joint Surg. 47B: 339-353, 1965.

Shurtleff, D. B., Sparkes, R. S., Clawson, D. K., Guntheroth, W. G. and Mottet, N. K.: Hereditary osteolysis with hypertension and nephropathy. J.A.M.A. 188: 363-368, 1964.

Thieffry, S. and Sorrel-Dejerine, J.: Forme speciale d'osteolyse essentialle hereditaire et familiale a stabilisation spontanee, survenant dans l'enfance. Presse Med. 66: 1858-1861, 1958.

Torg, J. S. and Steel, H. H.: Essential osteolysis with nephropathy: a review of the literature and case report of an unusual syndrome. J. Bone Joint Surg. 50A: 1629-1638, 1968.

Torg, J. S., Digeorge, A. M., Kirkpatrick, J. A., Jr. and Trujillo, M. M.: Hereditary multicentric osteolysis with recessive transmission: a new syndrome. J. Pediatr. 75: 243-252, 1969.

16640 OSTEOMAS OF MANDIBLE

Multiple smoothly outlined globoid osteomas occur on the jaw in Gardner syndrome (see POLYPOSIS III). Whether this tumor ever occurs as an inherited trait independent of intestinal polyps and other bony and soft-tissue tumors is not clear. Frangenheim (1914) described this type of tumor in a father and 3 of his children but intestinal polyps were not excluded.

Frangenheim, P.: Familiaere Hyperostosen der Kiefer. Beitr. Klin. Chir. 90: 139-152, 1914.

16650 OSTEOPATHIA STRIATA

The name of the condition refers to a feature of relatively little practical importance, longitudinal striations of osteosclerosis in the long bones. Osteosclerosis in the cranial and facial bones leads to disfigurement and to disability due to pressure on cranial nerves. Walker (1969) and Jones and Mulcahy (1968) described typical cases. Rucker and Alfidi (1964) described a patient with sclerotic bone disease which had the additional feature of striations. The father and grandfather were said to have the same disorder. The father died of severe aortic stenosis. Only one earlier case was found, that reported by Fairbank (1951).

Fairbank, T.: An Atlas of General Affections of the Skeleton. Baltimore: Williams and Wilkins, 1951.

Jones, M. D. and Mulcahy, N. D.: Osteopathia striata, osteopetrosis, and impaired hearing. A case report. Arch. Otolaryngol. 87: 116-118, 1968.

Rucker, T. N. and Alfidi, R. J.: A rare familial systemic affection of the skeleton, Fairbank's disease. Radiology 82: 63-66, 1964.

Walker, B. A.: Osteopathia striata with cataracts and deafness. The Clinical Delineation of Birth Defects. IV. Skeletal Dysplasias. New York: National Foundation, 1969. Pp. 295-297.

*16660 OSTEOPETROSIS ('MARBLE BONES,' OSTEOSCLEROSIS FRAGILIS GENERALISATA, ALBERS-SCHONBERG DISEASE)

Salzano (1961) estimated the frequency of the dominant form of osteopetrosis in Brazil to be about 1 in 100,000. Fragility of bones and dental abscess are leading complications. A more malignant form, inherited as a recessive, causes anemia and early death from interference with the bone marrow. Welford (1959) described 14 affected male members of five generations of a family. All affected persons had facial paralysis beginning usually at about the age of 12 years. Main clinical features are fractures and osteomyelitis, especially of the mandible. By X-ray the vertebral bodies have a characteristic 'sandwich' appearance resulting from sclerosis of the upper and lower plates with intervening less dense area. Long bones of the extremities may show a 'bone-within-bone' appearance. Osteosclerosis sometimes termed osteopetrosis is a feature of pycnodysostosis. Follow-up on the family reported by Ghormley (1922) was provided by McKusick (1961). Johnston et al. (1968) studied two families. In one pedigree, the disorder was twice nonpenetrant. Elevated acid phosphatase was a feature in all but one of the affected persons.

Ghormley, R. K.: A case of congenital osteosclerosis. Bull. Hopkins Hosp. 33: 444-446, 1922.

Ilha, D. O. and Salzano, F. M.: A roentgenologic and genetic study of a rare osseous dystrophy. Acta Genet. Med. Gemellol. 10: 340-352, 1961.

Johnston, C. C., Jr., Lavy, N., Lord, T., Vellios, F., Merritt, A. D. and Deiss, W. P., Jr.: Osteopetrosis. A clinical, genetic, metabolic, and morphologic study of the dominantly inherited, benign form. Medicine 47: 149-167, 1968.

McKusick, V. A. and colleagues: Medical genetics 1960. J. Chronic Dis. 14: 1-198, 1961 (fig. 67).

Salzano, F. M.: Osteopetrosis: review of dominant cases and frequency in a Brazilian state. Acta Genet. Med. Gemellol. 10: 353-358, 1961.

Welford, N. T.: Facial paralysis associated with osteopetrosis (marble bones). J. Pediatr. 55: 67-72, 1959.

*16670 OSTEOPOIKILOSIS

The term means literally 'spotted bones.' Circumscribed sclerotic areas occur near the ends of many bones. It is of no pathologic consequence. Spotty skin lesions also are found in many cases. These are connective tissue nevi. Berlin et al. (1967) showed that either the skin or the bone lesions can be absent in families in which some members have both. Striking pedigrees supporting autosomal dominant inheritance were published by Melnick (1959), Jonasch (1955) and Busch (1937) among others. Landberg and Akesson (1963) observed the bone lesions in father and son. Raque and Wood (1970) found dermato-osteopoikilosis in a brother and sister and in a son of the brother.

Berlin, R., Hedensio, B., Lilja, B. and Linder, L.: Osteopoikilosis — a clinical and genetic study. Acta Med. Scand. 181: 305-314, 1967.

Busch, K. F. B.: Familial disseminated osteosclerosis. Acta Radiol. 18: 693-714, 1937.

Danielsen, L., Midtgaard, K. and Christensen, H. E.: Osteopoikilosis associated with dermatofibrosis lenticularis disseminata. Arch. Dermatol. 100: 465-470, 1969.

Green, A. E., Ellswood, W. H. and Collins, J. R.: Melorheostosis and osteopoikilosis: with a review of the literature. Am. J. Roentgen. 87: 1096-1111, 1962.

Jonasch, E.: 12 Faelle von Osteopoikilie. Fortschr. Roentgenstr. 82: 344-353, 1955.

Landberg, T. and Akesson, H. O.: A study of osteopoikilosis. Acta Genet. Med. Gemellol. 12: 256-268, 1963.

Luzsa, G.: Osteopoikilia familiaris. Orv. Hetil. 103: 1267-1269, 1962.

Melnick, J. C.: Osteopathia condensans disseminata (osteopoikilosis). Study of a family of 4 generations. Am. J. Roentgen. 82: 229-238, 1959.

Raque, C. J. and Wood, M. G.: Connective-tissue nevus. Dermatofibrosis lenticularis disseminata with osteopoikilosis. Arch. Dermatol. 102: 390-396, 1970.

Schorr, W. F., Opitz, J. M. and Reyes, C. N.: The connective tissue nevus-osteopoikilosis syndrome. Arch. Dermatol. 106: 208-218, 1972.

Smith, A. D. and Waisman, M.: Connective tissue nevi: familial occurrence and association with osteopoikilosis. Arch. Dermatol. 81: 249-252, 1960.

*16675 OTODENTAL DYSPLASIA

Levin et al. (1972, 1975) described a new syndrome of sensorineural deafness and dental anomalies. A high frequency hearing loss varied in onset from early childhood to middle age. The maxillary deciduous canines and the deciduous and permanent molars were large and bulbous. Jorgenson et al. (1974) have studied a second family.

Jorgenson, R. J., March, S. J. and Farrington, F. H.: Columbia, S. Carolina, personal communication, 1974.

Levin, L. S. and Jorgenson, R. J.: Familial otodentodysplasia: a 'new' syndrome. (Abstract) Am. J. Hum. Genet. 24: 61A only, 1972.

Levin, L. S., Jorgenson, R. J. and Cook, R. A.: Otodental dysplasia: a 'new' ectodermal dysplasia. To be published, 1975.

Levin, L. S. and Jorgenson, R. J.: Otodental dysplasia: a previously undescribed syndrome. In, Bergsma, D. (ed.): Clinical Delineation of Birth Defects. XVI. Urinary System and Others. Baltimore: Williams and Wilkins, 1974. Pp. 310-312.

16680 OTOSCLEROSIS

Larsson (1960) reviewed all cases seen in the University of Goteborg Hospital from 1949 to 1957. In about 80 percent it was possible to verify a positive family history after examining sibs and parents. He concluded that autosomal dominant inheritance with penetrance between 25 and 40 percent accounts for the findings. Deafness interpreted as otosclerosis and beginning as early as age five in some cases was described by Kabat (1943) in nineteen members of four generations of a family. Otosclerosis is said to be rare in Japan (Shimizu, 1965). Morrison (1967) presented a survey of 150 English cases and their families. He concluded that otosclerosis is dominant with less than 50 percent penetrance. The risk to a child of an affected person is of the order of 25 percent.

Amidon, E. W.: Heredity and environment in otosclerosis. J. Hered. 39: 223-227, 1948.

Chumlea, B. J.: A pedigree of otosclerosis. J. Hered. 33: 98-99, 1942.

Kabat, C.: A family history of deafness. J. Hered. 34: 377-378, 1943.

Larsson, A.: Otosclerosis, a genetic and clinical study. Acta Otolaryngol. 154 (suppl.): 1-86, 1960.

MacGregor, A. G. and Harrison, R.: Congenital total color blindness associated with otosclerosis. Ann. Eugen. 15: 219-233, 1950.

Morrison, A. W.: Genetic factors in otosclerosis. Ann. Roy. Coll. Surg. Eng. 41: 202-237, 1967.

Shimizu, H.: Baltimore, Md.: personal communication, 1965.

16685 OUABAIN RESISTANCE

This is a cellular phenotype used in cell hybrid studies (Creagan, 1974). Mouse cells are naturally resistant.

Creagan, R. P.: New Haven, personal communication, 1974.

16690 OVALOCYTOSIS, HEREDITARY HEMOLYTIC

Cutting et al. (1965) reported seven affected members in three generations of a Caucasian family with three instances of male-to-male transmission. All 7 had 'full ovalocytes' and 6 had uncompensated hemolytic anemia which underwent remission with splenectomy. These writers suggested that there are two types of 'non-linked' elliptocytosis of which one type is hemolytic with predominant ovalocytes. They suggested this should be called ovalocytosis and 'elliptocytosis' reserved for the other conditions. See ELLIPTOCYTOSIS.

Cutting, H. O., McHugh, W. J., Conrad, F. G. and Marlow, A. A.: Autosomal dominant hemolytic anemia characterized by ovalocytosis. A family study of seven involved members. Am. J. Med. 39: 21-34, 1965.

16695 OVARIAN DERMOID CYSTS

Dermoid cysts are generally benign cystic tumors comprised of predominantly ectodermal elements. However, endodermal and mesodermal elements also may be included. These cysts are often filled with hair, skin, teeth, bones, neural tissue and sebaceous material. Plattner and Oxorn (1973) reported the presence of bilateral ovarian dermoid cysts in a mother and her only two daughters. This was the first report of such bilateral ovarian dermoid cysts occurring in consecutive generations of a family. These bilateral teratomas were surgically removed from the mother at age 22 and from both her daughters at age 23. The authors stated that the literature contained 18 cases in 6 families with a familial occurrence of dermoid cysts.

Plattner, G. and Oxorn, H.: Familial incidence of ovarian dermoid cysts. Canad. Med. Assoc. J. 108: 892-893, 1973.

16700 OVARIAN TUMOR

Jackson (1967) reported a Jamaican family in which grandmother, mother and daughter (i.e., members of 3 generations) developed ovarian tumors which in two were known to have been dysgerminomas. Lewis and Davison (1969) described a family in which 5 sisters (out of 6) and their mother had ovarian cancer. One of the five had a malignant ovarian cyst but subsequently died of colonic cancer. Prophylactic oophorectomy was performed in the sixth sister and in 5 females of the following generation. Liber (1950) described a family with histologically proven papillary adenocarcinoma of the ovary in 5 sisters and their mother. Li et al. (1970) reported a family in which 7 women (four of them sisters) were proved to have ovarian carcinoma and this form of malignancy was suspected in 3 others. Ovarian tumors also occur in the Peutz-Jeghers syndrome (q.v.), in cases of gonadal dysgenesis in which XY cells are present and in the basal cell nevus syndrome (q.v.). The ovarian tumor in the Peutz-Jeghers syndrome is characteristically a Sertoli tumor (Scully, 1970).

Jackson, S. M.: Ovarian dysgerminoma in three generations? J. Med. Genet. 4: 112-113, 1967.

Lewis, A. C. W. and Davison, B. C. C.: Familial ovarian cancer. Lancet II: 235-237, 1969.

Li, F. P., Rapoport, A. H., Fraumeni, J. F., Jr. and Jensen, R. D.: Familial ovarian carcinoma. J.A.M.A. 214: 1559-1561, 1970.

Liber, A. F.: Ovarian cancer in mother and five daughters. Arch. Pathol. 49: 280-290, 1950.

Scully, R. E.: Sex cord tumor with annular tubules — a distinctive ovarian tumor of the Peutz-Jeghers syndrome. Cancer 25: 1107-1121, 1970.

16705 OXYTOCIN

See 19233.

16710 PACHYDERMOPERIOSTOSIS (PRIMARY OR IDIOPATHIC HYPERTROPHIC OSTEOAR-THROPATHY)

The manifestations include clubbing of the fingers, thickening of the skin and periosteum of the distal part of the extremities, thickening and seborrhea of the skin of the face and forehead and hyperhidrosis (Vogl and Goldfischer, 1962). Simple digital clubbing (q.v.) may be a separate genetic defect. Rimoin (1965) observed affected persons in successive generations. Females were much more mildly affected than males. Heterogeneity in this condition and-or recessive inheritance is suggested by the considerable number of instances of affected sibs with apparently normal parents and the several examples of consanguineous parents (Leva, 1915; Simons, 1918; Shen and Yamanouchi, 1934).

Hambrick, G. W., Jr. and Carter, D. M.: Pachydermoperiostosis. Touraine-Solente-Gole syndrome. Arch. Dermatol. 94: 594-608, 1966.

Leva, J.: Ueber familiaere Akromegalie. Med. Klin. 11: 1266-1268, 1915.

Rimoin, D. L.: Pachydermoperiostosis (idiopathic clubbing and periostosis). Genetic and physiologic considerations. N. Engl. J. Med. 272: 923-931, 1965.

Shen, R. and Yamanouchi, N.: Ueber cutis gyrata und cutis veritis gyrata latens. Dermatol. Wschr. 98: 254 only, 1934.

Simons, A.: Familiaere Trommelschlaegelbildung und Knochenkypertrophie. Deutsch. Z. Nervenheilk. 59: 301-321, 1918.

Vogl, A. and Goldfischer, S.: Pachydermoperiostosis: primary or idiopathic osteoarthropathy. Am. J. Med. 33: 166-187, 1962.

*16720 PACHYONYCHIA CONGENITA

This dominantly inherited disorder is characterized by onychogryposis, hyperkeratosis of the palms, soles, knees and elbows, tiny cutaneous horns in many areas, and leukoplakia of the oral mucous membranes. Hyperhidrosis of the hands and feet is usually present. Jackson and Lawler (1951-52) reported 6 affected members of 3 generations. Murray (1921) found 7 affected in 3 generations. Kumer and Loos (1935) found 24 affected in 5 generations. The syndrome may be more frequent in Jews than in non-Jews. At birth some teeth are usually already erupted. In a Jewish kindred I have observed an apparent new mutation with transmission to a son of the male proband (McKusick, 1971). It is by no means certain that this is an entity separate from pachyonychia congenita as reported by others. Soderqvist and Reed (1968) described the same association but found that the cysts are epidermal cysts and suggested that steatocystoma is an inappropriate designation. They presented an interesting newspaper clipping with pictures which described neonatal teeth present in persons of three generations. The adult teeth were sound. In four generations of a family, Vineyard and Scott (1961) observed steatocystoma associated with pachyonychia congenita.

Akesson, H. O.: Pachyonychia congenita in six generations. Hereditas 58: 103-110, 1967.

Jackson, A. D. M. and Lawler, S. D.: Pachyonychia congenita. A report of six cases in one family, with a note on linkage data. Ann. Eugen. 16: 142-146, 1951-52.

Joseph, H. L.: Pachyonychia congenita. Arch. Dermatol. 90: 594-603, 1964.

Kumer, L. and Loos, H. O.: Ueber Pachyonychia congenita (Typus Riehl). Wien. Klin. Wschr. 48: 174-178, 1935.

McKusick, V. A.: Pachyonychia congenita in father and son. The Clinical Delineation of Birth Defects. XII. Skin, Hair and Nails. Baltimore: Williams and Wilkins, 1971. Pp. 274-275.

Murray, F. A.: Congenital anomalies of the nails. Four cases of hereditary hypertrophy of the nail bed associated with a history of erupted teeth at birth. Br. J. Dermatol. 33: 409-412, 1921.

Soderqvist, N. A. and Reed, W. B.: Pachyonychia congenita with epidermal cysts and other congenital dyskeratoses. Arch. Dermatol. 97: 31-33, 1968.

Vineyard, W. R. and Scott, R. A.: Steatocystoma multiplex with pachyonychia congenita. Eight cases in four generations. Arch. Dermatol. 84: 824-827, 1961.

Witkop, C. J., Jr. and Gorlin, R. J.: Four hereditary mucosal syndromes. Arch. Dermatol. 84: 762-771, 1961.

16725 PAGET DISEASE OF BONE

Reports of familial aggregation are rather numerous, including occurrence in successive generations. Montagu (1949) reviewed the reported families with multiple instances of Paget disease of bone and concluded that 'when inherited, it is transmitted as an incompletely dominant gene carried on an X chromosome.' McKusick (1960) reviewed 35 pedigrees reported to 1956 and added two others. In only one family, that of van Bogaert (1933), was there male-to-male transmission. All the persons affected by the bone disease and some members of the family not so affected also had retinitis pigmentosa, which may have been an independent, i.e., coincidental, genetic disorder. Jones and Reed (1967) observed 6 cases in 3 generations of a family. Evens and Bartter (1968) described 7 definite and two probable cases in one kindred.

Evens, R. G. and Bartter, F. C.: The hereditary aspects of Paget's disease (osteitis deformans). J.A.M.A. 205: 900-902, 1968.

Jones, J. V. and Reed, M. F.: Paget's disease: a family with six cases. Brit. Med. J. 2: 90-91, 1967.

McKusick, V. A.: Paget's disease of the bone. Heritable Disorders of Connective Tissue. St. Louis: C. V. Mosby Co., 1972 (3rd Ed.). Pp. 304-309.

Montagu, M. F. A.: Paget's disease (osteitis deformans) and heredity. Am. J. Hum. Genet. 1: 94-95, 1949.

Van Bogaert, L.: Ueber eine hereditaere und familiaere Form der Pagetschen ostitis deformans mit Chorioretinitis pigmentosa. Zbl. Ges. Neurol. Psychiat. 147: 327-345, 1933.

16730 PAGET DISEASE, EXTRAMAMMARY

extramammary Paget disease is a cancerous disease seen at various sites, most often in the anogenital region. The clinical features are usually those of eczematous eruptions with weeping and crust formation. This disease has been shown to be a skin manifestation of internal malignancy. Kuehn, Tennant and Brennerman (1973) described a case occurring in a father and son. The father, age 66, presented with extramammary Paget disease in the right scrotal area. No mention was made of other family history. Helwig and Graham (1963) in a study of 40 patients with Paget disease of the anogenital region did not find a family history of the disease in any of the cases.

Helwig, E. B. and Graham, F. N.: Anogenital (extramammary Paget's disease. Cancer 16: 387-403, 1963.

Kuehn, P. G., Tennant, R. and Brennerman, A. R.: Familial occurrence of extramammary Paget's disease. Cancer 31: 145-148, 1973.

16740 PAIN, SUBMANDIBULAR, OCULAR AND RECTAL, WITH FLUSHING

Hayden and Grossman (1959) described a syndrome consisting of very brief, excruciating pain of the submandibular, ocular and rectal areas with flushing of the surrounding skin. Autosomal dominant inheritance with variable penetrance of the components was suggested. Submandibular and ocular pain is a more consistent feature than rectal pain. They considered the condition a 'dysautonomia.' Dugan (1972) described affected individuals in 5 generations with male-to-male transmission. 'Intense searing pain' accompanied bowel movements. 'Jaw aches' also were frequent. Mann and Cree (1972) recorded some observations on another extensively affected family and gave graphic descriptions of the severe rectal pain. They concluded that the disorder is distinct from proctalgia fugax, first described by Thaysen (1935).

Dugan, R. E.: Familial rectal pain. (Letter) Lancet I: 854 only, 1972.

Hayden, R. and Grossman, M.: Rectal, ocular and submaxillary pain. A familial autonomic disorder related to proctalgia fugax. Report of a family. Am. J. Dis. Child. 97: 479-482, 1959.

Mann, T. P. and Cree, J. E.: Familial rectal pain. (Letter) Lancet I: 1016-1017, 1972.

Thaysen, T. E. H.: Proctalgia fugaz. A little known form of pain in the rectum. Lancet II: 243-246, 1935.

16750 PALATOPHARYNGEAL INCOMPETENCE

Congenital palatopharyngeal incompetence is characterized by cleft palate speech (rhinolalia aperta) in the absence of overt cleft palate. About a fourth of cases are 'unmasked' by adenoidectomy. Abnormalities of the uvula, soft palate and hard palate may be visible. Occasionally dominant inheritance may obtain, with great variability, making this essentially a multifactorial trait.

Pruzansky, S. and Mason, R.: Family studies of congenital palatopharyngeal incompetence. (Abstract) Proc. Third Intern. Cong. Hum. Genet. (Chicago, Sept. 5-10, 1966.).

16760 PALMARIS LONGUS MUSCLE, ABSENCE OF

At the wrist the tendon of the palmaris longus muscle is located in the middle of the ventral surface. It is flanked by the tendons of the flexor carpi ulnaris and flexor carpi radialis. Schaeffer (1953) recorded that the muscle was absent from 12.6 percent of the 310 limbs of 155 subjects and was bilaterally absent in 7.7 percent of subjects. The muscle is said to be absent more often in females and on the left side. For example, Thompson, McBatts and Danforth (1921) found the muscle missing in about 16 percent of males and 24 percent of females, these figures being based on studies of cadavers. Absence was thought to be a dominant trait, with incomplete penetrance and lateral variability. Thompson, McBatts and Danforth (1921) concluded that absence is dominant. Their study involved 81 families with a total of 188 children.

Schaeffer, J. P.: In, Human Anatomy. Morris (ed.) New York: Blakiston Co., 1953 (11th Ed.) Pp. 482-483.

Thompson, J. W., McBatts, J. and Danforth, C. H.: Hereditary and racial variations in the musculus palmaris longus. Am. J. Phys. Anthropol. 4: 205-218, 1921.

16770 PALMO-MENTAL REFLEX

The palmo-mental reflex is an ipsilateral or bilateral contraction of the mentalis muscle elicited by a scratch applied to the thenar eminence. In Japanese, Abe (1965) found it in one-third of 3-year-old children and one-sixth of the mothers, suggesting that about half the positive children become negative by adulthood. The reflex was much more often positive in mothers of children with the reflex than in mothers of 'negative' children. Further analysis of the data suggested dominant inheritance. The design of this study did not permit exclusion of X-linked dominance. A marked, slowly subsiding reflex in an adult may indicate cerebral disease.

Abe, K.: Genetic aspects of the palmo-mental reflex. Acta Genet. Statist. Med. 15: 327-336, 1965.

*16780 PANCREATITIS, HEREDITARY

Gross, Gambill and Ulrich (1962) described a kindred with affected persons in four generations. Four other families have been reported from the Mayo Clinic. A puzzling feature is the urinary excretion of lysine and cystine by about half the members of affected kindreds (with or without pancreatitis). Cystine urinary stones have not been observed. Singer and Cohen (1966) reported onset at about age 20 in a man whose younger sister and a cousin were similarly affected. The attacks were characterized by severe abdominal pains, fever and marked elevation of serum amylase. Except for the last, differentiation from familial Mediterranean fever (q.v.), also called 'familial paroxysmal peritonitis,' might be difficult. The aminoaciduria was almost certainly an incidental finding since family members without pancreatitis showed it and because other families with pancreatitis have not had this feature (Davidson et al., 1968). Robechek (1967) observed a family with 5 affected persons. He suggested that hypertrophy of the sphincter of Oddi together with a common ampulla of the biliary and pancreatic ducts may be the inherited factor. Mann and Rubin (1969) described a 17-month-old boy with steatorrhea whose 26-year-old brother and mother had steatorrhea and pancreatic calcification. Hereditary pancreatitis occurs with hyperparathyroidism in the multiple endocrine adenomatosis syndrome (q.v.). McElroy and Christiansen (1972) described a family in which 10 persons had definite pancreatitis and 16 others may have been affected. They pointed out that thrombosis in the portal or splenic vein occurs with significant frequency.

Carey, M. C. and Fitzgerald, O.: Hyperparathyroidism associated with chronic pancreatitis in a family. Gut 9: 700-703, 1968.

Davidson, P., Costanza, D., Swieconek, J. A. and Harris, J. B.: Hereditary pancreatitis: a kindred without gross aminoaciduria. Ann. Intern. Med. 68: 88-96, 1968.

Gross, J. B., Gambill, E. E. and Ulrich, J. A.: Hereditary pancreatitis. Description of a fifth kindred and summary of clinical features. Am. J. Med. 33: 358-364, 1962.

Gross, J. B., Ulrich, J. A. and Jones, J. D.: Urinary excretion of aminoacids in a kindred with hereditary pancreatitis and aminoaciduria. Gastroenterology 47: 41-48, 1964.

Kattwinkel, J., Lapey, A., Disant' Agnese, P. A., Edwards, W. A. and Huffy, M. P.: Hereditary pancreatitis: three new kindreds and a critical review of the literature. Pediatrics 51: 55-69, 1973.

Mann, T. P. and Rubin, J.: Familial pancreatic exocrine dysfunction with pancreatic calcification. Proc. R. Soc. Med. 62: 326 Only, 1969.

McElroy, R. and Christiansen, P. A.: Hereditary pancreatitis in a kinship associated with portal vein thrombosis. Am. J. Med. 52: 228-241, 1972.

Robechek, P. J.: Hereditary chronic relapsing pancreatitis. A clue to pancreatitis in general? Am. J. Surg. 113: 819-824, 1967.

Sibert, J. R.: Hereditary pancreatitis in a Newcastle family. Arch. Dis. Child. 48: 618-621, 1973.

Singer, M. and Cohen, F. B.: Hereditary chronic relapsing pancreatitis. J. Newark Beth Israel Hosp. 21: 121-126, 1966.

16790 PAPILLOMATOSIS, FAMILIAL CUTANEOUS

Baden (1965) described a confluent, reticular type of papillomatosis in two sisters and the daughter of one.

Baden, H. P.: Familial cutaneous papillomatosis. Arch. Dermatol. 92: 394-395, 1965.

16795 PAPILLOMATOSIS, FLORID, OF NIPPLE

Florid papillomatosis of the nipple is a benign disorder which simulates Paget disease of the nipple which has much more sinister implications. Mandelbaum (1972) described affected mother and daughter.

Mandelbaum, I.: Familial florid papillomatosis of the nipple. Ann. Surg. 175: 254-256, 1972.

*16800 PARAGANGLIOMATA

Kroll and colleagues (1964) found carotid body tumors in 12 members of a family in an autosomal dominant pattern of inheritance. Carotid body tumors and glomus jugulare tumors are considered to be chemodectomas, this being a term for tumors arising in chemoreceptor structures. Some would question the appropriateness of calling these paragangliomas. Resler et al. (1966) described a patient with bilateral carotid body tumors and a glomus jugulare tumor. They commented that familial carotid body tumors tend to be multiple. Familial glomus jugulare tumors are probably rare. The only reported family may be that with three affected sisters described in 1937 by Goekoop (cited by Rosen, 1952). Bartels (1949) found carotid body tumor in members of 3 successive generations. Wilson (1970) reviewed the familial reports and described a family with male-to-male transmission and a 'skipped generation.' Pratt (1973) reviewed the literature and reported 8 new cases of either unilateral or bilateral carotid body tumors in four generations of a kindred. In one generation of this family, 4 sisters had bilateral tumors and one brother had unilateral tumors. None of the 8 tumors reported were malignant.

Bartels, J.: De tumoren van het glomus jugulare. Thesis. Groningen, 1949.

Kroll, A. J., Alexander, B., Cochios, F. and Pechet, L.: Hereditary deficiencies of clotting factors VII and X associated with carotid-body tumors. N. Engl. J. Med. 270: 6-13, 1964.

Pratt, L. W.: Familial carotid body tumors. Arch. Otolaryng. 97: 334-336, 1973.

Resler, D. R., Snow, J. B. and Williams, G. R.: Multiplicity and familial incidence of carotid body and glomus jugulare tumors. Ann. Otol. 75: 114-122, 1966.

Rosen, S.: Glomus jugulare tumor of the middle ear with normal drum, improved biopsy technique. Ann. Otol. 61: 448-451, 1952.

Wilson, H.: Carotid body tumors: familial and bilateral. Ann. Surg. 171: 843-848, 1970.

16810 PARALYSIS AGITANS, JUVENILE, OF HUNT

Ramsey Hunt (1917) described a disorder with typical Parkinsonism beginning in the teens or earlier with tremor, mask-like facies, bradykinesia, dysarthria and rigidity. Progression is very slow. David B. Clark has seen the disorder in father and daughter (Ford, 1961). The substantia nigra is normal but degeneration and loss of large cells of the lenticular nuclei occur. Hunt's second case was the offspring of first cousins. She died at the age of 65 years. Autopsy showed pallido-pyramidal disease which is listed in the recessive catalog (q.v.).

Ford, F. R.: Hypertrophic interstitial poly-neuritis. Diseases of the Nervous System in Infancy, Childhood and Adolescence. Springfield, Ill.: Charles C Thomas, 1961 (4th Ed.). Pp. 369-399.

Hunt, J. R.: Progressive atrophy of the globus pallidus (primary atrophy of the pallidal system). Brain 40: 58-148, 1917.

Mjones, H.: Paralysis Agitans: a Clinical and Genetic Study. Copenhagen: E. Munksgaard, 1949.

16820 PARAMOLAR TUBERCLE OF BOLK

This is an extra small cusp located on the buccal side of the permanent molar teeth. Its significance is unknown.

Dahlberg, A. A.: Paramolar tubercle (Bolk). Am. J. Phys. Anthropol. 3: 97-103, 1945.

*16830 PARAMYOTONIA CONGENITA OF EULENBURG

Lajoie (1961) described a family with many affected members. The condition is manifested mainly by paralysis of muscles exposed to cold, is already evident in infancy, is not progressive, does not interfere with a reasonably normal social and economic life, and does not affect longevity. Hudson's family (1963) showed 17 affected in 5 generations. Drager, Hammill and Shy (1958) found thirty affected members in six generations of a family. The characteristics of this disease described by Eulenburg are (1) inheritance as a dominant with high penetrance; (2) myotonia, increased by exposure to cold; (3) intermittent flaccid paresis, not necessarily dependent on cold or myotonia; (4) lability of serum potassium; (5) non-progressive nature and (6) lack of atrophy or hypertrophy of muscles. Hudson (1963) commented on the phenotypic overlap of this condition with hypokalemic, eukalemic and hyperkalemic periodic paralysis, with myotonia congenita and with myotonic dystrophy. Six and possibly 9 generations had affected members in the French-Canadian family reported by Samaha (1964). Eating ice-cream or swimming in cold water was dangerous to affected members. Serum potassium levels were moderately increased and the patients were sensitive to administered potassium. Chlorothiazide was remarkably beneficial. Becker (1970) gave an extensive review of the subject and described studies in 18 kindreds.

Becker, P. E.: Paramyotonia congenita (Eulenburg). Fortschritte der Allgemeinen und Klinischen Humangenetik 3: 134, 1970.

Drager, G. A., Hammill, J. F. and Shy, G. M.: Paramyotonia congenita. Arch. Neurol. Psychiatry 80: 1-9, 1958.

Haynes, J. and Thrush, D. C.: Paramyotonia congenita: an electrophysiological study. Brain 95: 553-558, 1972.

Hudson, A. J.: Progressive neurological disorder and myotonia congenita associated with paramyotonia. Brain 86: 811-826, 1963.

Lajoie, W. J.: Paramyotonia congenita, clinical features and electromyographic findings. Arch. Phys. Med. 42: 507-512, 1961.

Magee, K. R.: Paramyotonia congenita: associated with cutaneous cold sensitivity and description of peculiar sustained postures after muscle contraction. Arch. Neurol. 14: 590-594, 1966.

Samaha, F. J.: Von Eulenburg's paramyotonia. Trans. Am. Neurol. Assoc. 89: 87-91, 1964.

Thomasen, E.: Myotonia. Thomsen's disease (myotonia congenita). Paramyotonia and Dystrophia Myotonica. A Clinical and Heredobiologic Investigation. Aarhus: Universitetsforlaget. 1948.

Thrush, D. C., Morris, C. J. and Salmon, M. V.: Paramyotonia congenita: a clinical, histochemical and pathological study. Brain 95: 537-552, 1972.

Langer et al. (1970) described 3 patients with a form of dwarfism in which deformities are recognized in the first 6 to 12 months of life. They named the disorder parastremmatic from the Greek term for twisted. Clinically the full syndrome is manifested by 10 years. Adult height is 90 to 110 cm. There are bizzare and symmetric deformities of the legs with severe genu valgum, bowing of the long bones, twisted thighs and shanks along the long axis, short neck, kyphoscoliosis, multiple contractures of major joints, clear cornea and normal cardiovascular system. Intelligence is also normal and there is no abnormal mucopolysac-chariduria. Radiographs show very coarse trabeculations with areas of irregular, dense stippling and streaking producing a 'flocky or wooly' appearance. In the pelvis this is seen as a lace-like border of the iliac crests. The metaphyses are clear and contain 'flocky' bone; severely deformed and radiolucent epiphyses are present. The evidence for dominant inheritance comes from the report of father and daughter by Rask (1963). Since the daughter was as severely affected as the father, the causative gene is probably autosomal.

Langer, L. O., Petersen, D. and Spranger, J.: An unusual bone dysplasia: parastremmatic dwarfism. Am. J. Roentgen. 110: 550-560, 1970.

Rask, M. R.: Morquio-Brailsford osteochondrodystrophy and osteogenesis imperfecta: report of a patient with both conditions. J. Bone Joint Surg. 45A: 561-570, 1963.

*16850 PARIETAL FORAMINA, SYMMETRICAL (FORAMINA PARIETALIA PERMAGNA)

Parietal foramina are symmetrical, oval defects in the parietal bone situated on each side of the saggital suture and separated from each other by a narrow bridge of bone. Goldsmith (1922) called this condition Catlin marks because he observed 16 instances in 5 generations of the Catlin family. This, like Hartnup disease, is one of the few examples of hereditary traits named for the family in which it was first observed. Lother (1959) described five cases in two generations. Many of the affected persons in Goldsmith's family had circumscribed aplasia of the scalp and the same was true of Lother's family. Kite (1961) observed association with seizures. The possibility of confusion with aboriginal trepination was pointed out by Powell (1970). Clefts of the lip and-or palate were present in cases reported by Hollender (1967), Irvine and Taylor (1936) and others. The frequency may be increased.

Goldsmith, W. M.: 'The Catlin mark': the inheritance of an unusual opening in the parietal bones. J. Hered. 13: 69-71, 1922.

Kite, W. C., Jr.: Seizures associated with the Catlin mark. Neurology 11: 345-348, 1961.

Hollender, L.: Enlarged parietal foramina. Oral Surg. 23: 447-453, 1967.

Irvine, E. D. and Taylor, F. W.: Hereditary and congenital large parietal foramina. Br. J. Radiol. 9: 456-462, 1936.

Lother, K.: Familiaeres Vorkommen von foramina parietalia permagna. Arch. Kinderheilk. 160: 156-168, 1959.

Murphy, J. and Gooding, C. A.: Evolution of persistently enlarged parietal foramina. Radiology 97: 391-392, 1970.

Powell, B. W.: Aboriginal trephination: case from southern New England? Science 170: 732-734, 1970.

*16860 PARKINSONISM

Spellman (1962) described a family in which multiple members in four generations had Parkinsonism beginning in the 30's and progressing rapidly to death in 2-12 years. Bell and Clark (1926) reviewed published pedigrees and published an additional one. Allan (1937) reported impressive pedigrees from North Carolina. It seems possible, indeed likely that Parkinsonism is heterogeneous with some Mendelian forms of the disease. We observed, for example one kindred strongly indicative of X-linked recessive inheritance (see 31150). However, analysis of the experience at the Mayo Clinic had Kondo et al. (1973) to conclude that irregular dominant transmission is untenable and that multifactorial inheritance with heritability of about 80 percent is more likely.

Allan, W.: Inheritance of shaking palsy. Arch. Intern. Med. 60: 424-436, 1937.

Bell, J. and Clark, A. J.: A pedigree of paralysis agitans. Ann. Eugen. 1: 455-462, 1926.

Kondo, K., Kurland, L. T. and Schull, W. J.: Parkinson's disease: genetic analysis and evidence of a multifactorial etiology. Mayo Clinic Proc. 48: 465-475, 1973.

Spellman, G. G.: Report of familial cases of Parkinsonism: evidence of a dominant trait in a patient's family. J.A.M.A. 179: 372-374, 1962.

16870 PARKINSONISM-DEMENTIA

It is not certain that this disorder, endemic among the natives of Guam, is genetic or, if genetic, is dominant.

Hirano, A., Kurland, L. T., Krooth, R. S. and Lessell, S.: Parkinsonism-dementia complex, an endemic disease on the Island of Guam. Brain 84: 642-661, 1961.

*16875 PAROTID BASIC PROTEIN

By acid-urea starch-gel electrophoresis, Azen (1972) demonstrated three phenotypes in the parotid saliva of black subjects. Inheritance is controlled by two co-dominant autosomal alleles. Only one heterozygote was found among 101 Caucasians. On the other hand the frequency of the two alleles in blacks are 0.84 for PB(1) and 0.16 for PB(2).

Azen, E. A.: Genetic polymorphism of basic proteins from parotid saliva. Science 176: 673-674, 1972.

Azen, E. A.: Properties of salivary basic proteins showing polymorphism. Biochem. Genet., In Press, 1973.

*16878 PAROTID PROLINE-RICH PROTEIN

By alkaline polyacrylamide gel electrophoresis, Azen (1973) demonstrated polymorphism of salivary protein found to be identical to previously identified proline-rich proteins (Oppenheim et al., 1971). These proteins have some similarities to collagen and others to enamel protein. Identification of polymorphism should stimulate search for relationship association between specific phenotype and oral disease. Furthermore, gene frequencies are such as to make this polymorphism useful as a marker trait in linkage studies.

Azen, E. A. and Oppenheim, F. G.: Genetic polymorphism of proline-rich human salivary proteins. Science 180: 1067-1069, 1973.

Oppenheim, F. G., Hay, D. I. and Fraublau, C.: Proline-rich proteins from human parotoid saliva. Isolation and partial characterization. Biochemistry 10: 4233-4238, 1971.

16880 PAROTIDOMEGALY, HEREDITARY BILATERAL

Marie et al. (1968) described six cases in 3 generations.

Marie, R., Marie, M., Grellet, M., Gouygou, C., Cariou, P., Gauthey, J. C. and Reverse, C.: Parotidomegalie bilaterale d'allure hereditaire. Dysplasie microkystique de la parotide: etude clinique, sialogrophique et anatomo-pathologique. Rev. Stomat. 68: 578-585, 1967.

16885 PATELLA APLASIA, COXA VARA, TARSAL SYNOSTOSIS

A seemingly unique syndrome was reported by Goeminne and Dujardin (1970). A mother had, in addition to absent patellas, severe coxa vara, hypoplasia of 'descending parts of the pubic arches' in the osseous pelvis, talocalcaneal synostosis and absence of one metatarsal bilaterally. A daughter had the full syndrome except for the tarsal synostosis. A son had only patella aplasia. Report of a similar family was found.

Goeminne, L. and Dujardin, L.: Congenital coxa vara, patella aplasia and tarsal synostosis. A new inherited syndrome. Acta Genet. Med. Gemellol. 19: 534-545, 1970.

*16890 PATELLA, CHONDROMALACIA OF

This disorder is characterized by well-localized pain when the patella is grated against the femoral condyles or when the knee is actively extended with the patella manually displaced distally. Rubacky (1963) described five families with multiple affected persons in multiple generations and male-to-male transmission. The association of patellar chondromalacia with recurrent dislocation of the patella (q.v.) is well known and the former is usually attributed to the latter. However, Rubacky (1963) suggested that the cause and effect relation may be the other way around, in some cases. This condition is probably not a form of osteodrondritis dissecans (q.v.), which can affect the patella.

Rubacky, G. E.: Inheritable chondromalacia of the patella. J. Bone Joint Surg. 45A: 1685-1688, 1963.

16900 PATELLA, FAMILIAL RECURRENT DISLOCATION OF

Carter and Sweetnan (1960) suggested that this is a dominant trait independent of familial joint laxity (q.v.).

Carter, C. and Sweetnan, R.: Recurrent dislocation of the patella and of the shoulder. Their association with familial joint laxity. J. Bone Joint Surg. 42B: 721-727, 1960.

16910 PATENT DUCTUS ARTERIOSUS (PDA)

Occasionally patent ductus arteriosus occurs in so many members of multiple generations of a family that simple autosomal dominant inheritance seems likely. For example, Burman (1961) described PDA in a girl, her father and two paternal aunts with the paternal grandfather and some other members of the family possibly also affected. Goodyear (1961) observed a family in which the mother had patent ductus arteriosus and two of her three children had persistent truncus arteriosus. An established exogenous cause of PDA is maternal rubella.

Burman, D.: Familial patent ductus arteriosus. Brit. Heart J. 23: 603-604, 1961.

Goodyear, J. E.: Persistent truncus arteriosus in two siblings. Br. Heart J. 23: 194-196, 1961.

Lynch, H. T., Grissom, R. L., Magnuson, C. R. and Krush, A.: Patent ductus arteriosus: study of two families. J.A.M.A. 194: 135-138, 1965.

16920 PECHET FACTOR (DYNIA FACTOR) DEFICIENCY

Pechet (1964, 1966) described a 'new' clotting defect in a 15-year-old boy, his mother, one brother and one sister. The proband had frequent traumatic hemorrhages. The relatives with laboratory abnormalities were asymptomatic. The maternal grandfather also showed a defect of clotting. The authors suggested that these persons lack a clotting factor which plays a role in the first phase of coagulation, following the activation of factor IX but before the activation of factor X.

Pechet, L., Cochios, F. and Deykin, D.: Further studies on the 'dynia' clotting abnormality. Thromb. Diath. Haemorrh. 17: 365-380, 1967.

Pechet, L., Goldstein, C. and Deykin, D.: A hitherto undescribed heredofamilial clotting defect. Blood 24: 854-855, 1964.

Pechet, L., Goldstein, C., Cochios, F. and Deykin, D.: A previously undescribed hereditary clotting abnormality. Thromb. Diath. Haemorrh. 20 (suppl.): 269-274, 1966.

D
O
M
I
N
A
N
T

Stoddard (1939) reported an extensively affected family with a pattern consistent with autosomal dominant inheritance. This deformity also occurs in the Marfan syndrome and some other hereditary disorders. Nowak (1936) traced pectus excavatum in 2-4 generations in 12 families. A generation was skipped in 5 families.

Nowak, H.: Die erbliche Trichterbrust. Deutsch. Med. Wschr. 62: 2003-2004, 1936.

Peiper, A.: Ueber die Erblichkeit der Trichterbrust. Klin. Wschr. 1: 1647 only, 1922.

Sainsbury, H. S. K.: Congenital funnel chest. Lancet II: 615-616, 1947.

Snyder, L. H. and Curtis, G. M.: An inherited 'hollow chest,' koilosternia, a new character dependent upon a dominant autosomal gene. J. Hered. 25: 445-447, 1934.

Stoddard, S. E.: The inheritance of 'hollow chest' 'cobbler's chest' due to heredity-not an occupational deformity. J. Hered. 30: 139-141, 1939.

*16940 PELGER-HUET ANOMALY

The nucleus of the granulocytes is hyposegmented, being rod-like, dumbbell, peanut-shaped or spectacle-like. In Spokane, Wash., Ludden and Harvey (1962) found 4 cases among 43,000 persons. Affected persons were of German or Dutch descent. In Cleveland, Skendzel and Hoffman (1962) found a frequency of 1 in 4785 routine smears. All figures in this country and also that of Davidson in England (1 in 6000) are lower than that of Nachtsheim (1 in 1020). This anomaly also is found in the rabbit. The homozygote in the rabbit has chondrodystrophy (Nachtsheim, 1950). Skeletal abnormality apparently does not occur in the human homozygote (Stobbe and Jorke, 1965). See also Haverkamp Begemann and van Lookeren Campagne (1952). See MUSCULAR DYSTROPHY, PROXIMAL, for information on linkage. Rioux et al. (1968) reported an extensively affected French-Canadian kindred. The nuclei of leukocytes had a pince-nez appearance.

Haverkamp Begemann, N. and Van Lookeren Campagne, A.: Homozygous form of Pelger-Huet's nuclear anomaly in man. Acta Haematatol. 7: 295-302, 1952.

Ludden, T. E. and Harvey, M.: Pelger-Huet anomaly of leukocytes. Report of a case and survey of incidence. Am. J. Clin. Pathol. 37: 302-304, 1962.

Nachtsheim, H.: The Pelger-anomaly in man and rabbit: mendelian character of the nuclei of the leucocytes. J. Hered. 41: 131-137, 1950.

Rioux, E., St.-Arneault, G. and Brosseau, C.: The Pelger-Huet anomaly of leukocytes: description of a Quebec kindred. Canad. Med. Assoc. J. 99: 621-624, 1968.

Rosse, W. F. and Gurney, C. W.: The Pelger-Huet anomaly in three families and its uses in determining the disappearance of transfused neutrophils from the peripheral blood. Blood 14: 170-186, 1959.

Skendzel, L. P. and Hoffman, G. C.: The Pelger anomaly of leukocytes: forty-one cases in seven families. Am. J. Clin. Pathol. 37: 294-301, 1962.

Stobbe, H. and Jorke, D.: Befunde an homozygoten pelger-merkmalstragern. Schweiz. Med. Wschr. 95: 1524-1529, 1965.

*16950 PELIZAEUS-MERZBACHER DISEASE (LATE FORM)

Zerbin-Rudin and Peiffer (1964) described a late form of this condition which showed autosomal dominant inheritance rather than X-linked inheritance typical of the form with early onset. The disease simulated disseminated sclerosis in some respects. It may be the same disorder as that reported by Camp and Lowenberg (1941).

Camp, C. D. and Lowenberg, K.: An American family with Pelizaeus-Merzbacher disease. Arch. Neurol. Psychiatry 45: 261-264, 1941.

Zerbin-Rudin, E. and Peiffer, J.: Ein genetischer Beitrag zur Frage der Spaetform der Pelizaeus-Merzbacherschen Krankheit. Humangenetik 1: 107-122, 1964.

*16960 PEMPHIGUS, BENIGN FAMILIAL (HAILEY-HAILEY DISEASE)

Recurrent eruption of vesicles and bullae involving predominantly the neck, groin and axillary regions is characteristic. Histological examination shows numerous acantholytic cells and the supra-basal type of blister formation, strikingly resembling those in pemphigus vulgaris malignus. Loewenthal (1959) thought that pyogenic bacteria act as a precipitating factor. This possibility is supported by the beneficial effects of antibiotics, use of which has converted this condition into a relatively insignificant disorder. In four cases of one family, Burns et al. (1967) and Wilson et al. (1968) found Candida albicans in the lesions and found that the fungus would induce lesions in previously uninvolved skin. Izumi et al. (1971) found neomycin to be a precipitating factor in one of their patients. Berger and Lynch (1971) suggested that environmental conditions resulting in maceration and sweating could induce lesions on areas not limited to the neck, axilla and groin.

Berger, R. S. and Lynch, P. J.: Familial benign chronic pemphigus. Arch. Dermatol. 104: 380-384, 1971.

Burns, R. A., Reed, W. B., Swatek, F. E. and Omieczynski, D. T.: Familial benign chronic pemphigus. Induction of lesions by Candida albicans. Arch. Dermatol. 96: 254-258, 1967.

Ellis, F. A.: Vesicular Darier's disease (so-called benign familial pemphigus). Arch. Dermatol. Syph. 61: 715-736, 1950.

Hailey, H. and Hailey, H.: Familial benign chronic pemphigus. Report of 13 cases in 4 generations of a family and report of 9 additional cases in 4 generations of a family. Arch. Dermatol. Syph. 39: 679-685, 1939.

Izumi, A. K., Shmunes, E. and Wood, M. G.: Familial benign chronic pemphigus. Arch. Dermatol. 104: 177-181, 1971.

Loewenthal, L. J. A.: Familial benign chronic pemphigus. The role of pyogenic bacteria. Arch. Dermatol. 80: 318-326, 1959.

Polano, M. K.: Pemphigus benignus familiaris (with special reference to the histopathological diagnosis). Dermatologica 135: 66-74, 1967.

Wilson, J. W., Burns, R. A., Reed, W. B. and Hagerman, R. D.: Penfigo familiar benigno cronico. Lesiones inducidas por 'Candida albicans.' Medicina Cutanea 3: 275-280, 1968.

Winer, L. H. and Leeb, A. J.: Benign familial pemphigus. Arch. Dermatol. 67: 77-83, 1953.

*16970 PEPSINOGEN

Pepsin is one of the main proteolytic enzymes secreted by the gastric mucosa. It consists of a single polypeptide chain and arises from its precursor, pepsinogen, by removal of a segment 41 amino acids long from the amino end. Pepsin is particularly effective in cleaving peptide bonds involving aromatic amino acids. Samloff and Townes (1970) showed that the pepsinogen-5 derived from the stomach and excreted in the urine is absent in some persons. Family and population data supported the view that absence of pepsinogen-5 is recessive, i.e., persons with the pepsinogen-5 band on electrophoresis are either homozygous or heterozygous for a particular allele. Samloff et al. (1973) found no instance of absent pepsinogen-5 among Japanese, Chinese and Filipinos. Among American whites and blacks a frequency of 14 percent was found.

Dayhoff, M. O.: Other proteases. Atlas of Protein Sequences and Structure 1972 (vol. 5). Washington: National Biomedical Research Foundation, 1972. Pp. D113-D126.

Samloff, I. M. and Townes, P. L.: Pepsinogens: genetic polymorphism in man. Science 168: 144-145, 1970.

Samloff, M., Liebman, S. M., Glober, G. A., Moore, J. O. and Indra, D.: Population studies of pepsinogen polymorphism. Am. J. Hum. Genet. 25: 178-180, 1973.

*16980 PEPTIDASE A

Lewis et al. (1968) have identified genetically variable peptidases determined by alleles at two separate and not closely linked structural loci (pep A and pep B). The peptidases studied are present in red cells and are capable of hydrolyzing di- and tri-peptides. Five distinct enzymes A, B, C, D and E have been identified. Lewis and Harris (1969) stated that peptidases A, B, C and D are products of separate gene loci and that E probably is also. By analysis of mouse-human somatic cell hybrids, Creagan et al. (1973) concluded that the structural locus for peptidase A is on chromosome no. 18. Cook et al. (1972) found no sign of close linkage of peptidases A, B, C and D. There were 'hints' of linkage between Pep B and Gm, between Pep C and Rh, and between Pep D, Lutheran and secretor. The second is noteworthy because of the assignment of both Pep C and Rh to chromosome no. 1.

Cook, P. J. L., Povey, S. and Robson, E. B.: Linkage studies on peptidases A, B, C and D in man. Ann. Hum. Genet. 36: 89-98, 1972.

Creagan, R., Tischfield, J., McMorris, F. A., Chen, S., Hirschi, M., Chen, T. R., Ricciuti, F. and Ruddle, F. H.: Assignment of the genes for human peptidase A to chromosome 18 and cytoplasmic glutamic oxaloacetate transaminase to chromosome 10 using somatic cell hybrids. Cytogenet. Cell Genet. 12: 187-198, 1973.

Lewis, W. H. P.: Common polymorphism of peptidase A. Electrophoretic variants associated with quantitative variation of red cell levels. Ann. Hum. Genet. 36: 267-271, 1973.

Lewis, W. H. P. and Harris, H.: Human red cell peptidases. Nature 215: 351-355, 1967.

Lewis, W. H. P. and Harris, H.: Molecular size estimates of human peptidases determined by separate gene loci. Ann. Hum. Genet. 33: 89-92, 1969.

Lewis, W. H. P., Corney, G. and Harris, H.: Pep A5-1 and pep A6-1: two new variants of peptidase A with features of special interest. Ann. Hum. Genet. 32: 35-42, 1968.

*16990 PEPTIDASE B

See PEPTIDASE A. The peptidase B locus is linked to the LDH-B locus (Ruddle et al., 1970). Both are situated on chromosome no. 12 (Chen et al., 1973).

Blake, N. M., Kirk, R. L., Lewis, W. H. P. and Harris, H.: Some further peptidase B phenotypes. Ann. Hum. Genet. 33: 301-305, 1970.

Chen, T.-R., McMorris, F. A., Creagan, R., Ricciuti, F., Tischfield, J. and Ruddle, F.: Assignment of the genes for malate oxidoreductase decarboxylating to chromosome 6 and peptidase B and lactate dehydrogenase B to chromosome 12 in man. Am. J. Hum. Genet. 25: 200-207, 1973.

Ruddle, F. H., Chapman, V. M., Chen, T.-R. and Klebe, R. J.: Linkage between human lactate dehydrogenase A and B and peptidase B. Nature 227: 251-257, 1970.

*17000 PEPTIDASE C

See PEPTIDASE A. Among the Babinga Pygmies Benerecetti (1970) found polymorphism of peptidase C and provided the first evidence on the genetics of this red cell enzyme. Three alleles were postulated, one of which is silent and has a frequency of 0.208 in the population studied. No abnormality was detected in persons with deficiency of the enzyme. Ruddle et al. (1972) assigned the peptidase C locus to chromosome 1 by human-mouse cell hybridization studies. Furthermore, phosphoglucomutase-1 is syntenic with peptidase C. By inference then, the Rh locus (which is linked to PGM-1) is on chromosome 1. Palmer and Schroder (1971) had suggested on the basis of a variant of chromosome 9 that the Rh locus is on that chromosome. Ruddle et al. (1972) could disprove that, since clones positive for peptidase C did not possess recognizable chromosome no. 9. By cell hybridization synteny of PGM(1) and peptidase C was demonstrated by Billardon et al. (1973). The somatic hybrid studies of Jongsma et al. (1973) assigned the pep C locus to the long arm. Assuming that each arm of chromosome no. 1 is 140 male cM in length, Cook et al. (1974) concluded that, measured from the centromere, map positions are as follows: PGD 1p124; Rh 1p109; PGM-1 1p079; Fy 1p010; PEP-C 1q030.

Benerecetti, S. A. S.: Studies of African Pygmies. III. Peptidase C polymorphism in Babinga Pygmies: a frequent erythrocytic enzyme deficiency. Am. J. Hum. Genet. 22: 228-231, 1970.

Billardon, C., Van Cong, N., Picard, J. Y., Dekaouel, C., Rebourcet, R., Weil, D., Feingold, J. and Frezal, J.: Linkage studies of enzyme markers in man-mouse somatic cell hybrids. Ann. Hum. Genet. 36: 273-284, 1973.

Cook, P. J. L., Robson, E. B., Buckton, K. E., Jacobs, P. A. and Polani, P. E.: Segregation of genetic markers in families with chromosome polymorphisms and structural rearrangements involving choromsome 1. Ann. Hum. Genet. 37: 261-274, 1974.

Jongsma, A., Van Someren, H., Westerveld, A., Hagemijer, A. and Pearson, P.: Localization of genes on human chromosomes by studies of human-Chinese hamster somatic cell hybrids. Assignment of PGM to chromosome C6 and regional mapping of the PGD, PGM, and pep-C genes on chromosome A1. Humangenetik 29: 195-202, 1973.

Palmer, C. G. and Schroder, J.: A familial variant of chromosome 9. J. Med. Genet. 8: 202-208, 1971.

Povey, S., Corney, G., Lewis, W. H. P., Robson, E. B., Parrington, J. M. and Harris, H.: The genetics of peptidase C in man. Ann. Hum. Genet. 35: 455-466, 1972.

Ruddle, F., Ricciuti, F., McMorris, F. A., Tischfield, J., Creagan, R., Darlington, G. and Chen, T.: Somatic cell genetic assignment of peptidase C and the Rh linkage group to chromosome A-1 in man. Science 176: 1429-1431, 1972.

*17010 PEPTIDASE D (PROLIDASE)

Lewis and Harris (1969) identified a number of electrophoretic variants of peptidase D of red cells.

Lewis, W. H. P. and Harris, H.: Peptidase D (prolidase) variants in man. Ann. Hum. Genet. 32: 317-322, 1969.

*17020 PEPTIDASE E

See PEPTIDASE A.

*17025 PEPTIDASE S

This peptidase has been found suitable for study in cell hybrids (Shows, 1973). Chromosomal assignment of the structural locus has not been achieved, however.

Lewis, W. H. and Harris, H.: Human red cell peptidases. Nature 215: 351-355, 1967.

Shows, T. B.: Buffalo, personal communication, 1973.

*17030 PERIODIC FEVER

Bouroncle and Doan (1957) described 12 cases of periodic fever in 6 sibships in 5 generations of a family. No abnormality was detected by clinical examinations during and between attacks or by many laboratory studies. In two brothers with periodic fever, Driessen et al. (1968) found that the non-esterified etiocholanolone level of the blood was raised not only during febrile attacks but also in fever-free periods. A sister had attacks of fever of unexplained origin accompanied by abdominal pain and rash but had no symptoms after menarche.

Bouroncle, B. A. and Doan, C. A.: 'Periodic fever.' Occurrence in five generations. Am. J. Med. 23: 502-506, 1957.

Driessen, O., Voute, P. A., Jr. and Vermeulen, A.: A description of two brothers with permanently raised non-esterified aetiocholanolone blood level. Acta Endocrinol. 57: 177-186, 1968.

*17040 PERIODIC PARALYSIS I (HYPOKALEMIC TYPE)

The classic picture is episodic weakness accompanied by low serum potassium levels. The attacks are aborted by administration of potassium or by exercise and are precipitated by insulin or glucose adminstration.

Cusins, P. J. and Van Rooyen, R. J.: Familial periodic paralysis. Seven cases in a Durban family. S. Afr. Med. J. 37: 1180-1183, 1963.

Pearson, C. M. and Kalyanaraman, K.: The periodic paralyses. In, Stanbury, J. B., Wyngaarden, J. B. and Fredrickson, D. S. (eds.): The Metabolic Basis of Inherited Disease. New York: McGraw-Hill, 1972 (3rd Ed.). Pp. 1181-1203.

Talbott, J. H.: Periodic paralysis: a clinical syndrome. Medicine 20: 85-143, 1941.

*17050 PERIODIC PARALYSIS II (HYPERKALEMIC TYPE)

Myotonic symptoms in periodic paralysis can be a clue that the disorder is of the hyperkalemic type. Ocular muscle myotonia is indicated by slow opening of the lids after forced active closure of the eyes. Potassium precipitates weakness. Gamstorp (1956, 1963) who first described hyperkalemic periodic paralysis (calling it adynamia episodica hereditaria) did not find myotonia in her cases. Whether two distinct entities are represented is not clear. Myotonia was present in Samaha's family (1965). Krull et al. (1966) claimed to have demonstrated a humoral substance, not potassium, originating from the contracting muscles of the forearm and producing striking generalized myotonia. Van'T Hoff (1962) found nine affected persons in four generations. All suffered from periodic attacks of weakness which could be induced by administering potassium and alleviated by administering calcium. Both between and during attacks, affected persons had myotonic lid lag lasting 15-20 seconds after elevation of the eyes. The family of Saunders et al. (1968) showed myotonic periodic paralysis with muscle wasting.

Armstrong, F. S.: Hyperkalemic familial periodic paralysis (adynamia episodica hereditaria). Ann. Intern. Med. 57: 455-461, 1962.

Gamstorp, I.: Adynamia episodica hereditaria and myotonia. Acta Neurol. Scand. 39: 41-58, 1963.

Gamstorp, I.: Adynamia episodica hereditaria. Acta Paediatr. 45 (suppl. 108): 1-126, 1956.

Herman, R. H. and McDowell, M. K.: Hyperkalemic paralysis (adynamia episodica hereditaria). Report of 4 cases and clinical studies. Am. J. Med. 35: 749-767, 1963.

Krull, G. H., Leijnse, B., De Vlieger, M., Vietor, W. P. J., Ter Braak, J. W. G. and Gerbrandy, J.: Myotonia produced by an unknown humoral substance. Lancet II: 668-672, 1966.

Layzer, R. B., Lovelace, R. E. and Rowland, L. P.: Hyperkalemic periodic paralysis. Arch. Neurol. 16: 455-472, 1967.

Samaha, F. J.: Hyperkalemic periodic paralysis. A genetic study, clinical observations, and report of a new method of therapy. Arch. Neurol. 12: 145-154, 1965.

Saunders, M., Ashworth, B., Emery, A. E. H. and Benedikz, J. E. G.: Familial myotonic periodic paralysis with muscle wasting. Brain 91: 295-304, 1968.

Van'T Hoff, W.: Familial myotonic periodic paralysis. Quart. J. Med. 31: 385-402, 1962.

*17060 PERIODIC PARALYSIS III (NORMOKALEMIC TYPE)

In the family reported by Poskanzer and Kerr (1961) 21 members were affected. In addition to normokalemia, favorable response to sodium chloride was an unusual feature. Danowski (1973) expressed doubts about the distinctness of the normokalemic and hyperkalemic types. Danowski et al. (1974) consider the normokalemic and hyperkalemic varieties of periodic paralysis to be one and the same entity.

Danowski, T. S.: Pittsburgh, personal communication, Aug., 1973.

Danowski, T. S., Fisher, E. R., Vidalon, C., Vester, J. W., Thompson, R., Nolan, S. and Stephan, T.: Clinical and ultrastructural observations in a kindred with normo-hyperkalemic periodic paralysis. Am. J. Med., in press, 1974.

Poskanzer, D. C. and Kerr, D. N. S.: A third type of periodic paralysis, with normokalemia and favorable response to sodium chloride. Am. J. Med. 31: 328-342, 1961.

17070 PERIPHERAL DYSOSTOSIS

Singleton, Daeschner and Teng (1960) reported a form of dysostosis limited essentially to the tubular bones of the hands and feet. The epiphyses in the fingers are conical in shape with their apex set into the metaphyseal ends of the phalanges (which look like the bottom of wine bottles). The cone-shaped epiphyses in the phalanges with a paucity of signs and symptoms elsewhere is characteristic. Bachman and Norman (1967) reported affected mother and her son and daughter; the mother, age 47, was 61.5 inches tall, had short fingers and suffered from severe osteoarthritis of the hips. This is probably a heterogeneous category in which one entity is the condition termed acrodysostosis (q.v.), in which pug nose, open mouth and prognathism, together with mental deficiency are additional features. Changes were almost limited to the hands and feet in the patient reported by Cohen and Van Creveld (1963). The facies were characterized by pug nose and sunken bridge but the skull did not suggest achondroplasia. Intelligence was considered normal.

Bachman, R. K. and Norman, A. P.: Hereditary peripheral dysostosis (three cases). Proc. R. Soc. Med. 60: 21 only, 1967.

Cohen, P. and Van Creveld, S.: Peripheral dysostosis. Br. J. Radiol. 36: 761-765, 1963.

Newcombe, D. S. and Keats, T. E.: Roentgenographic manifestations of hereditary peripheral dysostosis. Am. J. Roentgen. 106: 178-189, 1969.

Singleton, E. B., Daeschner, C. W. and Teng, C. T.: Peripheral dysostosis. Am. J. Roentgen. 84: 499-505, 1960.

17090 PERNICIOUS ANEMIA

In the relatives of thirty-four pernicious anemia probands, McIntyre and her associates (1959) tested the ability to absorb orally given doses of cobalt-60 labeled vitamin B12 (Schilling test). The relatives of pernicious anemia patients showed a negative correlation with age; control subjects did not. The relatives showed a tendency to bimodality. 48 percent of sibs and 32 percent of offspring had abnormal absorption. The authors suggested autosomal dominant inheritance. Wangel et al. (1968) suggested that the tendency to form autoantibodies against gastric parietal cells may be inherited as a dominant with incomplete penetrance. Later studies (McIntyre, 1968) yielded results which make a simple genetic hypothesis difficult to support.

McIntyre, P. A.: Genetic and auto-immune features of pernicious anemia. I. Unreliability of the Schilling test in detecting genetic predisposition to the disease. Johns Hopkins Med. J. 122: 181-183, 1968.

McIntyre, P. A., Hahn, R., Conley, C. L. and Glass, B.: Genetic factors in predisposition to pernicious anemia. Bull. Hopkins Hosp. 104: 309-342, 1959.

Wangel, A. G., Callender, S. T., Spray, G. H. and Wright, R.: A family study of pernicious anaemia. I. Autoantibodies, achlorhydria, serum pepsinogen and vitamin B12. Brit. J. Haemat. 14: 161-181, 1968. II. Intrinsic factor secretion, vitamin B12 absorption and genetic aspects of gastric autoimmunity. Brit. J. Haemat. 14: 183-204, 1968.

17095 PERNIOSIS (CHILBLAINS)

Harris (1947) concluded that tendency to excessive reaction to cold with development of severe perniosis may be inherited as an irregular dominant.

Harris, H.: A genetical factor in perniosis. Ann. Eugen. 14: 32-34, 1947.

17098 PERONEAL NERVE, ACCESSORY DEEP

Crutchfield and Gutmann (1973) found that the accessory deep peroneal nerve, a branch of the superficial peroneal nerve, partially innervated the extensor digitorum brevis muscle of at least one foot in 22 of 100 healthy unrealted persons. Five families studied because of a member with anomalous innervation yielded results they interpreted as indicating dominant inheritance.

Crutchfield, C. A. and Gutmann, L.: Hereditary aspects of accessory deep peroneal nerve. J. Neurol. Neurosurg. Psychiatry 36: 989-990, 1973.

17100 PEYRONIE DISEASE

This condition, a fibrous contracture of the penis, bears certain fundamental similarities to Dupuytren contracture of the hand and the two occur rather frequently in the same subject.

Murley, R. S.: Peyronie's disease. Br. Med. J. 1: 908 only, 1964.

Schourup, K.: Plastic induration of the penis. Acta Radiol. 26: 313-323, 1945.

17110 PHAGOCYTOSIS, PLASMA-RELATED DEFECT IN

Miller et al. (1968) described a familial disorder of phagocytosis due to a plasma-associated defect rather than a primary defect of polymorphonuclear leukocyte function. Leukocytes from the proband, incubated in her own plasma, showed greatly diminished ability to ingest yeast, rice-starch, or Staphylococcus aureus, but ingested the same particles normally in the presence of heterozygote plasma. Normal leukocytes showed impaired phagocytosis when incubated in plasma from the patient. The mother and many relatives had plasma which gave the same result. The father and two sibs were 'negative.' Both maternal grandparents and sibs of both of them were 'positive.' Consanguinity of these grandparents was considered possible but not proved. Infusion of fresh plasma corrected the deficiency of opsonization and was regularly followed by clinical improvement. The possibility of non-paternity was apparently not investigated. A priori, recessive inheritance would seem more likely, the proband being homozygous.

Miller, M. E., Seals, J., Kaye, R. and Levitsky, L.: A familial, plasma-associated defect of phagocytosis. A new cause of recurrent bacterial infections. Lancet II: 60-63, 1968.

*17120 PHENYLTHIOCARBAMIDE (PTC) TASTING

Supplementation of the standard test using quinine in the intermediate cases was suggested by Kalmus (1958). Ability to taste is dominant.

Harris, H. and Kalmus, H.: The measurement of taste sensitivity to phenylthiourea (PTC). Ann. Eugen. 15: 24-31, 1949.

Kalmus, H.: Improvements in the classification of the taster genotypes. Ann. Hum. Genet. 22: 222-230, 1958.

*17130 PHEOCHROMOCYTOMA

Adrenal medullary tumors occur sometimes with von Hippel-Lindau syndrome (q.v.), with neurofibromatosis (q.v.), and with familial endocrine adenomatosis. (See NEUROMATA, MUCOSAL, WITH ENDOCRINE TUMORS and see PHEOCHROMOCYTOMA WITH AMYLOID-PRODUCING MEDULLARY THYROID CARCINOMA, as examples of two other syndromes with pheochromocytoma as a feature.) Occurring as an isolated defect it probably is also inherited as a simple dominant in some families. The relation of the condition in the family reported by Hadorn (1963) is uncertain. Three sibs had adrenal tumors. A brother and sister suffered from tachycardia, sweating, hypertension and albuminuria. The sister had advanced hypertensive retinopathy and the brother had congestive heart failure. At autopsy the sister showed cerebral hemorrhage and bilateral adrenocortical tumors. A surviving sib developed similar symptoms. Pheochromocytoma was tentatively diagnosed. The regitine test was strongly positive, the urine contained large amounts of norepinephrine and pneumoperitoneum demonstrated an enlarged right adrenal. At operation a mixed tumor containing hypernephromatous and paraganglion tissue was found. The very large kindred studied by Tisherman et al. (1962) had at least 7 patients with pheochromocytoma. One or more cafe-au-lait spots (in 22 persons), extensive hemangiomas (in 2 persons) and angiomatosis retinae (in 2 persons) were discovered in members of the family. Pheochromocytoma was associated with congenital cataracts in one patient and with renal artery stenosis in another. Pheochromocytoma occurred in at least four members, including father and son, of a family studied by Swinton et al. (1972). They pointed out that hypercalcemia, corrected by adrenalectomy, can be associated with pheochromocytoma. This may be due to secretion of a calcitonin-like substance. The difficulties of discriminating this from multiple endocrine adenomatosis is obvious. Familial pheochromocytoma is usually bilateral and the patients are likely to show resistance to the vasopressor effects of tyramine (Engelman et al., 1968). Knudson and Strong (1972) have applied to pheochromocytoma Knudson's two mutation theory (see 18020) and concluded that it fits.

Carman, C. T. and Brashear, R. E.: Pheochromocytoma as an inherited abnormality: report of the tenth affected kindred and review of the literature. N. Engl. J. Med. 263: 419-423, 1960.

Cook, J. E., Ulrich, R. W., Sample, H. G., Jr. and Fawcett, N. W.: Peculiar familial and malignant pheochromocytomas of the organs of Zuckerkandl. Ann. Intern. Med. 52: 126-133, 1960.

Engelman, K., Horwitz, D., Ambrose, I. M. and Sjoerdsma, A.: Further evaluation of the tyramine test for pheochromocytoma. N. Engl. J. Med. 278: 705-709, 1968.

Hadorn, W.: Maligne Hypernephroide und paraganglionaere Mischgeschwuelste der Nebenniere bei drei Geschwistern. Helv. Med. Acta 30: 291-296, 1963.

Knudson, A. G., Jr. and Strong, L. C.: Mutation and cancer: neuroblastoma and pheochromocytoma. Am. J. Hum. Genet. 24: 514-532, 1972.

Strunge, P., Ingsrup, H. M., Lochte, J. J. and Zimmermann-Nielsen, C.: Bilateral phaeochromocytoma in two brothers. Acta Paediat. Scand. 61: 729-732, 1972.

Swinton, N. W., Clerkin, E. P. and Flint, L. D.: Hypercalcemia and familial pheochromocytoma. Correction after adrenalectomy. Ann. Intern. Med. 76: 455-457, 1972.

Tisherman, S. E., Gregg, F. J. and Danowski, T. S.: Familial pheochromocytoma. J.A.M.A. 182: 152-156, 1962.

Tradec, E., Maratka, Z. and Palecrova, M.: Le pheochromocytome avec caractere familial. J. Chir. 81: 479, 1961.

Von Doepp, C. E.: Das Phaeochromocytom als dominant vererbbare dysgenetische Geschwulst. Virchow Arch. Pathol. Anat. 335: 231-239, 1962.

*17140 PHEOCHROMOCYTOMA AND AMYLOID-PRODUCING MEDULLARY THYROID CARCINOMA (PTC SYNDROME) ;SIPPLE SYNDROME

Schimke and Hartmann (1965) described a syndrome of pheochromocytoma and medullary thyroid carcinoma with abundant amyloid stroma. A similar although perhaps distinct condition is described under NEUROMATA, MUCOSAL, WITH ENDOCRINE TUMORS. Steiner et al. (1967) described a family with 11 cases in successive generations. The pheochromocytomas were bilateral. Parathyroid adenoma was present in several. One patient had Cushing syndrome. Urbanski (1967) also found parathyroid adenoma to be part of the syndrome. Meyer and Abdel-Bari (1968) presented observations consistent with the view that medullary carcinoma is a thyrocalcitonin-producing neoplasm of parafollicular cells of the thyroid. Parathyroid hyperplasia or adenomas in some of these patients may be secondary to hypocalcemic effects of thyrocalcitonin. Johnston et al. (1970), as well as others, have shown calcitonin-secretion by medullary thyroid carcinoma. Steiner et al. (1967) referred to this disorder as 'multiple endocrine neoplasia, type II' to distinguish it from the multiple endocrine adenomatosis described by Wermer (q.v.), called type I by Steiner et al. (1967). Kaplan et al. (1970) showed that the adrenal medulla produces a calcitonin-like material indistinguishable from that of the thyroid by bio- and radioimmunoassay. They suggest that the parafollicular cells of the thyroid are of neural crest origin. The finding that medullary carcinoma of the thyroid arises from parafollicular cells and that like the cell of origin it sometimes produces thyrocalcitonin may account for the association of parathyroid hyperplasia and perhaps parathyroid adenoma. Poloyan et al. (1970) was impressed with the histologic similarity between the medullary thyroid cancer and pheochromocytoma metastases. Keiser et al. (1973), in a review pointed out that histaminase is useful in the identification of metastases of medullary carcinoma. In their opinion parathyroid adenomas are a primary feature of the disorder. Pearson et al. (1973) studied 21 members of a kindred with surgically confirmed multiple endocrine neoplasms. All 21 had medullary carcinoma of the thyroid. Adrenal pheochromocytomas were present in 10 and were bilateral in 6. Three had one or more parathyroid glands showing adenomatous hyperplasia and 10 showed chief cell hyperplasia. The thyroid cancer metastasized to other areas including the liver, lungs and bone in several of the patients. All patients had elevated peripheral thyrocalcitonin. Peripheral parathyroid hormone was elevated in only two; however, parathyroid hormone was elevated in the inferior thyroid vein of all patients examined.

Anderson, T. E., Spackman, T. J. and Schwartz, S. S.: Roentgen findings in intestinal ganglioneuromatosis. Its association with medullary thyroid carcinoma and pheochromocytoma. Radiology 101: 93-96, 1971.

Block, M. A., Horn, R. C., Jr., Miller, J. M., Barrett, J. L. and Brush, B. E.: Familial medullary carcinoma of the thyroid. Ann. Surg. 166: 403-412, 1967.

Cushman, P., Jr.: Familial endocrine tumors. Report of two unrelated kindred affected with pheochromocytomas, one also with multiple thyroid carcinomas. Am. J. Med. 32: 352-360, 1962.

Johnston, C. I., Martin, T. J. and Riddell, J.: Medullary thyroid carcinoma: a functional peptide secreting tumor. Aust. Ann. Med. 19: 50-53, 1970.

Kaplan, E. L., Arnaud, C. D., Hill, B. J. and Peskin; G. W.: Adrenal medullary calcitonin-like factor: a key to multiple endocrine neoplasia, type 2? Surgery 68: 146-149, 1970.

Keiser, H. R., Beaver, M. A., Doppman, J., Wells, S., Jr. and Buja, L. M.: Sipple's syndrome: medullary thyroid carcinoma, pheochromocytoma, and parathyroid disease. Ann. Intern. Med. 78: 561-579, 1973.

Lima, J. B. and Smith, P. D.: Sipple's syndrome (pheochromocytoma and thyroid carcinoma) with bilateral breast carcinoma. Am. J. Surg. 121: 732-735, 1971.

Meyer, J. S. and Abdel-Bari, W.: Granules and thyrocalcitonin-like activity in medullary carcinoma of the thyroid gland. N. Engl. J. Med. 278: 523-529, 1968.

Poloyan, E., Scanu, A., Straus, F. H., Pickleman, J. R. and Paloyan, D.: Familial pheochromocytoma, medullary thyroid carcinoma, and parathyroid adenomas. J.A.M.A. 214: 1443-1447, 1970.

Pearson, K. D., Wells, S. A. and Keiser, H. R.: Familial medullary carcinoma of the thyroid, adrenal phenochromocytoma and parathyroid hyperplasia. A syndrome of multiple endocrine neoplasia. Radiology 107: 249-256, 1973.

Sarosi, G. and Doe, R. P.: Familial occurrence of parathyroid adenomas, pheochromocytoma, and medullary carcinoma of the thyroid with amyloid stroma (Sipple's syndrome). Ann. Intern. Med. 68: 1305-1309, 1968.

Schimke, R. N. and Hartmann, W. H.: Familial amyloid-producing medullary thyroid carcinoma and pheochromocytoma, a distinct genetic entity. Ann. Intern. Med. 63: 1027-1039, 1965.

Sipple, J. H.: The association of pheochromocytoma with carcinoma of the thyroid gland. Am. J. Med. 31: 163-166, 1961.

Steiner, A. L., Goodman, A. D. and Powers, S. R., Jr.: Study of a kindred with pheochromocytoma, medullary thyroid carcinoma, hyperparathyroidism and Cushing's disease: multiple endocrine neoplasia, type II. Medicine 47: 371-409, 1968.

Tashjian, A. H., Jr. and Melvin, K. E. W.: Medullary carcinoma of the thyroid: thyrocalcitonin in plasma and tumor. N. Engl. J. Med. 279: 279-283, 1968.

Urbanski, F. X.: Medullary thyroid carcinoma, parathyroid adenoma, and bilateral pheochromocytoma. An unusual triad of endocrine tumors. J. Chronic Dis. 20: 627-636, 1967.

*17150 PHOSPHATASE, ACID, OF ERYTHROCYTE (ACP-1)

Hopkinson, Spencer and Harris (1963) described a new human polymorphism involving erythrocyte acid phosphatase as demonstrated in starch-gel electrophoresis. Three alleles, P(a), P(b) and P(c), are thought to be involved, their frequency being estimated to be about 0.35, 0.60 and 0.05, respectively. Another rare allele, P(r), was described by Giblett and Scott (1965). Weitkamp et al. (1969) presented data suggesting that the acid phosphatase locus may be on chromosome no. 2. Nguyen and Moullec (1971) believed that acid phosphatase and Lewis loci are linked. Renwick (1971) presented an analysis of the Weitkamp data supporting assignment to chromosome no. 2. Ferguson-Smith et al. (1973) presented evidence that the acid phosphatase locus is on the distal end of the short arm of chromosome no. 2 (somewhere between 2p23 and 2pter, according to the Paris terminology). A child lacking this segment was of phenotype B whereas the father and mother were homozygous phenotype B and A, respectively. Mace and Robson (1973) presented data consistent with loose linkage of red cell acid phosphatase and MNS blood group. There was also a hint of linkage between ACP and Kidd blood group. Hulten et al. (1966) described a family in which studies of a reciprocal translocation chromosome involving no. 2 suggested that the Kidd locus may be on one of the involved chromosomes. Swallow et al. (1973) showed that 'red cell' acid phosphatase is not limited to erythrocytes but can be demonstrated in other tissues, including cultured fibroblasts and lymphoblastoid cells where there is no possibility of contamination by blood. Cell hybrid studies confirmed the localization of acid phosphatase-1 on chromosome no. 2.

Ferguson-Smith, M. A., Newman, B. F., Ellis, P. M., Thomson, D. M. G. and Riley, I. D.: Assignment by deletion of human red cell acid phosphatase gene locus to the short arm of chromosome 2. Nature 243: 271-273, 1973.

Fisher, R. A. and Harris, H.: Studies on the separate isoenzymes of red cell acid phosphatase phenotypes A and B. Chromatographic separation of the isoenzymes. Ann. Hum. Genet. 34: 431-438, 1971.

Fuhrmann, W. and Lichte, K. H.: Human red cell acid phosphatase polymorphism. A study on gene frequency and forensic use of the system in cases of disputed paternity. Humangenetik 3: 121-126, 1966.

Giblett, E. R. and Scott, N. M.: Red cell acid phosphatase: racial distribution and report of a new phenotype. Am. J. Hum. Genet. 17: 425-432, 1965.

Herbich, J. and Meinhart, K.: The rare 'silent' allele P(O) or P(V) (P Vienna) of human red cell acid phosphatase, typed in a second family. Humangenetik 15: 345-348, 1972.

Herbich, J., Fisher, R. A. and Hopkinson, D. A.: Atypical segregation of human red cell acid phosphatase phenotypes: evidence for a rare 'silent' allele P(O). Ann. Hum. Genet. 34: 145-152, 1970.

Hopkinson, D. A., Spencer, N. and Harris, H.: Red cell acid phosphatase variants: a new human polymorphism. Nature 199: 969-971, 1963.

Hulten, M., Lindsten, J., Pen-Ming, L. M., Fraccaro, M., Mannini, A., Tiepolo, L., Robson, E. B., Heiken, A. and Tillinger, K. G.: Possible localization of the genes for the Kidd blood group on an autosome involved in a reciprocal translocation. Nature 211: 1067-1068, 1966.

Karp, G. W., Jr. and Sutton, H. E.: Some new phenotypes of human red cell acid phosphatase. Am. J. Hum. Genet. 19: 54-62, 1967.

Mace, M. and Robson, E. B.: Linkage data on ACP(1) and MNS. Intern. Workshop on Human Gene Mapping, New Haven, Conn., June, 1973.

Nguyen, Van-Cong and Moullec, J.: Linkage probable entre les groupes de phosphatase acide des globules rouges et le systeme Lewis. Ann. Genet. 14: 121-125, 1971.

Renwick, J. H.: Assignment and map-positioning of human loci using chromosomal variation. Ann. Hum. Genet. 35: 79-97, 1971.

Swallow, D. M., Povey, S. and Harris, H.: Activity of the 'red cell' acid phosphatase locus in other tissues. Ann. Hum. Genet. 37: 31-38, 1973.

Weitkamp, L. R., Janzen, M. K., Guttormsen, S. A. and Gershowitz, H.: Inherited pericentric inversion of chromosome number two: a linkage study. Ann. Hum. Genet. 33: 53-59, 1969.

Weitkamp, L. R., Johnston, E. and Guttormsen, S. A.: Genetic linkage of Pi and AcP(1). (Abstract) Am. J. Hum. Genet. 26: 92A only, 1974.

*17165 PHOSPHATASE, ACID, OF TISSUES (LYSOSOMAL ACID PHOSPHATASE; ACP-2 — BETA POLYPEPTIDE)

This appears to be chemically and presumably genetically distinct from red cell acid phosphatase (Lundin and Allison, 1966). It should be useful in both family and cellular studies of gene localization. Lysosomal acid phosphatase deficiency is described elsewhere (20095). The ACP-2 locus is syntenic with the LDH-A locus (15000) and therefore can be assigned to chromosome no. 11. Beckman et al. (1970) studied variants of this enzyme.

Beckman, G., Beckman, L. and Tarnvik, A.: A rare subunit variant shared by five acid phosphatase isozymes from human leukocytes and placentae. Hum. Hered. 20: 81-85, 1970.

Bruns, G. A. P. and Gerald, P. S.: Human acid phosphatase in somatic cell hybrids. Science 184: 480-482, 1974.

Harris, H., Hopkinson, D. A. and Robson, E. B.: The incidence of rare alleles determining electrophoretic variants: data on 43 enzyme loci in man. Ann. Hum. Genet. 37: 237-253, 1974.

Lundin, L. G. and Allison, A. C.: Acid phosphatases from different organs and animal forms compared by starch-gel electrophoresis. Acta Chem. Scand. 20: 2572-2579, 1966.

*17166 PHOSPHATASE, ACID, OF TISSUES (LYSOSOMAL ACID PHOSPHATASE; ACP-3 — ALPHA POLYPEPTIDE)

Swallow and Harris (1972) found a new variant in placental and leukocyte acid phosphatase. Their findings and those of Beckman (17165) suggested to them that the acid phsophatase is a dimer, that two dissimilar subunits (alpha and beta) can be present and that the three isozymes in placenta and leukocytes are alpha-alpha (A), and alpha-beta (B), and beta-beta (C) in composition. Their new variant appears to involve one subunit, that which they designate alpha.

Swallow, D. M. and Harris, H.: A new variant of the placental acid phosphatases. Its complications regarding their subunit structures and genetical determination. Ann. Hum. Genet. 36: 141 only, 1972.

17170 PHOSPHATASE, ALKALINE, BLOOD-GROUP-ASSOCIATED

Both the ABO and the secretor loci influence the appearance of alkaline phosphatase in the serum. Many uncertainties about the genetic control of alkaline phosphatase exist.

Beckman, L., Bjorling, G. and Heiken, A.: Human alkaline phosphatases and the factors controlling their appearance in serum. Acta Genet. Statist. Med. 16: 305-312, 1966.

Shreffler, D. C.: Genetic studies of blood group — associated variations in human serum alkaline phosphatase. Am. J. Hum. Genet. 17: 71-86, 1965.

17174 PHOSPHATASE, INTESTINAL ALKALINE

Harris et al. (1974) found no genetic variants by electrophoretic means.

Harris, H., Hopkinson, D. A. and Robson, E. B.: The incidence of rare alleles determining electrophoretic variants: data on 43 enzyme loci in man. Ann. Hum. Genet. 37: 237-253, 1974.

17176 PHOSPHATASE, LIVER ALKALINE

Harris et al. (1974) found no genetic variants by electrophoretic means.

Harris, H., Hopkinson, D. A. and Robson, E. B.: The incidence of rare alleles determining electrophoretic variants: data on 43 enzyme loci in man. Ann. Hum. Genet. 37: 237-253, 1974.

*17180 PHOSPHATASE, PLACENTAL ALKALINE

Boyer (1961, 1963) described an electrophoretic variant of alkaline phosphatase which appears in the serum during pregnancy in some but not all women and demonstrated its origin in the placenta. Since the human placenta is largely fetal in origin, the polymorphism may be a characteristic determined by the fetal genotype. Robson and Harris (1965) studied the genetics. Beckman et al. (1967) found a rare phenotype, absence of placental alkaline phosphatase, in twins and suggested that these twins might be homozygous for a 'silent allele.' The twins were also concordant for Crouzon craniofacial dysostosis, raising the question of a causal relationship.

Beckman, L., Beckman, G., Christodoulou, C. and Ifekwunigwe, A.: Variations in human placental alkaline phosphatase. Acta Genet. Statist. Med. 17: 406-412, 1967.

Beckman, L., Bjorling, G. and Christodoulou, C.: Pregnancy enzymes and placental polymorphism. Alkaline phosphatase. Acta Genet. Statist. Med. 16: 59-73, 1966.

Boyer, S. H.: Alkaline phosphatase in human sera and placenta. Science 134: 1002-1004, 1961.

Boyer, S. H.: Human organ alkaline phosphatases: discrimination by several means including starch gel electrophoresis of antienzyme-enzyme supernatant fluids. Ann. N.Y. Acad. Sci. 103: 938-950, 1963.

Donald, L. J. and Robson, E. B.: Rare variants of placental alkaline phosphatase. Ann. Hum. Genet. 37: 303-313, 1974.

Edwards, J. H. and Wingham, J.: Data on linkage between the locus determining placental alkaline phosphatase and other markers. Ann. Hum. Genet. 30: 233-237, 1967.

Robinson, J. C. and Goldsmith, L. A.: Genetically determined variants of serum alkaline phosphatase: a review. Vox Sang. 13: 289-307, 1967.

Robson, E. B. and Harris, H.: Genetics of the alkaline phosphatase polymorphism of the human placenta. Nature 207: 1257-1259, 1965.

17185 PHOSPHOFRUCTOKINASE (PFK) DEFICIENCY HEMOLYTIC ANEMIA

PFK may be the rate-limiting step in erythrocyte glycolysis under physiologic red cell pH. Waterbury and Frenkel (1972) found an intermediate level (60 percent of normal) of this enzyme in the red cells of a physician with chronic compensated hemolysis and in his mother and grandmother who lacked evidence of hemolysis. The proband had 9 percent reticulocytes. PFK of the proband showed markedly increased lability on in vitro storage. The absence of muscle disease and normal in vivo lactate production differentiated this family from type VII glycogen storage disease (23280).

Waterbury, L. and Frenkel, E. P.: Hereditary nonspherocytic hemolysis with erythrocyte phosphofructokinase deficiency. Blood 39: 415-425, 1972.

*17190 PHOSPHOGLUCOMUTASE-1: PGM(1)

By starch gel electrophoresis, Spencer, Hopkinson and Harris (1964) demonstrated polymorphism of phosphoglucomutase, the enzyme which catalyzes the transfer of a phosphate group between the 1- and 6-positions of glucose. Hopkinson and Harris (1965) presented evidence for the existence of two structural loci PGM(1) and PGM(2). Locus PGM(1) is thought to be responsible for electrophoretically slow-moving components and at least 5 alleles have been identified. Locus PGM(2) determines the electrophoretically fast-moving components and at least 3 alleles may exist at this locus. Evidence of a third structural locus controlling phosphoglucomutase was presented by Hopkinson (1966). The phosphoglucomutases are monomers. The existence of three genetic forms must mean that three separate enzymes have PGM specificity. This is not a situation in which polypeptide chains of different genetic origin combine in a single protein, as is the case with lactate dehydrogenase and hemoglobin. Parrington et al. (1968) found that the three PGM loci are not closely linked with each other. By the hamster-man cell hybridization method the PGM(1) locus was shown by Westerveld and Bootsma (1971) to be on the same chromosome as 6PGD (17220). By cell hybridization synteny of PGM(1) and peptidase C was demonstrated by Billardon et al. (1973). These loci are on chromosome no. 1. Douglas et al. (1973) demonstrated that the PGM-1 and 6PGD loci are on the distal end of the short arm of chromosome no. 1. Assuming that each arm of chromosome no. 1 is 140 male cM in length, Cook et al. (1974) concluded that, measrued from the centromere, map positions are as follows: PGD 1p124; Rh 1p109; PGM-1 1p079; Fy 1p010, PEP-C 1q030.

Billardon, C., Van Cong, N., Picard, J. Y., Dekaouel, C., Recourcet, R., Weil, D., Feingold, J. and Frezal, J.: Linkage studies of enzyme markers in man-mouse somatic cell hybrids. Ann. Hum. Genet. 36: 273-284, 1973.

Cook, P. J. L., Robson, E. B., Buckton, K. E., Jacobs, P. A. and Polani, P. E.: Segregation of genetic markers in families with chromosome polymorphisms and structural rearrangements involving chromosome 1. Ann. Hum. Genet. 37: 261-274, 1974.

Douglas, G. R., McAlpine, P. J. and Hamerton, J. L.: Regional localization of loci for human PGM(1) and 6PGD on human chromosome one by use of hybrids of Chinese hamster-human somatic cells. Proc. Nat. Acad. Sci. 70: 2737-2740, 1973.

Gedde-Dahl, T., Jr. and Monn, E.: Linkage relations of the phosphoglucomutase PGM(1) locus in man. Probable linkage to phenylthiocarbamid (PTC) taster locus. Acta Genet. Statist. Med. 17: 482-494, 1967.

Hopkinson, D. A. and Harris, H.: Rare phosphoglucomutase phenotypes. Ann. Hum. Genet. 30: 167-181, 1966.

Ishimoto, G.: Placental phosphoglucomutase in Japanese. Jap. J. Hum. Genet. 14: 183-188, 1969.

Quick, C. B., Fisher, R. A. and Harris, H.: Differentiation of the PGM(2) locus isozymes from those of PGM(1) and PGM(3) in terms of phosphopentomutase activity. Ann. Hum. Genet. 35: 445-454, 1972.

McAlpine, P. J., Hopkinson, D. A. and Harris, H.: Thermostability studies on the isoenzymes of human phosphoglucomutase. Ann. Hum. Genet. 34: 61-71, 1970.

Monn, E.: A new red cell phosphoglucomutase phenotype in man. Acta Genet. Statist. Med. 18: 123-127, 1967.

Parrington, J. M., Cruickshank, G., Hopkinson, D. A., Robson, E. B. and Harris, H.: Linkage

relationships between the three phosphoglucomutase loci PGM(1), PGM(2) and PGM(3). Ann. Hum. Genet.
32: 27-34, 1968.

Santachiara-Benerecetti.,Cattaneo, A. and Meera Khan, P.: Rare phenotypes of the PGM(1) and PGM(2) loci and a new PGM(2) variant allele in the Indians. Am. J. Hum. Genet. 24: 680-685, 1972.

Shinoda, T. and Matsunaga, E.: Polymorphism of red cell phosphoglucomutase among Japanese. Jap. J. Hum. Genet. 14: 316-323, 1970.

Spencer, N., Hopkinson, D. A. and Harris, H.: Phosphoglucomutase polymorphism in man. Nature 204: 742-745, 1964.

Westerveld, A. and Bootsma, D.: Personal communication to J. H. Renwick, 1971.

*17200 PHOSPHOGLUCOMUTASE-2: PGM(2)

See above description. By cell hybrid studies, PGM-2 was assigned to chromosome no. 4 (2nd International Workshop on Human Gene Mapping, Rotterdam, July, 1974).

Hopkinson, D. A. and Harris, H.: Evidence for a second 'structural' locus determining human phosphoglucomutase. Nature 208: 410-412, 1965.

*17210 PHOSPHOGLUCOMUTASE-3: PGM(3)

See above description. PGM(1) and PGM(3) are not closely linked (Hopkinson and Harris, 1968). The PGM-3 locus and the HL-A locus are linked (Lamm et al., 1970; Kissmeyer-Nielsen, 1970). Whereas PGM-1 and PGM-2 polymorphism is determined in red cells, PGM-3 is detected in white cells. The PGM-3 locus may be on chromosome no. 6. By study of human-hamster somatic cell hybrids, Jongsma et al. (1973) showed that chromosome no. 6 carries PGM-3. PGM-3 is linked to HL-A, the major histocompatibility locus must be on chromosome no. 6.

Hopkinson, D. A. and Harris, H.: A third phosphoglucomutase locus in man. Ann. Hum. Genet. 31: 359-368, 1968.

Jongsma, A., Van Someren, H., Westerveld, A., Hagemeijer, A. and Pearson, P.: Localization of genes on human chromosomes by studies of human-Chinese hamster somatic cell hybrids. Assignment of PGM to chromosome C6 and regional mapping of the PGD, PGM, and pep-C genes on chromosome A1. Humangenetik 20: 195-202, 1973.

Kissmeyer-Nielsen, F.: Aarhus, Denmark: personal communication, 1970.

Lamm, L. U., Kissmeyer-Nielsen, F. and Henningsen, K.: Linkage and association studies of two phosphoglucomutase loci (PGM-1 and PGM-3) to eighteen other markers. Hum. Hered. 20: 305-318, 1970.

Van Someren, H., Westerveld, A., Hagemeijer, A., Mees, J. R., Meera Khan, P. and Zaalberg, O. B.: Human antigen and enzyme markers in man-Chinese hamster somatic cell hybrids: evidence for synteny between the HL-A, PGM-3, ME-1, and IPO-B loci. Proc. Nat. Acad. Sci. 71: 962-965, 1974.

*17220 6-PHOSPHOGLUCONATE DEHYDROGENASE (6PGD), IN ERYTHROCYTE

Brewer and Dern (1964) reported deficiency of 6-PGD in 10 members of 4 generations of an American Negro family. They concluded that the inheritance is autosomal dominant, all 6-PGD-deficient persons observed being heterozygotes. However, no male-to-male transmission was observed: indeed, no offspring of affected males were tested. Against X-linkage is the fact that the average enzyme level in three 6-PGD-deficient males was somewhat higher than that in seven 6-PGD-deficient females. The opposite would be expected of an X-linked trait. The authors commented on the autosomal control of an enzyme which is closely related metabolically to G6PD, an enzyme controlled by an X-linked gene. In a survey of unrelated persons, Dern, Brewer, Tashian and Shows (1966) found in 3 of 873 American Negroes and 2 of 275 Caucasians a reduction in erythrocyte 6-phosphogluconate dehydrogenase (6-PGD) to the range of 42 to 65 percent of normal. Leukocyte enzyme was also reduced. No correlation was found between electrophoretic phenotype and the quantitative variation. The inheritance was clearly autosomal dominant.

Using starch-gel electrophoresis, Fildes and Parr detected two distinct types of human red cell 6-phosphogluconate dehydrogenase (6-PGD). Ten of 150 random blood samples showed two broad, less distinct bands in contrast to the single narrow, sharp band in the remainder. Inheritance appears to be autosomal, a point of particular note. Since the G6PD locus is X-linked, these two functionally related genes do not show clustering. Heterozygotes and homozygotes showed no quantitative difference in red blood cell 6-PGD activity. Deficiency of this enzyme, both with and without electrophoretic abnormality, has been observed (Parr, 1966). A possibility of linkage between the Rhesus and 6-PGD loci was found by Weitkamp et al. (1970). This has since been fully confirmed (Weitkamp et al., 1971). Weitkamp (1972) gave valid criticism of the conclusions of linkage studies of two groups. It is clear, however, that the Rhesus and 6-PGD loci are on chromosome no. 1. Douglas et al. (1973) demonstrated that the PGM-1 and 6PGD loci are on the distal end of the short arm of chromosome no. 1. Assuming that each arm of chromosome no. 1 is 140 male cM in length, Cook et al. (1974) concluded that measured from the centromere, map positions are as follows: PGD 1p124; Rh 1p109; PGM-1 1p079; Fy 1p010; PEP-C 1q030.

Blake, N. M. and Kirk, R. L.: New genetic variant of 6-phosphogluconate dehydrogenase in Australian aborigines. Nature 221: 278 only, 1969.

Bowman, J. E., Carson, P. E., Frischer, H. and De Garay, A. L.: Genetics of starch-gel electrophoretic variants of human 6-phosphogluconic dehydrogenase: population and family studies in the United States and in Mexico. Nature 210: 811-812, 1966.

Brewer, G. J. and Dern, R. J.: A new inherited enzymatic deficiency of human erythrocytes: 6-phosphogluconate dehydrogenase deficiency. Am. J. Hum. Genet. 16: 472-476, 1964.

Burgerhout, W., Van Someren, H. and Bootsma, D.: Cytological mapping of the genes assigned to the human A1 chromosome by use of radiation-induced chromosome breakage in a human-Chinese hamster hybrid cell line. Humangenetik 20: 159-162, 1973.

Cook, P. J. L., Robson, E. B., Buckton, K. E., Jacobs, P. A. and Polani, P. E.: Segregation of genetic markers in families with chromosome polymorphisms and structural rearrangements involving chromosome 1. Ann. Hum. Genet. 37: 261-274, 1974.

Davidson, R. G.: Electrophoretic variants of human 6-phosphogluconate dehydrogenase: population and family studies and description of a new variant. Ann. Hum. Genet. 30: 355-362, 1967.

Dern, R. J., Brewer, G. J., Tashian, R. E. and Shows, T. B.: Hereditary variation of erythrocytic 6-phosphogluconate dehydrogenase. J. Lab. Clin. Med. 67: 255-264, 1966.

Douglas, G. R., McAlpine, P. J. and Hamerton, J. L.: Regional localization of loci for human PGM-1 and 6PGD on human chromosme 1 by use of hybrids of Chinese hamster-human somatic cells. Proc. Natl. Acad. Sci. 70: 2737-2740, 1973.

Fildes, R. A. and Parr, C. W.: Human red-cell phosphogluconate dehydrogenases. Nature 200: 890-891, 1963.

Parr, C. W. and Fitch, L. I.: Inherited quantitative variations of human phosphogluconate dehydrogenase. Ann. Hum. Genet. 30: 339-353, 1967.

Parr, C. W.: Erythrocyte phosphogluconate dehydrogenase polymorphism. Nature 210: 487-489, 1966.

Parr, C. W.: Structural alleles at the same locus determining both electrophoretic variation and partial deficiency of erythrocyte phosphogluconate dehydrogenase in the human. (Abstract) Proc. Third Intern. Cong. Hum. Genet., (Chicago, Sept. 5-10), 1966. Pp. 75-76.

Ritter, H., Toriverdiau, G., Wendt, G. G. and Zilch, I.: Genetic and linkage analysis on 6-PGD. Humangenetik 14: 73-75, 1971.

Tariverdian, G., Ropers, H., Op'T Hof, J. and Ritter, H.: Zur Genetik der 6-Phosphogluconatdehydrogenase (ec: 1.1.1.44): Eine neue Variante F (Freiburg). Humangenetik 10: 355-357, 1970.

Weitkamp, L. R.: Genetic linkage relationships of the ADA and 6-PGD loci in 'Humangenetik.' (Letter) Humangenetik 15: 359-360, 1972.

Weitkamp, L. R., Guttormsen, S. A. and Greendyke, R. M.: Genetic linkage between a locus for 6-PDG and the Rh locus: evaluation of possible heterogeneity in the recombination fraction between sexes and among families. Am. J. Hum. Genet. 23: 462-470, 1971.

Weitkamp, L. R., Guttormsen, S. A., Shreffler, D. C., Sing, C. F. and Napier, J. A.: Genetic linkage relations of the loci for 6-phosphogluconate dehydrogenase and adenosine deaminase in man. Am. J. Hum. Genet. 22: 216-220, 1970.

Westerveld, A. and Meera Khan, P.: Evidence for linkage between human loci for 6-phosphogluconate dehydrogenase and phosphoglucomutase(1) in man-Chinese hamster somatic cell hybrids. Nature 236: 30-32, 1972.

*17225 PHOSPHOGLYCERIC ACID MUTASE

Phosphoglyceric acid mutase (PGAM; E.C.2.7.5.3) is widely distributed in mammalian tissues where it catalyzes the reversible reaction of 3-phosphoglycerate (3-PGA) to 2-phosphoglycerate (2-PGA) in the glycolytic pathway. Working with starch gel electrophoresis, Chen et al. (1974) described rare genetic variants of PGAM in red cells. (The same isozymes occur in white cells, liver, and spleen. A second set of isozymes in muscle kidney and thymus suggest the existence of a second PGAM locus.) The study of one family failed to exclude X-linkage but the finding of a heterozygous male indicated autosomal localization of the gene.

Chen, S.-H., Anderson, J., Giblett, E. R. and Lewis, M.: Phosphoglyceric acid mutase: rare genetic variants and tissue distribution. Am. J. Hum. Genet. 26: 73-77, 1974.

17230 PHOSPHOHEXOKINASE

From quantitative studies of red cell enzymes in cases of trisomy 21, Pantelakis et al. (1970) found suggestive evidence that the locus for phosphohexokinase is situated on chromosome 21.

Pantelakis, S. N., Karaklis, A. G., Alexiou, D., Vardas, E. and Valaes, T.: Red cell enzymes in trisomy 21. Am. J. Hum. Genet. 22: 184-193, 1970.

*17240 PHOSPHOHEXOSE ISOMERASE (GLUCOSEPHOSPHATE ISOMERASE)

Phosphohexose isomerase is also known as glucosephosphate isomerase and phosphoglucose isomerase. Baughan et al. (1968) found deficiency of erythrocyte glucosephosphate isomerase (GPI), which catalyzes the interconversion of glucose-6-phosphate and fructose-6-phosphate in an adolescent boy with life-long nonspherocytic hemolytic anemia. The autohemolysis pattern conformed to Dacie's type I. Both parents, a sib and five other relatives showed intermediate enzyme levels. The proband showed low enzyme in leukocytes and no detectable enzyme in plasma. Glucosephosphate isomerase is the catalyst specific to the second step of the Embden-Meyerhof glycolytic pathway. The deficiency occurs in leukocytes and plasma as well as erythrocytes but the only clinical manifestation is hemolytic anemia. Detter et al. (1968) found that the parents of a patient with hemolytic anemia had different electrophoretic variants of PHI, each associated with reduced enzyme activity. The definition of 'recessive' is strained, this becoming a situation like that in the Hb SC person. In the mouse the hemoglobin beta chain locus is loosely linked to that for glucosephosphate isomerase (recombination fraction, 32 percent). Even if homology exists in man, a linkage this loose would be hard to establish. Blume et al. (1972) described a patient with hemolytic anemia who was a genetic compound for two forms of GPI. The variant inherited from the mother had no detectable activity. That inherited from the father and designated GPI Los Angeles had residual activity and electrophoretic and thermolability peculiarities. A patient homozygous for GPI Winnepeg was also described. Blume and Beutler (1972) have developed a simple screening test for GPI deficiency. Paglia et al. (1969) found deficiency of red cell and leukocyte glucosephosphate isomerase in 3 sibs with hemolytic anemia. The anemia was ameliorated by splenectomy. Heterozygotes could be identified. Ritter et al. (1971) suggested that the PGI locus may be linked to the ABO locus. By cell hybridization the PHI locus is known to be on chromosome no. 19. Nakashima et al. (1973) described two Japanese families with nonspherocytic hemolytic anemia due to GPI deficiency. Each family demonstrated a 'new' variety of mutant enzyme with deficiency of catalytic function. Two electrophoretic variants, one with deficient activity and one with normal activity, were described by Beutler et al. (1974).

Baughan, M. A., Valentine, W. N., Paglia, M. D., Ways, P. O., Simon, E. R. and Demarsh, Q. B.: Hereditary hemolytic anemia associated with glucosephosphate isomerase (GPI) deficiency — a new enzyme defect of human erythrocytes. Blood 32: 236-249, 1968.

Beutler, E., Sigalove, W. H., Muir, W. A., Matsumoto, B. S. and West, C.: Glucosephosphate-isomerase (GPI) deficiency: GPI Elyria. Ann. Intern. Med. 80: 730-732, 1974.

Blume, K. G. and Beutler, E.: Detection of glucose-phosphate isomerase deficiency by a screening procedure. Blood 39: 685-687, 1972.

Blume, K. G., Hryniuk, W., Powars, D., Trinidad, F., West, C. and Beutler, E.: Characterization of two new variants of glucose-phosphate-isomerase deficiency with hereditary nonspherocytic hemolytic anemia. J. Lab. Clin. Med. 79: 942-949, 1972.

Detter, J. C., Ways, P. O., Giblett, E. R., Baughan, D. A., Hopkinson, D. A., Povey, S. and Harris, H.: Inherited variations in human phosphohexose isomerase. Ann. Hum. Genet. 31: 329-338, 1968.

Hutton, J. J.: Linkage analysis using biochemical variants in mice. Linkage of the hemoglobin beta-chain and glucosephosphate isomerase loci. Biochem. Genet. 3: 507-515, 1969.

Krone, W., Schneider, G., Schulz, D., Arnold, H. and Blume, K. G.: Detection of phosphohexose isomerase: deficiency in human fibroblast cultures. Humangenetik 10: 224-230, 1970.

McMorris, F. A., Chen, T. R., Ricciuti, F., Tischfield, J., Creagan, R. and Ruddle, F.: Chromosome assignments in man of the genes for two hexosphosphate isomerase. Science 179: 1129-1131, 1973.

Nakashima, K., Miwa, S., Oda, S., Oda, E., Matsumoto, N., Fukumoto, Y. and Yamada, T.: Electrophoretic and kinetic studies of glucosephosphate isomerase (GPI) in two different Japanese families with GPI deficiency. Am. J. Hum. Genet. 25: 294-301, 1973.

Paglia, D. E., Holland, P., Baughan, M. A. and Valentine, W. N.: Occurrence of defective hexosephosphate isomerization in human erythrocytes and leukocytes. N. Engl. J. Med. 280: 66-71, 1969.

Ritter, H., Tariverdian, G., Arnold, H., Blume, K. G., Schroter, W. and Wendt, G. G.: Evidence for linkage between the locus for the ABO-system and the locus for phosphoglucoseisomerase (PGI). Humangenetik 11: 349-350, 1971.

Schroter, W., Koch, H. H., Wonneberger, B. and Kalinowsky, W.: Glucose phosphate isomerase deficiency with congenital nonspherocytic hemolytic anemia: a new variant (type Nordhorn). I. Clinical and genetic studies. Pediatr. Res. 8: 18-25, 1974.

Tariverdian, G., Arnold, H., Blume, K. G., Lenkeit, U. and Lohr, G. W.: Zur Formalgenetik der Phosphoglucoseisomerase (ec: 5.3.1.9). Untersuchung einer Sippe mit Pgi-Defizienz. Humangenetik 10: 218-223, 1970.

Terrenato, L., Santolamazza, C., Piacentini, E., Ulizzi, L. and Stirati, G.: Two human red cell phosphohexose isomerase variants in a sample from the population of Rome. Humangenetik 14: 162-163, 1972.

Welch, S. G.: An immunological approach to the study of inherited differences in the activity of human erythrocyte phosphoglucose isomerase. Hum. Hered. 23: 164-174, 1973.

*17243 PHOSPHOPYRUVATE HYDRATASE (ENOLASE)

Giblett et al. (1973) observed an electrophoretic variant of red cell PPH among Cree Indians. Linkage was found with the Rhesus locus. Since the Rh locus has been assigned to chromosome no. 1 and since cell hybridization studies assign the PPH locus to chromosome no. 1, the new data are consistent.

Giblett, E. R., Chen, S.-H., Anderson, J. E. and Lewis, M.: A family study suggesting genetic linkage of phosphophyruvate hydratase (enolase) to the Rh blood group system. Intern. Workshop on Human Gene Mapping, New Haven, Conn., June, 1973. Cytogenet. Cell Genet. 13: 91-92, 1974.

17250 PHOTOMYOCLONUS, DIABETES MELLITUS, DEAFNESS, NEPHROPATHY, AND CEREBRAL DYSFUNCTION

Herrmann, Aguilar, and Sacks (1964) reported 14 members in five generations of a family with diabetes mellitus, nephropathy, epilepsy, and deafness. The proband, a 43-year-old woman, had photomyoclonic seizures for 20 years and progressive nerve deafness for seven years. Her terminal illness began six months before death with mild personality change, slowing and slurring of speech, followed by depression, mild diabetes, focal motor seizures affecting either side of the face, emaciation, and confusion. Terminally a coarse horizontal nystagmus and gross ataxia of the trunk and limbs appeared. Serial audiograms from preceding years were consistent with progressive cochlear degeneration. The kidneys at autopsy showed small foci of interstitial chronic inflammation. The renal tubules showed vacuolation and PAS-positive cytoplasmic granules. The brain showed diffuse neuronal degeneration and astrocytosis. Cerebellar granule cells were decreased. Neurons in the dentate and inferior olivary nucleus were decreased. Remaining neurons were ballooned by a PAS-positive, neutral fat positive material. Other nuclear groups were involved to a lesser degree. A female cousin of the proband had a similar illness with photomyoclonic seizures and progressive nerve deafness in early adult life. Progressive dementia began at age 40. Renal tests were normal. Diabetes and photic sensitivity were found in the two sibs of the proband, the mother of the proband and her sibs, the maternal grandmother and scattered other members of the kindred. 'Bright disease' occurred in three female relatives. Seven members in the family of the maternal grandfather, all male, succumbed in childhood or adolescence to a rapid neurological deterioration and dementia. The authors suggested the features of photomyoclonus, cochlear degeneration, diabetes, and nephropathy are inherited together as an autosomal dominant of variable penetrance. No instance of male-to-male transmission was observed.

Herrmann, C., Jr., Aguilar, M. J. and Sacks, O. W.: Hereditary photomyoclonus associated with diabetes mellitus, deafness, nephropathy, and cerebral dysfunction. Neurology 14: 212-221, 1964.

*17270 PICK DISEASE OF BRAIN (LOBAR ATROPHY)

Schenk (1959) followed up on a family with Pick disease (lobar atrophy) originally studied in 1938, at which time ten cases were identified in the family. Ten further cases were found in a dominant pattern of inheritance. See ALZHEIMER DISEASE.

Schenk, V. W. D.: Re-examination of a family with Pick's disease. Ann. Hum. Genet. 23: 325-333, 1959.

*17280 PIEBALD TRAIT

Keeler (1934) described a Louisiana Negro family in which the disorder could be traced back to a woman born in 1853. Sundfor (1939) described a family in which many persons had a white forelock often with unpigmented patches on the forehead, limbs, body, etc. The features are like those of Waardenburg syndrome (q.v.) except for absence of deafness and displaced inner canthus. Specifically the features are white forelock and absence of pigmentation of the medial portion of the forehead, eyebrows and chin and of the ventral chest, abdomen and extremities. The borders of unpigmented areas are hyperpigmented. Heterochromia iridis occurs in some. A defect in migration or differentiation of melanoblasts in hypopigmented areas was suggested by Comings and Odland (1965). Loewenthal (1959) assigned the name albinoidism to a dominantly inherited condition characterized by a white 'blaze' in the scalp hair, usually the forelock and-or patches of leukoderma. Epitheliomas occurred with increased frequency. The designation albinoidism is better reserved for the recessive condition simulating true albinism. White forelock and patches of leukoderma occur also in Waardenburg syndrome (q.v.) and in Fanconi anemia (a recessive). In mice aganglionic megacolon is associated with the piebald trait (Bielschowsky and Schofield, 1962), inherited probably as an autosomal recessive. Comings and Odland (1966) found the trait in 6 generations. A genetic defect in melanoblast differentiation was postulated. George Catlin (1796-1872), painter of the American Indians, painted an affected Mandan Indian. Multiple members of the group were said to have been affected. The statement that deafness does not occur in persons with the piebald trait as a pleiotropic effect of the gene may not be true. Reed et al. (1967) noted profound deafness with piebaldism in two patients. Some of the patients of Comings and Odland (1966) were deaf.

Bielschowsky, M. and Schofield, G. C.: Studies on megacolon in piebald mice. Aust. J. Exp. Biol. Med. Sci. 40: 395-403, 1962.

Comings, D. E. and Odland, G. F.: Electron microscope study of partial albinism. (Abstract) Clin. Res. 13: 265 only, 1965.

Comings, D. E. and Odland, G. F.: Partial albinism. J.A.M.A. 195: 510-523, 1966.

Cromwell, A. M.: Inheritance of white forelock in a mulatto family. J. Hered. 31: 94-96, 1940.

Fitch, L.: Inheritance of a white forelock: through five successive generations in the Logsdon family. J. Hered. 28: 413-414, 1937.

Froggatt, P.: An outline with bibliography of human pie-baldism and white forelock. Irish J. Med. Sci. 398: 86-94, 1951.

Jahr, H. M. and McIntyre, M. S.: Piebaldness, of familial white skin spotting (partial albinism). Am. J. Dis. Child. 88: 481-484, 1954.

Keeler, C. E.: The heredity of a congenital white spotting in Negroes. J.A.M.A. 103: 179-180, 1934.

Loewenthal, L. J. A.: Albinoidism with epitheliomatosis. Br. J. Dermatol. 71: 37-38, 1959.

Reed, W. B., Stone, V. M., Boder, E. and Ziprkowski, L.: Pigmentary disorders in association with congenital deafness. Arch. Dermatol. 95: 176-186, 1967.

Sundfor, H.: A pedigree of skin-spotting in man: 42 piebalds in a Norwegian family. J. Hered. 30: 67-77, 1939.

17285 PIEBALD TRAIT WITH NEUROLOGIC DEFECTS

Telfer et al. (1971) described two families in which cerebellar ataxia, impaired motor coordination and mental retardation of variable severity were associated with piebald traits. Some affected persons were deaf. There

were some dorsal areas of leukoderma as well as the usual ventral ones. Male-to-male transmission was noted.
The separateness from piebald trait without neurologic defects is not clear.

Telfer, M. A., Sugar, M., Jaeger, E. A. and Mulcahy, J.: Dominant piebald trait (white forelock and leukoderma) with neurological impairment. Am. J. Hum. Genet. 23: 383-389, 1971.

*17290 PIGMENTED PURPURIC ERUPTION

Gould and Farber (1966) described a family in which 6 persons in 3 generations (with one instance of male-to-male transmission) showed a bilaterally symmetrical pigmented and purpuric eruption beginning early in life. The condition may be the same as Schamberg disease (1901) which Baden (1964) observed in father and son.

Baden, H. P.: Familial Schamberg's disease. Arch. Dermatol. 90: 400 Only, 1964.

Gould, W. M. and Farber, E. M.: A familial pigmented purpuric eruption. Dermatologica 132: 400-408, 1966.

Schamberg, J. G.: A peculiar pigmentary disease of the skin. Br. J. Dermatol. 13: 1-5, 1901.

17300 PILONIDAL SINUS

Holmes and Turner (1969) observed 9 affected members in a family in a pattern consistent with autosomal dominant inheritance, although no male-to-male transmission was observed. However, father-son transmission was noted by Stone (1924).

Holmes, L. B. and Turner, E. A., Jr.: Hereditary pilonidal sinus. J.A.M.A. 209: 1525-1526, 1969.

Stone, H. B.: Pilonidal sinus (coccygeal fistula). Ann. Surg. 79: 410-414, 1924.

*17310 PITUITARY DWARFISM

Whether sexual ateleiosis (presumed or proved isolated growth hormone deficiency) is ever inherited as a dominant is not known. Persons who appear to have this condition have been observed in successive generations. Furthermore, dominant inheritance is a possible explanation for the findings in a family in which two midget parents with demonstrated isolated growth horomone deficiency have three offspring, two dwarfed and one of normal stature (Rimoin et al., 1966). One explanation is that at least one of the parents has different alleles each of which determines an ineffective growth hormone molecule and that through intracistronic crossing over a wild-type gene was reconstituted. Another possibility is that the father's condition is the result of new dominant mutation and that he transmitted the condition to the two affected offspring. Dominant inheritance seems possible in the case of those patients who have isolated growth hormone deficiency but do not have insulinopenia as is found in most such cases. Selle (1920) is said (Warkany et al., 1961) to have described a kindred in which 'primordial dwarfism' was transmitted through 3 generations, 10 persons being affected. Multigeneration kindreds were included in the review of Rischbieth and Barrington (1912). Whether these were instances of growth hormone deficiency is, of course, unknown. We (Merimee et al., 1969; Tyson, 1971) have observed a family with affected persons in four generations. Unlike type I isolated growth hormone deficiency, a recessive, insulin responses to glucose and to arginine are usually greater than normal. Sheikholislam and Stempfel (1972) reported isolated GH deficiency in a man and three daughters and a son. Three other children were unaffected. See also DWARFISM, LEVI OR 'SNUB-NOSED' TYPE (12710). Poskitt and Rayner (1974) described two families, each with a father and son affected by isolated growth hormone deficiency.

Poskitt, E. M. E. and Rayner, P. H. W.: Isolated growth hormone deficiency: two families with autosomal dominant inheritance. Arch. Dis. Child. 49: 55-59, 1974.

Merimee, T. J.: Studies in HGH-deficient dwarfs: the type II anomaly. Johns Hopkins Med. J. 131: 165-171, 1972.

Merimee, T. J., Hall, J. G., Rimoin, D. L. and McKusick, V. A.: A metabolic and hormonal basis for classifying ateliotic dwarfs. Lancet I: 963-965, 1969.

Poskitt, E. M. E. and Rayner, P. H. W.: Isolated growth hormone deficiency: two families with autosomal dominant inheritance. Arch. Dis. Child. 49: 55-59, 1974.

Rimoin, D. L., Merimee, T. J. and McKusick, V. A.: Growth hormone deficiency in man: an isolated recessively inherited defect. Science 152: 1635-1637, 1966.

Rischbieth, H. and Barrington, A.: Dwarfism. In, Pearson, K. (ed.): Treasury of Human Inheritance. London: Dulau and Co., 1912, vol. 1, pt. 7, sec. 15A, P. 355.

Selle, G.: Ueber Vererbung des echten Zwergwuchses. Inaug. Dissert., U. Of Jena, 1920.

Sheikholislam, B. M. and Stempfel, R. S., Jr: Hereditary isolated somatotropin deficiency: effects of human growth hormone administration. Pediatrics 49: 362-374, 1972.

Tyson, J. E. A.: Isolated growth hormone deficiency, type I (sexual ateleiosis, type I). The Clinical Delineation of Birth Defects. X. Endocrine System. Baltimore: Williams and Wilkins, 1971. Pp. 251-252.

Warkany, J., Monroe, B. B. and Sutherland, B. S.: Intrauterine growth retardation. Am. J. Dis. Child. 102: 249-279, 1961.

*17320 PITYRIASIS RUBRA PILARIS

The lesions were described as 'consisting of acuminate follicular plugging about the dorsal aspects of the hands and feet, and large plaquelike, scaling psoriasiform lesions of the extensor surfaces of the arms, legs and thighs as well as the neck and calves.' This disorder is 'characterized by scaly and horny productions situated chiefly in the sebaceous follicles and by a more or less generalized hyperemia' to use the words of DeVergie who first described it (Zeisler, 1923). He observed it in a man and his son and two daughters. Weiner and Levin (1943) found 39 cases in three generations. Beamer et al. (1972) contrasted the acquired and hereditary forms. The hereditary forms tend to be less severe and more limited in extent. The hereditary form does not show skin lesions at birth, a feature that distinguishes it from ichthyosiform dermatoses which it resembles.

Beamer, J. E., Newman, S. B., Reed, W. B. and Cram, D.: Pityriasis ruba pilaris. Cutis 10: 419-421, 1972.

Parish, L. C. and Woo, T. H.: Pityriasis rubra pilaris in Korea. Treatment with methotrexate. Dermatologica 139: 399-403, 1969.

Weiner, A. L. and Levin, A. A.: Pityriasis rubra pilaris of familial type: experience in the therapy with carotene and vitamin A. Arch. Dermatol. Syph. 48: 288-296, 1943.

Zeisler, E. P.: Pityriasis rubra pilaris — familial type. Arch. Dermatol. Syph. 7: 195-208, 1923.

17330 PLACENTAL ENZYMES

Numerous polymorphisms involving placental enzymes and other constituents are likely to be uncovered in the next few years. Some of these may be under the control of loci separate from those determining proteins with comparable function in extra-uterine life. The first polymorphism involving a placental protein, that of placental alkaline phosphatase (q.v.), was discovered by Boyer (1961).

Boyer, S. H. IV: Alkaline phosphatase in human sera and placenta. Science 134: 1002-1004, 1961.

17335 PLASMINOGEN

Plasminogen is the zymogen in the circulating blood from which plasmin is formed. It has a single chain with a molecular weight of about 81,000. Its conversion to the active form, plasmin, involves the proteolytic cleavage of an arg-val bond resulting in a molecule which has two chains held together by a disulfide bond. The heavier of the chains contains about 411 residues and the lighter one about 233 residues. The main function of plasmin is the digestion of fibrin in blood clots. Plasmin is a proteolytic enzyme with a specificity similar to that of trypsin.

Dayhoff, M. O.: Thrombin and plasmin. Atlas of Protein Sequence and Structure 1972 (vol. 5). Washington: National Biomedical Research Foundation, 1972. Pp. D100-D101 And D110.

*17350 PLATELET GROUPS — KO SYSTEM

In a long review Dausset and Tangun (1965) discussed antigens common to red cells, leukocytes and platelets, those limited to one of these and those shared by platelets and leukocytes. Ko and Zw (van der Weerdt et al., 1963) are two of the platelet systems. A third is Pl(E). Another, Duzo, is of uncertain relationship to the other three systems (van der Weerdt and van Loghem, 1972). The antiplatelet antibodies in idiopathic thrombocytopenic purpura (Karpatkin et al., 1972) might be useful in typing platelets. Transient neonatal thrombocytopenia can occur in multiple sibs on the basis of feto-maternal incompatibility for leukoplatelet antigens (Vaudour et al., 1974).

Dausset, J. and Tangun, Y.: Leucocyte and platelet groups and their practical significance. (Editorial) Vox Sang. 10: 641-659, 1965.

Hanna, N. and Nelken, D.: Detection, separation and characterization of organ specific antigens of human thrombocytes. Immunology 20: 533-543, 1971.

Karpatkin, S., Strick, N., Karpatkin, M. B. and Siskind, G. W.: Cumulative experience in the detection of antiplatelet antibody in 234 patients with idiopathic thrombocytopenic purpura, systemic lupus erythematosus and other clinical disorders. Am. J. Med. 52: 776-785, 1972.

Majsky, A. and Kreckova, M.: Un nouveau cas d'anticorps antiplaquettaire anti-Ko(a). Rev. Franc. Transfusion 11: 375, 1968.

Moulinier, J.: Iso-immunisation maternelle antiplaquettaires et purpura neonatal. Le systeme de groupe plaquettaire 'Duzo.' Proc. 6th Congr. Europ. Soc. Haemat. Karger, Basel

Shulman, N. R., Moor-Jankowski, J. and Hiller, M. C.: Platelet and leukocyte iso-antigens common to man and other animals. In Histocompatibility Testing 1965, Series Haematologica, vol 11, Munksgaard, Copenhagen (1965), p. 113.

Van der Weerdt, C. M. and Van Loghem, J. J.: Amsterdam, Holland: personal communication, 1972.

Van der Weerdt, C. M., Veenhoven-Von Riesz, L. E., Nijenhuis, L. E. and Van Loghem, J. J.: The zw blood group system in platelets. Vox Sang. 8: 513-530, 1963.

Van Loghem, J. J., Dorfmeyer, H., Van der Hart, M. and Schreuder, F.: Serological and genetical studies on a platelet antigen (zw). Vox Sang. 4: 161, 1959.

Vaudour, G., Leballe, J.-C., Beauvais, P., Costil, J. and Brissaud, H.-E.: Purpura thrombopenique neo-natal familial avec hemorragie cerebro-meningee par allo-immunisation foeto-maternelle. Arch. Franc. Pediat. 31: 37-57, 1974.

*17354 PLATELET GROUPS — PL(E) SYSTEM

See 17350.

17360 PNEUMOTHORAX, SPONTANEOUS

This is a complication of certain heritable disorders of connective tissue, particularly the Marfan syndrome and Ehlers-Danlos syndrome, but may occur as an isolated familial disorder without other stigmata of connective tissue disease (Boyd, 1957). Brock (1948) favored the presence of hereditary lung cysts as the anatomic substrate. Leman and Dines (1973) described 4 affected persons (a man and three daughters, including identical twins).

Berlin, R.: Familial occurrence of pneumothorax simplex. Acta Med. Scand. 137: 268-275, 1950.

Boyd, D. H. A.: Familial spontaneous pneumothorax. Scot. Med. J. 2: 220-221, 1957.

Brock, R. C.: Recurrent and chronic spontaneous pneumothorax. Thorax 3: 88-111, 1948.

Leman, C. B. and Dines, D. E.: Treatment of recurrent spontaneous familial pneumothorax. (Letters) J.A.M.A. 225: 1256 only, 1973.

17370 POIKILODERMA, HEREDITARY SCLEROSING

Weary et al. (1969) reported an apparently new disorder characterized by generalized poikiloderma accentuated in flexural areas and on extensor surfaces, sclerosis of the palms and soles, and in one patient late development of subcutaneous calcification. Clubbing of the fingers may be a feature. All seven patients were Negro. Six were from one family (mother and five affected children out of 10, by three different husbands).

Weary, P. E., Hsu, Y. T., Richardson, D. R., Caravati, C. M. and Wood, B. T.: Hereditary sclerosing poikiloderma. Report of two families with an unusual and distinctive genodermatosis. Arch. Derm. 100: 413-422, 1969.

17380 POLAND SYNDROME (OR POLAND SYNDACTYLY)

This condition consists of unilateral symbrachydactyly and ipsilateral aplasia of the sternal head of the pectoralis major muscle. Trier (1965) found two instances of parent and child with Poland syndrome. Fuhrmann et al. (1971) reported a family with father-son transmission and referred to other cases. Later information suggests that the grandfather may also have been affected (Fuhrmann, 1972). Females show aplasia of the breast and either sex may have patchy absence of axillary hair. David (1972) was impressed with a high frequency of 'potentially noxious social and physical ante-natal influence.' Of 10 patients, 5 were adopted and the mothers of the other 5 had probably attempted abortion in early pregnancy.

Brown, J. B. and McDowell, F.: Syndactylism with absence of the pectoralis major. Surgery 7: 599-601, 1940.

Clarkson, P.: Poland's syndactyly. Guy Hosp. Rep. 111: 335-346, 1962.

David, T. J.: Nature and etiology of the Poland anomaly. New Eng. J. Med. 287: 487-489, 1972.

Fuhrmann, W.: Giesen, Germany: personal communication, 1972.

Fuhrmann, W., Mosseler, U. and Neuss, H.: Zur Klinik und Genetik des Poland-syndroms. Deutsch. Med. Wschr. 96: 1076-1078, 1971.

Trier, W. C.: Complete breast absence. Case report and review of the literature. Plast. Reconstr. Surg. 36: 431-439, 1965.

*17385 POLIO VIRUS SUSCEPTIBILITY

Primates but not rodents are susceptible to poliomyelitis infection. Furthermore, human cells but not rodent cells are killed by polio virus in vitro. Human-mouse hybrids of at least one human chromosome is responsible. Miller et al. (1973) could show that chromosome no. 19 is correlated with susceptibility to polio virus.

Miller, O. J., Miller, D. A., Dev, V. G., Medrano, L. and Green, H.: Assignment of a polio sensitivity gene to human chromosome 19. Am. J. Hum. Genet. 25: 52A only, 1973.

Miller, D. A., Miller, O. J., Dev, V. G., Hashmi, S., Tantravahi, R., Medrano, L., and Green, H.: Human chromosome 19 carries a poliovirus receptor gene. Cell 1: 167-174, 1974.

*17390 POLYCYSTIC KIDNEYS

Ditlefsen and Tonjum (1960) described a family in which there were 15 verified and 2 suspected cases. Six of the patients suffered from cerebral hemorrhage. In one of the six, aneurysm of the middle cerebral artery was verified. Intracranial 'berry' aneurysm is a rather frequent associated malformation. Dalgaard (1963) found liver cysts in 43 percent of 173 autopsied cases in Denmark. In a review of cases, largely from the literature, Poinso et al. (1954) found that polycystic kidneys occurred in 53 percent of 224 cases of polycystic livers. Dalgaard (1963) said he has found a regular transition from polycystic liver degeneration to the solitary liver cyst in association with polycystic kidney. Ellis and Putschar (1968) presented the case of a 42-year-old woman with polycystic kidneys and portal hypertension for which splenorenal shunt was performed. Liver biopsy showed 'disseminated microcystic biliary hamartomas, with congenital fibrosis.' The mother died with hypertension, renal disease and stroke at age 64. Two of her sisters died of renal disease. Two sisters of the proband were said to have polycystic kidney disease. Emery et al. (1967) observed the coincidence of myotonic dystrophy (16090) and polycystic kidneys in at least 3 members of a family.

Dalgaard, O. Z.: Bilateral polycystic disease of the kidneys. A follow-up of two-hundred and eighty-four patients and their families. Copenhagen: E. Munksgaard, 1957. (also Acta. Med. Scand. 328 (suppl.): 1957).

Dalgaard, O. Z.: Bilateral polycystic disease of the kidneys. In, Strauss, M. B. and Welt, L. G. (eds.): Diseases of the Kidney. Boston: Little, Brown and Co., 1963. Pp. 907-910.

Ditlefsen, E. M. L. and Tonjum, A. M.: Intracranial aneurysms and polycystic kidneys. Acta Med. Scand. 168: 51-54, 1960.

Ellis, D. S. and Putschar, W. G. J.: Persistent fatigue, hepatosplenomegaly and portal hypertension. New Eng. J. Med. 278: 899-904, 1968.

Emery, A. E. H., Oleesky, S. and Williams, R. T.: Myotonic dystrophy and polycystic disease of the kidneys. J. Med. Genet. 4: 26-28, 1967.

Osathanondh, V. and Potter, E. L.: Pathogenesis of polycystic kidneys. Arch. Path. 77: 459-465, 1964.

Poinso, R., Monges, H. and Payan, H.: La Maladie Kystique du Foie. Expansion Scientifique Francaise, 1954.

*17400 POLYCYSTIC KIDNEYS, MEDULLARY TYPE

Goldman and colleagues (1966) described 17 affected members in five generations of a family. Fifteen had died in the second decade of life with rapid clinical deterioration after the onset of symptoms. The kidneys showed thin cortices, prominent glomerular hyalinization, numerous corticomedullary and intramedullary cysts lined by low cuboidal epithelium, and increase in medullary connective tissue. These are the findings also reported in sporadic cases of medullary cystic disease. Differences from the usual type of polycystic kidney include usual absence of flank pain, hypertension and hematuria and small kidneys by X-ray. In two extensively affected sibships on which Gardner (1971) provided follow-up information, the average age of onset of symptoms was 23 years in one and 35 years in a second. The average duration of illness was only 2.2 years. Thorn et al. (1944) who are credited with first discribing medullary cystic disease under the designation of 'salt-losing nephritis' noted the association of red and blond hair. Rayfield and McDonald (1972) reemphasized the association. Wrigley et al. (1973) described a family which differed from the usual medullary cystic disease in late onset and some other respects. The family reported by Whelton et al. (1974) illustrates occult affection of the mother of two severely affected persons.

Abeshouse, B. S. and Abeshouse, G. A.: Spongy kidney: a review of the literature and a report of five cases. J. Urol. 84: 252-267, 1960.

Butler, M. R., Devine, H. F. and O'Flynn, J. D.: Medullary sponge-kidney: review of the literature and presention of 33 cases. J. Irish Med. Ass. 66: 5-13, 1973.

Copping, G. A.: Medullary sponge kidneys: its occurrence in a father and daughter. Canad. M. Ass. J. 96: 608-611, 1967.

Dalgaard, O. Z.: Bilateral polycystic disease of the kidneys. In, Strauss, M. B. and Welt, L. G. (ed.): Diseases of the Kidney. Boston: Little, Brown and Co., 1963. Pp. 907-910.

Gardner, K. D., Jr.: Evolution of clinical signs in adult-onset cystic disease of the renal medulla. Ann. Intern. Med. 74: 47-54, 1971.

Goldman, S. H., Walker, S. R., Merigan, T. C., Jr., Gardner, K. D., Jr. and Bull, J. M. C.: Hereditary occurrence of cystic disease of the renal medulla. New Eng. J. Med. 274: 984-992, 1966.

Rayfield, E. J. and McDonald, F. D.: Red and blond hair in renal medullary cystic disease. Arch. Intern. Med. 130: 72-75, 1972.

Swenson, R. S., Kempson, R. L. and Freidland, G. W.: Cystic disease of the renal medulla in the elderly. J.A.M.A. 288: 1401-1404, 1974.

Thorn, G. W., Koepf, G. F. and Clinton, M.: Renal failure simulating adrenocortical insufficiency. New Eng. J. Med. 231: 76-85, 1944.

Whelton, A., Ozer, F. L., Bias, W., Williams, G. M. and Walker, W. G.: Renal medullary cystic disease: a family study. In, Bergsma, D. (ed.): Clinical Delineation of Birth Defects. XVI. Urinary System and Others. Baltimore: Williams and Wilkins, 1974. Pp. 154-156.

Wrigley, K. A., Sherman, R. L., Ennis, F. A. and Becker, L.: Progressive hereditary nephropathy. Arch. Intern. Med. 131: 240-244, 1973.

17410 POLYDACTYLY, IMPERFORATE ANUS, VERTEBRAL ANOMALIES

Say and Gerald (1968) found, among 186 cases of polydactyly, 10 who also had imperforate anus. Of the 10, 8 had severe skeletal anomalies, predominantly vertebral. None of the cases were familial. Mutations in mice that produce this triad were noted. Other cases have been reported by Filippi (1972) and by Kaufman et al. (1972). Filippi called it PIV syndrome.

Filippi, G.: The syndrome of polydactyly, imperforate anus and vertebral anomalies. The Clinical Delineation of Birth Defects. XIII. G. I. Tract Including Liver and Pancreas. Baltimore: Williams and Wilkins, 1972. Pp. 88-94.

Kaufman, R. L., Quinton, B. and Ternberg, J. L.: Imperforate anus, vertebral anomalies, and preaxial limb abnormalities. XIII. G. I. Tract Including Liver and Pancreas. Baltimore: Williams and Wilkins, 1972. Pp. 85-87.

Say, B. and Gerald, P. S.: A new polydactyly — imperforate-anus — vertebral-anomalies syndrome? (Letter) Lancet II: 688 only, 1968.

*17420 POLYDACTYLY, POSTAXIAL (PROBABLY AT LEAST TWO TYPES)

This form of polydactyly is about ten times more frequent in the Negro than in Caucasians (Frazier, 1960). From the study of various pedigrees of postaxial polydactyly it is suggested that two phenotypic and possibly genetically different varieties exist. In one of them, postaxial polydactyly type A, the extra digit is rather well formed and articulates with the fifth or an extra metacarpal. This type is inherited as a dominant trait with marked penetrance. In postaxial polydactyly (type B or pedunculated postminimi) the extra digit is not well formed and is frequently in the form of a skin tag. The genetics of this type is more complicated. Walker (1961) studied a pedigree with this trait and owing to lack of penetrance, suggested that the presence of two dominant genes would best explain the finding. The largest pedigree of postaxial polydactyly is that described by Odiorne (1943). Sverdrup (1922) studied a large kindred and noted the occurrence of both types A and B in the same pedigree and discussed the possibility of a genetic difference.

Castilla, E., Paz, J., Mutchinick, O., Munoz, E., Giorgiutti, E. and Gelman, Z.: Polydactyl: a genetic study in South America. Am. J. Hum. Genet. 25: 405-412, 1973.

Frazier, T. M.: A note on race-specific congenital malformation rates. Am. J. Obstet. Gynec. 80: 184-185, 1960.

Mohan, J.: Postaxial polydactyly in three Indian families. J. Med. Genet. 6: 196-200, 1969.

Odiorne, J. M.: Polydactylism in related New England families. J. Hered. 34: 45-56, 1943.

Sverdrup, A.: Postaxial polydactylism in six generations of a Norwegian family. J. Genet. 12: 217-240, 1922.

Walker, J. T.: A pedigree of extra-digit-v polydactyly in a Batutsi family. Ann. Hum. Genet. 25: 65-68, 1961.

17430 POLYDACTYLY, POSTAXIAL, WITH MEDIAN CLEFT OF UPPER LIP

Rischbieth (1910) pictured a Hindu patient with this combination. His brother was identically affected. Thurston had earlier (1909) reported these brothers. Rischbieth cited the family of Roux (1847) in which the father had unilateral harelip and six digits of all four limbs, whereas the son had double harelip and the same deformity of hands and feet.

Rischbieth, H.: Hare-lip and cleft palate. In, Treasury of Human Inheritance. London: Cambridge Univ. Press, 1910. Vol. I, part IV, plate J.

Roux, (NI): Bec-de-lievre unilateral. Gaz. Hop., P. 274, 1847.

Thurston, E. O.: A case of median hare-lip associated with other malformations. Lancet II: 996-997, 1909.

17440 POLYDACTYLY, PREAXIAL I ('THUMB POLYDACTYLY')

Preaxial polydactyly, i.e. polydactyly on the radial side of the hand, is a heterogeneous category. Four types are (1) thumb polydactyly, (2) polydactyly of triphalangeal thumb, (3) polydactyly of index finger, and (4) polysyndactyly. Preaxial polydactyly I, 'thumb polydactyly,' involves duplication of one or more of the skeletal components of a biphalangeal thumb. Severity varies from merely broadening of the distal phalanx with slight bifurcation at the tip to full duplication of the thumb including the metacarpals. This type is the most frequent form of polydactyly in many populations (Handforth, 1950). The genetics is not completely clear. Digby (1645) reported preaxial polydactyly, presumably of this type, in females in 5 generations. Pott (1884) observed 10 affected (6 females and 4 males) in 3 generations. Sinha (1918) found irregular segregation in a family with affected persons in 3 generations. In one generation, only 1 of 13 persons at risk were affected. De Marinis and Sobbota (1957) observed a girl with bilateral thumb polydactyly whose mother had radial deviation of the terminal phalanx (a feature which Pott also considered a manifestation of the same trait). No male-to-male transmission seems to have been documented.

De Marminis, F. and Sobbota, A.: On the inheritance and development of preaxial and postaxial types of polydactylism. Acta Genet. Med. Gemellol. 6: 85-93, 1957.

Digby, Sir Kenelm: The Immortality of Reasonable Souls. London: John Williams, 1645.

Handforth, J. R.: Polydactylism of hand in southern Chinese. Anat. Rec. 106: 119-125, 1950.

Pott, R.: Ein Beitrag zu den symmetrischen Missbildungen der Finger und Zehen. Jahrb. Kinderheilk. 21: 392-407, 1884.

Sinha, S.: Polydactylism and tooth color. J. Hered. 9: 96 only, 1918.

*17450 POLYDACTYLY, PREAXIAL II (POLYDACTYLY OF TRIPHALANGEAL THUMB)

The thumb in this malformation is opposable and possesses a normal metacarpal. Polydactyly consists of duplication of the distal phalanx giving a 'duck-bill' appearance. Reported families include the second in the paper by Haas (1939), and those described by Atwood and Pond (1917), Hefner (1940) and Ecke (1962). The proband of a family studied by Temtamy (1966) had opposable triphalangeal thumbs, all three phalanges being well developed, and in both feet had duplication of the great toes. The trait had passed through at least 6 generations.

Atwood, E. S. and Pond, C. P.: A polydactylous family. J. Hered. 8: 96 only, 1917.

Ecke, H.: Beitrag zu den doppelmissbildungen in bereich der finger. Bruns' Beitr. Klin. Chir. 205: 463-468, 1962.

Haas, S. L.: Three-phalangeal thumbs. Am. J. Roentgen. 42: 677-682, 1939.

Hefner, R. A.: Hereditary polydactyly: associated with extra phalanges in the thumb. J. Hered. 31: 25-27, 1940.

Temtamy, S. A.: The Genetics of Hand Malformations. Ph.D. Thesis, Johns Hopkins University, 1966.

*17460 POLYDACTYLY, PREAXIAL III ('INDEX FINGER POLYDACTYLY')

An historically notable example is the Scipion family in which the malformation was transmitted for over two thousand years (Manoiloff, 1931). The thumb is replaced by one or two triphalangeal digits, which may or may not be opposable (Swanson and Brown, 1962). The feet, in some cases, show preaxial polydactyly of the 1st or 2nd toes (Manoiloff, 1931; James and Lamb, 1963). A constant radiologic finding is distal epiphysis for the metacarpal of the accessory digits (Swanson and Brown, 1962).

James, J. I. R. and Lamb, D. W.: Congenital abnormalities of the limbs. Practitioner 191: 159-172, 1963.

Manoiloff, E. O.: A rare case of hereditary hexadactylism. Am. J. Phys. Anthrop. 15: 503-508, 1931.

Swanson, A. B. and Brown, K. S.: Hereditary triphalangeal thumb. J. Hered. 53: 259-265, 1962.

*17470 POLYDACTYLY, PREAXIAL IV (POLYSYNDACTYLY)

Although both preaxial polydactyly and syndactyly are cardinal features of this malformation, it is classified as a form of polydactyly because syndactyly does not occur in the absence of polydactyly (McClintic, 1935), the opposite not being true. On the other hand, synpolydactyly (q.v.) is here classified as a type of syndactyly because polydactyly (of the 3rd or 4th fingers and 5th toes) does not occur in the absence of syndactyly. In the hand the thumb shows only the mildest degree of duplication and syndactyly of various degrees affects fingers 3 and 4. The foot malformation is more constant and consists of duplication of part or all of the first or second toes and syndactyly affects all of the toes, especially the second and third. Thomsen (1927) described 10 affected females and 5 affected males in 5 generations. McClintic (1935) observed 15 affected in 5 generations, and Goodman (1965) 5 affected in 3 generations.

Goodman, R. M.: A family with polysyndactyly and other anomalies. J. Hered. 56: 37-38, 1965.

McClintic, B. S.: Five generations of polydactylism. J. Hered. 26: 141-144, 1935.

Thomsen, O.: Einige Eigenthuemlichkeiten der erblichen Poly- und Syndaktylie beim Menschen. Acta Med. Scand. 65: 609-644, 1927.

17480 POLYOSTOTIC FIBROUS DYSPLASIA

This disorder is also called Albright syndrome but should not be confused with Albright hereditary osteodystrophy, or pseudohypoparathyroidism (q.v.). There is little evidence of an hereditary basis. Hibbs and Rush (1952) reported the case of a 50-year-old woman with typical skin pigmentation and involvement of multiple bones. The daughter had no skin pigmentation (which is absent in some cases) but had a pathologic fracture of the left radius and radiologic and histologic changes interpreted as those of fibrous dysplasia. Firat and Stutzman (1968) described hyperthyroidism in one patient who also had pituitary gigantism and hyperparathyroidism in two others. The last two cases were mother and daughter. The fibrous dysplasia was limited to the jaw. Hyperthyroidism was noted by Lichtenstein and Jaffe (1942) as well as other authors and was present in a patient seen at this hospital.

Albright, F., Butler, A. M., Hampton, A. O. and Smith, P.: Syndrome characterized by osteitis fibrosa disseminata, areas of pigmentation and endocrine dysfunction, with precocious puberty in females. Report of five cases. New Eng. J. Med. 216: 727-746, 1937.

Albright, F., Scoville, B. and Sulkowitch, H. W.: Syndrome characterized by osteitis fibrosa disseminata, areas of pigmentation, and a gonadal dysfunction. Further observations including the report. Endocrinology 22: 411-421, 1938.

Firat, D. and Stutzman, L.: Fibrous dysplasia of the bone. Review of twenty-four cases. Am. J. Med. 44: 421-429, 1968.

Hall, R. and Warrick, C.: Hypersecretion of hypothalamic releasing hormones: a possible explanation of the endocrine manifestations of polyostotic fibrous dysplasia (Albright's syndrome). Lancet I: 1313-1316, 1972.

Hibbs, R. E. and Rush, H. P.: Albright's syndrome. Ann. Intern. Med. 37: 587-593, 1952.

Lichtenstein, L. and Jaffe, H. L.: Fibrous dysplasia of the bone. A condition affecting one, several or many bones, the graver cases of which may present abnormal pigmentation of skin, premature sexual development, hyperthyroidism or still other extraskeletal abnormalities. Arch. Path. 33: 777-816, 1942.

Wirth, W. A., Leavitt, D. and Enzinger, F. M.: Multiple intramuscular myxomas. Another extraskeletal manifestation of fibrous dysplasia. Cancer 27: 1167-1173, 1971.

*17490 POLYPOSIS COLI, JUVENILE TYPE

Veale et al. (1966) investigated the families of 11 patients. Juvenile polyps may be isolated or multiple, even very numerous. The histology and natural history of these polyps suggests they are hamartomas. Per se they probably are not precancerous. In four families multiple polyposis and-or colonic carcinoma occurred in relatives. For example, the father of an affected brother and sister had colonic cancer. In two instances a parent of a case of juvenile polyposis had colonic cancer and multiple polyposis. Smilow et al. (1966) described a 7-year-old boy with juvenile polyposis, his mother who at 10 years of age had noted a prolapsed polyp during defecation and his maternal grandfather who at age 60 had surgery for adenocarcinoma of the colon. Various polyps were present in the latter person, some resembling adenomatous polyps and others resembling the juvenile polyps found in the proband and his mother. In the proband's mother the lesions were so numerous that total colectomy and ileostomy were performed. Veale (1966) described juvenile polyps in two sisters and their mother. Haggitt and Pitcock (1970) described a girl who had onset of intermittent bright red rectal bleeding at age 3 years. Her father, an aunt and an uncle had 'well-differentiated adenocarcinoma with invasion of the submucosa.' The grandfather died at 42 of colonic cancer. Gathright and Cofer (1974) described the disorder in a mother and five sons. Three brothers and a sister in another family were affected.

Gathright, J. B., Jr., and Cofer, T. W., Jr.: Familial incidence of juvenile polyposis coli. Surg. Gynec. Obstet. 138: 185-188, 1974.

Haggitt, R. C. and Pitcock, J. A.: Familial juvenile polyposis of the colon. Cancer 26: 1232-1238, 1970.

Smilow, P. C., Pryor, C. A., Jr. and Swinton, N. W.: Juvenile polyposis coli: a report of three patients in three generations of one family. Dis. Colon Rectum 9: 248-254, 1966.

Veale, A. M., McColl, I., Bussey, H. J. R. and Morson, B. C.: Juvenile polyposis coli. J. Med. Genet. 3: 5-16, 1966.

17500 POLYPOSIS, FAMILIAL, OF ENTIRE GASTROINTESTINAL TRACT

Yonemoto et al. (1969) described a family with multiple cases consistent with dominant inheritance. One patient had a desmoid tumor of the abdominal wall. Whether distinct from Gardner syndrome or familial polyposis of the colon is unclear. Early development of symptoms is typical. Ravitch (1948) described a case. This was, however, a case of juvenile polyposis (Ravitch, 1974).

Ravitch, M. M.: Polypoid adenomatosis of entire gastro-intestinal tract. Ann. Surg. 128: 283-298, 1948.

Ravitch, M. M.: Pittsburgh, personal communication, 1974.

Yonemoto, R. H., Slayback, J. B., Byron, R. L., Jr. and Rosen, R. B.: Familial polyposis of the entire gastrointestinal tract. Arch. Surg. 99: 427-434, 1969.

*17510 POLYPOSIS, INTESTINAL, I (FAMILIAL POLYPOSIS OF THE COLON)

No extra-intestinal manifestations are associated with this form and the polyps are probably always limited to the colon. In extreme cases the colon becomes carpeted with myriads of polyps. This is a viciously premalignant condition. Carcinoma may arise in the teens or be postponed until the seventh decade. Bloody diarrhea and inanition may lead to the diagnosis of enteritis as the cause of death. Pierce (1968) reported the findings in a particularly extensively affected kindred. Veale (1965) could find no support for linkage with the MN locus which he had previously suggested. A possibility of linkage with Duffy blood group remained, however. Although some cases of familial polyposis of the entire gastrointestinal tract represent juvenile polyposis (17490), some seem to be adenomatous polyposis (e.g. Yonemoto et al., 1969).

Asman, H. B. and Pierce, E. R.: Familial multiple polyposis. A statistical study of a large Kentucky kindred. Cancer 25: 972-981, 1970.

Duhamel, J., Berthon, G. and Dubarry, J. J.: Etude mathematique de l'heredite de la polypose recto-colique. J. Genet. Hum. 9: 65-77, 1960.

McKusick, V. A.: Genetic factors in intestinal polyposis. J.A.M.A. 182: 271-277, 1962.

Pierce, E. R.: Some genetic aspects of familial polyposis of the colon in a kindred of 1,422 members. Dis. Colon Rectum 11: 321-329, 1968.

Pierce, E. R.: Pleiotropism and heterogeneity in hereditary intestinal polyposis. The Clinical Delineation of Birth Defects. XIII. G. I. Tract Including Liver and Pancreas. Baltimore: Williams and Wilkins, 1972. Pp. 52-62.

Veale, A. M.: Clinical and genetic problems in familial intestinal polyposis. Gut 1: 285-290, 1960.

Veale, A. M.: Intestinal polyposis. Eugenics Laboratory Memoirs, XL. London: Cambridge Univ. Press, 1965.

Yonemoto, R. H., Slayback, J. B., Byron, R. L., Jr. and Rosen, R. B.: Familial polyposis of the entire gastrointestinal tract. Arch. Surg. 99: 427-434, 1969.

*17520 POLYPOSIS, INTESTINAL, II (PEUTZ-JEGHERS SYNDROME)

Polyps may occur in any part of the gastrointestinal tract but jejunal polyps are a consistent feature. Intussusception and bleeding are the usual symptoms. Melanin spots of the lips, buccal mucosa and digits represent the second part of the syndrome. Malignant degeneration of the intestinal polyps is rare. The females are prone to develop ovarian tumor, especially granulosa cell tumor (Christian et al., 1964). Metastases in a malignant polyp in Peutz-Jeghers syndrome was reported by Williams and Knudsen (1965). In the family reported by Farmer et al. (1963) the father had only polyps, the son apparently only pigmentation and the daughter both polyps and pigmentation. A dissociation of signs was also noted by Kieselstein et al. (1969), who also found polycystic kidney disease in the same family. Sommerhaug and Mason (1970) added the ureter to the sites of polyps described in the Peutz-Jeghers syndrome. Previously described extra-intestinal sites include esophagus, bladder, renal pelvis, bronchus and nose. Dodds et al. (1972) found 15 cases of gastrointestinal carcinoma in Peutz-Jeghers syndrome: 5 in colon, 4 in duodenum, 4 in stomach, 1 in ileum and 1 in both jejunum and stomach.

Andre, R., Duhamel, G., Bruaire, M. and Tiollais, P.: Syndrome de Peutz-Jeghers avec polypose oesophagienne. Bull. Soc. Med. Hop. Paris 117: 505-510, 1966.

Bartholomew, L. G., Moore, C., Dahlin, D. C. and Waugh, J. M.: Intestinal polyposis associated with mucocutaneous pigmentation. Surg. Gynec. Obstet. 115: 1-11, 1962.

Christian, C. D., McLoughlin, T. G., Cathcart, E. S. and Eisenberg, M. M.: Peutz-Jeghers syndrome associated with functioning ovarian tumor. J.A.M.A. 190: 935-938, 1964.

Dodds, W. J., Schulte, W. J., Hensley, G. T. and Hogan, W. J.: Peutz-Jeghers syndrome and gastrointestinal malignancy. Am. J. Roentgen. 115: 374-377, 1972.

Farmer, R. G., Hawks, W. A. and Turnbull, R. B.: The spectrum of the Peutz-Jeghers syndrome. Report of 3 cases. Am. J. Dig. Dis. 8: 953-961, 1963.

Humphries, A. L. Jr., Shepherd, M. H. and Peters, H. J.: Peutz-jeghers syndrome with colonic adenocarcinoma and ovarian tumors. J.A.M.A. 197: 296-298, 1966.

Keen, G. and Murray, M. A.: Peutz-Jeghers syndrome: a further family history. Brit. Med. J. 1: 923-924, 1962.

Kieselstein, M., Herman, G., Wahrman, J., Voss, R., Gitelson, S., Feuchtwanger, M. and Kadar, S.: Mucocutaneous pigmentation and intestinal polyposis (Peutz-Jeghers syndrome) in a family of Iraqi Jews with polycystic kidney disease, with a chromosome study. Israel J. Med. Sci. 5: 81-90, 1969.

McAllister, A. J., Hicken, N. F., Latimer, R. G. and Condon, V. R.: Seventeen patients with Peutz-Jeghers syndrome in four generations. Am. J. Surg. 114: 839-843, 1967.

McKittrick, J. E., Lewis, W. M., Doane, W. A. and Gerwig, W. H.: The Peutz-Jeghers syndrome: report of two cases, one with 30-year follow-up. Arch. Surg. 103: 57-62, 1971.

Michalany, J. and Ferraz, M. D.: Peutz syndrome in a mulatto family. With special reference to the histological structure of the intestinal polyps. Gastroenterologia 97: 119-129, 1962.

Scully, R. E.: Sex cord tumors with annular tubules — a distinctive ovarian tumor of the Peutz-Jeghers syndrome. Cancer 25: 1107-1121, 1970.

Sheward, J. D.: Peutz-Jeghers syndrome in childhood: unusual radiological features. Brit. Med. J. 1: 921-923, 1962.

Sommerhaug, R. G. and Mason, T.: Peutz-Jeghers syndrome and ureteral polyposis. J.A.M.A. 211: 120-122, 1970.

Williams, J. P. and Knudsen, A.: Peutz-Jeghers syndrome with metastasizing duodenal carcinoma. Gut 6: 179-184, 1965.

*17530 POLYPOSIS, INTESTINAL, III (GARDNER SYNDROME)

Polyps of the colon and sometimes of the stomach and small intestine are associated with osseous and soft tissue tumors. Globoid osteomata of the mandible with overlying fibromata are characteristic. Osteomatous changes in the calvarium with associated fibromas (of the forehead, for example) are also observed. Sebaceous or epidermoid cysts occur on the back. Mesenteric fibromatosis may develop, especially after surgery (Simpson et al., 1964). The colonic polyps frequently undergo malignant degeneration. Oldfield's family (1954) had only sebaceous cysts with colonic polyposis. Whether this is the same mutation as that of the Gardner syndrome is unclear. The family reported by Oldfield (1954) were specifically stated to have multiple sebaceous cysts, or sebocystomatosis. In fact the same family had been previously reported by Ingram and Oldfield (1937) in connection with the skin tumors alone. Dramatic pictures were published. In the paper by Ingram and Oldfield (1937) the question of origin — retention vs. new formation-was discussed and the review of Benecke (1931) was cited together with his view that most so-called sebaceous cysts are more properly termed epidermoid cysts. In the family reported by Kenny and O'Neill (1958) the cysts were described as epidermoid. The pathologist described 'an oval cyst 5 x two and one half x two and one half cms. containing cheesy material. Microscopically, the lesion is an epidermoid cyst, similar to that removed from the patient's brother.' Fraumeni et al. (1968) described a family in which the father and a daughter had a malignant mesenchymal tumor, a son had polyposis coli, and another son had both polyposis coli and malignant mesenchymal tumor. (Fatal metastic carcinoma of the colon occurred in an 11-year-old boy, probably the youngest reported.) The relation of this family's disorder to Gardner syndrome was discussed. Marshall et al. (1967) reported a patient with Gardner syndrome (present also in multiple relatives) who developed adrenal carcinoma with Cushing syndrome. Camiel et al. (1968) described thyroid carcinoma in two sisters who also had Gardner syndrome which was probably present in at least 3 generations of the family. Smith (1968) also described patients with the association of colonic polyps and papillary carcinoma of the thyroid. Furthermore, Smith (1968) questioned that Gardner syndrome is distinct from familial multiple polyposis. The best evidence of distinctness is provided by large kindreds such as that of Asman and Pierce (1970) in which no extra-intestinal features were found and that of Gardner (1962) in which association of extra-bowel features was consistently found. Furthermore, restudy of an earlier reported kindred (Kelly and McKinnon, 1961) shows that the disorder is in fact Gardner syndrome with about 60 affected persons (Pierce et al., 1970). Hoffmann and Brooke (1970) described a family in which 6 persons in 3 generations had polyposis coli and a mother and son had sarcoma of bone leading to death from metastases at 28 and 13 years of age, respectively. No evidence of polyposis was found in either but special studies including autopsies were not done.

Asman, H. B. and Pierce, E. R.: Familial multiple polyposis: a statistical study of a large Kentucky kindred. Cancer 25: 972-981, 1970.

Benecke, E.: Ueber Epitheliome auf Atheromen (Epidermoide) und Dermoidcysten der Haut. Frankfurt. Z. Path. 42: 502-515, 1931.

Camiel, M. R., Mule, J. E., Alexander, L. L. and Benninghoff, D. L.: Association of thyroid carcinoma with Gardner's syndrome in siblings. New Eng. J. Med. 278: 1056-1058, 1968.

Chang, C. H., Platt, E. D., Thomas, K. E. and Watne, A. L.: Bone abnormalities in Gardner's syndrome. Am. J. Roentgen. 103: 645-652, 1968.

Fader, M., Kline, S. N., Spatz, S. S. and Zubrow, H. J.: Gardner's syndrome (intestinal polyposis, osteomas, sebaceous cysts) and a new dental discovery. Oral Surg. 15: 153-172, 1962.

Fraumeni, J. F., Jr., Vogel, C. L. and Easton, J. M.: Sarcomas and multiple polyposis in a kindred. A genetic variety of hereditary polyposis? Arch. Intern. Med. 121: 57-61, 1968.

Gardner, E. J.: Discovery of the Gardner syndrome. The Clinical Delineation of Birth Defects. XIII. G. I. Tract Including Liver and Pancreas. Baltimore: Williams and Wilkins, 1972. Pp. 48-51.

Gardner, E. J.: Follow-up study of a family group exhibiting dominant inheritance for a syndrome including intestinal polyps, osteomas, fibromas and epidermal cysts. Am. J. Hum. Genet. 14: 376-390, 1962.

Gorlin, R. J. and Chaudhry, A. P.: Multiple osteomatosis, fibromas, lipomas and fibrosarcomas of the skin and mesentery, epidermoid inclusion cysts of the skin, leiomyomas and multiple intestinal polyposis: an heritable disorder of connective tissue. New Eng. J. Med. 263: 1151-1158, 1960.

Haggitt, R. C. and Booth, J. L.: Bilateral fibromatosis of the breast in Gardner's syndrome. Cancer 25: 161-166, 1970.

Hoffmann, D. C. and Brooke, B. N.: Familial sarcoma of bone in a polyposis coli family. Dis. Colon Rectum 13: 119-120, 1970.

Ingram, J. T. and Oldfield, M. C.: Hereditary sebaceous cysts. Brit. Med. J. 1: 960-963, 1937.

Kelly, P. B. and McKinnon, D. A.: Familial multiple polyposis of the colon: review and description of a large kindred. McGill Med. J. 30: 67-85, 1961.

Kenny, P. J. and O'Neill, J.: Familial intestinal polyposis associated with further abnormalities of growth. Aust. New Zeal. J. Surg. 28: 145-150, 1958.

Lewis, R. J. and Mitchell, J. C.: Basal cell carcinoma in Gardner's syndrome. Acta Derm. Venerol. 51: 67-68, 1970.

MacDonald, J. M., Davis, W. C., Crago, H. R. and Berk, A. D.: Gardner's syndrome and periampullary malignancy. Am. J. Surg. 113: 425-430, 1967.

Marshall, W. H., Martin, F. I. R. and MacKay, I. R.: Gardner's syndrome with adrenal carcinoma. Aust. Ann. Med. 16: 242-244, 1967.

McKusick, V. A.: Genetic factors in intestinal polyposis. J.A.M.A. 182: 271-277, 1962.

Oldfield, M. C.: The association of familial polyposis of the colon with multiple sebaceous cysts. Brit. J. Surg. 41: 534-541, 1954.

Pierce, E. R., Weisbord, T. and McKusick, V. A.: Gardner's syndrome: formal genetics and statistical analysis of a large Canadian kindred. Clin. Genet. 1: 65-80, 1970.

Savage, P. T.: Polyposis coli associated with multiple tumours in other parts of the body (Gardner's syndrome). Proc. Roy. Soc. Med. 57: 402-403, 1964.

Schnur, P. L., David, E., Brown, P. W. Jr., Beahrs, O. H., Remine, W. H. and Harrison, E. G. Jr.: Duodenal cancer and Gardner syndrome. J.A.M.A. 223: 1229-1232, 1973.

Simpson, R. D., Harrison, E. G., Jr. and Mayo, C. W.: Mesenteric fibromatosis in familial polyposis: a variant of Gardner's syndrome. Cancer 17: 526-534, 1964.

Smith, W. G.: Familial multiple polyposis: research tool for investigating the etiology of carcinoma of the colon? Dis. Colon Rectum 11: 17-31, 1968.

Vanhoutte, J. J.: Polypoid lymphoid hyperplasia of the terminal ileum in patients with familial polyposis coli and with Gardner's syndrome. Am. J. Roentgen. 110: 340-342, 1970.

17540 POLYPOSIS, INTESTINAL, IV (SCATTERED, DISCRETE POLYPS)

Woolf, Richards and Gardner (1955) suggested that some families have scattered polyps as a dominant trait distinct from multiple polyposis of the colon. Studies of polyposis I families show, however, such wide variability in the number of polyps that it is difficult to accept the idea that a separate mutation exists. The evidence is, to say the least, inconclusive.

Woolf, C. M., Richards, R. C. and Gardner, E. J.: Occasional discrete polyps of the colon and rectum showing inherited tendency in a kindred. Cancer 8: 403-408, 1955.

17550 POLYPOSIS, SKIN PIGMENTATION, ALOPECIA AND FINGERNAIL CHANGES (CRONKITE-CANADA SYNDROME)

This syndrome was first described by Cronkite and Canada (1955) and later by Jarnum and Jensen (1966). Manousos and Webster (1966) reported the fourth patient. All cases have been sporadic. No evidence of a genetic basis is available. All have been adult. The prognosis is poor. The Cronkite-Canada syndrome is generalized intestinal polyposis with mucocutaneous pigmentation, atrophy of fingernails and alopecia (Cronkite and Canada, 1955; Dacruz, 1967). The etiology is unknown but it appears to be non-genetic. The pigmentation is diffuse, not spotted as in the Peutz-Jeghers syndrome.

Cronkite, L. W., Jr. and Canada, W. J.: Generalized gastrointestinal polyposis: an unusual syndrome of polyposis, pigmentation, alopecia and onychotrophia. New Eng. J. Med. 252: 1011-1015, 1955.

Dacruz, G. M. G.: Generalized gastrointestinal polyposis. An unusual syndrome of adenomatous polyposis, alopecia, onychorotrophia. Am. J. Gastroent. 47: 504-510, 1967.

Jarnum, S. and Jensen, H.: Diffuse gastrointestinal polyposis with ectodermal changes. A case with severe malabsorption and enteric loss of plasma proteins and electrolytes. Gastroenterology 50: 107-118, 1966.

Manousos, O. and Webster, C. V.: Diffuse gastrointestinal polyposis with ectodermal changes. Gut 7: 375-378, 1966.

*17570 POLYSYNDACTYLY WITH PECULIAR SKULL SHAPE (GREIG CEPHALO-POLYSYNDAC-TYLY SYNDROME)

Greig (1928) described digital malformations and peculiar skull shape in mother and daughter. The mother had syndactyly of both hands. The daughter had polysyndactyly and a peculiar skull shape in the form of expanded cranial vault leading to high forehead and bregma, with no evidence of precocious closure of cranial sutures. The daughter was of above average intelligence. The thumbs and great toes had bifid terminal phalanges. Temtamy (1966) studied a particularly instructive family in which 10 members of 4 generations in 6 sibships were affected in the pattern of a fully penetrant autosomal dominant trait. Hootnick and Holmes (1972) also reported a family and suggested that the family reported as a 'new' disorder designated frontodigital syndrome (13670) in fact had this condition.

Greig, D. M.: Oxycephaly. Edinb. Med. J. 33: 189-218, 1928.

Hootnick, D. and Holmes, L. B.: Familial polysyndactyly and craniofacial anomalies. Clin. Genet. 3: 128-134, 1972.

Temtamy, S. A.: Genetic Factors in Hand Malformations. Ph. D. Thesis, Johns Hopkins University, 1966.

17575 POPLITEAL CYST (BAKER CYST)

Toyama (1972) described three affected males, all first cousins, each in a different sibship. The relevant parents were two brothers and a sister all affected. Presumably there was no consanguinity in the family. Autosomal dominant inheritance with reduced penetrance would seem possible. Collaboration of a structural predisposition and repeated minor trauma may be involved in causation.

Toyama, W. M.: Familial popliteal cysts in children. Am. J. Dis. Child. 124: 586-587, 1972.

*17580 POROKERATOSIS OF MIBELLI

This is a rare hereditary keratoatrophoderma characterized by centrifugally spreading patches surrounded by narrow horny ridges and with central atrophy. The lesions are crater-like. More cases have been described in Italians than in other nationalities, according to some, although Bloom and Abramowitz (1943) were impressed with the wide ethnic distribution of cases including Negroes. They described the disorder in an Italian man and his two sons. The grandfather was said to be affected. Autosomal dominant inheritance, probably with some reduction in penetrance in females, seems quite certain. The prefix poro- comes from the Greek for callus. Mibelli (1860-1910), who described this condition, was an Italian dermatologist.

Bloom, D. and Abramowitz, E. W.: Porokeratosis mibelli: report of three cases in one family: histologic studies. Arch. Derm. Syph. 47: 1-15, 1943.

Cort, D. F.: Epithelioma arising in porokeratosis of Mibelli. Brit. J. Plastic Surg. 25: 318-328, 1972.

Harnden, D.: Birmingham, Eng., personal communication, May, 1973.

Reed, R. J. and Leone, P.: Porokeratosis — a mutant clonal keratosis of the epidermis. Histogenesis. Arch. Derm. 101: 340-347, 1970.

Saunders, T. S.: Porokeratosis. A disease of epidermal eccrine-sweat-duct units. Arch. Derm. 84: 980-988, 1961.

17585 POROKERATOSIS PLANTARIS, PALMARIS ET DISSEMINATA

In 8 persons in 4 generations, Guss et al. (1971) described a form of porokeratosis probably distinct from both the Mibelli type and DSAP. Characteristically, lesions appeared first on the palms and soles (in the late teens or early 20's) and subsequently on other parts of the body including areas not exposed to ultraviolet radiation. Porokeratosis is, in general, a chronic progressive disorder of keratinization with annular or gyrate plaques showing elevated borders. Palmar and plantar lesions are rare in the other two types. The family reported by Guss et al. (1971) showed a pedigree pattern consistent with either autosomal or X-linked dominant inheritance.

Guss, S. B., Osbourn, R. A. and Lutzner, M. A.: Porokeratosis plantaris, palmaris, et disseminata. A third type of porokeratosis. Arch. Derm. 104: 366-373, 1971.

*17590 POROKERATOSIS, DISSEMINATED SUPERFICIAL ACTINIC (DSAP)

Lesions occur almost only in sun-exposed areas of the skin. Lesions develop after age 16 and penetrance becomes almost complete by age 30 or 40. DSAP is much more frequent than porokeratosis of Mibelli from which it must be distinguished.

Anderson, D. E. and Chernosky, M. E.: Disseminated superficial actinic porokeratosis. Genetic aspects. Arch. Derm. 99: 408-412, 1969.

Chernosky, M. E. and Anderson, D. E.: Disseminated superficial actinic porokeratosis. Clinical studies and experimental production of lesions. Arch. Derm. 99: 401-407, 1969.

*17600 PORPHYRIA, ACUTE INTERMITTENT (SWEDISH TYPE OF PORPHYRIA)

Skin lesions do not occur in this disorder. Porphobilinogen is present in the urine at all times. Acute neuropathic attacks may be precipitated by barbiturates. Waldenstrom and Haeger-Aronsen (1963) estimated that there may be as many as 600 such cases in Sweden. With (1969) concluded that 'gene penetration' and drug sensitivity differ from family to family. 'Every porphyric family has its own characteristic disease.' Strand et al. (1970, 1971) found deficiency of uroporphyrinogen synthetase. Almost all enzymopathies are recessive because few enzymes are so rate-limiting as to cause a serious reduction in the rate of a metabolic pathway when the enzyme has 40-60 percent normal activity. Seemingly uroporphyrinogen synthetase is such an enzyme, however, so that AIP results in the heterozygote for deficiency. Strand et al. (1970) and Meyer et al. (1972) presented evidence that the defect concerns uroporphyrinogen I (URO)-synthetase activity as measured in liver and erythrocytes. This is a rare example of a dominant enzymopathy, i.e., an enzymopathy which leads to phenotypic effects when the mutant gene is present in only heterozygous state. Low URO-synthetase in red cells occurred in persons with no history of acute attacks and no increase in delta-aminolevulinic acid (ALA) and porphobilinogen (PBG) in urine. The deficient enzyme is also called porphobilinogen (PBG) deaminase.

Dean, G.: The porphyrias. A Story of Inheritance and Environment. Philadelphia: J. B. Lippincott Co., 1971 (2nd Ed.).

Drabkin, D. L.: Some historical highlights in knowledge of porphyrins and porphyrias. Ann. N.Y. Acad. Sci. 104: 658-665, 1963.

Goldberg, A. and Rimington, C.: Disease of Porphyrin Metabolism. Springfield, Ill.: Charles C Thomas, 1963.

Labbe, R. F.: Metabolic abnormality in porphyria. The result of impaired biological oxidation? Lancet 1: 1361-1364, 1967.

MacAlpine, I., Hunter, R., Rimington, C., Brooke, J. and Goldberg, A.: Porphyria — a rare royal malady. London: Brit. Med. Ass., 1968.

Meyer, U. A., Strand, L. J., Doss, M., Rees, A. C. and Marver, H. S.: Intermittent acute porphyria — demonstration of a genetic defect in porphobilinogen metabolism. New Eng. J. Med. 286: 1277-1282, 1972.

Sassa, S., Granick, S., Bickers, D. R., Bradlow, H. L. and Kappas, A.: A microassay for urophyrinogen I synthase, one of three abnormal enzyme activities in acute intermittent porphyria, and its application to the study of the genetics of this disease. Proc. Nat. Acad. Sci. 71: 732-736, 1974.

Stein, J. A. and Tschudy, D. P.: Acute intermittent porphyria. A clinical and biochemical study of 46 patients. Medicine 49: 1-16, 1970.

Strand, L. J., Felsher, B. F., Redeker, A. G. and Marver, H. S.: Heme biosynthesis in intermittent acute porphyria: decreased hepatic conversion of porphobilinogen to porphyrins and increased delta aminolevulinic acid synthetase activity. Proc. Nat. Acad. Sci. 67: 1315-1320, 1970.

Strand, L. J., Meyer, U. A., Felsher, B. F., Redeker, A. G. and Marver, H. S.: Decreased red cell uroporphyrinogen i synthetase activity in intermittent acute porphyria. J. Clin. Invest. 51: 2530-2536, 1972.

Sweeney, V. P., Pathals, M. A. and Asbury, A. K.: Acute intermittent porphyria. Increased ALA-synthetase activity during an acute attack. Brain 93: 369-380, 1970.

Tschudy, D. P.: Biochemical lesions in porphyria. J.A.M.A. 191: 718-730, 1965.

Waldenstrom, J. and Haeger-Aronsen, B.: Different patterns of human porphyria. Brit. Med. J. 2: 272-276, 1963.

Waldenstrom, J.: Studies on the incidence and heredity of acute porphyria in Sweden. Acta Genet. Statist. Med. 6: 122-131, 1956.

With, T. K.: Hereditary hepatic porphyrias. Gene penetration, drug sensitivity and subdivision in the light of systematic family studies. Acta Med. Scand. 186: 117-124, 1969.

17610 PORPHYRIA, HEPATIC-CUTANEOUS TYPE (PORPHYRIA CUTANEA TARDA)

This type occurs particularly in alcoholics, producing some of the same neurologic and cutaneous manifestations as are seen in other forms of porphyria. Genetically determined idiosyncrasy is suspected. Features include hyperpigmentation and scleroderma-like changes. Watson (1965) has observed affected brothers. Ziprkowski (1966) observed porphyria cutanea tarda in three successive generations. Venosection, originally performed because of confusion with hemochromatosis, seems to be beneficial. Phlebotomy was symptomatically and biochemically beneficial (Epstein and Redeker, 1968). Kushner et al. (1972) viewed PCT as an acquired disease, usually associated with alcoholic liver disease. They pointed out that it is the most frequent recognized disorder of porphyrin metabolism. They presented in vitro evidence to suggest that excessive synthesis of uroporphyrin I in this disease is due to inhibition of uroporphyrinogen III cosynthetase by ferrous iron.

Epstein, J. H. and Redeker, A. G.: Porphyria cutanea tarda: a study of the effect of phlebotomy. New Eng. J. Med. 279: 1301-1304, 1968.

Kushner, J. P., Lee, G. R. and Nacht, S.: The role of iron in the pathogenesis of porphyria cutanea tarda: an in vitro model. J. Clin. Invest. 51: 3044-3051, 1972.

Ramsey, C. A., Magnus, I. A., Turnbull, A. and Baker, H.: The treatment of porphyria cutanea tarda by venesection. Quart. J. Med. 43: 1-24, 1974.

Watson, C. J.: Minneapolis, Minn.: personal communication, 1965.

Ziprkowski, L., Krakowski, A., Crispin, M. and Szeinberg, A.: Porphyria cutanea tarda hereditaria. Israel J. Med. Sci. 2: 338-343, 1966.

*17620 PORPHYRIA, VARIEGATA (SOUTH AFRICAN TYPE OF PORPHYRIA)

Dean (1963) has described in an engaging manner his studies of porphyria in South Africa and comparative studies in Sweden, Holland, Turkey and elsewhere. The high frequency of the gene for porphyria variegata in South Africa is a cardinal example of founder effect. Dean estimates that about 8,000 persons in South Africa now suffer from porphyria inherited from either Gerrit Jansz, a Dutch settler in the Cape, or his wife, Ariaantje Jacobs, who was one of eight sent from an orphanage in Rotterdam to provide wives for Dutch settlers in the Cape. He estimates, furthermore, that one million of three million whites are descendants of 40 original settlers and their wives, a 12,000-fold increase. Affected persons show increased fecal excretion of protoporphyrin and coproporphyrin at all times. Porphyria variegata was observed in three families in Sweden by Hamnstrom et al. (1967). No genealogic connection with any of the 600 known cases of acute intermittent porphyria could be shown. MacAlpine et al. (1968) suggested that George III suffered from porphyria and that the disease can be traced back to Mary Queen of Scots. Identification of porphyria in two living persons in the kindred supported their suggestion. Presumably if barbiturates had been part of the pharmaceutical armamentarium 2 or 3 centuries ago the course of world history would have been quite different. Although the malady of George III was indistinguishable retrospectively from acute intermittent porphyria, the dermatologic manifestations and fecal findings in two living members of the family support the position that the royal porphyria was the variegate type. Cochrane and Goldberg (1968) reported studies of an extensive kindred of which the first author is a member.

Cochrane, A. L. and Goldberg, A.: A study of faecal porphyrin levels in a large family. Ann. Hum. Genet. 32: 195-208, 1968.

Dean, G.: The porphyrias. A Story of Inheritance and Environment. Philadelphia: J. B. Lippincott, Co., 1963.

Hamnstrom, B., Haeger-Aronsen, B., Waldenstrom, J., Hysing, B. and Molander, J.: Three Swedish families with porphyria variegata. Brit. Med. J. 2: 449-453, 1967.

MacAlpine, I., Hunter, R. and Rimington, C.: Porphyria in the royal houses of Stuart, Hanover and Prussia: a follow-up study of George III's illness. Brit. Med. J. 1: 7-17, 1968.

17625 POSTERIOR COLUMN ATAXIA

Biemond (1951) and Singh et al. (1973) described families with multiple members affected with ataxia due strictly to degeneration in the posterior columns. In Biemond's family the father, four of his children and his brother were affected. There was pregressive loss of vibration and postural sensibility and ataxia, with loss of muscle stretch reflexes and flexor plantar responses. Pain and temperature sensations were preserved. There were no signs of cerebellar or pyramidal tract involvement. Scoliosis was not mentioned. The age of onset of symptoms was between 19 and 30 years. In the family of Singh et al. (1973) the onset was in the first decade of life and scolisis was present. Four brothers were affected with ostensibly normal parents. The authers suggested that either interruption of motor efferent or propioceptive afferent nerve supply in the thoracic area can lead to scoliosis.

Biemond, A.: Les degenerations spino-cerebelleuses. Folia psychiat. Neerl. 54: 216-223, 1951.

Singh, N., Mehta, M. and Roy, S.: Familial posterior column ataxia (Biemond's) with scoliosis. Europ. Neurol. 10: 160-167, 1973.

P — R INTERVAL, SHORT see WOLFF-PARKINSON-WHITE SYNDROME (19420) see VENTRICULAR FIBRILLATION (19245)

17630 PREALBUMIN, POLYMORPHISM OF SERUM

Fagerhol and Braend (1965) demonstrated polymorphism by starch gel electrophoresis and presented family data supporting genetic control by three codominant alleles. Polymorphism of prealbumin is known in the mouse and pig (reviewed by Lush, 1966). The prealbumins, serum proteins which migrate faster than albumin in acidic starch gels, include alpha(1)-antitrypsin, thyroxine binding prealbumin and orosomucoid, an alpha(1)-acid glycoprotein (q.v.). Polymorphism of the first and last are known. The polymorphism of prealbumin which Fagerhol and Braend (1965, 1966) described was shown by Fagerhol and Laurell (1967) to be identical to alpha(1)-antitrypsin.

Fagerhol, M. K. and Braend, M.: Classification of human serum prealbumin after starch gel electrophoresis. Acta Path. Microbiol. Scand. 68: 434-438, 1966.

Fagerhol, M. K. and Braend, M.: Serum prealbumin: polymorphism in man. Science 149: 986-987, 1965.

Fagerhol, M. K. and Laurell, C. B.: The polymorphism of 'prealbumins' and alpha(1)-antitrypsin in human sera. Clin. Chim. Acta. 16: 199-203, 1967.

Lush, I. E.: The Biochemical Genetics of Vertebrates Except Man. Philadelphia: W. B. Saunders, 1966.

*17640 PRECOCIOUS PUBERTY

These cases are often misdiagnosed adrenogenital syndrome. Puberty may occur before 3 years of age. Male-to-male transmission has been observed. No peculiarity has been noted in females who can transmit the trait. Adult height is reduced. Rush et al. (1937) and Jacobsen and Macklin (1952) reported a family in which 27 males (but no females) in 4 generations showed sexual precocity. Wilkins (1965) stated that 'among girls we also have seen a familial tendency to sexual precocity and have had one family in which both sexes were affected.' Ferrier et al. (1961) observed affected brother and sister. Hampson and Money (1955) suggested that female sexual precocity may be transmitted through the male. Jungck et al. (1957) observed transmission of male precocity through females. The family of Beas et al. (1962) contained an affected brother and sister. This is so-called isosexual precocious puberty. A usual definition is onset of menarche in the female before age eight and one-half years, or pubertal changes in the male before age 10 years. It is a more frequent occurrence in females than in males, but familial occurrence seems rarer in females.

Beas, F., Zurbrugg, R. P., Leibow, S. G., Patton, R. G. and Gardner, L. I.: Familial male sexual precocity: report of the eleventh kindred found, with observations on blood group linkage and urinary C-19-steroid excretion. J. Clin. Endocr. 22: 1095-1102, 1962.

Ferrier, P., Shepard, T. H. and Smith, E. K.: Growth disturbances and values for hormone excretion in various forms of precocious sexual development. Pediatrics 28: 258-275, 1961.

Hampson, J. G. and Money, J.: Idiopathic sexual precocity in the female. Report of three cases. Psychosom. Med. 17: 16-35, 1955.

Jacobsen, A. W. and MacKlin, M. T.: Hereditary sexual precocity: report of a family with 27 affected members. Pediatrics 9: 682-694, 1952.

Jungck, E. C., Thrash, A. M., Ohlmacher, A. P., Knight, A. M., Jr. and Dyrenforth, L. Y.: Sexual precocity due to interstitial-cell tumor of the testis: report of 2 cases. J. Clin. Endocr. 17: 291-295, 1957.

Mortimer, E. A.: Familial constitutional precocious puberty in a boy three years of age. Report of a case. Pediatrics 13: 174-177, 1954.

Novak, E.: Constitutional type of female precocious puberty with a report of 9 cases. Am. J. Obstet. Gynec. 47: 20-42, 1944.

Rush, H. P., Bilderback, J. B., Slocum, D. and Rogers, A.: Pubertas praecox (macrogenitosomia). Endocrinology 21: 404-411, 1937.

Wilkins, L.: Diagnosis and Treatment of Endocrine Disorders in Childhood and Adolescence. Springfield, Ill.: Charles C Thomas, 1965 (3rd Ed.).

*17645 PRESACRAL TERATOMA

In studies of 23 cases of presacral teratoma, Ashcraft et al. (1974) obtained clear evidence of autosomal dominant inheritance. Adhesion to the dura and to the rectum and associatied boney defect in the sacrum were the rule. Abscess in the tumor was frequent. One case of metastases was observed. Invlovement of many persons in several generations with male-to-male transmission was observed.

Ashcraft, K. W., Holder, T. M. and Harris, D. J.: Familial presacral teratoma. To be published, 1974.

17650 PRESENILE DEMENTIA WITH SPASTIC PARALYSIS

Worster-Drought and colleagues (1933, 1940) described 9 affected persons in three generations. Onset occurred between 40 and 60 years with early onset of spasticity (increased DTR and tone). Muscular rigidity of extrapyramidal type was present. No tremors, spontaneous movements or sensory changes were observed. Mental deterioration was progressive, with survival as long as 13 years after onset. Paresis of pyramidal and extrapyramidal type is rare in Pick disease and occurs late. No male-to-male transmission was noted by Worster-Drought et al. (1940), although 12 persons in 3 generations were affected.

Worster-Drought, C., Greenfield, J. G. and McMenemey, W. H.: A form of familial presenile dementia with spastic paralysis (including pathological examination of a case). Brain 63: 237-254, 1940.

Worster-Drought, C., Hill, T. R. and McMenemey, W. H.: Familial presenile dementia with spastic paralysis. J. Neurol. Psychopath. 14: 27-34, 1933.

17660 PRESENILE DEMENTIA, KRAEPELIN TYPE

A nonspecific type of familial presenile dementia apparently distinct from both Alzheimer disease and Pick disease (q.v.) was described by Schaumburg and Suzuki (1968) in 6 persons in 3 generations with male-to-male transmission. The histologic changes corresponded to those described for Kraepelin disease. In 4 of the 6 persons onset was at a very early age: 28, 31, 33 and 34.

Schaumburg, H. H. and Suzuki, K.: Non-specific familial presenile dementia. J. Neurol. Neurosurg. Psychiat. 31: 479-486, 1968.

*17670 PROGNATHISM, MANDIBULAR

Mandibular prognathism was transmitted through many generations of the Hapsburg line as a simple dominant (Rubbrecht, 1930; Strohmayer, 1937). We have observed a dominant inheritance pattern in a Negro family. Involvement in four generations was described by Stiles and Luke (1953). An apparent conductor did not show the condition. Mandibular prognathism is a feature of the XXY, XXXY, and XXXXY syndromes and of interest is the progressive increase of this feature as the number of X chromosomes increased (Gorlin et al., 1965). Although the X chromosome has a role, the Mendelian trait is not X-linked.

Gorlin, R. J., Redman, R. S. and Shapiro, B. L.: Effect of X-chromosome anenploidy on jaw growth. J. Dental Res. 44: 269-282, 1965.

Grabb, W. C., Hodge, G. P., Dingman, R. O. and O'Neal, R. M.: The Hapsburg jaw. Plast. Reconstr. Surg. 42: 442-445, 1968.

Haecker, V.: Der Familientypus der Habsburger. Z. Abst. Vererb. 6: 61-89, 1911.

Rubbrecht, O.: Der Unterkieferprognathismus und dessen Verebung nach dem mendelschen Gesetz. Province Dentaire, p. 322, 1930.

Rubbrecht, O.: L'origin du type familial de la maison de Habsbourg. Bruxelles: G. Van Oest Et Cie, 1910.

Rubbrecht, O.: Study of the heredity of the anomalies of the jaws. Am. J. Orthodont. 25: 751-779, 1939.

Stiles, K. A. and Luke, J. E.: The inheritance of malocclusion due to mandibular prognathism. J. Hered. 44: 241-245, 1953.

Strohmayer, W.: Die Vererbung des Habsburger Familientypus. Nova Acta Leopoldina 5: 219-296, 1937.

17673 PROINSULIN

Insulin, synthesized by the beta cells of the islets of Langerhans, consists of two dissimilar polypeptide chains A and B which are linked by two disulfide bonds. However, unlike some other proteins made up of structurally distinct subunits, insulin is probably under the control of a single structural locus because both chains A and B are derived from a one-chain precursor, proinsulin. Proinsulin is converted to insulin by the enzymatic removal of a segment which connects the amino end of the A chain to the carboxyl end of the B chain.

Dayhoff, M. O.: Proinsulin. Atlas of Protein and Sequence and Structure 1972 (Vol. 5). Washington: National Biomedical Research Foundation, 1972. P. D208.

17675 PROLACTIN DEFICIENCY, ISOLATED

Isolated prolactin deficiency is a clear entity (Turkington, 1972) and it may be an autosomal recessive trait but this has not been established. The affected females are generally healthy but are unable to nurse following parturition and have no detectable prolactin secretion after stimulation with phenothiazine.

Turkington, R. W.: Phenothiazine stimulation test for prolactin reserve: the syndrome of isolated prolactin deficiency. J. Clin. Endocr. 34: 247-249, 1972.

17680 PRONATION-SUPINATION OF THE FOREARM, IMPAIRMENT OF

Thompson et al. (1968) described a family in which males in three successive generations had limitation in pronation and supination of the forearms. Radio-ulnar synostosis (q.v.) was not present.

Thompson, J. S., McLaughlin, P. R. and Heslin, D. J.: Impaired pronation-supination of the forearm: an inherited condition. J. Med. Genet. 5: 48-51, 1968.

17690 PROTEOLYTIC CAPACITY OF PLASMA

Jacobsen (1968) concluded that low proteolytic capacity is inherited as an autosomal dominant. Increased tendency to thrombosis did not occur in these persons.

Jacobsen, C. D.: Proteolytic capacity in human plasma. Genetics and clinical study. Scand. J. Clin. Lab. Invest. 21: 227-237, 1968.

*17700 PROTOPORPHYRIA, ERYTHROPOIETIC

Haeger-Aronsen (1963) found five cases in three generations of a Swedish family. It seems possible, however, that two of the cases are in fact heterozygotes and a father and his two daughters are homozygous. The mother of these daughters (a heterozygote by this line of thought) was apparently not tested. First described by Magnus et al. (1961), the condition is characterized by the sudden onset in childhood of itching, erythema and edema following exposure to ultraviolet light. Vesicles never develop. The most conspicuous biochemical change is a marked increase in the protoporphyrin and coproporphyrin content of red blood cells. The urinary excretion of porphyrins and their precursors is normal. Fecal excretion of coproporphyrin and protoporphyrin may be increased. It is of note that both of the British patients of Magnus et al. and one of Haeger-Aronsen's patients were operated on for gallstones at a relatively young age. Three generations were affected in the family studied by Lynch and Miedler (1965). Cripps (1966) claimed that patients with this condition have been incorrectly reported as examples of lipoid proteinosis. Rather numerous instances of parent-offspring involvement have been observed. Beta-carotene is an effective photoprotective agent (Matthews-Roth et al., 1970). Because of evidence they adduced for formation of protoporphyrin in at least the two tissues, Scholnick et al. (1971) proposed that the disorder be renamed erythrohepatic protoporphyria. Hovding et al. (1971) found evidence for dominant inheritance in two Norwegian families.

Cripps, D. J.: Erythropoietic protoporphyria (antea lipoid proteinosis) in sisters. Arch. Derm. 94: 682-686, 1966.

Donaldson, E. M., Donaldson, A. D. and Rimington, C.: Erythropoietic protoporphyria: a family study. Brit. Med. J. 1: 659-663, 1967.

Haeger-Aronsen, B. and Krook, G.: Erythropoietic protoporphyria. A study of known cases in Sweden. Acta Med. Scand. 445 (suppl.): 48-55, 1966.

Haeger-Aronsen, B.: Erythropoietic protoporphyria. A new type of inborn error of metabolism. Am. J. Med. 35: 450-454, 1963.

Hovding, G., Haavelsrud, O. I. and Wad, N.: Erythropoietic protoporphyria. Acta Derm. Venerol. 51: 383-386, 1971.

Lynch, P. J. and Miedler, L. J.: Erythropoietic protoporphyria. Report of a family and a clinical review. Arch. Derm. 92: 351-356, 1965.

Magnus, I. A., Jarrett, A., Prankerd, T. A. J. and Rimington, C.: Erythropoietic porphyria. A new protoporphyria syndrome with solar urticaria due to protoporphyrinaemia. Lancet II: 448-451, 1961.

Matthews-Roth, M. M., Pathak, M. A., Fitzpatrick, T. B., Harber, L. C. and Kass, E. H.: Beta-carotene as a photoprotective agent in erythropoietic protoporphyria. New Eng. J. Med. 282: 1231-1234, 1970.

Peterka, E. S., Fusaro, R. M., Runge, W. J., Jaffe, M. O. and Watson, C. J.: Erythropoietic protoporphyria. Clinical and laboratory features in seven new cases. J.A.M.A. 193: 1036-1042, 1965.

Reed, W. B., Wuepper, K. D., Epstein, J. H., Redeker, A., Simonson, R. J. and McKusick, V. A.: Erythropoietic protoporphyria. J.A.M.A. 214: 1060-1066, 1970.

Scholnick, P., Marver, H. S. and Schmid, R.: Erythropoietic protoporphyria: evidence for multiple sites of excess protoporphyrin formation. J. Clin. Invest. 50: 203-207, 1971.

17710 PRURITUS, HEREDITARY LOCALIZED

Comings and Comings (1965) described the entity in 8 members of three sibships in two generations in a pattern consistent with either autosomal or X-linked dominant inheritance. Onset was in the third decade and the itching was located in an area overlying the lower end of one scapula or the other.

Comings, D. E. and Comings, S. N.: Hereditary localized pruritus. Arch. Derm. 92: 236-237, 1965.

*17715 PSEUDOACHONDROPLASTIC DYSPLASIA I (FORMERLY PSEUDOACHONDROPLASTIC SPONDYLOEPIPHYSEAL DYSPLASIA)

The new term is that suggested in the Paris nomenclature (McKusick, Scott, 1971). The classification into four types, two dominant (I and III) and two recessive (II and IV), was suggested by Hall and Dorst (1969). The two dominant forms are distinguished on the basis of severity of radiographic findings and particularly the biochemical and morphologic characteristics of type III (McKusick, 1972). They might be allelic. In this class of disorders, dwarfism is delayed in onset and the head and face are not involved. The radiographic changes are quite different from those of true achondroplasia. Maroteaux and Lamy (1959) first clearly delineated the class and assigned the earlier term 'pseudoachondroplastic spondyloepiphyseal dysplasia.'

Hall, J. E. and Dorst, J. P.: Pseudoachondroplastic SED, recessive Maroteaux-Lamy type. The Clinical Delineation of Birth Defects. IV. Skeletal Dysplasias. New York: National Foundation, 1969. Pp. 254-259.

Maroteaux, P. and Lamy, M.: Les formes pseudo-achondroplasiques des dysplasies spondylo-epiphysaires. Presse Med. 67: 383-386, 1959.

McKusick, V. A.: Heritable Disorders of Connective Tissue. St. Louis: C. V. Mosby Co., 1972 (4th Ed.).

*17717 PSEUDOACHONDROPLASTIC DYSPLASIA III (FORMERLY PSEUDOACHONDROPLASTIC SPONDYLOEPIPHYSEAL DYSPLASIA)

This was probably the form which Maroteaux and Lamy (1959) dealt with in the main in their original description of this class of disorder, although they spoke of the 'formes' of pseudoachondroplasia. The distinctiveness of this type is indicated not only by the radiographic findings but also by cytoplasmic metachromasia of fibroblasts and unique electron microscopic changes in chondrocytes (Maynard et al., 1972).

Cooper, R. R., Ponseti, I. V. and Maynard, J. A.: Pseudoachondroplastic dwarfism. A rough-surfaced endoplasmic reticulum storage disorder. J. Bone Joint Surg. 55: 475-484, 1973.

Maroteaux, P. and Lamy, M.: Les formes pseudo-achondroplastiques des dysplasies spondylo-epiphysaires. Presse Med. 67: 383-386, 1959.

Maynard, J. A., Cooper, R. R. and Ponseti, I. V.: A unique rough surface endoplasmic reticulum inclusion in pseudoachondroplasia. Lab. Invest. 26: 40-44, 1972.

17720 PSEUDO-ALDOSTERONISM (LIDDLE SYNDROME)

Liddle et al. (1963) described hypertension associated with hypokalemic alkalosis not due to hyperaldosteronism but rather to a renal tubular peculiarity. Three generations had been affected with no known male-to-male transmission. See POTASSIUM AND MAGNESIUM DEPLETION in the recessive catalog. Liddle syndrome is characterized by hypoaldosteronism, hypokalemia, decreased renin and angiotensin. Gardner et al. (1970) presented evidence for a primary defect in membrane transport.

Gardner, J., Lapey, A., Simopoulos, A. and Bravo, E.: Evidence for a primary disturbance of membrane transport in Bartter's syndrome and Liddle's syndrome. (Abstract) J. Clin. Invest. 49: 32A only, 1970.

Liddle, G. W., Bledsoe, T. and Coppage, W. S., Jr.: A familial renal disorder simulating primary aldosteronism but with negligible aldosterone secretion. Trans. Ass. Am. Physicians 76: 199-213, 1963.

17730 PSEUDO-ARTHROGRYPOSIS (HEREDITARY CONGENITAL RIGIDITY OF ELBOWS AND KNEES)

Pasma and Wildervanck (1956) described a grandmother, her daughter and three granddaughters with rigidity of the elbows and knees. The grandmother showed bony ankylosis at the elbow and proximal fusion of the tibia and fibula. They pointed out a similarity to the cases in females in three generations described by Siwon (1928). In the latter family the rigidity appears to have been confined to the elbows. One patient was shown to have bilateral fusion of the humerus, radius and ulna as in one of the patients of Pasma and Wildervanck. See also PRONATION-SUPINATION OF FOREARM, IMPAIRMENT OF. See RADIO-ULNAR SYNOSTOSIS. See KUSKOKWIN SYNDROME.

Pasma, A. and Wildervanck, L. S.: Hereditary occurrence of congenital rigidity of the elbows and knees (congenital multiple 'pseudoarthrogryposis'). Arch. Chir. Neerl. 8: 43-56, 1956.

Siwon, P.: Kongenitale, hereditaere, doppelseitige Ankylosen der Ellenbogengelenke. Deutsch. Z. Chir. 209: 338-349, 1928.

*17740 PSEUDOCHOLINESTERASE TYPES, E(1) VARIANTS

Although succinylcholine sensitivity (pseudocholinesterase deficiency) is a recessive, methods for demonstrating the heterozygote and several different rare heterozygous phenotypes are known, hence inclusion here. Four allelic forms of the gene responsible for serum pseudocholinesterase are recognized. In addition to that determining the typical pseudocholinesterase, these are (1) gene for atypical form of enzyme less inhibited by dibucaine than the normal, (2) gene for form with normal dibucaine inhibition but less inhibition by fluoride than the normal, and (3) gene determining complete absence of cholinesterase activity ('silent gene'). In addition to the above alleles at the E(1) locus, a second separate locus called E(2) was described by Harris et al. (1963). Motulsky and Morrow (1968), using a rapid screening test, demonstrated a low frequency of heterozygotes among Congolese Africans, Japanese, Taiwanese, Filipinos and Eskimos. U.S. Caucasians, Greeks, Yugoslavs and East Indians had a relatively high frequency (2.8 to 3.3 percent). They predicted a low frequency of suxamethonium apnea in the low frequency groups. See TRANSFERRINS for reference to linkage between transferrin locus and pseudocholinesterase locus. The Cynthiana variant is associated with increased enzyme activity (Yoshida and Motulsky, 1969). Whether it is determined by the E(1) or E(2) locus is not known. Lubin et al. (1971) reported on findings using an autosomal screening method permitting study of one group of 2317 persons. Among Caucasians the ratio of male to female heterozygotes was 1.85 to 1.

Altland, K. and Goedde, H. W.: Heterogeneity in the silent gene phenotype of pseudocholinesterase of human serum. Biochem. Genet. 4: 321-338, 1970.

Das, P. K.: Further evidence on the heterogeneity of 'silent' serum cholinesterase variants. Hum. Hered. 23: 88 only, 1973.

Dietz, A. A., Lubrano, T. and Rubinstein, H. M.: Four families segregating for the silent gene for serum cholinesterase. Acta Genet. Statist. Med. 15: 208-217, 1965.

Goedde, H. W. and Baitsch, H.: On nomenclature of pseudocholinesterase polymorphism. Acta Genet. Statist. Med. 14: 366-369, 1964.

Harris, H., Hopkinson, D. A., Robson, E. B. and Whittaker, M.: Genetical studies on a new variant of serum cholinesterase detected by electrophoresis. Ann. Hum. Genet. 26: 359-382, 1963.

Lubin, A. H., Garry, P. J. and Owen, G. M.: Sex and population differences in the incidence of a plasma cholinesterase variant. Science 173: 161-164, 1971.

Motulsky, A. G. and Morrow, A.: Atypical cholinesterase gene E(1)(a): rarity in Negroes and most Orientals. Science 159: 202-203, 1968.

Whittaker, M.: Pseudocholinesterase variants: a study of fourteen families selected via the fluoride resistant phenotype. Acta Genet. Statist. Med. 17: 1-12, 1967.

Yoshida, A. and Motulsky, A. G.: A pseudocholinesterase variant (E cynthiana) associated with elevated plasma enzyme activity. Am. J. Hum. Genet. 21: 486-498, 1969.

*17750 PSEUDOCHOLINESTERASE TYPES, E(2) VARIANTS

See above. Merritt et al. (1973) presented data consistent with localization of the E(2) locus on chromosome no. 1 within mappable distance of the amylase loci (10470, 10471).

Merritt, A. D., Lovrien, E. W., Rivas, M. L., and Conneally, P. M.: Human amylase loci: genetic linkage with the Duffy blood group locus and assignment to linkage group I. Am. J. Hum. Genet. 1973, In press.

17760 PSEUDOCHOLINESTERASE, INCREASE IN PLASMA LEVEL OF

Neitlich (1966) described a kindred with increased plasma cholinesterase activity and decreased responsiveness to succinylcholinesterase.

Neitlich, H. W.: Increased plasma cholinesterase activity and succinylcholine resistance: a genetic variant. J. Clin. Invest. 45: 380-387, 1966.

17770 PSEUDOGLAUCOMA

This term applies to a condition characterized by normal intraocular tension with cupping of the optic disc and glaucomatous visual field defects. Sandvig (1961) described Norwegian families with a dominant inheritance pattern.

Sandvig, K.: Pseudoglaucoma of autosomal dominant inheritance. Acta Ophthal. 39: 33-43, 1961.

17780 PSEUDOPAPILLEDEMA

Hoyt and Pont (1962) described 28 patients who were first thought to have brain tumors. Identical twins were both affected. We have observed affected father and daughter. 'Buried drusen' were thought to be the cause. Jacquemin (1964) reported mother and two daughters. There may be more than one type of pseudopapilledema. Fite and Lewis (1966) described father and two sons with a type due apparently to 'hyperemia.' Singleton et al. (1973) reported 3 families demonstrating pseudopapilledema. This anomalous elevation of the optic disc was present in 1 member of each of 3 generations in one family and in 1 member of each of 2 generations in the other two families. There was no case of male-to-male transmission in these kindreds.

Chambers, J. W. and Walsh, F. B.: Hyaline bodies in the optic discs: report of 10 cases exemplifying importance in neurological diagnosis. Brain 74: 95-108, 1951.

Fite, J. D. and Lewis, A. D.: Familial anomaly simulating papilledema: a case report. J. Pediat. 68: 927-931, 1966.

Hoyt, W. F. and Pont, M. E.: Pseudopapilledema: anomalous elevation of optic disk. Pitfalls in diagnosis and management. J.A.M.A. 181: 191-196, 1962.

Jacquemin, P. J.: Oedeme papillaire familial et hereditaire. Ann. Oculist. 197: 449-460, 1964.

Lorentzen, S. E.: Drusen of optic disk, irregularly dominant hereditary affection. Acta Ophthal. 39: 626-643, 1961.

Lorentzen, S. E.: Drusen of the optic disk. A clinical and genetic study. Acta Ophthal. 90 (suppl.): 1-181, 1966.

Singleton, E. M., Kinsbourne, M. and Anderson, W. B., Jr.: Familial pseudopapilledema. S. Med. J. 66: 796-802, 1973.

*17785 PSEUDOXANTHOMA ELASTICUM

Based on the study of about 180 cases in England and Wales, Pope (1972) concluded that there is at least one autosomal dominant form of this disorder which has generally been considered to be a recessive (see 26480). He observed several families with affected persons in three generations with male-to-male transmission. Indeed, Pope (1972) suggests the existence of two autosomal dominant forms of PXE. Type I is characterized by classic peau d'orange skin changes, by severe vascular complications such as angina, claudication, and hypertension, and by severe choroiditis. Type II, which in Pope's experience was about four times more frequent than type I, is characterized by macular (or focal) changes in the skin, which is excessively stretchable, and by myopia, high arched palate, blue sclerae and loosejointedness in a significant proportion.

Pope, F. M.: Liverpool, England and Baltimore, Md.: personal communication, 1972.

Pope, F. M.: Autosomal dominant pseudoxanthoma elasticum. J. Med. Genet. 11: 152-157, 1974.

*17790 PSORIASIS

A very large family tree has been assembled in North Carolina (Abele et al., 1963). The authors concluded that penetrance was reduced to about 60 percent. The prevalence of arthritis was not increased in the psoriatic members of the kindred. Lomholt (1965) did a comprehensive study in the Faroe Islands. He found that 91 percent of patients had affected relatives. Transmission through many generations of the large kindred reported by Abele et al. (1963) supports dominant inheritance, the mode of inheritance espoused by Romanus (1945). Steinberg et al. (1951) suggested that homozygosity at two separate loci would best explain their family data. Russell et al. (1972) found that HL-A 13 was present in 12 of 44 unrelated persons with psoriasis and in 3 of 89 controls (a difference significant at a probability less than 0.0001. W17 was present in 10 of 44 unrelated patients and in 17 family members with psoriasis in 4 generations. Two sibs did not have either psoriasis or W17. The study was undertaken because psoriasis is aggravated by streptococcal infection and a protein of group A beta-hemolytic streptoccus cross-reacts with certain HL-A antigens. The finding of an HL-A and disease association is an indication of polygenic inheritance. Even if there is a single major gene the HL-A locus must also be a factor. White et al. (1972) likewise found an excess of W17 and HL-A 13 with a decrease in HL-A 12 in psoriatic patients. Burch and Rowell (1965) suggested the existence of several distinct genotypes in psoriasis, i.e., genetic heterogeneity. A twin study showed increased concordance in MZ twins (Farber and Nall, 1971). Watson et al. (1972) concluded the genetics is multifactorial. Psoriasis is rare in Eskimos, American Indians and Japanese, all of whom have a very low frequency of HL-A 13 and HL-A 17.

Abele, D. C., Dobson, R. L. and Graham, J. B.: Heredity and psoriasis. Study of a large family. Arch. Derm. 88: 38-47, 1963.

Burch, P. R. J. and Rowell, N. R.: Psoriasis: aetiological aspects. Acta Derm. Venerol. 45: 366-380, 1965.

Farber, E. M. and Nall, M. L.: Genetics of psoriasis: twin study. In Farber, E. M. and Cox, A. J.: Psoriasis (International Symposium). Stanford: Stanford Univ. Press, 1971. Pp. 7-13.

Farber, E. M., Nall, M. L. and Watson, W.: Natural history of psoriasis in 61 twin pairs. Arch. Derm. 109: 207-211, 1974.

Kimberling, W. and Dobson, R. L.: The inheritance of psoriasis. J. Invest. Derm. 60: 538-540, 1973.

Lomholt, G.: Psoriasis: prevalence, spontaneous course, and genetics. A Census Study on the Prevalence of Skin Disease on the Faroe Islands. Copenhagen: G. E. C. Gad, 1963.

Lomholt, G.: Psoriasis-Praevalenz, spontaner Verlauf und Vererbung. Eine Zensusuntersuchung von den Farinseln. Z. Haut Geschlechtskr. 38: 223-238, 1965.

Moll, J. M. H. and Wright, V.: Familial occurrence of psoriatic arthritis. Ann. Rheumatic Dis. 32: 181-201, 1973.

Romanus, T.: Psoriasis from a Prognostic and Hereditary Point of View. Dissertation, Uppsala, 1945.

Russell, T. J., Schultes, L. M. and Kuban, D. J.: Histocompatibility (HL-A) antigens associated with psoriasis. New Eng. J. Med. 287: 738-740, 1972.

Steinberg, A. G., Becker, S. W., Fitzpatrick, T. B. and Kierland, R. R.: A genetic and statistical study of psoriasis. Am. J. Hum. Genet. 3: 267-281, 1951. (A further note on the genetics of psoriasis. Am. J. Hum. Genet. 4: 373-375, 1952.)

Ward, J. H. and Stephens, F. E.: Inheritance of psoriasis in a Utah kindred. Arch. Derm. 84: 589-592, 1961.

Watson, W., Cann, H. W., Farber, E. M. and Nall, M. L.: The genetics of psoriasis. Arch. Derm. 105: 197-207, 1972.

White, S. H., Newcomer, V. D., Mickey, M. R. and Terasaki, P. I.: Disturbance of HL-A antigen frequency in psoriasis. New Eng. J. Med. 287: 740-743, 1972.

17800 PTERYGIUM OF CONJUNCTIVA AND CORNEA

When this term is used without further qualification it refers to a wing-shaped thickening in the conjunctiva in the interpalpebral fissure area. (Pterygium colli is webbed neck. Webbing in the popliteal (q.v.) or antecubital area is also referred to as pterygium.) Hilgers (1960) and Schwartz (1960) concluded that pterygium is in many instances a dominant trait. Environmental factors may influence penetrance. The disorder is more frequent in persons who work out-of-doors. Its frequency is probably the same in men and women working indoors. Although pterygium develops sometime fairly late in life in most cases, it is already evident at birth in rare instances (Schwartz, 1960). Murken and Dannheim (1965) concluded that the rare congenital type of pterygium is inherited as a dominant with 70 percent penetrance. Jacklin (1964) reported 6 affected persons (4 females, 2 males) in 3 generations of a family.

Hilgers, J. H. C.: Pterygium, its incidence, heredity and etiology. Am. J. Ophthal. 50: 635-644, 1960.

Jacklin, H. N.: Familial predisposition to pterygium formation. Report of a family. Am. J. Ophthal. 57: 481-482, 1964.

Murken, J. D. and Dannheim, R.: Zur Genetik des Pterygium corneae. Klin. Mbl. Angenheilk. 147: 574-579, 1965.

Schwartz, V. J.: Congenital pterygium. J.A.M.A. 174: 2078-2079, 1960.

17810 PTERYGIUM SYNDROME (PTERYGIUM COLLI SYNDROME)

Some females have webbed neck (pterygium colli), short stature and lymphedema — features suggesting the XO Turner syndrome — but have normal sexual development. Pulmonic stenosis is frequent in these cases. The etiology and pathogenesis are obscure. Chromosomal mosaicism seems to have been adequately excluded in many cases and familial incidence is not striking. We sometimes refer to this condition as the female pseudo-Turner syndrome. When the same situation occurs in males, it is sometimes referred to as the male Turner syndrome. Moldenhauer (1964) described a condition he called Nielson syndrome in 4 females of three generations of a family. The features were short stature, ptosis, cleft palate, camptodactyly, pterygium colli and vertebral anomalies. Fertility was normal. The difference from the Klippel-Feil syndrome and from the Bonnevie-Ullrich syndrome is not clear. Either X-linked or autosomal dominant inheritance could account for the findings. Dornstein (1966) described two unrelated males with what he termed pterygolymphangiectasia. In addition to pterygium colli, peripheral edema persisted to the third decade. The family history was unremarkable. In both, the genitalia were fully developed and sperm production was normal. Chromosome study in one yielded normal findings. To date only females have transmitted this disorder (Nora and Sinha, 1967; Polani et al., 1967). Alsev and Reinwein (1958) described brothers aged 16 and 19 who had webbing of the neck, congenital heart disease, lymphedema of late onset (Meige type) and cryptorchidism. Golden and Lakim (1959) reported as examples of the Marfan syndrome two brothers with web neck, fixed flexion of the knees and distal intraphalangeal joints, kyphoscoliosis, pectus excavatum and atrial septal defect which in one boy was confirmed by autopsy. The father had pectus excavatum and heart disease. Migeon and Whitehouse (1967) described two families each with two sibs with somatic features of the Turner syndrome. In one two brothers had webbing of the neck, coarctation of the aorta and cryptorchidism. In the second, a brother and sister were affected. Simpson et al. (1969) reported experiences which suggest that rubella embryopathy may result in the Turner phenotype thereby accounting for either the male Turner syndrome or the female pseudo-Turner syndrome. See the Noonan syndrome (16395), which probably is the same as the pterygium colli syndrome and is a preferred designation.

Alslev, J. and Reinwein, H.: Ueber das familiaere Vorkommen des sogenannten Ullrich-Turner-Syndromes und das Vorhandensein eines pterygium colli, eines Kryptorchismus und des Meige-Syndromes bei zwei Bruedern mit kongenitalen Vitien. Deutsch. Med. Wschr. 83: 601-604, 1958.

Dornstein, P.: Pterygolymphangiectasia. J. Albert Einstein Med. Cent. 14: 149-156, 1966.

Golden, R. L. and Lakim, H.: The forme fruste in Marfan's syndrome. New Eng. J. Med. 260: 797-801, 1959.

Kopits, E.: Die als 'Flughaut' bezeichneten Missbildungen und deren operative Behandlung (musculo-dysplasia congenita). Langenbeck. Arch. Klin. Chir. 37: 539-549, 1937.

Migeon, B. R. and Whitehouse, D.: Familial occurrence of the somatic phenotype of Turner's syndrome. Johns Hopkins Med. J. 120: 78-80, 1967.

Moldenhauer, E.: Zur Klinik des Nielson-Syndromes. Derm. Wschr. 150: 594-601, 1964.

Nora, J. J. and Sinha, A. K.: Hereditary Turner phenotypes. (Letter) Lancet II: 256 only, 1967.

Polani, P. E., Angell, R. and Polani, N.: Ullrich's syndrome. (Letter) Lancet II: 421 only, 1967.

Rossi, E. and Caflisch, A.: Le syndrome du pterygium status Bonnevie-Ullrich, dystrophia brevicolli congenita, syndrome de Turner et arthromyodysplasia congenita. Helv. Paediat. Acta 6: 119-148, 1951.

Rossi, E. and Howald, E.: Ueber die Erblichkeit des Status Bonnevie-Ullrich. Helv. Paediatr. Acta 2: 98-102, 1947.

Simpson, J. W., Nora, J. J., Singer, D. B. and McNamara, D. G.: Multiple valvular sclerosis in Turner phenotypes and rubella syndrome. Am. J. Cardiol. 23: 94-97, 1969.

17820 PTERYGIUM, ANTECUBITAL

Shun-Shin (1954) described 8 affected individuals in 3 generations of a Mauritian family. There was one instance of a 'skipped generation.' The web extended across the cubital fossa from the distal one-third of the upper arm to the proximal one-third of the forearm. Elbow extension was limited to 90 degrees, although flexion was unimpeded. Radiologically, posterior subluxation of the radial head (q.v.) and maldevelopment of the radio-ulnar joint were demonstrated.

Shun-Shin, M.: Congenital web formation. J. Bone Joint Surg. 36B: 268-271, 1954.

*17830 PTOSIS, HEREDITARY

Rodin and Barkan (1935) recognized four types: (1) hereditary congenital ptosis, (2) hereditary ptosis with external ophthalmoplegia, (3) hereditary non-congenital ptosis, and (4) hereditary ptosis with epicanthus. The second type is said to be most frequent. On the other hand, Duke-Elder (1963) stated that at least 8 types of congenital ptosis are recognizable of which 7 show a genetic basis. (1) Simple ptosis, due to failure of peripheral differentiation of muscles, transmitted as a dominant. The rectus superior muscle may be involved also. (2) Ptosis with blepharophimosis, also due to faulty peripheral differentiation and transmitted as a dominant. (3) Ptosis due to ophthalmoplegia (q.v.) usually of central origin. (4) Ptosis associated with myasthenia gravis and myotonia, both rare as congenital disorders. (5) Ptosis due to congenital sympathetic palsy. (6) Synkinetic ptosis (see MARCUS GUNN PHENOMENON). (7) Intermittent pseudo-ptosis associated with the retraction syndrome. The extensive Metcalf kindred in Lafayette, Tenn., has hereditary congenital ptosis (Briggs, 1919). The Georgia mountain family reported by Stuckey (1916) may have been related. The same condition was described by Usher (1925) as 'epicanthus and ptosis.' I doubt that the excess skin at the inner canthus in these 'slit-eyed people' should be called epicanthus. Blepharophimosis is present. See PURPURA SIMPLEX. Families with late onset ptosis such as that of Faulkner (1939) may have represented oculopharyngeal muscular dystrophy (q.v.). Congenital ptosis may be only unilateral. Epicanthus may be associated (Rank, Thompson, 1959).

Briggs, H. H.: Hereditary congenital ptosis with report of 64 cases conforming to the Mendelian rule of dominance. Am. J. Ophthal. 2: 408-417, 1919.

Duke-Elder, S.: Congenital Deformities. System of Ophthalmology Normal and Abnormal Development. St. Louis: C. V. Mosby Co., 3: (part 2) 1963.

Faulkner, S. H.: Familial ptosis with ophthalmoplegia externa starting late in life. Brit. Med. J. 1: 854 only, 1939.

Rank, B. K. and Thomson, J. A.: The genetic approach to hereditary congenital ptosis. Aust. New Zeal. J. Surg. 28: 274-279, 1959.

Rodin, F. H. and Barkan, H.: Hereditary congenital ptosis. Report of a pedigree and review of literature. Am. J. Ophthal. 18: 213-225, 1935.

Stuckey, H. P.: The slit-eyed people: constricted eyelids found in four generations of a Georgia family. J. Hered. 7: 147 only, 1916.

Usher, C. H.: A pedigree of epicanthus and ptosis. Ann. Eugen. 1: 128-138, 1925.

*17835 PUBIC BONE DYSPLASIA

Dysplasia and-or delayed ossification of the pubic bones at the symphysis, without other anomalies, was reported by Schey and Levin (1971) in an adult male and all three of his children (males). This condition may mimic diastasis of the pubic bones which is associated with genitourinary abnormalities, especially epispadias and extrophy of the urinary bladder. Cleidocranial dysplasia must also be considered in the differential diagnosis.

Schey, W. L. and Levin, B.: Familial pubic bone maldevelopment. Radiology 101: 147-150, 1971.

17840 PULMONARY EDEMA OF MOUNTAINEERS

Fred and colleagues (1962) described acute pulmonary edema precipitated in some persons at high altitude. Their two patients were both physicians who on one or more occasions were near death from pulmonary edema developed when skiing at altitudes of 6000 to 10,000 feet. The father of one of these, previously in good health, died at age 43 while mountain climbing and acute pulmonary edema was thought to be the cause. Hultgren and colleagues (1961) also noted familial occurrence. Cardiac catheterization during the acute episode showed normal left atrial and pulmonary vein pressures but elevation of pulmonary artery pressure. Pulmonary edema, it was proposed, results from increased vasomotor activity of the pulmonary venous capillaries or venules.

Fred, H. L., Schmidt, A. M., Bates, T. and Hecht, H. H.: Acute pulmonary edema of altitude. Clinical and physiologic observations. Circulation 25: 929-937, 1962.

Hultgren, H. N., Spickard, W. B., Hellriegel, K. and Houston, C. S.: High altitude pulmonary edema. Medicine 40: 289-313, 1961.

17850 PULMONARY FIBROSIS, IDIOPATHIC (SEE FIBROCYSTIC PULMONARY DYSPLASIA)

Jacox, Frymoyer and Bonanni (1964) described a family in which idiopathic pulmonary fibrosis had been observed in 8 definite and 3 probable instances in a dominant pedigree pattern. Apparent male-to-male transmission had occurred in one instance. Increase of a gamma globulin fraction was thought to be a possible integral part of the syndrome. Hughes (1964) described the disorder in a mother and two daughters. Danies and Potts (1964) observed affected brothers in whom clubbing of the fingers was present for many years before the development of respiratory symptoms. It is by no means certain that the condition in these reports is an entity separate from that referred to elsewhere as fibrocystic pulmonary dysplasia (q.v.). Wagley (1972) described a family in which three brothers and a sister had well-documented pulmonary fibrosis and their mother, two of their sibs and the son of one brother probably had pulmonary fibrosis.

Bonanni, P. P., Frymoyer, J. W. and Jacox, R. F.: A family study of idiopathic pulmonary fibrosis, a possible dysproteinemic and genetically determined disease. Am. J. Med. 39: 411-421, 1965.

Danies, G. M. and Potts, M. W.: Chronic diffuse interstitial pulmonary fibrosis in brothers. Guy. Hosp. Rep. 113: 36-44, 1964.

Hughes, E. W.: Familial interstitial pulmonary fibrosis. Thorax 19: 515-525, 1964.

Jacox, R. F., Frymoyer, J. W. and Bonanni, P. P.: A family study of idiopathic pulmonary fibrosis: a possible dysproteinemic and genetically determined disease. Trans. Ass. Am. Physicians 77: 232-238, 1964.

Swaye, P., Van Ordstrand, H. S., McCormick, L. J. and Wolpaw, S. E.: Familial Hamman-Rich syndrome: report of eight cases. Dis. Chest 55: 7-12, 1969.

Wagley, P. F.: A new look at the Hamman-Rich syndrome. Johns Hopkins Med. J. 131: 412-424, 1972.

*17860 PULMONARY HYPERTENSION, PRIMARY

Melmon and Braunwald (1963) observed two proved cases and 3 presumptive cases in three generations of a family. The family reported by Kuhn, Schaaf and Wagner (1963) may in fact be an example of the Lewis type of heart-hand syndrome (q.v.). Parry and Verel (1966) described the disorder in a mother and her two daughters and referred to at least two other reports of two generations being affected. X-linked dominance would account nicely for the preponderance of female cases. Kingdon et al. (1966) described the condition in brother and sister and their father, thus excluding, in this family at least, X-linkage. In affected members of a family with pulmonary hypertension, Inglesby et al. (1973) found elevated levels of antiplasmin. Recurrent pulmonary microembolization with impaired fibrinolysis has been postulated but not proved as the basis of this disorder.

Inglesby, T. V., Singer, J. W. and Gordon, D. S.: Abnormal fibrinolysis in familial pulmonary hypertension. Am. J. Med. 55: 5-14, 1973.

Kingdon, H. S., Cohen, L. S., Roberts, W. C. and Braunwald, E.: Familial occurrence of primary pulmonary hypertension. Arch. Intern. Med. 118: 422-426, 1966.

Kuhn, E., Schaaf, J. and Wagner, A.: Primary pulmonary hypertension, congenital heart disease and skeletal anomalies in three generations. Jap. Heart J. 4: 205-223, 1963.

Melmon, K. L. and Braunwald, E.: Familial pulmonary hypertension. New Eng. J. Med. 269: 770-775, 1963.

Parry, W. R. and Verel, D.: Familial primary pulmonary hypertension. Brit. Heart J. 28: 193-198, 1966.

Rogge, J. D., Mishkin, M. E. and Genovese, P. D.: The familial occurrence of primary pulmonary hypertension. Ann. Intern. Med. 65: 672-684, 1966.

Thompson, P. and McRae, C.: Familial pulmonary hypertension. Evidence of autosomal dominant inheritance. Brit. Heart J. 32: 758-760, 1970.

17870 PULMONARY VALVULAR DYSPLASIA

Koretzky et al. (1969) described an unusual type of pulmonary valvular dysplasia which showed a familial tendency with either affected parent and offspring or affected sibs. Although some relatives had pulmonary valvular stenosis of the standard dome-shaped variety, the valvular dysplasia in others was characterized by the presence of three distinct cusps and no commissural fusion. The obstructive mechanism was related to markedly thickened, immobile cusps, with disorganized myxomatous tissue. Other features were retarded growth, abnormal facies (triangular face, hypertelorism, low-set ears and ptosis of the eyelids), absence of ejection click and unusually marked right axis deviation by electrocardiogram.

Koretzky, E. D., Moller, J. H., Korns, M. E., Schwartz, C. J. and Edwards, J. E.: Congenital pulmonary stenosis resulting from dysplasia of valve. Circulation 40: 43-53, 1969.

17875 PULPAL DYSPLASIA ('PULP STONES')

By X-ray and by histologic study, calcified bodies are demonstrated within an enlarged pulp chamber. Richardson and Fantin (1970) observed the trait, which is of no pathologic significance, in three generations, with no male-to-male transmission.

Rao, S. R., Witkop, C. J. and Yamane, G. M.: Pulpal dysplasia. Oral Surg. 30: 682-689, 1970.

Richardson, A. S. and Fantin, J.: Anomalous dysplasia of dentine: report of case. J. Canad. Dent. Ass. 36: 189-191, 1970.

17880 PUPIL, EGG-SHAPED

White and Fulton (1937) described ovoid pupils which were large and reacted poorly to constricting stimuli in a woman of Russian-Jewish extraction and both her identical twin daughters.

*17890 PUPILLARY MEMBRANE, PERSISTENCE OF

Remnants of the pupillary membrane persist as strands and other irregular tissue in the region of the pupil. Cassady and Light (1957) described a family in which 11 persons in 4 generations showed remnants of the pupillary membrane. Four of these also had congenital cataract and 3 had increased corneal diameter.

Cassady, J. R. and Light, A.: Familial persistent pupillary membranes. Arch. Ophthal. 58: 438-448, 1957.

17900 PURPURA SIMPLEX

Purpura of the extremities, epistaxis, ecchymoses on slight trauma and menorrhagia are features. Tourniquet test is positive but all other tests of clotting are normal. In the family reported by Fisher et al. (1954) purpura and ptosis occurred together with male-to-male transmission in at least three generations. Among Davis' 27 families, 9 had 2 or more generations affected. Women were more often affected and he apparently had no instance of male-to-male transmission.

Davis, E.: Hereditary familial purpura simplex: review of 27 families. Lancet 1: 145-146, 1941.

Fisher, B., Zuckerman, G. H. and Douglass, R. C.: Combined inheritance of purpura simplex and ptosis in four generations of one family. Blood 9: 1199-1204, 1954.

17903 PYROPHOSPHATASE, ERYTHROCYTE INORGANIC

Among 3000 unrelated persons, Fisher et al. (1974) found no genetically determined variants.

Fisher, R. A., Turner, B. M., Dorkin, H. L. and Harris, H.: Studies on human erythrocyte inorganic pyrophosphatase. Ann. Hum. Genet. 37: 341-353, 1974.

*17905 PYRUVATE KINASE-3

At least three molecular forms with pyruvate kinase activity are known (Bigley et al., 1968). The form which is deficient in a type of hemolytic anemia (26620) is the red cell variety, PK-1. PK-2 is found in kidney. PK-3 is found in leukocytes but not in red cells or kidney. This form has been found to be syntenic with mannosephosphate isomerase (Shows, 1972). How many loci are involved in the genetic determination of the three forms of PK or whether they share common subunits is not known. The PK-3 and MPI loci are syntenic.

Bigley, R. H., Stenzel, P., Jones, R. T. et al.: Tissue distribution of human pyruvate kinase isozymes. Enzym. Biol. Clin. 9: 10-20, 1968.

Shows, T. B.: Linkage of loci for human pyruvate kinase and mannosephosphate isomerase in somatic cell hybrids. (Abstract) Am. J. Hum. Genet. 24: 13A only, 1972.

Shows, T. B.: Somatic cell genetics of enzyme markers associated with three human linkage groups. In, Davidson, R. L. (ed.): Proc. Conf. Somatic Cell Hybridization, Orlando, Fla., 1973.

17910 RADIAL DEFECTS (DEFICIENCY OF RADIAL RAYS AND RADIUS AND PHOCOMELIA)

Many of these cases are sporadic and in most of the reported familial instances it is impossible to exclude the heart-hand syndromes I and II, Fanconi panmyelophthisis, thrombocytopenia-absent radius and other syndromes with radial defects as a feature. In its grosser form the disorder consists of phocomelia due to lack of the radius and ulna and hypoplasia of the humerus with carpals and digits articulating with it, while milder cases show only underdevelopment of the thumb or the first metacarpal.

Reedy, J. J. and Bodner, L. M.: Dominant inheritance of radial hemimelia. J. Hered. 44: 254-256, 1953.

Temtamy, S. A.: Genetic Factors in Hand Malformations. Ph. D. Thesis, Johns Hopkins University, 1966.

17920 RADIAL HEADS, POSTERIOR DISLOCATION OF

Cockshott and Omololu (1958) described multiple cases of congenital posterior dislocation of the radial head in a family. Abbott (1892) observed seven cases in one family. Shun-Shin (1954) observed this disorder associated with antecubital webbing or pterygium (q.v.) in members of three generations of a family. Gunn and Pillay (1964) described congenital posterior dislocation of the head of the radius in a mother and daughter in Malaya. The mother's parents were consanguineous and she had married within a restricted group. A third unrelated patient came from first-cousin parents who were stated to be normal. The authors favored recessive inheritance.

Abbott, F. C.: Congenital dislocations of radius. Lancet I: 800 only, 1892.

Cockshott, W. P. and Omololu, A.: Familial congenital posterior dislocation of both radial heads. J. Bone Joint Surg. 40B: 483-486, 1958.

Gunn, D. R. and Pillay, V. K.: Congenital posterior dislocation of the head of the radius. Clin. Orthop. 34: 108-113, 1964.

Shun-Shin, M.: Congenital web formation. J. Bone Joint Surg. 36B: 268-271, 1954.

*17930 RADIO-ULNAR SYNOSTOSIS

Dominant inheritance through several lines in several generations was demonstrated by a family reported by Davenport, Taylor and Nelson (1924). Radio-ulnar synostosis is a feature of certain chromosome abnormalities, notably the triple X-Y syndrome (XXXY). See PRONATION-SUPINATION OF THE

FOREARM, IMPAIRMENT OF. Hansen and Andersen (1970) found a positive family history in 5 of 37 cases.

Davenport, C. B., Taylor, H. L. and Nelson, L. A.: Radio-ulnar synostosis. Arch. Surg. 8: 705-762, 1924.

Ferguson-Smith, M. A., Johnson, A. W. and Handmaker, S. D.: Primary amentia and micro-orchidism associated with the XXXY chromosome constitution. Lancet II: 184-187, 1960.

Hansen, O. H. and Andersen, N. O.: Congenital radio-ulnar synostosis. Report of 37 cases. Acta Orthop. Scand. 41: 225-230, 1970.

17940 RADIUS, APLASIA OF, WITH CLEFT LIP-PALATE

At least 18 cases have been reported (Immeyer, 1967). No information on its genetics is available.

Immeyer, F.: Lippen-Kiefer-Gaumenspalten bei thalidomidgeschaedigten Kindern. Acta Genet. Med. Gemellol. 16: 244-274, 1967.

17950 RAINDROP HYPOPIGMENTATION

Weary and Behlen (1965) described a distinctive bilateral, symmetrical, sharply localized hypopigmentation of the upper chest in a Negro woman and her four children. A single spot of depigmentation, with a shape suggesting a raindrop, was present below the mid-clavicle on each side. Either X-linked or autosomal dominant inheritance is possible.

Weary, P. E. and Behlen, C. H.: Unusual familial hypopigmentary anomaly. Arch. Derm. 92: 54-55, 1965.

*17960 RAYNAUD DISEASE ('HEREDITARY COLD FINGERS')

Lewis and Pickering (1933) described two working-class British families with multiple persons suffering from intermittent attacks of numb and white fingers. One family had 9 cases in two generations, the second 14 cases in 3 generations. Males and females were equally affected and several instances of male-to-male transmission were noted.

Lewis, T. and Pickering, G. W.: Observations upon maladies in which the blood supply to digits ceases intermittently or permanently, and upon bilateral gangrene of digits, observations relevant to so-called 'Raynaud's disease.' Clin. Sci. 1: 327-366, 1933.

*17965 RED CELL PERMEABILITY DEFECT

In three generations of a family Honig et al. (1971) demonstrated elliptocytosis with transverse slitlike areas of decreased density in the red cells. This was accompanied by no hemolysis in vivo and red cell survival was normal.

Honig, G. R., Lacson, P. S. and Maurer, H. S.: A new familial disorder with abnormal erythrocyte morphology and increased permeability of the erythrocytes. Pediat. Res. 5: 159-166, 1971.

*17970 RED CELL PHOSPHOLIPID DEFECT WITH HEMOLYSIS

In 8 members of a family from the Dominican Republic, Jaffe and Gottfried (1968) found a hemolytic disorder with mild hyperbilirubinemia and reticulocytosis of 6 to 15 percent but with little or no anemia, and was able to show an increase in lecithin. The pedigree suggested regular autosomal dominant inheritance. In a Polish-born Jewish family, Danon et al. (1962) described an electron microscopic abnormality of the red-cell membrane which probably was responsible for susceptibility to hemolysis on exposure to drugs and possibly viruses. Two sisters had similar findings. Questionable anomaly was found in the proband's son. Shohet et al. (1971) showed that there is a defect in the catabolism of membrane phosphatides and referred to the condition as high phophatidylcholine hemolytic anemia (HPCHA). The lipid defect of the red cell membrane is accompanied by excessive cation permeability and ouabain-sensitive pumping with excessive glycolytic energy diverted to the pump (Shohet et al., 1973).

Danon, D., De Vries, A., Djaldetti, M. and Kirschmann, C.: Episodes of acute haemolytic anaemia in a patient with familial ultrastructural abnormality of the red-cell membrane. Brit. J. Haemat. 8: 274-282, 1962.

Jaffe, E. R. and Gottfried, E. L.: Hereditary nonspherocytic hemolytic disease associated with an altered phospholipid composition of the erythrocytes. J. Clin. Invest. 47: 1375-1388, 1968.

Shohet, S. B., Livermore, B. M., Nathan, D. G. and Jaffe, E. R.: Hereditary hemolytic anemia associated with abnormal membrane lipids. I. Mechanism of accumulation of phosphatidyl choline. Blood 38: 445-456, 1971.

Shohet, S. B., Nathan, D. G., Livermore, B. M., Feig, S. A. and Jaffe, E. R.: Hereditary hemolytic anemia associated with anbormal membrane lipid. II. Ion permeability and transport abnormalities. Blood 42: 1-8, 1973.

*17980 RENAL TUBULAR ACIDOSIS I (CLASSIC, GRADIENT OR DISTAL TYPE)

Randall and Targgart (1961) observed renal tubular acidosis in members of several successive generations. All affected members showed both acidosis and nephrocalcinosis. Seedat (1964) presented a family with 8 affected in 4 generations. The proband was born of first-cousin parents. In another first-cousin marriage, 4 of his half-sibs were affected. Randall (1967) provided follow-up of the family reported by Targgart and him. The pedigree included four instances of male-to-male transmission. The features are nephrocalcinosis, fixed urinary specific gravity, fixed urinary pH of about 5.0, high serum chloride, low serum bicarbonate, osteomalacia, hypocalcemia. Alkalinization is effective therapy. Kolb (1967) showed me a pedigree with three generations affected and instances of male-to-male transmission. Seedat (1968) observed 18 affected persons in three generations. In the well-studied family reported by Gyory et al. (1968), 10 persons were affected by test, 3 others were (by genealogic connections) presumably affected and two others were reportedly affected. Male-to-male transmission occurred. Kuhlencordt et al. (1967) observed affected MZ twins whose parents were first-cousins and suggested that a form of this disorder is recessive. Thus, there may be more than one form of this disorder. See RTA II and RTA III in the recessive catalog. Renal tubular acidosis with perceptive deafness (q.v.) is a distinct entity. Morris (1970) suggested that at least three types of renal tubular acidosis can be recognized. In the classic type (RTA I) the bicarbonate threshold is normal, the defect is primarily in the distal tubule and inheritance is dominant. In RTA II the defect is in the proximal tubule, the bicarbonate threshold is low and inheritance is recessive. A third type of RTA is called 'dislocation' type and may also be recessively inherited.

A phenocopy of the genetic disorder is produced by amphotericin B (McCurdy et al., 1968). Richards and Wrong (1972) described proximal renal tubular acidosis in a mother and her three children. Buckalew et al. (1974) suggested that there are two autosomal dominant forms of RTA, one with hypercalcinuria and one without.

Buckalew, V. M., Jr.: Familial renal tubular acidosis. Ann. Intern. Med. 68: 1367-1368, 1968.

Buckalew, V. M., Purvis, M. L., Shulman, M. G., Herndon, C. N. and Rudman, D.: Hereditary renal tubular acidosis. Report of a 64 member kindred with variable clinical expression including idiopathic hypercalcinuria. Medicine, in press, 1974.

Gyory, A. Z. and Edwards, K. D. G.: Renal tubular acidosis. A family with an autosomal dominant genetic defect in renal hydrogen ion transport, with proximal tubular and collecting duct dysfunction and increased metabolism of citrate and ammonia. Am. J. Med. 45: 43-62, 1968.

Kolb, F. O.: San Francisco, Calif.: personal communication, 1967.

Kuhlencordt, F., Lenz, W., Seeman, N. and Zukschwerdt, L.: Renal tubular acidosis and bilateral nephrocalcinosis in uniovular twins. German Med. Monthly 12: 565-570, 1967.

McCurdy, D. K., Frederic, M. and Elkinton, J. R.: Renal tubular acidosis due to amphotericin B. New Eng. J. Med. 278: 124-131, 1968.

Morris, R. C.: Renal tubular acidosis. Mechanisms, classification and implications. New Eng. J. Med. 281: 1405-1413, 1970.

Musgrave, J. E., Bennett, W. M., Campbell, R. A. and Eisenberg, C. S.: Renal tubular acidosis. (Letter) Lancet II: 1364 only, 1972.

Randall, R. E., Jr. and Targgart, W. H.: Familial renal tubular acidosis. Ann. Intern. Med. 54: 1108-1116, 1961.

Randall, R. E., Jr.: Familial renal tubular acidosis revisited. (Letter) Ann. Intern. Med. 66: 1024-1025, 1967.

Richards, P. and Wrong, O. M.: Dominant inheritance in a family with familial renal tubular acidosis. Lancet II: 998-999, 1972.

Seedat, Y. K.: Familial renal tubular acidosis. (Letter) Ann. Intern. Med. 69: 1329 only, 1968.

Seedat, Y. K.: Some observations of renal tubular acidosis — a family study. S. Afr. Med. J. 38: 606-610, 1964.

Seldin, D. W. and Wilson, J. D.: Renal tubular acidosis. In, Stanbury, J. B., Wyngaarden, J. B. and Fredrickson, D. S. (eds.): The Metabolic Basis of Inherited Disease. New York: McGraw-Hill, 1972 (3rd Ed.). Pp. 1548-1566.

*17990 RETINAL APLASIA

Sorsby and Williams (1960) observed a family with multiple cases of retinal aplasia in which inheritance was autosomal dominant. 'Retinal aplasia' is the British term for what is called 'congenital amaurosis' on the continent. Much genetic heterogeneity undoubtedly exists, witness the demonstration of both autosomal dominant and autosomal recessive forms.

Sorsby, A. and Williams, C. E.: Retinal aplasia as a clinical entity. Brit. Med. J. 1: 293-297, 1960.

*18000 RETINAL ARTERIES, TORTUOSITY OF

Beyer (1958) described tortuous retinal arteries with foveal hemorrhage in a 43-year-old man and his 17-year-old son. A 12-year-old son showed early changes. Polycythemia was present in the 17-year-old. Werner and Gafner (1961) described tortuous arteries in a 47-year-old man and his son and 2 daughters. Cagianut and Werner (1968) observed four persons in one family with retinal arteriolar tortuosity and recurrent hemorrhages. Goldberg et al. (1972) described a family with 12 cases of retinal vascular tortuosity and-or retinal hemorrhage in five sibships, including three instances of father-to-son transmission. One of the 12 had retinal hemorrhage without tortuosity.

Beyer, E.: Familiaere Tortuositas der kleinen Netzhautarterien mit Makulablutung. (Familial tortuosity of the small retinal arteries with macular hemorrhage). Klin. Mbl. Augenheilk. 132: 532-539, 1958.

Cagianut, B. and Werner, H.: Zum Krankheitsbild der familiaeren Tortuositas der kleinen Netzhautarterien mit Maculablutung. Klin. Mbl. Augenheilk. 153: 533-542, 1968.

Cagianut, B.: Zum Krankheitsbild der familiaeren Tortuositas der kleinen Netzhautgefaesse. Ophthalmologica 156: 322-324, 1968.

Goldberg, M. F., Pollack, I. P. and Green, W. R.: Familial retinal arteriolar tortuosity with retinal hemorrhage. Am. J. Ophthal. 73: 183-191, 1972.

Werner, H. and Gafner, F.: Beitrag zur familiaeren Tortuositas der kleinen Netzhautarterien. Ophthalmologica 141: 350-356, 1961.

*18002 RETINAL CONE DEGENERATION

Krill et al. (1973) defined an autosomal dominant form of diffuse cone degeneration. The findings of electroretinogram were distinctive. Progressive loss of visual acuity, photophobia and defective color vision are the major complaints. Unlike retinitis pigemntosa (18010) loss of side vision and nightblindness are rare complaints. The most common macular lesion has a bull's eye appearance produced by a central area of uninvolved epithelium. Krill et al. (1973) published pedigrees of extensively affected families. The patients may be mis-labelled as total colorblindness. Berson et al. (1968), Davis and Hollenhorst (1955), Sloan and Brown (1962) and others have reported families.

Berson, E. L., Gouras, P. and Gunkel, R. D.: Progressive cone degeneration, dominantly inherited. Arch. Ophthal. 80: 77-83, 1968.

Davis, C. T. and Hollenhorst, R. W.: Hereditary degeneration of the macula (occurring in five generations). Am. J. Ophthal. 39: 637-643, 1955.

Sloan, L. L. and Brown, D. J.: Progressive retinal degeration with selective involvement of the cone mechanism. Am. J. Ophthal. 54: 629-641, 1962.

*18005 RETINAL DETACHMENT

Retinal detachment independent of myopia was transmitted as an autosomal dominant in the extensive kindred reported by McNiel and McPherson (1971). Presumably no features indicative of arthro-ophthalmopathy (10830) or other dominant syndromes with retinal detachment were present. Vogt (1940) found 19 families with retinal detachment in at least two generations. Some showed three generation involvement and one four generations.

McNiel, N. A. and McPherson, A.: The inheritance of detached retina in a Texas family. J. Hered. 62: 73-76, 1971.

Vogt, A., Wagner, H. and Schlaepfer, H.: Erbbiologie und Erbpathologie des Auges. In, Just, G. et al. (eds.): Handbuch der Erbbiologie des Menschen. Berlin: Springer, 1940. vol. 3, Pp. 659-662.

*18010 RETINITIS PIGMENTOSA (RP)

This is one of the simply inherited traits which appears in all three catalogs. Atypical RP occurs in the Flynn-Aird syndrome (q.v.). Dominant inheritance is noted in 3 or 4 percent of cases. Ayres (1886) reported 4 generations, Allan and Herndon (1944) 5 generations, Bordley (1908) 5 generations, Heuscher-Isler et al. (1949) 11 cases in 3 generations, Rehsteiner (1949) 16 cases in 4 generations, and so on. Constriction of the visual fields and night blindness are typical as well as the characteristic fundus changes including 'bone corpuscle' lumps of pigment. The most extensively affected family reported is probably that studied by Beckershaus (1925). The pathophysiology of retinitis pigmentosa was discussed by Dowling (1966), who presented experiments suggesting that exposure to bright light may accelerate the degenerative process. Sunga and Sloan (1967) described a family with 13 affected in 3 generations, including 2 instances of male-to-male transmission. They remarked on the wide variability in the rate of visual deterioration among individuals of the same family.

Allan, W. and Herndon, C. N.: Retinitis pigmentosa and apparently sex-linked idiocy in a single sibship. J. Hered. 35: 40-43, 1944.

Ammann, F., Klein, D. and Bohringer, H. R.: Resultats preliminaires d'une enquet sur la frequence et la distribution geographique des degenerescences tapeto-retiniennes en Suisse (etude de cinq cantons). J. Genet. Hum. 10: 99-127, 1961.

Ayres, S. C.: Retinitis pigmentosa. Am. J. Ophthal. 3: 81-90, 1886.

Beckershaus, F.: Dominante Vererbung der Retinitis pigmentosa. Klin. Mbl. Augenheilk. 75: 96-109, 1925.

Bordley, J.: A family of hemeralopes. Bull. Hopkins Hosp. 19: 278-281, 1908.

Dowling, J. E.: Night blindness. Sci. Am. 215 (no. 4): 78-84, 1966.

Heuscher-Isler, R., Gysin, W. and Hegner, H.: Beitrag zur Kasuistik der dominanten Vererbung der Retinitis pigmentosa. Ophthalmologica 118: 858-865, 1949.

Rehsteiner, K.: Ein weiterer schweizerischer Stammbaum von dominant vererbter Retinitis pigmentosa. Ophthalmologica 117: 51-59, 1949.

Sunga, R. N. and Sloan, L. L.: Pigmentary degeneration of the retina: early diagnosis and natural history. Invest. Ophthal. 6: 309-325, 1967.

*18020 RETINOBLASTOMA

Smith and Sorsby (1958) concluded that bilateral cases are most often familial. Many unilateral cases may be sporadic with a low risk (about 4 percent) to subsequent children or to offspring of the proband. In their opinion estimates of mutation rate of 2.3 x 10 (to the minus 5) as given by Falls and Neel (1951) are too high. Macklin (1959) demonstrated irregularities in the inheritance suggesting incomplete penetrance. In 10.5 percent of cases, affected persons were identified in collateral lines. Examples included (1) a bilateral case, his unilaterally affected brother and a bilaterally affected daughter of the latter person; (2) six bilaterally affected offspring of a woman who had one microphthalmic eye but refused examination; (3) several instances of two or more affected sibs with normal parents. The genetic nature of retinoblastoma and its dominant inheritance came to light early because early recognition and treatment of individual cases permitted survival. The genetic basis of other embryonic tumors, such as Wilms tumor, neuroblastoma and medulloblastoma, is beginning to be appreciated. In all of these tumors spontaneous regression ('cure') occurs in some cases. Macklin (1960) stated that in the U.S.A. the frequency of retinoblastoma is about one in 23,000 live births. Jensen and Miller (1971) found that at ages two to three years a peak of mortality occurred which was two and one-half times greater in Negroes than in whites. Whether this reflects a truly high frequency in Negroes or some other factor such as higher mortality from delayed diagnosis is not clear. Orye et al. (1971) found deletion of a distal part of the long arm of one chromosome 13 in a case of bilateral retinoblastoma. The broadest of the three Giemsa bands normally present on the long arm was missing. Grace et al. (1971) described a patient with typical 13q- syndrome plus retinoblastoma. The karyotype contained a ring D chromosome. In the patients of Orye et al. (1971) and that of Wilson et al. (1969), in which a 14q- karyotype was found, no clinical features of the type usually associated with 13q- were present. In 12 reported patients with a deletion of the long arm of a D chromosome, 7 had retinoblastoma, which in 3 instances was bilateral (Taylor, 1970; Gey, 1970). Knudson (1971) proposes that a two-mutation model best fits the data. In this view a fraction of cases are non-hereditary and result from two somatic mutational events in one cell. The remainder are hereditary cases, occurring in persons susceptible by reason of having inherited one of the mutational events. Cytogenetic evidence suggests that the locus or a locus for retinoblastoma is on the long arm of chromosome no. 13. Wilson et al. (1973) restudied their case of bilateral retinoblastoma and concluded with new banding techniques that this like all the other deleted D-chromosome cases was an instance of 13-q.

Eldridge, R., O'Meara, K. and Kitchin, D.: Superior intelligence in sighted retinoblastoma patients and their families. J. Med. Genet. 9: 331-335, 1972.

Falls, H. F. and Neel, J. V.: Genetics of retinoblastoma. Arch. Ophthal. 46: 367-389, 1951.

Francois, J.: Hereditary malignant tumor of the eye. Congenital Anomalies of The Eye. (Chapter 9), St. Louis: C. V. Mosby Co., 1968. Pp. 205-246.

Gey, W.: Dq-, multiple missbildungen und retinoblastom. Humangenetik 10: 362-365, 1970.

Grace, E., Drennan, J., Colver, D. and Gordon, R. R.: The 13q deletion syndrome. J. Med. Genet. 8: 351-357, 1971.

Jensen, R. D. and Miller, R. W.: Retinoblastoma: epidemiologic characteristics. New Eng. J. Med. 285: 307-311, 1971.

Knudson, A. G.: Mutation and cancer: statistical study of retinoblastoma. Proc. Nat. Acad. Sci. 68: 820-823, 1971.

Macklin, M. T.: A study of retinoblastoma in Ohio. Am. J. Hum. Genet. 12: 1-43, 1960.

Macklin, M. T.: Inheritance of retinoblastoma in Ohio. Arch. Ophthal. 62: 842-851, 1959.

Manchester, P. T., Jr.: Retinoblastoma among offspring of adult survivors. Arch. Ophthal. 65: 546-549, 1961.

Nirankari, M. S., Gulati, G. C. and Chaddah, M. R.: Retinoblastoma: genetics and report of a family. Am. J. Ophthal. 53: 523-532, 1962.

Orye, E., Delbeke, M. J. and Vandenabeele, B.: Retinoblastoma and D-chromosome deletions. (Letter) Lancet II: 1376 only, 1971.

Schappert-Kimmijser, (NI)., Hemmes, G. D. and Nijland, R.: The heredity of retinoblastoma. Ophthalmologica 151: 197-213, 1966.

Smith, S. M. and Sorsby, A.: Retinoblastoma: some genetic aspects. Ann. Hum. Genet. 23: 50-58, 1958.

Taylor, A. I.: Dq-, Dr and retinoblastoma. Humangenetik 10: 209-217, 1970.

Vogel, F.: Genetics of retinoblastoma. Modern Trends in Ophthalmology, 1968.

Vogel, F.: Genetics of retinoblastoma. In, Genetic Counseling. Heidelberg University, Science Library. Trans. by Sabine Kurth. New York: Springer Verlag, 1969.

Warburg, M.: Retinoblastoma. Chapter 18 in, Goldberg, M. F. (ed.): Genetic and Metabolic Eye Disease. Boston: Little, Brown and Co., Pp. 447-461.

Wilson, M. G., Melnyk, J. and Towner, J. W. J.: Retinoblastoma and deletion D(14) syndrome. J. Med. Genet. 6: 322-327, 1969.

Wilson, M. G., Towner, J. W. and Fujimoto, A.: Retinoblastoma and D-chromosome deletions. Am. J. Hum. Genet. 25: 57-61, 1973.

18030 RHEUMATOID ARTHRITIS

Occasional families show a considerable number of cases of this common disorder. A simple Mendelian mechanism cannot be proved, however. Indeed, some (Burch, O'Brien and Bunim, 1964) cannot demonstrate significant familial aggregation.

Burch, T. A., O'Brien, W. M. and Bunim, J. J.: Family and genetic studies of rheumatoid arthritis and rheumatoid factor in Blackfeet Indians. Am. J. Public Health 54: 1184-1190, 1964.

Gowans, J. D. C., Evangelista, I. and O'Sullivan, M. A.: Familial factors in rheumatoid arthritis. Arch. Intern. Med. 113: 744-747, 1964.

18040 RIBBING DISEASE (HEREDITARY MULTIPLE DIAPHYSEAL SCLEROSIS)

Ribbing (1949) described a family in which four of six sibs were affected. The diaphyseal osteosclerosis and hyperostosis were limited to one or more (up to four) of the long bones, the tibia being affected in all. The father, who was dead, had complained for many years of pains in the legs. Thus, the condition may be dominant; no X-ray studies of the father were available and Ribbing noted that the body had been cremated. Paul (1953) reported the same entity in 2 of 4 sibs, one of whom also had otosclerosis, which was present in several other members of the kindred. In an addendum, Paul noted that the infant son of one of his patients had difficulty walking and was found to have multiple sclerosing lesions of long bones. Again dominant inheritance is suggested.

Paul, L. W.: Hereditary multiple diaphyseal sclerosis (Ribbing). Radiology 60: 412-416, 1953.

Ribbing, S.: Hereditary, multiple, diaphyseal sclerosis. Acta Radiol. 31: 522-536, 1949.

*18042 RIBONUCLEIC ACID, 5S (5S RNA)

The descreteness of the gene(s) for 5S RNA is indicated by the complete sequencing data on 5S RNA and by their localization to the long arm of chromosome no. 1 through in situ annealing experiments. Steffensen (1974) further narrowed the localization to 1q41 or 1q42. 5S RNA is attached to 60S RNA and is thought to represent a common binding site for RNA.

Steffensen, D. M., Prensky, W. and Dufy, P.: Localization of the 5S ribosomal RNA genes in the human genome. First Intern. Workshop on Human Gene Mapping, New Haven, Conn., June, 1973.

Steffensen, D. M.: Urbana, Ill., personal communication, 1974.

*18045 RIBOSOMAL RNA

By in situ annealing methods, it is possible to demonstrate that DNA coding for ribosomal RNA is present on the satellited chromosomes, nos. 13, 14, 15, 21 and 22.

Atwood, K.: Columbia Univ., personal communication, 1973.

Evans, H. J.: Edinburgh, personal communication, 1973.

*18050 RIEGER SYNDROME (HYPODONTIA, MESOECTODERMAL DYSGENESIS OF IRIS AND CORNEA, AND MYOTONIC DYSTROPHY)

Hypodontia (partial anodontia) with malformation of the anterior chamber of the eye was recognized as a dominantly inherited disorder by Rieger (1935, 1941). The ocular features are microcornea with opacity, hypoplasia of the iris and anterior synechiae. In five generations of a family Busch and colleagues (1960) found myotonic dystrophy as a consistently associated feature. Pearce and Kerr (1965) studied a large kindred with many affected members and emphasized the variability in expression of the syndrome. A less well-known component of this syndrome is anal stenosis (Crawford, 1967; Brailey, 1890). It is interesting to note that Schachenmann et al. (1965) described a family in which the combination of coloboma of the iris, anal stenosis and renal malformation was inherited in a dominant manner and associated with a specific chromosome aberration. See CAT EYE SYNDROME (11545). Alkemade (1969) amply confirmed autosomal dominant inheritance. He pointed out characteristic facies consisting of broad nasal root with telecanthus and maxillary hypoplasia with protruding lower lip. A mother and 2 of her 3 children had severe developmental anomalies of the iris, associated with maldevelopment of the ear and maxilla, umbilical hernia and anal stenosis. Glaucoma occurred in all 3 patients. It is doubtful that Axenfeld anomaly should be considered a separate entity. It is one feature of Rieger syndrome. Feingold et al. (1969) observed 6 cases in 3 generations with male-to-male transmission.

Alkemade, P. P. H.: Dysgenesis mesodermalis of the iris and the cornea. A Study of Rieger's Syndrome and Peter's Anomaly. (Rotterdam Thesis) Van Gorcum, 1969.

Brailey, W. A.: Double microphthalmos with defective development of iris, teeth and anus. Glaucoma at an early age. Trans. Ophthal. Soc. U.K. 10: 139 only, 1890.

Busch, G., Weiskopf, J. and Busch, K.-T.: Dysgenesis mesodermalis et ectodermalis Rieger oder Rieger'sche krankheit. Klin. Mbl. Augenheilk. 36: 512-523, 1960.

Crawford, R. A.: Iris dysgenesis with other anomalies. Brit. J. Ophthal. 51: 438-440, 1967.

Feingold, M., Shiere, F., Fogels, H. R. and Donaldson, D.: Rieger's syndrome. Pediatrics 44: 564-569, 1969.

Pearce, W. G. and Kerr, C. B.: Inherited variation in Rieger's malformation. Brit. J. Ophthal. 49: 530-537, 1965.

Rieger, H.: Beitraege zur Kenntnis seltener Missbildungen der Iris: ueber Hypoplasie des Irisvorderblattes mit Verlagerung und Entrundung der Pupille. Graefe Arch. Ophthal. 133: 602-635, 1935.

Rieger, H.: Erbfragen in der Augenheilkunde. Graefe Arch. Ophthal. 143: 277-299, 1941.

Schachenmann, G., Schmid, W., Fraccaro, M., Mannini, A., Tiepolo, L., Perona, G. P. and Sartori, E.: Chromosomes in coloboma and anal atresia. Lancet II: 290 only, 1965.

*18060 RINGED HAIR (PILI ANNULATI)

On close inspection with the unaided eye alternating light and dark bands are visible on the hair. The light areas are due to inclusion of air in the cortex. The hair tends to break off at these points. See pedigree of Ashley and Jacques (1950) with six affected in four generations. Snell and Foley (1932) described 9 affected in four generations with an instance of male-to-male transmission.

Ashley, L. M. and Jacques, R. S.: Four generations of ringed hair. J. Hered. 41: 82-84, 1950.

Juon, M.: Eine Beobachtung familiaeren Auftretens von Pili annulati. Dermatologia 86: 117-122, 1942.

Snell, G. D. and Foley, F.: Inheritance of ringed hair. J. Hered. 23: 155-157, 1932.

18070 ROBINOW DWARFISM

Robinow et al. (1969) described a dwarf syndrome in six generations of a family but with no instance of male-to-male transmission. Normal vaginal delivery by affected females was possible. Interorbital distance was increased and the teeth were malaligned. Because of bulging forehead, depressed nasal bridge and short limbs achondroplasia is suggested but the spine and pelvic radiologic findings are nearly normal. Similarities to the Aarskog-Scott syndrome (30540) are noteworthy. The 'saddle scrotum' finding in the Aarskog-Scott syndrome may be the main differentiating feature. Waddington and Tucker (1973) and Vera-Roman (1973) emphasized the occurrence of small or absent penis and hemivertebrae. Waddington and Tucker (1973) described affected brother and sister with normal, non-consanguineous parents.

Robinow, M., Silverman, F. N. and Smith, H. D.: A newly recognized dwarfing syndrome. Am. J. Dis. Child. 117: 645-651, 1969.

Robinow, M.: Fetal face syndrome. In, Bergsma, D. (ed.): Birth Defects Atlas and Compendium. Baltimore: Williams and Wilkins, 1973. Pp. 410-411.

Robinow, M.: Syndrome's progress. Am. J. Dis. Child. 126: 150- , 1973.

Vera-Roman, J. M.: Robinow dwarfism syndrome accompanind by penile agenesis and hemivertebrae. Am. J. Dis. Child. 126: 206-208, 1973.

Waddlington, B., Tucker, V. L. and Schimke, N.: Mesomelic dwarfism with hemivertebrae and small genitalia (the Robinow syndrome). Am. J. Dis. Child. 126: 202-205, 1973.

*18080 ROUSSY-LEVY HEREDITARY AREFLEXIC DYSTASIA

This disorder usually begins in childhood but causes little disability. The condition was described independently in 1926 by Roussy and Levy, by Symonds and Shaw (who called it 'familial claw-foot with absent tendon jerks') and by Rombold and Riley (who called it an 'abortive type of Friedreich disease'). This condition resembles Charcot-Marie-Tooth disease in its dominant inheritance, clawfoot, weakness and atrophy of distal limb muscles especially the peronei, decreased excitability of muscles to galvanic and faradic stimulation, and some distal sensory loss. The syndrome differs in that it includes static tremor of the hands. Roussy and Levy (1926, 1934) stressed the absence of cerebellar signs, speech disturbances, Babinski sign and nystagmus. Low conduction velocity of peripheral nerves was a striking feature of the cases reported by Yudell et al. (1965). Rozanski (1951) described a family with affected members in four generations and with several instances of male-to-male transmission. Lapresle (1956) gave follow-up information on the family of Roussy and Levy.

Lapresle, J.: Contribution a l'etude de la dystasie areflexique hereditaire. Etat actuel de quatre des sept cas princeps de Roussy et Mlle. Levy, trente ans apres la premiere publication de ces auteurs. Sem. Hop. Paris 32: 2473-2482, 1956.

Rombold, C. R. and Riley, H. A.: The abortive type of Friedreich's disease. Arch. Neurol. Psychiat. 16: 301-312, 1926.

Roussy, G. and Levy, G.: A propos de la dystasie areflexique hereditaire. Rev. Neurol. 62: 763-773, 1934.

Roussy, G. and Levy, G.: Sept cas d'une maladie familiale particulaiere. Rev. Neurol. 45: 427-450, 1926.

Rozanski, J.: Hereditary areflexic dystasia: report on a family with Roussy-Levy disease in Israel. Mschr. Psychiat. Neurol. 122: 141-156, 1951.

Symonds, C. P. and Shaw, M. E.: Familial claw-foot with absent tendon jerks. Brain 49: 387-403, 1926.

Yudell, A., Dyck, P. J. and Lambert, E. H.: A kinship with the Roussy-Levy syndrome. Arch. Neurol. 13: 432-440, 1965.

*18090 RUTHERFURD SYNDROME

Houston and Shotts (1966) restudied the family reported by Rutherfurd in 1931. In five generations affected persons showed corneal dystrophy, hypertrophy of gums and failure of tooth eruption. Seven persons in 4 generations were affected with three instances of male-to-male transmission.

Houston, I. B. and Shotts, N.: Rutherfurd's syndrome. A familial oculo-dental disorder. A clinical and electrophysiologic study. Acta Paediat. Scand. 55: 233-238, 1966.

Rutherfurd, M. E.: Three generations of inherited dental defect. Brit. Med. J. 2: 9-11, 1931.

*18095 SALIVARY SUBSTANCE, CLOSTRIDUM BOTULINUM TYPE

Discovery of inherited blood group substances in the saliva has usually followed discovery of the antigen on red cells. This is primarily because the antibody for the red cell antigen is first discovered and investigated. Thereafter, when saliva is studied in hemagglutination-inhibition tests with the antibody, antigen might be identified. Such was the case in ABO (11030), Lewis (11110) and Sd (11175). Balding and Gold (1973) described a 'new' substance secreted in the saliva and recognized by using, not an antibody but a 'receptor specific protein', a hemoglutinin from clostridium botulinum, type C. They called the trait, Sal (CbC), and found reason to think that in Caucasians the frequency of the dominant allele is about 0.73. This may represent a hereditary saliva group which has no 'blood group' counterpart. Others may well exist.

Balding, P. and Gold, E. R.: A new saliva substance, probably inherited, and serologically independent of ABH, Lewis, and Sd blood group substances. J. Med. Genet. 10: 323-327, 1973.

18100 SARCOIDOSIS

Familial aggregation was studied by Buck and McKusick (1961) and by Allison (1964), among others. The familial aggregation in this disease of unknown etiology may have a non-genetic basis. The much greater frequency in U.S. Negroes than in U.S. whites suggests a genetic contribution to etiology. The family pattern does not conform to a simple Mendelian mode of inheritance. In Allison's family affected persons were two brothers out of 4 sibs and two of the 4 children of one of these. Willoughby (1971) described three sibs of whom two had sarcoidosis and one had Crohn disease. In a family of 9 sibs, Sharma et al. (1971) described sarcoidosis in 4. The mode of onset and clinical representation were acute in 3. The fourth was asymptomatic.

Allison, J. R., Jr.: Sarcoidosis. I. Familial occurrence. II. Pseudotumor cerebri and unusual skin lesions. Sth. Med. J. 57: 27-32, 1964.

Buck, A. A. and McKusick, V. A.: Epidemiologic investigations of sarcoidosis. III. Serum proteins, syphilis, association with tuberculosis: familial aggregation. Am. J. Hyg. 74: 174-188, 1961.

Sharma, O. P., Johnson, C. S. and Balchum, O. J.: Familial sarcoidosis. Report of four siblings with acute sarcoidosis. Am. Rev. Resp. Dis. 104: 255-257, 1971.

Willoughby, J. M. T., Mitchell, D. N. and Wilson, J. D.: Sarcoidosis and Crohn's disease in siblings. Am. Rev. Resp. Dis. 104: 249-254, 1971.

18110 SATELLITE ASSOCIATION RESULTING IN FAMILIAL CHROMOSOMAL MOSAICISM

Zellweger and Abbo (1965) described mosaicism in three successive generations. Clones with normal karyotype, D-G and D-D translocations, partial trisomy 21 and monosomy X were found. Because of an unusual frequency of satellite association they postulated the existence of a 'dominant gene' which leads to mosaicism of somatic origin. The family was described in full by Abbo, Zellweger and Cuany (1966), who in this publication concluded that inheritance of a postulated gene for increased satellite association from both parents might lead to mosaicism.

Abbo, G. N., Zellweger, H. and Cuany, R.: Satellite association (SA) in familial mosaicism. Helv. Paediat. Acta 21: 293-299, 1966.

Zellweger, H. V. and Abbo, G. N.: About a new gene as a cause of increased satellite association. (Abstract) J. Pediat. 67: 935 only, 1965.

Zellweger, H. V., Abbo, G. N. and Cuany, R.: Satellite association and translocation mongolism. J. Med. Genet. 3: 186-189, 1966.

18120 SC(1) TRAIT OF SALIVA

SC(1) is a component of saliva demonstrated immuno-electrophoretically. The precise mechanism of genetic control has not been determined although the importance of genetic factors has been demonstrated (Niswander et al., 1964) by family data and twin studies. Environmental influences seem rather strong. The component is lacking from serum.

Niswander, J. D., Shreffler, D. C. and Neel, J. V.: Genetic studies of quantitative variation in a component of human saliva. Ann. Hum. Genet. 27: 319-328, 1964.

18130 SCAPULA, CONTOUR OF VERTEBRAL BORDER OF

Graves (1921) found that about 54 percent of persons have a convex vertebral border, about 26 percent have a straight vertebral border and about 20 percent have a concave border.

Graves, W. W.: Method of recognizing scapular types in living. Arch. Intern. Med. 36: 51-61, 1925.

Graves, W. W.: Observations on age changes in the scapula: a primary note. Am. J. Phys. Anthrop. 5: 21-33, 1922.

Graves, W. W.: The relations of the scapular types to problems of human heredity, longevity, morbidity and adaptability in general. Arch. Intern. Med. 34: 1-26, 1924.

Graves, W. W.: The types of scapulae. A comparative study of some correlated characters in human scapulae. Am. J. Phys. Anthrop. 4: 111-128, 1921.

18140 SCAPULOPERONEAL AMYOTROPHY

Peroneal atrophy is accompanied by bilateral foot drop and talipes equinovarus. Following atrophy of the lower legs, the shoulder girdle is involved. Bulbar involvement is late. Autopsy shows muscular atrophy and involvement of caudal cranial nuclei. Palmer (1932) described a family with 8 persons affected, the earliest having onset about 1800. Palmer's case looks like Charcot-Marie-Tooth disease. Davidenkov (1939) suggested that cases reported by Wohlfart were the same as those he designated scapuloperoneal amyotrophy. Thus, scapuloperoneal amyopathy might be viewed as a dominant type of Wohlfart-Kugelberg-Welander juvenile muscular atrophy. See MUSCULAR AMYOTROPHY, JUVENILE, in this catalog. Emery et al. (1968) and Schuchmann (1970) reported sporadic childhood cases with EMG and biopsy evidence of neurogenic disease; motor nerve conduction velocities were borderline or normal, suggesting anterior horn cell pathology.

Davidenkov, S.: Scapuloperoneal amyotrophy. Arch. Neurol. Psychiat. 41: 694-701, 1939.

Emery, E. S., Fenichel, G. M. and Eng, G.: A spinal muscular atrophy with scapuloperoneal distribution. Arch. Neurol. 18: 129-133, 1968.

Kaeser, H. E.: Die familiaere scapuloperoneale Muskelatrophie. Deutsch. Z. Nervenheilk. 186: 379-394, 1964.

Palmer, H. D.: Familial scapuloperoneal amyotrophy. Arch. Neurol. Psychiat. 28: 473-477, 1932.

Schuchmann, L.: Spinal muscular atrophy of the scapulo-peroneal type. Z. Kinderheilk. 109: 118-123, 1970.

18145 SCHINZEL SYNDROME

Schinzel (1973) informed us of a Swiss kindred in which the proband, brother, father and nephew had ulnar ray defects, small penis, delayed puberty, and obesity and in the proband and his father anal atresia. The hand malformation varied from hypoplasia of the terminal phalanx of a stiff fifth finger to complete absence of fingers 4 and 5, including their metacarpals. The proband also had pyloric stenosis. The father had congential laryngeal stenosis from a subglottic cartilaginous web.

Schinzel, A.: Zurich, personal communication, 1973.

18150 SCHIZOPHRENIA

This may not be a single entity. Although the importance of genetic factors and the distinctness from maniac-depressive psychosis are indicated by twin studies, the mode of inheritance is unclear. Some (e.g., Garrone, 1962) suggest recessive inheritance. Others (e.g., Book, 1953, and Slater, 1958) favor irregular dominant inheritance. A priori, polygenic inheritance seems most likely, according to the rule that relatively frequent disorders such as this do not have simple monomeric genetic determination. Within the larger group there may be entities which behave in a simple Mendelian manner. Heston (1970) reviewed the evidence and concluded that it supports the autosomal dominant hypothesis. He points out that the definition of schizophrenia used by recent researchers is a broad one encompassing the schizoid state, the 'schizophrenic spectrum.' Schizoids and schizophrenics occur with about equal frequency among the cotwins of schizophrenic monozygotic twin probands, bringing the concordance rate close to 100 percent. About 45 percent of sibs, parents and offspring of schizophrenics are schizoid or schizophrenic, as are about 66 percent of the children of two schizophrenic parents. About 4 percent of the general population is affected with schizoid-schizophrenic disease. See review (Lancet, 1970). Elston et al. (1973) have attempted to demonstrate the operation of single genes through linkage studies. Kidd and Cavalli-Sforza (1973) favored recessive inheritance.

Annotation: Genetics of schizophrenia. (Editorial) Lancet I: 26 only, 1970.

Book, J. A.: Schizophrenia as a gene mutation. Acta Genet. Statist. Med. 4: 133-139, 1953.

Elston, R. C., Kringlen, E. and Namboodriri, K. K.: Possible linkage relationships between certain blood groups and schizophrenia of other psychoses. Behav. Genet. 3: 101-106, 1973.

Garrone, G.: Etude statistique et genetique de la schizophrenie a Geneve de 1901 a 1950. J. Genet. Hum. 11: 91-219, 1962.

Heston, L. L.: The genetics of schizophrenic and schizoid disease. Science 167: 249-256, 1970.

Karlsson, J. L.: A double dominant genetic mechanism for schizophrenia. Hereditas 65: 261-268, 1970.

Kidd, K. K. and Cavalli-Sforza, L. L.: An analysis of the genetics of schizophrenia. Soc. Biol. 20: 254-265, 1973.

Moran, P. A. P.: Class migration and the schizophrenic polymorphism. Ann. Hum. Genet. 28: 261-268, 1965.

Slater, E.: The monogenic theory of schizophrenia. Acta Genet. Statist. Med. 8: 50-56, 1958.

*18160 SCLERO-ATROPHIC AND KERATOTIC DERMATOSIS OF LIMBS (SCLEROTYLOSIS)

Huriez et al. (1968) described a 'new' geno-dermatosis in 44 members of three French kindreds. The characteristics were atrophic fibrosis of the skin of the limbs, hypoplasia of nails, and keratodermia of the palms and soles. Skin cancer and bowel cancer were frequent. Linkage with the MNS blood group locus has been established (Mennecier, 1967).

Huriez, C., Deminatti, M., Agache, P. and Mennecier, M.: A propos de 28 cas d'epidermolyse bulleuse dans 11 families dont une famile etudiee du point de une genetique, sans mise en evidence de linkage. Bull. Soc. Franc. Derm. Syph. 75: 750-755, 1968.

Huriez, C., Deminatti, M., Agache, P. and Mennecier, M.: Une genodysplasie non encore individualisee: la genodermatose sclero-atrophiante et keratodermique des extremites frequemment degenerative. Sem. Hop. Paris 44: 481-488, 1968.

Mennecier, M.: Individualisation d'une nouvelle entite: la genodermatose sclero-atrophiante et keratodermique des extremites frequemment degenerative. Etude clinique et genetique (possibilite de linkage avec le systeme MNSS). M.D. Thesis, U. de Lille, 1967.

18170 SCLEROCORNEA

In this congenital malformation of the cornea, the limits of the cornea and sclera are indistinct. A severe form is inherited as a recessive (q.v.). Sclerocornea is also a feature of cornea plana (q.v.).

18180 SCOLIOSIS, IDIOPATHIC

DeGeorge and Fisher (1967) could not find evidence for operation of simple genetic factors. High concordance in both monozygotic and dizygotic twins and an excess of propositi born to older mothers suggested to these workers that maternal factors predominate. Wynne-Davies (1968) favored either dominant or multifactorial inheritance. Dominant inheritance was suggested by Faber (1936), Garland (1934) who observed the condition in 5 generations, and Gilly et al. (1963). Male-to-male transmission is apparently rare and was specifically absent in 17 families studied by Cowell (1971), who suggested X-linked dominant inheritance. The 8 to 1 ratio of females to males supports this conclusion. Scoliosis occurs secondary to other hereditary disorders such as Marfan syndrome, dysautonomia, neurofibromatosis, Friedreich ataxia, muscular dystrophies, etc.

Cowell, H. R.: Genetic aspects of idiopathic scoliosis. J. Bone Joint Surg., In Press, 1971.

DeGeorge, F. V. and Fisher, R. L.: Idiopathic scoliosis: genetic and environmental aspects. J. Med. Genet. 4: 251-257, 1967.

Faber, A.: Untersuchungen ueber die Erblichkeit der Skoliose. Arch. Orthop. Unfallchir. 36: 217-296, 1936.

Garland, H. G.: Hereditary scoliosis. Brit. Med. J. 1: 328 only, 1934.

Gilly, R., Stagnara, P., Frederich, A., Dalloz, C., Robert, J. M. and Goldblatt, B.: Medical aspects of essential structural scoliosis in children. Lyon Med. 95: 79-95, 1963.

Wynne-Davies, R.: Familial idiopathic scoliosis. A family survey. J. Bone Joint Surg. 50A: 24-30, 1968.

*18190 SCROTAL TONGUE (LINGUA PLICATA)

The tongue is furrowed and grooved. Tobias (1945) reported two families, one with two generations and the other with four affected. Geographic tongue was an associated feature in the proband of one family. Seiler (1936) assembled the most extensive pedigree data supporting autosomal dominant inheritance.

Rolleri, F.: Ueber das Vorkommen der lingua plicata (Faltenzunge). Z. Menschl. Vererb. Konstitutionsl. 23: 587-593, 1939.

Seiler, A.: Zur Verbreitung und Vererbung der Faltenzunge (lingua plicata). Arch. Klaus Stift. Vererbungsforsch. 11: 541-569, 1936.

Tobias, N.: Scrotal tongue and its inheritance. Arch. Derm. Syph. 52: 266 only, 1945.

18195 SEA-BLUE HISTIOCYTE DISEASE, LEWIS TYPE

A recessive disorder with the morphologic peculiarity referred to as sea-blue histiocytes is referred to elsewhere (26960). Blankenship et al. (1973) suggested the existence of a dominant variety. Three sibs had splenomegaly, peripheral neuropathy, cafe-au-lait spots and elevated serum acid phosphatase levels. The father, who was not known to be related to the mother, showed elevated bone marrow acid phosphatase and abnormal histiocytes.

Blankenship, R. M., Greenburg, B. R., Lucas, R. N., Reynolds, R. D. and Beutler, E.: Familial sea-blue histiocytes with acid phosphatasemia. A syndrome resembling Gaucher disease: the Lewis variant. J.A.M.A. 225: 54-56, 1973.

18200 SEBORRHEIC KERATOSES

Butterworth and Strean (1962) described mother and daughter and stated that inheritance is autosomal dominant. Rieches (1952) described 7 families in which seborrheic keratosis was transmitted through two or three generations. The skin lesions of the basal cell nevus syndrome sometimes resemble seborrheic keratoses.

Butterworth, T. and Strean, L. P.: Clinical Genodermatology. Baltimore: Williams and Wilkins, 1962.

Rieches, A. J.: Seborrheic keratoses. Are they delayed hereditary nevi? Arch. Derm. Syph. 65: 596-600, 1952.

*18210 SECRETOR FACTOR

This might be considered either a physiologic trait or an honorary blood group. The so-called secretor has demonstrable ABH blood group antigen in the saliva and other body fluids. The non-secretor does not. Secretor is dominant. The secretor locus is linked to the Lutheran blood group locus.

Harper, P. S., Bias, W. B., Hutchinson, J. R. and McKusick, V. A. : ABH secretor status of the fetus: a genetic marker identifiable by amniocentesis. J. Med. Genet. 8: 438-440, 1971.

Race, R. R. and Sanger, R.: Blood Groups in Man. Philadelphia: F. A. Davis Co., 1968 (5th Ed.).

18220 SELLA TURCICA, BRIDGED

In a mother and three children Carey et al. (1968) observed osseous bridging between the anterior and posterior clinoids.

Carey, M. C., Fitzgerald, O. and McKiernan, E.: Osteogenesis imperfecta in twenty-three members of a kindred with heritable features contributed by a non-specific skeletal disorder. Quart. J. Med. 37: 437-449, 1968.

18223 SEPTO-OPTIC DYSPLASIA

There is no evidence for a Mendelian basis for this syndrome which features hypoplastic optic discs with characteristic double margin, absent septum-pellucidum and growth hormone deficiency.

Harris, R. J. and Haas, L.: Septo-optic dysplasia with growth hormone deficiency (de Morsier syndrome). Arch. Dis. Child. 47: 973-976, 1972.

18225 SMELL KETONE COMPOUNDS, ABILITY TO

Forrai et al. (1970) described polymorphism for ability to smell acetone and methylethylketone (MEK). The distribution of thresholds gave a bimodal curve for acetone and a trimodal curve for MEK.

Forrai, G., Szabados, T., Papp, E. S. and Bankovi, G.: Studies on the sense of smell to ketone compounds in a Hungarian population. Humangenetik 8: 348-353, 1970.

18230 'SNOW-CAPPED' TEETH

The incisal and occlusal surfaces of the teeth, especially the maxillary teeth, are opaque white. Expression is variable; hence, the condition is often confused with fluorosis. In the mildest expression only the incisors are affected. As the condition becomes more severe, posterior teeth are affected. This is thought to be a defect in maturation of enamel giving it an opaque, ground-glass appearance. The condition has been observed in areas essentially devoid of fluoride in drinking water and has occurred in family members over three generations who have resided in different geographic locations (Witkop and Rao, 1971).

Witkop, C. J., Jr. and Rao, S.: Inherited defects in tooth structure. In, Bergsma, D. (ed.): Clinical Delineation of Birth Defects. XI. Orofacial Structures. Baltimore: Williams and Wilkins, 1973. Pp. 153-184.

*18250 SORBITOL DEHYDROGENASE VARIANTS

Op't Hof (1969) stated that 'preliminary studies with human post-mortem liver specimens suggest that a polymorphism for SDH isoenzymes exists also in man.' Such was indeed found by Charlesworth (1972).

Charlesworth, D.: Starch-gel electrophoresis of four enzymes from human red blood cells: glyceraldehyde-3-phosphate dehydrogenase, fructoaldolase, glyoxalase II and sorbital dehydrogenase. Ann. Hum. Genet. 35: 477-484, 1972.

Op't Hof, J.: Isoenzymes and population genetics of sorbit dehydrogenase (ec: 1.1. 1.14) in Swine (Sus scrofa). Humangenetik 7: 258-259, 1969.

*18260 SPASTIC PARAPLEGIA

Probably in large part because of their exceptional length, the pyramidal tracts are unusually vulnerable to both acquired and genetic derangement. Autosomal dominant, autosomal recessive and X-linked recessive varieties of spastic paraplegia have been recognized and more than one recessive form exists. In the Amish of Lancaster County, Pa., a kindred with affected members in three generations was observed. In this closed community the origin of the De Novo mutation could be identified with considerable certainty. The disease was early in onset but very slowly progressive or even static. This same type of congenital stationary familial paraplegia was described in 7 members of two generations by Hohmann (1957). Schwarz (1956) reported several families including one originally reported by Bayley (1897) and now containing 22 affected persons in 6 generations. In contrast to the early onset, static form of disease in the Amish family, a family with many affected members I have studied on Deer Isle, Maine, has onset in the second or third decade and steady progression of neurologic defect.

Aagenaes (1959) described a family with thirty-one cases in four generations. Prognosis for life was good. Histopathologic changes were found bilaterally in the lateral corticospinal tracts in the thoracic cord and in the fasciculus gracilis. Although a majority of reported families have displayed recessive inheritance, 10-30 percent of families have a dominant pattern. The confusion of the spinocerebellar degenerations is illustrated by the fact that some members of Aagenaes' family had ataxia in addition to spastic paraplegia. The existence of two distinct autosomal dominant varieties of spastic paraplegia is indicated by the report of Thurmon and Walker (1970). One form, observed in a kindred on Deer Isle, Maine, had a very slowly progressive spastic paraplegia with onset usually in the late teens and with involvement limited to the legs with rectal and bladder disturbances late. The second form, observed in a Lancaster Co. (Pa.) Amish kindred, showed onset at the time the patient began to walk but was characterized by remarkably little progression and a normal lifespan. Behan and Maia (1974) studied six families. In two cases autopsy studies were performed. They concluded that distal axonal degeneration of the long ascending and descending tracts in the spinal cord is characteristic.

Aagenaes, O.: Hereditary spastic paraplegia. Acta Psychiat. Neurol. Scand. 34: 489-494, 1959.

Bayley, W. D.: Hereditary spastic paraplegia. J. Nerv. Ment. Dis. 24: 697-701, 1897.

Behan, W. M. H. and Maia, M.: Strumpell's familial spastic paraplegia: genetics and neuropathology. J. Neurol. Neurosurg. Psychiat. 37: 8-20, 1974.

Garland, H. G. and Astley, C. E.: Hereditary spastic paraplegia with amyotrophy and pes cavus. J. Neurol. Neurosurg. Psychiat. 13: 130-133, 1950.

Hariga, J. and Matthys, E.: De la paraplegie spasmodique de Strumpell-Lorrain a l'amyotrophie de Charcot-Marie-Tooth: (etude d'une famille). J. Genet. Hum. 10: 326-337, 1961.

Hohmann, H.: Die Diplegia spastica infantilis hereditaria und ihre Beziehungen zur familiaeren spastischen Spinalparalyse. Nervenarzt 28: 323-325, 1957.

Schwarz, G. A. and Liu, C. N.: Hereditary familial spastic paraplegia. Further clinical and pathologic observations. Arch. Neurol. Psychiat. 75: 144-162, 1956.

Thurmon, T. F. and Walker, B. A.: Two distinct types of autosomal dominant spastic paraplegia. The Clinical Delineation of Birth Defects. VI. Nervous System. Baltimore: Williams and Wilkins, 1971. Pp. 216-218.

Van Bogaert, L.: Etude genetique sur les paraplegies spasmodiques familiales. J. Genet. Hum. 1: 6-23, 1952.

18270 SPASTIC PARAPLEGIA WITH AMYOTROPHY OF HANDS

Silver (1966) described two unrelated English families with this combination which, he suggested, may represent a distinct type of spastic paraplegia. Wasting of the hand muscles was the first and most marked manifestation. See also AMYOTROPHIC DYSTONIC PARAPLEGIA.

Silver, J. R.: Familial spastic paraplegia with amyotrophy of the hands. Ann. Hum. Genet. 30: 69-75, 1966.

18280 SPASTIC PARAPLEGIA WITH ASSOCIATED EXTRAPYRAMIDAL SIGNS

Dick and Stevenson (1953) observed 7 cases of spastic paraplegia in 3 generations, with two instances of male-to-male transmission. Four of the affected had associated extrapyramidal signs.

Dick, A. P. and Stevenson, C. J.: Hereditary spastic paraplegia: report of a family with associated extrapyramidal signs. Lancet I: 921-923, 1953.

*18290 SPHEROCYTOSIS, HEREDITARY

MacKinney and colleagues (1962) and Morton and colleagues (1962) studied 26 families. They concluded that after the initial case in a family has been identified, four tests suffice for the diagnosis in other family members: smear, reticulocyte count, hemoglobin, bilirubin. The fragility test (increased osmotic fragility characterizes the disease) is unnecessary after the diagnosis has been made in the proband. Typical of other rare dominant traits in man, hereditary spherocytosis shows phenocopies, incomplete penetrance and incomplete ascertainment and may be genetically heterogeneous. It was estimated that prevalence is 2.2 per 10,000, that mutation rate is 0.000022 (2.2 x 10 'to the minus 5') and that about one-fourth of cases are sporadic. No evidence of reproductive compensation or of increased prenatal and infant mortality was found.

No enzyme defect has been identified (Miwa, Tanaka, Valentine, 1962) and indeed none would be expected, in view of the dominant inheritance. Jacob and Jandl (1964) are of the view that the primary defect is in the red cell membrane, which is abnormally permeable to sodium. A morphologically comparable disorder in the deer mouse Peromyscus is inherited as a recessive (Anderson, Huestis, Motulsky, 1960). Several observations suggest that more than one type of hereditary spherocytosis exists in man (review by Zail et al., 1967). Barry et al. (1968) pointed out that hemochromatosis is a serious complication of untreated spherocytosis. In a family with 6 persons affected in 3 generations, Wiley and Firkin (1970) found a form of hereditary spherocytosis with unusual features; other reports of atypical disease were reviewed. Chanmugam et al. (1971) found concordance for polycystic disease and hereditary spherocytosis in a father and three children. Three other children and four sibs of the father were thought to be free of both diseases. Of the several possible explanations, linkage is a particularly intriguing one. See ELLIPTOCYTOSIS for an example of exclusion of linkage with hereditary hemorrhagic telangiectasia on the basis of a small body of data. Jacob et al. (1971) identified an abnormal red cell membrane protein in spherocytosis. Jacob et al. (1971) demonstrated altered membrane protein in hereditary spherocytosis. Microfilamentous proteins resembling actin are important to the shape of the red cell. Comparable membrane proteins occur throughout phylogeny under circumstances suggesting a role in cell plasticity and shape. Furthermore, actin and myosin-like filamentous proteins occur in platelets. Kimberling and Lubs (1973) studied a family in which spherocytosis and a t(8p-; 12p) translocation segregated together. The lod score at theta of 0.0 was 3.01. The finding of peptidase B (16990) or LDH B (15010)) variants in spherocytosis families might permit direct confirmation of assignment to chromosome no.12+.At this writing (1973) no assignment to chromosome no. 8 has been proved.

Anderson, R., Huestis, R. R. and Motulsky, A. G.: Hereditary spherocytosis in the deer mouse. Its similarity to the human disease. Blood 15: 491-504, 1960.

Barry, M., Scheuer, P. J., Sherlock, S., Ross, C. F. and Williams, R.: Hereditary spherocytosis with secondary haemochromatosis. Lancet II: 481-485, 1968.

Chanmugam, D., Rasaretnam, R. and Karunaratne, K. E. S.: Hereditary spherocytosis and polycystic disease of the kidneys in four members of a family. Am. J. Hum. Genet. 23: 66 only, 1971.

Jacob, H. S. and Jandl, J. H.: Increased cell membrane permeability in the pathogenesis of hereditary spherocytosis. J. Clin. Invest. 43: 1704-1720, 1964.

Jacob, H. S.: Abnormalities in the physiology of the erythrocyte membrane in hereditary spherocytosis. Am. J. Med. 41: 734-741, 1966.

Jacob, H. S.: Dysfunction of the red blood cell membrane in hereditary spherocytosis. Brit. J. Haemat. 14: 99-104, 1968.

Jacob, H. S.: Hereditary spherocytosis: a disease of the red cell membrane. Seminars In Hemat. 2: 139-166, 1965.

Jacob, H. S., Amsden, T. and White, J.: Experimental production of hereditary spherocytosis (HS): role of defective membrane microfilaments in the disorder. (Abstract) J. Clin. Invest. 50: 48A only, 1971.

Jacob, H. S., Ruby, A., Overland, E. S. and Mazia, D.: Abnormal membrane protein of red blood cells in hereditary spherocytosis. J. Clin. Invest. 50: 1800-1805, 1971.

Jandl, J. H. and Cooper, R. A.: Hereditary spherocytosis. In, Stanbury, J. B., Wyngaarden, J. B. and Fredrickson, D. S. (eds.): The Metabolic Basis of Inherited Disease. New York: McGraw-Hill, 1972 (3rd Ed.). Pp. 1323-1337.

Kimberling, W. J. and Lubs, H. A.: Denver, Colo., personal communication, May 17, 1973.

MacKinney, A. A.: Hereditary spherocytosis. Clinical family studies. Arch. Intern. Med. 116: 257-265, 1965.

MacKinney, A. A., Morton, N. E., Kosower, N. S. and Schilling, R. F.: Ascertaining genetic carriers of hereditary spherocytosis by statistical analysis of multiple laboratory tests. J. Clin. Invest. 41: 554-567, 1962.

MacPherson, A. I. S., Richmond, J., Donaldson, G. W. K. and Muir, A. R.: The role of the spleen in congenital spherocytosis. Am. J. Med. 50: 35-41, 1971.

Miwa, S., Tanaka, K. R. and Valentine, W. N.: Enolase activity of erythrocytes in hereditary spherocytosis. Nature 195: 613-614, 1962.

Morton, N. E., MacKinney, A. A., Kosower, N., Schilling, R. F. and Gray, M. P.: Genetics of spherocytosis. Am. J. Hum. Genet. 14: 170-184, 1962.

Motulsky, A. G., Anderson, R., Sparkes, R. S. and Huestis, R. H.: Marrow transplantation in newborn mice with hereditary spherocytosis. A Model system. Trans. Ass. Am. Physicians 75: 64-72, 1962.

Wiley, J. S. and Firkin, B. G.: An unusual variant of hereditary spherocytosis. Am. J. Med. 48: 63-71, 1970.

Wiley, J. S.: Co-ordinated increase of sodium leak and sodium pump in hereditary spherocytosis. Brit. J. Haemat. 22: 529-542, 1972.

Zail, S. S., Krawitz, E., Viljoen, E., Kramer, S. and Metz, J.: Atypical hereditary spherocytosis: biochemical studies and sites of erythrocyte destruction. Brit. J. Haemat. 13: 323-334, 1967.

*18295 SPINAL ARACHNOIDITIS

Duke and Hashimoto (1974) described a Canadian kindred of Japanese ancestry in which six members of three generations had adult onset of progressive spastic paraparesis with prominent radicular pain and patchy numbness. Myelography showed obstruction to flow of contrast material in the thoracic area with multiple filling defects and fragmentation of the contrast material. Exploratory surgery showed band-like fibrous thickening of the spinal arachnoid. An analogy to Peyronie disease (17100) and Dupuytren contracture (12690) was made. Father-to-son transmission was noted.

Duke, R. J. and Hashimoto, S. A.: Familial spinal arachnoiditis, a new entity. Arch. Neurol. 30: 300-303, 1974.

*18300 SPINOCEREBELLAR ATAXIA AND PLAQUE-LIKE DEPOSITS

Seitelberger (1962) described a kindred with a unique neurologic disorder traced through 5 generations. Plaque-like deposits were found in the cerebral cortex, basal ganglia and (most extremely) all layers of the cerebellum. Clinically and pathologically the disorder most closely resembled kuru. However, in kuru the posterior white columns are spared and plaque-formation in the cerebral cortex is more intense.

Seitelberger, F.: Eigenartige familiaer-hereditaere Krankheit des Zentralnervensystems in einer Niedero-esterreichischeh Sippe (zugleich ein Beitrag zur Vergleichenden Neuropathologie des Kuru). Wien. Klin. Wschr. 74: 687-691, 1962.

*18305 SPINOCEREBELLAR ATAXIA WITH RIGIDITY AND PERIPHERAL NEUROPATHY

Ziegler et al. (1972) described a large kindred in which many persons were affected with a variable neurologic disorder: late onset cerebellar ataxia, muscular rigidity, bradykinesia, dysarthria, fasciculations, muscle atrophy, and spasticity appearing in various combinations in affected persons. There were many instances of male-to-male transmission. Pathologic studies in one case showed degeneration in spinocerebellar tracts, Purkinje cells and dentate nuclei of cerebellum, dorsal root ganglion cells and canda equina nerve roots. Peripheral neuropahty was present in several cases as evidenced by demylination found on sural nerve biopsy and by findings of nerve conduction studies. Several cases showed releif of rigidity when levo-dopa was administered. The two sisters reported by Sigwald et al. (1964) seem to have had a similar disorder, but the lack of evidence of dominant inheritance in that family leaves doubts as to the identity.

Sigwald, J., Lapresle, J., Raverdy, P. and Recondo, J.: Atrophie cerebrelleuse familiale avec association de lesions nigeriennes et spinales. Presse Med. 72: 557-562, 1964.

Ziegler, D. K., Schimke, R. N., Kepes, J. J., Ross, D. L. and Klinkerfuss, G.: Late onset ataxia, rigidity, and peripheral neuropahty. A familial syndrome with variable therapeutic responses to levo-dopa. Arch. Neurol. 27: 52-66, 1972.

18310 SPINOCEREBELLAR ATROPHY WITH PUPILLARY PARALYSIS

In a 37-year-old woman, her 14-year-old son and 6-year-old daughter, Sutherland, Tyrer and Eadie (1963) described spinocerebellar atrophy with absence of pupillary reaction to light or convergence, but preservation of accommodation reflexes.

Indemini, M. and Ammann, F.: Heredo-degenerescence spino-cerebelleuse (HDSC) associee au syndrome de Klinefelter. J. Genet. Hum. 10: 297-325, 1961.

Sutherland, J. M., Tyrer, J. H. and Eadie, M. J.: Atrophie spino-cerebelleuse familiale avec mydriase fixe. Rev. Neurol. 108: 439-442, 1963.

*18320 SPINO-PONTINE ATROPHY

Boller and Segarra (1969) observed 24 persons with late-onset ataxia in four generations of an Anglo-Saxon family. Taniguchi and Konigsmark (1971) described 16 affected persons in three generations of a Negro family. The pathologic findings were similar in the two families. The cerebellum was relatively spared and the inferior olives were normal. The spinal cord showed loss of myelinated fibers in the spinocerebellar tracts and posterior funiculi. There was also marked loss of nuclei basis ponti.

Boller, F. and Segarra, J. M.: Spino-pontine degeneration. European Neurol. 2: 356-373, 1969.

Taniguchi, R. and Konigsmark, B. W.: Dominant spino-pontine atrophy: report of a family through three generations. Brain 94: 349-358, 1971.

18330 SPLENO-GONADAL FUSION WITH LIMB DEFECTS AND MICROGNATHIA

An exceedingly bizarre syndrome is that of fusion of spleen and gonad with ectromelia. Hives and Eggum (1961) reported a ninth case. Seven were stillborn or died in infancy. The eighth died at age 10. Their patient was 15 years old. This may be a lethal dominant.

Hives, J. R. and Eggum, P. R.: Splenic-gonadal fusion causing bowel obstruction. Arch. Surg. 83: 887-889, 1961.

18340 SPLIT LOWER LIP

Herbst (1936) described a kindred in which 18 persons in four generations had a median groove or split in the lower lip. The upper lip was fleshy and moderately everted but only one of the examined persons had a median cleft of the upper lip. The maxilla was narrow and the teeth crowded and irregularly alligned. Gorlin (1968) thinks this may have been an example of lower lip pits.

Gorlin, R. J.: Minneapolis, Minn.: personal communication, 1968.

Herbst, E.: Erbliche Spaltbildungen der Unterlippe mit schweren Kieferdeformationen und Intelligenz-storeungen. Volk. Rasse. 11: 276-280, 1936.

18350 SPLIT-HAND AND FOOT WITH HYPODONTIA

Temtamy and McKusick (1971) described mother and son. See 12990.

Temtamy, S. A. and McKusick, V. A.: The Genetics of Hand Malformations. New York: National Foundation March of Dimes, 1975.

*18360 SPLIT-HAND DEFORMITY

Typical and atypical forms are recognized. Atypical cases are usually sporadic. Typical cases may be of the lobster-claw variety (absence of central rays) or monodactyly type (deficiency of radial rays with no cleft). Gradations between these types occur and cases of each type sometimes are found in the same family.

Features of genetic interest in reported families include regular dominant inheritance in three or more generations, lack of penetrance with skipped generations, markedly irregular 'dominant' inheritance, two or more affected offspring of normal parents, and anomalous segregation ratios in offspring of affected males. Vogel (1958) suggested that two varieties of split-hand deformity exist: (1) type with constant involvement of the feet and regular autosomal dominant inheritance, (2) type with inconsistent involvement of the feet and irregular inheritance. Birch-Jensen (1949) recognized two anatomical types: (1) typical lobster claw, and (2) monodactyly. The anatomical classification has no genetic significance because either type may occur in the same family or on different limbs of the same person (Temtamy, 1966). Absence of the central rays characterized the first anatomical type. The hand is divided into two parts by a cone-shaped cleft tapering proximally. The two parts of the hand can be apposed like a lobster claw. A comparable deformity of the feet may be present. In the second anatomical type, or monodactyly, the radial rays are absent with only the fifth digit remaining, as a rule. In Denmark Birch-Jensen (1949) estimated the frequency at birth to be about 1 in 90,000. About 70 pedigrees were reported prior to 1965 (Temtamy, 1966). Regular autosomal dominant inheritance through three or more generations was demonstrated by about 27 of the 70 pedigrees. Skipping of a generation was noted by at least 4 authors. Two or more affected sibs with both parents normal were noted by several authors (MacKenzie, Penrose, 1951; Graham, Badgley, 1955; Neugebauer, 1962; and others). Gonadal mosaicism was suggested by Auerbach (1956) as a possible explanation. In those pedigrees with inconstant involvement of the feet the genetics is less clear. A disturbed segregation ratio was found in the family first reported by McMullan and Pearson (1913) and brought up to date by Stevenson and Jennings (1960). A marked preponderance of affected sons of affected fathers suggested germinal selection to the latter workers. Ford (1963) raised the question of chromosomal aberration but could demonstrate none by the available methods. Anomalous segregation has also been observed with aniridia (q.v.) and with Alport syndrome (q.v.). Ray (1970) described two cases among the children of first-cousin, unaffected parents.

Auerbach, C.: A possible case of delayed mutation in man. Ann. Hum. Genet. 20: 266-269, 1956.

Birch-Jensen, A.: Congenital Deformities of the Upper Extremities. Copenhagen: Ejnar Munksgaard, 1949.

Ford, C. E.: Autosomal abnormalities. Sec. Intern. Conf. on Cong. Malformations, New York: National Foundation, 1963. P. 25.

Freire-Maia, A.: A recessive form of ectrodactyly: its implications in genetic counseling. J. Hered. 62: 53 Only, 1971.

Graham, J. B. and Badgley, C. E.: Split-hand with unusual complications. Am. J. Hum. Genet. 7: 44-50, 1955.

MacKenzie, H. J. and Penrose, L. S.: Two pedigrees of ectrodactyly. Ann. Eugen. 16: 88-96, 1951.

McMullen, G. and Pearson, K.: On the inheritance of the deformity known as split foot or lobster claw. Biometrika 9: 381-390, 1913.

Neugebauer, H.: Spalthand und -fuss mit familiaerer Besonderheit. Z. Orthop. 95: 500-506, 1962.

Ray, A. K.: Another case of split-foot mutation in two sibs. J. Hered. 61: 169-170, 1970.

Stevenson, A. C. and Jennings, L. M.: Ectrodactyly — evidence in favour of a disturbed segregation in the offspring of affected males. Ann. Hum. Genet. 24: 89-96, 1960.

Temtamy, S. A.: Genetic Factors in Hand Malformations. Ph. D. Thesis. Johns Hopkins University, 1966.

Vogel, F.: Verzoegerte Mutation beim Menschen: einige kritische Bemerkungen zuch. Auerbachs Arbeit (1956). Ann. Hum. Genet. 22: 132-137, 1958.

18370 SPLIT-HAND DEFORMITY WITH MANDIBULOFACIAL DYSOSTOSIS

Patterson and Stevenson (1964) studied a father with the full syndrome and his son who had only the split-foot deformity. See MANDIBULOFACIAL DYSOSTOSIS WITH LIMB ANOMALIES (NAGER ACROFACIAL DYSOSTOSIS).

Patterson, T. J. S. and Stevenson, A. C.: Craniofacial dysostosis and malformations of the feet. J. Med. Genet. 1: 112-114, 1964.

18380 SPLIT-HAND WITH CONGENITAL NYSTAGMUS, FUNDAL CHANGES, CATARACTS

In a father and daughter with split-hand split-foot deformity, Karsch (1936) found horizontal undulatory nystagmus, squint, fundal changes and cataract, which in the father appeared at a late age and in the daughter appeared earlier. Neugebauer (1962) described affected half sibs, a brother and sister ages 7 months and 42 months, respectively. The mother of the two children (by different husbands) was normal. Cataract was not present.

Karsch, J.: Erbliche Augenmissbildung in Verbindung mit Spalthand und -fuss. Z. Augenheilk. 89: 274-279, 1936.

Neugebauer, H.: Spalthand und -fuss mit familiaerer Besonderheit. Z. Orthop. 95: 500-506, 1962.

*18390 SPONDYLOEPIPHYSEAL DYSPLASIA, CONGENITAL TYPE

Spranger and Wiedemann (1966) suggested this designation for a disorder affecting particularly the vertebrae and juxta-truncal epiphyses. Four of 6 patients had progressive myopia. Three persons (mother and 2 sons) were affected in one family. They collected 14 cases from the literature. Bach et al. (1967) reported an isolated case. Platyspondyly, short limbs and cleft palate were evident at birth. Other malformations included myopia, hypoplasia of abdominal musculature, abdominal and inguinal hernias and mental retardation. Detachment of the retina occurs in some patients even without significant myopia. Roaf et al. (1967) reported 4 sporadic cases. Possibly the patient described by McKusick (1966) had this condition. Fraser (1968) observed dominant inheritance (his case M 13). Severe myopia in particular was a serious problem in the cases reported by Fraser et al. (1969). Mother and two children were affected in one of their families. Spranger and Langer (1970) reported 20 cases. In the affected newborn infant X-rays show lack of ossification of the os pubis, distal femoral and proximal tibial epiphyses, talus and calcaneus and flattening of vertebral bodies (Spranger and Langer, 1970).

Bach, C., Maroteaux, P., Schaeffer, P., Bitan, A. and Crumiere, C.: Dysplasia spondylo-epiphysaire congenitale avec anomalies multiples. Arch. Franc. Pediat. 24: 23-34, 1967.

Fraser, G. R. and Friedmann, A. I.: The Causes of Blindness in Childhood. Baltimore: Johns Hopkins Press, 1968.

Fraser, G. R., Friedmann, A. I., Maroteaux, P., Glen-Bott, A. M. and Mittwoch, V.: Dysplasia spondyloepiphysaria congenita and related generalized skeletal dysplasias among children with severe visual handicaps. Arch. Dis. Child. 44: 490-498, 1969.

McKusick, V. A.: Heritable Disorders of Connective Tissue. St. Louis: C. V. Mosby Co., 1972. (4th Ed.). P. 467.

Roaf, R., Longmore, J. B. and Forrester, R. M.: A childhood syndrome of bone dysplasia, retinal detachment and deafness. Develop. Med. Child. Neurol. 9: 464-473, 1967.

Spranger, J. and Langer, L. O., Jr.: Spondyloepiphyseal dysplasia congenita. Radiology 94: 313-322, 1970.

Spranger, J. and Wiedemann, H.-R.: Dysplasia spondyloepiphysaria congenita. (Letter) Lancet II: 642 only, 1966.

Spranger, J. and Wiedemann, H.-R.: Dysplasia spondyloepiphysaria congenita. Helv. Paediat. Acta 21: 598-611, 1966.

*18410 SPONDYLOEPIPHYSEAL DYSPLASIA, TARDA TYPE

A late form of SED producing marked dwarfism was observed in mother and son (1215027, 1215026). The radiographic changes were different from those of the X-linked SED. The dwarfing was marked, the mother being only about 4 feet tall. This condition is distinguished from brachyraphia (q.v.) by the fact that the arms are shortened to a degree about proportionate to the degree of shortening in the trunk. Felman (1969) described a Negro father and his son and daughter with epiphyseal and vertebral dysplasia producing severe scoliosis and truncal shortening as well as complete destruction of the femoral capital epiphyses and necks. The hands and feet were short and stubby. Clinically and radiologically the patients were normal at birth. Rubin (1964) presented (figs. 7.9-7.14) an instructive family in which platyspondyly accompanied changes in the epiphyses in the limbs. The family reported also by Moldauer et al. (1962), had seven affected persons in three generations with no male-to-male transmission. There may be more than one dominant form of spondyloepiphyseal dysplasia distinct from the pseudoachondroplastic types. It is clear, however, that there is at least one form. These cases have too much platyspondyly for it to be multiple epiphyseal dysplasia and the involvement of the bones of the limbs is not severe enough to fall into one of the pseudoachondroplasia groups.

Felman, A. H.: Multiple epiphyseal dysplasia. Three cases with unusual vertebral abnormalities. Radiology 93: 119-125, 1969.

Moldauer, M., Hanelin, J. and Bauer, W.: Familial precocious degenerative arthritis and the natural history of osteochondrodystrophy. In, Blumenthal, H. T. (ed.): Medical and Clinical Aspects of Aging. New York: Columbia U. Press, 1962. Pp. 226-233.

Rubin, P.: Dynamic Classification of Bone Dysplasias. Chicago: Year Book Medical Publishers, 1964.

18420 SPONDYLOLISTHESIS AND SPINA BIFIDA OCCULTA

Amuso and Mankin (1967) reported on a family in which five members in three generations had spondylolisthesis of the fifth lumbar vertebra on the first sacral in association with defects in the posterior spinous processes of the fifth lumbar vertebra and sacrum. Transmission from father to son occurred once. Shahriaree and Harkess (1970) found spondylolisthesis in a father and three sons. The defect was thought to concern the pars interarticularis.

Amuso, S. J. and Mankin, H. J.: Hereditary spondylolisthesis and spina bifida. Report of a family in which the lesion is transmitted as an autosomal dominant through three generations. J. Bone Joint Surg. 49A: 507-513, 1967.

Shahriaree, H. and Harkess, J. W.: A family with spondylolisthesis. Radiology 94: 631-633, 1970.

18430 SPONDYLOSIS, CERVICAL

Bull et al. (1969) from an X-ray study of the cervical spine in twins concluded that genetic factors are significant in degenerative changes in the cervical spine.

Bull, J., El Gammal, T. and Popham, M.: A possible genetic factor in cervical spondylosis. Brit. J. Radiol. 42: 9-16, 1969.

*18440 SPRENGEL DEFORMITY ('HIGH SCAPULA')

Congenital upward displacement of the scapula almost always occurs sporadically. However, Gottesleben (1927) observed 9 cases in 6 sibships of 3 generations of a family with male-to-male transmission. Schwarzweller (1937) found two affected sibs in two out of 9 families. In one of these the father had mild abnormality. Aubert and Arroyo (1967) observed the disorder in father and daughter. In another family reported by Perls (cited by Engel, 1943), a father and two sons had unilateral elevated scapulae. Wilson et al. (1971) reported a family in which affected persons were thought to have occurred in multiple sibships of five successive generations with instances of male-to-male transmission. Thus, there is probably a simple Mendelian form of Sprengel deformity, which represents a minority of cases.

Aubert, L. and Arroyo, H.: Maladie de Sprengel familiale. Marseille Med. 104: 287-290, 1967.

Engel, D.: The etiology of the undescended scapula and related syndromes. J. Bone Joint Surg. 25: 613-625, 1943.

Gottesleben, A.: Ueber den doppelseitigen und einseitigen Schulterblatthochstand. Arch. Klin. Chir. 144: 723-731, 1927.

Schwarzweller, F.: Der angeborene Schulterblatthochstand der Wirbelsaeule. (Eine erbbiologische Untersuchung ueber die Entstehung des angeborenen Schulterblatthochstandes). Z. Menschl. Vererb. Konstitutionsl. 20: 341-349, 1937.

Wilson, M. G., Milsity, V. G. and Shinno, N. W.: Dominant inheritance of Sprengel's deformity. J. Pediat., In Press, 1971.

*18450 STEATOCYSTOMA MULTIPLEX (SEBACEOUS CYSTS, MULTIPLE)

Noojin and Reynolds (1948) observed twelve cases in three generations. In typical cases the patient may exhibit 100 to 2000 round or oval cystic tumors widely distributed on the back, anterior trunk, arms, scrotum and thighs. Sebaceous cysts presenting mainly as wens of the scalp were reported by Stephens (1959) in a very large number of individuals in five generations in a dominant pedigree pattern. Sebaceous and other soft tissue tumors occur as part of Gardner syndrome (see POLYPOSIS III). Actually the so-called sebaceous cysts of Gardner syndrome are usually epidermoid cysts.

Noojin, R. O. and Reynolds, J. P.: Familial steatocystoma multiplex. Twelve cases in three generations. Arch. Derm. Syph. 57: 1013-1018, 1948.

Stephens, F. E.: Hereditary multiple sebaceous cysts. J. Hered. 50: 299-301, 1959.

18470 STEIN-LEVENTHAL SYNDROME

The fathers tend to be abnormally hairy, female sibs are hirsute and mothers and sisters often have oligomenorrhea. Culdoscopy has often shown signs of S-L, e.g., 8 of 12 sisters of cases showed ovarian changes consistent with that diagnosis (Cooper et al., 1968). Urinary steroid determinations also suggest a genetic basis. Ovarian hyperthecosis was the term used by Givens et al. (1971), who found 41 women (in 2 kindreds) who had hirsutism and-or oligomenorrhea. Ovarian histology performed in 8 showed hyperplasia of theca cells in atretic follicles, a paucity of primordial and developing follicles, and stromal hyperplasia. Elevated levels of androstenedione and-or testosterone and of luteinizing hormone were found. Estradiol and follicle-stimulating hormone were low. These levels tended to return to normal after bilateral wedge resection of the ovaries. Some men of the families had low plasma testosterone and had abnormally high LH-FSH ratio as in the women. The pedigrees were consistent with dominant inheritance probably autosomal because in one kindred the disorder was apparently transmitted through a father and son.

Borghi, A., Maiello, M. and Giusti, G.: Stein-Leventhal syndrome in sisters. The possible role of genetic factors in the 'polycistic ovary syndrome.' Acta. Genet. Med. Gem. 21: 79-93, 1972.

Cooper, H. E., Spellacy, W. N., Prem, K. A. and Cohen, W. D.: Hereditary factors in the Stein-Leventhal syndrome. Am. J. Obstet. Gynec. 100: 371-387, 1968.

Givens, J. R., Wiser, W. L., Coleman, S. A., Wilroy, R. S., Andersen, R. N., Fish, S. A. and Watson, B. S.: Familial ovarian hyperthecosis: a study of two families. Am. J. Obstet. Gynec. 110: 959-972, 1971.

18480 STERNUM, PREMATURE OBLITERATION OF SUTURES OF

Currarino and Silverman (1958) reported cases in which the sternal sutures were hypoplastic or closed prematurely leading to a characteristic deformity of the sternum which was abnormally short with an acute angulation in the normal position of the angle of Louis and depressed in its lower part. Associated manifestations in some cases included micrognathia, cryptorchidism, congenital heart malformation. Dorst (1966) observed the sternal anomaly in mother and daughter who were otherwise normal. The sternal deformity is seen in the male Turner syndrome, pterygium colli syndrome. It was also seen in brothers with multiple osteochondritis dissecans (q.v.).

Currarino, G. and Silverman, F. N.: Premature obliteration of the sternal sutures and pigeon-breast deformity. Radiology 70: 532-540, 1958.

Dorst, J. P.: Baltimore, Md.: personal communication, 1966.

18485 STIFF MAN SYNDROME, HEREDITARY FORM OF

Klein et al. (1972) described this disorder in 10 persons in 3 generations of a family. They had attacks of stiffness precipitated by surprise or minor physical contact and characterized by difficulty in making sudden movements but absence of sign of myotonia or myokymia. The electromyographic counterpart of stiffness was continuous activity at rest with normal action potentials. The continuous electrical activity was abolished by diazepam. X-linkage could not be excluded because there was no male-to-male transmission.

Klein, R., Haddow, J. E. and DeLuca, C.: Familial congenital disorder resembling stiff-man syndrome. Am. J. Dis. Child. 124: 730-731, 1972.

18490 STIFF SKIN SYNDROME

Esterly and McKusick (1971) described a disorder characterized by thickened and indurated skin of the entire body and limitation of joint mobility with flexion contractures. One patient they reported was a sporadic case but the other had an affected sister and mother. This may be the same disorder as that entered elsewhere as contractures with scleroderma-like changes (12110). The disorder named syndesmodysplastic dwarfism by Laplane et al. (1972), who observed the disorder in brothers, had similarities but was probably distinctive. For example, inheritance was probably recessive also the parana hard-skin syndrome (26053) is apparently distinct. This may be the same condition as that described under contractures with scleroderma-like changes (12110).

Esterly, N. B. and McKusick, V. A.: Stiff skin syndrome. Pediatrics 47: 360-369, 1971.

Laplane, R., Fontaine, J.-L., Lagardere, B. and Sambucy, F.: Nanisme syndesmodysplasique familial. Une entite morbide nouvelle. Arch. Franc. Pediat. 29: 831-838, 1972.

*18500 STOMATOCYTOSIS I

Lock, Smith and Hardisty (1961) described a 'new' hereditary red cell anomaly associated with hemolytic anemia. They referred to it as stomatocytosis becaused of a pale-staining band in the erythrocytes. Erythrocytes showed shortened survival and increased osmotic fragility. It is clear that there is more than one disorder manifested by stomatocytosis and hemolytic anemia. Stomatocytes are uniconcave with a slit-like rather than circular area of central pallor in stained preparations. The potassium-sodium disorder of erythrocytes (see 26390) shows stomatocytes and may be the same disorder as that listed here.

Lock, S. P., Smith, R. and Hardisty, R. M.: Stomatocytosis: a hereditary red cell anomaly associated with haemolytic anaemia. Brit. J. Haemat. 7: 303-314, 1961.

*18501 STOMATOCYTOSIS II

Miller et al. (1971) described a large kindred of Swiss-German origin in which three sibs appeared to be homozygous and 50 other persons heterozygous. All had stomatocytosis. The homozygotes had hemolytic anemia, decreased osmotic fragility, increase in intracellular sodium and marked increase in sodium pump rates. The heterozygotes had no anemia but had cholelithiasis and intermittent jaundice. Decreased fragility distinguishes it from other forms of stomatocytosis with hemolytic anemia.

*18505 STORAGE POOL PLATELET DISEASE

Weiss et al. (1969) described a kindred in which 10 members in 4 generations had a bleeding diathesis. There were several instances of male-to-male transmission. Six of the affected members were studied and found to have impaired release of platelet adenosine diphosphate (ADP). The platelets were smaller than normal. The major symptom was easy burising. Ingestion of asprin interferes with release of ADP even though the storage pool is normal. In a later paper on the same family Holmsen and Weiss (1970) postulated that these patients lack the storage, or non-metabolic, pool of ADP. Because of reduced release of ADP, collagen-induced platelet aggregation was impaired. By electron microscopy Weiss and Ames (1973) showed a marded decrease in platelet dense bodies. Since both serotonin and the storage pool of adenine nucleotrides are deficient in these platelets, the dense bodies may normally store them. Willis and Weiss (1973) showed that prostaglandin production is impaired in this disorder.

Holmsen, H. and Weiss, H. J.: Hereditary defect in the platelet release reaction caused by a deficiency in the storage pool of platelet adenine nucleotides. Br. J. Haematol. 19: 643-649, 1970.

Holmsen, H. and Weiss, H. J.: Further evidence for a deficient storage pool of adenine nucleotides in platelets from some patients with thrombocytopathia — storage pool disease. Blood 39: 197-209, 1972.

Weiss, H. J., Chervenick, P. A., Zalusky, R. and Factor, A.: A familial defect in platelet function associated with imparied release of adenosine diphosphate. New Eng. J. Med. 281: 1264-1270, 1969.

Weiss, H. J. and Ames, R. P.: Ultrastructural findings in storage pool disease and asprin-like defects of platelets. Am. J. Path. 71: 447-460, 1973.

Willis, A. L. and Weiss, H. J.: A congenital defect in platelet prostaglandin production associated with impaired hemostasis in storage pool disease. Prostaglandis 4: 793-796, 1973.

18510 STRABISMUS

Although the familial nature of strabismus has been recognized in the medical literature since Hippocrates (see Cantolino and Von Noorden, 1969), no simple Mendelian inheritance is established (Richter, 1967). Cantolino and Von Noorden (1969) arrived at the same conclusion from a family study of microtropia, the minor form of strabismus. Richter (1967) found lower risk in first-degree relatives with divergent strabismus than with convergent strabismus. When two first-degree relatives (e.g., two parents, one parent and a child, or two children) are affected the risk is about 1 in 4 and 1 in 2 for the two forms, respectively. A curious syndrome of cyclic strabismus (periodic esotrophia) has been described by Richter (1968) and by Friendly et al. (1973) among others. The eyes are alternately straight for 24 hours and crossed for 24 hours. Strabismus appears to be unusually frequent in the families of these patients (Friendly et al., 1973).

Cantolino, S. J. and Von Noorden, G. K.: Heredity in microtropia. Arch. Ophthalmol. 81: 753-759, 1969.

Friendly, D. S., Manson, R. A. and Albert, D. G.: Cyclic strabismus. A case study. Doc. Ophthalmol. 34: 189-202, 1973.

Richter, S.: Untersuchungen ueber die Hereditaet des Strabismus concomitans. Humangenetik 3: 235-243, 1967.

Richter, C. P.: Clock-mechanism esotrophia in children alternate-day squint. Johns Hopkins Med. J. 122: 218-223, 1968.

*18520 STRIAE DISTENSAE

I have observed transverse striae of the lumbar area in father and two sons. The striae appeared in their teens and faded as they grew older. Carr and Hamilton (1969) noted that such striae are more common in males. F. Parkes Weber (1935) called them idiopathic striae atrophicae of puberty. Striae distensae occur, especially in the deltoid, pectoral, hip and thigh areas, in the Marfan syndrome.

Carr, R. D. and Hamilton, J. F.: Transverse striae of the back. Arch. Dermatol. 99: 26-30, 1969.

McKusick, V. A.: Transverse striae distensae in the lumbar area in father and two sons. The Clinical Delineation of Birth Defects. XII. Skin, Hair and Nails. Baltimore: Williams and Wilkins, 1971. Pp. 260-261.

Weber, F. P.: 'Idiopathic' striae atrophicae of puberty. Lancet II: 885-886, and 1347 only, 1935.

18530 STURGE-WEBER SYNDROME

This condition, sometimes called the fourth phacomatosis, is characterized by nevus flammeus of the face and angioma of the meninges. Unlike the other phacomatoses (tuberous sclerosis, neurofibromatosis and von Hippel-Lindau disease), no clear evidence of heredity has been discovered. Sometimes (see Bonse, 1951, and Nonnenmacher, 1955) the Klippel-Trenaunay-Weber syndrome (q.v.), which also does not seem to Mendelize, is associated. See KLIPPEL-TRENAUNAY-WEBER SYNDROME.

Bonse, G.: Roentgenbefunde bei einer Phakomatose (Sturge-Weber kombiniert mit Klippel-Trenaunay). Fortschr. Roentgenstr. 74: 727, 1951.

Furukawa, T., Igata, A., Toyokura, Y. and Ikeda, S.: Sturge-Weber and Klippel-Trenaunay syndrome with nevus of OTA and ITO. Arch. Dermatol. 102: 640-645, 1970.

Nonnenmacher, H.: Augenaerztliche Betrachtungen zum Symptomenkomplex morbus Sturge-Weber, Klippel-Trenaunay und Parkes-Weber. Klin. Mbl. Augenheilk. 126: 154-164, 1955.

18540 SUBGLOTTIC BAR

Howie, Ladefoged and Stark (1961) described subglottic bar in a grandfather, mother and two daughters (4 persons in three generations). Severe dyspnea with respiratory infection in a 6-year-old brought the condition to attention. All four had a harsh, quivering, high-pitched, weak voice and three had suffered from respiratory distress with inspiratory stridor. Imperfect adduction of the vocal cords was an associated finding.

Howie, T. O., Ladefoged, P. and Stark, R. E.: Congenital subglottic bars found in 3 generations of one family. Folia Phoniat. 13: 56-61, 1961.

18545 SUBLUXATION OF LENSES, LATE

'Simple' autosomal dominant forms of ectopia lentis, i.e., forms unassociated with extra-ocular manifestations apparently exist in two forms, congenital (see 12960) and late.

*18550 SUPRAVALVAR AORTIC STENOSIS

Eisenberg and colleagues (1964) reported 22 cases involving 3 generations of each of two families. Some had associated pulmonary valvular or peripheral arterial stenosis. None had unusual facies. A similar condition which may be the result of fetal hypercalcemia is characterized by elfin facies (anteverted nostrils and patulous lips) and mental retardation with supravalvar aortic stenosis. It is apparently non-familial and a phenocopy of familial supravalvar aortic stenosis. Pulmonary artery stenosis was noted in mother and son by Gyllensward et al. (1957). Lewis et al. (1969) described a sibship in which 5 of 9 sibs had supravalvar aortic stenosis with peculiar facies but normal intelligence. Antia et al. (1967) commented on the lack of clear distinction between the familial supravalvar aortic stenosis with normal facies and mentality and the non-familial type with abnormal facies and mental retardation. McDonald et al. (1969) described an arteriopathy, with multiple pulmonary and systemic arterial stenoses, in a mother and three daughters. Two had supravalvar aortic stenosis. The familial occurrence of pulmonary arterial stenoses is documented (McCue et al., 1965) and their occurrence after maternal rubella is well established (Rowe, 1963). It can be argued that supravalvar aortic stenosis is an inadequate or inappropriate designation. Strong et al. (1970) observed sudden death following premedication for cardiac catheterization in an 11-month-old male. Postmortem showed severe fibromuscular dysplasia of both systemic and pulmonary arteries. A sister had signs of mild pulmonary artery and supravalvular aortic stenosis. The mother had signs of mild aortic stenosis. Sibs were reported by Wooley et al. (1961). Beuren (1972) presented compelling evidence that supravalvular aortic stenosis and idiopathic hypercalcemia (23800) are one and the same disorder.

Antia, A. U., Wiltse, H. E., Rowe, R. D., Pitt, E. L., Levin, S., Ottesen, O. E. and Cooke, R. E.: Pathogenesis of the supravalvular aortic stenosis syndrome. J. Pediat. 71: 431-441, 1967.

Beuren, A. J.: Supravalvular aortic stenosis: a complex syndrome with and without mental retardation. Clinical Delineation of Birth Defects. XV. Cardiovascular System. Baltimore: Williams and Wilkins Co., 1972. Pp. 45-56.

Eisenberg, R., Young, D., Jacobson, B. and Boito, A.: Familial supravalvar aortic stenosis. Am. J. Dis. Child. 108: 341-347, 1964.

Garcia, R. E., Friedman, W. F., Kaback, M. M. and Rowe, R. D.: Idiopathic hypercalcemia and supravalvular aortic stenosis: documentation of a new syndrome. New Eng. J. Med. 271: 117-120, 1964.

Gyllensward, A., Lodin, H., Lundberg, A. and Moller, T.: Congenital, multiple peripheral stenosis of the pulmonary artery. Pediatrics 19: 399-410, 1957.

Jorgensen, G. and Beuren, A. J.: Genetische Untersuchungen bei supravalvularen Aortenstenosen. Humangenetik 1: 497-515, 1965.

Lewis, A. J., Ongley, P. A., Kincaid, O. W. and Ritter, D. G.: Supravalvular aortic stenosis. Report of a family with peculiar somatic features and normal intelligence. Dis. Chest 55: 372-379, 1969.

Logan, W. F., Jones, E. W., Walker, E., Coulshed, N. and Epstein, E. J.: Familial supravalvar aortic stenosis. Brit. Heart J. 27: 547-559, 1965.

McCue, C. M., Robertson, L. W., Lester, R. G. and Mauck, H. P., Jr.: Pulmonary artery coarctations. A report of 20 cases with review of 319 cases from the literature. J. Pediat. 67: 222-238, 1965.

McCue, C. M., Spicuzza, T. J., Robertson, L. W. and Mauck, H. P., Jr.: Familial supravalvular aortic stenosis. J. Pediat. 73: 889-895, 1968.

McDonald, A. H., Gerlis, L. M. and Somerville, J.: Familial arteriopathy with associated pulmonary and systemic arterial stenosis. Brit. Heart J. 31: 375-385, 1969.

Morrison, R. C. and McNalley, M. C.: The spectrum of abnormalities in supravalvular aortic stenosis. (Abstract) Am. J. Cardiol. 19: 143 only, 1967.

Page, H. L., Jr., Vogel, J. H. K., Pryor, R. and Blount, S. G., Jr.: Supravalvular aortic stenosis. Unusual observations in three patients. Am. J. Cardiol. 23: 270-277, 1969.

Rowe, R. D.: Maternal rubella and pulmonary artery stenoses. Report of eleven cases. Pediatrics 32: 180-185, 1963.

Strong, W. B., Perrin, E., Liebman, J. and Silbert, D. R.: Systemic and pulmonary artery dysplasia associated with unexpected death in infancy. J. Pediat. 77: 233-238, 1970.

Williams, J. C., Barratt-Boyes, B. G. and Lowe, J. B.: Supravalvular aortic stenosis. Circulation 24: 1311-1318, 1961.

Wooley, C. F., Hosier, D. M., Booth, R. W., Molnar, W., Sirak, H. D. and Ryan, J. M.: Supravalvular aortic stenosis. Clinical experiences with four patients including familial occurrence. Am. J. Med. 31: 717-725, 1961.

18560 SYMPHALANGISM OF TOES

Garn et al. (1965) described fusion across the interphalangeal joints of the toes as an isolated inherited anatomical variant, often secondary to absence of secondary ossification centers of the feet. The hands are not comparably involved. It is rare for all of the toes to be involved.

Garn, S. M., Rohmann, C. G. and Silverman, F. N.: Missing secondary ossification centers of the foot. Inheritance and developmental meaning. Ann. Radiol. 8: 629-644, 1965.

*18570 SYMPHALANGISM, DISTAL

A separate dominant mutation produces ankylosis of the distal interphalangeal joints. See recessive catalog for the SYMPHALANGISM-DWARFISM SYNDROME. Proximal symphalangism occurs with the recessive disorder diastrophic dwarfism (q.v.). Symphalangism also occurs among the multiple digital anomalies of brachydactyly, type C (q.v.).

Steinberg, A. G. and Reynolds, E. L.: Further data on symphalangism. J. Hered. 39: 23-27, 1948.

Wildervanck, L. S.: Erfelijkheid van stijve distale vinger en teengewrichten. Ned. Tijdschr. Geneesk. 96: 3115-3122, 1952.

*18580 SYMPHALANGISM, PROXIMAL (HEREDITARY ABSENCE OF THE PROXIMAL INTER-PHALANGEAL JOINTS)

Cushing (1916) described a large American family with many affected members and assigned the designation symphalangism. Fusion of carpal and tarsal bones is also a feature. (See CALCANEO-NAVICULAR COALATION.) This trait was thought to enjoy the distinction of being traced through more generations than almost any other, having been identified in the first Earl of Shrewsbury who lived in the 15th century (Drinkwater, 1917). After a re-examination of the evidence, however, Elkington and Huntsman (1967) concluded that the Earl probably did not have symphalangism and the mutation is of more recent origin in that kindred. In the family reported by Vesell (1960) mother and daughter had conductive deafness. The mother was apparently the new mutation. Strasburger and colleagues (1965) followed up on Cushing's family. Conductive deafness with early onset occurred sufficiently often in affected members of this large kindred to suggest that it is an effect of the same gene. Wildervanck et al. (1967) observed two accessory bones in the feet of multiple affected persons in one family.

Cushing, H.: Hereditary anchylosis of proximal phalangeal joints (symphalangism). Genetics 1: 90-106, 1916.

Drinkwater, H.: Phalangeal anarthrosis (synostosis, ankylosis) transmitted through 14 generations. Proc. Roy. Soc. Med. 10: 60-68, 1917.

Elkington, S. G. and Huntsman, R. G.: The Talbot fingers: a study in symphalangism. Brit. Med. J. 1: 407-411, 1967.

Gorlin, R. J., Kietzer, G. and Wolfson, J.: Stapes fixation and proximal symphalangism. Z. Kinderheilk. 108: 12-16, 1970.

Strasburger, A. K., Hawkins, M. R., Eldridge, R., Hargrave, R. L. and McKusick, V. A.: Symphalangism: genetic and clinical aspects. Bull. Hopkins Hosp. 117: 108-127, 1965.

Vesell, E. S.: Symphalangism, strabismus and hearing loss in mother and daughter. New Eng. J. Med. 263: 839-842, 1960.

Wildervanck, L. S., Goedhard, G. and Meijer, S.: Proximal symphalangism of fingers associated with fusion of os naviculare and talus and occurrence of two accessory bones in the feet (os paranaviculare and os tibiale externum) in a European-Indonesian-Chinese family. Acta Genet. Statist. Med. 17: 166-177, 1967.

*18590 SYNDACTYLY, TYPE I (ZYGODACTYLY)

From the medical literature and from our own experience we concluded that there are at least 5 phenotypically different types of syndactyly involving the hands with or without foot involvement. All are inherited as autosomal dominant traits and within any pedigree there is uniformity of type of syndactyly, allowing for the variation characteristic for dominant traits. These genetic types of syndactyly have to be differentiated from syndactyly associated with congenital bands for which there is no evidence of a genetic basis. In this common type of syndactyly, sometimes called zygodactyly, there is usually webbing between the 3rd and 4th fingers, either complete or partial and occasionally associated with fusion of the distal phalanges of these fingers. Other fingers are sometimes also involved but the 3rd and 4th fingers are the most commonly affected. In the feet there is usually webbing between the 2nd and 3rd toes, either complete or partial. Sometimes the hands are only affected and sometimes only the feet. Lueken (1938) reported this type of syndactyly in 18 males and 29 females of 5 generations illustrating the various degrees of expressivity of the same gene. Schofield (1921) presented a pedigree which suggested holandric inheritance to Castle (1922). Stern (1957) was unable, however, to obtain further evidence of same and suggested that inheritance is autosomal dominant. Straus (1926) supported this mode of inheritance. Hsu (1965) described bilateral syndactyly in 6 generations of a Chinese family. Of the 31 descendants of one syndactylous woman, 22 were affected. Skin and bony fusion of the distal phalanges of the third, fourth and fifth fingers were present. At least one person also showed union of the third, fourth and fifth toes.

Castle, W. E.: The Y-chromosome type of sex-linked inheritance in man. Science 55: 703-704, 1922.

Hsu, C.-K.: Hereditary syndactylia in a Chinese family. Chin. Med. J. 84: 482-485, 1965.

Lueken, K. G.: Ueber eine Familie mit Syndaktylie. Z. Menschl. Vererb. Konstitutionsl. 22: 152-159, 1938.

Schofield, R.: Inheritance of webbed toes. J. Hered. 12: 400-401, 1921.

Stern, C.: The problem of complete Y-linkage in man. Am. J. Hum. Genet. 9: 147-166, 1957.

Straus, W. L., Jr.: The nature and inheritance of webbed toes in man. J. Morph. 41: 427-439, 1926.

*18600 SYNDACTYLY, TYPE II (SYNPOLYDACTYLY)

In the hands there is usually syndactyly of the 3rd and 4th fingers associated with polydactyly of all components or of part of the 4th finger in the web. In the feet there is polydactyly of the 5th toe included in a web of syndactyly of the 4th and 5th toes. The most extensive pedigree is that described by Thomsen (1927) showing 31 affected males and 11 affected females in 7 generations. Other kindreds were reported by Alvord (1947), and Pipkin and Pipkin (1946) among others. Cross et al. (1968) observed a kindred with 27 affected persons. Two persons transmitted the gene without showing any effects themselves. All persons with clinically evident malformation in the hand showed anomalous palmar dermatoglyphics. No linkage with any of 12 loci was demonstrable. An excess of affected males has been a consistent feature. Cross et al. (1968) found, in the literature and in their kindred, 133 females and 174 males affected.

Alvord, R. M.: Zygodactyly and associated variations in a Utah family. J. Hered. 38: 49-53, 1947.

Cross, H. E., Lerberg, D. B. and McKusick, V. A.: Type II syndactyly. J. Med. Genet. 20: 368-380, 1968.

Pipkin, S. B. and Pipkin, A. C.: Two new pedigrees of zygodactyly. Variation of expression of polydactyly. J. Hered. 37: 93-96, 1946.

Thomsen, O.: Einige Eigentuemlichkeiten der erblichen Poly- und Syndaktylie bei Menschen. Acta Med. Scand. 65: 609-644, 1927.

Wood, V. E.: Treatment of central polydactyly. Clin. Orthop. 74: 196-205, 1971.

*18610 SYNDACTYLY, TYPE III (RING AND LITTLE FINGER SYNDACTYLY)

In this type there is syndactyly between the 4th and 5th fingers, usually complete and bilateral. Usually it is soft tissue syndactyly but occasionally the distal phalanges are fused. In this type the 5th finger is short with absent or rudimentary middle phalanx. The feet are not affected in this type. The largest pedigree is that described by Johnston and Kirby (1955) of seven affected males and seven affected females in five generations.

Johnston, O. and Kirby, V. V.: Syndactyly of the ring and little finger. Am. J. Hum. Genet. 7: 80-82, 1955.

18620 SYNDACTYLY, TYPE IV (HASS TYPE)

This type of syndactyly has been reported only by Haas, occurring in a mother and her two children. The syndactyly is complete, affecting the fingers of both hands with six metacarpals and six digits, and is associated with flexion of the fingers, giving the hands a cup-shaped form. In contradistinction to the type of syndactyly in Apert syndrome there was no bone fusion. There was no mention of the condition of the feet and there were no associated malformations.

Haas, S. L.: Bilateral complete syndactylism of all fingers. Am. J. Surg. 50: 363-366, 1940.

*18630 SYNDACTYLY, TYPE V (SYNDACTYLY WITH METACARPAL AND METATARSAL FUSION)

The characteristic finding in this rare type of syndactyly is the presence of an associated metacarpal and metatarsal fusion. The metacarpals and metatarsals most commonly fused are the 4th and 5th or the 3rd and 4th. Soft tissue syndactyly usually affects the 3rd and 4th fingers and the 2nd and 3rd toes. Syndactyly is usually more extensive and complete. Kemp and Ravn (1932) described this anomaly in five generations.

Kemp, T. and Ravn, J.: Ueber erbliche Hand- und Fussdeformitaeten in einem 140-koepfigen Geschlecht, nebst einigen Bemerkungen ueber Poly- und Syndaktylie beim Menschen. Acta Psychiat. Neurol. 7: 275-296, 1932.

*18640 SYNOSTOSES (TARSAL, CARPAL AND DIGITAL)

Pearlman, Edkin and Warren (1964) described mother and daughter with multiple carpal and tarsal synostoses (carpal and tarsal coalition) as well as radial-head subluxation, aplasia or hypoplasia of the middle phalanges and metacarpophalangeal synostoses. The latter synostoses seem comparable to those which occur in the two more distal joints in the two forms of symphalangism (q.v.). Although the authors felt this to be the disorder described by Nievergelt (see NIEVERGELT SYNDROME), this is almost certainly not the case but a distinct entity is involved. Bersani and Samilson (1957) described a mother and her daughter and son with massive synostosis of tarsal bones. No specific statement was made about the state of the carpal bones. Wray and Herndon (1963) observed calcaneonavicular coalition in three generations. Fusion of carpal and tarsal bones occurs in symphalangism (q.v.). Isolated fusion of carpal and tarsal bones was described by Kewesch (1934).

Bersani, F. A. and Samilson, R. L.: Massive familial tarsal synostosis. J. Bone Joint Surg. 39A: 1187-1190, 1957.

Kewesch, E. L.: Ueber hereditaere Verschmelzung der Hand-und Fusswurzelknochen. Fortschr. Roentgenstr. 50: 550- , 1934.

Pearlman, H. S., Edkin, R. E. and Warren, R. F.: Familial tarsal and carpal synostosis with radial-head subluxation (Nievergelt's syndrome). J. Bone Joint Surg. 46A: 585-592, 1964.

Wray, J. B. and Herndon, C. N.: Hereditary transmission of congenital coalition of the calcaneus to the navicular. J. Bone Joint Surg. 45A: 365-372, 1963.

Fuhrmann et al. (1966) described mother and son with bilateral dysplasia and synostosis of the elbow joint, synostoses in the fingers, wrist and foot, and short middle phalanges and metacarpals. The combination was described in father and daughter and father and son by earlier authors.

Fuhrmann, W. G., Steffens, C. and Rompe, U.: Dominant erbliche doppelseitige Dysplasie und Synostose des Ellenbogengelenks mit symmetrischer brachymesophalangie und Brachymetakarpie sowie Synostosen im Finger-, Hand- und Fusswurzelbereich. Humangenetik 3: 64-75, 1966.

*18655 SYNOSTOSIS, CARPAL, WITH DYSPLASTIC ELBOW JOINTS AND BRACHYDACTYLY

Liebenberg (1973) described four males and six females in five generations of a white family with upper limb deformities affecting the fingers, wrists and elbows. Male-to-male transmission suggested autosomal dominant inheritance. Affected members had dysplasia of all bony components of the elbow causing flexion deformity and an appearance resembling anterior dislocation. At the wrist, anomalies were triquetro-pisiform fusion, small capitate, trapezium and trapezoid, enlarged triquetrum and hamate, and slight flexion and radial deviation. The fingers had short club-shaped distal phalanges and small grooved nails. One affected member had bilateral fifth finger camptodactyly. There were no other bony fusions, tarsal coalition or clubfeet, thus differentiating this disorder from others characterized by carpal synostosis with more extensive bony fusions (see 18640 and 18650). The disorder is also distinct from Banki syndrome (10930) characterized by lunato-triquetral fusion, brachymetacarpy and leptometacarpy with normal elbows. In some ways it resembles synostoses, multiple, with brachydactyly (18650).

Liebenberg, F.: A pedigree with unusual anamolies of the elbows, wrists and hands in five generations. S. Afr. Med. J. 47: 745-747, 1973.

18660 SYRINGOMAS, MULTIPLE

Multiple syringomas or sweat gland tumors occur particularly on the face and around the eyes. They are not to be confused with milia, which are intraepithelial cysts. Familial occurrence is, it seems, a commonplace observation of dermatologists and autosomal dominant inheritance is likely (Reed, 1967). Reed (1970) described a family in which 7 females and 1 male in 4 generations were affected.

Reed, W. B.: Burbank, Calif.: personal communication, 1967.

Reed, W. B.: Genetische Aspekte in der Dermatologie. Hautarzt 21: 8-16, 1970.

18670 SYRINGOMYELIA, LUMBOSACRAL

Greenfield (1954) stated that some cases, in fact, probably have Denny Brown 'hereditary sensory radicular neuropathy' (q.v.). Ostertag (1930) found dominant inheritance of syringomyelia in rabbits. Curtius (1939) suggested that the same mode of inheritance occurs in man. Mulvey and Riely (1942) described a family with affected persons in 3 generations. They recognized that this was probably not true syringomyelia.

Barraquer, L. U. and De Gispert, I.: Die Syringomyelie, eine familiaere und hereditaere Krankheit (13 Falle in 2 Generationen derselben Familie). Deutsch. Z. Nervenheilk. 141: 146-157, 1936.

Curtius, F.: Status dysraphicus und Myelodysplasie. Fortschr. Erbpathol. 3: 199-258, 1939.

Goldbladt, A.: Syringomyelie bei Mutter und Tochter: zugleich ein Beitrag zur Pathologie des Sympathicus. Deutsch. Med. Wschr. 36: 1523-1526, 1910.

Greenfield, J. G.: The Spino-Cerebellar Degenerations. Oxford: Blackwell, 1954.

Karplus, J. P.: Syringomyelie bei Vater und Sohn. Med. Klin. 11: 1344-1347, 1915.

Kino, F.: Ueber heredo-familiaere Syringomyelie (zugleich ein Beitrag zur topischen Gliederung im Querschnitt des Vordenhorns). Z. Ges. Neurol. Psychiat. 107: 1-15, 1927.

Mulvey, B. E. and Riely, L. A.: Familial syringomyelia and status dysraphicus. Ann. Intern. Med. 16: 966-994, 1942.

Ostertag, B.: Die Syringomyelie als erbbiologisches Problem. Verh. Deutsch. Ges. Path. 25: 166-174, 1930.

Tenner, J.: Syringomyelie bei Vater und Tochter. Deutsch. Z. Nervenheilk. 106: 13-25, 1928.

Van Epps, C. and Kerr, H. D.: Familial lumbosacral syringomyelia. Radiology 35: 160-173, 1940.

*18680 T-ANTIGEN OF SV40

Croce et al. (1973) demonstrated that the gene(s) for the T-antigen of SV40 is located on chromosome no. 7. (Transformation of mammalian cells by Simian Virus 40 is associated with integration of the viral genome in the cellular DNA and by expression of several viral functions such as SV40 tumor (T) antigen. It is not known whether the SV40 T antigen(s) are virus-coded or coded by the cell genome and expressed as a result of viral DNA integration.)

Croce, C. M., Girardi, A. J. and Koprowski, H.: Assignment of the T-antigen gene of Simian virus 40 to human chromosome no. 7. Proc. Nat. Acad. Sci. 70: 3617-3620, 1973.

*18685 TARSAL FUSION

An autosomal dominant form of tarsal bone fusions (without carpal fusion), displaying high penetrance, was demonstrated by Wynne-Davies and her colleagues (1973). Croce (1974) found evidence that the entire SV-40 genome is integrated into one chromosome no. 7.

Wynne-Davies, R.: Edinburgh, personal communication, 1973.

18690 TEETH, GENETIC VARIATION AND DISORDER OF

The dominant or probably dominant mutations affecting the teeth include dentinogenesis imperfecta, osteogenesis imperfecta, enamel dysplasia, 'shovel-shaped' incisors, long incisors, absent lateral incisors, Carabelli tubercles, absence of upper permanent canines, anodontia, enamel hypoplasia, dentine hypoplasia, pigmented hypomaturation of teeth, hypoplasia of teeth, paramolar tubercle of Bolk, diastema, microdontia. A particularly good review is that of Witkop and Rao (1971).

Krogman, W. M.: Oral structures genetically and anthropologically considered. Ann. N.Y. Acad. Sci. 85: 17-41, 1960.

Lasker, G. W.: Genetic analysis of racial traits of the teeth. Cold Spring Harbor Symposia Quant. Biol. 15: 191-202, 1950.

Witkop, C. J. and Rao, S.: Inherited defects in tooth structure. The Clinical Delineation of Birth Defects. XI. Orofacial Structures. Baltimore: Williams and Wilkins, 1971. Pp. 153-184.

*18700 TEETH, ODD SHAPES OF

Robbins and Keene (1964) presented a 19-year-old boy whose teeth showed partial pegging, deep lingual pits, exaggeration of middle labial lobes of the canines, and reduced premolar size. One sib was normal. In 5 generations, 10 persons showed odd shaped teeth, 16 were normal and 8 were unknown.

Robbins, I. M. and Keene, H. J.: Multiple morphologic dental anomalies. Report of a case. Oral Surg. 17: 683-690, 1964.

18705 TEETH, PRESENT AT BIRTH (NATAL TEETH)

Sibert and Porteous (1974) observed natal teeth in 6 members of a kindred. Limrick (1893) first observed this in a mother, her son and her sister's daughter. Natal teeth occur with Ellis-van Creveld syndrome (22550), pachyonychia congenita (16720), and Hallermann-Streiff syndrome (23410).

Limrick, O. E. B.: Born with teeth. (Letter) Lancet II: 965 only, 1893.

Sibert, J. R. and Porteous, J. R.: Erupted teeth in the newborn. 6 members of a family. Arch. Dis. Child. 39: 492-493, 1974.

18710 TEETH, SUPERNUMERARY

Finn (1967) presented a pedigree in which all females (numbering 14) were affected and all males (numbering 3) were unaffected, in five sibships in three generations. The author suggested X-linked dominant inheritance with female limitation, or female-limited autosomal dominant inheritance. In some of the affected females the supernumerary teeth occurred in the midline of the maxilla, so-called mesiodens.

Finn, S. B.: Clinical Pedodontics. Philadelphia: W. B. Saunders Co., 1967.

18720 TELANGIECTASES OF BRAIN

Michael and Levin (1936) described a Swedish family in which a mother, her two brothers and three daughters had multiple telangiectases of the brain. Convulsions and migraine attacks were observed. Autopsy in one case demonstrated calcification in the vascular lesions of the brain.

Michael, J. C. and Levin, P. M.: Multiple telangiectases of brain: discussion of hereditary factors in their development. Arch. Neurol. Psychiat. 36: 514-529, 1936.

*18726 TELANGIECTASIA, HEREDITARY BENIGN

Ryan and Wells (1971) described 7 kindreds in each of which several persons had widespread telangiectases. The areas affected were predominantly the face, upper limbs and upper trunk. The telangiectases were venular and associated with upper dermal atrophy.

Ryan, T. J. and Wells, R. S.: Hereditary benign telangiectasia. Trans. St. John'S Derm. Soc. 57: 148-156, 1971

*18730 TELANGIECTASIA, HEREDITARY HEMORRHAGIC, OF RENDU, OSLER AND WEBER

The tip of the tongue and mucosal surface of the lips are frequent sites of telangiectases which also occur on the face, conjunctiva, ears, fingers, and mucosa of the nasopharynx, gastrointestinal tract and bladder. Bleeding from all these sites is a major problem. Cirrhosis of the liver occurs in some cases. Pulmonary arteriovenous fistula with polycythemia and clubbing occur in some cases. Over half the cases of pulmonary arteriovenous fistula are on the basis of this disorder. Snyder and Doan (1944) reported a possible instance of homozygosity, a stillborn offspring of two affected parents had extensive angiomatous malformation of the viscera. An important phenocopy is the CRST syndrome (calcinosis, Raynaud syndrome, sclerodactyly, telangiectasia), a probable 'collagen vascular disease.' The mucosal and cutaneous telangiectases are indistinguishable from those of the hereditary disorder (Winterbauer, 1964). Tunte (1964) studied 18 families. Liver disease was twice as frequent in affected members as in unaffected ones. The frequency of the condition was estimated to be 1 or 2 in 100,000. The mutation rate was estimated to be 2×10^{-6} to 3×10^{-6}. Reported instances of familial epistaxis (e.g., Lane, 1916) probably represent this disorder. By angiographic methods various types of visceral angiodysplasias have been demonstrated (Halpern et al., 1968). These include arterial aneurysm, arteriovenous communication including discrete A-V fistula, conglomerate masses of angiectasia, phlebectasia and angioma. Michaeli et al. (1968) described a 47-year-old woman with O-R-W disease and hepatic portocaval shunts of sufficient magnitude to cause repeated episodes of encephalopathy. The liver was not scarred.

Bacardi, R., Guardia, J., Rius, J. M., Angel, J. and Martinez, J. M.: Maladie de Rendu-Osler-Weber avec atteinte hepatique (telangiectasie hepatique). Presse Med. 79: 1023-1024, 1971.

Bergqvist, N., Hessen, I. and Hey, M.: Arteriovenous pulmonary aneurysms in Osler's disease. Acta Med. Scand. 171: 301-309, 1962.

Burckhardt, D., Stalder, G. A., Ludin, H. and Bianchi, L.: Hyperdynamic circulatory state due to Osler-Weber-Rendu disease with intrahepatic arterio-venous fistulas. Am. Heart J. 85: 797-800, 1973.

Davis, D. G. and Smith, J. L.: Retinal involvement in hereditary hemorrhagic telangiectasia. Arch. Ophthal. 85: 618-623, 1971.

Feizi, O.: Hereditary hemorrhagic telangiectasia presenting with portal hypertension and cirrhosis of the liver. A case report. Gastroenterology 63: 660-664, 1972.

Halpern, M., Turner, A. F. and Citron, B. P.: Hereditary hemorrhagic telangiectasia. A visceral angiodysplasia associated with gastrointestinal hemorrhage. Radiology 90: 1143-1149, 1968.

Harrison, D. F. N.: Hereditary haemorrhagic telangiectasia and oral contraceptives. (Letter) Lancet I: 721 only, 1970.

Hodgson, C. H., Burchell, H. B., Good, C. A. and Clagett, O. T.: Hereditary hemorrhagic telangiectasia and pulmonary arteriovenous fistula: survey of a large family. New Eng. J. Med. 261: 625-636, 1959.

Lane, W. C.: Hereditary nose-bleed. J. Hered. 7: 132-134, 1916.

Michaeli, D., Ben-Bassat, I., Miller, H. I. and Deutsch, V.: Hepatic telangiectases and portosystemic encephalopathy in Osler-Weber-Rendu disease. Gastroenterology 54: 929-932, 1968.

Mirra, J. M. and Arnold, W. D.: Skeletal hemagiomatosis in association with hereditary hemorrhagic telangiectasia. A case report. J. Bone Joint Surg. 55: 850-854, 1973.

Rowley, P. T., Kurnick, J. and Cheville, R.: Hereditary haemorrhagic telangiectasia: aggravation by oral contraceptive? (Letter) Lancet I: 474-475, 1970.

Snyder, L. H. and Doan, C. A.: Clinical and experimental studies in human inheritance: is the homozygous form of multiple telangiectasia lethal? J. Lab. Clin. Med. 29: 1211-1216, 1944.

Trell, E., Johansson, B. W., Linell, F. and Ripa, J.: Familial pulmonary hypertension and multiple abnormalities of large systemic arteries in Osler's disease. Am. J. Med. 53: 50-63, 1972.

Tuente, W.: Klinik und Genetik der Oslerschen Krankheit. Z. Menschl. Vererb. Konstitutionsl. 37: 221-250, 1964.

Whicker, J. H. and Lake, C. F.: Hemilateral rhinotomy in the treatment of hereditary hemorrhagic telangiectasia. Arch. Otolaryng. 96: 319-321, 1972.

Winterbauer, R. H.: Multiple telangiectasia, Raynaud's phenomenon, sclerodactyly and subcutaneous calcinosis. A syndrome mimicking hereditary hemorrhagic telangiectasia. Bull. Hopkins Hosp. 114: 361-383, 1964.

18735 TELECANTHUS

Pryor (1969) gave normal values for various interpupillary measurements. Juberg and Hirsch (1971) described primary telecanthus, increased separation of the medial canthi without abnormal separation of the orbits, in 5 females and 3 males of five generations. There was no instance of male-to-male transmission. The phenotype is that displayed by Jacqueline Kennedy Onassis. One instance of non-penetrance was observed. Bilateral cleft lip and cleft palate occurred in some. Mental retardation and dental agenesis may be occasional manifestations of the gene.

Juberg, R. C. and Hirsch, R.: Expressivity of heritable telecanthus in five generations of a kindred. Am. J. Hum. Genet. 23: 547-554, 1971.

Pryor, H. B.: Objective measurement of interpupillary distance. Pediatrics 44: 973-977, 1969.

*18737 TENDO CALCANEUS, SHORT

Hall et al. (1967) reported 33 cases of congenital short tendo calcaneus causing those affected to walk on their toes. There was no evidence in these cases for any underlying neuromuscular disease. Familial occurrence was noted in several cases, including an affected father and son, two affected brothers and an affected brother and sister. Levine (1973) reported 5 cases in 2 generations of a kindred. A mildly affected father, who had had a mildly affected sister, produced 2 severely affected sons and one mildly affected daughter. The inheritance may be autosomal dominant with variable expressivity.

Hall, J. E., Slater, R. B. and Bhalla, S. K.: Congenital short tendo calcaneus. J. Bone Joint Surg. 49B: 695-697, 1967.

Levine, M. S.: Congenital short tendo calcaneus. Am. J. Dis. Child. 125: 858-859. 1973.

18740 TESTICULAR TORSION

Cunningham (1960) observed testicular torsion in three brothers, ages 14, 15 and 21. The father and two other brothers had hypermobility of the testicle but had not suffered acute torsion. The anatomic peculiarity is presumably inherited and is either autosomal dominant (obviously male-limited), or Y-linked.

18750 TETRALOGY OF FALLOT

Pitt (1962) described a family in which 11 persons had either tetralogy of Fallot or one of its components. The diagnosis was confirmed at operation or autopsy in five of the 11. The large study of Boon et al. (1972) lead to the conclusion that heritability is about 54 percent and that in sibs the recurrence risk is about 1 percent for Fallot tetralogy and about 2 percent for any cardiac defect.

Boon, A. R., Farmer, M. B. and Roberts, D. F.: A family study of Fallot's tetralogy. J. Med. Genet. 9: 179-192, 1972.

Pitt, D. B.: A family study of Fallot's tetrad. Aust. Ann. Med. 11: 179-183, 1962.

18775 THORACIC DYSOSTOSIS, ISOLATED

Rabushka et al. (1973) described a family in which the father and all five children had a constricted, bell-shaped throrax with foreshortened and deformed ribs and pectus excavatum. Clinically, there were repeated respiratory illnesses but no fatalities. No changes elsewhere in the skeleton were described. The changes in the ribs were identical to those in osteodysplasty of Melnick and Needles (16610). Because of the possibility that the new disorder is an allelic variant of osteodysplasia, no asterisk is used here.

Rabushka, S. E., Love, L. and Kadison, H. I.: Isolated thoracic dysostosis. Radiology 106: 161-165, 1973.

*18780 THROMBASTHENIA OF GLANZMANN AND NAEGELI

In one family studied by Gross and colleagues (1960) three generations had affected members. Clinically petechiae, bleeding from mucous membrane, prolonged bleeding after injury, and severe anemia were features. Studies revealed prolonged bleeding time, abnormal capillary fragility, normal or increased number of platelets, with giant platelets. Alteration in the concentration of several platelet enzymes were found. Of 13 families studied by Caen et al. (1966), only one seemed to have dominant inheritance with probable transmission through four generations with male-to-male transmission. In the hands of Booyse et al. (1972) microquantitation of thrombosthenin by radial immunodiffusion and specific immunohistochemical antibody staining technique indicated absence of the surface-localized thrombosthenin in platelets from Glanzmann's thrombasthenic patients. In addition ADP and ATP induced changes of the surface of normal platelets could not be demonstrated. In von Willebrand disease (19340), factor VIII is low and the platelets show faulty adhesion to glass. In hereditary thrombopathy, availability of platelet factor 3 is reduced and platelets do not aggregate on exposure to collagen. Crowell and Eisner (1972) described a family with a combination of these abnormalities in affected persons in several successive generations (without male-to-male transmission).

Booyse, F., Kisieleski, D., Seeler, R. and Rafelson, M., Jr.: Possible thrombosthenin defect in Glanzmann's thrombasthenia. Blood 39: 377-381, 1972.

Caen, J. P., Castaldi, P. A., Leclerc, J. C., Inceman, S., Larriere, M. J., Probst, M. and Bernard, J.: Congenital bleeding disorders with long bleeding time and normal platelet count. I. Glanzmann's thrombasthenia (report of fifteen patients). Am. J. Med. 41: 11-26, 1966.

Crowell, E. B., Jr. and Eisner, E. V.: Familial association of thrombopathia and antihemophilic factor (AHF, factor VIII) deficiency. Blood 40, 227-233, 1972.

Gross, R., Gerok, W., Lohr, G. W., Vogell, W., Walker, H. D. and Theopold, W.: Ueber die Natur der Thrombasthenie: Thrombopathie Glanzmann Naegeli. Klin. Wschr. 38: 193-206, 1960.

*18790 THROMBASTHENIA-THROMBOCYTOPENIA, HEREDITARY

Quick and Hussey (1962) differentiated this disorder from von Willebrand disease by a negative tourniquet test and poor prothrombin consumption. Bleeding time is prolonged. Onset is in infancy with a hemophilia-like picture. Platelets are normal in numbers. The disorder is not influenced by splenectomy. Seip (1964) observed autosomal dominant transmission in two families. Marrow preparations showed normal or increased megakaryocytes with little or no signs of active thrombopoiesis. No response to adrenal steroids or splenectomy was noted. Most instances seem to be recessive (q.v.) making it unclear what condition was present in the family described above. Seip and Kjaerheim (1965) studied a mother and her only son. Symptoms and signs were present from birth. Bleeding time exceeded 30 minutes. Platelet counts varied from 60,000 to 120,000. Electron microscopy showed liked vacuoles in the platelets and some had abnormal granules.

Kurstjens, R., Bolt, C., Vossen, M. and Haanen, C.: Familial thrombopathic thrombocytopenia. Brit. J. Haemat. 15: 305-317, 1968.

Quick, A. J. and Hussey, C. V.: Hereditary thrombasthenia-thrombocytopenia. J. Lab. Clin. Med. 60: 1006 only, 1962.

Seip, M. and Kjaerheim, A.: A familial platelet disease — hereditary thrombasthenic-thrombopathic thrombocytopenia. Scand. J. Clin. Lab. Invest. 17 (suppl. 84): 159-169, 1965.

Seip, M.: Hereditary hypoplastic thrombocytopenia. Sangre 9: 382-384, 1964.

*18800 THROMBOCYTOPENIA

Seip (1963) described a mother and her two sons with thrombocytopenia. Platelet antibodies were not demonstrated. One son had bilateral aplasia of the 12th rib and mild right hydronephrosis. The other son had frequent episodes of hematuria and recurrent hydronephrosis. Ata, Fisher and Holman (1965) found undue bleeding in 10 members of 6 sibships in 5 generations of a family. Inheritance was thought to be autosomal dominant with incomplete penetrance in females. Splenectomy performed in 3 affected persons

310

D
O
M
I
N
A
N
T

corrected thrombocytopenia. The only affected woman recovered spontaneously. Harms and Sachs (1965) described 3 sisters, their mother and their maternal grandmother with chronic idiopathic thrombocytopenia and platelet auto-antibodies associated with a diminution of clotting factor IX. A particularly convincing pedigree studied by Bithell et al. (1965) had 8 proven cases of thrombocytopenia in three generations. In addition, a history of hemorrhagic diathesis was given by 7 other persons so that the involved spanned at least 4 generations, involving at least 11 sibships. Murphy et al. (1969) described a family with five cases of thrombocytopenia in three generations, with no example of male-to-male transmission. Shortened platelet lifespan was demonstrated and was shown to be an intrinsic property of the platelet. Morphologic and biochemical studies failed to elucidate the nature of the defect. Other apparently dominant pedigrees were reported by Bethard and Boyer (1964) and Wooley (1956). The disorder reported by Grottum and Solum (1969) may be distinctive. Giant platelets were associated with abnormal composition of the platelet membrane, namely decreased content of sialic acid.

Ata, M., Fisher, O. D. and Holman, C. A.: Inherited thrombocytopenia. Lancet I: 119-123, 1965.

Bethard, W. F. and Boyer, J. L.: Familial thrombocytopenia. (Abstract) J. Lab. Clin. Med. 64: 842 only, 1964.

Bithell, T. C., Didisheim, P., Cartwright, G. E. and Wintrobe, M. M.: Thrombocytopenia inherited as an autosomal dominant trait. Blood 25: 231-240, 1965.

Grottum, K. A. and Solum, N. O.: Congenital thrombocytopenia with giant platelets: a defect in the platelet membrane. Brit. J. Haemat. 16: 277-290, 1969.

Harms, D. and Sachs, V.: Familial chronic thrombocytopenia with platelet autoantibodies. Acta Haemat. 34: 30-35, 1965.

Kurstjens, R., Bolt, C. and Haanen, C. A.: Familiale thrombocytopenia. Nederl. T. Geneesk. 111: 1897-1898, 1967.

Murphy, S., Oski, F. A. and Gardner, F. H.: Hereditary thrombocytopenia with an intrinsic platelet defect. New Eng. J. Med. 281: 857-862, 1969.

Myllyla, G., Pelkonen, R., Ikkala, E. and Apajalahti, J.: Hereditary thrombocytopenia: report of three families. Scand. J. Haemat. 4: 441-452, 1967.

Quick, A. J. and Hussey, C. V.: Hereditary thrombopathic thrombocytopenia. Am. J. Med. Sci. 245: 643-653, 1963.

Seip, M.: Hereditary hypoplastic thrombocytopenia. Acta Paediat. 52: 370-376, 1963.

Wooley, E. J. S.: Familial idiopathic thrombocytopenic purpura. Brit. Med. J. 1: 440 only, 1956.

18805 THROMBOPHILIA

Margolis and Corrigan (1972) described a family in which a mother and son, who had a history of repeated thrombotic episodes, showed abnormal platelet aggregation in response to various agents.

Margolis, H. S. and Corrigan, J. J., Jr.: Abnormal platelet aggregation and thrombosis — a familial disorder. (Abstract) Pediat. Res. 6: 367 only, 1972.

18810 THUMB DEFORMITY

Bilbrey (1966) described thumb deformity of the type seen with the heart-hand syndrome. The thumb was either absent or hypoplastic. The published X-rays do not demonstrate whether the metacarpal of the thumb when present had an epiphyseal ossification center at each end. No cardiac anomaly was detected in any of the 13 affected persons in 3 generations. The pedigree contained no instance of male-to-male transmission.

Bilbrey, G. L.: Isolated congenital familial thumb deformities. Report of a family. New Eng. J. Med. 274: 1057-1060, 1966.

18820 THUMBNAILS, ABSENT

Strandskov (1939) observed absent thumbnails in a woman, two of her three daughters and in a son of one of the daughters. Thus the findings were equally consistent with autosomal and X-linked dominance. He was of the opinion that the mutation is separate and distinct from the nail-patella mutation. No skeletal abnormalities were detected in his family, but no X-ray information was available, it seems. Absent thumbnails in female members of three generations of a family (V. D., 845898) proved on further study to be the nail-patella syndrome (Schleutermann, 1968).

Schleutermann, D. A.: Baltimore, Md.: personal communication, 1968.

Strandskov, H. H.: Inheritance of absence of thumb nails. J. Hered. 30: 53-54, 1939.

*18830 THYMIDINE KINASE

Genetic variation in this enzyme has not been identified in man. However, localization of the gene has been achieved by hybridization experiments. Weiss and Green (1967) found that fusion of mouse cells lacking this enzyme with normal human cells could be achieved, that progressive loss of human chromosomes from the hybrid occurred with passage of time and that at a stage when only one human chromosome remained the cell still had the capacity to synthesize thymidine kinase. The assumption was that the remaining chromosome, now identified as chromosome 17, Migeon, Miller, (1968; Miller et al., 1971), carries the thymidine kinase locus. Ruddle's group has evidence that TK is on the long arm of chromosome 17 (Boone et al. 1972). McDougall et al. (1971) showed that adeno 12 virus causes a gap in the long arm of chromosome 17. Since the adeno 12 virus causes a 2 or 3 fold increase in TK the gap may represent the TK locus and may be comparable to a puff. By study of a 11-17 translocation in mouse-man hybrid cells, Franche and Busby (1974) located the TK locus to the region distal to q21. Presumably this is the location of the thymidine kinase locus. By cell hybridization studies Croce (1974) found that the structural genes for both galactokinase and thymidine kinase are on the same chromosome (one resembling the human E-17) in the African green monkey. This is another striking example of chromosomal homology.

Croce, C. M.: Philadelphia, personal communication, 1974.

Franche, U. and Busby, N.: Intrachromosomal mapping of human thymidine kinase locus. (Abstract) Clin. Res. 22: 217A only, 1974.

McDougall, J. K., Kucherlapati, R. and Ruddle, F. H.: Localization and induction of the human thymidine kinase gene by adenovirus 12. Nature N.B. 245: 172-175, 1973.

McDougall, J. K.: Adenovirus induced chromosome aberrations in human cells. J. Gen. Virol. 12: 43-51, 1971.

McDougall, J. K.: Effects of adenoviruses on the chromosomes of normal human cells and cells trisomic for an E chromosome. Nature 225: 456-458, 1970.

Migeon, B. R. and Miller, C. S.: Human-mouse somatic cell hybrids with single human chromosome (group E): link with thymidine kinase activity. Science 162: 1005-1006, 1968.

Miller, O. J., Allderdice, P. W. and Miller, D. A.: Human thymidine kinase gene locus: assignment to chromosome 17 in a hybrid of man and mouse cells. Science 173: 244-245, 1974.

Vause, K. E. and McDougall, J. K.: Identification of group 'E' chromosome abnormalities in human cells. J. Med. Genet. 10: 70-73, 1973.

Weiss, M. and Green, H.: Human-mouse hybrid cell lines containing partial complements of human chromosomes and functioning human genes. Proc. Nat. Acad. Sci. 58: 1104-1111, 1967.

18840 THYMUS AND PARATHYROIDS, ABSENCE OF (DIGEORGE SYNDROME)

This is a congenital anomaly in development of derivatives of the 3rd and 4th pharyngeal pouches. Deformities of the ear, nose, mouth and aortic arch are often associated. Transplantation of fetal thymus has been successfully accomplished, with dramatic reconstruction of the immune mechanism. The possibility of new autosomal dominant mutation should be investigated by determination of mean paternal age. The only familial cases seem to be those of Steele et al. (1972). A white girl and her maternal half-brother were affected, and their mother was shown to have hypoparathyroidism and diminished cell-mediated immunity. The girl and a boy had different fathers and died at about 11 weeks and 4 months, respectively. At age 2 the mother had secondary vaccinia following routine immunization. At age 7 she was hospitalized for 6 months for 'severe chicken pox.' At age 24 tetany and hypocalcemia responsive to parathyroid hormone were documented and treated with oral calcium supplement. Absolute lymphocyte counts were low and in vitro lymphocyte stimulation by phytohemagglutinin and pokeweed was defective. Goldman and Goldblum (1973) suggested that the familial occurrence reported by Steele et al. (1972) may be due to transplacental transmission of antibodies from the mother. Patients with DiGeorge syndrome have a characteristic appearance, including low-set ears.

Cleveland, W. W., Fogel, B. J., Brown, W. T. and Kay, H. E. M.: Foetal thymic transplant in a case of DiGeorge's syndrome. Lancet II: 1211-1214, 1968.

DiGeorge, A. M.: Congenital absence of the thymus and its immunologic consequences: concurrence with congenital hypoparathyroidism. In Good, R. A. (ed.).: Immunologic Deficiency Diseases. New York: National Foundation, 1968. Pp. 116-123.

Goldman, A. S. and Goldblum, R. M.: Familial thymic aplasia-genetic defect or maternal effect. (Letter) New Eng. J. Med. 288: 108 only, 1973.

Steele, R. W., Limas, C., Thurman, G. B., Bauer, H. and Bellanti, J. A.: Familial thymic aplasia: attempted reconstruction with fetal thymus in a millipore diffusion chamber. (Abstract) Pediat. Res. 6: 380 only, 1972.

Steele, R. W., Limas, C., Thruman, G. B., Schuelein, M., Baur, H. and Bellanti, J. A.: Familial thymic aplasia. Attempted reconstitution with fetal thymus in a millipore diffusion chamber. New Eng. J. Med. 287: 787-791, 1972.

18850 THYROID AUTOANTIBODIES

Hall, Owen and Smart (1964) studied six families in which the father had thyroid autoantibody and the mother did not. In each case female children had thyroid autoantibodies. Transplacental transmission was thus ruled out and genetic transmission was suggested.

Hall, R., Owen, S. G. and Smart, G. A.: Paternal transmission of thyroid autoimmunity. Lancet II: 115 only, 1964.

*18860 THYROXINE-BINDING GLOBULIN (TBG) OF SERUM, VARIANTS OF

In addition to the usual X-linked form of decreased or increased TBG, an autosomal dominant form appears to exist. Persons with the autosomal form show an increase in TBG level with administration of estrogen, suggesting that the mutation may concern a regulator gene rather than a structural gene. For review, see Rivas et al. (1971). Electrophoretic variants of TBG were described by Thorson et al. (1966) and there may be both autosomal and X-linked varieties. Evidence for autosomal dominant transmission of TBG deficiency was presented by Nicoloff et al. (1964) and by Kraemer and Wiswell (1968). In the last report three brothers had absent TBG, and their father, paternal uncle and paternal grandmother had low values whereas the mother and several other relatives on her side had normal values.

Kraemer, E. and Wiswell, J. G.: Familial thyroxine-binding globulin deficiency. Metabolism 17: 260-262, 1968.

Nicoloff, J. T., Dowling, J. T. and Patton, D. D.: Inheritance of decreased thyroxine-binding by the thyroxine-binding globulin. J. Clin. Endocr. 24: 294-298, 1964.

Rivas, M.: Indianapolis, Ind.: personal communication, 1968.

Rivas, M., Merritt, A. D. and Oliner, L.: Genetic variants of thyroxine binding globulin (TBG). The Clinical Delineation of Birth Defects. X. The Endocrine System. Baltimore: Williams and Wilkins, 1971. Pp. 34-41.

Thorson, S. C., Tauxe, W. N. and Taswell, H. F.: Evidence for the existence of two thyroxine-binding globulin moieties: correlation between paper and starch-gel electrophoretic patterns utilizing thyroxine-binding globulin-deficient sera. J. Clin. Endocr. 26: 181-188, 1966.

Torkington, P., Harrison, R. J., MacLagan, N. F. and Burston, D.: Familial thyroxine-binding globulin deficiency. Brit. Med. J. 3: 27-29, 1970.

18870 TIBIA VARA (BLOUNT DISEASE, OR OSTEOCHONDROSIS DEFORMANS TIBIAE)

Little is known about this condition which bears some similarity to osteochondritis of various sites (q.v.) and which may be heterogeneous. Blount (1937) suggested the existence of an infantile type with onset in the first year or two of life and an adolescent type developing just before puberty. Tobin's description (1957) of tibia vara beginning at puberty with osteochondritis dissecans of the knees in father and two sons strengthens the view that the two disorders are fundamentally identical.

Blount, W. P.: Tibia vara: osteochondrosis deformans tibiae. J. Bone Joint Surg. 19A: 1-29, 1937.

Tobin, W. J.: Familial osteochondritis dissecans with associated tibia vara. J. Bone Joint Surg. 39A: 1091-1105, 1957.

18874 TIBIA, ABSENCE OF, WITH POLYDACTYLY

Dankmeyer (1935) reported familial occurrence and predominant involvement of the right lower limb. Ollerenshaw (1925) reported identical twin sisters with unilateral (left) absent tibia and polydactyly. 10 older sibs were healthy. Pratt (1971) described congenital cardiac malformations in association with absent tibia and polydactyly. Pfeiffer et al. (1971) described a boy with tibial agenesis, fibula duplication, mirror foot and normal upper limbs whose mother had the same anomalies on the left but only prehallucal polydactyly on the right. (See 13575). They offered a classification. See TIBIA, HYPOPLASIA OF, WITH POLYDACTYLY.

Dankmeyer, J.: Congenital absence of the tibia. Anat. Rec. 62: 179-194, 1935.

Ollerenshaw, R.: Congenital defects of the long bones of the lower limbs. A contribution to the study of their causes, effects and treatment. J. Bone Joint Surg. 7: 528-552, 1925.

Pfeiffer, R. A. and Roeskau, M.: Agenesie der Tibia, Fibulaverdopplung und spiegelbildliche Polydaktylie (Diplopodie) bei Mutter und Kind. Z. Kinderheilk. 111: 38-50, 1971.

Pratt, A. D., Jr.: Apparent congenital absence of the tibia with lethal congenital cardiac disease. Am. J. Dis. Child. 122: 452-454, 1971.

18877 TIBIA, HYPOPLASIA OF, WITH POLYDACTYLY

Eaton and McKusick (1969) reported a family in which four persons in three successive generations had bilateral hypoplasia of the tibia with polydactyly in the feet and hands. Since the tibia may be late in ossifying it is not certain that this trait is different from that separately listed as 'tibia, absence of, with polydactyly.'

Eaton, G. O. and McKusick, V. A.: A seemingly unique polydactyly-syndactyly syndrome in four persons in three generations. The Clinical Delineation of Birth Defects. III. Limb Malformations. New York: National Foundation, 1969. Pp. 221-225.

Reber, M.: Un syndrome osseux peu commun associant une heptadactylie et une aplasie des tibias. J. Genet. Hum. 16: 15-39, 1967-8.

*18880 TIBIAL TORSION, BILATERAL MEDIAL

Blumel et al. (1957) reported a family with 8 affected persons in four generations. No male-to-male transmission was observed. Bowlegs are the main clinical feature. Matsoukas et al. (1972) described autosomal dominant inheritance of congenital lateral bowing in the proximal diaphyso-metaphyseal area of the tibia. They termed it tibial scoliosis. The deformity was present from birth, was bilateral and did not correct itself during growth. Male-to-male transmission was observed. It seems, from the photographs and X-rays, possible that this was the same condition as that reported by Blumel et al. (1957). Fitch (1974) observed 6 affected persons in three generations, with one instance of father-to-son transmission.

Blumel, J., Eggers, G. W. and Evans, E. B.: Eight cases of hereditary bilateral tibial torsion in four generations. J. Bone Joint Surg. 39A: 1198-1202, 1957.

Fitch, N.: Male-to-male transmission of tibial torsion. Am. J. Hum. Genet..26: 662 only, 1974.

Matsoukas, J., Pantazopoulos, T., Mitsou, A. and Hartofilakidis-Garofalidis, G.: Hereditary scoliosis of tibiae (a new entity?). Am. J. Hum. Genet., in press, 1972.

18890 TOE, FIFTH ROTATED

I have observed two kindreds in which rotation of the fifth toes on their long axis, with laterally facing nail, was transmitted as an autosomal dominant.

18900 TOE, FIFTH, NUMBER OF PHALANGES IN

The fifth toe may show either two or three phalanges (Venning, 1954). Sib pairs showed a correlation coefficient of 0.28.

Venning, P.: Sib correlations with respect to the number of phalanges on the fifth toe. Ann. Eugen. 18: 232-254, 1953-1954.

18910 TOE, MISSHAPEN

Garber (1950) reported five persons in three generations with toes peculiarly positioned in relation to each other. There was male-to-male transmission.

Garber, M. J.: Misshapen toes in three generations of the G family. J. Hered. 41: 215-216, 1950.

Larson, C. A.: Garber's toe deformity. Report of a kindred. Acta Genet. Statist. Med. 4: 414-416, 1953.

18920 TOES, RELATIVE LENGTH OF 1ST AND 2ND

Kaplan (1964) claims the relative length of the hallux and second toe is simply inherited, long hallux being recessive. In Cleveland Caucasoids the frequency of the dominant and recessive phenotypes was 24 percent and 76 percent respectively. Usually the first toe is longest, although in the Ainu the second toe is said to be longest in 90 percent of persons. In Sweden Romanus (1949) found the second toe longest in 2.95 percent of 8,141 men. Romanus thought that long second toe is dominant with reduced penetrance. Beers and Clark (1942) described a family in which long second toe occurred in 10 persons in 3 generations.

Beers, C. V. and Clark, L. A.: Tumors and short-toe — a dihybrid pedigree: a family history showing the inheritance of hemangioma and metatarsus activitus. J. Hered. 33: 366-368, 1942.

Kaplan, A. R.: Genetics of relative toe lengths. Acta Genet. Med. Gemellol. 13: 295-304, 1964.

Romanus, T.: Heredity of a long second toe. Hereditas 35: 651-652, 1949.

18930 TONGUE CURLING, FOLDING, OR ROLLING

Sturtevant (1940) described two classes, 'roller' and 'non-roller,' the roller phenotype being dominant. However, Sturtevant (1965) cited Matlock as finding a high frequency of discordance in monozygotic twins, suggesting little genetic basis for the trait. Hsu (1948) described the ability to fold up the tip of the tongue as a recessive. Liu and Hsu (1949) and Lee (1955) demonstrated independence of the two traits. The clover-leaf tongue (ability to fold the tongue in a particular configuration) may be yet another distinct trait (Whitney, 1950), inherited probably as a dominant. Hirschhorn (1970) emphasized that ample time for learning must be allowed in doing family studies of tongue gymnastic ability.

Gahres, E. E.: Tongue rolling and tongue folding and other hereditary movements of the tongue. J. Hered. 43: 221-225, 1952.

Hirschhorn, H. H.: Transmission and learning of tongue gymnastic ability. Am. J. Phys. Anthrop. 32: 451-454, 1970.

Hsu, T. C.: Tongue upfolding: a newly reported heritable character in man. J. Hered. 39: 187-188, 1948.

Komai, T.: Notes on lingual gymnastics. Frequency of tongue rollers and pedigrees of tied tongues in Japan. J. Hered. 42: 293-297, 1951.

Lee, J. W.: Tongue-folding and tongue-rolling in an American Negro population sample. J. Hered. 46: 289-291, 1955.

Liu, T. T. and Hsu, T. C.: Tongue-folding and tongue-rolling in a sample of the Chinese population. J. Hered. 40: 19-21, 1949.

Matlock, P.: Identical twins discordant in tongue-rolling. J. Hered. 43: 24 Only, 1952.

Sturtevant, A. H.: A History of Genetics. New York: Harper, Row, 1965. P. 127.

Sturtevant, A. H.: A new inherited character in man. Proc. Nat. Acad. Sci. 26: 100-102, 1940.

Urbanowski, A. and Wilson, J.: Tongue curling. J. Hered. 38: 365-366, 1947.

Vogel, F.: Ueber die Faehigkeit, die Zunge um die Laengsachse zu rollen. Acta Genet. Med. Gemellol. 6: 225-230, 1957.

Whitney, D. D.: Clover-leaf tongues. J. Hered. 41: 176 only, 1950.

18950 TOOTH-AND-NAIL SYNDROME (DYSPLASIA OF NAILS WITH HYPODONTIA)

Changes are limited largely to teeth (some of which are missing) and nails (which are poorly formed early in life, especially toenails). This condition is distinguished from anhidrotic ectodermal dysplasia by autosomal dominant inheritance and little involvement of hair and sweat glands. The teeth are not as severely affected. Witkop (1965) stated that the condition is frequent among Dutch Mennonites in Canada. He presented a pedigree supporting autosomal dominant inheritance. The teeth are not affected in the autosomal dominant hidrotic ectodermal dysplasia. Giancanti et al. (1974) reported a single case. The main features were hypoplastic nails and hypodontia. Eyebrows and eyelashes were normal, but the scalp hair was fine. The patient showed bilateral polycystic ovaries. Redpath and Winter (1969) probably reported cases.

Giansanti, J. S., Long, S. M. and Rankin, J. L.: The 'tooth and nail' type of autosomal dominant ectodermal dysplasia. Oral Surg. 37: 576-582, 1974.

Redpath, T. H. and Winter, G. B.: Autosomal dominant ectodermal dysplasia with significant dental defects. Brit. Dent. J. 126: 123-128, 1969.

Witkop, C. J.: Genetic disease of the oral cavity. Oral Pathology. Tiecke, R. W. (ed.): New York: McGraw-Hill, 1965.

Witkop, C. J., Jr.: In, Tiecke, R. W. (ed.): Oral Pathology. New York: McGraw-Hill Book Co., 1965. Pp. 810-814.

18960 TORTICOLLIS

Male-to-male transmission (Isigkeit, 1931; Garceau, 1962) and transmission through 3 or more generations (Armstrong et al., 1965) has been reported. Facial asymmetry may be a partial manifestation.

Armstrong, D., Pickrell, K., Fetter, B. and Pitts, W.: Torticollis: an analysis of 271 cases. Plast. Reconstr. Surg. 35: 14-25, 1965.

Garceau, G. J.: Congenital muscular torticollis (hematoma, fact or myth). Rhode Island Med. J. 45: 401-404, 1962.

Isigkeit, E.: Untersuchungen ueber Hereditaet orthopaedischer Leiden: der angeborene Schiefhals. Arch. Orthop. Unfallchir. 30: 459-494, 1931.

*18970 TORUS PALATINUS AND TORUS MANDIBULARIS

The study of Suzuki and Sakai (1960) suggests that the two anomalies are equivalent, i.e., due to the same gene, and that the inheritance is autosomal dominant with reduced penetrance. A study by Johnson, Gorlin and Anderson (1965) supported dominant inheritance of torus mandibularis. They found that 85.7 and 89.7 percent, respectively, of children with torus palatinus or torus mandibularis had at least one parent with one or the other anomaly. A sex predilection was noted, males having torus only 70 percent as often as females.

Johnson, C. C., Gorlin, R. J. and Anderson, V. E.: Torus mandibularis: a genetic study. Am. J. Hum. Genet. 17: 433-439, 1965.

Suzuki, M. and Sakai, T.: A familial study of torus palatinus and torus mandibularis. Am. J. Phys. Anthrop. 18: 263-272, 1960.

18980 TOXEMIA OF PREGNANCY

Humphries (1960) made the first systematic study of hypertensive toxemia of pregnancy in mother-daughter pairs delivered at The Johns Hopkins Hospital. Toxemia occurred in 28 percent of daughters of women who had toxemia in the pregnancy in which they were delivered as compared with 13 percent in a comparison group. Chesley et al. (1968) did a similar study with very similar results. In cases in which 2 or more daughters of an eclamptic woman have been tested by pregnancy, toxemia developed in the first pregnancy of at least 1 daughter in 53 percent of the families.

Chesley, L. C., Annitto, J. E. and Cosgrove, R. A.: The familial factor in toxemia of pregnancy. Obstet. Gynec. 32: 303-311, 1968.

Humphries, J. O.: Occurrence of hypertensive toxemia of pregnancy in mother-daughter pairs. Bull. Johns Hopkins Hosp. 107: 271-277, 1960.

18986 TRACHEOESOPHAGEAL FISTULA

Engel et al. (1970) gave the first report of childbearing by a woman who had had correction of esophageal atresia and tracheoesophageal fistula during infancy. The report was of further significance because the child likewise had esophageal atresia and tracheoesophageal fistula.

Engel, P. M. A., Vos, L. J. M., De Vries, J. A. and Kuijjer, P. J.: Esophageal atresia with tracheoesophageal fistula in mother and child. J. Pediat. Surg. 5: 564-565, 1970.

18990 TRACHEOESOPHAGEAL FISTULA WITH ESOPHAGEAL ATRESIA

Engel et al. (1970) described affected mother and daughter. See 21580. Schimke et al. (1972) reviewed the literature on esophageal atresia with or without tracheoesophageal fistula and reported a kindred with two proved and three probable cases. Affected sibs were reported by several authors and parental consanguinity in at least one report (Grieve and McDermott, 1939). Mendelian inheritance is unlikely. Dennis et al. (1973) reported esophageal atresia in a boy, his mother and his mother's sister. They reviewed the literature and concluded that etiology is probably multifactorial.

Dennis, N. R., Nicholas, J. L. and Kovar, I.: Oesophageal atresis: 3 cases in 2 generations. Arch. Dis. Child. 48: 980-982, 1973.

Engel, M. A., Vos, L. J. M., De Vries, J. A. and Kuijjer, P. J.: Esophageal atresia with tracheoesophageal fistula in mother and child. J. Pediat. Surg. 5: 564-565, 1970.

Grieve, J. C. and McDermott, J. G.: Congenital atresia of the oesophagus in two brothers. Canad. Med. Ass. J. 41: 185-186, 1939.

Schimke, R. N., Leape, L. L. and Holder, T. M.: Familial occurrence of esophageal atresia: a preliminary report. The Clinical Delineation of Birth Defects. XIII. G. I. Tract Including Liver and Pancreas. Baltimore: Williams and Wilkins, 1972. Pp. 22-23.

*19000 TRANSFERRIN

Transferrin, the iron-binding protein of serum, is a beta-globulin. Polymorphism was first demonstrated by Smithies using starch gel electrophoresis. Eighteen or more types have been identified. Robson et al. (1966) presented evidence of linkage between the transferrin locus and the serum cholinesterase locus E(1). Serum transferrin consists of a single polypeptide chain with a molecular weight of about 77,000. Lactotransferrin, found in milk of many mammals including man, is structurally similar to serum transferrin but is presumably coded by a different gene.

Dayhoff, M. O.: Transferrin. Atlas of Protein Sequence and Structure 1972 (vol. 5). Washington: National Biomedical Research Foundation, 1972. Pp. D310 and D317.

Parker, W. C. and Bearn, A. G.: Additional genetic variation of human serum transferrin. Science 137: 854-856, 1962.

Robson, E. B., Sutherland, I. and Harris, H.: Evidence for linkage between the transferrin locus (TF) and the serum cholinesterase locus E(1) in man. Ann. Hum. Genet. 29: 325-336, 1966.

Wang, A.-C. and Sutton, H. E.: Human transferrins C and D(1): chemical difference in a peptide. Science 149: 435-437, 1965.

Wang, A.-C., Sutton, H. E. and Howard, P. N.: Human transferrins C and D(Chi): an imino-acid difference. Biochem. Genet. 1: 55-60, 1967.

Wang, A.-C., Sutton, H. E. and Riggs, A.: A chemical difference between human transferrins B2 and C. Am. J. Hum. Genet. 18: 454-458, 1966.

*19010 TREMBLING CHIN

Wadlington (1958) found the condition in eight members of three generations, with no associated neurologic or other abnormalities. Anxiety or emotional upset was a trigger mechanism and tranquilizing and anticonvulsant agents reduced the attacks. Attacks were observed as early as two months of age. There was no instance of male-to-male transmission and all three daughters of the one male with children were affected. Trembling of the chin occurs as part of the oral-facial-digital syndrome (q.v.). Other families of trembling chin were reported by Grossman (1957), Frey (1930) and Ganner (1938), and those reported by Stocks (1922-23) and by Goldsmith (1927) as facial spasm (q.v.) were probably trembling chin. Male-to-male transmission occurred in some of these families. The condition was probably first reported by Massaro (1894), who described 26 cases in 5 generations. Laurance et al. (1968) described two families. The condition ameliorates with age. Also see FACIAL TIC.

Frey, E.: Ein streng dominant erbliches Kinnmuskelzittern (Beitrag zur Evforschung der menschlichen Affektausserungen). Deutsch. Z. Nervenheilk. 115: 9-26, 1930.

Ganner, H.: Erbliches Kinnzittern in einer Tiroler Talschaft. Z. Ges. Neurol. Psychiat. 161: 259-266, 1938.

Goldsmith, J. B.: Inheritance of 'facial spasm,' and effect of modifying factor associated with high temperature. J. Hered. 18: 185-187, 1927.

Grossman, B.: Trembling of the chin — an inheritable dominant character. Pediatrics 19: 453-455, 1957.

Laurance, B. M., Matthews, W. B. and Diggle, J. H.: Hereditary quivering of the chin. Arch. Dis. Child. 43: 249-251, 1968.

Stocks, P.: Facial spasm inherited through four generations. Biometrika 14: 311-315, 1922-23.

Wadlington, W. B.: Familial trembling of the chin. J. Pediat. 53: 316-321, 1958.

19020 TREMOR OF INTENTION, ATAXIA AND LIPOFUSCINOSIS

Feldman et al. (1969) described three persons in three successive generations with this combination. Autopsy at age 80 in one case showed intracytoplasmic lipofuscin granules in the inferior olivary nuclei and hepatocytes. The affected persons had premature graying.

Feldman, R. G., Iseri, O. A., Gottlieb, L. S. and Greenberg, J. P.: Familial intention tremor, ataxia, and lipofuscinosis. Liver biopsy studies. Neurology 19: 503-509, 1969.

*19030 TREMOR, HEREDITARY ESSENTIAL

Larsson and Sjogren (1960) did a thorough study of hereditary essential tremor in a parish of Sweden. In all, 210 cases were ascertained. The age of onset was on the average about 50 years and somewhat later in women than in men. The age of onset showed high intrafamilial correlation. 'Anticipation' was not observed. Fine rapid tremor of the hands was usually the first symptom. Tremor of the arms, tongue (with dysarthria), head, legs and trunk developed later, usually in the order listed. Mild extrapyramidal symptoms in the form of rigidity and stiffness of gait occurred frequently, but the clinical picture was easily distinguishable from Parkinsonism. Mental deterioration was not a feature. With two exceptions, all 210 cases could be traced back to four ancestral couples. The inheritance was autosomal dominant. From observation of about 15 presumed homozygous individuals, it was concluded that there is no difference from the disease in heterozygotes. It was estimated that more than 9 percent of the males and 6 to 6.5 percent of females of the parish carry the gene for essential tremor. The authors could find no reason to suspect selective fertility, selective mortality, or assortative mating as factors in the high gene frequency observed. Rather, chance variations that occurred when the population was small — about 150 persons in the late 1700's — seem to have been responsible. Kehrer (1965) described a family in which members of 3 successive generations had tremor of the hands and face and in two patients studied in detail, cerebral atrophy demonstrable by pnuemoencephalography. He suggested that this represents a distinct entity.

Kehrer, H. E.: Ueber hereditaeren essentiellen Tremor mit Hirnatrophie. Arch. Psychiat. Nervenkr. 207: 6-22, 1965.

Larsson, T. and Sjogren, T.: Essential tremor. A clinical and genetic population study. Acta Psychiat. Neurol. Scand. 36 (suppl. 144): 1-176, 1960.

Schade, H.: Vererbungsfragen bei einer Familie mit essentiellem hereditaeren Tremor. Z. Menschl. Vererb. Konstitutionsl. 33: 355-364, 1966.

Winkler, G. F. and Young, R. R.: Control of familial, senile or essential tremor by propranolol. New Eng. J. Med. 290: 984-988, 1974.

19033 TRICHOMEGALY

Unusually long eyelashes is a morphologic trait which is observed in multiple relatives and has been reported in association with a variety of medical problems as indicated by Goldstein and Hutt (1972), who found it with cataract in a brother and sister who also had hereditary spherocytosis. Gray (1944) reported father and daughter.

Goldstein, J. H. and Hutt, A. E.: Trichomegaly, cataract, and hereditary spherocytosis in two siblings. Am. J. Ophthal. 73: 333-335, 1972.

Gray, H.: Trichomegaly, or movie lashes. Stanford Med. Bull. 2: 157, 1944.

*19035 TRICHORHINOPHALANGEAL SYNDROME

This syndrome is entered also in the recessive catalog. That a recessive form also exists cannot be excluded. However, autosomal dominant inheritance seems unequivocal in light of a family in which we have now observed affected grandfather, son and grandson (Murdoch, 1969; McKusick, 1972). The earliest affected male died at age 43 years of a cerebrovascular accident. Beals (1973) described a family in which the father and two of four children, a male and a female, were affected.

Beals, R. K.: Tricho-rhino-phalangeal dysplasia. Report of a kindred. J. Bone Joint Surg. 55: 821-826, 1973.

Giedion, A., Burdea, M., Fruchter, Z., Meloni, T. and Trosc, V.: Autosomal dominant transmission of the tricho-rhino-phalangeal syndrome. Report of 4 unrelated families, review of 60 cases. Helv. Paediat. Acta 28: 249-259, 1973.

McKusick, V. A.: Heritable Disorders of Connective Tissue. St. Louis: C. V. Mosby Co., 1972 (4th Ed.).

Murdoch, J. L.: Tricho-rhino-phalangeal dysplasia with possible autosomal dominant transmission. The Clinical Delineation of Birth Defects. II. Malformation Syndromes. New York: National Foundation, 1969. Pp. 218-220.

19040 TRIGEMINAL NEURALGIA (TIC DOULOUREUX)

Auld and Buermann (1965) observed six affected sibs. Only one sib was unaffected. No comment on parental consanguinity was made. Harris (1936) observed 9 cases in 3 generations. Allan (1938) described the condition in a 32-year-old man, his maternal uncle and his maternal grandmother.

Allan, W.: Familial occurrence of tic douloureux. Arch. Neurol. Psychiat. 40: 1019-1020, 1938.

Auld, A. W. and Buermann, A.: Trigeminal neuralgia in six members of one generation. Arch. Neurol. 13: 194 only, 1965.

Harris, W.: Bilateral trigeminal tic: its association with heredity and disseminated sclerosis. Ann. Surg. 103: 161-172, 1936.

19043 TRIGLYCERIDE STORAGE DISEASE, TYPE II

Galton et al. (1974) described patients with obesity resulting from a defect in triglyceride breakdown. In the form of triglyceride storage disease they called type II, both the beta-adrenergic receptor and adenyl cyclase were intact as judged by a normal increment in tissue levels of cyclic-AMP on treatment with isoprenaline. However cyclic-AMP did not activate triglyceride-lipase with the expected release of glycerol from the tissues. The defect was found in a 60-year-old woman, her daughter and her eldest sister, whereas her non-identical twin sister and brother showed the same as did obese control subjects. In type I disease noradrenaline poorly stimulated the activity of adenyl cyclase in tissues, suggesting a defect either in the beta-adrenergic receptor or in adenyl cyclase itself. Type III disease is Wolman disease (27800).

Galton, D. J., Gilbert, C., Reclkess, J. P. D. and Kaye, J.: Triglyceride storage disease. A group of inborn errors of triglyceride metabolism. Quart. J. Med. 43: 63-71, 1974.

19045 TRIOSEPHOSPHATE ISOMERASE

Electrophoretic variants have been identified by the Galton Laboratory group (Hopkinson, Harris, 1971). Sparkes et al. (1969) suggested that the locus may be on the short arm of chromosome no. 5. See 27580. No asterisk is used here because the entry in the recessive catalog is asterisked. Cell hybridization studies suggest that the TPI locus may be on chromosome no. 12.

Hendrickson, R. J., Snapka, R. M., Sawyer, T. H. and Gracy, R. W.: Studies on human triosephosphate isomerase. II. Characterization of the enzyme from patients with the Cri Du Chat Syndrome. Am. J. Hum. Genet. 25: 433-438, 1973.

Hopkinson, D. A. and Harris, H.: Recent work on isozymes in man. Ann. Rev. Genet. 5: 5-32, 1971.

Peters, J., Hopkinson, D. A. and Harris, H.: Genetic and non-genetic variations of triose phosphate isomerase isozymes in human tissues. Ann. Hum. Genet. 36: 297-312, 1973.

Sparkes, R. S., Carrel, R. E. and Paglia, D. E.: Probable localization of a triosephosphate isomerase gene to the short arm of a number 5 human chromosome. Nature 224: 367-398, 1969.

19050 TRIPHALANGEAL THUMB WITH DOUBLE PHALANGES

Ecke (1962) described triphalangy of the thumb with doubling of the two distal phalanges in a grandfather, son and grandson.

Ecke, H.: Beitrag zu den Doppelmissbildungen im Bereich der Finger. Beitr. Klin. Chir. 205: 463-468, 1962.

*19060 TRIPHALANGEAL THUMB, NON-OPPOSABLE

Swanson and Brown (1962) described a family in which 30 persons in 5 generations had five digits of each hand triphalangeal and apparently lacked a true thumb. The 'thumb' could not be opposed. No associated internal malformations were detected. Triphalangeal thumb of this type occurs in some cases of the Holt-Oram syndrome (q.v.), although the thumb when present is opposable in the family I reported. Whereas in the cases of Swanson and Brown the metacarpal of the triphalangeal thumb had only a distal epiphysis as is normal for metacarpals II-V, the metacarpal I in the Holt-Oram syndrome shows both a proximal and a distal epiphysis. In three of the affected persons Swanson and Brown (1962) found polydactylism.

Swanson, A. B. and Brown, K. S.: Hereditary triphalangeal thumb. J. Hered. 53: 259-265, 1962.

19080 TRISTICHIASIS (THREE ROWS OF EYELASHES)

A dominant pedigree pattern was referred to by Danforth (1925) and by Loeffler (1940). See DISTRICHIASIS.

Danforth, C. H.: Studies on hair, with special reference to hypertrichosis. Arch. Derm. Syph. 11: 494-508, 1925.

Loeffler, L.: Erbbiologie des menschlichen Hautorgans. In, Handbuch der Erbbiologie des Menschen. Berlin: Springer Verlag, 1940. Pp. 391-406.

*19090 TRITANOPIA

Kalmus (1955) concluded that tritanopia is autosomal dominant with incomplete manifestation. The minimum frequency in Great Britain was estimated as 1 in 13,000 and according to Kalmus is probably higher. Defective blue vision is characteristic. An X-linked form also is known (30400). Krill et al. (1971) suggested that congenital tritanopia and hereditary dominant optic atrophy are identical conditions, i.e., tritanopia is merely a manifestation of optic atrophy.

Kalmus, H.: Diagnosis and Genetics of Defective Colour Vision. Oxford: Pergamon Press, 1965. Pp. 58-59.

Kalmus, H.: The familial distribution of congenital tritanopia with some remarks on some similar conditions. Ann. Hum. Genet. 20: 39-56, 1955.

Krill, A. E., Smith, V. C. and Pokorny, J.: Further studies supporting the identity of congenital tritanopia and hereditary dominant optic atrophy. Invest. Ophthal. 10: 457-465, 1971.

19100 TROCHLEA OF THE HUMERUS, APLASIA OF

Mead and Martin (1963) described a Negro family in which a mother and four children had aplasia of the trochlea of the humerus (that part which articulates with the ulna). Three of the children were by one father and one by another. He could find no identical case in the literature. The deformity was bilaterally symmetrical. The patient held the elbows in flexion and the forearms in pronation. The humerus was shortened. A web of soft tissue stretched across the antecubital space. The elbows could not be extended beyond a right angle but could be flexed to about 30-0. Pronation was moderately limited; supination was normal. The biceps brachii appeared to be either hypoplastic or absent. One of the affected children had a cleft palate. Whereas the lateral part of the distal humerus including the capitellum was essentially normal, the medial part had no trochlea or medial epicondyle. The ulna was displaced and did not articulate with the humerus. The authors suggested that this is a 'new' mutation both in the sense of having occurred first in the mother and of not having been described previously. Because of the high illegitimacy rate in Negroes, new mutation is difficult to defend. It is also rash to suggest the disorder has never been reported. Certainly this must be a very rare anomaly.

Mead, C. A. and Martin, M.: Aplasia of the trochlea — an original mutation. J. Bone Joint Surg. 45A: 379-383, 1963.

*19110 TUBEROUS (OR TUBEROSE) SCLEROSIS

The preferred designation for this syndrome refers to the changes observed in the brain. Adenoma sebaceum and epiloia are synonyms which refer to the cutaneous features. Rhabdomyoma of the myocardium and mixed tumor of the kidney also occur. Fitzpatrick et al. (1968) pointed out the diagnostic usefulness of white macules shaped like the leaf of a mountain ash in patients with tuberous sclerosis. The white macule is probably present at birth in most cases, thus permitting early diagnosis. They may be evident only under Wood light. Kidney lesions are in the form of angiomyolipoma (Anderson and Tannen, 1969). Teplick (1969) stated that adenoma sebaceum is absent in half the cases — surely too high an estimate. He described a 53-year-old woman of normal intelligence with bone and pulmonary lesions misinterpreted as those of sarcoid. Bundey et al. (1970) described affected father and three children without adenoma sebaceum. Adenoma sebaceum is a misnomer. Facial angiofibroma more accurately describes the lesions. Contrary to the findings with other dominants such as achondroplasia (10080), Apert syndrome (10120), and fibrodysplasia ossificans (13510), no increase in parental age has been found in sporadic (presumably new mutation) cases (Nevin and Pearce, 1968). Larbre et al. (1971) described aortic aneurysm in a child with tuberous sclerosis.

Anderson, D. and Tannen, R. L.: Tuberous sclerosis and chronic renal failure. Potential confusion with polycystic kidney disease. Am. J. Med. 47: 163-168, 1969.

Bjornberg, A.: Adenoma sebaceum. Review, case reports and discussion of eugenic aspects. Acta Derm. Venerol. 41: 213-223, 1961.

Borberg, A.: Clinical and Genetic Investigations into Tuberous Sclerosis and Recklinghausen's Neurofibromatosis. Copenhagen: Munksgaard, 1951.

Bundey, S., Dutton, G. and Wells, R. S.: Tuberose sclerosis without adenoma sebaceum. J. Ment. Def. Res. 14: 243-249, 1970.

De la Cruz, F. F. and Laveck, G. D.: Tuberous sclerosis: a review and report of eight cases. Am. J. Ment. Defic. 67: 369-380, 1962.

Dwyer, J. M., Hickie, J. B. and Garvan, J.: Pulmonary tuberous sclerosis. Report of three patients and a review of the literature. Quart. J. Med. 40: 115-126, 1971.

Fitzpatrick, T. B., Szabo, G., Hori, Y., Simone, A. A., Reed, W. B. and Greenberg, M. H.: White leaf-shaped macules. Arch. Derm. 98: 1-6, 1968.

Hudolin, V.: La sclerose tubereuse (compte rendu des cas Yougoslaves). J. Genet. Hum. 10: 128-155, 1961.

Lagos, J. C. and Gomez, M. R.: Tuberous sclerosis: reappraisal of a clinical entity. Mayo Clin. Proc. 42: 26-49, 1967.

Larbre, F., Loire, R., Guibaud, P., Lauras, B. and Weill, B.: Clinical and anatomical observation of aorta aneurysm during Bourneville's disease. Arch. Franc. Pediat. 28: 975-984, 1971.

Milledge, R. D., Gerald, B. E. and Carter, W. J.: Pulmonary manifestations of tuberous sclerosis. Am. J. Roentgen. 98: 734-738, 1966.

Nevin, N. C. and Pearce, W. G.: Diagnostic and genetical aspects of tuberous sclerosis. J. Med. Genet. 5: 273-280, 1968.

Nickel, W. R. and Reed, W. B.: Tuberous sclerosis. Special reference to the microscopic alterations in the cutaneous hamartomas. Arch. Derm. 85: 209-226, 1962.

Scheig, R. L. and Bornstein, P.: Tuberous sclerosis in the adult. An unusual case without mental deficiency or epilepsy. Arch. Intern. Med. 108: 789-795, 1961.

Schull, W. J. and Crowe, F. W.: Neurocutaneous syndromes in a kindred: a case of simultaneous occurrence of tuberous sclerosis and neurofibromatosis. Neurology 3: 904-909, 1953.

Stevenson, A. C. and Fisher, O. D.: Frequency of epiloia in Northern Ireland. Brit. J. Prev. Soc. Med. 10: 134-135, 1956.

Teplick, J. G.: Tuberous sclerosis. Extensive roentgen findings without usual clinical picture: a case report. Radiology 93: 53-55, 1969.

19115 TUFTSIN DEFICIENCY

Three families were observed in which members had deficiency of the tetrapeptide tuftsin (thr — lys — - pro — arg) and a history of repeated and severe infections. Tuftsin is presumably synthesized in the spleen and its absence after splenectomy leads to problems with infection. In each of the two families reported by Constantopoulos et al. (1972), one child had recurrent infections and one parent had low tuftsin levels but was asymptomatic. Tuftsin stimulates the phagocytic activity of polymorphonuclear leukocytes. It is activated in the spleen and bound to a carrier leukokinin molecule, a gamma-globulin which coats the polymorph. Tuftsin is absent in splenectomized humans and dogs. Congenital familial deficiency has been observed in at least four families (Constantopoulos and Najjar, 1973).

Constantopoulos, A., Najjar, V. A. and Smith, J. W.: Tuftsin deficiency: a new syndrome with defective phagocytosis. J. Pediat. 80: 564-572, 1972.

Constantopoulos, A. and Najjar, V. A.: Tuftsin deficiency syndrome. A report of two new cases. Acta Paediat. Scand. 62: 645-648, 1973.

19120 TUNE DEAFNESS

Seashore (1940) reviewed the complexity of the problem of the inheritance of musical ability. Kalmus (1949) studied tune deafness in a group of Continental and British students at University College in London. He found a bimodal distribution in population investigations, with frequent segregation in families and sib pairs. He suggested this might be caused by a unit gene substitution, possibly a dominant.

Kalmus, H.: Tune deafness and its inheritance. Hereditas 35: 605 only, 1949.

Seashore, C. E.: Musical inheritance. Scientific Monthly 50: 351-356, 1940.

*19140 ULNA AND FIBULA, HYPOPLASIA OF

Pfeiffer (1966) and Reinhardt and Pfeiffer (1967) studied a kindred with 14 persons affected by hypoplasia of ulna and fibula in the pattern of a regular autosomal dominant. See MESOMELIC DWARFISM OF HYPOPLASTIC ULNA, FIBULA AND MANDIBLE TYPE. Also see NIEVERGELT SYNDROME.

Reinhardt, K. and Pfeiffer, R. A.: Ulno-fibulare Dysplasie. Eine autosomal-dominant vererbte Mikromesomelie aehnlich dem Nievergeltsyndrom. Fortschr. Roentgenstr. 107: 379-391, 1967.

Pfeiffer, R. A.: Beitrag zur erblichen Verkurzung von Ulna und Fibula. In, Wiedemann, H.-R. (Ed.): Dysostosen. Stuttgart: Gustav Fischer Verlag, 1966.

*19150 UNDRITZ ANOMALY (HYPERSEGMENTATION OF THE NUCLEI OF THE POLYMORPHO-NUCLEAR LEUKOCYTES)

Hypersegmentation of the nuclei of neutrophiles was known in rabbits as a genetic trait before the description in man by Undritz. Undritz (1958) observed a possible instance of homozygosity in an offspring of two affected parents. Hypersegmentation was extreme. Barbier (1958) observed the anomaly in three generations of a family. One patient developed hypersegmentation of the nuclei of lymphocytes, monocytes and plasma cells during a bout of Henoch-Schoenlein purpura. Undritz (1954) also described hypersegmentation of the eosinophiles, a genetic trait possibly distinct from hypersegmentation of the neutrophiles. He observed the trait in otherwise normal mother and daughter. Inherited variations in leukocytes were usefully reviewed by Davidson (1961).

Barbier, F.: Un cas particulier d'hypersegmentation constitutionnelle des noyaux des neutrophiles chez l'homme. Acta Haemat. 19: 121-125, 1958.

Davidson, W. M.: Inherited variations in leucocytes. Brit. Med. Bull. 17: 190-195, 1961.

Undritz, E.: Eine neue Sippe mit erblich-konstitutioneller Hochsegmentierung der Neutrophilenkerne. Schweiz. Med. Wschr. 88: 1000-1001, 1958.

Undritz, E.: Les malformations hereditaires des elements figures du sang. Sang 25: 296-324, 1954.

*19155 URETER, BIFID OR DOUBLE

Atwell et al. (1974) found a high frequency of unilateral or bilateral bifid or double ureter among the sibs and parents of 30 probands with this finding. When a bifid pelvi-calyceal system was included, 20 of the 30 families had affected first degree relatives. Male-to-male transmission was observed.

Atwell, J. D., Cook, P. L., Howell, C. J., Hyde, I. and Parker, B. C.: Familial incidence of bifid and double ureters. Arch. Dis. Child. 49: 390-393, 1974.

19160 URETER, CANCER OF

Burkland and Juzek (1966) reported cancer of the right ureter in mother and son.

Burkland, C. E. and Juzek, R. H.: Familial occurrence of carcinoma of the ureter. J. Urol. 96: 697-701, 1966.

19170 URIC ACID UROLITHIASIS

De Vries, Frank and Atsmon (1962) presented evidence, based on three extensively studied families, that uric acid urolithiasis can be inherited as an autosomal dominant trait independent of gout. In these families no gout and hyperuricemia were found. Cases of this type have rather long been recognized and have been referred to by Henneman as 'idiopathic uric acid stone formers.' The familial nature has apparently not been previously recognized. Recognition of the disorder as familial is important to its prevention. Oral alkalinization and high fluid intake will often dissolve stones already formed and can be depended on to prevent stone formation. Henneman et al. (1962) suggested that elderly Italian or Jewish patients are most likely to get into trouble with uric acid stones despite normal serum and urine concentrations of uric acid. Constant acidity of the urine and low ammonium excretion may be involved in pathogenesis.

De Vries, A., Frank, M. and Atsmon, A.: Inherited uric acid lithiasis. Am. J. Med. 33: 880-892, 1962.

Henneman, P. H., Wallach, S. and Dempsey, E. F.: The metabolic defect responsible for uric acid stone formation. J. Clin. Invest. 41: 537-542, 1962.

*19173 URIDINE MONOPHOSPHATE KINASE

This enzyme, UMPK, catalyzes the first step in the production of the pyrimidine nucleoside triphosphates required for RNA and DNA synthesis, namely the phosphorylation of uridine monophosphate to uridine diphosphate. Giblett et al. (1974) found genetic polymorphism of UMPK by means of starch gel electrophoresis. Evidence for three alleles — UMPK-1, UMPK-2, and UMPK-3 — at an autosomel locus was provided by family studies. The UMPK-1 allele was associated with about three times the catalytic activity of the UMPK-2 allele, so that UMPK-2 homozygotes are relatively deficient of the enzyme. Two of three UMPK-2 homozygotes were children with prolonged respiratory infection. Possbily the ability of immunocompetent lymphocytes to respond to appropriate stimuli is impaired in the UMPK-2 homozygote in a manner similar to the immune defect resulting from adenosine deaminase deficiency.

Giblett, E. R., Anderson, J. E., Chen, S.-H., Teng, Y.-S. and Cohen, F.: Uridine monophosphate kinase: a new genetic polymorphism with possible clinical implications. Am. J. Hum. Genet. 26: 627-635, 1974.

*19175 URIDYL DIPHOSPHATE GLUCOSE PYROPHOSPHATE

The structural locus for this enzyme has been assigned to chromosome no. 1 by somatic cell studies.

Burgerhout, W., Van Someren, H. and Bootsma, D.: Cytological mapping of the gene assigned to the human A1 chromosome by the use of radiation induced chromosome breakage in a human-Chinese hamster hybrid cell line.. Humangenetik, in press, 1973.

*19177 URIDYLDIPHOSPHOGLUCOSE PYROPHOSPHORYLASE (UGPP)

According to cell hybridization studies, this locus may be on chromosome no. 1 (Van Someren, 1973).

Van Someren, H.: Intern. Workshop on Human Gene Mapping, New Haven, Conn., June, 1973.

19180 URINARY BLADDER, ATONY OF

Gundrum (1922) described 9 (8 male, 1 female) cases in three generations. Most performed catheterization daily on themselves.

Gundrum, F. F.: Familial bladder atony. J.A.M.A. 78: 411-412, 1922.

*19190 URTICARIA, DEAFNESS AND AMYLOIDOSIS

Muckle and Wells (1962) described a family in which urticaria, progressive perceptive deafness and amyloidosis were combined in a dominantly inherited syndrome. Five generations were affected. Autopsy in two patients showed absent organ of Corti, atrophy of the cochlear nerve and amyloid infiltration of the kidneys. Amyloidosis is a complication of urticaria due to cold sensitivity (q.v.). Black (1969) described affected persons in three generations of a family and emphasized limb pains as a feature.

Black, J. T.: Amyloidosis deafness, urticaria and limb pains: a hereditary syndrome. Ann. Intern. Med. 70: 989-994, 1969.

Muckle, T. J. and Wells, M.: Urticaria, deafness and amyloidosis: a new heredo-familial syndrome. Quart. J. Med. 31: 235-248, 1962.

19195 URTICARIA, FAMILIAL LOCALIZED HEAT

Michaelsson and Ros (1971) described a delayed heat urticaria, limited to the area of contact, in a 48-year-old female, two of her three children, one of her two sisters, and four of the latter's five children. Repeated heat exposure showed a decrease in response. Local pretreatment with lidocaine completely inhibited whealing. Oral antihistamines lessened the urticarial response. A higher percentage of basophils were degranulated in vitro in the experimental subject than in the controls. Acetylcholine as an allergen was postulated.

Michaelsson, G. and Ros, A.-M.: Familial localized heat urticaria of delayed type. Acta Derm. Venerol. 51: 279-283, 1971.

19200 UTERINE ANOMALIES

Holmes (1956) reported a mother with uterus arcuatus who delivered a stillborn female in whom uterus bicornis unicollis was demonstrated at autopsy. Similar uterine anomalies were described in mother and daughter by Stevenson et al. (1959) and in sisters by Drescher (1966) and Nykiforuk (1938).

Drescher, H.: Zur Frage gehaeuften familiaeren Vorkommens von Uterusmissbildungen. Zbl. Gynaek. 88: 1673-1675, 1966.

Holmes, J. A.: Congenital abnormalities of the uterus and pregnancy. Brit. Med. J. 1: 1144-1147, 1956.

Nykiforuk, N. E.: Uterus didelphys. Canad. Med. Ass. J. 38: 175 only, 1938.

Stevenson, A. C., Dudgeon, M. Y. and McClure, H. I.: Pregnancies in women resident in Belfast. II. Abortions, hydatiform moles and ectopic pregnancies. Ann. Hum. Genet. 23: 395-411, 1959.

19210 UVULA, BIFID (SPLIT UVULA, CLEFT UVULA)

The uvula is split into two lobes by a central fissure. About 1 percent of Caucasians and 10 percent of American Indians and Japanese show it in some degree. The frequency in sibs and parents of affected persons is said to be about 18 percent.

Meskin, L. H., Gorlin, R. J. and Isaacson, R. J.: Abnormal morphology of the soft palate. II. The genetics of cleft uvula. Cleft Palate J. 2: 40-45, 1965.

19220 VARICOSE VEINS

Dominant inheritance with reduced penetrance was suggested by Arnoldi (1958). He thought that late menarche is related to varicosity. Varicose veins are about twice as frequent in females as in males and no male-to-male transmission was indicated in his illustrative pedigree. Possible X-linked dominance should be considered. Varicose veins are frequent in some genetic disorders such as the Marfan syndrome. Hauge and Gundersen (1969) presented a family study of 249 probands, with the conclusion that multifactorial inheritance seems 'very probable.'

Arnoldi, C. C.: The heredity of venous insufficiency. Danish Med. Bull. 5: 169-176, 1958.

Hauge, M. and Gundersen, J.: Genetics of varicose veins of the lower extremities. Hum. Hered. 19: 573-580, 1969.

Leu, H. J.: Familial congenital absence of valves in the deep leg veins. Humangenetik 22: 347-349, 1974.

19230 VASCULAR HELIX OF UMBILICAL CORD

Malpas and Symonds (1966) found in Liverpool, Eng., that of 652 cords the helix was right-handed in 133 and left-handed in 519. Although a genetic basis for the difference was suggested, family data are yet to be collected.

Malpas, P. and Symonds, E. M.: The direction of the helix of the human umbilical cord. Ann. Hum. Genet. 29: 409-410, 1966.

19231 VASCULITIS, HEREDITARY INFLAMMATORY, WITH PERSISTENT NODULES

This condition was described by Reed et al. (1972) in three generations of a family. Lesions were of two types: 1) multiple small to medium-sized nodules on the arms, legs and buttocks; 2) multiple larger, firm nodules, resembling rheumatoid nodules, over bony prominences. The lesions were present from birth or early life. Exposure to sunlight aggravated the lesions, whereas chloroquine suppressed them completely. Histology showed lymphocytic vasculitis without necrosis, extending deep into the fat. A relationship to the lupus erythematosus LE was postulated. 'Rheumatoid arthritis' and discoid LE were present in the family. No male-to-male transmission was observed.

19233 VASOPRESSIN

The hypothalamus produces two main peptide hormones which are stored in the posterior pituitary (neurohypophysis). From the functional point of view these peptides are of two main types (with some overlap): pressor hormones and uterine- contracting hormones. All are nonapeptides (i.e. have 9 amino acids) and have a disulfide bond between the cysteines at positions 1 and 6. Vasopressin and oxytocin (16705), produced in the hypothalamus, are, respectively, examples of pressor and antidiuretic peptide hormones.

Dayhoff, M. O.: Hormones, active peptides and toxins. Atlas of Protein Sequence and Structure 1972 (vol. 5). Washington: National Biomedical Research Foundation, 1972. Pp. D173-D227.

19235 VATER ASSOCIATION

Vater is a mnemonically useful acronym for vertebral defects, anal atresia, tracheoesophageal fistula with esophageal atresia and radial dysplasia. This combination of associated defects was pointed out by Quan and Smith (1972). All cases have been sporadic, with no recognized teratogen or chromosomal abnormality.

Kaufman, R. L., Quinton, B. and Ternberg, J. L.: Imperforate anus, vertebral anomalies and preaxial limb abnormalities. The Clinical Delineation of Birth Defects. XIII. G. I. Tract Including Liver and Pancreas. Baltimore: Williams and Wilkins, 1972. Pp. 85-87.

Quan, L. and Smith, D. W.: The vater association: vertebral defects, anal atresia, tracheoesophageal fistula with esophageal atresia, radial dysplasia. The Clinical Delineation of Birth Defects. XIII. G. I. Tract Including Liver and Pancreas. Baltimore: Williams and Wilkins, 1972. Pp. 75-78.

19240 VEINS, PATTERN OF, ON ANTERIOR THORAX

Spuhler (1950) found two alternative patterns. (1) In the transverse type, the superficial veins radiate laterally from the pectoral venous plexus toward the axillary region. (2) In the longitudinal type the veins radiate in a fan-like pattern downward and laterally from the point where the anterior jugular vein turns beneath the sternocleidomastoid muscle. In a study in the Navajo Indians, the transverse pattern appeared to behave as a dominant.

Spuhler, J. N.: Genetics of three normal morphological variations: pattern of superficial veins of the anterior thorax, peroneus tertius muscle, and number of vallate papillae. Cold Spring Harbor Symposia Quant. Biol. 15: 175-188, 1950.

19245 VENTRICULAR FIBRILLATION, PAROXYSMAL FAMILIAL

McRae et al. (1974) described a family in which three brothers had syncopal attacks and died suddenly at ages 17, 12, and 12 years. Autopsy in two of them showed no abnormality. A fourth brother had syncopal episodes and proved paroxysmal ventricular fibrillation. Important electrocardiographic changes were short P-R interval and prominent gamma wave. Fibrillation was induced by stressful emotional stimuli, but could not be induced by exercise. Propranolol was found to be effective prophylactic medication. The mother had experienced 25 episodes of syncope between ages 15 and 25. Each episode was precipitated by an emotionally stressful event causing fright or anger. The mother, like her son, had a short P-R interval.

McRae, J. R., Wagner, G. S., Rogers, M. C. and Canent, R. V.: Paroxysmal familial ventricular fibrillation. J. Pediat. 84: 515-518, 1974.

*19250 VENTRICULAR FIBRILLATION WITH PROLONGED Q-T INTERVAL

Ward (1964) observed syncope due to ventricular fibrillation in a brother and sister whose resting electrocardiogram showed abnormal prolongation of the Q-T interval. The mother, although asymptomatic, had a prolonged Q-T interval also. Her sister had attacks of syncope and died in one of these at the age of 30 years. This disorder appears to be distinct from the recessively inherited syndrome described by Jervell and Lange-Nielsen (see DEAF-MUTISM III). Deafness is not a feature. Similar families were reported by Romano et al. (1963) and by Barlow et al. (1964). Transmission through three generations was described by Garza et al. (1970). Propranolol effectively prevented ventricular arrhythmia. Multiple generation involvement was reported also by Barlow et al. (1964) and by Romano (1965). Male-to-male transmission has, it seems, not been adequately documented. Gamstorp et al. (1964) reported a family with prolonged Q-T interval and cardiac arrhythmias without deafness but unlike the families mentioned above hypokalemia and beneficial effects of administration of potassium were noted. Gale et al. (1970) also suggested that adrenergic beta-blockade is the best method of treatment. In a non-familial case, Moss and McDonald (1971) observed benefit from sympathetic denervation of the heart.

Barlow, J. B., Bosman, C. K. and Cochrane, J. W. C.: Congenital cardiac arrhythmia. Lancet II: 531 only, 1964.

Gale, G. E., Bosman, C. K., Tucker, R. B. K. and Barlow, J. B.: Hereditary prolongation of Q-T interval. Study of two families. Brit. Heart J. 32: 505-509, 1970.

Gamstorp, I., Nilsen, R., Westling, H.: Congenital cardiac arrhythmia. (Letter) Lancet II: 965 only, 1964.

Garza, L. A., Vick, R. L., Nora, J. J. and McNamara, D. G.: Heritable Q-T prolongation without deafness. Circulation 41: 39-48, 1970.

Moss, A. J. and McDonald, J.: Unilateral cervico-thoracic sympathetic ganglionectomy for the treatment of long Q-T interval syndrome. New Eng. J. Med. 285: 903-904, 1971.

Romano, C.: Congenital cardiac arrhythmia. (Letter) Lancet I: 658-659, 1965.

Romano, C., Gemme, G. and Pongiglione, R.: Aritmie cardiache rare dell' eta pediatrica. II. Accessi sincopali per fibrillazione ventricolare parossistica. (Presentazione del primo caso della letteratura pediatrica Italiana). Clin. Pediat. 45: 656-683, 1963.

Van der Straaten, P.J.C. and Bruins, C. L. D.: A family with heritable electrocardiographic Q-T prolongation. J. Med. Genet. 10: 158-160, 1973.

Ward, O. C.: A new familial cardiac syndrome in children. J. Irish Med. Ass. 54: 103-106, 1964.

*19260 VENTRICULAR HYPERTROPHY, HEREDITARY

This condition has been called muscular subaortic stenosis but more generalized ventricular hypertrophy is often an earlier and more impressive feature and obstruction to outflow from the right ventricle can also occur. Study of the families of probands with the full-blown condition shows that an atrial heart sound ('presystolic gallop') and EKG changes of ventricular hypertrophy are the earliest signs. Sudden death occurs in some cases. Braunwald and colleagues (1964) reported in detail on 64 patients. Multiple cases were observed in 11 families, which contained in all at least 41 definite or probable cases. In the family reported by Horlick et al. (1966), 10 persons in four generations were thought to have been affected. Pare and colleagues (1961) described this disorder in 30 out of 87 members of a French-Canadian kindred. The genealogic survey was carried back to the original emigrant from France in the 1600's. The pattern of occurrence over five generations and 160 years since the death of the man believed to be the first instance of the heart disease indicates autosomal dominant inheritance. As pointed out by Nasser et al. (1967) among others, outflow obstruction may be absent in some affected members of families in which others do have outflow obstruction. Elevated paternal age of sporadic (possible fresh mutation) cases was observed by Jorgensen (1968). Asymmetric septal hypertrophy (ASH) and hypertrophic obstructive cardiomyopathy (HOCAM) are other synonyms. The family study of Clark et al. (1973), using echocardiography, indicated that 28 of 30 probands (93 percent) had an affected parent. This agrees well with estimates of the extent to which this disorder, on the average reduces reproductive fitness.

Braunwald, E., Lambrew, C. T., Rockoff, S. D., Ross, J., Jr. and Morrow, A. G.: Idiopathic hypertrophic subaortic stenosis. I. A description of the disease based on an analysis of 64 patients. Circulation 30 (suppl. 4): 3-119, 1964.

Clark, C. E., Henry, W. L. and Epstein, S. E.: Familial prevalance and genetic transmission of idiopathic hypertrophic subaortic stenosis. New Eng. J. Med. 289: 709-714, 1973.

Criley, J., Lewis, K. B., White, R. I., Jr. and Ross, R. S.: Pressure gradients without obstruction: a new concept of 'hypertrophic subaortic stenosis.' Circulation 32: 881-887, 1965.

Hardarson, T., Curiel, R., De la Calzada, C. S. and Goodwin, J. F.: Prognosis and mortality of hypertrophic obstructive cardiomyopahty. Lancet II: 1462-1467, 1973.

Horlick, L., Petkovich, N. J. and Bolton, C. F.: Idiopathic hypertrophic subvalvular stenosis. A study of a family involving four generations. Clinical, hemodynamic and pathologic observations. Am. J. Cardiol. 17: 411-418, 1966.

Jorgensen, G.: Genetische Untersuchungen bei funktionell-obstruktiver subvalvulaerer Aortenstenose (irregulaer hypertrophische Kardiomyopathie). Humangenetik 6: 13-28, 1968.

Manchester, G. H.: Muscular subaortic stenosis. New Eng. J. Med. 269: 300-306, 1963.

Nasser, W. K., Williams, J. F., Mishkin, M. E., Childress, R. H., Helmen, C., Merritt, A. D. and Genovese, P. D.: Familial myocardial disease with and without obstruction to left ventricular outflow: clinical, hemodynamic and angiographic findings. Circulation 35: 638-652, 1967.

Pare, J. A. P., Fraser, R. G., Pirozynski, W. J., Shanks, J. A. and Stubington, D.: Hereditary cardiovascular dysplasia. A form of familial cardiomyopathy. Am. J. Med. 31: 37-62, 1961.

Powell, W. J., Whiting, R. B., Dinsmore, R. E. and Sanders, C. A.: Symptomatic prognosis in patients with idiopathic hypertrophic subaortic stenosis (IHSS). Am. J. Med. 55: 15-24, 1973.

Wood, R. S., Taylor, W. J., Wheat, M. W. and Schiebler, G. L.: Muscular subaortic stenosis in childhood. Report of occurrence in three siblings. Pediatrics 30: 749-758, 1962.

19270 VENULAR INSUFFICIENCY, SYSTEMIC

Seijffers, Groen and Davis (1964) described what they termed systemic venular insufficiency in a 40-year-old Ashkenazi Jew. Marked cyanosis and swelling of the head and neck followed bending over and the hands and feet were similarly affected when in the dependent position. Small veins and venules in conjunctiva showed marked dilation. Erection did not occur but could be induced by manual compression of the root of the penis. The authors suggested a venous defect, either absence of valves or absence of smooth muscle

Seijffers, M. J., Groen, J. J. and Davis, E.: Systemic venular insufficiency. Am. J. Med. 36: 158-166, 1964.

19280 VERTEBRAL FUSION, POSTERIOR LUMBOSACRAL, WITH BLEPHAROPTOSIS

Faulk et al. (1970) described a mother and two daughters with congenital ptosis and posterior fusion of lumbosacral vertebrae. The mother's mother had ptosis and 'had never been able to place her feet flat on the floor' because of 'tightness of the heel cords.' Serum lactic dehydrogenase activity was elevated in the mother and one daughter studied.

Faulk, W. P., Epstein, C. J. and Jones, M. D.: Familial posterior lumbosacral vertebral fusion and eyelid ptosis. Am. J. Dis. Child. 119: 510-512, 1970.

*19290 VERTEBRAL HYPOPLASIA WITH LUMBAR KYPHOSIS

Beals (1969) observed multiple cases of vertebral hypoplasia leading to kyphosis in the upper lumbar area, in multiple generations of a family, with male-to-male transmission. The familial cases reported by van Assen (1930) and by Bauer (1933) may have been the same condition.

Bauer, H.: Ueber angeborene Wirbelsaeulenmissbildungen, insbesondere angeborene Kyphosen. Ztschr. Orthop. Chir. 58: 354-381, 1933.

Beals, R. K.: Familial vertebral hypoplasia and kyphosis. J. Bone Joint Surg. 51: 190-196, 1969.

Van Assen, J.: Angeborene Kyphose. Acta Chir. Scand. 67: 14-33, 1930.

19300 VESICOURETERAL REFLUX

Mulcahy et al. (1970) described a high familial incidence. The disorder is rare in Negroes. Burger (1972) found 23 families with two or more affected first-degree relatives and added seven more containing a total of 20 affected first-degree relatives. The anatomic substrate was thought to be abnormally short intravesical ureter. Mother and at least one child were affected in four families.

Burger, R. H.: Congenitally short ureterovesical junction causing primary reflux — a common familial and hereditary trait. (Abstract) Pediat. Res. 6: 418 only, 1972.

Mulcahy, J. J., Kelalis, P. P., Stickler, G. B. and Burke, E. C.: Familial vesicoureteral reflux. J. Urol. 104: 762-764, 1970.

19305 VIBRATORY ANGIOEDEMA

Persons in at least four generations showed local erythematous and edematous lesions following loci stimulati of a vibratory or frictional nature. Facial or generalized erythema and headache accompanied severe local reactions. Elevated plasma amine levels were found in the venous blood returning from a limb subjected to appropriate stimualtion.

Patterson, R., Mellies, C. J., Blankenship, M. L. and Pruzansky, J. J.: Vibratory angioedema: a hereditary type of physical hypersensitivity. J. Allergy Clin. Immunol. 50: 174-182, 1972.

19307 VIRUS (RD114) RNA COMPLEMENTARITY

From in situ hybridization studies Price et al. (1973) suggested that a D-group chromosome contains on its long arm DNA complementary to the RNA of the oncogenic virus RD114.

Price, P. M., Hirschhorn, K., Gabelman, N. and Waxman, S.: In situ hybridization of RD114-virus RNA with human metaphase chromosomes. Proc. Natl. Acad. Sci. 70: 11-14, 1973.

*19310 VITAMIN-D-RESISTANT RICKETS

Autosomal dominant inheritance in some families was suggested by Prader et al. (1961). However, later observations led Prader to conclude that his 'hereditare pseudo-mangelrachitis' is an autosomal recessive (see PSEUDO-VITAMIN D DEFICIENCY RICKETS). Harrison et al. (1966) mentioned affected brother and two sisters, whose father had hypophosphatemia, severe osteomalacia and stunting of growth and whose mother was normal (also see Bianchine et al., 1971). They emphasized that serum phosphorus is likely to be at a normal level at birth and during early life. Wilson et al. (1965) reported a family study initiated from a female proband with typical vitamin-D-resistant rickets. Only the proband was clinically affected, but, although the parents had normal blood phosphorus, many more remote relatives had hypophosphatemia. Father-to-son transmission of hypophosphatemia was observed. Although the normal parents and their relationship as second cousins suggested autosomal recessive inheritance, the authors favored autosomal dominance with reduced penetrance. It is certainly possible for more than one genetic variety of vitamin-D-resistant rickets to exist. Pak et al. (1972) reported a presumably autosomal dominant form of vitamin-D-resistant rickets. In both this and the X-linked form (30780), Brickman et al. (1973) found that 1,25-dihydroxycholecalciferol is ineffective.

Bianchine, J. W., Stambler, A. A. and Harrison, H. E.: Familial hypophosphatemic rickets showing autosomal dominant inheritance. The Clinical Delineation of Birth Defects. X. The Endocrine System. Baltimore: Williams and Wilkins, 1971. Pp. 287-294.

Brickman, A. S., Coburn, J. W., Kurokawa, K., Bethune, J. E., Harrison, H. E. and Norman, A. W.: Actions of 1,25 dihydroxycholecalciferol in patients with hypophosphatemic, vitamin-D-resistant rickets. New Eng. J. Med. 289: 495-498, 1973.

Deluca, H. F.: Vitamin D. New Eng. J. Med. 281: 1103-1104, 1969.

Harrison, H. E., Harrison, H. C., Lifshitz, F. and Johnson, A. D.: Growth disturbance in hereditary hypophosphatemia. Am. J. Dis. Child. 112: 290-297, 1966.

Matsuda, I., Sugai, M. and Ohsawa, T.: Laboratory findings in a child with pseudo-vitamin D deficiency rickets. Helvet. Paediat. Acta 24: 329-336, 1969.

Pak, C. Y. C., Deluca, H. F., Bartter, F. C., Henneman, D. H., Frame, B., Simopoulos, A. and Delea, C. S.: Treatment of vitamin D-resistant rickets with 25-hydroxycholecalciferol. Arch. Intern. Med. 129: 894-899, 1972.

Prader, A., Illig, R. and Heierli, E.: Eine besondere Form der primaren vitamin-d-resistenten Rachitis mit Hypocalcamie und autosomal-dominantem Erbgang: die hereditare Pseudo-mangelrachitis. Helv. Paediat. Acta 16: 452-468, 1961.

Wilson, D. R., York, S. E., Jaworski, Z. F. and Yendt, E. R.: Studies in hypophosphatemic vitamin D-refractory osteomalacia in adults. Oral phosphate supplements as an adjunct to therapy. Medicine 44: 99-134, 1965.

19320 VITILIGO

Vitiligo differs from piebald trait (q.v.) in onset after birth, absence of predilection for ventral skin and tendency to progress or regress. Few pedigrees have been reported, but Lerner (1959) suggested autosomal dominant inheritance.

Lerner, A. B.: Vitiligo. J. Invest. Derm. 32: 285-310, 1959.

*19325 VOLVULUS OF MIDGUT

Smith (1972) documented 8 cases of midgut volvulus in one kindred. The propositus, a male, his two sons and three daughters, as well as his two grandchildren demonstrated this midgut malrotation syndrome. The midgut volvulus caused great discomfort to those affected. Six of the affected have undergone a total of 24 operative procedures to alleviate problems caused by the malrotation of the midgut. The clinical course of the five sibs showed normal growth and development followed by the appearance of abdominal distension, pain and constipation, by the age of six. The two affected grandchildren died at the age of 4-weeks, one of post-operative complications to repair the volvulus and the other due to multiple congenital defects.

This kindred also demonstrated a thick disc of fibromuscular tissue on the antrum of the stomach of three of the patients and major obstetrical abnormalities in 10 of 19 pregnancies produced by the five affected sibs.

Smith, S. L.: Familial midgut volvulus. Surgery 72: 420-426, 1972.

*19330 VON HIPPEL-LINDAU SYNDROME

The cardinal features are angiomata of the retina and hemangioblastoma of the cerebellum. Hemangioma of the spinal cord has also been observed. Pheochromocytoma occurs in some patients. The combination of hypertension with angioma may lead to subarachnoid hemorrhage. Hypernephroma-like renal tumors occur in some patients. Polycythemia may be due to either the hemangioblastoma of the cerebellum or the hypernephroma. Hemangiomas of the adrenals, lungs and liver and multiple cysts of the pancreas and kidneys have been observed in some instances. The condition of arteriovenous aneurysm of retina and mid-brain with facial nevus, described by Bonnet and others (1938) and by Wyburn-Mason (1943) is of uncertain relationship to this condition. Metastatic renal cancer occurs in some instances (Kranes and Balogh, 1966). Goldberg and Duke (1968) examined the eyes of an affected 51-year-old Negro male whose mother died of cerebellar tumor at age 26 years. The same case was described by McKusick et al. (1961). In addition to the association of tumors of the brain and adrenal medulla which occur in neurofibromatosis and in von Hippel-Lindau disease, cerebellar tumors sometimes produce paroxysmal hypertension like that of pheochromocytoma. Urinary catecholamines are normal in such cases (Cameron, Doig, 1970). Shokeir (1970) described a pedigree he interpreted as indicative of autosomal dominant inheritance with incomplete penetrance. I have observed a skipped generation in the large kindred reported by Silver (1954). In another kindred Shokeir (1970) suggested autosomal recessive inheritance but incomplete penetrance of the dominant disorder seems equally plausible.

Bonnet, P., Dechaume, J. and Blanc, E.: L'anevrisme cirsoide de la retine l'anevrisme racemeux, ses relations avec l'anevrisme cirsoide de la face et l'anevrisme cirsoid du cerveau. Bull. Soc. Franc. Ophtal. 51: 521-524, 1938.

Brown, D. G., Hilal, S. K. and Tenner, M. S.: Wyburn-Mason syndrome. Arch. Neurol. 28: 67-68, 1973.

Cameron, S. J. and Doig, A.: Cerebellar tumors presented with clinical features of phaeochromocytoma. Lancet I: 492-494, 1970.

Chapman, R. C. and Diaz-Perez, R.: Pheochromocytoma associated with cerebellar hemangioblastoma. J.A.M.A. 182: 1014-1017, 1962.

Christoferson, L. A., Gustafson, M. B. and Petersen, A. G.: Von Hippel-Lindau's disease. J.A.M.A. 178: 280-282, 1961.

Goldberg, M. F. and Duke, J. R.: Von Hippel-Lindau disease: histopathologic findings in a treated and untreated eye. Am. J. Ophthal. 66: 693-705, 1968.

Hennessy, T. G., Stern, W. E. and Herrick, S. E.: Cerebellar hemangioblastoma: erythropoietic activity by radioiron assay. J. Nuclear Med. 8: 601-606, 1967.

Kaplan, C., Sayre, G. P. and Greene, L. F.: Bilateral nephrogenic carcinomas in Lindau-von Hippel disease. J. Urol. 86: 36-42, 1961.

Kranes, A. and Balogh, K., Jr.: Liver disease in a patient with von Hippel-Lindau disease. New Eng. J. Med. 275: 950-959, 1966.

McKusick, V. A. and colleagues: Medical Genetics 1960. J. Chronic Dis. 14: 1-198, 1961. Fig. 71.

Nibbelink, D. W., Peters, B. H. and McCormick, W. F.: On the association of pheochromocytoma and cerebellar hemangioblastoma. Neurology 19: 455-460, 1969.

Otenasek, F. J. and Silver, M. L.: Spinal hemangioma (hemangioblastoma) in Lindau's disease. Report of six cases in a single family. J. Neurosurg. 18: 295-300, 1961.

Rho, Y. M.: Von Hippel-Lindau's disease: a report of 5 cases. Canad. Med. Ass. J. 101: 135-142, 1969.

Sander, S., Normann, T. and Mathisen, W.: Pheochromocytoma associated with von-Hippel-Lindau's disease in a family. Scand. J. Urol. Nephrol. 4: 259-263, 1970.

Schechterman, L.: Lindau's disease: report of an unusual case and two additional cases in a Negro family. Med. Ann. D.C. 30: 64-76, 1961.

Sharp, W. V. and Platt, R. L.: Familial pheochromocytoma: association with von-Hippel-Lindau's disease. Angiology 22: 141-146, 1971.

Shokeir, M. H. K.: Von Hippel-Lindau syndrome: a report on three kindreds. J. Med. Genet. 7: 155-157, 1970.

Silver, M. L.: Hereditary vascular tumors of the nervous system. J.A.M.A. 156: 1053-1056, 1954.

Thomas, M. and Burnside, R. M.: Von Hippel-Lindau disease. Am. J. Ophthal. 51: 140-146, 1961.

Wise, K. S. and Gibson, J. A.: Von Hippel-Lindau's disease and phaeochromocytoma. Brit. Med. J. 1: 441 Only, 1971.

Wyburn-Mason, R.: Arteriovenous aneurysm of mid-brain and retina, facial naevi and mental changes. Brain 66: 163-203, 1943.

*19340 VON WILLEBRAND DISEASE

Von Willebrand (1931) discovered a hemorrhagic condition in persons living on the Aland Islands in the Sea of Bothnia between Sweden and Finland and called it 'pseudohemophilia.' The main difference from classic hemophilia was prolonged bleeding time. Main problems were gastrointestinal, urinary and uterine bleeding. Hemarthroses were rare. The condition ameliorated with age. Later Jergens (1937) working with Willebrand and using the capillary thrombometer suggested the designation, 'constitutional thrombopathy.' In 1953, Alexander and Goldstein discovered low anti-hemophilic globulin (Factor VIII) in this disorder. Thereafter the condition became known as 'vascular hemophilia.' In recent years the main developments have been the demonstrations (1) that the platelet is intrinsically normal but has reduced adhesiveness because of the Factor VIII deficiency and (2) that plasma from persons with classical hemophilia will correct both the vascular defect and the Factor VIII deficiency. In a family which appeared to contain both homozygotes and heterozygotes for the Von Willebrand gene, Barrow et al. (1965) found that hemophilic plasma resulted in about 8 times as great synthesis of AHG in heterozygotes as in homozygotes. They interpreted this as suggesting the presence of two subunits of AHG which are under separate genetic control. Several observations (Cornu, et al., 1963; Biggs and Matthews, 1963) are pertinent to the nature of the AHG defect in Von Willebrand disease. (1) Blood from a patient with hemophilia A will correct the clotting defect in Von Willebrand disease. (2) The converse is not true. Blood from a patient with Von Willebrand disease will not correct the clotting defect in hemophilia A. (3) The bleeding tendency in Von Willebrand disease is corrected promptly by normal blood. (4) After administration of hemophilia A blood to Von Willebrand patients there is a delay of several hours before the level of AHG reaches normal. These observations are consistent with the following schema: at least two biochemical steps are involved in the synthesis of AHG. The first step under control of an autosomal locus produces the Willebrand factor which is concerned with platelet adhesiveness and therefore with vascular integrity. The Willebrand factor is also the substrate for the second step which is under X-chromosome control and which results in AHG. The above schema conceives, therefore, a chain of biochemical processes, each under separate genetic control — the type of system of which many instances have now been demonstrated. Telangiectasia and Von Willebrand disease occurred in a mother and daughter reported by Quick (1967). The difficult topic of diagnostic criteria was reviewed by Weiss (1968). A phenocopy of Von Willebrand disease in a patient with systemic lupus erythematosus was reported by Simone et al. (1968). Homozygotes have been observed (Veltkamp and van Tilburg, 1973).

Alexander, B. and Goldstein, R.: Dual hemostatic defect in pseudohemophilia. (Abstract) J. Clin. Invest. 32: 551 only, 1953.

Barrow, E. M., Heindel, C. C., Roberts, H. R. and Graham, J. B.: Heterozygosity and homozygosity in von Willebrand's disease. Proc. Soc. Exp. Biol. Med. 118: 684-687, 1965.

Bennett, B., Ratnoff, O. D. and Levin, J.: Immunological studies in von Willebrand's disease. Evidence that the antihemophilic Factor (AHF) produced after transfusions lacks an antigen associated with normal AHF and the inactive material produced by patients with classic hemophilia. J. Clin. Invest. 51: 2597-2601, 1972.

Biggs, R. and Matthews, J. M.: The treatment of haemorrhage in von Willebrand's disease and the blood level of Factor VIII (AHG). Brit. J. Haemat. 9: 203-214, 1963.

Blomback, M., Jorpes, J. E. and Nilsson, I. M.: Von Willebrand's disease. Am. J. Med. 34: 236-241, 1963.

Cornu, P., Larrieu, M. J., Caen, J. P. and Bernard, J.: Transfusion studies in von Willebrand's disease: effect on bleeding time and Factor VIII. Brit. J. Haemat. 9: 189-202, 1963.

Dodds, W. J.: Canine von Willebrand's disease. J. Lab. Clin. Med. 76: 713-721, 1970.

Firkin, B., Firkin, F. and Stott, L.: Von Willebrand's disease type b: a newly defined bleeding diathesis Aust. New Zeal. J. Med. 3: 225-229, 1973.

Hagedorn, B.: Von Willebrand's disease. J.A.M.A. 216: 991-995, 1971.

Nevanlinna, H. R., Ikkala, E. and Vuopio, P.: Von Willebrand's disease. Acta Haemat. 27: 65-77, 1962.

Peake, I. R., Bloom, A. L. and Giddings, J. C.: Inherited variants of Factor-VII related protein in Von Willebrand's disease. J. Med. 291: 113-117, 1974.

Quick, A. J.: Telangiectasia: its relationship to the Minot-von Willebrand syndrome. Am. J. Med. Sci. 254: 585-601, 1967.

Raccuglia, G. and Neel, J. V.: Congenital vascular defect associated with platelet abnormality and antihemophilic factor deficiency. Blood 15: 807-829, 1960.

Simone, J. V., Cornet, J. A. and Abildgaard, C. F.: Acquired von Willebrand's syndrome in systemic lupus erythematosus. Blood 31: 806-812, 1968.

Strauss, H. S. and Bloom, G. E.: Von Willebrand's disease: use of a platelet-adhesiveness test in diagnosis and family investigation. New Eng. J. Med. 273: 171-181, 1965.

Veltkamp, J. J. and Van Tilburg, N. H.: Detection of heterozygotes for recessive von Willebrand's disease by the assay of antihemophilic-factor-like antigen. New Eng. J. Med. 289: 882-885, 1973.

Von Willebrand, E. A.: Ueber hereditaere Pseudohaemophilie. Acta Med. Scand. 76: 521-550, 1931.

Weiss, H. J.: Von Willebrand's disease — diagnostic criteria. Blood 32: 668-679, 1968.

*19350 WAARDENBURG SYNDROME

The features are wide bridge of the nose owing to lateral displacement of the inner canthus of each eye, pigmentary disturbance (frontal white blaze of hair, heterochromia iridis, white eye lashes, leukoderma), and cochlear deafness. The severity varies widely and some affected persons escape deafness. Lateral displacement of the inner canthi is seen also in the orodigitofacial syndrome (X-linked). The disorder has been described in the American Negro (Hansen, Ackaouy and Crump, 1965) and the Maori (Houghton, 1964) as well as in Europeans. Cleft palate and-or lip occurs in some cases. Premature graying of the hair is an effect of the gene. The fundus may be albinotic completely or partially and depigmented areas like piebald trait (q.v.) may be present elsewhere. In the state of South Australia, the Waardenburg syndrome is a leading cause of deafness and 'enjoys' a position comparable to porphyria in South Africa having been introduced by early settlers who have many descendants (Fraser, 1967). The white forelock may be present at birth and later disappear (Feingold et al., 1967). An affected Chinese family was reported by Chew et al. (1968). The work of Bosher and Hallpike (1966) on an animal analog might have important implications for prevention of deafness. Their work with deaf white cats suggested that destruction of the inner ear mechanism occurs in the first days of extra-uterine life and was correlated with an inability to regulate properly the constitution of the endolymphatic fluid. The cat, like man, may escape deafness in one or both ears. If we knew more of the factors that lead to retention of hearing we might be able to prevent deafness. Skipped generations and the occurrence of bilateral cleft lip were documented by Giacoia and Klein (1969). Laestadius et al. (1969) provided normal standards for the measurement of inner canthal and outer canthal distance. Standards were also presented by Christian et al. (1969). Klein's name is sometimes combined with Waardenburg's in the eponymic designation of this disorder, on the basis of a patient which Klein (1949) described with 'partial albinism,' blue eyes, deaf-mutism, undeveloped muscles and fused joints in the arms, skeletal dysplasia etc. This was rather clearly a separate disorder.

Bosher, S. K. and Hallpike, C. S.: Observations on the histogenesis of the inner ear degeneration of the deaf white cat and its possible relationship to the aetiology of certain unexplained varieties of human congenital deafness. J. Laryng. 80: 222-235, 1966.

Chew, K. L., Chen, A. J. and Tan, K. H.: A Chinese family with Waardenburg's syndrome. Am. J. Ophthal. 65: 174-182, 1968.

Christian, J. C., Bixler, D., Blythe, S. C. and Merritt, A. D.: Familial telecanthus with associated congenital anomalies. The Clinical Delineation of Birth Defects. II. Malformation Syndromes. New York: National Foundation, 1969. Pp. 82-85.

David, T. J. and Warin, R. P.: Waardenburg's syndrome in two siblings, both parents and their maternal grandmother. Proc. Roy. Soc. Med. 65: 601-602, 1972.

Feingold, M., Robinson, M. J. and Gellis, S. S.: Waardenburg's syndrome during the first year of life. J. Pediat. 71: 874-876, 1967.

Fraser, G. R.: Adelaide, Australia: personal communication, 1967.

Giacoia, J. P. and Klein, S. W.: Waardenburg's syndrome with bilateral cleft lip. Am. J. Dis. Child. 117: 344-348, 1969.

Goldberg, M. F.: Waardenburg's syndrome with fundus and other anomalies. Arch. Ophthal. 76: 797-810, 1966.

Hansen, A. C., Ackaouy, G. and Crump, E. P.: Waardenburg's syndrome: report of a pedigree. J. Nat. Med. Ass. 57: 8-12, 1965.

Houghton, N. I.: Waardenburg's syndrome with deafness as the presenting symptom. Report of two cases. New Zealand J. Med. 63: 83-89, 1964.

Klein, D.: Albinisme partiel (leucisme) avec surdi-mutite, blepharophimosis et dysplasie myo-osteo-articulaire. Helvet. Paediat. Acta 5: 38-58, 1950.

Laestadius, N. D., Aase, J. M. and Smith, D. W.: Normal inner canthal and outer orbital dimensions. J. Pediat. 74: 465-468, 1969.

McKusick, V. A.: Congenital deafness and Hirschsprung's disease. (Letter) New Eng. J. Med. 288: 691 only, 1973.

Settelmayer, J. R. and Hogan, M.: Waardenburg's syndrome — report of a case in a non-Dutch family. New Eng. J. Med. 264: 500-501, 1961.

Simpson, J. L., Falk, C. T., Morillo-Cucci, G., Allen, F. H., Jr. and German, J.: Analysis for possible linkage between the loci for the Waardenburg syndrome and various blood groups and serological traits. Humangenetik 23: 45-50, 1974.

19360 WEYERS OLIGODACTYLY SYNDROME

This syndrome is characterized by the association of deficiency of ulna and ulnar rays, antecubital pterygia, reduced sternal segments, and malformation of the kidney and spleen with cleft lip, cleft palate. The two reported cases were sporadic.

Weyers, H.: Das Oligodactylie syndrom des Menschen und seine Parallelmutation bei der Hausmaus. Ann. Paediat. 189: 351-370, 1957.

*19370 WHISTLING FACE-WINDMILL VANE HAND SYNDROME (CRANIOCARPOTARSAL DYSTROPHY: FREEMAN-SHELDON SYNDROME)

In craniocarpotarsal dystrophy, a syndrome first described by Freeman and Sheldon (1938), certain skeletal malformations are associated with facial characteristics. The skeletal malformations are mainly, in the hands, camptodactyly with ulnar deviation, in the feet, talipes equinovarus, and in the skull, an abnormal X-ray appearance of the floor of the anterior cranial fossa. The facial characteristics are deep-sunken eyes with hypertelorism, increased philtrum length, small nose and nostrils and a small mouth. Rintala (1968) described a case. He accepted only Freeman and Sheldon's and Otto's as 'genuine.' Steep anterior cerebral fossa was striking in his patient. He also pointed out in his and the other patients vertical 'folds of skin in the jaw.' In a study of genetic factors in hand malformations Temtamy (1966) noted the occurrence of this syndrome in two generations of three different families. Jacquemain (1966) described congenital windmill vane position of the hand: bilateral ulnar deviation and contracture of fingers II-V at the metacarpophalangeal joints with adduction of thumbs. The deformity resembled that of rheumatoid arthritis. Clubfoot was also present. They found that 7 were affected in four generations. 14 of 23 cases in the literature were familial and cases occurred in successive generations with father-to-son transmission. The defect was thought to concern the palmar fascia. This type of deformity, especially when combined with clubfoot, might mistakenly be called arthrogryposis multiplex congenita. Weinstein and Gorlin (1969) gave a full clinical description and referred to observation of affected father and daughter by Fraser (personal communication). They also suggested 'dysplasia' as more appropriate than 'dystrophy.' Cervenka, Figalova and Gorlin (1969) provided normal standards for the measurement of oral intercommissural distance in children. Fraser et al. (1970) reported the syndrome in father and son. Dramatic pictures of Fraser and Pashayan's example of affected father and son have been published (Gellis and Feingold, 1970). Autosomal dominant inheritance was well documented by Aalam (1972).

Aalam, M. and Kuhhirt, M.: Angeborene Windmuehlenfluegeldeformitaet der Finger. Z. Orthop. 110: 395-398, 1972.

Burian, F.: The 'whistling face' characteristic in a compound cranio-facio-corporal syndrome. Brit. J. Plast. Surg. 16: 140-143, 1963.

Cervenka, J., Figalova, P. and Gorlin, R. J.: Cranio-carpo-tarsal dysplasia or the whistling face syndrome. II. Oral intercommissural distance in children. Am. J. Dis. Child. 117: 434-435, 1969.

Cervenka, J., Gorlin, R. J., Figalova, P. and Farkasova, J.: Craniocarpotarsal dysplasia or whistling face syndrome. Arch. Otolaryng. 91: 183-187, 1970.

Fraser, F. C., Pashayan, H. and Kadish, M. E.: Cranio-carpo-tarsal dysplasia. Report of a case in father and son. J.A.M.A. 211: 1374-1376, 1970.

Freeman, E. A. and Sheldon, J. H.: Cranio-carpotarsal dystrophy: undescribed congenital malformation. Arch. Dis. Child. 13: 277-283, 1938.

Gellis, S. S., Feingold, M. and Gorlin, R. J.: Picture of the month. Oral-facial-digital syndrome. Am. J. Dis. Child. 120: 241-242, 1970.

Jacquemain, B.: Die angeborene Windmuehlenfluegelstellung als erbliche Kombinationsmissbildung. Z. Orthop. 102: 146-154, 1966.

Lundblom, A.: On congenital ulnar deviation of the fingers of familial occurrence ('deviation des doigts en coup de vent'). Acta Orthop. Scand. 3: 393-404, 1932.

Otto, F. M.: Die cranio-carpo-tarsal Dystrophie (Freeman and Sheldon) ein rasuistischer Beitrag. Z. Kinderheilk. 73: 240-250, 1953.

Rintala, A. E.: Freeman-Sheldon's syndrome, cranio-carpo-tarsal dystrophy. Acta Paediat. Scand. 57: 553-556, 1968.

Sharma, R. N. and Tandon, S. N.: 'Whistling face' deformity in compound cranio-facio-corporal syndrome. Brit. Med. J. 4: 33 Only, 1970.

Temtamy, S. A.: Genetic Factors in Hand Malformations. Ph. D. Thesis, Johns Hopkins University, 1966.

Weinstein, S. and Gorlin, R. J.: Cranio-carpo-tarsal dysplasia or the whistling face syndrome. I. Clinical considerations. Am. J. Dis. Child. 117: 427-433, 1969.

*19380 WHITE HAIR, PREMATURE

Hare (1929) described 9 cases in 5 generations with male-to-male transmission. Onset of whitening was in the teens.

Hare, H. J. H.: Premature whitening of the hair. J. Hered. 20: 31-32, 1929.

*19390 WHITE SPONGE NEVUS OF CANNON

This disorder is manifested by thickened spongy fold mucosa in the mouth with a white opalescent tint. It may be the same as the condition referred to by Zegarelli, Everett and Kutscher (1961) as white folded hyperplasia of the mucous membranes. It is differentiated from benign intraepithelial dyskeratosis (q.v.) by the presence of vaginal and anal lesions and the absence of conjunctival involvement and the characteristic cell-within-cell histologic change. Scott (1966) found three generations affected. Haye and Whitehead (1968) reported on 7 cases in 3 generations with male-to-male transmission. Verma (1967) described the disorder in Asiatic Indians.

Browne, W. G., Izatt, M. M. and Renwick, J. H.: White sponge naevus of the mucosa: clinical and linkage data. Ann. Hum. Genet. 32: 271-282, 1969.

Haye, K. R. and Whitehead, F. I. H.: Hereditary leukokeratosis of the mucous membranes. Brit. J. Derm. 80: 529-533, 1968.

Scott, C. R.: Hereditary leukokeratosis, white mouth. J. Pediat. 68: 768-772, 1966.

Verma, B. S.: Hereditary mucosal keratosis. Indian J. Med. Sci. 21: 310-313, 1967.

Witkop, C. J. and Gorlin, R. J.: Four hereditary mucosal syndromes. Arch. Derm. 84: 762-771, 1961.

Zegarelli, E. V., Everett, F. G. and Kutscher, A. H.: Familial white folded dysplasia of the mucous membranes. An atlas of oral lesions. Oral Surg. 14: 1436-1443, 1961.

19400 WIDOW'S PEAK

A pointed frontal hairline may be inherited as a dominant. For picture see P. 359 of Winchester. Smith and Cohen (1973) pointed out an association between ocular hypertelorism and widow's peak.

Smith, D. W. and Cohen, M. M.: Widow's peak scalp-hair anomaly and it's relation to ocular hypertelorism. Lancet II: 1127-1128, 1973.

Winchester, A. M.: Genetics. Boston: Houghton Mifflin Co., 1958 (2nd Ed.).

19410 WISDOM TEETH, ABSENCE OF

Gruneberg (1936) described a family in which a mother and four of five children lacked some or all wisdom teeth. The evidence for simple dominant inheritance is meager.

Gruneberg, H.: Two independent inherited tooth anomalies in one family. J. Hered. 27: 225-228, 1936.

19420 WOLFF-PARKINSON-WHITE SYNDROME

The features of this electrocardiographic syndrome are short PR interval and prolonged QRS, specifically with a slurred-up stroke of the R wave called a delta wave. The patients are prone to paroxysmal supra-ventricular tachycardia. The familial occurrence of the Wolff-Parkinson-White syndrome has been reported many times (Harnischfeger, 1959). In at least two reported families it has been associated with familial cardiomyopathy (Massumi, 1967). Schneider (1969) observed affected mother and son.

Harnischfeger, W. W.: Hereditary occurrence of the pre-excitation (Wolff-Parkinson-White) syndrome with re-entry mechanism and concealed conduction. Circulation 19: 28-40, 1959.

Massumi, R. A.: Familial Wolff-Parkinson-White syndrome with cardiomyopathy. Am. J. Med. 43: 951-955, 1967.

Schneider, R. G.: Familial occurrence of Wolff-Parkinson-White syndrome. Am. Heart J. 78: 34-36, 1969.

*19430 WOOLLY HAIR

The hair is short, tightly curled and woolly, resembling that of a Negro. Mohr (1932) considered Negro admixture very unlikely in the Norwegian kindred with many persons affected. Anderson (1936) and Schokking (1934) also reported Caucasian families with many affected. Anderson (1936), who had close familiarity with Negro hair, felt that the woolly hair was different.

Anderson, E.: An American pedigree for woolly hair. J. Hered. 27: 444 Only, 1936.

Mohr, O. L.: Woolly hair, a dominant mutant character in man. J. Hered. 23: 345-352, 1932.

Sanders, J.: Eine Familie mit Kraushaar. Genetica 18: 97-104, 1936.

Schokking, C. P.: Another woolly hair mutation in man. J. Hered. 25: 337-340, 1934.

19440 XERODERMA PIGMENTOSUM

In addition to the usual severe, recessively inherited xeroderma pigmentosum, the existence of a milder form behaving as a dominant has been claimed by Anderson and Begg (1950) who described 11 affected persons in 5 sibships of four generations of a Scottish family by the name of MacPherson. The patients showed freckling and multiple skin cancers as in the recessive form but did not get trouble as early in life and survived longer. Indeed, Anderson and Begg examined one affected member of the family who was 74 years of age. No affected member was said to have died of the disease.

Anderson, T. E. and Begg, M.: Xeroderma pigmentosum of mild type. Brit. J. Derm. 62: 402-407, 1950.

AUTOSOMAL RECESSIVE PHENOTYPES

Features are celiac syndrome, pigmentary degeneration of the retina, progressive ataxic neuropathy, and a peculiar 'burr-cell' malformation of the red cells called acanthocytosis (sometimes incorrectly written 'acanthrocytosis'). Intestinal absorption of lipids is defective, serum cholesterol very low and serum beta lipoprotein absent. Few cases have to date been discovered and almost all have been Jews. Autopsy (Sobrevilla et al., 1964) and biopsy of peripheral nerves show extensive central and peripheral demyelination. Lees (1967) demonstrated that the lipid-free apoprotein of beta-lipoprotein is present in abetalipoproteinemia. The defect must concern formation of the complete macromolecule. See LIPID TRANSPORT DEFECT OF INTESTINE for a disorder with some of the same features as abetalipoproteinemia.

Dische, M. R. and Porro, R. S.: The cardiac lesions in Bassen-Kornzweig syndrome. Report of a case, with autopsy findings. Am. J. Med. 49: 568-571, 1970.

Dodge, J. T., Cohen, G., Kayden, H. J. and Phillips, G. B.: Peroxidative hemolysis of red blood cells from patients with abetalipoproteinemia (acanthocytosis). J. Clin. Invest. 46: 357-368, 1967.

Fredrickson, D. S., Gotto, A. M. and Levy, R. I.: Familial lipoprotein deficiency. In, Stanbury, J. B., Wyngaarden, J. B. and Fredrickson, D. S. (eds.): The Metabolic Basis of Inherited Disease. New York: McGraw-Hill, 1972 (3rd Ed.). Pp. 493-530.

Isselbacher, K. J., Scheig, R., Plotkin, G. R. and Caulfield, J. B.: Congenital beta-lipoprotein deficiency: an hereditary disorder involving a defect in the absorption and transport of lipids. Medicine 43: 347-361, 1964.

Lees, R. S.: Immunological evidence for the presence of Beta protein (apoprotein of beta-lipoprotein) in normal and abetalipoproteinemia plasma. J. Lipid. Res. 8: 396-405, 1967.

Mier, M., Schwartz, S. O. and Boshes, B.: Acanthocytosis, pigmentary degeneration of the retina and ataxic neuropathy: a genetically determined syndrome with associated metabolic disorder. Blood 16: 1586-1608, 1960.

Salt, H. B., Wolff, O. H., Lloyd, J. K., Fosbrooke, A. S., Cameron, A. H. and Hubble, D. V.: On having no beta-lipoprotein. A syndrome comprising a-beta-lipoproteinaemia, acanthocytosis and steatorrhoea. Lancet II: 325-329, 1960.

Schwartz, J. F., Rowland, L. P., Eder, H., Marks, P. A., Osserman, E. F., Hirschberg, E. and Anderson, H.: Bassen-Kornzweig syndrome. Deficiency of serum beta-lipoprotein. Arch. Neurol. 8: 438-454, 1963.

Sobrevilla, L. A., Goodman, M. L. and Kane, C. A.: Demyelinating central nervous system disease, macular atrophy and acanthocytosis (Bassen-Kornzweig syndrome). Am. J. Med. 37: 821-832, 1964.

20013 ABSENT EYEBROWS AND EYELASHES WITH MENTAL RETARDATION (PSEUDOPRO-GERIA SYNDROME)

Hall et al. (1974) reported two brothers with mental retardation, absence of eyebrows and eyelashes, progressive spastic quadroplegia, micrcephaly, glaucoma, small and beaked nose. One had had a 'cervical spinal cyst' removed at age 1 year and the second had occipital cranium bifidum occulatum. The parents were unrelated. They and three brothers were normal.

Hall, B. D., Berg, B. O., Rudolph, R. S. and Epstein, C. J.: Pseudoprogeria — Hallermann-Streiff (PHS) syndrome. Birth Defects Orig. Art. Ser. 10 (7): 137-146, 1974.

*20015 ACANTHOCYTOSIS

Cederbaum et al. (1971) observed a family in which three sibs had developed progressive chorea and dementia and had acanthocytes in the peripheral blood. A brother and sister had died at ages 32 and 39 and the proband was a 41-year-old-male. Both parents were healthy but consanguineous. Two children of the proband were healthy. They suggested that the same disorder may have been present in the family of Critchley et al. (1967, 1970). Although in that family the disorder was thought to be dominant (10050), the inheritance could be recessive.

Cederbaum, S., Heywood, D., Aigner, R. and Motulsky, A.: Progressive chorea, dementia and acanthocytosis: a genocopy of Huntington's chorea. Clin. Res. 19: 177 only, 1971.

*20020 ACATALASEMIA

Acatalasia was first discovered in Japan by Takahara, an otolaryngologist, who, in cases of progressive oral gangrene, found that peroxide applied to the ulcerated areas did not froth in the usual manner. Heterozygotes have an intermediate level of catalase in the blood. The frequency of the gene, although relatively high in Japan, is variable. The frequency of heterozygotes is 0.09 percent in Hiroshima and Nagasaki but is of the order of 1.4 percent in other parts of Japan (Hamilton et al., 1961). Acatalasia has been detected in Switzerland (Aebi et al., 1962), and in Israel (Szeinberg et al., 1963). In both of the latter situations the homozygotes showed some residual catalase activity suggesting that this may be a different mutation than that responsible for the Japanese disease in which catalase activity is zero and no cross-reacting material has been identified. Hamilton and Neel (1963) presented evidence that at least two forms of acatalasia exist in Japan. In an extensive kindred with acatalasia in two sibships, heterozygotes showed catalase values overlapping with the normal. Hypocatalasia has also been found in the guinea pig, dog and domestic fowl (see review by Lush, 1966). Electrophoretic variants of red cell catalase have been described (see dominant catalog). These may be determined by genes allelic with that for acatalasemia. Shibata et al. (1967) found that an immunologically reactive but enzymatically inactive protein about one-sixth the size of active catalase is present in red cells of acatalasemics.

R
E
C
E
S
S
I
V
E

Aebi, H. and Suter, H.: Acatalasia. In, Stanbury, J. B., Wyngaarden, J. B. and Fredrickson, D. S. (eds.): The Metabolic Basis of Inherited Disease. New York: McGraw-Hill, 1972 (3rd Ed.). Pp. 1710-1729.

Aebi, H., Baggiolini, M., Dewald, B., Lauber, E., Sutter, H., Micheli, A. and Frei, J.: Obervations in two Swiss families with acatalasia. Enzym. Biol. Clin. 4: 121-151, 1964.

Aebi, H., Jeunet, F., Richterich, R., Suter, H., Butler, R., Frei, J. and Marti, H. R.: Observations in two Swiss families with acatalasia. Enzym. Biol. Clin. 2: 1-22, 1962.

Baur, E. W.: Catalase abnormality in a Caucasian family in the United States. Science 140: 816-817, 1963.

Feinstein, R. N., Howard, J. B., Braun, J. T. and Seaholm, J. E.: Acatalasemic and hypocatalasemic mouse mutants. Genetics 53: 923-933, 1966.

Hamilton, H. B. and Neel, J. V.: Genetic heterogeneity in human acatalasia. Am. J. Hum. Genet. 15: 408-419, 1963.

Hamilton, H. B., Neel, J. V., Kobara, T. Y. and Ozaki, K.: The frequency in Japan of carriers of the rare 'recessive' gene causing acatalasemia. J. Clin. Invest. 40: 2199-2208, 1961.

Lush, I. E.: The Biochemical Genetics of Vertebrates Except Man. Philadelphia: W. B. Saunders, 1966.

Matsubara, S., Suter, H. and Aebi, H.: Fractionation of erythrocyte catalase from normal, hypocatalatic and acatalatic humans. Humangenetik 4: 29-41, 1967.

Shibata, Y., Higashi, T., Hirai, H. and Hamilton, H. B.: Immunochemical studies on catalase. II. An anticatalase reacting component in normal hypocatalasic, and acatalasic human erythrocytes. Arch. Biochem. 118: 200-209, 1967.

Szeinberg, A., De Vries, A., Pinkhas, J., Djaldetti, M. and Ezra, R.: A dual hereditary red blood cell defect in one family: hypocatalasemia and glucose-6-phosphate dehydrogenase deficiency. Acta Genet. Med. Gem. 12: 247-255, 1963.

*20030 ACETOPHENETIDIN SENSITIVITY

Shahidi (1967) described a 17-year-old girl with severe methemoglobinemia and hemolysis following ingestion of acetophenetidin. The activity of G6PD, 6PGD, diaphorase, and glutathione reductase was normal, as was also the concentration of reduced glutathione. Hemoglobin was physically normal. Previously unknown metabolites of acetophenetidin were found in the urine. A 38-year-old sister showed the same abnormality. Inadequate deethylation was suggested with increased hydroxylation of acetophenetidin to hydroxypheneti-din which was thought to be responsible for methemoglobin production. Phenobarbital administration had adverse effects possibly by stimulation of the hydroxylation process. The parents were not related. The family was of German extraction (Shahidi, 1967).

Shahidi, N. T.: Acetophenetidin sensitivity. Am. J. Dis. Child. 113: 81-82, 1967.

Shahidi, N. T.: Acetophenetidin — induced methemoglobinemia. Ann. N.Y. Acad. Sci. 151: 822-832, 1968.

Shahidi, N. T.: Milwaukee, Wis.: personal communication, 1967.

20040 ACHALASIA, FAMILIAL ESOPHAGEAL

Thibert et al. (1965) described two families each with two affected sibs under 16 years of age. Cloud et al. (1966) observed the disorder in 4 full-blooded Apache Indian sibs less than 6 years old. Polonsky and Guth (1970) reported the condition in two sibs, and possibly a third, all less than 5 years old. Dayalan et al. (1972) reported 3 documented and 4 probable cases of achalasia cardia among a sibship of 8. The parents were of an uncle-niece consanguineous marriage. Koivukangas et al. (1973) found Sjogren syndrome and achalasia in two sisters. (This Sjogren syndrome consists of the triad of keratoconjunctivitis sicca, xerostomia, and rheumatoid arthritis or other connective tissue disease.) Vaughan and Williams (1973) described two male sibs, ages 8 and 2, with achalasia. Both presented with pulmonary complications caused by their achalasia.

Cloud, D. T., Jr., White, R. F., Linkner, L. M. and Taylor, L. C.: Surgical treatment of esophageal achalasia in children. J. Pediat. Surg. 1: 137-144, 1966.

Dayalan, N., Chettur, L. and Ramakrishnan, M. S.: Achalasia of the cardia in sibs. Arch. Dis. Child. 47: 115-118, 1972.

Koivukagas, T., Simila, S., Heikkinen, E., Rasanen, O. and Wasz-Hachert, O.: Sjogren's syndrome and achalasis of the cardia in two siblings. Pediat. 51: 943-945, 1973.

Polonsky, L. and Guth, P. H.: Familial achalasia. Am. J. Digest. Dis. 15: 291-295, 1970.

Thibert, F., Chicoine, R., Chartier-Ratelle, G.: Forme familiale de l'achalasie de l'oesophage chez l'enfant. Un. Med. Canada 94: 1293-1300, 1965.

Vaughan, W. H. and Williams, J. L.: Familial achalasia with pulmonary complications in children. Radiology 107: 407-410, 1973.

*20050 ACHEIROPODY (BRAZILIAN TYPE)

Absence of hands and feet has probably been observed only in multiple members of an inbred Brazilian kindred of Portuguese ancestry. The hands and feet are missing so that the arms and legs end as stumps. Toledo et al. (1972) gave further data on the kindred together with an updated pedigree.

Bohomoletz, M.: Further light on the handless and footless family of Brazil. Eugen. News 15: 143-145, 1930.

Koehler, O.: Die Hand- und Fusslosen brasilianischen Geschwister. Ein Beitrag zur Frage der Erbbedingheit angeborener Missbildungen. Z. Menschl. Vererb. Konstitutionsl. 19: 670-690, 1936.

Quelce-Salgado, A., Freire-Maia, N. and Koehler, R. A.: Marilia and Curitiba, Brazil: personal communication, 1966.

Toledo, S. P. A. and Saldanha, P. H.: A radiological and genetic investigation of acheiropody in a kindred including six cases. J. Genet. Hum. 17: 81-94, 1969.

*20060 ACHONDROGENESIS, TYPE I (PARENTI-FRACCARO OR LETHAL TYPE)

Two quite distinct disorders have been given the name achondrogenesis. That described by Parenti (1936) and by Fraccaro (1952) is a severe chondrodystrophy characterized radiographically by deficient ossification in the lumbar vertebrae and absent ossification in the sacral, pubic and ischial bones and clinically by stillbirth or early death (Maroteaux and Lamy, 1968; Langer et al., 1969). Houston (1970) has observed 4 sibs with achondrogenesis out of a family of 9. Enchondral ossification was lacking between resting cartilage cells. There is almost certainly heterogeneity within achondrogenesis I. Laxova et al. (1973) described a family in which three stillborn sibs (2 males, 1 female) from a first-cousin marriage were affected. Fibroblast cultures showed numerous large intracellular lipid inclusions. The mother showed the same to a lesser degree. The use of the finding in prenatal diagnosis was discussed. Wiedemann et al. (!974) pointed out the importance of distinguishing hypophosphatasia (24150).

Fraccaro, M.: Contributo allo studio delle malattie del mesenchima osteopoietico. L'Acondrogenesi. Folia Hered. Path. 1: 190-208, 1952.

Houston, C. S.: Saskatoon, Saskatchewan, Canada: personal communication, 1970.

Houston, C. S., Awen, C. F. and Kent, H. P.: Fatal neonatal dwarfism. J. Canad. Ass. Radiol. 23: 45-61, 1972.

Langer, L. O., Jr., Spranger, J. W., Greinacher, I. and Herdman, R. C.: Thanatophoric dwarfism. A condition confused with achondroplasia in the neonate, with brief comments on achondrogenesis and homozygous achondroplasia. Radiology 92: 285-294, 1969.

Laxova, R., O'Hara, P. T., Ridler, M. A. C. and Timothy, J. A. D.: Family with probable achondrogenesis and lipid inclusions in fibroblasts. Arch. Dis. Child. 48: 212-216, 1973.

Maroteaux, P. and Lamy, M.: Le diagnostic des nanismes chondro-dystrophiques chez les nouveau-nes. Arch. Franc. Pediat. 25: 241-262, 1968.

Parenti, G. C.: La anosteogenesi (una varieta della osteogenesi imperfetta). Pathologica 28: 447-462, 1936.

Saldino, R. M.: Lethal short-limbed dwarfism: achondrogenesis and thanatophoric dwarfism. Am. J. Roentgen. 112: 185-197, 1971.

Wiedemann, H.-R., Remagen, W., Hienz, H. A., Gorlin, R. J. and Maroteaux, P.: Achondrogenesis within the scope of connately manifested generalized skeletal dysplasias. Z. Kinderheilk, 116: 223-251, 1974.

*20061 ACHONDROGENESIS, TYPE IB

Spranger et al. (1974) distinguishes two forms of achondrogenesis, which they call types I and II and which we call here types IA and IB because 'achondrogeneisi, type II' is used for a quite different disorder (20070). Type IA is the classic variety described by Parenti, Fraccaro, and Houston et al. (see 20060) for references). It also is the type in which the ribs tend to be thin often with multiple fractures leading Harris et al. (1972) to refer to it as pseudoachondrogenesis with fractures. Indeed it might be confused with the broad-bone form of osteogenesis imperfecta (25940). Type IB achondrogenesis (type II of Spranger et al.) is characterized by virtual absence of ossification in the vertebral column, sacrum and public bones. Saldino (see 20060) reported on this form. In both forms the trunk is short with prominent abdomen and hydropic appearance. Micromelia is striking. In both death occurs in utero or the early neonatal period.

Harris, R., Patton, I. T. and Barson, A. J.: Pseudo-achondrogenesis with fractures. Clin. Genet. 3: 435-441, 1972.

*20070 ACHONDROGENESIS, TYPE II (GREBE OR BRAZILIAN TYPE)

Grebe (1952, 1955) described the disorder in 7- and 11-year-old sisters, offspring of a consanguineous mating. The same disorder was found in Brazil by Quelce-Salgado (1964). In these cases all four limbs are markedly shortened and end in tiny digits. The trunk and head are normal. A case with childhood and adult radiographic studies was presented by Scott (1969).

Grebe, H.: Chondrodysplasie. Rome: Inst. Greg. Mendel, 1955. Pp. 300-303.

Grebe, H.: Die Achondrogenesis: ein einfach rezessives Erbmerkmal. Folia Hered. Path. 2: 23-28, 1952.

Quelce-Salgado, A.: A new type of dwarfism with various bone aplasias and hypoplasias of the extremities. Acta Genet. Statist. Med. 14: 63-66, 1964.

Scott, C. I.: Discussion. The Clinical Delineation of Birth Defects. IV. Skeletal Dysplasias. New York: National Foundation, 1969. Pp. 14-16.

20080 ACHONDROPLASIA

Whether achondroplasia completely indistinguishable from the achondroplasia which is demonstrably dominant is ever inherited as a recessive is a mooted matter. Documentation of the diagnosis is inadequate in most reports of possible recessive inheritance. Cohn and Weinberg (1956) reported affected twins with an affected sib. (This may have been achondrogenesis, q.v.). Chiari (1913) reported affected half-sibs. The father was the same. I have observed two cousins with undoubted achondroplasia, a male and female. The mothers are sisters. Most dominants show sufficient variability to account for observations such as these on the basis of reduced penetrance but such is not the case with achondroplasia. Gonadal mosaicism (or spermatogonial mutation) is a possible explanation for affected sibs from normal parents. Affected cousins could be coincidence of two mutations. Durr (1968) described an achondroplastic-like disorder in two sibs. Retardation of growth, micromelia and square iliac wings resembled achondroplasia. Spine and other pelvic changes of achondroplasia were missing.

Chiari, H.: Ueber familiare Chondrodystrophia foetalis. Munchen. Med. Wschr. 60: 248-249, 1913.

Cohn, S. and Weinberg, A.: Identical hydrocephalic achondroplastic twins. Subsequent delivery of single sibling with same abnormality. Am. J. Obstet. Gynec. 72: 1346-1348, 1956.

Durr, D. K.: Eine neue Dysostoseform mit Mikromelie bei zwei Geschwistern. Helv. Paediat. Acta 23: 184-194, 1968.

*20090 'ACHONDROPLASIA' AND SWISS-TYPE AGAMMAGLOBULINEMIA

Davis (1967) stated that at least five cases are known to him. The case he personally described was a female infant whose parents were Jewish but not known to be related. The child died at 2 months of age. Gatti et al. (1969) described affected brother and sister. They suggested that other cases had been reported by McKusick and Cross (1966), Davis (1966), Fulginiti et al. (1967), Alexander and Dunbar (1968). Say et al. (1972) reported two affected Turkish sibs. The skeletal dysplasia in these cases may be best classified as a metaphyseal chondrodysplasia. Differentiation from a cartilage-hair hypoplasia (21230) is not completely certain. I saw a family studied by Mathies (1972) in which the skeletal changes are typical of CHH including 'metaphyseal dysostosis' by X-ray, excessively long fibulas, Harrison grooves, etc. The hair was light in color and required cutting less often than one would expect but its caliber appeared normal. All three children were affected. The oldest had secondary vaccinia after routine vaccination and is reported by Fulginiti (1968) — see case M. N., p. 135. Mandi et al. (1971) found a profound disturbance in endochondral ossification in albino rats thymectonized 36-48 hours after birth. Other manifestations of runting were present. Main laboratory findings are lymphopenia, agammaglobulinemia and, by X-ray, thymic hypoplasia. These and the clinical course are like those in Swiss-type agammeglobulinemia (20250).

Alexander, W. J. and Dunbar, J. S.: Unusual bone changes in thymic alymphoplasia. Ann. Radiol. 11: 389-394, 1968.

Davis, J. A.: A case of Swiss-type agammaglobulinaemia and achondroplasia. Brit. J. Med. 2: 1371-1374, 1966.

Davis, J. A.: Swiss-type agammaglobulinaemia and achondroplasia. (Letter) Brit. Med. J. 3: 110 only, 1967.

Fulginiti, V. A., Hathaway, W. E., Pearlman, D. S. and Kempe, C. H.: Agammaglobulinaemia and achondroplasia. (Letter) Brit. Med. J. 2: 242 only, 1967.

Fulginiti, V. A., Kempe, C. H., Hathaway, W. E., Pearlman, D. S., Sieber, O. F., Jr., Eller, J. J., Joyner, J. J. and Robinson, A.: Immunologic Deficiency Diseases in Man. Birth Defects Orig. Art. Series. vol. 4 (no. 1): 129-151, 1968.

Gatti, R. A., Platt, N., Pomerance, H. H., Hong, R., Langer, L. O., Kay, H. E. M. and Good, R. A.: Hereditary lymphopenic agammaglobulinemia associated with a distinctive form of short — limbed dwarfism and ectodermal dysplasia. J. Pediat. 75: 675-684, 1969.

Mandi, B., Hadhazy, C., Mandi, A. and Glant, T.: Effect of postnatal thymectomy on enchondral ossification. Acta Morph. Acad. Sci. Hung. 19: 259-268, 1971.

Mathies, A. W.: Los Angeles, Calif.: personal communication, 1972.

McKusick, V. A. and Cross, H. E.: Ataxia-telangiectasia and Swiss-type agammaglobulinemia. Two genetic disorders of the immune mechanism in related Amish sibships. J.A.M.A. 195: 739-745, 1966.

Say, B., Tinazteppe, B. and Tinazteppe, K.: Thymic dysplasia associated with dyschondroplasia in an infant. Am. J. Dis. Child. 123: 240-244, 1972.

*20095 ACID PHOSPHATASE DEFICIENCY

Nadler and Egan (1970) discovered this disorder. The clinical features are intermittent vomiting, hypotonia, lethargy, opisthotonos, terminal bleeding and death in early infancy. Lysosomal acid phosphatase is deficient in cultured fibroblasts and multiple tissues. Prenatal diagnosis was possible. The parents were first cousins. After treatment with phytohemagglutinin, lymphocytes from heterozygotes and controls could be distinguished. It may be lysosomal acid phosphatase which has been found to be polymorphic (see 17160).

Nadler, H. L. and Egan, T. J.: Deficiency of lysosomal acid phosphatase. A new familial metabolic disorder. New Eng. J. Med. 282: 303-307, 1970.

*20100 ACROCEPHALOPOLYSYNDACTYLY TYPE II (ACPS II, CARPENTER SYNDROME)

Carpenter (1909) described two sisters and a brother with acrocephaly, peculiar facies, brachydactyly, and syndactyly in the hands, and preaxial polydactyly and syndactyly of the toes. Temtamy (1966) could find 9 other reported cases and added one. In older patients obesity, mental retardation and hypogonadism have been noted. In all cases the parents have been normal. Parental consanguinity was suspected in one case. In the dominant catalog, see ACPS I and see POLYSYNDACTYLY WITH PECULIAR SKULL SHAPE. The case of acrocephalosyndactyly with foot polydactyly reported by Owen (1952) probably represented this entity, as do also the sibs reported by Schonenberg and Scheidhauer (1966). One patient thought to have this condition by Palacios and Schimke (1969) was 49-years-old. Eaton et al. (1974) reported affected sibs.

Carpenter, G.: Case of acrocephaly with other congenital malformations. Proc. Roy. Soc. Med. 2: 45-53, 199-201, 1909.

Eaton, A. P., Sommer, A., Kontras, S. B. and Sayers, M. P.: Carpenter syndrome — acrocephalopolysyndactyly type II. Birth Defects Orig. Art. Ser. 10: 249-260, 1974.

Owen, R. H.: Acrocephalosyndactyly: a case with congenital cardiac abnormalities. Brit. J. Radiol. 25: 103-106, 1952.

Palacios, E. and Schimke, R. N.: Craniosynostosis — syndactylism. Am. J. Roentgen. 106: 144-155, 1969.

Schonenberg, H. and Scheidhauer, E.: Uber zwei ungewohnliche Dyscranio-dysphalangien bei Geschwistern (atypische Akrocephalosyndaktylie und fragliche Dysencephalia splanchnocystica). Mschr. Kinderheilk. 114: 322-327, 1966.

Temtamy, S. A.: Carpenter's syndrome: acrocephalopolysyndactyly. An autosomal recessive syndrome. J. Pediat. 69: 111-120, 1966.

*20110 ACRODERMATITIS ENTEROPATHICA

The disorder is characterized by intermittent simultaneous occurrence of diarrhea and dermatitis with failure to thrive. Alopecia of the scalp, eyebrows and eyelashes is a usual feature. The skin lesions are bullous. Noteworthy is the cure by diodoquin, or diiodohydroxyquinoline (Dillaha and colleagues, 1953; Bloom and Sobel, 1955). Moynahan et al. (1963) found a deficiency of succinic dehydrogenase in intestinal mucosal cells by histochemical methods. One of two cases showed electron microscopic abnormality. Cash and Berger (1969) found defective interconversion of unsaturated fatty acids, in particular, in the synthesis of essential fatty acids. Rodin and Goldman (1969) described autopsy findings, including pancreatic islet hyperplasia, absence of the thymus and of germinal centers and plasmocytosis of lymph nodes and spleen.

Bloom, D. and Sobel, N.: Acrodermatitis enteropathica successfully treated with diodoquin. J. Invest. Derm. 24: 167-177, 1955.

Cash, R. and Berger, C. K.: Acrodermatitis enteropathica: defective metabolism of unsaturated fatty acids. J. Pediat. 74: 717-729, 1969.

Dillaha, C. J., Lorincz, A. L. and Aavik, O. R.: Acrodermatitis enteropathica. Review of the literature and report of a case successfully treated with diodoquin. J.A.M.A. 152: 509-512, 1953.

Lindstrom, B.: Familial acrodermatitis enteropathica in an adult. Acta Dermatovener. 43: 522-527, 1963.

Margileth, A. M.: Acrodermatitis enteropathica. Case report and review of literature. Am. J. Dis. Child. 105: 285-291, 1963.

Moynahan, E. J., Johnson, F. R. and McMinn, R. M. H.: Acrodermatitis enteropathica: demonstration of possible intestinal enzyme defect. Proc. Roy. Soc. Med. 56: 300-301, 1963.

Rodin, A. E. and Goldman, A. S.: Autopsy findings in acrodermatitis enteropathica. Am. J. Clin. Path. 51: 315-322, 1969.

Stevenson, J. R., Fidone, G. S. and Leland, L. S.: Acrodermatitis enteropathica. Arch. Derm. 89: 224-228, 1964.

Vedder, J. S.: Acrodermatitis enteropathica (Danbolt-Closs) in five siblings: efficacy of diodoquin in its management. J. Pediat. 48: 212-219, 1956.

20120 ACROGERIA

Gottron (1940) reported a brother and sister, 16-and 19-years-old, whose hands and feet had appeared old since infancy because of thin skin. General physical and mental development were normal. Less severe skin atrophy was present elsewhere. Huttova et al. (1967) also described affected sibs. The Ehlers-Danlos syndrome is often mis-diagnosed. Indeed this may be the ecchymotic, arterialor sack variety of Ehlers-Danlos syndrome (E-D IV). Some of the features are seen in mandibulacral dysplasia, a probably dominant disorder.

Calvert, H. T.: Acrogeria (Gottron type). Brit. J. Derm. 69: 69 only, 1957.

Gottron, H.: Familiare akrogerie. Arch. Derm. Syph. 181: 571-583, 1940.

Huttova, M., Rusnak, M. and Lysa, G.: Akrogeria. Cesk. Pediat. 22: 233-237, 1967.

*20125 ACROMESOMELIC DWARFISM

The forearms, hands and feet are predominantly involved. Adult height is about 120 cm. The radius is curved and the head is often dislocated posteriorly. The metacarpals, metatarsals and phalanges are particularly short. The phalanges are almost square. Despite some resemblances to pseudoachondroplastic dysplasia, epiphyseal and metaphyseal changes of pseudoachondroplasia are missing. In one case reported by Maroteaux et al. (1971) the parents were normal and first-cousins. In a second family two sisters were affected.

Maroteaux, P.: Acromesomelic dwarfism. In, Kaufmann, H. J.(ed.): Intrinsic Diseases of Bone. Vol. 4 of Progress in Pediatric Radiology. Basel S. Karger, 1973. Pp. 563-565.

Maroteaux, P., Martinelli, B. and Campailla, E.: Le nanisme acromesomelique. Presse Med. 79: 1839-1842, 1971.

Giaccai (1952) found four cases among the children of an Arab man who married two first cousins. By the first, one of the children was affected and by the second, three out of five were affected. The spinal cord was normal at autopsy. He concluded that the abnormality resides in peripheral sensory nerves. See INSENSITIVITY TO PAIN. Rimoin et al. (1972) have a well-studied family. See Van Bogaert-Hozay syndrome.

Giaccai, L.: Familial and sporadic neurogenic acro-osteolysis. Acta Radiol. 38: 17-29, 1952.

Hozay, J.: Sur une dystrophie familiale particuliere (inhibition precoce de la croissance et osteolyse non mutilante acrales avec dysmorphie faciale). Rev. Neurol. 89: 245-258, 1953.

Rimoin, D. L., Reed, W. B. and Hollister, D.: Torrance, Calif.: personal communication, 1972.

Van Bogaert, L.: Familial ulcers, mutilating lesions of the extremities and acro-osteolysis. Brit. Med. J. 2: 367-371, 1957.

20140 ACTH DEFICIENCY

Hung and Migeon (1968) described a 34-month-old Negro boy with apparent isolated ACTH deficiency. The adrenal medulla was unresponsive to insulin-induced hypoglycemia. Treatment of the adrenocortical insufficiency restored responsiveness. The enzyme phenylethanolamine-N-methyl transferase (PNMT) is localized to the adrenal medulla and catalyzes the N-methylation of norepinephrine to epinephrine. The activity of this enzyme is controlled by glucocorticoids. No familial cases have, it seems, been reported.

Hung, W. and Migeon, C. J.: Hypoglycemia in a two-year-old boy with adrenocorticotropic hormone (ACTH) deficiency (probably isolated) and adrenal medullary unresponsiveness to insulin-induced hypoglycemia. J. Clin. Endocr. 28: 146-152, 1968.

O'Dell, W. D., Green, G. M. and Williams, R. H.: Hypoadrenotropism: the isolated deficiency of adrenotropic hormone. J. Clin. Endocr. 20: 1017-1028, 1960.

20150 ADDISON DISEASE AND SPASTIC PARAPLEGIA

Harris-Jones and Nixon (1955) described two brothers in whom Addison disease was first recognized at 39 and 40 and who subsequently developed spastic paraplegia. No autopsy was performed. A similar case was reported by Penman (1960) in a 28 year old woman. The late onset and the occurrence in a female patient probably indicates that this is a disorder distinct from Addison disease and cerebral sclerosis, a well-established X-linked recessive. On the other hand, the brothers reported by Harris-Jones and Nixon (1955) may have suffered from an allelic form of the X-linked disorder (30010).

Harris-Jones, J. N. and Nixon, P. G. F.: Familial Addison's disease with spastic paraplegia. J. Clin. Endocr. 15: 739-744, 1955.

Penman, R. W. B.: Addison's disease in association with spastic paraplegia. Brit. Med. J. 1: 402 only, 1960.

*20155 ADDUCTED THUMBS SYNDROME

Christian et al. (1971) described three sibships in an Amish kindred with members affected by a new syndrome they chose to designate the 'adducted thumbs syndrome.' All six parents shared a common ancestral couple. Three Amish children and an unrelated child had cleft palate, arthrogryposis, craniostenosis, swallowing difficulties and microcephaly. Neuropathologic study of one of the Amish patients, who died at 18 days of age, showed dysmyelination with excessive myelin-dependent gliosis, myelin solubilization and transient formation of phospholipid-containing placques on the surface of the brain during fixation in formalin.

Christian, J. C., Andrews, P. A., Conneally, P. M. and Muller, J.: The adducted thumbs syndrome. An autosomal recessive disease with arthrogryposis, dysmyelination, craniostenosis, and cleft palate. Clin. Genet. 2: 95-103, 1971.

20160 ADENYLATE KINASE DEFICIENCY, ANEMIA DUE TO

In two offspring of second-cousin Arab parents Szeinberg et al. (1969) found marked AK deficiency with intermediate levels in the presumed heterozygotes. Severe anemia was present in both. Presumably this mutation is at the same locus as that which controls the polymorphism of AK (10300).

Boivin, P., Galand, C., Hakim, J., Simony, D. and Seligman, M.: Deficit congenital en adenylate-kinase erythrocytaire. (Letter) Presse Med. 78: 1443 only, 1970.

Szeinberg, A., Gavendo, S. and Cahane, D.: Erythrocyte adenylate-kinase deficiency. (Letter) Lancet I: 315-316, 1969.

Szeinberg, A., Kahana, D., Gavendo, S., Zaidman, J. and Ben-Ezzer, J.: Hereditary deficiency of adenylate kinase in red blood cells. Acta Haemat. 42: 111-126, 1969.

*20171 ADRENAL HYPERPLASIA I (WITH DEFECT IN ENZYME PRIOR TO DELTA 5-PREGNENO-LONE; LIPOID HYPERPLASIA OF ADRENAL CORTEX WITH MALE PSEUDOHERMAPHRO-DITISM; 20, 21 DESMOLASE DEFICIENCY)

The several types of adrenal hyperplasia are numbered I through V in order of the steps in the synthetic pathway. This form of adrenal hyperplasia is characterized in the male by various degrees of hypospadias or even almost complete failure of the external genitalia to undergo masculine development. It is believed that the genetic defect involves an enzyme necessary for the synthesis of both testicular and adrenocortical hormones. Probably the testes are unable to secrete the fetal male 'inductor' hormone which results in normal masculine genital organogenesis. The nature of the defect was stated to be unknown by Bongiovanni and Root (1963). The defect is now known to concern 20, 21 desmolase, which converts cholesterol to pregnenolone. The first clue to the genetic basis of this syndrome was the observation of consanguinity in the parents of cases (Prader and Siebenmann, 1957).

Bongiovanni, A. M. and Root, A. W.: The adrenogenital syndrome. New Eng. J. Med. 268: 1283-1289, 1351, and 1391-1399, 1963.

Camacho, A. M., Kowarski, A., Migeon, C. J. and Brough, A. J.: Congenital adrenal hyperplasia due to a deficiency of one of the enzymes involved in the biosynthesis of pregnonole. J. Clin. Endocr. 28: 153-161, 1968.

Prader, A. and Anders, G. J. P. A.: Zur Genetik der kongenitalen Lipoidhyperplasie der Nebennieren. Helv. Paediat. Acta 17: 285-289, 1962.

Prader, A. and Siebenmann, R. E.: Nebenniereninsuffizienz bei kongenitaler Lipoidhyperplasie der Nebennieren. Helv. Paediat. Acta 12: 569-595, 1957.

*20181 ADRENAL HYPERPLASIA II (WITH DEFECT IN 3-BETA-HYDROXYSTEROID DEHYDRO-GENASE)

Virilization is much less marked or does not occur in this type, suggesting that the gene — determined defect involves the testis as well as the adrenal. Males with the defect have hypospadias. Indeed, this form of adrenal hyperplasia can cause male pseudohermaphroditism. Salt loss is frequent cause of death. Death may occur even with adequate adrenal replacement therapy, perhaps because of the enzyme deficiency in other organs. (For another genetic disorder of the adrenal with salt loss, see ALDOSTERONE SYNTHESIS, DEFECT IN.)

Bongiovanni, A. M.: The adrenogenital syndrome with deficiency of 3-beta-hydroxysteroid dehydrogenase. J. Clin. Invest. 41: 2086-2092, 1962.

Hamilton, W. and Brush, M. G.: Four clinical variants of congenital adrenal hyperplasia. Arch. Dis. Child. 39: 66-72, 1964.

*20191 ADRENAL HYPERPLASIA III (WITH DEFECT IN 21-HYDROXYLASE)

All forms of adrenal hyperplasia show signs of excessive secretion of adrenal androgens in the form of virilization and rapid somatic advance. In some cases vomiting and dehydration resembling Addisonian crisis develop within a few weeks after birth and lead to rapid deterioration and death. Hypoglycemia sometimes occurs. Recurrent fever also may occur and may be related to etiocholanolone, although this remains to be clarified. Hypertension occurs in this form in addition to the other features. Even after being present for several years it is relieved by steroid therapy. All types of adrenal hyperplasia were reviewed exhaustively by Bongiovanni and Root (1963). Prader and colleagues (1962) reported an enormous interlocking Swiss kindred. Two types of 21-hydroxylase defect appear to occur, one mild and one severe. In the severe form, aldosterone production is curtailed and aldosterone antagonists accumulate leading to severe salt wasting and Addisonian crisis. In females virilization is usually evident at birth. Indeed some affected females are reared as males. In the male the condition is often not recognized until late infancy or childhood. Other features of the adrenogenital syndrome are salt and water loss, hypertension, possibly fever, and Addisonian crisis. The common denominator of the several forms, in both males and females, is excessive secretion of adrenal androgens. (See PRECOCIOUS PUBERTY OF MALE in dominant catalog for simulating condition.) In the canton of Zurich, Switzerland, Prader (1958) estimated the frequency to be 1 in 5041 live births, giving a frequency of carriers of 1 in 35. Childs, Grumbach and Van Wyk (1956) had estimated the frequency in Maryland to be 1 in 67,000 births. A remarkable and possibly significant feature from the point of view of selection and gene frequency is the finding of Lewis et al. (1968) that intelligence is increased in the adrenogenital syndrome. Merkatz et al. (1969) could not diagnose the disorder early in pregnancy by amniocentesis and hormone assay of the amniotic fluid. Galal et al. (1969) concluded that the two clinical forms of 21-hydroxylase deficiency (with and without salt-losing) correlate with the extent of the defect in the cortisol pathway. In Toronto Qazi and Thompson (1972) estimated the minimum frequency of salt-losing C-21 hydroxylase deficiency as 1 per 26,292. Presumably it is a salt-losing variety of 21-hydroxylase deficiency which is present in relatively high frequency in Eskimos of Alaska (Hirschfeld and Fleshman, 1969). Other recessive conditions of high frequency among the Alaskan Eskimos include Kuskokwin disease (20820), methemoglobinemia (25080), and pseudocholinesterase deficiency (27240).

Bongiovanni, A. M.: Disorders of adrenocortical steroid biogenesis. In, Stanbury, J. B., Wyngaarden, J. B. and Fredrickson, D. S. (eds.): The Metabolic Basis of Inherited Disease. New York: McGraw-Hill, 1972 (3rd Ed.). Pp. 857-885.

Bongiovanni, A. M. and Root, A. W.: The adrenogenital syndrome. New Eng. J. Med. 268: 1283-1289, 1342-1351, And 1391-1399, 1963.

Childs, B., Grumbach, M. M. and Van Wyk, J. J.: Virilizing adrenal hyperplasia: genetic and hormonal studies. J. Clin. Invest. 35: 213-222, 1956.

Galal, O. M., Rudd, B. T. and Drayer, N. M.: Evaluation of deficiency of 21-hydroxylation in patients with congenital adrenal hyperplasia. Arch. Dis. Child. 43: 410-414, 1969.

Hirschfeld, A. J. and Fleshman, J. K.: An unusually high incidence of salt — losing congenital adrenal hyperplasia in the Alaskian Eskimo. J. Pediat. 75: 492-494, 1969.

Lewis, V. G., Money, J. and Epstein, R.: Concordance of verbal and nonverbal ability in the adrenogenital syndrome. Johns Hopkins Med. J. 122: 192-195, 1968.

Merkatz, I. R., New, M. I., Peterson, R. E. and Seaman, M. P.: Prenatal diagnosis of adrenogenital syndrome by amniocentesis. J. Pediat. 75: 977-982, 1969.

Prader, A.: Die Haufigkeit des kongenitalen adrenogenitalen Syndroms. Helv. Paediat. Acta 13: 426-431, 1958.

Prader, A., Anders, G. J. P. A. and Habich, H.: Zur Genetik des kongenitalen adrenogenitalen Syndroms (virilisierende Nebennierenhyperplasia). Helv. Paediat. Acta 17: 271-284, 1962.

Qazi, Q. H. and Thompson, M. W.: Incidence of salt — losing form of congenital virilizing adrenal hyperplasia. Arch. Dis. Child. 47: 302-303, 1972.

*20201 ADRENAL HYPERPLASIA IV (WITH DEFECT IN 11-BETA-HYDROXYLASE)

When the defect involves the enzyme system concerned in hydroxylation of C11, 11-deoxycorticosterone, a potent salt-retainer, accumulates, leading to arterial hypertension. The nature of the defect was first demonstrated by Eberlein and Bongiovanni (1956) on the basis of the accumulated steroids.

Eberlein, W. R. and Bongiovanni, A. M.: Plasma and urinary corticosteroids in the hypertensive form of adrenal hyperplasia. J. Biol. Chem. 223: 85-94, 1956.

Visser, H. K. A.: Inherited variation in the biosynthesis of adrenal corticosteroids in man. In, Endocrine Genetics. Spickett, S. G. (ed.): Mem. Soc. Endocrinology, 1967. Pp. 145-178.

*20211 ADRENAL HYPERPLASIA V (WITH DEFECT IN 17-HYDROXYLASE)

New and Peterson (1967) described what they suggested is a new form of adrenal hyperplasia in a 12 year old boy. Features included (1) classic signs of primary hyperaldosteronism (mild hypertension, hypokalemic alkalosis, low plasma renin, hypervolemia and fixed hyperaldosterone levels in blood uninfluenced by sodium restriction or excess), (2) low normal plasma cortisol and corticosterone, (3) elevated plasma ACTH, (4) fall in aldosterone production and in blood pressure during treatment with glucocorticoids, (5) normal rise of plasma testosterone to chorionic gonadotropin. The father and two normotensive sibs showed no abnormality on multiple testing but the hypertensive mother had abnormal aldosterone regulation. Thus X-linked recessive inheritance is possible. A 17-hydroxylase defect in the kidney but not the testis was postulated. A deficiency of adrenal 17-hydroxylation activity was demonstrated in a single patient by Biglieri et al. (1966). A similar defect in the gonad was suggested. Production of excessive corticosterone and deoxycorticosterone resulted in hypertension and hypokalemic alkalosis. Aldosterone synthesis was almost totally absent. Amenorrhea was present. Stature was normal. Although there were no other cases in the family and parental consanguinity was not noted, recessive inheritance is possible, indeed likely. Goldsmith et al. (1967) reported a second case in whom the defect in 17-alpha-hydroxylation may have been less complete than in the first case. Again a single person was affected — a 26-year-old woman with hypertension, primary amenorrhea and lack of secondary sexual characteristics. Mallin (1969) described affected sisters. 17-hydroxylase is necessary for both cortisol and estrogen synthesis. Because of lack of these hormones increase in ACTH and FSH occurs. Excessive synthesis of deoxycorticosterone and corticosterone produce hypertension. Estrogen lack results in primary amenorrhea and absent sexual maturation. Ovarian enlargement and infarction from twisting also occur. Therapy with dexamethasone and estrogen lowers blood pressure and produces feminization. New (1970) reported the first affected male. The clinical features were pseudohermaphroditism with ambiguous external genitalia and prominent breast development at puberty. Unlike the previously reported female cases this male patient did not demonstrate severe hypertension or hypokalemia.

Biglieri, E. G., Herron, M. A. and Brust, N.: 17-hydroxylation deficiency in man. J. Clin. Invest. 45: 1946-1954, 1966.

Goldsmith, O., Solomon, D. H. and Horton, R.: Hypogonadism and mineralocorticoid excess: 17-hydroxylase deficiency. New Eng. J. Med. 277: 673-677, 1967.

Mallin, S. R.: Congenital adrenal hyperplasia secondary to 17-hydroxylase deficiency. Ann. Intern. Med. 70: 69-76, 1969.

New, M. I. and Peterson, R. E.: A new form of congenital adrenal hyperplasia. J. Clin. Endocr. 27: 300-305, 1967.

New, M. I.: Male pseudohermaphroditism due to 17 alpha-hydroxylase deficiency. J. Clin. Invest. 49: 1930-1941, 1970.

*20220 ADRENAL UNRESPONSIVENESS TO ACTH

Migeon and colleagues (1968) have described an entity of adrenal unresponsiveness to ACTH. Features are hypoglycemia, hyperpigmentation, feeding problems in infancy, low urinary 17-OHCS, normal tolerance to salt deprivation, and no elevation of 17-OHCS excretion or plasma cortisol concentration with administration of ACTH. Two of their patients were brothers. Sibs of two other patients were probably affected. Affected male and female sibs have been reported (Shepard, Landing, Mason, 1959). Franks and Nance (1970) observed the condition in two sisters and a brother, offspring of first cousin parents, and reviewed 8 other familial cases. An excess of males and a deficiency of consanguinity suggested the existence of both autosomal and X-linked recessive forms. Plasma ACTH levels were greatly elevated. Kelch et al. (1972) reported three families. They pointed out that variable adrenal pathology family to family and the possibility of both autosomal and X-linked forms suggest heterogeneity in this condition.

Franks, R. C. and Nance, W. E.: Hereditary adrenocortical unresponsiveness to ACTH. Pediatrics 45: 43-48, 1970.

Kelch, R. P., Kaplan, S. L., Biglieri, E. G., Daniels, G. H., Epstein, C. J. and Grumbach, M. M.: Hereditary adrenocortical unresponsiveness to adrenocorticotripic hormone. J. Pediat. 81: 726-736, 1972.

R
E
C
E
S
S
I
V
E

Migeon, C. J., Kenny, F. M., Kowarski, A., Snipes, C. A., Spaulding, J. S., Finkelstein, J. W. and Blizzard, R. M.: The syndrome of congenital adrenocortical unresponsiveness to ACTH. Report of six cases. Pediat. Res. 2: 501-513, 1968.

Shepard, T. H., Landing, B. H. and Mason, D. G.: Familial Addison's disease. Case reports of two sisters with corticoid deficiency unassociated with hypoaldosteronism. Am. J. Dis. Child. 97: 154-162, 1959.

Stempfel, R. S., Jr. and Engel, F. L.: A congenital, familial syndrome of adrenocortical insufficiency without hypoaldosteronism. J. Pediat. 57: 443-451, 1960.

20230 ADRENOCORTICAL CARCINOMA

Fraumeni and Miller (1967) mentioned affected sibs. Mahloudji et al. (1970) observed affected brother and sister who were products of a consanguineous union. Nichols (1968) also described affected brother and sister.

Fraumeni, J. F., Jr. and Miller, R. W.: Adrenocortical neoplasms with hemihypertrophy, brain tumors, and other disorders. J. Pediat. 70: 129-138, 1967.

Mahloudji, M., Ronaghi, H. and Dutz, W.: Familial adrenal cortical carcinoma. To be published, 1970.

Nichols, J.: Adrenal cortex. In, Bloodworth, J. M. B. (ed.): Baltimore: Williams and Wilkins Co., 1968.

*20240 AFIBRINOGENEMIA, CONGENITAL

Relatively few cases have been reported. However, the high proportion with consanguineous parents and-or affected sibs makes recessive inheritance very likely. The blood is completely incoagulable, yet some of the affected persons have remarkably little trouble with bleeding. In some cases the disorder was detected at birth because of excess bleeding from the umbilical stump. A partial deficiency of fibrinogen has been observed in parents and other heterozygotes. In two brothers reported by Lemoine et al. (1963) congenital afibrinogenemia was associated with osseous and hepatic lesions, thought to be of hemorrhagic origin.

Bommer, W., Kunzer, W. and Schroer, H.: Kongenitale Afibrinogenamie. Ann. Paediat. 200: 46-59, 1963.

Bronnimann, R.: Kongenitale Afibrinogenamie. Acta Haemat. 11: 40-51, 1954.

Lawson, H. A.: Congenital afibrinogenemia: report of a case. New Eng. J. Med. 248: 552-554, 1953.

Lemoine, P., Harousseau, H., Guimbretiere, J., Lenne, Y. and Angebaud, Y.: Afibrinemie congenitale chez deux freres avec lesions osseuses et hepatiques. Arch. Franc. Pediat. 20: 463-483, 1963.

Prichard, R. W. and Vann, R. L.: Congenital afibrinogenaemia: report on a child without fibrinogen and review of the literature. Am. J. Dis. Child. 88: 703-710, 1954.

Werder, E.: Kongenitale Afibrinogenamie. Helv. Paediat. Acta 18: 208-229, 1963.

*20250 AGAMMAGLOBULINEMIA, SWISS OR ALYMPHOCYTOTIC TYPE

In addition to the more frequent X-linked variety, a presumed autosomal recessive form has been described by several authors. Good (1963) referred to the latter as the Swiss type of agammaglobulinemia. Unlike the X-linked variety, the patient is unusually susceptible to fungal and viral as well as pyogenic pathogens and lacks delayed hypersensitivity as well as showing failure of antibody production. Furthermore, the thymus is very small and shows lack of lymphoid cells and Hassall corpuscles, whereas it may be quite normal in the X-linked form. Cooper, Peterson and Good (1965) have suggested that both the thymus system responsible for cellular immunity and the tonsillar system responsible for immunoglobulin production are absent in this disorder whereas only the latter is affected in Bruton type agammaglobulinemia (X-linked form). Only the thymus system may be defective in the disorder described under IMMUNE DEFECT DUE TO ABSENCE OF THYMUS (q.v.). See ATAXIA-TELANGIECTASIA for possible relationship to that disorder. This disorder is relatively frequent among Mennonites living in southern Manitoba (Haworth et al., 1967). Heterogeneity in the autosomal recessive immune disorders is indicated by the report of Lipsey et al. (1967) of three families with multiple sibs with an immune disorder which defies classification. The three probands died in the first three years of life of pneumonia.

Comings, D. E.: A third gamma-globulin chain? (Letter) Lancet II: 786, 1963.

Cooper, M. D., Peterson, R. D. and Good, R. A.: 'New' concept of the cellular basis of immunity. (Abstract) J. Pediat. 67: 907-908, 1965.

Greenwood, R. D., Traisman, H. S., Rice, H. M. and Oh-Paik, S. G.: Swiss type agammaglobulinemia in the United States. Autosomal recessive lymphopenic thymic dysplasia with agammaglobulinemia. Am. J. Dis. Child. 121: 30-34, 1971.

Gitlin, D., Janeway, C. A., Apt, C. and Craig, J. M.: Agammaglobulinemia. In, Laurence, H. S. (ed.): Cellular and Humoral Aspects of Hypersensitive States. New York: Hoeber-Harper, 1959.

Gitlin, D., Rosen, F. S. and Janeway, C. A.: Undue susceptibility to infection. Pediat. Clin. N. Am. 9: 405-423, 1962.

Good, R. A.: Immunologic competence — its development and relation to thymus function. Sec. Intern. Conf. on Cong. Malformations, 1963.

Good, R. A., Kelly, W. D., Rotstein, J. and Varco, R. L.: Agammaglobulinemia, hypogammaglobulinemia, Hodgkin's disease and sarcoidosis. Progr. Allerg. 6: 187-319, 1962.

Haworth, J. C., Hoogstraten, J. and Taylor, H.: Thymic alymphoplasia. Arch. Dis. Child. 42: 40-54, 1967.

Hitzig, W. H. and Willi, H.: Hereditare lympho-plasmocytare dysgenesie ('alymphocytose mit agammaglobulinamie'). Schweiz. Med. Wschr. 91: 1625-1633, 1961.

Hitzig, W. H.: The Swiss type of agammaglobulinemia. In, Good, R. A. (ed.): Immunologic Deficiency Diseases. New York: National Foundation, 1968. Pp. 82-90.

Lawton, A. R., Bockman, D. E., Cooper, M. D.: Treatment of autosomal recessive lymphopenic agammaglobulinemia by transplantation of matched allogeneic bone marrow. Am. J. Med. 54: 98-110, 1973.

Lipsey, A. I., Kahn, M. J. and Bolande, R. P.: Pathologic variants of congenital hypogammaglobulinemia: an analysis of 3 patients dying of measles. Pediatrics 39: 659-674, 1967.

Rosen, F. S., Gitlin, D. and Janeway, C. A.: Alymphocytosis, agammaglobulinaemia, homografts, and delayed hypersensitivity: report of a case. Lancet 2: 380-381, 1962.

Tobler, R. and Cottier, H.: Familiare Lymphopenie mit Agammaglobulinaemie und schwerer Moniliasis. Helv. Paediat. Acta 13: 313-338, 1958.

20260 AGENESIS OF CEREBRAL WHITE MATTER

Waggoner et al. (1942) described six sisters in a sibship of 11 with agenesis of the white matter and idiocy, surviving to adulthood. The family was of Finnish extraction. No parental consanguinity was known.

Waggoner, R. W., Lowenberg-Scharenberg, K. and Schilling, M. E.: Agenesis of white matter with idiocy. Am. J. Ment. Defic. 47: 20-24, 1942.

*20270 AGRANULOCYTOSIS, INFANTILE GENETIC, OF KOSTMANN

In addition to Kostmann agranulocytosis, recessively inherited neutropenic syndromes include (1) neutropenia, congenital, with eosinophilia, (2) Chediak-Higashi syndrome, and (3) Fanconi pancytopenic syndrome. Hedenberg (1959) found that addition of sulfur-containing amino acids to tissue cultures led to maturation of white cells. L'Esperance et al. (1973) showed that the disease could be reproduced in tissue culture. Experiments such as Hedenburg's should be repeated using this technique. Barak et al. (1971) also cultured marrow cells from a patient with this disease.

Andrews, J. P., McClellan, J. T. and Scott, C. H.: Lethal congenital neutropenia with eosinophilia occurring in two siblings. Am. J. Med. 29: 358-362, 1960.

Barak, Y., Paran, M., Levin, S. and Sachs, L.: Blood 38: 74-80, 1971.

Hedenberg, F.: Infantile agranulocytosis of probably congenital origin. Acta Paediat. 48: 77-84, 1959.

Kostmann, R.: Infantile genetic agranulocytosis (agranulocytosis infantilis hereditaria): a new recessive lethal disease in man. Uppsala: Almuvist and Wiksells Boktryckeri, 1956.

L'Esperance, P. L., Brunning, R. and Good, R. A.: Congenital neutropenia: in vitro growth of colonies mimicking the disease. Proc. Nat. Acad. Sci. 70: 669-672, 1973.

20280 ALACRIMIA CONGENITA

Kruger (1954) described brother and sister with ptosis, distichiasis, conjunctivitis, keratitis, and alacrimia congenita. The father and another brother were said to have defective lacrimation. A nuclear defect was postulated.

Kruger, K. E.: Angeborenes Fehlen der Tranensekretion in einer Familie. Klin. Mbl. Augenheilk. 124: 711-713, 1954.

20290 ALANINURIA WITH MICROCEPHALY, DWARFISM, ENAMEL HYPOPLASIA, DIABETES MELLITUS

Stimmler et al. (1970) described two sisters born in 1963 and 1964 with microcephaly at birth, low birth weight, severe mental retardation and dwarfism, small teeth, and diabetes mellitus. Excessive quantities of alanine were found in the urine. Alanine, pyruvate and lactate were elevated in the blood. Pyruvate was thought to be a source of the alanine. The authors contrasted the findings with those in the condition described by Haworth et al. (1967) and in Leigh subacute necrotizing encephalopathy with lactic acidosis (Worsley et al., 1965). The main differences were elevated plasma chloride and lack of hyperalaninemia in the other two conditions.

Haworth, J. C., Ford, J. D. and Younoszai, M. K.: Familial chronic acidosis due to an error in lactate and pyruvate metabolism. Canad. Med. Ass. J. 97: 773-779, 1967.

Stimmler, L., Jensen, N. and Toseland, P.: Alaninuria, associated with microcephaly, dwarfism, enamel hypoplasia, and diabetes mellitus in two sisters. Arch. Dis. Child. 45: 682-685, 1970.

Worsley, H. E., Brookfield, R. W., Elwood, J. S., Noble, R. L. and Taylor, W. H.: Lactic acidosis with necrotizing encephalopathy in two sibs. Arch. Dis. Child. 40: 492-501, 1965.

20300 ALAR-NASAL CARTILAGES, COLOBOMA OF, WITH TELECANTHUS

Rimoin (1969) described two sisters with an identical malformation of the nose consisting mainly of hypoplasia and coloboma of the alar cartilages. Both also showed telecanthus. The parents and other relatives were unaffected and no parental consanguinity was reported.

Rimoin, D. L.: Hypoplasia and coloboma of the alar-nasal cartilages with pseudohypertelorism in sibs. The Clinical Delineation of Birth Defects. II. Malformation Syndromes. New York: National Foundation, 1969. Pp. 224-225.

*20310 ALBINISM I

Amelanic melanocytes are present in the skin of albinos. These contain granules similar to the premelanosomes of normal melanocytes. The nature of the basic defect is unknown. In mice the non-alpha hemoglobin locus is linked to the albinism locus. Therefore, the family with both albinism and sicklemia, reported by Massie and Hartmann (1957), is of interest. Froggatt (1960) estimated a phenotype frequency of 1 in 10,000 in Northern Ireland. First-cousin marriages occurred in 4.5 percent of the parents. An excess of males was almost exclusively in the probands and the sex ratio of secondary cases was about 1: therefore, bias of ascertainment probably accounted for the excess of males. The mutation rate was estimated to be between 3.3 and 7 x 10-5 per gene per generation. Abnormal iris translucency, occurring in 70 percent of the parents and children of albinos, was interpreted as a heterozygous manifestation. Keeler (1953) in describing albinism in the Caribe Cuna Indians commented on the abundant straight white down consisting of hairs up to two and one half cm in length which develops on the body and extremities. It is not clear that this indicates genetic distinctness but may somehow be related to the exposure of the subjects. Partial albinism in association with deaf-mutism occurs as a dominant trait in Waardenburg syndrome (q.v.). Pipkin and Pipkin (1942) claimed dominant inheritance for total albinism without other features in one family, but a quasidominant pedigree pattern of the usual recessive forms seems quite likely. Working with albino melanomas and tyrosinase inhibitor in animals, Chian and Wilgram (1967) found that the inhibitor is effective against soluble tyrosinase but not against tyrosinase aggregated into melanosomes. In one type of albino mutation, tyrosinase apparently could not aggregate because of genetic alteration in its protein carrier and therefore was vulnerable to the effects of the inhibitor. These workers suggested that a similar situation may obtain in some type of albinism of man. See 25830 for information on linkage. In a wide variety of animals, the albinism gene is known to have a pleiotrophic effect on the visual pathways (Guillery, 1974). Some of the optic nerve fibers go to the wrong side of the brain. This structural abnormality, the mechanism of which is unknown, can be associated with crossed eyes in albino animals. Evidence on whether a similar structural abnormality occurs in human albinos is not available.

Chian, L. T. Y. and Wilgram, G. F.: Tyrosinase inhibition: its role in suntanning and in albinism. Science 155: 198-200, 1967.

Fitzpatrick, T. B. and Quevedo, W. C., Jr.: Albinism. In, Stanbury, J. B., Wyngaarden, J. B. and Fredrickson, D. S. (eds.): The Metabolic Basis of Inherited Disease. New York: McGraw-Hill, 1972 (3rd Ed.). Pp. 326-337.

Froggatt, P.: Albinism in Northern Ireland. Ann. Hum. Genet. 24: 213-238, 1960.

Guillery, R. W.: Visual pathways in albinos. Scientific American 230 (No. 5): 44-54, 1974.

Hanhart, E.: Uber 18 lebende und 13 verstorbene Albinos in einem Dorf des Piemont nebst weiteren Beitragen zur Populationsgenetik des Albinismus universalis. Arch. Klaus Stift. Vererbungsforsch. 27: 178-188, 1952.

Keeler, C. E.: The Caribe Cuna Moon-child and its heredity. J. Hered. 44: 163-171, 1953.

Massie, R. W. and Hartmann, R. C.: Albinism and sicklemia in a Negro family. Am. J. Hum. Genet. 9: 127-132, 1957.

Pipkin, A. C. and Pipkin, S. B.: Albinism in Negroes. J. Hered. 33: 419-427, 1942.

Sears, M. L.: Browning of the lens in generalized albinism. Am. J. Ophthal. 77: 819-823, 1974.

R
E
C
E
S
S
I
V
E

*20320 ALBINISM II

The evidence for a second non-allelic form of recessive albinism was provided by a family reported by Trevor-Roper (1952, 1963). Two albino parents had four normally pigmented children. Assuming paternity (and blood groups provided no reason to question it), it is possible that the father had X-linked ocular albinism and a light complexion. However, if such were the case, his daughters, necessarily heterozygous for the X-linked gene, should have had the mosaic pigmentary pattern characteristic of the fundus oculi in the heterozygote. Such was not found. The existence of more than one locus may also be supported by the fact that the rate of parental consanguinity is higher than would be expected if only one locus were involved. Finally, applying the chemical method of Kugelman and Van Scott (1961), Witkop (1962) found suggestive evidence of separate forms of albinism. Witkop (1966) examined Trevor-Roper's family and found that whereas the mother did not show pigmentation in the Kugelman-Van Scott test, the father did show pigment.

It seems clear that there is a separate recessively inherited condition called albinoidism characterized by ocular albinism, nystagmus, myopia and reduced pigmentation generally. The deficiency in pigmentation is striking early in life, but as the affected person grows older the hair and skin darken. Heterozygotes do not show the mosaic pigmentary pattern of the fundus as do the carriers for X-linked ocular albinism. Probably in the family reported by Trevor-Roper the mother had true albinism and the father had albinoidism. Klein (1961) referred to albinoidism as universal incomplete albinism. Nance et al. (1970) described a distinctive form of recessive albinism in an Amish isolate. Affected persons showed profound generalized albinism at birth but developed normal skin pigmentation and yellow hair by age two, although persistent ocular albinism and nystagmus permitted diagnosis in the adult. Results of hair-bulb incubation studies were considered to be intermediate between those of tyrosinase-positive and tyrosinase-negative albinism. Abundant phaeomelanin but little eumelanin was found naturally in these Amish patients who were referred to as representing the yellow mutant (ym). The allelic relationship to other forms of albinism is unknown. Witkop (1971) suggested that the 'yellow type albino' (ym — yellow mutant) may be quite distinct from both tyrosinase-positive and tyrosinase-negative albinism, indeed perhaps determined by a separate locus.

Klein, D.: Les diverses formes hereditaires de l'albinisme. Bull. Acad. Suisse. Sci. (Bull. Schweiz. Akad. Med. Wiss.) 17: 351-364, 1961.

Kugelman, T. P. and Van Scott, E.: Tyrosinase activity in melanocytes of human albinos. J. Invest. Derm. 37: 73-76, 1961.

McKusick, V. A. and colleagues: Medical genetics 1963. J. Chronic Dis. 17: 1077-1215, 1964.

Nance, W. E., Jackson, C. E. and Witkop, C. J., Jr.: Amish albinism: a distinctive autosomal recessive phenotype. Am. J. Hum. Genet. 22: 579-586, 1970.

Nance, W. E., Witkop, C. J. and Rawls, R. F.: Genetic and biochemical evidence for two forms of oculocutaneous albinism in man. The Clinical Delineation of Birth Defects. VIII. Eye. Baltimore: Williams and Wilkins, 1971. Pp. 125-128.

Trevor-Roper, P. D.: Marriage of two complete albinos with normally pigmented offspring. Brit. J. Ophthal. 36: 107-110, 1952, And Proc. Roy. Soc. Med. 56: 21-24, 1963.

Waardenburg, P. J.: Genetics and ophthalmology. Springfield, Ill.: Charles C Thomas, 1: 732 only, 1961.

Witkop, C. J., Jr.: Albinism. Chapter 2 in, Harris, H. and Hirschhorn, K. (eds.): Advances in Human Genetics. New York: Plenum Press, 1971. vol. 2, Pp. 61-142.

Witkop, C. J., Jr.: Dental problems of an hereditary nature. In, Witkop, C. J. (ed.): Genetics and Dental Health. New York: McGraw-Hill, 1962.

Witkop, C. J., Jr., Van Scott, E. J. and Jacoby, G. A.: Evidence for two forms of autosomal recessive albinism in man. Proc. Sec. Intern. Cong. Hum. Genet. (Rome, Sept. 6-12, 1961.) 2: 1064-1065, 1963.

*20330 ALBINISM WITH HEMORRHAGIC DIATHESIS AND PIGMENTED RETICULOENDOTHELIAL CELLS

Hermansky and Pudlak (1959) described two unrelated albinos with lifelong bleeding tendency and peculiar pigmented reticular cells in the bone marrow as well as in lymph node and liver biopsies. One was male and one female: both were 33 years old. The female has since died and was found to have large amounts of the pigment in reticuloendothelial cells everywhere and in the walls of small blood vessels (Hermansky, 1963). Two families, each with two sibs affected with this syndrome, have come to Hermansky's attention (1963). This syndrome is clearly different from the Chediak-Higashi syndrome (q.v.) because no qualitative changes of leukocytes are found in Hermansky syndrome and no pigmented macrophages are found in the Chediak-Higashi syndrome. Report of a family by Verloop et al. (1964) supports this conclusion. Logan et al. (1971) described a patient with albinism and bleeding diathesis in whom a defect in platelet ADP-release was demonstrated. Prolonged bleeding time and defective platelet aggregation were found. Two other albino patients with a defect in ADP-release had been reported, as well as 12 albino patients with prolonged bleeding. In 6 of 7 in whom the bone marrow was studied, histiocytes were found to contain abnormal granules.

Hermansky, F. and Pudlak, P.: Albinism associated with hemorrhagic diathesis and unusual pigmented reticular cells in the bone marrow: report of two cases with histochemical studies. Blood 14: 162-169, 1959.

Hermansky, F.: Prague, Czechoslovakia: personal communication, 1963.

Logan, L. J., Rapaport, S. I. and Maher, I.: Albinism and abnormal platelet function. New Eng. J. Med. 284: 1340-1345, 1971.

Verloop, M. C., Von Wieringen, A., Vuylsteke, J., Hart, H. C. and Huizinga, J.: Albinismus, hemorrhagische Diathese und anormale Pigmentzellen im Knockenmark. Med. Klin. 59: 408-412, 1964.

White, J. G., Edson, J. R., Desnick, S. J. and Witkop, C. J.: Studies of platelets in a variant of the Hermansky-Pudlak syndrome. Am. J. Path. 63: 319-332, 1971.

20333 ALBRIGHT HEREDITARY OSTEODYSTROPHY

Althought X-linked dominant inheritance has been favored (see 30080), some evidence is available for an autosomal recessive form (Cederbaum and Lippe, 1973).

Cederbaum, S. D. and Lippe, B. M.: Probable autosomal recessive inheritance in a family with Albright's hereditary osteodystrophy and an evaluation of the genetics of the disorder. Am. J. Hum. Genet. 25: 638-645, 1973.

*20335 ALDOLASE A DEFICIENCY

Beutler et al. (1973) described a daughter of first-cousin parents who had nonspherocytic hemolytic anemia, mental retardation and increased hepatic glycogen due, apparently, to deficiency of red cell aldolase. Muscle and red cell aldolase is type A. Liver aldolase, deficient in fructose intolerance (22960), is type B. In brain aldolase C occurs together with aldolase A (Penhoet, 1966). Puzzlingly, both parents had normal levels of red cell aldolase. They were related as first-cousins.

Beutler, E., Scott, S., Bishop, A., Margolis, N., Matsumoto, F. and Kuhl, W.: Red cell aldolase deficiency and hemolytic anemia: a new syndrome. Trans. Assoc. Am. Phys. 86: 154-166, 1973.

Penhoet, E., Rajkumar, T. and Rutter, W. I.: Multiple forms of fructose diphosphate aldolase in mammalian tissues. Proc. Nat. Acad. Sci. 56: 1275-1282, 1966.

*20340 ALDOSTERONE DEFICIENCY, DUE TO, DEFECT IN 18-HYDROXYLASE OR 18-DEHYDROGENASE

Visser and Cost (1964) described three infants with a typical clinical picture consisting of dehydration, occasional vomiting, poor feeding, failure to gain weight, intermittent fever, hypernatremia, and hypokalemia. DOCA was successful in the treatment of these cases. All six parents of the three patients shared a

R
E
C
E
S
S
I
V
E

great-grandparental ancestral couple in common. The total urinary excretion of 17-ketosteroids, 17 ketogenic steroids and 17-hydroxycorticosteroids was normal. No aldosterone was detected. Autopsy in one infant showed the adrenals to be grossly normal, but on microscopic examination the zona glomerulosa showed tubular and empty areas. The findings suggested a defect in 18-oxidation, which would be expected to affect biosynthesis of aldosterone at the step between corticosterone and aldosterone. David et al. (1968) concluded that the enzymatic defect is in the dehydrogenation of 18-hydroxycorticosterone to aldosterone. The clinical manifestations may be subtle. Growth retardation was the leading feature in two infant Puerto Rican sibs reported by David et al. (1968). Abnormality in serum electrolytes was transient in one. Rappaport et al. (1968) observed two brothers with a salt-losing syndrome due to 18-OH-dehydrogenase deficiency. Spontaneous improvement occurred.

David, R., Golan, S. and Drucker, W.: Familial aldosterone deficiency: enzyme defect, diagnosis and clinical course. Pediatrics 41: 403-412, 1968.

Rappaport, R., Dray, F., Legrand, J. C. and Royer, P.: Hypoaldosteronisme congenital familial par defaut de la 18-OH-dehydrogenase. Pediat. Res. 2: 456-463, 1968.

Ulick, S., Gautier, E., Vetter, K. K., Markello, J. R., Yaffe, S. and Lowe, C. U.: An aldosterone biosynthetic defect in a salt-losing disorder. J. Clin. Endocr. 24: 669-672, 1964.

Visser, H. K. A. and Cost, W. S.: A new hereditary defect in the biosynthesis of aldosterone: urinary C(21)-corticosteroid pattern in three related patients with a salt-losing syndrome, suggesting an 18-oxidation defect. Acta Endocr. 47: 589-612, 1964.

20345 ALEXANDER DISEASE

Wohlwill et al. (1959) described a sibship of 9, of whom 1 sister and 3 brothers had large heads called hydrocephalic and died at ages 4, 5, 6 and 3, respectively. Alexander disease was proven histologically in the last. Alexander described the disorder in 1949. It is characterized clinically by development of megalencephaly in infancy accompanied by progressive spasticity and dementia. Histologically it is characterized by numerous homogeneous eosinophilic masses which form elongated tapered rods up to 30 microns in length, which are scattered throughout the cortex and white matter and which are most numerous in the subpial, perivascular and subependymal regions. Demyelination is present, usually as a prominent feature. A few cases have had hydrocephalus. The eosinophilic deposits are morphologically identical to Rosenthal fibers which are commonly found in astrocytomas, optic nerve gliomas and states of chronic reactive gliosis. Herndon et al. (1970) expressed the view that Rosenthal fibers found in this situation are the result of degenerative changes in the cytoplasm and cytoplasmic processes of astrocytic glial cells.

Alexander, W. S.: Progressive fibrinoid degeneration of fibullary astrocytes associated with mental retardation in a hydrocephalic infant. Brain 72: 373-381, 1949.

Herndon, R. N., Rubinstein, L. J., Freeman, J. N. and Mathieson, G.: Light and electron microscopic observations on Rosenthal fibers in Alexander's disease and in multiple sclerosis. Neuropath. Exp. Neurol. 29: 524-551, 1970.

Wohlwill, F. J., Bernstein, J. and Yarovlev, P. I.: Dysmyelinogenic leukodystrophy. J. Neuropath. Exp. Neurol. 18: 359-383, 1959.

*20350 ALKAPTONURIA

Alkaptonuria enjoys the historic distinction of being one of the first conditions in which Mendelian recessive inheritance was proposed (by Garrod, 1902, on the suggestion of Bateson) and of being one of the four conditions in the charter group of inborn errors of metabolism. The manifestations are urine that turns dark on standing and alkalinization, black ochronotic pigmentation of cartilage and collagenous tissues and arthritis, especially characteristic in the spine. Sandler et al. (1970) raised the question of whether Parkinsonism occurs in increased frequency with alkaptonuria, either as a complication or as a distinct syndromal entity separate from ordinary alkaptonuria. Lustberg et al. (1970) presented evidence that ascorbic acid in high doses decreases binding of C(14)-homogentisic acid in connective tissues of rats with experimental alkaptonuria. Long-term therapy in young patients with alkaptonuria is indicated. Alkaptonuria is unusually frequent in the Dominican Republic (Milch, 1960) and in Slovakia (Cervenansky et al., 1959).

Abe, Y., Oshima, N., Hatanaka, R., Amako, T. and Hirohata, R.: Thirteen cases of alkaptonuria from one family tree with special reference to osteo-arthrosis alkaptonurica. J. Bone Joint Surg. 42A: 817-831, 1960.

Cervenansky, J., Sitaj, S. and Urbanek, T.: Alkaptonuria and ochronosis. J. Bone Joint Surg. 41A: 1169-1182, 1959.

Garrod, A. E.: The incidence of alkaptonuria: a study in chemical individuality. Lancet II: 1616-1620, 1902.

Knox, A. E.: Sir Archibald Garrod's 'inborn errors of metabolism.' II. Alkaptonuria. Am. J. Hum. Genet. 10: 95-124, 1958.

La Du, B. N.: Alcaptonuria. In, Stanbury, J. B., Wyngaarden, J. B. and Fredrickson, D. S. (eds.): The Metabolic Basis of Inherited Disease. New York: McGraw-Hill, 1972 (3rd Ed.). Pp. 308-325.

Lustberg, T. J., Schulman, J. D. and Seegmiller, J. E.: Decreased binding of (14)C-homogentisic acid induced by ascorbic acid in connective tissues of rats with experimental alkaptonuria. Nature 228: 770-771, 1970.

Milch, R. A.: Studies of alcaptonuria: inheritance of 47 cases in eight highly inter-related Dominican kindreds. Am. J. Hum. Genet. 12: 76-85, 1960.

R
E
C
E
S
S
I
V
E

344

Reginato, A., Riera, M., Martinez, V. and Ruiz, F.: Alkaptonuria, ochronotic arthropathy and aortic stenosis. Rev. Med. Chile 100: 529-533, 1972.

Sandler, M., Karoum, F. and Ruthven, C. R. J.: Parkinsonism with alkaptonuria: a new syndrome? (Letter) Lancet II: 770 only, 1970.

20360 ALOPECIA-EPILEPSY-OLIGOPHRENIA SYNDROME OF MOYNAHAN (FAMILIAL CONGENITAL ALOPECIA, EPILEPSY, MENTAL RETARDATION AND UNUSUAL EEG)

In the family reported by Moynahan (1962) two brothers were affected. The alopecia consisted of a delay in the growth of hair. The father of the boys had been bald until age 2 and a maternal aunt until age 4.

Moynahan, E. J.: Familial congenital alopecia, epilepsy, mental retardation with unusual electroencephalograms. Proc. Roy. Soc. Med. 55: 411-412, 1962.

*20370 ALPERS DIFFUSE DEGENERATION OF CEREBRAL GRAY MATTER (POLIODYSTROPHIA CEREBRI PROGRESSIVA) WITH HEPATIC CIRRHOSIS

The illness usually begins in early life with convulsions. A progressive neurologic disorder characterized by spasticity, myoclonus and dementia ensues. Status epilepticus is often the terminating development. The cases, in brother and sister, reported by Ford et al. (1951) are thought to be in this category. (See MYOCLONIC EPILEPSY for reference to same cases reported by Morse.) Familial cases were also reported by Palinsky et al. (1954), by Christensen and Hojgaard (1964) and by Blackwood et al. (1963).

It is now realized that progressive neuronal degeneration can follow convulsions and anoxic episodes from other causes. Cardiorespiratory arrest, hypotension, cyanosis and the vascular changes observed in the exposed brain by neurosurgical investigators of epilepsy are likely to lead to brain damage in which the cerebellum participates as well as the cerebrum. (Cerebellar damage due to convulsions must be distinguished from that due to dilantin used in their treatment.) Alpers disease may be a non-specific entity, only some cases of which have a specific genetic basis. In the family reported by Alberca-Serrano et al. (1965) four of 6 sibs were affected. The parents were unrelated. Several relatives of the father may have had the same disorder, which had the picture of encephalitis progressing to infantile spastic diplegia. Post-mortem study in one showed 'diffuse anoxic encephalopathy.' All the cases had reacted to infections with violent convulsions. The authors suggested that this represents a familial susceptibility and that the cerebral damage was secondary to anoxia. Wefring and Lamvik (1967) described brother and sister who developed convulsions at ages 11 and 14 months, followed by progressive hypotonia, dementia and jaundice 4 and 2 weeks before death at the age of 15 and 20 months. In addition to the typical findings of Alpers disease, the liver showed extensive atrophy with fibrosis, inflammation and bile duct proliferation. Blackwood et al. (1963) also described sibs with this combination, which may represent a separate entity.

Alberca-Serrano, R., Fabiani, F., Deneve, V. and Macken, J.: Familial spastic diplegia due to anoxic encephalopathy (Alpers). A contribution to the study of vascular fragilities of the nervous system of genetic type. J. Neurol. Sci. 2: 419-433, 1965.

Alpers, B. J.: Diffuse progressive degeneration of gray matter of cerebrum. Arch. Neurol. Psychiat. 25: 469-505, 1931.

Blackwood, W., Buxton, P. H., Cumings, J. N., Robertson, D. J. and Tucker, S. M.: Diffuse cerebral degeneration in infancy (Alpers' disease). Arch. Dis. Child. 38: 193-204, 1963.

Christensen, E. and Hojgaard, K.: Poliodystrophia cerebri progressiva infantilis. Acta Neurol. Scand. 40: 21-40, 1964.

Ford, F. R., Livingston, S. and Pryles, C. V.: Familial degeneration of the cerebral gray matter in childhood with convulsions, myoclonus, spasticity, cerebral ataxia, choreoathetosis, dementia, and death in status epilepticus. Differentiation of infantile and juvenile types. J. Pediat. 39: 33-43, 1951.

Palinsky, M., Kozinn, P. J. and Zahtz, H.: Acute familial infantile heredodegenerative disorder of the central nervous system. J. Pediat. 45: 538-545, 1954.

Wefring, K. W. and Lamvik, J. O.: Familial progressive poliodystrophy with cirrhosis of the liver. Acta Paediat. Scand. 56: 295-300, 1967.

*20375 ALPHA-METHYLACETOACETICACIDURIA

Daum et al. (1971) described a disorder at the sixth step in the catabolism of isoleucine, for the conversion of alpha-methylacetoacetate to propionate. As in many of the other inborn errors of branched-chain amino acid catabolism, the presenting clinical feature was recurrent severe metabolic acidosis. Both parents and a sib had increased amounts of alpha-methyl-beta-hydroxybutyric acid in the urine and this was increased by administration of isoleucine. The proband also showed excessive alpha-methylacetoacetate in the urine. Scriver (1972) suggested the designation used here. Hillman and Keating (1974) described a female patient with the 'ketotic hyperglycinemia syndrome' (see 23200 and 25100) and normal propionate and methylmalonate metabolism but markedly impaired catabolism of isoleucine. Studies of her urine and cultured fibroblasts suggested a defect in the beta-ketothiolase reaction which cleaves alpha-methylaceto-acetyl CoA to propionyl CoA and acetyl CoA. This is another potentially treatable condition of young infants with vomiting and acidosis. Hillman and Keating's patient was more severely affected than that of Daum et al. (1973). The M family of Daum et al. (1973) was consanguineous. The parents of the case reported by Hillman and Keating (1974) were not related (Hillman, 1974).

Daum, R. S., Lamm, P. H., Mamer, O. A. and Scriver, C. R.: A 'new' disorder of isoleucine catabolism. Lancet II: 1289-1290, 1971.

of isoleucine catabolism causing accumulation of alpha-methylacetoacetate and alpha-methyl-beta-hydrox-
ybutyrate and intermittent metabolic acidosis. Pediat. Res. 7: 149-160, 1973.

Hillman, R. E. and Keating, J. P.: Beta-ketothiolase deficiency as a cause of the 'ketotic hyperglycinemia
syndrome.' Pediatrics 53: 221-225, 1974.

Hillman, R. E.: St. Louis, personal communication, 1974.

Scriver, C. R.: Montreal, Canada: personal communication, 1972.

*20380 ALSTROM SYNDROME

Although this recessive disorder bears many similarities to the Laurence-Moon-Biedl syndrome (q.v.),
Alstrom et al. (1959) claims it is a distinct entity because there is no mental defect, polydactyly or
hypogonadism. The presence of retinitis pigmentosa, deafness, obesity and diabetes mellitus are elements of
similarity. The retinal lesion causes nystagmus and early loss of central vision in contrast to loss of peripheral
vision first, in other pigmentary retinopathies. Weinstein et al. (1969) described the condition of two brothers
with a disorder which they suggested 'resembles that described by Alstrom and his co-workers.' In spite of
the presence of small testes and elevated urinary gonadotropin levels, secondary sexual characteristics were
normal. Associated findings were blindness, deafness, obesity, and several metabolic abnormalities including
hyperuricemia and elevated serum triglyceride and pre-beta-lipoprotein. Autosomal recessive and X-linked
recessive inheritance cannot be distinguished and even male-limited autosomal dominant inheritance is
possible. However, the pedigree data of Alstrom make both X-linked recessive and autosomal dominant
inheritance unlikely. Goldstein and Fialkow (1973) described three affected sisters and pointed out that a
slowly progressive chronic nephropathy is a usual feature. The diabetes mellitus which occurs in this
condition is the result of resistance to the action of insulin. Target organ unresponsiveness to the action of
other polypeptide hormones, including vasopressin and gonadotropins, is suspected. Goldstein and Fialkow
(1973) pointed out that acanthosis nigricans is also a feature. They concluded that autosomal recessive
inheritance is indisputable.

Alstrom, C. H., Hallgren, B., Nilsson, L. B. and Asander, H.: Retinal degeneration combined with
obesity, diabetes mellitus and neurogenous deafness. A specific syndrome (not hitherto described) distinct
from the Laurence-Moon-Biedl syndrome. A clinical endocrinological and genetic examination based on a
large pedigree. Acta Psychiat. Neurol. Scand. 34 (suppl. 129): 1-35, 1959.

Goldstein, J. L. and Fialkow, P. J.: The Alstrom syndrome. Report of three cases with further delineation
of the clinical, pathophysiological, and genetic aspects of the disorder. Medicine 52: 53-71, 1973.

Weinstein, R. L., Kliman, B. and Scully, R. E.: Familial syndrome of primary testicular insufficiency with
normal virilization, blindness, deafness and metabolic abnormalities. New Eng. J. Med. 281: 969-977, 1969.

*20390 ALYMPHOCYTOSIS, PURE (THYMIC DYSPLASIA WITH NORMAL IMMUNOGLOBULINS AND IMMUNOLOGIC DEFICIENCY)

Nezelof (1968) lists the characteristics of this disorder as severe lymphopenia, tissue alymphocytosis, thymic
hypoplasia, fatal course, normal or subnormal serum immunoglobulins and presence of plasma cells. He
presented a pedigree strongly suggestive of autosomal recessive inheritance. Fireman et al. (1966) reported
a case. Whereas both cellular and humoral immune mechanisms are affected in the Swiss type
agammaglobulinemia and only the humoral mechanism in the Bruton (X-linked) type, only the cellular
mechanism is affected in this condition.

Fireman, P., Johnson, H. A. and Gitlin, D.: Presence of plasma cells and gamma-1-M-globulin synthesis
in a patient with thymic alymphoplasia. Pediatrics 37: 485-492, 1966.

Nezelof, C.: Thymic dysplasia with normal immunoglobulins and immunologic deficiency: pure
alymphocytosis. In, Good, R. A. (ed.): Immunologic Deficiency Diseases. New York: National Foundation,
1968. Pp. 104-115.

*20400 AMAUROSIS CONGENITA OF LEBER I

Alstrom (1957) found that a single disorder inherited as an autosomal recessive was responsible for 10 percent
of blindness in Sweden. Total blindness or greatly impaired vision with loss of central vision was present.
Early in life fundus changes were lacking, but by age 50 years widespread atrophy exposed white areas of
sclera. Cataract and keratoconus were associated. Keratoconus was of diagnostic usefulness. No
manifestations except in the eye were discovered. 'It was not until combined genealogic and genetico-statisti-
cal studies had been made, and clinical data collected over a long period that the congenital development
and affinity of these apparently heterogeneous cases could be established with some degree of probability'
(Alstrom, 1957). Striking pedigrees were presented. In Holland, Schappert-Kimmijser, Henkes and Van den
Bosch (1959) studied 227 cases and also presented pedigrees typical of autosomal recessive inheritance.
Among the causes of profound visual impairment of childhood, amaurosis congenita is comparable to
recessive congenital deafness as the cause of profound deafness of childhood. Undoubtedly great
heterogeneity exists. Probably a minimum of 6 different loci and possibly many more exist, homozygosity
at any one of which can result in the same phenotype. Separate entities are beginning to be separated on the
basis of associated abnormalities especially neurologic. See RENAL DYSPLASIA and RETINAL
APLASIA.

Congenital nystagmus and cerebral (or cortical) blindness were terms often assigned to these cases in the
past before the chorioretinal site of abnormality was appreciated. Sometimes it is confused with retinitis
pigmentosa. Retinal aplasia is the term most frequently used in England. Congenital absence of the rods and
cones is a designation often used in the U.S.A. Photophobia is frequently present and in young children may

be associated with forceful digging of the fingers and fists into the orbits. This may be responsible for the keratoconus. In a family reported by Rahn et al. (1968) there were cigarette-paper scars and stretchable skin suggesting Ehlers-Danlos syndrome.

Alstrom, C. H.: Heredo-retinopathia congenitalis monohybrida recessiva autosomalis. Hereditas 43: 1-178, 1957.

Gillespie, F. D.: Congenital amaurosis of Leber. Am. J. Ophthal. 61: 874-880, 1966.

Rahn, E. K., Meadow, E., Falls, H. F., Knaggs, J. C. and Proux, D. J.: Leber's congenital amaurosis with Ehlers-Danlos-like syndrome. Study of an American family. Arch. Ophthal. 79: 135-141, 1968.

Schappert-Kimmijser, J., Henkes, H. E. and Van den Bosch, J.: Amaurosis congenita (Leber). Arch. Ophthal. 61: 211-218, 1959.

*20410 AMAUROSIS CONGENITA OF LEBER II

One reason for suspecting the existence of two forms of the disease is a pedigree published by Waardenburg (1963) which shows all normal children from two affected parents. The mother had two affected sisters and the father was the product of a first-cousin marriage (Waardenburg and Schappert-Kimmijser, 1963). Keratoconus (or keratoglobus), a frequent feature of this condition, was not present in either parent but was found in one of the mother's affected sisters. This condition, is, of course, not to be confused with Leber optic atrophy.

Waardenburg, P. J. and Schappert-Kimmijser, J.: Genetics and Ophthalmology. Waardenburg, P. J., Franceschetti, A. and Klein, D. (eds.): Springfield, Ill.: Charles C Thomas, 2: 1579 only, 1963.

Waardenburg, P. J. and Schappert-Kimmijser, J.: On various recessive biotypes of Leber's congenital amaurosis. Acta Ophthal. 41: 317-320, 1963.

*20420 AMAUROTIC FAMILY IDIOCY, JUVENILE TYPE (BATTEN DISEASE IN ENGLAND, VOGT-SPIELMEYER DISEASE ON THE CONTINENT)

The first manifestation is often rapid deterioration of vision and a slower but progressive deterioration of intellect. Seizures and psychotic behavior developed later. The fundi show pigmentary degeneration. Kyphoscoliosis may develop. Onset is at age 5-10 years. Brain biopsy and rectal biopsy usually make the diagnosis by demonstration of nerve cells heavily laden with lipid. The relatively high frequency in non-Jewish northern Europeans (e.g., Swedes) emphasizes the fact that this form is distinct from Tay-Sachs disease, which, of course, it differs from greatly in clinical behavior. Vacuolation of the lymphocytes is a well established feature of the homozygote (McKusick et al., 1963). What is not so certain is vacuolation in heterozygotes. Rayner (1963) claims that about 1 percent of lymphocytes are vacuolated in heterozygotes. Bessman and Baldwin (1962) found imidazole aminoaciduria in five patients and some of their immediate relatives in three unrelated families. Potentially the method might be useful for detection of heterozygotes and for identifying heterogeneity in this category of disease. Strouth, Zeman and Merritt (1966) found azurophilic cytoplasmic granules in the peripheral leukocytes in 12 out of 16 patients. Furthermore, both parents and two-thirds of normal sibs showed these granulations which resemble those of the Alder anomaly (q.v.). The cases with absent leukocyte granulations may represent a different entity. Anatomic features are (1) severe widespread neuronal degeneration resulting in simple retinal atrophy and in massive loss of brain substance, the average brain weight being about 600 gm, and (2) accumulation of lipofuscin in neuronal perikaryon. The lipofuscin accumulation has been demonstrated by electron microscopy (Zeman and Donahue, 1963; Gonatas and Terry et al., 1963). Although the similar name assigned because of some histologic similarity to Tay-Sachs disease might suggest biochemical relatedness, there is no evidence that Batten disease is a ganglioside lipidosis as is Tay-Sachs disease. Danes and Bearn (1968) showed that both homozygotes and heterozygotes can be identified on the basis of metachromasia in skin fibroblasts in cell culture. Seitelberger et al. (1967) called the condition 'myoclonic variant of cerebral lipidosis.' Dayan and Trickey (1970) found large amounts of lipofuscin in the thyroid. By electron microscopy, Dolman and Chang (1972) found curvilinear bodies not only in the central and autonomic nervous system but also in the cells of virtually every organ examined.

Bessman, S. P. and Baldwin, R.: Imidazole aminoaciduria in cerebromacular degeneration. Science 135: 789-791, 1962.

Danes, B. S. and Bearn, A. G.: Metachromasia and skin-fibroblast cultures in juvenile familial amaurotic idiocy. Lancet II: 855-856, 1968.

Dayan, A. D. and Trickey, R. J.: Thyroid involvement in juvenile amaurotic idiocy (Batten's disease). Lancet II: 296-297, 1970.

Dolman, C. L. and Chang, E.: Visceral lesions in amaurotic familial idiocy with curvilinear bodies. Arch. Path. 94: 425-430, 1972.

Gonatas, N. K., Terry, R. D., Winkler, R., Korey, S. R., Gomez, C. J. and Stein, A.: A case of juvenile lipidosis: the significance of electron microscopic and biochemical observations of a cerebral biopsy. J. Neuropath. Exp. Neurol. 22: 557-580, 1963.

Gordon, N. S., Marsden, H. B. and Noronha, M. J.: Neuronal ceroid lipofuscinosis (Batten's disease). Arch. Dis. Child. 47: 285-291, 1972.

Harlem, O. K.: Juvenile cerebroretinal degeneration (Spielmeyer-Vogt). Am. J. Dis. Child. 100: 918-923, 1960.

Levenson, J., Lindahl-Kiessling, K. and Rayner, S.: Carnosine excretion in juvenile amaurotic idiocy. Lancet II: 756-757, 1964.

R
E
C
E
S
S
I
V
E

Rayner, S.: Juvenile amaurotic idiocy in Sweden with particular reference to the occurrence of vacuoles in the lymphocytes of homo- and heterozygotes. Uppsala: University of Uppsala, 1962.

Rayner, S.: Juvenile amaurotic idiocy in Sweden. Proc. 11th Intern. Cong. Genet., The Hague, 1963. p. 283.

Seitelberger, F., Jacob, H. and Schnabel, R.: The myoclonic variant of cerebral lipidosis. In, Aronson, S. M. and Volk, B. W. (eds.): Inborn Disorders of Sphingolipid Metabolism. Oxford: Perganon Press, 1967. Pp. 43-74.

Sjogren, T.: Die juvenile amaurotische Idiotie. Klinische und erblichkeitsmedizinische Untersuchungen. Hereditas 14: 197-426, 1931.

Strouth, J. C., Zeman, W. and Merritt, A. D.: Leukocyte abnormalities in familial amaurotic idiocy. New Eng. J. Med. 274: 36-38, 1966.

Zeman, W. and Donahue, S.: Fine structure of the lipid bodies in juvenile amaurotic idiocy. Acta Neuropath. 3: 144-149, 1963.

Zeman, W. and Strouth, J. C.: Leukocytic hypergranulation versus lymphocytic vacuolization as markers for heterozygotes and with Batten-Spielmeyer-Vogt disease. In, Aronson, S. M. and Volk, B. W. (eds.): Inborn Disorders of Sphingolipid Metabolism. Oxford: Pergamon Press, 1967. Pp. 475-484.

20430 AMAUROTIC IDIOCY, ADULT TYPE (KUF DISEASE)

The existence of this type is questionable, in the opinion of some. The case of Kufs (1925) had onset at age 26 and death at age 38. Fine, Barron and Hirano (1960) found reports of 18 complete histologic descriptions. Cases with the anatomic characteristics listed for the juvenile form may have late onset, making it possible that the adult and juvenile forms are in fact one entity (Zeman and Hoffman, 1962). Chou and Thompson (1970) reported the morphologic changes in a man who was well until age 17 and died at age 32. A sister was said to have died of a similar clinical picture (seizures, intellectual deterioration, lack of motor control, development of athetoid movements). The parents were well and were related as first cousins.

Chou, S. M. and Thompson, H. G.: Electron microscopy of storage cytosomes in Kufs' disease. Arch. Neurol. 23: 489-501, 1970.

Fine, D. I., Barron, K. D. and Hirano, A.: Central nervous system lipidosis in an adult with atrophy of the cerebellar granular layer. A case report. J. Neurol. 19: 355-369, 1960.

Kufs, H.: Uber eine Spatform der amaurotischen Idiotie und ihre heredofamiliaren Grundlagen. Zbl. Ges. Neurol. Psychiat. 95: 169-188, 1925.

Zeman, W. and Hoffman, J.: Juvenile and late forms of amaurotic idiocy in one family. J. Neurol. Neurosurg. Psychiat. 25: 352-362, 1962.

*20440 AMAUROTIC IDIOCY, CONGENITAL FORM

Norman and Wood (1941) described a single case, a female infant who died at 18 days. The parents were not related. (Tay-Sachs disease does not become evident before three months at the earliest.) In this case the intracellular granular inclusions were insoluble. Two other sibs had similar clinical and histologic findings (Brown and colleagues, 1954). Another case may be that of Epstein (1917) in which manifestation appeared in the second week of postnatal life. Hagberg et al. (1965) found a disialoganglioside, G(D3), not previously identified, in tissue from congenital amaurotic idiocy. Chemical studies in one case from the family reported by Norman and Wood (1941) showed a threefold increase in cholesterol in the brain, which weighed only 65 gm (normal 360 gm) (Brown et al., 1954). This finding distinguishes the disorder from both Tay-Sachs disease (27280) and the neuronal ceroid-lipofuscinoses. Since the infants died shortly after birth when neither vision nor intellect could be evaluated, the term 'congenital amaurotic idiocy' is meaningless.

Brown, N. J., Corner, B. D. and Dodgson, M. C. H.: A second case in the same family of congenital familial cerebral lipoidosis resembling amaurotic family idiocy. Arch. Dis. Child. 29: 48-54, 1954.

Epstein, J.: Amaurotic family idiocy. New York J. Med. 106: 887-889, 1917.

Hagberg, B., Hultqvist, G., Ohman, R. and Svennerholm, L.: Congenital amaurotic idiocy. Acta Paediat. Scand. 54: 116-130, 1965.

Norman, R. M. and Wood, N.: A congenital form of amaurotic family idiocy. J. Neurol. Psychiat. 4: 175-190, 1941.

20450 AMAUROTIC IDIOCY, LATE INFANTILE TYPE (JANSKY-BIELSCHOWSKY)

No fundus change or optic atrophy is observed. The cherry red spot is typical of the infantile form (Tay-Sachs) and retinitis pigmentosa is typical of the juvenile form (Spielmeyer-Vogt-Batten). More cerebellar involvement occurs in the late infantile form than in the others. Hassin (1926) reviewed the pathology. Seitelberger, Vogel and Stepan (1957) collected 28 cases from the world's literature. On the basis of electron microscopic findings Gonatas et al. (1968) suggested that two cases they studied and 4 cases reported by others represented a different type of late infantile amaurotic idiocy. Some cases reported as this entity may be instances of generalized gangliosidosis (Donahue et al., 1967).

Donahue, S., Zeman, W. and Watanabe, I.: Electron microscopic observations in Batten's disease. In, Aronson, S. M. and Volk, B. W. (eds.): Inborn Disorders of Sphingolipid Metabolism. Oxford: Pergamon Press, 1967. Pp. 3-22.

R
E
C
E
S
S
I
V
E

Gonatas, N. K., Gambetti, P. and Baird, H.: A second type of late infantile amaurotic idiocy with multilamellar cytosomes. J. Neuropath. Exp. Neurol. 27: 371-389, 1968.

Hassin, G. B.: Amaurotic family idiocy: late infantile type (Bielschowsky) with the clinical picture of decerebrate rigidity. Arch. Neurol. Psychiat. 16: 708-727, 1926.

Seitelberger, F., Vogel, G. and Stepan, H.: Spatinfantile amaurotische Idiotie. Arch. Psychiat. Nervenkr. 196: 154-190, 1957.

Volk, B. W., Wallace, B. J., Schneck, L. and Saifer, A.: Late infantile amaurotic idiocy. Ultramicroscopic and histochemical studies on a case. Arch. Path. 78: 483-500, 1964.

*20460 AMAUROTIC IDIOCY, LATE INFANTILE, WITH MULTILAMELLAR CYTOSOMES

Elfenbein and Cantor (1969) suggested this designation, based on the striking morphologic feature, for a disorder with onset between 2-and-a-half and 4 years, seizures, myoclonus, dementia, blindness with pigmentary changes in the fundus. They noted familial occurrence as did also Richardson and Bornhofen (1968) and Gonatas et al. (1968).

Elfenbein, I. B. and Cantor, H. E.: Late infantile amaurotic idiocy with multilamellar cytosomes: an electron microscopic study. J. Pediat. 75: 253-264, 1969.

Gonatas, N. K., Gambetti, P. and Baird, H.: A second type of late infantile amaurotic idiocy with multilamellar cytosomes. J. Neuropath. Exp. Neurol. 27: 371-389, 1968.

Richardson, M. E. and Bornhofen, J. H.: Early childhood cerebral lipidosis with prominent myoclonus. Ultrastructural and histochemical studies of a cerebral biopsy. Arch. Neurol. 18: 34-43, 1968.

*20470 AMELOGENESIS IMPERFECTA, PIGMENTED HYPOMATURATION TYPE

For a general discussion of this and other genetic abnormalities of the teeth and related structures see Witkop (1965). Only two families have been studied. In one a brother and sister were affected. Parents and more remote relatives were unaffected. The parents were first cousins once removed. Both the primary and the secondary dentition were affected. The teeth had a shiny agar jelly appearance and the enamel was softer than normal. The usual radiographic contrast between enamel and dentine was lacking. Histologically a brown pigment which is probably not derived from blood pigments but is of unknown nature was demonstrable in the middle layers of enamel.

Witkop, C. J.: Genetic disease of the oral cavity. In, Tiecke, R. W. (ed.): Oral Pathology. New York: McGraw-Hill, 1965.

Witkop, C. J., Kuhlmann, W. and Sauk, J.: Autosomal recessive pigmented hypomaturation amelogenesis imperfecta. Oral Surg. Oral Med. Oral Path. 36: 367-382, 1973.

20480 AMINOACIDURIA WITH MENTAL DEFICIENCY, DWARFISM, MUSCULAR DYSTROPHY, OSTEOPOROSIS AND ACIDOSIS

Stransky, Bayani-Sioson, and Lee (1962) described a family in which 5 of 7 sibs had this combination. The mother and two normal sibs had mild aminoaciduria.

Stransky, E., Bayani-Sioson, P. S. and Lee, W.: A peculiar type of familial mental deficiency, probably due to metabolic disturbance. A preliminary report. Philipp. Med. Assoc. J. 38: 903-908, 1962.

20490 AMYLOIDOSIS, CUTANEOUS BULLOUS

De Souza (1963) reported 4 affected sibs (1 male, 3 female). Onset was between 10 and 13 years. The lesions were mainly around the joints and were bullous in nature.

De Souza, A. R.: Amiloidose cutanea bulhosa familial. Observacao de 4 casos. Rev. Hosp. Clin. Fac. Med. S. Paulo 18: 413-417, 1963.

20500 AMYOTONIA CONGENITA (OPPENHEIM DISEASE)

Much uncertainty exists as to what Oppenheim had in mind and what this entity is — if indeed it exists at all. The best discussion is that of Greenfield, Cornman and Shy (1958) under the heading of 'the floppy infant.' When the primary defect resides in the spinal cord the condition is infantile muscular atrophy (q.v.), otherwise known as Werdnig-Hoffmann disease or infantile spinal amyotrophy. Possibly the term amyotonia congenita should be reserved for those conditions in which the primary abnormality resides in muscle and the disorder is essentially non-progressive. Certainly there are multiple causes, e.g., glycogen storage disease, the atonic-astatic syndrome of Foerster, and the congenital nonprogressive myopathy (q.v.) described by Batten and by Turner. Nemaline myopathy and central core diseases (q.v.) are other entities producing floppy infants.

Greenfield, J. G., Cornman, T. and Shy, G. M.: The prognostic value of the muscle biopsy in the 'floppy infant.' Brain 81: 461-484, 1958.

*20510 AMYOTROPHIC LATERAL SCLEROSIS, JUVENILE

In an Amish isolate we (Gragg et al., 1971) have observed two brothers with onset in the first decade of the ALS symptom complex: distal muscular atrophy, increased deep tendon reflexes, spasticity and fasciculations. Refsum and Skillicon (1954) described the same picture in two brothers and a sister. Onset was between 3 and 5 years. They stated that the condition was indistinguishable from amyotrophic lateral sclerosis.

Gragg, G. W., Fogelson, M. H. and Zwirecki, R. J.: Juvenile amyotrophic lateral sclerosis in two brothers from an inbred community. In Bergsma D. (ed.) The Clinical Delineation of Birth Defects. VI. Nervous System. Baltimore: Williams and Wilkins, 1971. Pp. 222-225.

20520 AMYOTROPHIC LATERAL SCLEROSIS, JUVENILE, WITH DEMENTIA

Hoffmann (1894) described slowly progressive juvenile amyotrophic lateral sclerosis with concomitantly progressive dementia in 4 sibs. Staal and Went (1968) described 7 sibs (out of 15), offspring of a first-cousin marriage, affected by the same disorder. Three boys and 4 girls were affected. Death had occurred in 5 of 7 sibs at intervals varying from 9 to 21 years after onset of symptoms which started at about age 10 years.

Hoffmann, J.: Ueber einen eigenartigen Symptomencomplex, eine Combination von angenborenem Schwachsinn mit progressiver Muskelatrophie, als weiterer Beitrag zu den erblichen Nervenkrankheiten. Deutsch. Z. Nervenheilk. 6: 150-166, 1894.

Staal, A. and Went, L. N.: Juvenile amyotrophic lateral sclerosis-dementia complex in a Dutch family. Neurology 18: 800-806, 1968.

*20530 ANALBUMINEMIA

Analbuminemia is a completely recessive condition. Serum albumin has a normal level in heterozygotes. The homozygotes have remarkably little inconvenience attributable to the lack of serum albumin. The disorder was first reported in 1954 by Bennhold and colleagues of Tubingen. It must be very rare. See review by Ott (1962). Whether the mutation is at the same locus as those responsible for the electrophoretic variants of albumin (see dominant catalog) is unknown.

Bennhold, H. and Kallee, E.: Comparative studies on the half-life of 1131 labelled albumins and nonradioactive human serum albumin in a case of analbuminemia. J. Clin. Invest. 38: 863-872, 1959.

Bennhold, H., Peters, H. and Roth, E.: Uber einen Fall von kompletter Analbuminaemie ohne wesentliche klinische Krankheitszeichen. Verh. Deutsch. Ges. Inn. Med. 60: 630-634, 1954.

Ott, H.: Analbuminemia. In, Erbliche Stoffwechselkrankheiten. Linneweh, F. (ed.): Munich: Urban und Schwarzenberg, 1962. p. 44.

*20540 ANALPHALIPOPROTEINEMIA (TANGIER DISEASE)

The disorder has been found among inhabitants of Tangier Island in the Chesapeake Bay, most of whom are descendants of first settlers of 1686. Characteristics are very large tonsils which have a very characteristic gross and histologic appearance, enlarged liver, spleen and lymph nodes, and hypocholesterolemia. The thymus is loaded with lipid which can be shown to consist of cholesterol esters. Heterozygotes show low alpha-lipoproteins in the serum. Other affected families have been discovered in Missouri and in Kentucky. In Britain Kocen et al. (1967) described the condition in a 37 year old air force corporal who showed widespread dissociated loss of pain and temperature sensation and progressive muscle wasting and weakness. They commented that whereas the characteristic pharyngeal appearance had been the presenting feature in children, adolescents had presented with relapsing peripheral neuropathy and adults with hypersplenism or with precocious coronary artery disease. Engel et al. (1967) found recurrent neuropathy and intestinal lipid storage as features. Lux et al. (1972) demonstrated a marked reduction in one of the two major apoproteins of high density lipoprotein — apo-lp-gln-i. Since no immunochemical difference could be demonstrated between this apoprotein of Tangier disease and that of normals, they concluded that Tangier disease may be a mutation in a gene which regulates the synthesis of apo-lp-gln-i.

Clifton-Bligh, P., Nestel, P. J. and Whyte, H. M.: Tangier disease: report of a case and studies of lipid metabolism. New Eng. J. Med. 286: 567-571, 1972.

Engel, W. K., Dorman, J. D., Levy, R. I. and Fredrickson, D. S.: Neuropathy in Tangier disease. Alpha-lipoprotein deficiency manifesting as familial recurrent neuropathy and intestinal lipid storage. Arch. Neurol. 17: 1-9, 1967.

Fredrickson, D. S., Gotto, A. M. and Levy, R. I.: Lipoprotein deficiency. In, Stanbury, J. B., Wyngaarden, J. B. and Fredrickson, D. S. (eds.): The Metabolic Basis of Inherited Disease. New York: McGraw-Hill, 1972 (3rd Ed.). Pp. 493-530.

Fredrickson, D. S.: The inheritance of high density lipoprotein deficiency (Tangier disease). J. Clin. Invest 43: 228-236, 1964.

Kocen, R. S., Lloyd, J. K., Lascelles, P. T., Fosbrooke, A. S. and Williams, D.: Familial alpha-lipoprotein deficiency (Tangier disease) with neurological abnormalities. Lancet I: 1341-1345, 1967.

Lux, S. E., Levy, R. I., Gotto, A. M. and Fredrickson, D. S.: Studies on the protein defect in Tangier disease. Isolation and characterization of an abnormal high density lipoprotein. J. Clin. Invest. 51: 2502-2519, 1972.

20550 ANAL-SACRAL ANOMALIES

Aaronson (1970) described two brothers and a sister with anterior sacral meningocele, anal canal duplication cyst and covered anus. The parents were not related.

Aaronson, I.: Anterior sacral meningocele, anal canal duplication cyst and covered anus occurring in one family. J. Pediat. Surg. 5: 559-563, 1970.

20560 ANEMIA AND TRIPHALANGEAL THUMBS

Aase and Smith (1969) observed 2 brothers with congenital anemia and triphalangeal thumbs. In one, ventricular septal defect was thought to be present. The shoulders were narrow and sloping. They considered it an entity distinct from Fanconi panmyelopathy, thrombocytopenia with absent radius, and the Holt-Oram syndrome. It may be distinct also from the Blackfan-Diamond syndrome (20590), which, however is an

R
E
C
E
S
S
I
V
E

ill-defined condition. Indeed, Diamond et al. (1961, ref. in 20590) observed triphalangeal thumbs in one of 30 patients.

Aase, J. M. and Smith, D. W.: Congenital anemia and triphalangeal thumbs: a new syndrome. J. Pediat. 74: 471-474, 1969.

Jones, B. and Thompson, H.: Triphalangeal thumbs associated with hypoplastic anemia. Pediatrics 52: 609-612, 1973.

Murphy, S. and Lubin, B.: Triphalangeal thumbs and congenital erythroid hypoplasia: report of a case with unusual features. J. Pediat. 81: 987-989, 1972.

20570 ANEMIA, AUTOIMMUNE HEMOLYTIC

Dobbs (1965) reported brother and sister with 'Coombs positive' hemolytic anemia. Another sister seems to have died of autoimmune hemolytic anemia. Positive latex fixation, positive Wassermann test and negative T. pallidum test was found in both parents and the father had hypergammaglobulinemia. Others have reported familial autoimmune hemolytic anemia with abnormalities of gamma globulin.

Dobbs, C. E.: Familial auto-immune hemolytic anemia. Arch. Intern. Med. 116: 273-276, 1965.

Fialkow, P. J., Fudenberg, H. and Epstein, W. V.: 'Acquired' antibody hemolytic anemia and familial aberrations in gamma globulins. Am. J. Med. 36: 188-199, 1964.

Kissmeyer-Nielsen, F., Hansen, K. and Kieler, J.: Immuno-hemolytic anemia with familial occurrence. Acta Med. Scand. 144: 35-39, 1952.

20580 ANEMIA, CHLORAMPHENICOL-INDUCED

Nagao and Mauer (1969) described identical twins with chloramphenicol-induced aplastic anemia. Dameshek (1969), in an accompanying editorial, reviewed evidence for a genetic susceptibility to drug-induced bone marrow suppression.

Dameshek, W.: Chloramphenicol aplastic anemia in identical twins — a clue to pathogenesis. (Editorial) New Eng. J. Med. 281: 42-43, 1969.

Nagao, T. and Mauer, A. M.: Concordance for drug-induced aplastic anemia in identical twins. New Eng. J. Med. 281: 7-11, 1969.

20590 ANEMIA, CONGENITAL HYPOPLASTIC, OF BLACKFAN AND DIAMOND (CHRONIC CONGENITAL AREGENERATIVE ANEMIA, ERYTHROGENESIS IMPERFECTA, 'PURE RED CELL ANEMIA')

R
E
C
E
S
S
I
V
E

Familial cases have been reported by Burgert, Kennedy and Pease (1954) and by Diamond, Allen and Magill (1961). This disorder is sometimes encountered in the newborn, is progressive and is non-regenerative. There is no erythroblastosis, hemolysis or hepatosplenomegaly (until many transfusions have been given). Leukocytes and platelets are usually normal. Occasionally cortisone is effective. In some an abnormality of tryptophane metabolism, manifested by urinary excretion of anthranilic acid, has been found. Hirschman et al. (1969) reported two brothers with aplastic anemia similar to Fanconi anemia but without associated congenital anomalies. Both responded to androgen therapy. Both showed increased chromosomal breakage as in Fanconi anemia. One had a stable translocation chromosome in bone marrow cells. The other's skin fibroblasts showed increased susceptibility to 'malignant' transformation by SV40 virus, as in Fanconi anemia. Skin fibroblasts of the mother and a sister, both normal, also showed increased susceptibility to 'malignant' transformation. The father was, it seems, not studied from this point of view. See 20560 for the syndrome of triphalangeal thumbs with congenital hypoplastic anemia. Dominant inheritance is suggested by at least five reported families. Lawton et al. (1974) described father and son with documented anemia from infancy. The father's anemia remitted at age 6 years but he continued to have macrocytosis, reticulocytosis, he continued to have raised fetal hemoglobin. Forare (1963) observed affected brother and sister with the same father but different mothers. Falter and Robinson (1972) described affected mother and daughter. Hamilton et al. (1974) described affected mother and daughter. In addition, Wallmann described a father and daughter with erythroid hypoplasia but the ages of onset (34 and 6 years, respectively) were beyond the usual limits of the Diamond-Blackfan syndrome.

Altman, K. I. and Miller, G.: A disturbance of tryptophan metabolism in congenital hypoplastic anemia. Nature 172: 868 only, 1953.

Bloom, G. E., Warner, S., Gerald, P. S. and Diamond, L. K.: Chromosome abnormalities in constitutional aplastic anemia. New Eng. J. Med. 274: 8-14, 1966.

Burgert, E. O., Jr., Kennedy, R. L. J. and Pease, G. L.: Congenital hypoplastic anemia. Pediatrics 13: 218-226, 1954.

Diamond, L. K., Allen, D. W. and Magill, F. B.: Congenital (erythroid) hypoplastic anemia: a 25 year study. Am. J. Dis. Child. 102: 403-415, 1961.

Falter, M. L. and Robinson, M. G.: Autosomal dominant inheritance and aminoaciduria in Blackfan-Diamond anemia. J. Med. Genet. 9: 64-66, 1972.

Hamilton, P. J., Dawson, A. A. and Galloway, W. H.: Congenital erythroid hyperplastic anaemia in mother and daughter. Arch. Dis. Child. 49: 71-73, 1974.

Hunter, R. E. and Hakami, N.: The occurrence of congenital hypoplastic anemia in half-brothers. J. Pediat. 81: 346-348, 1972.

Kass, A. and Sundal, A.: Anaemia hypoplastica congenita (anaemia typus Josephs-Diamond-Blackfan). Report of a case treated with adrenocorticotropin with effect. Acta Paediat. 42: 265-274, 1953.

Lawton, J. W. M., Aldrich, J. E. and Turner, T. L.: Congenital erythroid hypoplastic anemia: autosomal dominant transmission. Am. J. Med., in press, 1974.

Mott, M. G., Apley, J. and Raper, A. B.: Congenital (erythroid) hypoplastic anaemia: modified expression in males. Arch. Dis. Child. 44: 757- , 1969.

Pearson, H. A. and Cone, T. E., Jr.: Congenital hypoplastic anemia. Pediatrics 19: 192-200, 1957.

*20600 ANEMIA, FAMILIAL PYRIDOXINE-RESPONSIVE

Unlike the clinically similar disorder reported by Cooley and by Rundles and Falls and transmitted as an X-linked recessive, the condition in the family described by Cotton and Harris (1962) was clearly autosomal recessive.

Cotton, H. B. and Harris, J. W.: Familial pyridoxine-responsive anemia. (Abstract) J. Clin. Invest. 41: 1352 only, 1962.

20610 ANEMIA, HYPOCHROMIC MICROCYTIC

Shahidi, Nathan and Diamond (1964) described hypochromic microcytic anemia in a brother and sister of French-Canadian extraction. An error in iron metabolism was characterized by high serum iron, massive hepatic iron deposition and absence of stainable bone marrow iron stores. No defect in transferrin or in the qualitative aspects of heme synthesis could be shown. The parents and two other sibs were normal. Despite adequate transferrin-iron complex, delivery of iron to the erythroid bone marrow was apparently insufficient for the demands of hemoglobin synthesis.

Shahidi, N. T., Nathan, D. G. and Diamond, L. K.: Iron deficiency anemia associated with an error of iron metabolism in two siblings. J. Clin. Invest. 43: 510-521, 1964.

20630 ANEMIA, NONSPHEROCYTIC HEMOLYTIC, ASSOCIATED WITH ABNORMALITY OF RED-CELL MEMBRANE

In a Polish-born Jewish family, Danon et al. (1962) described an electron microscopic abnormality of the red-cell membrane which probably was responsible for susceptibility to hemolysis on exposure to drugs and possibly viruses. Two sisters had similar findings. Questionable anomaly was found in the proband's son.

Danon, D., De Vries, A., Djaldetti, M. and Kirschmann, C.: Episodes of acute haemolytic anaemia in a patient with familial ultrastructural abnormality of the red-cell membrane. Brit. J. Haemat. 8: 274-282, 1962.

20640 ANEMIA, NONSPHEROCYTIC HEMOLYTIC, POSSIBLY DUE TO DEFECT IN PORPHYRIN METABOLISM

From Berne, Tonz, Mereu and Kaser (1961) reported two brothers, age 7 and 14 years, with hemolytic disease already manifest in the first weeks of life. Chronic jaundice, severe anemia and splenomegaly were features. Splenectomy was of some benefit. Several enzymes of the erythrocyte were normal, but pyruvate kinase activity was not measured. The urine consistently showed an increased amount of porphobilinogen and delta-aminolevulinic acid. A defect in porphyrin metabolism (i.e., heme synthesis) was suggested. Since the ancestors of the Amish cases of pyruvate kinase deficiency (q.v.) first reported by Bowman and Procopio originated in the canton Berne, studies of pyruvate kinase are particularly pertinent.

Tonz, O., Mereu, T. R. and Kaser, H.: Familiaere, nicht-sphaerocytaere haemolytische Anaemie mit Ausscheidung von Porphyrinpraekursoren. Helv. Paediat. Acta 16: 111-133, 1961.

20650 ANENCEPHALY

Penrose (1957) concluded that recessive cases exist. Multiple affected sibs were reported by several authors, e.g., Iffy (1963) who observed three affected sibs and quoted the description by Martin (1840) of 6 affected sibs. A striking geographic variation may be in part due to ethnic genetic differences (Masterson, 1962). Concordantly affected presumably monozygotic twins were reported by Taber and Elwell (1960), Josephson and Waller (1933) and Labate and Calvelli (1952). Discordance in monozygotic twins was reported by Grebe (1949), and Pedlow (1961) and Litt and Strauss (1935). Horne's patient (1958) had 4 anencephalic offspring of which the last was sired by a man other than the husband. In single families (Stevenson, 1960; Martin, 1840), six sibs have been affected. Dumoulin and Gordon (1959) reported a patient who in addition to producing 3 normal and 2 anencephalic infants had uniovular twins, one of which was anencephalic. Record and McKeown (1950) estimated that the empiric risk of recurrence is about 2 percent. Yen and MacMahon (1968) studied the recurrence of anencephaly in families and concluded that the findings were explained by a persistent environmental factor as adequately as by genetic factors. Christakos and Simpson (1969) described anencephaly in three sibs. Spina bifida (27100) and anencephaly are generally considered one entity. Fuhrmann et al. (1971) described 5 children with one or the other abnormality among 8 children of two related families. The two fathers had married two sisters and each union was a third-cousin marriage.

Christakos, A. C. and Simpson, J. L.: Anencephaly in three siblings. Obstet. Gynec. 33: 267-270, 1969.

Coleman, J. U.: Repeat anencephaly. Canad. Med. Ass. J. 79: 395-397, 1958.

Dumoulin, J. G. and Gordon, M. E.: Anencephaly in twins. J. Obstet. Gynaec. Brit. Comm. 66: 964-968, 1959.

Fuhrmann, W., Seeger, W. and Bohm, R.: Apparently monogenic inheritance of anencephaly and spina bifida in a kindred. Humangenetik 13: 241-243, 1971.

Grebe, H.: Anencephalie bei einem Paarling von eineiigen Zwillingen. Virchow. Arch. Path. Anat. 316: 116-124, 1949.

Horne, H. W.: Anencephaly in four consecutive pregnancies. Report of a case. Fertil. Steril. 9: 67-68, 1958.

Iffy, L.: Thrice recurring anencephalus. Brit. J. Clin. Pract. 17: 83-84, 1963.

Josephson, J. E. and Waller, K. B.: Anencephaly in identical twins. Canad. Med. Ass. J. 29: 34-37, 1933.

Labate, J. S. and Calvelli, G. J., Jr.: Anencephalic twins with rupture of the uterus. New York J. Med. 52: 2662 only, 1952.

Litt, S. and Strauss, H. A.: Monoamniotic twins, one normal, other anencephalic: multiple true knots in cords. Am. J. Obstet. Gynec. 30: 728-730, 1935.

Martin, J.: Succession of monstrous births occurring in the same female. Med. Exam. 5: 23, 1840.

Masterson, J. G.: Empiric risk, genetic counseling and preventive measures in anencephaly. Acta Genet. Statist. Med. 12: 219-229, 1962.

Pedlow, P. R. B.: Anencephaly in a mono-amniotic twin. Brit. Med. J. 2: 997-998, 1961.

Penrose, L. S.: Genetics of anencephaly. J. Ment. Defic. Res. 1: 4-15, 1957.

Record, R. G. and McKeown, T.: Congenital malformation of the central nervous system. III. Risk of malformation in sibs of malformed individuals. Brit. J. Prev. Soc. Med. 4: 217-220, 1950.

Stevenson, A. C.: The relation of hydramnios with congenital malformations. In, Wolstenholme, G. E. W. and O'Connor, C. M. (eds.): Ciba Foundation Symposium on Congenital Malformations. Boston: Little, Brown and Co., 1960. p. 259.

Taber, K. W. and Elwell, W. J., Jr.: Monozygotic anencephalic twins. Maryland Med. J. 9: 14 only, 1960.

Yen, S. and MacMahon, B.: Genetics of anencephaly and spina bifida? Lancet II: 623-626, 1968.

*20657 ANGIOMATOSIS, DIFFUSE CORTICO-MENINGEAL, OF DIVRY AND VAN BOGAERT

Features in addition to the cortico-meningeal angiomatosis were meyelination of the white substance of the centrum ovale with hemianopsia, and 'marbled skin' resulting from a telangiectatic network. Three affected brothers were described by Divry and Van Bogaert (1946). Martin et al. (1973) studied two sibs, a male and a female, who demonstrated this condition. Both presented similar symptoms of epileptic seizures during the second decade, visual field defects, migranes with focal paresthesias, mental disturbances and progressive dementia. Surgery to relieve these symptoms was unsuccessful. Necroscopy revealed diffuse capillaro-venous non-calcifying leptomeningeal angiomatoses in the depths of the sulci becoming more prominent toward the occipital lobes. All the abnormally proliferated vessels showed fibrotic changes. The brain showed diffuse anoxic cortical encephalopathy with areas of atrophy and secondary degeneration of the white matter. These changes became most severe in the parietal-occipital-temporal areas. The brain stem showed signs of fibrillary gliosis of some nuclei and tracts, particularly the vestibular and reticular nuclei, trigemenal spinal tracts and pyrmidal tracts. These patients had no other physical abnormalities or marbling of the skin.

Divry, P. and Van Bogaert, L.: Une maladie familiale caracterisee par une angiomatose diffuse cortico-meningee non calcifiante et une demyelinisation progressive de la substance blanche. J. Neurol. Neurosurg. Psychiat. 9: 41-54, 1946.

Martin, J. J., Navarro, C., Roussel, J. M. and Michielssen, P.: Familial capillaro-venous leptomeningeal angiomatosis. Europ. Neurol. 9: 202-215, 1973.

*20660 ANHIDROSIS

Anhidrotic ectodermal dysplasia is usually inherited as an X-linked disorder. Mahloudji and Livingston (1967) described an Iranian sibship in which a boy and two girls had anhidrosis without dental, facial, brain or other anomalies characteristic of the X-linked disorder. The parents were first cousins. See ECTODER-MAL DYSPLASIA, ANHIDROTIC, in this catalog.

Mahloudji, M. and Livingston, K. E.: Familial and congenital simple anhidrosis. Am. J. Dis. Child. 113: 477-479, 1967.

20670 ANIRIDIA, CEREBELLAR ATAXIA AND MENTAL DEFICIENCY

Gillespie (1965) described brothers and sisters with this combination which has apparently not been reported previously, although cerebellar ataxia, mental deficiency and congenital cataracts are known in the Marinesco-Sjogren syndrome. It is likely that Gillespie's patients represent a separate mutation. The karyotype was normal in his patients. Sarsfield reported a further example of the above syndrome complex occurring in a male, the second child of normal parents. Bilateral partial aniridia was noted at birth and developmental milestones were subsequently delayed. Although muscle biopsies and nerve conduction times were normal, there was persistent hypotonia with normal tendon reflexes, normal sensation but gross uncoordination and attention tremor and scanning speech. There was some improvement in motor performance with age but mental retardation was evident. All lab investigations including karyotype were normal.

Gillespie, F. D.: Aniridia, cerebellar ataxia, and oligophrenia in siblings. Arch. Ophthal. 73: 338-341, 1965.

Sarsfield, J. K.: The syndrome of congenital cerebellar ataxia, aniridia and mental retardation. Develop. Med. Child. Neurol. 13: 508-511, 1971.

R
E
C
E
S
S
I
V
E

Littman and Levin (1964) observed an affected brother and sister with no other anomaly and with no affected relatives. Timmer and Wildervanck (1969) described congenital complete anonychia in a girl whose parents were somewhat more closely related than second cousins. Conclusive evidence for recessive inheritance was presented by Mahloudji and Amidi (1971). Hopsu-Hava and Jansen (1973) described anonychia congenita in a Finnish family. Four of ten sibs, two males and two females, were affected. These affected sibs had no other physical abnormalities. Both parents were descendants of a 17th-century churchman.

Hopsu-Hava, V. K. and Jansen, C. T.: Anonychia congenita. Arch. Derm. 107: 752-753, 1973.

Littman, A. and Levin, S.: Anonychia as a recessive autosomal trait in man. J. Invest. Derm. 42: 177-178, 1964.

Mahloudji, M. and Amidi, M.: Simple anonychia. Further evidence for autosomal recessive inheritance. J. Med. Genet. 8: 478-480, 1971.

Timmer, J. and Wildervanck, L. S.: Anonychia congenita totalis van vingers en tensen. Nederl. T. Geneesk. 113: 395-397, 1969.

*20690 ANOPHTHALMOS, TRUE OR PRIMARY

This anomaly is due to failure of formation of the optic pit. Only the ectodermal elements are missing. It is always bilateral. In almost all instances the parents are related. For example, Cecchetto (1920) reported a pedigree in which two brothers, each married to a first cousin, had a child with bilateral anophthalmos. The common grandparents were also first cousins. Hesselberg (1951) reported affected children from first-cousin parents. Sorsby (1934) discovered early reports of affected sibs with normal parents. Ashley (1947) reported affected Japanese brother and sister. Sometimes differentiation of extreme microphthalmos (q.v.) and of cryptophthalmos (21900) from anophthalmos is difficult.

Ashley, L. M.: Bilateral anophthalmos in a brother and sister. J. Hered. 38: 174-176, 1947.

Cecchetto, E.: Dell'anoftalmo congenito familiare. Arch. Ottal. 27: 114-119, 1920.

Hesselberg, C.: Congenital bilateral anophthalmia. Acta Ophthal. 29: 183-189, 1951.

Joseph, R.: A pedigree of anophthalmos. Brit. J. Ophthal. 41: 541-543, 1957.

Sorsby, A.: Anophthalmos: unpublished manuscript by James Briggs giving first account of familial occurrence of condition. Brit. J. Ophthal. 18: 469-472, 1934.

20695 ANORCHIA, CONGENITAL

Hall et al. (1974) observed two unrelated sibships each with two boys with anorchia. In one family the boys were identical twins, one with bilateral anorchia, the other with left sided anorchia only. In the second family both boys had left sided involvement only. Concordantly affected twins have been reported by others (e.g. Farrington, 1967) and affected brothers have been reported by Abeyaratne et al., 1969; Bobrow, 1970).

Abeyaratne, M. R., Aherne, W. A. and Scott, J. E. S.: The vanishing testis. Lancet II: 822-824, 1969.

Bobrow, M.: Bilateral absence of testes. Lancet II: 266 only, 1970.

Hall, J. G., Morgan, A. and Blizzard, R. M.: Familial congenital anorchia. In press, 1974.

20700 ANOSMIA FOR ISOBUTYRIC ACID

Amoore (1967) studied anosmia for the sweat-like odor of isobutyric acid. The frequency was about 2.5 percent. No family studies were reported. By analogy to Daltonism, he suggested it be called Davism in honor of Alfred Davis who described it.

Amoore, J. E.: Specific anosmia: a clue to the olfactory code. Nature 214: 1095-1098, 1967.

20710 ANOTIA AND MEATAL ATRESIA

Ellwood et al. (1968) described two sibs with bilateral anotia and meatal atresia. In a second unrelated family, one sib had unilateral microtia and bilateral meatal atresia whereas the other had unilateral microtia and meatal atresia.

Ellwood, L. C., Winter, S. T. and Dar, H.: Familial microtia with meatal atresia in two sibships. J. Med. Genet. 5: 289-291, 1968.

20730 ANTITHROMBIN, FAMILIAL HEMORRHAGIC DIATHESIS DUE TO

Brown and colleagues (1963) have described a hemorrhagic diathesis apparently due to the presence of an antithrombin as the primary defect. The disorder occurred in a Mohawk Indian kindred. Recessive inheritance is not completely certain. See 10730 for a discussion of antithrombin III deficiency.

Brown, G. M., Diamant, N. E., Galbraith, P. R. and Wilson, W. E. C.: A familial hemorrhagic diathesis due to an antithrombin. Blood 21: 298-305, 1963.

20740 ANTITRYPSIN DEFICIENCY OF PLASMA

Laurell and Eriksson (1963) described absence of alpha-1-antitrypsin from the plasma in patients with degenerative lung disease leading to death in middle life. Family studies indicate recessive inheritance. The heterozygotes are free of disease but can be identified chemically. Several workers have confirmed these findings. Of 12 patients with destructive lung disease present prior to age forty, two were judged by Tarkoff et al. (1968) to be homozygous for the deficiency and one heterozygous. Among 103 patients with obstructive lung disease Kueppers et al. (1969) found 5 homozygotes and 25 heterozygotes for the deficiency gene. They suggested that especially in males heterozygosity may predispose to chronic obstructive lung disease. Lieberman (1969) presented evidence indicating that heterozygotes also have a predisposition to lung disease. The importance of prompt treatment of respiratory infections and avoidance of proteolytic aerosols, smoking and employment entailing exposure to respiratory irritants was emphasized as preventive measures in these families. Bell (1970) pointed out that the emphysematous changes involve primarily the lower lung fields. Gans et al. (1969) described familial infantile liver cirrhosis in presumed homozygotes for alpha(1)-antitrypsin deficiency. Stevens et al. (1971) concluded that heterozygotes may develop emphysema qualitatively like that in homozygotes but at a later age. An adult with antitrypsin deficiency and combined liver and lung disease was reported by Gherardi (1971). See the study of 12 cases of combined disease by Berg and Erikkson (1972). This entry has no asterisk because the locus is already represented by entry no. 10740.

Bell, R. S.: The radiographic manifestations of alpha-1 antitrypsin deficiency. An important recognizable pattern of chronic obstructive pulmonary disease (COPD). Radiology 95: 19-24, 1970.

Berg, N. O. and Eriksson, S.: Liver disease in adults with alpha-1-antitrypsin deficiency. New Eng. J. Med. 287: 1264-1267, 1972.

Eriksson, S.: Studies in alpha 1-antitrypsin deficiency. Acta Med. Scand. 177 (suppl. 432): 1-85, 1965.

Falk, G. A. and Briscoe, W. A.: Alpha-1-antitrypsin deficiency in chronic obstructive pulmonary disease. (Editorial) Ann. Intern. Med. 72: 427-429, 1970.

Falk, G. A. and Briscoe, W. A.: Chronic obstructive pulmonary disease and heterozygous alpha-1-anti-trypsin deficiency. (Editorial) Ann. Intern. Med. 72: 595-596, 1970.

Gans, H., Sharp, H. L. and Tan, B. H.: Antiprotease deficiency and familial infantile liver cirrhosis. Surg. Gynec. Obstet. 129: 289-299, 1969.

Gherardi, G. J.: Alpha(1)-antitrypsin deficiency and its effect on the liver. Hum. Path. 2: 173-175, 1971.

Guenter, C. A., Welch, M. H. and Hammarsten, J. F.: Alpha-1-antitrypsin deficiency and pulmonary emphysema. Ann. Rev. Med. 22: 283-292, 1971.

Hepper, N. G., Black, L. F., Gleich, G. J. and Kueppers, F.: The prevalence of alpha(1)-antitrypsin deficiency in selected groups of patients with chronic obstructive lung disease. Mayo Clin. Proc. 44: 697-710, 1969.

Kueppers, F., Briscoe, W. A. and Bearn, A. G.: Hereditary deficiency of serum alpha 1-antitrypsin. Science 146: 1678-1679, 1964.

Kueppers, F., Fallat, R. and Larson, R. K.: Obstructive lung diseases and alpha-antitrypsin deficiency gene heterozygosity. Science 165: 899-901, 1969.

Laurell, C.-B. and Eriksson, S.: The electrophoretic alpha-1-globulin pattern of serum in alpha-1-antitrypsin deficiency. Scand. J. Clin. Lab. Invest. 15: 132-140, 1963.

Lieberman, J.: Heterozygous and homozygous alpha-1-antitrypsin deficiency in patients with pulmonary emphysema. New Eng. J. Med. 281: 279-284, 1969.

Lopez, V., Oetliker, O., Colombo, J. P. and Butler, R.: Ein Fall von familiarem alpha-1-Antitrypsinman-gel. Helv. Paediat. Acta 19: 296-303, 1964.

Pierce, J. A., Eisen, A. Z. and Dhingra, H. K.: Relationship of antitrypsin deficiency to the pathogenesis of emphysema. Trans. Ass. Am. Phys. 82: 87-97, 1969.

Sharp, H. L., Bridges, R. A., Krivit, W. and Freier, E. F.: Cirrhosis associated with alpha-1-antitrypsin deficiency: a previously unrecognized inherited disorder. J. Lab. Clin. Med. 73: 934-939, 1969.

Stevens, P. M., Hnilica, V., Johnson, P. C. and Bell, R. L.: Pathophysiology of hereditary emphysema. Ann. Intern. Med. 74: 672-680, 1971.

Talamo, R. C., Allen, J. D., Kahan, M. G. and Austen, K. F.: Hereditary alpha(1)-antitrypsin deficiency. New Eng. J. Med. 278: 345-351, 1971, 1968.

Talamo, R. C. and Feingold, M.: Infantile cirrhosis with hereditary alpha-1-antitrypsin deficiency. Am. J. Dis. Child. 125: 845-849, 1973.

Tarkoff, M. P., Kueppers, F. and Miller, W. F.: Pulmonary emphysema and alpha(1)-antitrypsin deficiency. Am. J. Med. 45: 220-228, 1968.

Townley, R. G., Ryning, F., Lynch, H. and Brody, A. W.: Obstructive lung disease in hereditary alpha-1-antitrypsin deficiency. J.A.M.A. 214: 325-331, 1970.

20750 ANUS, IMPERFORATE

Families with multiple affected sibs, both male and female, have been reported (Van Gelder and Kloepfer, 1961; Winkler and Weinstein, 1970). See X-linked catalog.

Van Gelder, D. W. and Kloepfer, H. W.: Familial anorectal anomalies. Pediatrics 27: 334-336, 1961.

Winkler, J. M. and Weinstein, E. D.: Imperforate anus and heredity. J. Pediat. Surg. 5: 555-558, 1970.

20760 AORTIC ARCH SYNDROME ('YOUNG FEMALE ARTERITIS,' 'PULSELESS DISEASE,' OR TAKAYASU'S ARTERITIS)

We have observed Japanese sisters with aortic arch syndrome. This common disease in Japanese is not strikingly familial. The racial concentration of cases is not necessarily genetic. The disease is relatively

R
E
C
E
S
S
I
V
E

frequent throughout the Orient, for example in India among Caucasoid people of that country. Several studies suggest an autoimmune basis. A modest familial aggregation may have the same basis as that observed in other types of possible autoimmune disease, such as Hashimoto struma (q.v.).

Hirsch, M. S., Aikat, B. K. and Basu, A. K.: Takayasu's arteritis. Report of five cases with immunologic studies. Bull. Hopkins Hosp. 115: 29-64, 1964.

Ikeda, M.: Immunologic studies on Takayasu's arteritis. Jap. Cir. J. 30: 87-89, 1966.

Ito, I.: Aortitis syndrome with reference to detection of anti-aorta antibody from patients' sera. Jap. Circ. J. 30: 75-78, 1966.

*20770 APLASIA CUTIS CONGENITA (CONGENITAL DEFECT OF SKIN, CONGENITAL DEFECT OF SKULL AND SCALP)

The scalp is the most frequent site. Lesions on the trunk or extremities appear as areas in which the absent skin is represented by a thin transparent membrane through which underlying structures are visible. Bone underlying the involved skin, especially skull, shows a disturbance of development. This and the site of predilection leads to the designation 'congenital defect of skull and scalp' sometimes used. Recessive inheritance is suggested by the findings in some families: Gedda et al. (1963) reported the condition in a boy and girl from consanguineous parents. In other families dominant inheritance with reduced penetrance is equally possible (Rauschkolb and Enriquez, 1962). A defect in the skin of the scalp is sometimes found in cases of D1 trisomy (Lee, 1964) and those of deletion of chromosome 4 or 5 (Hirschhorn et al., 1965). A similar condition with absence defect of the limbs is described in the catalog of dominants.

De Vink, L. P. H. J.: Kongenitaler Hautdefekt bei einem Neugeborenen. Arch. Gynaek. 167: 291-299, 1938.

Gedda, L., Muratore, A. and Bernardi, A.: La gangrena asettica della teca cranica come aplasia circoscritta ereditaria del neonato. Acta Genet. Med. Gem. 12: 117-133, 1963.

Greig, D. M.: Localized congenital defects of the scalp. Edinb. Med. J. 38: 341-358, 1931.

Hirschhorn, K., Cooper, H. L. and Firschein, I. L.: Deletion of short arms of chromosome 4-5 in a child with defects of midline fusion. Humangenetik 1: 479-482, 1965.

Lee, C. S. N.: Baltimore, Md.: personal communication, 1964.

Rauschkolb, R. R. and Enriquez, S. I.: Aplasia cutis congenita. Arch. Derm. 86: 54-57, 1962.

Rogatz, J. L. and Davidson, H.: Congenital defect of skin in newborn infant. Am. J. Dis. Child. 65: 916-919, 1943.

*20780 ARGININEMIA

Terheggen et al. (1969) described two sisters, aged 18 months and 5 years, with spastic paraplegia, epileptic seizures and severe mental retardation. The parents were related. Arginine levels were high in the blood and spinal fluid of the patients and showed intermediate elevations in both parents and two healthy sibs. Arginase activity in red cells was very low in the patients and intermediate in the parents. The observation that research workers with the Shope virus have low blood arginine led to the use of Shope virus in treatment of this disorder (Rodgers, 1970). The ability of this DNA virus to restore arginase activity in the affected children and the clinical effects of the same remain to be determined. In 1971 another affected girl was born into the family observed by Terheggen et al. (1972). However, Rogers et al. (1973) has reported an induction of arginase activity by inoculation of the Shope virus into tissue cultures of an argininemic patient's fibroblasts.

Rogers, S.: Oak Ridge, Tenn.: personal communication. 1970.

Rogers, S., Lowenthal, A., Terheggen, H. G. and Columbo, J. P.: Induction of arginase activity with the Shope papilloma virus in tissue culture cells from an argininemic patient. J. Exper. Med. 137: 1091-1096, 1973.

Terheggen, H. G., Lavinha, F., Colombo, J. P., Van Sande, M. and Lowenthal, A.: Familial hyperargininemia. J. Genet. Hum. 20: 69-84, 1972.

Terheggen, H. G., Schwenk, A., Lowenthal, A., Van Sande, M. and Colombo, J. P.: Argininaemia with arginase deficiency. (Letter) Lancet II: 748-749, 1969.

Terheggen, H. G., Schwenk, A., Lowenthal, A., Van Sande, M. and Colombo, J. P.: Hyperargininamie mit arginasedefekt. Eine Neue Familiare Stoffwechselstorung. I. Klinische Befunde. Z. Kinderheilk. 107: 298-312, 1970.

*20790 ARGININOSUCCINICACIDURIA

Onset is in the first weeks of life. Features include mental and physical retardation, liver enlargement, skin lesions, dry and brittle hair showing trichorrhexis nodosa microscopically and fluorescing red, convulsions and episodic unconsciousness. Brittle hair may be found only on a low protein diet (Coryell et al., 1964), because this has not been an impressive feature in this country. The patients cannot make arginine which, however, is probably supplied adequately by the usual diet in the U.S. In Britain, where the average protein intake is less ample, hair changes are the rule. Lewis and Miller (1970) described the neuropathologic changes. Astrocyte transformation to Alzheimer type II glia may be a consistent feature of any form of hyperammonemia. Postmortem liver showed marked deficiency of argininosuccinatelyase. Deficiency of argininosuccinase was demonstrated in cultured fibroblasts from patients (Shih et al., 1969). Two forms of argininosuccinicaciduria, possibly allelic, have been recognized: an early-onset, or malignant, type and a late-onset type (Shih and Efron, 1972).

RECESSIVE

Coryell, M. E., Hall, W. K., Thevaos, T. G., Welter, D. A., Gatz, A. J., Horton, B. F., Sisson, B. D., Looper, J. W., Jr. and Farrow, R. T.: Familial study of human enzyme defect, argininosuccinic aciduria. Biochem. Biophys. Res. Commun. 14: 307-312, 1964.

Goodman, S. I., Mace, J. W., Turner, B. and Garrett, W. J.: Antenatal diagnosis of argininosuccinic aciduria. Clin. Genet. 4: 236-240, 1973.

Kint, J. and Carton, D.: Deficient argininosuccinase activity in brain in argininosuccinicaciduria. (Letter) Lancet II: 635 only, 1968.

Levin, B.: Arginosuccinic aciduria. Am. J. Dis. Child. 113: 162-165, 1967.

Levin, B., MacKay, H. M. and Oberholzer, V. G.: Argininosuccinic aciduria. An inborn error of amino acid metabolism. Arch. Dis. Child. 36: 622-632, 1961.

Lewis, P. D. and Miller, A. L.: Argininosuccinic aciduria. Case report with neuropathological findings. Brain 93: 413-422, 1970.

Moser, H. W., Efron, M. L., Brown, H., Diamond, R. and Neumann, C. G.: Argininosuccinic aciduria: report of two cases and demonstration of intermittent elevation of blood ammonia. Am. J. Med. 42: 9-26, 1967.

Shih, V. E. and Efron, M. L.: Urea cycle disorders. In, Stanbury, J. B., Wyngaarden, J. B. and Fredrickson, D. S. (eds.): The Metabolic Basis of Inherited Disease. New York: McGraw-Hill, 1972 (3rd Ed.). Pp. 370-392.

Shih, V. E., Littlefield, J. W. and Moser, H. W.: Argininosuccinase deficiency in fibroblasts cultured from patients with argininosuccinic aciduria. Biochem. Genet. 3: 81, 1969.

20795 ARNOLD-CHIARI MALFORMATION

This deformity consists of elongation of the cerebellar tonsils and herniation through the foramen magnum into the spinal canal. Lindenberg and Walker (1971) described this malformation, with autopsy confirmation, in two successively born daughters of non-consanguineous parents. Both children had lumbar meningomyelocele. Hydrocephalus was also present.

Lindenberg, R. and Walker, B. A.: Arnold-Chiari malformation in sibs. The Clinical Delineation of Birth Defects. VI. Nervous System. Baltimore: Williams and Wilkins, 1971. Pp. 234-236.

*20800 ARTERIAL CALCIFICATION, GENERALIZED, OF INFANCY

This lesion has been noted in multiple sibs (Hunt and Leys, 1957; Menton and Fetterman, 1948). It may be fundamentally a defect of elastic fiber. Calcification occurs particularly in the internal elastic lamina. Material with the staining properties of mucopolysaccharide accumulates around the elastic fibers. Fine calcium incrustation of the lamina is the minimal lesion. Later the lamina is ruptured and occlusive changes in the intima take place. Death from myocardial infarction usually occurs in the first six months. Calcification in a peripheral artery with EKG changes of occlusive coronary artery disease suggests the diagnosis. Witzleben (1970) suggested that calcification has been overemphasized and is really only a secondary phenomenon. 'Infantile coronary sclerosis' is too restrictive in its topographic implications. He suggested 'occlusive infantile arteriopathy' as the preferred term.

Bird, T.: Idiopathic arterial calcification in infancy. Arch. Dis. Child. 49: 82-89, 1974.

Hunt, A. C. and Leys, D. G.: Generalized arterial calcification in infancy. Brit. Med. J. 1: 385-386, 1957.

McKusick, V. A.: Heritable Disorders of Connective Tissue. St. Louis: C. V. Mosby Co., 1972 (3rd Ed.). Pp. 310-311 and fig. 103.

Menton, M. L. and Fetterman, G. G.: Coronary sclerosis in infancy. Report of three autopsied cases, two in siblings. Am. J. Clin. Path. 18: 805-810, 1948.

Moran, J. J. and Becker, S. M.: Idiopathic arterial calcification of infancy: report of 2 cases occurring in siblings, and review of the literature. Am. J. Clin. Path. 31: 517-529, 1959.

Witzleben, C. L.: Idiopathic infantile arterial calcification — a misnomer? Am. J. Cardiol. 26: 305-309, 1970.

20805 ARTERIAL TORTUOSITY

From Ankara, Turkey, Ertugrel (1967) described a 10-year-old girl with generalized tortuosity and elongation of all major arteries including the aorta. Telangiectases of the cheeks, high palate, aortic regurgitation and histologic fragmentation of the internal elastic membrane of arteries were noted. Three brothers were well. The parents were also healthy. No comment on consanguinity was made. The same condition may have been present in the boy reported by Beuren et al. (1969). Multiple pulmonary artery stenoses were present. The child reported by Lees et al. (1969) had tortuous systemic arteries and multiple pulmonary artery stenoses, but the skin was considered excessively stretchable consistent with the Ehlers-Danlos syndrome. The sibs reported by Welch et al. (1971) had features suggesting cutis laxa (q.v.) with arterial tortuosity of severe degree. The parents were consanguineous. The father and many of his relatives had joint laxity interpreted as the benign hypermobile form of Ehlers-Danlos syndrome.

Beuren, A. J., Hort, W., Kalbfleisch, H., Muller, H. and Stoermer, J.: Dysplasia of the systemic and pulmonary arterial system with tortuosity and lengthening of the arteries. A new entity, diagnosed during life, and leading to coronary death in early childhood. Circulation 39: 109-115, 1969.

Ertugrel, A.: Diffuse tortuosity and lengthening of the arteries. Circulation 36: 400-407, 1967.

R
E
C
E
S
S
I
V
E

Lees, M. H., Menashe, V. D., Sunderland, C. O., Morgan, C. L. and Dawson, P. J.: Ehlers-Danlos syndrome associated with multiple pulmonary artery stenoses and tortuous systemic arteries. J. Pediat. 75: 1031-1036, 1969.

Welch, J. P., Aterman, K., Day, E. and Roy, D. L.: Familial aggregation of a 'new' connective tissue disorder, a nosologic problem. The Clinical Delineation of Birth Defects. XII. Skin, Hair and Nails. Baltimore: Williams and Wilkins, 1971. Pp. 204-213.

20807 ARTERIOHEPATIC DYSPLASIA

Watson and Miller (1973) described a syndrome of pulmonary artery stenoses and neonatal obstructive jaundice. The facies tended to be odd: namely, flat with high wide cheekbones and prominent forehead and chin. Five families, some with two or more affected sibs, were described. None of the parents were consanguineous. An infectious etiology is possible.

Watson, G. H. and Miller, V.: Arteriohepatic dysplasia: familial pulmonary arterial stenosis with neonatal liver disease. Arch. Dis. Child. 48: 459-466, 1973.

*20810 ARTHROGRYPOSIS MULTIPLEX CONGENITA

Like amyotonia congenita, arthrogryposis is really a syndrome. Genetic forms seem to be rare. Several discordant monozygotic twin pairs have been described. The possibility of infection of the fetus by a virus with neuromyal tropism (e.g., coxsackie) should be investigated epidemiologically, virologically and immunologically.

Frischknecht and colleagues (1960) described three affected sibs and suggested instead of arthrogryposis the designation 'neuroarthromyodysplasia' because at autopsy changes were found to involve the spinal cord and the Betz cells. Swinyard (1963) has also reported familial cases. Weissman and colleagues (1963) described an arthrogryposis-like picture consisting of flexion contractures at the elbows or knees and no dislocation of the hips. Bargeton et al. (1961) reported autopsy findings in one of two brothers, the offspring of first-cousin parents. The primary lesions were neurologic. Ek (1958) had affected sisters. In addition to the forms of arthrogryposis due to loss of motor neurons in the anterior horn of the spinal cord and due to congenital muscular dystrophy, Bargeton et al. (1961) described a third type which is familial and characterized by focal collagenous proliferation in the anterior spinal roots. Pena et al. (1968) studied two Puerto Rican families, each with two affected children. At least one of the four affected children was female. The accumulated experience appears to indicate the existence of at least one form of recessively inherited arthrogryposis (hence the asterisk). Probably these represent only a small proportion of the whole. Srivastava (1968) reported as arthrogryposis two brothers with multiple hemivertebrae and fusion of several vertebral bodies. Flexion contracture of the elbows and knees was present. However, arthrogryposis does not seem a justified diagnosis. Laitinen and Hirvensalo (1966) observed affected sibs. Three sibs were apparently affected in a family reported by Pena et al. (1968). Histologic abnormalities were found in the spinal cord. Lebenthal et al. (1970) reported further observations of the kindred studied by Weissman et al. They found 23 cases in an inbred Arab group and concluded that the disorder is of the myopathic type in these cases. Six of the patients had congenital heart disease. The Drachman hypothesis that arthrogryposis is caused by immobilization of fetal limbs during the period of formation of joints received support from the finding of arthrogryposis in the offspring of a woman who received tubocurarine in early pregnancy for treatment of tetanus (Jago, 1970). Arthrogryposis, apparently recessively inherited, is known in sheep (Roberts, 1929) and in cattle (Hutt, 1934), although this designation is not used. It seems quite certain that at least one autosomal recessive form of arthrogryposis multiplex congenita exists and perhaps at least two forms with this mode of inheritance, a neuropathic and a myopathic form.

Bargeton, E., Nezelof, C., Guran, P. and Job, J.-C.: Etude anatomique d'un cas d'arthrogrypose multiple congenitale et familiale. Rev. Neurol. 104: 479-489, 1961.

Crowe, M. W. and Pike, H. T.: Congenital arthrogryposis associated with ingestion of tobacco stalks by pregnant sows. J. Am. Vet. Med. Ass. 162: 453-455, 1973.

Drachman, D. B. and Banker, B. Q.: Arthrogryposis multiplex congenita. Case due to disease of the anterior horn cells. Arch. Neurol. 5: 77-93, 1961.

Drachman, D. B. and Coulombre, A. J.: Experimental clubfoot and arthrogryposis multiplex congenita. Lancet II: 523-526, 1962.

Ek, J. I.: Cerebral lesions in arthrogryposis multiplex congenita. Acta Paediat. 47: 302-316, 1958.

Frischknecht, W., Bianchi, L. and Pilleri, G.: Familiare arthrogryposis multiplex congenita. Helv. Paediat. Acta 15: 259-279, 1960.

Hutt, F. B.: A hereditary lethal muscle contracture in cattle. J. Hered. 25: 41-46, 1934.

Jago, R. H.: Arthrogryposis following treatment of maternal tetanus with muscle relaxants. Case report. Arch. Dis. Child. 45: 277-279, 1970.

Laitinen, O. and Hirvensalo, M.: Arthrogryposis multiplex congenita. Ann. Paediat. Fenn. 12: 133-138, 1966.

Lebenthal, E., Shochet, S. B., Adam, A., Seelenfreund, M., Fried, A., Najenson, T., Sandbank, U. and Matoth, Y.: Arthrogryposis multiplex congenita — 23 cases in an Arab kindred. Pediatrics 46: 891-899, 1970.

Pena, C. E., Miller, F., Budzilovich, G. N. and Feigin, I.: Arthrogryposis multiplex congenita: report of two cases of a radicular type with familial incidence. Neurology 18: 926-930, 1968.

Roberts, J. A. F.: The inheritance of a lethal muscle contracture in sheep. J. Genet. 21: 57-69, 1929.

Rosenmann, A. and Arad, I.: Arthrogryposis multiplex congenita: neurogenic type with autosomal recessive inheritance. J. Med. Genet. 11: 91-94, 1974.

Srivastava, R. N.: Arthrogryposis multiplex congenita. Case report of two siblings. Clin. Pediat. 7: 691-694, 1968.

Swinyard, C. A.: Multiple congenital contractures (arthrogryposis) nature of the syndrome and hereditary considerations. Proc. Sec. Intern. Cong. Hum. Genet. (Rome, Sept. 6-12, 1961.) 3: 1397-1398, 1963.

Weissman, S. L., Khermosh, C. and Adam, A.: Arthrogryposis in an Arab family. In, Goldschmidt, E. (ed.): Genetics of Migrant and Isolate Populations. Baltimore: Williams and Wilkins, 1963. P. 313.

*20820 ARTHROGRYPOSIS-LIKE DISORDER

Petajan et al. (1969) described an arthrogryposis-like syndrome in the Eskimo. They called it Kuskokwim disease for the Kuskokwim Delta area where it was observed. Multiple joint contractures affected predominantly the knees and ankles with atrophy and compensatory hypertrophy of associated muscle groups. The familial pattern strongly suggested autosomal recessive inheritance.

Petajan, J. H., Momberger, G. L., Aase, J. M. and Wright, D. G.: Arthrogryposis syndrome (Kuskokwim disease) in the Eskimo. J.A.M.A. 209: 1481-1486, 1969.

Wright, D. G. and Aase, J.: The Kuskokwim syndrome: an inherited form of arthrogryposis in the Alaskan Eskimo. The Clinical Delineation of Birth Defects. III. Limb Malformations. New York: National Foundation, 1969. Pp. 91-95.

20830 ASCITES, CHYLOUS

Lee and Young (1953) described chylous ascites in two female sibs under one year of age. One also had swelling of one arm evident at one week and the entire body somewhat later and developed bilateral glaucoma in the first 6 months of life. Both this patient and the younger sister had spontaneous clearing of the manifestations. Chylous ascites and chylous pleural effusions probably occur at times with hereditary lymphedema, but this condition in its various forms is usually dominant.

Lee, C.-H. and Young, J. R.: Chylous ascites in siblings. J. Pediat. 42: 83-86, 1953.

*20840 ASPARTYLGLYCOSAMINURIA

In a 32-year-old female and her 20-year-old brother with mental retardation Pouitt et al. (1968) found urinary excretion of abnormal amounts of 2-acetamido-1-(beta prime-l-aspartamido)-1, 2-dideoxyglucose. An enzyme responsible for hydrolyzing this compound is normally present in seminal fluid but was absent in that of the brother. A generalized lack of this enzyme was postulated. Both sibs had thick sagging skin of the cheeks, a finding not present in normal members of the family. Palo and Mattsson (1970) reported 11 cases. The parents of one patient were first cousins. They estimated that there are at least 130 cases in the total population of 4.5 million in Finland. PKU has a very low incidence in Finland (Palo, 1967). Other recessive disorders which seem to have a relatively high frequency in Finland include congenital nephrosis (q.v.). The Finnish cases showed, in addition to severe mental retardation, sagging cheeks, broad nose and face, short neck, cranial asymmetry, scoliosis, periodic hyperactivity, and vacuolated lymphocytes. Diarrhea and frequent infections were problems in infancy. This disorder was first reported by Jenner and Pouitt (1967). Aspartylglycosaminuria is a lysosomal disease. The enzyme deficient in these cases is N-aspartyl-beta-glycosaminidase.

Autio, S., Palo, J. and Perheentupa, J.: Aspartylglycosaminuria: a gargoyle-like syndrome with autosomal recessive inheritance. In, Bergsma, D. (ed.): Clinical Delineation of Birth Defects. XVI. Urinary System and Others. Baltimore: Williams and Wilkins, 1974. Pp. 193-200.

Palo, J. and Mattsson, K.: Eleven new cases of aspartylglycosaminuria. J. Ment. Defic. Res. 14: 168-173, 1970.

Palo, J.: Prevalence of phenylketonuria and some other metabolic disorders among mentally retarded patients in Finland. Acta Neurol. Scand. 43: 573-579, 1967.

Pouitt, R. J., Jenner, F. A. and Merskey, H.: Aspartylglycosaminuria: an inborn error of metabolism associated with mental defect. Lancet II: 253-255, 1968.

*20850 ASPHYXIATING THORACIC DYSTROPHY OF THE NEWBORN (JEUNE SYNDROME; THORACIC-PELVIC-PHALANGEAL DYSTROPHY)

Most cases have a fatal outcome in the newborn period. Involvement of the rib cage is responsible for asphyxia. Changes here and in the extremities are rather similar to those of the Ellis-van Creveld syndrome. Indeed polydactyly was present in a case of Pirnar and Neuhauser (1966). The latter authors observed three affected brothers. Dysplasia of the fingernails is not present in this condition. Chronic nephritis is a complication (Wahlers, 1966). Hanissian et al. (1967) reported two families each with two affected brothers. One family was Negro. These authors thought the family reported by Shapira et al. (1965) had this condition. Langer (1968) pointed out that in those cases with polydactyly differentiation from Ellis-van Creveld syndrome may not be possible on radiologic grounds alone. Polydactyly is an inconstant feature of this and when present usually affects the feet also. (Polydactyly of the hands is a constant feature in EvC but the feet are uncommonly affected.) Nail dysplasia and peculiar upper lip (features of EvC) are not seen in this condition. The main visceral abnormality is renal in this condition, whereas it is cardiac in EvC. Shokeir (1970) described five related affected persons of Norwegian extraction. Cystic renal changes (Potter's type IV) were described. Shokeir et al. (1971) presented strong evidence for recessive inheritance in a Norwegian kindred and raised the possibility that chest deformity may be a manifestation of the gene in the heterozygote. Finegold et al. (1971) reported on a case with hypoplastic lungs with marked reduction in the number of alveoli at autopsy finding. Barnes et al. (1971) reported successful thoracic reconstruction in a child whose sib had died of the disorder and whose mother was thought to have been affected (Barnes et al., 1969).

Barnes, N. D., Hull, D. and Symons, J. S.: Thoracic dystrophy. Arch. Dis. Child. 44: 11-17, 1969.

Barnes, N. D., Hull, D., Milner, A. D. and Waterston, D. J.: Chest reconstruction in thoracic dystrophy. Arch. Dis. Child. 46: 833-837, 1971.

Finegold, M. J., Katzew, H., Genieser, N. B. and Becker, M. H.: Lung structure in thoracic dystrophy. Am. J. Dis. Child. 122: 153-159, 1971.

Gruskin, A. B., Baluarte, H. J., Cote, M. L. and Elfenbein, I. B.: The renal disease of thoracic asphyxiant dystrophy. In, Bergsma, D. (ed.): Clinical Delineation of Birth Defects. XVI. Urinary System and Others. Baltimore: Williams and Wilkins, 1974. Pp. 44-50.

Hanissian, A. S., Riggs, W. W., Jr. and Thomas, D. A.: Infantile thoracic dystrophy — a variant of Ellis-van Creveld syndrome. J. Pediat. 71: 855-864, 1967.

Herdman, R. C. and Langer, L. O.: The thoracic asphyxiant dystrophy and renal disease. Am. J. Dis. Child. 116: 192-201, 1968.

Jeune, M., Beraud, C. and Carron, R.: Dystrophie thoracique asphyxiante de caractere familial. Arch. Franc. Pediat. 12: 886-891, 1955.

Karjoo, M., Koop, C. E., Cornfield, D. and Holtzapple, P. G.: Pancreatic exodrine enzyme deficiency associated with asphyxiating thoracic dystrophy. Arch. Dis. Child. 48: 143-146, 1973.

Langer, L. O., Jr.: Thoracic-pelvic-phalangeal dystrophy: asphyxiating thoracic dystrophy of the newborn, infantile thoracic dystrophy. Radiology 91: 447-456, 1968.

Maroteaux, P. and Savart, P.: La dystrophie thoracique asphyxiante: etude radiologique et rapports avec le syndrome d'Ellis et van Creveld. Ann. Radiol. 7: 332-338, 1964.

Pirnar, T. and Neuhauser, E. B. D.: Asphyxiating thoracic dystrophy of the newborn. Am. J. Roentgen. 98: 358-364, 1966.

Shapira, E., Fischel, E., Moses, S. and Levin, S.: Syndrome of incomplete regional achondroplasia (ilium and ribs) with abdominal muscle dysplasia. Arch. Dis. Child. 40: 694-697, 1965.

Shokeir, M. H. K.: Asphyxiating thoracic chondrodystrophy: association with urinary malformations and evidence for heterozygous expression. (Abstract) Am. J. Hum. Genet. 22: 18A-19A, 1970.

Shokeir, M. H. K., Houston, C. S. and Awen, C. F.: Asphyxiating thoracic chondrodystrophy: association with renal disease and evidence for possible heterozygous expression. J. Med. Genet. 8: 107-112, 1971.

Wahlers: Cited by Lenz, W.: Symposion uber generalisierte Anomalien des Skeletes. Mschr. Kinderheilk. 114: 157-158, 1966.

R
E
C
E
S
S
I
V
E

*20853 ASPLENIA WITH CARDIOVASCULAR ANOMALIES (IVEMARK SYNDROME)

Parental consanguinity in three instances and four instances of multiple affected sibs (Simpson and Zellweger, 1973) support autosomal recessive inheritance. Hypoplasia of the spleen is sometimes the finding rather than aplasia.

Simpson, J. and Zellweger, H.: Familial occurrence of Ivemark syndrome with splenic hypoplasia and asplenia in sibs. J. Med. Genet. 10: 303-304, 1973.

20855 ASTHMA, NASAL POLYPS, ASPIRIN INTOLERANCE (ASA TRIAD)

Lockey et al. (1973) observed two families. In one consanguinity suggested recessive inheritance. The late onset and discordance in a pair of identical twins suggested that environmental factors may be important also. Miller (1971) reported affected sisters. Von Maur and Van Metre (1973) described a family in which autosomal dominant inheritance of aspirin asthma was suggested. In addition to mode of inheritance, differences from earlier reports included an earlier age of onset, lack of nasal polyps and sinusitis, and milder asthma. Other studies have suggested recessive inheritance (e.g. Miller, 1971; Lockey et al. 1973).

Lockey, R. F., Rucknagel, D. L. and Vanselow, N. A.: Familial occurrence of asthma nasal polyps and aspirin intolerance. Ann. Intern. Med. 78: 57-63, 1973.

Miller, F. F.: Aspirin-induced bronchial asthma in sisters. Ann. Allergy 29: 263-265, 1971.

Von Maur, K. and Van Metre, T. E., Jr.: Familial occurrence of aspirin intolerance. In press, 1973.

20860 ASTHMA, SHORT STATURE AND ELEVATED IGA

Sly and Heimlich (1967) reported identical female twins with this combination. The mother and some of the sibs were thought also to have abnormalities of immunoglobulins.

Sly, R. M. and Heimlich, E. M.: Identical twins with short stature, elevated IgA and asthma. Ann. Allerg. 25: 578-586, 1967.

20870 ATAXIA WITH MYOCLONUS EPILEPSY AND PRESENILE DEMENTIA

In a brother and sister, Skre and Loken (1970) described a disorder with clinical features of Friedreich ataxia and in the late stages myoclonus epilepsy and progressive dementia. Neuropathologic studies showed spinocerebellar degeneration as in Friedreich ataxia, cerebral involvement as in subacute presenile dementia, and peripheral neuropathy as in Charcot-Marie-Tooth disease.

Skre, H. and Loken, A. C.: Myoclonus epilepsy and subacute presenile dementia in heredo-ataxia. A clinical, electroencephalographic, and pathological study with a discussion of classification and etiology. Acta Neurol. Scand. 46: 18-42, 1970.

*20880 ATAXIA, INTERMITTENT, WITH PYRUVATE DEHYDROGENASE (DECARBOXYLASE) DEFICIENCY

Blass et al. (1970) described a deficiency of pyruvate decarboxylase in an 8 year old boy who had suffered 2 to 6 episodes of ataxia each year since the age of 16 months. Most attacks followed nonspecific febrile illness or other stresses. Chorioathetosis as well as cerebellar ataxia was present during the episodes. Serum pyruvic acid and alanine levels were elevated. The father's fibroblasts and leukocytes showed partially defective pyruvate decarboxylase and values in the mother were at the lower limit of normal. Pyruvate dehydrogenase is a multi-enzyme complex. The patient of Blass et al. (1970) was reminiscent of a boy reported by Lonsdale et al. (1969). The latter patient likewise showed intermittent ataxia and choreoathetose, precipitated by acute infections. Both patients showed conspicuous abnormalities of eye movement. Thiamine in large doses appeared to benefit Lonsdale's patient.

Blass, J. P., Avigan, J. and Uhlendorf, B. W.: A defect in pyruvate decarboxylase in a child with an intermittent movement disorder. J. Clin. Invest. 49: 423-432, 1970.

Blass, J. P., Kark, R. A. P. and Engel, W. K.: Clinical studies of a patient with pyruvate dehydroxylase deficiency. Arch. Neurol. 25: 449-460, 1971.

Lonsdale, D., Faulkner, W. R., Price, J. M. and Smeby, R. R.: Intermittent cerebellar ataxia associated with hyperpyruvic acidemia, hyperphemylalaminemia and hyperalaninuria. Pediatrics 43: 1025-1034, 1969.

Willems, J. L., Monnens, L. A. H., Trijbels, J. M. G., Sengers, R. C. A. and Veerkamp, J. H.: Pyruvate decarboxylase deficiency in liver. (Letter) New Eng. J. Med. 290: 406-407, 1974.

20885 ATAXIA-DEAFNESS-RETARDATION (ADR) SYNDROME

Berman et al. (1973) described three Negro brothers with progressive ataxia, hearing loss, mental retardation and signs of both upper and lower motor neuron disease, all beginning in infancy. This is different from the Richards-Rundle syndrome (24510), although the two syndromes share the ataxia, deafness and retardation.

Berman, W., Haslem, R. H. A., Konigsmark, B. W., Capute, A. J. and Migeon, C. J.: A new familial syndrome with ataxia, hearing loss, and mental retardation. Arch. Neurol. 29: 258-261, 1973.

*20890 ATAXIA-TELANGIECTASIA

The features are progressive cerebellar ataxia, telangiectases especially of the conjunctiva, and proneness to sinopulmonary infection. The nature of the basic defect is a mystery. A defect of the immune mechanism and hypoplasia of the thymus is demonstrated. In two Amish sibships, of which the four parents shared a common ancestral couple, ataxia telangiectasia occurred in one and Swiss-type agammaglobulinemia (q.v.) in the second, suggesting to McKusick and Cross (1966) a possible relationship of these two disorders of the immune mechanism. Patients with this disorder tend to develop lymphatic malignancy. Hecht et al. (1966) observed lymphocytic leukemia in patients with ataxia-telangiectasia. A non-leukemic sib and two unrelated patients with ataxia-telangiectasia had multiple chromosomal breaks and impaired responsiveness to phytohemagglutinin. Leukemia and chromosomal abnormalities occur in at least two other Mendelian disorders, Fanconi pancytopenia and Bloom disease. Telangiectases can be inconspicuous and patients may be diagnosed as 'Friedreich ataxia' for many years. The oldest patients known to me are now 41 and 37 years old. Haerer et al. (1969) described a Negro sibship of 12, of whom 5 had ataxia-telangiectasia, of whom 2 died of mucinous adenocarcinoma of the stomach at ages 21 and 19 years. Hagberg et al. (1970) described a disorder suggesting ataxia-telangiectasia in all respects except that no telangiectases were present. Two sibs with unrelated parents were affected. Although they considered it a distinct entity, the evidence is not completely convincing. The possibility of heteroalleles at the ataxia-telangiectasia loci might be suggested. Waldmann and McIntire (1972) showed raised alpha-fetoprotein in the blood of patients with AT. This, they felt, suggests immaturity of the liver and is consistent with the view that the primary defect is in tissue differentiation, specifically a defect in the interaction necessary for differentiation of gut-associated organs such as the thymus and liver.

Ammann, A. J., Cain, W. A., Ishizaka, K., Hong, R. and Good, R. A.: Immunoglobulin E deficiency in ataxia-telangiectasia. New Eng. J. Med. 281: 469-472, 1969.

Boder, E. and Sedgwick, R. P.: Ataxia-telangiectasia: a familial syndrome of progressive cerebellar ataxia, oculocutaneous telangiectasia and frequent pulmonary infection. Pediatrics 21: 526-554, 1958.

Feigin, R. D., Vietti, T. J., Wyatt, R. G., Kaufman, D. G. and Smith, C. H.: Ataxia telangiectasia with granulocytopenia. J. Pediat. 77: 431-438, 1970.

Haerer, A. F., Jackson, J. F. and Evers, C. G.: Ataxia-telangiectasia with gastric adenocarcinoma. J.A.M.A. 210: 1884-1887, 1969.

Hagberg, A., Hansson, O., Liden, S. and Nilsson, K.: Familial ataxic diplegia with deficient cellular immunity. A new clinical entity. Acta Paediat. Scand. 59: 545-550, 1970.

Hecht, F., Koler, R. D., Rigas, D. A., Dahnke, G. S., Case, M. P., Tisdale, V. and Miller, R. W.: Leukemia and lymphocytes in ataxia-telangiectasia. (Letter) Lancet II: 1193 only, 1966.

R
E
C
E
S
S
I
V
E

Korein, J., Steinman, P. A. and Senz, E. H.: Ataxia-telangiectasia: report of a case and review of the literature. Arch. Neurol. 4: 272-280, 1961.

Levin, S. and Perlov, S.: Ataxia-telangiectasia in Israel, with observations on its relationship to malignant disease. Israel J. Med. Sci. 7: 1535-1541, 1971.

Lisker, R. and Cobo, A.: Chromosome breakage in ataxia — telangiectasia. (Letter) Lancet I: 618 only, 1970.

McFarlin, D. E., Strober, W. and Waldmann, T. A.: Ataxia — telangiectasia. Medicine 51: 281-314, 1972.

McKusick, V. A. and Cross, H. E.: Ataxia-telangiectasia and Swiss-type agammaglobulinemia. Two genetic disorders of the immune mechanism in related Amish sibships. J.A.M.A. 195: 739-745, 1966.

Miller, M. E. and Chatten, J.: Ovarian changes in ataxia telangiectasia. Acta Paediat. Scand. 56: 559-561, 1967.

Peterson, R. D. A., Kelly, W. D. and Good, R. A.: Ataxia-telangiectasia: its association with a defective thymus, immunological-deficiency disease and malignancy. Lancet I: 1189-1193, 1964.

Reye, C. and Mosman, N. S. W.: Ataxia-telangiectasia. Am. J. Dis. Child. 99: 238-247, 1960.

Schalch, D. S., McFarlin, D. E. and Barlow, M. H.: An unusual form of diabetes mellitus in ataxia telangiectasia. New Eng. J. Med. 282: 1396-1402, 1970.

Shuster, J., Hart, Z., Stimson, C. W., Brough, A. J. and Poulik, M. D.: Ataxia — telangiectasia with cerebellar tumor. Pediatrics 37: 776-786, 1966.

Sourander, P., Bonnevier, J. O. and Olsson, Y.: A case of ataxia telangiectasia with lesions in the spinal cord. Acta Neurol. Scand. 42: 354-366, 1966.

Tadjoedin, M. K. and Fraser, F. C.: Heredity of ataxia telangiectasia (Louis-Bar syndrome). Am. J. Dis. Child. 110: 64-68, 1965.

Waldmann, T. A. and McIntire, K. R.: Serum-alpha-fetoprotein levels in patients with ataxia-telangiectasia. Lancet II: 1112-1115, 1972.

20900 ATAXIC DIPLEGIA AND DEFECTIVE CELLULAR IMMUNITY

Hagberg et al. (1970) described affected brother and sister. The sister had vaccinia gangrenosa, at age 15 months, which was successfully drug-treated. She died of generalized varicella at age four and one half. The brother died at five of brain abscess.

Hagberg, B., Hansson, O., Liden, S. and Nilsson, K.: Familial ataxic diplegia with deficient cellular immunity. A new clinical entity. Acta Paediat. Scand. 59: 545-550, 1970.

Silverstein, M. N. and Ellefson, R. D.: The syndrome of the sea-blue histiocyte. Sem. Hemat. 9: 299-308, 1972.

*20910 ATONIC-ASTATIC SYNDROME OF FOERSTER

Manifestations are oligophrenia, pronounced muscular hypotonia, static ataxia, astasia, abasia and slow, monotonous speech. Van Rossum (1959) described an affected brother and sister from consanguineous parents. Consanguinity has been described in two other reports.

Van Rossum, A.: Foerster's atonic-astatic syndrome. Recent Neurological Research, Elsevier, 1959.

20920 ATOPIC HYPERSENSITIVITY

Asthma, hay fever and eczema are embraced by this term. The genetics is certainly not simple. Tips (1954) thought that each of the three forms of atopy is determined by homozygosity at a single and separate locus. The study of Lubs (1972) suggests, however, a more general increased risk of allergic manifestations. Others (Cooke and Vander Veer, 1916; Coca, 1928; Schwartz, 1952) have proposed dominant inheritance. Demonstration of immune response genes in man (14685) gives support to the heritability of atopy (and tends to support dominant inheritance).

Clarke, J. A., Jr., Donnally, H. H. and Coca, A. F.: Studies in specific hypersensitiveness. J. Immun. 15: 9-11, 1928.

Cooke, R. A. and Vander Veer, A., Jr.: Human sensitization. J. Immun. 1: 201-305, 1916.

Lubs, M.-L. E.: Empiric risks for genetic counseling in families with allergy. J. Pediat. 80: 26-31, 1972.

Rajka, G.: Prurigo Besnier (atopic dermatitis) with special reference to the role of allergic factors. I. The influence of atopic hereditary factors. Acta Dermatovener. 40: 285-306, 1960.

Schwartz, M.: Heredity in Bronchial Asthma. Copenhagen: Munksgaard, 1952.

Tips, R. L.: A study of the inheritance of atopic hypersensitivity in man. Am. J. Hum. Genet. 6: 328-343, 1954.

*20930 ATRANSFERRINEMIA

Heilmeyer and colleagues (1961) described total absence of transferrin in a 7-year-old girl whose presenting complaint was severe hypochromic anemia. Death occurred from heart failure. Severe hemosiderosis of the heart and liver was found at autopsy. Low normal transferrin levels were found in both parents, who were not known to be related (personal communication). About half-normal levels of transferrin in both parents supported recessive inheritance (Goya et al., 1972). Treatment with human serum transferrin was reported by Goya et al. (1972). Goya et al. (1972) described a patient with only a trace of transferrin in the blood by immunological methods, who responded well to parenteral administration of transferrin.

Goya, N., Miyazaki, S., Kodate, S. and Ushio, B.: A family of congenital atransferrinemia. Blood 40: 239-245, 1972.

Heilmeyer, L., Keller, W., Vivell, O., Keiderling, W., Betke, K., Wohler, F. and Schultze, H. E.: Kongenitale atransferrinamie bei einem sieben Jahre alten Kind. Deutsch. Med. Wschr. 86: 1745-1751, 1961.

20940 ATRIAL SEPTAL DEFECT, PRIMUM TYPE

Yao et al. (1968) observed four sibs with atrial septal defect of the primum type. Five other sibs and the parents were normal. Familial aggregation of secundum ASD has been reported rather frequently (e.g., Nora and Meyer, 1966), but the experience of Yao et al. is unusual. Sanchez Cascos (1972), among others, concluded inheritance is multifactorial. He made the interesting observation that although 64 percent of ASD cases are female, the recurrence risk to sibs is greater when the proband is male. This is like the finding in ankylosing spondylitis (10630) where also familial incidence is greater when the proband is of the less frequently involved sex. Ostium primum type of atrial septal defect occurs in over half of patients with the Ellis-van Creveld syndrome (22550).

Nora, J. J. and Meyer, T. C.: Familial nature of congenital heart disease. Pediatrics 37: 329-334, 1966.

Sanchez Cascos, A.: Genetics of atrial septal defect. Arch. Dis. Child. 47: 581-588, 1972.

Yao, J., Thompson, M. W., Trusler, G. A. and Trimble, A. S.: Familial atrial septal defect of the primum type: a report of four cases in one sibship. Canad. Med. Ass. J. 98: 218-219, 1968.

*20950 ATRICHIA WITH PAPULAR LESIONS

Almost complete absence of hair and papillary lesions over most of the body were features. The patients are born with hair which falls out and is not replaced. Histologic studies show malformation of the hair follicles. Damste and Prakken (1954) described a kindred in which three sisters and two sons of their mother's first cousin were affected. Loewenthal and Prakken (1961) described another case, the daughter of third cousins.

Damste, T. J. and Prakken, J. R.: Atrichia with papular lesions: variant of congenital ectodermal dysplasia. Dermatologica 108: 114-122, 1954.

Loewenthal, L. J. A. and Prakken, J. R.: Atrichia with papular lesions. Dermatologica 122: 85-89, 1961.

R
E
C
E
S
S
I
V
E

20960 ATRIOVENTRICULAR DISSOCIATION

Wagner and Hall (1967) reported two brothers and a sister with congenital atrioventricular dissociation. They emphasized that this is distinct from A-V block. In dissociation the abnormality seems to be 'lazy' sino-atrial pacemaker with the A-V node taking over intermittently by default. In A-V block an impediment to A-V conduction exists. See HEART BLOCK. See NODAL RHYTHM.

Wagner, C. W., Jr. and Hall, R. J.: Congenital familial atrioventricular dissociation: report of three siblings. Am. J. Cardiol. 19: 593-596, 1967.

*20970 ATROPHODERMIA VERMICULATA (FOLLICULITIS ULERYTHEMATOSA, ATROPHO-DERMA RETICULATA, HONEYCOMB ATROPHY, ATROPHODERMIA RETICULATA SYM-METRICA FACIEI, ETC.)

The skin changes are usually limited to the face and consist of symmetrical small crowded areas of skin atrophy producing pits with sharp edges and an overall worm-eaten appearance. Association with congenital heart block, coarctation of the aorta and other defects has been described by Kooij and Venter (1959) and Carol and colleagues (1940) reported familial occurrence with heart anomaly.

Carol, W. L. L., Godfried, E. G., Prakken, J. R. and Prick, J. J. G.: V. Recklinghausensche Neurofibromatosis, Atrophodermia vermiculata und kongenitale Herzanomalie als Hauptkennzeichen eines familiar-hereditaren Syndroms. Dermatologica 81: 345-365, 1940.

Kooij, R. and Venter, J.: Atrophodermia vermiculata with unusual localisation and associated congenital anomalies. Dermatologia 118: 161-167, 1959.

Mackee, G. M. and Cipollaro, A. C.: Folliculitis ulerythematosa reticulata. Arch. Derm. Syph. 57: 281-292, 1948.

Savatard, L.: Honeycomb atrophy. Brit. J. Derm. 55: 259-266, 1943.

20980 AUSTRALIA ANTIGEN

Blumberg et al. (1965) described an antigen in the serum of an Australian Aborigine which reacted with an antibody in certain hemophilic patients who had received multiple transfusions. The same antigen appeared in the serum of some leukemia patients. Blumberg et al. (1966) found reasonably good agreement of family data with the expectations that individuals homozygous for a gene tentatively designated Au(1) have the antigen detectable by double diffusion methods, whereas persons heterozygous for the gene or lacking it entirely do not have the antigen. Blumberg et al. (1967) found that the Australia antigen is more common in patients with lepromatous leprosy than in patients with tuberculoid leprosy or in non-leprosy controls. Association with hepatitis has also been demonstrated. Au(1) has been found in the serum of 38-58 percent of patients with acute hepatitis (London et al., 1969) but in less than 0.1 percent of healthy North Americans. The viral nature of the Australia antigen is suggested by electron-microscopic studies (Bayer et al., 1968). With fluorescent antibody techniques Au(1) has been detected consistently in the nuclei of liver cells from hepatitis patients with Au(1) in their serum (Millman et al., 1969). Australia antigen is found in the sera of patients with acute and chronic hepatitis and may actually be a form of virus. It is very common in tropical areas and persons in these areas with the antigen appear to be hepatitis carriers. The antigen is detected by immunodiffusion in agar gel (Ouchterlony method). Family studies by Blumberg et al. (1969) again suggested recessive inheritance of susceptibility to infection as manifested by presence of the Australia antigen.

Alter, H. J. and Blumberg, B. S.: Further studies on a 'new human' isoprecipitin system (Australia antigen). Blood 27: 297-309, 1966.

Bayer, M. E., Blumberg, B. S. and Werner, B.: Particles associated with Australia antigen in the sera of patients with leukaemia, Down's syndrome and hepatitis. Nature 218: 1057-1059, 1968.

Blumberg, B. S., Alter, H. J. and Visnich, S.: A 'new' antigen in leukemia sera. J.A.M.A. 191: 541-546, 1965.

Blumberg, B. S., Friedlaender, J. S., Woodside, A., Sutnick, A. I. and London, W. T.: Hepatitis and Australia antigen: autosomal recessive inheritance of susceptibility to infection in humans. Proc. Nat. Acad. Sci. 62: 1108-1115, 1969.

Blumberg, B. S., Melartin, L., Guinto, R. S. and Werner, B.: Family studies of a human serum isoantigen system (Australia antigen). Am. J. Hum. Genet. 18: 594-608, 1966.

Blumberg, B. S., Melartin, L., Lechat, M. and Guinto, R. S.: Association between lepromatous leprosy and Australia antigen. Lancet II: 173-176, 1967.

Blumberg, B. S., Sutnick, A. I. and London, W. T.: Australia antigen as a hepatitis virus. Variation in host response. Am. J. Med. 48: 1-8, 1970.

London, W. T., Sutnick, A. I. and Blumberg, B. S.: Australia antigen and acute viral hepatitis. Ann. Intern. Med. 70: 55-59, 1969.

Millman, I., Zavatone, V., Gerstley, B. J. S. and Blumberg, B. S.: Australia antigen detected the nuclei of liver cells of patients with viral hepatitis by the flourescent antibody technique. Nature 222: 181-184, 1969.

Wright, R., McCollum, R. W. and Klatskin, G.: Australia antigen in acute and chronic liver disease. Lancet II: 117-121, 1969.

*20990 BARDET-BIEDL SYNDROME

Ammann (1970) pointed out that the syndrome usually called Laurence-Moon-Biedl-Bardet syndrome (mental retardation, pigmentary retinopathy, polydactyly, obesity, hypogenitalism) was present in Biedl's (1922) and Bardet's (1920) patients, but that those of Laurence and Moon had a distinct disorder with paraplegia and without polydactyly and obesity (see LAURENCE-MOON SYNDROME). As indicated by Ammann's study, residual heterogeneity may exist even after the Laurence-Moon syndrome is separated off. Clearly Biemond syndrome II (iris coloboma, hypogenitalism, obesity, polydactyly and mental retardation) is distinct, as is also Alstrom syndrome (retinitis pigmentosa, obesity, diabetes mellitus and perceptive deafness). Renal abnormalities appear to have a high frequency in this syndrome (Alton and McDonald, 1973).

Alton, D. J. and McDonald, P.: Urographic findings in Laurence-Moon-Biedl syndrome. Radiology, in press, 1973.

Ammann, F.: Investigations cliniques et genetiques sur le syndrome de Bardet-Biedl en Suisse. J. Genet. Hum. 18 (suppl.): 1-310, 1970.

Bardet, G.: Sur un syndrome d'obesite infantile avec polydactylie et retinite pigmentaire. (Contribution a l'etude des Formes Cliniques de l'Obesite Hypophysaire). Thesis, Paris, No. 479, 1920.

Bell, J.: The Laurence-Moon syndrome. In, Penrose, L. S. (ed.): Treasury of Human Inheritance. Cambridge: Univ. Press, vol. 5 (part III): 51-96, 1958.

Biedl, A.: Ein Geschwisterpaar mit adiposo-genitaler Dystrophie. Deutsch. Med. Wschr. 48: 1630 Only, 1922.

Ciccarelli, E. C. and Vesell, E. S.: Laurence-Moon-Biedl syndrome. Report of an unusual family. Am. J. Dis. Child. 101: 519-524, 1961.

Kalbian, V. V.: Laurence-Moon-Biedl syndrome in an Arab boy: familial incidence. J. Clin. Endocr. 16: 1622-1625, 1956.

*21000 BEHR SYNDROME (BEHR COMPLICATED FORM OF INFANTILE HEREDITARY OPTIC ATROPHY)

Behr's description was published in 1909. Onset is in early infancy and the features are (1) bilateral optic atrophy, with field defects, generally temporal and rarely complete, (2) neurologic signs (increased tendon reflexes, Babinski sign, slight incoordination with ataxia and spastic gait, mental deficiency, nystagmus), and (3) static condition for many years following a period of progression. Involvement of multiple brothers and sisters with normal parents and parental consanguinity suggests recessive inheritance. Van Bogaert and Andre-Van Leeuwen (1942) reported necropsy findings, but in their pedigree mild manifestations were evident in heterozygotes.

Behr, C.: Die komplizierte, hereditarfamiliare Optikusatrophie des Kindesalters: ein bisher nicht beschriebener Symptomenkomplex. Klin. Mbl. Augenheilk. 47: 138-160, 1909.

Franceschetti, A. and Bamatter, F.: Atrophie optique infantile associee a des troubles generaux (syndrome de Behr). Schweiz. Med. Wschr. 21: 285-286, 1940.

Van Bogaert, L. and Andre-Van Leeuwen, M.: Premiere observation anatomo-clinique de l'atrophie optique heredofamiliale compliquee de Behr. Bull. Acad. Roy. Med. Belg. 7: 218-225, 1942.

21010 BETA-AMINOISOBUTYRIC ACID (BAIB), URINARY EXCRETION OF

BAIB is a non-protein amino acid, i.e. it is not a constituent amino acid of any protein. Not only is the urinary excretion of BAIB a genetic trait, but also it is excreted in leukemia and by mongoloid idiots (Wright, Fink, 1957). Yanai et al. (1969), from an extensive study in Japan, concluded that high excretion is recessive. Heterozygotes excreted more BAIB than did homozygous low excretors.

De Grouchy, J. and Sutton, H. E.: A genetic study of beta-aminoisobutyric acid excretion. Am. J. Hum. Genet. 9: 76-80, 1957.

Gartler, S. M., Firschein, I. L. and Kraus, B. S.: An investigation into the genetics and racial variation of BAIB excretion. Am. J. Hum. Genet. 9: 200-207, 1957.

Wright, S. W. and Fink, K.: The excretion of beta-aminoisobutyric acid in normal, mongoloid mentally and non-mongoloid defective children. Am. J. Ment. Defic. 61: 530-533, 1957.

Yanai, J., Kakimoto, Y., Tsujio, T. and Sano, I.: Genetic study of beta-aminoisobutyric acid excretion by Japanese. Am. J. Hum. Genet. 21: 115-132, 1969.

*21020 BETA-HYDROXYISOVALERIC ACIDURIA AND BETA-METHYLCROTONYL-GLYCINURIA

Like maple syrup urine disease and isovaleric acidemia this is an inborn error of the leucine degradation pathway. The patient had no tendency to metabolic acidosis, a feature of the other two conditions. The main manifestations were muscular hypotonia and atrophy, probably of spinal origin. The disorder was gradually progressive despite a diet which reduced excretion of the abnormal metabolites. A single patient was studied. The two parents and two sibs excreted one of the abnormal metabolites and were judged to be heterozygous. Tanaka and Isselbacher (1970) supported the suggestion that the metabolic block is at the stage of beta-methylcrotonyl CoA carboxylase (one of several enzymes which contain biotin as an essential functional group) by showing that in the experimental animal biotin deficiency is accompanied by beta-hydroxyisovaleric aciduria. Eldjarn et al. (1972) gave a full report of their single case whose clinical features suggested Werdnig-Hoffmann disease. Biotin was of no therapeutic value. Although a diet low in leucine resulted in immediate reduction in the urinary excretion of abnormal metabolites and elimination of the peculiar smell, the patient was not improved clinically. Gompertz et al. (1971) identified a biotin-responsive form of this disorder.

Eldjarn, L., Jellum, E., Stokke, O., Pande, H. and Waaler, P. E.: Beta-hydroxyisovaleric aciduria and beta-methylcrotonylglycinuria: a new inborn error of metabolism. Lancet I: 521-522, 1970.

Gompertz, D., Draffan, G. H., Watts, J. L. and Hull, D.: Biotin -responsive beta-methylcrotonyl-glycinuria. Lancet II: 22-24, 1971.

Stokke, O., Eldjarn, L., Jellum, E., Pande, H. and Waalter, P. E.: Beta-methylcrotonyl-CoA carboxylase deficiency: a new metabolic error in leucine degeneration. Pediatrics 49: 726-735, 1972.

Tanaka, K. and Isselbacher, K. J.: Experimental beta-hydroxyisovaleric aciduria induced by biotin deficiency. (Letter) Lancet II: 930-931, 1970.

*21025 BETA-SITOSTEROLEMIA

Bhattacharyya and Connor (1973) described two intellectually normal female students with tendonous and tuberous xanthoma and elevation of beta-sitosterol and two other plant sterols (campesterol and stigmasterol) in the blood. Abnormally great intestinal absorption was the proposed mechanism.

Bhattacharyya, A. K. and Connor, W. E.: Beta-sitosterol and xanthomatosis: a newly described lipid storage disease in two sisters. (Abstract) J. Clin. Invest. 52: 9A only, 1973.

Bhattacharyya, A. K. and Connor, W. E.: Beta-sitosterolemia and xanthomatosis. A newly described lipid storage disease in two sisters. J. Clin. Invest. 53: 1033-1043, 1974.

21030 BIEMOND CONGENITAL AND FAMILIAL ANALGESIA

Biemond (1955) described 11-year-old fraternal twins (male and female) with loss of pain sensation, diminished touch and temperature sense, and absent tendon reflexes. Postmortem showed deficient development in the posterior root ganglia, gasserian ganglion, posterior roots, posterior horns of the spinal gray matter and posterior columns. The spinothalamic tracts could not be demonstrated. In a child (D.D., 762247) incorrectly diagnosed as dysautonomia, Freytag and Lindenberg (1967) found 'absence of posterior ascending tracts, severe reduction in the number of neurons in peripheral sensory and autonomic ganglia and a hypoplasia of the pyramidal tracts.'

Biemond, A.: Investigation of the brain in a case of congenital and familial analgesia. Proc. 11Th Intern. Cong. Neuropath. London: Sept., 1955.

Freytag, E. and Lindenberg, R.: Neuropathologic findings in patients of a hospital for the mentally deficient. A survey of 359 cases. Johns Hopkins Med. J. 121: 379-392, 1967.

21035 BIEMOND SYNDROME II

The features of this syndrome, which resembles Laurence-Moon-Biedl-Bardet (LMBB) syndrome, are iris coloboma, mental retardation, obesity, hypogenitalism and postaxial polydactyly. The 3 brothers described by Blumel and Kniker (1959) as LMBB may have had this condition. Hydrocephalus and hypospadias were also present. Irregular autosomal dominant inheritance is suggested by the segregation of iris coloboma for

RECESSIVE

four generations in the family reported by Grebe (1953) and the occurrence of postaxial polydactyly of the toes in the father and a paternal aunt of the sibs described by Blumel and Kniker.

Biemond, A.: Het syndroom van Laurence-Biedl en een aanverwant, nieuw syndroom. Nederl. T. Geneesk. 78: 1801-1814, 1934.

Blumel, J. and Kniker, W. T.: Lawrence-Moon-Bardet-Biedl syndrome. Review of the literature and a report of five cases including a family group with three affected males. Texas Rep. Biol. Med. 17: 391-410, 1959.

Grebe, H.: Contribution au diagnostic differential du syndrome de Bardet-Biedl. J. Genet. Hum. 2: 127-144, 1953.

21040 BIFID NOSE (MEDIAN FISSURE OF NOSE, MEDIAN CLEFT NOSE)

Khoo Boo-Chai (1965) described 3 cases in sibs of Asiatic Indian descent. Esser (1939) reported four affected sibs (2 males, 2 females) and an affected male first-cousin. Ocular hypertelorism (sometimes a dominant) is occasionally associated with bifid nose but the genetics of the combination is unknown.

Esser, E.: Median fissure of the nose. Plast. Chir. 1: 40-50, 1939.

Glanz, S.: Hypertelorism and the bifid nose. Sth. Med. J. 59: 631-635, 1966.

Khoo Boo-Chai: The bifid nose, with report of 3 cases in siblings. Plast. Reconstr. Surg. 36: 626-628, 1965.

21050 BILIARY ATRESIA, EXTRAHEPATIC

Krauss (1964) noted the reports of 5 sibships in which two or more sibs were affected. Renal and cardiac malformations were associated in Krauss' cases. Sweet (1932) found 3 cases in one family and two of the 3 had right ventricular hypertrophy (one with VSD and PDA). Other familial cases have been reported by Hopkins (1941), Rumber (1961) and Whitten and Adie (1952). The report of biliary atresia probably due to ascending cholangitis as part of an intrauterine infection by Listeria monocytogenes indicates a possible basis for familial occurrence of biliary atresia (Becroft, 1972). Listeria infection has been observed in successive pregnancies .

Becroft, D. M. O.: Biliary atresia associated with prenatal infections by Listeria monocytogenes. Arch. Dis. Child. 47: 656-660, 1972.

Hopkins, N. K.: Congenital absence of common duct: three cases in one family. J. Lancet 61: 90-91, 1941.

Krauss, A. N.: Familial extrahepatic biliary atresia. J. Pediat. 65: 933-937, 1964.

Rumber, W.: Uber die kongenitale Gallenwegsatresie Zum familiaren Vorkommen und zur Genese dieser Fehlbildung. Arch. Kinderheilk. 164: 238-248, 1961.

Sweet, L. K.: Congenital malformation of the bile ducts. A report of three cases in one family. J. Pediat. 1: 496-501, 1932.

Whitten, W. W. and Adie, G. C.: Congenital biliary atresia. Report of three cases: two occurring in one family. J. Pediat. 40: 539-548, 1952.

21055 BILIARY MALFORMATION WITH RENAL TUBULAR INSUFFICIENCY

Lutz-Richner and Landolt (1973) described two male sibs with second-cousin parents and an identical syndrome leading to death at the age of about 4 months. Features were extrahepatic and intrahepatic biliary hyperplasia, tubular renal failure with generalized nonspecific aminoaciduria, proteinuria, glycosuria and chronic metabolic acidosis, failure to thrive and predisposition to infections.

Lutz-Richner, A. R. and Landolt, R. F.: Familiare Gallengangmissbildungen mit tubularer Niereninsuffizienz. Helv. Paediat. Acta. 28: 1-12, 1973.

*21060 BIRD-HEADED DWARF (NANOCEPHALY OR SECKEL TYPE DWARFISM)

This condition was given its two names by Virchow. Seckel (1960) produced the definitive publication based on two personally observed cases and thirteen more reliable plus eleven less reliable cases from the literature. In addition to dwarfism of 'low birth weight' type, the features are small head, large eyes, beaklike protrusion of the nose, narrow face and receding lower jaw. Mental retardation is not as marked as might be expected in view of the very small brain. Multiple occurrence in the same sibship, increased frequency of parental consanguinity, occurrence in both sexes and normal parents suggest autosomal recessive inheritance. Affected sisters were reported by Black (1961). Harper et al. (1967) reported brother and sister who strikingly resembled Seckel's cases 1 and 2, two other reported cases and the three sibs reported by McKusick et al. (1967).

Bixler, D. and Antley, R. M.: Microcephalic dwarfism in sisters. Birth Defects Orig. Art. Ser. 10 (7): 161-165, 1974.

Black, J.: Low birth weight dwarfism. Arch. Dis. Child. 36: 633-644, 1961.

Harper, R. G., Orti, E. and Baker, R. K.: Bird-headed dwarfs (Seckel's syndrome). A familial pattern of developmental, dental, skeletal, genital and central nervous system anomalies. J. Pediat. 70: 799-804, 1967.

McKusick, V. A., Mahloudji, M., Abbott, M. H., Lindenberg, R. and Kepas, D.: Seckel's bird-headed dwarfism. New Eng. J. Med. 277: 279-286, 1967.

Sauk, J. J., Litt, R., Espiritu, C. E. and Delaney,. J. R.: Familial bird-headed dwarfism (Seckel's syndrome). J. Med. Genet. 10: 196-198, 1973.

R
E
C
E
S
S
I
V
E

Seckel, H. P. G.: Bird-headed dwarfs. Studies in Developmental Anthropology Including Human Proportions. Springfield, Ill.: Charles C Thomas, 1960.

21070 BIRD-HEADED DWARFISM, MONTREAL TYPE

In Montreal Fitch et al. (1970) described a patient with a form of bird-headed dwarfism clearly distinct from Seckel type. There were signs of premature senility, namely premature graying and loss of scalp hair, redundant and wrinkled skin of the palms. Other features included mental retardation, ptosis and cryptorchidism. Birth weight was normal. Although some features suggested the syndromes of Werner, Seckel, Hallermann-Streiff, Noonan, etc., the authors considered that differences from all these existed, justifying its listing as a separate entity. We (Smith et al., 1970) agree, having observed an affected brother and sister, and propose autosomal recessive inheritance. To take care of the problem of nomenclature I suggest we borrow the practice of the hemoglobinologists and call this the Montreal type of bird-headed dwarfism.

Fitch, N., Pinsky, L. and Lachance, R. C.: A form of bird-headed dwarfism with features of premature senility. Am. J. Dis. Child. 120: 260-264, 1970.

Smith, W. K. and McKusick, V. A.: Baltimore, unpublished observations, 1970.

21075 BLOND HAIR

Strikingly blond hair may be recessive. I know of families in which both parents and many other sibs of the blond child are relatively dark haired, although both parents have very blond relatives. Red hair (26630) also seems to be recessive.

21080 BLOOD GROUPS

All blood groups are co-dominant with rare exceptions. Blood type A(1) is dominant to blood type A(2), so that the A(1) A(2) heterozygote types as A(1). A(1), A(2) and B blood types are dominant to blood type O. The Bombay phenotype (q.v.) is due to a recessive gene. In addition various blood group phenotypes which are thought to be the result of genetic deletion behave as recessives. These include the Rh-phenotype with no Rh antigens (Vos et al., 1961) and the K(O) phenotype in which no antigen of the Kell system is demonstrable (Nunn et al., 1966). Examples are also known in the Duffy and Lutheran systems.

Nunn, H. D., Giles, C. M. and Dormandy, K. M.: A second example of anti-Ku in a patient who has the rare Kell phenotype, K(O). Vox Sang. 11: 611-619, 1966.

Vos, G. H., Vos, D., Kirk, R. L. and Sanger, R.: A sample of blood with no detectable Rh antigens. Lancet I: 14-15, 1961.

*21090 BLOOM SYNDROME (DWARFISM WITH SKIN CHANGES)

The dwarfism is of the 'low birth weight' type, i.e., although full term the child is abnormally small. The cutaneous feature is rash from sensitivity to sunlight. Szalay (1963) provided the first evidence of a genetic basis. He described (1) an isolated case, the child of first-cousin parents; and (2) two affected sibs. Multiple seemingly non-specific chromosomal breaks have been observed in these cases as in Fanconi anemia (q.v.) and may be related causally to the high frequency of leukemia (German et al., 1965). Nine of 13 families were Jewish. Landau et al. (1966) described a patient whose parents were second-cousins and who showed low gamma-A and gamma-M serum proteins. Ferrara et al. (1967) described the disease in a 'Chinese-American.' However, the diagnosis was later (Ferrara, 1972) revised to focal dermal hypoplasia (30560). Twelve of 21 families first discovered with Bloom syndrome were Ashkenazic and in these only one parental couple was consanguineous. On the other hand, 6 of the other 9 non-Jewish unions were consanguineous. The Jewish gene appeared to have originated in a local area of eastern Europe. In a later tabulation of cases, German (1969) found that 10 of 21 families were Ashkenazic.

Bloom, D.: The syndrome of congenital telangiectatic erythema and stunted growth. J. Pediat. 68: 103-113, 1966.

Ferrara, A.: Goltz's syndrome. (Letter) Am. J. Dis. Child. 123: 262, 1972.

Ferrara, A., Fontana, V. J. and Numsen, G.: Bloom's syndrome in Oriental male. New York J. Med. 67: 3258-3262, 1967.

German, J.: Bloom's syndrome. I. Genetical and clinical observations in the first twenty-seven patients. Am. J. Hum. Genet. 21: 196-227, 1969.

German, J., Archibald, R. and Bloom, D.: Chromosomal breakage in a rare and probably genetically determined syndrome of man. Science 148: 506-507, 1965.

Landau, J. W., Sasaki, M. S., Newcomer, V. D. and Norman, A.: Bloom's syndrome. The syndrome of telangiectatic erythema and growth retardation. Arch. Derm. 94: 687-694, 1966.

Sawitsky, A., Bloom, D. and German, J.: Chromosomal breakage and acute leukemia in congenital telangiectatic erythema and stunted growth. Ann. Intern. Med. 65: 487-495, 1966.

Szalay, G. C.: Dwarfism with skin manifestations. J. Pediat. 62: 686-695, 1963.

21100 BLUE DIAPER SYNDROME (FAMILIAL HYPERCALCEMIA WITH NEPHROCALCINOSIS AND INDICANURIA)

Hypercalcemia and nephrocalcinosis are associated with a defect in the intestinal transport of tryptophan. Bacterial degradation of the tryptophan leads to excessive indole production and thus to indicanuria which, on oxidation to indigo blue, causes a peculiar bluish discoloration of the diaper. Drummond, Michael, Ulstrom and Good (1964) reported two affected brothers. Although almost certainly recessive, the disorder

R
E
C
E
S
S
I
V
E

discoloration of the stools by a pigment elaborated by Pseudomonas aeruginosa.

Drummond, K. N., Michael, A. F., Ulstrom, R. A. and Good, R. A.: The blue diaper syndrome: familial hypercalcemia with nephrocalcinosis and indicanuria. A new familial disease, with definition of the metabolic abnormality. Am. J. Med. 37: 928-948, 1964.

Libit, S. A., Ulstrom, R. A. and Doeden, D.: Fecal Pseudomonas aeruginosa as a cause of the blue diaper syndrome. J. Pediat. 81: 546-547, 1972.

*21110 BOMBAY PHENOTYPE

All human bloods, with exceedingly rare exceptions, carry the red cell H antigen. It is present in greatest amount on type O red cells and least on (A1B) cells. The antigen is now regarded as an intermediate stage in a series of syntheses ending, in the presence of the A or B genes, in the production of the corresponding A and B antigens. The first examples of blood completely lacking H were found in Bombay by Bhende and colleagues (1952). These individuals are recognized by the presence of anti-H in the serum, in addition to anti-A and anti-B, as in type O persons. By family studies Levine and colleagues (1955) and Aloysia et al. (1961) showed that the Bombay phenotype, called by them OH, is due to the presence in homozygous state of a rare recessive gene. Yunis et al. (1969) found seven affected persons in three generations including a homozygous X heterozygous mating. They proposed that there are two kinds of Bombay genotypes.

Aloysia, M., Gelb, A. G., Fudenberg, H., Hamper, J., Tippett, P. and Race, R. R.: The expected 'Bombay' group O(H-A1) and O(H-A2). Transfusion 1: 212-217, 1961.

Bhende, Y. M., Deshpande, C. K., Bhatia, H. M., Sanger, R., Race, R. R., Morgan, W. T. J. and Watkins, W. M.: A 'new' blood group character related to the ABO system. Lancet I: 903-904, 1952.

Hrubisko, M., Laluha, J., Mergancova, O. and Zakovicova, S.: New variants in the ABOH blood group system due to interaction of recessive genes controlling the formation of H antigen in erythrocytes: the 'Bombay-like' phenotypes O HM, OB HM, OAB HM. Vox Sang. 19: 113-122, 1970.

Levine, P., Robinson, E., Celano, M., Briggs, O. and Falkinburg, L.: Gene interaction resulting in suppression of blood group substance B. Blood 10: 1100-1108, 1955.

Yunis, E. J., Svardal, J. M. and Bridges, R. A.: Genetics of the Bombay phenotype. Blood 33: 124-132, 1969.

21120 BOWEN SYNDROME OF MULTIPLE MALFORMATIONS

Bowen and colleagues (1964) described two families, each with two sibs displaying features suggesting autosomal trisomy, particularly trisomy 17-18. However, no chromosomal abnormality was identified. Cardinal features were failure to thrive, absent or weak sucking and swallowing, finger flexion, congenital glaucoma, malformed ears, small mandible, heart malformations, enlarged clitoris, hypospadias, agenesis of the corpus callosum and death at an early age. No parental consanguinity was demonstrated in either family. One family was Negro, the other white. See FRASER SYNDROME (21900) for a comparable, although seemingly distinct, syndrome of malformations in sibs. It now seems clear that the second of the families reported by Bowen et al., that contributed by Zellweger, had cerebro-hepato-renal syndrome (q.v.). The nature of the defect in the first family is not certain.

Bowen, P., Lee, C. N. S., Zellweger, H. and Lindenburg, R.: A familial syndrome of multiple congenital defects. Bull. Hopkins Hosp. 114: 402-414, 1964.

21130 BOWING OF LEGS, ANTERIOR, WITH DWARFISM (WEISMANN-NETTER SYNDROME; TOXOPACHYOSTEOSE DIAPHYSAIRE TIBIO-PERONIERE)

The presenting manifestations are dwarfism and sabre shins, mental retardation, mild upper extremity involvement and dural calcification. Familial incidence has been noted by Larcan et al. (1963). Hoefnagel (1969) and Keats and Alavi (1970) have reported cases in this country.

Alavi, S. M. and Keats, T. F.: Toxopachyosteose diaphysaire tibio-peroniere: Weismann-Netter syndrome. Am. J. Roentgen. 118: 314-317, 1973.

Hoefnagel, D.: Malformation syndromes with mental deficiency. The Clinical Delineation of Birth Defects. II. Malformation Syndromes. New York: National Foundation, 1969. Pp. 11-14.

Keats, T. E. and Alavi, M. S.: Toxopachyosteose diaphysaire tibio-peroniere (Weismann-Netter syndrome). Am. J. Roentgen. 109: 568-574, 1970.

Krewer, B.: Dysmorphie jambiere de Weismann-Netter (toxo-pachy-osteose diaphysaire tibio-peroniere) chez deux vrais jumeaux. Presse Med. 69: 419-420, 1961.

Larcan, A., Cayotte, J. L., Gaucher, A. and Bertheau, J. M.: La toxopachyosteose de Weismann-Netter. Ann. Med. 2: 1724-1732, 1963.

Stuve, A. and Wiedemann, H.-R.: Angeborene Verbiegungen langer Rohrenknochen — eine geschwister-beobachtung. Z. Kinderheilk. 111: 184-192, 1971.

21135 BOWING, CONGENITAL, OF LONG BONES WITH ASSOCIATED SKELETAL AND OTHER DEFECTS

This is a disorder of the newborn characterized by congenital bowing and angulation of long bones, together with other skeletal and extraskeletal defects. The scapulae are very small and the pelvis and spine show changes. Cleft palate, micrognathia, flat face and hypertelorism are also features. Most patients die in the neonatal period of respiratory distress. Stuve and Wiedemann (1971) observed affected sisters. Campomelic dwarfism is a proposed synonym (Maroteaux et al., 1971). Congenital bowing of the legs occurs in osteogenesis imperfecta congenita and in hypophosphatasia (Weller, 1959). 'Simple' idiopathic congenital bowing of the legs also occurs (Angle, 1954; Caffey, 1947). Cutaneous dimpling can occur with any prenatal bowing. Lee et al. (1972) described three cases emphasizing the tracheobronchial hypoplasia as a significant factor in the neonatal respiratory deaths. The designations campomelic and camptomelic come from the bowing of the legs, especially the tibias. Eleven pairs of ribs are usually present. The inferior part of the scapula is hypoplastic.

Angle, C. R.: Congenital bowing and angulation of the long bones. Pediatrics 13: 257-268, 1954.

Bain, A. D. and Barrett, H. S.: Congenital bowing of the long bones: report of a case. Arch. Dis. Child. 34: 516-524, 1959.

Caffey, J. P.: Prenatal bowing and thickening of tubular bones, with multiple cutaneous dimples in arms and legs: a congenital syndrome of mechanical origin. Am. J. Dis. Child. 74: 543-562, 1947.

Cremin, B. J., Orsmond, G. and Beighton, P.: Autosomal recessive inheritance in campomelic dwarfism. (Letter) Lancet I: 488-489, 1973.

Lee, F. A., Issacs, H., Strauss, J.: The 'camptomelic' syndrome. Short life-span dwarfism with respiratory distress, hypotonia, peculiar facies, and multiple skeletal and cartilaginous deformities. Am. J. Dis. Child. 124: 485-496, 1972.

Maroteaux, P., Spranger, J., Opitz, J. M., Kucera, J., Lowry, R. B., Schimke, N. and Kagan, S. M.: Le syndrome campomelique. Presse Med. 22: 1157-1162, 1971.

Stuve, A. and Wiedemann, H.-R.: Congenital bowing of the long bones in two sisters. (Letter) Lancet I: 495 only, 1971.

Weller, S. D. V.: Hypophosphatasia with congenital dimples. Proc. Roy. Soc. Med. 52: 637 only, 1959.

21138 BRACHIO-SKELETAL-GENITAL SYNDROME

Among the children of a first-cousin couple, Elsahy and Waters (1971) described three boys with an identical syndrome of mental retardation, maxillary hypoplasis, mandibular prognathism (relative or absolute), dental cysts, broad nasal bridge, hypertelorism, bifid uvula or partial cleft plate, pectus excavatum, fused cervical spinous process, penoscrotal hypospadias, and Schmorl nodes.

Elsahy, N. I. and Waters, W. R.: The brachio-skeletal-genital syndrome. A new hereditary syndrome. Plastic Reconstr. Surg. 48: 542-550, 1971.

21140 BRONCHIECTASIS

Danielson et al. (1967) found 4 of 5 sibs (2 male, 2 female) affected with bronchiectasia of the middle lobe.

Danielson, G. K., Hanson, C. W. and Cooper, E. C.: Middle lobe bronchiectasis. Report of an unusual familial occurrence. J.A.M.A. 201: 605-608, 1967.

21145 BRONCHOMALACIA

In four of five brothers, Agosti et al. (1974) observed chronic respiratory distress in early infancy and showed in one that it was due to bronchial flaccidity. Because of the bronchomalasia, first and second generation bronchi almost collapsed during expiration. Air trapping and respiratory distress simulated bronchial asthma. The parents were not known to be related but had the same surname and originated from the same small village in Italy.

Agosti, E., DeFilippi, G., Fior, R. and Chiussi, F.: Generalized famialial bronchomalacia. Acta Paediat. Scand. 63: 616-618.

21150 BULBAR PALSY, PROGRESSIVE, OF CHILDHOOD (FAZIO-LONDE DISEASE)

Londe (1894) reported affected 5-and 6-year-old brothers whose parents were first-cousins. Marinesco (1915) described it in a 12-year-old girl and her 8-year-old brother. Pyramidal tracts were not involved. Fazio's cases are said (Gomez, Clermont, Bernstein, 1962) to have been a mother and her four-and-one-half-year-old son. See AMYOTROPHIC LATERAL SCLEROSIS.

Gomez, M. R., Clermont, V. and Bernstein, J.: Progressive bulbar paralysis in childhood (Fazio-Londe's disease). Report of a case with pathologic evidence of nuclear atrophy. Arch. Neurol. 6: 317-323, 1962.

Londe, P.: Paralysie bulbaire progressive, infantile et familiale. Rev. Med. 14: 212-254, 1894.

Marinesco, G.: Sur deux cas de paralysie bulbaire progressive infantile et familiale. Comp. Rend. Soc. Biol. 78: 481-483, 1915.

21155 BUNDLE BRANCH BLOCK

Husson et al. (1973) described a family in which a girl had complete heart block at age 2 years and died at age 10 with ventricular fibrillation. A brother had right bundle branch block at age 15 years and complete heart block at age 17. A sister age 17 years had prolonged intraventricular conduction time with incomplete right bundle branch block. Thus, complete heart block and bundle branch block may be, at times, expressions of one and the same genotype.

Husson, G. S., Blackman, M. S., Rogers, M. C., Bharati, S. and Levi, M.: Familial congenital bundle branch system disease. Am. J. Cardiol. 32: 365-369, 1973.

*21160 BYLER DISEASE (FATAL INTRAHEPATIC CHOLESTASIS)

R
E
C
E
S
S
I
V
E

In the old order Amish, Clayton and his colleagues (1965) have demonstrated a variety of intrahepatic cholestasis which leads to death in the first decade of life. It appears to be different from the more benign type of intrahepatic cholestasis (q.v.). Features are (1) early onset of loose, foul-smelling stools; (2) 'attacks' of jaundice possibly related to infection; (3) hepatosplenomegaly; (4) dwarfism; and (5) in 4 of 6 cases, death between 17 months and 8 years. One mother had extreme pruritus without jaundice in the last trimester of each of 4 pregnancies. Two fathers had reduced maximum excretion of BSP. Cholestyramine, a bile-salt-sequestering exchange resin, reduced the hyperbilirubinemia. Because the bile showed an increased proportion of dihydroxy bile salts, as well as the early onset of changes in the stool and the response to cholestyramine, a defect in bile salt metabolism was postulated. Serum cholesterol was low. A familial cholestatic disorder which is probably different was studied by Kaye (see KAYE DISEASE). The same condition was probably described by Gray and Saunders (1966) in two sisters, offspring of unrelated parents (mother-Welsh, father-Irish), who died under 3 years of age. Toussaint and Gros (1966) reported affected brothers. The same condition may have been present in the patient reported by Hirooka and Ohno (1968). See 24330. Williams et al. (1972) described three affected sibs. Landing (1972) suggests that hepatoma may be a terminal event in some of these patients.

Ballow, M., Margolis, C. Z., Schachtel, B. and Hsia, Y. E.: Progressive familial intrahepatic cholestasis. Pediatrics 51: 998-1005, 1973.

Clayton, R. J., Iber, F. L., Ruebner, B. H. and McKusick, V. A.: Byler's disease. Fatal familial intrahepatic cholestasis in an Amish kindred. (Abstract) J. Pediat. 67: 1025-1028, 1965.

Gray, O. P. and Saunders, R. A.: Familial intrahepatic cholestatic jaundice in infancy. Arch. Dis. Child. 41: 320-328, 1966.

Hirooka, M. and Ohno, T.: A case of familial intrahepatic cholestasis. Tohoku J. Exp. Med. 94: 293-306, 1968.

Juberg, R. C., Holland-Moritz, R. M., Henley, K. S. and Gonzalez, C. F.: Familial intrahepatic cholestasis with mental and growth retardation. Pediatrics 38: 819-836, 1966.

Landing, B. H.: Los Angeles, Calif.: personal communication, 1972.

Linarelli, L. D., Williams, C. N. and Phillips, M. J.: Byler's disease: fatal intrahepatic cholestasis. J. Pediat. 81: 484-492, 1972.

Toussaint, W. and Gros, H.: Familiarer Icterus durch intrahepatische Cholestase. Deutsch. Z. Verdau. Stoffwechselkr. 26: 23-31, 1966.

Williams, C. N., Kaye, R., Baker, L., Hurwitz, R. and Senior, J. R.: Progressive familial cholestatic cirrhosis and bile acid metabolism. J. Pediat. 81: 493-500, 1972.

*21170 B12-BINDING ALPHA GLOBULIN, DEFICIENCY OF

In two Puerto Rican-Corsican brothers in their 40's, low vitamin B12 and low B12-binding alpha globulin were found in the blood. No symptoms were attributable thereto. Three children of one of the men had normal valves.

Carmel, R. and Herbert, V.: Deficiency of vitamin B12-binding alpha globulin in two brothers. Blood 33: 1-12, 1969.

21175 C SYNDROME

Opitz et al. (1969) described a brother and sister with a malformation syndrome which included unusual facies, polydactyly, cardiac abnormality and in the boy cryptorchidism. Preus et al. (1973) described two similar cases who were unrelated.

Opitz, J. M., Johnson, R. C., McCreadie, S. R. and Smith, D. W.: The C syndrome of multiple congenital anomalies. The Clinical Delineation of Birth Defects. II. Malformation Syndromes. New York: National Foundation, 1969. Pp. 161-166.

Preus, M., Alexander, W. J. and Fraser, F. C.: The 'C' syndrome. The Clinical Delineation of Birth Defects. XVII. Malformation Syndromes (cont.). Baltimore: Williams and Wilkins, 1973.

21180 CALCIFICATION OF JOINTS AND ARTERIES

Sharp (1954) described a family in which two of four sibs from a first-cousin marriage displayed calcification of joint structures and arteries of an unusual type. The remaining two sibs and the son and daughter of one of the severely affected sibs seemed to show a milder form of the disorder affecting only arteries. Two previously reported sporadic cases were noted.

Sharp, J.: Heredo-familial vascular and articular calcification. Ann. Rheum. Dis. 13: 15-27, 1954.

*21190 CALCINOSIS, TUMORAL, WITH HYPERPHOSPHATEMIA

Baldursson et al. (1969) observed four affected sibs out of twelve in a Negro family. Hyperphosphatemia was documented as early as twenty-one months of age in one of them in whom tumoral calcinosis appeared at four years. A majority of the cases of this condition reported in the Anglo-American literature have been in Negroes. Other familial cases have been reported by Barton and Reeves (1961) and Harkess and Peters (1967). Dodge, Travis and Assemi (1965) described three sibs with heterotopic calcification, hyperphosphatemia, unresponsiveness to parathyroid hormone, and elevated renal tubular maximum for phosphate reabsorption. Stigmata of Albright osteodystrophy (X-linked) were not present. Some reported patients have had angioid streaks of the retina (McPhaul, Engel, 1961). This is consistent with the view that angioid streaks in pseudoxanthoma elasticum, sickle cell anemia and Paget disease are due to a brittle state of Bruch membrane produced by deposition of calcium, iron and perhaps other cations. Ghormley (1942) reported multiple affected sibs. McPhaul and Engel (1961) reported affected brothers and in another family the proband's paternal grandfather was thought to have been affected and he was related to a family reported as pseudoxanthoma elasticum. From Beirut, Najjar et al. (1968) described two sibs with periarticular calcified masses, increased blood phosphorus, normal blood calcium, calcified vessels and skin changes of PXE. The parents may have been related. An aunt was said to have heterotopic calcification. I suspect that this is a disorder distinct from ordinary PXE, although with many similar features. In a review of the radiologic findings of PXE, James et al. (1969) pictured a large calcified mass in the region of the elbow. The patient probably had the entity discussed here. This condition was called lipocalcinogranulomatose by Teutschlender (1935). The designation 'tumoral calcinosis' was proposed by Inclan et al. (1943). Collard (1966) described 2 affected sisters in a sibship of 5. Calcification of the media was limited to arteries of the leg. The parents were normal and unrelated. Large calcified tophus-like nodules were situated around the joints of the fingers and toes. Although rheumatic symptoms had begun at age 20 in both, the sisters were in their 50's at the time of report. Mozaffarian et al. (1972) proposed treatment with a low-phosphorus diet combined with large oral doses of aluminum hydroxide. Affected sibs were reported by Duret (1899) in the first description and by Wilber and Slatopolsky (1968).

Baldursson, H., Evans, E. B., Dodge, W. F. and Jackson, W. T.: Tumoral calcinosis with hyperphosphatemia. A report of a family with incidence in four siblings. J. Bone Joint Surg. 51B: 913-925, 1969.

Barton, D. L. and Reeves, R. J.: Tumoral calcinosis. Report of 3 cases and review of the literature. Am. J. Roentgen. 86: 351-358, 1961.

Collard, M.: Une forme familiale de lipocalcigranulomatose avec calcinose arterielle. J. Raidol. Electr. 47: 31-40, 1966.

Dodge, W. F., Travis, L. B. and Assemi, M.: Familial heterotopic calcification and hyperphosphatemia unresponsive to parathyroid extract. (Abstract) J. Pediat. 67: 944-945, 1965.

Ghormley, R. K.: Multiple calcified bursae and calcified cysts in soft tissues. Trans. West. Surg. Ass. 51: 292-309, 1942.

Harkess, J. W. and Peters, H. J.: Tumoral calcinosis. A report of six cases. J. Bone Joint Surg. 49A: 721-731, 1967.

Inclan, A., Leon, P. and Camejo, M. G.: Tumoral calcinosis. J.A.M.A. 121: 490-495, 1943.

James, A. E., Jr., Eaton, S. B., Blazek, J. V., Donner, M. W. and Reeves, R. J.: Roentgen findings in pseudoxanthoma elasticum (PXE). Am. J. Roentgen. 106: 642-647, 1969.

McPhaul, J. J., Jr. and Engel, F. L.: Heterotopic calcification, hyperphosphatemia and angioid streaks of the retina. Am. J. Med. 31: 488-492, 1961.

Mozaffarian, G., Lafferty, F. W. and Pearson, O. H.: Treatment of tumoral calcinosis with phosphorus deprivation. Ann. Intern. Med. 77: 741-745, 1972.

Najjar, S. S., Farah, F. S., Kurban, A. K., Melhem, R. E. and Khatchadourian, A. K.: Tumoral calcinosis and pseudoxanthoma elasticum. J. Pediat. 72: 243-247, 1968.

Teutschlender, D.: Uber progressive Lipogranulomatose der Muskulatur. Klin. Wschr. 14: 451-453, 1935.

Teutschlaender, O.: Die Lipoidocalcinosis oder Lipoidkalkgicht (Lipocalcinogranulomatose). Beitr. Path. Anat. 110: 402-432, 1949.

21193 CAMPTODACTYLY WITH FIBROUS TISSUE HYPERPLASIA AND SKELETAL DYSPLASIA

Goodman et al. (1972) described this combination in two sisters and a brother from unaffected first-cousin, Iranian-Jewish parents. The brother was referred at age 19 for possible Marfan syndrome. At age 7 patent ductus arteriosus was ligated. The nose in all three affected sibs was broad with flaring nostrils. The facial appearance differed from that of unaffected sibs. Skeletal anomalies in all three included scoliosis, arachnodactyly and hammer toes.

Goodman, R. M., Katznelson, M. B.-M. and Manor, E.: Camptodactyly: occurrence in two new genetic syndromes and its relationship to other syndromes. J. Med. Genet. 9: 203-212, 1972.

21196 CAMPTODACTYLY WITH MUSCULAR HYPOPLASIA, SKELETAL DYSPLASIA AND ABNORMAL PALMAR CREASES

Goodman et al. (1972) described a brother and sister with this combination. The sister had bilateral clubbed feet. The brother had an inguinal hernia. Interphalangeal finger creases were completely absent in both. The parents, Moroccan Jews, were not known to be related.

Goodman, R. M., Katznelson, M. B.-M. and Manor, E.: Camptodactyly: occurrence in two new genetic syndromes and its relationship to other syndromes. J. Med. Genet. 9: 203-212, 1972.

21200 CANCER OF THE BREAST, FAMILIAL

Cady (1970) described a family in which three sisters had bilateral breast cancer. Together with reports in the literature, this suggested to him the existence of families with a particular tendency to early onset and bilateral breast cancer. The genetic basis might, of course, be multifactorial.

Cady, B.: Familial bilateral cancer of the breast. Ann. Surg. 172: 264-272, 1970.

*21205 CANDIDIASIS, FAMILIAL CHRONIC MUCOCUTANEOUS (FCMC)

Wells et al. (1972) investigated 46 patients with chronic oral candidiasis. Within the series they recognized a 'new' syndrome, present in 22 cases. The nails and skin were sometimes affected. Eighteen cases in 8 kindreds were studied. Parental consanguinity was demonstrated in four of these. A group of severely affected patients probably have a distinct disorder which may be non-genetic, although new autosomal dominant mutation cannot be excluded. FCMC is distinct from candidiasis with endocrinopathy (24030). A late onset group of cases of oral candidiasis appeared to be non-genetic. Of 14 fully investigated patients with FCMC, 10 were found to have iron deficiency. Higgs and Wells (1972) discussed a familial form and suggested a relationship to transferin type (which remains to be proved).

Higgs, J. M. and Wells, R. S.: Chronic muco-cutaneous candidiasis: associated abnormalities of iron metabolism. Brit. J. Derm. 86 (suppl. 8): 88-102, 1972.

Wells, R. S., Higgs, J. M., McDonald, A., Valdimarsson, H. and Holt, P. J. L.: Familial chronic muco-cutaneous candidiasis. J. Med. Genet. 9: 302-310, 1972.

21208 CARDIAC LIPIDOSIS, FAMILIAL

Deacon et al. (1973) described brother and sister with a form of infantile cardiomyopathy characterized by accumulation of lipid in the sarcoplasm of myocardial fibers. Only sporadic cases had been reported previously (Reid et al., 1968). In Deacon's cases onset was at birth and 4 weeks of age and death at 19 days and 4 months from congestive heart failure. Both had microcephaly. Severe mitochondrial changes were found in the myocardial fibrils in addition to the accumulation of neutral fat. The parents were thought to be non-consanguineous.

Deacon, J. S. R., Gilbert, E. F., Viseskul, C., Herrmann, J., Angevine, J. M., Opitz, J. M. and Albert, A. E.: Familial cardiac lipidosis. Birth Defects Orig. Art. Ser. 10: 181-195, 1973.

Reid, J. D., Hadju, S. I. and Attah, E.: Infantile cardiomyopathy: a previously unrecognized type with histiocytoid reaction. J. Pediat. 73: 335-339, 1968.

21210 CARDIO-AUDITORY SYNDROME OF SANCHEZ CASCOS

A 'new' cardio-auditory syndrome was found in 12 deaf children by Sanchez Cascos et al. (1969). All but 2 had X-ray evidence of left ventricular hypertrophy, most had electrocardiographic changes of biventricular hypertrophy and most showed a high proportion of whorls in the dermatoglyphs. One of the 12 was a girl. One of the parental pairs was consanguineous. Six of the 12 were in 3 sibships.

Sanchez Cascos, A., Sanchez-Harguindey, L. and De Rabago, P.: Cardio-auditory syndromes. Cardiac and genetic study of 511 deaf-mute children. Brit. Heart J. 31: 26-33, 1969.

*21220 CARNOSINEMIA

Perry et al. (1967) described two unrelated children with a progressive neurologic disorder characterized by severe mental defect and myoclonic seizures. Both excreted carnosine in the urine, even when all source of the dipeptide was excluded from the diet. Both had unusually high concentrations of homocarnosine in the cerebrospinal fluid. When fed a dietary source of anserine, the children excreted anserine in the urine but not its hydrolysis product, methylhistidine. Perry et al. suggested that one and perhaps both had a defect in carnosinase activity. One child, of German and Dutch ancestry, was the offspring of first-cousin parents. The other child was of Chinese ancestry. Perry et al. (1968) found that the enzyme of normal human serum that hydrolyzes the dipeptides carnosine and anserine into their constituent amino acids was almost absent in the two patients. No comment was made on the level of enzyme in the parents. Carnosine is a dipeptide of alanine and histidine. Scriver et al. (1968) commented on the possible relationship of the mental retardation that occurs with hyper-beta-carnosinemia (q.v.) and phenylketonuria. In the case of the affected Dutch child reported by Heeswijk et al. (1969) the parents were consanguineous and showed decreased serum carnosinase activity. A new family with this rare anomaly was reported by Terplan and Cares (1972). Two brothers ages 7 and 4 had died. A sister aged 6 was normal but had chemical changes. The parents have low carnosinase activity. Autopsy on the older boy showed severe axonal degeneration, numerous 'spheroids' in the grey matter, demyelinization, fibrosis and loss of Purkinje fibers.

Heeswijk, P. J., Trijbels, J. M. F., Schretlen, A. M., Munster, P. J. J. and Monnens, L. A. H.: A patient with a deficiency of serum-carnosinase activity. Acta Paediat. Scand. 58: 584-592, 1969.

Perry, T. L., Hansen, S. and Love, D.: Serum-carnosinase deficiency in carnosinaemia. Lancet I: 1229-1230, 1968.

Perry, T. L., Hansen, S., Tischler, B., Bunting, R. and Berry, K.: Carnosinemia: metabolic disorder with neurologic disease and mental defect. New Eng. J. Med. 277: 1219-1227, 1967.

Scriver, C. R., Allen, R. J., Tourtellotte, W. W., Adriaenssens, K., Lowenthal, A. and Mardens, Y.: Carnosinaemia. (Letter) Lancet I: 1249 only, 1968.

Terplan, K. L. and Cares, H. L.: Histopathology of the nervous system in carnosinase enzyme deficiency with mental retardation. Neurology 22: 644-654, 1972.

*21240 CATARACT AND CONGENITAL ICHTHYOSIS

Pinkerton (1958) described Japanese sibs with cortical cataract and ichthyosis. The parents were not affected by either disorder and were not related. Jancke (1950) reported three affected sisters.

Jancke, G.: Cataracta syndermatotica und Ichthyosis congenita. Klin. Mbl. Augenheilk. 117: 286-290, 1950.

Pinkerton, O. D.: Cataract associated with congenital ichthyosis. Arch. Ophthal. 60: 393-396, 1958.

*21250 CATARACT, CONGENITAL OR JUVENILE

Cataract occurs as a feature of several of the other entities in this catalog: galactosemia, cerebral cholesterinosis, chondrodystrophia calcificans congenita, congenital amaurosis, Rothmund syndrome, Marinesco-Sjogren syndrome, Crome syndrome, Refsum syndrome, retinitis pigmentosa, etc. In addition cataract sometimes occurs as an isolated defect with recessive inheritance. For example, Saebo (1949) studied 17 families with cases of congenital or juvenile cataracts. Two or more sibs were affected in 8 families. In 9 families the parents were related, being first-cousins in 5. In one family the proband had retinitis pigmentosa (q.v.), of which cataract is a known complication. In another family the proband had retinitis pigmentosa and deaf-mutism (Usher syndrome, q.v.). Recessively inherited cataract seems to be unusually frequent in Japan (Nakajima, 1964). Yamaguchi et al. (1972) presented evidence suggesting linkage of the I-blood group locus and a recessive form of congenital cataract. In each of four Japanese families, two sibs were both homozygous for 'little eye' (no pun intended), and affected with a recessive form of cataract. Recessively inherited congenital cataract was found rather frequently in Cyprus by Merin et al. (1972). There are probably many different disorders represented by the category called recessive congenital cataract. Galactokinase deficiency (23020) and epimerase deficiency (23035) are examples of two recently found disorders that may present as seemingly isolated congenital cataract.

Francois, J.: Heredity in Ophthalmology. St. Louis: C. V. Mosby Co., 1961. p. 356.

Gianferrari, L., Cresseri, A. and Maltarello, A.: Ricerche sulla ereditarieta dell'idroftalmo e della cataratta congenita in paesi delle prealpi orobiche. Acta Genet. Med. Gem. 3: 1-15, 1954.

Joseph, R.: Congenital total cataract — possibly recessive. Brit. J. Ophthal. 41: 444-445, 1957.

Klein, D.: Cataracte congenitale familiale: consanguinite des parents. J. Genet. Hum. 5: 283-284, 1956.

Merin, S., Lapithis, A. G., Horovitz, D. and Michaelson, I. C.: Childhood blindness in Cyprus. Am. J. Ophthal. 74: 538-542, 1972.

Nakajima, A.: Population genetic study of blinding diseases in Japan. Proc. 2nd. Intern. Cong. Hum. Genet., Rome, 1961. vol. 3, p. 1961, 1964.

Saebo, J.: An investigation into the mode of heredity of congenital and juvenile cataracts. Brit. J. Ophthal. 33: 601-629, 1949.

Yamaguchi, H., Okubo, Y. and Tanaka, M.: A note on possible close linkage between the Ii blood locus and a congenital cataract locus. Proc. Japan Acad. 48: 625-628, 1972.

21255 CATARACT, MICROPHTHALMIA AND NYSTAGMUS

Harman (1910) reported this association in 9 persons in 5 generations of a family (see 15685). Zeiter (1963) saw the triad together with extreme miosis in 7 members of 3 generations. Temtamy and Shalash (1973) suggested autosomal recessive inheritance on the basis of an affected boy and girl with first-cousin parents.

Harman, N.: Ten pedigrees of congenital and infantile cataract, lamellar, coralliform, discoid, posterior polar with microphthalmia. Trans. Ophthal. Soc. U.K. 30: 251, 1910.

Temtamy, S. A. and Shalash, B. A.: Genetic heterogeneity of the syndrome: microphthalmos with congenital cataract. The Clinical Delineation of Birth Defects. XVI. Urinary System and Others. Baltimore: Williams and Wilkins, 1974. Pp. 292-293.

Zeiter, H. J.: Congenital microphthalmus. A pedigree of 4 affected siblings and an additional report of 44 sporadic cases. Am. J. Ophthal. 55: 910-922, 1963.

21260 CATARACT, NUCLEAR

Although usually inherited as a dominant (q.v.), nuclear cataract may be inherited as a recessive in the pedigrees reported by Rados (1947) and others.

Rados, A.: Central pulverulent (discoid) cataract and its hereditary transmission. Arch. Ophthal. 38: 57-77, 1947.

21270 CATARACT, TOTAL NUCLEAR

Although usually inherited as a dominant (q.v.), 'recessive pedigrees' are reported.

Bane, W. M.: Congenital cataracts. Am. J. Ophthal. 27: 651 only, 1944.

Saebo, J.: An investigation into the mode of heredity of congenital and juvenile cataracts. Brit. J. Ophthal. 33: 601-629, 1949.

Wagner, H.: Recessive vererbter angeborener Star. Klin. Mbl. Augenheilk. 104: 337-338, 1940.

21275 CELIAC ARTERY STENOSIS FROM COMPRESSION BY MEDIAN ARCUATE LIGAMENT OF DIAPHRAGM

Dodinval and Dreze (1972) described a mother and daughter with this finding. The celiac artery was malpositioned congenitally. Both suffered from abdominal pains which were relieved by appropriate surgery.

Dodinval, P. and Dreze, C.: Stenose du tronc coeliaque chez une mere et sa fille par compression due au ligament arque median du diaphragme (lere observation familiale). J. Genet. Hum. 20: 49-67, 1972.

*21280 CEPHALIN LIPIDOSIS

From England Baar and Hickmans (1956) reported on a brother and sister with mental retardation and slow deterioration, marked splenomegaly with absence of glandular involvement or bone changes, and death at 4 and 6 years. The reticuloendothelial cells of the liver and spleen and the nerve cells of the cerebral cortex

R
E
C
E
S
S
I
V
E

and spinal cord showed extensive lipid deposition. The lipid was identified as inosamine phosphatide. No similar cases had been previously reported.

Baar, H. S. and Hickmans, E. M.: Cephalin-lipidosis: a new disorder of lipid metabolism. Acta Med. Scand. 155: 49-64, 1956.

21290 CEREBELLAR ATAXIA, INFANTILE, WITH PROGRESSIVE EXTERNAL OPHTHALMOPLE-GIA

In the family described by Franceschetti and colleagues (1945) four of five sibs had cerebellar ataxia (which was considered to be of the Pierre Marie type) combined with ophthalmoplegia. The parents were normal and not related. See 16450 for a dominant form of cerebellar ataxia with external ophthalmoplegia.

Franceschetti, A., De Morsier, G. and Klein, D.: Ueber eine neue mit Ophthalmoplegia externa progressiva kombinierte infantile Form von zerebellarer Heredoataxie (P. Marie) bei vier Geschwistern. Arch. Klaus Stift. Vererbungsforch. 20 (suppl.): 59-81, 1945.

21300 CEREBELLAR HYPOPLASIA

Two pairs of affected sibs have been reported (Crouzon, 1929; Sarrouy et al., 1957). In addition Norman and Urich (1958) noted parental consanguinity in an isolated case. See CEREBELLO-PARENCHYMAL ATROPHY IV.

Crouzon, O.: Atrophie Cerebelleuse Idiotique, in Etudes sur les Maladies Familiales Nerveuses et Dystrophiques. Paris, 1929. Pp. 90-111.

Friede, R. L.: Arrested cerebellar development, a type of cerebellar degeneration in amaurotic idiocy. J. Neurol. Neurosurg. Psychiat. 27: 41-45, 1964.

Norman, R. M. and Urich, H.: Cerebellar hypoplasia associated with systemic degeneration in early life. J. Neurol. Neurosurg. Psychiat. 21: 159-166, 1958.

Sarrouy, C., Raffi, A. and Boineau, N.: A propos de deux cas d'hypoplasic cerebelleuse dans une meme fratrie. Arch. Franc. Pediat. 14: 449-460, 1957.

*21310 CEREBELLO-PARENCHYMAL DISORDER II (CPD II; LATE ONSET RECESSIVE TYPE)

Ataxia and dysarthria developed in the fourth or fifth decades of life. Richter (1940) described three affected sibs and Thorpe (1935) described two. Autopsies showed absent Purkinje cells but only mild loss of granule cells and dentate neurones. The inferior olivary nuclei and the pons were normal.

Richter, R.: Clinico-pathologic study of parenchymatous cortical cerebellar atrophy: report of familial case. J. Nerv. Ment. Dis. 91: 37-46, 1940.

Thorpe, F. T.: Familial degeneration of the cerebellum in association with epilepsy. A report of two cases, one with pathological findings. Brain 58: 97-114, 1935.

*21320 CEREBELLO-PARENCHYMAL DISORDER III (CPD III; CONGENITAL CEREBELLAR GRANULAR CELL HYPOPLASIA AND MENTAL RETARDATION)

Jervis (1954) also observed the disorder in both of monozygotic twins. Mental deficiency and cerebellar ataxia are congenital. The cerebellum is small with severe loss of granule cells and with heterotopic Purkinje cells. Infection of the fetal rat by rat virus (Margolis and Kelham, 1968) and of the fetal kitten by panleukopenia virus (Kelham and Margolis, 1966) results in a similar picture of granule cell hypoplasia. Norman (1940) described three affected sibs in one family and two in another. Scherer (1933) described two affected sibs, and Jervis (1950) three affected sibs. See 25830. Skre and Berg (1974) concluded that this disorder and albinism (20310) are genetically linked. They observed an inbred kindred in which the two traits occurred together presumably because of linkage disequelibrium rather than pleiotropism.

Jervis, G. A.: Concordant primary atrophy of cerebellar granules in monozygotic twins. Acta Genet. Med. Gem. 3: 153-162, 1954.

Jervis, G. A.: Early familial cerebellar degeneration. (Report of three cases in one family). J. Nerv. Ment. Dis. 111: 398-407, 1950.

Kelham, L. and Margolis, G.: Viral etiology of spontaneous ataxia of cats. Am. J. Path. 48: 991-1011, 1966.

Margolis, G. and Kilham, L.: Virus-induced cerebellar hypoplasia. Res. Publ. Ass. Res. Nerv. Ment. Dis. 44: 113-146, 1968.

Norman, R. M.: Primary degeneration of the granular layer of the cerebellum: an unusual form of familial cerebellar atrophy occurring in early life. Brain 63: 365-379, 1940.

Scherer, H. J.: Beitrage zur pathologischen Anatomie des Kleinhirns: genuine Kleinhirnatrophien. Zbl. Neurol. Psychiat. 145: 335-405, 1933.

Skre, H. and Berg, K.: Cerebellar ataxia and total albinism: a kindred suggesting pleiotropism or linkage. Clin. Genet. 5: 196-204, 1974.

21330 CEREBELLO-PARENCHYMAL DISORDER IV (CPD IV; CEREBELLAR VERMIS AGENESIS)

De Haene (1955) collected from the literature 4 cases of total and 7 cases of partial agenesis of the vermis of the cerebellum, and added the only familial example: 3 brothers (one autopsy) died at age 4-8 years, the illness being characterized by tremor and hypotonia. Andermann (1968) tells me of 4 French-Canadian sibs with this condition. Respiration was characterized by alternating hyperpnea as in Cheyne-Stokes respiration.

R
E
C
E
S
S
I
V
E

Joubert et al. (1969) described four French-Canadian sibs with this abnormality. By autopsy or pneumoencephalogram the vermis was shown to be completely or partially absent in all four. One also had an occipital meningomyelocele. Symptoms included episodic hyperpnea, abnormal eye movements and psychomotor retardation. The oldest living sib was 8 years old. The parents were distantly related. See CEREBELLAR HYPOPLASIA.

De Haene, A.: Agenesie partielle du vermis du cervelet a caractere familial. Acta Neurol. Belg. 55: 622-628, 1955.

Joubert, M., Eisenring, J. J., Robb, J. P. and Andermann, F.: Familial agenesis of the cerebellar vermis. A syndrome of episodic hyperpnea, abnormal eye movements, ataxia, and retardation. Neurology 19: 813-825, 1969.

21340 CEREBELLO-PARENCHYMAL DISORDER V (CPA V; SPINODENTATE ATROPHY: DYS-SYNERGIA CEREBELLARIS MYOCLONICA OF HUNT)

Ramsey Hunt (1921) described twin brothers with a cerebellar disturbance combined with severe myoclonic jerks brought on by muscular effort. Autopsy in one of them who died at age 36 years showed marked loss of dentate neurones and their fibers in the superior cerebellar peduncles. Hunt described several other cases with affected relatives and without autopsy.

Hunt, J. R.: Dyssynergia cerebellaris myoclonica — primary atrophy of the dentate system: a contribution to the pathology and symptomatology of the cerebellum. Brain 44: 490-538, 1921.

21350 CEREBRAL ANGIOPATHY, DYSHORIC

Richard and colleagues (1965) studied the brain of 18 members of 8 families in which one member had histologically confirmed angiopathy. Of 6 sibships studied, 5 had more than one affected sib. Parent-child pairs were studied but in no instance were both involved. This condition, described by Oppenheim, is characterized by arteriolocapillary degeneration particularly in the occipital cortex and the calcarine area.

Richard, J., De Ajuriaguerra, J. and Constantinidis, J.: L'incidence familiale de l'angiopathie dyshorique du cortex cerebral. Int. J. Neuropsychiat. 1: 118-124, 1965.

21360 CEREBRAL CALCIFICATION, NON-ARTERIOSCLEROTIC

This condition was probably first described by Fahr in 1930. Melchior, Benda and Yakovlev (1960) described families with affected sibs, 3 out of 10 in one and 2 out of 4 in the second. The clinical evolution is that of a degenerative rather than a developmental disorder. Progressive deterioration of mentality and loss of motor accomplishments take place and symmetrical spastic paralysis and sometimes athetosis appear, progressing to a decerebrate state. The head is small and round. Optic atrophy may be present. Mineral deposits are distributed throughout the cerebral cortex, basal ganglia, dentate nucleus, subthalamus and red nucleus with cell loss in these areas. Calcification probably occurs in areas of demyelination and lipid deposition. Hallervorden (1950) observed sibs as did also Beyme (1945) and Foley (1951). Jervis (1954) described the pathologic findings in two cases who were microcephalic idiots with muscular hypertonicity and choreo-athetosis. Calcification was found in the basal ganglia, cerebellum and cerebral cortex and the centrum ovale showed extensive demyelination. Bowman (1954) described two affected male sibs. One died at 33 months and one at 31 months. Calcification was demonstrated at autopsy but not by X-ray during life. Lowenthal (1948) reviewed 32 cases in the literature of which 3 were familial. In some cases hypoparathyroidism may be present. Pilleri (1966) reported clinico-anatomic studies of a 64-year-old male with Fahr disease, or nonarteriosclerotic, idiopathic intracerebral calcification of the blood vessels. The disorder was diagnosed radiologically in three generations of the family. Clinical features included fits, pyramidal symptoms, cerebellar dysarthria and psychic changes. Calcification involved the media and adventitia of brain vessels of all sizes and calcium concretions lay free in the tissues. Male-to-male transmission was not proved. Almost certainly more than one genetic variety of non-arteriosclerotic cerebral calcification exists. Babbitt et al. (1968) described this disorder, called by them 'familial cerebrovascular ferrocalcinosis' in two sisters and a brother.

Beyme, F.: Uber das Gehirn einer familiar Oligophrenen mit symmetrischen Kalkablagerungen besonders in den Stammganglien. Schweiz. Arch. Neurol. Psychiat. 56: 161-190, 1945.

Babbitt, D. P., Tang, T., Dobbs, J. and Berk, R.: Idiopathic familial cerebrovascular ferrocalcinosis (Fahr's disease) and review of differential diagnosis of intracranial calcification in children. Am. J. Roentgen. 105: 352-358, 1968.

Bowman, M. S.: Familial occurrence of 'idiopathic' calcification of cerebral capillaries. Am. J. Path. 30: 87-97, 1954.

Fahr, T.: Idiopathische Verkalkung der Hirngefasse. Zbl. Allg. Path. 50: 129-133, 1930.

Foley, J.: Calcification of the corpus striatum and dentate nuclei occurring in a family. J. Neurol. Neurosurg. Psychiat. 14: 253-261, 1951.

Hallervorden, I.: Uber diffuse symmetrische Kalkablagerungen bei einem Krankheitsbild mit Mikrocephalie und Meningoencephalitis. Arch. Psychiat. 184: 579-600, 1950.

Jervis, G. A.: Microcephaly with extensive calcium deposits and demyelination. J. Neuropath. Exp. Neurol. 13: 318-329, 1954.

Lowenthal, A.: La calcification vasculaire intracerebrale non arteriosclereuse de Fahr. Est-elle la manifestation cerebrale d'une perturbation des fonctions parathyroidiennes? Acta Neurol. Psychiat. Belg. 48: 613-631, 1948.

R
E
C
E
S
S
I
V
E

Melchior, J. C., Benda, C. E. and Yakovlev, P. I.: Familial idiopathic cerebral calcifications in childhood.
Am. J. Dis. Child. 99: 787-803, 1960.

Pilleri, G.: A case of morbus Fahr (non arteriosclerotic, idiopathic intracerebral calcification of the blood vessels) in three generations. A clinico-anatomical contribution. Psychiat. Neurol. 152: 43-58, 1966.

*21370 CEREBRAL CHOLESTERINOSIS (CEREBROTENDINOUS XANTHOMATOSIS)

Van Bogaert and colleagues (1937) described affected cousins. Onset was at age 12 or 13 years. When examined in their 30's the patients demonstrated cerebellopyramidal signs, myoclonus of the soft palate, mental debility, cataracts, xanthelasmata and tendon xanthomata. At autopsy many deposits were found in the white matter of the cerebellum and the cerebral peduncles. Menkes et al. (1968) described brother and sister, ages 60 and 57 years, respectively. The brother had slowly progressive ataxia in later years. Cataracts were removed in his 20's and he had enlarged Achilles tendons from childhood. Serum cholesterol was normal. He died of myocardial infarction. The cerebellar white matter was demyelinated and contained cholesterol deposits. The sister had had progressive enlargement of Achilles tendons, minimal mental retardation and unsteadiness of gait. Bilateral cataracts were removed at age 24 years. Serum cholesterol was normal. Menkes and his colleagues (1968) speculated that the defect concerns transport of cholesterol out of cells. Cholesterol can be synthesized in many tissues but oxidation is virtually limited to the liver. Whereas tendon xanthomata and cataracts may appear early, neurologic impairment may be a late development. Philippart and Van Bogaert (1969) gave follow-up on a member of the first family described by Van Bogaert. The disorder is characterized by progressive cerebellar ataxia after puberty, juvenile cataracts, systemic spinal cord involvement and a pseudobulbar phase leading to death. The deposited material is cholestanol. The diagnosis can be made by demonstrating cholestanol in abnormal amounts in the serum and tendon of persons suspected of being affected. Harlan and Still (1968) described Negro brother and sister with multiple tendinous and tuberous xanthomas despite plasma lipids which were quantitatively and qualitatively normal. Evidence of xanthomatous involvement of the lungs was found in the male. The authors suggested that normolipemic xanthomatosis is a distinct entity inherited as an autosomal recessive and that it should be classified as a reticuloendotheliosis. Swanson (1968) suggested that this may be the same entity as cerebrotendious xanthomatosis. Although neurological manifestations were not evident, these may be late in appearing. Lung involvement occurs with cerebrotendinous xanthomatosis. Setoguchi et al. (1974) found that bile acid production in this disorder (abbreviated by them CTX) is subnormal, yet the activity of cholesterol 7-alpha-hydroxylase, the rate-determining enzyme of bile acid synthesis, is elevated.

Giampalmo, A.: Les lipidoses cholesteriniques du systeme nerveux. Acta Neurol. Belg. 54: 786-808, 1954.

Harlan, W. R., Jr. and Still, W. J.: Hereditary tendinous and tuberous xanthomatosis without hyperlipidemia. A new lipid-storage disorder. New Eng. J. Med. 278: 416-422, 1968.

Menkes, J. H., Schimschock, J. R. and Swanson, P. D.: Cerebrotendinous xanthomatosis: the storage of cholestanol within the nervous system. Arch. Neurol. 19: 47-53, 1968.

Philippart, M. and Van Bogaert, L.: Cholestanolosis (cerebrotendinous xanthomatosis). A follow-up study on the original family. Arch. Neurol. 21: 603-610, 1969.

Salen, G.: Cholestanol deposition in cerebrotendinous xanthomatosis. A possible mechanism. Ann. Intern. Med. 75: 843-851, 1971.

Schimschock, J. R., Alvord, E. C., Jr. and Swanson, P. D.: Cerebrotendinous xanthomatosis: clinical and pathological studies. Arch. Neurol. 18: 688-698, 1968.

Schneider, C.: Uber eine eigenartige Hirnerkrankung (vaskulare Lipoidose). Allg. Z. Psychiat. 104: 144-163, 1936.

Setoguchi, T., Salen, G., Tint, G. S. and Mosbach, E. H.: A biochemical abnormality in cerebrotendinous xanthomatosis. Impairment of bile acid biosynthesis associated with incomplete degradation of the cholesterol side chain. J. Clin. Invest. 53: 1393-1401, 1974.

Swanson, P. D.: Cerebrotendinous xanthomatosis. (Letter) New Eng. J. Med. 278: 857 only, 1968.

Van Bogaert, L., Scherer, H. J. and Epstein, E.: Une forme cerebrale de la cholesterinose generalisee. Paris: Masson, 1937.

Van Bogaert, L., Scherer, H. J., Froehlich, A. and Epstein, E.: Une deuxieme observation de cholesterinose tendineuse symetrique avec symptomes cerebraux. Ann. Med. 42: 69-101, 1937.

R
E
C
E
S
S
I
V
E

21380 CEREBRAL GIGANTISM (SOTOS SYNDROME)

Except for a concordant set of identical twins (Hook and Reynolds, 1967), most cases have been sporadic. (I have observed the case of an affected boy whose father, not available for study, is described as having similar features.) The reported cases may represent new dominant mutations. Large size with large hands and feet are present from birth. Growth is rapid in the first years of life but final height may not be excessive. Bone age is advanced. The skull is large with moderate prognathism. Mild dilation of the cerebral ventricles, nonspecific EEG changes and seizures have been observed. Poor coordination and mental retardation are features. The differential diagnosis should include the XYY syndrome. Bejar et al. (1970) studied two patients finding abnormal dermatoglyphics, normal growth hormone levels, and high levels of valine, isoleucine and leucine in the blood. The glycine-to-valine ratio seemed particularly useful in distinguishing patients from controls. Hooft et al. (1968) described cerebral gigantism in two first-cousins. Nevo et al. (1974) described affected brother and sister and their affected double first-cousin, in an inbred Arab family in Israel. Two of the three showed generalized edema and flexion contractures of the feet at birth.

Bejar, R. L., Smith, G. F., Park, S., Spellacy, W. N., Wolfson, S. L. and Nyhan, W. L.: Cerebral gigantism: concentrations of amino acids in plasma and muscle. J. Pediat. 76: 105-111, 1970.

Hooft, C., Schotte, H. and Van Hooren, G.: Familial cerebral gigantism. Acta Paediat. Belg. 22: 173-186, 1968.

Hook, E. B. and Reynolds, J. W.: Cerebral gigantism: endocrinological and clinical observations of six patients including a congenital giant, concordant monozygotic twins, and a child who achieved adult gigantic size. J. Pediat. 70: 900-914, 1967.

Nevo, S., Zeltzer, M., Benderly, A. and Levy, J.: Evidence for autosomal recessive inheritance in cerebral gigantism. J. Med. Genet. 11: 158-165, 1974.

Sotos, J. F., Dodge, P. R., Muirhead, D., Crawford, J. D. and Talbot, N. B.: Cerebral gigantism in childhood: a syndrome of excessively rapid growth with acromegalic features and a nonprogressive neurologic disorder. New Eng. J. Med. 271: 109-116, 1964.

Stephenson, J. N., Mellinger, R. C. and Manson, G.: Cerebral gigantism. Pediatrics 41: 130-138, 1968.

21390 CEREBRAL SCLEROSIS LIKE PELIZAEUS-MERZBACHER DISEASE

Fahmy et al. (1969) observed a brother and sister (out of a sibship of 11), offspring of first-cousin parents, who had a slowly progressive neurologic disorder beginning its manifestations in early childhood. Electron microscopic studies of sural nerve showed unique rod-shaped bodies in Schwann cells. The clinical picture was similar to that of the Pelizaeus-Merzbacher syndrome, an X-linked disorder.

Fahmy, A., Carter, T., Paulson, G. and Nance, W. E.: A 'new' form of hereditary cerebral sclerosis. Arch. Neurol. 20: 468-478, 1969.

*21400 CEREBRO-COSTO-MANDIBULAR SYNDROME

In a female and two male sibs, McNicholl et al. (1970) described a syndrome of mental retardation, palatal defects (short hard palate with central hole, absent soft palate, absent uvula), micrognathia, glossoptosis, severe costovertebral abnormalities. A barking cough in one suggested tracheal cartilage abnormality as in the case of Smith et al. (1966) which bore other similarities. The condition has also been designated rib gap defects with micrognathia (Miller et al., 1972). The 'gaps' occur in the posterior portion of the ribs and may lead to 'flail chest.'

McNicholl, B., Egan-Mitchell, B., Murray, J. P., Doyle, J. F., Kennedy, J. D. and Crome, L.: Cerebro-costo-mandibular syndrome. A new familial developmental disorder. Arch. Dis. Child. 45: 421-424, 1970.

Miller, K. E., Allen, R. P. and Davis, W. S.: Rib gap defects with micrognathia. Am. J. Roentgenol. 114: 253-256, 1972.

Smith, D. W., Theiler, K. and Schachenmann, G.: Rib-gap defect with micrognathia, malformed tracheal cartilages, and redundant skin: a new pattern of defective development. J. Pediat. 69: 799-803, 1966.

*21410 CEREBRO-HEPATO-RENAL SYNDROME (ZELLWEGER SYNDROME)

Smith, Opitz and Inhorn (1965) described a Caucasian brother and sister who died at 8 and 10 weeks of age with aberrant development of the skull, face, ears, eyes, hands and feet, polycystic kidneys with adequate functional renal parenchyma and intrahepatic biliary dysgenesis. Jaundice developed before death. The karyotype was normal. Passarge and McAdams (1967) described 5 sisters out of a sibship of 13 with severe, generalized hypotonia and absent Moro response, characteristic craniofacial abnormalities, cortical renal cysts and hepatomegaly. The brain in two studied histologically showed sudanophilic leukodystrophy. The authors considered this to be the same entity as that reported by Smith, Opitz and Inhorn (1965) and perhaps the same as that described by Bowen et al. (1964). They proposed cerebro-hepato-renal syndrome as an appropriate designation. Bowen et al. (1964) described two families each with two sibs who displayed an unusual malformation syndrome. Opitz et al. (1969) described further cases, suggested that only one of the two sets of sibs (that contributed by Zellweger) had the cerebro-hepato-renal syndrome, and made the important observation that serum iron level and iron binding capacity were high in one well-studied case and should provide an easy method for diagnosis of this disorder. A defect in the placental iron transfer mechanism was postulated. Chondral calcification, most marked in the patellas, is a feature pointed out by Poznanski et al. (1970). The change is somewhat like that of chondrodystrophia calcificans congenita. Patton et al. (1972) described two cases with the additional features of TSHT cell hyperplasia and thymic anomalies. Abnormalities of iron metabolism were not present. Goldfischer et al. (1973) presented evidence of abnormality in peroxisomes and mitochondria, the two organelles principally concerned with cellular respiration.

Bowen, P., Lee, C. S. N., Zellweger, H. and Lindenburg, R.: A familial syndrome of multiple congenital defects. Bull. Johns Hopkins Hosp. 114: 402-414, 1964.

Goldfischer, S., Moore, C. L., Johnson, A. B., Spiro, A. J., Wisniewski, H. K., Ritch, R. H., Norton, W. T., Rapin, I. and Gartner, L. M.: Peroxisomal and mitochondrial defects in the cerebro-hepato-renal syndrome. Science 182: 62-64, 1973.

Opitz, J. M., ZuRhein, G. M., Vitale, L., Shahidi, N. T., Howe, J. J., Chou, S. M., Shanklin, D. R., Sybers, H. D., Dood, A. R. and Gerritsen, T.: The Zellweger syndrome (cerebro-hepato-renal syndrome). The Clinical Delineation of Birth Defects. II. Malformation Syndromes. New York: National Foundation, 1969. Pp. 144-160.

Passarge, E. and McAdams, A. J.: Cerebro-hepato-renal syndrome. A newly recognized hereditary

disorder of multiple congenital defects, including sudanophilic leukodystrophy, cirrhosis of the liver, and
polycystic kidneys. J. Pediat. 71: 691-702, 1967.

Patton, R. G., Christie, D. L., Smith, D. W. and Beckwith, J. B.: Cerebro-hepato-renal syndrome of
Zellweger. Am. J. Dis. Child. 124: 840-844, 1972.

Poznanski, A. K., Nosanchuk, J. S., Baublis, J. and Holt, J. F.: The cerebro-hepato-renal syndrome
(CHRS): (Zellweger's syndrome). Am. J. Roentgen. 109: 313-322, 1970.

Smith, D. W., Opitz, J. M. and Inhorn, S. L.: A syndrome of multiple developmental defects including
polycystic kidneys and intrahepatic biliary dysgenesis in 2 siblings. J. Pediat. 67: 617-624, 1965.

21420 CEROID STORAGE DISEASE

Oppenheimer and Andrews (1959) reported two cases: (1) a white 4-year-old male from West Virginia
(B2644; aut. 24455) who died from liver failure and had ceroid deposits of liver, spleen and intestinal mucosa;
and (2) a white 22-month-old female who at autopsy had ceroid limited largely to hepatic macrophages.
Landing and Shirkey (1957) described two children who may have had the same disorder. No evidence for
or against a genetic basis is available. The sister and two brothers reported by Nelson et al. (see 24750) may
have had the same condition. The isolated cases reported by Jonas (1966) and by Ryan et al. (1970) may
have the same or a related condition.

Jonas, O.: Ceroid storage in a child with a Niemann-Pick type syndrome. Med. J. Aust. 2: 551-554, 1970.

Landing, B. H. and Shirkey, H. S.: A syndrome of recurrent infection and infiltration of viscera by
pigmented lipid histiocytes. Pediatrics 20: 431-447, 1957.

Oppenheimer, E. H. and Andrews, E. C., Jr.: Ceroid storage disease in childhood. Pediatrics 23:
1091-1102, 1959.

Ryan, G. B., Anderson, R. M., Menkes, J. H. and Dennett, X.: Lipofuscin (ceroid) storage disease of
the brain. Neuropathological and neurochemical studies. Brain 93: 617-628, 1970.

21430 CERVICAL VERTEBRAL FUSION

C5-C6 fusion may be recessively inherited. Lubs, Gunderson and Greenspan (1963) found two of eleven sibs
with this type of fusion and a third with narrowing of the interspace. The parents were probably
consanguineous.

Gunderson, C. H., Greenspan, R. H., Glaser, G. H. and Lubs, H. A., Jr.: The Klippel-Feil syndrome:
genetic and clinical reevaluation of cervical fusion. Medicine 46: 491-512, 1967.

Lubs, H. A., Jr., Gunderson, C. H. and Greenspan, R. H.: Genetic reevaluation of fused cervical vertebrae
(Klippel-Feil anomaly). Clin. Res. 11: 179 only, 1963.

*21440 CHARCOT-MARIE-TOOTH PERONEAL MUSCULAR ATROPHY

The autosomal recessive form is less frequent than the dominant and X-linked recessive forms. This is one
of the conditions used by Allan (1939) to illustrate the 'law' that recessive disorders are more severe than
dominant ones and that X-linked disorders tend to be intermediate in severity. This disorder may be
unusually frequent in the hill folk of the western part of North Carolina where Allan worked. Contrary to
the usual rarity of the recessive form, he found 8 young girls with the disorder in the North Carolina
orthopedic hospital which catered to patients under the age of 16 years. The eight came from six families
with both parents normal. In 4 of the 6 families the parents were cousins. Beighton (1971) described 9,
possibly 10 cases of recessive C-M-T disease in an inbred Amish group. Identical twins were concordantly
affected.

Allan, W.: Relation of hereditary pattern to clinical severity as illustrated by peroneal atrophy. Arch.
Intern. Med. 63: 1123-1131, 1939.

Beighton, P. H.: Recessively inherited Charcot-Marie-Tooth syndrome in identical twins. The Clinical
Delineation of Birth Defects. VII. Muscle. Baltimore: Williams and Wilkins, 1971. P. 105.

*21450 CHEDIAK-HIGASHI SYNDROME

The features are decreased pigmentation of hair and eyes, called partial albinism, photophobia, nystagmus,
large eosinophilic, peroxidase-positive inclusion bodies in the myeloblasts and promyelocytes of the bone
marrow, neutropenia, abnormal susceptibility to infection and peculiar malignant lymphoma. Death occurs
before the age of 7 years. Hermansky and Pudlak (1959) described two unrelated albinos with life-long
bleeding tendency and peculiar pigmented reticular cells in the bone marrow. One was male, one female, both
were 33-years-old. This may represent a distinct entity, possibly inherited as a recessive. (See ALBINISM
WITH HEMORRHAGIC DIATHESIS AND PIGMENTED RETICULO-ENDOTHELIAL CELLS.)

Kritzler and colleagues (1964) found the karyotype normal in a 16-year-old patient. Glycolipid inclusions
were described in histiocytes, renal tubular epithelium and neurons. Heterozygotes were identifiable by the
presence of a granular anomaly of the lymphocytes. The patient died of massive gastrointestinal hemorrhage.

Padgett et al. (1964) described the Chediak-Higashi syndrome in mink and cattle. In these species also it
is autosomal recessive. Leukemia and lymphoma have been observed (Efrati and Jonas, 1958).

Windhorst, Zelickson and Good (1966) found large lysosomal granules in leukocytes and giant melanosomes
in melanocytes. For this reason Leader et al. (1966) have referred to the condition as 'hereditary

leukomelanopathy.' Sheramata et al. (1971) described three brothers aged 31, 34 and 38, who had this disorder and a neurologic picture resembling spino-cerebellar degeneration.

Blume, R. S. and Wolff, S. M.: The Chediak-Higashi syndrome: studies in four patients and a review of the literature. Medicine 51: 247-280, 1972.

Chediak, M.: Nouvelle anomalie leucocytaire de caractere constitutionnel et familial. Rev. Hemat. 7: 362-367, 1952.

Efrati, P. and Jonas, W.: Chediak's anomaly of leukocytes in malignant lymphoma associated with leukemic manifestations: case report with necropsy. Blood 13: 1063-1073, 1958.

Gilloon, J. R., Pease, G. L. and Mills, S. D.: Chediak-Higashi anomaly of the leukocytes. Report of a case. Mayo Clin. Proc. 35: 635-640, 1960.

Hermansky, F. and Pudlak, P.: Albinism associated with hemorrhagic diathesis and unusual pigmented reticular cells in the bone marrow: report of two cases with histochemical studies. Blood 14: 162-169, 1959.

Kanfer, J. N., Blume, R. S., Yankee, R. A. and Wolff, S. M.: Sphingolipid metabolism in leukocytes in Chediak-Higashi syndrome. New Eng. J. Med. 279: 410-413, 1968.

Kritzler, R. A., Terner, J. Y., Lindenbaum, J., Magidson, J., Williams, R., Preisig, R. and Phillips, G. B.: Chediak-Higashi syndrome. Cytologic and serum lipid observations in a case and family. Am. J. Med. 36: 583-594, 1964.

Leader, R. W., Padgett, G. A. and Gorham, J. R.: Hereditary leukomelanopathy (Chediak-Higashi syndrome of man, mink and cattle). In, D. C. Gajdusek, C. J. Gibbs, Jr. and M. Alpers (eds.). Slow, Latent and Temperate Virus Infections. Pp. 393-399, 1966.

Padgett, G. A., Leader, R. W., Gorham, J. R. and O'Mary, C. C.: The familial occurrence of the Chediak-Higashi syndrome in mink and cattle. Genetics 49: 505-512, 1964.

Page, A. R., Berendes, H., Warner, J. and Good, R. A.: The Chediak-Higashi syndrome. Blood 20: 330-343, 1962.

Sadan, N., Yaffe, D., Rozenszajn, L. and Efrati, P.: Chediak's disease: clinical, cytological and hereditary aspects. (Abstract) Israel J. Med. Sci. 1: 850 only, 1965.

Sheramata, W., Kott, H. S. and Cyr, D. P.: The Chediak-Higashi-Steinbrinck syndrome. Arch. Neurol. 25: 289-294, 1971.

Spencer, W. H. and Hogan, M. J.: Ocular manifestations of Chediak-Higashi syndrome. Report of a case with histopathologic examination of ocular tissues. Am. J. Ophthal. 50: 1197-1203, 1962.

Stegmaier, O. C. and Schneider, L. A.: Chediak-Higashi syndrome: dermatologic manifestations. Arch. Derm. 91: 1-8, 1965.

Tay, C. H., Lopez, C. G. and Lazarus, A. R.: The Chediak-Higashi syndrome. Med. J. Aust. 2: 1024-1028, 1970.

White, J. G.: The Chediak-Higashi syndrome: a possible lysosomal disease. Blood 28: 143-156, 1966.

Windhorst, D. B., White, J. G., Zelickson, A. S., Clawson, C. C., Dent, P. B., Pollara, B. and Good, R. A.: The Chediak-Higashi anomaly and the Aleutian trait in mink: homologous defects of lysosomal structure. Ann. N.Y. Acad. Sci. 155: 818-846, 1968.

Windhorst, D. B., Zelickson, A. S. and Good, R. A.: Chediak-Higashi syndrome: hereditary gigantism of cytoplasmic organelles. Science 151: 81-83, 1966.

21460 CHEILOSIS-SEBORRHEA-AMINOACIDURIA

Menano and his colleagues (1960), of Lisbon, described a child from healthy and apparently unrelated parents who had cheilosis-like mucosal and cutaneous lesions, seborrheic dermatitis and aminoaciduria. A brother and the mother had similar aminoaciduria but were free of the other manifestations. Until further observations are reported, the nature of this syndrome, if such it is, remains unclear.

Menano, H., Relvas, M. E., Ferraz, F., Halpern, M. and Teixeira, F.: Cheilosis-like mucous and cutaneous lesions, seborrheic dermatitis and hereditary aminoaciduria. Helv. Paediat. Acta 15: 487-494, 1960.

*21470 CHLORIDE DIARRHEA, FAMILIAL

Voluminous watery stools containing an excess of chloride are present from a few weeks of age. The children are often premature and hydramnios may complicate pregnancy. Potassium chloride is the main therapy. Pasternack and Perheentupa (1966) described vascular changes resembling those of hypertensive angiopathy in seven children ages 1 to 42 months at the time of biopsy. All were normotensive. Kidney and muscle were biopsied. This disorder was described first by Gamble et al. (1945) and Darrow (1945). Both sexes have been affected and two sibs appear to have been affected in several families (Kelsey, 1954; Perheentupa et al., 1965).

Darrow, D. C.: Congenital alkalosis with diarrhea. J. Pediat. 26: 519-532, 1945.

Gamble, J. L., Fahey, K. R., Appleton, J. and MacLachlan, E. A.: Congenital alkalosis with diarrhea. J. Pediat. 26: 509-518, 1945.

Gorden, P. and Levitin, H.: Congenital alkalosis with diarrhea: a sequel to Darrow's original description. Ann. Intern. Med. 78: 876-882, 1972.

Kelsey, W. M.: Congenital alkalosis with diarrhea. Am. J. Dis. Child. 88: 344-347, 1954.

R
E
C
E
S
S
I
V
E

Norio, R., Perheentupa, J., Launiala, K. and Hallman, N.: Congenital chloride diarrhea, an autosomal recessive disease. Genetic study of 14 Finnish and 12 other families. Clin. Genet. 2: 182-192, 1971.

Pasternack, A. and Perheentupa, J.: Hypertensive angiopathy in familial chloride diarrhoea. Lancet II: 1047-1049, 1966.

Perheentupa, J., Eklund, J. and Kojo, N.: Familial chloride diarrhoea ('congenital alkalosis with diarrhoea'). Acta Paediat. Scand. 159 (suppl.): 119-120, 1965.

Turnberg, L. A.: Abnormalities in intestinal electrolyte transport in congenital chloridorrhoea. Gut 12: 544-551, 1971.

Yssing, M. and Friis-Hansen, B.: Congenital alkalosis with diarrhea. Acta Paediat. Scand. 55: 341-344, 1966.

21480 CHOANAL ATRESIA, POSTERIOR

This is a threat to life because young infants cannot establish the habit of mouth breathing. Ransome (1964) found 12 families with two or more members affected. One of these, in which 4 of 5 sibs were affected, was described by him. Most cases of multiple affected relatives have concerned sibs. However, the first reported, that by Lang (1912), involved in addition to the proband, the mother, sister and maternal aunt and perhaps a brother. Fendel (1966) described affected sibs. Grahne and Kaltiokallio (1966) observed affected sisters. The condition is said to occur twice as often in girls as in boys and more frequently in the right side than the left side. Fitch (1973) told me of a case of bilateral posterior choanal atresia associated with bilateral optic coloboma. It probably is a multifactorial trait, like cleft palate and cleft lip. The fact that both affected successive generations and affected single generations have been reported supports this (Lang, 1912; Phelps, 1926; and McGovern, 1950).

Dirlewanger, A.: Hereditares Vorkommen von Choanalatresien. Pract. Otorhinolaryng. 28: 211-218, 1966.

Fendel, K.: Zur familiaren Haufung der angeborenen Choanalatresie. Z. Laryng. Rhinol. Otol. 45: 67-73, 1966.

Fitch, N.: Montreal, personal communication, Sept. 6, 1973.

Grahne, B. and Kaltiokallio, K.: Congenital choanal atresis and its heredity. Acta Otolaryng. 62: 193-200, 1966.

Lang, J.: Ueber Choanenatresie (Hereditat derselben). Mschr. Ohrenheilk. 46: 970-1001, 1912.

McGovern, F. H.: Congenital choanal atresia. Laryngoscope 60: 815-831, 1950.

Phelps, K. A.: Congenital occlusion of the choanae. Ann. Otol. Rhinol. Laryn. 35: 143-151, 1926.

Ransome, J.: Familial incidence of posterior choanal atresia. J. Laryng. 78: 551-554, 1964.

*21490 CHOLESTASIS AND LYMPHEDEMA

In a Norwegian kindred Aagenaes et al. (1970) described a syndrome of hereditary recurrent cholestasis and lymphedema. Jaundice became evident soon after birth and recurred in episodes throughout life. Edema in the legs began at about school age and progressed. It was shown to be due to hypoplasia of the lymphatic vessels of the legs. Sixteen individuals in 7 interconnected sibships appear to have been affected. One instance of affected mother and daughter may have resulted from the fact that the father was a heterozygote.

Aagenaes, O., Cuderman, B., Sigstad, H., Leonard, A. S., Krivit, W. and Sharp, H. L.: Clinical and experimental relationships between cholestasis and abnormal hepatic lymphatics. (Abstract) Pediat. Res. 4: 377 only, 1970.

Aagenaes, O., Sigstad, H. and Bjorn-Hansen, R.: Lymphoedema in hereditary recurrent cholestasis from birth. Arch. Dis. Child. 45: 690-695, 1970.

Aagenaes, O.: Hereditary recurrent cholestasis with lymphoedema-two new families. Acta Paediat. Scand. 63: 465-471, 1974.

Sharp, H. L. and Krivit, W.: Hereditary lymphedema and obstructive jaundice. J. Pediat. 78: 491-496, 1971.

21500 CHOLESTEROL ESTER STORAGE DISEASE OF LIVER

Schiff et al. (1968) described cholesterol ester storage disease of the liver in teen-age brother and sister whose livers were orange in color. Four younger sibs showed milder changes. The parents were not related to their knowledge. Tissue accumulation of cholesterol esters and triglycerides occurs in both this disease and Wolman disease. The chemical and enzymatic abnormalities are similar. The marked difference in phenotypic expression is unexplained but is comparable to the difference between Hurler and Scheie syndromes, the late infantile and adult forms of metachromatic leukodystrophy, and the classic and visceral forms (A and B) of Niemann-Pick disease. Each of these is presumably a pair of allelic disorders. For this reason no asterisk is placed by this entry, only an asterisk with Wolman disease (27800).

Schiff, L., Schubert, W. K., McAdams, A. J., Spiegel, E. L. and O'Donnell, J. F.: Hepatic cholesterol ester storage disease, a familial disorder. I. Clinical aspects. Am. J. Med. 44: 538-546, 1968.

Sloan, H. R. and Fredrickson, D. S.: Cholesteryl ester storage diseases: studies of the chemical and biochemical abnormalities. (Abstract) Pediat. Res. 6: 376 only, 1972.

R E C E S S I V E

Sloan, H. R. and Fredrickson, D. S.: Enzyme deficiency in cholesteryl ester storage disease. J. Clin. Invest. 51: 1923-1926, 1972.

21503 CHOLESTEROL PNEUMONIA

Pelz et al. (1972) described cholesterol pneumonia in brother and sister, who died at 9.5 and 4 months, respectively. Tachypnea, cough and cyanosis were symptoms.

Pelz, L., Hobusch, D., Erfurth, F. and Richter, K.: Familiare Cholesterin-pneumonie. Helvet. Paediat. Acta. 27: 361-370, 1972.

21505 CHONDRODYSPLASIA CALCIFICANS METAPHYSEALIS

Van Creveld et al. (1971) reported two unrelated cases of a new form of metaphyseal chondrodysplasia, characterized clinically by dwarfism and progressive deformity and radiographically by metaphyseal dysplasia with massive deposits of calcified densities, extensive defects of ossification and proliferation of cartilage. Epiphyses also show changes. Although the Jansen type of metaphyseal chondrodysplasia is superficially suggested, the ribs and the iliac, tarsal and carpal bones are much more affected in the new disorder, which shows changes in all metaphyses. One of the cases, a child, showed excessive mucopolysacchariduria.

Van Creveld, S., Kozlowski, K., Pietron, K. and Van der Valk, A.: Metaphyseal chondrodysplasia calcificans. A report of two cases. Brit. J. Radiol. 44: 773-779, 1971.

*21510 CHONDRODYSPLASIA PUNCTATA (CHONDRODYSTROPHIA CALCIFICANS CONGENITA, CHONDRODYSTROPHIA CALCIFICANS PUNCTATA, CONRADI DISEASE)

R E C E S S I V E

This is a rare disorder of the bones of the fetus and newborn, characterized by the presence of stippled foci of calcification within hyaline cartilage and associated with dwarfing, congenital cataract and various malformations. Several families of affected sibs are reported and the frequency of parental consanguinity is rather high. Doubtlessly there are a number of different entities which have the same cartilaginous changes, e.g., Rosenfield et al. (1962) found them in a case of trisomy 18. The evolution of this disorder of early life into multiple epiphyseal dysplasia was observed by Silverman (1961) and the inheritance seems to be dominant. Thus it is possible that a quite different entity is represented. Skin changes like ichthyosiform erythroderma have been reported, as well as contractures. Melnick (1965) observed a case in the offspring of a father-daughter mating. Fifteen year follow-up was provided by Comings et al. (1968). Saddle nose secondary to involvement of the facial bones is present in about 40 percent of cases according to Fritsch and Manzke (1963). In Australia this feature has led to the condition being called the koala bear syndrome (Danks, 1970). It was the suggestion of a group convened in Paris by the European Society of Pediatric Radiology that the disorder be called chondrodysplasia punctata (Maroteaux, 1970). Spranger et al. (1970) concluded that punctata intra- and extracartilaginous calcification may be found in a variety of hereditary and nonhereditary conditions. Punctate calcifications may occur, for example, in Zellweger syndrome (q.v.). They suggested that Zellweger syndrome was present in the cases reported as instances of chondrodystrophia calcificans by De Lange and Janssen (1949), Gekle (1963), Philips (case 2, 1957), and Putschar (1951). The second form is called rhizomelic type because of severe, symmetrical proximal shortening of the limbs. There are marked metaphyseal changes, cataracts in about 72 percent of cases, skin changes in about 27 percent. Inheritance is clearly recessive. A disorder simulating chondrodystrophia punctata is produced by maternal ingestion of anticoagulant (dicoumarol or Warfarin) in early pregnancy.

Allansmith, M. and Senz, E.: Chondrodystrophia congenita punctata (Conradi's disease). Am. J. Dis. Child. 100: 109-116, 1960.

Bodian, E. L.: Skin manifestations of Conradi's disease. Chondrodystrophia congenita punctata. Arch. Derm. 94: 743-748, 1966.

Comings, D. E., Papazian, C. and Schoene, H. R.: Conradi's disease (chondrodystrophia calcificans congenita, congenital stippled epiphyses). J. Pediat. 72: 63-69, 1968.

Danks, D. M.: Melbourne, Australia: personal communication, 1970.

De Lange, C. and Janssen, T.: Congenital chondrodystrophia calcicans of infant in association with other abnormalities: case. Mschr. Kindergeneesk. 17: 67-74, 1949.

Fraser, F. C. and Scriver, J. B.: A hereditary factor in chondrodystrophia calcificans congenita. New Eng. J. Med 250: 272-277, 1954.

Fritsch, H. and Manzke, H.: Beitrag zur Chondrodystrophia calcificans connata (Conradi-Hunermann-Syndrom). Arch. Kinderheilk. 169: 235-254, 1963.

Gekle, D.: Ein Beitrag zum Problem der Chondrodystrophia calcificans congenita. Arch. Kinderheilk. 169: 267-273, 1963.

Josephson, B. M. and Oriatti, M. D.: Chondrodystrophia calcificans congenita: report of a case and review of the literature. Pediatrics 28: 425-435, 1961.

Maroteaux, P.: Nomenclature internationale des maladies osseuses constitutionelles. Ann. Radiol. 13: 455-464, 1970.

Melnick, J. C.: Chondrodystrophia calcificans congenita (chondrodysplasia epiphysialis punctata, stippled epiphyses). Am. J. Dis. Child. 110: 218-225, 1965.

Philips, L. I.: Chondrodystrophia calcificans congenita. New Zeal. J. Med. 56: 22-27, 1957.

Putschar, W. G. J.: Chondrodystrophia calcificans congenita (dysplasia epiphysialis punctata). Bull. Hosp. Joint Dis. 11: 514-527, 1951.

Rosenfield, R. L., Breibart, S., Isaacs, H., Klevit, H. D. and Mellman, W. J.: Trisomy of chromosomes 13-15 and 17-18: its association with infantile arteriosclerosis. Am. J. Med. Sci. 244: 763-779, 1962.

Silverman, F. N.: Dysplasies epiphysaires: entite proteiforme. Ann. Radiol. 4: 833-867, 1961.

Spranger, J. W., Opitz, J. M. and Bidder, V.: Heterogeneity of chondrodysplasia punctata. Humangenetik 11: 190-212, 1971.

Tasker, W. G., Mastri, A. R. and Gold, A. P.: Chondrodystrophia calcificans congenita (dysplasia epiphysalis punctata). Recognition of the clinical picture. Am. J. Dis. Child. 119: 122-127, 1970.

21520 CHONDRODYSTROPHY, JOINT DISLOCATION, GLAUCOMA, AND MENTAL RETARDATION

These were the features of two sisters, ages 8 and 20 months, reported by Desbuquois et al. (1966). Dislocation of the patellae and hips was present. Dwarfing was severe.

Desbuquois, G., Grenier, B., Michel, J. and Rossignol, C.: Nanisme chondrodystrophique avec ossification anarchique et poly-malformations chez deux soeurs. Arch. Franc. Pediat. 23: 573-587, 1966.

21525 CHONDROITIN-6-SULFATURIA, DEFECTIVE CELLULAR IMMUNITY, NEPHROTIC SYNDROME

Schimke et al. (1971) described a girl who excreted about 100 mg. of acid mucopolysaccharide daily, and showed a non-progressive form of nephrotic syndrome with proteinuria and a defect of cellular immunity. Clinical features included short stature, low birth weight, disseminated herpetic infection, truncal shortening, corneal opacities, demineralization of bones.

Schimke, R. N., Horton, W. A. and King, C. R.: Chondroitin-6-sulphaturia, defective cellular immunity, and nephrotic syndrome. (Letter) Lancet II: 1088-1089, 1971.

21530 CHONDROSARCOMA

Schajowicz and Bessone (1967) described three brothers who respectively developed chondrosarcoma of the pelvic bone at 18 years, of the fibula and femur at 16 years and of the femur at 17 years. Two brothers and a sister were living and well. Karyotypes were normal. See OSTEOGENIC SARCOMA.

Schajowicz, F. and Bessone, J. E.: Chondrosarcoma in 3 brothers. A pathological and genetic study. J. Bone Joint Surg. 49A: 129-141, 1967.

21540 CHORDOMA

Foote and others (1958) described middle-aged brother and sister with sacro-coccygeal chordoma. Recurrence and metastases occurred in both.

Foote, R. F., Ablin, G. and Hall, W.: Chordoma in siblings. Calif. Med. 88: 383-386, 1958.

21545 CHOREA, FAMILIAL BENIGN

Both a dominant (see 11870) and a recessive form may exist. Nutting et al. (1969) described three affected sibs out of 5 with phenotypically normal, nonconsanguineous parents. Chun et al. (1973) described four affected sibs out of 7, again with normal, unrelated parents. Reduced penetrance in one parent is possible.

Chun, R. W. M., Daly, R. F., Mansheim, B. J., Jr. and Wolcott, G. J.: Benign familial chorea with onset in childhood. J.A.M.A. 225: 1603-1607, 1973.

Nutting, P. A., Cole, B. R. and Schimke, R. N.: Benign recessively inherited choreoathetosis. J. Med. Genet. 6: 408-410, 1969.

*21550 CHOROIDAL SCLEROSIS

Waardenburg (1952) described central choroidal sclerosis in two daughters of a first-cousin marriage. Many others have reported sibs with central choroidal sclerosis and several instances of parental consanguinity are on record (e.g., Sorsby and Crick, 1953). Krill and Archer (1971) described brother and sister with choriocapillaris atrophy throughout most of the posterior eyegrounds.

Krill, A. E. and Archer, D.: Classification of the choroidal atrophies. Am. J. Ophthal. 72: 562-585, 1971.

Sorsby, A. and Crick, R. P.: Central areolar choroidal sclerosis. Brit. J. Ophthal. 37: 129-139, 1953.

Waardenburg, P. J.: Angio-sclerose familiale de la choroide. J. Genet. Hum. 1: 83-93, 1952.

21555 CIRCUMVALLATE PLACENTA SYNDROME

Deacon et al. (1974) reported three sisters who died neonatally of respiratory insufficiency. All three pregnancies were complicated by polyhydramnios, and each infant showed cutaneous and intracranial hemorrhage, marked central nervous system depression and skeletal abnormalities (ovetubulation of ribs and long bones of the limbs). Since the third infant had a circumvallate placenta, the authors suggested that this might be a primary and gene-determined defect. Familial occurrence of circumvallate placenta was reported by Hunt (1953) and by Morgan (1955).

Deacon, J. S. R., Gilbert, E. F., Viseskul, C., Herrmann, J. and Opitz, J. M.: Polyhydramnios and neonatal hemorrhage in three sisters. Birth Defects Orig. Art. Ser. 10 (7): 41-49, 1974.

Hunt, A. B.: Discussion. Am. J. Obstet. Gynec. 65: 497 only, 1953.

R
E
C
E
S
S
I
V
E

Morgan, J.: Circumvallate placenta. J. Obstet. Gynaec. Brit. Comm. 62: 899-900, 1955.

21560 CIRRHOSIS, FAMILIAL

Aside from Wilson disease, type IV glycogen storage disease and galactosemia (q.v.), well known causes of familial cirrhosis, families with multiple affected sibs and normal parents have been observed (Iber, Maddrey, 1965). The group is probably heterogeneous and in some instances non-genetic factors may be responsible for the familial aggregation. Iber and Maddrey (1965) reviewed 13 reported families and 8 of their own, each with two or more affected members. They pointed out that with one exception the multiple cases were in the same generation. Within a given family age of onset, clinical course and biopsy findings were very similar but there were wide differences between families. Also see WILSON DISEASE and INTRAHEPATIC CHOLESTASIS. Baber (1956) described cases of congenital cirrhosis with generalized aminoaciduria. Some of these patients may be examples of Wilson disease. Others may have tyrosinemia (Zetterstrom 1963, Gentz et al., 1965). See TYROSINEMIA. In India, so-called Indian childhood cirrhosis (Sen syndrome) affects multiple sibs (Chaudhuri and Chaudhuri, 1965). Yet another cause of congenital cirrhosis is deficiency of alpha-1-antitrypsin (20740).

Baber, M. D.: Case of congenital cirrhosis of the liver with renal tubular defects akin to those in the Fanconi syndrome. Arch. Dis. Child. 31: 335-339, 1956.

Chaudhuri, A. and Chaudhuri, K. C.: The karyotype in infantile cirrhosis of the liver (Sen's syndrome). Indian J. Pediat. 32: 209-218, 1965.

Gentz, J., Jagenburg, R. and Zetterstrom, R.: Tyrosinemia: an inborn error of tyrosine metabolism with cirrhosis of the liver and multiple renal tubular defects. J. Pediat. 66: 670-696, 1965.

Iber, F. L. and Maddrey, W. C.: Familial hepatic diseases with cirrhosis or without portal hypertension. Progr. Liver Dis. 2: 290-302, 1965.

Maddrey, W. C. and Iber, F. L.: Familial cirrhosis. A clinical and pathological study. Ann. Intern. Med. 61: 667-679, 1964.

Miller, M. C.: Familial cirrhosis with hepatoma. Am. J. Dig. Dis. 12: 633-638, 1967.

Zetterstrom, R.: Tyrosinosis. Ann. N.Y. Acad. Sci. 111: 220-226, 1963.

*21570 CITRULLINURIA (CITRULLINEMIA)

Severe vomiting spells beginning at the age of 9 months and mental retardation were features of the first case, offspring of first-cousin parents. McMurray and colleagues (1962) found citrulline in very high concentration in serum, spinal fluid and urine. The amino acid gets its name from its high concentration in the watermelon citrullus vulgaris. Visakorpi (1962) also described a case of citrullinuria. Vomiting and ammonia intoxication are other manifestations. The enzyme defect concerns argininosuccinic acid synthetase. Tedesco and Mellman (1967) found that the enzyme has an altered Michaelis constant.

McMurray, W. C., Mohyuddin, F., Rossiter, R. J., Rathbun, J. C., Valentine, G. H., Koegler, S. J. and Zarfas, D. E.: Citrullinuria: a new aminoaciduria associated with mental retardation. Lancet I: 138 only, 1962.

McMurray, W. C., Rathbun, J. C., Mohyuddin, F. and Koegler, S. J.: Citrullinuria. Pediatrics 32: 347-357, 1963.

Mohyuddin, F., Rathbun, J. C. and McMurray, W. C.: Studies on amino acid metabolism in citrullinuria. Am. J. Dis. Child. 113: 152-156, 1967.

Morrow, G. III., Barness, L. A. and Efron, M. L.: Citrullinemia with defective urea production. Pediatrics 40: 565-574, 1967.

Tedesco, T. A. and Mellman, W. J.: Argininosuccinate synthetase activity and citrulline metabolism in cells cultured from a citrullinemic subject. Proc. Nat. Acad. Sci. 57: 829-834, 1967.

Van der Zee, S. P. M., Trijbels, J. M. F., Monnens, L. A. H., Hommes, F. A. and Schretlen, E. D. A. M.: Citrullinaemia with rapidly fatal neonatal course. Arch. Dis. Child. 46: 847-851, 1971.

Vidailhet, M., Levin, B., Dautrevaux, M., Paysant, P., Gelot, S., Badonnel, Y., Pierson, M. and Niemann, N.: Citrullinemia. Arch. Franc. Pediat. 28: 521-532, 1971.

Visakorpi, J. K.: Citrullinuria. (Letter) Lancet I: 1357-1358, 1962.

Wick, H., Bachmann, C., Baumgartner, R., Brechbuhler, T., Colombo, J. P., Wiesmann, U., Mihatsch, M. J. and Ohnacker, H.: Variants of citrullinaemia. Arch. Dis. Child. 48: 636-641, 1973.

21580 CLEFT LARYNX, POSTERIOR

Zachary and Emery (1961) reported three cases of lack of fusion of the posterior larynx and persistence of common tracheoesophagus. Two of these were sibs, the mother having two other normal children. One was male, the sex of the second was not stated. In sporadic cases males and females are affected about equally often. Finlay (1949) and Crooks (1954) described a family of 5 girls, four of whom had laryngeal stridor. At least two had cleft larynx. Ordinary tracheo-esophageal fistula (18990) shows little familial aggregation. Phelan et al. (1973) described a remarkable kindred in which two brothers married two sisters. Each married couple had three affected children. They made the proposal of autosomal dominant inheritance, but this would seem improbable requiring lack of penetrance in three individuals one parent of each sibship and one parent of those two.

Crooks, J.: Non-inflammatory laryngeal stridor in infants. Arch. Dis. Child. 29: 12-17, 1954.

R
E
C
E
S
S
I
V
E

Finlay, H. V. L.: Familial congenital stridor. Arch. Dis. Child. 24: 219-223, 1949.

Phelan, P. D., Stocks, J. G., Williams, H. E. and Danks, D. M.: Familial occurrence of congenital laryngeal clefts. Arch. Dis. Child. 48: 275-278, 1973.

Zachary, R. B. and Emery, J. L.: Failure of separation of larynx and trachea from the esophagus. Persistent esophagotrachea. Surgery 49: 525-529, 1961.

21590 CLEFT LIP WITH OR WITHOUT CLEFT PALATE

As an isolated malformation cleft lip with or without cleft palate behaves as an entity distinct from cleft palate alone (q.v.). It appears to have complex genetics. Curtis, Fraser and Warburton (1961) estimated that the risk of recurrence in subsequently born children is 4 percent if one child has it, 4 percent if one parent has it, 17 percent if one parent and one child has it and 9 percent if two children have it. The syndrome of cleft lip with or without cleft palate in association with mucous pits of the lower lip is inherited as an autosomal dominant.

Curtis, E. J., Fraser, F. C. and Warburton, D.: Congenital cleft lip and palate. Am. J. Dis. Child. 102: 853-857, 1961.

21610 CLEFT LIP-PALATE WITH ABNORMAL THUMBS AND MICROCEPHALY

Juberg and Hayward (1968) described a syndrome with oral, cranial and digital manifestations in 5 of 6 children of normal, unrelated parents. Two brothers had cleft lip and palate, microcephaly, hypoplasia and distal placement of the thumbs and elbow deformities limiting extension. One of the brothers had toe anomalies as did 3 of the 4 sisters. Among the sisters microcephaly, stiff thumbs and forme fruste cleft lip were observed.

Juberg, R. C. and Hayward, J. R.: A new familial syndrome of oral, cranial, and digital anomalies. J. Pediat. 74: 755-762, 1968.

21620 CLEFT PALATE ALONE

Cleft palate as an isolated malformation behaves as an entity distinct from cleft lip with or without cleft palate. Curtis, Fraser and Warburton (1961) estimated that the risk of recurrence in subsequently born children is about 2 percent if one child has it, 6 percent if one parent has it and 15 percent if one parent and one child have it. As for cleft lip with or without cleft palate, as well as many other relatively frequent congenital malformations, the genetics is apparently complex.

Curtis, E. J., Fraser, F. C. and Warburton, D.: Congenital cleft lip and palate. Am. J. Dis. Child. 102: 853-857, 1961.

21630 CLEFT PALATE, DEAFNESS, OLIGODONTIA

In a sibship of Swedish extraction, Gorlin et al. (1971) observed two sisters with cleft soft palate, severe oligodontia of the deciduous teeth, no permanent dentition, bilateral conductive deafness due to fixation of the footplate of the stapes, short halluces with wide space between the first and second toes, and coalition of bones in the foot.

Gorlin, R. J., Schlorf, R. A. and Paparella, M. M.: Cleft palate, stapes fixation and oligodontia. The Clinical Delineation of Birth Defects. XI. Orofacial Structures. Baltimore: Williams and Wilkins, 1971. P. 87 only.

21635 COATS DISEASE, DEAFNESS, MUSCLE WEAKNESS, MENTAL RETARDATION

Small (1968) described a family in which four of 7 sibs had retinal changes ranging from tortuous vessels to exudative retinitis, moderate to severe hearing loss, muscular weakness and mental retardation.

Small, R. G.: Coats' disease and muscular dystrophy. Trans. Am. Acad. Ophthal. Otolaryng. 72: 225-231, 1968.

*21640 COCKAYNE SYNDROME

MacDonald, Fitch and Lewis (1960) described affection of 3 out of 5 sibs. Characteristics are dwarfism, precociously senile appearance, pigmentary retinal degeneration, optic atrophy, deafness, marble epiphyses in some digits, sensitivity to sunlight and mental retardation. The most striking pedigree is that of Paddison, Moossy, Derbes and Kloepfer (1963). In 1971, through the courtesy of kloepfer, I had an opportunity to see two affected males, then ages 29 and 24, from this pedigree. They were markedly dwarfed with 'hollow eyes.' They could not close the eyes completely so that severe corneal changes contributed to the visual impairment. Head and body hair was of normal male quality and distribution. The face required shaving several times a week. Neill and Dingwall (1950) described a progeria-like syndrome characterized by dwarfism, microcephaly, severe mental retardation, 'pepper-and-salt' chorioretinitis, and intracranial calcification. The parents were not closely related. It now seems likely that the diagnosis was the Cockayne syndrome. Death from early atherosclerosis occurred in these sibs as in progeria (Neill, 1966). Norman (1963) examined the brain of the two sibs. Massive pericapillary calcification was present in the putamina, thalami and cerebellar white matter superficial to the dentate nuclei. In the larger vessels the calcification was mainly in the adventitial coat.

Cotton, R. B., Keats, T. E. and McCoy, E. E.: Abnormal blood glucose regulation in Cockayne's syndrome. Pediatrics 46: 54-60, 1970.

Fujimoto, W. Y., Greene, M. L. and Seegmiller, J. E.: Cockayne's syndrome: report of a case with hyperlipoproteinemia, hyperinsulinemia, renal disease, and normal growth hormone. J. Pediat. 75: 881-884, 1969.

R
E
C
E
S
S
I
V
E

Lanning, M. and Simila, S.: Cockayne's syndrome. Report of a case with normal intelligence. Z. Kinderheilk. 109: 70-75, 1970.

MacDonald, W. B., Fitch, K. D. and Lewis, I. C.: Cockayne's syndrome: a heredo-familial disorder of growth and development. Pediatrics 25: 997-1007, 1960.

Moosa, A. and Dubowitz, V.: Peripheral neuropathy in Cockayne's syndrome. Arch. Dis. Child. 45: 674-677, 1970.

Neill, C. A. and Dingwall, M. M.: A syndrome resembling progeria: a review of two cases. Arch. Dis. Child. 25: 213-223, 1950.

Neill, C. A.: Baltimore, Md.: personal communication, 1966.

Norman, R. M. and Tingey, A. H.: Syndrome of micrencephaly, strio-cerebellar calcifications, and leucodystrophy. J. Neurol. Neurosurg. Psychiat. 29: 157-163, 1966.

Norman, R. M.: Malformations of the nervous system, birth injury and diseases of early life. In, Blackwood and others (eds.): Greenfield's Neuropathology. Baltimore: Williams and Wilkins, 1963. P. 350.

Paddison, R. M., Moossy, J., Derbes, V. J. and Kloepfer, H. W.: Cockayne's syndrome. A report of five new cases with biochemical, chromosomal, dermatologic, genetic and neuropathologic observations. Derm. Trop. 2: 195-203, 1963.

Pfeiffer, R. A. and Bachmann, K. D.: An atypical case of Cockayne's syndrome. Clin. Genet. 4: 28-32, 1973.

Rowlatt, U.: Cockayne's syndrome. Report of case with necropsy findings. Acta Neuropath. 14: 52-61, 1969.

*21650 COGAN CONGENITAL OCULAR MOTOR APRAXIA

Congenital ocular motor apraxia, first reported by Cogan (1952), is a condition characterized by (1) defective or absent horizontal voluntary eye movements and (2) defective or absent horizontal ocular attraction movements. Vassella et al. (1972) provided observations on three patients and summarized the findings on the 33 previously reported cases in the literature. Random eye movements and voluntary vertical gaze are usually retained by the affected individuals. Compensation for the defective horizontal eye movements is accomplished through rotating the head sharply laterally to forcefully bring the eyes to view the desired object. The eyes tend to deviate in the opposite direction from this movement because of the vestibular reflex necessitating even a greater head swing. Thus, the most noticable feature of the condition in young patients is jerking movements of the head. The disease is not progressive, and older patients may be able to compensate by an over-shooting thrust of the eyeballs rather than by head jerks. The site of the brain lesion in congenital ocular motor apraxia is speculative. Some evidence does exist for the heritability of the disorder. Robles (1966) reported identical twins with the condition. Sachs (1967) and Arthius (1971) observed the disorder in sibs, with Sachs' case being of consanguineous parents. Twenty-three of 34 cases have been males. Vassella et al. has reported a case occurring in two generations. The father (affected) and mother were first cousins. Thus, this may also be an instance of recessive inheritance.

Arthius, M.: Comparaison des troubles de la mobilite oculaire dans l'ataxie telangiectasie et le syndrome de Cogan. Film presented at the reunion de la Section Mediterraneenne du Groupement d'Etude Europeenne de Neurologie Infantile, Paris, July 2-3, 1971.

Cogan, D. G.: A type of congenital ocular motor apraxia presenting jerky head movements. Trans. Am. Acad. Ophthal. Otolaryng. 56: 853-862, 1952.

Robles, J.: Congenital ocular motor apraxia in identical twins. Arch. Ophthal. 75: 746-749, 1966.

Sachs, R.: Apraxie oculo-motrice congenitale de Cogan. A propos de trois nouveaux cas dont deux dans la meme fratrie. Ann. Oculist. 200: 266-274, 1967.

Vassella, F., Lutschg, J. and Mumenthaler, M.: Cogan's congenital ocular motor apraxia in two successive generations. Develop. Med. Child. Neurol. 14: 788-796, 1972.

21660 COLLAGENOMA, FAMILIAL CUTANEOUS

Henderson et al. (1968) described three brothers with numerous skin nodules on the back. These consisted of thickened dermis due to increased collagenous tissue. One brother had idiopathic myocardopathy, a second had atrophy of the left iris and severe high frequency sensorineural hearing loss, and the third had recurrent vasculitis. Thus, the cutaneous abnormality may be merely part of a systemic disorder. It seems not to have been previously reported.

Henderson, R. R., Wheeler, C. E., Jr. and Abele, D. C.: Familial cutaneous collagenoma. Arch. Derm. 98: 23-27, 1968.

21680 COLOBOMA OF MACULA AND SKELETAL ANOMALIES

Phillips and Griffiths (1969) described a brother and sister with bilateral macular coloboma, cleft palate, hallux valgus and other abnormalities. The parents were not related. The ocular trait was like that described by Sorsby as a dominant and listed here as 'coloboma of the macula with type B brachydactyly' (q.v.). Although digital abnormalities were present in the sibs reported by Phillips and Griffiths, they were of relatively mild type and different nature than those in Sorsby's family.

Phillips, C. I. and Griffiths, D. L.: Macular coloboma and skeletal abnormality. Brit. J. Ophthal. 53: 346-349, 1969.

RECESSIVE

The British expression 'day-blindness' is a good one because the cones are missing and the subjects see better at night. This term is parallel to night-blindness. The largest pedigree is that of a family residing on the Island of Fur in the Limfjord in the north of Denmark (Holm and Lodberg, 1940; Franceschetti, Francois and Babel, 1963).

Franceschetti, A., Francois, J. and Babel, J.: Les heredo-degenerescences chorio-retiniennes (degenerescences tapeto-retiniennes) Paris: Masson, 2: 1252-1254, 1963.

Hanhart, E.: Uber den Zusammenhang 48 neuer Beobachtungen von totaler Farbenblindheit (Acromatopsie) mit den 21 bisher publizierten schweizer Fallen und die Haldanesche Lokalisation des betreffenden Gens im X-Chromosom. Arch. Klaus Stift. Vererbungsforch. 23: 465 only, 1948.

Harrison, R., Hoefnagel, D. and Hayward, J. N.: Congenital total color blindness. Arch. Ophthal. 64: 685-692, 1960.

Holm, E. and Lodberg, C. V.: Family with total color-blindness. Acta Ophthal. 18: 224-258, 1940.

*21695 COMPLEMENT COMPONENT C1R, DEFICIENCY OF

Day et al. (1972) observed two sibs with C'1r deficiency. The brother (18 years old) had shown lupus-like features for 5 years. The sister (24 years old) had had arthralgia and recurrent rhinobronchitis from early childhood. Three sibs had died, one at 12 with symptoms like the male and two in infancy, probably from infection. Laboratory findings suggested the existence of an alternative pathway for activation of the terminal portion of the complement cascade which does not use the usual early components.

Day, N. K., Geiger, H., Stroud, R., DeBracco, M., Mancado, B., Windhorst, D. B. and Good, R. A.: C'1r deficiency: an inborn error associated with cutaneous and renal disease. J. Clin. Invest. 51: 1102-1108, 1972.

Moncada, B., Day, N. K. B., Good, R. A. and Windhorst, D. B.: Lupus-erythematosus-like syndrome with a familial defect of complement. New Eng. J. Med. 286: 689-693, 1972.

*21700 COMPLEMENT COMPONENT-2, DEFICIENCY OF

Klemperer et al. (1966, 1967) found multiple affected persons in a kindred. No gene product was detected in those with the deficiency (homozygotes). In heterozygotes a partial deficiency of C'2 was found. Restudy of Silverstein's family demonstrated identical findings. None of the homozygotes have been unduly sensitive to bacterial infection or had other evident abnormality. By means of monospecific antiserum, Polley (1968) showed that homozygotes have no second component of complement and heterozygotes have an intermediate amount. Thus, the defect is failure of synthesis rather than synthesis of an inactive analog. See VARIANTS OF C2 in dominant catalog. These may concern one and the same locus.

Austen, K. F.: Inborn errors of the complement system of man. New Eng. J. Med. 276: 1363-1367, 1967.

Austen, K. F., Becker, E. L., Bero, C. E., Borsos, T., Dalmasso, A. P. and Dias Da Silva, D.: Nomenclature of complement. Bull. World Health Organ. 39: 935-938, 1968.

Klemperer, M. R., Austen, K. F. and Rosen, F. S.: Hereditary deficiency of second component of complement (C-prime-2) in man: further observations on a second kindred. J. Immunol. 98: 72-78, 1967.

Klemperer, M. R., Woodworth, H. C., Rosen, F. S. and Austen, K. F.: Hereditary deficiency of second component of complement (C-prime-2) in man. J. Clin. Invest. 45: 880-890, 1966.

Polley, M. J.: Inherited C-prime-2 deficiency in man: lack of immunochemically detectable C-prime-2 protein in serums from deficient individuals. Science 161: 1149-1151, 1968.

Ruddy, S. and Austen, K. F.: Inherited abnormalities of the complement system in man. In, Steinberg, A. G. and Bearn, A. G. (eds.): Progress in Medical Genetics, chapter 3 vol. 7, 1970. Pp. 69-95.

Silverstein, A. M.: Essential hypocomplementemia. Report of a case. Blood 16: 1338-1341, 1960.

*21708 COMPLEMENT COMPONENT-6, DEFICIENCY OF

Leddy et al. (1974) and Heusinkveld et al. (1974) described deficiency of the sixth component of complement in an 18-year-old woman in good general health. Her serum lacked hemolytic complement activity. The action of an abnormal inhibitor was excluded. Both parents and five of six sibs had about half the normal levels of functional C6. Unlike C6 deficiency in rabbits, no abnormality of clotting was demonstrated.

Heusinkveld, R. S., Leddy, J. P., Klemperer, M. R. and Breckenridge, R. T.: Hereditary deficiency of the sixth component complement in man. II. Studies of hemostasis. J. Clin. Invest. 53: 554-558, 1974.

Leddy, J. P., Frank, M. M., Gaither, T., Baum, J. and Klemperer, M. R.: Hereditary deficiency of the sixth component of complement in man. I. Immunochemical, biologic, and familial studies. J. Clin. Invest. 53: 544-553, 1974.

21710 CONSTRICTING BANDS, CONGENITAL ('AMNIOTIC BANDS')

Temtamy (1966) could find no evidence of a clear or simple genetic basis. Since the work of Streeter (1930) the causative role of amniotic bands has been discounted and the malformations, both the bands and the associated absence deformities, are thought to result from tissue necrosis probably on a vascular basis. However, the work of Torpin (1968) makes a modified form of the amniotic band theory plausible. A considerable body of observations indicates that rupture of the amnion and constriction of members which are displaced through holes in the amnion are involved. Amputated parts have been recovered in some instances.

Streeter, G. L.: Focal deficiencies in fetal tissues and their relation to intra uterine amputation. Contrib. Embryol. Carnegie Inst. Washington 22: (No. 126) 1-144, 1930.

Temtamy, S. A.: Genetic Factors in Hand Malformations. Ph. D. Thesis, Johns Hopkins University, 1966.

Torpin, R.: Fetal Malformations Caused by Amnion Rupture during Gestation. Springfield, Ill.: Charles C Thomas, 1968.

21720 CONVULSIVE DISORDER, FAMILIAL, WITH PRENATAL OR EARLY ONSET

In utero onset was noted by Badr El-Din (1960), who described the condition in sibs as a familial convulsive disorder. Other features were mental retardation, generalized hypertonus, reflex myoclonus and death in the first year. Winkelman and Moore (1942) described a single case with antenatal onset. Liu and Sylvester (1960) reported a disorder beginning near or before birth and characterized by mental deterioration, fits, spasticity, paralysis, deafness and blindness. The parents were not related and two brothers were affected. The condition could, of course, be X-linked as well as autosomal recessive. See also JOSEPH SYNDROME, which has convulsions of early onset as one feature. Intrauterine convulsions also occur in pyridoxine dependency (Bejsovec et al., 1967), which is discussed elsewhere.

Badr El-Din, M. K.: A familial convulsive disorder with an unusual onset during intrauterine life. A case report. J. Pediat. 56: 655-657, 1960.

Bejsovec, M., Kulenda, Z. and Ponca, E.: Familial intrauterine convulsions in pyridoxine dependency. Arch. Dis. Child. 42: 201-207, 1967.

Liu, M. C. and Sylvester, P. E.: Familial diffuse progressive encephalopathy. Arch. Dis. Child. 35: 345-351, 1960.

Winkelman, N. W. and Moore, M. T.: Progressive degenerative encephalopathy (report of case in infancy with antenatal onset simulating 'swayback' of lambs). J. Neuropath. Exp. Neurol. 1: 127 Only, 1942.

*21730 CORNEA PLANA

In 1925 Felix described two affected brothers from an uncle-niece mating. In 1961 Forsius reported a study in Finland in which 19 cases were found in 9 families in patterns consistent with autosomal recessive inheritance. Eriksson et al. (1973) pointed out that the autosomal recessive form has more severe manifestations than the dominant form (12140), in terms of reduced visual activity, extreme hyperopia (usually plus 10 d. or more), hazy corneal limbus, opacities in the corneal parenchyma, and marked arcus senilis (often detected at an early age).

Eriksson, A. W., Lehmann, W. and Forsius, H.: Congenital cornea plana in Finland. Clin. Genet. 4: 301-310, 1973.

Felix, C. H.: Congenitale familiare cornea plana. Klin. Mbl. Augenheilk. 74: 710-716,, Springfield, Ill.: 1925. (Pedigree, Fig. 345, P. 448 of Waardenburg, P. J., Franceschetti, A. and Klein, D. (eds.): Genetics and Ophthalmology, vol. I. Charles C Thomas, 1961.)

Forsius, H.: Studien uber Cornea plana congenita bei 19 Kranken in 9 Familien. Acta Ophthal. 39: 203-221, 1961.

21740 CORNEAL DYSTROPHY AND PERCEPTIVE DEAFNESS

Harboyan et al. (1971) described three sibs from a consanguineous mating with late onset, perceptive deafness and corneal clouding like that of congenital hereditary corneal dystrophy (q.v.).

Harboyan, G., Mamo, J., Der Kaloustian, V. M. and Karam, F.: Congenital corneal dystrophy. Progressive sensorineural deafness in a family. Arch. Ophthal. 85: 27-32, 1971.

*21750 CORNEAL DYSTROPHY, BAND-SHAPED (BAND KERATOPATHY)

Streiff and Zwahlen (1946) observed the rare hereditary form of band-shaped corneal dystrophy in three of 9 children of a first-cousin mating. The opacity began at puberty in two but was already present at birth in the third. The opacity forms a well-delimited band across the cornea at the level of the pupil and occupying the region of the palpebral fissure. It is denser centrally and consists of many small grayish elements like tapioca grains. Corneal diagrams and the pedigree are reproduced by Waardenburg (1961). Band keratopathy may occur in hypercalcemia, Still juvenile arthritis, tuberous sclerosis, Fanconi syndrome, hypophosphatasia, etc. Brother and sister, ages 11 and 16, were reported by Fuchs (1939). On the other hand father and son were reported by Glees (1950).

Fuchs, A.: Ueber primaere guertelfoermige Hornhauttruebung. Klin. Mbl. Augenheilk. 103: 300-309, 1939.

Glees, M.: Ueber familiaeres Auftreten der primaeren, bandfoermigen Hornhautdegeneration. Klin. Mbl. Augenheilk. 116: 185-187, 1950.

Streiff, E. B. and Zwahlen, P.: Une famille avec degenerescence en bandelette de la cornee. Ophthalmologica III: 129-134, 1946. (See Also fig. 392 in, Waardenburg, P. J., Franceschetti, A. and Klein, D. (eds.): Genetics And Ophthalmology. Springfield, Ill.: Charles C Thomas, 1: 485 only, 1961.).

21760 CORNEAL DYSTROPHY, CENTRAL TYPE

Francois (1958) described a brother and sister, ages 50 and 35, respectively, with what he considered to be a 'new' type of hereditary corneal dystrophy. They referred to it as 'dystrophie corneenne nuageuse centrale.'

Francois, J.: L'Heredite en Ophtalmologie. Paris: Masson, 1958.

R
E
C
E
S
S
I
V
E

Maumenee (1960) reported several cases in which family histories suggested recessive inheritance. In each of two families a brother and sister were affected. One was a Negro family (L. M. 644879 and F. M. 644875) and the other was a West Virginian white family (J. M. 354118 and W. M. 354126). In view of the degree of corneal clouding, vision is often remarkably good. Redmond (1946) described 3 affected daughters of normal but consanguineous parents.

Maumenee, A. E.: Congenital hereditary corneal dystrophy. Am. J. Ophthal. 50: 1114-1124, 1960.

Redmond, S. P.: Three sisters showing congenital opacities in the cornea. Trans. Ophthal. Soc. U.K. 66: 367-368, 1946.

Waardenburg, P. J., Franceschetti, A. and Klein, D. S.: Genetics and Ophthalmology. Springfield, Ill.: Charles C Thomas, 1: 485 only, 1961.

*21780 CORNEAL DYSTROPHY, MACULAR TYPE (GROENOUW TYPE II)

The differentiation from the granular and lattice types (see dominant catalog) was discussed by Jones and Zimmerman (1961). Onset occurs in the first decade, usually between ages 5 and 9. The disorder is progressive. Minute, gray, punctate opacities develop. Corneal sensitivity is usually reduced. Painful attacks with photophobia, foreign body sensations, and recurrent erosions occur in most patients. Acid mucopolysaccharides are demonstrable in corneal fibroblasts. Klintworth and Vogel (1964) suggested that this is a localized mucopolysaccharide.

Blum, J. D.: Relations entre les degenerescences heredo-familiales et les opacites congenitales de la cornee (etude clinique et genealogique). Ophthalmologica 109: 123-136, 1944.

Goldberg, M. F., Maumenee, A. E., and McKusick, V. A.: Corneal dystrophies associated with abnormalities of mucopolysaccharide metabolism. Arch. Ophthal. 74: 516-520, 1965.

Jones, S. T. and Zimmerman, L. E.: Histopathologic differentiation of granular, macular and lattice dystrophies of the cornea. Am. J. Ophthal. 51: 394-410, 1961.

Klintworth, G. K. and Vogel, F. S.: Macular corneal dystrophy. An inherited acid mucopolysaccharide storage disease of the corneal fibroblast. Am. J. Path. 45: 565-586, 1964.

21790 CORNELIA DE LANGE SYNDROME (TYPUS DEGENERATIVUS AMSTELODAMENSIS)

In 1933 in Amsterdam, Cornelia de Lange described two infant girls with mental deficiency and other features. The facies are curious, with eyebrows growing across the base of the nose (synophrys), hair growing well down onto the forehead, and low on the neck, unusually long eyelashes, depressed bridge of nose which has uptilted tip and forward-directed nostrils, small widely spaced teeth, small head and low-set ears. 'The hands are characteristic, with flat spade-like appearance and short tapering fingers, the fifth especially so and curved inwards. A single deep transverse crease was seen over the palms' (Schlesinger and colleagues, 1963). The thumbs appear to arise from a position abnormally far proximal. The thenar eminence is inconspicuous so that the thumb suggests a lobster claw. Large joints show limitation of motion. At times absence deformity, usually of one arm only, is severe so that only a single finger remains on a short arm. A case was reported by Ullrich (1951).

In some instances (e.g., Borghi et al., 1954), multiple sibs have been affected with both parents normal. Although Ptacek et al. (1963) suggested dominant inheritance, Opitz (1964) later thought recessive inheritance likely. No chromosomal abnormality has been related to the syndrome. The large number of De Lange cases found to have one or another type of chromosomal aberration may be fortuitous, may indicate a predisposition to chromosomal change induced in some way by a point mutation (as in Bloom syndrome and in Fanconi panmyelopathy), or may indeed have cause-and-effect relationship. According to Craig and Luzzatti (1965), 11 out of 38 patients in whom the chromosomes have been studied showed abnormalities. They felt this was more than chance association. Falek, Schmidt and Jervis (1966) described three affected sibs and their affected first cousins. Patients showed 46 chromosomes with loss of one small acrocentric of the G group and an additional metacentric chromosome resembling, but somewhat smaller than, the 16th chromosome. Six phenotypically normal relatives including one parent of each of the two affected sibships had the same anomalous chromosome as the affected children but in addition an apparent deletion of one chromosome 3. The authors suggested that the Cornelia De Lange syndrome is due to excessive chromosome 3 material. The anomalous chromosome was interpreted as combining one G chromosome with a fragment from one chromosome 3. McArthur and Edwards (1967) found normal chromosomes in all 20 of their cases. However, they expressed the opinion that the condition is most likely related to a chromosomal deficiency which is not readily detectable. This would explain both the usual sporadic nature and the occasional familial occurrence. Broholm et al. (1968) described a patient with Cornelia De Lange syndrome and a B-D translocation inherited from the normal mother. The patient was thought to be partially trisomic for a group D chromosome. Pashayan et al. (1969) concluded that the recessive hypothesis can be rejected. The empiric recurrence risk in a sib of an affected child was estimated to be between 2 and 5 percent. Familial occurrence and parental consanguinity were noted by Pearce et al. (1967). Opitz (1971) found normal parental age (average paternal and maternal age 30.6 and 28.9 years, respectively), suggesting a new dominant mutation. Beratis et al. (1971) described three affected sibs with normal karyotypes and normal, non-consanguineous parents.

Beratis, N. G., Hsu, L. Y. and Hirschhorn, K.: Familial de Lange syndrome. Report of three cases in a sibship. Clin. Genet. 2: 170-176, 1971.

Borghi, A., Giusti, G. and Bigozzi, U.: Nanismo degenerativo tipo di Amsterdam (typus Amstelodamensis — malattia di Cornelia de Lange): presentazione di un caso e considerazioni di ordine genetico. Acta Genet. Med. Gem. 3: 365-372, 1954.

Broholm, K.-A., Eeg-Olofsson, O. and Hall, B.: An inherited chromosome aberration in a girl with signs of de Lange syndrome. Acta Paediat. Scand. 57: 547-552, 1968.

Craig, A. P. and Luzzatto, L.: Translocation in de Lange's syndrome. Lancet II: 445-446, 1965.

De Lange, C.: Sur un type nouveau de degeneration (typus Amstelodamensis). Arch. Med. Enf. 36: 713-719, 1933.

Falek, A., Schmidt, R. and Jervis, G. A.: Familial de Lange syndrome with chromosome abnormalities. Pediatrics 37: 92-101, 1966.

McArthur, R. G. and Edwards, J. H.: de Lange syndrome: report of 20 cases. Canad. Med. Ass. J. 96: 1185-1198, 1967.

Motl, M. L. and Opitz, J. M.: Studies of malformation syndromes XXVA. Phenotypic and genetic studies of the Brachmann-de Lange syndrome. Hum. Hered. 21: 1-16, 1971.

Opitz, J. M.: Comment. In, Gellis, S. S. (ed.): Year Book of Pediatrics, 1971. Chicago: Year Book Medical Publishers, 1971. P. 489.

Opitz, J. M., Segal, A. T., Lehrke, R. L., Nadler, H. L.: The etiology of the Brachmann-de Lange syndrome. The Clinical Delineation of Birth Defects. New York: National Foundation, 1964. Pp. 22-23.

Pashayan, H., Whelan, D., Guttman, S. and Fraser, F. C.: Variability of the de Lange syndrome: report of 3 cases and genetic analysis of 54 families. J. Pediat. 75: 853-858, 1969.

Payne, H. W. and Maeda, W. K.: The Cornelia de Lange syndrome: clinical and cytogenetic interpretations. Canad. Med. Assoc. J. 93: 577-586, 1965.

Pearce, P. M., Pitt, D. B. and Roboz, P.: Six cases of the de Lange's syndrome: parental consanguinity in two. Med. J. Aust. 1: 502-506, 1967.

Ptacek, L. J., Opitz, J. M., Smith, D. W., Gerritsen, T. and Waisman, H. A.: The Cornelia de Lange syndrome. J. Pediat. 63: 1000-1020, 1963.

Schlesinger, B., Clayton, B., Bodian, M. and Jones, K. V.: Typus degenerativus Amstelodamensis. Arch. Dis. Child. 38: 349-357, 1963.

Smith, G. F.: A study of the dermatoglyphs in the de Lange syndrome. J. Ment. Defic. Res. 10: 241-247, 1966.

Ullrich, O.: Typus Amstelodamensis (Cornelia de Lange). Ergebn. Inn. Med. Kinderheilk. 2: 454-458, 1951.

RECESSIVE

*21800 CORPUS CALLOSUM, AGENESIS OF

Naiman and Fraser (1955) described two sisters and Ziegler (1958) described two brothers with agenesis of the corpus callosum associated with mental and physical retardation. An X-linked form (q.v.) described by Menkes et al. had additional developmental abnormalities of the brain. Andermann et al. (1972) have observed a family with two brothers who showed associated anterior horn cell disease and a clinical syndrome of mental retardation, areflexia and paraparesis. The clinical picture was the same as in the sisters reported by Naiman and Fraser (1955) and the two families were French-Canadian from the same region of Quebec (Charlevoix County). Shapira and Cohen (1973) reported two affected sisters whose parents were more closely related than first cousins.

Andermann, F., Andermann, E., Joubert, M., Karpati, G., Carpenter, S. and Melancon, D.: Familial agenesis of the corpus callosum with anterior horn cell disease. A syndrome of mental retardation, areflexia, and paraplegia. Trans. Am. Neurol. Ass., Chicago, June, 1972.

Naiman, J. L. and Fraser, F. C.: Agenesis of the corpus callosum. A report of two cases in siblings. Arch. Neurol. Psychiat. 74: 182-185, 1955.

Shapira, Y. and Cohen, T.: Agenesis of the corpus callosum in two sisters. J. Med. Genet. 10: 266-269, 1973.

Ziegler, E.: Boesartige familiaere fruehinfantile Krampfkrankheit, teilweise verbunden mit familiaerer Balkenaplasie. Helv. Paediat. Acta 13: 169-184, 1958.

*21810 CRANIAL NERVES, CONGENITAL PARESIS OF

Stark (1940) observed congenital weakness of cranial nerves III, IV and VII in two sisters and a brother from a consanguineous mating. Thomas (1898) described congenital facial paralysis in two brothers who also had malformed external ears. Cadwalader (1922) reported affected sibs from a first-cousin marriage.

Cadwalader, W. B.: Two cases of agenesis (congenital paralysis) of the cranial nerves. Am. J. Med. Sci. 163: 744-748, 1922.

Henderson, J. L.: The congenital facial diplegia syndrome: clinical features, pathology and aetiology. A review of 61 cases. Brain 62: 381-403, 1939.

Stark, T.: Ueber kongenitale und progressive Ophthalmoplegien (unter Beruecksichtigung des 'infantilen Moebiusschen Kernschwunds'). Zbl. Ges. Ophthal. 43: 148-149, 1940.

Thomas, H. M.: Congenital facial paralysis. J. Nerv. Ment. Dis. 25: 571-593, 1898.

In the offspring of Jewish first-cousins, Currie (1970) described 4 sibs (3 brothers and a sister) of 5 who suffered recurrent episodes of Bell palsy and external ophthalmoplegia. All 4 had Bell palsy to a total of 7 episodes. Three had a total of 4 episodes of ocular palsy. One brother had proved diabetes and one had latent diabetes. One had polycythemia. The episodes were characteristic of those in diabetics. The lack of iridoplegia with the third nerve palsy distinguishes the ocular palsy from that of berry aneurysm. This is probably just a chance familial aggregation of cranial neuropathy in diabetes.

Currie, S.: Familial oculomotor palsy with Bell's palsy. Brain 93: 193-198, 1970.

*21830 CRANIODIAPHYSEAL DYSPLASIA

Cranial and facial hyperostosis results in a characteristic clinical and radiographic appearance. The diaphyses of the bones are generally expanded. Halliday (1949) and Stransky (1962) reported isolated cases very similar in findings. Facial and cranial thickening and distortion are particularly striking in this form. Most cases have been mentally retarded. Unlike the situation in the craniometaphyseal dysplasias (q.v.), the long bones do not show metaphyseal flaring but show diaphyseal endostosis and a shape like a policeman's nightstick. Affected male and female sibs were reported by De Souza (1927) and the parents of Halliday's case (1949) were related. Joseph et al. (1958), who first suggested the designation of progressive craniodiaphyseal dysplasia, described a patient with a picture they considered identical to that described by Halliday.

De Souza, O.: Leontiasis ossea. Porto Alegre (Brazil) Faculdade de Med. Rev. Dos. Cursos. 13: 47-54, 1927.

Halliday, J.: Rare case of bone dystrophy. Brit. J. Surg. 37: 52-63, 1949.

Joseph, R., Lefebvre, J., Guy, E. and Job, J.-C.: Dysplasie cranio-diaphysaire progressive. Ses relations avec la dysplasie diaphysaire progressive de Camurati-Engelmann. Ann. Radiol. 1: 477-490, 1958.

Stransky, E., Mabilangan, L. and Lara, R. T.: On Paget's disease with leontiasis ossea and hypothyreosis, starting in early childhood. Ann. Paediat. 199: 399-408, 1962.

*21840 CRANIOMETAPHYSEAL DYSPLASIA

Both dominant and recessive forms have been identified (see 12300). The recessive form is more severe than the dominant form. Nasal obstruction is usually complete and involvement of cranial nerves is the rule. Case 4 of Jackson et al. (1954) was blind from optic atrophy at 15 months. Deafness and facial palsy are the rule. Affected sibs were described by Millard et al. (1967) and by Lehmann (1957) and parental consanguinity was recorded by Lievre and Fischgold (1956). Pyle disease is metaphyseal dysplasia with little cranial involvement (see 26590).

Jackson, W. P. U., Hanelin, J. and Albright, F.: Metaphyseal dysplasia, epiphyseal dysplasia, diaphyseal dysplasia, and related conditions: familial metaphyseal dysplasia and craniometaphyseal dysplasia: their relation to leontiasis ossea and osteopetrosis: disorders of 'bone remodeling.' Arch. Intern. Med. 94: 871-885, 1954.

Lehmann, E. C. H.: Familial osteodystrophy of the skull and face. J. Bone Joint Surg. 39B: 313-315, 1957.

Lievre, J. A. and Fischgold, H.: Leontiasis ossea chez l'enfant (osteopetrose partielle probable). Presse Med. 64: 763-765, 1956.

Millard, D. R., Maisels, D. D., Batstone, J. H. F. and Yates, B. W.: Craniofacial surgery in craniometaphyseal dysplasia. Am. J. Surg. 113: 615-621, 1967.

*21850 CRANIOSTENOSIS

In the Amish of Holmes County (Ohio), Cross (1969) observed multiple cases of craniostenosis in a pedigree pattern consistent with autosomal recessive inheritance. Most other reports have suggested dominant inheritance (q.v.). However, Duguid (1929) found it in 4 sibs. Gillot et al. (1960) found craniostenosis in a brother and sister whose parents and three sibs were unaffected. Gaudier et al. (1967) reviewed the subject and reported a series of cases which included an affected brother and sister. Craniostenosis is a feature of hypophosphatasia (q.v.). Armendares (1970) also presented evidence supporting recessive inheritance. He pointed out that the particular deformity of the skull is dependent on which sutures close first and the exact type of skull deformity resulting from the primary process of premature closure of the sutures varies not only between families but even within families.

Armendares, S.: On the inheritance of craniostenosis. Study of thirteen families. J. Genet. Hum. 18: 121-134, 1970.

Cross, H. E. and Opitz, J. M.: Craniosynostosis in the Amish. J. Pediat. 75: 1037-1044, 1969.

Duguid, H.: An instance of familial scaphocephaly. J. Ment. Sci. 75: 704-706, 1929.

Gaudier, B., Laine, E., Fontaine, G., Castier, C. and Farriaux, J.-P.: Les craniosynostoses (etude de vingt observations). Arch. Franc. Pediat. 24: 775-792, 1967.

Gillot, F., Marchioni, J. and Reibel, C.: Craniostenose familiale. Pediatrie 15: 695-697, 1960.

21855 CRANIOSYNOSTOSIS WITH FIBULAR APLASIA

Lowry (1972) described brothers with this combination. The parents were related.

Lowry, R. B.: Congenital absence of the fibula and craniosynostosis in sibs. J. Med. Genet. 9: 227-229, 1972.

R
E
C
E
S
S
I
V
E

*21860 CRANIOSYNOSTOSIS WITH RADIAL DEFECTS (CRANIOSYNOSTOSIS-RADIAL APLASIA SYNDROME)

Baller (1950) described a female with oxycephaly and absent radius. The parents were third cousins. Gerold (1959) described a brother and sister, aged 16 years and 2 days, with tower skull, radial aplasia and slight ulnar hypoplasia.

Baller, F.: Radiusaplasie und Inzucht. Z. Menschl. Vererb. Konstitutionsl. 29: 782-790, 1950.

Gerold, M.: Frakturheilung bei einem seltenen Fall kongenitaler Anomalie der oberen Gliedmassen. (Healing of a fracture in an unusual case of congenital anomaly of the upper extremities). Zbl. Chir. 84: 831-834, 1959.

Greitzer, L. J., Jones, K. L., Schnall, B. S. and Smith, D. W.: Craniosynostosis-radial aplasia syndrome. J. Pediat. 84: 723-727, 1974.

*21870 CRETINISM, ATHYREOTIC

Athyreotic cretinism is not as clearly Mendelizing as is goitrous cretinism. There is some familial aggregation which may be of the same type as is seen with many common congenital malformations. It is noteworthy that whether goiter is present or not is dependent on age and treatment. Under certain circumstances a patient who has the same defect as in one of the types of goitrous cretinism may appear to be athyreotic (Beierwaltes, 1964). Blizzard and others (1960) have suggested that maternal autoantibodies may be responsible for destruction of the fetal thyroid. They observed the birth of two successive cretins from a mother with autoantibodies. Antibodies were implicated in the familial cases of Sutherland et al. (1960). This could be a non-genetic mechanism of familial occurrence of athyreotic cretinism. Although usually these cases, like those of panhypopituitarism, are sporadic, in 152 cases in Wilkins' clinic one pair of sibs was found (1965). Ainger and Kelley (1955) reported three sibs, and Sutherland and colleagues (1960) three sibs. Females are affected about twice as often as males. Myotonia and muscular pseudohypertrophy occur in some of these patients, the so-called Kocher-Debre-Semelaigne syndrome. Athyreotic cretinism is probably as heterogeneous a category as goitrous cretinism. The justification for marking this item with an asterisk comes from the evidence that at least one form of athyreotic cretinism is inherited as a recessive. In an inbred Amish group (Cross and colleagues, 1968), we have observed two sisters with cretinism and the Kocher-Debre-Semelaigne syndrome. Although no thyroid was palpable, sensitive scanning techniques showed the presence of a small amount of thyroid tissue in the neck. Thus, 'agoitrous cretinism' is a better designation than athyreotic cretinism. Greig et al. (1966) described two pairs of monozygotic twins with the co-twins both affected in each case. One pair was considered athyreotic and the other had residual thyroid and ectopic tissue, respectively. In another instance a mother and child were affected. The father was unknown and presumably incest was possible, making recessive inheritance likely in that instance also. The authors referred to the condition as thyroid dysgenesis.

Ainger, L. E. and Kelley, V. C.: Familial athyreotic cretinism: report of 3 cases. J. Clin. Endocr. 15: 469-475, 1955.

Beierwaltes, W. H.: Genetics of thyroid disease. In, Hazard, J. B. and Smith, D. E. (eds.): The Thyroid. Baltimore: Williams and Wilkins, 1964.

Blizzard, R. M., Chandler, R. W., Landing, B. H., Pettit, M. D. and West, C. D.: Maternal autoimmunization to thyroid as a probable cause of athyrotic cretinism. New Eng. J. Med. 263: 327-336, 1960.

Cross, H. E., Hollander, C. S., Rimoin, D. L. and McKusick, V. A.: Familial agoitrous cretinism accompanied by muscular hypertrophy. Pediatrics 41: 413-420, 1968.

Greig, W. R., Henderson, A. S., Boyle, J. A., McGirr, E. M. and Hutchison, J. H.: Thyroid dysgenesis in two pairs of monozygotic twins and in a mother and child. J. Clin. Endocr. 26: 1309-1316, 1966.

Najjar, S. S. and Nachman, H. S.: The Kocher-Debre-Semelaigne syndrome. Hypothyroidism with muscular 'hypertrophy.' J. Pediat. 66: 901-908, 1965.

Sutherland, J. M., Esselborn, V. M., Burket, R. L., Skillman, T. B. and Benson, J. T.: Familial nongoitrous cretinism apparently due to maternal antithyroid antibody. New Eng. J. Med. 263: 336-341, 1960.

Wilkins, L.: Diagnosis and Treatment of Endocrine Disorders in Childhood and Adolescence. Springfield, Ill.: Charles C Thomas, 1965 (3rd Ed.).

*21880 CRIGLER-NAJJAR SYNDROME

Intense jaundice appears in the first days of life and persists thereafter. Some affected infants die in the first weeks or months of life with kernicterus. Others have survived with little or no neurologic defect. The level of bilirubin in the blood is in the vicinity of 20 mg percent with most of it indirect reacting. Childs, Sidbury and Migeon (1959) concluded that tests using sodium salicylate show impairment of glucuronide conjugation in heterozygotes. One of the affected sibships in the inbred kindred reported by Crigler and Najjar (1952) included a case of Morquio syndrome. Direct demonstration of the enzyme defect was provided by Szabo and colleagues (1962). The same group found reduced urinary excretion of menthol following oral loading dose in both parents, three grandparents and six sibs of a case. The values were midway between those of normal controls and the very low values observed in affected persons. Both parents had normal bilirubin tolerance tests. Bilirubin is linked to glucuronic acid by an ester bond whereas menthol and other test substances, such as para-aminophenol, salicylamide and 4-methyl umbelliferone, have an ether bond. Sugar (1961) described a patient who survived to adulthood, married and had two children of whom one was severely affected. Further insight into the natural history of this disease was afforded by the observations of Blumenschein et al. (1968). A male member of the kindred originally studied by Crigler and Najjar was normal, apart from his jaundice, for all his life until age 16 when he developed neurologic disability progressing to death after 6 months. Gardner and Konigsmark (1969) described the histopathologic findings in that patient. See HYPERBILIRUBINEMIA, ARIAS TYPE, in dominant catalog for discussion of another defect involving glucuronyl transferase. Blumenschein et al. (1968) described the clinical features. Some presumed cases of Crigler-Najjar syndrome have been said to respond to phenobarbital with lowering of serum bilirubin (Karon et al., 1970). Serum bilirubin concentrations of newborn infants can be reduced by exposure to sunlight or artificial blue light. This measure was found effective in a case of presumed Crigler-Najjar syndrome (Karon et al., 1970).

Blumenschein, S. D., Kallen, R. J., Storey, B., Natzschka, J. C., Odell, G. B. and Childs, B.: Familial nonhemolytic jaundice with late onset of neurological change. Pediatrics 42: 786-792, 1968.

Childs, B., Sidbury, J. B. and Migeon, C. J.: Glucuronic acid conjugation by patients with familial nonhemolytic jaundice and their relatives. Pediatrics 23: 903-913, 1959.

Crigler, J. F., Jr. and Najjar, V. A.: Congenital familial nonhemolytic jaundice with kernicterus. Pediatrics 10: 169-179, 1952.

Gardner, W. A., Jr. and Konigsmark, B. W.: Familial nonhemolytic jaundice: bilirubinosis and encephalopathy. Pediatrics 43: 365-376, 1969.

Karon, M., Imach, D. and Schwartz, A.: Effective phototherapy in congenital nonobstructive, nonhemolytic jaundice. New Eng. J. Med. 282: 377-380, 1970.

Sugar, P.: Familial nonhemolytic jaundice. Congenital with kernicterus. Arch. Intern. Med. 108: 121-127, 1961.

Szabo, L. and Ebrey, P.: Studies on the inheritance of Crigler-Najjar's syndrome by the menthol test. Acta Paediat. Acad. Sci. Hung. 4: 153-158, 1963.

Szabo, L., Kovacs, Z. and Ebrey, P.: Congenital non-haemolytic jaundice. (Letter) Lancet I: 322 only, 1962.

*21890 CROME SYNDROME

Crome, Duckett and Franklin (1963) described two female infants with an identical disorder — congenital cataracts, epileptic fits, mental retardation, small stature, and death (at 4 and 8 months). Postmortem showed renal tubular necrosis and encephalopathy. The parents were first cousins. Similarities to Marinesco-Sjogren syndrome (q.v.), and to Lowe syndrome were pointed out. The latter is an X-linked recessive. The former is autosomal recessive but renal change has not been described and survival to a later age is usual.

Crome, L., Duckett, S. and Franklin, A. W.: Congenital cataracts, renal tubular necrosis and encephalopathy in two sisters. Arch. Dis. Child. 38: 505-515, 1963.

*21900 CRYPTOPHTHALMOS WITH OTHER MALFORMATIONS

In each of the two sibships Fraser (1962) observed two sisters affected at birth by various combinations: (a) cryptophthalmos; (b) absent or malformed lacrimal ducts; (c) middle and outer ear malformations; (d) high palate; (e) cleavage along the midplane of nares and tongue; (f) hypertelorism; (g) laryngeal stenosis; (h) syndactyly; (i) wide separation of symphysis pubis; (j) displacement of umbilicus and nipples; (k) primitive mesentry of small bowel; (l) maldeveloped kidneys; (m) fusion of labia and enlargement of clitoris; and (n) bicornuate uterus and malformed fallopian tubes. In each sibship one sister was stillborn and the other viable. Sex chromatin was positive in both surviving infants. Neither set of parents was consanguineous. See BOWEN SYNDROME for a comparable but probably distinct syndrome of multiple congenital malformations.

Gupta and Saxema (1962) reported cryptophthalmos in two offspring of consanguineous parents. In one it was unilateral and death occured at 1 month. In the second the cryptophthalmos was bilateral and was accompanied by congenital deafness, undescended testes, small penis with hypospadias and other deformities. The older literature on cryptophthalmos with associated malformations is reviewed by Duke-Elder (1963). Francois (1969) described affected brother and sister and gave a comprehensive review pointing out the rather frequent examples of parental consanguinity (about 15 percent of cases) and of familial cases. Syndactyly is a feature of many of the cases. An isolated case was reported by Ide and Wollschlaeger (1969). The parents were not related. Azevedo et al. (1973) reported four cases in two sibships, each with consanguinous parents. Syndactyly and other malformations were present in some.

Azevedo, E. S., Biondi, J. and Ramalho, M.: Cryptophthalmos in two families from Bahia, Brazil. J. Med. Genet. 10: 389-392, 1973.

Duke-Elder, S.: System of Ophthalmology, Normal and Abnormal Development. St. Louis: C. V. Mosby Co. 3: (part 2) 1963. Pp. 829-834.

Francois, J.: Syndrome malformatif avec cryptophtalmie. Acta Genet. Med. Gem. 18: 18-50, 1969.

Fraser, G. R.: Our genetical 'load.' A review of some aspects of genetical variation. Ann. Hum. Genet. 25: 387-415, 1962.

Fraser, G. R.: XX chromosomes and renal agenesis. (Letter) Lancet I: 1427 only, 1966.

Gupta, S. P. and Saxema, R. C.: Cryptophthalmos. Brit. J. Ophthal. 46: 629-632, 1962.

Ide, C. H. and Wollschlaeger, P. B.: Multiple congenital abnormalities associated with cryptophthalmia. Arch. Ophthal. 81: 638-644, 1969.

RECESSIVE

Goltz, Hult, Goldfarb and Gorlin (1965) described affected brothers and suggested recessive inheritance because of other reported instances of affected sibs as well as parental consanguinity. One child had multiple diverticula (esophagus, duodenum, ileum, bladder). The other had pulmonary emphysema and died at 18 months from cor pulmonale. The authors suggested 'generalized elastolysis' as a more satisfactory designation. Death from pulmonary emphysema was also described by Christiaens et al. (1954). Hayden et al. (1968) described a 4-year-old patient with cutis laxa and congenital pulmonary artery stenosis. A deficiency of elastic fibers in the skin was reported. Hajjar and Joyner (1968) described a 6-month-old Puerto Rican child with advanced pulmonary emphysema. Serum copper level was low and urinary excretion high, consistent with the theory that deficiency of serum copper produces a low elastase inhibitor substance with increased destruction of elastic fibers (Goltz et al., 1965). The Negro patient of Maxwell and Esterly (1969) had pulmonary emphysema. Hernias have been an important feature of many cases (Schreiber and Tilley, 1961; Cashman, 1957; Goltz et al., 1965). Welch et al. (1971) described three sons of a consanguineous mating who had features suggesting cutis laxa of the malignant form. Unusual features were tortuous arteries and arterial aneurysms. The father and many of his relatives had the benign hypermobile form of Ehlers-Danlos syndrome. Beighton (1972) reported a case with first-cousin parents and a case resulting from a father-daughter mating. Sestak (1962) reported affected brother and sister whose parents were first cousins once removed and who had a common ancestor of the two parents reported affected. One of these sibs was pictured by Cashman (1957). A dominant form of cutis laxa (12370) is characterized by freedom from the pulmonary and other internal complications.

Beighton, P. H.: The dominant and recessive forms of cutis laxa. J. Med. Genet. 9: 216-221, 1972.

Beighton, P. H., Bull, J. C. and Edgerton, M. T.: Plastic surgery in cutis laxa. Brit. J. Plast. Surg. 23: 285-290, 1970.

Cashman, M. E.: Cutis laxa. Proc. Roy. Soc. Med. 50: 719-720, 1957.

Christiaens, L., Marchand-Alphant, A. and Fovet, A.: Emphyseme congenital et cutix laxa. Presse Med. 62: 1799-1801, 1954.

Goltz, R. W., Hult, A. M., Goldfarb, M. and Gorlin, R. J.: Cutis laxa, a manifestation of generalized elastolysis. Arch. Derm. 92: 373-387, 1965.

Hajjar, B. A. and Joyner, E. N.: Congenital cutis laxa with advanced cardiopulmonary disease. J. Pediat. 73: 116-119, 1968.

Hayden, J. G., Talner, N. S. and Klaus, S. N.: Cutis laxa associated with pulmonary artery stenosis. J. Pediat. 72: 506-509, 1968.

Maxwell, E. and Esterly, N. B.: Cutis laxa. Am. J. Dis. Child. 117: 479-482, 1969.

Schreiber, M. M. and Tilley, J. C.: Cutis laxa. Arch. Derm. 84: 266-272, 1961.

Sestak, Z.: Ehlers-Danlos syndrome and cutis laxa: an account of families in the Oxford area. Ann. Hum. Genet. 25: 313-321, 1962.

Welch, J. P., Aterman, K., Day, E. and Roy, D. L.: Familial aggregation of a 'new' connective-tissue disorder: a nosologic problem. The Clinical Delineation of Birth Defects. XII. Skin, Hair and Nails. Baltimore: Williams and Wilkins, 1971. Pp. 204-213.

21920 CUTIS LAXA WITH BONE DYSTROPHY

Fittke (1942) described a ten-and-one-half-month-old female whose skin from birth had been in loose redundant folds. The face was spared, however. On stretching, the skin returned only slowly to its original position. The skeletal system showed widely persistent fontanelles, slight oxycephaly, and dislocation of one hip. The parents were not known to be related but lived in the area of Europe where most persons were related in some degree. The mother, age 25 years, had long suffered from 'weak knee joints.' An-8-year old cousin of the proband showed the same skin changes, as well as pigeon breast, static scoliosis, and flat feet. The fontanelles had not closed until the third year. The case of Debre et al. (1937) may be identical.

Debre, R., Marie, J. and Seringe, P.: 'Cutis laxa' avec dystrophies osseuses. Bull. Soc. Med. Hop. Paris 53: 1038-1039, 1937.

Fittke, H.: Ueber eine ungewoehnliche Form 'multipler Erbabartung' (Chalodermie und Dysostose). Z. Kinderheilk. 63: 510-523, 1942.

21930 CUTIS VERTICIS GYRATA AND MENTAL DEFICIENCY

McDowall (1893) first described this association which may not be rare since Akesson (1964) found 47 cases in a survey of institutionalized mental defectives in Sweden. See ACROMEGALOID CHANGES, etc., in dominant catalog.

Akesson, H. O.: Cutis verticis gyrata and mental deficiency in Sweden. I. Epidemiologic and clinical aspects. Acta Med. Scand. 175: 115-127, 1964.

Akesson, H. O.: Cutis verticis gyrata and mental deficiency in Sweden. II. Genetic Aspects. Acta Med. Scand. 177: 459-464, 1965.

McDowall, T. W.: Case of abnormal development of the scalp. J. Ment. Sci. 39: 62-64, 1893.

21940 CYANOSIS AND HEPATIC DISEASE

Silverman et al. (1968) observed 2 children, brother and sister, who developed dyspnea, cyanosis and digital clubbing 11 and 18 months after episodes of hepatitis. Pulmonary arteriovenous fistulae too small to be demonstrated by angiography were postulated.

Silverman, A., Cooper, M. D., Moller, J. H. and Good, R. A.: Syndrome of cyanosis, digital clubbing, and hepatic disease in siblings. J. Pediat. 72: 70-80, 1968.

*21950 CYSTATHIONINURIA

During a survey by paper chromatography of amino acids in the urine of patients in an institution for mental defectives, Harris, Penrose and Thomas (1959) discovered a case with abnormal excretion of cystathionine. An inborn error involving the cleavage of cystathionine to give cysteine and homoserine was suggested. The subject was a severely retarded female aged 64 years at the time of study. Another case was studied at The New York Hospital. Other clinical manifestations have been clubfoot, developmental defects about the ears, convulsions and thrombocytopenia. Urinary lithasis also occurs. Frimpter (1965) has shown that the defect involves cystathionase which does not properly bind its coenzyme, pyridoxal phosphate. In vitro studies suggested that high pyridoxine would be therapeutically beneficial. Mongeau et al. (1967) described the case of a two-year-old boy with normal mentality, thrombocytopenia and urinary calculi. The relation of the latter two features to the metabolic defect was problematical. Both parents (who were apparently unrelated) showed cystathioninuria after methionine loading test. With administration of pyridoxine, cystathioninuria was diminished in the proband. Schneiderman (1967) studied two mentally retarded brothers who excreted large amounts of cystathionine after methionine ingestion. The mother and another brother excreted lesser but abnormal amounts after methionine loading. The father was not tested. Perry et al. (1968) discovered cystathioninuria in a brother and sister when the brother's urine was by chance subjected to two-dimensional paper chromatography for amino acids. Both children were normal. The parents excreted cystathionine only after methionine loading. The authors suggested that mental defect and other disorders reported in association with cystathioninuria may have been coincidental. Whelan and Scriver (1968) also found cystathioninuria as an apparently benign inborn error. The case of Tada et al. (1968) did not respond to B6.

Frimpter, G. W.: Cystathioninuria: nature of the defect. Science 149: 1095-1096, 1965.

Frimpter, G. W.: Cystathioninuria, sulfite oxidase deficiency, and 'beta-mercaptolactate-cysteine disulfiduria. In, Stanbury, J. B., Wyngaarden, J. B. and Fredrickson, D. S. (eds.): The Metabolic Basis of Inherited Disease. New York: McGraw-Hill, 1972 (3rd Ed.). Pp. 413-425.

Frimpter, G. W., Haymovitz, A. and Horwith, M.: Cystathioninuria. New Eng. J. Med. 268: 333-339, 1963.

Harris, H., Penrose, L. S. and Thomas, D. H. H.: Cystathioninuria. Ann. Hum. Genet. 23: 442-453, 1959.

Lyon, I. C. T., Procopis, P. G. and Turner, B.: Cystathioninuria in a well baby population. Acta Paediat. Scand. 60: 324-328, 1971.

Mongeau, J.-G., Hilgartner, M., Worthen, H. G., and Frimpter, G. W.: Cystathioninuria: study of an infant with normal mentality, thrombocytopenia, and renal calculi. J. Pediat. 69: 1113-1120, 1967.

Perry, T. L., Hardwick, D. F., Hansen, S., Love, D. L. and Israels, S.: Cystathioninuria in two healthy siblings. New Eng. J. Med. 278: 590-592, 1968.

Schneiderman, L. J.: Latent cystathioninuria. J. Med. Genet. 4: 260-263, 1967.

Scott, C. R., Dassell, S. W., Clark, S. H., Chiang-Teng, C. and Swedberg, K. R.: Cystathioninemia: a benign genetic condition. J. Pediat. 76: 571-577, 1970.

Shaw, K. N. F., Lieberman, E., Koch, R. and Donnell, G. N.: Cystathioninuria. Am. J. Dis. Child. 113: 119-128, 1967.

Tada, K., Yoshida, T., Yokoyama, Y., Sato, T., Nakagawa, H. and Arakawa, T.: Cystathioninuria not associated with vitamin B6 dependency: a probably new type of cystathioninuria. Tohoku J. Exp. Med. 95: 235-242, 1968.

Whelan, D. T. and Scriver, C. R.: Cystathioninuria and renal iminoglycinuria in a pedigree. A perspective on counseling. New Eng. J. Med. 278: 924-927, 1968.

21960 CYSTIC DISEASE OF LUNG

A strikingly high frequency of cystic disease of the lung has been observed in 'Oriental' (non-Ashkenazi) Jews in Israel, particularly in Yemenites (Racz et al., 1965). The disease manifests itself relatively early in life, even in the first decade in some and recurrent infection is the principal feature. Family studies have not been reported. See FIBROCYSTIC PULMONARY DYSPLASIA in the dominant catalog. The genetics of this disorder is unclear. However, the observations of a relatively high frequency in Oriental Jews in Israel (Baum et al., 1966) and in the Maori of New Zealand (Hinds, 1958) are noteworthy.

Baum, G. L., Racz, I., Bubis, J. J., Molho, M. and Shapiro, B. L.: Cystic disease of the lung. Report of eighty-eight cases, with an ethnologic relationship. Am. J. Med. 40: 578-602, 1966.

Hinds, J. R.: Bronchiectasis in the Maori. New Zeal. Med. J. 57: 328-332, 1958.

Racz, I. and Baum, G. L.: The relationship of ethnic origin to the prevalence of cystic lung disease in Israel. A preliminary report. Am. Rev. Resp. Dis. 91: 552-555, 1965.

*21970 CYSTIC FIBROSIS (MUCOVISCIDOSIS)

Manifestations relate not only to the disruption of exocrine function of the pancreas but also to intestinal glands (meconium ileus), biliary tree (biliary cirrhosis), bronchial glands (chronic broncho-pulmonary infection with emphysema), and sweat glands (high sweat electrolyte with depletion in a hot environment).

Attempting total ascertainment of cases in white children born alive in Ohio during the years 1950 through 1953, Steinberg and Brown (1960) estimate the phenotype frequency to be about 1 in 3,700, a value only about one-fourth that of some earlier estimates. Cystic fibrosis even at this lower estimate is the most frequent lethal genetic disease of childhood. The gene frequency was estimated to be about .016 and about 3 percent of white persons are heterozygotes. In Connecticut Honeyman and Siker (1965) arrived at higher estimates of 1 in 489 (maximal) and 1 in 1863 (minimal).

Roberts (1960) collected family data which appeared to him inconsistent with the quarter ratio expected of a recessive trait. Bulmer (1961) pointed out, however, that when proper correction is made for ascertainment bias the observed proportions may agree with those expected for a recessive trait. Recessive inheritance was first shown by Lowe, May and Reed (1949). The observation of Spock et al. (1967) that patients have a factor in serum which inhibits the action of cilia in explants of rabbit tracheal mucosa may prove very important. Serum from heterozygotes contained an amount of the factor intermediate between none (the normal situation) and the level in patients. Danes and Bearn (1968) found, in skin fibroblasts from both homozygotes and heterozygotes, cytoplasmic intravesicular metachromasia of a type readily distinguished from that of mucopolysaccharidoses. Smith et al. (1968) found cystic fibrosis in a child with cri-du-chat syndrome. Only the mother was heterozygous by Spock test. They suggested that loss of part of the short arm of the chromosome 5 derived from the father had occurred and that the deleted portion carried the cystic fibrosis locus. Danes and Bearn (1968) found vesicular metachromasia in the fibroblasts of both parents suggesting that the reported experience cannot be taken as evidence of localization of the CF gene on the short arm of chromosome 5. Danes and Bearn (1969) described a morphologic change in the fibroblasts and furthermore suggested that homozygosity at either of two different loci can produce cystic fibrosis. In type I the fibroblasts show discrete metachromatic cytoplasmic vesicles and normal mucopolysaccharide content. In type II, fibroblast metachromasia is present in both vesicles and granules and is evenly distributed through the cytoplasm; mucopolysaccharide content of the cells is markedly increased. Kaplan et al. (1968) found that males with cystic fibrosis are infertile because of failure of normal development of the vas deferens. Oppenheimer and Esterly (1969) concluded that the changes in the transport ducts of the male genital system are responsible for infertility and are not a developmental anomaly but degenerative change due to obstruction like that which occurs in the pancreas and salivary glands. Formerly known as cystic fibrosis of the pancreas, this entity has increasingly been labelled simply 'cystic fibrosis.' Oppenheimer et al. (1970) suggested that characteristics of cervical mucus may account for infertility in females with cystic fibrosis. Perhaps it should not be surprising that some patients with cystic fibrosis have no pancreatic lesions (Oppenheimer, 1972). A deficiency of arginine esterase has been suggested by Rao and Nadler (1974), who reported absence of one of three isozymes in various cases of cystic fibrosis. Their hypothesis is that the ciliary factor and related substances is present because of failure of degradation when the enzyme is deficient.

Brusilow, S. W.: Cystic fibrosis in adults. Ann. Rev. Med. 21: 99-104, 1970.

Bulmer, M. G.: Fibrocystic disease of the pancreas: a comment. Ann. Hum. Genet. 25: 163-164, 1961.

Danes, B. S. and Bearn, A. G.: A genetic cell marker in cystic fibrosis of the pancreas. Lancet I: 1061-1063, 1968.

Danes, B. S. and Bearn, A. G.: Cystic fibrosis of the pancreas. A study in cell culture. J. Exp. Med. 129: 775-794, 1969.

Danes, B. S. and Bearn, A. G.: Cystic fibrosis: an improved method for studying white blood-cells in culture. (Letter) Lancet II: 437 only, 1969.

Danes, B. S. and Bearn, A. G.: Cystic fibrosis: distribution of mucopolysaccharides in fibroblast cultures. Biochem. Biophys. Res. Commun. 36: 919-924, 1969.

Danes, B. S. and Bearn, A. G.: Localisation of the cystic-fibrosis gene. (Letter) Lancet II: 1303 only, 1968.

Danks, D. M., Allan, J. and Anderson, C. M.: A genetic study of fibrocystic disease of the pancreas. Ann. Hum. Genet. 28: 323-356, 1965.

Di Sant'Agnese, P. A. and Talamo, R. C.: Pathogenesis and physiopathology of cystic fibrosis of the pancreas: fibrocystic disease of the pancreas (muco-viscidosis). New Eng. J. Med. 277: 1287-1274 And 1344-1352, 1967.

Harris, R. L. and Riley, H. D., Jr.: Cystic fibrosis in the American Indian. Pediatrics 41: 733-738, 1968.

Honeyman, M. S. and Siker, E.: Cystic fibrosis of the pancreas: an estimate of the incidence. Am. J. Hum. Genet. 17: 461-465, 1965.

Kaplan, E., Shwachman, H., Perlmutter, A. D., Rule, A., Khaw, K.-T. and Holsclaw, D. S.: Reproductive failure in males with cystic fibrosis. New Eng. J. Med. 279: 65-69, 1968.

Lobeck, C. C.: Cystic fibrosis. In, Stanbury, J. B., Wyngaarden, J. B. and Fredrickson, D. S. (eds.): The Metabolic Basis of Inherited Disease. New York: McGraw-Hill, 1972 (3rd Ed.). Pp. 1605-1626.

Lowe, C. U., May, C. D. and Reed, S. C.: Fibrosis of the pancreas in infants and children: a statistical study of clinical and hereditary features. Am. J. Dis. Child. 78: 349-374, 1949.

Mangos, J. A. and McSherry, N. R.: Studies on the mechanism of inhibition of sodium transport in cystic fibrosis of the pancreas. Pediat. Res. 2: 378-384, 1968.

Oppenheimer, E. H. and Esterly, J. R.: Observations on cystic fibrosis of the pancreas. V. Developmental changes in the male genital system. J. Pediat. 75: 806-811, 1969.

Oppenheimer, E. H. and Esterly, J. R.: Observations on cystic fibrosis of the pancreas. VI. The uterine 395 cervix. J. Pediat. 77: 991-995, 1970.

Oppenheimer, E. H.: Absence of pancreatic lesions in cystic fibrosis. The Clinical Delineation of Birth Defects. XIII. G. I. Tract Including Liver and Pancreas. Baltimore: Williams and Wilkins, 1972. Pp. 108-113.

Oppenheimer, E. H., Case, A. L., Esterly, J. R. and Rothberg, R. M.: Cervical mucus in cystic fibrosis: a possible cause of infertility. Am. J. Obstet. Gynec. 108: 673-674, 1970.

Rao, G. J. S., Posner, L. A. and Nadler, H. L.: Deficiency of kallikrein activity in plasma of patients with cystic fibrosis. Science 177: 610-611, 1972.

Rao, G. J. S. and Nadler, H. L.: Arginine esterase in cystic fibrosis of the pancreas. Pediat. Res. 8: 684-686, 1974.

Roberts, G. B. S.: Familial incidence of fibrocystic disease of the pancreas. Ann. Hum. Genet. 24: 127-135, 1960.

Smith, D. W., Docter, J. M., Ferrier, P. E., Frias, J. L. and Spock, A.: Possible localisation of the gene for cystic fibrosis of the pancreas to the short arm of chromosome 5. Lancet II: 309-312, 1968.

Spock, A., Heick, H. M. C., Cress, H. and Logan, W. S.: Abnormal serum factor in patients with cystic fibrosis of the pancreas. Pediat. Res. 1: 173-177, 1967.

Steinberg, A. G. and Brown, D. C.: On the incidence of cystic fibrosis of the pancreas. Am. J. Hum. Genet. 12: 416-424, 1960.

Wright, S. W. and Morton, N. E.: Genetic studies on cystic fibrosis in Hawaii. Am. J. Hum. Genet. 20: 157-162, 1968.

*21980 CYSTINOSIS I (EARLY ONSET NEPHROPATHIC TYPE: INFANTILE TYPE)

The fact that plasma levels are well below saturation indicates that the defect is a cellular one. Within the cell cystine is compartmentalized with acid phosphatase and is membrane-bound as demonstrated by electron microscopy. Ferritin accumulates in the same organelle which appears to be the lysosome. An abnormality in heterozygotes was demonstrated by Schneider et al. (1967) who found the concentration of free cystine to be about 6 times normal in the leukocytes of parents of patients. The features resulting from accumulation of cystine in the kidney are those of the Fanconi syndrome (q.v.). Teree et al. (1970) studied physiologically and anatomically two male sibs with cystinosis . Microdissection of the kidney tubules suggested that the morphologic abnormality of the proximal tubule is 'acquired' and progressive. Mahoney et al. (1970) found that renal transplants in four children with cystinosis did not develop glomerular and tubular epithelial cellular changes of cystinosis. Schneider et al. (1974) showed that cystinosis can be diagnosed in the 18-week-old fetus on the basis of an increased content of nonprotein cystine in culture aminotic-fluid cells.

R
E
C
E
S
S
I
V
E

Mahoney, C. P., Striker, G. E., Hickman, R. O., Manning, G. B. and Marchioro, T. L.: Renal transplantation for childhood cystinosis. New Eng. J. Med. 283: 397-402, 1970.

Schneider, J. A., Bradley, K. and Seegmiller, J. E.: Increased cystine in leukocytes from individuals homozygous and heterozygous for cystinosis. Science 157: 1321-1322, 1967.

Schneider, J. A., Verroust, F. M., Kroll, W. A., Garvin, A. J., Horger, E. O., III., Wong, V. G., Spear, G. S., Jacobson, C., Pellett, O. L. and Becker, F. L. A.: Prenatal diagnosis of cystinosis. New Eng. J. Med. 290: 878-882, 1974.

Schulman, J. D. and Bradley, K. H.: Cystinosis: therapeutic implications of in vitro studies of cultured fibroblasts. J. Pediat. 78: 833-836, 1971.

Schulman, J. D., Fujimoto, W. Y., Bradley, K. H. and Seegmiller, J. E.: Identification of heterozygous genotype for cystinosis in utero by a new pulse-labeling technique: preliminary report. J. Pediat. 77: 468-470, 1970.

Shulman, J. D. (ed.): Cystinosis. Washington: U. S. Government Printing Office, 1973.

Spear, G., Slusser, R. J., Tousimis, A. J., Taylor, C. G. and Schulman, J. D.: Cystinosis. An ultrastructural and electron probe study of the kidney with unusual findings. Arch. Path. 21: 206-221, 1971.

Teree, T. M., Friedman, A. B., Kent, L. M. and Fetterman, G. H.: Cystinosis and proximal tubular nephropathy in siblings. Progressive development of the physiological and anatomical lesion. Am. J. Dis. Child. 119: 481-487, 1970.

Weinberg, T.: Cystine storage disease. Report of a case. Am. J. Clin. Path. 29: 54-60, 1958.

Worthen, H. G. and Good, R. A.: The de Toni-Fanconi syndrome with cystinosis: clinical and metabolic study of two cases in a family and a critical review of the nature of the syndrome. Am. J. Dis. Child. 100: 653-688, 1960.

*21990 CYSTINOSIS II (LATE ONSET NEPHROPATHIC TYPE; JUVENILE OR ADOLESCENT TYPE)

This form of cystine nephropathy manifests itself first at age 10 or 12 years with proteinuria due to glomerular damage rather than with the manifestations of tubular damage which occur first in cystinosis I. There is no excess aminoaciduria and stature is normal. Photophobia, late development of pigmentary retinopathy and chronic headaches are features. White cells show high cystine content in heterozygotes for cystinosis II, just as they do in cystinosis I. Spear et al. (1971) described glomerular changes in renal biopsies from a case of late-onset nephropathic cystinosis. Clinically the disorder shows a slowly progressive glomerular insufficiency rather than the prominent Fanconi syndrome, electrolyte and water disturbances, growth arrest and rickets typical of cystinosis I. The patient was the only affected person in the family and the parents were not related (as one would expect if cystinosis II is the genetic compound of cystinosis I and cystinosis III).

Goldman, H., Scriver, C. R., Aaron, K., Delvin, E. and Canlas, Z.: Adolescent cystinosis: comparisons with infantile and adult forms. Pediatrics 47: 970-988, 1971.

Spear, G. S., Slusser, R. J., Shulman, J. D. and Alexander, F.: Polykaryocytosis of the visceral glomerular epithelium in cystinosis with description of an unusual clinical variant. Johns Hopkins Med. J. 129: 83-99, 1971.

*22000 CYSTINOSIS III (BENIGN TYPE; ADULT TYPE)

A benign form of cystinosis has been described in a few cases. For example, Leitman et al. (1966) observed three affected sibs from cousin parents. The ages of patients were 53, 50 and 42 years. Crystals of cystine were demonstrated in the cornea, buffy coat of the blood and bone marrow. No aminoaciduria or impairment of renal function was found. Cogan et al. (1958) also had an asymptomatic adult with cystine demonstrable in cornea and bone marrow. Although the patients with adult cystinosis show characteristic crystals in the cornea, conjunctiva, circulating white cells and bone marrow, no evidence of renal tubular dysfunction is found. Some reported cases of familial crystalline corneal dystrophy may be examples of this condition. Deposits resembling those of cystinosis occur in the cornea in patients with dysproteinemia such as in multiple myeloma (Burki, 1958). Schneider et al. (1968) reported studies of 3 further adult cystinosis cases. The intracellular deposits of free cystine appear to be unavailable for sustaining normal metabolism since fibroblasts from either the childhood or the adult type are not viable in a cystine-free medium. The intracellular content of cystine is lower in the adult form than in the childhood form, yet higher than in the heterozygote for the childhood form. Retinal lesions occur in the childhood form but not the adult form and may be responsible for the photophobia which is much more a feature of the childhood form. An abnormality in heterozygotes was demonstrated by Schneider et al. (1967) who found the concentration of free cystine to be about 6 times normal in the leukocytes of parents of patients. Brubaker et al. (1970) described brother and sister, ages 16 and 11 years, respectively. Since they had no proteinuria or other clinical abnormality except for crystalline corneal deposits, their disorder fits the 'adult' type rather than the juvenile or adolescent type. The genetic relationship of the three types is unknown. It is possible that types I and III are homozygous states for alleles and that type II is the genetic compound.

Brubaker, R. F., Wong, V. G., Schulman, J. D., Seegmiller, J. E. and Kuwabara, T.: Benign cystinosis. The clinical, biochemical and morphologic findings in a family with two affected siblings. Am. J. Med. 49: 546-550, 1970.

Burki, E. and Rohner, M.: Ein seltener Fall von kristalliner Hornhautdegeneration. A rare case of crystalline corneal degeneration. Ophthalmologica 129: 211-217, 1955.

Burki, E.: A case of corneal changes in multiple myeloma (plasmacytoma) — ueber Hornhautveraenderunger bei einem Fall von multiplem Myelom (Plasmocytom). Ophthalmologica 135: 565-572, 1958.

Cogan, D. G., Kuwabara, T., Hurlbut, C. S. and McMurray, V.: Further observations on cystinosis in the adult. J.A.M.A. 166: 1725-1726, 1958.

Leitman, P. S., Frazier, P. D., Wong, V. G., Shotton, D. and Seegmiller, J. E.: Adult cystinosis — a benign disorder. Am. J. Med. 40: 511-517, 1966.

Schneider, J. A., Bradley, K. and Seegmiller, J. E.: Increased cystine in leukocytes from individuals homozygous and heterozygous for cystinosis. Science 157: 1321-1322, 1967.

Schneider, J. A., Wong, V. G., Bradley, K. and Seegmiller, J. E.: Biochemical comparisons of the adult and childhood forms of cystinosis. New Eng. J. Med. 279: 1253-1257, 1968.

*22010 CYSTINURIA I, II, III (AT LEAST 3 ALLELES AT ONE LOCUS)

In cystinuria I the homozygote excretes relatively large amounts of cystine, lysine, arginine and ornithine in the urine. Heterozygotes (e.g., parents) have no abnormal aminoaciduria. Urinary stones form in all three types of cystinuria because of the limited solubility of this amino acid.

Cystinuria II is incompletely recessive because heterozygotes have a moderate degree of aminoaciduria, mainly cystine and lysine, and may occasionally form cystine stones. Observations in kindreds in which both cystinuria I and cystinuria II are segregating demonstrate that the genes for these are allelic (Hershko et al., 1965).

In cystinuria III, intestinal transport of all dibasic amino acids is retained by heterozygotes and homozygotes excrete cystine in slight excess.

Rosenberg (1966) and others observed families in which persons doubly heterozygous (I-II, I-III, or II-III) had full-blown cystinuria. The findings are best explained on the basis of allelism of the genes responsible for the 3 types. Actually, 'genetic compound' is a term preferable to 'double heterozygote' when the mutant genes are allelic. Scriver et al. (1970) presented evidence indicating that cystinuria patients are at increased risk for impaired cerebral function.

Bostrom, H. and Tottie, K.: Cystinuria in Sweden. II. The incidence of homozygous cystinuria in Swedish school children. Acta Paediat. 48: 345-352, 1959.

Bostrom, H.: Cystinuria in Sweden III. The prognosis of homozygous cystinuria. Acta Chir. Scand. 116: 287-295, 1959.

R
E
C
E
S
S
I
V
E

Fariss, B. L. and Kolb, F. O.: Factors involved in crystal formation in cystinuria. Reduction in cystine cystalluria with chlordiazepoxide and during nephrotic syndrome. J.A.M.A. 205: 846-848, 1968.

Harris, H., Mittwoch, U., Robson, E. B. and Warren, F. L.: Phenotypes and genotypes in cystinuria. Ann. Hum. Genet. 20: 57-91, 1955.

Hershko, C., Ben-Ami, E., Paciorkovski, J. and Levin, N.: Allelomorphism in cystinuria. Proc. Tel. Hashomer. Hosp. 4: 21-23, 1965.

Knox, W. E.: Sir Archibald Garrod's inborn errors of metabolism. I. Cystinuria. Am. J. Hum. Genet. 10: 3-32, 1958.

Rosenberg, L. E.: Cystinuria: genetic heterogeneity and allelism. Science 154: 1341-1343, 1966.

Rosenberg, L. E., Downing, S., Durant, J. L. and Segal, S.: Cystinuria: biochemical evidence for three genetically distinct diseases. J. Clin. Invest. 45: 365-371, 1966.

Rosenberg, L. E., Durant, J. L. and Holland, J. M.: Intestinal absorption and renal extraction of cystine and cysteine in cystinuria. New Eng. J. Med. 273: 1239-1245, 1965.

Scriver, C. R., Whelan, D. T., Clow, C. L. and Dallaire, L.: Cystinuria: increased prevalence in patients with mental disease. New Eng. J. Med. 283: 783-786, 1970.

Thier, S. O. and Segal, S.: Cystinuria. In, Stanbury, J. B., Wyngaarden, J. B. and Fredrickson, D. S. (eds.): The Metabolic Basis of Inherited Disease. New York: McGraw-Hill, 1972 (3rd Ed.). Pp. 1504-1519.

*22015 DALMATIAN HYPOURICEMIA

Greene et al. (1972) reported brother and sister with low serum urate concentration due to an isolated defect in renotubular reabsorption of urate such as occurs in the Dalmatian coachhound (see 24205).

Greene, M. L., Marcus, R., Aurbach, G. D., Kazam, S. and Seegmiller, J. E.: Hypouricemia due to isolated renal tubular defect. Dalmatian dog mutation in man. Am. J. Med. 53: 361-367, 1972.

*22020 DANDY-WALKER SYNDROME

The primary defect is atresia of the foramina of Luschka and Magendie. The fourth ventricle becomes dilated into a large cyst in the posterior fossa. Clement Benda (1954) apparently introduced the designation Dandy-Walker syndrome. Furthermore he reported familial occurrence. D'Agostino, Kernohan and Brown (1963) found the condition in sibs who also had polycystic kidneys.

Benda, C. E.: The Dandy-Walker syndrome or the so-called atresia of the foramen of Magendie. J. Neuropath. Exp. Neurol. 13: 14-29, 1954.

D'Agostino, A. N., Kernohan, J. W. and Brown, J. R.: The Dandy-Walker syndrome. J. Neuropath. Exp. Neurol. 22: 450-470, 1963.

22030 DEAF-MUTISM AND FAMILIAL MYOCLONUS EPILEPSY

Latham and Munro (1937) reported a family in which the parents were second cousins and 5 out of 8 sibs had congenital deafness with myoclonus epilepsy which began at age 10-12 years. Probably no other such families have been reported. See MYOCLONUS, CEREBELLAR ATAXIA and DEAFNESS.

Latham, A. D. and Munro, T. A.: Familial myoclonus epilepsy associated with deaf-mutism in a family showing other psychobiological abnormalities. Ann. Eugen. 8: 166-175, 1937.

*22040 DEAF-MUTISM AND FUNCTIONAL HEART DISEASE (PROLONGED Q-T INTERVAL IN EKG AND SUDDEN DEATH)

In the report of Levine and Woodworth (1958) no note on parental consanguinity was recorded. There was but one case, the proband, in the family. In Jervell and Lange-Nielsen's report (1957) 4 of 6 children were described as affected and the parents were not related. Fraser, Froggatt and Murphy (1964) estimated that the prevalence in children ages 4-15 in England, Wales and Ireland is between 1.6 and 6 per million. They suggested that heterozygous persons may show slight or moderate prolongation of the Q-T interval. Also see VENTRICULAR FIBRILLATION in dominant catalog. In studies of the temporal bones of two children who died with this condition, Friedmann, Fraser and Froggatt (1966) found a striking anomaly in the form of PAS-positive hyaline nodules throughout both the cochlear and the vestibular portions of the membranous labyrinth in, or adjacent to, the terminal vessels of the vascular stria.

Fraser, G. R. and Froggatt, P.: The syndrome of congenital deafness with abnormal electrocardiogram. Heredity 15: 454, 1960.

Fraser, G. R., Froggatt, P. and James, T. N.: Congenital deafness associated with electrocardiographic abnormalities, fainting attacks and sudden death. Quart. J. Med. 33: 361-385, 1964.

Fraser, G. R., Froggatt, P. and Murphy, T.: Genetical aspects of the cardioauditory syndrome of Jervell and Lange-Nielsen (congenital deafness and electrocardiographic abnormalities). Ann. Hum. Genet. 28: 133-157, 1964.

Friedmann, I., Fraser, G. R. and Froggatt, P.: Pathology of the ear in the cardioauditory syndrome of Jervell and Lange-Nielsen (recessive deafness with electrocardiographic abnormalities). J. Laryng. 80: 451-470, 1966.

Furlanello, F., Macca, F. and Dal Palu, C.: Observation on a case of jervell and lang-neilsen syndrome in an adult. Brit. Heart J. 34: 648, 1972.

Jervell, A. and Lange-Nielsen, F.: Congenital deaf-mutism, functional heart disease with prolongation of Q-T interval and sudden death. Am. Heart J. 54: 59-68, 1957.

Levine, S. A. and Woodworth, C. R.: Congenital deaf-mutism, prolonged qt interval, syncopal attacks and sudden death. New Eng. J. Med. 259: 412-417, 1958.

*22050 DEAF-MUTISM AND ONYCHODYSTROPHY

Feinmesser and Zelig (1961) reported two affected sisters from a consanguineous mating. The association might, of course, be merely the coincidence of two rare recessives. Goodman et al. (1969) observed mother and son with sensorineural deafness and onychodystrophy. The father also had sensorineural deafness, presumably of a type different from that in his wife. In the mother the right thumb was triphalangic. The left thumb was biphalangic but a rudimentary third phalanx appeared to be fused with the middle phalanx. This may be a dominant trait distinct from that reported by Feinmesser and Zelig (1961). Walbaum et al. (1970) described a brother and sister with mental retardation, perceptive deafness, dysplasia of the finger nails, triphalangeal thumbs, hypoplasia of the terminal phalanges, and 'decapsalidic' fingerprints, i.e., an arch pattern on each finger. The parents were normal and unrelated. They pointed out similarities to the cases of Feinmesser and Zelig (1961) and of Goodman et al. (1969). Moghadam and Statten (1972) observed triphalangeal thumbs (with hypoplastic terminal phalanges), absent or hypoplastic fingernails and deafness in mother and son of Filipino extraction.

Feinmesser, M. and Zelig, S.: Congenital deafness associated with onychodystrophy. Arch. Otolaryng. 74: 507-508, 1961.

Goodman, R. M., Lockareff, S. and Gwinup, G.: Hereditary congenital deafness with onychodystrophy. Arch. Otolaryng. 90: 474-477, 1969.

Moghadam, H. and Statten, P.: Hereditary sensorineural hearing loss associated with onychodystrophy and digital malformations. Canad. Med. Assoc. J. 107: 310-311, 1972.

Walbaum, R., Fontaine, G., Lienhardt, J. and Piquet, J. J.: Surdite familiale avec osteo-onycho-dysplasie. J. Genet. Hum. 18: 101-108, 1970.

22060 DEAF-MUTISM AND SPLIT HANDS AND FEET

Wildervanck (1963) observed the association in two sons of unrelated parents. Birch-Jensen (1949) mentioned a sporadic case of the association. G. R. Fraser (personal communication) has seen a brother and sister with this combination.

Birch-Jensen, A.: Congenital deformities of the upper extremities. Op. Ex. Domo Biol. Hered. Hum. U. Hafniensis. 19: 1949.

Wildervanck, L. S.: Deafness associated with split hands and feet in two siblings. A new syndrome. Proc. 11th. Intern. Cong. Genet. The Hague, 1963. Pp. 286-287.

*22070 DEAF-MUTISM I (CONGENITAL DEAFNESS)

Because of the presence of deafness from birth speech does not develop unless the affected child has special training, hence the popular term deaf-mutism for congenital deafness. Many, especially those involved in teaching the deaf, disapprove of the term and appropriately so because mutism is not an immutable part of the phenotype.

Fraser (1964) estimated that half of severe childhood deafness was due to simple Mendelian inheritance and that 87 percent of this group is autosomal recessive. Three recessive syndromes were identifiable: Pendred syndrome (10 percent of the hereditary group), Usher syndrome (2 percent) and deafness with unique EKG changes (1 percent). The existence of several genetic forms is supported by the diversity of findings in the ears of deaf-mutes. Ormerod (1960) recognized the following types, beginning with the most complete form of deafness: (1) Michel type — complete lack of development of internal ear. (2) Mondini-Alexander type — development only of a single nerved tube representing the cochlea and similar immaturity of the vestibular canals. (3) Bing-Siebenmann type — bony labyrinth well formed but membranous part and particularly the sense organ poorly developed. This type is often associated with retinitis pigmentosa and-or mental retardation. (4) Scheibe cochleo-saccular type. In this form, which is the most frequent one, the vestibular part is developed and functioning. Malformation is restricted to the membranous cochlea and saccule. This type occurs in Waardenburg syndrome, a dominant. (5) Siebenmann type — changes mainly in middle ear and often due to thyroid hormone deficiency. The middle ear is involved in myxomatous change which may be embryonic persistence. (6) Microtia and atresia of the meatus — abnormality limited to the external ear.

By ingenious mathematical analysis Morton (1960) arrived at the conclusion that recessive inheritance is responsible for 68 percent of congenital deafness, that homozygosity at any one of 35 loci can result in this phenotype and that 16 percent of the normal population are carriers of a gene for deaf-mutism.

As early as 1862 Boudin noted the association between consanguinity and deaf-mutism.

Boudin, M.: De la necessite des croisements et du danger des unions consanguine dans l'espece humaine et parmi les animaux. Rec. Med. Chir. et Pharm. Milit. 7: 193-197, 1862.

Chung, C. S., Robinson, O. W. and Morton, N. E.: A note on deafmutism. Ann. Hum. Genet. 23: 357-366, 1959.

Deraemaeker, R.: Recessive congenital deafness in a north Belgian province. Acta Genet. Statist. Med. 10: 295-304, 1960.

Fraser, G. R.: Profound childhood deafness. J. Med. Genet. 1: 118-151, 1964.

Hanhart, E.: Die 'sporadische' Taubstummheit als Prototyp einer einfach rezessiven Mutation. Z. Menschl. Vererb. Konstitutionsl. 21: 609-671, 1938.

Lindenov, H.: The etiology of deaf-mutism with special reference to heredity. Op. Ex. Domo Biol. Hered. Hum. U. Hafniensis. 8: 1-268, 1945.

Morton, N. E.: The mutational load due to detrimental genes in man. Am. J. Hum. Genet. 12: 348-364, 1960.

Ormerod, F. C.: The pathology of congenital deafness. J. Laryng. 74: 919-950, 1960.

Slatis, H. M.: Comments on the inheritance of deaf mutism in Northern Ireland. Ann. Hum. Genet. 22: 153-157, 1957.

Stevenson, A. C. and Cheeseman, E. A.: Hereditary deaf mutism, with particular reference to Northern Ireland. Ann. Hum. Genet. 20: 177-231, 1956.

*22080 DEAF-MUTISM II (CONGENITAL DEAFNESS)

Direct genetic evidence for the existence of at least two non-allelic, recessive, phenotypically indistinguishable forms of deaf-mutism is provided by the rather frequent pedigrees of the type reported by Stevenson and Cheeseman (1956). In only 5 of 32 hereditary deaf by hereditary deaf matings were all children deaf. From this the authors concluded that there are probably six separate loci for recessive deaf-mutism assuming that the mutant genes at each have a similar frequency. See comments of Slatis (1957). Chung, Robinson and Morton (1959) also supported the notion of multiple recessive forms of deaf-mutism. The existence as listed below of no fewer than six recessive syndromes with deaf-mutism as the main feature but with various associated features is further corroboration. Mengel et al. (1968) presented an instructive pedigree in which two congenital deaf parents had all normal-hearing offspring. One parent came from a Mennonite group with numerous cases of congenital deafness in a recessive pattern. The other parent came from an Amish group which also contained several persons with apparently recessively inherited congenital deafness.

Chung, C. S., Robinson, O. W. and Morton, N. E.: A note on deaf mutism. Ann. Hum. Genet. 23: 357-366, 1959.

Mengel, M. C., Konigsmark, B. W. and McKusick, V. A.: Two types of congenital recessive deafness. Eye Ear Nose Throat Monthly 48: 301-305, 1968.

Slatis, H. M.: Comments on the inheritance of deaf mutism in Northern Ireland. Ann. Hum. Genet. 22: 153-157, 1958.

Stevenson, A. C. and Cheeseman, E. A.: Hereditary deaf mutism, with particular reference to Northern Ireland. Ann. Hum. Genet. 20: 177-231, 1956.

22090 DEAF-MUTISM WITH TOTAL ALBINISM

Ziprkowski and Adam (1964) described a Sephardic Jewish family from Morocco in which two children in each of two families with consanguineous parents had the association mentioned. The two sibships are related to each other and shared a pair of great-great-grandparents in common. In one sibship three sibs of the two doubly affected sibs had only congenital deafness. Thus it is not completely certain that the association is a monomeric syndrome. Dominant and X-linked recessive forms of congenital deafness with albinism, total or partial, were reviewed by these authors.

Ziprkowski, L. and Adam, A.: Recessive total albinism and congenital deafmutism. Arch. Derm. 89: 151-155, 1964.

22100 DEAF-MUTISM, SEMILETHAL

Pfandler (1960) studied deaf-mutism in several populations of Switzerland and found that the proportion of affected sibs was far less than the expected 0.25 (6.25 to 16.7 percent). He suggested that a semilethal effect of the gene could explain the findings. The data showed a deficiency of deaf-mute females. An alternative hypothesis — the necessary coincidence of homozygosity at two separate loci — did not fit the data satisfactorily. Mental defect and hypogonadism also occurred in these cases. It is possible that this series was contaminated by sporadic cases of non-genetic or non-recessive causation.

Pfaendler, U.: Une forme semiletale de la surdimutite recessive dans differentes populations de la Suisse orientale. Bull. Acad. Suisse Sci. Med. 16: 255-277, 1960.

22110 DEAFNESS AND ATOPIC DERMATITIS

Konigsmark et al. (1968) observed cochlear deafness and atypical atopic dermatitis in two brothers and a sister. The atypical features of atopic dermatitis were somewhat late onset (9-11 years) and location on the hands and forearms.

Konigsmark, B. W., Hollander, M. B. and Berlin, C. I.: Familial neural hearing loss and atopic dermatitis. J.A.M.A. 204: 953-957, 1968.

22120 DEAFNESS, COCHLEAR, WITH MYOPIA AND INTELLECTUAL IMPAIRMENT

Eldridge et al. (1968), in a survey of mental retardation in an inbred Amish community, observed four of seven sibs in a family (2 males, 2 females) with the above combination. The extent of intellectual impairment was difficult to evaluate. Sensory deprivation might be a main factor.

Eldridge, R., Berlin, C. I., Money, J. W. and McKusick, V. A.: Cochlear deafness, myopia, and intellectual impairment in an Amish family. A new syndrome of hereditary deafness. Arch. Otolaryng. 88: 49-54, 1968.

*22130 DEAFNESS, CONDUCTIVE, WITH MALFORMED EXTERNAL EAR

In two sibships in a Mennonite isolate, Mengel et al. (1969) observed 6 persons with conductive deafness and malformed, low-set external ear. The four parents shared a common ancestral couple. At operation malformation of the ossicles was demonstrated in the middle ear. Mental retardation and hypogonadism may be additional features.

Mengel, M. C., Konigsmark, B. W., Berlin, C. I. and McKusick, V. A.: Conductive hearing loss and malformed low-set ears, as a possible recessive syndrome. J. Med. Genet. 6: 14-21, 1969.

22140 DEAFNESS, NERVE TYPE, WITH MESENTERIC DIVERTICULA OF SMALL BOWEL AND PROGRESSIVE NEUROPATHY

Hirschowitz et al. (1971) described three sisters from a sibship of six, who had progressive nerve deafness beginning at 8, 3 and 9 years, respectively, and becoming complete or nearly complete by ages 10, 5 and 18 years. Vestibular function remained normal. Progressive sensory neuropathy without peripheral trophic changes was also present. Tachycardia and loss of the carotid sinus reflex may indicate involvement of the cardiac vagus. Involvement of the vagus nerve led to progressive loss of gastric motility. Two of the sisters were demonstrated to have multiple diverticula with jejunoileal ulceration from which the eldest sister died at age 18 years. Malabsorption of fat and intestinal loss of serum protein occurred. A surviving sister had marked acanthosis nigricans. This appears to be an entity distinct from others such as Refsum syndrome and hereditary sensory radicular neuropathy (q.v.).

Hirschowitz, B. I., Groll, A. and Ceballos, R.: Hereditary nerve deafness in 3 sisters with absent gastric motility, small bowel diverticulitis and ulceration and progressive sensory neuropathy. The Clinical Delineation of Birth Defects. XIII. G. I. Tract Including Liver and Pancreas. Baltimore: Williams and Wilkins, 1972. Pp. 27-41.

22150 DEAFNESS, NEURAL, CONGENITAL MODERATE

Konigsmark et al. (1970) described congenital moderate neural hearing loss in three sibships with apparent recessive inheritance. They concluded that this type had not been described previously.

Konigsmark, B. W., Mengel, M. C. and Haskins, H.: Familial congenital moderate neural hearing loss. J. Laryng. 84: 495-505, 1970.

22160 DEAFNESS, NEURAL, EARLY ONSET

Mengel et al. (1967) found severe deafness in 16 members of a kindred. By history all were born with at least some hearing but suffered progressive severe loss in later childhood. Sonographic and speech analysis gave further evidence of some hearing in early childhood. Audiologic tests suggested cochlear location of the defect. Although successive generations were affected in some instances, consanguinity and recessive inheritance were thought to account for the finding. Barr and Wedenberg (1964) described this disorder in four of seven sibs.

Barr, B. and Wedenberg, E.: Prognosis of perceptive hearing loss in children with respect to genesis and use of hearing aid. Acta Otolaryng. 59: 462-474, 1964.

Mengel, M. C., Konigsmark, B. W., Berlin, C. I. and McKusick, V. A.: Recessive early-onset neural deafness. Acta Otolaryng. 64: 313-326, 1967.

22170 DEAFNESS, NEURAL, WITH ATYPICAL ATOPIC DERMATITIS

Konigsmark et al. (1968) found this combination in 3 of 4 sibs. The atopic dermatitis was atypical in late age of onset and distribution (ulnar aspects of forearms and antecubital fossae). The hearing loss was cochlear, was first noted between ages 3 and 5 years and was sufficiently mild that it caused no difficulty in school.

Konigsmark, B. W., Hollander, M. B. and Berlin, C. I.: Familial neural hearing loss and atopic dermatitis. J.A.M.A. 204: 953-957, 1968.

22175 DEAFNESS, NEUROSENSORY, WITH PITUITARY DWARFISM

Winkelmann et al. (1972) described two sisters with inner ear deafness and asexual ateleiotic dwarfism. Deficiency of growth hormone and gonadotropin was demonstrated by radioimmunoassay. The parents were not known to be related. Possibly this 'syndrome' is the result of mutation at two linked loci.

Wiekelmann, W., Bethge, H. and Pfeiffer, R. A.: Hypothalamo-hypophysaerer Minderwuchs mit Innenohrschwerhoerigkeit bie zwei Schwestern. Internist 13: 52-56, 1972.

*22180 DERMO-CHONDRO-CORNEAL DYSTROPHY OF FRANCOIS

The features are (1) skeletal deformity of the hands and feet; (2) xanthomatous nodules on the pinnae, dorsal surface of the metacarpophalangeal and interphalangeal joints, posterior surface of the elbows, nose, etc.; and (3) corneal dystrophy. Francois (1949) observed two affected sibs and the parents of Jensen's case were related. Remky and Engelbrecht (1967) described the disorder in both of unlike-sex twins. They identified a hypercholesterolemic early stage, involvement of the entire skeleton except the vertebrae and skull and abnormal EEG with seizures.

Francois, J. and Detrait, C.: Dystrophie dermo-chondro-corneenne familiale. Ann. Paediat. 174: 145-174, 1950.

Francois, J.: Dystrophie dermo-chondro-corneenne familiale. Ann. Oculist. 182: 409-442, 1949.

Remky, H. and Engelbrecht, G.: Dystrophia dermo-chondro-cornealis (Francois). Klin. Mbl. Augenheilk. 151: 319-331, 1967.

Wiedemann, H.-R.: Zur Francois'schen Krankheit. Aerztl. Wschr. 13: 905-909, 1958.

22190 DETACHMENT OF RETINA, CONGENITAL

Norrie disease, an X-linked condition, is a form of congenital, solid detachment of the retina. An autosomal recessive form of congenital retinal detachment is suggested by the reports of Weve (1938) and of Joannides and Protonotarios (1965). See 26810. Parental consanguinity was noted by Weve (1938) among others. The parents came from an isolate in other reports (e.g., Joannides and Protonotarios, 1965).

Joannides, T. and Protonotarios, P.: Decollement faciforme de la retine chez un frere et une soeur. Ann. Oculist. 198: 904-911, 1965.

Weve, H.: Ablatio falciformis congenita (retinal fold). Brit. J. Ophthal. 22: 456-470, 1938.

22200 DIABETES INSIPIDUS

X-linked and autosomal dominant forms of diabetes insipidus are known in man. Autosomal recessive diabetes insipidus due to a defect in vasopressin synthesis by the posterior pituitary is known in the rat (Valtin et al., 1965).

Valtin, H., Sawyer, W. H. and Sokol, H. W.: Neurohypophysial principles in rats homozygous and heterozygous for hypothalamic diabetes insipidus (Brattleboro strain). Endocrinology 77: 701-706, 1965.

22210 DIABETES MELLITUS

Although the important genetic factor in diabetes is obvious, the mode of inheritance is obscure. Recessive, dominant and multifactorial hypotheses have been advanced. Multiple distinct entities probably exist under this heading. Nilsson (1964) commented on the difficulties of distinguishing dominant and recessive inheritance when gene frequency is high. He considered most likely autosomal recessive inheritance with a gene frequency of about 0.30 and a life-time penetrance of about 70 percent for males and 90 percent for females. A gene frequency of about 0.05 and a penetrance of 25-30 percent would be required to account for the findings on a dominant hypothesis. Using synalbumin insulin antagonism as a test, Vallance-Owen (1966) studied 9 families containing 16 overt cases of diabetes mellitus and concluded that the state of synalbumin positivity is a dominant. Most recent workers favor a multifactorial hypothesis for diabetes (Neel, 1969; Steinberg et al., 1970). In a large series of identical twins Tattersall and Pyke (1972) found a much higher concordance for diabetes when diabetes developed in the index twin after the age of 40 than when it developed before 40. This suggests that late-onset diabetes has a larger genetic component than the early onset variety, a conclusion contrary to what one might guess. Vinik et al. (1974) suggested that the defect in diabetes may be 'blindness' of both alpha and beta cells to glucose, i.e., a recptor defect.

Neel, J. V.: Current concepts of the genetic basis of diabetes mellitus and the biological significance of the diabetic predisposition. In, Diabetes Int. Congress Series, vol. 72S. Amsterdam: Excerpta Med. Foundation, 1969. P. 68.

Neel, J. V., Fajans, S. S., Conn, J. W. and Davidson, R. T.: Diabetes mellitus. Genetics and Epidemiology of Chronic Diseases. Neel, J. V., Shaw, M. W. and Shull, W. J. (eds.): Washington, D. C.: Government Printing Office, 1965.

Nilsson, S. E.: On the heredity of diabetes mellitus and its interrelationship with some other diseases. Acta Genet. Statist. Med. 14: 97-124, 1964.

Pyke, D. A.: The genetics of diabetes. Postgrad. Med. J. 46: 604-606, 1970.

Renold, A. E., Stauffacher, W. and Cahill, G. F., Jr.: Diabetes mellitus. In, Stanbury, J. B., Wyngaarden, J. B. and Fredrickson, D. S. (eds.): The Metabolic Basis of Inherited Disease. New York: McGraw-Hill, 1972 (3rd Ed.). Pp. 83-118.

Simpson, N. E.: Multifactorial inheritance. A Possible hypothesis for diabetes. Diabetes 13: 462-471, 1964.

Steinberg, A. G., Rushforth, N. B., Bennett, P. H., Burch, T. A. and Miller, M.: On the genetics of diabetes mellitus. In, Proc. Nobel Symposium XIII: On the Pathogenesis of Diabetes Mellitus. New York: Wiley, 1970. P. 237.

Tattersall, R. B. and Pyke, D. A.: Diabetes in identical twins. Lancet II: 1120-1125, 1972.

Vallance-Owen, J.: The inheritance of essential diabetes mellitus from studies of synalbumin insulin antagonist. Diabetologia 2: 248-252, 1966.

Vinik, A. I., Kalk, W. J. and Jackson, W. P. U.: A unifying hypothesis for hereditary and acquired diabetes. Lancet I: 485-486, 1974.

*22230 DIABETES MELLITUS, JUVENILE, WITH OPTIC ATROPHY

Hearing loss also occurs in some cases. Wolfram and Wagener (1938) found juvenile diabetes mellitus and optic atrophy in 4 of 8 sibs. Tyrer (1943) observed three affected out of 8 sibs. Tyrer (1943) observed three affected out of 4 offspring of a first-cousin marriage. Rose et al. (1966) reviewed these and other reports and described several cases including two unrelated cases, each the sons of a consanguineous mating. They suggested that homozygosity for a gene with pleiotropic effects may be involved and that because of clinical heterogeneity more than one locus may be involved. All seven patients described by Rose et al. (1966) were

RECESSIVE

male. Affected females were described by others, e.g., Wolfram and Tyrer. Rorsman and Soderstrom (1967) described a family in which three sisters and a brother developed diabetes mellitus and optic atrophy in their teens. In one the optic atrophy appeared before the diabetes mellitus. Diabetes mellitus, diabetes insipidus and optic atrophy were associated in a family recently studied here (D.R., 1264444). Starnes and Welsh (1970) noted association of renal calculi. The stones were predominantly calcium oxalate in one case. Raiti, Plotkin and Newns (1963) reported two sisters with both diabetes mellitus and diabetes insipidus. The association in the same patient is rare and no other instance of familial occurrence of the association has been reported. Diabetes mellitus developed at age 9 and age 5 years. Autosomal recessive inheritance was suggested. Histiocytosis X is an 'acquired' cause of double diabetes. Nevin (1974) tells me of a sibship of 10 of whom two girls aged 14 and 11 years have juvenile diabetes mellitus and optic atrophy. The younger girl also has diabetes insipidus. Shaw and Duncan (1958) described two sisters and a niece with optic atrophy, nerve deafness and diabetes mellitus. All three features had their onset in the first year of life. Ikkos et al. (1970) described first-cousin parents.

Hurley, P. J., Hitchcock, G. C. and Wilson, J. D.: Histiocytosis X and double diabetes. Aust. Ann. Med. 16: 250-254, 1967.

Nevin, N. C.: Belfast, Northern Ireland, personal communication, 1974.

Niemeyer, G. and Marquardt, J. L.: Retinal function in a unique syndrome of optic atrophy, juvenile diabetes mellitus, diabetes insipidus, neurosensory hearing loss, autonomic dysfunction, and hyperalaninuria. Invest. Ophthal. 11: 617-624, 1972.

Raiti, S., Plotkin, S. and Newns, G. H.: Diabetes mellitus and insipidus in two sisters. Brit. Med. J. 2: 1625-1629, 1963.

Rorsman, G. and Soderstrom, N.: Optic atrophy and juvenile diabetes mellitus with familial occurrence. Acta Med. Scand. 182: 419-425, 1967.

Rose, F. C., Fraser, G. R., Friedmann, A. I. and Kohner, E. M.: The association of juvenile diabetes mellitus and optic atrophy: clinical and genetical aspects. Quart. J. Med. 35: 385-405, 1966.

Sauer, H., Chuden, H., Gotterburen, H., Schmitz-Valckenberg, P. and Seitz, D.: Familiares Vorkmen von Diabetes, Opticusatrophie und Innenohrschwerhorigkeit. Dtsch. Med. Wschr. 98: 243-250, 1973.

Shaw, D. A. and Duncan, L. J. P.: Optic atrophy and nerve deafness in diabetes mellitus. J. Neurol. Psychiat. 21: 47-49, 1958.

Starnes, C. W. and Welsh, J. D.: Intestinal sucrase-isomaltase deficiency and renal calculi. New Eng. J. Med. 282: 1023-1024, 1970.

Stevens, P. R. and MacFadyen, W. A. L.: Familial incidence of juvenile diabetes mellitus, progressive optic atrophy, and neurogenic deafness. Brit. J. Ophthal. 56: 496-500, 1972.

Tyrer, J.: A case of infantilism with goitre, diabetes mellitus, mental defect and bilateral primary optic atrophy. Med. J. Aust. 2: 398-401, 1943.

Wolfram, D. J. and Wagener, H. P.: Diabetes mellitus and simple optic atrophy among siblings: report of four cases. Proc. Mayo Clin. 13: 715-718, 1938.

*22240 DIAPHRAGM, UNILATERAL AGENESIS OF

Passarge et al. (1968) reported unilateral agenesis of the diaphragm in a brother and sister and found four reports of multiple affected sibs in the literature. A sibship with at least three affected was reported by Ten Kate and Anders (1970). Seeming parental consanguinity has never been observed. Daentl and Passarge (1972) found that two or more sibs had been affected in nine unrelated families and found probable consanguinity in one. They suggested that tentatively one should quote 'up to 25 percent risk of recurrence to parents who have had one child with this defect.'

Daentl, D. L. and Passarge, E.: Familial agenesis of the diaphragm. The Clinical Delineation of Birth Defects. XIII. G. I. Tract Including Liver and Pancreas. Baltimore: Williams and Wilkins, 1972. Pp. 24-26.

Passarge, E., Halsey, H. and German, J.: Unilateral agenesis of the diaphragm. Humangenetik 5: 226-230, 1968.

Ten Kate, L. P. and Anders, G. J. P. A.: Unilateral agenesis of the diaphragm. (Letter) Humangenetik 8: 366-367, 1970.

22250 DIASTEMATOMYELIA

In this condition the spinal cord is divided longitudinally in the antero-posterior plane by a fibrous or bony structure. The cases are usually isolated but affected sisters were reported by Kapsalakis (1964). Gardner (1973) described a family in which three sisters had diastematomyelia and other dysraphic malformations in various combinations.

Gardner, W. J.: The dysraphic states from syringomyelia to anencephaly. Amsterdam: Excepta Medica, 1973. Pp. 89-94.

Kapsalakis, Z.: Diastematomyelia in two sisters. J. Neurosurg. 21: 66-67, 1964.

*22260 DIASTROPHIC DWARFISM

The patients show scoliosis, a form of clubbed foot bilaterally, malformed pinnae with calcification of the cartilage, premature calcification of the costal cartilages and cleft palate in some cases. Particularly characteristic is the 'hitchhiker' thumb due to deformity of the first metatarsal. The term diastrophic was

R
E
C
E
S
S
I
V
E

crust by which mountains, continents, ocean basins, etc., are formed. Cases have been described under many different designations in the past. See the case described by Mau (1958) in his section on 'multiple congenital malformations and contractures.' These cases have frequently been placed in the wastebasket of arthrogryposis multiplex congenita in hospital diagnostic files. Many cases of so-called achondroplasia with clubfoot are examples of diastrophic dwarfism (e.g. Kite, 1964). The foot deformity is relatively refractory to surgical treatment. Langer (1967) refers to an entity which phenotypically is a mild form of diastrophic dwarfism as 'diastrophic variant.' Bony changes are qualitatively similar but less severe. Soft tissue changes are absent or mild and the clubfoot is not as resistant to treatment as in regular diastrophic dwarfism. Consanguinity was noted in the reports of Taybi (1963) and Jager and Refior (1969). Known to me are two affected women each of whom had a normal child delivered by caesarian and a 50-year-old affected man with two normal teen-age daughters.

Jager, M. and Refior, H. J.: Diastrophischer Zwergwuchs. Z. Orthop. 106: 830-840, 1969.

Kite, J. H.: The Clubfoot. New York: Grune and Stratton, 210-218, 1964.

Lamy, M. and Maroteaux, P.: Le nanisme diastrophique. Presse Med. 68: 1977-1980, 1960.

Langer, L. O., Jr.: Diastrophic dwarfism in early infancy. Am. J. Roentgen. 93: 399-404, 1965.

Langer, L. O., Jr.: Minneapolis, Minn.: personal communication, 1967.

Mau, H.: Wesen und Bedeutung der enchondralen Dysostosen. Stuttgart: Georg Thieme Verlag, 1958. P. 108 Ff.

McKusick, V. A. and Milch, R. A.: The clinical behavior of genetic disease: selected aspects. Clin. Orthop. 33: 22-39, 1964.

Taybi, H.: Diastrophic dwarfism. Radiology 80: 1-10, 1963.

Walker, B. A., Scott, C. I., Hall, J. G., Murdoch, J. L. and McKusick, V. A.: Diastrophic dwarfism. Medicine 51: 41-60, 1971.

*22270 DIBASICAMINOACIDURIA II

Oyanagi et al. (1970) described severe mental retardation, physical retardation, mild intestinal malabsorption syndrome, and increased urinary excretion of lysine, ornithine and arginine in two Japanese sisters with second-cousin parents. Cystine excretion was always within normal limits. This disorder seems to be particularly frequent in Finland. Kekomaki et al. (1967) described an affected male age 23 years and his affected 15-year-old sister. Both refused protein-rich food. Institution of cow's milk at age 1 year resulted in prolonged watery diarrhea and retardation of physical development. With increase in protein in his teens the male grew but mental function deteriorated and typical attacks of stupor and asterixis occurred, accompanied by hyperammonemia. The liver was enlarged and fatty. In their first report in 1965, Perheentupa and Visakorpi described two affected infant sibs. Blood urea is low. Lysine and arginine are increased in the urine. In a group of children including several pairs of sibs one of which had consanguineous parents, Kekomaki et al. (1967) described vomiting, diarrhea, failure to thrive, hepatomegaly, diffuse cirrhosis, low blood urea, hyperammonemia and leukopenia. Symptoms were aggravated by high protein intake and relieved by protein restriction. An excess of ornithine, arginine and lysine, but not of cystine, was excreted in the urine. Intestinal absorption of arginine and lysine was normal. A low concentration of arginine relative to lysine in body fluids was thought responsible for the hyperammonemia and reduced urea synthesis. An asymptomatic dibasicaminoaciduria behaving as a dominant was described in French-Canadians by Whelan and Scriver (1968). Malmquist et al. (1971) stated that 13 cases of familial protein intolerance had been observed in Finland. In Sweden they described a patient who came from Finland. Intellectual impairment, X-ray evidence of brain atrophy and marked skeletal fragility were features. Administration of l-alanine resulted in elevation of blood ammonia and glucose. Urea cycle function appeared to be normal and the defect was thought to concern the mechanisms by which amino nitrogen is transferred to the urea-synthesizing system. The studies of Norio et al. (1971), who called the condition 'lysinuric protein intolerance,' left no doubt of the recessive inheritance. Kihara et al. (1973) suggested that the disease in Japanese reported by Oyanagi et al. (1970) may be a different disorder from that reported in Finland.

RECESSIVE

Kekomaki, M., Toivakka, E., Hakkinen, V. and Salaspuro, M.: Familial protein intolerance with deficient transport of basic amino acids. Acta Med. Scand. 183: 357-359, 1968.

Kekomaki, M., Visakorpi, J. K., Perheentupa, J. and Saxen, L.: Familial protein intolerance with deficient transport of basic amino acids. An analysis of 10 patients. Acta Paediat. Scand. 56: 617-630, 1967.

Kihara, H., Valente, M., Porter, M. T. and Fluharty, A. L.: Hyperdibasicaminoaciduria in a mentally retarded homozygote with a peculiar response to phenothiazines. Ped. 51: 223-229, 1973.

Malmquist, J., Jagenburg, R. and Lindstedt, G.: Familial protein intolerance: possible nature of enzyme defect. New Eng. J. Med. 284: 997-1002, 1971.

Norio, R., Perheentupa, J., Kekomaki, M. and Visakorpi, J. K.: Lysinuric protein intolerance, an autosomal recessive disease. A genetic study of 10 Finnish families. Clin. Genet. 2: 214-222, 1971.

Oyanagi, K., Miura, R. and Yamanouchi, T.: Congenital lysinuria: a new inherited transport disorder of dibasic amino acids. J. Pediat. 77: 259-266, 1970.

Perheentupa, J. and Visakorpi, J. K.: Protein intolerance with deficient transport of basic amino acids. Another inborn error of metabolism. Lancet II: 813-816, 1965.

Perheentupa, J. and Simell, O.: Lysinuric protein intolerance. Clinical Delineation of Birth Defects. XVI. Urinary System and Others. Baltimore: Williams and Wilkins, 1974. Pp. 201-207.

Whelan, D. T. and Scriver, C. R.: Hyperdibasicaminoaciduria: an inherited disorder of amino acid transport. Pediat. Res. 2: 525-534, 1968.

22275 DIPHENYLHYDANTOIN, DEFECT IN HYDROXYLATION OF

Diphenylhydantoin is poorly excreted by the kidney. Removal from the body depends on its hydroxylation. Kutt et al. (1964) found a family in which three members had reduced ability to hydroxylate diphenylhydantoin. The proband, who developed toxicity on usual doses of the drug, showed accumulation of the drug and much less hydroxylated derivative than normal in the urine. A defect in the hydroxylation of diphenylhydantoin can be produced by simultaneous administration of isoniazid (INH) which inhibits hydroxylation by liver microsomes (Kutt et al., 1968). Patients who show intolerance to diphenylhydantoin when receiving INH at the same time are patients who are the slow acetylators (24340) of INH (Kutt et al., 1970; Brennan et al., 1970).

Brennan, R. W., Dehejia, H., Kutt, H., Verebely, K. and McDowell, F.: Diphenylhydantoin intoxication attendant to slow inactivation of isoniazid. Neurology 20: 687-693, 1970.

Kutt, H., Brennan, R., Dehejia, H. and Verebely, K.: Diphenylhydantoin intoxication. A complication of isoniazid therapy. Am. Rev. Resp. Dis. 101: 377-383, 1970.

Kutt, H., Verebely, K. and McDowell, F.: Inhibition of diphenylhydantoin metabolism in rat and in rat liver microsome by antitubercular drugs. Neurology 18: 706-710, 1968.

Kutt, H., Wolk, M., Scherman, R. and McDowell, F.: Insufficient parahydroxylation as a cause of diphenylhydantoin toxicity. Neurology 14: 542-548, 1964.

*22280 DIPHOSPHOGLYCERATE MUTASE DEFICIENCY OF ERYTHROCYTE, ANEMIA DUE TO

Schroter (1965) described severe hemolytic anemia in an infant. Although the proband's blood could not be studied because of multiple transfusions, the erythrocytes of the consanguineous parents, the sister and the father's mother showed activity of 2,3-diphosphoglycerate mutase about half of normal. The family of Bowdler and Prankerd (1964) is puzzling in that father and son had hemolytic anemia for which splenectomy was performed. In father and son, Labie et al. (1970) found a decrease in DPGM by about 50 percent. An increase in oxygen affinity of hemoglobin was observed. Schroter (1965) observed heterozygotes in 3 generations including both parents of a homozygous child with hemolytic anemia. Chen et al. (1971) described a genetically determined electrophoretic variant of 2, 3-diphosphoglycerate mutase in a Canadian Eskimo family. The findings in heterozygotes were consistent with the view that the protein is a dimer of two identical subunits.

Bowdler, A. J. and Prankerd, T. A. J.: Studies in congenital non-spherocytic haemolytic anaemias with specific enzyme defects. Acta Haemat. 31: 65-78, 1964.

Chen, S. H., Anderson, J. E. and Giblett, E. R.: 2, 3-diphosphoglycerate mutase: its demonstration by electrophoresis and the detection of a genetic variant. Biochem. Genet. 5: 481-486, 1971.

Labie, D., Leroux, J.-P., Najman, A. and Reyrolle, C.: Familial diphosphoglyceratemutase deficiency. Influence on the oxygen affinity curves of hemoglobin. Febs Letters 9: 37-40, 1970.

Lohr, G. W. and Waller, H. D.: Zur Biochemie einiger angeborener Hamolytischer Anamien. Folia Haemat. 8: 377-397, 1963.

Schroter, W.: Kongenitale nichtspharocytare hamolytische Anamie bei 2,3-Diphosphoglyceratmutase-mangel der Erythrocyten im fruhen Sauglingsalter. Klin. Wschr. 43: 1147-1153, 1965.

*22290 DISACCHARIDE INTOLERANCE I (CONGENITAL SUCROSE-ISOMALTOSE MALABSORPTION: CONGENITAL SUCROSE INTOLERANCE)

Dahlqvist (1967) gave a useful review of the small intestinal disaccharidases in man. He recognizes six of these, so presumably six unitary defects plus many combined defects might occur. The six are maltase IA, maltase IB (invertase), maltase II, maltase III, lactase (which may be two enzymes) and trehalase. Maltose and lactose are well tolerated in 'sucrose intolerance.' Presumably the defect concerns intestinal invertase. See Durand (1964) for a symposium on this whole group of disorders. Peterson and Herber (1967) found that intestinal sucrase deficiency is a cause of diarrhea in adults and present in a frequency of almost 0.2 percent. Enzyme of fungal origin is effective treatment. Involvement of multiple sibs (Kerry and Townley, 1965) and consanguineous parents (Jansen et al., 1965) support recessive inheritance. Homozygotes have severe enzyme deficiency with clinical symptoms throughout life. Heterozygotes have intermediate enzyme values and no symptoms in adulthood, but may have mild symptoms in infancy. Rather numerous examples of affected sibs and several instances of consanguineous parents are recorded. A form symptomatic in adults and late in onset was described by Jansen et al. (1965). Ten percent of Greenland Eskimos have sucrose intolerance (McNair et al., 1972) and the frequency is probably increased in Alaskan Eskimos (Ament et al., 1973).

Ament, M. E., Perera, D. R. and Esther, L. J.: Sucrase-isomaltase deficiency a frequently misdiagnosed disease. J. Pediat. 83: 721-727, 1973.

Antonowicz, I., Lloyd-Still, J. D., Khaw, K. T. and Shwachman, H.: Congenital sucrase-isomaltase deficiency. Observations over a period of 6 years. Pediatrics 49: 847-853, 1972.

Dahlqvist, A.: Localization of the small-intestinal disaccharidases. Am. J. Clin. Nutr. 20: 81-88, 1967.

Davidson, M.: Disaccharide intolerance. Pediat. Clin. N. Am. 14: 93-107, 1967.

R
E
C
E
S
S
I
V
E

Greene, H. L., Stifel, F. B. and Herman, R. H.: Dietary stimulation of sucrase in a patient with sucrase-isomaltase deficiency. Biochem. Med. 6: 409-418, 1972.

Holzel, A.: Sugar malabsorption due to deficiencies of disaccharidase activities and of monosaccharide transport. Arch. Dis. Child. 42: 341-352, 1967.

Jansen, W., Que, G. S. and Veeger, W.: Primary combined saccharase and isomaltase deficiency. Report of two adult siblings of consanguineous parentage. Arch. Intern. Med. 116: 879-885, 1965.

Kerry, K. R. and Townley, R. R. W.: Genetic aspects of intestinal sucrase-isomaltase deficiency. Aust. Paediat. J. 1: 223-235, 1965.

McNair, A., Hyer, E. G., Jarnum, S. and Orridl, L.: Sucrose malabsorption in Greenland. Brit. Med. J. 1: 19 only 1972.

Peterson, M. L. and Herber, R.: Intestinal sucrase deficiency. Trans. Ass. Am. Physicians 80: 275-283, 1967.

Prader, A. and Auricchio, S.: Defects of intestinal disaccharide absorption. Ann. Rev. Med. 16: 345-358, 1965.

*22300 DISACCHARIDE INTOLERANCE II (CONGENITAL LACTOSE INTOLERANCE)

Cellobiose intolerance would be expected as well as that for lactose. Sucrose, maltose and starch are well tolerated. Affected sibs were described by Holzel et al. (1959), Weijers and Van De Kamer (1964), and Launiala et al. (1969). No instance of parental consanguinity has been reported and no stigma of heterozygosity has been noted. In a breastfed infant who developed watery diarrhea on the third day of life, Levin et al. (1970) demonstrated absent lactase in a specimen of duodenal mucosa which was histologically normal and showed normal maltase isomaltase and sucrase activities. Convincing direct demonstration of absent lactase in biopsies obtained in infancy, has been achieved only twice before, according to the authors. A sister of the proband was probably identically affected. Sahi et al. (1973) presented extensive family data supporting recessive inheritance.

Dahlqvist, A.: Specificity of the human intestinal disaccharidases and implications for hereditary disaccharide intolerance. J. Clin. Invest. 41: 463-470, 1962.

Darling, S., Mortensen, O. and Sondergaard, G.: Lactosuria and amino-aciduria in infancy: a new inborn error of metabolism? Acta Paediat. 49: 281-290, 1960.

Holzel, A., Schwarz, V. and Sutcliffe, K. W.: Defective lactose absorption causing malnutrition in infancy. Lancet I: 1126-1128, 1959.

Launiala, K., Perheentupa, J. and Hallman, N.: Congenital sugar malabsorption. In, Gardner, L. I. (ed.): Endocrine and Genetic Diseases of Childhood. Philadelphia: W. B. Saunders Co., 1969. Pp. 830-843.

Levin, B., Abraham, J. M., Burgess, E. A. and Wallis, P. G.: Congenital lactose malabsorption. Arch. Dis. Child. 45: 173-177, 1970.

Sahi, T., Isokoski, M., Jussila, J., Launiala, K. and Pyorala, K.: Recessive inheritance of adult-type lactose malabsorption. Lancet II: 823-825, 1973.

Weijers, H. A. and Van de Kamer, J. H.: Fermentative diarrhoeas. In, Durand, P. (ed.): Disorders Due to Intestinal Defective Carbohydrate Digestion and Absorption. Rome: Il Pensiero Scientifico, 1964.

R
E
C
E
S
S
I
V
E

*22310 DISACCHARIDE INTOLERANCE III (ADULT LACTASE DEFICIENCY)

Several studies (Cuatrecasas et al., 1965; Friedland, 1965) of the oral lactose tolerance test have found diarrhea and flat blood-glucose curves in a considerable proportion of adults, especially in Negroes. Intestinal lactase activity is lost with age in rats, pigs and rabbits. Man may be polymorphic with regard to the loss or retention of lactase activity in adulthood. The genetic control of this and its relationship to lactase deficiency evident in infancy (see DISACCHARIDE INTOLERANCE II) has not been worked out. Lactose intolerance is much more frequent in Negroes than in Caucasoids (Bayless and Rosensweig, 1966). Isolated lactase deficiency of adulthood is also more frequent in the American Indian than Caucasians (Welsh et al., 1967). Lactose intolerance is also present in a great majority of adult Orientals (Huang and Bayless, 1968). The intolerance usually first appears in the late teens. Perhaps this represents failure of development of a normal post-weaning lactose digesting system. Cook (1967) found that the deficiency developed in the first four years and sometimes in the first 6 months in Africans. Rosensweig et al. (1967) found three groups as to lactase level and suggested that these correspond to three genotypes. Some heterozygotes in their classification had milk and lactose induced symptoms. Work of Semenza et al. (1965) suggests the existence of two separate lactases which may be under separate genetic control.

The form of intestinal lactase deficiency present in adults was called primary hypolactasia by Ferguson and Maxwell (1967) as contrasted with hereditary alactasia, the disorder causing diarrhea in infancy (see DISACCHARIDE INTOLERANCE II). These authors described affected brother and sister. In patients with intestinal malabsorption (e.g. tropical sprue) Gray et al. (1969) found that, of the two lactases with different pH optima found in normal intestine, only enzyme I with a pH optimum of 6.0 and molecular weight of 280,000 was absent. Similar studies in adult intestinal lactase deficiency without malabsorption are indicated. Baer (1970) suggested that the development of yogurt was a compensation for the intestinal lactase deficiency in countries with a large frequency of the disorder. Welsh (1970) reviewed reports of a high frequency in American Negroes, Africans, Asians, Greek Cypriots, Australian Aborigines and South

American Indians. Ferguson and Maxwell (1967) observed two affected children with normal parents. The family data of Welsh (1970) indicate a genetic basis but give no conclusive indication of the mode of inheritance. From the findings in children of African-European matings Kretchmer (1972) concluded that lactose tolerance, which on a world-wide basis is the rare condition, is dominant. Flatz and Rotthauwe (1973) suggested that the present day higher frequency of adult lactose tolerance in some populations is due not to a non-specific nutritional advantage of milk but rather to a specific advantage, namely, lactose induced enhancement of calcium absorption.

Baer, D.: Lactase deficiency and yogurt. Social Biol. 17: 143 only, 1970.

Bayless, T. M. and Rosensweig, N. S.: A racial difference in incidence of lactase deficiency. A survey of milk intolerance and lactase deficiency in healthy adult males. J.A.M.A. 197: 968-972, 1966.

Bayless, T. M. and Rosensweig, N. S.: Incidence and implications of lactase deficiency and milk intolerance in white and Negro populations. Johns Hopkins Med. J. 121: 54-64, 1967.

Bayless, T. M.: Intestinal lactase deficiency. The Clinical Delineation of Birth Defects. XIII. G. I. Tract Including Liver and Pancreas. Baltimore: Williams and Wilkins, 1972. Pp. 4-11.

Bryant, G. D., Chu, Y. K. and Lovitt, R.: Incidence and aetiology of lactose intolerance. Med. J. Aust. 1: 1285-1288, 1970.

Cook, G. C.: Lactase activity in newborn and infant baganda. Brit. Med. J. 1: 527-530, 1967.

Cuatrecasas, P., Lockwood, D. H. and Caldwell, J. R.: Lactase deficiency in the adult. A common occurrence. Lancet I: 14-18, 1965.

De Ritis, F., Balestrieri, G. G., Ruggiero, G., Filosa, E. and Auricchio, S.: High frequency of lactase activity deficiency in small bowel of adults in the Neapolitan area. Enzym. Biol. Clin. 11: 263-267, 1970.

Ferguson, A. and Maxwell, J. D.: Genetic aetiology of lactose intolerance. Lancet II: 188-190, 1967.

Flatz, G. and Rotthauwe, H. W.: Lactose nutrition and natural selection. Lancet II: 1973.

Frieland, N.: 'Normal' lactose tolerance test. Arch. Intern. Med. 116: 886-888, 1965.

Gilat, T., Banaroya, Y., Gelman-Malachi, E. and Adam, A.: Genetics of primary adult lactase deficiency. Gastroenterology 64: 562-568, 1973.

Gilat, T., Kuhn, R., Gelman, E. and Mizrahy, O.: Lactase deficiency in Jewish communities in Israel. Am. J. Dig. Dis. 15: 895-904, 1970.

Gray, G. M., Santiago, N. A., Colver, E. H. and Genel, M.: Intestinal beta-galactosidases. II. Biochemical alteration in human lactase deficiency. J. Clin. Invest. 48: 729-735, 1969.

Huang, S.-S. and Bayless, T. M.: Lactose intolerance in healthy children. New Eng. J. Med. 276: 1283-1287, 1967.

Huang, S.-S. and Bayless, T. M.: Milk and lactose intolerance in healthy Orientals. Science 160: 83-84, 1968.

Jussila, J., Isokoski, M. and Launiala, K.: Prevalence of lactose malabsorption in a Finnish rural population. Scand. J. Gastroent. 5: 49-56, 1970.

Kretchmer, N.: Lactose and lactase — a historical perspective. Gastroenterology 61: 805-813, 1971.

Kretchmer, N.: Lactose and lactase. Scientific American 227 (no. 4): 70-78, 1972.

Rosensweig, N. S., Huang, S.-S. and Bayless, T. M.: Transmission of lactose intolerance. (Letter) Lancet II: 777 only, 1967.

Semenza, G., Auricchio, S. and Rubino, A.: Multiplicity of human intestinal disaccharidases. I. Chromatographic separation of maltases and of two lactases. Biochim. Biophys. Acta 96: 487-497, 1965.

Welsh, J. D.: Isolated lactase deficiency in humans: report on 100 patients. Medicine 49: 257-277, 1970.

Welsh, J. D., Rohrer, V., Knudsen, K. B. and Paustian, F. F.: Isolated lactase deficiency: correlation of laboratory studies and clinical data. Arch. Intern. Med. 120: 261-269, 1967.

R
E
C
E
S
S
I
V
E

22320 DISSEMINATED SCLEROSIS (MULTIPLE SCLEROSIS)

MacKay and Myrianthopoulos (1966) found that concordance is slightly higher in monozygotic than in dizygotic twins and that multiple sclerosis is about 20 times more frequent among relatives of probands than in the general population. The frequency declined as the relationship to the proband became more remote. They concluded that the family data consistent with autosomal recessive inheritance with reduced penetrance but that exogenous factors must be very strong. On the other hand, the concordance rate in monozygotic twins is so low that it is difficult to think that genetic factors are of great importance. There appear to be rare forms of multiple sclerosis or multiple sclerosis-like diseases which are genetic.

Ekbom, K.: Familial multiple sclerosis associated with narcolepsy. Arch. Neurol. 15: 337-344, 1966.

MacKay, R. P. and Myrianthopoulos, N. C.: Multiple sclerosis in twins and their relatives. Final report. Arch. Neurol. 15: 449-462, 1966.

22330 DISSEMINATED SCLEROSIS WITH NARCOLEPSY

Ekbom (1966) described four families in which multiple members had multiple sclerosis. In 3 of the 4 families one or more affected persons also had narcolepsy. No consanguinity was found.

22333 DIVERTICULOSIS OF BOWEL, HERNIA, RETINAL DETACHMENT

Clunie and Mason (1962) described a unique disorder in 3 brothers whose parents were first cousins. All had recurrent femoral and-or inguinal hernias and diverticula of the large and small bowel or urinary bladder. Two of the brothers had a Marfanoid habitus. A sister had diverticula. Severe myopia, internal strabismus and retinal detachment were present the the 3 brothers.

Clunie, G. J. A. and Mason, J. M.: Visceral diverticula and the Marfan syndrome. Brit. J. Surg. 50: 51-52, 1962.

22335 DOHLE BODIES AND LEUKEMIA

Goudsmit et al. (1971) reported a family in which two sisters and three brothers had Dohle bodies. Two of these 5 died of acute myeloblastic leukemia and two others had iron-resistant anemia. The parents and another sib did not have Dohle bodies. No statement concerning parental consanguinity was made. Dohle bodies of polymorphoneuclear leukocytes are also seen in the May-Hegglin anomaly (15510).

Goudsmit, R., Leeuwen, A. M. and James, J.: Dohle bodies and acute myeloblastic leukemia in one family: a new familial disorder. Brit. J. Haemat. 20: 557-562, 1971.

*22337 DUBOWITZ SYNDROME

Three patients with a malformation syndrome were reported by Dubowitz (1965). The four patients had intrauterine growth retardation, short stature, microcephaly, mild mental retardation with behavior problems, eczema and unusual and distinctive facies. A variety of minor malformations, such as pilonidal dimples, submucous clefts, high pitched voice and sparse hair were also seen. Two of the four cases were full sibs with nonconsanguineous parents. An older sib of Dubowitz's original report was probably affected but studies were not done at her death. Grosse et al. (1971) added two more cases. Features were intrauterine growth retardation (with primordial shortness of stature), microcephaly, variable degrees of eczema and mental retardation, and characteristic facies (blepharophimosis, micrognathia, apparent hypertelorism). Opitz et al. (1973) concluded that eczema may be absent, stature may be normal, and intelligence may also be normal, although head circumference is always below the third percentile. They observed first cousin parents. In the review of Opitz et al. (1973), first-cousin parents in 1 of 7 families and two affected sibs in at least 4 families were noted.

Dubowitz, V.: Familial low birthweight dwarfism with an unusual facies and a skin eruption. J. Med. Genet. 2: 12-17, 1965.

Grosse, R., Gorlin, J. and Opitz, J. M.: The Dubowitz syndrome. Z. Kinderheilk. 110: 175-187, 1971.

Opitz, J. M., Pfeiffer, R. A., Hermann, J. P. R. and Kushnick, T.: Studies of malformation syndromes of man, XXIV B: the Dubowitz syndrome. Further observations. Z. Kinderheilk. 116: 1-12, 173.

*22340 DUODENAL ATRESIA

Mishalany et al. (1970) described two children with duodenal atresia, all four parents of whom were descendents from one couple, being related as first cousins. In 1971 the same authors reported that a third affected child had been born in this kindred. See JEJUNAL ATRESIA. Der Kaloustian et al. (1974) reported yet another affected child.

Der Kaloustian, V. M., Slim, M. S. and Mishalany, H. G.: Familial congenital duodenal atresia (cont.). (Letter) Pediatrics 54: 118 only, 1974.

Mishalany, H. G., Der Kaloustian, V. M. and Ghandour, M.: Familial congenital duodenal atresia. Pediatrics 46: 629-632, 1970.

Mishalany, H. G., Der Kaloustian, V. M. and Ghandour, M. H.: Familial congenital duodenal atresia. (Letter) Pediatrics 47: 633-634, 1971.

22350 DWARFISM, LOW BIRTH-WEIGHT TYPE, WITH UNRESPONSIVENESS TO GROWTH HORMONE

Van Gemund et al. (1969) described two boys who were offspring of first-cousin parents and 'small for dates' at birth showed marked dwarfism, severe mental retardation, and congenital deafness. One relative was congenitally deaf with normal stature and intellect. A maternal uncle was an imbecile and dwarfed without deafness. Insulin-induced hypoglycemia evoked excessively high levels of immunoreactive HGH. They did not show increased sensitivity to fatty acid levels. Orally administered glucose suppressed HGH and evocated insulin secretion. Exogenous HGH did not decrease urinary nitrogen excretion or increase urinary hydroxyproline excretion. Growth promoting effects of exogenosis testosterone were intact. Unresponsiveness to somatotropic effects of HGH were postulated. The consanguinity suggests autosomal recessive inheritance. Since a maternal uncle had dwarfism and mental retardation, X-linked recessive inheritance is a possibility.

Van Gemund, J. J., Laurent de Angulo, M. S. and Vangelderen, H. H.: Familial prenatal dwarfism with elevated serum immuno-reactive growth hormone levels and end-organ unresponsiveness. Maandschr. Kindergeneesk. 37: 372-382, 1969.

22354 DWARFISM, MENTAL RETARDATION, EYE ABNORMALITY

Mollica et al. (1972) described two sisters and a brother with short stature, mental retardation, small head, and ocular abnormalities (iris hypoplasia, nuclear cataracts, severe myopia). Birth weights were not given. The parents, apparently unrelated, were from the same small village in Sicily.

Mollica, F., Pavone, L. and Antener, I.: Short stature, mental retardation and ocular alterations in three siblings. Helv. Paediat. Acta 27: 463-469, 1972.

22355 DWARFISM, PROPORTIONATE, WITH HIP DISLOCATION

McKusick (1966) reported on a woman with proportionate dwarfism and bilateral dislocated hips whose great-grandmothers through both her mother and her father were also dwarfed. The patient died following surgery for rheumatic heart disease. Fuhrmann (1972) told me of sisters with proportionate dwarfism and dislocation of the hip. The vertebral bodies showed columnization (greater height than AP dimension).

Fuhrmann, W.: Giessen, Germany: personal communication, 1972.

McKusick, V. A.: Medical Genetics 1961-1963. Oxford: Pergammon Press, 1966. Fig. 35, opposite P. 294. (Also J. Chron. Dis. 16: 457-634, 1963.)

22360 DWARFISM, 'SNUB-NOSED' TYPE

Levi (1910) described a variety of low-birth-weight dwarfs with normal proportions as 'microsomie essentielle.' Black (1961) referred to them as 'snub-nosed dwarfs.' Von Verschuer and Conradi (1938) suggested recessive inheritance. The low birth weight is probably not well documented and these may be instances of sexual ateleiosis (q.v.). I have seen an isolated case of what appears to be 'snub-nosed' dwarfism (D.M., 1550681). The patients pointed out that 'snub-nosed' may not be an acceptable designation for laymen. Low-birth-weight Levi dwarfism may be better. Levi (1910) pictured (see Black, 1961) affected father and son. Hence, autosomal dominant inheritance is possible.

Black, J.: Low birth weight dwarfism. Arch. Dis. Child. 36: 633-644, 1961.

Levi, E.: Contribution a la connaissance de la microsomie essentielle heredo-familiale: distinction de cette forme clinique d'avec les nanismes, les infantilismes et les formes mixtes de ces differentes dystrophies. N. Iconog. Salpet. 23: 522-570, 1910.

Von Verschuer, O. F. and Conradi, L.: Eine Sippe mit rezessiv erblichem primordialem Zwergwuchs. Z. Menschl. Vererb. Konstitutionsl. 22: 261-267, 1938.

22380 DYGGVE-MELCHIOR-CLAUSEN DISEASE

Among the children from uncle-niece marriage in Greenland, Dyggve et al. (1962) found three children with a condition resembling Hurler syndrome and Morquio syndrome in some respects. The fingers were clawed with limitation in extension. The patients were mentally retarded and the urine showed mucopolysaccharide. The spine showed generalized platyspondyly. Irregularities of the iliac crest gave an appearance of a lace border around it. The patient shown in family 12 (plate XII) of Hobaek's Norwegian study is probably identical.

Dyggve, H. V., Melchior, J. C. and Clausen, J.: Morquio-Ullrich's disease. An inborn error of metabolism? Arch. Dis. Child. 37: 525-534, 1962.

Hobaek, A.: Problems of Hereditary Chondrodysplasias. Oslo, Norway: Oslo U. Press, 1961.

*22390 DYSAUTONOMIA (RILEY-DAY SYNDROME)

Features are lack of tearing, emotional lability, paroxysmal hypertension, increased sweating, cold hands and feet, corneal anesthesia, erythematous blotching of the skin, and drooling. Almost all cases are Ashkenazi Jews. Brown, Beauchemin and Linde (1964) described the pathological findings in two Jewish sibs with this disease, namely, demyelination in the medulla, pontine reticular formation and dorso-longitudinal tracts, and degeneration, pigmentation and loss of cells in autonomic ganglia. Yatsu and Zussman (1964) provided follow-up on one of the 5 cases reported by Riley and Day in 1949. The patient died suddenly at age 31. In Israel, as in the United States, most cases are Ashkenazic Jews from Poland (Goldstein-Nieviazhski and Wallis, 1966). Rare non-Jewish cases have been well documented (Burke, 1966). Conditions which have been confused with dysautonomia include Biemond congenital and familial analgesia and neuropathy, congenital sensory, with anhidrosis. Goodall et al. (1971) demonstrated a decrease in synthesis of noradrenaline. Weinshilboum and Axelrod (1971) found decreased dopamine-beta-hydroxylase (DBH), the enzyme which converts dopamine to norepinephrine. Some dysautonomic children had no plasma DBH activity and their mothers had decreased activity.

Aguayo, A. J., Nair, C. P. V. and Bray, G. M.: Peripheral nerve abnormalities in the Riley-Day syndrome. Findings in a sural nerve biopsy. Arch. Neurol. 24: 106-116, 1971.

Brown, W. J., Beauchemin, J. A. and Linde, L. M.: A neuropathological study of familial dysautonomia (Riley-Day syndrome) in siblings. J. Neurol. Neurosurg. Psychiat. 27: 131-139, 1964.

Brunt, P. W. and McKusick, V. A.: Familial dysautonomia. A report of genetic and clinical studies, with a review of the literature. Medicine 49: 343-374, 1970.

Burke, V.: Familial dysautonomia. Aust. Paediat. J. 2: 58-63, 1966.

Gitlow, S. E., Bertani, L. M., Wilk, E., Li, B. L. and Dziedzic, S.: Excretion of catecholamine metabolites by children with familial dysautonomia. Pediatrics 46: 513-522, 1970.

Goldstein-Nieviazhski, C. and Wallis, K.: Riley-Day syndrome (familial dysautonomia). Survey of 27 cases. Ann. Paediat. 206: 188-194, 1966.

Goodall, M., Gitlow, S. E. and Alton, H.: Decreased noradrenaline (norepinephrine) synthesis in familial dysautonomia. J. Clin. Invest. 50: 2734-2740, 1971.

Hutchison, J. H. and Hamilton, W.: Familial dysautonomia in two siblings. Lancet 1: 1216-1218, 1962.

McKusick, V. A., Norum, R. A., Farkas, H. J., Brunt, P. W. and Mahloudji, M.: The Riley-Day syndrome — observations on genetics and survivorship. Israel J. Med. Sci. 3: 372-379, 1967.

Pearson, J., Finegold, M. J. and Budzilovich, G.: The tongue and taste in familial dysautonomia. Pediatrics 45: 739-745, 1970.

Riley, C. M.: Familial autonomic dysfunction. J.A.M.A. 149: 1532-1535, 1952.

Weinshilboum, R. M. and Axelrod, J.: Reduced plasma dopamine-beta-hydroxylase activity in familial dysautonomia. New Eng. J. Med. 285: 938-942, 1971.

Yatsu, F. and Zussman, W.: Familial dysautonomia (Riley-Day syndrome). Case report with post-mortem findings of a patient at age 31. Arch. Neurol. 10: 459-463, 1964.

22400 DYSAUTONOMIA-LIKE DISORDER

Schmidt et al. (1970) concluded that the disorder they observed in two daughters of a Sephardic uncle-niece marriage was a disorder distinct from familial dysautonomia, which, of course, occurs mainly in Ashkenazic Jews. In these patients mental retardation and normal taste, fungiform papillae, histamine test and urinary VMA excretion differentiate the condition. See NEUROPATHY, CONGENITAL SENSORY, WITH ANHIDROSIS, another dysautonomia like condition.

Schmidt, R., Alkan, W. J., Moses, S. W., Mundel, G. and Roizen, S.: A clinical entity simulating familial dysautonomia in a North African Jewish family. J. Pediat. 76: 283-288, 1970.

*22410 DYSERYTHROPOIETIC ANEMIA, HEMPAS TYPE OR TYPE II

Verwilghen et al. (1969) reported two families. De Lozzio et al. (1962) studied an affected woman with two affected sisters. The parents could not be examined. They demonstrated endopolyploidy by chromosome studies of bone marrow. The karyotype of skin cells was normal. They pointed out that several instances are known in plants and animals where the mitotic process is influenced by mutant genes. Crookston et al. (1969) observed 5 patients (including two sisters) with what appears to be the same disorder: anemia characterized by multiple nuclei in erythroblasts, ineffective erythropoiesis and lysis of red cells by acidified serum from some but not all persons. The Crookstons (1972) suggested the designation HEMPAS, an acronym for hereditary erythroblastic multinuclearity with positive acidified-serum test (also called HAM test). This appears to be the commonest form of inherited dyserythropoietic anemia. See 10560 and 22412 for two distinct forms, which do not have a positive acidified-serum test. This is called type II hereditary dyserythropoietic anemia in the classification of Wendt and Heimpel referred to in entry 22412. Enquist et al. (1972) described 3 cases in a sibship of 10. They described the occurrence of Gaucher-like histiocytes in bone marrow, resembling those seen in chronic myelogenous leukemia and thalassemia. They made the important observation that heterozygotes may show some of the serologic abnormalities of HEMPAS without clinical disease. Increased susceptibility to lysis by anti-I antibody (11080) is a feature of HEMPAS.

Crookston, J. H. and Crookston, M. C.: Hereditary anemia with multinuclear erythroblasts ('HEMPAS'). The Clinical Delineation of Birth Defects. XIV. Blood. Baltimore: Williams and Wilkins, 1972.

Crookston, J. H., Crookston, M. C., Burnie, K. L., Francombe, W. H., Dacie, J. V., Davis, J. A. and Lewis, S. M.: Hereditary erythroblastic multinuclearity associated with a positive acidified-serum test: a type of congenital dyserythropoietic anaemia. Brit. J. Haemat. 17: 11-26, 1969.

De Lozzio, C. B., Valencia, J. I. and Acame, E.: Chromosomal study in erythroblastic endopolyploidy. Lancet I: 1004-1005, 1962.

Roberts, P. D., Wallis, P. G. and Jackson, A. D. M.: Haemolytic anaemia with multinucleated normoblasts in the marrow. (Letter) Lancet I: 1186 only, 1962.

Verwilghen, R., Verhaegen, H., Waumans, P. and Beert, J.: Ineffective erythropoiesis with morphologically abnormal erythroblasts and unconjugated hyperbilirubinaemia. Brit. J. Haemat. 17: 27-33, 1969.

Verwilghen, R. L., Lewis, S. M., Dacie, J. V., Crookston, J. H. and Crockston, M. C.: Hempas: congenital dyserythropoietic anaemia (type II). Quart. J. Med. 42: 257-278, 1973.

*22412 DYSERYTHROPOIETIC ANEMIA, TYPE I

In 1967 Wendt and Heimpel described dizygotic twins both affected with a macrocytic form of dyserythropoietic anemia in which the bone marrow contained megaloblastoid erythroblasts with characteristic chromatin bridges between the nuclei. These authors gave the classification of dyserythropoietic anemia which is followed here. See 22410 and 10560 for the other two types.

Wendt, F. and Heimpel, H.: Kongenitale dyserythropoietische Anamie bei einem zweieiigen Zwillingspaar. Med. Klin. 62: 172-177, 1967.

22420 DYSGENESIS MESODERMALIS CORNEAE ET SCLERAE

Bertelsen (1968) described a brother and sister with first-cousin parents and markedly blue sclerae and thin cornea. In the girl, rupture of the cornea occurred in both eyes after slight indirect trauma. Megalocornea, deep anterior chambers and severe myopia were present. No signs of osteogenesis imperfecta were present in the patients or family. This may be the 'ocular form' of the Ehlers-Danlos syndrome (22541).

Bertelsen, T. I.: Dysgenesis mesodermalis corneae et sclerae. Rupture of both corneae in a patient with blue sclerae. Acta Ophthal. 46: 486-491, 1968.

*22430 DYSOSTEOSCLEROSIS

R
E
C
E
S
S
I
V
E

Spranger et al. (1968) used this term to distinguish a syndrome chiefly characterized by osteosclerosis and platyspondyly. The affected children are usually short and have a tendency to fracture. Cranial nerve compression occurs in some. Macular atrophy of the skin, flattened fingernails, and poorly calcified or chalky enamel has been noted. The calvarium, especially in the frontal area, and the base of the skull are sclerotic. The vertebral bodies are flattened, deformed and diffusely dense. While the rest of the long bones are sclerotic, widely splayed submetaphyseal portions are clear with irregularly coarse trabecular pattern. Affected sibs have been reported by Ellis (1934), Field (1939) and Stehr (1942). Parental consanguinity was noted by Spranger et al. (1968) and by Ellis (1934) and Field (1939).

Ellis, R. W. B.: Osteopetrosis (marble bones: Albers-Schonberg's disease: osteosclerosis fragilis generalisata: congenital osteosclerosis). Proc. Roy. Soc. Med. 27: 1563-1571, 1934.

Field, C. E.: Albers-Schonberg disease. Atypical case. Proc. Roy. Soc. Med. 32: 320-324, 1939.

Spranger, J. W., Albrecht, C., Rohwedder, H. J. and Wiedemann, H.-R.: Die Dysosteosklerose: eine Sonderform der generalisierten Osteosklerose. Fortschr. Roentgenstr. 109: 504-512, 1968.

Stehr, L.: Pathogenese und Klinik der Osteosklerosen. Arch. Orthop. Unfall-Chir. 41: 156-182, 1942.

22440 DYSOSTOSIS, ENCHONDRAL, OF NIERHOFF-HUBNER TYPE

The features are micromelia with normal stature at birth, sometimes microcephaly, severe epiphyseal and metaphyseal disturbances in the long bones, vertebrae and ribs. Of 6 sibs, a female and 2 males, died at the age of a few weeks. All showed clonic convulsions, and at autopsy leptomeningeal hemorrhages. Spranger (1974) subsequently determined that the disorder in these sibs was hypophosphatasia (24150).

Rupprecht, E. and Doerfel, E.: Enchondrale Dysostose Typ Nierhoff-Huebner bei 3 Geschwistern. Arch. Kinderheilk. 173: 64-73, 1966.

Spranger, J.: Kiel, personal communication, July 29, 1974.

*22450 DYSTONIA MUSCULORUM DEFORMANS

Santangelo (1934) observed 3 of 5 children affected, from a marriage of unaffected second cousins. Eldridge (1967) concluded, from a study of a large series of cases and their families in the United States that a recessive form is particularly frequent in Jews and differs from the autosomal dominant form in earlier age of onset and more consistent grade of severity. Eldridge et al. (1970) presented evidence favoring increased intelligence in this disorder. If a definite although perhaps more difficult to demonstrate superiority of intelligence were to occur in heterozygotes, the relatively high frequency of the dystonia gene in Jews might have its explanation therein.

Eldridge, R.: Bethesda, Md.: personal communication, 1967.

Eldridge, R., Harlan, A., Cooper, I. S. and Riklan, M.: Superior intelligence in recessively inherited torsion dystonia. Lancet I: 65-67, 1970.

Santangelo, G.: Contributo clinico alla conoscenza delle forme familiari della dysbasia lordotica progressiva (spasmo di torsione). G. Psychiat. Neuropat. 62: 52-77, 1934.

22455 DYSTONIA WITH 'RINGBINDEN'

A non-progressive disorder with multiple mild flexion contractures developing in infancy was described in two brothers by Fenichel et al. (1971). Motor strength was normal. Lower limb tendon reflexes were exaggerated but plantar responses were flexor. Associated findings were borderline normal intelligence, speech defect, choreic movements of the outstretched hands, normal cranial nerve, sensory and cerebellar functions, and EEG's indicating paroxysmal disorder. CPK was elevated in the younger boy. Muscle biopsies showed decreased fiber size, especially of the atpase positive type (A fibers), increased amounts of PAS positive material, and 'Ringbinden,' without typical myopathic or neuropathic changes. The authors interpreted the findings as the result of a primary cerebral disorders.

Fenichel, G. M., Olson, W. H. and Kilroy, A. W.: Hereditary dystonia associated with unique features in skeletal muscle. Arch. Neurol. 25: 552-559, 1971.

22460 DYSTONIA, PERIODIC

Smith and Heersema (1941) observed episodic dystonic movements of 5-10 seconds duration induced by movement in three unrelated sibships of Polish and Lithuanian extraction. Four, one and two sibs were affected. See FAMILIAL PAROXYSMAL CHOREO-ATHETOSIS for a somewhat similar condition inherited as a dominant. Also see DYSTONIA in the dominant catalog.

Smith, L. A. and Heersema, P. H.: Periodic dystonia. Proc. Mayo Clin. 16: 842-846, 1941.

22470 EBSTEIN ANOMALY

Gueron et al. (1966) described a brother and sister with Ebstein anomaly, a congenital malformation of the heart, which consists of downward placement of the tricuspid valve such that part of the right ventricle becomes incorporated into the pretricuspid chamber. Associated deformity of the tricuspid leaflets and defect of the atrial septum are frequent. Donegan et al. (1968) found Ebstein anomaly in a 6-year-old boy and his maternal uncle. Gouffault et al. (1960) found Ebstein malformation in one sib and a comparable deformity of the mitral valve in a sister. The same combination of Ebstein anomaly in one sib and comparable mitral anomaly in another was apparently present in the family reported by Yamauchi and Cayler (1964).

Donegan, C. C., Jr., Moore, M. M., Wiley, T. M., Jr., Hernandez, F. A., Green, J. R., Jr. and Schiebler, G. L.: Familial Ebstein's anomaly of the tricuspid valve. Am. Heart J. 75: 375-379, 1968.

Gouffault, J., Ledamany, L. and Lenegre, J.: Un type particulier d'anomalie congenitale de la valve mitrale. Arch. Mal. Coeur. 53: 1175-1181, 1960.

Gueron, M., Hirsch, M., Stern, J., Cohen, W. and Levy, M. J.: Familial Ebstein's anomaly with emphasis on the surgical treatment. Am. J. Cardiol. 18: 105-111, 1966.

Yamauchi, T. and Cayler, G. G.: Ebstein's anomaly in the neonate. A clinical study of three cases observed from birth through infancy. Am. J. Dis. Child. 107: 165-172, 1964.

22480 ECTODERMAL DYSPLASIA AND NEURISENSORY DEAFNESS

Mikaelian et al. (1970) described brother and sister whose parents were first cousins and who had hidrotic ectodermal dysplasia, sensorineural hearing loss (due probably to a defect of the cells of organ of Corti which are of ectodermal origin) and contracture of the fifth fingers. The sister also had thoracic scoliosis.

Mikaelian, D. O., Der Kaloustian, V. M., Shahin, N. A. and Barsoumian, V. M.: Congenital ectodermal dysplasia with hearing loss. Arch. Otolaryng. 92: 85-89, 1970.

*22490 ECTODERMAL DYSPLASIA, ANHIDROTIC

A rare autosomal recessive form of anhidrotic ectodermal dysplasia is suggested by the findings of Passarge, Nuzum and Schubert (1966) in inbred people of eastern Kentucky. Phenotypically the features were indistinguishable from those in males with the X-linked form. The existence of an autosomal recessive form is further supported strongly by the report by Gorlin et al. (1970) of a female with the full-blown syndrome and by their review of reported cases in females and of parental consanguinity.

Crump, I. A. and Danks, D. M.: Hypohidrotic ectodermal dysplasia. A study of sweatpores in the X-linked form and in a family with probable autosomal recessive inheritance. J. Pediat. 78: 466-473, 1971.

Gorlin, R. J., Old, T. and Anderson, V. E.: Hypohidrotic ectodermal dysplasia in females. A critical analysis and argument for genetic heterogeneity. Z. Kinderheilk. 108: 1-11, 1970.

Passarge, E., Nuzum, C. T. and Schubert, W. K.: Anhidrotic ectodermal dysplasia as autosomal recessive trait in an inbred kindred. Humangenetik 3: 181-185, 1966.

22500 ECTODERMAL DYSPLASIA, CLEFT LIP AND PALATE, HAND AND FOOT DEFORMITY AND MENTAL RETARDATION

Rosselli and Gulienetti (1961) described four patients with anhidrosis, hypotrichosis, microdontia, dysplasia of nails, cleft lip and palate, deformity of the fingers and toes, and malformation in the genitourinary system. Popliteal and perineal pterygium was also described. Syndactyly was the predominant digital deformity. Two were brother and sister whose parents were second cousins. A family observed by Bowen had 3 affected sibs out of 10. Cleft lip and palate, popliteal pterygium and digital and genital anomalies also occur apparently as a dominant (q.v.). The dominant EEC syndrome (12990) has similar features.

Bowen, P.: Edmonton, Alberta, Canada: personal communication, 1967.

Bowen, P. and Armstrong, H. B.: Cleft lip-palate, ectodermal dysplasia, hand-foot anomalies and oligophrenia. In, Bergsma, D. (ed.): Birth Defects. Atlas and Compendium. New York: National Foundation-March of Dimes, 1973. P. 262.

Rosselli, D. and Gulienetti, R.: Ectodermal dysplasia. Brit. J. Plast. Surg. 14: 190-204, 1961.

22510 ECTOPIA LENTIS

An autosomal recessive form of uncomplicated ectopia lentis may occur. This is not as well established, however, as is ectopia lentis with ectopia of the pupil (q.v.). See also WEILL-MARCHESANI SYNDROME and HOMOCYSTINURIA.

McKusick, V. A.: Primordial dwarfism and ectopia lentis. Am. J. Hum. Genet. 7: 189-198, 1955.

*22520 ECTOPIA LENTIS ASSOCIATED WITH ECTOPIA OF THE PUPIL

The lens and the pupil are usually displaced in opposite directions. Whether simple ectopia lentis is an entity separate from this is somewhat doubtful since simple and 'associated' forms are said to occur in the same family (Franceschetti, 1927; Diethelm, 1947). The recessive inheritance of combined ectopia lentis and ectopia pupillae has been well established (Siemens, 1920).

Diethelm, W.: Ueber Ectopia lentis ohne Arachnodaktylie und ihre Beziehungen zur Ectopia lentis et pupillae. Ophthalmologia 114: 16-32, 1947.

Franceschetti, A.: Ectopia lentis et pupillae congenita als rezessives Erbleiden und ihre Manifestierung durch Konsanguinitaet. Klin. Mbl. Augenheilk. 78: 351-362, 1927.

Francois, J.: Heredity in Ophthalmology. St. Louis: C. V. Mosby Co., 1961. p. 164, fig. 101.

Siemens, H. W.: Ueber die Aetiologie der Ectopia lentis et pupillae. Graefe. Arch. Ophthal. 109: 359-383, 1920.

Waardenburg, P. J.: Ueber das Erblichkeitsmoment bei der angeborenen Ektopie der Pupille und der Linse. Genetica 6: 337-382, 1924.

22530 ECTRODACTYLY (ABSENCE OF FINGERS) (SEE SPLIT-HAND)

Klein (1932) described an affected boy and girl born from the mating between a man and the daughter of his half-brother. When hereditary, this trait usually behaves as a dominant.

Klein, I. J.: Hereditary ectrodactylism in siblings. Am. J. Dis. Child. 43: 136-142, 1932.

R
E
C
E
S
S
I
V
E

*22540 EHLERS-DANLOS SYNDROME, TYPE VI (PROTO-COLLAGEN LYSYL HYDROXYLASE DEFICIENCY; OCULAR FORM OF E-D)

In two sisters with features somewhat suggesting the Ehlers-Danlos syndrome Pinnell et al. (1972) found deficiency of hydroxylysine in collagen with storkiometric replacement by lysine, and Krane et al. (1972) found deficiency of collagen lysyl hydroxylase. Hydroxylysine is important to cross-linking of collagen. Skin collagen was abnormally soluble. Clinical features included severe scoliosis from an early age, recurrent joint dislocations, stretchable skin, premature rupture of fetal membranes, floppiness in early life leading to the diagnosis of amyotonia congenita in one. The same patient, aged 9 years, had had one eye enucleated after an automobile accident. I mentioned this because I have a patient who appears to have the same defect (Lichtenstein, Nigra and Martin, 1972). This patient appears in fig. 5-12 of Heritable Disorders of Connective Tissue (McKusick, 1966) and was reported earlier in the ophthalmologic literature (Durham, 1953). On the basis of this patient Beighton (1970) raised the possibility of an autosomal recessive form of the Ehlers-Danlos syndrome, in which skin and joint changes like those of the dominant form occur but in addition serious ocular complications, particularly retinal detachment, are a conspicuous feature. He described affected brother and sister with normal parents. The affected male had four unaffected children. Mechanic (1972), looking at collagen in a clinically unspecified case of Ehlers-Danlos syndrome, found a deficiency of hydroxylysinonorleucine and other crosslinks and suggested a crosslinkage defect in this disease. Elsas et al. (1974) described a patient with apparent benefit from ascorbic acid.

Beighton, P. H.: Serious ophthalmological complications in the Ehlers-Danlos syndrome. Brit. J. Ophthal. 54: 263-268, 1970.

Durham, D. G.: Cutis hyperelastica (Ehlers-Danlos syndrome) with blue scleras, microcornea, and glucoma. Arch. Opthal. 49: 220, 1953.

Elsas, L. J., Hollins, B. and Pinnell, S. R.: Hydroxylysine-deficient collagen disease: effect of ascorbic acid. (Abstract) Am. J. Hum. Genet. 26: 28A only, 1974.

Krane, S. M., Pinnell, S. R. and Erbe, R. W.: Lysyl-protocollagen hydroxylase deficiency in fibroblasts from siblings with hydroxylysine-deficient collagen. Proc. Nat. Acad. Sci. 69: 2899-2903, 1972.

Lichtenstein, J. R., Nigra, T. P. and Martin, G. R.: Bethesda and Baltimore, Md.: personal communication, 1972.

Mechanic, G.: Crosslinking of collagen in a heritable disorder of connective tissue: Ehlers-Danlos syndrome. Biochim. Biophys. Res. Commun. 47: 267-272, 1972.

Pinnell, S. R., Krane, S. M., Kenzora, J. E. and Glimcher, M. J.: Heritable disorder with hydroxylysine-deficient collagen. Hydroxylysine-deficient collagen disease. New Eng. J. Med. 286: 1013-1020, 1972.

*22541 EHLERS-DANLOS SYNDROME, TYPE VII (PROCOLLAGEN PROTEASE DEFICIENCY; ARTHROCHALASIS MULTIPLEX CONGENITA)

In dermatosparaxis, a heritable disorder of connective tissue, in cattle and sheep, deficiency of the enzyme which cleaves the 'registration peptide' off the N-terminal end of collagen after it has been secreted from the fibroblasts has been demonstrated by Lapiere et al. (1971) and by Grant and Prockop (1972), respectively. The same defect has been demonstrated by Lichtenstein et al. (1973) in three patients with severe loosejointedness and mild stretchability and bruisability of the skin studied in this department. This should, like collagen lysyl hydroxylase deficiency (22540), be considered a form of the Ehlers-Danlos syndrome. Based on the three cases observed here, other clinical features of the disorder are short stature, epicanthal folds, depressed nasal bridge and micrognathia.

Hass, J. and Hass, R.: Arthrochalasis multiplex congenita. J. Bone Joint Surg. 40A: 663-674, 1958.

Lapiere, C. M., Lenaers, A. and Kohn, L. D.: Procollagen peptidase: an enzyme excising the coordination peptides of collagen. Proc. Nat. Acad. Sci. 68: 3054-3058, 1971.

Lichtenstein, J. R., Martin, G. R., Kohn, L. D., Byers, P. H. and McKusick, V. A.: Defect in conversion of procollagen to collagen in a form of Ehlers-Danlos syndrome. Science 182: 298-299, 1973.

*22550 ELLIS-VAN CREVELD SYNDROME (CHONDROECTODERMAL DYSPLASIA)

The largest pedigree is that observed by McKusick and colleagues (1964) in an inbred religious isolate, the Old Order Amish, in Lancaster County, Pennsylvania. Almost as many persons are known in this one kindred as are reported in all the medical literature. Features are dwarfism with most striking shortening in the distal part of the extremities, polydactyly, fusion of the hamate and capitate bones of the wrist, dystrophy of the fingernails, change in the upper lip variously called 'partial hare-lip,' 'lip-tie,' etc., and cardiac malformation, usually septal defects and often single atrium. Mesoectodermal dysplasia seems a better designation than chondroectodermal dysplasia. Blackburn and Belliveau (1971) reported two sibs with single atrium and hypoplastic left heart syndrome.

Alvarez-Borja, A.: Ellis-Van Creveld syndrome. Report of two cases. Pediatrics 26: 301-309, 1960.

Blackburn, M. G. and Belliveau, R. E.: Ellis-Van Creveld syndrome. A report of previously undescribed anomalies in two siblings. Am. J. Dis. Child. 122: 267-270, 1971.

Donlan, M. A., Murphy, J. J. and Brakel, C. A.: Ellis-Van Creveld syndrome associated with complete situs inversus. Clin. Pediat. 8: 366-368, 1969.

Douglas, W. F., Schonholtz, G. J. and Geppert, L. J.: Chondroectodermal dysplasia (Ellis-Van Creveld syndrome). Am. J. Dis. Child. 97: 473-478, 1959.

RECESSIVE

Hirokawa, K. and Suzuki, S.: Ellis-Van Creveld syndrome: report of an autopsy case. Acta Path. Jap. 17: 139-143, 1967.

Husson, G. S. and Parkman, P.: Chondroectodermal dysplasia (Ellis-Van Creveld syndrome) with a complex cardiac malformation. Pediatrics 28: 285-292, 1961.

McKusick, V. A., Egeland, J. A., Eldridge, R. and Krusen, D. E.: Dwarfism in the Amish. I. The Ellis-Van Creveld syndrome. Bull. Hopkins Hosp. 115: 306-336, 1964.

Walls, W. L., Altman, D. H. and Winslow, O. P.: Chondroectodermal dysplasia (Ellis-Van Creveld syndrome). Report of a case and review of the literature. Am. J. Dis. Child. 98: 242-248, 1959.

*22560 EMG SYNDROME (EXOMPHALOS-MACROGLOSSIA-GIGANTISM SYNDROME; BECK-WITH-WIEDEMANN SYNDROME)

The enlarged tongue, together with omphalocele or other umbilical abnormalities, permits recognition of the disorder at birth. Because many of the affected infants have hypoglycemia in the first days of life, anticipation of this complication can prevent serious neurologic sequelae. Visceromegaly, adrenocortical cytoanegaly and dysplasia of the renal medulla are conspicuous features. Adrenal carcinoma or nephroblastoma occurs with increased frequency. Wiedemann (1964) reported three affected sibs and Irving (1967) observed a family with two affected sibs and an affected second cousin. I have seen this disorder in a Negro child and Thorburn et al. (1970) described 6 cases in Jamaican Negroes and estimated an incidence of 1 in 13,700 births.

Beckwith, J. B.: Macroglossia, omphalocele, adrenal cytomegaly, gigantism, and hyperplastic visceromegaly. The Clinical Delineation of Birth Defects. II. Malformation Syndromes. New York: National Foundation, 1969. Pp. 188-196.

Filippi, G. and McKusick, V. A.: The Beckwith-Wiedemann syndrome (the exomphalos-macroglossia-gigantism syndrome): report of two cases and review of the literature. Medicine 49: 279-298, 1970.

Irving, I. M.: Exomphalos with macroglossia: a study of eleven cases. J. Pediat. Surg. 2: 499-507, 1967.

Irving, I. M.: The 'E.M.G.' syndrome (exomphalos, macroglossia, gigantism). Progr. Pediat. Surg. 1: 1-16, 1970.

Reddy, J. K., Schimke, R. N., Chang, C. H. J., Svoboda, D. J., Slaven, J.: Beckwith-Wiedemann syndrome. Wilms' tumor, cardiac hamartoma, persistent visceromegaly, and glomeruloneogenesis in a 2-year-old boy. Arch. Path. 94: 523-532, 1972.

Thorburn, M. J., Wright, E. S., Miller, C. G. and Smith-Read, E. H. M.: Exomphalos-macroglossia-gigantism syndrome in Jamaican infants. Am. J. Dis. Child. 119: 316-321, 1970.

Wiedemann, H.-R.: Complexe malformatif familial avec hernie ombilicale et macroglossie — un 'syndrome nouveau'? J. Genet. Hum. 13: 223-232, 1964.

Wiedemann, H.-R.: Das EMG-Syndrome: Exomphalos, Makroglossie, Gigantismus und Kohlenhydratstoffwechselstoerung. Z. Kinderheilk. 106: 171-185, 1969.

Wiedemann, H.-R., Spranger, J. W., Mogharei, M., Kubler, W., Tolksdorf, M., Bontemps, M., Drescher, J. and Gunschera, H.: Ueber das Syndrom Exomphalos-Makroglossie-Gigantismus, ueber generalisierte Muskelhypertrophie, progressive Lipodystrophie und Miescher-Syndrom im Sinne diencephaler Syndrome. Z. Kinderheilk. 102: 1-36, 1968.

22570 ENCEPHALOMALACIA, MULTILOCULAR

Crome and Williams (1960) observed multilocular encephalomalacia in an infant who died at one month of age. A sib was living at age 6 years but may have had the same abnormality manifested by microcephaly, spastic diplegia and idiocy. It is not certain that this is a distinct entity.

Crome, L. and Williams, C.: The problem of familial multilocular encephalomalacia. Acta Paediat. 49: 175-184, 1960.

*22600 ENDOCARDIAL FIBROELASTOSIS

The reports of endocardial fibroelastosis in sibs include those of Vestermark (1962), Winter and colleagues (1960), Zanker and Fisher (1960) and McKusick and colleagues (1962). Moller et al. (1966) described endocardial fibroelastosis in a young woman who died of heart failure during the postpartum period and in the child who was born of that pregnancy and died at 11 months of age. Either genetic causation or viral infection was suggested. Among the children of first-cousin parents Rafinski et al. (1967) observed three who died of endocardial fibroelastosis at ages of 10, 11 and 13 years, which is longer survival than is usual. Although the accumulated experience strongly supports the existence of an autosomal recessive variety of endocardial fibroelastosis, many cases may occur on a non-genetic basis. Hunter and Keay (1973) found 9 of 16 affected sibs in 4 families and suggested autosomal dominant inheritance with incomplete penetrance as the basis for their findings. EFE is called primary or secondary according to whether malformations are not or are associated. Weinberg and Himelfarb (1943) first introduced the term EFE, although the disorder had been described under other designations before. Hunter and Keay (1973) described a family in which two sisters had five affected children, one having affected children by different husbands. Autosomal dominant inheritance with incomplete penetrance was suggested.

Hunter, A. S. and Keay, A. J.: Primary endocardial fibroelastosis. An inherited condition. Arch. Dis. Child. 48: 66-69, 1973.

Lee, M. O., Liebman, J., Steinberg, A. G., Perrin, E. V. and Whitman, V.: Familial occurrence of endocardial fibroelastosis in three siblings, including identical twins. Pediatrics 51: 402-411, 1973.

McKusick, V. A. and colleagues: Medical genetics 1961. J. Chronic Dis. 15: 417-572, 1962 (fig. 18).

Moller, J. H., Fisch, R. O., From, A. H. L. and Edwards, J. E.: Endocardial fibroelastosis occurring in a mother and son. Pediatrics 38: 918-921, 1966.

Rafinski, T., Golenia, A., Wozniewicz, B. and Wlad, S.: Familial endocardial fibroelastosis. J. Pediat. 70: 574-576, 1967.

Vestermark, S.: Primary endocardial fibroelastosis in siblings. Acta Paediat. 51: 94-96, 1962.

Weinberg, T. and Himelfarb, A. J.: Endocardial fibroelastosis (so-called fetal endocarditis): a report of two cases occurring in siblings. Bull. Johns Hopkins Hosp. 72: 299-306, 1943.

Winter, S. T., Moses, W. S., Cohen, N. J. and Naftalin, J. M.: Primary endocardial fibroelastosis in two sisters. Am. J. Dis. Child. 99: 529-533, 1960.

Zanker, T. and Fisher, R. S.: Endocardial fibroelastosis in siblings. Maryland Med. J. 9: 60-65, 1960.

22610 ENDOCARDIAL FIBROELASTOSIS AND COARCTATION OF ABDOMINAL AORTA

Hallidie-Smith and Olsen (1968) described a girl and her two affected brothers. Mitral regurgitation was present. The parents were not related.

Hallidie-Smith, K. A. and Olsen, E. G. J.: Endocardial fibro-elastosis, mitral incompetence, and coarctation of abdominal aorta. A report of 3 sibs. Brit. Heart J. 30: 850-858, 1968.

*22620 ENTEROKINASE DEFICIENCY

Hadorn et al. (1969) described a female infant with diarrhea, failure to thrive and hypoproteinemic edema who was shown to have deficiency of the intestinal enterokinase which activates pancreatic proteolytic enzymes (trypsin, chymotrypsin and carboxypeptidase-A). The parents were not studied.

Hadorn, B., Tarlow, M. J., Lloyd, J. and Wolff, O. H.: Intestinal enterokinase deficiency. Lancet I: 812-813, 1969.

Tarlow, M. J., Hadorn, B., Arthurton, M. W. and Lloyd, J. K.: Intestinal enterokinase deficiency. A newly-recognized disorder of protein digestion. Arch. Dis. Child. 45: 651-655, 1970.

*22630 ENTEROPATHY, PROTEIN-LOSING

R
E
C
E
S
S
I
V
E

In the family described by Sheba et al. (1968) inheritance appeared clearly to be autosomal recessive. Intestinal lymphangiectasia was suspected but not proved. See LYMPHANGIECTASIA, INTESTINAL (15280). In a later publication they (Shani et al., 1974) concluded that intestinal lymphangiectasia was not present. The kindred was from an inbred Christian Arab group living in Israel. Eight of 28 children in two sibships were affected. The parents were in each case related as first-cousins-once-removed and the two affected sibships were first-cousins through their mothers and second-cousins through their fathers. Affected children showed edema, growth retardation, diarrhea, abdominal pain and clubbing. Ascites and death occurred in four; an autopsy, performed in two of these, showed hepatic vein stenosis which caused a Budd-Chiari syndrome. Lymphocyte counts were normal. Iron-deficiency anemia and hympoproteinemia were shown by all eight.

Sheba, C., Shami, M., Frand, M., Theodor, E. and Rotem, Y.: Familial protein losing enteropathy. Proc. Tel-Hashomer Hosp. 7: 62-66, 1968.

Shani, M., Theodore, E., Frand, M. and Goldman, B.: A family with protein-losing enteropathy. Gastroenterology 66: 433-445, 1974.

22640 EPIDERMODYSPLASIA VERRUCIFORMIS

Sullivan and Ellis (1939) found that of the 16 previously reported families, four had consanguineous parents. The lesions often resemble verrucae planae. The mucous membranes, hair and nails are not affected. Malignant degeneration, usually of the superficial basal cell type, is frequent. Characteristic changes in the epidermal cells with peculiar vacuolization are observed.

Ellis (1953) stated that this disorder occurs most frequently in Orientals. It is by no means proved that this is a Mendelizing disorder. The view that epidermodysplasia verruciformis is an extensive form of viral verrucae planae is supported by successful autoinnoculation and heteroinnoculation experiments. Lutz (1957) who was one of the first to describe the condition, accepted that it is not an entity but suggested that genetic predisposition may account for the extensiveness of the eruption of warts. Familial aggregation was described by Midana (1949) and by Jablonska et al. (1966). Hermann (1955) found parental consanguinity. Baker (1968) as well as others demonstrated, by electron microscopy, particles suggesting papovavirus.

Baker, H.: Epidermodysplasia verruciformis with electron microscopic demonstration of virus. Proc. Roy. Soc. Med. 61: 589-590, 1968.

Ellis, F.: In discussion of Barker and Sachs. Arch. Derm. 67: 443-455, 1953.

Hermann, H.: Epidermodysplasia verruciformis: Erb- und Erscheinungsbild. Z. Menschl. Vererb. Konstitutionsl. 32: 409-417, 1955.

Jablonska, S. and Formas, I.: Weitere positive Ergebnisse mit Auto- und Heteroinokulation bei Epidermodysplasia verruciformis Lewandowsky-Lutz. Dermatologica 118: 86-93, 1959.

Jablonska, S., Fabjanska, L. and Formas, I.: On the viral etiology of epidermodysplasia verruciformis. Dermatologica 132: 369-385, 1966.

Lutz, W.: Zur Epidermodysplasia verruciformis. Dermatologica 115: 309-314, 1957.

Midana, A.: Sulla questione dei rapporti tra epidermodysplasia verruciformis e verrucosi generalizzata. Dermatologica 99: 1-23, 1949.

Sullivan, M. and Ellis, F. A.: Epidermodysplasia verruciformis (Lewandowsky and Lutz). Arch. Derm. Syph. 40: 422-432, 1939.

*22650 EPIDERMOLYSIS BULLOSA DYSTROPHICA NEUROTROPHICA (EPIDERMOLYSIS BULLOSA WITH CONGENITAL DEAFNESS)

This 'new' entity was delineated by Gedde-Dahl (1970). The features are onset of localized traumatic blistering in late childhood or adolescence, onset of nail manifestations several years before the skin manifestations, diffuse and slowly progressive skin atrophy of hands, feet, elbows, knees, palms and soles with loss of dermal ridge pattern of fingers, occasional blistering of oral mucosa and congenital, slowly progressive perceptive deafness.

Gedde-Dahl, T., Jr.: Epidermolysis bullosa. A Clinical, Genetic and Epidemiological Study. Oslo, Norway, 1970.

*22660 EPIDERMOLYSIS BULLOSA DYSTROPHICA

There may be five varieties of epidermolysis bullosa (Davison, 1965): (1) dominant epidermolysis bullosa simplex, (2) dominant epidermolysis bullosa of Cockayne, (3) dominant epidermolysis bullosa dystrophica, (4) recessive epidermolysis bullosa dystrophica, and (5) recessive epidermolysis bullosa letalis. This severe and destructive form of epidermolysis bullosa may be present at birth or appears in infancy. Hands, feet, elbows and knees are sites of predilection. Bullae also develop on the mucosal surfaces and even the conjunctiva and cornea may be involved. The impressive kindred reported by Hofman is diagrammed on page 279 of von Verschuer (1959). Bauer et al. (1974) demonstrated elevated collagenase in the lesions and in unaffected skin of patients with recessive epidermolysis bullosa dystrophica.

Bauer, E. A., Gedde-Dahl, T. and Eisen, A. Z.: Rose of human skin collagenase in dystrophic epidermolysis bullosa. (Abstract) Clin. Res. 22: 326A only, 1974.

Book, J.: Frequence de mutation de la chondrodystrophie et de l'epidermolyse bulleuse dans une population du sud de la Suede. J. Genet. Hum. 1: 24-26, 1952.

Davison, B. C. C.: Epidermolysis bullosa. J. Med. Genet. 2: 233-242, 1965.

Didolkar, M. S., Gerner, R. E. and Moore, G. E.: Epidermolysis bullosa dystrophica and epithelioma of the skin: review of published cases and report of an additional patient. Cancer 33: 198-202, 1974.

Heinrichsbauer, F.: Ein weiterer Beitrag zur Frage angeborener Hautdefekte. (Uber ein familiaeres letales Krankheitsbild mit Blasenbildung und angeborenen Defekten der Haut). Arch. Gynaek. 134: 673-692, 1928.

Robinson, M. M.: Epidermolysis bullosa hereditaria. Urol. Cutan. Rev. 50: 545-561, 1946.

Schnyder, U. W. and Eichhoff, D.: Zur Klinik und Genetik der dominant-dystrophischen Epidermolysis bullosa hereditaria. Arch. Derm. 218: 62-90, 1963.

Sorsby, A.: (ed.) Clinical Genetics. St. Louis: C. V. Mosby Co., 1953. P. 136.

Sorsby, A., Roberts, J. A. F. and Brain, R. T.: Essential shrinking of conjunctiva in hereditary affection allied to epidermolysis bullosa. Docum. Ophthal. 5-6: 118-150, 1951.

Von Verschuer, O. F.: Genetik des Menschen. Lehrbuch der Humangenetik. Berlin: Urban und Schwarzenberg, 1959.

*22670 EPIDERMOLYSIS BULLOSA LETALIS

Roberts and colleagues (1960) described three cases in branches of a French-Canadian family from an area in Nova Scotia with much inbreeding. The infants were born with bullous lesions and died at 20, 24 and 42 days, respectively, despite meticulous nursing care, antibiotics, corticosteroids and increased dietary protein. Loss of serum protein and electrolytes and dermal sepsis seemed to have been responsible for death.

Klunker (1963) thought it doubtful that the two forms of epidermolysis bullosa here listed are separate and distinct. Even if distinct, their allelic versus non-allelic relationship is, of course, unknown. Davison (1965) also found 'lethal' cases in the same sibship as cases with the dysthrophic form. Cross et al. (1968) studied an extensively involved kindred. The consistently lethal behavior suggests that it may indeed be distinct. Congenital absence of skin in localized areas is probably due to intrauterine trauma and bullae. The hands and feet are relatively spared. Except for dystrophic nails the patients can completely recover after age two years if therapy with massive steroids and prevention and therapy of infections are adequate.

Bergenholtz, A. and Olsson, O.: Epidermolysis bullosa hereditaria. I. Epidermolysis bullosa hereditaria letalis. A survey of the literature and report of 11 cases. Acta Dermatovener. 48: 220-241, 1968.

Cross, H. E., Wells, R. S. and Esterly, J. R.: Inheritance in epidermolysis bullosa letalis. J. Med. Genet. 5: 189-196, 1968.

Davison, B. C. C.: Epidermolysis bullosa. J. Med. Genet. 2: 233-242, 1965.

Klunker, W.: Zur nosologischen Stellung der Epidermolysis bullosa hereditaria letalis Herlitz (mit Kasuistik). Arch. Klin. Exp. Derm. 216: 74-100, 1963.

Pearson, R. W., Potter, B. and Strauss, F.: Epidermolysis bullosa hereditaria letalis. Arch. Derm. 109: 349-355, 1974.

R
E
C
E
S
S
I
V
E

Roberts, M. H., Howell, D. R. S., Bramhall, J. L. and Reubner, B.: Epidermolysis bullosa letalis: report of three cases with particular reference to the histopathology of the skin. Pediatrics 25: 283-290, 1960.

22680 EPILEPSY, PHOTOGENIC, WITH SPASTIC DIPLEGIA AND MENTAL RETARDATION

Daly, Siekert and Burke (1959) found 3 of 4 sibs affected.

Daly, D., Siekert, R. G. and Burke, E. C.: A variety of familial light sensitive epilepsy. Electroenceph. Clin. Neurophysiol. 11: 141-145, 1959.

*22690 EPIPHYSEAL DYSPLASIA

Juberg and Holt (1968) described three sisters and a brother with multiple epiphyseal dysplasia. The parents were normal and not related. This experience and some reported in the literature, including instances of parental consanguinity, led them to support recessive inheritance for one form of multiple epiphyseal dysplasia.

Hunt, D. D., Ponseti, I. V., Pedrini-Mille, A. and Pedrini, V.: Multiple epiphyseal dysplasia in two siblings. J. Bone Joint Surg. 49A: 1611-1627, 1967.

Juberg, R. C. and Holt, J. F.: Inheritance of multiple epiphyseal dysplasia, tarda. Am. J. Hum. Genet. 20: 549-563, 1968.

Watt, J. K.: Multiple epiphyseal dysplasia. A report of four cases. Brit. J. Surg. 39: 533-535, 1952.

22695 EPIPHYSEAL DYSPLASIA OF FEMORAL HEADS, MYOPIA, DEAFNESS

In three sons of third-cousin parents Pfeiffer et al. (1973) described a syndrome of femoral capital epiphyseal dysplasia, severe myopia and deafness. Stature was normal. Although the femoral heads showed the most striking epipsyseal dysplasia, the changes were apparently not limited to that site. The authors find no reported case that seemed identical to these.

Pfeiffer, R. A., Junemann, G., Polster, and Bauer, H.: Epiphyseal dysplasia of the femoral head, severe myopia and perceptive hearing loss in three brothers. Clin. Genet. 4: 141-144, 1973.

22700 ERYTHEMA OF ACRAL REGIONS

In a brother and sister and a paternal first-cousin of theirs, Bryan and Coskey (1967) described an asymptomatic, papular and placque-like erythema appearing in infancy and involving the external ears and limbss. In the sibship of the affected sibs, four had clubfoot and dental anomalies.

Bryan, H. G. and Coskey, R. J.: Familial erythema of acral regions. Arch. Derm. 95: 483-486, 1967.

22710 ERYTHRODERMIA DESQUAMATIVA OF LEINER

Simon, Becker and Wiedemann (1965) described three male sibs with erythroderma, severe diarrhea and reduced resistance to infection. Death occurred at the age of 2, 6 and 9 months. Postmortem findings included lymphatic hypoplasia and increase in reticular cells of the lymph nodes.

Simon, C., Becker, V. and Wiedemann, H.-R.: Uber ein unter dem Bilde der Erythrodermia desquamativa Leiner verlaufenes todliches Leiden bei drei Brudern. Z. Kinderheilk. 94: 12-24, 1965.

*22720 EUNUCHOIDISM, FAMILIAL HYPOGONADOTROPHIC

In some families both males and females are affected (Biben and Gordan, 1955) and only members of one generation (Hurxthal, 1943). Le Marquand (1954) described three affected brothers and two affected sisters in the same family. The parents were not related. It is likely that there is a recessively inherited monotropic pituitary defect, limited to gonadotropin, comparable to the monotropic defect of growth hormone demonstrated in sexual ateliotic dwarfs ('midgets'). Ewer (1968) observed affected brother and 2 sisters from a marriage of second cousins once removed. Another sib, a male, deceased, was probably affected. Absence of secondary sex characteristics and relatively long extremities were the only findings. Clomiphene administration has no effect (Ewer, 1968).

Biben, R. L. and Gordan, G. S.: Familial hypogonadotropic eunuchoidism. J. Clin. Endocrin. 15: 931-942, 1955.

Ewer, R. W.: Familial monotropic pituitary gonadotropin insufficiency. J. Clin. Endocr. 28: 783-788, 1968.

Hurxthal, L. M.: Sublingual use of testosterone in 7 cases of hypogonadism: report of 3 congenital eunuchoids occurring in one family. J. Clin. Endocr. 3: 551-556, 1943.

Le Marquand, H. S.: Congenital hypogonadotrophic hypogonadism in five members of a family, three brothers and two sisters. Proc. Roy. Soc. Med. 47: 442-446, 1954.

Spitz, I. M., Diamant, Y., Rosen, E., Bell, J., Ben-David, M., Polishuk, W. and Rabinowitz, D.: Isolated gonadotropin deficiency. A heterogenous syndrome. New Eng. J. Med. 290: 10-15, 1974.

22723 EXUDATIVE VITREORETINOPATHY, FAMILIAL

This disorder was first described by Criswick and Schepens (1969) on the basis of six patients in two kindreds. The findings bore some similarities to retrolental fibroplasia and to Coats disease. The changes were slowly progressive. Affected children were otherwise healthy. None was premature or treated neonatally with oxygen. Posterior vitreous detachment with organized membranes were found in all quadrants. Vitreoretinal traction was produced by the membranes and resulted in displacement of the macula. Snowflake opacies were scattered through the vitreous. Localized retinal detachments and recurrent vitreous hemorrhages from peripheral new vessels were noted. A brother and sister in one family were affected. In the other family three brothers and their maternal uncle were affected. A distant male relative related through females was blind, making X-linked recessive inheritance a possibility. This may be the same as congenital falciform retinal detachment (22190), or pseudoglioma (26420).

Criswick, V. G. and Schepens, C. L.: Familial exudative vitreoretinopathy. Am. J. Ophthal. 68: 578-594, 1969.

22725 EYE COLOR

This is almost certainly a polygenic trait. The early view that blue is a simple recessive has been repeatedly shown to be wrong by observation of brown-eyed offspring of two blue-eyed parents.

Davenport, G. C. and Davenport, C. B.: Heredity of eye color in man. Science 26: 589-592, 1907.

Rufer, V., Bauer, J. and Soukup, F.: On the heredity of eye colour. Acta Univ. Carol. Med. 16: 429-434, 1970.

22727 FACIAL ABNORMALITIES, KYPHOSCOLIOSIS AND MENTAL RETARDATION

Jammes et al. (1973) described two brothers with a new mental retardation syndrome characterized by macrocephaly, hypertelorism, downward slanted palpebral slits, protruding tongue, kyphoscoliosis and marked difficulty walking. No parental consanguinity was noted.

Jammes, J., Mirhossen, S. A. and Holmes, L. B.: Syndrome of facial abnormalities, kyphoscoliosis and severe mental retardation. Clin. Genet. 4: 203-209, 1973.

*22728 FACIAL ECTODERMAL DYSPLASIA

Setleis et al. (1963) described five children in three apparently unrelated Puerto Rican families who had an aged leonine appearance with puckered skin about the eyes, absent eyelashes on both lids or multiple brows on the upper lids and none on the lower lids, eyebrows which slanted sharply upward laterally and a rubbery feel of the nose and chin. Some of the patients showed bilateral temporal marks superficially like forceps marks and like the lesions seen in focal facial dermal dysplasia, a dominant disorder (13650).

Setleis, H., Kramer, B., Valcarcel, M..and Einhorn, A. H.: Congenital ectodermal dysplasia of the face. Pediatrics 32: 540-548, 1963.

22729 FACIO-OCULO-ACUSTICO-RENAL (FOAR) SYNDROME

Murdoch amd Mengel (1971) and Holmes and Schepens (1972) separately reported on a brother and sister with a syndrome of ocular and facial anomalies, telecanthus, perceptive deafness, epiphyseal dysplasia of the femoral heads and proteinuria. Myopia and both telecanthus and true hypertelorism were present. Confusion with Waardenburg syndrome was possible. Fraser (1974) described a single case. In his patient the urine contained 250 mgm. of protein per 100 ml.

Fraser, G.: The Causes of Profound Deafness in Childhood. A Study of 3535 Individuals With Severe Auditory Handicaps Present at Birth or of Childhood Onset. Baltimore: Johns Hopkins University Press, 1974.

Holmes, L. B. and Schepens, C. L.: Syndrome of ocular and facial anomalies, telecanthus and deafness. J. Pediat. 81: 552-555, 1972.

Murdoch, J. L. and Mengel, M. C.: An unusual eye-ear syndrome with renal abnormality. Clinical Delineation of Birth Defects. IX. Ear. New York: National Foundation — March of Dimes, 1971. P. 136.

Ozer, F. L.: A possible 'new' syndrome with eye and renal abnormalities. In, Bergsma, D. (ed.): Clinical Delineation of Birth Defects. XVI. Urinary System and Others. Baltimore: Williams and Wilkins, 1974. P. 168 only.

22730 FACTOR V AND FACTOR VIII, COMBINED DEFICIENCY OF

Congenital hemorrhagic disorders characterized by deficiency of two clotting factors comprise a disputed group. Combined deficiency of factors V and VIII is supported by relatively convincing laboratory data. Seven patients in 5 families have been described. At least three of five parental matings were consanguineous (Jones et al., 1962). Up to 1958 (Seibert et al., 1958) four cases in three families had been described. All four were males. Two were brothers and the parents were consanguineous in two instances but the third set of parents came from the same small Yugoslavian village.

Jones, J. H., Rizza, C. R., Hardisty, R. M., Dormandy, K. M., and MacPherson, J. C.: Combined deficiency of factor V and factor VIII (antihemophilic globulin). A report of three cases. Brit. J. Heamat. 8: 120-128, 1962.

Seibert, R. H., Margolius, A., Jr. and Ratnoff, O. D.: Observations on hemophilia, parahemophilia and coexistent hemophilia and parahemophilia. Alterations in the platelets and the thromboplastin generation test. J. Lab. Clin. Med. 52: 449-462, 1958.

*22740 FACTOR V DEFICIENCY (OWREN PARAHEMOPHILIA; LABILE FACTOR DEFICIENCY)

The diagnosis of this hemorrhagic diathesis is made by the prolonged one-stage prothrombin time which is completely corrected by the addition of fresh deprothrombinized rabbit plasma. Bleeding times and clotting times are consistently prolonged. Clinical bleeding is usually mild. Heterozygotes have lowered levels of factor V but probably never have abnormal bleeding. Parental consanguinity was described by Kingsley (1954), and by Seibert, Margolius and Ratnoff (1958).

Friedman, I. A., Quick, A. J., Higgins, F., Hussey, C. V. and Hickey, M. E.: Hereditary labile factor (factor V) deficiency. J.A.M.A. 175: 370-374, 1961.

R E C E S S I V E

Kingsley, C. S.: Familial factor V deficiency: the pattern of heredity. Quart. J. Med. 23: 323-329, 1954.

Seibert, R. H., Margolius, A., Jr. and Ratnoff, O. D.: Observations on hemophilia, parahemophilia and coexistent hemophilia and parahemophilia. Alterations in the platelets and the thromboplastin generation test. J. Lab. Clin. Med. 52: 449-462, 1958.

*22750 FACTOR VII DEFICIENCY (HYPOPROCONVERTINEMIA)

Recessive inheritance is established by the demonstration of lower-than-normal levels of factor VII in both parents (Kupfer, Hanna and Kinne, 1960). See review by Marder and Shulman (1964). The Dubin-Johnson syndrome (23750) shows association with deficiency of factor VII. The mechanism of the association is not clear.

Denson, K. W. E., Conrad, J. and Samama, M.: Genetic variants of factor VII. (Letter) Lancet I: 1234 only, 1972.

Glueck, H. I. and Sutherland, J. M.: Inherited factor-VII defect in Negro family. Pediatrics 27: 204-213, 1961.

Hitzig, W. H. and Zollinger, W.: Kongenitaler Faktor-VII Mangel. Familienuntersuchung und physiologische Studien ueber den Faktor VII. Helv. Paediat. Acta 13: 189-203, 1958.

Kupfer, H. G., Hanna, B. L. and Kinne, D. R.: Congenital factor VII deficiency with normal Stuart activity: clinical, genetic and experimental observations. Blood 15: 146-163, 1960.

Marder, V. J. and Shulman, N. R.: Clinical aspects of congenital factor VII deficiency. Am. J. Med. 37: 182-194, 1964.

Spurling, N. W., Burton, L. K., Peacock, R. and Pilling, T.: Hereditary factor-VII deficiency in the beagle. Brit. J. Haemat. 23: 59-68, 1972.

*22760 FACTOR X DEFICIENCY (DEFICIENCY OF STUART-PROWER FACTOR)

The bleeding tendency is manifested by prolonged nasal and mucosal hemorrhage, menorrhagia, hematuria and occasionally hemarthrosis. Mr. Stuart and Miss Prower were the first persons shown to have this abnormality. Mr. Stuart was the product of an aunt-nephew mating. Girolami et al. (1970) described a hemorrhagic disorder which may be the result of an abnormal factor X. Polymorphism of factors IX and X were suggested by the findings of Lester et al. (1972).

Bachmann, F.: Familienuntersuchungen beim kongenitalen Stuart-Prower-Factor Mangel. Arch. Klaus Stift. Vererbungsforsch. 33: 27-78, 1958.

Dodds, W. J.: Canine factor X (Stuart-Prower factor) deficiency. J. Lab. Clin. Med. 82: 560-566, 1973.

Girolami, A., Lazzarin, M., Scarpa, R. and Brunetti, A.: Further studies on the abnormal factor X (factor X friuli) coagulation disorder: a report of another family. Blood 37: 534-541, 1971.

Girolami, A., Molaro, G., Lazzarin, N., Scarpa, R. and Brunetti, A.: Congenital haemorrhagic condition similar but not identical to factor X deficiency. A haemorrhagic state due to an abnormal factor X? Scand. J. Haemat. 7: 91-99, 1970.

Girolami, A., Molaro, G., Lazzarin, N., Scarpa, R. and Brunetti, A.: A 'new' congenital haemorrhagic condition due to the presence of an abnormal factor X (factor X friuli): study of a large kindred. Brit. J. Haemat. 19: 179-192, 1970.

Girolami, A., Nicolini, R., Furlani, E. and Bareggi, G.: Abnormal factor X (factor X friuli) coagulation disorder. Acta Haemat. 49: 114-122, 1973.

Lester, R. H., Elston, R. C. and Graham, J. B.: Variations in levels of blood clotting factors IX and X in a population of normal men: possible genetic polymorphisms. Am. J. Hum. Genet. 24: 168-180, 1972.

Roos, J. and Huizinga, J.: Genetic investigation of the Stuart coagulation defect. Acta Genet. Statist. Med. 9: 115-122, 1959.

*22765 FANCONI PANCYTOPENIA (CONSTITUTIONAL INFANTILE PANMYELOPATHY)

Usually all marrow elements are affected with resulting anemia, leukopenia and thrombopenia. Pigmentary changes in the skin and malformations of the heart, kidney and extremities (aplasia of the radius, thumb deformity) are associated features. Leukemia is a fatal complication (Garriga and Crosby, 1959) and may occur in family members lacking full-blown features. This particular point mutation apparently predisposes to multiple chromosomal breaks (Bloom et al., 1966). Bloom syndrome (q.v.) is another single gene disorder accompanied by chromosomal breakage and predisposition to leukemia. Lohr et al. (1965) in two brothers and a third unrelated patient found marked reduction of red cell, leukocyte and platelet hexokinase activity. This is apparently a different defect from the hexokinase deficiency (q.v.) which is limited to red cells and which results in hemolytic anemia alone. A consistent defect in hexokinase cannot be considered as proved (Brunetti et al., 1966). Radius-platelet hypoplasia (q.v.) is a separate entity. Zaizov et al. (1969) described two sisters and a brother with pancytopenia like that of Fanconi syndrome but without congenital malformations. Chromosomal changes like those of Fanconi syndrome were present and patchy areas of hyperpigmentation were noted in two of the sibs. Swift et al. (1974) concluded that male heterozygotes for Fanconi anemia have a risk of malignant neoplasm 3.4 times that of the general population. O'Brien (1974) believes that exonuclease deficiency is the defect. The deficiency has not been demonstrated directly. He and his associates have shown that skin-derived fibroblasts are deficient in excising ultra-violet induced thymine dimers and covalently bound products of dimethylbenzanthracene from their DNA. They are normal with respect to their ability to produce single strand scissions after ultra-violet inadiation and to conduct unscheduled DNA synthesis and repair replication. They also found that DNA from Fanconi cells sediments anomalously in sucrose gradients.

Bernstein, M. S., Hunter, R. L. and Yachnin, S.: Hepatoma and peliosis hepatis developing in a patient with Fanconi's anemia. New Eng. J. Med. 284: 1135-1136, 1971.

Bloom, G. E., Warner, S., Gerald, P. S. and Diamond, L. K.: Chromosome abnormalities in constitutional aplastic anemia. New Eng. J. Med. 274: 8-14, 1966.

Brunetti, P., Neuci, G. G., Vaccaro, R., Puxeddu, A. and Migliorini, E.: Fanconi's anaemia. (Letter) Lancet II: 1194-1195, 1966.

Fanconi, G.: Familial constitutional panmyelocytopathy, Fanconi's anemia (F.A.). I. Clinical aspects. Sem. Hemat. 4: 233-240, 1966.

Garriga, S. and Crosby, W. H.: The incidence of leukemia in families of patients with hypoplasia of the marrow. Blood 14: 1008-1014, 1959.

Lohr, G. W., Waller, H. D., Anschutz, F. and Knopp, A.: Biochemische Defekte in den Blutzellen bei familiaerer Panmyelopathie (Typ Fanconi). Humangenetik 1: 383-387, 1965.

McDonald, R. and Goldschmidt, B.: Pancytopenia with congenital defects (Fanconi's anaemia). Arch. Dis. Child. 35: 367-372, 1960.

O'Brien, R. L.: Los Angeles and Geneva, personal communication, Feb. 6, 1974.

Schmid, W.: Familial constitutional panmyeloctyopathy, Fanconi's anemia (F. A.). II. A discussion of the cytogenetic findings in Fanconi's anemia. Sem. Hemat. 4: 241-249, 1967.

Schmid, W., Scharer, K., Baumann, T. and Fanconi, G.: Chromosomenbruechigkeit bei der familiaeren Panmyelopathie (typus Fanconi). Schweiz. Med. Wschr. 95: 1461-1464, 1965.

Swift, M. R. and Hirschhorn, K.: Fanconi's anemia: inherited susceptibility to chromosome breakage in various tissues. Ann. Intern. Med. 65: 496-503, 1966.

Swift, M. R. and Sholman, L.: Diabetes mellitus and the gene for Fanconi's anemia. Science 178: 308-310, 1972.

Swift, M., Cohen, J. and Pinlchham, R.: Maximum-likelihood method for estimating the disease predisposition of heterozygotes. Am. J. Hum. Genet. 26: 304-317, 1974.

Zachmann, M., Illig, R. and Prader, A.: Fanconi's anemia with isolated growth hormone deficiency. (Letter) J. Pediat. 80: 159 only, 1972.

Zaizov, R., Matoth, Y. and Mamon, Z.: Familial aplastic anaemia without congenital malformations. Acta Paediat. Scand. 58: 151-156, 1969.

*22770 FANCONI SYNDROME I (CHILDHOOD AND INFANTILE FORM WITHOUT CYSTINOSIS)

The main features of the Fanconi syndrome are rickets or osteomalacia, which is resistant to vitamin D in the usual doses, glucosuria, generalized aminoaciduria and hyperphosphaturia in spite of normal or reduced plasma concentrations of these substances, and usually chronic acidosis, hypouricemia and hypokalemia. Clay, Darmady and Hawkins (1953) described a characteristic swan-neck deformity of the proximal renal tubule. In an Iraqi Jewish family, Klajman and Arber (1967) found glycosuria and aminoaciduria in a woman and her son. Her husband was a first cousin. Two other sons had glycosuria, aminoaciduria and low serum alkaline phosphatase. Another son had only glycosuria and two other sons had only low alkaline phosphatase. A phenocopy of the genetic Fanconi syndrome is produced by ingestion of degraded ('outdated') tetracycline (Brodehl et al., 1968).

Brodehl, J., Gellissen, K., Hagge, W. and Schumacher, H.: Reversibles renales Fanconi-syndrom durch toxisches Abbauprodukt des Tetrazyklins. Helv. Paediat. Acta 23: 373-383, 1968.

Clay, R. D., Darmady, E. M. and Hawkins, M.: The nature of the renal lesion in the Fanconi syndrome. J. Path. Bact. 65: 551-558, 1953.

Harrison, H. E.: The Fanconi syndrome. J. Chronic Dis. 7: 346-355, 1958.

Klajman, A. and Arber, I.: Familial glycosuria and amino-aciduria associated with low serum alkaline phosphatase. Israel J. Med. Sci. 3: 392-396, 1967.

Schneider, J. A. and Seegmiller, J. E.: Cystinosis and the Fanconi syndrome. In, Stanbury, J. B., Wyngaarden, J. B. and Fredrickson, D. S. (eds.): The Metabolic Basis of Inherited Disease. New York: McGraw-Hill, 1972 (3rd Ed.). Pp. 1581-1604.

*22780 FANCONI SYNDROME II ('ADULT' FORM WITHOUT CYSTINOSIS)

Dent and Harris's family (1956) is the most convincing for recessive inheritance. Four out of five sibs were affected. The disease presents at about age 40. The bones become tender and show 'looser zones' by X-ray. Loss of height and muscle weakness are noted. The urine contains large amounts of amino acids and glucose as in the childhood form. No cystinosis is demonstrable. Serum phosphorus is low and phosphatase elevated. Hunt et al. (1966) described a family in which persons in four generations appear to have had retarded growth, rickets, hypophosphatemia, hypokalemia, acidosis, aminoaciduria, proteinuria and glycosuria. Autopsy and biopsies showed no cystine deposits in tissues. Inheritance was thought to be dominant.

Dent, C. E. and Harris, H.: Hereditary forms of rickets and osteomalacia. J. Bone Joint Surg. 38B: 204-226, 1956.

Hunt, D. D., Stearns, G., McKinley, J. B., Froning, E., Hicks, P. and Bonfiglio, M.: Long-term study of a family with Fanconi syndrome without cystinosis (de Toni-Debre-Fanconi syndrome). Am. J. Med. 40: 492-510, 1966.

Wilson, D. R. and Yendt, E. R.: Treatment of the adult Fanconi syndrome with oral phosphate supplements and alkali. Report of two cases associated with nephrolithiasis. Am. J. Med. 35: 487-511, 1963.

22785 FANCONI-LIKE SYNDROME

In two brothers Abels and Reed (1973) described a disorder with both similarities to and differences from the Fanconi syndrome. One brother died in his mid-twenties after a prolonged course characterized by pancytopenia, recurrent infections, low IgA, chronic lung infections complicated by multiple bilateral pneumothroaces, osteomyelitis and multiple cutaneous malignancies with lymph node metastases. The other brother had severe pancytopenia responsive to methyltestosterone therapy. Poon et al. (1974) showed that cells from patients with Fanconi anemia are deficient in their ability to excise UV induced pyrimidine dimers from their DNA. They are capable, however, of single strand break production and unscheduled DNA synthesis. From this they inferred deficiency in an exonuclease which specifically recognizes and excises distortions in the tertiary structure of DNA.

Abels, D. and Reed, W. B.: Fanconi-like syndrome. Immunologic deficiency, pancytopenia, and cutaneous malignancies. Arch. Derm. 107: 419-423, 1973.

Poon, P. K., O'Brien, R. L. and Parker, J. W.: Defective DNA repair in Fanconi's anemia. Nature, in press, 1974.

*22800 FARBER LIPOGRANULOMATOSIS

In the few reported cases manifestations appeared in the first few weeks of life and consisted of irritability, hoarse cry and nodular, erythematous swellings of the wrists and other sites, particularly those subject to trauma. Severe motor and mental retardation is evident. Death occurs by 2 years of age. The histologic appearance is granulomatous. In the nervous system both neurones and glial cells are swollen with stored material with the characteristics of nonsulfonated acid mucopolysaccharide (Abul-Haj and colleagues, 1962). Parental consanguinity has been identified in no instance. However, in one case parents had the same family name in ancestors, and two of 3 families seen at Children's Hospital, Boston, were of Portuguese extraction. The family with two affected sibs had father from the Azores Islands and mother from the Madeira Islands. The parents of the other family were both born in the Azores (Crocker et al., 1967). Clausen et al. (1970) proposed that an enzymatic defect in glycolipid degradation is the basic fault. Sugita et al. (1972) suggested that the basic defect is a deficiency of ceramidase. No activity of this enzyme could be demonstrated in kidney and cerebellum. The same enzyme normally catalyzes the synthesis and degradation of ceramide.

Abul-Haj, S. K., Martz, D. G., Douglas, W. F. and Geppert, L. J.: Farber's disease. Report of a case with observations on its histiogenesis and notes on the nature of the stored material. J. Pediat. 61: 221-232, 1962.

Clausen, J. and Rampini, S.: Chemical studies of Farber's disease. Acta Neurol. Scand. 46: 313-322, 1970.

Crocker, A. C., Cohen, J. and Farber, S.: The 'lipogranulomatosis' syndrome: review, with report of patient showing mild involvement. In, Aronson, S. M. and Volk, B. W. (eds.): Inborn Disorders of Sphingolipid Metabolism. Oxford: Pergamon Press, 1967. Pp. 485-503.

Farber, S., Cohen, J. and Uzman, L. L.: Lipogranulomatosis: a new lipo-glyco-protein 'storage' disease. J. Mount Sinai Hosp. N.Y. 24: 816-837, 1957.

Sugita, M., Dulaney, J. T. and Moser, H. W.: Ceramidase deficiency in Farber's disease (lipogranulomatosis). Science 178: 1100-1102, 1972.

22810 FATTY METAMORPHOSIS OF VISCERA

Peremans et al. (1967) described a sibship of 14 children, offspring of first cousins once removed, among whom 5 children showed progressive muscular hypotonia, lethargy, coma and death in the first days of life. A sixth child was found to have hypocalcemia and hypoglycemia. At autopsy, the heart, liver and kidneys were grossly very pale and histologically these and other organs showed loading of parenchymal cells with sudanophilic material. Autopsy in two of the other infants also showed pallor of viscera. The relationship to the condition described by Utian et al. (1964) and Reye et al. (1963) was unclear. Satran et al. (1969) described two brothers and a sister who died at ages 4 days, 19 days and 12 weeks of fatty liver disease marked by a severe hemorrhagic disorder. They suggested that the disorder reported by Peremans et al. (1966) may be the same. Wadlington and Riley (1973) described a family in which five male sibs died in the first two weeks of life after an illness characterized by jaundice and kernicterus. Liver tissue obtained at autopsy in one showed a striking increase in total lipids and fatty acids.

Peremans, J., Degraef, P. J., Strubbe, G. and De Block, G.: Familial metabolic disorder with fatty metamorphosis of the viscera. J. Pediat. 69: 1108-1112, 1967.

Rasanen, O., Korhonen, M., Simila, S., Autere, T. and Hakosalo, J.: Fatal familial steatosis of the liver and kidney in two siblings. Z. Kinderheilk. 110: 267-275, 1971.

Reye, R. D. K., Morgan, G. and Baral, J.: Encephalopathy and fatty degeneration of the viscera. A disease entity in children. Lancet II: 749-752, 1963.

Satran, L., Sharp, H. L., Schenken, J. R. and Krivit, W.: Fatal neonatal hepatic steatosis: a new familial disorder. J. Pediat. 75: 39-46, 1969.

Utian, H. L., Wagner, J. M. and Sichel, R. J. S.: White liver disease. Lancet II: 1043-1045, 1964.

R
E
C
E
S
S
I
V
E

Wadlington, W. B. and Riley, H. D., Jr.: Familial disease characterized by neonatal jaundice, and probable hepatosteatosis and kernicterus: a new syndrome? Pediat. 51: 192-198, 1973.

22820 FEMUR-FIBULA-ULNA (FFU) SYNDROME

Neither familial occurrence nor associated exogenous factors have been identified. When cases of femoral defects associated with malformations of the arms are collected, a highly specific pattern of rare arm defects are found, such as amelia, peromelia at the lower end of the humerus, humeroradial synostosis, defects of the ulna and ulnar rays (Kuhne et al., 1967). This disorder of the femurs has been called PFFD (proximal focal femoral deficiency) in this country (Aitken, 1969) and is probably heterogeneous.

Aitken, G. T.: Proximal femoral focal deficiency, a congenital anomaly. A symposium. Washington: National Academy of Science, 1969.

Kuhne, D., Lenz, W., Petersen, D. and Schonenberg, H.: Defekt von Femur und Fibula mit Amelie, Peromelie oder ulnaren Strahldefekten der Arme. Ein Syndrom. Humangenetik 3: 244-263, 1967.

22830 FERTILE EUNUCH

McCullagh, Beck and Schaffenburg's (1953) patient had a brother with eunuchoidal features who refused examination. A deficiency of ICSH (interstitial cell stimulating hormone) was postulated. Luteinizing hormone (LH) in the male is also known as ICSH (interstitial cell stimulating hormone). The clinical picture is one of androgenic insufficiency with 'normal' spermatogenesis. The semen shows abnormalities of sperm count, morphology and mobility but at least two patients are said to have fathered children. Isolated deficiency of LH, in the presence of normal concentrations of FSH, was documented by radio-immuno-assay by Faiman et al. (1968).

Faiman, C., Hoffman, D. L., Ryan, R. J. and Albert, A.: The 'fertile eunuch' syndrome: demonstration of isolated luteinizing hormone deficiency by radio-immuno-assay technique. Mayo Clin. Proc. 43: 661-667, 1968.

McCullagh, E. P., Beck, J. C. and Schaffenburg, C. A.: Syndrome of eunuchoidism with spermiogenesis, normal urinary FSH and low or normal ICSH: ('fertile eunuchs'). J. Clin. Endocr. 13: 489-509, 1953.

22840 FEVER, FAMILIAL LIFELONG PERSISTENT

Herman et al. (1969) described twin brothers of Lebanese extraction with persistent fever of 102 degrees F. without diurnal variation. The family contained multiple consanguineous marriages. Hormonal and sweat studies yielded normal findings. Adrenosteroid and uronic acids which inhibit beta-glucuronidase decreased the temperature. The authors suggested that beta-glucuronidase is important in controlling the level of free intrahepatic etiocholanolone and that these patients had an abnormality of the enzyme such that it is more active, perhaps because of undersensitivity to natural inhibitors.

Herman, R. H., Overholt, E. L. and Hagler, L.: Familial life-long persistent fever of unknown origin responding to dexamethasone and uronic acids. Am. J. Med. 46: 142-153, 1969.

*22850 FIBRIN-STABILIZING FACTOR (FIBRINASE, OR FACTOR XIII) DEFICIENCY

Several families have been reported from Switzerland and Finland. Wound healing is poor. Hemorrhage from the umbilical cord and intracranial hemorrhage have been observed. By means of a technique with enhanced sensitivity, Duckert (1964) demonstrated partial deficiency in presumptive heterozygotes. Urea-solubility of the fibrin clot is an in vitro characteristic. All the 'usual' clotting tests are normal, but the diagnosis is made easily by the urea solubility test. Butten (1967) described a case both of whose parents as well as several other relatives were by test apparently heterozygous. Fisher et al. (1966) described an affected Moroccan woman who was offspring of an uncle-niece mating. Parents and sibs were apparently normal. Ratnoff and Steinberg (1968) pointed out that, although the evidence for autosomal recessive inheritance in some families is quite convincing, the possibility of X-linked recessive inheritance in other families is suggested by the data. Zahir (1969) observed an affected female the offspring of a first-cousin marriage. Both parents had low factor XIII levels. Deficiency of FSF can be either autosomal recessive or X-linked recessive. Like hemoglobin the FSF molecule is a tetramer of two different types of polypeptide chains, alpha and beta (Schwartz et al., 1971). Aguercif et al. (1971) described a seven-year-old French girl who had ecchymoses and muscular hematomas following minor trauma. Factor XIII activity was found deficient. Immunodiffusion showed a protein with antigenicity of factor XIII.

Aguercif, M., Nigg, O. M., Lopez, J. M. and Bouvier, C. A.: Congenital factor-XIII-activity deficiency with immnologically characterized FSF-like-protein. Nouv. Rev. Franc. Hemat. 11: 841-848, 1971.

Amris, C. J. and Ranek, L.: A case of fibrin-stabilizing factor (FSF) deficiency. Thromb. Diath. Haemorrh. 14: 332-340, 1965.

Butten, A. F. H.: Congenital deficiency of factor XIII (fibrin-stabilizing factor). Report of a case and review of the literature. Am. J. Med. 43: 751-761, 1967.

Duckert, F.: Factor XIII deficiency. Proc. 10th Intern. Congr. Soc. Haematol., Stockholm, 1964.

Duckert, F., Jung, E. and Shmerling, D. H.: A hitherto undescribed congenital haemorrhagic diathesis probably due to fibrin stabilizing factor deficiency. Thromb. Diath. Haemorrh. 5: 179-186, 1960.

Fisher, S., Rikover, M. and Naor, S.: Factor 13 deficiency with severe hemorrhagic diathesis. Blood 28: 34-39, 1966.

Ikkala, E. and Nevanlinna, H. R.: Congenital deficiency of fibrin stabilizing factor. Thromb. Diath. Haemorrh. 7: 567-571, 1962.

Lorand, L., Urayama, T., Atencio, A. C. and Hsia, D. Y.-Y.: Inheritance of deficiency of fibrin-stabilizing factor (factor XIII). Am. J. Hum. Genet. 22: 89-95, 1970.

McDonagh, J., McDonagh, R. P., Myllyla, G. and Ikkala, E.: Factor XIII deficiency: a genetic study of two affected kindreds in Finland. Blood 43: 327-332, 1974.

Ratnoff, O. D. and Steinberg, A. G.: Inheritance of fibrin-stabilizing-factor deficiency. Lancet I: 25-26, 1968.

Schwartz, M. L., Pizzo, S. V., Hill, R. L. and McKee, P. A.: The subunit structures of human plasma and platelet factor XIII (fibrin-stabilizing factor). J. Biol. Chem. 246: 5851-5854, 1971.

Schmerling, D. H., Jung, E. and Duckert, F.: Eine neue familiaere Koagulopathie infolge Mangels an fibrinstabilisierendem Faktor. Helv. Paediat. Acta 15: 471-478, 1960.

Zahir, M.: Congenital deficiency of fibrin-stabilizing factor. Report of a case and family study. J.A.M.A. 207: 751-753, 1969.

*22860 FIBROMATOSIS, JUVENILE

Both males and females are affected and in at least two instances (Drescher et al., 1967; Enjoji et al., 1968) two affected sibs have been reported. The disorder is characterized by multiple subcutaneous tumors, particularly of the scalp, appearing at about age 2 years and slowly growing, causing deformities. Nodular or diffuse hypertrophy of the gums is also observed. The tumors recur after removal. Histologically they demonstrate an abundance of homogeneous, amorphous, acidophilic ground substance in which spindle shaped cells form minute streaks. Gingival fibromatosis is associated. In 1873 Murray and in 1903 Whitfield and Robinson reported three affected sibs whose unaffected parents were first cousins. Microscopic and ultrastructural features have been described.

Drescher, E., Woyke, S., Markiewicz, C. and Tegi, S.: Juvenile fibromatosis in siblings (fibromatosis hyalinica multiplex juvenilis). J. Pediat. Surg. 2: 427-430, 1967.

Enjoji, M., Kato, N., Kamikarzuru, K. and Arima, E.: Juvenile fibromatosis of the scalp in siblings. Acta Med. Univ. Kagoshima (suppl. 10): 145-151, 1968.

Whitfield, A. and Robinson, A. H.: A further report on the remarkable series of cases of molluscum fibrosum in children communicated to the society by Dr. John Murray in 1873. Med.-Chir. Trans. London 86: 293, 1903.

Woyke, S., Wenancjusz, D. and Olszewski, W.: Ultrastructure of a fibromatosis hyalinica multiplex juvenilis. Cancer 26: 1157-1168, 1970.

22870 FIBROMUSCULAR HYPERPLASIA OF THE RENAL ARTERIES

This change, leading to hypertension, occurs almost only in females, manifesting itself in early adulthood as a rule. Hansen, Holten and Thorberg (1965) reported affected sisters. A 25-year-old patient with this anomaly had a hypertensive 22-year-old brother (Wood, Borges, 1963). Other visceral arteries are affected in some patients. Halpern, Sanford and Viamonte (1965) described affected sisters but gave no information on the parents or other sibs.

Halpern, M. M., Sanford, H. S. and Viamonte, M., Jr.: Renal-artery abnormalities in three hypertensive sisters. Probable familial fibromuscular hyperplasia. J.A.M.A. 194: 512-513, 1965.

Hansen, J., Holten, C. and Thorberg, J. V.: Hypertension in two sisters caused by so-called fibromuscular hyperplasia of the renal arteries. Acta Med. Scand. 178: 461-474, 1965.

Najafi, H.: Fibromuscular hyperplasia of the external iliac arteries. An unusual cause of intermittent claudication. Arch. Surg. 92: 394-396, 1966.

Wood, C. and Borges, F. J.: Perimuscular fibrosis of renal arteries with hypertension. Arch. Intern. Med. 112: 79-91, 1963.

22880 FIBROSCLEROSIS, MULTIFOCAL

Comings et al. (1967) reported two brothers, offspring of a first-cousin marriage, who had different combinations of retroperitoneal fibrosis, mediastinal fibrosis, sclerosing cholangitis, Riedel sclerosing thyroiditis and pseudotumor of the orbit. One of the brothers had fibrotic contracture of the fingers.

Comings, D. E., Skubi, K. B., Van Eyes, J. and Motulsky, A. G.: Familial multifocal fibrosclerosis. Findings suggesting that retroperitoneal fibrosis, mediastinal fibrosis, sclerosing cholangitis, Riedel's thyroiditis and pseudotumor of the orbit may be different manifestations of a single disease. Ann. Intern. Med. 66: 884-892, 1967.

22890 FIBULA APLASIA AND COMPLEX BRACHYDACTYLY

This syndrome seems to have been described only by Grebe (1955) who reported a brother and sister, from a first-cousin marriage, who had shortening of various metacarpals, small carpals, trapezoid middle phalanx of the index finger, with radial deviation, almost complete absence of the fibula bilaterally and tibio-tarsal dislocation (Volkmann deformity). The toes were short and laterally deviated.

Grebe, H.: Chondrodysplasie. Rome: Int. Greg. Mendel, 1955. Pp. 300-303.

*22900 FLETCHER FACTOR DEFICIENCY

Hathaway et al. (1965) described a Kentucky kindred in which four sibs of the name Fletcher showed a previously undescribed coagulation defect. Although they had no abnormal bleeding tendency, their blood showed much prolonged activated partial thromboplastin time and delayed thromboplastin generation but normal prothrombin time. Plasmas deficient in factor VIII, IX, XI and XII corrected the abnormality. Hattersley and Hayse (1970) reported three unrelated cases. Research by Saito et al. (1972) suggests that the Fletcher factor deficiency is associated with an inhibitor to the clot-promoting activities of glass-like surfaces. Wuepper (1973) presented data indicating identity of Fletcher factor and prekallikrein. Weiss et al. (1974) presented evidence consistent with the identity of Fletcher factor and prekallikrein.

Hathaway, W. E. and Alsever, J.: The relation of 'Fletcher factor' to factor XI and XII. Brit. J. Haemat. 18: 161-169, 1970.

Hathaway, W. E., Belhasen, L. P. and Hathaway, H. S.: Evidence for a new plasma thromboplastin factor. I. Case report, coagulation studies and physiochemical properties. Blood 26: 521-532, 1965.

Hattersley, P. G. and Hayse, D.: Fletcher factor deficiency: a report of three unrelated cases. Brit. J. Haemat. 18: 411-416, 1970.

Saito, H., Ratnoff, O. D., Donaldson, V. H., Abilgaard, C. C. and Hattersley, P. G.: Fletcher factor. (Letter) Blood 39: 745-747, 1972.

Weiss, A. S., Gallin, J. I. and Kaplan, A.: Fletcher factor deficiency. A diminished rate of Hageman factor activation caused by absence of prekallikrein with abnormalities of coagulation, fibrinolysis, chemotactic activity, and kiningeneration. J. Clin. Invest. 53: 622-633, 1974.

Wuepper, K. D.: Prekallikrein deficiency in man. J. Exp. Med. 138: 1345-1355, 1973.

22903 FOLIC ACID REDUCTASE, DEFICIENCY OF

Walters (1967) reported a case of congenital megaloblastic anemia responsive to N(5)-formyltetrahydrofolic acid administration but not to folic acid. A liver specimen was found deficient in folic acid reductase activity. The patient showed no neurologic abnormality.

Walters, T. R.: Congenital megaloblastic anemia responsive to N(5)-formyl tetrahydrofolic acid administration. (Abstract) J. Pediat. 70: 686-687, 1967.

*22905 FOLIC ACID, TRANSPORT DEFECT INVOLVING

Luhby et al. (1965) observed affected sisters, and Lanzkowsky (1970) described a 20-year-old sporadic case. The patients had an isolated defect in intestinal absorption of folic acid and a defect in transport of folic acid into the cerebrospinal fluid. Recurrent megaloblastic anemia, mental retardation, convulsions, and movement disorder (ataxia in Luhby's cases, athetosis in Lanzkowsky's) were manifestations. Basal ganglion calcification was described in Lanzkowsky's cases. The seizures were said to be reduced by folic acid in Luhby's cases but aggravated by folic acid in Lanzkowsky's. Parental folic acid corrected the anemia.

Lanzkowsky, P.: Congenital malabsorption of folate. Am. J. Med. 48: 580-583, 1970.

Luhby, A. L., Cooperman, J. M. and Pesci-Bourel, A.: A new inborn error of metabolism: folic acid responsive megaloblastic anemia, ataxia, mental retardation, and convulsions. J. Pediat. 67: 1052 only, 1965.

Santiago-Borrero, P. J., Santini, R. Jr., Perez-Santiago, E. and Maldonado, N.: Congenital isolated defect of folic acid absorption. J. Pediat. 82: 450-455, 1973.

R
E
C
E
S
S
I
V
E

22907 FOLLICLE-STIMULATING HORMONE, ISOLATED DEFICIENCY OF

Rabin et al. (1972) described a 22-year-old woman with primary amenorrhea, high LH, on biopsy of the ovaries primordial follicles which had not matured to the stage of antral formation, undetectable serum FSH. The defect was thought to be at the level of the pituitary, not the hypothalamus. FSH, LH and TSH (thyroid stimulating hormone) are glycoproteins secreted by basophil cells. Immunohistochemical and ultrastructural work indicates that a distinctive cell produces each of the three hormones. (See 22830 for isolated deficiency of LH and 27510 for isolated deficiency of TSH.) Pierce (1971) showed that TSH, LH and HCG (human chorionic gonadotropin) are made up of two dissimilar subunits. The alpha subunits are very similar, possess little biologic activity and probably account for most of the immunologic cross-reactivity of the three molecules. Specificity of hormone action is endowed by the beta subunit, which is different for each hormone. FSH probably has the same general structure. Thus, a defect in synthesis of the beta chain of FSH might be the basis of the deficiency in the patient of Rabin et al. (1972). Exclusion of the alternative possibility, a defect in the hypothalamic factor responsible for release of FSH from the pituitary, could be achieved perhaps with LRH (luteinizing-hormone-releasing hormone) administration. LRH appears to cause the release of both LH and FSH (Reichlin, 1972).

Pierce, J. G.: The subunits of pituitary thyrotropin — their relationship to other glycoprotein hormones. Endocrinology 89: 1331-1344, 1971.

Rabin, D., Spitz, I., Bercovici, B., Bell, J., Laufer, A., Benveniste, R. and Polishuk, W.: Isolated deficiency of follicle-stimulating hormone. Clinical and laboratory features. New Eng. J. Med. 287: 1313-1317, 1972.

Reichlin, S.: Anterior pituitary — six glands and one. (Editorial) New Eng. J. Med. 287: 1351-1352, 1972.

*22910 FORMIMINOTRANSFERASE DEFICIENCY

Mental retardation is the main clinical feature. The ferric chloride test is positive due to formiminoglutamic acid in the urine. The features are marked mental and physical retardation, anemia, megaloblastic bone marrow and biochemical evidence of disturbed folic acid metabolism. Two related patients, both Japanese, have been described. Very large amounts of FIGLU were excreted in the urine. The level of folic acid in the blood is increased. Hyperfolicacidemia followed histidine loading. The single case described by Arakawa et al. (1965) had hypersegmentation of the nuclei of neutrophils. This may have been fortuitous association of an independent trait, since the father and his sister and mother showed the same finding but were otherwise normal. See UNDRITZ ANOMALY, a dominant. Heterogeneity in this category is indicated by the report by Niederwiesser et al. (1974) of two sisters who had FIGLU in the urine with normal serum folic acid levels. They differed from reported cases of postulated formininotransferase deficiency in a 10-fold increase in FIGLU excretion with histidine loading, normal hematologic findings, normal serum folic acid and lack of mental retardation in one.

Arakawa, T. S., Fujii, M. and O'Hara, K.: Erythrocyte formiminotransferase activity in formininotransferase deficiency syndrome. Tohoku J. Exp. Med. 88: 195-202, 1966.

Arakawa, T. S., Ohara, K., Takahashi, Y., Ogasawara, J., Hayashi, T., Chiba, R., Wada, Y., Tada, K., Mizuno, T., Okamura, T. and Yoshida, T.: Formiminotransferase-deficiency syndrome: a new inborn error of folic acid metabolism. Ann. Paediat. 205: 1-11, 1965.

Arakawa, T. S., Tamura, T., Higashi, O., Ohara, K., Tanno, K., Honda, Y., Narisawa, K., Konno, T., Wada, Y., Sato, Y. and Mizuno, T.: Formiminotransferase deficiency syndrome associated with megaloblastic anemia responsive to pyridoxine or folic acid. Tohoku J. Exp. Med. 94: 3-16, 1968.

Arakawa, T., Tamura, T., Ohara, K., Narisawa, K., Tanno, K., Honda, Y. and Higashi, O.: Familial occurrence of formiminotransferase deficiency syndrome. Tohoku J. Exp. Med. 96: 211-217, 1968.

Arakawa, T., Yoshida, T., Konno, T. and Honda, Y.: Defect of incorporation of glycine-1-(14)C into urinary uric acid in formiminotransferase deficiency syndrome. Tohoku J. Exp. Med. 106: 213-218, 1972.

Niederwieser, A., Giliberti, P., Matasovic, A., Pluznik, S., Steinmann, B. and Baerlocher, K.: Folic acid non-dependent formininoglutamic aciduria in two siblings. Clin. Chim. Acta 54: 293-316, 1974.

*22920 FRAGILITAS OCULI (CORNEAL FRAGILITY, KERATOGLOBUS, BLUE SCLERAE) WITH JOINT HYPEREXTENSIBILITY

A seemingly distinctive disorder with clearly autosomal recessive inheritance has been described by Stein et al. (1968) in two Tunisian Jewish brothers with consanguineous parents, by Hyams et al. (1969) in a Tunisian Jewish boy who may be related to the patients of Stein et al. (1968) because 'the two families come from the same town in Tunisia,' by Badtke (1941) in two sisters with related parents from south Tyrol, by Tucker in a brother and sister with first-cousin parents, and by Arkin in a 17-year-old boy. The features include blue sclerae; large cloudy, thin, bulging cornea, noted from early in life, and mimicking buphthalmos but accompanied by normal intraocular pressure; fragility of the cornea with repeated rupture; dental abnormalities somewhat like those of osteogenesis imperfecta; abnormal proclivity to fracture of bones; long slender hyperextensible fingers; hernia. The Tunisian cases of Stein et al. (1968) and Hyams (1969) had red hair, a sufficiently unusual finding in this group to suggest to the authors that it is a part of the syndrome. In keratoglobus the thinning of the cornea is generalized or in the periphery, whereas in keratoconus it is mainly central. Two affected sibs with first-cousin parents were reported by Greenfield et al. (1973). The ocular form of the Ehlers-Danlos syndrome (E-D VI) also shows fragilitas oculi (see 22540).

Arkin, W.: Blue scleras with keratoglobus. Am. J. Ophthal. 58: 678-682, 1964.

Badtke, G.: Ueber einen eigenartigen fall von keratokonus und blauen skleren bei geschwistern. Klin. Mbl. Augenheilk. 106: 585-592, 1941.

Greenfield, G., Stein, R. R. and Goodman, R. M.: Blue sclerae and keratocanus: key features of a distinct heritable disorder of connective tissue. Clin. Genet. 4: 8-16, 1973.

Hyams, S. W., Kar, H. and Neumann, E.: Blue sclerae and keratoglobus. Ocular signs of a systemic connective tissue disorder. Brit. J. Ophthal. 53: 53-58, 1969.

Stein, R., Lazar, M. and Adam, A.: Brittle cornea. A familial trait associated with blue sclera. Am. J. Ophthal. 66: 67-69, 1968.

22925 FREESIA FLOWERS, INABILITY TO SMELL

This may be an autosomal recessive trait.

McWhirter, K.: Ethnography of specific anosmia. Canad. J. Genet. Cytol. 11: 479 only, 1969.

*22930 FRIEDREICH ATAXIA

This is one of the rare hereditary spinocerebellar degenerations. The spinocerebellar tracts, dorsal columns, pyramidal tracts and, to a lesser extent, the cerebellum and medulla are involved. The disorder is usually manifest before adolescence and is generally characterized by incoordination of limb movements, dysarthria, nystagmus, diminished or absent tendon reflexes, Babinski sign, impairment of position and vibratory senses, scoliosis, pes cavus and hammer toe. The triad of hypoactive knee and ankle jerks, signs of progressive cerebellar dysfunction and pre-adolescent onset is commonly regarded as sufficient for diagnosis. Cardiac manifestations are conspicuous in some cases (Boyer, Chisholm and McKusick, 1962). Hewer (1968) found that one-half of 82 fatal cases of Friedreich ataxia died of heart failure and nearly three-quarters had evidence of cardiac dysfunction in life. 23 percent had diabetes and 4 developed diabetic ketosis terminally. One case had an affected parent. Age at death varied from the first (3 cases) to the eighth (1 case) decade with a mean of 36.6 years. Muscular subaortic stenosis has been described in cases of Friedreich ataxia (Elias, 1972; Boehm et al. 1970).

Boehm, T. M., Dickerson, R. B. and Glasser, S. P.: Hypertrophic subaortic stenosis occurring in a patient with Friedreich ataxia. Am. J. Med. Sci. 260: 279-284, 1970.

Boyer, S. H., IV, Chisholm, A. W. and McKusick, V. A.: Cardiac aspects of Friedreich's ataxia. Circulation 25: 493-505, 1962.

R
E
C
E
S
S
I
V
E

Elias, G.: Muscular subaortic stenosis and Friedreich's ataxia. Am. Heart J. 84: 843 only, 1972.

Hartman, J. M. and Booth, R. W.: Friedreich's ataxia: a neurocardiac disease. Am. Heart J. 60: 716-720, 1960.

Heck, A. F.: A study of neural and extraneural findings in a large family with Friedreich's ataxia. J. Neurol. Sci. 1: 226-255, 1964.

Hewer, R. L.: Study of fatal cases of Friedreich's ataxia. Brit. Med. J. 3: 649-652, 1968.

Hughes, J. T., Brownell, B. and Hewer, R. L.: The peripheral sensory pathway in Friedreich's ataxia. An examination by light and electron microscopy of the posterior nerve roots, posterior root ganglia, and peripheral sensory nerves in cases of Friedreich's ataxia. Brain 91: 803-818, 1969.

Koennicke, W.: Friedreichsche Ataxie und Taubstummheit. Zbl. Ges. Neurol. Psychiat. 53: 161-164, 1919-20.

*22950 FRUCTOSE AND GALACTOSE INTOLERANCE

In 1961 Dormandy and Porter reported the above combination in two sisters. Unlike fructose intolerance patients, both were fond of candy and showed no nausea or vomiting after fructose ingestion. Both galactose and fructose induced severe hypoglycemia. Galactose-1-phosphate uridyl transferase, the enzyme deficient in galactosemia, was normal. In both patients serum insulin by immuno-assay was in the same high range as is found in patients with beta islet cell adenomas (Samols and Dormandy, 1963). Turner et al. (1972) gave a full follow-up. The proband presented originally with a long history of 'epilepsy,' treated with anticonvulsants and punctuated by episodes of confusion attributed to overdosage of anticonvulsants. By 1972 hyperinsulinism had disappeared and fructose and galactose intolerance could no longer be demonstrated. The other sib had died.

Dormandy, T. L. and Porter, R. J.: Familial fructose and galactose intolerance. Lancet I: 1189-1194, 1961.

Samols, E. and Dormandy, T. L.: Insulin response to fructose and galactose. Lancet I: 478-479, 1963.

Turner, R. C., Spathis, G. S., Nabarro, J. D. N. and Dormandy, T. L.: Familial fructose and galactose intolerance. (Letter) Lancet II: 872 only, 1972.

*22960 FRUCTOSE INTOLERANCE, HEREDITARY (FRUCTOSEMIA)

Most of the recognized cases have been severely ill infants with recurrent hypoglycemia and vomiting, occurring at the time of weaning when fructose or sucrose is added to the diet and resulting in marked malnutrition. However, a three-year-old brother of a severely affected infant was found to have hepatomegaly and hypoglycemic shock was precipitated by an oral test dose of fructose, although he was clinically healthy (Perheentupa and Pitkanen, 1962). He had a marked aversion to sweets and fruit. Froesch et al. (1963) described two adults, ages 33 and 39 years, with the same condition. In addition to the aversion to fructose-containing foods, remarkable absence of dental caries was noted. The defect resides in the liver aldolase, which splits fructose-1-phosphate. By analogy to galactosemia the term fructosemia was suggested by Levin et al. (1963). The patient reported by Mass et al. (1966) had renal tubular acidosis as an independent recessive (q.v.) or as a complication of the fructosemia. Wolf et al. (1959) recorded cases in father and son but the mother may have been heterozygous. Swales and Smith (1966) described an affected 21-year-old man. Evidence for genetic heterogeneity was considered convincing by Levin et al. (1968). Both structural and controller mutations may exist, as well as more than one type of structural mutation. One of their cases and a previously reported one had a near normal ratio of fructose-1-phosphate aldolase to fructose diphosphate aldolase, suggesting a controller mutation. Kohlin and Melin (1968) reported adult cases. Perheentupa and Raivio (1967) discussed hyperuricemia in this disorder. Nordmann et al. (1968) have studied the immunologic and kinetic properties of the liver and suggest that a mutation of the structural gene is responsible for the abnormal fructose-1 phosphate aldolase activity in fructosemia. The question of genetics of this disorder seems to have been settled by Raivio (1967), who showed that parents of patients with this disorder had normal fructose-1-phosphate activity. These data are consistent only with an autosomal recessive trait in which the enzyme activity of carriers is entirely intact.

Cornblath, M., Rosenthal, I. M., Reisner, S. H., Wybregt, S. H. and Crane, R. K.: Hereditary fructose intolerance. New Eng. J. Med. 269: 1271-1278, 1963.

Froesch, E. R., Wolf, H. P., Baitsch, H., Prader, A. and Labhart, A.: Hereditary fructose intolerance: an inborn defect of hepatic fructose-1-phosphate splitting aldolase. Am. J. Med. 34: 151-167, 1963.

Kohlin, P. and Melin, K.: Hereditary fructose intolerance in four Swedish families. Acta Paediat. Scand. 57: 24-32, 1968.

Kranhold, J. F., Loh, D. and Morris, R. C., Jr.: Renal fructose-metabolizing enzymes: significance in hereditary fructose intolerance. Science 165: 402-403, 1969.

Levin, B., Oberholzer, V. G., Snodgrass, G. J. A. I., Stimmler, L. and Wilmers, M. J.: Fructosaemia. An inborn error of fructose metabolism. Arch. Dis. Child. 38: 220-230, 1963.

Levin, B., Snodgrass, G. J. A. I., Oberholzer, V. G., Burgess, E. A. and Dobbs, R. H.: Fructosaemia: observations on seven cases. Am. J. Med. 45: 826-838, 1968.

Mass, R. E., Smith, W. R. and Walsh, J. R.: The association of hereditary fructose intolerance and renal tubular acidosis. Am. J. Med. Sci. 251: 516-523, 1966.

Nikkila, E. A., Somersalo, O., Pitkanen, E. and Perheentupa, J.: Hereditary fructose intolerance, an inborn deficiency of liver aldolase complex. Metabolism 11: 727-731, 1962.

R
E
C
E
S
S
I
V
E

Nordmann, Y., Schapira, F. and Dreyfus, J.-C.: A structurally modified liver aldolase in fructose intolerance: immunological and kinetic evidence. Biochem. Biophys. Res. Comm. 31: 884-889, 1968.

Perheentupa, J. and Pitkanen, E.: Symptomless hereditary fructose intolerance. (Letter) Lancet I: 1358-1359, 1962.

Perheentupa, J. and Raivio, K.: Fructose-induced hyperuricaemia. Lancet II: 528-531, 1967.

Raivio, K., Perheentupa, J. and Nikkila, E. A.: Aldolase activities in the liver in parents of patients with hereditary fructose intolerance. Clin. Chim. Acta 17: 275-279, 1967.

Rennert, O. M. and Greer, M.: Hereditary fructosemia. Neurology 20: 421-425, 1970.

Swales, J. D. and Smith, A. D. M.: Adult fructose intolerance. Quart. J. Med. 35: 455-473, 1966.

Wolf, H., Zschocke, D., Wedemeyer, F. W. and Huebner, W.: Angeborene hereditaere Fructose-Intoleranz. Klin. Wschr. 37: 693-696, 1959.

*22970 FRUCTOSE-1, 6-DIPHOSPHATASE, HEPATIC DEFICIENCY OF

Baker and Winegrad (1970) described a girl with hypoglycemia and metabolic acidosis on fasting. The defect was impaired gluconeogenesis due to deficiency of hepatic fructose-1, 6-diphosphatase. A sib had died of a clinically similar ailment. The patient of Baerlocher et al. (1971) had consanguineous parents and two sisters had died apparently of the same disorder. Greene et al. (1972) treated two cases with folate with benefit. The enzymatic diagnosis can be made from study of white blood cells. Rat liver fructose-1,6-diphosphatase is a tetramer and like hemoglobin has two different types of subunits, alpha and beta (Sia et al., 1969). If the same is true in man, there is opportunity for at least two non-allelic varieties of FDP deficiency. In the case reported by Hulsmann and Fernandez (1971) the parents were related and two sibs were also affected.

Baerlocher, K., Gitzelmann, R., Nussli, R. and Dumermuth, G.: Infantile lactic acidosis due to hereditary fructose 1, 6-diphosphatase deficiency. Helv. Paediat. Acta 26: 489-506, 1971.

Baker, L. and Winegrad, A. I.: Fasting hypoglycaemia and metabolic acidosis associated with deficiency of hepatic fructose-1, 6-diphosphatase activity. Lancet II: 13-16, 1970.

Greene, H. L., Stifel, F. B. and Herman, R. H.: Hypoglycemia due to fructose-1,6-diphosphatase deficiency and the treatment of two patients with folate. (Abstract) Pediat. Res. 6: 432 only, 1972.

Greene, H. L., Stifel, F. B. and Herman, R. H.: 'Ketotic hypoglycemia' due to hepatic fructose-1,6-diphosphatase deficiency. Am. J. Dis. Child. 124: 415-420, 1972.

Hulsmann, W. C. and Fernandez, J.: A child with lactacidemia and fructose diphosphatase deficiency in the liver. Pediat. Res. 5: 633-637, 1971.

Melancon, S. B. and Nadler, H. L.: Detection of fructose-1,6-diphosphatase deficiency with use of white blood cells. (Letter) New Eng. J. Med. 286: 731-732, 1972.

Pagliara, A. S., Karl, I. E., Keating, J. P., Brown, B. I. and Kipnis, D. M.: Hepatic fructose-1,6-diphosphatase deficiency. A cause of lactic acidosis and hypoglycemia in infancy. J. Clin. Invest. 51: 2115-2123, 1972.

Sia, C. L., Traniello, S., Pontremoli, S. and Horecker, B. L.: Studies on the subunit structure of rabbit liver fructose diphosphatase. Arch. Biochem. Biophys. 132: 325-330, 1969.

*22980 FRUCTOSURIA

This is a benign, asymptomatic defect of intermediary metabolism. There is no evidence of a renal defect. The enzyme involved is thought to be hepatic fructokinase.

Froesch, E. R.: Essential fructosuria and hereditary fructose intolerance. In, Stanbury, J. B., Wyngaarden, J. B. and Fredrickson, D. S. (eds.): The Metabolic Basis of Inherited Disease. New York: McGraw-Hill, 1972 (3rd Ed.). Pp. 131-148.

Lasker, M.: Essential fructosuria. Hum. Biol. 13: 51-63, 1941.

*22990 FUCHS ATROPHIA GYRATA CHORIOIDEAE ET RETINAE

This very rare disorder is characterized by slowly progressive atrophy of the choroid, pigment epithelium and retina. Francois and his colleagues observed a patient (born of a consanguineous marriage) in whom Alder anomaly of the leukocytes was present not only in the patient but also in both parents and in other members of the family through four generations. These workers suggested that the leukocyte anomaly is a heterozygous expression of the gene which in the homozygous state produces Fuchs atrophy. In a later publication, however, Francois et al. (1966) reported failure to find the Alder anomaly in 9 patients with the eye anomaly.

Francois, J.: Heredity in Ophthalmology. St. Louis: C. V. Mosby Co., 1961.

Francois, J.: Progress in Ophthalamic Genetics. In, Steinberg, A. G. and Bearn, A. G. (eds.): Progress in Medical Genetics. New York: Grune and Stratton, 1962 (vol. 2). Pp. 331-365.

Francois, J., Barbier, F. and De Rouck, A.: A propos des conducteurs du gene de l'atrophia gyrata chorioideae et retinae de fuchs. Acta Genet. Med. Gem. 15: 34-35, 1966.

Francois, J., Barbier, F. and De Rouck, A.: Les conducteurs du gene de l'atrophia gyrata chorioideae et retinae de fuchs (anomalie d'Alder). Acta Genet. Med. Gem. 9: 74-91, 1960.

*23000 FUCOSIDOSIS

Van Hoof and Hers (1968) found a deficiency of alpha-fucosidase activity in the liver of patients with a Hurler-like disorder described by Durand et al. (1967, 1968). Fucose accumulated in all tissues (Durand et al., 1968). The patient of Bernard et al. (1966) was female. Durand et al. (1968) called the condition fucosidosis. The Belgian patient studied by Loeb et al. (1969) is probably related to the two Italian patients reported by Durand et al. (1969). Patel et al. (1972) described a different phenotype resulting from deficiency of alpha-l-fucosidase. The patient showed unusual survival (to 16 years) and from age 4 had angiokeratoma of the skin as in Fabry disease. Differing from Fabry disease was severe mental and physical retardation and normal renal function. This is, presumably, an example of allelism with production of quite different clinical picture. Compare the Hurler and Scheie syndromes (25280). Patel et al. (1972) described a 20-year-old male with severe mental and physical retardation, anhidrosis and inability to control body temperature, and angiokeratoma carporis diffusum. Urinary and leukocyte alpha-l-fucosidase was then 10 percent of normal, obligate heterozygotes had intermediate values. The patient was not Hurler-like in appearance. Yet another phenotype with deficiency of alpha-l-fucosidase was reported by Schafer et al. (1971) who found deficiency of this enzyme in a 9-year old-child with an unusual spondylometaphyseoepiphyseal dysplasia. In the rat alpha-l-fucosidase has a tetrameric structure, with two structurally different subunits, alpha and beta, like hemoglobin (Carlsen and Pierce, 1972). If the same is true in man, there is opportunity for at least two non-allelic varieties of fucosidosis. Gatti et al. (1973) emphasized heterogeneity in fucosidosis. Patients with this disorder have difficulty in degrading fucose-containing blood group H and Lewis substances.

Carlsen, R. B. and Pierce, J. G.: Purification and properties of an alpha-l-fucosidase from rat epididymis. J. Biol. Chem. 247: 23-32, 1972.

Durand, P., Borrone, C. and Della Cella, G.: Fucosidosis. J. Pediat. 75: 665-674, 1969.

Durand, P., Borrone, C., Della Cella, G. and Philippart, M.: Fucosidosis. (Letter) Lancet I: 1198 only, 1968.

Durand, P., Philippart, M., Borrone, C. and Della Cella, G.: A new glycolipid storage disease. (Abstract) Pediat. Res. 1: 416 only, 1967.

Epinette, W. W., Norins, A. L. and Drew, A. L.: Angiokeratoma corporis diffusum. Arch. Derm. 107: 754-757, 1973.

Gatti, R., Borrone, C., Trias, X., and Durand, P.: Genetic heterogeneity in fucosidosis. (Letter) Lancet II: 1024 only, 1973.

Leroy, J. G.: Fucosidosis? (Letter) Lancet II: 408-409, 1968.

Loeb, H., Tondeur, M., Jonniaux, G., Mockel-Pohl, S. and Vamos-Hurwitz, E.: Biochemical and ultrastructural studies in a case of mucopolysaccharidosis f (fucosidosis). Helv. Paediat. Acta 24: 519-537, 1969.

Patel, V., Watanabe, I. and Zeman, W.: Deficiency of alpha-l-fucosidase. Science 176: 426-427, 1972.

Schafer, I. A., Powell, D. W. and Sullivan, J. C.: Lysosomal bone disease. (Abstract) Pediat. Res. 5: 391-392, 1971.

Van Hoof, F. and Hers, H. G.: Mucopolysaccharidosis by absence of alpha-fucosidase. (Letter) Lancet I: 1198 only, 1968.

Zielke, K., Okada, S. and O'Brien, J. S.: Fucosidosis: diagnosis by serum assay of alpha-l-fucosidase. J. Lab. Clin. Med. 79: 164-169, 1972.

Zielke, K., Veath, M. L. and O'Brien, J. S.: Fucosidosis: deficiency of alpha-l-fucosidase in cultured skin fibroblasts. J. Exp. Med. 136: 197-199, 1972.

23010 FUNDUS FLAVIMACULATUS

This is probably a genetic disorder and probably autosomal recessive. Klein and Krill (1967) observed a 'familial incidence . . . in 10 of 27 patients.' The 10 familial cases included four pairs of affected sibs with ostensibly normal parents who were, however, not examined in most instances. No parental consanguinity was described. In one instance the father and two daughters were affected. In the instance of an affected brother and sister, the father was Negro and the mother white. Thus the inheritance is in doubt. This disorder derives its name from the occurrence of many yellow spots rather uniformly distributed over the fundus.

Klien, B. A. and Krill, A. E.: Fundus flavimaculatus: clinical, functional and histopathologic observations. Am. J. Ophthal. 64: 3-23, 1967.

*23020 GALACTOKINASE DEFICIENCY

In two sibs of a consanguineous Gypsy family, Gitzelmann (1967) found juvenile cataract related to galactokinase deficiency. Fanconi had previously reported the cases as instances of 'galactose diabetes.' Galactose-1-phosphate uridyltransferase activity in red cell was normal. No mental retardation was present. Several close relatives had reduced red cell galactokinase activity suggesting that they are heterozygotes. Mental retardation was present in some of Cotton's cases (1967). In Buffalo, N.Y., Mayes and Guthrie (1968) found 6 heterozygotes among 642 persons. The ethnic extraction was not given. Cook et al. (1971) described a case in a newborn ascertained because of hyperbilirubinemia with resolution of the cataract on dietary management. The cataracts in galactosemia and galactokinase deficiency are secondary to accumulation of galacitol in the lenses. Tedesco et al. (1972) presented evidence that American blacks have an allele in high frequency which causes a decrease in red cell galactokinase activity. It is probably distinct from the allele that causes, in the homozygous state, galactokinase deficiency as presently known. Several black families were shown to segregate for low, intermediate and high levels. Electrophoretic polymorphism of galactokinase has not yet been discovered (Vigneron, 1971). Ruddle (1973) has found that the locus is on chromosome no. 17

R
E
C
E
S
S
I
V
E

428   close to the thymidine kinase locus. Sun et al. (1973) had tentatively proposed that the galactokinase locus, as well as the next one in the metabolic chain, galactose-1-phosphate uridyltransferase, is located on chromosome no. 2. By cell hybridization studies Croce (1974) found that the structural genes for galactokinase and thymidine kinase are on the same chromosome (one resembling the human E-17) in the African green monkey. This is another striking example of chromosomal homology.

Beutler, E., Matsumoto, F., Kuhl, W., Krill, A., Levy, N., Sparkes, R. and Degnan, M.: Galactokinase deficiency as a cause of cataracts. New Eng. J. Med. 288: 1203-1206, 1973.

Cook, J. G. H., Don, N. A. and Mann, T. P.: Hereditary galactokinase deficiency. Arch. Dis. Child. 46: 465-469, 1971.

Cotton, J.-B.: Deficit hereditaire en galactokinase. Pediatrie 22: 609-611, 1967.

Croce, C. M.: Philadelphia, personal communication, 1974.

Gitzelmann, R.: Hereditary galactokinase deficiency, a newly recognized cause of juvenile cataracts. Pediat. Res. 1: 14-23, 1967.

Kaloud, H. and Sitzmann, F. C.: The galactokinase deficiency in two human populations: Styria (Austria) and Franconia (Bavaria). A comparative investigation on gene frequency. Z. Kinderheilk. 116: 185-192, 1974.

Kerr, M. M., Logan, R. W., Cant, J. S. and Hutchison, J. H.: Galactokinase deficiency in a newborn infant. Arch. Dis. Child. 46: 864-866, 1971.

Levy, N. S., Krill, A. E. and Beutler, E.: Galactokinase deficiency and cataracts. Am. J. Ophthal. 74: 41-48, 1972.

Mayes, J. S. and Guthrie, R.: Detection of heterozygotes for galactokinase deficiency in a human population. Biochem. Genet. 2: 219-230, 1968.

Oberman, A. E., Wilson, W. A., Fraiser, S. D., Donnell, G. N. and Bergren, W. R.: Galactokinase-deficiency cataracts in identical twins. Am. J. Ophthal. 74: 887-892, 1972.

Pickering, W. R. and Howell, R. R.: Galactokinase deficiency: clinical and biochemical findings in a new kindred. J. Pediat. 81: 50-55, 1972.

Ruddle, F. H.: New Haven, Conn., personal communication, 1973.

Sun, N. C., Chang, C. C. and Chu, E. H. Y.: Chromosome assignment of the human gene for galactose-1-phosphate uridyltransferase. Am. J. Hum. Genet. 25: 77A, 1973.

Tedesco, T. A., Bonow, R., Miller, K. and Mellman, W. J.: Galactokinase: evidence for a new racial polymerization. Science 178: 176-178, 1972.

Thalhammer, O., Gitzelmann, R. and Pantlitschko, M.: Hypergalactosemia and galactosuria due to galactokinase deficiency in a newborn. Pediatrics 42: 441-445, 1968.

Vigneron, C.: Electrophoresis of erythrocyte galactokinase. Enzyme 12: 426-432, 1971.

R E C E S S I V E

23030 GALACTORRHEA

Wider et al. (1969) described 3 sisters with non-puerperal galactorrhea occurring after treatment with oral contraceptive. Although all 3 had oligo-ovulation the evidence suggested independent control of ovulation and lactation: galactorrhea continued in one sister while she took an oral contraceptive containing estrogen-progesterone while presumably suppressed production of plasma gonadotropin by measures which stimulated the release of gonadotropins. Two of the sisters conceived after ovulations which occurred despite continuing ovulation.

Wider, J. A., Marshall, J. R. and Ross, G. T.: Familial galactorrhea in three sisters with oligo-ovulations. J.A.M.A. 209: 669-671, 1969.

*23035 GALACTOSE EPIMERASE DEFICIENCY

Glucose-1-phosphate and UDP-galactose are formed by the gal-1-P uridyltransferase reaction deficient in classic galactosemia. The interconversion of UDP-galactose and UDP-glucose is catalyzed by UDP-galactose 4-epimerase. The reaction is important to infants who receive a fifth of their daily caloric intake in the form of galactose. Also since the reaction produces galactose from glucose, galactose is not an essential component of food in man. Galactose-free diet is possible in galactokinase deficiency (23020) and in galactosemia (23040). Epimerase deficiency makes the individual dependent on exogenous galactose for necessary precursors for the synthesis of glycoproteins and glycolipids. Gitzelmann (1972) reported epimerase deficiency in a healthy infant. Elevated blood galactose was detected in a screening program. The parents had an intermediate level of enzymatic activity. The prognosis in the child is uncertain. Kalckar (1965) predicted some of the consequences of epimerase deficiency. This condition is almost certainly an autosomal recessive. However, only one case has been observed thus far.

Gitzelmann, R.: Deficiency of uridine diphosphate galactose 4-epimerase in blood cells of an apparently healthy infant. Helvet. Paediat. Acta 27: 125-130, 1972.

Gitzelmann, R. and Steinmann, B.: Uridine diphosphate galactose 4-epimerse deficiency. II. Clinical follow-up, biochemical studies and family investigation. Helv. Paediat. Acta. 28: 497-510, 1973.

Kalckar, H. M.: Galactose metabolism and cell 'sociology.' Science 150: 305-313, 1965.

*23040 GALACTOSEMIA

Cardinal features are hepatomegaly, cataracts and mental retardation. The defect concerns galactose-1-phosphate uridyl transferase. Beutler, Baluda, Sturgeon and Day (1965) have suggested that some persons with intermediate levels of the enzyme are not heterozygotes for the usual galactosemia but rather are homozygotes for what they term the Duarte variant. Heterozygotes for this variant have about 75 percent normal activity. This new form was discovered in the course of a screening program. Another type of galactosemia has been called the Negro variant. The difference in behavior of the metabolism of galactose in those patients may be due to the development of an alternative pathway (Cuatrecasas and Segal, 1966). Other relevant observations on the Negro variant were reported by Baker et al. (1967), Mellman et al. (1965), and Hsia (1967). Mellman et al. (1965) showed that the heterozygous parents of the Negro variant show nearly normal enzyme levels in white cells whereas classically galactosemic heterozygotes have about 50 percent activity in both red cells and white cells. Heterogeneity was demonstrated by the studies of Segal and Cuatrecasas (1968). In Massachusetts Shih et al. (1971), on the basis of a screening of newborns, found only two cases of galactosemia among 374,341 births. Both infants died with Escherichia coli sepsis in the neonatal period. Tedesco and Mellman (1971) demonstrated that in galactosemia gal-1-P uridyl transferase is immunologically intact although enzymatically defective. Thus, a structural gene mutation is involved. Nadler et al. (1970) found restoration of enzyme activity when cells from two patients with galactosemia were hybridized. Although they interpreted this as evidence of interallelic complementation, interlocus complementation seems possible. Patients with the Duarte variant of galactosemia are usually healthy, despite functional and structural abnormality in their galactose-1-phosphate uridyl transferase. An 8-month-old boy who had jaundice and liver enlargement during the first 2 months was reported by Kelly et al. (1972). He was homozygote for the Duarte variant. Both parents and two sisters were carriers. Surgical biopsy of the liver showed marked fatty infiltration, periportal fibrosis and cirrhosis. His subsequent development was normal. Improvement, the authors suggested, may have been due to maturation of the enzyme. Two similar cases have been reported. Sun et al. (1973) tentatively proposed that the galactose-1-phosphate uridyltransferase locus, as well as the preceding one in the metabolic pathway, galactokinase, is located on chromosome no. 2. Sun et al. (1974) concluded, from the study of Chinese hamster-human somatic cell hybrids, that the structural gene for gal-1-P uridyltransferase is located on chromosone no. 1. By study of cell hybrids, Tedesco (1973) concluded that the structural locus for galactose-1-phosphate uridyltransferase may be on chromosome no. 3.

Baker, L., Mellman, W. J., Tedesco, T. A. and Segal, S.: Galactosemia: symptomatic and asymptomatic homozygotes in one Negro sibship. J. Pediat. 68: 551-558, 1967.

Beutler, E., Baluda, M. C., Sturgeon, P. and Day, R.: A new genetic abnormality resulting in galactose-1-phosphate uridyltransferase deficiency. Lancet I: 353-354, 1965.

Cuatrecasas, P. and Segal, S.: Galactose conversion to d-xylulose: an alternate route of galactose metabolism. Science 153: 549-550, 1966.

Dawson, S. P., Hickman, R. O. and Kelley, V. C.: Galactosemia. A genetic study of four generations by enzyme assay. Am. J. Dis. Child. 100: 69-73, 1960.

Gitzelmann, R., Poley, J. R. and Prader, A.: Partial galactose-1-phosphate uridyltransferase deficiency due to a variant enzyme. Helv. Paediat. Acta 22: 252-257, 1967.

Haschemian, G. and Menne, F.: Beobachtungen einer familie mit galaktosamie 'duarte-variante.' Humangenetik 15: 223-226, 1972.

Hill, H. Z. and Puck, T. T.: Detection of inborn errors of metabolism: galactosemia. Science 179: 1136-1139, 1973.

Hsia, D. Y.-Y.: Clinical variants of galactosemia. Metabolism 16: 419-437, 1967.

Hsia, D. Y.-Y.: Galactosemia. (Conference 1967). Springfield, Ill.: Charles C Thomas, 1969.

Kelly, S., Desjardins, L. and Khera, S. A.: A duarte variant with clinical signs. J. Med. Genet. 9: 129, 1972.

Mellman, W. J., Tedesco, T. A. and Baker, L.: A new genetic abnormality. (Letter) Lancet I: 1395-1396, 1965.

Nadler, H. L., Chacko, C. M. and Rachmeler, M.: Interallelic complementation in hybrid cells derived from human diploid strains deficient in galactose-1-phosphate uridyl transferase activity. Proc. Nat. Acad. Sci. 67: 976-982, 1970.

Ng, W. G., Bergren, W. R. and Donnell, G. N.: A new variant of galactose-1-phosphate uridyltransferase in man: the Los Angeles variant. Ann. Hum. Genet. 37: 1-8, 1973.

Segal, S. and Cuatrecasas, P.: The oxidation of C(14) galactose by patients with congenital galactosemia. Evidence for a direct oxidative pathway. Am. J. Med. 44: 340-347, 1968.

Segal, S.: Disorders of galactose metabolism. In, Stanbury, J. B., Wyngaarden, J. B. and Fredrickson, D. S. (eds.): The Metabolic Basis of Inherited Disease. New York: McGraw-Hill, 1972 (3rd Ed.). Pp. 174-195.

Shih, V. E., Levy, H. L., Karolkewicz, V., Houghton, S., Efron, M. L., Isselbacher, K. J., Beutler, E. and MacCready, R. A.: Galactosemia screening of newborns in Massachusetts. New Eng. J. Med. 284: 753-757, 1971.

Sun, N. C., Chang, C. C. and Chu, E. H. Y.: Chromosome assignment of the human gene for galactose-1-phosphate uridyltransferase. Am. J. Hum. Genet. 25: 77A, 1973.

Sun, N. C., Chang, C. C. and Chu, E. H. Y.: Chromosome assignment of the human gene for galactose-1-phosphate uridyltransferase. (Gene mapping, Chinese-hamster cells, cell fusion). Proc. Nat. Acad. Sci. 71: 404-407, 1974.

RECESSIVE

Tedesco, T. A. and Mellman, W. J.: Galactosemia: evidence for a structural gene mutation. Science 172: 727-728, 1971.

Tedesco, F. J.: Philadelphia, personal communication, 1974.

Walker, F. A., Hsia, D. Y.-Y., Slatis, H. M. and Steinberg, A. G.: Galactosemia: a study of twenty-seven kindreds in North America. Ann. Hum. Genet. 25: 287-311, 1962.

*23045 GAMMA-GLUTAMYL-CYSTEINE SYNTHETASE DEFICIENCY, HEMOLYTIC ANEMIA DUE TO

Some patients with hemolytic anemia and low red-cell glutathione have deficiency of glutathione synthetase, the second enzyme involved in synthesis of glutathione (see 23190). Konrad et al. (1972) described a brother and sister of German descent with hemolytic anemia due to deficiency of the first enzyme of glutathione synthesis, gamma-glutamyl-cysteine synthetase. There was no known consanguinity in the family. Obligatory heterozygotes had an intermediate level of enzyme. Glutathione levels of red cells were normal in heterozygotes. Both affected sibs had late onset spinocerebellar degeneration.

Konrad, P. N., Richards, F., Valentine, W. N. and Paglia, D. E.: Gamma-glutamyl-cysteine synthetase deficiency: a cause of hereditary hemolytic anemia. New Eng. J. Med. 286: 557-561, 1972.

*23050 GANGLIOSIDOSIS, GENERALIZED GM(1), TYPE I

Landing (1964) first described this entity which has been variously called 'Hurler variant,' 'pseudo-Hurler disease,' and 'Tay-Sachs disease with visceral involvement.' O'Brien et al. (1965) suggested the designation 'generalized gangliosidosis.' The features are (1) severe cerebral degeneration leading to death within the first two years of life, (2) accumulation of ganglioside in neurons, and in hepatic, splenic and other histiocytes, and in renal glomerular epithelium, and (3) the presence of skeletal deformities resembling Hurler disease. The ganglioside stored is different from that in Tay-Sachs disease. It was identified as a Gm(1) ganglioside by O'Brien et al. (1965). Scott et al. (1967) described affected sibs. Renal biopsy showed storage of an acid mucopolysaccharide rather than a glycolipid in vacuoles of the glomerular epithelium. The vacuoles were thought to represent lysosomes. They suggested that neuro-visceral lipidosis or generalized gangliosidosis, as it has been called, may be closely related to the Hurler syndrome which it resembles clinically and radiologically. Okada and O'Brien (1968) demonstrated that beta-galactosidase deficiency is the fundamental fault in generalized gangliosidosis. The same enzyme cleaves the terminal galactose from the oligosaccharide moiety of Gm(1) and breaks down mucopolysaccharide. Grossman and Danes (1968) demonstrated X-ray features resembling those of Hurler syndrome, increased synthesis and storage of mucopolysaccharides by skin fibroblasts, and marked metachromasia of fibroblasts in both parents supporting autosomal recessive inheritance. Caffey (1951) probably described the first cases, interpreting them as gargoylism with prenatal onset. O'Brien (1969) found that all three isoenzymes of acid beta-galactosidase, A, B and C, were grossly deficient in all tissues. Theoretically, family studies of the linkage of the beta-galactosidase locus could be performed in families of patients with generalized gangliosidosis (Singer and Schafer, 1972).

Baker, H. J., Jr., Lindsey, J. R., McKhann, G. M. and Farrell, D. F.: Neuronal Gm(1) gangliosidosis in a siamese cat with beta-galactosidase deficiency. Science 174: 838-839, 1971.

Caffey, J. P.: Gargoylism (Hunter-Hurler disease, dysostosis multiplex, lipochondrodystrophy): prenatal and neonatal bone lesions and their early postnatal evolution. Bull. Hosp. Joint Dis. 12: 38-66, 1951.

Emery, J. M., Green, W. R., Wyllie, R. G. and Howell, R. R.: Gm(1)-gangliosidosis. Ocular and pathological manifestations. Arch. Ophthal. 85: 177-187, 1971.

Grossman, H. and Danes, B. S.: Neurovisceral storage disease: features and mode of inheritance. Am. J. Roentgen. 103: 149-153, 1968.

Kaback, M. M., Sloan, H. R., Sonneborn, M., Herndon, R. M. and Percy, A. K.: Gm(1) gangliosidosis type I: in utero detection and fetal manifestations. J. Pediat. 82: 1037-1041, 1973.

Landing, B. H., Silverman, F. N., Craig, J. M., Jacoby, M. D., Lahey, M. E. and Chadwick, D. L.: Familial neurovisceral lipidosis. An analysis of eight cases of a syndrome previously reported as 'Hurler-variant,' 'pseudo-Hurler disease' and 'Tay-Sachs disease with visceral involvement.' Am. J. Dis. Child. 108: 503-522, 1964.

MacBrinn, M. C., Okada, S., Ho, M. W., Hu, C. C. and O'Brien, J. S.: Generalized gangliosidosis: impaired cleavage of galactose from a mucopolysaccharide and a glycoprotein. Science 163: 946-947, 1969.

O'Brien, J. S.: Generalized gangliosidosis. J. Pediat. 75: 167-186, 1969.

O'Brien, J. S., Stern, M. B., Landing, B. H., O'Brien, J. K. and Donnell, G. N.: Generalized gangliosidosis: another inborn error of ganglioside metabolism? Am. J. Dis. Child. 109: 338-346, 1965.

Okada, S. and O'Brien, J. S.: Generalized gangliosidosis: beta-galactosidase deficiency. Science 160: 1002-1004, 1968.

Pinsky, L., Miller, J., Shanfield, B., Watters, G. and Wolfe, L. S.: Gm(1) gangliosidosis in skin fibroblast culture: enzymatic differences between types 1 and 2 and observation on a third variant. Am. J. Hum. Genet. 26: 563-577, 1974.

Scott, C. R., Lagunoff, D. and Trump, B. F.: Familial neuro-visceral lipidosis. J. Pediat. 71: 357-366, 1967.

Singer, H. S. and Schafer, I. A.: Clinical and enzymatic variations in Gm-1 generalized gangliosidosis. Am. J. Hum. Genet. 24: 454-463, 1972.

RECESSIVE

Thomas, G. H.: Beta-d-galactosidase in human urine: deficiency in generalized gangliosidosis. J. Lab. Clin. Med. 74: 725-731, 1969.

*23060 GANGLIOSIDOSIS, GENERALIZED GM(1), TYPE II, OR LATE INFANTILE TYPE

This disorder differs clinically and chemically from type I. Only B and C isoenzymes of beta-galactosidase are deficient (O'Brien, 1969). Gm(1) gangliosides accumulate in the brain but not in the viscera. Instead the viscera show excessive amounts of undersulfated keratansulfate-like mucopolysaccharide (Suzuki et al., 1969; first patient). The patients of Kint et al. (1969) and Wolfe et al. (1970) apparently had type II Gm(1)-gangliosidosis. Clinically the disorder develops later than type I gangliosidosis. Whereas type I is usually evident at birth and the affected infant rarely survives beyond the age of two years, clinical symptoms do not develop in type II until the second year of life and survival to 10 years has been observed. The initial description was made by Derry et al. (1968) in two sibs of French-Canadian ancestry. Differences in the beta-galactosidase in the two forms were found by Singer and Schafer (1972). Galjaard (1974) presented data from heterokaryotes indicating that the two varieties of Gm(1)-gangliosidosis (beta-galactosidase deficiency) may be determined by allelic genes because complementation was not observed. He studied two other types of beta-galactosidase deficiency which did complement types 1 and 2 but did not complement each other. Because of these findings, the asterisk has been removed from this entry (23060). When the second complementation group of beta-galactosidase deficiency is better characterized a separate entry will be made. Asterisks may be improper for entry 23060 because evidence is strong for a single polypeptide chain without subunits in beta-galactosidase A, and because cross-reacting protein to anti-A enzyme is found in tissues of pateints with all types (O'Brien, 1974).

Derry, D. M., Fawcett, J. S., Andermann, F. and Wolfe, L. S.: Late infantile systemic lipidosis (major monosialogangliosidosis delineation of two types). Neurology 18: 340-347, 1968.

Galjaard, H.: Rotterdam, personal communication, 1974.

Kint, J. A., Dacremont, G. and Vlietinck, R.: Type II Gm(1) gangliosidosis? Lancet II: 108-109, 1969.

O'Brien, J. S.: Five gangliosidoses. (Letter) Lancet II: 805 only, 1969.

O'Brien, J. S., Ho, M. W., Veath, M. L., Wilson, J. F., Myers, G., Opitz, J. M., ZuRhein, G. M., Spranger, J. W., Hartmann, H. A., Haneberg, B. and Grosse, F. R.: Juvenile Gm1 gangliosidosis: clinical, pathological, chemical and enzymatic studies. Clin. Genet. 3: 411-434, 1972.

O'Brien, J. S.: LaJolla and Berne, personal communication, Sept. 9, 1974.

Singer, H. S. and Schafer, I. A.: Clinical and enzymatic variations in Gm(1) generalized gangliosidosis. Am. J. Hum. Genet. 24: 454-463, 1972.

Suzuki, K., Suzuki, K. and Kamoshita, S.: Chemical pathology of Gm(1)-gangliosidosis (generalized gangliosidosis). J. Neuropath. Exp. Neurol. 28: 25-73, 1969.

Wolfe, L. S., Callahan, J., Fawcett, J. S., Andermann, F. and Scriver, C. R.: Gm(1)-gangliosidosis without chondrodystrophy or visceromegaly. Neurology 20: 23-43, 1970.

*23070 GANGLIOSIDOSIS, GM(2), TYPE III, OR JUVENILE TYPE

Six patients in four families have been observed (Suzuki et al., 1970; O'Brien, 1971). All have been of non-Jewish origin, as in the case of Sandhoff disease (type II Gm(2)-gangliosidosis). Onset occurs with ataxia between ages 2 and 6 years. Thereafter deterioration to decerebrate rigidity takes place. Blindness occurred late in the course in only some patients, unlike the situation in Tay-Sachs and Sandhoff diseases in which blindness is an invariable and early development. Death usually occurs between ages 5 and 15 years. The disorder is probably often misdiagnosed Batten-Spielmeyer-Vogt disease. The defect in this disorder is a partial deficiency of hexosaminidase A, the component deficient in Tay-Sachs disease.

O'Brien, J. S.: Ganglioside storage diseases. In, Harris, H. and Hirschhorn, K. (eds.): Advances in Human Genetics, 1971.

Suzuki, K., Suzuki, K., Rapin, I., Suzuki, Y. and Ishii, N.: Juvenile Gm(2)-gangliosidosis. Clinical variant of Tay-Sachs disease or a new disease. Neurology 20: 190-204, 1970.

Suzuki, Y. and Suzuki, K.: Partial deficiency of hexosaminidase component a in juvenile Gm(2)-gangliosidosis. Neurology 20: 848-851, 1970.

23075 GANGLIOSIDOSIS, GM(3)

Max et al. (1974) described an infant with a previously undescribed lipid storage disease. The clinical signs included poor physical and motor development, coarse facies, macroglossia, gingiva hypertrophy, stubby hands and feet, large inguinal hernias, hepatosplenomegaly and normal fundi. The infant was limp and unresponsive from soon after birth. Death occurred at 14 weeks. An accumulation of ganglioside Gm(3) was demonstrated in the liver and brain, with total absence of higher ganglioside homologs. The authors suggested that the defect is in the ganglioside biosynthesis, not degradation. The parents were of European Jewish descent and not known to be related. A maternal uncle died at 10 weeks with clinical and autopsy findings seemingly identical to the proband's. Thus, X-linked recessive inheritance is possible. This is the first identified example of a synthetic disorder of sphingogomyelin. The enzyme deficient is Gm(3)-UDP-N-acetyl-galactosaminyl transferase.

Max, S. R., Maclaren, N. K., Brady, R. O., Bradley, R. M., Rennels, M. B., Tanaka, J., Garcia, J. H. and Cornblath, M.: Gm(3) hematoside sphinoglipodystrophy. New Eng. J. Med. 291: 929-931, 1974.

*23080 GAUCHER DISEASE TYPE I (NON-CEREBRAL, JUVENILE)

The several forms of Gaucher disease are cerebroside lipidoses. The disease has been diagnosed as early as the first week of life and as late as 86 years. The classification followed here is that of Knudson and Kaplan (1962). An instructive pedigree was reported by Herrlin and Hillborg (1962). Serum acid phosphatase (which unlike the prostatic enzyme is not inhibited by L-tartrate) is elevated. Wiedemann and collaegues (1965) found typical Gaucher cells in the bone marrow of two clinically normal parents and a normal sister of two affected children and in the two clinically normal parents and two normal sisters of an affected young man. Brady et al. (1965) demonstrated a deficiency of glucoserbroside splitting enzyme in the spleen of Gaucher disease. This enzyme, normally present in large amounts in the spleen, is thought to be involved in the break-down of gluboside, an important lipoid constituent of red cells. Danes and Bearn (1968) found giant fibroblasts containing metachromatic material in both affected persons and heterozygotes for the chronic noncerebral form.

Brady, R. O.: The sphingolipidoses. New Eng. J. Med. 275: 312-318, 1966.

Brady, R. O., Kanfer, J. N. and Shapiro, D.: Metabolism of glucocerebrosides. II. Evidence of an enzymatic deficiency in Gaucher's disease. Biochem. Biophys. Res. Commun. 18: 221-225, 1965.

Crocker, A. C. and Landing, B. H.: Phosphatase studies in Gaucher's disease. Metabolism 9: 341-362, 1960.

Danes, B. S. and Bearn, A. G.: Gaucher's disease: a genetic disease detected in skin fibroblast cultures. Science 161: 1347-1348, 1968.

Davies, G. T. and Foreman, H. M.: Haemorrhagic pericardial effusion in adult Gaucher's disease. Brit. Heart J. 32: 855-858, 1970.

Fredrickson, D. S. and Sloan, H. R.: Glucosyl ceramide lipidoses: Gaucher's disease. In, Stanbury, J. B., Wyngaarden, J. B. and Fredrickson, D. S. (eds.): The Metabolic Basis of Inherited Disease. New York: McGraw-Hill, 1972 (3rd Ed.). Pp. 730-759.

Herrlin, K.-M. and Hillborg, P. O.: Neurological signs in a juvenile form of Gaucher's disease. Acta Paediat. 51: 137-154, 1962.

Hsia, D. Y.-Y., Naylor, J. and Bigler, J. A.: Gaucher's disease: report of two cases in father and son and review of the literature. New Eng. J. Med. 261: 164-169, 1959.

Kampine, J. P., Brady, R. O. and Kanfer, J. N.: Diagnosis of Gaucher's disease and Niemann-Pick disease with small samples of venous blood. Science 155: 86-88, 1967.

Knudson, A. G., Jr. and Kaplan, W. D.: Genetics of the sphingolipidoses. In, Aaronson, S. M. and Volk, B. W. (eds.): Cerebral Sphingolipidoses. A symposium on Tay-Sachs disease. New York: Academic Press. 1962. Pp. 395-411.

Wiedemann, H.-R., Gerken, H., Graucob, E. and Hansen, H.-G.: Recognition of heterozygosity in sphingolipidoses. (Letter) Lancet I: 1283 only, 1965.

R
E
C
E
S
S
I
V
E

23090 GAUCHER DISEASE TYPE II (INFANTILE, CEREBRAL)

This form does not show a preponderant Jewish incidence. We have observed Negro cases. Drukker et al. (1970) described a case in a Sephardic-Jewish infant. The disorder led to death at the age 48 hours from intracranial hemorrhage. Death usually occurs before the age of one year. Enlargement of the abdomen from hepatosplenomegaly and neurologic signs such as retroflexion of the head, strabismus, dysphagia, choking spells and hypertonicity are features.

Drukker, A., Sacks, M. I. and Gatt, S.: The infantile form of Gaucher's disease in an infant of Jewish Sephardic origin. Pediatrics 45: 1017-1023, 1970.

Schneider, E. L., Ellis, W. G., Brady, R. O., McCulloch, J. R. and Epstein, C. J.: Infantile (type II) Gaucher's disease: in utero diagnosis and fetal pathology. J. Pediat. 81: 1134-1139, 1972.

23100 GAUCHER DISEASE TYPE III (JUVENILE AND ADULT, CEREBRAL)

Hematologic abnormalities with hypersplenism, bone lesions, skin pigmentation and pingueculae occur in this form. This type is particularly frequent in Jews. For references, see GAUCHER DISEASE, TYPE I. Partial manifestation in heterozygotes has led some to propose dominant inheritance. Desnick et al. (1971) demonstrated that both homozygotes and heterozygotes can be identified by chemical analysis of the sediment from a 24-hour urine collection. Individual neutral glycosphingolipids were separated by thin-layer chromatography and quantitatively estimated by gas-liquid chromatography. Other glycosphingolipids which could be diagnosed by this method included Krabbe leukodystrophy, lactosylceramidosis, Fabry disease, Sandhoff disease and metachromatic leukodystrophy. Beutler et al. (1971) demonstrated deficiency of beta-glucosidase activity in fibroblasts from homozygotes with the adult form of Gaucher disease and found an intermediate level of enzyme activity in heterozygote. Note that only one asterisk is assigned to the three forms of Gaucher disease because the same enzyme is deficient in each and until evidence to the contrary is available we are forced to conclude that the mutations responsible for the several forms are allelic. As suggested by Fredrickson and Sloan (1972), genetic compounds would be expected on the basis of this hypothesis and may indeed be the basis of some cases not typical of one of the three classic types. Miller et al. (1973) described a Negro family in which three sibs had enzymatically proved Gaucher disease and neurologic manifestations including seizures. This may be an allelic variant.

Beutler, E. and Kuhl, W.: The diagnosis of the adult type of Gaucher's disease and its carrier state by demonstration of deficiency of beta-glucosidase activity in peripheral blood leukocytes. J. Lab. Clin. Med. 76: 747-755, 1970.

Beutler, E., Kuhl, W., Trinidad, F., Teplitz, R. and Nadler, H.: Beta-glucosidase activity in fibroblasts from homozygotes and heterozygotes for Gaucher's disease. Am. J. Hum. Genet. 23: 62-66, 1971.

Desnick, R. J., Dawson, G., Desnick, S. J., Sweeley, C. C. and Krivit, W.: Diagnosis of glycosphingolipidoses by urinary-sediment analysis. New Eng. J. Med. 284: 739-744, 1971.

Fredrickson, D. S. and Sloan, H. R.: Glucosyl ceramide lipidoses: Gaucher's disease. In, Stanbury, J. B., Wyngaarden, J. B. and Fredrickson, D. S. (eds.): The Metabolic Basis of Inherited Disease. New York: McGraw-Hill, 1972 (3rd Ed.). Pp. 730-759.

Ho, M. W., Seck, J., Schmidt, D., Veath, M. L., Johnson, W., Brady, R. O. and O'Brien, J. S.: Adult Gaucher's disease: kindred studies and demonstration of a deficiency of acid beta-glucosidase in cultured fibroblasts. Am. J. Hum. Genet. 24: 37-45, 1972.

Miller, J. D., McCluer, R. and Kanfer, J. N.: Gaucher's disease: neurologic disorder in adult siblings. Ann. Intern. Med. 78: 883-887, 1973.

23105 GELEOPHYSIC DWARFISM

Spranger et al. (1971) suggested this designation because of the happy faces of the affected children. They further suggested that the disorder is a 'focal' mucopolysaccharidosis. In addition to the facial appearance three unrelated children showed dysostosis-multiplex-like changes predominantly in the hands and feet and an apparently focal accumulation of acid mucopolysaccharides in the liver and possibly the cardiovascular system. Small hands and feet were evident at birth. The upper lip was long and thick with 'ironing out' of the philtrum. The nasal bridge was depressed. Joint contractures affected particularly the fingers. Hepatomegaly and cardiomegaly were present. Urinary excretion of mucopolysaccharides was normal.

Spranger, J. W., Gilbert, E. F., Tuffli, G. A., Rossiter, F. P. and Opitz, J. M.: Geleophysic dwarfism — a 'focal' mucopolysaccharidosis? (Letter) Lancet I: 97-98, 1971.

*23110 GIANT CELL HEPATITIS, NEONATAL

Increased parental consanguinity suggested autosomal recessive inheritance. However, only 12 of 71 sibs of index cases were also affected. It was suggested that in some with the appropriate genotype the disease is manifested so severely or so mildly that the diagnosis is not made. An apparent excess of affected males may be further evidence of failure of manifestation of the genotype. Alternatively the cases analyzed may include more than one disease. Feinberg (1960) reported two pairs of male sibs and Laurendeau, Hill and Manning (1961) observed two affected sisters. The disorder is sometimes loosely labeled 'neonatal hepatitis.'

Cassady, G., Morrison, A. B. and Cohen, M. M.: Familial 'giant-cell hepatitis' in infancy. Clinical, pathologic, and genetic studies on a large family. Am. J. Dis. Child. 107: 456-469, 1964.

Danks, D. and Bodian, M.: A genetic study of neonatal obstructive jaundice. Arch. Dis. Child. 38: 378-390, 1960.

Feinberg, R.: Perinatal idiopathic hemochromatosis: giant cell hepatitis interpreted as an inborn error of metabolism. Am. J. Clin. Path. 33: 480-491, 1960.

Laurendeau, T., Hill, J. E. and Manning, G. B.: Idiopathic neonatal hemochromatosis in siblings. An inborn error of metabolism. Arch. Path. 72: 410-423, 1961.

R
E
C
E
S
S
I
V
E

*23130 GLAUCOMA, CONGENITAL (BUPHTHALMOS)

The ocular globe is usually large as a result of the increased intra-ocular pressure dating from intrauterine life, hence the term buphthalmos, meaning 'ox eye.' In only about half of cases are both eyes involved and males are affected somewhat more often than females. The canal of Schlemm is present and communicates normally with the veins as is proved by demonstrable filling of the canal with blood when the jugular veins are compressed. The defect is thought to involve the permeability of the trabeculum to aqueous humor. Autosomal recessive inheritance is quite certain in a significant proportion of cases. The syndrome of congenital glaucoma with mental retardation and decreased renal ammonium production (Lowe syndrome) is inherited as an X-linked recessive. Autosomal recessive glaucoma occurs in the rabbit (Hanna et al., 1962).

Barkan, O. and Ferguson, W. J., Jr.: Congenital glaucoma. Pediat. Clin. N. Am. 5: 225-229, 1958.

Graham, M. V. and Crick, R. P.: Bilateral congenital buphthalmos in two sisters. Brit. J. Ophthal. 42: 370-371, 1958.

Hanna, B. L., Sawin, P. B. and Sheppard, L. B.: Recessive buphthalmos in the rabbit. Genetics 47: 519-529, 1962.

Westerlund, E.: Clinical and genetic studies on the primary glaucoma diseases. Op. ex. Domo Biol. Hered. Hum. U. Hafniensis 12: 11-207, 1947.

23140 GLAUCOMA, CONGENITAL, WITH MENTAL RETARDATION

We have observed three sibs (2 males, 1 female) with congenital glaucoma and severe mental retardation (214487, 261714). One of the males, the oldest of the 3 affected sibs, died at age 32 of coronary occlusion.

*23150 GLAUCOMA, JUVENILE

There is some question what should be classified as juvenile glaucoma. Most cases may be either congenital glaucoma with late onset or open-angle or closed-angle glaucoma with early onset. Waardenburg (1950) suggested that recessive inheritance of some cases of glaucoma is proved by (1) a high frequency of parental consanguinity, (2) the presence of the disease in about 25 percent of sibs of probands, (3) the presence of the disease in all children of a marriage between two affected persons, and (4) the occurrence of glaucoma in collaterals of both parents in some families. Beiguelman and Prado (1963) reported a Brazilian pedigree as convincing evidence for recessive inheritance of juvenile glaucoma.

Beiguelman, B. and Prado, D.: Recessive juvenile glaucoma. J. Genet. Hum. 12: 53-54, 1963.

Waardenburg, P. J.: Ueber das familiaere Vorkommen und den Erbgang des praesenilen und senilen Glaukoms. Genetica 25: 79-125, 1950.

*23160 GLUCOSE-GALACTOSE MALABSORPTION

A picture clinically indistinguishable from intestinal disaccharidase deficiency is produced by intestinal monosaccharidase deficiency. Because of the deficiency glucose and galactose are not absorbed. Fructose and xylose are normally absorbed. This disorder is a transport defect. In vitro the intestinal mucosa is incapable of taking up glucose even to the concentration of the medium. Occurrence in both sexes, familial incidence, and at least three instances of parental consanguinity are consistent with autosomal recessive inheritance.

Anderson, C. M., Kerry, K. R. and Townley, R. R. W.: An inborn defect of intestinal absorption of certain monosaccharides. Arch. Dis. Child. 40: 1-6, 1965.

Elsas, L. J. and Lambe, D. W., Jr.: Familial glucose-galactose malabsorption: remission of glucose intolerance. J. Pediat. 83: 226-232, 1973.

Elsas, L. J., Hillman, R. E., Patterson, J. H. and Rosenberg, L. E.: Renal and intestinal hexose transport in familial glucose-galactose malabsorption. J. Clin. Invest. 49: 576-585, 1970.

Lebenthal, E., Garti, R., Mathoth, Y., Cohen, B. E. and Katzenelson, D.: Glucose-galactose malabsorption in an Oriental-Iraqi Jewish family. J. Pediat. 78: 844-850, 1971.

Lindquist, B., Meeuwisse, G. W. and Melin, K.: Osmotic diarrhoea in genetically transmitted glucose-galactose malabsorption. Acta Pediat. 52: 217-219, 1963.

Meeuwisse, G. W. and Dahlqvist, A.: Glucose-galactose malabsorption. A study with biopsy of the small intestinal mucosa. Acta Paediat. Scand. 57: 273-280, 1968.

Meeuwisse, G. W.: Glucose-galactose malabsorption. Studies on the intermediate carbohydrate metabolism. Helvet. Paediat. Acta 25: 13-24, 1970.

Schneider, A. J., Kintner, W. B. and Stirling, C. E.: Glucose-galactose malabsorption. Report of a case with autoradiographic studies of a mucosal biopsy. New Eng. J. Med. 274: 305-312, 1966.

23165 GLUTAMATE-ASPARTATE TRANSPORT DEFECT

Teijema et al. (1974) described a child with a defect in renal and probably intestinal transport of two acidic amino acids, glutamic and aspartic acids. The patient also had moderate hyperprolinemia. Hypoglycemia was a feature.

Teijema, Hl L., Van Gelderan, H. H., Giesberts, M. A. H. and Laurent de Angulo, M. S. L.: Dicarboxylic amino aciduria: an inborn error of glutamic and aspartate transport with metabolic implications, in combination with a hyperprolinemia. Metabolism 23: 115-123, 1974.

*23167 GLUTARIC ACIDEMIA

Goodman et al. (1974) described glutaric aciduria and acidemia in a brother and sister with a neurodegenerative disorder beginning at about 6 months of age and characterized by opisthotonus, dystonia and athetoid posturing. Deficiency of glutaryl-CoA dehydrogenase.

Goodman, S. I., Moe, P. G. and Markey, S. P.: Glutaric aciduria: a 'new' inborn error of amino acid metabolism. (Abstract) Am. J. Hum. Genet. 26: 36A only, 1974.

*23170 GLUTATHIONE PEROXIDASE DEFICIENCY, HEMOLYTIC ANEMIA DUE TO

Necheles et al. (1968) observed hemolytic disease of the newborn with hyperbilirubinemia and Heinz bodies, associated with partial deficiency of red cell glutathione peroxidase. The clinical manifestations were self-limited and evidence of hemolysis had disappeared by 3 months of age, although the enzyme deficiency persisted. Sibs were affected in some instances and one parent had comparably depressed enzyme level and a history of neonatal jaundice. Necheles et al. (1969) found low levels of glutathione peroxidase in an 18-year-old Puerto Rican male with compensated hemolytic anemia. Both parents and one sib had intermediate enzyme levels. By electrophoretic means, Beutler and West (1974) demonstrated polymorphism of red cell glutathione peroxidase in Afro-Americans. Since no male-to-male transmission was noted, X-linkage could not be excluded but is unlikely.

Beutler, E. and West, C.: Red cell glutathione peroxidase polymorphism in Afro-Americans. Am. J. Hum. Genet. 26: 255-258, 1974.

Boivin, P., Galand, C. and Hakim, J.: Anemie hemolytique avec deficit en glutathion-peroxydase chez un adulte. Enzymol. Biol. Clin. 10: 68-80, 1969.

Necheles, T. F., Boles, T. A. and Allen, D. M.: Erythrocyte glutathione-peroxidase deficiency and hemolytic disease of the newborn infant. J. Pediat. 72: 319-324, 1968.

Necheles, T. F., Maldonado, N., Barquet-Chediak, A. and Allen, D. M.: Homozygous erythrocyte glutathione-peroxidase deficiency: clinical and biochemical studies. Blood 33: 164-169, 1969.

Necheles, T. F., Steinberg, M. H. and Cameron, D.: Erythrocyte glutathione-peroxidase deficiency. Brit. J. Haemat. 19: 605-612, 1970.

R
E
C
E
S
S
I
V
E

Nishimura, Y., Chida, N., Hayashi, T. and Arakawa, T. S.: Homozygous glutathione-peroxidase deficiency of erythrocytes and leukocytes. Tohoku J. Exp. Med. 108: 207-218, 1972.

Steinberg, M. H. and Necheles, T. F.: Erythrocyte glutathione peroxidase deficiency. Biochemical studies on the mechanisms of drug-induced hemolysis. Am. J. Med. 50: 542-546, 1971.

Steinberg, M. H., Brauer, M. J. and Necheles, T. F.: Acute hemolytic anemia associated with erythrocyte glutathione-peroxidase deficiency. Arch. Intern. Med. 125: 302-303, 1970.

*23180 GLUTATHIONE REDUCTASE, HEMOLYTIC ANEMIA DUE TO DEFICIENCY OF, IN RED CELLS

Lohr and Waller (1962) observed a 'new' form of enzyme-deficiency hemolytic anemia. Glutathione reductase was deficient. Reduced glutathione (GSH) was low as a consequence. (This condition is apparently distinct from that described by Oort et al. (1961) in which GSH was also low, but glucose-6-phosphate dehydrogenase and glutathione reductase were normal.) Lohr (1963) observed 10 homozygotes and 5 heterozygotes in a family distribution consistent with autosomal recessive inheritance. Blume et al. (1968) studied a kindred with many persons who were demonstrably heterozygous by chemical test. Hampel et al. (1969) found a markedly increased frequency of chromosomal aberrations in a patient with pancytopenia and absent GR-II band in the electropherogram. The mother was hematologically normal but had absent GR-II band and a moderate increase in the frequency of chromosomal aberrations. Addition of chloramphenicol to the cultures increased the number of damaged chromosomes in both the mother and the son. Staal et al. (1969) described a variety of glutathione reductase anemia in which the variant enzyme had diminished affinity for flavin adenine dinucleotide. The patient's anemia was corrected by vitamin B2. Administration of flavin compounds to normal individuals or addition to hemolysates of most normal persons causes an increase in activity of glutathione reductase (Beutler, 1969). Long (1972) had observed two variant forms of red cell glutathione reductase which appear to bind far more avidly than the common form of the enzyme. Fajnholc et al. (1971) found red cell GR deficiency in a patient with systemic lupus erythematosus. The deficiency was correctable in vivo with riboflavin and in vitro with flavin adenine nucleotide. The same deficiency was found in the mother and some of her relatives (who were asymptomatic) but not in the father and his relatives. Enzyme kinetics were normal. These workers concluded that the defect was not in the apoenzyme. Thus, the locus concerned may be different from that involved with the electrophoretic variants of GR (13830).

Beutler, E.: Effect of flavin compounds on glutathione reductase activity: in vivo and in vitro studies. J. Clin. Invest. 48: 1957-1966, 1969.

Blume, K. G., Gottwik, M., Lohr, G. W. and Rudiger, H. W.: Familienuntersuchungen zum Glutathionreduktasemangel menschlicher Erythrocyten. Humangenetik 6: 163-170, 1968.

Carson, P. E., Brewer, G. J. and Ickes, C.: Decreased glutathione reductase with susceptibility to hemolysis. (Abstract) J. Lab. Clin. Med. 58: 804 only, 1961.

Fajnholc, N. E., Kaminsky, E., Machtey, I, and De Vries, A.: Hereditary erythrocyte glutathione reductase deficiency. Rev. Europ. Clin. Biol. 16: 987-991, 1971.

Hampel, K. E., Lohr, G. W., Blume, K. G. and Rudiger, H. W.: Spontane und chloramphenicolinduzierte Chromosomenmutationen und biochemische Befunde bei zwei Faellen mit Glutathionreduktasemangel (NAD(P)H: glutathione oxidoreductase, e.C.1.6.4.2). Humangenetik 7: 305-313, 1969.

Kurz, R. and Hohenwallner, W.: Familiaerer Glutathionreduktasemangel und Stoerung der Glutathion-synthese im Erythrozyten. Helv. Paediat. Acta 25: 542-552, 1970.

Lohr, G. W. and Waller, H. D.: Eine neue enzymopenische haemolytische Anaemie mit Glutathionreduktase-Mangel. Med. Klin. 57: 1521-1525, 1962.

Lohr, G. W. and Waller, H. D.: Zur Biochemie einiger angeborener haemolytischer Anaemien. Folia Haemat. 8: 377-397, 1963.

Lohr, G. W.: Marburg, Germany: personal communication, 1963.

Long, W. K.: Austin, Texas: personal communication, 1972.

Oort, M., Loos, J. H. and Prins, H. K.: Hereditary absence of reduced glutathione in the erythrocytes — a new clinical and biochemical entity. Vox Sang. 6: 370-373, 1961.

Staal, G. E. J., Helleman, P. W., De Wael, J. and Veeger, C.: Purification and properties of an abnormal glutathione reductase from human erythrocytes. Biochem. Biophys. Acta 185: 63-69, 1969.

R
E
C
E
S
S
I
V
E

*23190 GLUTATHIONE SYNTHETASE DEFICIENCY OF ERYTHROCYTES, HEMOLYTIC ANEMIA DUE TO

Mohler et al. (1970) described a man of Scottish extraction with hemolytic anemia due to deficiency of glutathione synthetase. (Two separate enzymes are involved in glutathione synthesis. The coupling of glutamic acid and cysteine is catalyzed by glutamyl-cysteine synthetase and glycine is added to form the tripeptide through the enzymatic action of glutathione synthetase.) Four children of the proband, one of three of his sibs and both parents had intermediate levels of enzyme. Presumably the family of Oort et al. (1961) and of Prins et al. (1966) had the same condition as did also that of Boivin et al. (1966). In the family reported by Prins and colleagues (1963), three out of 12 sibs from consanguineous (second cousin) parents had absence of glutathione in the erythrocytes. The clinical picture was that of nonspherocytic hemolytic anemia. Glyoxylase activity, which is dependent on glutathione as a cofactor, was also deficient. Other enzymes were increased, presumably due to the younger average age of erythrocytes. In a later report on the kindred 5 cases in 2 sibships with all 4 parents traced to a common ancestral couple were described. Glutathione (gamma-glutamyl-cysteinyl-glycine) was less than 10 percent of normal in presumed homozygotes.

436

Boivin, P., Galand, C., Andre, R. and Debray, J.: Anemies hemolytiques congenitales avec deficit isole en glutathion reduit par deficit en glutathion synthetase. Nouv. Rev. Franc. Hemat. 6: 859-865, 1966.

Mohler, D. N., Majerus, P. W., Minnich, V., Hess, C. E. and Garrick, M. D.: Glutathione synthetase deficiency as a cause of hereditary hemolytic disease. New Eng. J. Med. 283: 1253-1257, 1970.

Oort, M., Loos, J. A. and Prins, H. K.: Hereditary absence of reduced glutathione in the erythrocytes — a new clinical and biochemical entity. Vox Sang. 6: 370-373, 1961.

Prins, H. K., Oort, M., Loos, J. A., Zurcher, C. and Beckers, T.: Congenital nonspherocytic hemolytic anemia, associated with glutathione deficiency of the erythrocytes. Hematologic, biochemical and genetic studies. Blood 27: 145-166, 1966.

Zurcher, C.: Glutathione deficiency. In, Beutler, E. (ed.): Hereditary Disorders of Erythrocyte Metabolism. New York: Grune and Stratton, 1967.

*23200 GLYCINEMIA (HYPERGLYCINEMIA WITH KETOACIDOSIS AND LEUKOPENIA); PROPIONICACIDEMIA

The features are episodic vomiting, lethargy and ketosis, neutropenia, periodic thrombocytopenia, hypogammaglobulinemia, developmental retardation and intolerance to protein. Outstanding chemical features are hyperglycinemia and hyperglycinuria. This disorder is not to be confused with hereditary glycinuria which has been described only in one family (De Vries et al. 1957) and is presumably transmitted as a dominant because affected members occurred in three successive generations. (The possibility of quasi-dominant pedigree pattern should be investigated by inquiry into the possibility of consanguinity and the presence of a partial defect in the presumably normal spouses.) The defect resides in the renal tubule. To avoid confusion and to parallel the usage with galactosemia, I prefer to call this disease glycinemia and the disorder in the Bulgarian-Jewish family glycinuria, paralleling the usage with cystinuria. Soriano et al. (1967) suggested that in the disorder first described by Childs et al. (1961) a generalized defect in utilization of amino acids results in excessive deamination of certain amino acids in muscle, with consequent hyperammonemia and ketoacidosis. In a second group of patients whose disorder is also termed hyperglycinemia, ketoacidosis, neutropenia and thrombocytopenia have not been observed and glycine is the only amino acid present in excess in serum and urine. See HYPERGLYCINEMIA, ISOLATED. Also see METHYLMALONIC ACIDURIA. Hsia et al. (1969) demonstrated deficient propionate carboxylation as the basic defect in ketotic hyperglycinemia. In a male Pakistani offspring of first-cousin parents, Gompertz et al. (1970) described acidosis and ketosis due to propionicacidemia, leading to death at 8 days. A sib had died at 2 weeks of age with metabolic acidosis and ketonuria. The defect was found to involve mitochondrial propionyl-CoA carboxylase. The same condition was described by Hommes et al. (1968). Hsia et al. (1971) showed that 'ketotic hyperglycinemia' is the same as propionicacidemia and is the result of a defect in propionyl-CoA carboxylase. They studied fibroblasts from a sister of the boy in whom this disorder was first described by Childs et al. (1961). Clinical and biochemical similarities between the condition and methylmalonicaciduria had suggested that it also had a defect in the propionate-methylmalonate-succinate pathway. Patients with this disorder have a characteristic facies with very puffy cheeks and exaggerated Cupid's bow upper lip. Protein restriction is effective therapy. In a sister of the original case reported by Childs et al. (1961), Brandt et al. (1972) demonstrated that with low protein diet growth and intelligence developed normally to age 9 years. Indeed intelligence was superior.

R
E
C
E
S
S
I
V
E

Ando, T., Rasmussen, K., Nyhan, W. L., Donnell, G. N. and Barnes, N. D.: Propionicacidemia in patients with ketotic hyperglycinemia. J. Pediat. 78: 827-832, 1971.

Barnes, N. D., Hull, D., Balgobin, L. and Gompertz, D.: Biotin-responsive propionicacidaemia. Lancet II: 244-245, 1970.

Brandt, I. K., Hsia, Y. E., Clement, D. H. and Provence, S. A.: Propionicacidemia (ketotic hyperglycinemia): dietary treatment resulting in normal growth and development. (Abstract) Am. J. Hum. Genet. 24: 23A only, 1972.

Brandt, I. K., Hsia, E., Clement, D. H. and Provence, S. A.: Propionicacidemia (ketotic hyperglycinemia): dietary treatment resulting in normal growth and development. Pediatrics 53: 391-395, 1974.

Childs, B., Nyhan, W. L., Borden, M., Bard, L. and Cooke, R. E.: Idiopathic hyperglycinemia and hyperglycinuria: a new disorder of amino acid metabolism. Pediatrics 27: 522-538, 1961.

De Vries, A., Kochwa, S., Lazebnik, J., Frank, M. and Djaldetti, M.: Glycinuria, a hereditary disorder associated with nephrolithiasis. Am. J. Med. 23: 408-415, 1957.

Gompertz, D., Bau, D. C. K., Storrs, C. N., Peters, T. J. and Hughes, E. A.: Localisation of enzymic defect in propionicacidaemia. Lancet I: 1140-1143, 1970.

Hommes, F. A., Kuipers, J. R. G., Elema, J. D., Jansen, J. F. and Jonxis, J. H. P.: Propionicacidemia, a new inborn error of metabolism. Pediat. Res. 2: 519-524, 1968.

Hsia, Y. E., Scully, K. J. and Rosenberg, L. E.: Defective propionate carboxylation in ketotic hyperglycinaemia. Lancet I: 757-758, 1969.

Hsia, Y. E., Scully, K. J. and Rosenberg, L. E.: Inherited propionyl-coa carboxylase deficiency in 'ketotic hyperglycinemia.' J. Clin. Invest. 50: 127-130, 1971.

Landes, R. D., Avery, G. B., Walker, F. A. and Hsia, Y. E.: Propionyl-coa carboxylase deficiency (propionicacidemia): another cause of hyperammonemia. (Abstract) Pediat. Res. 394 only, 1972.

Nyhan, W. L.: Treatment of hyperglycinemia. Am. J. Dis. Child. 113: 129-133, 1967.

Nyhan, W. L.: Nonketotic hyperglycinemia. In, Stanbury, J. B., Wyngaarden, J. B. and Fredrickson, D. S. (eds.): The Metabolic Basis of Inherited Disease. New York: McGraw-Hill, 1972 (3rd Ed.). Pp. 464-475.

Nyhan, W. L., Borden, M. and Childs, B.: Idiopathic hyperglycinemia: a new disorder of amino-acids metabolism. II. The concentrations of other amino-acids in the plasma and their modification by the administration of leucine. Pediatrics 27: 539-550, 1961.

Nyhan, W. L., Chisolm, J. J., Jr. and Edwards, R. O., Jr.: Idiopathic hyperglycinuria. III. Report of a second case. J. Pediat. 62: 540-545, 1963.

Rampini, S., Vischer, D., Curtius, H. C., Anders, P. W., Tancredi, F., Frischknecht, W. and Prader, A.: Hereditare hyperglycinamie. Helv. Paediat. Acta 22: 135-159, 1967.

Soriano, J. R., Taitz, L. S., Finberg, L. and Edelmann, C. M., Jr.: Hyperglycinemia with ketoacidosis and leukopenia. Pediatrics 39: 818-828, 1967.

23210 GLYCOGEN STORAGE DISEASE LIMITED TO HEART (ANTOPOL DISEASE)

In 1940 Antopol and colleagues described two brothers who died in the second decade of life with heart failure and showed at autopsy, in one so studied, glycogen storage disease limited to the myocardium. Mehrizi and Oppenheimer (1960) reported two related cases which appear to represent the identical disease (J.H.H. cases B46872 and A70767). Antopol's case had excessive deposits of glycogen in skeletal muscle also and comments on skeletal muscle were not made in the cases of Mehrizi and Oppenheimer. Thus, it is not certain that this entity is distinct from one of the other glycogenoses.

Antopol, W., Boas, E. P., Levison, W. and Tuchman, L. R.: Cardiac hypertrophy caused by glycogen storage disease in a 15-year-old boy. Am. Heart J. 20: 546-556, 1940.

Mehrizi, A. and Oppenheimer, E. H.: Heart failure associated with unusual deposition of glycogen in the myocardium. Bull. Hopkins Hosp. 107: 329-336, 1960.

*23220 GLYCOGEN STORAGE DISEASE I (VON GIERKE DISEASE; HEPATORENAL FORM OF GLYCOGEN STORAGE DISEASE; GLUCOSE-6-PHOSPHATASE DEFICIENCY; HEPATORENAL GLYCOGENOSIS)

The liver and kidney are involved. The basic defect resides in glucose-6-phosphatase. Hypoglycemia is a major problem. Lipidemia also occurs and may lead to xanthoma formation. Rare survival to adulthood has been observed. Hyperuricemia has been observed in a considerable number of patients and in some clinical gout has occurred. Inhibited tubular secretion of uric acid due to hyperlacticacidemia and ketonemia has been postulated. Senior and Loridan (1968) found that the effects of glycerol administered by mouth on levels of glucose and of lactate, together with the response to epinephrine or glucagon permitted differentiation of the several types of hepatic glycogenosis (I, II, III and IV). They proposed the existence of a second type of von Gierke disease in which, although glucose-6-phosphatase activity is present on in vitro assay, glucose is not liberated from glucose-6-phosphate in vivo. They referred to this as 'functional deficiency of G6P.' They pointed out that some mutants in neurospora show impaired enzyme function in the intact fungus despite normal activity in homogenates. The glycogen storage diseases represent a notable example of genetic heterogeneity. Glycogenosis I in particular illustrates pleiotropism with simulation of primary gout and xanthomatosis.

Fine, R. N., Wilson, W. A. and Donnell, G. N.: Retinal changes in glycogen storage disease type I. Am. J. Dis. Child. 115: 328-331, 1968.

Howell, R. R.: The glycogen storage diseases. In, Stanbury, J. B., Wyngaarden, J. B. And Fredrickson, D. S. (eds.): The Metabolic Basis of Inherited Disease. New York: McGraw-Hill, 1972 (3rd Ed.). Pp. 149-173.

Howell, R. R.: The interrelationship of glycogen storage disease and gout. Arth. Rheum. 8: 780-785, 1965.

Senior, B. and Loridan, L.: Functional differentiation of glycogenoses of the liver: with respect to the use of glycerol. New Eng. J. Med. 279: 965-970, 1968.

Senior, B. and Loridan, L.: Liver glycogenoses: metabolism of intravenously administered glycerol. New Eng. J. Med. 279: 958-965, 1968.

Sidbury, J. B., Jr.: The genetics of the glycogen storage disease. In, Steinberg, A. G. and Bearn, A. G. (eds.): Progress in Medical Genetics. Grune and Stratton, Vol. 4, 1965. Pp. 32-58.

Spencer-Peet, J., Norman, M. E., Lake, B. D., McNamara, J. and Patrick, A. D.: Hepatic glycogen storage disease. Clinical and laboratory findings in 23 cases. Quart. J. Med. 40: 95-114, 1971.

*23230 GLYCOGEN STORAGE DISEASE II (POMPE DISEASE; CARDIAC FORM OF GENERAL-IZED GLYCOGENOSIS; CARDIOMEGALIA GLYCOGENICA DIFFUSA; ETC.)

The defect involves acid-alpha-1,4-glucosidase and involvement is generalized. The affected children are prostrate, appear imbecilic, and are markedly hypotonic with large hearts. The tongue is enlarged. Neurologic disorders may result from extensive CNS involvement. The liver is rarely enlarged (except as a result of heart failure) and hypoglycemia and acidosis do not occur as they do in type I. See Field, R. A.: loc. cit. Pompe disease may be of more than one type. In the classical cases death occurs in the first year and cardiac involvement is striking. Indeed, Pompe reported this condition in 1932 as 'idiopathic hypertrophy of the heart' and 'cardiomegalia glycogenica' is a synonym..However, Smith, Zellweger and Afifi (1967) reported a boy with amyotonic form of disease and survival to the age of almost 11 years. The heart was not involved significantly. Alpha-1, 4-glucosidase was absent from liver and muscle. There were heavy glycogen deposits and an anomalous polysaccharide with short outer chains was identified. Smith, Amick and Sidbury (1966) reported a similar case in a boy who survived to the age of 4.5 years. Although this form of glycogen storage

R E C E S S I V E

438

disease has long been known, the enzyme defect was elucive. The above named enzyme, also called acid maltase, is a lysosomal enzyme with a pH optimum of 4.5-5. Whereas the glycogen is distributed rather uniformly in the cytoplasm in the other glycogenoses, it is enclosed in lysosomal membranes in this form. Hudgson et al. (1968) reported the case of a Portuguese girl who died at age 19 and that of a living 44 year old housewife. Other experiences suggesting the existence of more than one type of glycogenosis II were reported by Swaiman et al. (1968). Zellweger et al. (1965) described brothers age 15 and 4.5 years with minimal manifestations limited to skeletal muscle. A deficiency of muscle alpha-1,4-glucosidase was demonstrated. Muscle showed abnormal accumulations of glycogen. A maternal uncle may have been affected also. Muscle enzyme studies in the parents might differentiate autosomal from X-linked inheritance. Angelini et al. (1972) showed that the adult form of the disease can be diagnosed in cultured skin fibroblasts. Theoretically, family studies of the linkage of the acid-glucosidase locus could be performed in families of the patient with Pompe disease.

Angelini, C., Engel, A. G. and Titus, J. L.: Adult acid maltase deficiency. Abnormalities in fibroblasts cultured from patients. New Eng. J. Med. 287: 948-951, 1972.

Hirschhorn, K., Nadler, H. L., Waithe, W. I., Brown, B. I. and Hirschhorn, R.: Pompe's disease: detection of heterozygotes by lymphocyte stimulation. Science 166: 1632-1633, 1969.

Hudgson, P., Gardner-Medwin, D., Worsfold, M., Pennington, R. J. T. and Walton, J. N.: Adult myopathy from glycogen storage disease due to acid maltase deficiency. Brain 91: 435-462, 1968.

Salafsky, I. S. and Nadler, H. L.: Deficiency of acid alpha glucosidase in the urine of patients with Pompe disease. J. Pediat. 82: 294-298, 1973.

Smith, H. L., Amick, L. D. and Sidbury, J. B., Jr.: Type II glycogenosis. Am. J. Dis. Child. 3: 475-481, 1966.

Smith, J., Zellweger, H. and Afifi, A. K.: Muscular form of glycogenosis, type II (Pompe). Neurology 17: 537-549, 1967.

Swaiman, K. F., Kennedy, W. R. and Sauls, H. S.: Late infantile acid maltase deficiency. Arch. Neurol. 18: 642-648, 1968.

Zellweger, H., Brown, B. I., McCormick, W. F. and Jun-Bi, T.: A mild form of muscular glycogenosis in two brothers with alpha-1,4-glucosidase deficiency. Ann. Paediat. 205: 413-437, 1965.

R
E
C
E
S
S
I
V
E

*23240 GLYCOGEN STORAGE DISEASE III (FORBES DISEASE; CORI DISEASE; LIMIT DEXTRINOSIS)

Liver and heart muscle show predominant effects. The defect concerns debrancher enzyme (amylo-1, 6-glucosidase). The clinical features are somewhat like type I but milder and involvement of heart and skeletal muscle adds other features. In Israel 73 percent of glycogen storage disease was of this type and all were non-Ashkenazi, being mainly of North African extraction, in which group the minimal estimate of frequency was 1 in 5,420 (Levin et al., 1967). See Field, R. A.: loc. cit.

Brunberg, J. A., McCormick, W. F. and Schochet, S. S., Jr.: Type III glycogenosis. An adult with diffuse weakness and muscle wasting. Arch. Neurol. 25: 171-178, 1971.

Garancis, J. C., Panares, R. R., Good, T. A. and Kuzma, J. F.: Type 3 glycogenosis. A biochemical and electron microscopic study. Lab. Invest. 22: 468-477, 1970.

Levin, S., Moses, S. W., Chayoth, R., Jadoga, N. and Steinitz, K.: Glycogen storage disease in Israel. A clinical, biochemical and genetic study. Israel J. Med. Sci. 3: 397-410, 1967.

Waaler, P. E., Garatun-Tjeldsto, O. and Moe, P. J.: Genetic studies in glycogen storage disease type III. Acta Paediat. Scand. 59: 529-535, 1970.

*23250 GLYCOGEN STORAGE DISEASE IV (ANDERSEN DISEASE; BRANCHER DEFICIENCY; AMYLOPECTINOSIS; FAMILIAL CIRRHOSIS WITH DEPOSITION OF ABNORMAL GLYCOGEN)

The liver shows the main involvement, resulting from a defect of amylo(1,4 to 1,6) transglucosidase (brancher enzyme). Very few cases have been identified but the evidence of recessive inheritance is strong: affected sibs, parental consanguinity, partial enzyme deficiency in both parents. Levin et al. (1968) described a case of this rare form of glycogenosis, alternatively called amylopectinosis. It is distinguished from the more common types by early development of cirrhosis with portal hypertension, ending in severe liver failure, as well as positive results in the simple test with iodine (formation of a blue colored complex of glycogen and iodine).

Howell, R. R., Kaback, M. M. and Brown, B. I.: Type IV glycogen storage disease: branching enzyme deficiency in skin fibroblasts and possible heterozygote detection. J. Pediat. 78: 638-642, 1971.

Levin, B., Burgess, E. A. and Mortimer, P. E.: Glycogen storage disease type IV, amylopectinosis. Arch. Dis. Child. 43: 548-555, 1968.

Schochet, S. S., Jr., McCormick, W. F. and Zellweger, H.: Type IV glycogenosis (amylopectinosis). Light and electron microscopic observations. Arch. Path. 90: 354-363, 1970.

Sidbury, J. B., Jr., Mason, J., Burns, W. B., Jr. and Ruebner, B. H.: Type IV glycogenosis. Report of a case proven by characterization of glycogen and studied at necropsy. Bull. Johns Hopkins Hosp. 111: 157-181, 1962.

*23260 GLYCOGEN STORAGE DISEASE V (MCARDLE DISEASE; MYOPHOSPHORYLASE DEFICIENCY GLYCOGENOSIS)

Skeletal muscle is involved exclusively in a deficiency of muscle phosphorylase. The disorder may present as intermittent myoglobinuria. A. S. (718935) is a Johns Hopkins Hospital case of the disease. McArdle's original patient was a 30 year old man who experienced first pain and then weakness and stiffness with exercise of any muscle including the masseters. Symptoms disappeared promptly with rest. Blood lactate does not increase after exercise.

A deficiency of phosphofructokinase (see GLYCOGEN STORAGE DISEASE VII) produces the same clinical picture. This is not surprising since the enzyme deficiency results in inability to metabolize through fructose to lactose. A different condition may have been reported by di Sant'Agnese and colleagues (1962) in a two-and-one-half-year-old child with hypotonia and palatal paralysis without cardiomegaly or hepatomegaly. Striated muscle showed an excessive accumulation of glycogen which had normal chemical structure. Debrancher enzyme was normal. Unfortunately phosphorylase activity was not determined. The possibility of more than one form of muscle phosphorylase deficiency is also suggested by the case of Mellick, Mahler and Hughes (1962).

This is a cause of myoglobinuria. The phases of the disease are (1) in childhood and adolescence, intermittent dark urine, (2) in early adult life, cramping muscle pain on exertion, occasionally followed by transient myoglobinuria, and (3) in the fourth (or fifth) decade, persistent and progressive weakness and wasting of muscle, with absent or rare myoglobinuria. Engel, Eyerman and Williams (1963) observed onset of first manifestations at age 49 in a sister and brother. The sister had progressive generalized muscular weakness without cramps and had complete absence of enzyme. The brother had muscle cramps after exercise and about 35 percent normal activity of phosphorylase. Neither had myoglobinuria. Dawson, Spong and Harrington (1968) suggested a test for detection of asymptomatic heterozygotes based on the development of brief painful cramps during exercise. Grunfeld et al. (1972) found evidence for the existence of two forms of the disease, i.e., CRM-positive and CRM-negative forms. They also observed renal failure from acute rhabdomyolysis in two patients. The cramps are 'electrically silent,' i.e., show no activity on electromyography. Interpretation of the ailment as psychoneurosis is frequent.

Cochran, P., Huges, R. R., Buxton, P. H. and Yorke, R. A.: Myophosphorylase deficiency (McArdle's disease) in two interrelated families. J. Neurol. Neurosurg. Psychiatry. 36: 217-224, 1973.

Dawson, D. M., Spong, F. L. and Harrington, J. F.: McArdle's disease: lack of muscle phosphorylase. Ann. Intern. Med. 69: 229-236, 1968.

Di Sant'Agnese, P. A., Anderson, D. H. and Metcalf, K. M.: Glycogen storage disease of the muscles. J. Pediat. 61: 438-442, 1962.

Engel, W. K., Eyerman, E. L. and Williams, H. E.: Late-onset type of skeletal-muscle phosphorylase deficiency. A new familial variety with completely and partially affected subjects. New Eng. J. Med. 268: 135-137, 1963.

Grunfeld, J.-P., Ganeval, D., Chanard, J., Fardeau, M. and Dreyfus, J.-C.: Acute renal failure in McArdle's disease: report of two cases. New Eng. J. Med. 286: 1237-1241, 1972.

Howell, R. R.: The glycogen storage diseases. In, Stanbury, J. B., Wyngaarden, J. B. and Fredrickson, D. S. (eds.): The Metabolic Basis of Inherited Disease. New York: McGraw-Hill, 1972 (3rd Ed.). Pp. 149-173.

Lehoczky, T., Halasy, M., Simon, G. and Harmos, G.: Glycogenic myopathy. A case of skeletal muscle-glycogenosis in twins. J. Neurol. Sci. 2: 366-384, 1965.

Mellick, R. S., Mahler, R. F. and Hughes, B. P.: McArdle's syndrome. Phosphorylase-deficient myopathy. Lancet I: 1045-1048, 1962.

Rowland, L. P., Lovelace, R. E., Schotland, D. L., Araki, S. and Carmel, P.: The clinical diagnosis of McArdle's disease. Identification of another family with deficiency of muscle phosphorylase. Neurology 16: 93-100, 1966.

Schmid, R. and Hammaker, L.: Hereditary absence of muscle phosphorylase (McArdle's syndrome). New Eng. J. Med. 264: 223-225, 1961.

Schmid, R. and Mahler, R.: Chronic progressive myopathy with myoglobinuria: demonstration of a glycogenolytic defect in the muscle. J. Clin. Invest. 38: 2044-2058, 1959.

*23270 GLYCOGEN STORAGE DISEASE VI (HERS DISEASE; PHOSPHORYLASE DEFICIENCY GLYCOGEN-STORAGE DISEASE OF LIVER)

The clinical picture is one of mild to moderate hypoglycemia, mild ketosis, growth retardation and prominent hepatomegaly. Heart and skeletal muscle are not affected. The prognosis seems to be excellent. Wallis et al. (1966) determined erythrocyte glycogen concentration and leukocyte phosphorylase activity in 17 members of 4 generations of the family of a boy with biopsy-proved glycogen storage disease of type VI. The findings clearly indicate autosomal recessive inheritance. Hers and Van Hoof (1968) suggested that type VI is a 'waiting room' from which new entities will be separated in the future. The class will be reserved for those with liver phosphorylase deficiency as the primary defect. Deficiency of phosphorylase kinase is an X linked defect (see GLYCOGEN STORAGE DISEASE VIII in the X-linked catalog).

Hers, H. G. and Van Hoof, F.: Glycogen storage diseases: type II and type VI glycogenosis. In, Dickens, F., Randle, P. J. and Whelan, W. J. (eds.): Carbohydrate Metabolism and its Disorders. New York: Academic Press, 1968.

Hers, H. G.: Etudes enzymatiques sur fragments hepatiques: application a la classification des glycogenoses. Rev. Int. Hepat. 9: 35-55, 1959.

RECESSIVE

Wallis, P. G., Sidbury, J. B., Jr. and Harris, R. C.: Hepatic phosphorylase defect. Studies on peripheral blood. Am. J. Dis. Child. 111: 278-282, 1966.

Williams, H. E. and Field, J. B.: Low leukocyte phosphorylase in hepatic phosphorylase-deficient glycogen storage disease. J. Clin. Invest. 40: 1841-1845, 1961.

*23280 GLYCOGEN STORAGE DISEASE VII (PHOSPHOFRUCTOKINASE DEFICIENCY GLYCOGEN DISEASE OF MUSCLE)

Layzer et al. (1967) provided strong evidence for recessive inheritance by demonstrating partial deficiency of enzyme activity in erythrocytes of both parents of an affected 18-year-old male. Parents were not known to be related. The only previously described family was that reported from Japan by Tarui et al. (1967). Muscle cramps with exertion and myoglobinuria with extreme exertion are features as in McArdle disease (glycogen storage disease V). That the clinical manifestations are identical is not surprising since in both production of lactate is interfered with. PFK of muscle and erythrocyte are immunologically related but not identical (Layzer et al., 1969). Recognizable hemolysis occurs in this disease. The genetic defect may involve a subunit common to both the muscle and the red cell enzyme. The classification of the glycogenoses is a matter of dispute. Hug (1974), for example, assigns number VIII to a form of phosphorylase deficiency with brain involvement and number IX to phosphorylase kinase deficiency.

Hug, G.: Cincinnati, personal communication, 1974.

Layzer, R. B., Rowland, L. P. and Bank, W. J.: Physical and kinetic properties of human phosphofructokinase from skeletal muscle and erythrocytes. J. Biol. Chem. 244: 3823-3831, 1969.

Layzer, R. B., Rowland, L. P. and Ranney, H. M.: Muscle phosphofructokinase deficiency. Arch. Neurol. 17: 512-523, 1967.

Nishikawa, M., Tsukiyama, K., Enomoto, T., Tarui, S., Okuno, G., Ueda, K., Ikura, T., Tsujii, T., Sugase, T., Suda, M. and Tanaka, T.: A new type of skeletal muscle glycogenosis due to phosphofructokinase deficiency. Proc. Jap. Acad. 41: 350-353, 1965.

Tarui, S., Okuno, G., Ikura, Y. and Shima, K.: Phosphofructokinase deficiency in skeletal muscle: a new type of glycogenosis. Biochem. Biophys. Res. Commun. 19: 517-523, 1967.

23290 GLYCOPROTEIN STORAGE DISEASE

Zugibe et al. (1969) described a 52-year-old man with gout and marked splenomegaly. Reticuloendothelial cells in the spleen and bone marrow contained large eosinophilic granules when stained with hematoxylin and eosin. Urinary hexosamine levels were elevated in the proband and some close relatives.

Zugibe, F. T., Gilbert, E. F. and Gaziano, D.: Glycoprotein storage disease, a new entity. Am. J. Med. 47: 135-140, 1969.

23300 GLYCOPROTEIN: LACK OF BETA(2)-GLYCOPROTEIN I

Haupt et al. (1968) described a family in which two brothers had complete absence of what they termed beta(2)-glycoprotein I. Both parents, a sister, and both children of one of the brothers had half-normal levels of the protein.

Haupt, H., Schwick, H. G. and Storiko, K.: Ueber einen erblichen beta(2)-Glycoprotein Mangel. Humangenetik 5: 291-293, 1968.

*23310 GLYCOSURIA, RENAL (ALSO SEE FANCONI SYNDROME)

This trait has often been considered a dominant (Hjarne, 1927). Although it is incompletely recessive, i.e. heterozygotes may show mild glycosuria, consistent heavy glycosuria is a feature of the homozygote (Khachadurian, 1964). The physiologic defect is low renal threshold for glucose. The clinical picture is loss of 50-60 gms. of glucose in the urine daily despite a normal glucose tolerance test. A relation to diabetes mellitus has been suspected but not completely established. Monasterio et al. (1964) did microdissection and electron microscopy in two cases. Abnormality was limited to the proximal tubules which showed vacuolization, accumulation of abnormal PAS-positive material and changes in the brush border. Elsas and Rosenberg (1969) clarified the situation by pointing out that type A (low threshold and low glucose Tm) and type B (low threshold but normal Tm) may be observed in the same family, that both parents may be completely normal or may show abnormality in the renal tubular transport of glucose, and that defective reabsorption of glucose by the kidney need not be accompanied by abnormalities in intestinal glucose transport. Several different mutations are probably involved in renal glycosuria, as in the case in cystinuria. Elsas et al. (1971) provided clear evidence of autosomal recessive inheritance of type A renal glycosuria. They found a family in which both parents and a sib of the affected persons had an intermediate type of defect (i.e., a similar kinetic pattern with a less marked defect).

Elsas, L. J., Busse, D. and Rosenberg, L. E.: Autosomal recessive inheritance of renal glycosuria. Metabolism 20: 968-975, 1971.

Elsas, L. J. and Rosenberg, L. E.: Familial renal glycosuria: a genetic reappraisal of hexose transport by kidney and intestine. J. Clin. Invest. 48: 1845-1854, 1969.

Elsas, L. J., Hillman, R. E., Patterson, J. H. and Rosenberg, L. E.: Renal and intestinal hexose transport in familial glucose-galactose malabsorption. J. Clin. Invest. 49: 576-585, 1970.

Gjone, E.: Idiopatisk renal glykosuria in 3 generationer with high incidence. Nord. Med. 59: 306-307, 1958.

Hjarne, V.: Study of orthoglycaemic glycosuria with particular reference to its hereditability. Acta Med. Scand. 67: 422-571, 1927.

Khatchadurian, A. K. and Khachadurian, L. A.: The inheritance of renal glycosuria. Am. J. Hum. Genet. 16: 189-194, 1964.

Monasterio, G., Oliver, J., Muiesan, G., Pardelli, G., Marinozzi, V. and MacDowell, M.: Renal diabetes as a congenital tubular dysplasia. Am. J. Med. 37: 44-61, 1964.

Scriver, C. R.: Familial iminoglycinuria. In, Stanbury, J. B., Wyngaarden, J. B. and Fredrickson, D. S. (eds.): The Metabolic Basis of Inherited Disease. New York: McGraw-Hill, 1972 (3rd Ed.). Pp. 1520-1535.

*23320 GLYOXALASE II (HYDROXYACYL-GLUTATHIONE HYDROLASE) DEFICIENCY

Valentine et al. (1970) described a family in which homozygotes and heterozygotes for deficiency of glyoxalase II (hydroxyacyl-glutathione hydrolase) could be demonstrated in three generations of a family. Homozygotes had no clinical or hematologic abnormality, and elliptocytosis (which was segregating independently in the family) was not worsened by the presence of the enzyme defect.

Valentine, W. N., Paglia, D. E., Neerhout, R. C. and Konrad, P. N.: Erythrocyte glyoxalase II deficiency with coincidental hereditary elliptocytosis. Blood 36: 797-808, 1970.

*23325 GOLDBERG SYNDROME

Goldberg et al. (1971) described three children (two boys and a girl) in a Mexican family with first cousin parents who have a new disorder characterized by the presence of dwarfism, gargoyle facies, mental retardation, seizures, corneal clouding, macular cherry-red spot, beta-galactosidase deficiency in skin, dysostosis multiplex, and hearing loss. The absence of clinically enlarged viscera, vacuolated blood cells and mucopolysacchariduria was likewise distinctive. The combination of features of a mucopolysaccharidosis and a sphingolipidosis suggests this should be considered a mucolipidosis. Berard-Badier et al. (1970) described a 17-year-old patient (case 3) who had corneal opacities, a cherry-red spot and the same type of vacuolation of the Kupffer cells as that in the family studied by Goldberg et al.

Berard-Badier, M., Adechy-Benkoel, L., Chamlian, A. et al.: Etude ultrastructurale du parenchyme hepatique dans les mucopolysaccharidoses. Path. Biol. (Paris) 18: 117-128, 1970.

Goldberg, M. F., Cotlier, E., Fichenscher, L. G., Kenyon, K., Enat, R. and Borowsky, S. A.: Macular cherry-red spot, corneal clouding, and beta-galactosidase deficiency. Clinical, biochemical, and electron microscopic study of a new autosomal recessive storage disease. Arch. Intern. Med. 128: 387-398, 1971.

*23330 GONADAL DYSGENESIS, XX TYPE

Elliott, Sandler and Rabinowitz (1959) reported the condition in 3 sisters who had normal stature and sex chromatin but had never menstruated and had severe osteoporosis. The parents were first cousins in the case of the two affected sisters (with normal stature and sex-chromatin positivity) reported by Klotz, Merger and Avril (1956). Christakos et al. (1969) observed gonadal dysgenesis in three sisters whose parents were second cousins. Each had a normal female 46-XX karotype. Somatic features of Turner syndrome were not found. All three had elevated gonadotropins and laparotomy on the two older sisters showed streak gonads and unstimulated Mullerian structures. Gonadal dysgenesis, often with somatic abnormalities, has been reported in sibs by several other authors and in some of these reports the parents were consanguineous. Simpson and German (1970) pointed out that only affected sibs have been described and parental consanguinity is frequent. See 30610 for discussion of the XY female type of gonadal dysgenesis.

Boczkowski, K.: Pure gonadal dysgenesis and ovarian dysplasia in sisters. Am. J. Obstet. Gynec. 106: 626-628, 1970.

Christakos, A. C., Simpson, J. L., Younger, J. B. and Christian, C. D.: Gonadal dysgenesis as an autosomal recessive condition. Am. J. Obstet. Gynec. 104: 1027-1030, 1969.

Elliott, G. A., Sandler, A. and Rabinowitz, D.: Gonadal dysgenesis in three sisters. J. Clin. Endocr. 19: 995-1003, 1959.

Klotz, H. P., Merger, R. and Avril, J.: Syndrome de Turner chez deux soeurs issues de cousins germains. Consideration pathogeniques. Ann. Endocr. 17: 43-46, 1956.

Perez-Ballester, B., Greenblatt, R. B. and Byrd, J. R.: Familial gonadal dysgenesis. Am. J. Obstet. Gynec. 107: 1262-1263, 1970.

Simpson, J. L., Christakos, A. C., Horwith, M. and Silverman, F. S.: Gonadal dysgenesis in individuals with apparently normal chromosomal complements: tabulation of cases and compilation of genetic data. The Clinical Delineation of Birth Defects. X. Endocrine System. Baltimore: Williams and Wilkins, 1971. Pp. 215-228.

23340 GONADAL DYSGENESIS, XX TYPE, WITH DEAFNESS

Two families have been reported in which multiple members with XX gonadal dysgenesis all had deafness as well, suggesting the existence of two recessive forms of this disorder (Christakos et al., 1969; Perez-Ballester et al., 1970).

Christakos, A. C., Simpson, J. L., Younger, J. B. and Christian, C. D.: Gonadal dysgenesis as an autosomal recessive condition. Am. J. Obstet. Gynec. 104: 1027-1030, 1969.

Perez-Ballester, B., Greenblatt, R. B. and Byrd, J. R.: Familial gonadal dysgenesis. Am. J. Obstet. Gynec. 107: 1262-1263, 1970.

R
E
C
E
S
S
I
V
E

23350 GORLIN SYNDROME (CRANIOFACIAL DYSOSTOSIS, HYPERTRICHOSIS, HYPOPLASIA OF LABIA MAJORA, DENTAL AND EYE ANOMALIES, PATENT DUCTUS ARTERIOSUS, NORMAL INTELLIGENCE)

Gorlin, Chaudhry and Moss (1960) described sisters with this combination of features. The parents were not known to be related. The same sisters were reported by Feinberg (1960) as instances of the Weill-Marchesani syndrome (q.v.), which is clearly an incorrect diagnosis. Gorlin (1974) has seen no further cases of this syndrome and knows of no others in the literature.

Feinberg, S. B.: Congenital mesodermal dysmorpho-dystrophy (brachymorphic type). Radiology 74: 218-224, 1960.

Gorlin, R. J., Chaudhry, A. P. and Moss, M. L.: Craniofacial dysostosis, patent ductus arteriosus, hypertrichosis, hypoplasia of labia majora, dental and eye anomalies — a new syndrome? J. Pediat. 56: 778-785, 1960.

Gorlin, R. J.: Minneapolis, personal communication, 1974.

23360 GRANULOCYTOPENIA WITH IMMUNOGLOBULIN ABNORMALITY

Lonsdale et al. (1967) described three brothers who died at ages 12 months, 6 years, and 41 months from overwhelming infection. The bone marrow picture indicated maturation arrest and in two patients episodes of leukocytosis of unknown cause punctuated the course. Total gamma globulins were low in the serum.

Lonsdale, D., Deodhar, S. D. and Mercer, R. D.: Familial granulocytopenia and associated immunoglobulin abnormality. Report of three cases in young brothers. J. Pediat. 71: 790-801, 1967.

*23370 GRANULOMATOUS DISEASE DUE TO LEUKOCYTE MALFUNCTION

In addition to the well-established X-linked form, an autosomal recessive form appears to exist. Baehner and Nathan (1968) observed a 17-year-old female, offspring of first-cousins, who showed a clinical course and leukocyte behavior in vitro like those in affected males with the X-linked disease. Chromosomes were normal. The nitro blue tetrazolium test of leukocytes was normal in all relatives. Azimi et al. (1968), furthermore, described three Negro sisters with the same abnormality. In both families, parents showed normal leukocyte function. Other female patients have been reported. Holmes et al. (1970) presented evidence that leukocyte glutathione peroxidase activity is defective in females with chronic granulomatous disease. Deficiency of red cell glutathione peroxidase leads to hemolytic anemia, a feature absent in the present cases. In two patients with CGD, Curnutte et al. (1974) found low levels of superoxide production. Superoxide is a highly reactive compound produced with oxygen is reduced by a single electron. It is generated during the normal catalytic function of a number of enzymes including xanthine oxidase and cytochrome P-450. It may be produced in tissues exposed to ionizing radiation and in the oxidation of hemoglobin to methemoglobin. Living organisms have an enzyme, superoxide dismutase (18547), capable of destroying superoxide. Bacteria killed by oxygen usually lack this enzyme. The fact that bacterial killing by polymorphonuclear leukocytes is oxygen-dependent prompted the study by Curnutte et al. (1974). Both of their patients were male (Babior, 1974).

Azimi, P. H., Bodenbender, J. G., Hintz, R. L. and Kontras, S. B.: Chronic granulomatous disease in three female siblings. J.A.M.A. 206: 2865-2870, 1968.

Babior, B. M.: Boston, personal communication, March 26, 1974.

Baehner, R. L. and Nathan, D. G.: Quantitative nitroblue tetrazolium test in chronic granulomatous disease. New Eng. J. Med. 278: 971-976, 1968.

Curnutte, J. T., Dana, B. A. and Babior, B. M.: Defective superoxide production by granulocytes from patients with chronic granulomatous disease. New Eng. J. Med. 290: 593-597, 1974.

Koch, C., Sogaard, H. and Christensen, M. F.: Inheritance of chronic granulomatous disease in females. Report of a female patient and the leucocyte function studies in the family. Acta Paediat. Scand. 62: 659-665, 1966.

Holmes, B., Park, B. H., Malaevista, S. E., Quie, P. G., Nelson, D. L. and Good, R. A.: Chronic granulomatous disease in females. A deficiency of leukocyte glutathione peroxidase. New Eng. J. Med. 283: 217-221, 1970.

23380 GROUPED PIGMENTATION OF THE MACULA

Grouped pigmentation of the retina limited strictly to the foveal area was described by Loewenstein and Steel (1941) and by Chan (1951). Forgacs and Bozin (1966) reported the first familial incidence, two affected sisters. They complained of metamorphopsia and showed pigmented spots surrounded by a clear halo in the foveal area. Forsius et al. (1970) doubted that the disorder in the sisters was grouped pigmentation of the macula and pointed to the lack of familial incidence in several studies including his own. Furthermore, he found no parental consanguinity. He concluded that the anomaly is the result of an embryonic accident.

Chan, E.: Melanosis retinae. Chinese Med. J. 69: 431-432, 1951.

Forgacs, J. and Bozin, I.: Manifestation familiale de pigmentations groupees de la region maculaire. Ophthalmologica 152: 364-368, 1966.

Forsius, H., Eriksson, A., Nuutila, A., Vainio-Mattila, B. and Krause, U.: A genetic study of three rare retinal disorders: dystrophia retinae dysacusis syndrome, X-chromosomal retinoschisis and grouped pigments of the retina. The Clinical Delineation of Birth Defects. VIII. Eye. Baltimore: Williams and Wilkins, 1970.

Loewenstein, A. and Steel, J.: Special case of melanosis fundi: bilateral congenital group pigmentation of the central area. Brit. J. Ophthal. 25: 417-423, 1941.

23390 GYNECOMASTIA, HEREDITARY

Some families suggest autosomal recessive inheritance because of involvement of two or more brothers with both parents normal but consanguineous. However, because of male limitation the recessive pattern could result by chance of transmission through females for several generations.

Ljungberg, T.: Hereditary gynaecomastia. Acta Med. Scand. 168: 371-379, 1960.

*23400 HAGEMAN FACTOR DEFICIENCY

No symptoms occur. The deficiency is usually discovered because of the practice in some hospitals of routinely performing whole blood clotting times before surgical operations (McCain, Chernoff and Graham, 1959). Ratnoff and Steinberg (1962) analyzed data on 55 cases in 37 families. Parental consanguinity was present in at least two instances. Some heterozygotes show partial deficiency. The Japanese case reported by Miwa et al. (1968) had first-cousin parents. Josso and de Grouchy (1968) presented evidence that the Hageman locus may be on the short arm of a group C chromosome, probably No. 6. Egeberg (1970) described four Norwegian families with deficient factor XII (about half normal). Unlike the usual experience of no abnormality, they showed a slight to moderate bleeding tendency and a high incidence of cerebral apoplexy occurring at a relatively early age. Some of the patients had attacks of local edema, severe headache, abdominal pain and various forms of allergy. Localization of the Hageman factor locus on the short arm of chromosome 6 was suggested by de Grouchy et al. (1968).

De Grouchy, J., Veslot, J., Bonnette, J. and Roidot, M.: Case of (q) 6p- chromosomal aberration. Am. J. Dis. Child. 115: 93-99, 1968.

Egeberg, O.: Factor XII defect and hemorrhage. Evidence for a new type of hereditary hemostatic disorder. Thromb. Diath. Haemorrh. 23: 432-440, 1970.

Josso, F. and De Grouchy, J.: Localisation probable d'un locus Hageman (facteur XII) sur un autosome. Ann. Genet. 11: 95-97, 1968.

McCain, K. F., Chernoff, A. I. and Graham, J. B.: Establishment of the inheritance of Hageman defect as an autosomal recessive trait. Hemophilia and Other Hemorrhagic States. Brinkhous, K. M. (ed.): Chapel Hill: University Of North Carolina Press, 1959. Pp. 179-191.

Miwa, S., Asai, I., Tsukada, T., Shimizu, M., Teramura, K. and Sunaga, Y.: Hageman factor deficiency. Report of a case found in a Japanese girl. Acta Haemat. 39: 36-41, 1968.

Ratnoff, O. D. and Steinberg, A. G.: Further studies on the inheritance of Hageman trait. J. Lab. Clin. Med. 59: 980-985, 1962.

Ratnoff, O. D., Busse, R. J., Jr. and Sheon, R. P.: The demise of John Hageman. New Eng. J. Med. 279: 760-761, 1968.

Thompson, J. H., Jr., Spittel, J. A., Jr., Pascuzzi, C. A. and Owen, C. A., Jr.: Laboratory and genetic observations in another family with Hageman trait. Mayo Clin. Proc. 35: 421-427, 1960.

*23405 HAIR-BRAIN SYNDROME (AMISH BRITTLE HAIR SYNDROME)

Among the Amish Allen (1971) and subsequently Jackson et al. (1974) delineated a syndrome characterized by short stature, intellectual impairment, brittle hair and decreased fertility. Twenty-five cases in an autosomal recessive pedigree pattern were identified. Impairment of linear growth and intellect were relatively mild in most. Microscopically, hairs showed an irregular, grooved surface lacking in scales. The sulfur content of the hair was about half normal.

Allen, R. J.: Neurocutaneous syndromes in children. Postgrad. Med. 50: 83 only, 1971.

Jackson, C. E., Weiss, L., and Watson, J. H. L.: 'Brittle' hair with short stature, intellectual impairment and decreased fertility: an autosomal recessive syndrome in an Amish kindred. Pediatrics 54: 201-212, 1974.

23410 HALLERMANN-STREIFF SYNDROME

This is also called the dyscephalic syndrome of Francois. The features are bird-like facies with hypoplastic mandible and beaked nose, proportionate dwarfism, hypotrichosis, microphthalmia and congenital cataract. Teeth are already present at birth. Affected monozygotic twins and affected sibs are known. Some of the features suggest bird-headed dwarfism (q.v.). Forsius and de la Chapelle (1964) found normal chromosomes in two cases. The only reported familial cases may be those of Bueno (1966) who found this syndrome in two out of three sibs resulting from a consanguineous marriage. Karyotypes were normal. On the other hand Fraser and Friedmann (1967) supported dominant inheritance with almost all cases being the result of fresh mutation. They pointed to the probable cases in father and daughter reported by Guyard et al. (1962). The father was married to a distant relative, however. Dental features were discussed by Caspersen and Warburg (1968).

Bueno-Sanchez, M.: Sindrome de Hallerman-Streiff-Francois. A proposito de una presentacion familiar. Boll. Soc. Vasco-Navarra 1: 21-35, 1966.

Carones, A. V.: Francois's dyscephalic syndrome. Ophthalmologica 142: 510-518, 1961.

Caspersen, I. and Warburg, M.: Hallermann-Streiff syndrome. Acta Ophthal. 46: 385-390, 1968.

Falls, H. F. and Schull, W. J.: Hallermann-Streiff syndrome. A dyscephaly with congenital cataracts and hypotrichosis. Arch. Ophthal. 63: 409-420, 1960.

Fraser, G. R. and Friedmann, A. I.: The Causes of Blindness in Childhood. A Study of 776 Children With Severe Visual Handicaps. Baltimore: Johns Hopkins Press, 1967. P. 89.

Forsius, H. and De la Chapelle, A.: Dyscephalia oculo-mandibulo-facialis. Two cases in which the chromosomes were studied. Ann. Paediat. Fenn. 10: 280-287, 1964.

Guyard, M., Perdriel, G. and Ceruti, F.: On 2 cases of cranial dysostosis with 'bird head.' Bull. Soc. Ophtal. Franc. 62: 443-447, 1962.

Hoefnagel, D. and Benirschke, K.: Dyscephalia mandibulo-oculo-facialis (Hallermann-Streiff syndrome). Arch. Dis. Child. 40: 57-61, 1965.

*23420 HALLERVORDEN AND SPATZ, SYNDROME OF

The original description by the authors whose names are attached to this syndrome concerned a sibship of 12 in which 5 sisters showed clinically increasing dysarthria and progressive dementia, and at autopsy brown discoloration of the globus pallidus and substantia nigra was observed. Familial cases have been reported by others as well. About 30 cases were reported by Meyer (1958). Clinically the condition is characterized by progressive rigidity, first in the lower and later in the upper extremities. An equinovarus deformity of the foot has been the first sign in several cases. Involuntary movements of choreic or athetoid type sometimes precede or accompany rigidity. Both involuntary movements and rigidity may involve muscles supplied by cranial nerves, resulting in difficulties in articulation and swallowing. Mental deterioration and epilepsy occur in some. Onset is in the first or second decade and death usually before the age of 30 years.

Hallervorden, J. and Spatz, H.: Eigenartige Erkrankung im extrapyramidalen System mit besonderer Beteiligung des globus pallidus und der Substantia nigra. Ein Beitrag zu den Beziehungen zwischen diesen beiden Zentren. Zbl. Ges. Neurol. Psychiat. 79: 254-302, 1922.

Meyer, A.: The Hallervorden-Spatz syndrome. In, Greenfield, J. G. (ed.): Neuropathology. London: Edward Arnold Ltd., 1958. P. 525 ff.

23430 HALO NEVI (LEUKODERMA ACQUISITUM CENTRIFUGUM OF SUTTON)

Chisa (1965) reported affected brother and sister and Kopf, Morrill and Silberberg (1965) had affected sisters.

Chisa, N.: Multiple halo nevi in siblings. Arch. Derm. 92: 404-405, 1965.

Kopf, A. W., Morrill, S. D. and Silberberg, I.: Broad spectrum of leukoderma acquisitum centrifugum. Arch. Derm. 92: 14-35, 1965.

23440 'HAPPY PUPPET' SYNDROME

Bower (1967) coined the name, the 'happy puppet' syndrome, for a condition characterized by severe motor and intellectual retardation, ataxia, hypotonia, epilepsy and unusual facies characterized by a large mandible and open-mouthed expression revealing the tongue. A total of 8 cases have been described. Angelman (1965) reported 3 with optic atrophy. Six 'happy puppet' children have demonstrated excessive laughter on occipital groove, a great facility for protruding the tongue, abnormal choroidal pigmentation and characteristic EEG discharges. Two cases showed jerky movements and trouble walking. The walking problem may be due to poor balance. One, a 9-year-old boy noticed as an infant to be 'floppy,' could take only a few steps without support. Both patients had major convulsions and showed periods of flapping their arms up and down with the elbows flexed. The EEG pattern seen in these two cases and in Bower's cases consisted of high amplitude bilateral spike-and-wave activity which was symmetrical, synchronous and most often monorhythmic having a slow wave component at 2 cycles per sec. chromosomes have been normal in 5 cases. Berg and Pakula (1972) reported two siblings, one affected and one unaffected. However, the unaffected sib showed abnormal EEG patterns.

Angelman, H.: 'Puppet children.' A report of three cases. Dev. Med. Child Neurol. 7: 681 only, 1965.

Berg, J. M. and Pakula, Z.: Angelman's ('happy puppet') syndrome. Am. J. Dis. Child. 123: 72-77, 1972.

Bower, B. D. and Jeavons, P. M.: The 'happy puppet' syndrome. Arch. Dis. Child. 42: 298-301, 1967.

Moore, J. R. and Jeavons, P. M.: The 'happy puppet' syndrome: two new cases and a review of five previous cases. Neuropadiat. 4: 172-179, 1973.

*23450 HARTNUP DISEASE

First described by Baron, Dent, Harris, Hart and Jepson (1956), this disorder is characterized by a pellagra-like light-sensitive rash, cerebellar ataxia, emotional instability and aminoaciduria. The defect involves the intestinal and renal transport of certain neutral alpha-amino acids (Scriver, 1965). In the United States, cases of the full-blown clinical disorder are not seen, probably because of super-adequate diet. Pomeroy et al. (1968) reported the first instance of affected persons (one male, one female) who had children. In Colombia Lopez et al. (1969) described two affected brothers whose parents were double second cousins. Two other deceased brothers were probably affected also. Genetic heterogeneity probably exists because cases have been described in which only the urinary characteristics of Hartnup disease were present, and no evidence of an intestinal transport defect (Srikantia et al., 1964). Seakins and Ersser (1967) described a patient in whom the intestinal transport defect was partially evident only under loading conditions. Lysine transport was impaired, whereas histidine transport was not. Hartnup disease was found to have about the same frequency in Massachusetts as phenylketonuria, i.e., 1 in 14,219 births (Levy et al., 1972).

Baron, D. N., Dent, C. E., Harris, H., Hart, E. W. and Jepson, J. B.: Hereditary pellagra-like skin rash with temporary cerebellar ataxia, constant renal amino-aciduria and other bizarre biochemical features. Lancet II: 421-433, 1956.

Borrie, P. F. and Lewis, C. A.: Hartnup disease. Proc. Roy. Soc. Med. 55: 231-232, 1962.

Jepson, J. B.: Hartnup disease. In, Stanbury, J. B., Wyngaarden, J. B. and Fredrickson, D. S. (eds.): The Metabolic Basis of Inherited Diseases. New York: McGraw-Hill, 1972 (3rd Ed.). Pp. 1486-1503.

Levy, H. L., Madigan, P. M. and Shih, V. E.: Massachusetts metabolic screening program. I. Technique and results of urine screening. Pediatrics 49: 825-836, 1972.

Lopez, G. F., Velez, A. H. and Toro, G. G.: Hartnup disease in two Colombian siblings. Neurology 19: 71-76, 1969.

Milne, M. D., Crawford, M. A., Girao, C. B. and Loughridge, L. W.: The metabolic disorder in Hartnup disease. Quart. J. Med. 29: 407-421, 1960.

Pomeroy, J., Efron, M. L., Dayman, J. and Hoefnagel, D.: Hartnup disorder in a New England family. New Eng. J. Med. 278: 1214-1216, 1968.

Scriver, C. R.: Hartnup disease. A genetic modification of intestinal and renal transport of certain neutral alpha-amino acids. New Eng. J. Med. 273: 530-532, 1965.

Seakins, J. W. and Ersser, R. S.: Effects of amino acid loads on a healthy infant with the biochemical features of Hartnup disease. Arch. Dis. Child. 42: 682-688, 1967.

Srikantia, S. G., Venkatachalam, P. S. and Reddy, V.: Clinical and biochemical features of a case of Hartnup disease. Brit. Med. J. 1: 282-285, 1964.

23460 HEART BLOCK AND OPHTHALMOPLEGIA

Ross et al. (1969) described the association of chronic progressive external ophthalmoplegia and complete heart block and noted four earlier reports of the same. Apparently no familial cases have been reported. Rosenberg et al. (1968) reviewed syndromes involving ophthalmoplegia.

Rosenberg, R. N., Schotland, D. L., Lovelace, R. E. and Rowland, L. P.: Progressive ophthalmoplegia: report of cases. Arch. Neurol. 19: 362-376, 1968.

Ross, A., Lipschutz, D., Austin, J. and Smith, J., Jr.: External ophthalmoplegia and complete heart block. New Eng. J. Med. 280: 313-315, 1969.

*23470 HEART BLOCK, CONGENITAL

A rather large number of families with multiple affected sibs and normal parents have been reported. Latta and Crittenden (1964) studied the hearts of two sibs (the 7th and 8th offspring) who died neonatally of congenital heart block. In neither was an atrioventricular node found, nor were myocardial fibers present in the lower part of the interatrial septum. Both hearts showed foci of calcification, fibrosis, increased vascularization and a few small accumulations of inflammatory cells. Thus, fetal infection could have been responsible. In another family Crittenden, Latta and Ticinovich (1964) described four of eight sibs with congenital heart block. A fifth may have been affected. One died at age 14 and the others died in the neonatal period. The parents were normal and of Czechoslovakian ancestry. No mention of consanguinity was made. Cannom and Hancock (1974) described a distinctive syndrome of cardiomyopathy, probably congenital, with mitral regurgitation, complete heart block and atrial arrhythmia in four unrelated male patients. The disorder is relatively benign. No familial occurrence was observed. Congenital cardiomyopathy may be the basis for other instances of congenital complete heart block which might appear in an otherwise normal heart. This appears particularly likely in cases of associated atrial arrhythmia and atrioventricular block.

Aylward, R. D.: Congenital heart-block. The occurrence of two cases of congenital heart-block in one family is so unusual as to deserve being placed on record. Brit. Med. J. 1: 943 only, 1928.

Cannom, D. S. and Hancock, E. W.: A syndrome of congenital cardiomyopathy with mitral regurgitation, complete heart block and atrial arrhythmia. Am. J. Med. 56: 261-268, 1974.

Crittenden, I. H., Latta, H. and Ticinovich, D. A.: Familial congenital heart block. Am. J. Dis. Child. 108: 104-108, 1964.

Latta, H. and Crittenden, I. H.: Acquired lesions of the conduction system in familial congenital heart block. Lab. Invest. 13: 214-221, 1964.

Lynch, R. J. and Engle, M. A.: Familial congenital complete heart block. Am. J. Dis. Child. 102: 210-217, 1961.

Osler, W.: On the so-called Stokes-Adams disease (slow pulse with syncopal attacks). Lancet II: 516-524, 1903.

Sarachek, N. S. and Leonard, J. J.: Familial heart block and sinus bradycardia: classification and natural history. Am. J. Cardiol. 29: 451-458, 1972.

Wallgren, G. and Agorio, E.: Congenital complete a-v block in three siblings. Acta Paediat. 49: 49-56, 1960.

23475 HEART, MALFORMATION OF

Stevenson et al. (1971) described single ventricle in two sisters.

Stevenson, C., Franken, E. A., Ha-Upala, S. and Christian, J. C.: Familial occurrence of single ventricle. Arch. Dis. Child. 46: 730-731, 1971.

23480 HEMANGIOMATOSIS, CUTANEOUS, WITH ASSOCIATED FEATURES

Gluszcz, Polis and Waleszkowski (1963) described four sibs with cutaneous hemangiomatosis, acrocyanosis, hyperflexibility of joints and phimosis. Some showed slight abnormalities of the vertebral bodies and ocular hypertelorism. In two (a female age 15 and a male age 19) tumors resembling cerebellar angioblastoma of von Hippel-Lindau disease were removed from the cervico-thoracic portion of the spinal canal.

Gluszcz, A., Polis, Z. and Waleszkowski, J.: Familial syndrome of general dysplasia of the connective tissue and of the vascular system associated with angioblastoma of the spinal canal. Pol. Med. J. 2: 924-936, 1963.

23500 HEMIHYPERTROPHY

Fraumeni et al. (1967) described affected brother and sister and recorded that their maternal uncle was said to have had one leg longer than the other since childhood. They reviewed 6 other examples of familial occurrence. These included instances of successive generations affected.

Fraumeni, J. F., Jr., Geiser, C. F. and Manning, M. D.: Wilms' tumor and congenital hemihypertrophy: report of five new cases and review of literature. Pediatrics 40: 886-899, 1967.

*23520 HEMOCHROMATOSIS, JUVENILE

Debre and colleagues (1958) concluded that the biochemical defect of idiopathic hemochromatosis is present in heterozygotes and that whether the disease develops is dependent on other influences on iron metabolism. They suggest that juvenile hemochromatosis resulting from consanguineous marriages may represent the homozygous state of the gene. The pedigree of Nussbaumer, Plattner and Rywlin (1952) is reproduced by Sorsby (1953). The inheritance of the adult-onset hemochromatosis may be dominant (Williams, Scheuer, Sherlock, 1962). Hemochromatosis is, for that reason, included also in the dominant catalog, but without an asterisk, because by the prevailing hypothesis, the same gene is responsible. Saddi and Feingold (1974) reported a study of 96 pedigrees, which, they concluded, support autosomal recessive inheritance. Consanguinity was increased among the parents. No parent or offspring was affected. Segregation analysis was consistent with autosomal recessive inheritance if reduced penetrance in females was assumed.

Debre, R., Dreyfus, J.-C., Frezal, J., Labie, D., Lamy, M., Maroteaux, P., Schapira, F. and Schapira, G.: Genetics of haemochromatosis. Ann. Hum. Genet. 23: 16-30, 1958.

Felts, J. H., Nelson, J. R., Herndon, C. N. and Spurr, C. L.: Hemochromatosis in two young sisters. Case studies and a family survey. Ann. Intern. Med. 67: 117-123, 1967.

Nussbaumer, T., Plattner, H. C. and Rywlin, A.: Hemochromatose juvenile chez trois soeurs et un frere avec consanguinite des parents: etude anatomoclinique et genetique du syndrome endocrinohepato-myocardique. J. Genet. Hum. 1: 53-59, 1952.

Saddi, R. and Feingold, J.: Idiopathic haemochromatosis: an autosomal recessive disease. Clin. Genet. 5: 234-241, 1974.

Sorsby, A.: Clinical Genetics. St. Louis: C. V. Mosby Co., 1953. P. 206.

Williams, R., Scheuer, P. J. and Sherlock, S.: The inheritance of idiopathic haemochromatosis. A clinical and liver biopsy study of 16 families. Quart. J. Med. 31: 249-265, 1962.

23530 HEMOGLOBIN A2, COMPLETE ABSENCE OF

This occurs in the homozygote for the 'persistent fetal hemoglobin gene,' for the Hb Lepore gene, or for the delta thalassemia gene.

23535 HEMOLYTIC ANEMIA ('RH-NULL DISEASE')

Rh null persons, those without any representative of the Rh antigens or of the Rh-associated antigen LW, have hemolytic anemia which is usually compensated (Schmidt and Vos, 1967). From this it is deduced that the Rh antigens or LW antigens or both are essential to the integrity of the red-cell membrane. Chown et al. (1971) described an offspring of a cousin marriage who had continuous hyperbilirubinemia punctuated by episodic acute hemolysis.

Chown, B., Lewis, M., Kaita, H. and Lowen, B.: A new cause of haemolytic anaemia? (Letter) Lancet I: 396 only, 1971.

Schmidt, P. J. and Vos, G. H.: Multiple phenotypic abnormalities associated with Rh-null. Vox Sang. 13: 18-20, 1967.

23540 HEMOLYTIC-UREMIC SYNDROME

In two sisters, Hagge and colleagues (1967) found intravascular hemolysis, thrombocytopenia and azotemia. Repeated attacks ended in renal failure and death at age 8 years. The second recovered completely after one attack. Concordant monozygotic twins have also been reported (Campbell and Carre, 1965). The features are acute renal failure, thrombocytopenia and hemolytic anemia associated with distorted erythrocytes ('burr cells'). Gianantonio et al. (1968) observed 75 cases in Argentina where the disorder seems unusually frequent and assembled some evidence for viral etiology. At any rate Mendelian inheritance of a significant proportion of cases seems very unlikely. Chan et al. (1969) found the disorder in two adopted, unrelated sibs.

Bergstein, J., Michael, A., Jr., Kjellstrand, C., Simmons, R. and Najarian, J.: Hemolytic-uremic syndrome in adult sisters. Transplantation 17: 487-490, 1974.

Campbell, S. and Carre, I. J.: Fatal haemolytic uraemic syndrome and idiopathic hyperlipaemia in monozygotic twins. Arch. Dis. Child. 40: 654-658, 1965.

R
E
C
E
S
S
I
V
E

Chan, J. C. M., Eleff, M. G. and Campbell, R. A.: The hemolytic-uremic syndrome in nonrelated adopted siblings. J. Pediat. 75: 1050-1053, 1969.

Gianantonio, C. A., Vitacco, M., Mendilaharzu, F. and Gallo, G.: The hemolytic-uremic syndrome. Renal status of 76 patients at long-term follow-up. J. Pediat. 72: 757-765, 1968.

Hagge, W. W., Holley, K. E., Burke, E. C. and Stickler, G. B.: Hemolytic-uremic syndrome in two siblings. New Eng. J. Med. 277: 138-139, 1967.

23550 HEMOSIDEROSIS, PULMONARY, WITH DEFICIENCY OF GAMMA-A GLOBULIN

Idiopathic pulmonary hemosiderosis has not been shown to be familial. That a generalized dysfunction of the macrophages system may be involved in some cases and that the defect may be genetically determined is suggested by the finding in some cases of deficiency of gamma-A globulin and of histologic alterations in the lymphoreticular organs compatible with an immune deficiency disorder.

Krieger, I. and Brough, J. A.: Gamma-A deficiency and hypochromic anemia due to defective iron mobilization. New Eng. J. Med. 276: 886-894, 1967.

*23560 HERMAPHRODITISM, TRUE

Milner et al. (1958) reported two 'brothers' who had hypospadias and both testicular and ovarian tissue bilaterally. Familial cases have also been reported by Rosenberg, Clayton and Hsu (1963), who found a normal female karyotype in several tissues examined. The autosomal inheritance of this disorder is one of the numerous pieces of information indicating that genes controlling sexual development and differentiation are not limited to the sex chromosomes.

Milner, W. A., Garlick, W. B., Fink, A. J. and Stein, A. A.: True hermaphrodite siblings. J. Urol. 79: 1003-1009, 1958.

Rosenberg, H. S., Clayton, G. W. and Hsu, T. C.: Familial true hermaphrodism. J. Clin. Endocr. 23: 203-206, 1963.

*23570 HEXOKINASE DEFICIENCY HEMOLYTIC ANEMIA

Valentine et al. (1967) described a child with anemia present from birth and deficiency of red cell hexokinase. The father and one sib had low levels. The mother's level was also low but within the range of normal. The deficiency apparently did not involve leukocytes and platelets and is different from the hexokinase deficiency identified in Fanconi pancytopenia (q.v.). Necheles et al. (1970) found, however, associated deficiency of leukocyte hexokinase. As listed in the dominant catalog, there is electrophoretic polymorphism of hexokinase due presumably to alleles at the same locus.

Altay, C., Alper, C. A. and Nathan, D. C.: Normal and variant isoenzymes of human blood cell hexokinase and the isoenzyme patterns in hemolytic disease. Blood 36: 219-227, 1970.

Keitt, A. S.: Hemolytic anemia with impaired hexokinase activity. J. Clin. Invest. 48: 1997-2007, 1969.

Necheles, T. F., Rai, U. S. and Cameron, D.: Congenital nonspherocytic hemolytic anemia associated with an unusual erythrocyte hexokinase abnormality. J. Lab. Clin. Med. 76: 593-602, 1970.

Valentine, W. N., Oski, F. A., Paglia, D. E., Baughan, M. A., Schneider, A. S. and Naiman, J. L.: Hereditary hemolytic anemia with hexokinase deficiency. Role of hexokinase in erythrocyte aging. New Eng. J. Med. 276: 1-11, 1967.

*23580 HISTIDINEMIA

A false positive ferric chloride urine test for phenylketonuria occurs in these cases. Of note is the occurrence of a pin-pointed cerebral defect involving speech. A majority of cases show retardation, however, and treatment with histidine-restriction is worthwhile in the opinion of Wadman et al. (1967). The cases reported by Woody et al. (1965) had a partial histidase deficiency, indicating heterogeneity in this condition. Rosenblatt et al. (1970) described histidinemia discovered in a 17 year-old French-Canadian girl after renal transplant for chronic glomerulonephritis. The histidase activity of the transplanted kidney was not adequate to correct the metabolic defect. Bruckman et al. (1970) raised a question of dominant inheritance in a family because the reported father of three affected sibs was chemically normal and apparently not heterozygous. The mother and three children were apparent homozygotes. Kacser et al. (1973) described histidinemia in mice and presented evidence that the metabolic defect in the mother may have a teratogenic effect on the fetus.

Auerbach, V. H., DiGeorge, A. M., Baldridge, R. C., Tourtellotte, C. D. and Brigham, M. P.: Histidinemia: a deficiency in histidase resulting in the urinary excretion of histidine and of imidazolepyruvic acid. J. Pediat. 60: 487-497, 1962.

Bruckman, C., Berry, H. K. and Dasenbrock, R. J.: Histidinemia in two successive generations. Am. J. Dis. Child. 119: 221-227, 1970.

Kappelman, M., Thomas, G. H. and Howell, R. R.: Histidinemia in a Negro child. Am. J. Dis. Child. 122: 212-214, 1971.

Kacser, H. K., Bulfield, G. and Wallace, M. E.: Histidinaemia mutant in the mouse. Nature: 77-79, 1973.

La Du, B. N.: Histidinemia: current status. Am. J. Dis. Child. 113: 88-92, 1967.

La Du, B. N., Howell, R. R., Jacoby, G. A., Seegmiller, J. E., Sober, E. K., Zannoni, V. G., Canby, J. P. and Ziegler, L. K.: Clinical and biochemical studies on two cases of histidinemia. Pediatrics 32: 216-227, 1963.

Neville, B. G. R., Bentovim, A., Clayton, B. E. and Sheperd, J.: Histidinaemia: study of relation between clinical and biological findings in 7 subjects. Arch. Dis. Child. 47: 190-200, 1972.

Neville, B. G. R., Harris, R. F., Stern, D. J. and Stern, J.: Maternal histidinaemia. Arch. Dis. Child. 46: 119-121, 1971.

Popkin, J. S., Clow, C. L.: Scriver, C. R. and Grove, J.: Is hereditary histidinemia harmful? Lancet I: 721-722, 1974.

Rosenblatt, D., Mohyuddin, F. and Scriver, C. R.: Histidinemia discovered by urine screening after renal transplantation. Pediatrics 46: 47-53, 1970.

Wadman, S. K., Van Sprang, F. J., Van Stekelenburg, G. K. and De Bree, P. K.: Three new cases of histidinemia. Clinical and biochemical Data. Acta Paediat. Scand. 56: 485-492, 1967.

Woody, N. C., Snyder, C. H. and Harris, J. A.: Histidinemia. Am. J. Dis. Child. 110: 606-613, 1965.

*23590 HISTIOCYTOSIS, FAMILIAL LIPOCHROME

In three sisters in a sibship of 9 Ford and colleagues (1962) observed lipochrome granulation of the histiocytes, pulmonary infiltration, hyperglobulinemia, transient polyarthritis and susceptibility to infection. No abnormality was seen in plasma cells or lymphocytes. The hyperglobulinemia involved gamma- and alpha (2)-globulins. The authors suggested that the primary defect caused the lipochrome deposition and that the other features were secondary to the deposits. The ages of the sisters were 26, 21 and 16 years. Pincus and Klebanoff (1971) demonstrated a defect in the conversion of iodide to a trichloroacetic acid-precipitable-form by phagocytizing leukocytes. A defect was also shown in chronic granulomatous disease and in myeloperoxidase deficiency but not in Job syndrome.

Ford, D. K., Price, G. E., Culling, C. F. and Vassar, P. S.: Familial lipochrome pigmentation of histiocytes with hyperglobulinemia, pulmonary infiltration, splenomegaly, arthritis and susceptibility to infection. Am. J. Med. 33: 478-489, 1962.

Pincus, S. H. and Klebanoff, S. J.: Quantitative leukocyte iodination. New Eng. J. Med. 284: 744-750, 1971.

23600 HODGKIN DISEASE

Manigand and colleagues (1964) described a brother and sister with Hodgkin disease and reviewed the literature on familial occurrence.

Manigand, G., Macrez, C., Chome, J., Bosson, C. H., Delamare, J. and Deparis, M.: Maladie de Hodgkin familiale. Presse Med. 72: 1871-1874, 1964.

*23610 HOLOPROSENCEPHALY, FAMILIAL ALOBAR (ARHINENCEPHALY)

DeMyer, Zeman and Palmer (1963) described two sisters with alobar holoprosencephaly associated with median cleft lip and palate. A paternal aunt may have been identically affected. Chromosomes were normal. Holoprosencephaly with a different array of extra-cephalic malformations occurs with 13-15 trisomy. Hintz et al. (1968) also observed affected sibs. Cohen and Gorlin (1969) described a Chippewa Indian sibship in which one sib had cyclopia and four others had cleft lip and-or palate. The parents were related. Consanguinity was also noted in the cases of Klopstock (1921) and Grebe (1954). DeMyer (1963) pointed out that there is a spectrum of holoprosencephalic disorders representing impaired midline cleavage of the embryonic forebrain. In cyclopia, the most extreme form, a single eye globe with varying degrees of doubling of intrinsic ocular structures, arhinia and a blind-ending proboscis located above the median eye are found. In ethmocephaly the features are extreme orbital hypotelorism, arhinia, and a blind-ended proboscis located between the eyes. In cebocephaly, orbital hypotelorism is associated with single-nostril nose. Premaxillary agenesis is characterized by a median pseudocleft, agenesis of nasal bones and primary palate, and ocular hypotelorism. Ellis (1865) reported twins with cyclops. Klopstock (1921) reported two brothers. Three children were affected in the family reported by Dominok and Kirchmair (1961). Pfitzer and Muntefering (1968) observed 4 affected children whose mothers were relatives and had the same anomalous karyotype, thought to represent balanced translocation. Dallaire et al. (1971) described multiple affected persons in several different sibships of a French-Canadian kindred. Holmes et al. (1974) pointed out the heterogeneity in cebocephaly, since some cases have autosomal trisomy, e.g., trisomy 13 (McKusick, 1961) whereas others are apparently caused by a single gene. James and Van Leeuwen (1970) and Holmes et al. (1974) described sibs with cebocephaly.

Cohen, M. M., Jr. and Gorlin, R. J.: Genetic considerations in a sibship of cyclopia and clefts. The Clinical Delineation of Birth Defects. II. Malformation Syndromes. New York: National Foundation, 1969. Pp. 113-118.

Dallaire, L., Fraser, F. C. and Wiglesworth, F. W.: Familial holoprosencephaly. The Clinical Delineation of Birth Defects. XI. Orofacial Structures. Baltimore: Williams and Wilkins, 1971. Pp. 136-142.

DeMyer, W., Zeman, W. and Palmer, C. D.: Familial alobar holoprosencephaly (arhinencephaly) with median cleft lip and palate. Report of patient with 46 chromosomes. Neurology 13: 913-918, 1963.

Dominok, G. W. and Kirchmair, H.: Familial incidence of malformations of the arhinencephalia group. Z. Kinderheilk. 85: 19-30, 1961.

Ellis, R.: On a rare form of twin monstrosity. Trans. Obstet. Soc. 7: 160-164, 1865.

Grebe, H.: Familienbefunde bei letalen Anomalien der Koerperform. Acta. Genet. Med. Gem. 3: 93-111, 1954.

Holmes, L. B., Driscoll, S. and Atkins, L.: Genetic heterogenity of cebocephaly. J. Med. Genet. 11: 35-40, 1974.

Hintz, R. L., Menking, M. and Sotos, J. F.: Familial holoprosencephaly with endocrine dysgenesis. J. Pediat. 72: 81-87, 1968.

James, E. and Van Leeuwen, G.: Familial cebocephaly. Case description and survey of the anomaly. Clin. Pediat. 9: 491-493, 1970.

Klopstock, A.: Familiaeres Vorkommen von Cyklopie und Arrhinencephalie. Mschr. Geburtsh. Gynaek. 56: 59-71, 1921.

McKusick, V. A.: Medical Genetics 1960. J. Chr. Dis. 14: 1-198, 1961.

Pfitzer, P. and Muntefering, H.: Cyclopism as a hereditary malformation. Nature 217: 1071-1072, 1968.

*23620 HOMOCYSTINURIA

This disorder was discovered in 1962, independently by Gerritsen, Vaughn and Waisman in Madison, Wis., and by Carson et al. in Belfast, Northern Ireland. The patients of both groups were studied because of mental retardation. It is now known that about one-third of subjects have normal intelligence. Ectopia lentis is a constant feature in patients over age 10 but because of its progressive nature may be absent in younger patients. Skeletal features suggesting Marfan syndrome, generalized osteoporosis and thrombotic lesions of arteries and veins are other features. Methionine as well as homocystine is elevated in the urine. The defect concerns cystathionine synthetase. See SULFO-CYSTEINURIA. The disorder has been observed in Japan (Tada et al., 1967) and in persons of many different ethnic extractions living in the United States (Schimke et al., 1965). Spaeth and Barbour (1967) described a silver-nitroprusside test which is almost completely specific for homocystine. Uhlendorf and Mudd (1968) found that fibroblasts derived from skin and cells in amniotic fluid, grown in tissue culture, have cystathionine synthetase activity, although the enzyme is not detectable in intact normal skin. Fibroblasts grown from the skin of homocystinuric persons are deficient in the enzyme. The observations of Ratnoff (1968) may have bearing on the mechanism of the thrombotic accidents. Carey et al. (1968) pointed out that 27 cases had been found in Ireland. Carey et al. (1968) suggested that folic acid in pharmacologic doses is therapeutically valuable in this disease. Decrease in urinary excretion of homocystine and increase in methionine was noted during treatment. Kelly and Copeland (1968) suggest that there is an alternative pathway for metabolism of homocysteine through homolanthionine. In addition to cystathionine synthetase deficiency, three 'causes' of homocystinuria are known. These are (1) defect in vitamin B12 metabolism (27740); (2) deficiency of N(5,10)-methylenetetrahydrofolate reductase (23625) and (3) selective intestinal malabsorption of vitamin B12 (26110). Rat liver cystathionine synthetase has a tetrameric structure of two different subunits, like hemoglobin (Kashiwamata et al., 1970). If the same is true in man, there is opportunity for non-allelic genetic heterogeneity in homocystinuria. Heterogeneity is clear in the differentiation of vitamin B6 responsive and non-responsive cases, but whether the basis of this is allelic or non-allelic is not known.

Barber, G. W. and Spaeth, G. L.: Pyridoxine therapy in homocystinuria. (Letter) Lancet I: 337 only, 1967.

Carey, M. C., Donovan, D. E., Fitzgerald, O. and McAuley, F. D.: Homocystinuria. A clinical and pathological study of nine subjects in six families. Am. J. Med. 45: 7-25, 1968.

Carey, M. C., Fennelly, J. J. and Fitzgerald, O.: Homocystinuria. II. Subnormal serum folate levels, increased folate clearance and effects of folic acid therapy. Am. J. Med. 45: 26-31, 1968.

Carson, N. A. J. and Neill, D. W.: Metabolic abnormalities detected in a survey of mentally backward individuals in Northern Ireland. Arch. Dis. Child. 37: 505-513, 1962.

Carson, N. A. J., Cusworth, D. C., Dent, C. E., Field, C. M. B., Neill, D. W. and Westall, R. G.: Homocystinuria: a new inborn error of metabolism associated with mental deficiency. Arch. Dis. Child. 38: 425-436, 1963.

Field, C. M. B., Carson, N. A. J., Cusworth, D. C., Dent, C. E. and Neill, D. W.: Homocystinuria, a new disorder of metabolism. (Abstract) Proc. 10th Intern. Congr. Pediat., Lisbon, 1962. Pp. 274-275.

Frimpter, G. W.: Homocystinuria: vitamin B6 dependent or not? (Editorial) Ann. Intern. Med. 71: 209-211, 1969.

Gerritsen, T., Vaughn, J. G. and Waisman, H. A.: The identification of homocystine in the urine. Biochem. Biophys. Res. Commun. 9: 493-496, 1962.

Goldstein, J. L., Campbell, B. K. and Gartler, S. M.: Cystathionine synthase activity in human lymphocytes: induction by phytohemagglutinin. J. Clin. Invest. 51: 1034-1037, 1972.

Goldstein, J. L., Campbell, B. K. and Gartler, S. M.: Homocystinuria: heterozygote detection using phytohemagglutinin-stimulated lymphocytes. J. Clin. Invest. 52: 218 only, 1973.

Hooft, C., Carton, D. and Samyn, W.: Pyridoxine treatment in homocystinuria. (Letter) Lancet I: 1384 only, 1967.

Kaeser, A. C., Rodnight, R. and Ellis, B. A.: Psychiatric and biochemical aspects of a case of homocystinuria. J. Neurol. Neurosurg. Psychiat. 32: 88-93, 1969.

Kashiwamata, S., Kotake, Y. and Greenberg, D. M.: Studies of cystathionine synthase of rat liver: dissociation into two components by sodium dodecyl sulfate disc electrophoresis. Biochem. Biophys. Acta 212: 501-503, 1970.

RECESSIVE

Kelly, S. and Copeland, W.: Preliminary report: a hypothesis in the homocystinuric's response to pyridoxine. Metabolism 17: 794-795, 1968.

Komrower, G. M.: Dietary treatment of homocystinuria. Am. J. Dis. Child. 113: 98-100, 1967.

McCully, K. S. and Ragsdale, B. D.: Production of arteriosclerosis by homocystinuria. Am. J. Path. 61: 1-12, 1970.

Mudd, S. H., Edwards, W. A., Loeb, P. M., Brown, M. S. and Laster, L.: Homocystinuria due to cystathionine synthase deficiency: the effect of pyridoxine. J. Clin. Invest. 49: 1762-1773, 1970.

Mudd, S. H., Levy, H. L., Abeles, R. H.: A derangement in B12 metabolism leading to homocystinemia, cystathioninemia and methylmalonic aciduria. Biochem. Biophys. Res. Commun. 35: 121-126, 1969.

Perry, T. L., Hansen, S., Love, D. L., Crawford, L. E. and Tischler, B.: Treatment of homocystinuria with a low-methionine diet, supplemental cystine and a methyl donor. Lancet II: 474-478, 1968.

Ratnoff, O. D.: Activation of Hageman factor by L-homocystine. Science 162: 1007-1009, 1968.

Schimke, R. N., McKusick, V. A., Huang, T. and Pollack, A. D.: Homocystinuria: studies of 20 families with 38 affected members. J.A.M.A. 193: 711-719, 1965.

Shelley, W. B., Rawnsley, H. M. and Morrow, G. III: Pyridoxine-dependent hair pigmentation in association with homocystinuria. Arch. Derm. 106: 228-230, 1972.

Shih, V. E. and Efron, M. L.: Pyridoxine-unresponsive homocystinuria. New Eng. J. Med. 283: 1206-1208, 1970.

Shipman, R. T., Townley, R. R. W. and Danks, D. M.: Homocystinuria, Addisonian pernicious anaemia, and partial deletion of a G chromosome. Lancet II: 693-694, 1969.

Spaeth, G. L. and Barber, G. W.: Prevalence of homocystinuria among the mentally retarded: evaluation of a specific screening test. Pediatrics 40: 586-589, 1967.

Tada, K., Yoshida, T., Hirono, H. and Arakawa, T.: Homocystinuria: amino acid pattern of the liver. Tohoku J. Exp. Med. 92: 325-332, 1967.

Uhlendorf, B. W. and Mudd, S. H.: Cystathionine synthase in tissue culture derived from human skin: enzyme defect in homocystinuria. Science 160: 1007-1009, 1968.

Wong, P. K. W., Schwarz, V. and Komrower, G. M.: The biosynthesis of cystathionine in patients with homocystinuria. Pediat. Res. 2: 149-160, 1968.

*23625 HOMOCYSTINURIA DUE TO DEFICIENCY OF N(5,10)-METHYLENETETRAHYDROFO-LATE REDUCTASE ACTIVITY

Freeman et al. (1972) studied a 15-year-old mildly retarded Negro female with a two year history of progressive withdrawal, hallucinations, delusions, and catatonia unresponsive to psychotherapy. Homocystinuria without elevation of plasma methionine was found. Psychotic symptoms gradually disappeared with administration of pyridoxine and folic acid. A sister has the same chemical findings but no symptoms. Cystathionine synthetase and the enzymes methylating homocysteine were normal in liver and fibroblasts. A decrease was shown in methylenetetrahydrofolate reductase, the enzyme synthesizing N(5)-methyltetrahydrofolate. Shih et al. (1972) described the case of a 16-year-old boy with proximal muscle weakness, waddling gait and episodes of flinging movements of the upper limbs. Folic acid reduced the homocystinuria. Flavin adenine dinucleotide, which had no effect in Freeman's cases, reduced the homocystinuria. Thus, Shih's patient may have had an allelic disorder. Preliminary results of enzymatic studies in Freeman's case were reported by Mudd et al. (1972).

Freeman, J. M., Finkelstein, J. D., Mudd, S. H. and Uhlendorf, B. W.: Homocystinuria presenting as reversible 'schizophrenia.' A new defect in methionine metabolism with reduced methylene-tetrahydrofolate-reductase activity. (Abstract) Pediat. Res. 6: 423 only, 1972.

Freeman, J. M., Finkelstein, J. D. and Mudd, S. H.: Folate responsive homocystinuria and 'schizophrenia': a defect in methylation due to deficient 5, 10-methylenetetrahydrofolate reductase activity. In press, Sept., 1974.

Mudd, S. H., Uhlendorf, B. W., Freeman, J. M., Finkelstein, J. D. and Shih, V. E.: Homocystinuria associated with decreased methylenetetrahydrofolate reductase activity. Biochem. Biophys. Res. Commun. 46: 905-912, 1972.

Shih, V. E., Salem, M. Z., Mudd, S. H., Uhlendorf, B. W. and Adams, R. D.: A new form of homocystinuria due to N(5,10)-methylenetetrahydrofolate reductase deficiency. (Abstract) Pediat. Res. 6: 395 only, 1972.

*23630 HOOFT DISEASE

Hooft (1962) of Ghent, Belgium, described a family in which two sisters had retarded physical development, erythemato-squamous eruption, opaque leukonychia, mental retardation and low serum lipids. One had tapetoretinal degeneration. Acanthocytosis and disturbance of intestinal absorption (see ABETALIPOPRO-TEINEMIA) were not present.

Francois, J. and De Blond, R.: Degenerescence tapeto-retinienne associee a un syndrome hypolipidemique. Acta Genet. Med. Gem. 12: 145-157, 1963.

Hooft, C., De Laey, P., Herpol, J., De Loore, F. and Verbeeck, J.: Familial hypolipidaemia and retarded development without steatorrhoea. Another inborn error of metabolism? Helv. Paediat. Acta 17: 1-23, 1962.

In two of 3 sons of third cousin parents Keutel et al. (1970) described humeroradial synostosis. No precisely identical cases were found in the literature.

Keutel, J., Kindermann, I. and Mockel, H.: Eine wahrscheinlich autosomal recessiv vererbte Skeletmissbildung mit Humeroradialsynostose. Humangenetik 9: 43-53, 1970.

*23660 HYDROCEPHALUS

This abnormality can, of course, have many causes such as Arnold-Chiari malformation, atresia of foramen of Magendie, stenosis of aqueduct of Sylvius (an X-linked trait), toxoplasmosis, hydranencephaly, etc. Furthermore, it develops in infancy or childhood in achondroplasia (a dominant) and in Hurler disease. Schockaert and Janssens (1952) observed four sibs, including a female, with hydrocephalus. Abdul-Karim et al. (1964) reported two instances of consanguineous unions each of which resulted in three affected sibs. I have knowledge of an Amish family in which one female and two male sibs have hydrocephalus. Mehne's family (1961) was non-Amish, living in Indiana. Borle (1953) reviewed the instances of familial hydrocephalus and Gellman (1959) reviewed those of hydrocephalus in twins. A sex-linked recessive variety of stenosis of the aqueduct of Sylvius has become familiar in recent years through the work of Edwards (1961).

Abdul-Karim, R., Iliya, F. and Iskandar, G.: Consecutive hydrocephalus. Report of two cases. Obstet. Gynec. ·24: 376-378, 1964.

Borle, A.: Sur l'etiologie de l'hydrocephalie congenitale a propos d'un cas d'hydrocephalie concordante chez des jumeaux univitellins. J. Genet. Hum. 2: 157-202, 1953.

Edwards, J. H.: The syndrome of sex-linked hydrocephalus. Arch. Dis. Child. 36: 486-493, 1961.

Gellman, V.: Congenital hydrocephalus in monovular twins. Arch. Dis. Child. 34: 274-276, 1959.

Mehne, R. G.: Three hydrocephalic newborns — each of a successive pregnancy of a white female. Arch. Pediat. 78: 67-71, 1961.

Schockaert, R. and Janssens, J.: Hydrocephalies congenitales repetees. Bruxelles Med. 32: 2011-2019, 1952.

*23670 HYDROMETROCOLPOS

This malformation develops as a result of transverse vaginal membrane and excessive cervical secretions in response to maternal hormone. McKusick and colleagues (1964) have evidence that at least one form is inherited as an autosomal recessive. Birth of another affected female in a third sibship closely related to one of the two reported in 1964 further strengthens the conclusion (McKusick et al., 1968). Hydrometrocolpos has been described in the Ellis-van Creveld syndrome (Akoun and Bagard, 1956). Dangy et al. (1971) found hydrometrocolpos secondary to vaginal atresia and bilateral postaxial hexadactyly in an offspring of first-cousin parents. A comparable disorder, imperforate vagina, is autosomal recessive in the mouse (Gowen and Heidenthal, 1942; Chase 1944). If the membrane which closes the vagina is removed surgically, the mouse is fully viable and fertile. Untreated the malformation leads to death about the time of puberty. Kaufman et al. (1972) suggested that postaxial polydactyly and-or congenital heart disease may sometimes accompany hydrometrocolpos. In the kindred of McKusick et al. (1964) one of the girls with hydrometrocolpos had postaxial polydactyly and another girl in the same sibship had polydactyly and congenital heart disease without hydrometrocolpos.

Akoun, R. and Bagard, M.: La maladie d'Ellis-van Creveld. Algerie Med. 60: 769-772, 1956.

Chase, E. B.: Inheritance of imperforate vagina of the mouse. J. Hered. 35: 363-364, 1944.

Dangy, C. I., Aptekar, R. G. and Cann, H. M.: Hereditary hydrometrocolpos with polydactyly in infancy. Pediatrics 47: 138-141, 1971.

Gowen, J. W. and Heidenthal, G.: Imperforate vagina in the mouse, its inheritance and relation to endocrine function. J. Exp. Zool. 89: 433-450, 1971.

Kaufman, R. L., Hartmann, A. F. and McAlister, W. H.: Family studies in congenital heart disease II: a syndrome of hydrometrocolpos, postaxial polydactyly and congenital heart disease. Clinical Delineation of Birth Defects. XV. Cardiovascular System. Baltimore: Williams and Wilkins Co., 1972. Pp. 85-87.

McKusick, V. A., Bauer, R. L., Koop, C. E. and Scott, R. B.: Hydrometrocolpos as a simply inherited malformation. J.A.M.A. 189: 813-816, 1964.

McKusick, V. A., Weilbaecher, R. G. and Gragg, G. W.: Recessive inheritance of a congenital malformation syndrome. J.A.M.A. 204: 113-118, 1968.

23680 HYDROXYKYNURENINURIA

Komrower, et al. (1964) described a female patient, an only child, who excreted large amounts of kynurenine, 3-hydroxykynurenine and xanthurenic acid in the urine. Absence of kynureninase was postulated resulting in a block in the pathway from tryptophan to nicotinic acid. Under these circumstances tryptophan is no longer a source of nicotinic acid and deficiency of the vitamin can develop. The mother excreted 3-4 times normal amounts of xanthurenic acid. The father's excretion was at the upper limit of normal.

Komrower, G. M. and Westall, R.: Hydroxykynureninuria. Am. J. Dis. Child. 113: 77-80, 1967.

Komrower, G. M., Wilson, V., Clamp, J. R. and Westall, R. G.: Hydroxykynureninuria. A case of abnormal tryptophane metabolism probably due to a deficiency of kynureninase. Arch. Dis. Child. 39: 250-256, 1964.

Benson et al. (1969) described hydroxylysinuria in a 19-year-old man and his 16-year-old sister who both had myoclonic and major motor seizures and were mentally retarded. The parents were related. The clinical features were similar in a patient reported by Parker et al. (1970).

Benson, P. F., Swift, P. N. and Young, V. K.: Hydroxylysinuria. (Abstract) Arch. Dis. Child. 44: 134-135, 1969.

Parker, C. E., Shaw, K. N. F., Jacobs, E. E. and Gutenstein, M.: Hydroxylysinuria. (Letter) Lancet I: 1119-1120, 1970.

*23700 HYDROXYPROLINEMIA

Mental retardation and microscopic hematuria are clinical features. A defect in hydroxyproline oxidase is proposed (Efron, Bixby, Pryles, 1965). Prior to the discovery of this disorder the same enzymes were thought to be involved in proline and hydroxyproline breakdown (see HYPERPROLINEMIA). Even when only one case was reported, a female, this condition was thought to be an autosomal recessive because of its nature as an inborn error of metabolism and because the parents were thought to have been sibs. Pelkonen and Kivirikko (1970) described hydroxyprolinemia in a brother and sister. No clinical abnormality was present and the authors suggested that hydroxyprolinemia is like cystathioninuria a 'non-disease.' However, Scriver and Efron (1972) described another case with mental retardation observed by Noel Raine in Birmingham, Eng. In vivo studies indicate a deficiency of the enzyme which oxidizes hydroxyproline to delta(1)-pyrro-line-3-hydroxy-5-carboxylic acid.

Efron, M. L., Bixby, E. M. and Pryles, C. V.: Hydroxyprolinemia. II. A rare metabolic disease due to deficiency of enzyme 'hydroxyproline oxidase.' New Eng. J. Med. 272: 1299-1309, 1965.

Pelkonen, R. and Kivirikko, K. I.: Hydroxyprolinemia: an apparently harmless familial metabolic disorder. New Eng. J. Med. 283: 451-456, 1970.

Scriver, C. R. and Efron, M. L.: Disorders of proline and hydroxyproline metabolism. In, Stanbury, J. B., Wyngaarden, J. B. and Fredrickson, D. S. (eds.): The Metabolic Basis of Inherited Disease. New York: McGraw-Hill, 1972 (3rd Ed.). Pp. 351-369.

Scriver, C. R.: Membrane transport in disorders of imino-acid metabolism. Am. J. Dis. Child. 113: 170-174, 1967.

23710 HYMEN, IMPERFORATE

McIlroy and Ward (1930) reported three sisters ages 20, 16 and 14 who had not menstruated and all had imperforate hymen. The two older sibs had hematocolpos. Hydrometrocolpos of congenital type (q.v.) is due to transverse vaginal septum different from the hymen.

McIlroy, L. and Ward, I. V.: Three cases of imperforate hymen occurring in one family. Proc. Roy. Soc. Med. 23: 633-634, 1930.

*23720 HYPERAMMONEMIA I (ORNITHINE TRANSCARBAMYLASE DEFICIENCY)

Russell (1962) described two cousins with chronic ammonia intoxication and mental deterioration. By liver biopsy the activity of hepatic ornithine transcarbamylase was shown to be very low. A defect is presumed to be present in urea synthesis at the level of conversion of ornithine to citrulline. (See also LYSINE INTOLERENCE AND CITRULLINURIA.) Four forms of hyperammonemia corresponding to each of the enzymes required for the Krebs-Henseleit urea cycle have now been recognized. The genetic interpretation of ornithine transcarbamylase deficiency is complicated by the report of Levin et al. (1969) of a typically affected female infant whose mother had an aversion to protein and raised plasma ammonia levels, whereas the father was normal. The authors pointed to the rarity of male cases of the condition. In another infant, a male, Levin et al. (1969) found what they considered a variant of the usual hyperammonemia caused by ornithine transcarbamylase deficiency, presumably due to a different enzymatic change. Enzyme activity was 25 percent of normal, rather than 5-7 percent of normal as in other cases, and other properties of the enzyme showed differences from the normal. The clinical picture was milder than in the usual cases. Bruton et al. (1970) described astrocyte transformation to Alzheimer type II glia, a feature of any form of hyperammone-mia. Shih and Efron (1972) call this hyperammonemia II and call carbamyl phosphate synthetase deficiency hyperammonemia I. Campbell et al. (1971) suggested that an X-linked gene may code for ornithine-transcar-bamylase so that mutation leads to partial deficiency in heterozygous females and total absence of the enzyme in hemizygous males. (Many, e.g., Shih and Efron, 1972, call OTC deficiency hyperammonemia II and CPS deficiency hyperammonemia I. This has some justification in the fact that CPS is earlier than OTC in the metabolic pathways from ammonia to urea.) Thaler et al. (1974) described a 'novel protein tolerant variant' of ornithine transcarbamylase deficiency in a child with the clinical picture of Reye syndrome (encephalopa-thy with fatty visceral degeneration).

Bruton, C. J., Corsellis, J. A. N. and Russell, A.: Hereditary hyperammonaemia. Brain 93: 423-434, 1970.

Campbell, A. G. M., Rosenberg, L. E., Snodgrass, P. J. and Nuzum, C. T.: Lethal neonatal hyperammonaemia due to complete ornithine-transcarbamylase deficiency. (Letter) Lancet II: 217-218, 1971.

Herrin, J. T. and McCredie, D. A.: Peritoneal dialysis in the reduction of blood ammonia levels in a case of hyperammonaemia. Arch. Dis. Child. 44: 149-151, 1969.

Hopkins, I. J., Connelly, J. F., Dawson, A. G., Hird, F. J. R. and Maddison, T. G.: Hyperammonaemia due to ornithine transcarbamylase deficiency. Arch. Dis. Child. 44: 143-148, 1969.

R
E
C
E
S
S
I
V
E

Levin, B., Abraham, J. M., Oberholzer, V. G. and Burgess, E. A.: Hyperammonaemia: a deficiency of liver ornithine transcarbamylase. Occurrence in mother and child. Arch. Dis. Child. 44: 152-161, 1969.

Russell, A., Levin, B., Oberholzer, V. G. and Sinclair, L.: Hyperammonaemia. A new instance of an inborn enzymatic defect of the biosynthesis of urea. Lancet II: 699-700, 1962.

Shih, V. E. and Efron, M. L.: Urea cycle disorders. In, Stanbury, J. B., Wyngaarden, J. B. and Fredrickson, D. S. (eds.): The Metabolic Basis of Inherited Disease. New York: McGraw-Hill, 1972 (3rd Ed.). Pp. 370-392.

Sunshine, P., Lindenbaum, J. E., Levy, H. L. and Freeman, J. M.: Hyperammonemia due to a defect in hepatic ornithine transcarbamylase. Pediatrics 50: 100-111, 1972.

Thaler, M. M., Hoogenraad, N. J. and Boswell, M.: Reye's syndrome due to a novel protein-tolerent variant of ornithine-transcarbamylase deficiency. Lancet II: 438-440, 1974.

*23730 HYPERAMMONEMIA II (CARBAMYL PHOSPHATE SYNTHETASE DEFICIENCY)

A second type of hyperammonemia has a defect in the preceding step of the urea cycle, involving carbamyl phosphate synthetase. Serum urea nitrogen may be very low in these cases. The patients show an amazing tolerance to high ammonia levels. Defects in the ammonia cycle are especially likely to be accompanied by ammonia intoxication. Defects have been identified at all 5 steps. See HYPERAMMONEMIA I, ARGININEMIA, CITRULLINEMIA and ARGININOSUCCINACIDURIA. A remarkable feature of patients with these disorders is their dislike of protein-containing foods, a phenomenon akin to the avoidance of milk by galactosemics. The only known patient with this disorder was the one reported by Freeman et al. (1970) until Russell's report ( ) of a probable case. Many of the features of this disorder are identical to those of ketotic hyperglycinemia, or propionicacidemia (23200). In E. coli carbamylphosphate synthetase is a dimer of two structurally different polypeptides, alpha and beta (Trotta et al., 1971). If the same is true in man, there is opportunity for non-allelic heterogeneity of this form of hyperammonemia. A family with three affected sibs was reported by Hommes et al. (1969) and by Ebels (1972). Gelehrter and Snodgrass (1974) reported a case and commented on the fact that it is mitochondrial carbamyl phosphate synetase which is deficient in this condition, not the soluble form.

Ebels, E. J.: Neuropathological observations in a patient with carbamyl-phosphate-synthetase deficiency and in two sibs. Arch. Dis. Child. 47: 47-51, 1972.

Freeman, J. M., Nicholson, J. F., Schimke, R. T., Rowland, L. P. and Carter, S.: Congenital hyperammonemia: association with hyperglycinemia and decreased levels of carbamyl phosphate synthetase. Arch. Neurol. 23: 430-437, 1970.

Gelehrter, T. D. and Snodgrass, P. J.: Lethal neonatal deficiency of carbamyl phosphate synthetase. New Eng. J. Med. 290: 430-433, 1974.

Hommes, F. A., De Groot, C. J., Wilmink, C. W. and Jonxis, J. H. P.: Carbamylphosphate synthetase deficiency in an infant with severe cerebral damage. Arch. Dis. Child. 44: 688-693, 1969.

Trotta, P. P., Burt, M. E., Haschemeyer, R. H. and Meister, A.: Reversible dissociation of carbamyl phosphate synthetase into a regulated synthesis subunit and a subunit required for glutamine utilization. Proc. Nat. Acad. Sci. 68: 2599-2603, 1971.

23740 HYPER-BETA-ALANINEMIA

Scriver, Pueschel and Davies (1966) described a somnolent convulsing male infant who had hyper-beta-alaninemia. Beta amino acids (beta-alanine, beta-amino-isobutyric acid and taurine) were excreted in excess in the urine, as a result probably of an interaction between beta-alanine and a specific cellular transport system with preference for beta-amino compounds. GABA (gamma-amino-butyric acid) was also present in the urine but this was independent of plasma levels of alanine. Postmortem tissues had elevated levels of beta-alanine and carnosine. The authors suggested a defect in beta-alanine-alpha-ketoglutarate transaminase which could expand the free beta-alanine pool and increase tissue carnosine. Beta alanine is a central nervous system depressant. Inhibition of GABA transaminase and displacement of GABA from central nervous system binding sites may account for GABA-uria and convulsions. The parents were healthy and not related. Three half sibs were normal. One infant died four hours after birth with 'breathing trouble.' A fifth pregnancy ended in miscarriage.

Scriver, C. R., Pueschel, S. and Davies, E.: Hyper-beta-alaninemia associated with beta-aminoaciduria and gamma-aminobutyricaciduria, somnolence and seizures. New Eng. J. Med. 274: 635-643, 1966.

*23750 HYPERBILIRUBINEMIA II (DUBIN-JOHNSON SYNDROME)

The usefulness of inbred groups for the study of rare recessives is nicely illustrated by this disorder which occurs with a minimal frequency of 1 per 1300 among Iranian Jews (Shani et al., 1970). The characteristics of the disorder are hyperbilirubinemia, deposition of melanin (or at least melanin-like pigment) in otherwise normal liver cells, in some hepatomegaly and abdominal pain, prolonged retention of sulfobromophthalein (which may show a higher concentration at 60 to 90 minutes than at 45 minutes) and otherwise normal liver function.

Shani et al. (1970) studied 101 patients with the Dubin-Johnson syndrome (DJS) ascertained in Israel between 1955 and 1969. Age at onset of jaundice varied from 10 weeks to 56 years. Penetrance is reduced in females. Sixty-four of the cases were Iranian Jews. Parents of affected sibships were consanguineous in 45 per cent of cases as compared with a frequency of 26 per cent among Iranian Jews generally. Segregation analysis yielded results consistent with autosomal recessive inheritance with reduced penetrance. The authors suggested that minor abnormalities may occur in heterozygotes. This suggestion is supported by the findings of Butt et al. (1966), who performed an extensive family study with liver biopsies and other examinations in many relatives.

In the Israel group of cases of DJS, Seligsohn et al. (1970) reported a striking association with deficiency of factor VII. The association was limited to Iranian Jews. I wonder if this may indicate that the DJS and factor VII loci are closely linked and that the two mutant genes are in coupling in a majority of the Iranian Jewish group, not having yet attained equilibrium of linkage phase. Before the report of Shani et al. (1970), the Dubin-Johnson syndrome has been described twice in mother and son (Beker and Read, 1958; Wolf et al., 1960), but at least 7 instances of multiple affected sibs with normal parents are on record (Du and Rogers, 1967). Furthermore, Calderon and Goldgraber (1961) described a Peruvian patient whose parents were first cousins. Du and Rogers (1967) described three affected sisters whose clinically normal parents were first cousins once removed. Three offspring of one affected sister had normal livers (by inspection at laparotomy in two and by autopsy in the third). Arias (1971) gave a useful review of all hereditary hyperbilirubinemias. Adam (1972) questions the linkage interpretation (although he has no alternative explanation) because the association has been seen not only in Iranian Jews but also in Iraqi and Moroccan Jews, in Ashkenazim and perhaps in other Europeans. Furthermore, he points out that the family (no. 55) reported by Shani, Seligsohn et al. (1970) shows several recombinants among the children of a woman who must have been doubly heterozygous in coupling because her mother was doubly homozygous. Wolkoff et al. (1973) found that urinary coproporphyrin I is a good indicator of the homozygote and heterozygote. Normals excreted 24.8 percent of urinary coproporphyrin as coproporphyrin I, whereas homozygotes and heterozygotes excreted 88.9 and 31.6 percent, respectively. The standard errors of these means were 1.3, 1.3 and 1.2 percent, respectively.

Adam, A.: Tel Aviv, Israel: personal communication, 1972.

Arias, I. M.: Inheritable and congenital hyperbilirubinemia. Models for the study of drug metabolism. New Eng. J. Med. 285: 1416-1421, 1971.

Beker, S. and Read, A. E.: Familial Dubin-Johnson syndrome. Gastroenterology 35: 387-389, 1958.

Butt, H. R., Anderson, E., Foulk, W. T., Baggenstoss, A. H., Schoenfield, L. J. and Dickson, E. R.: Studies of chronic idiopathic jaundice (Dubin-Johnson syndrome). II. Evaluation of a large family with the trait. Gastroenterology 51: 619-630, 1966.

Calderon, A. and Goldgraber, M. B.: Chronic idiopathic jaundice: a case report. Gastroenterology 40: 244-247, 1961.

Du, J. N. H. and Rogers, A. G.: Dubin-Johnson syndrome: a family with three affected sisters. Canad. Med. Ass. J. 97: 1225-1226, 1967.

Seligsohn, U., Shani, M., Ramot, B., Adam, A. and Sheba, C.: Dubin-Johnson syndrome in Israel. II. Association with factor-VII deficiency. Quart. J. Med. 39: 569-584, 1970.

Shani, M., Seligsohn, U., Gilon, E., Sheba, C. and Adam, A.: Dubin-Johnson syndrome in Israel. I. Clinical, laboratory, and genetic aspects of 101 cases. Quart. J. Med. 39: 549-567, 1970.

Wolf, R. L., Pizette, M., Richman, A., Dreiling, D. A., Jacobs, W., Fernandez, O. and Popper, H.: Chronic idiopathic jaundice. A study of two afflicted families. Am. J. Med. 28: 32-41, 1960.

Wolkoff, A. W., Cohen, L. E. and Arias, I. M.: Inheritance of the Dubin-Johnson syndrome. New Eng. J. Med. 288: 113-117, 1973.

*23780 HYPERBILIRUBINEMIA, SHUNT

Israels, Suderman and Ritzmann (1959) described what they called shunt hyperbilirubinemia: excess bilirubin appears to be derived from a source other than circulating erythrocytes through an alternative pathway of bilirubin production. Clinical manifestations — jaundice and splenomegaly — have their onset in the second decade. They observed three affected sibs and a fourth case in Mennonites living in Canada. The authors suggested that these patients might be related to those described by Kalk (1955) at Kassel, which is not far from Krefeld, formerly a German Mennonite center. Israels and his colleagues (1963) confirmed their earlier work that the underlying mechanism is an increased production of bilirubin from the early breakdown of heme or its precursors. The liver appears to be capable of direct synthesis of bilirubin ('early labelling bilirubin') without the intermediacy of hemoglobin. The condition may be rather frequent. It should be suspected whenever fecal urobilinogen is markedly increased in the absence of signs of hemolysis.

Israels, L. G., Suderman, H. J. and Ritzmann, S. E.: Hyperbilirubinemia due to an alternate path of bilirubin production. Am. J. Med. 27: 693-702, 1959.

Israels, L. G., Yamamoto, T., Skanderbeg, J. and Zipursky, A.: Shunt bilirubin: evidence for two components. Science 139: 1054-1055, 1963.

Kalk, H. and Wildhirt, E.: Die posthepatitische Hyperbilirubinaemie. Z. Klin. Med. 153: 354-387, 1955.

Kalk, H.: Ueber die posthepatitische Hyperbilirubinaemie. (Der sog. erworbene raemolytische Ikterus nach Hepatitis). Gastroenterologia 84: 207-225, 1955.

23790 HYPERBILIRUBINEMIA, TRANSIENT FAMILIAL NEONATAL

The cause may be steroidal substances in the plasma and milk of the mother which inhibit conjugation of bilirubin (Lucey, Arias and McKay, 1960). The same condition may be present in Yemenite Jews (Sheba). Occasionally, severe neonatal unconjugated hyperbilirubinemia occurs without evident etiologic explanation. Lucey, Arias and McKay (1960) and Arias and colleagues (1965) suggested that some of these cases may have a familial basis. The latter authors found, furthermore, a high level of a maternal serum substance which

E
C
E
S
S
I
V
E

inhibits formation of the glucuronide of direct-reacting bilirubin and O-aminophenol by rat liver slices and homogenates. The inhibitor was present in these mothers in concentrations four to ten times that in other pregnant mothers. The inhibitor is probably a progestational steroid. (This entity is distinct from the severe and prolonged unconjugated hyperbilirubinemia which occurs in breast-fed but not in bottle-fed infants of mothers whose breast milk contains a sterol which inhibits hepatic glucuronyl transferase activity in vitro. The latter state may also have a genetic basis.) Arias and colleagues (1965) made reference to observations on five mothers who gave birth to a total of 16 infants, each of whom had severe transient neonatal hyperbilirubinemia. Three of the 16 died of kernicterus and one was left with quadriplegic cerebral palsy. The mothers do not show hyperbilirubinemia, probably because of a large functional reserve. This is an interesting genetic disease of which there are few examples — one in which the genotype of the mother is responsible for the disease in the infant. Another example is mental retardation in the offspring of women with phenylketonuria (Mabry, et al., 1963). The ethnic background of these mothers and the presence or absence of consanguinity in their parents would be of interest. Transient nonhemolytic unconjugated hyperbilirubinemia is observed in breast-fed but not bottle-fed babies of mothers whose breast milk contains pregnane-3 (alpha), 20 (beta)-diol that competitively inhibits hepatic glucuronyl transferase activity in vitro. Serum from these mothers contains no more inhibitory substance than does normal pregnancy serum. Kernicterus has not been observed, probably because severe jaundice does not develop until the 7th to 10th day, when the infant's blood-brain barrier has become relatively impermeable to unconjugated bilirubin. This is another phenotype of the infant which is dependent on the maternal genotype.

Arias, I. M. and Gartner, L. M.: Production of unconjugated hyperbilirubinaemia in full-term new-born infants following administration of pregnane-3 (alpha), 20 (beta)-diol. Nature 203: 1292-1293, 1964.

Arias, I. M., Gartner, L. M., Seifter, S. and Furman, M.: Prolonged neonatal unconjugated hyperbilirubinemia associated with breast feeding and a steroid, pregnane-3 (alpha), 20 (beta)-diol, in maternal milk that inhibits glucuronide formation in vitro. J. Clin. Invest. 43: 2037-2047, 1964.

Arias, I. M., Wolfson, S., Lucey, J. F. and McKay, R. J., Jr.: Transient familial neonatal hyperbilirubinemia. J. Clin. Invest. 44: 1442-1450, 1965.

Lucey, J. F., Arias, I. M. and McKay, R. J., Jr.: Transient familial neonatal hyperbilirubinemia. Am. J. Dis. Child. 100: 787-789, 1960.

Mabry, C. C., Denniston, J. C., Nelson, T. L. and Nelson, C. D.: Maternal phenylketonuria: a cause of mental retardation in children without the metabolic defect. New Eng. J. Med. 269: 1404-1408, 1963.

Newman, A. J. and Gross, S.: Hyperbilirubinemia in breast-fed infants. Pediatrics 32: 995-1001, 1963.

Sheba, C.: Tel-Aviv, Israel: personal communication, 1964.

23800 HYPERCALCEMIA, IDIOPATHIC

Suspicion of a genetic basis of hypercalcemia was provided by the family reported first in 1959 and later in 1963. Two sisters were affected. The authors (Smith et al., 1959; Kenny et al., 1963) suggested that the defect may concern vitamin D inactivation. The parents had normal serum calcium levels. The mother, but not the father, became hypercalcemic with a small dose of added vitamin D (Blizzard, 1963; Ehrhardt and Money, 1967). It is possible, therefore, that the condition is dominant, not recessive.

Hooft and his colleagues (1961) described a family in which a child had idiopathic hypercalcemia and the father had sarcoidosis with hypercalcemia. See discussion of hypercalcemia in connection with SUPRAVAL-VAR AORTIC STENOSIS in the dominant catalog. Although both aortic and pulmonary stenosis occur with both rubella and hypercalcemia, aortic stenosis is more frequent with hypercalcemia and pulmonary stenosis with rubella (Varghese et al., 1969). A probably different form of familial hypercalcemia was described by Foley et al. (1972). Predominantly females in four generations of the family were affected, with no male-to-male transmission. The parathyroid glands were normal on surgical exploration. Immuno-assayable parathyroid hormone levels were normal in the serum. Urinary calcium excretion was low. Serum phosphate levels were normal or low for the age. A defect in the parathyroid receptor mechanism which responds to elevated serum calcium was postulated.

Blizzard, R. M.: Baltimore, Md.: personal communication, 1963.

Ehrhardt, A. A. and Money, J.: Hypercalcemia — a family study of psychologic functioning. Johns Hopkins Med. J. 121: 14-20, 1967.

Foley, T. P., Jr., Hanison, H. C., Arnaud, C. D. and Harrison, H. E.: Familial benign hypercalcemia. J. Pediat. 81: 1060-1067, 1972.

Hooft, C., Vermassen, A., Eeckels, R. and Vanheule, R.: Familial incidence of hypercalceamia. Extreme hypersensitivity to vitamin D in an infant whose father suffered from sarcoidosis. Helv. Paediat. Acta 16: 199-210, 1961.

Kenny, F. M., Aceto, T., Jr., Purisch, M., Harrison, H. E., Harrison, H. C. and Blizzard, R. M.: Metabolic studies in a patient with idiopathic hypercalcemia of infancy. J. Pediat. 62: 531-537, 1963.

Smith, D. W., Blizzard, R. M. and Harrison, H. E.: Idiopathic hypercalcemia. A case report with assays of vitamin D in the serum. Pediatrics 24: 258-269, 1959.

Varghese, P. J., Izukawa, T. and Rowe, R. D.: Supravalvular aortic stenosis as part of rubella syndrome, with discussion of pathogenesis. Brit. Heart J. 31: 59-62, 1969.

23810 HYPERCALCIURIA

De Luca and Guzzetta (1965) reported four brothers, the products of their mother's first four pregnancies, with hypercalciuria. Two younger sibs, girls, were normal. The parents were not related. A defect of the renal tubule was postulated. Whether genetic and, if so, whether autosomal are not proved. See RENAL TUBULAR ACIDOSIS (17980) for a discussion of hypercalcinuria with that condition.

De Luca, R. and Guzzetta, F.: Idiopathic hypercalciuria in children. Observations in 4 brothers. Pediatria 73: 613-640, 1965.

23820 HYPERCYSTINURIA, ISOLATED

A renal tubular defect limited to cystine and therefore distinct from that in the several forms of classical cystinuria was described by Brodehl et al. (1967). Two sibs were affected. The parents were not related.

Brodehl, J., Gellissen, K. and Kowalewski, S.: Isolierter Defekt der tubulaeren Cystin-Rueckresorption in einer Familie mit idiopathischem Hypoparathyroidismus. Klin. Wschr. 45: 38-40, 1967.

*23830 HYPERGLYCINEMIA, ISOLATED

Unlike glycinemia with ketoacidosis and leukopenia (q.v.), episodic ketoacidosis with vomiting, neutropenia and thrombocytopenia does not occur and glycine is the only amino acid elevated in serum and urine. Glycine is the only amino acid harmful to these patients. Some have died in the newborn period after a course characterized by lethargy, weak cry, generalized hypotonia, absent reflexes, and periodic myoclonic jerks (Balfe et al., 1965). The few who attain an older age show severe mental retardation (Mabry and Karam, 1963; Gerritsen et al., 1965). Sibs with this condition have been reported. Gerritsen et al. (1965) described abnormally low oxalate excretion in the urine and postulated a defect in glycine oxidase. Tada et al. (1969) concluded that the primary lesion in hyperglycinemia of the non-ketotic variety is in the glysine cleavage reaction. Baumgartner et al. (1969) showed that nonketotic variety can have a fulminant early onset. The defect concerns the enzyme involved in the conversion of glycine to CO_2, NH_3 and hydroxymethyltetrahydrofolic acid. DeGroot et al. (1970) described two affected sisters with consanguineous parents and presented evidence indicating that the defect lies in glycine decarboxylase, rather than glycine oxidase.

Balfe, J. W., Levison, H., Hanley, W. B., Jackson, S. H. and Sass-Kortsak, A.: Hyperglycinemia and glycinuria in a newborn. (Abstract) Canad. Med. Ass. J. 92: 347 only, 1965.

Baumgartner, R., Ando, T. and Nyhan, W. L.: Nonketotic hyperglycinemia. J. Pediat. 75: 1022-1030, 1969.

DeGroot, C. J., Troelstra, J. A. and Hommes, F. A.: Nonketotic hyperglycinemia: an in vitro study of the glycine-serine conversion in liver of three patients and the effect of dietary methionine. Pediat. Res. 4: 238-243, 1970.

Gerritsen, T., Kaveggia, E. and Waisman, H. A.: A new type of idiopathic hyperglycinemia with hypo-oxaluria. Pediatrics 36: 882-891, 1965.

Mabry, C. C. and Karam, F. A.: Idiopathic hyperglycinemia and hyperglycinuria. (Abstract) Sth. Med. J. 56: 1444 only, 1963.

Tada, K., Narisawa, K., Yoshida, T., Konno, T., Yokoyama, Y., Nakagawa, H., Tanno, K., Mochizuki, K. and Arakawa, T.: Hyperglycinemia: a defect in glycine cleavage reaction. Tohoku J. Exp. Med. 98: 289-296, 1969.

23840 HYPERLIPIDEMIA V (FAMILIAL HYPERPREBETALIPOPROTEINEMIA, CARBOHYDRATE-INDUCIBLE HYPERLIPEMIA)

The cholesterol is not as markedly elevated as in type III. Triglycerides are markedly elevated. Like type III, the hyperlipemia is carbohydrate-inducible, PHLA is normal and the glucose tolerance test may be abnormal.

23850 HYPERLIPIDEMIA VI (FAMILIAL HYPERCHYLOMICRONEMIA WITH HYPERPREBETALIPOPROTEINEMIA, MIXED HYPERLIPEMIA, COMBINED FAT AND CARBOHYDRATE-INDUCED HYPERLIPEMIA)

On a regular diet both chylomicra and pre-beta-lipoproteins are increased. Alpha- and beta-lipoproteins are normal or low. Features are occult or mild diabetes mellitus, bouts of abdominal pain, and eruptive xanthoma. Fredrickson and Lees (1966) observed parental consanguinity. Hence, this may be a recessive.

Fredrickson, D. S. and Levy, R. I.: Familial hyperlipoproteinemia. In, Stanbury, J. B., Wyngaarden, J. B. and Fredrickson, D. S. (eds.): The Metabolic Basis of Inherited Disease. New York: McGraw-Hill, 1972 (3rd Ed.). Pp. 545-614.

Nixon, J. C., Martin, W. G., Kalab, M. and Monahan, G. J.: Type V hyperlipoproteinemia. A study of a patient and family. Clin. Biochem. 2: 389-398, 1969.

*23860 HYPERLIPOPROTEINEMIA I (FAMILIAL HYPERCHYLOMICRONEMIA, IDIOPATHIC HYPERLIPERMIA OF BURGER-GRUTZ TYPE, ESSENTIAL FAMILIAL HYPERLIPEMIA)

Holt and his colleagues (1939) first reported the familial occurrence of this syndrome. Boggs and colleagues (1957) described three affected sibs from a first cousin mating. Massive hyperchylomicronemia occurs when the patient is on a normal diet and disappears completely in a few days on fat-free feeding. On a normal diet alpha and beta lipoproteins are low. A defect in removal of chylomicrons (fat induction) and of other triglyceride-rich lipoproteins (carbohydrate induction) is present. Decreased plasma postheparinlipolytic activity (PHLA) is demonstrated. Low tissue activity of lipoprotein lipase is suspected. The full blown disease, manifested by attacks of abdominal pain, hepatosplenomegaly, eruptive xanthomas, and lactescence of the plasma, is a recessive. Heterozygotes may show slight hyperlipemia and reduced PHLA. Precocious atherosclerosis seems not to be a feature. This condition was called fat-induced hypertriglyceridemia by Nevin and Slack (1968). Adipose tissue in heterozygotes shows intermediate levels of lipoprotein lipase. Schreibman

R
E
C
E
S
S
I
V
E

Berger, H., Richter, A., Gilardi, A. and Wagner, H.: Essential familial hyperlipaemia in a 2-year-old child. Ann. Paediat. 199: 445-466, 1962.

Boggs, J. D., Hsia, D. Y.-Y., Mais, R. F. and Bigler, J. A.: The genetic mechanism of idiopathic hyperlipemia. New Eng. J. Med. 257: 1101-1108, 1957.

Franklin, S. M.: Splenomegaly with lipaemia. Proc. Roy. Soc. Med. 30: 711 Only, 1937.

Fredrickson, D. S. and Levy, R. I.: Familial hyperlipoproteinemia. In, Stanbury, J. B., Wyngaarden, J. B. and Fredrickson, D. S. (eds.): The Metabolic Basis of Inherited Disease. New York: McGraw-Hill, 1972 (3rd Ed.). Pp. 545-614.

Holt, L. E., Jr., Aylward, F. X. and Timbers, H. G.: Idiopathic familial lipemia. Bull. Hopkins Hosp. 64: 279-314, 1939.

Nevin, N. C. and Slack, J.: Hyperlipidaemic xanthomatosis II: mode of inheritance in 55 families with essential hyperlipidaemia and xanthomatosis. J. Med. Genet. 5: 9-28, 1968.

Schreibman, P. H., Arons, D. L., Saudek, C. D. and Arky, R. A.: Abnormal lipoprotein lipase in familial exogenous hypertriglyceridemia. J. Clin. Invest. 52: 2074-2082, 1973.

Wessler, S. and Avioli, L. A.: Familial hyperlipoproteinemia. J.A.M.A. 207: 929-937, 1969.

*23870 HYPERLYSINEMIA

Ghadimi et al. (1965) found hyperlysinemia in two unrelated mentally retarded patients. The level of lysine in the CSF was also elevated. Blood levels rose abnormally with lysine loading. A block in the metabolism of lysine was postulated. The patients were aged 2 and 27 years. Impaired sexual development, lax ligaments and muscles, convulsions in early life and perhaps mild anemia were features. Woody (1964) found elevated lysine in the blood and spinal fluid of a physically and mentally retarded girl with convulsions, muscular and ligamentous asthenia, and normocytic, normochromic anemia which responded to dietary restriction of lysine. This worker suggested that incorporation of lysine into protein was defective. An ostensibly normal cousin also had hyperlysinuria. The parents of the proband were related. Dancis et al. (1969) demonstrated reduced lysine-ketoglutarate reductase activity in skin fibroblasts from 3 affected sibs. In view of the ligamentous laxity, it is of interest that subluxation of the lenses developed in some of the patients (Woody, 1971; Smith et al. 1971)). The hyperlysinemia in the cases studied by Davis et al. (1969) was more marked than that in other reported cases such as that of Ghadimi et al. (1965) yet the latter cases were more severely retarded. The relationship to these other reported cases and to the entity discussed elsewhere as lysine intolerance awaits elucidation. Saccharopinuria (Carson et al., 1968) is presumably a distinct disorder involving the lysine metabolic pathway and showing hyperlysinemia. One of the cases of Ghadimi et al. (1965) was the product of father-daugher incest. Woody's cases are inbred Louisiana Cajuns.

R
E
C
E
S
S
I
V
E

Carson, N. A. J., Scally, B. G., Neill, D. W. and Carre, I. J.: Saccharopinuria: a new born error of lysine metabolism. Nature 218: 679 only, 1968.

Choremis, C., Yannakos, D., Papadatos, C. and Baroutsou, E.: Osteitis deformans (Paget's disease) in an 11-year-old boy. Helv. Paediat. Acta 13: 185-188, 1958.

Dancis, J., Hutzler, J., Cox, R. P. and Woody, N. C.: Familial hyperlysinemia with lysine-ketoglutarate reductase insufficiency. J. Clin. Invest. 48: 1447-1452, 1969.

Ghadimi, H., Binnington, V. I. and Pecora, P.: Hyperlysinemia associated with mental retardation. New Eng. J. Med. 273: 723-729, 1965.

Smith, T. H., Holland, M. G. and Woody, N. C.: Ocular manifestations of familial hyperlysinemia? Trans. Am. Acad. Ophthal. Otolaryng. 75: 355-360, 1971.

Woody, N. C. and Pupene, M. B.: Derivation of pipecolic acid from L-lysine by familial hyperlysinemics. Pediat. Res. 5: 511-513, 1971.

Woody, N. C.: Hyperlysinemia. Am. J. Dis. Child. 108: 543-553, 1964.

Woody, N. C.: New Orleans, La.: personal communication, 1971.

Woody, N. C., Hutzler, J. and Dancis, J.: Further studies of hyperlysinemia. Am. J. Dis. Child. 112: 577-580, 1960.

Woody, N. C. and Pupene, M. B.: Excretion of hypusine by children and by patients with familial hyperlysinemia. Pediat. Res. 7: 994-995, 1973.

23875 HYPERLYSINURIA WITH HYPERAMMONEMIA

Brown et al. (1972) described a physically and mentally retarded child with dibasicaminoaciduria and hyperammonemia. Oral loading tests showed diminished capacity for absorbing lysine. Fasting blood arginine and lysine concentrations were low. Post-prandial hyperammonemia was thought to be due to deficiency of arginine to serve as substrate for urea cycle activity. The defect in intestinal absorption distinguishes this disorder from familial protein intolerance (12600, 22270).

Brown, J. H., Fabre, L. F., Jr., Farrell, G. L. and Adams, E. D.: Hyperlysinuria with hyperammonemia. Am. J. Dis. Child. 124: 127-132, 1972.

23880 HYPERMETABOLISM DUE TO DEFECT IN MITOCHONDRIA

Luft and colleagues (1962) observed a 35 year old patient with a BMR of 150 to 200 percent since at least 7 years of age, yet normal thyroid function. Studies of mitochondria from skeletal muscle showed a defect of coupling between oxidation and phosphorylation. The parents were not related and no other cases were recognized in the family. However, the possibility of a genetic basis was raised.

Luft, R., Ikkos, D., Palmieri, G., Ernster, L. and Afzelius, B.: A case of severe hypermetabolism of nonthyroid origin with a defect in the maintenance of mitochondrial respiratory control: a correlated clinical, biochemical, and morphological study. J. Clin. Invest. 41: 1776-1804, 1962.

23890 HYPERMETHIONINEMIA

Perry et al. (1965) described three sibs (2 females and a male) in one sibship who died in the third month after an illness characterized by irritability and progressive somnolence, and terminally by a tendency to bleed and hypoglycemia. A peculiar odor was noted. Pathologic changes included hepatic cirrhosis, renal tubular dilatation and pancreatic islet hypertrophy. Biochemical studies showed generalized aminoaciduria, very marked elevation of methionine in the serum and a disproportionately high urinary excretion of methionine. Alpha-keto-gamma-methiolbutyric acid was present in the urine and may account for the peculiar odor. The hypertrophy of the islets of Langerhans was probably due to stimulation by methionine or one of its metabolites. It seems likely that the disorder was tyrosinemia (q.v.) since hypermethioninemia occurs secondary to liver failure in that condition (Scriver et al., 1967).

Perry, T. L., Hardwick, D. F., Dixon, G. H., Dolman, C. L. and Hansen, S.: Hypermethioninemia: a metabolic disorder associated with cirrhosis, islet cell hyperplasia, and renal tubular degeneration. Pediatrics 36: 236-250, 1965.

Scriver, C. R., Larochelle, J. and Silverberg, M.: Hereditary tyrosinemia and tyrosyluria in a French-Canadian geographic isolate. Am. J. Dis. Child. 113: 41-46, 1967.

*23900 HYPEROSTOSIS CORTICALIS DEFORMANS JUVENILIS (JUVENILE PAGET DISEASE, CHRONIC CONGENITAL IDIOPATHIC HYPERPHOSPHATASEMIA)

Caffey (1961) and Rubin (1964) presented cases. Bakwin and Eiger (1956) and Bakwin, Golden and Fox (1964) described a familial disorder manifesting itself from early in life by large head and expanded and bowed extremities. Alkaline phosphatase was elevated. The long bones are greatly expanded with osteoporosis and coarse trabeculations. The calvarium is markedly thickened with islands of increased bone density. Muscular weakness may be striking. In Bakwin's family two sisters were severely affected. The parents were first cousins and the mother was mildly affected. The findings in her would probably have escaped detection if X-rays had not been made. The authors thought this to be the same as the condition described in two sisters by Swoboda (1958) as hyperostosis corticalis deformans juvenilis and by Choremis et al. (1958) as Paget disease in an 11-year-old boy. Of interest is the presence of angioid streaks in one of Bakwin's patients. Fanconi (1964) described the X-ray and histologic changes in a young Brazilian male and suggested the designation osteochalasia desmalis familiaris. Since the basic disorder is unknown, another label is not warranted. The condition called familial osteoectasia by Stemmermann (1966) appears to be the same. His cases were in brother and sister, age 2 and 3, of Puerto Rican ancestry. Bakwin, Golden and Fox (1964) observed this disorder in two sisters of Puerto Rican parentage. Both had retinal degeneration. In one the changes included angioid streaks. Brother and sister of mixed Hawaiian, Filipino and Puerto Rican ancestry were described by Eyring and Eisenberg (1968). Fragile bones, premature loss of teeth and dwarfism were features. Increased bone formation and destruction were thought to be present. Both acid and alkaline phosphatases and leucine amino peptidase were elevated. Increased hydroxyproline in blood and urine and hyperuricemia were also demonstrated. Caffey (1973) reviewed the findings in 14 patients distributed in 10 families.

Bakwin, H. and Eiger, M. S.: Fragile bones and macrocranium. J. Pediat. 49: 558-564, 1956.

Bakwin, H., Golden, A. and Fox, S.: Familial osteoectasia with macrocranium. Am. J. Roentgen. 91: 609-617, 1964.

Caffey, J. P.: Pediatric X-ray Diagnosis. Chicago: Year Book Medical Publishers, (4th Ed.), 1961.

Caffey, J.: Familial hyperphosphatasemia with ateliosis and hypermetabolism of growing membranous bone: review of the clinical, radiographic and chemical features. In, Kaufmann, H. J. (ed.): Intrinsic Diseases of Bones. Vol. 4 of Progress in Pediatric Radiology. Basel: S. Karger, 1973. Pp. 438-468.

Fanconi, G., Moreira, G., Uehlinger, E. and Giedion, A.: Osteochalasia desmalis familiaris. Hyperostosis corticalis deformans juveniles, chronic idiopathic hyperphosphatasia and macrocranium. Helv. Paediat. Acta 19: 279-295, 1964.

Rubin, P.: Chronic idiopathic hyperphosphatasemia, congenital. (Syndrome: juvenile Paget's disease, hyperostosis corticalis deformans juveniles, hyperphosphatasia). Dynamic Classification of Bone Dysplasias. Chicago: Year Book Medical Publishers, 1964. Pp. 340-344.

Swoboda, H.: Hyperostosis corticalis deformans juvenilis: ungewohnliche generalisierte Osteopathie bei zwei Geschwistern. Helv. Paediat. Acta 13: 292-312, 1958.

Stemmermann, G. N.: An histologic and histochemical study of familial osteoectasia (chronic idiopathic hyperphosphatasia). Am. J. Path. 48: 641-651, 1966.

*23910 HYPEROSTOSIS CORTICALIS GENERALISATA (VAN BUCHEM DISEASE: HYPERPHOS-PHATASEMIA TARDA)

Van Buchem and colleagues (1962) found osteosclerosis of the skull, mandible, clavicles, ribs and diaphysis of the long bones beginning during puberty and sometimes leading to optic atrophy and perceptive deafness

RECESSIVE

from nerve pressure. The same disorder was probably reported earlier by Garland (1946) as 'generalized leontiasis ossea' and by Halliday (1949) as bone dystrophy.

Garland, L. H.: Generalized leontiasis ossea. Am. J. Roentgen. 55: 37-43, 1946.

Halliday, J.: A rare case of bone dystrophy. Brit. J. Surg. 37: 52-63, 1949.

Van Buchem, F. S. P., Hadders, H. N., Hansen, J. F. and Woldring, M. G.: Hyperostosis corticalis generalisata: report of seven cases. Am. J. Med. 33: 387-397, 1962.

*23920 HYPERPARATHYROIDISM, NEONATAL FAMILIAL PRIMARY

Hillman and colleagues (1964) described neonatal primary hyperparathyroidism in two male sibs, offspring of first cousin parents. Philips (1948) had earlier reported one of the sibs. Goldbloom et al. (1972) observed two affected sisters. Early diagnosis and parathyroidectomy is necessary to permit survival.

Corbeel, L., Casaer, P., Malvaux, P., Lormans, J. and Boorgeois, N.: Hyperparathyroidie congenitale. Arch. Franc. Pediat. 25: 879-891, 1968.

Goldbloom, R. B., Gillis, D. A. and Prasad, M.: Hereditary parathyroid hyperplasia: a surgical emergency of early infancy. Pediatrics 49: 514-523, 1972.

Hillman, D. A., Scriver, C. R., Pedvis, S. and Shragovitch, I.: Neonatal familial primary hyperparathyroidism. New Eng. J. Med. 270: 483-490, 1964.

Philips, R. N.: Primary diffuse parathyroid hyperplasia in an infant of four months. Pediatrics 2: 428-434, 1948.

*23930 HYPERPHOSPHATASIA WITH MENTAL RETARDATION

Three sibs and a first cousin had severe mental retardation, seizures, various neurologic abnormalities and greatly elevated alkaline phosphatase. Both pairs of parents were consanguineous. The alkaline phosphatase present in excess seemed to be of hepatic origin.

Mabry, C. C., Bautista, A., Kirk, R. F. H., Dubilier, L. D., Braunstein, H. and Koepke, J. A.: Familial hyperphosphatasia with mental retardation, seizures, and neurologic deficits. J. Pediat. 77: 74-85, 1970.

23940 HYPERPIPECOLATEMIA

In a child with a degenerative neurological disease and hepatomegaly, Gatfield et al. (1968) found grossly elevated blood concentrations of pipecolic acid with mild generalized aminoaciduria. Pipecolic acid is an intermediate in lysine catabolism. However, the patient showed no delay in clearing lysine from the blood, indicating, as does other evidence, that the main lysine catabolic pathway is not via a pipecolic acid. Autopsy revealed widespread demyelination in the central nervous system.

Gatfield, P. D., Taller, E., Hinton, G. G., Wallace, A. C., Abdelnour, G. M. and Haust, M. D.: Hyperpipecolatemia: a new metabolic disorder associated with neuropathy and hepatomegaly: a case study. Canad. Med. Ass. J. 99: 1215-1233, 1968.

*23950 HYPERPROLINEMIA, TYPE I

Scriver, Schafer and Efron (1961) and Schafer, Scriver and Efron (1962) described a family in which the male proband and three sibs had elevated plasma levels of L-proline. Probably the anomaly bore no relation to two other genetic defects in the same family: familial nephropathy and photogenic epilepsy. The amino-aciduria includes hydroxyproline and glycine as well as proline, presumably because these three amino acids share a renal tubular active transport mechanism which is overloaded by the high level of proline in the glomerular filtrate. Two types of hyperprolinemia appear to exist. In type I referred to above the defect involves the enzyme proline oxidase (Efron, 1965). Renal abnormalities occur in this form. In type II, characterized by mental retardation and convulsions, the enzyme defect concerns delta-1-pyrroline-5-carboxylate (PC) dehydrogenase and the substance normally acted on by this enzyme is excreted in the urine. The family of Efron (1965) was Italian. That of Scriver et al. (1961) and Schafer et al. (1962) was Scotch-Irish. Perry et al. (1968) reported hyperprolinemia of type I in two generations of a consanguineous American Indian family. Hereditary renal abnormalities occurred in members of 3 generations. The proband later developed Wilms tumor. Marked elevations of plasma proline occur in homozygotes and normal or moderately elevated levels in heterozygotes, in the view of the authors. Both genotypes are accompanied by renal abnormalities. Mental retardation is not a feature of type I hyperprolinemia. Goyer et al. (1968) observed hereditary nephritis, neurosensory hearing loss, prolinuria and ichthyosis in various combinations in 23 members of a kindred. The relation to the hyperprolinurias and to Alport syndrome is not clear. The patient reported by Rokkones et al. (1968) had uncle-niece parents. Selkoe (1969) described a second type of hyperprolinemia with only mild mental retardation and without renal disease. The enzyme involved seems to be delta prime-pyrroline-5-carboxylic acid dehydrogenase. Emery et al. (1968) described an affected 18-year-old girl who was mentally retarded and had a retarded sister who had died probably of the same disorder.

Blake, R. L., Grillo, R. V. and Russell, E. S.: Increased taurine excretion in hereditary hyperprolinemia of the mouse. Life Sci. 14: 1285-1290, 1974.

Efron, M. L.: Familial hyperprolinemia. Report of second case, associated with congenital renal malformation, hereditary hematuria and mild mental retardation, with demonstration of enzyme defect. New Eng. J. Med. 272: 1243-1254, 1965.

Emery, F. A., Goldie, L. and Stern, J.: Hyperprolinaemia type 2. J. Ment. Defic. Res. 12: 187-195, 1968.

Goyer, R. A., Reynolds, J., Jr., Burke, J. and Burkholder, P.: Hereditary renal disease with neurosensory hearing loss, prolinuria and ichthyosis. Am. J. Med. Sci. 256: 166-179, 1968.

Perry, T. L., Hardwick, D. F., Lowry, R. B. and Hansen, S.: Hyperprolinaemia in two successive generations of a North American Indian family. Ann. Hum. Genet. 31: 401-408, 1968.

Rokkones, T. and Loken, A. C.: Congenital renal dysplasia, retinal dysplasia and mental retardation associated with hyperprolinuria and hyper-OH-prolinuria. Acta Paediat. Scand. 57: 225-229, 1968.

Schafer, I. A., Scriver, C. R. and Efron, M. L.: Familial hyperprolinemia, cerebral dysfunction and renal anomalies occurring in a family with hereditary nephropathy and deafness. New Eng. J. Med. 267: 51-60, 1962.

Scriver, C. R. and Efron, M. L.: Disorders of proline and hydroxyproline metabolism. In, Stanbury, J. B., Wyngaarden, J. B. and Fredrickson, D. S. (eds.): The Metabolic Basis of Inherited Disease. New York: McGraw-Hill, 1972 (3rd Ed.). Pp. 351-369.

Scriver, C. R., Schafer, I. A. and Efron, M. L.: New renal tubular amino-acid transport system and a new hereditary disorder of amino-acid metabolism. Nature 192: 672-673, 1961.

Selkoe, D. J.: Familial hyperprolinemia and mental retardation. A second metabolic type. Neurology 19: 494-502, 1969.

*23951 HYPERPROLINEMIA, TYPE II

See above.

Valle, D. L. and Phang, J. M.: Type 2 hyperprolinemia: absence of delta-1-pyrroline-5-carboxylic acid dehydrogenase activity. Science 185: 1053-1054, 1974.

23960 HYPERSEROTONEMIA

Southern et al. (1959) described a 49-year-old woman who from early childhood had severe rage reactions with episodes of flushing of the face, neck and arms. Hand tremor, slurred speech and ataxia began at age 32. Blood serotonin was markedly elevated. 5-hydroxyindoleacetic acid was normal in the urine but increased after administration of serotonin. Administration of reserpine aggravated the symptoms. Scriver and Efron (1972) concluded that renal disease was only a coincidental occurrence in type I hyperprolinemia. The enzyme defect has been demonstrated in vitro for type I but not for type II.

Southern, A. L., Warner, R. R. P., Christoff, N. I. and Weiner, H. E.: An unusual neurologic syndrome associated with hyperserotonemia. New Eng. J. Med. 260: 1265-1268, 1959.

23970 HYPERTELORISM, CRYPTORCHIDISM, DIGITAL CONTRACTURES, STERNAL DEFORMITY, AND OSTEOCHONDRITIS DISSECANS

This combination of abnormalities has been noted in two brothers. Osteochondritis dissecans occurred at multiple sites (knee, elbow, etc.). Early fusion of the manubrium and corpus sterni occurred. The ears were floppy. Familial osteochondritis dissecans have been thought to be dominant (q.v.). Ptosis was present in one of the brothers. Gorlin (1967) has shown me a family in which two boys and their mother have manifestations like those in the sibs reported by Hanley et al. (1967). The boys had different fathers. Hence, the inheritance may be dominant. Welch (1971) has evaluated two brothers with this syndrome.

Gorlin, R. J.: Minneapolis, Minn.: personal communication, 1967.

Hanley, W. B., McKusick, V. A. and Barranco, F. T.: Osteochondritis dissecans with associated malformations in two brothers. A review of familial aspects. J. Bone Joint Surg. 49A: 925-937, 1967.

Welch, J. P.: Halifax, Nova Scotia: personal communication, 1971.

23980 HYPERTELORISM, MICROTIA, FACIAL CLEFTING (HMC) SYNDROME

Bixler, Christian and Gorlin (1969) described two sisters who had hypertelorism, microtia, and clefting of the lip, palate and nose. In addition, they showed psychomotor retardation, atretic auditory canals, microcephaly, and ectopic kidneys. Both had congenital heart malformations, as did also several relatives on the mother's side. The parents were normal and unrelated.

Bixler, D., Christian, J. C. and Gorlin, R. J.: Hypertelorism, microtia and facial clefting: a new inherited syndrome. The Clinical Delineation of Birth Defects. II. Malformation Syndromes. New York: National Foundation, 1969. P. 7781.

Edgerton, M. T., Udvarhelyi, G. B. and Knox, D. L.: The surgical correction of ocular hypertelorism. Ann. Surg. 172: 473-496, 1970.

23990 HYPERTROPHIC NEUROPATHY AND CATARACT

Gold and Hogenkuis (1968) observed this combination in 2 sisters and their brother of Hindu extraction. Spinal fluid protein was moderately elevated. Severe distal sensory and motor loss was present.

Gold, G. N. and Hogenkuis, L. A. H.: Hypertrophic interstitial neuropathy and cataracts. Neurology 18: 526-533, 1968.

24000 HYPERURICEMIA, INFANTILE, WITH ABNORMAL BEHAVIOR AND NORMAL HYPOXANTHINE GUANINE PHOSPHORIBOSYL TRANSFERASE

Nyhan et al. (1969) reported a 3-year-old boy with mental retardation, dysplastic teeth, failure to cry with tears, absent speech and autistic behavior. HGPT was normal, whereas the activity of adenine phosphoribosyltransferase was increased. Nothing is known about its genetics.

R
E
C
E
S
S
I
V
E

Nyhan, W. L., James, J. A., Teberg, A. J., Sweetman, L. and Nelson, L. G.: A new disorder of purine metabolism with behavioral manifestations. J. Pediat. 74: 20-27, 1969.

24010 HYPERURICEMIA, LIPODYSTROPHY AND NEUROLOGIC DEFECT

Meador (1966) informed me of three sibs (2 female, 1 male), whose parents are probably related and who show loss of fat on the lower part of the body with abundant fat on the upper part, especially around the neck, pyramidal tract disease, pes cavus, and hyperuricemia with clinical gout. The approximate ages were 28, 24 and 18.

Meador, C.: Birmingham, Ala.: personal communication, 1966.

*24020 HYPOADRENOCORTICISM, FAMILIAL

The isolated form is less frequent than that combined with other endocrinopathy, particularly hypoparathyroidism. A noteworthy feature is the lack of hypoaldosteronism (Stempfel and Engel, 1960; Shepard, Landing and Mason, 1959). Androgen metabolism could not be tested. These cases may well have a defect limited to corticoid metabolism. Some of these cases may with more validity be classed as adrenal unresponsiveness to ACTH (q.v.). Berlin (1952) reported Addison disease in brother and sister, the latter having also pernicious anemia. Brochner-Mortensen (1956) described Addison disease in two brothers and two of their maternal uncles. Meakin, Nelson and Thorn (1959) described two brothers with onset of adrenal insufficiency at age 3-4 years. Addison disease falls into the same category as pernicious anemia, systemic lupus erythematosus, myasthenia gravis, Hashimoto thyroiditis, athyreotic cretinism, in which an autoimmune basis is suggested by some evidence and in which familial aggregation occurs. In all these conditions, the role of a single genetic locus in etiology is unclear. Williams and Freeman (1965) reported adrenal cortical hypofunction without salt loss in 3 of 4 children of second cousin parents. O'Donohoe and Holland (1968) described autopsy-proven adrenal hypoplasia in a sister of two affected males. Lemli and Smith (1968) reported affected sisters.

Berlin, R.: Addison's disease. Familial incidence and occurrence in association with pernicious anemia. Acta Med. Scand. 144: 1-6, 1952.

Boyd, J. F. and MacDonald, A. M.: Adrenal cortical hypoplasia in siblings. Arch. Dis. Child. 35: 561-568, 1960.

Brochner-Mortensen, K.: Familial occurrence of Addison's disease. Acta Med. Scand. 156: 205-209, 1956.

Lemli, L. and Smith, D. W.: Idiopathic adrenal insufficiency in two siblings. Maandschr. Kindergeneesk. 34: 63, 1968.

Louria, D. B., Shannon, D., Johnson, G., Caroline, L., Okas, A. and Taschdjian, C.: The susceptibility to moniliasis in children with endocrine hypofunction. Trans. Ass. Am. Physicians 80: 236-249, 1967.

Meakin, J. W., Nelson, D. H. and Thorn, G. W.: Addison's disease in two brothers. J. Clin. Endocr. 19: 726-731, 1959.

Mitchell, R. G. and Rhaney, K.: Congenital adrenal hypoplasia in siblings. Lancet I: 488-492, 1959.

O'Donohoe, N. V. and Holland, P. D. J.: Familial congenital adrenal hypoplasia. Arch. Dis. Child. 43: 717-723, 1968.

Shepard, T. H., Landing, B. H. and Mason, D. G.: Familial Addison's disease: case reports of two sisters with corticoid deficiency unassociated with hypoaldosteronism. Am. J. Dis. Child. 97: 154-162, 1959.

Stempfel, R. S., Jr. and Engel, F. L.: A congenital, familial syndrome of adrenocortical insufficiency without hypoaldosteronism. J. Pediat. 57: 443-451, 1960.

Williams, H. E. and Freeman, M.: Primary familial Addison's disease. Aust. Pediat. J. 1: 93-97, 1965.

*24030 HYPOADRENOCORTICISM, WITH HYPOPARATHYROIDISM AND SUPERFICIAL MONILIASIS

Moniliasis usually precedes symptoms and signs of endocrinopathy. Furthermore, hypoparathyroidism usually reveals itself before adrenal insufficiency. See HYPOPARATHYROIDISM.

An infectious etiology was suggested by Kunin and colleagues (1963) who pointed out that hepatitis has occurred in a number of these cases before the development of endocrinopathy.

Hung, Migeon and Parrott (1963) found circulating adrenal antibodies in two sibs with Addison disease. A third sib had died from Addison disease. One of the affected sibs also had hypoparathyroidism, pernicious anemia and superficial moniliasis. The authors suggested the disorder may not be inherited as a simple Mendelian recessive but may be auto-immune in nature. Shannon et al. (1966) made the novel suggestion that a genetic defect of the integument is primary and predisposes to development of chronic moniliasis, and that an absorption product of Candida albicans acts directly as a toxin or indirectly as a cross-reacting antigen to give progressive tissue damage. If true, the theory makes it urgent to eradicate the fungus from these patients. Heterogeneity in this group of cases (Addison disease without hypoparathyroidism, Addison disease with hypoparathyroidism, hypoparathyroidism without Addison disease, Schmidt syndrome) was suggested by the analysis of Spinner et al. (1968). Foz et al. (1970) made a brief note of a sibship, offspring of first-cousin parents, containing two female sibs with idiopathic Addison disease. One also had primary hypoparathyroidism and one had oral candidiasis. Malabsorption and diarrhea can be very striking and even dominate the clinical picture (Prader, 1972).

R
E
C
E
S
S
I
V
E

Castells, S., Fikrig, S., Inamdar, S. and Orti, E.: Familial moniliasis, defective delayed hypersensitivity, and adrenocorticotropic hormone deficiency. J. Pediat. 79: 72-79, 1971.

Craig, J. M., Schiff, L. H. and Boone, J. E.: Chronic moniliasis associated with Addison's disease. Am. J. Dis. Child. 89: 669-684, 1955.

Foz, M., Mirada, A. and Guardia, J.: Endocrine disorders in a family. (Letter) Lancet II: 269 only, 1970.

Gass, J. D. M.: The syndrome of keratoconjunctivitis, superficial moniliasis, idiopathic hypoparathyroidism and Addison's disease. Am. J. Ophthal. 54: 660-674, 1962.

Hiekkala, H.: Idiopathic hypoparathyroidism, adrenal insufficiency and moniliasis in children. Ann. Paediat. Fenn. 10: 213-222, 1964.

Hung, W., Migeon, C. J. and Parrott, R. H.: A possible autoimmune basis for Addison's disease in three siblings, one with idiopathic hypoparathyroidism, pernicious anemia and superficial moniliasis. New Eng. J. Med. 269: 658-663, 1963.

Kenny, F. M. and Holliday, M. D.: Hypoparathyroidism, moniliasis, Addison's and Hashimoto's disease. Hypercalcemia treated with intravenously administered sodium sulfate. New Eng. J. Med. 271: 708-713, 1964.

Kunin, A. S., MacKay, B. R., Burns, S. L. and Halberstam, M. J.: The syndrome of hypoparathyroidism and adrenocortical insufficiency, a possible sequel of hepatitis: case report and review of the literature. Am. J. Med. 34: 856-866, 1963.

Prader, A.: Zurich, Switzerland: personal communication, 1972.

Shannon, D. C., Johnson, G. and Austen, K. F.: Genetic and clinical aspects of the syndrome of chronic moniliasis and endocrine deficits. Soc. Pediat. Res. (April 29-30, 1966) 101 only, 1966.

Spinner, M. W., Blizzard, R. M. and Childs, B.: Clinical and genetically heterogeneity in idiopathic Addison's disease and hypoparathyroidism. J. Clin. Endocr. 28: 795-804, 1968.

Sweetnam, W. P.: Juvenile familial endocrinopathy. Lancet I: 463-465, 1966.

Whitaker, J. A., Landing, B. H., Esselborn, V. M. and Williams, R. R.: Syndrome of familial juvenile hypoadrenocorticism, hypoparathyroidism and superficial moniliasis. J. Clin. Endocr. 16: 1374-1387, 1956.

*24040 HYPOASCORBEMIA

As far as is known, man lacks the ability to synthesize ascorbic acid, through lack of the enzyme L-gulonolactone oxidase which most other mammals possess. As Stone (1967) points out hypoascorbemia is an inborn error of metabolism. Borrowing a term from the blood groups we might say that it is a 'public' inborn error of metabolism. The mechanism whereby an organism loses a particular metabolic function which is of no use in a particular environment was discussed by King and Jukes (1969). The accumulation of random mutations in the gene for the relevant enzyme might be expected to destroy the functional capacity of the enzyme, most mutations being disruptive. If the enzyme is not required in the particular environment, the constraint of selection is removed. Primates and the guinea pig, by this hypothesis, have lost the capacity to synthesize ascorbic acid because of the adequacy of dietary intake. An intraspecies example of this phenomenon may be the loss of adult intestinal lactase in people who do not consume milk.

Chatterjee, I. B.: Evolution and the biosynthesis of ascorbic acid. Science 182: 1271-1271, 1973.

King, J. L. and Jukes, T. H.: Non-Darwinian evolution. Science 164: 788-798, 1969.

Pauling, L.: Evolution and the need for ascorbic acid. Proc. Nat. Acad. Sci. 67: 1643-1648, 1970.

Stone, I.: The genetic disease, hypoascorbemia. A fresh approach to an ancient disease and some of its medical implications. Acta Genet. Med. Gem. 16: 52-62, 1967.

*24050 HYPOGAMMAGLOBULINEMIA

Wollheim (1961) described two females with 'acquired' hypogammaglobulinemia who came from different parts of Sweden but were remotely related. He suggested that a recessive genetic factor may be involved in 'acquired' hypogammaglobulinemia. Kamin et al. (1968) found that phytohemagglutinin-induced incorporation of labelled precursors into DNA and RNA by lymphocytes is significantly diminished in cells of adults with so-called 'acquired' agammaglobulinemia. The difference was independent of the characteristics of the culture-medium, indicating a cellular abnormality. They suggested that this is the first laboratory test that detects the carrier state in a genetically determined disorder that becomes manifest in adult life. Cooper et al. (1971) found normal numbers of B lymphocytes bearing membrane-bound immunoglobulins and germinal centers were normally found in antigen-stimulated lymph nodes. They postulated that although the B lymphocytes in such patients have surface recognition antigens, they lack the mechanism for plasma cell differentiation. Wilson and Nossal (1971) concluded that circulating lymphocytes are of two types: B (bursa) with a high density of surface immunoglobulins and T (thymus) with a low density.

Charache, P., Rosen, F. S., Janeway, C. A., Craig, J. M. and Rosenberg, H. A.: Acquired agammaglobulinemia in siblings. Lancet I: 234-237, 1965.

Cooper, M. D., Lawton, A. R. and Bockman, D. E.: Agammaglobulinaemia with B lymphocytes. Specific defect of plasma-cell differentiation. Lancet II: 791-794, 1971.

Kamin, R. M., Fudenberg, H. H. and Douglas, S. D.: A genetic defect in 'acquired' agammaglobulinemia. Proc. Nat. Acad. Sci. 60: 881-885, 1968.

Wilson, J. D. and Nossal, G. J. V.: Identification of human T and B lymphocytes in normal peripheral blood and in chronic lymphocytic leukemia. Lancet II: 788-791, 1971.

Wollheim, F. A.: Inherited 'acquired' hypogammaglobulinaemia. Lancet I: 316-317, 1961.

Wollheim, F. A.: Primary 'acquired' hypogammaglobulinemia: genetic defect or acquired disease? In, Immunologic Deficiency Diseases in Man. (Birth Defects Original Article Series, vol. IV, no. 1). New York: National Foundation, 1968.

24055 HYPOGLYCEMIA WITH ABSENT PANCREATIC ALPHA CELLS

McQuarrie et al. (1950) observed the conditions in sibs. Gotlin and Silver (1970) measured high insulin levels.

Gotlin, R. W. and Silver, H. K.: Neonatal hypoglycaemia, hyperinsulinism, and absence of pancreatic alpha-cells. (Letter) Lancet II: 1346 only, 1970.

McQuarrie, I., Bell, E. T., Zimmerman, B. and Wright, W. S.: Deficiency of alpha cells of pancreas as possible etiological factor in familial hypoglycemosis. (Abstract) Fed. Proc. 9: 337 only, 1950.

*24060 HYPOGLYCEMIA WITH DEFICIENCY OF GLYCOGEN SYNTHETASE IN THE LIVER

In a well-studied family, Lewis, Spencer-Peet and Stewart (1963) demonstrated that infantile hypoglycemia was due to a deficiency of glycogen synthetase in the liver. The cases were probably of the same type as those reported by Broberger and Zetterstrom (1961) because urinary excretion of catecholamines was not influenced by hypoglycemia. The observations of Lewis et al. (1963) are particularly convincing evidence for autosomal recessive inheritance of this one form, although iron-clad proof awaits demonstration of a partial deficiency in both parents. See FRUCTOSE-1,6-PHOSPHATASE, HEPATIC DEFICIENCY OF (another cause of 1,6-hypoglycemia). Howell (1972) doubted that the deficiency of glycogen synthetase is primary. He suggested that the low level of glycogen synthetase is due to low levels of insulin which normally stimulates the enzyme. He pointed out that with feeding glycogen is synthesized and glucagon is effective. The exact defect remains unknown but presumably concerns gluconeogenesis. Dykes and Spencer-Peet, (1972) restudied the family. They pointed out that elevation of blood lactate after administration of glucose or more particularly of galactose is a useful diagnostic test. The level of enzyme activity in cultured fibroblasts was not commented on.

Broberger, O. and Zetterstrom, R.: Hypoglycemia with an inability to increase the epinephrine secretion in insulin-induced hypoglycemia. J. Pediat. 59: 215-222, 1961.

Dykes, J. R. W. and Spencer-Peet, J.: Hepatic glycogen synthetase deficiency: further studies on a family. Arch. Dis. Child. 47: 558-563, 1972.

Howell, R. R.: Glycogen storage diseases. In, Stanbury, J. B., Wyngaarden, J. B. and Fredrickson, D. S. (eds.): The Metabolic Basis of Inherited Disease. New York: McGraw-Hill, 1972 (3rd. Ed.). Pp. 149-173.

Lewis, G. M., Spencer-Peet, J. and Stewart, K. M.: Infantile hypoglycaemia due to inherited deficiency of glycogen synthetase in liver. Arch. Dis. Child. 38: 40-48, 1963.

24065 HYPOGLYCEMIA, KETOTIC, OF CHILDHOOD

Ketotic hypoglycemia is the commonest form of hypoglycemia in'childhood. Pagliara et al. (1971) presented evidence that the 'cause' is deficiency of alanine as a gluconeogenic precursor rather than a defect in hepatic gluconeogenesis.

Pagliara, A., Karl, I., Devivo, D., Feigin, R. and Kipnis, D.: Hypoalaninemia: the cause of ketotic hypoglycemia of childhood. (Abstract) J. Clin. Invest. 50: 73A only, 1971.

*24080 HYPOGLYCEMIA, LEUCINE INDUCED

Several types of familial infantile hypoglycemia have been reported, including those precipitated by leucine (Cochrane et al., 1956; DiGeorge and Auerbach, 1960). Ebbin et al. (1967) observed symptomatic hypoglycemia with leucine sensitivity in a mother and daughter. Other cases of adults with leucine sensitivity have had islet adenomas which apparently were not present in this case, however.

Cochrane, W. A., Payne, W. W., Simpkiss, M. J. and Woolf, L. I.: Familial hypoglycemia precipitated by amino acids. J. Clin. Invest. 35: 411-422, 1956.

DiGeorge, A. M. and Auerbach, V. H.: Leucine-induced hypoglycemia: a review and speculations. Am. J. Med. Sci. 240: 792-801, 1960.

Ebbin, A. J., Huntley, C. and Tranquada, R. E.: Symptomatic leucine sensitivity in a mother and daughter. Metabolism 16: 926-932, 1967.

McQuarrie, I.: Idiopathic spontaneously occurring hypoglycemia in infants. Clinical significance of problems and treatment. Am. J. Dis. Child. 87: 399-428, 1954.

24090 HYPOGLYCEMIA, NEONATAL, SIMULATING FOETOPATHIA DIABETICA

Hansson and Redin (1963) observed two female offspring from first-cousin parents who had neonatal hypoglycemia and an appearance like Cushing disease. Although these features suggested those of the baby born of a diabetic mother, the glucose tolerance test was normal in the mother.

Hansson, G. and Redin, B.: Familial neonatal hypoglycemia. A syndrome resembling foetopathia diabetica. Acta Paediat. 52: 145-152, 1963.

24100 HYPOGONADISM WITH LOW-GRADE MENTAL DEFICIENCY AND MICROCEPHALY

Kraus-Ruppert (1958) described three brothers from a consanguineous mating. Syndactyly of the second to fourth toes and eunuchoidism were also present. The testes showed no spermatogenesis and the interstitium was occupied mainly by connective tissue.

Kraus-Ruppert, R.: Zur Frage ererbter diencephaler Stoerungen (infantiler Eunuchoidismus sowie Mikrocephalie bei rezessivem Erbgang). Z. Menschl. Vererb. Konstitutionsl. 34: 643-656, 1958.

24110 HYPOGONADISM, MALE

Familial male hypogonadism is a highly heterozygous category from which some disorders such as Reifenstein syndrome, Kallman syndrome, isolated gonadotropin deficiency and some other entities can be separated presently. The presence of an autosomal recessive form is suggested by the occurrence of parental consanguinity (Nowakowski and Lenz, 1961). Ferriman (1954) described a possibly distinct form in two sons of first-cousin parents. First degree hypospadias, small penis, gynecomastia, markedly diminished secondary sexual characters and normal sized testes were described. In all except the parental consanguinity suggesting recessive inheritance, the disorder resembles Reifenstein syndrome clinically.

Ferriman, D. G.: Familial hypogonadism. Proc. Roy. Soc. Med. 47: 439-442, 1954.

Nowakowski, H. and Lenz, W.: Genetic aspects in male hypogonadism. Recent Progr. Hormone Res. 17: 53-95, 1961.

*24120 HYPOKALEMIC ALKALOSIS (BARTTER SYNDROME)

Bartter syndrome (Bartter et al., 1962) is an unusual form of secondary hyperaldosteronism in which hypertrophy and hyperplasia of the juxtaglomerular cells are associated with normal blood pressure and hypokalemic alkalosis in the absence of edema. Cannon et al. (1968) reviewed the subject and pointed out that affected twins were reported by Campbell et al. (1966) and affected sibs by Trygstad et al. (1967). Evidence for a primary defect in membrane transport was presented by Gardner et al. (1970), on the basis of studies of sodium content and outflux of erythrocytes. Sutherland et al. (1970) described the disorder in three sibs (including a pair of female twins) and in the offspring of an incestuous (father-daughter) mating. Arant et al. (1970) reported on two brothers with features of Bartter syndrome but with severe azotemia at the onset and in one of them renal osteodystrophy. Renal biopsy showed only mild hyperplasia of juxtaglomerular cells and severe glomerulonephritis. Over three fourths of affected families in the United States are Negro (Hall, 1971). Most of the patients have shown retardation of growth and mental development, but the patient of Tarm et al. (1973) represented an exception. Erkelens and van Eps (1973) described a patient with erythrocytosis in addition to the Bartter syndrome. They interpreted this as evidence that both renin and erythropoietin are produced in the juxtaglomerular apparatus.

Arant, B. S., Brackett, N. C., Jr., Young, R. B. and Still, W. J. S.: Case studies of siblings with juxtaglomerular hyperplasia and secondary aldosteronism associated with severe azotemia and renal rickets — Bartter's syndrome or disease? Pediatrics 46: 344-361, 1970.

Bartter, F. C., Pronove, P., Gell, J. R., Jr. and MacCardle, R. C.: Hyperplasia of the juxtaglomerular complex with hyperaldosteronism and hypokalemic alkalosis. A new syndrome. Am. J. Med. 33: 811-828, 1962.

Campbell, R. A., Blair, H. R., Klevit, H. D. and Goodnight, S. H.: Hypokalemic alkalosis and normopiesis with elevated aldosterone excretion in an 8-year-old twin girl. (Abstract) Soc. Pediat. Res., Atlantic City, 1966. P. 111.

Cannon, P. J., Leeming, J. M., Sommers, S. C., Winters, R. W. and Laragh, J. H.: Juxtaglomerular cell hyperplasia and secondary hyperaldosteronism (Bartter's syndrome): a re-evaluation of the pathophysiology. Medicine 47: 107-131, 1968.

Erkelens, D. W. and Statius van Eps, L. W.: Bartter's syndrome and erythrocytosis. Am. J. Med. 55: 711-719, 1973.

Gardner, J., Lapey, A., Simopoulos, A. and Bravo, E.: Evidence for a primary disturbance of membrane transport in Bartter's syndrome and Liddle's syndrome. (Abstract) J. Clin. Invest. 49: 32A only, 1970.

Hall, B. D.: Preponderance of Bartter syndrome among blacks. (Letter) New Eng. J. Med. 285: 581 only, 1971.

Mace, J., Hambidge, K. M., Gotlin, R. and Dubois, R.: Bartter's syndrome in Blacks. (Letter) New Eng. J. Med. 285: 1488 only, 1971.

Sutherland, L. E., Hartroft, P., Balis, J. V., Bailey, J. D. and Lynch, M. J.: Bartter's syndrome. A report of four cases, including three in one sibship, with comparative histologic evaluation of the juxtaglomerular apparatuses and glomeruli. Acta Paediat. Scand. (suppl. 201): 24, 1970.

Tarm, F., Juncos, L. L., Anderson, C. F. and Donadio, J. V., Jr.: Bartter's syndrome: an unusual presentation. Mayo Clin. Proc. 48: 280-283, 1973.

Trygstad, C. W., Mangos, J. A., Hansen, M. R. and Lobeck, C. C.: Familial hypokalemic alkalosis with growth failure. Am. Pediat. Soc., Atlantic City, 1967. P. 66.

24130 HYPOMAGNESEMIA, PRIMARY

Friedman, Hatcher and Watson (1967) described convulsions in infants in the neonatal period. Primary hypomagnesemia due possibly to a defect in intestinal absorption was thought to be present. Associated hypocalcemia was corrected by administration of magnesium alone. The genetic basis of the defect was suggested by its persistence over a period of months and by the fact that the parents were first cousins.

Friedman, M., Hatcher, G. and Watson, L.: Primary hypomagnesaemia with secondary hypocalcaemia in an infant. Lancet I: 703-705, 1967.

*24140 HYPOPARATHYROIDISM

Some reports suggest recessive inheritance. Affected sibs were born of consanguineous parents (Sutphin et al., 1943; Chaptal et al., 1960). Bronsky et al. (1968) described two brothers who developed idiopathic hypoparathyroidism when 11 and 21 years old. A sister, who died when 19 years old, may also have been affected. Six other families, in which more than one member was affected, were found in the literature. Congenital absence of the parathyroid and thymus glands (III and IV pharyngeal pouch syndrome, or DiGeorge syndrome, q.v.) is always a sporadic condition (Taitz et al., 1966). Familial cases of Sutphin et al. (1943) showed moniliasis also (see HYPOADRENOCORTICISM WITH HYPOPARATHYROIDISM AND SUPERFICIAL MONILIASIS). Recessive inheritance was simulated in the family of Buchs (1961) in which three brothers had congenital hypoparathyroidism apparently as a response to maternal hyperparathyroidism. See entry 14620 for description of the converse situation. The report of Niklasson (1970) may concern autosomal recessive isolated hypoparathyroidism.

Bronsky, D., Kiamko, R. T. and Waldstein, S. S.: Familial idiopathic hypoparathyroidism. J. Clin. Endocr. 28: 61-65, 1968.

Buchs, S.: Angeborener Hypoparathyreoidismus von drei Bruedern infolge Hyperparathyreoidismus der Mutter. Schweiz. Med. Wschr. 91: 660, 1961.

Chaptal, J., Jean, R., Bonnet, H., Guillaumot, R. and Morel, G.: Hypoparathyroidie familiale. Etudes clinique, biologique et therapeutique. Arch. Franc. Pediat. 17: 866-878, 1960.

Niklasson, E.: Familial early hypoparathyroidism associated with hypomagnesaemia. Acta Paediat. Scand. 59: 715, 1970.

Sutphin, A., Albright, F. and McCune, D. J.: Five cases (three in siblings) of idiopathic hypoparathyroidism associated with moniliasis. J. Clin. Endocr. 3: 625-634, 1943.

Taitz, L. S., Zarate-Salvador, C. and Schwartz, E.: Congenital absence of the parathyroid and thymus glands in an infant (III and IV pharyngeal pouch syndrome). Pediatrics 38: 412-418, 1966.

*24150 HYPOPHOSPHATASIA (PHOSPHOETHANOLAMINURIA)

In most cases hypophosphatasia is a grave and usually fatal disorder of infancy. However, Bethune and Dent (1960) described two sisters in their 40's with skeletal trouble dating from childhood. This may be the same disorder as the grave one of infancy, for we may just now be recognizing the spectrum of severity which the disease can show. The heterozygote can be recognized by low serum levels of alkaline phosphatase (Rathbun et al., 1961). Pimstone, Eisenberg and Silverman (1966) pointed out that premature shedding of teeth may be the only overt manifestation. Almost certainly several genetically distinct types of hypophosphatasia exist but the details have not been fully elucidated. Three more or less distinct types can be identified: (1) Type 1 with onset in utero or in early postnatal life, craniostenosis, severe skeletal abnormalities, hypercalcemia, death in the first year or so of life. (2) Type 2 with later, more gradual development of symptoms, moderately severe 'rachitic' skeletal changes and premature loss of teeth. (3) Type 3 with no symptoms, the condition being determined on routine studies. Eisenberg and Pimstone (1967) described a 50 year old woman with hypophosphatasia but provided no family data. In 1940 Macey reported two brothers with very low values for serum phosphatase who had 'rickets' in childhood and femoral pseudofractures in adulthood. O'Duffy (1970) reported on the occurrence of attacks of monoarthritis and wide-spread calcification of articular cartilage in a 51 year old woman with hypophosphatasia. Warshaw et al. (1971) demonstrated that long-chain triglycerides cause a rise in serum alkaline phosphatase in hypophosphatasia. Medium-chain triglycerides which are absorbed by the portal route cause no such rise. Residual phosphatase activity in this disorder is probably intestinal in origin to a significant extent, a conclusion supported by the finding of normal intestinal alkaline phosphatase by biopsy. Mehes et al. (1972) studied an inbred Hungarian village where among 198 school children they found 3 homozygotes and 12 heterozygotes for the juvenile form of hypophosphatasia. Study of the families brought to light 19 further cases. The study would suggest that the severe infantile form and the mild juvenile type are separate. There was no instance of the infantile form in this group. Heterozygotes excreted phosphoethanolamine in the urine and suffered early loss of teeth. Scriver and Cameron (1969) described a female infant with classic clinical features of hypophosphatasia but consistently normal levels of alkaline phosphatase in plasma by the usual tests which use high substrate concentrations. It was found that at low substrate concentrations the patient's plasma hydrolyzed phosphoethanolamine more slowly than did normal plasma. This may be an allelic form of hypophosphatasia.

Bartter, F. C.: Hypophosphatasia. In, Stanbury, J. B., Wyngaarden, J. B. and Fredrickson, D. S. (eds.): The Metabolic Basis of Inherited Disease. New York: McGraw-Hill, 1972 (3rd Ed.). Pp. 1295-1304.

Bethune, J. E. and Dent, C. E.: Hypophosphatasia in the adult. Am. J. Med. 28: 615-622, 1960.

Eisenberg, E. and Pimstone, B.: Hypophosphatasia in an adult. A case report. Clin. Orthop. 52: 199-212, 1967.

Macey, H. B.: Multiple pseudofractures: report of a case. Proc. Staff Meet. Mayo Clinic 15: 789-791, 1940.

Mehes, K., Klujber, L., Lassu, G. and Kajtar, P.: Hypophosphatasia: screening and family investigations in an endogamous Hungarian village. Clin. Genet. 3: 60-66, 1972.

O'Duffy, J. D.: Hypophosphatasia associated with calcium pyrophosphate dihydrate deposits in cartilage. Report of a case. Arthritis Rheum. 13: 381-388, 1970.

R
E
C
E
S
S
I
V
E

Pimstone, B., Eisenberg, E. and Silverman, S.: Hypophosphatasia: genetic and dental studies. Ann. Intern. Med. 65: 722-729, 1966.

Rathbun, J. C., MacDonald, J. W., Robinson, H. M. C. and Wanklin, J. M.: Hypophosphatasia: a genetic study. Arch. Dis. Child. 36: 540-542, 1961.

Scriver, C. R. and Cameron, D.: Pseudohypophosphatasia. New Eng. J. Med. 281: 604-606, 1969.

Teree, T. M. and Klein, L.: Hypophosphatasia: clinical and metabolic studies. J. Pediat. 72: 41-50, 1968.

Warshaw, J. B., Littlefield, J. W., Fishman, W. H., Inglis, N. R. and Stolbach, L. L.: Serum alkaline phosphatase in hypophosphatasia. J. Clin. Invest. 50: 2137-3142, 1971.

24155 HYPOPLASTIC LEFT HEART SYNDROME

Shokeir (1971) described thirteen patients in five families. Parental consanguinity was present in three sibships. In all affected infants, the course of the disease was inexorably progressive and ultimately fatal. Holmes et al. (1973) found a frequency of the hypoplastic left heart syndrome among sibs most consistent with multifactorial inheritance. The possibility of a subtype with autosomal recessive inheritance remains.

Holmes, L. B., Rose, V., Child, A. H. and Kratzer, W.: Commentary on the inheritance of the hypoplastic left heart syndrome. Clinical Delineation of Birth Defects. XVI. Urinary System and Others. Baltimore: Williams and Wilkins, 1974. Pp. 228-230.

Shokeir, M. H. K.: Hypoplastic left heart syndrome: an autosomal recessive disorder. Clin. Genet. 2: 7-14, 1971.

24160 HYPOPROTEINEMIA, HYPERCATABOLIC

Waldmann et al. (1968) described two sibs, a 34-year-old woman and 17-year-old man, who were products of a first-cousin marriage and showed marked reduction of serum IgG and of albumin. IgM and IgA were normal or slightly elevated. The rate of catabolism of IgG was increased five fold over the normal. Excessive gastrointestinal loss was excluded as the cause of the hypoproteinemia.

Waldmann, T. A.: Disorders of immunoglobulin metabolism. New Eng. J. Med. 281: 1170-1177, 1969.

Waldmann, T. A., Miller, E. J. and Terry, W. D.: Hypercatabolism of IgG and albumin: a new familial disorder. (Abstract) Clin. Res. 16: 45 only, 1968.

*24170 HYPOPROTHROMBINEMIA

In the report of Josso and colleagues (1962) two offspring of a first-cousin mating were affected. Debastos, Reno and Carrea (1964) described three affected sibs with consanguineous parents. A fourth sib died of umbilical bleeding. In a patient reported by Quick and Hussey (1962), Lanchantin et al. (1968) found no identifiable protein thus distinguishing the disorder from that in which immunoassayable but biologically inactive protein is present (see DYSPROTHROMBINEMIA).

Debastos, O., Reno, R. S. and Carrea, O. T.: A study of three cases of familial congenital hypoprothrombinemia (factor II deficiency). Thromb. Diath. Haemorrh. 11: 497-505, 1964.

Girolami, A.: The hereditary transmission of congenital 'true' hypoprothrombinaemia. Brit. J. Haemat. 21: 695-704, 1971.

Josso, F., Monasterio De Sanchez, J., Lavergne, J. M., Menache, D. and Soulier, J. P.: Congenital abnormality of the prothrombin molecule (factor II) in four siblings: prothrombin Barcelona. Blood 38: 9-16, 1971.

Josso, P., Prou-Wartelle, O. and Soulier, J. P.: Etude d'un cas d'hypoprothrombinemie congenitale. Nouv. Rev. Franc. Hemat. 2: 647-672, 1962.

Kattlove, H. E., Shapiro, S. S. and Spivack, M.: Hereditary prothrombin deficiency. New Eng. J. Med. 282: 57-61, 1970.

Lanchantin, G. F., Hart, D. W., Friedmann, J. A., Saavedra, N. V. and Mehl, J. W.: Amino acid composition of human plasma prothrombin. J. Biol. Chem. 243: 5479-5485, 1968.

Pool, J. G., Desai, R. and Kropatkin, M.: Severe congenital hypoprothrombinemia in a Negro boy. Thromb. Diath. Haemorrh. 8: 235-240, 1962.

Quick, A. J. and Hussey, C. V.: Hereditary hypoprothrombinemias. Lancet 1: 173-177, 1962.

24180 HYPOTHALAMIC HAMARTOMAS

In a case of hypothalamic hamartoma, Marcuse et al. (1953) reported that one sib had internal hydrocephalus and died within a day after operation and another sib ran a clinical course similar to the proband's dying without autopsy at age 2 months. A double first cousin of the proband had a clinical course like the proband's: postmortem at age 5 months showed 'mature glioma of the brain stem.' The proband died at 6 months.

Marcuse, P. M., Burger, R. A. and Salmon, G. W.: Hamartoma of the hypothalamus. Report of two cases with associated developmental defects. J. Pediat. 43: 301-308, 1953.

*24190 HYPOTRICHOSIS ('HAIRLESSNESS')

Isolated alopecia or hypotrichosis is rare. The disorder is characterized by failure to replace the intrauterine hair which is shed shortly before or after birth. Pubic and axillary hair do not develop at puberty. No abnormality of teeth, nails or sweat glands is present. Sly and Treister (1967) observed the condition in 6 of 13 sibs. This and 13 previously reported families supported autosomal recessive inheritance. Recessive

hairlessness has been observed in the deer mouse, house mouse, rat and rabbit. Landes and Logan (1956)
described a recessive form of hypotrichosis.

Landes, E. and Langer, I.: Ein Beitrag zur Hypotrichosis congenita. Hautarzt 7: 413-415, 1956.

Sly, W. S. and Treister, M.: Isolated congenital hypotrichosis: recessive hairlessness in man. To be published.

24200 HYPOTRICHOSIS, SYNDACTYLY AND RETINITIS PIGMENTOSA

Albrectsen and Svendsen (1956) reported brother and sister, offspring of first cousin parents with this combination. The boy showed partial ectrodactyly as well as syndactyly.

Albrectsen, B. and Svendsen, I. B.: Hypotrichosis, syndactyly and retinal degeneration in two siblings. Acta Dermatovener. 36: 96-101, 1956.

*24205 HYPOURICEMIA, HYPERCALCINURIA, AND DECREASED BONE DENSITY

Sperling et al. (1974) described this combination. Renal clearance of uric acid was greatly increased. Two brothers and a sister were affected, together with two grandchildren, two of them being products of a first-cousin marriage of obligatory heterozygotes. Renal hypouricemia has been reported by Green et al. (1972) and by Khachadurian and Arslanian (1973). Hypouricemia occurs with xanthine oxidase deficiency (27830), Wilson disease (27790) and Fanconi syndrome (13460).

Green, M. L., Marcus, R. and Aurbach, G. D.: Hypouricemia due to isolated renal tubular defect. Dalmation dog mutation in man. Am. J. Med. 53: 361-367, 1972.

Khachadurian, A. K. and Arslanian, M. J.: Hypouricemia due to renal uricosuria. A case study. Ann. Intern. Med. 78: 547-550, 1973.

Sperling, O., Weinberger, A., Oliver, I., Liberman, U. A. and De Vries, A.: Hypouricemia, hypercalcinuria, and decreased bone density: a hereditary syndrome. Ann. Intern. Med. 80: 482-487, 1974.

*24210 ICHTHYOSIFORM ERYTHRODERMA, BROCQ CONGENITAL, NON-BULLOUS FORM

In the case of Wile (1924) three males were affected. They were the offspring of matings in which two brothers married two sisters, who were their first cousins. The subject was reviewed by MacKee and Rosen (1917). Arce and Berchmans (1969) described ichthyosiform dermatosis in 13 members of an inbred Brazilian kindred.

Heimendinger and Schnyder (1962) distinguished two types of congenital ichthyosiform erythroderma, one inherited as an autosomal dominant and the other as an autosomal recessive trait. The recessive form is non-bullous and is associated with growth retardation, oligophrenia, spastic paralysis, genital hypoplasia, hypotrichia and shortened life-expectancy. In the autosomal dominant or bullous form (q.v.), however, life-expectancy is not shortened and the associated symptoms include only seborrhea of the head and probably polydipsia. Both types begin at birth and are localized mostly on the flexor surfaces. For classification of the ichthyoses, see ICHTHYOSES in the dominant catalog.

Arce, B. and Berchmans, M.: An ichthyosiform dermatosis with clinical forms of congenital ichthyosiform erythroderma and ichthyosis vulgaris. Hum. Hered. 19: 121-125, 1969.

Heimendinger, J. and Schnyder, U. W.: Bullose 'Erythrodermie ichthyosiforme congenitale' in zwei Generationen. Helv. Paediat. Acta 17: 47-55, 1962.

MacKee, G. M. and Rosen, I.: Erythrodermie congenitale ichthyosiforme: report of a case with a discussion of the clinical and histological features and a review of the literature. J. Cutan. Dis. 35: 235-251, and 511-540, 1917.

Wile, U. J.: Familial study of three unusual cases of congenital ichthyosiform erythrodermia. Arch. Derm. Syph. 10: 487-498, 1924.

24215 ICHTHYOSIFORM ERYTHRODERMIA, CORNEAL INVOLVEMENT, DEAFNESS

Desmons et al. (1971) described 3 sibs with ichthyosiform erythrodermia and deafness among the six children of a first-cousin marriage. Corneal involvement, which is frequent in sporadic cases, was not noted by Desmons et al. (1971). On the other hand, the patients of Desmons et al. (1971) all showed hepatomegaly, hepatic cirrhosis and glycogen storage in middle age. Other reported cases had not reached middle age.

*24220 ICHTHYOSIFORM ERYTHRODERMA, UNILATERAL, WITH IPSILATERAL MALFORMATIONS ESPECIALLY ABSENCE DEFORMITY OF LIMBS

Falek et al. (1968) described sibs with the combination and other familial cases are known.

Cullen, S. I., Harris, D. E., Carter, C. H. and Reed, W. B.: Congenital unilateral ichthyosiform erythroderma. Arch. Derm. 99: 724-729, 1969.

Falek, A., Heath, C. W., Jr., Ebbin, A. J. and McLean, W. R.: Unilateral limb and skin deformities with congenital heart disease in two siblings: a lethal syndrome. J. Pediat. 73: 910-913, 1968.

Lewis, R. G. and Messner, D. G.: Prosthetic fitting of congenital unilateral ichthyosiform erythroderma. A case report. Inter-Clinic Inform. Bull. 9 (no. 11): 1-6, 1970.

Shear, C. S., Nyhan, W. L., Frost, P. and Weinstein, G. D.: Syndromes of unilateral ectromelia, psoriasis and central nervous system anomalies. The Clinical Delineation of Birth Defects. XII. Skin, Hair and Nails. Baltimore: Williams and Wilkins, 1971. Pp. 197-203.

*24230 ICHTHYOSIS CONGENITA (LAMELLAR EXFOLIATION, OR DESQUAMATION OF THE NEWBORN, COLLODION FETUS, ETC.)

The infant with this disorder may die of complications (sepsis, protein and electrolyte loss) in the first months of life or the skin disorder may heal completely. Sometimes a condition like ordinary ichthyosis simplex is present for the rest of the patient's life. (See picture, Sorsby, 1953.) Nix et al. (1963) described 9 cases among 22 offsprings of three couples of German extraction. All six parents had a common ancestral couple. They concluded that the 'harlequin fetus' is the result of a separate recessive gene.

Belisario, C. and Panero, C.: Su di un caso di 'collodion-skin.' Riv. Clin. Pediat. 69: 312-324, 1962.

Nix, T. E., Jr., Kloepfer, H. W. and Derbes, V. J.: Ichthyosis, lamellar exfoliative type. Derm. Trop. 2: 142-152, 1963.

Shelmire, J. B., Jr.: Lamellar exfoliation of the newborn. Arch. Derm. 71: 471-475, 1955.

Smeenk, G.: Two families with collodion babies. Brit. J. Derm. 78: 81-86, 1966.

Sorsby, A.: (ed.) Clinical Genetics. St. Louis: C. V. Mosby Co. 1953. P. 136.

Von Reuss, A. R.: The Diseases of the Newborn. New York: William And Wood Co., 1922.

24240 ICHTHYOSIS CONGENITA WITH BILIARY ATRESIA

Gould (1854) described two sibs with this combination.

Gould, A. A.: Ichthyosis in an infant: hemorrhage from umbilicus: death. Am. J. Med. Sci. 27: 356 only, 1854.

24250 ICHTHYOSIS CONGENITA, 'HARLEQUIN FETUS' TYPE

Nix et al. (1963) claimed that this is a recessive disorder distinct from the lamellar exfoliative type of congenital ichthyosis. It carries a more grave prognosis (Shelmire, 1955). Evidence for recessive inheritance was provided by several family reports (Bustamante and Tejeda, 1950; Kingery, 1926; Lattuada and Parker, 1951; Smith, 1880; Thomson and Wakeley, 1921).

Bustamente, W. and Tejeda, M.: Ichthyosis fetalis gravis in two successive pregnancies. J. Pediat. 36: 501-504, 1950.

Kingery, L. B.: Ichthyosis congenita with unusual complications. Arch. Derm. Syph. 13: 90-105, 1926.

Lattuada, H. P. and Parker, M. S.: Congenital ichthyosis. Am. J. Surg. 82: 236-239, 1951.

Nix, T. E., Jr., Kloepfer, H. W. and Derbes, V. J.: Ichthyosis, lamellar exfoliative type. Derm. Trop. 2: 142-152, 1963.

Shelmire, J. B., Jr.: Lamellar exfoliation of newborn. Arch. Derm. 71: 471-475, 1955.

Smith, R. W.: A case of intrauterine ichthyosis. Am. J. Obstet. Gynec. 13: 458-461, 1880.

Thomson, M. S. and Wakeley, C. P. G.: The harlequin foetus. J. Obstet. Gynec. Brit. Emp. 28: 190-203, 1921.

*24260 IMINOGLYCINURIA

The imino acids, proline and hydroxyproline, share a renal tubular reabsorptive mechanism with glycine. Rosenberg et al., (1968) found increased amounts of all three substances in the urine of a 6-year-old boy with congenital nerve deafness. Both parents had hyperglycinuria without iminoaciduria. No defect in intestinal transport of these substances was found. These authors, as well as Whelan and Scriver (1968) concluded that iminoglycinuria is the homozygous form of the trait that presents as hyperglycinuria in the heterozygote. It is a benign inborn error of amino acid transport. See also HYPERPROLINEMIA, HYDROXY-PROLINEMIA, GLYCINEMIA and GLYCINURIA. Genetic heterogeneity in iminoglycinuria is suggested by the facts that some apparent homozygotes show a defect in intestinal absorption of L-proline whereas others do not (Goodman et al., 1967; Scriver, 1968), and that some obligate heterozygotes show hyperglycinuria with glycine loading, whereas others do not (Scriver, 1968). Scriver (1968) observed the instructive case of an apparent homozygote's child whose father had hyperglycinuria and mother did not. He suggested that this child was a 'compound' carrying two different mutant alleles. Similar compounds for cystinuria have been observed. Scriver also suggested plausibly that glycinuria (q.v. in dominant catalog) is the heterozygous state of iminoglycinuria. Iminoglycinuria may be more frequent in Ashkenazic Jews than others. See 13850 for discussion of another type of iminoglycinuria.

Goodman, S. I., McIntyre, C. A., Jr. and O'Brien, D.: Impaired intestinal transport of proline in a patient with familial iminoaciduria. J. Pediat. 71: 246-249, 1967.

Procopis, P. G. and Turner, B.: Iminoaciduria: a benign renal tubular defect. J. Pediat. 79: 419-422, 1971.

Rosenberg, L. E., Durant, J. L. and Elsas, L. J.: Familial iminoglycinuria: an inborn error of renal tubular transport. New Eng. J. Med. 278: 1407-1413, 1968.

Scriver, C. R.: Renal tubular transport of proline, hydroxyproline, and glycine. III. Genetic basis for more than one mode of transport in human kidney. J. Clin. Invest. 47: 823-835, 1968.

Tancredi, F., Guazzi, G. and Auricchio, S.: Renal iminoglycinuria without intestinal malabsorption of glycine and imino acids. J. Pediat. 76: 386 only, 1970.

Whelan, D. T. and Scriver, C. R.: Cystathioninuria and renal iminoglycinuria in a pedigree. A perspective on counseling. New Eng. J. Med. 278: 924-927, 1968.

R
E
C
E
S
S
I
V
E

The possibility of a separate entity distinct from Bruton type agammaglobulinemia in which the tonsillar system is absent and from Swiss-type agammaglobulinemia (q.v.) in which both the thymus and the tonsillar systems are absent has been postulated by Cooper, Peterson and Good (1965). In this entity the defect may be limited to the thymus system which is responsible for cellular immunity. The cases of Allibone et al. (1964) and Nezelof et al. (1964) may be examples. Fulginiti et al. (1967) observed two sisters in one family and a brother and sister in another family with thymic dysplasia (similar to that seen in Swiss-type agammaglobulinemia), lymphopenia and normal immunoglobulins. Three died before age 2 years of recurrent pseudomonas and monilia infections. The living child displayed impaired delayed hypersensitivity. No skin reactions to mumps, parainfluenza or monilia antigens were observed. Repeated attempts to produce sensitivity to fluorodinitrobenzene failed and a skin graft from the mother showed no skin rejection. Nezelof et al. (1964) first reported this syndrome. Some of these patients have changes of metaphyseal dysostosis (Fulginiti et al., 1967), suggesting a relationship to cartilage-hair hypoplasia (q.v.) in which susceptibility to viral infections may be present. Furthermore a patient thought to have Swiss-type agammaglobulinemia had 'achondroplasia' (McKusick and Cross, 1966). This association of dwarfism probably represents a distinct entity (see 'ACHONDROPLASIA' WITH SWISS-TYPE AGAMMAGLOBULINEMIA). Nahmias et al. (1967) observed marked susceptibility to measles with death from giant cell pneumonia. Autopsy showed plasma cells but no small lymphocytes and no thymus. In the Negro sibship they described 3 girls and 1 boy who were definitely affected and another girl may have been affected. Humoral immunity is normal but cellular immunity is deficient, findings precisely opposite to those of congenital agammaglobulinemia (Kretschmer et al., 1968).

Allibone, E. C., Goldie, W. and Marmion, B. P.: Pneumocystis carinii pneumonia and progressive vaccinia in siblings. Arch. Dis. Child. 39: 26-34, 1964.

Cooper, M. D., Peterson, R. D. A. and Good, R. A.: A new concept of the cellular basis of immunity. (Abstract) J. Pediat. 67: 907-908, 1965.

Fulginiti, V. A., Hathaway, W. E., Pearlman, D. S. and Kempe, C. H.: Agammaglobulinemia and achondroplasia. (Letter) Brit. Med. J. 1: 242 only, 1967.

Fulginiti, V. A., Hathaway, W. E., Pearlman, D. S., Blackburn, W. R., Reiquam, C. W., Githens, J. H., Claman, H. N. and Kempe, C. H.: Dissociation of delayed-hypersensitivity and antibody-synthesizing capacities in man. Report of two sibships with thymic dysplasia, lymphoid tissue depletion, and normal immunoglobulins. Lancet II: 5-8, 1967.

Kretschmer, R., Say, B., Brown, D. and Rosen, F. S.: Congenital aplasia of the thymus gland (DiGeorge's syndrome). New Eng. J. Med. 279: 1295-1301, 1968.

McKusick, V. A. and Cross, H. E.: Ataxia-telangiectasia and Swiss-type agammaglobulinemia. Two genetic disorders of the immune mechanisms in related Amish sibships. J.A.M.A. 195: 739-745, 1966.

Miller, M. E. and Schieken, R. M.: Thymic dysplasia. A separate entity from 'Swiss agammaglobulinemia.' Am. J. Med. Sci. 253: 741-750, 1967.

Nahmias, A. J., Griffith, D., Salbury, C. and Yoshida, K.: Thymic aplasia: with lymphopenia, plasma cells, and normal immunoglobulins. J.A.M.A. 201: 729-734, 1967.

Nezelof, C., Jammet, M.-L., Lortholary, P., Labrune, B. and Lamy, M.: L'hypoplasie hereditaire du thymus: sa place et sa responsabilite dans une observation d'aplasie lymphocytaire, normoplasmocytaire et normoglobulinemique du nourrisson. Arch. Franc. Pediat. 21: 897-920, 1964.

R
E
C
E
S
S
I
V
E

24275 IMMUNE DEFECT WITH DEFICIENCY OF ADENOSINE DEAMINASE

Giblett et al. (1972) described two girls in separate families with impaired cellular immunity and absent red cell adenosine deaminase. One child, aged 22 months, showed recurrent respiratory infections, candidiasis and marked lymphopenia from birth. The other, aged 3 and one-half years, was allegedly normal in the first 2 years of life. Mild upper respiratory infections began at age 24 months and progressed to severe pulmonary insufficiency and hepatosplenomegaly by age 30 months. The parents of the first child were related and the second child had a sister who died in consequence of a major immunologic defect (Hong et al., 1970). Supporting recessive inheritance is the finding that both pairs of parents had an intermediate level of red cell ADA. Possibly a different allele is present in the two families because in the first family the parents showed about a 50 percent level of ADA whereas it was about two-thirds normal in the second pair. Since most of lymphocyte ADA is of the same electrophoretic type as red cell ADA, a connection between the deficiency and the immune defect is plausible. This entry is not asterisked because of the uncertainty that it represents a locus distinct from that indicated by the electrophoretic variation in ADA (10270). This is a form of combined immunodeficiency disease (CID), i.e., there is dysfunction of both B and T lymphocytes with impaired cellular immunity and decreased production of immunoglobulins. This is sometimes called the Swiss type of agammaglobulinemia. There are undoubtedly multiple forms which witness the occurrence of both autosomal recessive (20250) and X-linked recessive (30040) forms. CID with ADA deficiency is one of the autosomal types. There are boney changes in the patients with CID with ADA deficiency suggesting that this may be the defect in at least some cases of reported 'achondroplasia and Swiss-type agammaglobulinemia' (20090). Note also that cartilage-hair hypoplasia (25025) has a defect in cellular immunity in association with skeletal changes.

Chen, S.-H., Scott, C. R. and Giblett, E. R.: Adenosine deaminase: demonstration of a 'silent' gene associated with combined immunodeficiency disease. Am. J. Hum. Genet. 26: 103-107, 1974.

Dissing, J. and Knudsen, B.: Adenosine-deaminase deficiency and combined immunodeficiency syndrome. (Letter) Lancet II: 1316 only, 1972.

Giblett, E. R., Anderson, J. E., Cohen, F., Pollara, B. and Meuwissen, H. J.: Adenosine-deaminase deficiency in two patients with severely impaired cellular immunity. Lancet I: 1067-1069, 1972.

Hirschhorn, R., Levytska, V. and Parkman, R.: A mutant form of adenosine deaminase in severe combined immunodeficiency. (Abstract) J. Clin. Invest. 53: 33A only, 1974.

Hong, R., Galti, R., Rathburn, J. C. and Good, R. A.: Thymic hypoplasia and thyroid dysfunction. New Eng. J. Med. 282: 470-474, 1970.

Scott, C. R., Chen, S.-H. and Giblett, E. R.: Deletion of the carrier state in combined immunodeficiency disease associated with deaminase deficiency. J. Clin. Invest. 53: 1194-1196, 1974.

Van der Weyden, M. B. and Kelley, W. N.: Adenosine deaminase deficiency in severe combined immunodeficiency: evidence for a posttranslational defect. (Abstract) J. Clin. Invest. 53: 81-82A, 1974.

Yount, J., Nichols, P., Ochs, H. D., Hammar, S. P., Scott, C. R., Chen, S.-H., Giblett, E. R. and Wedgwood, R. J.: Absence of erythrocyte adenosine deaminase associated with severe combined immunodeficiency. J. Pediat. 84: 173-177, 1974.

*24280 IMMUNE DEFECT WITH LYMPHOTOXIC FACTOR

Kretschmer et al. (1969) described a brother and sister who died in childhood with an illness characterized by recurrent infections, eczema and episodic lymphopenia. The boy showed dysgammaglobulinemia, impaired cellular immunity and immunologic amnesia like that in animals treated with antilymphocyte serum. A complement-dependent lymphotoxic factor was demonstrated in the boy's serum during an episode of lymphopenia. Postmortem examination in both showed depletion of small lymphocyte from thymus-dependent areas of peripheral lymphoid organs. The autosomal inheritance and lack of thrombocytopenia distinguish this disorder from the Wiskott-Aldrich syndrome (q.v.). At least 9 other cases have been reported (e.g., Stoop et al., 1962).

Kretschmer, R., August, C. S., Rosen, F. S. and Janeway, C. A.: Recurrent infections, episodic lymphopenia and impaired cellular immunity: further observations on 'immunologic amnesia' in two siblings. New Eng. J. Med. 281: 285-290, 1969.

Stoop, J. W., Ballieux, R. E. and Weyers, H. A.: Paraproteinemia with secondary immune globulin deficiency in infants. Pediatrics 29: 97-104, 1962.

24285 IMMUNE DEFICIENCY DISEASE

R
E
C
E
S
S
I
V
E

This disorder is characterized by partial deficiency of both humoral and cellular systems, the principle finding being a severe deficiency of IgM. Clinically the defect is manifested by difficulty in containing both bacterial and viral infections. Infections by encapsulated extracellular pathogens such as pneumococcus are frequent. Septicemia is common in patients with IgM deficiency. IgM predominates during a primary antibody response. In this disorder antibody response to primary immunization is defective. Record et al. (1973) described intrahepatic sclerosing cholangitis in a girl with this disorder and probably in two others. The mother had died of septicemia following a hysterectomy at age 43 and a maternal aunt had died of fulminant hepatitis at age 21.

Record, C. O., Eddleston, A. L. W. F., Shilkin, K. B. and Williams, R.: Intrahepatic sclerosing cholangitis associated with a familial immunodeficinecy syndrome. Lancet II: 18-20, 1973.

24290 INDOLYLACROYL GLYCINURIA WITH MENTAL RETARDATION

Mellman et al. (1963) found indolylacroyl glycinuria in the urine of five mentally retarded sibs. The mother also excreted the substance. Tryptophane loading orally or intravenously did not increase the excretion but oral neomycin caused disappearance of the substance from the urine in four of the five sibs. The substance would appear to be derived from the bowel where it is probably a product of bacterial action and may find its way into the blood and urine because of a specific transmucosal transport defect as in Hartnup disease.

Mellman, W. J., Barness, L. A., Tedesco, T. A. and Besselman, D.: Indolylacroyl glycine excretion in a family with mental retardation. Clin. Chim. Acta 8: 843-847, 1963.

*24300 INSENSITIVITY TO PAIN (INDIFFERENCE TO PAIN; CONGENITAL ANALGIA) (ALSO SEE NEUROPATHY, SENSORY. ALSO SEE BIEMOND CONGENITAL AND FAMILIAL ANALGESIA)

Saldanha and his colleagues (1964) described two families. In one, three brothers out of ten sibs and in the other two sibs out of eleven were affected. The parents of the probands were normal and in one case were consanguineous (f=0.0703). Recessive inheritance was proposed. However, a chromosomal aberration (mosaicism) was also detected (Becak et al. 1963). Insensitivity to pain is a feature of familial dysautonomia (q.v.) with which this pure form should not be confused.

Some cases classed as insensitivity to pain may have congenital sensory neuropathy, which may be merely a mild form of acro-osteolysis (q.v.). When familial, sensory neuropathy is said to show dominant inheritance. Winkelmann, Lambert and Hayles (1962) reviewed the subject of congenital absence of pain with a useful discussion of differential diagnosis.

Fanconi and Ferrazzini (1957) described an affected brother and sister from consanguineous parents and parental consanguinity has been noted in other cases (Thiemann, 1961). Saldanha, Schmidt and Leon (1964) described two families with three out of 10 offspring of unrelated parents in one and two affected in the second with first-cousin parents. Although the patients do not react to painful stimuli, they are otherwise neurologically normal. Absent corneal reflexes and slight mental retardation have also been described. In several but not all of these patients, Becak, Becak and Andrade (1964) found mosaicism of cells with normal karyotype and cells trisomic for a chromosome in the 13-15 group. Gilley and colleagues (1964) described 2 affected sibs who were born of normal parents and were normally intelligent. Bertoye and colleagues (1964) observed the disorder in the child of consanguineous parents. In a case of indifference to pain reported by Ogden et al. (1959) the parents were first cousins. Blau and Mutton (1967) could demonstrate no chromosomal abnormality. Silverman and Gilden (1959) described a family in which two of eight children of consanguineous parents were affected. Gaudier et al. (1969) described affected brothers. Osuntokun et al. (1968) described brother and half-sister who presumably had different fathers, both normal, and who had congenital indifference to pain. They referred to the condition as pain asymbolia and noted the association of auditory imperception.

Becak, W., Becak, M. L. and Andrade, J. D.: A genetical investigation of congenital analgesia. I. Cytogenetic studies. Acta Genet. Statist. Med. 14: 133-142, 1964.

Becak, W., Becak, M. L. and Schmidt, B. J.: Chromosome trisomy of group 13-15 in two cases of generalised congenital analgesia. (Letter) Lancet I: 664-665, 1963.

Bertoye, A., Carron, R., Rosenberg, D., Cotton, J.-B. and Michel, M.: A propos d'une observation d'indifférence congénitale a la douleur (analgesie congenitale universelle). Hypothese pathogenique. Pediatrie 19: 605-608, 1964.

Blau, J. N. and Mutton, D. E.: Chromosome studies in the 'sensory syndrome.' Acta Genet. 17: 226-233, 1967.

Bourland, A. and Winkelmann, R. K.: Study of cutaneous innervation in congenital anesthesia. Arch. Neurol. 14: 223-227, 1966.

Fanconi, G. and Ferrazzini, F.: Kongenitale Analgie (kongenitale generalisierte Schmerzindifferenz). Helv. Paediat. Acta 12: 79-115, 1957.

Gaudier, B., Bourlond, A., Nuyts, J.-P., Ryckewaert, P. H., Lefebvre, P. and Ryckewaert-Sandor, L.: L'indifférence congénitale a la douleur. A propos de deux nouvelles observations. Arch. Franc. Pediat. 26: 1027-1040, 1969.

Gilly, R., Chevallier, G., Foray, G., Rambaud, G. and Raveau, J.: Indifference congenitale a la douleur. Observation familiale, particularites cliniques et biologiques. Pediatrie 19: 609-614, 1964.

Ogden, T. E., Robert, F. and Carmichael, E. A.: Some sensory syndromes in children: indifference to pain and sensory neuropathy. J. Neurol. Neurosurg. Psychiat. 22: 267-276, 1959.

Osuntokun, B. O., Odeku, E. L. and Luzzatto, L.: Congenital pain asymbolia and auditory imperception. J. Neurol. Neurosurg. Psychiat. 31: 291-296, 1968.

Saldanha, P. H., Schmidt, B. J. and Leon, N.: A genetical investigation of congenital analgesia. II. Clinico-genetical studies. Acta Genet. Statist. Med. 14: 143-158, 1964.

Silverman, F. N. and Gilden, J. J.: Congenital insensitivity to pain. A neurologic syndrome with bizarre skeletal lesions. Radiology 72: 176-190, 1959.

Thiemann, H. H.: Analgia congenita (angeborene universelle Schmerzindifferenz). Arch. Kinderheilk. 164: 255-262, 1961.

Winkelmann, R. K., Lambert, E. H. and Hayles, A. B.: Congenital absence of pain. Report of a case and experimental studies. Arch. Derm. 85: 325-339, 1962.

24305 INSENSITIVITY TO PAIN, WITH ANHIDROSIS

Swanson et al. (1965) described two brothers with congenital insensitivity to pain and anhidrosis (despite normal appearing sweat glands on skin biopsy). Temperature sensation was also defective. One of the brothers died after a 24-hour illness during which his temperature reached 109 degrees F. Almost complete absence of the first order afferent system considered responsible for pain and temperature was found at autopsy.

Swanson, A. G., Buchan, G. C. and Alvord, E. C., Jr.: Anatomic changes in congenital insensitivity to pain. Absence of small primary sensory neurons in ganglia, roots, and Lissauer's tract. Arch. Neurol. 12: 12-18,,1965.

24310 INTERNAL CAROTID ARTERIES, HYPOPLASIA OF

Austin and Stears (1971) reported hypoplasia of both internal carotid arteries in two and possibly three brothers from a sibship of 11. Symptoms began at ages 18, 30 and 33 years and were attributable to cerebral ischemia. One became demented.

Austin, J. H. and Stears, J. C.: Familial hypoplasia of both internal carotid arteries. Arch. Neurol. 24: 1-10, 1971.

*24315 INTESTINAL ATRESIA, MULTIPLE

Jejunal atresia is listed elsewhere (24360) as a distinct recessive. It seems quite certain that multiple intestinal atresia is a separate entity because of the wide distribution of involvement — from stomach to anus. The best evidence for autosomal recessive inheritance was provided by Dallaire and Perreault (1973) who found 5 French-Canadian cases in three sibships with common ancestry. Two of the three sibships had demonstrably consanguineous parents. Intraluminal calcifications were demonstrable radiographically. Whether duodenal atresia (22340) is a separate entity is not certain. Atresia of the ileum was reported by Blank (1965) in two brothers with cystic fibrosis. Two other sibs had cystic fibrosis without intestinal atresia.

R E C E S S I V E

Blank, C., Okmian, L. and Robbe, H.: Mucoviscidosis and intestinal atresia. A study of four cases in the same family. Acta Pediat. Scand. 54: 557-565, 1965.

Dallaire, L. and Perreault, G.: Hereditary multiple intestinal atresia. The Clinical Delineation of Birth Defects. XVI. Urinary System and Others. Baltimore: Williams and Wilkins, 1974. Pp. 259-264.

24320 INTRACRANIAL HYPERTENSION, IDIOPATHIC

Buchheit et al. (1969) described two sisters with idiopathic intracranial hypertension with papilledema (pseudotumor cerebri).

Buchheit, W. A., Burton, C., Haag, B. and Shaw, D.: Familial papilledema and idiopathic intracranial hypertension. New Eng. J. Med. 280: 938-942, 1969.

24330 INTRAHEPATIC CHOLESTASIS

Kuhn (1963) described two teen-age brothers with repeated attacks of jaundice accompanied by itching and hepatomegaly. Progression to biliary cirrhosis was suspected in one. He suggested that the same condition was described by Tygstrup (1960) in two distantly related 15-year-old boys living in a small village in the Faroe Islands. Onset in these was in the first two years of life. Cholestasis was demonstrated by liver biopsy and direct cholangiography. Kaye (1965) studied three sibs with intrahepatic cholestasis in which itching predated jaundice which began by 2 or 3 years. One sib died at about 7 years of age and 2 were still alive at ages of about 10 and 5. Cholestyramine had no benefit. These patients were reported by Williams et al. (1972) and probably had Byler disease (21160). Somayaji et al. (1968) reported sisters who developed cholestatic jaundice following the taking of an oral contraceptive agent. One of them had had pruritus during the latter part of each of three pregnancies. Intrahepatic cholestasis of pregnancy has been reported in sisters by Svanborg and Ohlsson (1959), Cahill (1962) and Fast and Roulston (1964). Mother and two daughters were affected in the report of Holzbach and Sanders (1965). Mothers of patients with Byler disease (q.v.) had severe pruritus in late pregnancy raising the possibility that cholestasis of pregnancy may be a manifestation of the heterozygous state of the gene which in the homozygote produces a fatal form of cholestasis (McKusick and Clayton, 1968). Conceivably, this milder form of intrahepatic cholestasis is due to homozygosity for an allele of the gene responsible for the Byler disease, fatal intrahepatic cholestasis (21160). Numerous examples of mild and severe forms of disease are suspected to be allelic because a defect in one and the same enzyme has been found.

Cahill, K. M.: Hepatitis in pregnancy. Surg. Gynec. Obstet. 114: 545-552, 1962.

Da Silva, L. C. and De Brito, T.: Benign recurrent intrahepatic cholestasis in two brothers. A clinical light and electron microscopy study. Ann. Intern. Med. 65: 330-341, 1966.

Fast, B. B. and Roulston, T. M.: Idiopathic jaundice of pregnancy. Am. J. Obstet. Gynec. 88: 314-321, 1964.

Holzbach, R. T. and Sanders, J. H.: Recurrent intrahepatic cholestasis of pregnancy. Observations on pathogenesis. J.A.M.A. 193: 542-544, 1965.

Kaye, R.: Comments. J. Pediat. 67: 1027-1028, 1965.

Kuhn, H. A.: Intrahepatic cholestasis in two brothers. German Med. Monthly 8: 185-188, 1963.

McKusick, V. A. and Clayton, R. J.: Cholestasis of pregnancy. (Letter) New Eng. J. Med. 278: 566 only, 1968.

Somayaji, B. N., Paton, A., Price, J. H., Harris, A. W. and Flewett, T. H.: Norethisterone jaundice in two sisters. Brit. Med. J. 2: 281-283, 1968.

Svanborg, A. and Ohlsson, S.: Recurrent jaundice of pregnancy. A clinical study of twenty-two cases. Am. J. Med. 27: 40-49, 1959.

Tygstrup, N.: Intermittent possibly familial intrahepatic cholestatic jaundice. Lancet I: 1171-1172, 1960.

Williams, C. N., Kaye, R., Baker, L., Hurwitz, R. and Senior, J. R.: Progressive familial cholestatic cirrhosis and bile acid metabolism. J. Pediat. 81: 493-500, 1972.

*24340 ISONIAZID (INH) INACTIVATION

The anti-tuberculosis agent, INH, is rendered therapeutically inactive by acetylation. Most, perhaps all populations of the world are polymorphic for 'rapid inactivation' versus 'slow inactivation.' The 'slow inactivator' person is homozygous. The rapid inactivator person may be either homozygous or heterozygous. Sunahara's method permits separation of the homozygotes and heterozygotes, i.e., three genotypes in all. The rapid vs. slow acetylation of sulfadiazine in rabbits (Frymoyer and Jacox, 1963) is similar. The polymorphism in acetylation extends to the acetylation of sulfamethazine which can be used as a test (Parker, 1969).

Evans, D. A. P., Manley, K. A. and McKusick, V. A.: Genetic control of isoniazid metabolism in man. Brit. Med. J. 2: 485-491, 1960.

Frymoyer, J. W. and Jacox, R. F.: Studies of genetically controlled sulfadiazine acetylation in rabbit livers: possible identification of the heterozygous trait. J. Lab. Clin. Med. 62: 905-909, 1963.

Parker, J. M.: Human variability in the metabolism of sulfamethazine. Hum. Hered. 19: 402-409, 1969.

Schloot, W. and Goedde, H. W.: Studies on the polymorphism of isoniazid (INH) acetylation in rhesus monkeys (Macaca mulatta). Acta Genet. Statist. Med. 18: 394-398, 1968.

Sunahara, S., Urano, M. and Ogawa, M.: Genetical and geographic studies on isoniazid inactivation. Science 134: 1530-1531, 1961.

R
E
C
E
S
S
I
V
E

About 1.4 percent of Caucasians and 9.1 percent of Negroes cannot smell the sweaty odor of isovaleric acid.

Amoore, J. E.: Specific anosmia: a clue to the olfactory code. Nature 242: 1095-1098, 1967.

Whissell-Buechy, D. and Amoore, J. E.: Odour-blindness to musk: simple recessive inheritance. Nature 242: 271-273, 1973.

*24350 ISOVALERICACIDEMIA

Budd et al. (1967) observed brother and sister who starting before age 6 months showed retarded psychomotor development, a peculiar odor resembling sweaty feet, an aversion to dietary protein, and pernicious vomiting, leading to acidosis and coma. The odor is due to isovaleric acid, an intermediary of leucine. The defect concerns IVA-CO a dehydrogenase. The unusual smell was identified as isovaleric acid by experts of the Arthur D. Little Co., Industrial Consultants, Cambridge, Mass. In the metabolic pathways this disorder is closely related to maple syrup urine disease. See also SIDBURY SYNDROME. Ando et al. (1971) showed that isovaleric acidemia can produce hyperglycinemia and leukopenia, as well as episodic ketoacidosis, thus resembling propionicacidemia and methylmalonicacidemia.

Ando, T., Klingberg, W. G., Ward, A. N., Rasmussen, K. and Nyhan, W. L.: Isovaleric acidemia presenting with altered metabolism of glycine. Pediat. Res. 5: 478-486, 1971.

Budd, M. A., Tanaka, K., Holmes, L. B., Efron, M. L., Crawford, J. D. and Isselbacher, K. J.: Isovaleric acidemia: clinical feature of a new genetic defect of leucine metabolism. New Eng. J. Med. 277: 321-327, 1967.

Efron, M. L.: Isovaleric acidemia. Am. J. Dis. Child. 113: 74-76, 1967.

Newman, C. G. H., Wilson, B. D. R., Callaghan, P. and Young, L.: Neonatal death associated with isovalericacidaemia. Lancet II: 439-441, 1967.

Tanaka, K., Budd, M. A., Efron, M. L. and Isselbacher, K. J.: Isovaleric acidemia: a new genetic defect of leucine metabolism. Proc. Nat. Acad. Sci. 56: 236-242, 1966.

Tanaka, K., Orr, J. and Isselbacher, K. J.: Identification of b-hydroxyisovaleric acid in the urine of a patient with isovaleric acidemia. Biochim. Biophys. Acta 152: 638-641, 1968.

*24360 JEJUNAL ATRESIA ('APPLE PEEL' SYNDROME)

In this condition, because of agenesis of the mesentery, the distal small bowel comes straight off the caecum and twists around the marginal artery, suggesting a maypole or apple peel at operation. Mishalany and Najjar (1968) observed 3 affected out of 16 liveborn offspring of first cousin parents and Blyth and Dickson (1969) observed two affected sibs in each of two families. See DUODENAL ATRESIA (22340). Mishalany and Der Kaloustian (1971) described multiple-level intestinal atresia in two sons of distantly related parents. Rickham and Karplus (1971) had two families with affected sibs.

Blyth, H. M. and Dickson, J. A. S.: Apple peel syndrome (congenital intestinal atresia). A family study of seven index patients. J. Med. Genet. 6: 275-277, 1969.

Mishalany, H. G. and Der Kaloustian, V. M.: Familial multiple-level intestinal atresia: report of two siblings. J. Pediat. 79: 124 only, 1971.

Mishalany, H. G. and Najjar, F. B.: Familial jejunal atresia: three cases in one family. J. Pediat. 73: 753-755, 1968.

Rickham, P. P. and Karplus, M.: Familial and hereditary intestinal atresia. Helvet. Paediat. Acta 26: 561-564, 1971.

*24370 JOB SYNDROME

The book of Job records that 'Satan . . . . . smote Job with sore boils from the sole of his foot unto his crown' (Job 2:7). For this reason Davis et al. (1966) gave the name Job syndrome to a disorder affecting two unrelated girls. Both had had life-long histories of indolent ('cold') staphylococcal abscesses. A defect in local resistance to staphylococcal infection was suggested. Thompson (1968) informed me of affected sibs in a southern Italian family with possibly consanguineous parents. These patients like Davis' had fair skin and red hair. Sherry (1968) observed a Negro child with characteristic features but the usual Negro hair. Two sisters with Job syndrome reported by Davis et al. in 1966 were reported by White et al. (1969) to have normal leukocyte functions which are defective in chronic granulomatous disease. Bannatyne et al. (1969) described two affected sisters whose parents were second cousins. Despite the fact that their parents were dark-skinned and dark-haired southern Italian immigrants, the proband had red hair, fair skin and reddish-brown eyes. A sister was clinically well but had a mild leukocyte defect demonstrated in vitro and had red hair. In four females with Job syndrome, Hill et al. (1974) found a profound defect in neutrophil granulocyte chemotaxis and very high serum IgE levels.

Bannatyne, R. M., Skowron, P. N. and Weber, J. L.: Job's syndrome, a variant of chronic granulomatous disease. J. Pediat. 75: 236-242, 1969.

Davis, S. D., Schaller, J. and Wedgwood, R. J.: Job's syndrome. Recurrent, 'cold,' staphylococcal abscesses. Lancet I: 1013-1015, 1966.

Hill, H. R., Ochs, H. D., Quie, P. G., Clark, R. A., Pabst, H. F., Klebanoff, S. J. and Wedgwood, R. J.: Defect in neutrophil granulocyte chemotaxis in Job's syndrome of recurrent 'cold' staphylococcal abcesses. Lancet II: 617-619, 1974.

Sherry, M. N.: Washington, D.C.: personal communication, 1968.

R
E
C
E
S
S
I
V
E

Thompson, M. W.: Toronto, Canada: personal communication, 1968.

White, L. R., Iannetta, A., Kaplan, E. L., Davis, S. D. and Wedgwood, R. J.: Leucocytes in Job's syndrome. (Letter) Lancet I: 630 only, 1969.

24380 JOINT LAXITY (ARTHROCHALASIS MULTIPLEX CONGENITA)

Extreme joint laxity with multiple recurrent joint dislocations was observed in three sibs, the offspring of third cousin parents (McKusick, 1966). The parents were said to be unaffected but were not examined. Epicanthus, depressed nasal bridge, micrognathia and diaphragmatic hernia occur in some of these patients. The disorder was observed by Capotorti and Antonelli (1966) in an inbred kindred. Fragility of the skin is lacking in these patients. Stretchability and bruisability are minimal. The proband in the above family with third cousin parents has been found to have deficiency of procollagen protease (26405).

Capotorti, L. and Antonelli, M.: Sindrome di Ehlers-Danlos. Quattro casi accertati e due probabli in una famiglia con piu matrimoni fra consanguinei. Acta Genet. Med. Gem. 15: 273-295, 1966.

Hass, J. and Hass, R.: Arthrochalasis multiplex congenita. Congenital flaccidity of the joints. J. Bone Joint Surg. 40A: 663-674, 1958.

McKusick, V. A.: Heritable Disorders of Connective Tissue. St. Louis: C. V. Mosby Co., 1966 (3rd Ed.). figs. 5-11.

24390 JORDANS ANOMALY OF LEUKOCYTES

Jordans (1953) found fat-containing cytoplasmic vacuoles in the leukocytes of two brothers with progressive muscular dystrophy. Rozenszajn et al. (1966) found them in two sisters with ichthyosis.

Jordans, G. H. W.: The familial occurrence of fat containing vacuoles in the leukocytes diagnosed in two brothers suffering from dystrophia musculorum progressiva (Erb). Acta Med. Scand. 145: 419-423, 1953.

Rozenszajn, L., Klajman, A., Yaffe, D. and Efrati, P.: Jordans' anomaly in white blood cells. Report of case. Blood 28: 258-265, 1966.

24400 JOSEPH SYNDROME

The features are convulsions of early onset, elevated spinal fluid protein, aminoaciduria (proline, hydroxyproline, glycine). Several disorders, e.g., maple syrup urine disease, would fit this syndrome. It is not clear that it is a distinct entity.

Jonxis, J. H. P.: Hereditary aminoaciduria. In, Steinberg, A. G. and Bearn, A. G. (eds.): Progress in Medical Genetics. New York: Grune and Stratton, 2: 1962.

Joseph, R., Ribierre, M., Job, J.-C. and Girault, M.: Maladie familiale associant des convulsions a debut tres precoce, une hyperalbuminorachie et une hyperaminoacidurie. Arch. Franc. Pediat. 15: 374-387, 1958.

24410 JUMPING FRENCHMAN OF MAINE (SEE ALSO HYPER-REFLEXIA, HEREDITARY)

Beard (1878) first studied this disorder, an exaggerated startle reflex. Stevens (1966) has written on it. Beard thought it familial and a disorder particularly of French-Canadians. Stevens cited a personal communication describing five affected sibs, offspring of a French-Canadian fishing guide in Wedgport, Nova Scotia.

Beard, G. M.: Remarks upon 'jumpers or jumping Frenchmen.' J. Nerv. Ment. Dis. 5: 526, 1878.

Stevens, H.: Jumping Frenchmen of Maine. Arch. Neurol. 12: 311-314, 1966.

24420 KALLMANN SYNDROME (HYPOGONADOTROPIC HYPOGONADISM AND ANOSMIA)

This entity is discussed also in the X-linkage catalog. Midline cranial anomalies (cleft lip, cleft palate and imperfect fusion) are also features. Rosen (1965) examined a large kindred with a high rate of consanguinity and found 5 cases of hypogonadism, 3 of anosmia and 6 of midline anomalies. Two persons had two defects and 2 showed all three. Both males and females were affected and the pedigree suggested autosomal recessive inheritance. Tagatz et al. (1970) described three unrelated females with hypogonadotropic hypogonadism and anosmia. No relative was affected and the parents in each case were unrelated. Induction of ovulation with resulting normal term pregnancy was achieved in two of the patients with exogenous gonadotropins.

Rosen, S. W.: The syndrome of hypogonadism, anosmia and midline cranial anomalies. Proc. 47th Meet. Endocr. Soc., 1965.

Tagatz, G., Fialkow, P. J., Smith, D. and Spadoni, L.: Hypogonadotropic hypogonadism associated with anosmia in the female. New Eng. J. Med. 283: 1326-1329, 1970.

24430 KALLMANN SYNDROME WITH FACIAL CLEFTING

Rosen (1965) presented evidence for a recessive form of Kallmann syndrome (hypogonadotrophic hypogonadism and anosmia) which has facial clefting as an additional feature. Rosen's patients came from a consanguineous French-Canadian family. The same or a related disorder may be that reported by Hintz et al. (1968).

Hintz, R. L., Menking, M. and Sotos, J. F.: Familial holoprosencephaly with endocrine dysgenesis. J. Pediat. 72: 81-87, 1968.

Rosen, S. W.: The syndrome of hypogonadism, anosmia and midline cranial anomalies. Proc. 47th Meeting Endocr. Soc., 1965.

24435 KAPPA-CHAIN DEFICIENCY

In a female offspring of an uncle-niece marriage, Bernier et al. (1972) observed deficient synthesis of

R
E
C
E
S
S
I
V
E

Bernier, G. M., Gunderman, J. R. and Ruymann, F. B.: Kappa-chain deficiency. Blood 40: 795-805, 1972.

*24440 KARTAGENER SYNDROME (DEXTROCARDIA, BRONCHIECTASIS AND SINUSITIS)

Kartagener and Stucki (1962) found 334 cases in the literature and added two more. Gorham and Merselis (1959) concluded that the disorder is inherited as a recessive with incomplete penetrance. Family studies were done by Knox, Murray and Strang (1960) and by Cook et al. (1962). Knox et al. (1960) suggested linkage with the Rhesus locus. Probably all familial cases have been confined to sibs, although Torgersen (1947) suggested dominant inheritance. Moreno et al. (1965) found the full syndrome in two of 5 offspring of first-cousin parents. Another sib had bronchiectasis as did also the father and the other two children were 'chronic coughers.' Holmes et al. (1968) found low serum levels of gamma A globulin in some cases. It is likely that the Kartagener syndrome is a Mendelian subgroup of situs inversus viscerum (27010), which for the most part has no simple Mendelian basis (Torgersen, 1950). There is no association with left-handedness.

Cook, C. D., Geller, F., Hutchison, G. B., Gerald, P. S. and Allen, F. H., Jr.: Blood grouping in three families with Kartagener's syndrome. Am. J. Hum. Genet. 14: 290-294, 1962.

Gorham, G. W. and Merselis, J. G., Jr.: Kartagener's triad: a family study. Bull. Hopkins Hosp. 104: 11-16 1959.

Hartline, J. V. and Zelkowitz, P. S.: Kartagener's syndrome in childhood. Am. J. Dis. Child. 121: 349-352, 1971.

Holmes, L. B., Blennerhassett, J. B. and Austen, K. F.: A reappraisal of Kartagener's syndrome. Am. J. Med. Sci. 255: 13-28, 1968.

Kartagener, M. and Stucki, P.: Bronchiectasis with situs inversus. Arch. Pediat. 79: 193-207, 1962.

Knox, G., Murray, S. and Strang, L. B.: A family with Kartagener's syndrome: linkage data. Ann. Hum. Genet. 24: 137-140, 1960.

Logan, W. D., Jr., Abbott, O. A. and Hatcher, C. R., Jr.: Kartagener's triad. Dis. Chest 48: 613-616, 1965.

Moreno, J., Ortega, L. and Montero, E.: Sindrome de Kartagener. Referencia de dos casos familiares con analysis citogenetico. An. Desarrollo 13: 207-213, 1965.

Torgersen, J.: Familial transposition of viscera. Acta Med. Scand. 126: 319-322, 1946.

Torgersen, J.: Genic factors in visceral asymmetry and in the development and pathologic changes of the lungs, heart and abdominal organs. Arch. Path. 47: 566-593, 1949.

Torgersen, J.: Situs inversus, asymmetry, and twinning. Am. J. Hum. Genet. 2: 361-370, 1950.

Torgersen, J.: Transposition of viscera-bronchiectasis, and nasal polyps. A genetical analysis and contributions to the problem of constitution. Acta Radiol. 28: 17-24, 1947.

24450 KERATOCONUS

Hamilton (1938) claimed that certain of his pedigrees strongly supported autosomal recessive inheritance. Keratoconus is a feature of amaurosis congenita (q.v.). Indeed it is an occasional feature of mongolism. In this and other conditions including amaurosis congenita of Leber, eye rubbing may be an important factor in the causation of keratoconus. It is unproved that keratoconus occurs as an isolated Mendelizing disorder.

Hamilton, J. B.: Significance of heredity in ophthalmology. Preliminary survey of hereditary eye diseases in Tasmania. Brit. J. Ophthal. 22: 83-108, 1938.

Van der Hoeve, J.: Vererbbarkeit des Keratokonus. Z. Augenheilk. 52: 321-336, 1924.

24460 KERATOCONUS POSTICUS CIRCUMSCRIPTUS

Haney and Falls (1961) described affected brother and sister with associated manifestations in the form of retarded mental and physical growth, hypertelorism, corneal nebulae, short 'bull neck,' stubby limbs and digits. They quoted the following description of the corneal lesion: '.....the appearance one might expect if into the posterior surface of a plastic corner one had excavated a subsidiary small basin-like depression by pressing into it a marble of much smaller curvature than that of the corneal surface itself.' The parents denied consanguinity. Curiously the authors suggested autosomal dominant inheritance with poor penetrance. It is true that Jacobs (1957) reported keratoconus posticus in father and son. He made no mention of associated manifestations.

Haney, W. P. and Falls, H. F.: The occurrence of congenital keratoconus posticus circumscriptus in two siblings presenting a previously unrecognized syndrome. Am. J. Ophthal. 52: 53-57, 1961.

Jacobs, H. B.: Posterior conical cornea. Brit. J. Ophthal. 41: 31-39, 1957.

*24480 KERATOSIS PALMO-PLANTARIS WITH CORNEAL DYSTROPHY (RICHNER-HANHART SYNDROME)

The names of Richner (1938) and Hanhart (1948) are associated with this disorder. The parents of Hanhart's patient (1947) were second cousins. Richner (1938) described skin lesions in brother and sister. Only the brother had corneal lesions. Waardenburg (1961) described children of a first-cousin marriage, one with the full syndrome and one with only corneal changes. Hanhart's patients (1947) also had severe mental and somatic retardation. The pedigree he reported is reproduced by Waardenburg. Ventura et al. (1965) described the syndrome in two sons of first cousin-parents. This rare disorder is characterized clinically by herpetiform corneal ulcers, palmo-plantar keratoses and mental retardation. Goldsmith et al. (1972) demonstrated

R
E
C
E
S
S
I
V
E

tyrosinemia and phenylaceticacidemia in this disorder. Their patient was the 14-year-old son of consanguineous Italian parents. The urine contained excessive P-hydroxyphenyllactic acid. Urinary P-hydroxyphenylpyruvic acid was normal. Clinical and biochemical improvement followed accompanied low phenylalanine-low tyrosine diet. They suggested that soluble tyrosine aminotransferase may be deficient. See 27660 for further information on tyrosine transaminase deficiency.

Goldsmith, L. A., Kang, E., Biefang, D. C., Jimbow, K., Gerald, P. S. and Baden, H. P.: Tyrosinemia with plantar and palmar keratosis and keratitis. J. Pediat. 83: 798-805, 1973.

Hanhart, E.: Neue Sonderformen von Keratosis palmo-plantaris, u.a. eine regelmassig-dominante mit systematisierten Lipomen, ferner 2 einfach-rezessive mit Schwachsinn und Z.T. mit Hornhautveraenderungen des Auges (Ektodermatosyndrom). Dermatologica 94: 286-308, 1947.

Ventura, G., Biasini, G. and Petrozzi, M.: Cheratomia palmoplantare dissipatum associato a lesioni corneali in due fratelli. Boll. Oculist. 44: 497-510, 1965.

Waardenburg, P. J., Franceschetti, A. and Klein, D.: In, Genetics and Ophthalmology. Springfield, Ill.: Charles C Thomas, 1: 515-517, 1961.

*24500 KERATOSIS PALMO-PLANTARIS WITH PERIODONTOPATHIA (PAPILLON-LEFEVRE SYNDROME)

Both the milk teeth and the permanent teeth are lost prematurely. The skin lesions are very similar or identical to those of mal de Meleda (q.v.). Gorlin, Sedano and Anderson (1964) suggested that calcification of the dura mater is a third component of the syndrome. Schopf et al. (1971) described keratosis palmo-plantaris with hypodontia, hypotrichosis and cysts of the eyelids in sisters whose parents were first cousins. The deciduous teeth were lost early and the permanent dentition in one patient consisted only of two incisors and a molar. Palmo-plantar keratosis and fragility of the nails began at about age 12. At age 25 the head hair became sparce and body hair was lost completely. Cysts of both upper and lower eyelids were noted at age 60. The cysts were thought to be derived from the glands of Moll. This may be the Papillon-Lefevre syndrome.

Gorlin, R. J., Sedano, H. and Anderson, V. E.: The syndrome of palmar-plantar hyperkeratosis and premature periodontal destruction of the teeth. A clinical and genetic analysis of the Papillon-Lefevre syndrome. J. Pediat. 65: 895-908, 1964.

Greither, A.: Keratosis palmo-plantaris mit Periodontopathie (Papillon-Lefevre). Dermatologica 119: 248-263, 1959.

Jansen, L. H. and Dekker, G.: Hyperkeratosis palmo-plantaris with periodontosis (Papillon-Lefevre). Dermatologica 113: 207-219, 1956.

Schopf, E., Schulz, H.-J. and Passarge, E.: Syndrome of cystic eyelids, palmo-plantar keratosis, hypodontia and hypotrichosis as a possible autosomal recessive trait. The Clinical Delineation of Birth Defects. XII. Skin, Hair and Nails. Baltimore: Williams and Wilkins, 1971. Pp. 219-221.

Ziprkowski, L., Raymon, Y. and Brish, M.: Hyperkeratosis palmoplantaris with periodontosis (Papillon-Lefevre). Arch. Derm. 88: 207-209, 1963.

24505 KETOACIDOSIS OF INFANCY (SUCCINYL-COA: 3-KETOACID COA-TRANSFERASE DEFICIENCY)

By study of cultured fibroblasts and post mortem tissue from a Negro male infant who died at age 6 months from severe, intermittent ketoacidosis, Tildon and Cornblath (1972) found no measurable activity of succinyl CoA: 3-ketoacid CoA-transferase. Other causes of ketoacidosis in the neonate include diabetes mellitus, type I glycogen storage disease (23220), glycinemia (23200), methylmalonic aciduria (25100) and lactic acidosis (24540). Family information would be of interest.

Tildon, J. T. and Cornblath, M.: Succinyl-CoA: 3-ketoacid CoA-transferase deficiency. A cause for ketoacidosis in infancy. J. Clin. Invest. 51: 493-498, 1972.

*24510 KETOACIDURIA WITH MENTAL DEFICIENCY AND OTHER FEATURES (RICHARDS-RUNDLE SYNDROME)

Richards and Rundle (1959) described a family in which 5 of 13 offspring of a marriage of first cousins once removed had ketoaciduria, mental retardation, under-development of secondary sex characteristics, deafness, ataxia, and peripheral muscle wasting. See also the report of Matthews (1950). The condition progressed in childhood but eventually became static. It represented no risk to life. Richards and Rundle found in the literature a description of a brother and sister who probably had the same condition (Koennecke, 1920). Sylvester (1972) studied two of the sibs reported by Richards and Rundle. The neuropathologic findings suggested the Roussy-Levy syndrome (18080).

Berman, W., Haslam, R. H. A., Konigsmark, B. W. and Capute, A. J.: Progressive ataxia, hearing loss and mental retardation in three brothers (variant Richards-Rundle syndrome). In, Bergsma, D. (ed.): Clinical Delineation of Birth Defects. XVI. Urinary System and Others. Baltimore: Williams and Wilkins, 1974. Pp. 345-346.

Koennecke, W.: Friedreichsche Ataxie und Taubstummheit. Z. Neurol. Psychiat. 53: 161-165, 1920.

Matthews, W. B.: Familial ataxia, deaf-mutism, and muscular wasting. J. Neurol. Psychiat. 13: 307-311, 1950.

Richards, B. W. and Rundle, A. T.: A familial hormonal disorder associated with mental deficiency, deaf mutism and ataxia. J. Ment. Defic. Res. 3: 33-55, 1959.

Sylvester, P. E.: Spino-cerebellar gegeneration, hormone disorder, hypogonadism, deaf-mutism and mental deficiency. J. Ment. Defic. Res. 16: 203-214, 1972.

24515 KEUTEL SYNDROME

Among the children of first cousins once removed, Keutel et al. (1972) found a brother and sister with an apparently distinctive syndrome: multiple peripheral pulmonary stenoses, neural hearing loss, short terminal phalanges, and calcification and-or ossification of the cartilage in the external ears, nose, larynx, trachea and ribs.

Keutel, J., Jorgensen, G. and Gabriel, P.: A new autosomal recessive syndrome: peripheral pulmonary stenoses, brachytelephalangism, neural hearing loss and abnormal cartilage calcifications-ossification. Clinical Delineation of Birth Defects. XV. Cardiovascular System. Baltimore: Williams and Wilkins Co., 1972. Pp. 60-68.

*24520 KRABBE DISEASE (GLOBOID CELL SCLEROSIS)

Onset occurs at 4-6 months of age. Definitive diagnosis in this disorder which clinically can be so similar to several other encephalopathies of infancy is made by finding characteristic 'globoid cells' in brain tissue. Nelson and colleagues (1963) observed three affected sibs. A somewhat similar state was described in 3 adult sibs by Ferraro (1927), but this may be a genetically distinct condition. See discussion of Menkes (1963) and of Norman et al. (1961). D'Agostino et al (1963) concluded that the initial histologic manifestation of the disease is the presence of PAS-positive material extracellularly and cerithin in microglial cells, which later appear as globoid cells. First cousin parents were noted by Van Gehuchten (1956). Many have described affected sibs. Although deficiency of cerebroside-sulfatide sulfotransferase was earlier reported in Krabbe disease (Bachhawat et al., 1967), Suzuki and Suzuki (1970) found deficiency of galactocerebroside beta-galactosidase which they felt is etiologic and better accounts for the morphologic and biochemical features of the disorder. Suzuki et al. (1971) has succeeded in demonstrating an intermediate level of activity of galactocerebroside beta-galactosidase in serum, white cells and fibroblasts of heterozygotes. Suzuki (1972) tells me of two patients with morphologically and enzymatically proved Krabbe disease who have survived unusually long — into the teens in the oldest — and may represent an allelic form. Young et al. (1972) found deficiency of the same enzyme, galactocerebrosidase in a case of late onset. Crome et al. (1973) described a late onset variety which is probably allelic to the usual form.

Andrews, J. M., Cancilla, P. A., Grippo, J. and Menkes, J. H.: Globoid cell leukodystrophy (Krabbe's disease): morphological and biochemical studies. Neurology 21: 337-352, 1971.

Austin, J.: Studies in globoid (Krabbe) leukodystrophy. I. The significance of lipid abnormalities in white matter in 8 globoid and 13 control patients. Arch. Neurol. 9: 207-231, 1963.

Austin, J., Suzuki, K., Armstrong, D., Brady, R. O., Bachhawat, B. K., Schlenker, J. and Stumpf, D.: Studies in globoid (Krabbe) leukodystrophy (gld). V. Controlled enzymic studies in ten human cases. Arch. Neurol. 23: 502-512, 1970.

Bachhawat, B. K., Austin, J. and Armstrong, D.: A cerebroside sulphotransferase deficiency in a human disorder of myelin. Biochem. J. 104: 15C-17C, 1967.

Crome, L., Hanefeld, F., Patrick, D. and Wilson, J.: Late onset globoid cell leucodystrophy. Brain 96: 841-848, 1973.

D'Agostino, A. N., Sayre, G. P. and Hayles, A. B.: Krabbe's disease. Globoid cell type of leukodystrophy. Arch. Neurol. 8: 82-96, 1963.

Farrell, D. F., Perry, A. K., Kaback, M. M. and McKhann, G. M.: Globoid cell (Krabbe) leukodystrophy: heterozygote detection in cultured skin fibroblasts. Am. J. Hum. Genet. 25: 604-609, 1973.

Ferraro, A.: Familial form of encephalitis periaxialis diffusa. J. Nerv. Ment. Dis. 66: 329-354, 1927.

Krabbe, K.: A new familial infantile form of diffuse brain-sclerosis. Brain 39: 74-114, 1916.

Menkes, J. H.: Metabolic disease of the nervous system. In, Brennemann, J. (ed.): Practice of Pediatrics. Hagerstown: W. F. Pryor Co. 4: 1963.

Nelson, E., Aurebeck, G., Osterberg, K., Berry, J., Jabbour, J. T. and Bornhofen, J. H.: Ultrastructural and chemical studies on Krabbe's disease. J. Neuropath. Exp. Neurol. 22: 414-434, 1963.

Norman, R. M., Oppenheimer, D. R. and Tingey, A. H.: Histological and chemical findings in Krabbe's leucodystrophy. J. Neurol. Neurosurg. Psychiat. 24: 223-232, 1961.

Suzuki, K. and Suzuki, Y.: Globoid cell leucodystrophy (Krabbe's disease): deficiency of galactocerebroside beta-galactosidase. Proc. Nat. Acad. Sci. 66: 302-309, 1970.

Suzuki, K.: Bronx, N. Y.: personal communication, 1972.

Suzuki, Y. and Suzuki, K.: Krabbe's globoid cell leukodystrophy: deficiency of galactocerebrosidase in serum, leukocytes, and fibroblasts. Science 171: 73-74, 1971.

Van Gehuchten, P.: Sur l'origine des cellules globoides dans un cas de sclerose diffuse. Rev. Neurol. 94: 253-258, 1956.

Wenger, D. A., Sattler, M. and Hiatt, W.: Globoid cell leukodystrophy: deficiency of lactosyl ceramide beta-galactosidase. Proc. Nat. Acad. Sci. 71: 854-857, 1974.

Young, E., Wilson, J., Patrick, A. D. and Crome, L.: Galactocerebrosidase deficiency in globoid cell leucodystrophy of late onset. Arch. Dis. Child. 47: 449-450, 1972.

Reproduction of the disease clinically and histopathologically in chimpanzees injected with material from the brain of human cases (Gajdusek et al., 1966) seems to establish kuru as being due to a 'slow virus.' Whether significant genetic factors are also involved remains uncertain. 'Scrapie' is a chronic neurologic disease of the sheep in which a 'slow virus' has been demonstrated but genetic factors may also be involved. Bennett et al. (1959) had suggested that affected males were homozygous and affected females either homozygous or heterozygous for a single gene for kuru.

Beck, E., Daniel, P. M., Alpers, M., Gajdusek, D. C. and Gibbs, C. J., Jr.: Experimental 'kuru' in chimpanzees. A pathological report. Lancet II: 1056-1059, 1966.

Bennett, J. H., Rhodes, F. A. and Robson, H. N.: A possible genetic basis for kuru. Am. J. Hum. Genet. 11: 169-187, 1959.

Gajdusek, D. C., Gibbs, C. J., Jr. and Alpers, M.: Experimental transmission of a kuru-like syndrome to chimpanzees. Nature 209: 794-796, 1966.

Gajdusek, D. C., Gibbs, C. J., Jr. and Alpers, M.: Transmission and passage of experimental 'kuru' to chimpanzees. Science 155: 212-214, 1967.

*24540 LACTIC ACIDOSIS, FAMILIAL INFANTILE

Erickson (1965) reported affected brother and sister with relatives who died in infancy perhaps of the same condition. The diagnosis is suggested by discrepancy between total cations and anions in the blood. Mental retardation is present. Treatment consists of replacing glucose with galactose and of administered bicarbonate. Lactic acidosis occurs in glycogen storage disease I (q.v.). Worsley et al. (1965) described two brothers who presented in the second year of life with ataxia, muscle twitching and intermittent hyperpnea at rest. The condition progressed with mental deterioration, loss of scalp hair and death about 6 months after onset. Widespread necrotizing encephalopathy was found at autopsy. Spontaneous increases in lactic acid in the blood were apparently responsible for the hyperpnea. Renal aminoaciduria and lowered serum phosphate were also found. They suggested that this is the first description of familial lactic acidosis in young children. Haworth, Ford and Younoszai (1967) described an American Indian family in which three sibs were mentally retarded and had convulsions, other neurologic abnormalities, muscular hypotonia, obesity and signs and symptoms of metabolic acidosis. Blood lactate and pyruvate levels were elevated. Five other Indians died before 2 years of age with symptoms suggesting the same disorder. Binkiewicz et al. (1972) observed two sibs with severe physical and mental retardation and lactate levels about 4 times normal. Pyruvate was essentially normal. Metabolic findings suggesting impaired oxidation of NADH2 were described. This suggested decreased effectiveness of the mitochondrial respiratory chain such as occurs in the petite mutant mitochondrial disorder of yeast. Brunette et al. (1973) studied a thiamine-responsive case of lactic acidosis. Pyruvate dehydrogenase activity (which is thiamine-dependent) was normal in leukocytes and cultured skin fibroblasts. Hepatic pyruvate carboxylase activity (which is biotin-dependent) was found to comprise more than one component. Partial deficiency was demonstrated with loss of activity confined to the low Km component. The causes of familial lactic acidosis are rather numerous, although each entity is rare. Pyruvate carboxylase deficiency (26615) and pyruvate dehydrogenase deficiency (20880) are two causes. The clinical picture in some cases is that of Leigh necrotizing encephalopathy (25600). Hyperalainemia (20290) is a feature of many of the forms of familial lactic acidosis, because of the intimate inter-relationship of alanine, pyruvate and lactate metabolism.

Binkiewicz, A., Jungas, R. L., Hochman, H. and Senior, B.: Familial idiopathic lactic acidosis — petite mutant disease in man? (Abstract) Pediat. Res. 6: 395 only, 1972.

Brunette, M. G., Delvin, E., Hazel, B. and Scriver, C. R.: Thiamine-responsive lactic acidosis in a patient with low Km pyruvate carboxylase activity in liver. Pediatrics 50: 702-711, 1972.

Erickson, R. J.: Familial infantile lactic acidosis. J. Pediat. 66: 1004-1016, 1965.

Haworth, J. C., Ford, J. D. and Younoszai, M. K.: Familial chronic acidosis due to an error in lactate and pyruvate metabolism. Canad. Med. Ass. J. 97: 773-779, 1967.

Lie, S. O., Loken, A. C., Stromme, J. H. and Aagenaes, O.: Fatal congenital lactic acidosis in two siblings I. Clinical and pathological studies. Acta Paediat. Scand. 60: 129-137, 1971.

Skrede, S., Stromme, J. H., Stokke, O., Lie, S. O. and Eldjarn, L.: Fatal congenital lactic acidosis in two siblings. II. Biochemical studies in vivo and vitro. Acta Paediat. Scand. 60: 138-145, 1971.

Worsley, H. E., Brookfield, R. W., Elwood, J. S., Noble, R. L. and Taylor, W. H.: Lactic acidosis with necrotizing encephalopathy in two sibs. Arch. Dis. Child. 40: 492-501, 1965.

*24550 LACTOSYLCERAMIDOSIS

Lactosylceramide accumulates in the viscera and nervous system in this disorder and lactosylceramide galactosyl hydrolase is deficient. Both the accumulation and the enzyme deficiency are demonstrable in cultured fibroblasts. Only one patient has been observed, a Negro girl, but the presence of partial deficiency in both parents supports recessive inheritance. Retardation in psychomotor development was evident by age 25 months.

Dawson, G. and Stein, A. O.: Lactosyl ceramidosis: catabolic enzyme defect of glycosphingolipid metabolism. Science 170: 556-558, 1970.

Dawson, G., Matalon, R. and Stein, A. O.: Lactosylceramidosis: lactosylceramide galactosyl hydrolase deficiency and accumulation of lactosylceramide in cultured skin fibroblasts. J. Pediat. 79: 423-429, 1971.

R
E
C
E
S
S
I
V
E

Lenn, N. J.: Lactosylceramidosis: light and electron microscopic observations. Neurology 23: 791-797, 1973.

*24560 LARSEN SYNDROME

Larsen, Schottstaedt and Bost (1950) called attention to a syndrome of multiple congenital dislocations and characteristic facies (prominent forehead, depressed nasal bridge, wide-spaced eyes). Clubfoot, bilateral dislocation of elbows, hips and knees (most characteristically, anterior dislocation of the tibia on the femur), and short metacarpals with cylindrical fingers lacking the usual tapering were the skeletal features of note. Cleft palate, hydrocephalus and abnormalities of spinal segmentation were found in some. These authors found no similar cases in the families. See P. 126 of Gorlin and Pindborg (1964). Several instances of multiple affected sibs are known to me. Steel (1966) has observed three affected sibs and Rimoin (1970) showed me a family with multiple affected sibs. The sibs reported by Block and Peck (1965) may have had this condition. Congenital dislocation of the knees with unilateral cataract and unilateral undescended testis was present in a newborn male. A sister was born with bilateral dislocation of the knees and hips and cleft palate. One of the earliest reports may have been that of McFarland (1929). Latta et al. (1971) made a point of a juxtacalcaneal accessory bone which may be specific for this entity. The mother of their patient had a saddle nose which developed at age 18 after tennis-ball trauma. Autosomal dominant inheritance is suggested by McFarlane's report (1947) of a woman with saddle nose, congenital dislocation of the knees and hyperextensibility of the elbows. By each of three different mates she produced an affected child with bilateral knee dislocations.

Bloch, C. and Peck, H. M.: Bilateral congenital dislocation of the knees. J. Mt. Sinai Hosp. 32: 607-614, 1965.

Gorlin, R. J. and Pindborg, J. J.: Syndromes of the Head and Neck. New York: Blakiston Division, McGraw-Hill Book Co., 1964.

Larsen, L. J., Schottstaedt, E. R. and Bost, F. C.: Multiple congenital dislocations associated with characteristic facial abnormality. J. Pediat. 37: 574-581, 1950.

Latta, R. J., Graham, C. B., Aase, J. M., Scham, S. M. and Smith, D. W.: Larsen's syndrome: a skeletal dysplasia with multiple joint dislocations and unusual facies. J. Pediat. 78: 291-298, 1971.

McFarlane, A. L.: A report on four cases of congenital genu recurvatum occurring in one family. Brit. J. Surg. 34: 388-391, 1947.

McFarland, B. L.: Congenital dislocation of the knee. J. Bone Joint Surg. 11: 281-285, 1929.

Rimoin, D. L.: St. Louis, Mo.: personal communication, 1970.

Steel, H. M.: Philadelphia, Penn.: personal communication, 1966.

*24580 LAURENCE-MOON SYNDROME

The features in the four sibs reported by Laurence and Moon (1866) and later by Hutchinson (1882, 1900) were mental retardation, pigmentary retinopathy, hypogenitalism and spastic paraplegia. It represents an entity distinct from that described by Bardet and Biedl (see BARDET-BIEDL SYNDROME). Unfortunately most authors have adopted the designation suggested by Solis-Cohen and Weiss (1925), Laurence-Moon-Biedl-Bardet syndrome. The Laurence-Moon syndrome (strictu sensu) is the same as the disorder reported by Kapuscinski (1934). The family reported by Bowen et al. (1965) probably had this syndrome.

Bowen, P., Ferguson-Smith, M. A., Mosier, D., Lee, C. S. N. and Butler, H. G.: The Laurence-Moon syndrome. Association with hypogonadotrophic hypogonadism and sex-chromosome aneuploidy. Arch. Intern. Med. 116: 598-604, 1965.

Hutchinson, J.: On retinitis pigmentosa and allied affections, as illustrating the laws of heredity. Ophthal. Rev. 1: 2-7 and 26-30, 1882.

Hutchinson, J.: Slowly progressive paraplegia and disease of the choroids with defective intellect and arrested sexual development. Arch. Surg. 11: 118-122, 1900.

Kapuscinski, W.: Ueber familiaere Aderhautentartung mit ataktischen Stoerungen. Ber. Dtsch. Ophthal. Ges. 50: 13-19, 1934.

Laurence, J. Z. and Moon, R. C.: Four cases of retinitis pigmentosa occurring in the same family and accompanied by general imperfection of development. Ophthal. Rev. 2: 32-41, 1866.

Solis-Cohen, S. and Weiss, E.: Dystrophia adiposogenitalis with atypical retinitis pigmentosa and mental deficiency: the Laurence-Biedl syndrome. Am. J. Med. Sci. 169: 489-505, 1925.

Stiggelbout, T.: The (Laurence Moon) Bardet Biedl syndrome. Assen, The Netherlands: Van Gorcum, 1969.

24585 LAZY LEUKOCYTE SYNDROME

Miller et al. (1971) described two unrelated children, a boy and a girl, with episodes of recurrent stomatitis, gingivitis, otitis media and fevers. A severe neutropenia was found. Bone marrow studies showed normal numbers of mature, morphologically normal neutrophils. A poor neutrophil response was obtained upon stimulation with both epinephrine and endotoxin, as well as upon induced inflammation by the Rebuck skin window technique. Leukocyte phaocytosis and bacterio-acidal activity were normal. Both random mobility and chemotactic function were defective. See neutrophil chemotactic defect (16282) for description of a disorder limited to chemotaxis. At least four other cases are known to Miller (1974). None is familial and no parental consanguinity is know.

Miller, M. E., Oski, F. A. and Harris, M. B.: Lazy-leukocyte syndrome. A new disorder of neutrophil function. Lancet I: 665-669, 1971.

Miller, M. E.: Los Angeles, personal communication, June 25, 1974.

Miller, M. E.: Pathology of chemotaxis and random mobility. Seminars Hemat., in press, Jan., 1975.

*24590 LECITHIN: CHOLESTEROL ACYLTRANSFERASE (LCAT) DEFICIENCY (NORUM DISEASE)

In Norway Norum and Gjone (1967) described a possibly 'new' error of lipid metabolism in sisters with normochromic anemia, proteinuria and corneal deposits of lipid. Total serum cholesterol was elevated, almost all of it being free cholesterol. Lack of plasma cholesterol-lecithin acyltransferase was postulated. Gjone and Norum (1968) reported the clinical features in 3 adult sisters who showed only traces of esterified cholesterol in the serum. All had proteinuria and anemia. Total cholesterol, triglyceride and phospholipid were increased. Lysolecithin of serum was decreased. Foam cells were present in the bone marrow and in the glomerular tufts of the kidney. The tonsils were normal. The liver was not enlarged and there was no evidence of liver disease which might account for a defect in cholesterol esterification. Teisberg (1973) showed me data suggesting close linkage of the alpha-haptoglobin locus and the LCAT locus. In three sibships LCAT deficiency seemed to travel with the alpha-Hp-1 allele. The lod score was about 2.9 at a recombination fraction of 0. The linkage disequilibrium strongly favored close linkage. The mutation was thought to have occurred in rural Norway at least 250-300 years ago. Because of a high degree of inbreeding the frequency of the gene is higher.

Gjone, E. and Norum, K. R.: Familial serum cholesterol ester deficiency. Clinical study of a patient with a new syndrome. Acta Med. Scand. 183: 107-112, 1968.

Gjone, E., Torsvik, H. and Norum, K. R.: Familial plasma cholesterol ester deficiency. A study of erythrocytes. Scand. J. Clin. Lab. Invest. 21: 327-332, 1968.

Nordoy, A. and Gjone, E.: Familial plasma lecithin: cholesterol acyltransferase deficiency. Scand. J. Lab. Invest. 27: 263-268, 1971.

Norum, K. R. and Gjone, E.: Familial serum-cholesterol esterification failure. A new inborn error of metabolism. Biochim. Biophys. Acta 144: 698-700, 1967.

Teisberg, P.: Oslo, Norway, personal communication, Nov. 3, 1973.

*24600 LEG, ABSENCE DEFORMITY OF, WITH CONGENITAL CATARACT

In two distantly related Amish boys, McKusick et al. (1968) observed absence deformity of one leg, congenital cataract and progressive scoliosis. All four parents shared at least two ancestral couples in common.

McKusick, V. A., Weilbaecher, R. G. and Gragg, G. W.: Recessive inheritance of a congenital malformation syndrome. J.A.M.A. 204: 113-118, 1968.

24610 LEIOMYOMATA OF SKIN

Kloepfer and colleagues (1958) described three half-first-cousins with multiple leiomyomata of the skin. The parents and common grandparent were not known to be affected, but all critical individuals were not examined. In this type of anomaly one would, as the authors point out, anticipate dominant inheritance, probably with reduced penetrance. See 15080.

Kloepfer, H. W., Krafchuk, J., Derbes, V. and Burks, J.: Hereditary multiple leiomyoma of the skin. Am. J. Hum. Genet. 10: 48-52, 1958.

*24620 LEPRECHAUNISM

Among the children of second cousins once removed, Donohue and Uchida (1954) observed two sisters with the following features — apparent cessation of growth at about the seventh month of gestation, peculiar facies creating a gnomelike appearance and leading to the designation, and severe endocrine disturbance indicated by emaciation, enlargement of breasts and clitoris and histologic changes in the ovaries, pancreas and breasts. Three abortions (one child at 4 months, the others earlier) had been experienced by this mother. The patients died at 46 and 66 days of age, respectively. Patterson and Watkins (1962) described a probable case in a male. The four previously described cases had been female. Follow-up observations (Patterson, 1969) suggest that this may have been a different disorder. There were clinical signs of Cushing disease and at autopsy the adrenals were found to be much enlarged. Before the patient died at the age of almost 8 years, severe changes in the bones, of an unusual type, had developed. Serum alkaline phosphatase was always low, but no phosphoethanolamine was demonstrated in the urine. Two affected sisters were reported by Lakatos and colleagues (1963). Salmon and Webb (1963) observed consanguineous parents of a case. Dekaban (1965) found normal chromsomes. See SEIP SYNDROME. Der Kaloustian et al. (1971) described two unrelated cases each born of consanguineous parents.

Dekaban, A.: Metabolic and chromosomal studies in leprechaunism. Arch. Dis. Child. 40: 632-636, 1965.

Der Kaloustian, V. M., Kronfol, N. M., Takla, R., Habash, A., Khazin, A. and Najjar, S. S.: Leprechaunism. A report of two new cases. Am. J. Dis. Child. 122: 442-445, 1971.

Donohue, W. L. and Uchida, I.: Leprechaunism: a euphuism for a rare familial disorder. J. Pediat. 45: 505-519, 1954.

Evans, P. R.: Leprechaunism. Arch. Dis. Child. 30: 479-483, 1955.

R
E
C
E
S
S
I
V
E

Kuhlkamp, F. and Helwig, H.: Das Krankheitsbild des kongenitalen Dysendokrinismus oder Leprechaunismus. Z. Kinderheilk. 109: 50-63, 1970.

Lakatos, I., Kallo, A. and Szijarto, L.: Leprechaunism (Donohue syndrome). Orv. Hetil. 104: 1075-1080, 1963.

Patterson, J. H. and Watkins, W. L.: Leprechaunism in a male infant. J. Pediat. 60: 730-739, 1962.

Patterson, J. H.: Presentation of a patient with leprechaunism. The Clinical Delineation of Birth Defects. IV. Skeletal Dysplasias. New York: National Foundation, 1969. Pp. 117-121.

Salmon, M. A. and Webb, J. N.: Dystrophic changes associated with leprechaunism in male infant. Arch. Dis. Child. 38: 530-535, 1963.

Summitt, R. L. and Favara, B. E.: Leprechaunism (Donohue's syndrome): a case report. J. Pediat. 74: 601-610, 1969.

24630 LEPROSY, VULNERABILITY TO

Beiguelman (1968) reviewed the evidence for an inherited basis of vulnerability to leprosy and the familial pattern of the Mitsuda (late lepromin) reaction. The following observations suggest the heritability of leprosy: (1) The disease fails to manifest itself in most exposed persons, even heavily exposed persons. (2) The frequency of leprosy among relatives of index cases is higher when the subjects are from a consanguineous marriage. (3) Different racial stocks living in the same area show different prevalence rates. (4) Even in populations with a high frequency, familial aggregation is demonstrable, i.e., the distribution in sibships is not random. (5) The distribution of polar types (typical lepromatous or malignant versus typical tuberculoid or benign) is not at random among affected sib pairs. (6) One polar form cannot be converted into the other by environmental agents. Beiguelman and Quagliato (1965) studied the familial distribution of the Mitsuda reaction and presented evidence which can be interpreted as supporting monogenic determination.

Beiguelman, B. and Quagliato, R.: Nature and familial character of the lepromin reactions. Int. J. Leprosy 33: 800-807, 1965.

Beiguelman, B.: Some remarks on the genetics of leprosy resistance. Acta Genet. Med. Gem. 17: 584-594, 1968.

*24640 LETTERER-SIWE DISEASE

Kloepfer (1971) has an unpublished pedigree of an inbred kindred suggesting autosomal recessive inheritance. Christie and colleagues (1954) described the disease in sibs who were never in contact, thus tending to discredit an infectious hypothesis. Rogers and Benson (1962) reported affected sibs and reviewed the literature. Falk and Gellei (1963) also observed a family. Schoeck, Peterson and Good (1963) described two sibs with Letterer-Siwe disease (acute disseminated histiocytosis X). Ten other families with multiple affected sibs were reviewed, including Farquhar 'familial hemophagocytic reticulosis' (q.v.) and Nelson 'generalized lymphohistiocytic infiltration' (q.v.), which Schoeck and his colleagues suggest are all the same entity. In a survey of deaths from Letterer-Siwe disease in a five year period in the U.S., Glass and Miller (1968) found five sib pairs among 270 deaths, a pair of concordant like-sex twins, and a peak of mortality under 1 year of age. (Freundlich et al. (1972) reported 2 families with multiple cases of consanguineous parents). Hirsch and Kong (1973) reported a father and son with histiocytosis X of the lung. The father presented with cough and exertional dyspnea, whereas the son was asymptomatic. Biopsies confirmed histiocytosis X (eosinophilic granuloma) in both. Neither father nor son had any evidence of disseminated histiocytosis. I have information from Cook (1967) concerning eight cases of histiocytosis X occurring in two sibships in an inbred Mennonite group in Waterloo County, Ontario. In each case the parents were related as second-cousins and all four parents shared in common a grandparental couple. In two cases treatment with adrenocorticosterioids was begun early and both patients survived. The other cases pursued an identical course. They were well until ages 818 weeks, following which they developed general irritability, especially on being touched or moved. There was pallor, dyspenia, distended abdomen, fever and in the terminal stages usually jaundice. Medical investigations showed hepatosplenomegaly, anemia, neutropenia and thrombocytopenia. Autopsy showed histiocytic infiltration of the liver, spleen and lymph nodes. There was no persistent skin rash and no bone lesions were identified. The course of the ilness in all six fatal cases was rapid, ranging from 2-5 weeks. None of the children had contact with each other.

Christie, A., Batson, R., Shapiro, J., Riley, H. D., Laughmiller, R. and Stahlman, M.: Acute disseminated (non-lipid) reticuloendotheliosis. Acta Paediat. 43 (suppl. 100): 65-76, 1954.

Cook, M. S.: Toronto, personal communication, 1967.

Falk, W. and Gellei, B.: Letterer-Siwe disease (non-lipoid reticuloendotheliosis). In, Goldschmidt, E. (ed.): Genetics of Migrant and Isolate Populations. Baltimore: Williams and Wilkins, 1963. P. 312. (See also, The familial occurrence of Letterer-Siwe disease. Acta Paediat. 46: 471-480, 1957.)

Freundlich, E., Amit, S., Montag, Y., Suprun, H. and Nevo, S.: Familial occurrence of Letterer-Siwe disease. Arch. Dis. Child. 47: 122-125, 1972.

Glass, A. G. and Miller, R. W.: U.S. mortality from Letterer-Siwe disease, 1960-1964. Pediatrics 42: 364-367, 1968.

Hirsch, M. S. and Kong, C. H.: Familial pulmonary histiocytosis X. Am. Rev. Resp. Dis. 107: 831-835, 1973.

Juberg, R. C., Kloepfer, H. W. and Oberman, H. A.: Genetic determination of acute disseminated histiocytosis X (Letterer-Siwe syndrome). Pediatrics 45: 753-765, 1970.

Kloepfer, H. W.: New Orleans, La.: personal communication, 1971.

Rogers, D. L. and Benson, T. E.: Familial Letterer-Siwe disease. Report of a case. J. Pediat. 60: 550-554, 1962.

Schoeck, V. W., Peterson, R. D. A. and Good, R. A.: Familial occurrence of Letterer-Siwe disease. Pediatrics 32: 1055-1063, 1963.

*24650 LEUKOMELANODERMA, INFANTILISM, MENTAL RETARDATION, HYPODONTIA, HYPOTRICHOSIS

In the family reported by Berlin (1961) two males and two females were affected out of 12 offspring of a cousin marriage.

Berlin, C.: Congenital generalized melanoleucoderma associated with hypodontia, hypotrichosis, stunted growth and mental retardation occurring in two brothers and two sisters. Dermatologica 123: 227-243, 1961.

24655 LICHTENSTEIN SYNDROME

Lichtenstein (1971) described a 'new' syndrome comprising frequent infections due to a leukocyte and immune defect (neutropenia, IgA deficiency), bony abnormalities (peripheral osteoporosis) with tendency to fracture, failure of fusion of posterior spinal arches, subluxation at C1-C2 resulting in long-tract signs, metacarpophalangeal camptodactyly with ulnar deviation of the fingers and Simian crease, giant cyst of the lung, and unusual facies ('carp mouth,' synophrys, anteverted nostrils). Lichtenstein (1971) observed the syndrome in both of female monozygotic twins.

Lichtenstein, J. R.: A 'new' syndrome with neutropenia, immune deficiency, and multiple congenital anomalies (spondylolysis, open posterior cervical arches, ulnar deviation of fingers, carp mouth). In press, 1971.

*24660 LIPASE, CONGENITAL ABSENCE OF PANCREATIC

Sheldon (1964) described two unrelated sibships with a brother and sister in one, and two brothers in another, showing congenital absence of pancreatic lipase. Rey et al. (1966) described a single case. In none were the parents related.

Rey, J., Frezal, J., Royer, P. and Lamy, M.: L'absence congenitale de lipase pancreatique. Arch. Franc. Pediat. 23: 5-14, 1966.

Sheldon, W.: Congenital pancreatic lipase deficiency. Arch. Dis. Child. 39: 268-271, 1964.

24670 LIPID TRANSPORT DEFECT OF INTESTINE

Anderson et al. (1961), Lamy et al. (1967) and Silverberg et al. (1968) described cases. Two brothers were affected (Lamy et al., 1967). Parental consanguinity was noted by Silverberg et al. (1968). Intestinal symptoms and a failure of fat transport occur as in abetalipoproteinemia but neither acanthocytosis or neuro-ocular symptoms occur and low-density lipoproteins are present in the plasma. As in abetalipoproteinemia, there is failure of chylomicron formation. The nature of the defect is unknown, as is also the genetic relationship to abetalipoproteinemia, e.g. whether the genes are allelic.

Anderson, C. M., Townley, R. R. W., Freeman, M. and Johansen, P.: Unusual causes of steatorrhoea in infancy and childhood. Med. J. Aust. 2: 617-622, 1961.

Lamy, M., Frezal, J., Rey, J., Jos, J., Nezelof, C., Herrault, A. and Cohen-Solal, J.: Diarrhee chronique par trouble du transfert intra-cellulaire des lipides. Arch. Franc. Pediat. 24: 1079 only, 1967.

Silverberg, M., Kessler, J., Neumann, P. Z. and Wiglesworth, F. W.: An intestinal lipid transport defect. A possible variant of hypo-beta-lipoproteinemia. (Abstract) Gastroenterology 54: 1271-1272, 1968.

*24680 LIPIDOSIS, JUVENILE DYSTONIC

DeLeon et al. (1969) described two females and a male in a Negro kindred with a juvenile form of cerebral lipidosis. Clinical features were onset between age 4 and 9 years, dementia progressing to complete amentia and an akinetic mute state, grand mal and minor motor seizures, progressive dystonia of posture with tendency to flexion of the arms, hyperextension of the spine and extension of the legs, but without torsion dystonia, clumsiness and mild atypical ataxia, some intention tremor and athetosis, grasp reflexes and severe reflex trismus in the final stages, tendency to hyperreflexia but preservation of fair strength and normal plantar reflexes until late. Notably absent were retinal degeneration, myoclonus, prominent pyramidal or bulbar involvement and hepatosplenomegaly. In one case foam histiocytes were demonstrated in the bone marrow. Cerebral sphingolipids in biopsy-obtained material were normal. Electronmicroscopic findings supported the distinctness of this entity (Elfenbein, 1968). The case reported by Kidd (1967) is thought to be identical.

DeLeon, G. A., Kaback, M. M., Elfenbein, I. B., Percy, A. K. and Brady, R. O.: Juvenile dystonia lipidosis. Johns Hopkins Med. J. 125: 62-77, 1969.

Elfenbein, I. B.: Dystonic juvenile idiocy without amaurosis. A new syndrome. Johns Hopkins Med. J. 123: 205-221, 1968.

Kidd, M.: An electronmicroscopic study of a case of atypical cerebral lipidosis. Acta Neuropath. 9: 70-78, 1967.

*24710 LIPOID PROTEINOSIS OF URBACH AND WIETHE (LIPOPROTEINOSIS; HYALINOSIS CUTIS ET MUCOSAE)

The association of early hoarseness with an unusual skin eruption suggests this diagnosis. Cutaneous and

R
E
C
E
S
S
I
V
E

mucosal infiltrations may take protean forms. Lipids of the blood may be elevated. Definitive information on the biological behavior, e.g., age of onset, prognosis, etc., is not available. Most of the cases have been described on an ad hoc basis by dermatologists or laryngologists. Multiple cases, male and female, in sibships and frequent parental consanguinity make recessive inheritance very likely. Papular infiltration of the margin of the lids producing 'itchy eyes,' and infiltration in the tongue and its frenulum, in the larynx leading to hoarseness and in the skin (e.g., elbows and axilla) is characteristic. Erythropoietic protoporphyria (q.v.) is sometimes mis-diagnosed lipoid proteinosis. The gene is said to be unusually frequent in South Africa. A disturbance in mucopolysaccharide metabolism was suggested by Moynahan (1966). In the family reported by Rosenthal and Duke (1967), a mother, 3 sons and a daughter were affected but the father was a first cousin of the mother. Thus quasi-dominant pedigree pattern resulting from consanguinity is likely. Almost a quarter of all reported cases of lipoid proteinosis have been in residents of South Africa. Recessive inheritance is well documented by the study of Gordon et al. (1969) of numerous cases in an inbred South African community. Newton et al. (1971) reported an affected brother and sister of Lebanese extraction whose parents were second cousins and who manifested neuropyschiatric symptoms including seizures, memory defects and rage attacks. The authors stressed the presence of specific intracranial calcifications which they considered pathognomonic of the disease. By electronmicroscopy they found filamentous-like material in skin lesions but its composition could not be defined.

Beurey, J., Neimann, N., Pierson, M., Tridon, P., Sapelier and Medlin, P.: Maladie Durbach-Wiethe familiale avec indifference a la douleur. Arch. Belg. Derm. Syph. 19: 310-312, 1964.

Blodi, F. C., Whinery, R. D. and Hendricks, C. A.: Lipid-proteinosis (Urbach-Wiethe) involving the lids. Trans. Am. Ophthal. Soc. 58: 155-166, 1960.

Burnett, J. W. and Marcy, S. M.: Lipoid proteinosis. Am. J. Dis. Child. 105: 81-84, 1963.

Caplan, R. M.: Lipoid proteinosis: a review including some new observations. Univ. Mich. Med. Bull. 28: 365-377, 1962.

Gordon, H., Gordon, W., Botha, V. and Edelstein, I.: Lipoid proteinosis. The Clinical Delineation of Birth Defects. XII. Skin, Hair and Nails. Baltimore: Williams and Wilkins, 1971. Pp. 164-177.

Gordon, H., Gordon, W. and Botha, V.: Lipoid proteinosis in an inbred Namaqualand community. Lancet I: 1032-1035, 1969.

Hewson, S. E.: Lipidproteinosis (Urbach-Wiethe syndrome). Brit. J. Ophthal. 47: 242-245, 1963.

Heyl, T.: Genealogy of lipoid proteinosis. (Letter) Lancet II: 162-163, 1969.

Laymon, C. W. and Hill, E. M.: An appraisal of hyalinosis cutis et mucosae. Arch. Derm. 75: 55-65, 1957.

Moynahan, E. J.: Hyalinosis cutis et mucosae (lipoid proteinosis). Demonstration of a new disorder of macopolysaccharide metabolism. Proc. Roy. Soc. Med. 59: 1125-1126, 1966.

Newton, F. H., Rosenberg, R. N., Lampert, P. W. and O'Brien, J. S.: Neurological involvement in Urbach-Wiethe's disease (lipoid proteinosis): a clinical, ultrastructrual, and chemical study. Neurology 21: 1205-1213, 1971.

Rosenthal, A. R. and Duke, J. R.: Lipoid proteinosis: case report of direct lineal transmission. Am. J. Ophthal. 64: 1120-1124, 1967.

Scott, F. P. and Findlay, G. H.: Hyalinosis cutis et mucosae (lipoid proteinosis). S. Afr. Med. J. 34: 189-195, 1960.

Urbach, E. and Wiethe, C.: Lipoidosis cutis et mucosae. Virchow. Arch. Path. Anat. 273: 285-319, 1929.

R
E
C
E
S
S
I
V
E

*24720 LISSENCEPHALY SYNDROME

Lissencephaly means 'smooth brain,' i.e., brain without convolutions or gyri. Miller (1963) described this condition in a brother and sister who were the fifth and sixth children of unrelated parents. The features were microcephaly, small mandible, bizarre facies, failure to thrive, retarded motor development, dysphagia, decorticate and decerebrate postures, and death at 3 and 4 months. Autopsy showed anomalies of the brain, kidney, heart and gastrointestinal tract. The brains were smooth with large ventricles and a histologic architecture more like normal fetal brain of 3-4 months gestation. Dieker et al. (1969) described two affected brothers and an affected female maternal first cousin. They also emphasized that this should be termed the lissencephaly syndrome because malformations of the heart, kidneys and other organs are associated, as well as polydactyly, unusual facial appearance.

Reznik and Alberca-Serrano (1964) described two brothers with congenital hypertelorism, mental defect, intractable epilepsy, progressive spastic paraplegia and death at ages 19 and 9 years. The mother showed hypertelorism and short-lived epileptiform attacks. Autopsy showed lissencephaly with massive neuronal heterotopies and large ventricular cavities of embryonic type. (The findings in the mother make X-linked recessive inheritance a possibility.) The patients of Reznik and Alberca-Serrano (1964) may have suffered from a disorder distinct from that of Miller (1963) and Dieker et al. (1969). All these cases are idiots. None learned to speak. They may walk by 3 to 5 years but spastic diplegia with spastic gait is evident. As in other forms of stationary fore-brain developmental anomalies, decerebrate posturing with head retraction emerges in the first year of life.

Dieker, H., Edwards, R. H., ZuRhein, G., Chou, S. M., Hartman, H. A. and Opitz, J. M.: The lissencephaly syndrome. The Clinical Delineation of Birth Defects. II. Malformation Syndromes. New York: Nation Foundation, 1969. Pp. 53-64.

Miller, J. Q.: Lissencephaly in 2 siblings. Neurology 13: 841-850, 1963.

Reznik, M. and Alberca-Serrano, R.: Forme familiale d'hypertelorisme avec lissencephalie se presentant cliniquement sous forme d'une arrieration mentale avec epilepsie et paraplegie spasmodique. J. Neurol. Sci. 1: 40-58, 1964.

24730 LIVER CANCER

Kaplan and Cole (1965) described primary liver cancer in 3 brothers. Recessive inheritance is, of course, not proved. X-linked recessive inheritance is as plausible as autosomal recessive.

Kaplan, L. and Cole, S. L.: Fraternal primary hepatocellular carcinoma in three males, adult siblings. Am. J. Med. 39: 305-311, 1965.

24740 LOW BIRTH WEIGHT DWARFISM WITH SKELETAL DYSPLASIA

Taybi and Linder (1967) described brother and sister, of Italian extraction with first-cousin parents, who had low birth weight dwarfism, dysplasia of the osseous skeleton including the skull, microcephaly, and death at ages 1 month and 1 year. Autopsy was done in both. Extensive malformation of the brain was present. Taybi (1974) was aware of no other similar case.

Taybi, H. and Linder, D.: Congenital familial dwarfism with cephaloskeletal dysplasia. Radiology 89: 275-281, 1967.

Tayli, H.: Oakland, Calif., personal communication, 1974.

24743 LYMPHOBLASTIC TRANSFORMATION, INHIBITION OF

In cases of mucocutaneous candidiasis, Paterson et al. (1971) found that the patients' plasma inhibited in the vitro proliferative resonse of their own lymphocytes to various antigens.

Paterson, P. Y., Semo, R., Blumerschein, G. and Swelstad, J.: Mucocutaneous candidiasis, anergy and a plasma inhibitor of cellular immunity: reversal after amphotericin B therapy. Clin. Exp. Immunol. 9: 595-602.

24745 LYMPHOBLASTIC TRANSFORMATION, INTRINSIC DEFECT IN

In a patient with chronic mucocutaneous candidiasis, Buckley et al. (1968) found a decrease in the number of lymphocytes capable of transformation in response to in vitro phytothemagglutinin stimulation.

Buckley, R. H., Lucas, Z. J., Hattler, B. G., Jr., Zmijewski, C. M. and Amos, D. B.: Defective cellular immunity associated with chronic mucocutaneous moniliasis and recurrent staphylococcal botryomycosis immunologial reconstruction by allogenic bone marrow. Clin. Exp. Immunol. 3: 153-169, 1968.

24750 LYMPHOHISTIOCYTIC INFILTRATION, GENERALIZED

Nelson and colleagues (1961) claim that the disorder they describe is quite different from Letterer-Siwe disease (q.v.) and presumably also from histophagocytic (or hemophagocytic) reticulosis (q.v.). Chediak-Higashi syndrome (q.v.) has only partial similarity. Mozziconacci and colleagues (1965) described two brothers, ages 6 and 8, with this fatal disease characterized by high and irregular fever, hepatosplenomegaly, purpura, and later jaundice, polyneuritis, meningeal reaction, choked disks, moderate anemia and severe granulocytopenia. The possible relationship to ceroid storage disease (21420) is only speculative.

Landing, B. H., Strauss, L., Crocker, A. C., Braunstein, H., Henley, W. L., Will, J. R. and Sanders, M.: Thrombocytopenic purpura with histiocytosis of the spleen. New Eng. J. Med. 265: 572-576, 1961.

Mozziconacci, P., Nezelof, C., Attal, C., Girard, F., Pham-Huu-Trung, (NI)., Weil, J., Desbuquois, B. and Gadot, M.: La lympho-histiocytose familiale. Arch. Franc. Pediat. 22: 385-408, 1965.

Nelson, P., Santamaria, A., Olson, R. L. and Nayak, N. C.: Generalized lymphohistiocytic infiltration. A familial disease not previously described and different from Letterer-Siwe disease and Chediak-Higashi syndrome. Pediatrics 27: 931950, 1961.

24760 LYMPHOHISTIOCYTOSIS OF NERVOUS SYSTEM

Price et al. (1971) described four out of 12 sibs with a progressive neurologic disease characterized by diffuse lymphohistiocytic infiltrations of the central nervous system in association with multiple foci of parenchymal destruction. The range of age at death was 15 months to 12 years. The spinal fluid showed pleocytosis and increased protein. Histologically the disorder resembled familial hemophagocytic reticulosis or familial erythrophagocytic lymphohistiocytosis but unlike these conditions the process was largely confirmed to the CNS.

Price, D. L., Woolsey, J. E., Rosman, N. P. and Richardson, E. P., Jr.: Familial lymphohistiocytosis of the nervous system. Arch. Neurol. 24: 270-283, 1971.

24763 LYMPHOID SYSTEM DETERIORATION, PROGRESSIVE

Seeger et al. (1970) described brother and sister with a 'new' immunologic disorder, characterized by defective cellular and humoral immunity, associated bone marrow aplasia, deficiency of IgG and IgM with normal IgA. One patient developed graft-versus-host reaction as a complication of blood transfusion. Lymphopenia and candidiasis developed. The progressive nature beginning in the second year of life was emphasized.

Seeger, R. C., Amman, A. J., Good, R. A. and Hong, R.: Progressive lymphoid system deterioration: a new familial lymphopenic immunological deficiency disease. Clin. Exp. Immun. 6: 169-180, 1970.

24765 LYMPHOKINE DEFICIENCY

Chronic mucocutaneous candidiasis can have many causes, e. g. (1) failure of lymphocytes to transform in response to antigen, either because of an intrinsic defect (24757) or because of an inhibiting serum factor

(24755); (2) failure of production of lymphokine; (3) unresponsiveness of monocytes to lymphokine (25225). Deficient production of lymphokine despite normal lymphoblastic transformation was demonstrated by Lehner et al. (1972).

Lehner, T., Wilton, J. M. A. and Ivanyi, L.: Immunodeficiencies in chronic mucocutaneous candidiasis. Immunology 22: 775-787, 1972.

*24780 LYMPHOPENIC HYPERGAMMAGLOBULINEMIA, ANTIBODY DEFICIENCY, AUTO-IMMUNE HEMOLYTIC ANEMIA AND GLOMERULONEPHRITIS

Schaller et al., (1966) described an infant with these features plus marked lymphoid hypoplasia, absence of lymphoid elements and Hassall corpuscles from thymus and plasmocytosis. She died at 6 months with pneumocystis carinii pneumonia. Two sibs succumbed apparently from the same ailment.

Schaller, J., Davis, S. D., Ching, Y. C., Lagunoff, D., Williams, C. P. S. and Wedgwood, R. J.: Hypergammaglobulinaemia, antibody deficiency, autoimmune haemolytic anaemia, and nephritis in an infant with a familial lymphopenic immune defect. Lancet II: 825-829, 1966.

*24790 LYSINE INTOLERANCE

Colombo and colleagues (1964) described episodic vomiting, rigidity and coma in an infant, relieved by low protein diet. During coma, ammonia was high in the blood and the amino acids lysine and arginine were also high. Defect in degradation of lysine was proposed. Lysine is a potent competitive inhibitor of arginase. As a result urea synthesis and ammonia detoxication are interfered with. Colombo et al. (1967) demonstrated a defect in L-lysine: NAD-oxido-reductase activity in liver. This apparently is responsible for accumulation of lysine. Hyperlysinemia (q.v.) is a separate entity.

Colombo, J. P., Burgi, W., Richterich, R. and Rossi, E.: Congenital lysine intolerance with periodic ammonia intoxication: a defect in L-lysine degradation. Metabolism 16: 910-925, 1967.

Colombo, J. P., Richterich, R., Donath, A., Spahr, A. and Rossi, E.: Congenital lysine intolerance with periodic ammonia intoxication. Lancet I: 1014-1015, 1964.

Colombo, J. P., Vassella, F., Humbel, R. and Burgi, W.: Lysine intolerance with periodic ammonia intoxication. Am. J. Dis. Child. 113: 138-141, 1967.

24800 MACROCEPHALY (MEGELENCEPHALY)

Walsh (1957) described three affected sibs with normal parents. At least two of the three were female. Mental defect and optic atrophy were present. In another family two sibs may have been affected. Of course, a large head occurs with hydrocephalus and with gargoylism and is also a feature of Canavan disease. Weil (1933) described the case of a male in which at autopsy the brain (at age 7 years) weighed 1856 gm. The precentral area was underdeveloped as were also skeletal musculature and the adrenal medullas. Mental development had been normal until age 6. A brother had a large head but was well at age 12 years. The possibility of X-linked recessive macrocephaly was raised by Waisman (1967). Differentiation from X-linked stenosis of the aqueduct of Sylvius is necessary. De Almeida and Debarros (1964) observed parental consanguinity.

De Almeida, G. and Debarros, N.: Megalencefalia: consideracones a respecto de 7 casos diagnosticados en vida. Arq. Neuropsiquiat. 22: 25, 1964.

DeMyer, W.: Megalencephaly in children: clinical syndromes, genetic patterns, and differential diagnosis from other causes of megalocephaly. Neurology 22: 634-643, 1972.

Waisman, H. A.: Madison, Wis.: personal communication, 1967.

Walsh, F. B.: Clinical Neuro-ophthalmology. Baltimore: Williams and Wilkins, 1957 (2nd Ed.). Pp. 402-404.

Weil, A.: Megalencephaly with diffuse glioblostomatosis of the brain stem and the cerebellum. Arch. Neurol. Psychiat. 30: 795-809, 1933.

24810 MACROSOMIA ADIPOSA CONGENITA

Christiansen (1929) described a Danish kindred in which 7 infants (6 females, 1 male), the offspring of sisters by presumably unrelated husbands, developed gross obesity beginning soon after birth. Precocious skeletal development was evident in the ossification centers and teeth. Marked voracity was a feature. Relative eosinophilia and low vitality with death of five of the children in the first year were noted. Adrenocortical adenomas were found at autopsy. The nature of the disorder is obscure.

Christiansen, T.: Macrosomia adiposa congenita. A new dysendocrine syndrome of familial occurrence. Endocrinology 13: 149-163, 1929.

*24820 MACULAR DEGENERATION, JUVENILE

Degeneration limited to the macular area of the retina was described in multiple sibs by Ford (1961) and by Walsh (1957). Typically onset is in early or middle childhood. Sometimes the condition has been called central retinitis pigmentosa or retinitis pigmentosa with macular involvement. However, ordinary retinitis pigmentosa does not affect the macula. Homozygosity at any one of several loci is probably capable of producing this phenotype. Krill and Deutman (1972) gave a useful evaluation. They concluded that recessive macular dystrophy was the disorder described and beautifully illustrated by Stargardt (1909) and the same as the disorder which was renamed fundus flavimaculatus (see 23010) by Franceschetti (1963). Onset is in the first two decades of life. The possibility of a rarer autosomal dominant form, indistinguishable phenotypically, was suggested by Krill and Deutman (1972).

RECESSIVE

Ford, F. R.: Diseases of the Nervous System in Infancy, Childhood and Adolescence. Springfield, Ill.: Charles C Thomas, 1961. Pp. 358-359.

Franceschetti, A.: Ueber tapeto-retinale Degenerationen in Kindesalter. In, Entwicklung und Fortschitt in der Augenkeilkunde. Stuttgart: Enke Verlag, 1963. Pp. 107-120.

Krill, A. E. and Deutman, A. F.: The various categories of juvenile macular degeneration. Trans. Am. Ophtlal. Soc. 70: 220-245, 1972.

Stargardt, K.: Ueber familiare, progressive Degeneration in der Makulagegend des Auges. Graefe Arch. Ophthal. 71: 534-549, 1909.

Walsh, F. B.: Clinical Neuro-ophthalmology. Baltimore: Williams and Wilkins, 1957 (2nd Ed.). Pp. 673-674.

Wright, R. E.: Familial macular degeneration. Brit. J. Ophthal. 19: 160-165, 1935.

*24830 MAL DE MELEDA (KERATOSIS PALMO-PLANTARIS TRANSGRADIENS OF SIEMENS)

Congenital symmetrical cornification of the palms and soles with ichthyotic changes elsewhere characterize this disorder which derives its name from its relatively high frequency among inhabitants of the Island of Meleda, Dalmatia, Yugoslavia. Bosnjakovic (1938) studied the family in Mljet (or Meleda). Schnyder et al. (1969) provided more recent observations. Hyperhidrosis, perioral erythema and lichenoid plaques were also noted. Franceschetti et al. (1972) also made a recent study.

Bosnjakovic, S.: Vererbungsverhaeltnisse bei der sog. Krankheit von Mljet ('Mal de Meleda'). Acta Dermatovenen. 19: 88-122, 1938.

Franceschetti, A., Peinhart, V. and Schnyder, U. W.: La maladie de Meleda. J. Genet. Hum. 20: 267-296, 1972.

Niles, H. D. and Klumpp, M. M.: Mal de Meleda: review of the literature and report of four cases. Arch. Derm. Syph. 39: 409-421, 1939.

Salamon, T. and Lazovic, O.: Contribution au probleme de la maladie de Mljet (mal de Meleda). J. Genet. Hum. 10: 172-201, 1961.

Schnyder, U. W., Franceschetti, A., Ceszarovic, B. and Segedin, J.: La maladie de Meleda autochtone. Ann. Derm. Syph. 96: 517-530, 1969.

24837 MANDIBULOACRAL DYSPLASIA

Young et al. (1971) and Sensenbrenner and Fiorelli (1971) each described a teen-age male with hypoplastic mandible producing severe dental crowding, acroosteolysis, stiff joints and atrophy of the skin over hands and feet. The boys had an 'Andy Grump' appearance. The clavicles were hypoplastic. Persistently wide cranial sutures and multiple Wormian bones were noted. The patients are somewhat short of stature (Cohen et al. 1973). Cleiodocranial dysplasia (11960) and acrogeria (20120) are other diagnoses entertained in these cases. Patients with this condition have been mistakenly diagnosed as having the Werner syndrome. Recessive inheritance seems quite certain with observation by Welsh (1974) of what I believe is the same disorder in two males and two females from a sibship of 14.

Cohen, L. K., Thurmon, T. F. and Salvaggio, J.: Werner syndrome. Cutis 12: 76-80, 1973.

Welsh, O.: Monterry, Mexico, personal communication, 1974.

Young, L. W., Radebaugh, J. F., Rubin, P., Sensenbrenner, J. A. and Fiorelli, G.: New syndrome manifested by mandibular hypoplasia, acroosteolysis, stiff joints and cutaneous atrophy (mandibuloacral dysplasia) in two unrelated boys. In Bergsma, D. (ed.): Clinical Delineation of Birth Defects. XI. Orofacial Structures. Baltimore: Williams and Wilkins, 1971. Pp. 291-297

24840 MANDIBULOFACIAL DYSOSTOSIS WITH MENTAL DEFICIENCY

Jancar (1961) described a family with possible recessive inheritance. The changes in the head were reminiscent of those of trisomy 17-18. However, in one of the affected males no abnormality of the chromosomes was detected.

Jancar, J.: Mandibulo-facial dysostosis (Berry-Franceschetti syndrome). J. Irish Med. Ass. 48: 145-148, 1961.

*24850 MANNOSIDOSIS

Ockerman (1967) described a boy who represented an isolated case of an apparently 'new' disorder. Susceptibility to infection, vomiting, coarse features, macroglossia, flat nose, large clumsy ears, widely spaced teeth, large head, big hands and feet, tall stature, slight hepatosplenomegaly, muscular hypotonia, lumbar gibbus, radiographic skeletal abnormalities, dilated cerebral ventricles, lenticular opacities, hypogammaglobulinemia, 'storage cells' in the bone marrow, and vacuolated lymphocytes in the bone marrow and blood were features. Histologic study showed storage of material (not acid mucopolysaccharide) in cerebral cortex, brain stem, spinal medulla, neurohypophysis, retina and myenteric plexus. Total mannose in the liver was strikingly increased. Alpha-mannosidase activity in all tissues studied was abnormally low whereas other acid hydrolases had higher activities than normal. Only one patient has been observed. He died at the age of four and one half years during an attack of increased intracranial pressure. Mannosidosis is known in cattle where the disorder is a recessive (Jolly, 1972). Hocking et al. (1972) described mannosidosis in cattle. The disease is manifest by head tremor, aggressive tendency, ataxia, failure to thrive and early death. Ockerman et al. (1973) referred to identification of the disease in two Hungarian sisters and three Finnish boys including two brothers. A procedure for the study of low-molecular-weight urinary compounds containing mannose was useful in the study of these cases. Normal liver alpha-mannosidosidase exists in at least 3 forms, separable by DEAE cellulose chromatography. The A and B forms are most active at pH 4.4 whereas form C is most active at pH 6.0. In two cases of mannosidosis, Carroll et al. (1972) found that forms A and B were missing.

Autio, S., Norden, N. E., Ockerman, P. A., Riekkinen, P., Rapola, J. and Louhimo, T.: Mannosidosis: clinical, fine-structural and biochemical findings in three cases. Acta Paediat. Scand. 62: 555-565, 1973.

Carroll, M., Dance, N., Masson, P. K., Robinson, D. and Winchester, B. G.: Human mannosidosis-the enzymic defect. Biochem. Biophys. Res. Commun. 49: 579-583, 1972.

Hocking, J. D., Jolly, R. D. and Batt, R. D.: Deficiency of alpha-mannosidase in Angus cattle. An inherited lysosomal storage disease. Biochem. J. 128: 69-78, 1972.

Hultberg, B.: Properties of alpha-mannosidase in mannosidosis. Scand. J. Clin. Lab. Invest. 26: 155-160, 1970.

Jolly, R. D.: Massey University, Palmerston North, New Zealand, 1972.

Kjellmann, B., Gamstorp, I., Brun, A., Ockerman, P. A. and Palmgren, B.: Mannosidosis: a clinical and histopathologic study. J. Pediat. 75: 366-373, 1969.

Ockerman, P. A.: A generalized storage disorder resembling Hurler's syndrome. Lancet II: 239-241, 1967.

Ockerman, P. A.: Mannosidosis: isolation of oligosaccharide storage material from brain. J. Pediat. 75: 360-365, 1969.

Ockerman, P. A., Autio, S. and Norder, N. E.: Diagnosis of mannosidosis. Lancet I: 207-208, 1973.

*24860 MAPLE SYRUP URINE DISEASE (BRANCHED-CHAIN KETOACIDURIA)

Features are mental and physical retardation, feeding problems and a maple syrup odor to the urine. The keto acids of leucine, isoleucine and valine are present in the urine, suggesting a block in oxidative decarboxylation. A mild variant has been reported which may be a separate entity (Morris et al., 1961). The keto acid of isoleucine (alpha-keto-beta-methylvalinic acid) is responsible for the characteristic odor. In two sibs of each of two families, Dancis, Hutzler and Rokkones (1967) observed a variant of MSUD. The children suffered from a transient neurologic disorder associated with elevation of branched-chain amino acids and their keto acids in, and a distinctive odor to, the urine. Late onset of symptoms and clinical normality between attacks differentiated the condition from regular MSUD. However, one sib of each family died during an attack. The level of leukocyte keto acid decarboxylase activity seemed to be higher than in the classic form of the disease. One must take the lymphocyte count into account in testing for heterozygotes. The relevant enzyme is in the lymphocytes and lymphocytopenia or lymphocytosis can give false positive or false negative tests for heterozygosity. Two Norwegian families with the intermittent form were described by Goedde et al. (1970). In this form only one parent shows decreased enzyme activity, as a rule. Schulman et al. (1970) described a patient affected with a variant. MSUD is sometimes effectively treated with thiamine. It is, therefore, a vitamin-response inborn error of metabolism. Variants for the intermittent type are usually mentally and neurologically normal except during episodes. Van der Horst and Wadman (1971) described an intermittent form with severe episodes of acidosis with mental retardation that was partially reversed on dietary therapy. Scriver et al. (1970) described a variant in which the hyperaminoacidemia was completely corrected by thiamine hydrochloride (10 mg. per day) without dietary restriction. In summary, there are four clinical variants of MSUD (Wong et al., 1972): (1) the classic form, a severe disorder; (2) the intermittent form (Dancis et al., 1967); (3) the intermediate form (Schulman et al., 1970); (4) the thiamine-responsive form. The relationship of the four to each other, e.g., whether allelic or non-allelic, is unknown. Lyons et al. (1973) sought heterogeneity in maple syrup urine disease by the study of heterokaryons derived from cultured fibroblasts of different patients. Fibroblasts from one patient consistently complemented (resulted in increase in the level of branched-chain keto acid decarboxylase), those from other particular patients showed lower enzyme activity than either parent. Correlation with clinical expression could not be made.

Dancis, J. and Levitz, M.: Abnormalities of branched-chain amino acid metabolism. In, Stanbury, J. B., Wyngaarden, J. B. and Fredrickson, D. S. (eds.): The Metabolic Basis of Inherited Disease. New York: McGraw-Hill, 1972 (3rd Ed.). Pp. 426-439.

Dancis, J., Hutzler, J. and Levitz, M.: The diagnosis of maple syrup disease (branched chain ketoaciduria) by the in vitro study of the peripheral leukocyte. Pediatrics 32: 234-238, 1963.

Dancis, J., Hutzler, J. and Rokkones, T.: Intermittent branched-chain ketonuria. Variant of maple-syr-up-urine disease. New Eng. J. Med. 276: 84-89, 1967.

Dancis, J., Levitz, M. and Westall, R. G.: Maple syrup urine disease: branched-chain ketoaciduria. Pediatrics 25: 72-79, 1960.

Goedde, H. W., Langenbeck, U. and Brackertz, D.: Detection of heterozygotes in maple syrup urine disease: role of lymphocyte count. Humangenetik 6: 189-190, 1968.

Goedde, H. W., Langenbeck, U., Brackertz, D., Keller, W., Rokkones, T., Halvorsen, S., Kiil, R. and Merton, B.: Clinical and biochemical-genetic aspects of intermittent branched-chain ketoaciduria. Report of two Scandinavian families. Acta Paediat. Scand. 59: 83-87, 1970.

Kalyanaraman, K., Chamukuttan, S., Arjundas, G., Gajanan, N. and Ramamurthi, B.: Maple syrup urine disease (branched-chain keto-aciduria). Variant type manifesting as hyperkinetic behaviour and mental retardation. Report of two cases. J. Neurol. Sci. 15: 209-218, 1972.

Kiil, R. and Rokkones, T.: Late manifesting variant of branched-chain ketoaciduria: (maple syrup urine disease). Acta Paediat. 53: 356-364, 1964.

Lyons, L. B., Cox, R. P. and Dancis, J.: Complementation analysis of maple syrup urine disease in heterokaryons derived from cultured human fibroblasts. Nature 243: 533-535, 1973.

Morris, M. D., Fisher, D. A. and Fiser, R.: Late-onset branched-chain ketoaciduria: (maple syrup urine disease). J. Lancet 86: 149-152, 1966.

Morris, M. D., Lewis, B. D., Doolan, P. D. and Harper, H. A.: Clinical and biochemical observations on an apparently nonfatal variant of branched-chain ketoaciduria (maple syrup urine disease). Pediatrics 28: 918-923, 1961.

Norton, P. M., Roitman, E., Snyderman, S. E. and Holt, L. E., Jr.: A new finding in maple-syrup-urine disease. Lancet I: 26-27, 1962.

Schulman, J. D., Lustberg, T. J., Kennedy, J. L., Museles, M. and Seegmiller, J. E.: A new variant of maple syrup urine disease (branched-chain ketoaciduria). Clinical and biochemical evaluation. Am. J. Med. 49: 118-124, 1970.

Scriver, C. R., MacKenzie, S., Clow, C. L. and Delvin, E.: Thiamine-responsive maple-syrup-urine disease. Lancet I: 310-312, 1971.

Snyderman, S. E.: The therapy of maple syrup urine disease. Am. J. Dis. Child. 113: 68-73, 1967.

Valman, H. B., Patrick, H. B., Seakins, A. D., Platt, J. W. and Gompertz, D.: Family with intermittent maple syrup urine disease. Arch. Dis. Child. 48: 225-228, 1973.

Van der Horst, J. L. and Wadman, S. K.: A variant form of branched-chain keto aciduria. Case report. Acta Paediat. Scand. 60: 594-599, 1971.

Wong, P. W. K., Justice, P., Smith, G. F. and Hsia, D. Y.-Y.: A case of classical maple syrup urine disease, 'thiamine non-responsive.' Clin. Genet. 3: 27-33, 1972.

Woody, N. C. and Harris, J. A.: Family screening studies in maple syrup urine disease (branched-chain ketoaciduria). J. Pediat. 66: 1042-1048, 1965.

*24870 MARDEN-WALKER SYNDROME

Marden and Walker (1966) described an infant with blepharophimosis, micrognathia, immobile facies, kyphoscoliosis, limb contractures, pigeon breast and arachnodactyly. There was microcystic disease of the kidney. The infant died at three months of age. In some respects the case resembled the sibs with myotonia myopathy, etc. (q.v.) described by Aberfeld et al. (1965). Fitch et al. (1971) reported a case similar in facial appearance to Marden and Walker's. Their patient's severe joint contractures largely disappeared by 6 months of age. Pneumoencephalography showed cerebellar and brain stem hypoplasia. Temtamy (1972) has shown me identical cases in two first-cousin males who in each instance had first-cousin parents.

Marden, P. M. and Walker, W. A.: A new generalized connective tissue syndrome. Am. J. Dis. Child. 112: 225-228, 1966.

Fitch, N., Karpati, G. and Pinsky, L.: Congenital blepharophimosis, joint contractures, and muscular hypotonia. Neurology 21: 1214-1220, 1971.

Temtamy, S. A.: Cairo, Egypt: personal communication, 1972.

*24880 MARINESCO-SJOGREN SYNDROME

Cerebellar ataxia, congenital cataracts, retarded somatic and mental maturation are the cardinal features. Alter and his colleagues (1962) suggested the designation 'hereditary oligophrenic cerebellolental degeneration.' Garland and Moorhouse (1953) published a striking pedigree. A dominantly inherited syndrome of cataract and ataxia is also known. In a boy almost 5 years old Todorov (1965) found the brain lesions limited almost exclusively to the cerebellum which showed massive cortical atrophy. Many of the Purkinje cells which remained were vacuolated or binucleated.

Alter, M., Talbert, O. R. and Croffead, G.: Cerebellar ataxia, congenital cataracts and retarded somatic and mental maturation. Report of cases of Marinesco-Sjogren syndrome. Neurology 12: 836-847, 1962.

Franceschetti, A., Klein, D., Wildi, E. and Todorov, A.: Le syndrome de Marinesco-Sjogren. Premiere verification anatomique. Arch. Suisses Neur. Neurochir. Psychiat. 97: 234-240, 1966.

Garland, H. and Moorhouse, D.: An extremely rare recessive hereditary syndrome including cerebellar ataxia, oligophrenia, cataract, and other features. J. Neurol. Neurosurg. Psychiat. 16: 110-116, 1953.

Sjogren, T.: Hereditary congenital spinocerebellar ataxia accompanied by congenital cataract and oligophrenia. A genetic and clinical investigation. Confin. Neurol. 10: 293-308, 1950.

Sjogren, T.: Hereditary congenital spinocerebellar ataxia combined with congenital cataract and oligophrenia. Acta Psychiat. Neurol. Scand. 46 (suppl.): 286-289, 1947.

Todorov, A.: Le syndrome de Marinesco-Sjogren: premiere etude anatomo-clinique. J. Genet. Hum. 14: 197-233, 1965.

*24890 MAST SYNDROME

In an Ohio Amish isolate Cross and McKusick (1967) found 20 cases of a recessively inherited form of presenile dementia which they termed Mast syndrome. Onset in the late teens or twenties and slow progression with development of spastic paraparesis and basal ganglion manifestations were features.

Cross, H. E. and McKusick, V. A.: The Mast syndrome: a recessively inherited form of presenile dementia with motor disturbances. Arch. Neurol. 16: 1-13, 1967.

R
E
C
E
S
S
I
V
E

This condition is also called dysencephalia splanchnocystica and Gruber syndrome (1934). Opitz and Howe (1969) suggested it be called Meckel syndrome because of Meckel's clear description (1822). Although a great variety of malformations have been observed and no single malformation is invariably present or unique to Meckel syndrome, a frequent and particularly memorable combination is sloping forehead, posterior exencephalocele, polydactyly and polycystic kidneys. Death occurs in the perinatal period. Numerous examples of affected sibs, concordance in presumably monozygotic twins (Stockard, 1921), roughly equal occurrence in males and females, and parental consanguinity in some instances (Tucker et al., 1966; Walbaum et al., 1967) make autosomal recessive inheritance quite certain. See editorial (1970) for biographical information on Meckel. Simopoulos et al. (1967) described three male sibs with polycystic kidneys, internal hydrocephalus and postaxial polydactyly. The parents were not related. Hsia et al. (1971) described seven cases in two sibships: two sets of monozygotic twins in one and three sibs in another. Although many of the features suggest trisomy 13, occipital encephalocele has apparently never been observed in the chromosomal aberration. Meckel and Passarge (1972) reported two affected sisters.

Anon.: Editorial: Johann Friedrich Meckel, the younger (1781-1833). J.A.M.A. 214: 138-139, 1970.

Gruber, G. B.: Beitrage zur Frage 'gekoppelter' Missbildungen. (Akrocephalo-Syndactylie und Dysencephalia Splanchnocystica). Beitr. Path. Anat. 93: 459-476, 1934.

Hsia, Y. E., Bratu, M. and Herbordt, A.: Genetics of the Meckel syndrome (dysencephalia splanchnocystica). Pediatrics 48: 237-247, 1971.

Meckel, S. and Passarge, E.: Encephalocele, polycystic kidneys, and polydactyly as an autosomal recessive trait similating certain other disorders: the Meckel syndrome. Ann. Genet. 14: 97-103, 1971.

Meckel, J. F.: Beschreibung zweier durch sehr ahnliche Bildungsabweichungen entstellter Geschwister. Deutsch. Arch. Physiol. 7: 99-172, 1822.

Naffah, J., Ghosn, G. and Gharios, N.: Three new cases of Meckel's syndrome or Gruber's dysencephalia splanchnocystica in siblings. Arch. Fran. Pediat. 29: 1069-1082, 1972.

Opitz, J. M. and Howe, J. J.: The Meckel syndrome (dysencephalia splanchnocystica, the Gruber syndrome). The Clinical Delineation of Birth Defects. II. Malformation Syndromes. New York: National Foundation, 1969. Pp. 167-179.

Simopoulos, A. P., Brennan, G. G., Alwan, A. and Fidis, N.: Polycystic kidneys, internal hydrocephalus and polydactylism in newborn siblings. Pediatrics 39: 931-934, 1967.

Stockard, C. R.: Developmental rate and structural expression: an experimental study of twins, 'double monsters' and single deformities, and the interaction among embryonic organs during their origin and development. Am. J. Anat. 28: 115277, 1921.

Tucker, C. C., Finley, S. C., Tucker, E. S. and Finley, W. H.: Oral-facial-digital syndrome, with polycystic kidneys and liver: pathological and cytogenetic studies. J. Med. Genet. 3: 145-147, 1966.

Walbaum, R., Dehaene, P. and Duthoit, F.: Polydactylie familiale avec dysplasie neuro-cranienne. Ann. Genet. 10: 39-41, 1967.

R
E
C
E
S
S
I
V
E

*24910 MEDITERRANEAN FEVER, FAMILIAL

This disease occurs mainly in Armenians and Sephardic Jews (those who left Spain during the Inquisition and settled in various countries bordering the Mediterranean). Features include short recurrent bouts of fever accompanied by pain in the abdomen, chest or joints and an erysipelas-like erythema. The sedimentation rate is increased, but the white count is usually normal. Many of the patients have been subjected to one or more needless laparotomies. Amyloidosis is a complication and may develop without overt crises of the above description. Sohar and his colleagues (1967) estimated that in some Jewish groups the phenotype frequency is 1 in 2720 and that the minimal estimates for gene frequency and heterozygote frequency are 1 in 52 and 1 in 26, respectively. The possibility that the disorder in Armenians is distinct from that in Sephardic Jews is suggested by the alleged rarity of amyloidosis and efficacy of low-fat diet in Armenian cases. This condition is called 'familial paroxysmal peritonitis' by Siegal (1964) who was the first to delineate the disorder clearly in this country and who has observed rather numerous cases in Ashkenazi Jews. The number of Ashkenazic cases observed in Israel by Sohar et al. (1967) is sufficient to make it not surprising that a fair number of cases are observed in the large Ashkenazic group in the United States. In Turkey many cases of FMF are observed in persons without known Armenian ancestry (Sokmen, 1959).

Under the term periodic peritonitis, Reimann et al. (1954) described many cases from Lebanon, most of them Armenian. In one remarkable family, survivors of the seige of Musa Dagh, 20 affected persons occurred in five generations. There were 3 instances of skips in the pedigree. Conceivably high gene frequency and small breeding group can account for the findings. Certainly the distribution of cases in the United States is much more suggestive of recessive than of dominant inheritance. Reich and Franklin (1970) described a 79-year-old Sicilian with intestinal amyloidosis whose daughter and grandaughter had attacks of fever and abdominal pain. The Italian extraction, long survival and 3 generation involvement is unusual for FMF. Goldfinger (1972) claims benefit from colchicine in reducing painful attacks in FMF. A beneficial effect of colchicine was demonstrated by Wolff et al. (1974).

Dormer, A. E. and Hale, J. F.: Familial Mediterranean fever, a cause of periodic fever. Brit. Med. J. 1: 87-89, 1962.

Ehrenfeld, E. N., Eliakim, M. and Rachmilewitz, M.: Recurrent polyserositis (familial Mediterranean fever: periodic disease). A report of fifty-five cases. Am. J. Med. 31: 107-123, 1961.

Goldfinger, S. E.: Colchicine for familial Mediterranean fever. (Letter) New Eng. J. Med. 287: 1302 only, 1972.

Heller, H., Sohar, E., Gafni, J. and Heller, J.: Amyloidosis in familial Mediterranean fever. Arch. Intern. Med. 107: 539-550, 1961.

Hurwich, B. J., Schwartz, J. and Goldfarb, S.: Record survival of siblings with familial Mediterranean fever, phenotypes 1 and 2. Arch. Intern. Med. 125: 308-311, 1970.

Lawrence, J. S. and Mellinkoff, S. M.: Familial Mediterranean fever. Trans. Ass. Am. Physicians 72: 111-121, 1959.

Ozdemir, A. I. and Sokmen, C.: Familial Mediterranean fever among the Turkish people. Am. J. Gastroent. 51: 311-316, 1969.

Reich, C. B. and Franklin, E. C.: Familial Mediterranean fever in an Italian family. Arch. Intern. Med. 125: 337-340, 1970.

Reimann, H. A., Moadie, J., Semerdijian, S. and Sahyoun, P. F.: Periodic peritonitis-heredity and pathology. Report of seventy-two cases. J.A.M.A. 154: 1254-1259, 1954.

Siegal, S.: Familial paroxysmal polyserositis. Analysis of fifty cases. Am. J. Med. 36: 893-918, 1964.

Sohar, E., Gafni, J., Pras, M., and Heller, H.: Familial Mediterranean fever. A survey of 470 cases and review of literature. Am. J. Med. 43: 227-253, 1967.

Sokmen, C.: Comment. Trans. Ass. Am. Physicians 72: 120-121, 1959.

Wolff, S. M., Dinarello, C. A., Dale, D. C., Goldfinger, S. E. and Alling, D. W.: Colchicine therapy of familial Mediterranean fever. (Abstract) Clin. Res. 22: 567A only, 1974.

24920 MEGACOLON, AGANGLIONIC (HIRSCHSPRUNG DISEASE)

In mice aganglionic megacolon is associated with piebald trait and inherited apparently as an autosomal recessive (Bielschowsky and Schofield, 1962). We know of a human case of heterochromia iridis and megacolon (R.C., 943266), congenital deafness also being present. Boggs and Kidd (1958) described sibs with absence of the innervation of the entire intestinal tract below the ligament of Treitz. It is noteworthy that Bodian and Carter (1963) found that in Hirschsprung disease, of which Boggs and Kidd's cases represent a variety, cases with extensive involvement of the gut were more likely to be familial. For the series of Hirschsprung disease as a whole they could not demonstrate simple Mendelian inheritance. Hirschsprung disease is probably multifactorial (polygenetic) in its causation. All multifactorial traits have a 'sliding' risk. Not only does the recurrence risk increase as the number of affected sibs increases, but it also is greater when involvement is more severe. Thus it is not unexpected that cases with more extensive involvement are more likely to be familial. Passarge (1967) arrived at a similar conclusion. Empiric risk figures were as follows: 7.2 percent for the sibs of an affected female, 2.6 percent for the sibs of an affected male. In at least four instances, parent-child involvement is known (Ehrenpreis, 1970). In all four cases, the parent was the mother. Aganglionic megacolon is clearly a heterogeneous category. It is a frequent finding in cases of trisomy 21 (mongolism). Six of 63 probands in the Passarge (1967) study were cases of mongolism. Skinner and Irvine (1973) described four unrelated patients with Hirschsprung, disease and profound congenital deafness. There were no stigmata of Waardenburg, syndrome, which is sometimes accompanied by megacolon (see 19350).

Bielschowsky, M. and Schofield, G. C.: Studies on megacolon in piebald mice. Aust. J. Exp. Biol. Med. Sci. 40: 395-403, 1962.

Bodian, M. and Carter, C. O.: A family study of Hirschsprung's disease. Ann. Hum. Genet. 26: 261-277, 1963.

Boggs, J. D. and Kidd, J. M.: Congenital abnormalities of intestinal innervation: absence of innervation of jejunum, ileum and colon in siblings. Pediatrics 21: 261-266, 1958.

Ehrenpreis, T.: Hirschsprung's Disease. Chicago: Year Book Medical Publishers, Inc., 1970.

Lane, P. W.: Association of megacolon with two recessive spotting genes in the mouse. J. Hered. 57: 29-31, 1966.

Passarge, E.: Genetic heterogeneity and recurrence risk of congenital intestinal aganglionosis. The Clinical Delineation of Birth Defects. XIII. G. I. Tract Including Liver and Pancreas. Baltimore: Williams and Wilkins, 1972. Pp. 63-67.

Passarge, E.: The genetics of Hirschsprung's disease. Evidence for heterogeneous etiology and a study of sixty-three families. New Eng. J. Med. 276: 138-143, 1967.

Skinner, R. and Irvine, D.: Hirschsprung disease and congenital deafness. J. Med. Genet. 10: 337-339, 1973.

24925 MEGALOBLASTIC ANEMIA DUE TO DIHYDROFOLATE REDUCTASE DEFICIENCY

Walters (1967) described an infant with megaloblastic anemia who responded to parenteral administration of 100 micrograms of N(5)-formyltetrahydrofolate but not to the same dose of folic acid. These findings suggested an abnormality in dihydrofolate reductase activity, a thesis confirmed by hepatic biopsy.

Walters, T. R.: Congenital megaloblastic anemia responsive to N(5)-formyltetrahydrofolic acid administration. J. Pediat. 70: 686-687, 1967.

24927 MEGALOBLASTIC ANEMIA, THIAMINE-RESPONSIVE

R
E
C
E
S
S
I
V
E

Rogers et al. (1969) described an 11-year-old girl with megaloblastic anemia responsive only to thiamine.
She also had diabetes mellitus, aminoaciduria, and sensorineural deafness.

Rogers, L. E., Porter, F. S. and Sidbury, J. B., Jr.: Thiamine-responsive megalobalstic anemia. J. Pediat. 74: 494-504, 1969.

24930 MEGALOCORNEA

Autosomal dominant inheritance is much rarer than X-linked recessive (q.v.). Megalocornea is an occasional feature of the Marfan syndrome.

Alaerts, L.: Familial megalocornea. Bull. Soc. Belg. Opthal. 92: 322-326, 1949.

Bonhomme, F.: Un cas de megalocornee. Bull. Soc. Ophtal. Franc. 49: 184-190, 1937.

Gredig, C.: Eine neue Vererbungsart der Megalocornea. Arch. Klaus Stift. Vererbungsforsch. 2: 79-89, 1926.

Klar, R.: Beitrage zur Frage der Megalokornea auf grund von Untersuchungen eines staroperierten Patienten und siener Sippe. Klin. Mbl. Augenheilk..104: 286-299, 1940.

24940 MELANOSIS, NEUROCUTANEOUS

This rare condition, associated skin and meningeal pigmentation, is potentially highly malignant. Death usually occurs in early childhood. No certain evidence of a Mendelian basis has been found. The condition is thought to be a congenital dysplasia of the neural crest.

Fox, H., Emery, J. L., Goodbody, R. A. and Yates, P. O.: Neuro-cutaneous melanosis. Arch. Dis. Child. 39: 508-516, 1964.

Reed, W. B., Becker, S. W., Becker, S. W., Jr. and Nickel, W. R.: Giant pigmented nevi melanoma, and leptomeningeal melanocytosis: a clinical and histopathological study. Arch. Derm. 91: 100-119, 1965.

Tveten, L.: Primary meningeal melanosis. A clinico-pathological report of two cases. Acta Path. Microbiol. Scand. 63: 1-10, 1965.

24950 MENTAL RETARDATION

Mental retardation is a leading feature of many phenotypes listed here, e.g., amaurotic idiocy, cystathioninuria, galactosemia, hyperglycinemia, ketoaciduria with mental deficiency and other features, aminoaciduria and other features, aniridia, atonia-astatic syndrome, cerebellar atrophy, cutis verticis gyrata, megaloblastic anemia, homocystinuria, the Laurence-Moon-Biedl syndrome, microcephaly, phenylketonuria, the Sjogren-Larsson syndrome, Smith syndrome, the mucopolysaccharidoses, methemoglobinemia and the several defects of thyroid hormone synthesis. In addition, studies in mental institutions such as those of Priest and colleagues (1961) and of Wright and colleagues (1959) show that mental retardation of unclassified type occurs in multiple sibs in a considerable number of cases. Some of these doubtless represent rare recessive disorders. Study of this group may reveal 'new' recessive diseases. See TRICHOMEGALY, etc.

Breg (1962) has in his classification of mental defect a waste-basket group, 'hereditary cerebral maldevelopment, not clinically classifiable.' Most of these cases are, he thinks, autosomal recessive disorders. Two or more sibs show intellectual impairment, usually in the low or middle grade range without other clinical or laboratory manifestations that permit further classification. Among 3,500 admissions to an institution for mental defectives he found 53 cases he so classified. In the same group 25 cases of phenylketonuria, 3 of goitrous cretinism, 39 of cerebral degenerative diseases (including the lipidoses and scleroses) and 20 of primary microcephaly were observed.

The study of Carson and Neill (1962) is illustrative of the type of chemical investigations which can be used to detect metabolic errors in an inbred population and specifically in cases of mental retardation. McMurray (1962) also reviewed the biochemical defects that have been identified in patients with mental retardation.

Morton (1960) arrived at the conclusion that homozygosity at any one of 69 loci may result in low-grade mental defect, that about 8 percent of such cases are recessive and that about a third of normal persons are heterozygous for a gene for low-grade mental defect. An estimate of 114 loci was arrived at by Dewey, Barrai, Morton and Mi (1965). Karlsson and colleagues (1961) used the same approach of studying families with multiple affected sibs. In the family reported by Friedman and Roy (1944) all 6 children of parents who were first cousins once removed but of normal intelligence were severely retarded with internal strabismus, hyperactive tendon reflexes and positive Babinskis. The mother was said to have an abnormal electroencephalogram, nystagmus and external strabismus. Maternal phenylketonuria (q.v.) can result in mental retardation in multiple sibs and the mother may appear normal. Dekaban (1958) described a family in which both parents had undifferentiated mental retardation as did also all three of their children. A brother of the father was also retarded. All four grandparents were of normal intelligence. He suggested that an accumulation of pedigrees in which both parents are affected would help elucidate the category of undifferentiated mental retardation.

Breg, W. R.: Genetic aspects of mental retardation. Quart. Rev. Pediat. 17: 9-23, 1962.

Carson, N. A. J. and Neill, D. W.: Metabolic abnormalities detected in a survey of mentally backward individuals in Northern Ireland. Arch. Dis. Child. 37: 505-513, 1962.

Dekaban, A. S.: Mental deficiency. Recessive transmission to all children by parents similarly affected. Arch. Neurol. Psychiat. 79: 123-131, 1958.

RECESSIVE

Dewey, W. J., Barrai, I., Morton, N. E. and Mi, M. P.: Recessive genes in severe mental defect. Am. J. Hum. Genet. 17: 237-256, 1965.

Friedman, A. P. and Roy, J. E.: An unusual familial syndrome. J. Nerv. Ment. Dis. 99: 42-44, 1944.

Karlsson, J. L., Kihara, H., Grant, J. and Nelson, T. L.: Metabolic disorders leading to mental deficiency. I. Screening for excessive urinary excretion of nitrogenous compounds. J. Ment. Defic. Res. 5: 17-29, 1961.

McMurray, W. C.: Biochemical genetics and mental retardation. Canad. Med. Ass. J. 87: 486-490, 1962.

Morton, N. E.: The mutational load due to detrimental genes in man. Am. J. Hum. Genet. 12: 348-364, 1960.

Priest, J. H., Thuline, H. C., Laveck, G. D. and Jarvis, D. B.: An approach to genetic factors in mental retardation. Studies of families containing at least two siblings admitted to a state institution for the retarded. Am. J. Ment. Defic. 66: 42-50, 1961.

Wright, S. W., Tarjan, G. and Eyer, L.: Investigation of families with two or more mentally defective siblings: clinical observations. Am. J. Dis. Child. 97: 445-456, 1959.

24960 MENTAL RETARDATION SYNDROME (MIETENS-WEBER TYPE)

Mietens and Weber (1966) described, in 4 of six offspring of unaffected parents, a syndrome consisting of mental retardation, corneal opacity, nystagmus, strabismus, small pinched nose, flexion contracture of the elbows, dislocation of head of radius, abnormally short ulna and radius, and clinodactyly. The parents were second cousins.

Mietens, C. and Weber, H.: A syndrome characterized by corneal opacity, nystagmus, flexion contracture of the elbows, growth failure, and mental retardation. J. Pediat. 69: 624-629, 1966.

24963 MENTAL RETARDATION, BUENOS AIRES TYPE

Among the children of a consanguineous mating, Mutchinick (1972) described two with an apparently distinctive syndrome of mental and physical retardation, peculiar facies and heart and renal malformations. True microcephaly and Seckel bird-headed dwarfism were suggested but for one or another reason did not satisfy the features of these cases.

Mutchinick, O.: A syndrome of mental and physical retardation, speech disorders, and peculiar facies in two sisters. J. Med. Genet. 9: 60-63, 1972.

R
E
C
E
S
S
I
V
E

*24965 MERCAPTOLACTATE-CYSTEINE DISULFIDURIA

Only one patient has been observed, but the fact that the parents were brother and sister strongly supports recessive inheritance. The patient, a male aged 45, had a low IQ, grand mal seizures, flattened nasal bridge and excessively arched palate. He was placid and hypokinetic (Ampola et al., 1969). The condition is likely to be recessive considering its nature as an inborn error of metabolism. Autosomal recessive inheritance is supported by the observation of two affected sisters by Baerlocher (1972). The cases were detected on a screening for cystinuria in the regular schools. The girls were only mildly, if at all, retarded. Their disorder may be different from that in the earlier reported case because response to methionine-loading was different.

Ampola, M. G., Efron, M. L., Bixby, E. M. and Meshorer, E.: Mental deficiency and a new aminoaciduria. Am. J. Dis. Child. 117: 66-70, 1969.

Baerlocher, K.: Zurich, Switzerland: personal communication, 1972.

Crawhall, J. C., Parker, R., Sneddon, W. and Young, E. P.: Beta-mercaptolactate-cysteine disulfatide in the urine of a mentally retarded patient. Am. J. Dis. Child. 117: 71-82, 1969.

*24970 MESOMELIC DWARFISM OF THE HYPOPLASTIC ULNA, FIBULA AND MANDIBLE TYPE

In the course of studies of inbred groups in northern Sweden, Book observed a severe form of chondrodystrophy which may be different from others listed here. The parents of the proband were first cousins. Heterozygotes in this kindred were short (the father was 160 cm and the mother 150 cm) and had relatively short fingers and broad hands, but otherwise were not strikingly abnormal. Chondrohypoplasia was the designation Book used for the heterozygotes. Book (1950) thought the disorder most closely resembled that in the family reported by Brailsford (1935). In this family children of normal but short parents were affected. Blockey and Lawrie (1963) described 2 affected sibs (a brother and a sister), the offspring of normal parents. There was no mention of parental consanguinity. The limb malformation is aplasia or severe hypoplasia of the ulna and fibula, thickened and curved radius and tibia. Other than displacement deformities of the hands and feet, their skeletal structures are normal. This entity can be designated micromelic dwarfism. Blockey and Lawrie (1963), mistakenly I think, considered their cases instances of Nievergelt syndrome, a dominant (q.v.). Langer (1967) studied two cases and referred to the entity as 'mesomelic dwarfism of the hypoplastic ulna, fibula, mandible type.' Hypoplasia of the mandible was a feature not emphasized in other reports. Mesomelic is a non-specific term which refers to shortening most striking in the forearm and lower leg. This is a characteristic of dyschondrosteosis (q.v.) and of the Ellis-van Creveld syndrome (q.v.). Espiritu et al. (1974) suggested that this phenotype may sometimes be produced by homozygosity for the dyschondrosteosis (12730) gene.

Blockey, N. J. and Lawrie, J. H.: An unusual symmetrical distal limb deformity in siblings. J. Bone Joint Surg. 45B: 745-747, 1963.

Book, J. A.: A clinical and genetical study of disturbed skeletal growth (chondrohypoplasia). Hereditas 36: 161-180, 1950.

Brailsford, J. F.: Dystrophies of the skeleton. Brit. J. Radiol. 8: 533-569, 1935.

Espiritu, C., Chen, H. and Woolley, P. V., Jr.: Probable homozygosity for the dyschondrosteosis gene (two cases of autosomal dominant mesomelic dwarfism of the hypoplastic mandible, ulna and fibula type). To be published, 1974.

Langer, L. O., Jr.: Mesomelic dwarfism of the hypoplastic ulna, fibula, mandible type. Radiology 89: 654-660, 1967.

24980 METACHROMATIC LEUKODYSTROPHY AND AMAUROTIC IDIOCY, COMBINED FEATURES OF

Mossakowski, Mathieson and Cumings (1961) found three affected sibs in a French-Canadian family in whom histologic and chemical features of both diseases were present.

Mossakowski, M., Mathieson, G. and Cumings, J. N.: On the relationship of metachromatic leucodystrophy and amaurotic idiocy. Brain 84: 585-604, 1961.

*25000 METACHROMATIC LEUKODYSTROPHY, ADULT

At least two forms of metachromatic leukodystrophy (MLD) can be distinguished. The late infantile form has its onset before age 30 months and the adult form begins after age 16. In addition, onset was between 4 and 15 years in a group difficult to classify. In the adult form initial symptoms have usually been psychiatric leading to a diagnosis of schizophrenia. Disorders of movement and posture appear late. Differences from the late infantile form also include ability to demonstrate metachromatic material in paraffin- or celloidin-embedded sections in the adult form and probably greater sulfatide excess in the gray than in the white matter in this form. The relation of the adult form to the presumed X-linked cerebral sclerosis of Scholz (q.v.) is unclear. The gallbladder is usually non-functional. Betts et al. (1968) described a man who was 28 when admitted to a psychiatric hospital for 'acute schizophrenia' and 35 when he died of bronchopneumonia. Muller et al. (1969) and Pilz and Muller (1969) described two unrelated women with this disorder. Affected sibs were recorded by Austin et al. (1968), among others. Percy and Kaback (1971) found no difference in enzyme levels between the infantile and adult-onset types. Some other factor must account for the difference in age of onset. Porter et al. (1971) reported that cultured fibroblasts from late-onset metachromatic leukodystrophy hydrolyzed appreciable amounts of exogenous cerebroside sulfate, whereas fibroblasts from patients with the early onset form hydrolyzed none. Studies of cell-free preparations showed no cerebroside sulfatase activity.

Austin, J., Armstrong, D., Fouch, S., Mitchell, C., Stumpf, D., Shearer, L. and Briner, O.: Metachromatic leukodystrophy (MLD). VIII. MLD in adults: diagnosis and pathogenesis. Arch. Neurol. 18: 225-240, 1968.

Betts, T. A., Smith, W. T. and Kelly, R. E.: Adult metachromatic leukodystrophy (sulphatide lipidosis) simulating acute schizophrenia. Report of a case. Neurology 18: 1140-1142, 1968.

Muller, D., Pilz, H. and Ter Meulen, V.: Studies on adult metachromatic leukodystrophy. I. Clinical, morphological and histochemical observations in two cases. J. Neurol. Sci. 9: 567-584, 1969.

Percy, A. K. and Kaback, M. M.: Infantile and adult-onset metachromatic leukodystrophy. Biochemical comparisons and predictive diagnosis. New Eng. J. Med. 285: 785-787, 1971.

Pilz, H. and Muller, D.: Studies on adult metachromatic leukodystrophy. II. Biochemical aspects of adult cases of metachromatic leukodystrophy. J. Neurol. Sci. 9: 585-595, 1969.

Porter, M. T., Fluharty, A. L., Trammell, J. and Kihara, H.: A correlation of intracellular cerebroside sulfatase activity in fibroblasts with latency in metachromatic leukodystrophy. Biochem. Biophys. Res. Commun. 44: 660-666, 1971.

Sourander, P. and Svennerholm, L.: Sulphatide lipidosis in the adult with the clinical picture of progressive organic dementia with epileptic seizures. Acta Neuropath. 1: 384-396, 1962.

Van Bogaert, L. V. and Dewulf, A.: Diffuse progressive leukodystrophy in the adult with production of metachromatic degenerative products (Alzheimer-Baroncini). Arch. Neurol. Psychiat. 42: 1083-1097, 1939.

25010 METACHROMATIC LEUKODYSTROPHY, LATE INFANTILE (METACHROMATIC LEUKOENCEPHALOPATHY; METACHROMATIC FORM OF DIFFUSE CEREBRAL SCLEROSIS; SULFATIDE LIPIDOSIS)

This condition was first described by Greenfield in 1933. Onset is usually in the second year of life and death occurs before five years in most. Clinical features are motor symptoms, rigidity, mental deterioration and in some convulsions. Early development is normal but onset occurs before 30 months of age. The cerebrospinal fluid protein is usually over 100 mg. percent.

Galactosphingosulfatides strongly metachromatic, doubly refractile in polarized light and pink with PAS are found in excess in the white matter of the central nervous system, in the kidney and in the urinary sediment (Austin, 1960). The defect may concern the lysosomal enzyme arylsulfatase A (Austin, et al. 1964). Masters et al. (1964) described four cases in two families. Progressive physical and mental deterioration began a few months after birth. Megacolon with attacks of abdominal distension was observed. Sufficient difference from the usual cases existed as to suggest to the authors that more than one entity is encompassed by metachromatic leukodystrophy. A curious feature of later bedridden stages of the disease is marked genu recurvatum. The first manifestations appearing before the second birthday, include hypotonia, muscle weakness and unsteady gait, suggesting a myopathy or neuropathy. Austin's test to demonstrate absence of arylsulfatase A (ASA) activity in the urine is useful in the early diagnosis (Greene et al., 1967). Since the metachromatic material is cerebroside sulfate, MLD is a sulfatide lipidosis. See SULFATIDOSIS, JUVENILE, for a disorder which combines features of a mucopolysaccharidosis with those of metachromatic leukodystrophy. Stumpf et al. (1971) presented evidence to suggest that the abnormality in arylsulfatase A

R E C E S S I V E

is qualitatively different in the late infantile and juvenile forms of metachromatic leukodystrophy. Kaback and Howell (1970) demonstrated profound deficiency of arylsulfatase A in cultured skin fibroblasts of patients and an intermediate deficiency in carriers. Normally enzyme levels were low in mid-trimester amniotic cells: hence homozygotes cannot be reliably identified by amniocentesis. Note that only one asterisk is assigned to the metachromatic leukodystrophies, adult and late infantile forms, for the reason that the enzymatic evidence indicates that these are allelic disorders. With both artificial and natural substrate no difference in degree of deficiency of arylsulfatase A was found (Percy and Kaback, 1971). However, when the degradation of natural substrate by fibroblasts from the two forms of the disease was studied, a distinctive difference was found (Porter and Fluharty, 1971). Gustavson and Hagberg (1971) described 13 cases of late-infantile MLD from 11 families. Two pairs of families were related to each other and three sets of parents were consanguineous. Arylsulfatase A and B are probably quite different in amino acid composition but amino acid assays have not been performed on type B for lack of samples of proven homogeneity (Nicholls and Roy, 1971).

Austin, J. H.: Metachromatic form of diffuse cerebral sclerosis. III. Significance of sulfatide and other lipid abnormalities in white matter and kidney. Neurology 10: 470-483, 1960.

Austin, J. H.: Some recent findings in leukodystrophies and in gargoylism. In, Aronson, S. M. and Volk, B. W. (eds.): Inborn Disorders of Sphingolipid Metabolism. Oxford: Pergamon Press, 1967. Pp. 359-387.

Austin, J., McAfee, D. and Shearer, L.: Metachromatic form of diffuse cerebral sclerosis. IV. Low sulfatase activity in the urine of nine living patients with metachromatic leukodystrophy (MLD). Arch. Neurol. 12: 447-455, 1965.

Austin, J., McAfee, D., Armstrong, D., O'Rourke, M., Shearer, L. and Bachhawat, B. K.: Abnormal sulphatase activities in two human diseases (metachromatic leukodystrophy and gargoylism). Biochem. J. 93: 15C-17C, 1964.

Black, J. W. and Cumings, J. N.: Infantile metachromatic leukodystrophy. J. Neurol. Neurosurg. Psychiat. 24: 233-239, 1961.

Cravioto, H., O'Brien, J., Lockwood, R., Kasten, F. H. and Booker, J.: Metachromatic leukodystrophy (sulfatide lipidoses) cultured in vitro. Science 156: 243-245, 1967.

Greene, H., Hug, G. and Schubert, W. K.: Arylsulfatase a in the urine and metachromatic leukodystrophy. J. Pediat. 71: 709-711, 1967.

Greenfield, J. G.: Form of progressive cerebral sclerosis in infants associated with primary degeneration of interfascicular glia. Proc. Roy. Soc. Med. 26: 690-697, 1933.

Gustavson, K.-H. and Hagberg, B.: The incidence and genetics of metachromatic leukodystrophy in northern Sweden. Acta Paediat. Scand. 60: 585-590, 1971.

Hagberg, B., Sourander, P. and Svennerholm, L.: Sulfatide lipidosis in childhood. Am. J. Dis. Child. 104: 644-656, 1962.

Jervis, G. A.: Infantile metachromatic leukodystrophy: (Greenfield's disease). J. Neuropath. Exp. Neurol. 19: 323-341, 1960.

Kaback, M. M. and Howell, R. R.: Infantile metachromatic leukodystrophy: heterozygote detection in skin fibroblasts and possible applications to intrauterine diagnosis. New Eng. J. Med. 282: 1336-1340, 1970.

Masters, P. L., MacDonald, W. B., Ryan, M. M. P. and Cumings, J. N.: Familial leucodystrophy. Arch. Dis. Child. 39: 345-355, 1964.

Moser, H. W.: Sulfatide lipidosis: metachromatic leukodystrophy. In, Stanbury, J. B., Wyngaarden, J. B. and Fredrickson, D. S. (eds.): The Metabolic Basis of Inherited Disease. New York: McGraw-Hill, 1972 (3rd Ed.). Pp. 688-729.

Nicholls, R. G. and Roy, A. G.: Arysulfatases. In, Boyer, P. D. (ed.): The Enzymes. New York: Academic Press, 1971. Vol. 5, Pp. 21-41.

Percy, A. K. and Brady, R. O.: Metachromatic leukodystrophy: diagnosis with samples of venous blood. Science 161: 594-595, 1968.

Porter, M. T., Fluharty, A. L. and Kihara, H.: Correction of abnormal cerebroside sulfate metabolism in cultured metachromatic leukodystrophy fibroblasts. Science 172: 1262-1265, 1971.

Porter, M. T., Fluharty, A. L., Trammell, J. and Kihara, H.: A correlation of intracellular cerebroside sulfatase activity in fibroblasts with latency in metachromatic leukodystrophy. Biochem. Biophys. Res. Commun. 44: 660-666, 1971.

Stumpf, D. and Austin, J.: Metachromatic leukodystrophy (MLD). IX. Qualitative and quantitative differences in urinary arylsulfatase A in different forms of MLD. Arch. Neurol. 24: 117-124, 1971.

R
E
C
E
S
S
I
V
E

*25020 METACHROMATIC LEUKODYSTROPHY, JUVENILE

Schutta et al. (1966) recognized a form of metachromatic leukodystrophy with onset between ages 4 and 10 years, as compared with the more frequent late infantile form with onset between ages 12 and 24 months. Lyon et al. (1961) described affected brothers with onset at 7 years and at 4 years and with marked elevation of protein in the cerebrospinal fluid. Porter et al. (1971) corrected the metabolic defect in cultured fibroblasts by addition of arylsulfatase A to the medium. Moser (1972) suggested that juvenile cases of MLD, especially those of late juvenile onset, should be classed with the adult form. An alternative possibility is that some of these cases with phenotype intermediate between those of the late infantile and adult forms represent genetic compounds. The same very low levels of arylsulfatase A are found in the three forms, infantile, juvenile and adult. The reason for the differences in age of onset is unknown.

Lyon, G., Arthuis, M. and Thieffry, S.: Leucodystrophie metachromatique infantile familiale. Etude de deux observations, dont une avec examen anatomique et chimique. Rev. Neurol. 104: 508-533, 1961.

Moser, H. W.: Sulfatide lipidosis: metachromatic leukodystrophy. In, Stanbury, J. B., Wyngaarden, J. B. and Fredrickson, D. S.: The Metabolic Basis of Inherited Disease. New York: McGraw-Hill, 1972 (3rd. Ed.). Pp. 688-729.

Porter, M. T., Fluharty, A. L. and Kihara, H.: Correction of abnormal cerebroside sulfate metabolism in cultured metachromatic leukodystrophy fibroblasts. Science 172: 1263-1265, 1971.

Schutta, H. S., Pratt, R. T. C., Metz, H., Evans, K. A. and Carter, C. O.: A family study of the late infantile and juvenile forms of metachromatic leukodystrophy. J. Med. Genet. 3: 86-91, 1966.

*25025 METAPHYSEAL CHONDRODYSPLASIA, MCKUSICK TYPE (FORMERLY CALLED CARTILAGE-HAIR HYPOPLASIA)

This disorder was first recognized as a syndrome in the Old Order Amish, a religious isolate, but has more recently been identified in other groups. The skeletal feature is short-limbed dwarfism. By X-ray the changes are of the type called metaphyseal dysostosis by the radiologists. Biopsy shows hypoplasia of cartilage to be the nature of the abnormality. The hair is fine, sparse and light-colored. Microscopically it has an abnormally small caliber. Autosomal recessive inheritance seems quite certain although penetrance is reduced (when dwarfism is taken as the phenotype for ascertainment). The relationship of the syndrome described by Burgert, Dower and Tauxe (1965), with aregenerative anemia and celiac syndrome, is unclear. Unexplained features present in some cases include anemia, malabsorption, Hirschsprung disease, and susceptibility to chicken pox. Some of these features resemble those of the patients with pancreatic insufficiency and neutropenia reported by Burke et al. (1967) and some of their patients had metaphyseal changes. See also the reports of Burgert et al. (1965) and of Theodorou and Adams (1963). Kelling et al. (1973) suggested that there may be decreased reactivity of some disulfide bands in hair leading to its abnormal biophysical and biochemical characteritics.

Burgert, E. O., Jr., Dower, J. C. and Tauxe, W. N.: A new syndrome — aregenerative anemia, malabsorption (celiac), dyschondroplasia and hyperphosphatemia. (Abstract) J. Pediat. 67: 711-712, 1965.

Burke, V., Colebatch, J. H., Anderson, C. M. and Simons, M. J.: Association of pancreatic insufficiency and chronic neutropenia in childhood. Arch. Dis. Child. 42: 147-157, 1967.

Coupe, R. L. and Lowry, R. B.: Abnormality of the hair in cartilage-hair hypoplasia. Dermatologica 141: 329-334, 1970.

Halle, M. A., Collipp, P. J. and Roginsky, M.: Cartilage-hair hypoplasia in childhood. New York J. Med. 70: 2705-2708, 1970.

Hong, R., Ammann, J., Haung, S. W., Levy, R. L., Davenport, G., Bach, M. L., Bach, F. H., Bortin, M. M. and Kay, H. E. M.: Cartilage-hair hypoplasia: effect of thymus transplants. Clin. Immun. Immunopath. 1: 15-25, 1972.

Kelling, C., Goldsmith, L. A. and Baden, H. P.: Biophysical and biochemical studies of the hair in cartilage-hair hypoplasia. Clin. Genet. 4: 500-506, 1973.

Lowry, R. B., Wood, B. J., Birkbeck, J. A. and Padwick, P. H.: Cartilage-hair hypoplasia. A rare and recessive cause of dwarfism. Clin. Pediat. 9: 44-46, 1970.

Lux, S. E., Johnston, R. B., Jr., August, C. S., Say, B., Penchaszadeh, V. B., Rosen, F. S. and McKusick, V. A.: Neutropenia and abnormal cellular immunity in cartilage-hair hypoplasia. New Eng. J. Med. 282: 234-236, 1970.

McKusick, V. A., Eldridge, R., Hostetler, J. A., Egeland, J. A. and Ruangwit, U.: Dwarfism in the Amish. II. Cartilage-hair hypoplasia. Bull. Hopkins Hosp. 116: 285-326, 1965.

Theodorou, S. D. and Adams, J.: An unusual case of metaphyseal dysplasia. J. Bone Joint Surg. 45B: 364-369, 1963.

25030 METAPHYSEAL CHONDRODYSPLASIA, PENA TYPE

This is one of the group of disorders formerly termed metaphyseal dysostosis. Pena (1965) and Lenz (1967) described affected sibs, the parents being normal. The metaphyses of the long bones had an extensive sponge-like appearance radiologically and showed histologically numerous islands of cartilage reminiscent of enchondromatosis. Vaandrager (1960) described concordant one-egg twins. Kozlowski and Sikorska (1970) described a case.

Kozlowski, K. and Sikorska, B.: Dysplasia metaphysaria Typ Vaandrager-Pena. Z. Kinderheilk. 108: 165-170, 1970.

Lenz, W.: Diagnosis in medical genetics. In, Crow, J. F. and Neel, J. V. (eds.): Proc. 3rd. Intern. Cong. Hum. Genet., Sept. 1966. Baltimore: Johns Hopkins Press, 1967. Pp. 29-36.

Pena, J.: Disostosis metafisaria. Una revision. Con aportacion de una observacion familiar. Una forma nueva de la enfermedad? Radiologia 47: 3-22, 1965.

Vaandrager, G. J.: Metafysaire dysostosis? Nederl. T. Geneesk. 104: 547-552, 1960.

25040 METAPHYSEAL CHONDRODYSPLASIA, SPAHR TYPE

RECESSIVE

This is one of the group of disorders formerly called metaphyseal dysostosis. Spahr and Spahr-Hartmann (1961) described four sibs with metaphyseal dysostosis. The parents were normal but consanguineous. Bowing of the legs was striking and at least one required bilateral osteotomy.

Spahr, A. and Spahr-Hartmann, I.: Dysostose metaphysaire familiale. Etude de 4 cas dans une fratrie. Helv. Paediat. Acta 16: 836-849, 1961.

25050 METAPHYSEAL MODELING ABNORMALITY, SKIN LESIONS AND SPASTIC PARAPLE-GIA

Roy, Maroteaux et al. (1968) described a 14-year-old girl with defective metaphyseal modeling as in Pyle disease, increased bone density, plaque-like skin lesions, and signs of spastic paraplegia. The parents were not related.

Roy, C., Maroteaux, P., Kremp, L., Courtecuisse, V. and Alagille, D.: Un nouveau syndrome osseux avec anomalies cutanees et troubles neurologiques. Arch. Franc. Pediat. 25: 893-906, 1968.

*25060 METATROPIC DWARFISM

Maroteaux, Spranger and Wiedemann (1966) described a chondrodystrophy which at birth is likely to be called achondroplasia because of the short limbs and later in life Morquio syndrome because of the relatively short spine and severe scoliosis. The designation for the condition was chosen to convey the change or reversal in body proportions. The manifestations are already present at birth, with generalized epi-metaphyseal disturbance of ossification. Kyphoscoliosis is progressive and severe. Anisospondyly, halberd-shaped pelvis and hyperplastic femoral trochanters are features. The coccyx is unusually long resulting in a tail. At birth it may be called hyperplastic type of achondroplasia. The ends of the femurs and humeri are trumpeted. The two brothers reported by Michail et al. (1956) probably had this condition which appears to be autosomal recessive. The disorder described by Kniest (1952) has some similarity to metatropic dwarfism but must be considered a separate entity which might be called metatropic dwarfism, type II, or Kniest syndrome.

Jenkins, P., Smith, M. B., McKinnell, J. S.: Metatropic dwarfism. Brit. J. Radiol. 43: 561-565, 1970.

Kniest, W.: Zur Abgrenzung der Dysostosis enchondralis von der Chondrodystrophie. Z. Kinderheilk. 43: 633-640, 1952.

Larose, J. H. and Gay, B. B., Jr.: Metatropic dwarfism. Am. J. Roentgen. 106: 156-161, 1969.

Maroteaux, P., Spranger, J. W. and Wiedemann, H.-R.: Der metatropische Zwergwuchs. Arch. Kinderheilk. 173: 211-226, 1966.

Michail, J., Matsovkas, J., Theodorou, S. and Houliaras, K.: Maladie de Morquio (osteochondrodystrophie polyepiphysaire deformante) chez deux freres. Helv. Paediat. Acta 11: 403-413, 1956.

25065 METHANE PRODUCTION

Bond et al. (1970) made the following observations: Methane (CH4) in man is derived solely from the metabolism of the colonic flora. Respiratory CH4 excretion is a simple but reliable indicator of intestinal CH4 production. In the adult population about one-third excrete large amounts of CH4 whereas the others excrete very little. No adult changed his excretion status over a period of one year. Children below the age of 3 excrete no CH4. If both parents excrete CH4 all offspring over age 7 excrete CH4. The concordance between marriage partners was random. 11 of 12 identical twins and 14 of 16 fraternal twins were concordant. The genetics of this trait are unclear.

Bond, J. H., Engel, R. R. and Levitt, M. D.: Methane production in man. (Abstract) Gastroenterology 58: 1035 only, 1970.

*25070 METHEMOGLOBIN REDUCTASE (TPNH-) (DEFICIENCY OF NADPH-DEPENDENT MET-HEMOGLOBIN REDUCTASE)

In recessively inherited methemoglobinemia (see below), DPNH-methemoglobin reductase is deficient. Sass et al. (1967) found a Negro male with TPNH-methemoglobin reductase deficiency. The case was detected when the patient's red cells were found to be abnormal with the methylene-blue screening test which is ordinarily an indication of G6PD-deficiency but by actual assay G6PD activity was found normal. Administration of primaquine for 30 days produced no hemolysis. Five close relatives including the mother had intermediate levels of TPNH-methemoglobin reductase consistent with heterozygous status. The father was dead. As one would predict from knowledge of the relative activities of the TPNH- and DPNH-methemoglobin reductases, methemoglobinemia was not present in the presumed homozygote. Bloom and Zarkowsky (1970) also reported such a patient. (The new terminology for TPN is NADPH). Their patient in comparison with methemoglobinemia cases, demonstrated that NADPH-reductase (also called NADPH dehydrogenase) is separate and distinct from NADH reductase.

Bloom, G. E. and Zarkowsky, H. S.: Heterogeneity of the enzyme defect in congenital methemoglobinemia. New Eng. J. Med. 281: 919-922, 1970.

Sass, M. D., Caruso, C. J. and Farhangi, M.: TPNH-methemoglobin reductase deficiency: a new red-cell enzyme defect. J. Lab. Clin. Med. 70: 760-767, 1967.

Schwartz, J. M., Paress, P. S., Ross, J. M., Dipillo, F. and Rizek, R.: Unstable variant of NADH methemoglobin reductase in Puerto Ricans with hereditary methemoglobinemia. J. Clin. Invest. 51: 1594-1601, 1972.

*25080 METHEMOGLOBINEMIA DUE TO DEFICIENCY OF METHEMOGLOBIN-REDUCTASE (DIAPHORASE): DEFICIENCY OF NADH-DEPENDENT METHEMOGLOBIN REDUCTASE

RECESSIVE

This disorder demonstrates very well that the clinical disorders resulting from enzyme deficiencies, i.e., inborn errors of metabolism, are inherited as recessives, whereas structural defects, such as brachydactyly and structural anomalies of nonenzymatic proteins, are usually inherited as dominants. The form of methemoglobin with electrophoretically atypical hemoglobin (of which there are several types) is dominant (see Hb M).

Mental deficiency occurs only with the enzyme-deficient recessive form of the disorder (Hitzenberger, 1932; Worster-Drought, White and Sargent, 1953; Jaffe, 1963).

Muller and colleagues (1963) described 3 sibs with methemoglobinemia. They showed deficient ability of erythrocytes to utilize glucose for methemoglobin reduction but normal reduction of lactate. They concluded that two enzyme-deficient forms of methemoglobinemia may exist just as there are two methemoglob-in-reducing systems normally present in red cells, viz., nicotinamide-adenine dinucleotide phosphate (NADPH2) reductase or nicotinamide-adenine dinucleotide (NADH2) reductase. Muller et al. (1963) suggested that their family suffered from a defect in the former system. The enzyme type of methemoglobine-mia has unprecedentedly high frequency in the Athabaskan Indians (Eskimos) of Alaska (Scott, 1960; Scott et al., 1963). Balsamo, Hardy and Scott (1964) also observed diaphorase deficiency in Navajo Indians. Since the Navajo Indians and the Athabaskan Indians of Alaska are the same linguistic stock, the finding may illustrate the usefulness of rare recessive genes in tracing relationships of ethnic groups. Ozsoylu (1967) reported enzyme-deficiency methemoglobinemia in 3 generations and proposed dominant inheritance. However, consanguinity was present to account for a quasi-dominant pattern. The author thought this possibility was excluded by a normal diaphorase activity in two individuals who would need to be heterozygotes to account for the pattern. Enterogenous methemoglobinemia might be confused with the genetic form. Rossi et al. (1966) described a case with methemoglobinemia for 14 years before cure by a course of neomycin. West et al. (1967) provided electrophoretic evidence of anomalous enzyme structure in a case of methemoglobinemia. Cohen et al. (1968) suggested that methemoglobinemia induced by malarial prophylaxis (by chloroquine, primaquine and diamino-diphenylsulfone) was an indication of the presence of the heterozygous state. Electrophoretic variants of NADH diaphorase without methemoglobinemia have also been found, with a family pattern consistent with co-dominant inheritance. Bloom and Zarkowsky (1970) described three varieties: total absence of detectable enzyme activity, decreased quantities of presumably normal enzyme and decreased quantities of structurally variant enzyme. They added two new structural variants of NADH-methemoglobin reductase to the one originally described by Kaplan and Beutler (1967). Treatment with methylene blue (100-300 mg. orally per day) or ascorbic acid (500 mg. a day) is of cosmetic value (Waller, 1970). Additional electrophoretic variants of red cell NADH diaphorase were described by Hopkinson et al. (1970).

Balsamo, P., Hardy, W. R. and Scott, E. M.: Hereditary methemoglobinemia due to diaphorase deficiency in Navajo Indians. J. Pediat. 65: 928-930, 1964.

Bloom, G. E. and Zarkowsky, H. S.: Heterogeneity of the enzyme defect in congenital methemoglobine-mia. New Eng. J. Med. 281: 919-922, 1970.

Cawein, M. J., Behlen, C. H., Lappat, E. J. and Cohn, J. E.: Hereditary diaphorase deficiency and methemoglobinemia. Arch. Intern. Med. 113: 578-585, 1964.

Cohen, R. J., Sachs, J. R., Wicker, D. J. and Conrad, M. E.: Methemoglobinemia provoked by malarial chemoprophylaxis in Vietnam. New Eng. J. Med. 279: 1127-1131, 1968.

Fialkow, P. J., Browder, J. A., Sparkes, R. S. and Motulsky, A. G.: Mental retardation in methemoglobinemia due to diaphorase deficiency. New Eng. J. Med. 273: 840-845, 1965.

Giblett, E. R. and Detter, J. C.: Inherited NADH diaphorase variation without methemoglobinemia. Am. Soc. Hum. Genet., San Francisco, Oct., 1969.

Hitzenberger, K.: Autotoxic cyanosis due to intraglobular methemoglobinemia. Wein. Arch. Med. 23: 85-96, 1932.

Hopkinson, D. A., Corney, G., Cook, P. J. L., Robson, E. B. and Harris, H.: Genetically determined electrophoretic variants of human red cell NADH diaphorase. Ann. Hum. Genet. 34: 1-10, 1970.

Hsieh, H.-S. and Jaffe, E. R.: Electrophoretic and functional variants of NADH-methemoglobin reductase in hereditary methemoglobinemia. J. Clin. Invest. 50: 196-202, 1971.

Jaffe, E. R.: The reduction of methemoglobin in erythrocytes of a patient with congenital methemoglobi-nemia, subjects with erythrocyte glucose-6-phosphate dehydrogenase deficiency, and normal individuals. Blood 21: 561-572, 1963.

Kaplan, J. C. and Beutler, E.: Electrophoresis of red cell NADH- and NADPH- diaphorases in normal subjects and patients with congenital methemoglobinemia. Biochem. Biophys. Res. Commun. 29: 605-610, 1967.

Muller, J., Murawski, K., Szymanowska, Z., Koziorowski, A. and Radwan, L.: Hereditary deficiency of NADPH 2-methaemoglobin reductase. Acta Med. Scand. 173: 243-247, 1963.

Ozsoylu, S.: Hereditary methemoglobinemic cyanosis due to diaphorase deficiency in three successive generations. Acta Haemat. 37: 276-283, 1967.

Rossi, E. C., Bryan, G. T., Schilling, R. F. and Clatanoff, D. V.: Remission of chronic methemoglobine-mia following neomycin therapy. Am. J. Med. 40: 440-447, 1966.

Scott, E. M. and Wright, R. C.: The absence of close linkage of methemoglobinemia and other loci. Am. J. Hum. Genet. 21: 194-195, 1969.

Scott, E. M.: The relationship of diaphorase of human erythrocytes to inheritance of methemoglobinemia. J. Clin. Invest. 39: 1176-1179, 1960.

Scott, E. M., Lewis, M., Kaita, H., Chown, B. and Giblett, E. R.: The absence of close linkage of methemoglobinemia and blood group loci. Am. J. Hum. Genet. 15: 493-494, 1963.

Townes, P. L. and Morrison, M.: Investigation of the defect in a variant of hereditary methemoglobinemia. Blood 19: 60-74, 1962.

Waller, H. D.: Inherited methemoglobinemia (enzyme deficiencies). Humangenetik 9: 217-218, 1970.

West, C. A., Gomperts, B. D., Huehns, E. R., Kessel, I. and Ashby, J. R.: Demonstration of an enzyme variant in a case of congenital methaemoglobinaemia. Brit. Med. J. 4: 212-214, 1967.

Worster-Drought, C., White, J. C. and Sargent, F.: Familial, idiopathic methaemoglobinaemia associated with mental deficiency and neurological abnormalities. Brit. Med. J. 2: 114-118, 1953.

25085 METHIONINE ADENOSYLTRANSFERASE DEFICIENCY

Gaull and Tallan (1974) studied an infant found to have hypermethioninemia on newborn screening. Liver biopsy showed a deficiency of methionine adenosyltransferase.

Gaull, G. E. and Tallen, H. H.: Methionine adenosyltransferase deficiency: new enzymatic defect associated with hypermethionemia. Science 186: 59-60, 1974.

*25090 METHIONINE MALABSORPTION SYNDROME

Smith and Strang (1958) described a disorder they called oasthouse urine disease. The infant had white hair, hyperpnea, convulsions and mental retardation. The urine had a characteristic and unique odor like that of an oasthouse (building for drying hops). Although phenylpyruvic acid was found in the urine, the odor was different from that of phenylketonuria. The defect was thought to concern the utilization of the alpha-keto acids of all essential amino acids as a result of which alpha-keto acids, their amino acic precursors or hydroxy acid derivatives accumulated in the blood and overflowed in the urine. The unusual odor was thought to be produced by alpha hydroxybutric acid, but could be some other substance rather like it. Efron described the amino acid in the urine. No further cases have been discovered (Strang, 1963). The case of Hooft and colleagues (1964) may be of the same disorder. The disorder seems to combine the features of phenylketonuria and of methionine malabsorption. The ferric chloride test is positive. The case of Hooft et al. (1965) was in a girl with mental retardation, diarrhea, convulsions, polypnea, blue eyes, and strikingly white hair. The manifestations in the patient described by Hooft et al. (1968) were diarrhea, convulsions, peculiar smell, and mental retardation. Both parents and three sibs showed abnormal excretion of alpha-hydroxybutyric acid after methionine load, a presumed manifestation of heterozygosity. They considered this disorder different from 'oasthouse disease' of Smith and Strang.

Efron, M. L.: Aminoaciduria. New Eng. J. Med. 272: 1058-1067, 1107-1113, 1965.

Hooft, C., Timmermans, J., Snoeck, J., Antener, I., Oyaert, W. and Van der Hende, C. H.: Methionine malabsorption in a mentally defective child. Lancet II: 20 only, 1964.

Hooft, C., Timmermans, J., Antener, I., Oyaert, W. and Van der Hende, C. H.: Methionine malabsorption syndrome. Ann. Paediat. 205: 73-104, 1965.

Hooft, C., Carton, D., Snoeck, J., Timmermans, J., Antener, I., Van der Hende, C. and Oyaert, W.: Further investigations in the methionine malabsorption syndrome. Helv. Paediat. Acta 23: 334-349, 1968.

Jepson, J. B., Smith, A. J. and Strang, L. B.: An inborn error of metabolism with urinary excretion of hydroxyacids, ketoacids and aminoacids. (Letter) Lancet II: 1334-1335, 1958.

Smith, A. J. and Strang, L. B.: An inborn error of metabolism with the urinary excretion of alpha-hydroxy-butyric acid and phenylpyruvic acid. Arch. Dis. Child. 33: 109-113, 1958.

*25100 METHYLMALONICACIDURIA I (VITAMIN B12 UNRESPONSIVE)

Rosenberg et al. (1968) described an 8-month-old boy with profound metabolic acidosis, developmental retardation and an unusual biochemical triad: methylmalonic aciduria, long chain ketonuria and intermittent hyperglycinemia. Valine, isoleucine or high protein intake accentuated the biochemical abnormalities. Rosenberg et al. (1968) presented indirect evidence that the defect concerns methylmalonyl-CoA isomerase, a vitamin B12 dependent enzyme which converts methylmalonyl-CoA to succinyl-CoA. Furthermore they found that their patient responded to vitamin B12 administration. Thus, in some but not all patients, the characteristic and potentially lethal episodes of ketoacidosis can be avoided. Barness et al. (1968) also pointed out that some cases of methylmalonic aciduria respond to vitamin B12 and others do not. Furthermore, of those not responsive to B12, some have hyperglycinemia and some do not. The conversion of methylmalonate to succinate involves two enzymes only one of which is B12-dependent. Morrow et al. (1969) provided enzymatic proof of two forms of the disease. Methylmalonyl-CoA carbonylmutase activity was essentially absent from the liver in a vitamin B12-unresponsive case, whereas in a vitamin B12-responsive case the liver showed in vitro normal enzymatic activity with added coenzyme and essentially no activity without added coenzyme. Methylmalonyl CoA mutase requires 5 prime-deoxyadenosylcobalamin, a coenzyme form of vitamin B12. The work of Rosenberg et al. (1969) suggests that the primary defect in B12-responsive methymalonic aciduria is impaired ability to convert B12 to the coenzyme (because of deficiency of deoxyadenosyl transferase), whereas the B12-unresponsive form has a defect in the apoenzyme.

R
E
C
E
S
S
I
V
E

Barness, L. A. and Morrow, G., III: Methylmalonic aciduria — a newly discovered inborn error. Ann. Intern. Med. 69: 633-635, 1968.

Hsia, Y. E., Lilljeqvist, A. C. and Rosenberg, L. E.: Vitamin B12-dependent methylmalonic aciduria amino acid toxicity, long chain ketonuria, and protective effect of vitamin B12. Pediatrics 46: 497-507, 1970.

Morrow, G., III, Barness, L. A., Cardinale, G. J., Abeles, R. H. and Flaks, J. G.: Congenital methylmalonic acidemia: enzymatic evidence for two forms of the disease. Proc. Nat. Acad. Sci. 63: 191-197, 1969.

Oberholzer, V. G., Levin, B., Burgess, E. A. and Young, W. F.: Methylmalonic aciduria. An inborn error of metabolism leading to chronic metabolic acidosis. Arch. Dis. Child. 42: 492-504, 1967.

Rosenberg, L. E., Lilljeqvist, A. C. and Hsia, Y. E.: Methylmalonic aciduria: an inborn error leading to metabolic acidosis, long-chain ketonuria and hyperglycinemia. New Eng. J. Med. 278: 1319-1322, 1968.

Rosenberg, L. E., Lilljeqvist, A. C. and Hsia, Y. E.: Methylmalonic aciduria: metabolic block localization and vitamin B12 dependency. Science 162: 805-807, 1968.

Rosenberg, L. E., Lilljeqvist, A. C., Hsia, Y. E. and Rosenbloom, F. M.: Vitamin B12 dependent methylmalonic-aciduria: defective B12 metabolism in cultured fibroblasts. Biochem. Biophys. Res. Comm. 37: 607-614, 1969.

*25110 METHYLMALONICACIDURIA II (VITAMIN B12 RESPONSIVE)

See METHYLMALONICACIDURIA I for evidence of the existence of two enzymatically distinct forms of methylmalonicaciduria.

*25112 METHYLMALONICACIDURIA III

Kang et al. (1972) described a single infant with methylmalonicaciduria due to deficiency of methylmalonyl-CoA racemase. Scriver (1974) studied cases.

Kang, E. S., Snodgrass, P. J. and Gerald, P. S.: Methylmalonyl-CoA racemase defect: another cause of methylmalonic aciduria. (Abstract) Pediat. Res. 6: 393 only, 1972.

Scriver, C. R.: Montreal, personal communication, 1974.

25115 METHYLTETRAHYDROFOLATE CYCLOHYDROLASE DEFICIENCY

It is not certain that this is a distinct entity (Arakawa, 1970).

Arakawa, T.: Congenital defects in folate utilization. Am. J. Med. 48: 594-598, 1970.

Arakawa, T., Fujii, M., O'Hara, K., Watanabe, S., Karahashi, M., Kobayashi, M. and Hirano, H.: Mental retardation with hyperfolic acidemia not associated with formiminoglutamic aciduria: cyclohydrolase deficiency syndrome. Tohoku J. Exp. Med. 88: 341-352, 1966.

*25120 MICROCEPHALY

Microcephaly is a heterogeneous state (Cowie, 1960). Care must be taken to distinguish microcephaly secondary to degenerative brain disorder from true microcephaly which is inherited as an autosomal recessive. Microcephaly is produced, furthermore, by exposure of the human fetus to X-rays (Plummer, 1952). In true microcephaly there is no neurologic defect and no skeletal or other malformation. A well-integrated extrovert personality is maintained. In the Netherlands the frequency of true microcephaly was placed at about 1 in 250,000 by Van den Bosch (1959). The most extensive pedigree yet reported is that assembled by Kloepfer and colleagues (1964). The consistent association of chorioretinopathy in the microcephalic patients reported by McKusick et al. (1966) may indicate the existence of a separate entity. Schmidt et al. (1968) observed the same association in multiple members of a family. Koch (1963) also found such a case in a population-based study of microcephaly. The differentiation of primary and secondary microcephaly was investigated by Qasi and Reed (1972).

Brandon, M. G. W., Kirman, B. H. and Williams, C. E.: Microcephaly in one of monozygous twins. Arch. Dis. Child. 34: 56-59, 1959.

Cowie, V.: The genetics and sub-classification of microcephaly. J. Ment. Defic. Res. 4: 42-47, 1960.

Davies, H. and Kirman, B. H.: Microcephaly. Arch. Dis. Child. 37: 623-627, 1962.

Hanhart, E.: Ueber einfache Rezessivitaet bei Mikrocephalia vera, spuria et combinata und das herdweise Vorkommen der Mikrocephalia vera in Schweizer Isolaten. Acta Genet. Med. Gem. 7: 445-524, 1958.

Kloepfer, H. W., Platou, R. V. and Hansche, W. J.: Manifestations of a recessive gene for microcephaly in a population isolate. J. Genet. Hum. 13: 52-59, 1964.

Koch, G.: Genealogisch-demographische Untersuchungen ueber Mikrocephalie in Westfalen. Forschungsberichte des Landes Nordrhein-Westfalen, No. 1963, P. 99, 1968.

Koch, G.: Genetics of microcephaly in man. Acta Genet. Med. Gem. 8: 75-86, 1959.

Komai, T., Kishimoto, K. and Ozaki, Y.: Genetic study of microcephaly based on Japanese material. Am. J. Hum. Genet. 7: 51-65, 1955.

McKusick, V. A., Stauffer, M., Knox, D. L. and Clark, D. B.: Chorioretinopathy with hereditary microcephaly. Arch. Ophthal. 75: 597-600, 1966.

Plummer, G.: Anomalies occurring in children exposed in utero to the atomic bomb in Hiroshima. Pediatrics 10: 687-693, 1952.

RECESSIVE

Qasi, Q. H. and Reed, T. E.: A problem in diagnosis of primary versus secondary microcephaly. (Abstract) Am. J. Hum. Genet. 24: 35A only, 1972.

Qasi, Q. H. and Reed, T. E.: A problem in diagnosis of primary versus secondary microcephaly. Clin. Genet. 4: 46-52, 1973.

Schmidt, B., Jaeger, W. and Neubauer, H.: Ein Mikrozephalie-Syndrome mit atypischer tapetoretinaler Degeneration bei 3 Geschwistern. Klin. Mbl. Augenheilk. 150: 188-196, 1968.

Van den Bosch, J.: Microcephaly in the Netherlands: a clinical and genetical study. Ann. Hum. Genet. 23: 91-116, 1959.

25125 MICROCEPHALY WITH CERVICAL SPINE FUSION ANOMALIES

Zackai et al. (1972) described brothers from a consanguineous marriage who had microcephaly, mild mental retardation, short stature and skeletal anomalies. The facies were similar to those in Seckel syndrome. One brother had fusion C6-7 with instability at C2-3 producing spinal cord compression. The other brother had fusion at C2-3 and C7-T1.

Zackai, E. H., Sly, W. S. and McAlister, W. H.: Microcephaly, mild mental retardation, short stature, and skeletal anomalies in siblings. Am. J. Dis. Child. 124: 111-119, 1972.

25130 MICROCEPHALY, HIATUS HERNIA AND NEPHROTIC SYNDROME

Galloway and Mowat (1968) observed a brother and sister with this combination. Death from nephrosis occurred at 20 and 28 months, respectively. Parental consanguinity could not be demonstrated.

Galloway, W. H. and Mowat, A. P.: Congenital microcephaly with hiatus hernia and nephrotic syndrome in two sibs. J. Med. Genet. 5: 319-321, 1968.

Greene, M. L., Lietman, P. S., Rosenberg, L. E. and Seegmiller, J. E.: Trimethadione (tridione (R)) — induced nephrotic syndrome. Report of a case with unique ultrastructural renal pathology. Am. J. Med. 54: 265-271, 1973.

25140 MICROCOLON

Caresano and Borghi (1966) described microcolon in two newborn males of an Italian family. Microcolon occurs with agangliosis of the entire colon and part of the small intestine and with obstruction of the small intestine as in congenital atresia or meconium ileus. Thus, a familial aggregation of microcolon might result from the well-known occurrence of meconium ileus with cystic fibrosis of the pancreas. Lee and MacMillan (1950) claim that it can rarely be considered a primary entity.

Caresano, A. and Borghi, A.: Il microcolon: a propito di due osservazioni nella medesima famiglia. Quad. Radiol. 31: 173-185, 1966.

Hunt, H. B.: Roentgenological aspects of the congenitally small colon and of intestinal occlusions: with report of five cases. Am. J. Roentgen. 41: 564-574, 1939.

Lee, C. M., Jr. and MacMillan, B. G.: The fallacy in the diagnosis of microcolon in the newborn. Radiology 55: 807-813, 1950.

25150 MICROPHTHALMIA AND MENTAL DEFICIENCY

This combination suggests Norrie disease, an X-linked disorder (q.v.). Sjogren and Larsson (1949) described the association as an autosomal recessive syndrome. Pinsky et al. (1965) described three sisters with microphthalmos, severe mental retardation and spastic cerebral palsy. Balci et al. (1974) described this condition in a girl whose parents were first-cousins. Corneal opacities were present and glycinuria was found.

Balci, S., Say, B. and Firat, T.: Corneal opacity, microphthalmia, mental retardation, microcephaly and generalized muscular spasticity associated with hyperglycinemia. Clin. Genet. 5: 36-39, 1974.

Pinsky, L., DiGeorge, A. M., Harley, R. D. and Baird, H. W., III: Microphthalmos, corneal opacity, mental retardation, and spastic cerebral palsy. An oculocerebral syndrome. J. Pediat. 67: 387-398, 1965.

Sjogren, T. and Larsson, T.: Microphthalmos and anophthalmos with or without coincident oligophrenia. A clinical and genetic-statistical study. Acta Psychiat. Neurol. Scand. 56 (suppl.): 1-103, 1949.

*25160 MICROPHTHALMOS

Gill and Harris (1959) reported a family with two cases of microphthalmos, in the proband and in her great-aunt. Wolff (1930) described a family of 10 children whose parents were first cousins and among whom 3 males and two females had microphthalmos, high grade hyperopia (up to + 20d) and glaucoma. In extreme instances differentiation from anophthalmos (q.v.) may be impossible without histologic study. The eye is generally small without gross congenital malformations. Holst (1950) observed 6 cases in two related sibships. Nanophthalmos is a synonym for microphthalmos. Both dominant and recessive forms are known.

Ashley, L. M.: Bilateral anophthalmos in brother and sister. J. Hered. 38: 174-176, 1947.

Gill, E. G. and Harris, R. B.: Congenital microphthalmos with cyst formation. Virginian Med. Monthly 86: 33-36, 1959.

Holst: Blindhetsarsaker I Norge (Oslo), 1950. Cited by Sorsby, A.: System of Ophthalmology, Normal and Abnormal Development. St. Louis: C. V. Mosby Co., 3: (part 2) 1963. P. 490.

Joseph, R.: A pedigree of anophthalmos. Brit. J. Ophthal. 41: 541-543, 1957.

R E C E S S I V E

McMillan, L.: Anophthalmia and maldevelopment of the eyes: four cases in the same family. Brit. J. Ophthal. 5: 121-122, 1921.

Wolff, E.: A microphthalmic family. Proc. Roy. Soc. Med. 23 (part I): 623-626, 1930.

25170 MICROPHTHALMOS WITH HYPERMETROPIA, RETINAL DEGENERATION, MACRO-PHAKIA AND DENTAL ANOMALIES

In a sibship of 7 without parental consanguinity, Franceschetti and Gernet (1965) found four (three males, one female) with marked microphthalmos, diagnosed with the echogram (ultrasonogram), with cornea of normal size. Associated features were high grade hypermetropia, macrophakia, retinal degeneration and dental anomalies. Two had glaucoma.

Franceschetti, A. and Gernet, H.: Diagnostic ultrasonique d'une microphtalmie sans microcornee, avec macrophakie, haute hypermetropie associee a une degenerescence tapeto-retinienne, une disposition glaucomateuse et des anomalies dentaires (nouveau syndrome familial). Arch. Ophtal. (Paris) 25: 105-116, 1965.

25175 MICROSPHEROPHAKIA

Small round lens as an isolated abnormality appears to be a recessive. Affected sibs have been reported by Fleischer (1916), Gil (1928) and Franceschetti (1930), among others, and parental consaguinity by Fleischer (1916) and Franceschetti (1930).

Fleischer, B.: Abnorme Kleinheit und Kugelgestalt der Linse bei zwei Geschwisterpaaren. Arch. Augenheilk. 80: 248, 1916.

Franceschetti, A.: Ueber Mikrophakie und deren Erbgang. Klin. Mbl. Augenheilk. 85: 285, 1930.

Gil, R. R.: Familiare Microphakie. Klin. Mbl. Augenheilk. 85: 285, 1928.

25180 MICROTIA WITH MEATAL ATRESIA

Ellwood et al. (1968) reported (1) brother and sister with bilateral anotia with meatal atresia and (2) two brothers, one with unilateral microtia and bilateral meatal atresia and the other with unilateral microtia and meatal atresia. The first sibship had had first-cousin parents. The evidence for recessive inheritance is inconclusive.

Ellwood, L. C., Winter, S. T. and Dar, H.: Familial microtia with meatal atresia in two sibships. J. Med. Genet. 5: 289-291, 1968.

25190 MITOCHONDRIAL ABNORMALITIES WITH MYOPATHY

Several probably distinct myopathies with morphologic and-or biochemical abnormalities of the mitochondria have been described. (See HYPERMETABOLISM DUE TO DEFECT IN MITOCHONDRIA. See PLEOCONIAL MYOPATHY. See MYOPATHY WITH GIANT ABNORMAL MITOCHONDRIA.) Coleman et al. (1967) described two patients with progressive proximal and subsequently distal muscle fatigability and weakness at ages 5 to 10 years. Unusually large mitochondria, with high activities of oxidative enzymes, and abnormal accumulation of neutral fat were demonstrated by muscle biopsy. The muscle mitochondria contained anomalous quadrilaminar structures (Price et al., 1967). Van Wijngaarden et al. (1967) gave a follow-up on the patient of Luft et al. (see HYPERMETABOLISM DUE TO DEFECT IN MITOCHONDRIA) and described another case of myopathy with mitochondrial abnormality.

Coleman, R. F., Nienhuis, A. W., Brown, W. J., Munsat, T. L. and Pearson, C. M.: New myopathy with mitochondrial enzyme hyperactivity. J.A.M.A. 199: 624-630, 1967.

Price, H. M., Gordon, G. B., Munsat, T. L. and Pearson, C. M.: Myopathy with atypical mitochondria in type I skeletal muscle fibers. A histochemical and ultrastructural study. J. Neuropath. Exp. Neurol. 26: 475-497, 1967.

Van Wijngaarden, G. K., Bethlem, J., Meijer, A. E. F. H., Hulsmann, W. C. and Feltkamp, C. A.: Skeletal muscle disease with abnormal mitochondria. Brain 90: 577-592, 1967.

25195 MITOCHONDRIAL MYOPATHY WITH LACTIC ACIDOSIS

Hackett et al. (1973) described two sisters with signs of growth failure, severe muscle weakness, and moderate neural deafness. Light microscopy of skeletal muscle showed areas of 'granular necrosis' which by electronmicroscopy were found to be produced by large and numerous mitochondria. Hyperalaninemia and hyperalaninuria were demonstrated and an oral alanine load was more slowly cleared than normal. They also had elevated pyruvate concentration in the blood and severe lactic acidosis which in one girl was fatal at age 11 years. The girls were asymptomatic until ages 6 and 8 years. One sister was alive at age 20. No statement about parental consanguinity was made. See 23880, 25200, 25540, and 26290 for other 'mitochondrial myopathies.'

Hackett, T. N., Jr., Bray, P. F., Ziter, F. A., Nyhan, W. L. and Creer, K. M.: A metabolic myopathy associated with chronic lactic acidemia, growth failure, and nerve deafness. J. Pediat. 83: 426-431, 1973.

25200 MITOCHONDRIAL MYOPATHY WITH SALT CRAVING

Spiro et al. (1970) described a 13-year-old boy who was floppy at birth, showed delayed motor milestones, was found to have severe salt craving and non-progressive myopathy. Ultrastructural abnormalities consisting of increased numbers of large mitochondria aligned with lipid bodies were noted in biopsied skeletal muscle fibers. No other members of the family were affected.

Spiro, A. J., Prineas, J. W. and Moore, C. L.: A new mitochondrial myopathy in a patient with salt craving. Arch. Neurol. 22: 259-269, 1970.

*25205 MIXED DISULFIDURIA I

Crawhall et al. (1971) described a 49-year-old male patient, the product of brother-sister incest, who excreted the mixed disulfide, beta-mercaptolactone-cysteine. The structure of the disulfide is indicated by its name: in one half of the molecule the -NH2 of cysteine is replaced by -OH. The patient had been found in the course of screening mentally retarded patients with the nitroprusside test. Administration of cysteine but not of methionine increased excretion of the mixed disulfide. Niederwieser et al. (1973) found the same material in the urine of two mentally normal sisters aged 11 and 13 years.

Crawhall, J. C., Bir, K., Purkiss, P. and Stanbury, J. B.: Sulfur amino acids as precursors of beta-mercaptolactate cysteine disulfide in human subjects. Biochem. Med. 5: 109-115, 1971.

Crawhall, J. C., Purkiss, P. and Stanbury, J. B.: Metabolism of isotopically labelled sulfur amino acids in a patient excreting beta-mercaptolactate-cysteine disulfide. (Abstract) J. Clin. Invest. 50: 22A only, 1971.

Niederwieser, A., Giliberti, P. and Baerlocher, K.: Beta-mercaptolactate cysteine disulfiduria in two normal sisters. Isolation and characterization of beta-mercaptolactate cysteine disulfide: Clin. Chim. Acta 43: 405-416, 1973.

*25210 MOHR SYNDROME (OFD SYNDROME II)

Otto L. Mohr (1941) described a family in which four males of a sibship of five boys and two girls showed a syndrome which was detailed in the case of one affected male whom he personally observed. The features were poly-, syn-, and brachydactyly, lobate tongue with papilliform protuberances, high arched palate, angular form of the alveolar process of the mandible, supernumerary sutures in the skull, and an episodic neuromuscular disturbance. Three of the four affected males had died prior to the time of report. One of these had cleft palate. No similarly affected persons in previous generations were known. The parents were not related. Mohr suggested that the syndrome is due to a recessive, sub-lethal, X-linked gene. Obviously the evidence for this suggestion was feeble. Claussen (1946) provided a follow-up of the kindred with description of an affected male cousin. Furthermore, the parents of the new case were related. He suggested autosomal recessive inheritance, which seems to be supported by Gorlin's (1967) observation of the same syndrome in two sisters. In several respects the Mohr syndrome resembles oral-facial-digital syndrome. Rimoin and Edgerton (1967) described three affected sibs (two male, one female) and suggested that this might be called the oral-facial-digital syndrome II. In addition to the different mode of inheritance, the Mohr syndrome shows none of the skin and hair changes of the X-linked oral-facial-digital syndrome I but does show conductive hearing loss and bilateral hallucal polysyndactyly not present in OFD I. Gustavson et al. (1971) reported two affected sisters.

R
E
C
E
S
S
I
V
E

Claussen, O.: Et arvelig syndrom omfattende tungemissdannelse og polydaktyli. Nord. Med. 30: 1147-1151, 1946.

Gorlin, R. J.: Minneapolis, Minn.: personal communication, 1967.

Gustavson, K.-H., Kreuger, A. and Petersson, P. O.: Syndrome characterized by lingual malformation, polydactyly, tachypnea, and psychomotor retardation (Mohr syndrome). Clin. Genet. 2: 261-266, 1971.

Mohr, O. L.: A hereditary lethal syndrome in man. Avh. Norske Videnskad. Oslo 14: 1-18, 1941.

Pfeiffer, R. A., Majewski, F. and Mannkopf, H.: Das syndrome Von Mohr und Claussen. Klin. Padiat. 184: 224-229, 1972.

Rimoin, D. L. and Edgerton, M. T.: Genetic and clinical heterogeneity in the oral-facial-digital syndromes. J. Pediat. 71: 94-102, 1967.

25220 MONILETHRIX

Extensively affected kindreds with the pattern of dominant inheritance have been reported. However, Hanhart (1955) claimed recessive inheritance for a kindred he studied. Working also in Zurich, Salamon and Schnyder (1962) suggested that one out of five families might have a recessive form of the disorder. Recessive inheritance cannot be considered as proved, however.

Hanhart, E.: Erstmaliger Hinweis auf das Vorkommen eines monohybridrezessiven Erbgangs bei Monilethrix (Moniletrichosis). Arch. Klaus Stift. Vererbungsforsch. 30: 1-11, 1955.

Salamon, T. and Schnyder, U. W.: Ueber die Monilethrix. Arch. Klin. Exp. Derm. 215: 105-136, 1962.

25225 MONOCYTE CHEMOTACTIC DISORDER

In a 9-year-old girl with chronic mucocutaneous candidiasis and cutaneous anergy Snyderman (1973) found that mononuclear leukocytes failed to migrate in vitro toward two chemotactic stimuli, leukocyte-derived chemotactic factor and C5A. After treatment with transfer factor, the patient's monocytes responded to both chemotactic factors. There is no information on the genetics of this presumably genetic disorder, but autosomal recessive inheritance is a reasonable presumption. Deficiency of leukocyte myeloperoxidase has been found with disseminated candidiasis (25460). In other cases chronic mucocutaneous candidiasis has been related to a deficiency of lymphokine (24765) or a defect in lymphocyte transformation either intrinsic (24757) or resulting from inhibition by a serum factor (24755).

Snyderman, R., Altman, L. C., Frankel, A. and Blaese, R. M.: Defective mononuclear leukocyte chemotaxis: a previously unrecognized immune dysfunction. Studies in a patient with chronic mucocutaneous candidiasis. Ann. Inter. Med. 78: 509513, 1973.

Some patients have a disorder qualitatively like mucopolysaccharidosis IV (q.v.) but milder. Slight corneal clouding occurs. This is the condition present in the patient shown by McKusick (1960, P. 91). The patient has a normal child. Two male first cousins are identically affected. These patients come from an inbred Early American group in which at least 4 other rare recessives have been found: Crigler-Najjar syndrome, homocystinuria, bird-headed dwarfism, and metachromatic leukodystrophy. Many forms of spondyloepiphyseal dysplasia have been incorrectly labelled Morquio syndrome. There are, however, some cases which seem legitimately termed Morquio syndrome in which keratosulfate is not excreted in the urine. The condition or conditions in this group of patients may still be the result of a disturbance in mucopolysaccharide metabolism. Danes and Bearn (1967) studied 8 families, each with at least one case of Morquio syndrome. In 6 families with the disorder limited to the skeleton, no metachromasia was found in fibroblasts. In one of the other families corneal clouding, Reilly bodies and severe mental retardation accompanied the skeletal features and in a second 'shoe-shaped' sella turcica and widened humeral shafts accompanied the usual features of Morquio syndrome. Both these two families did show fibroblast metachromasia. Conceivably this is a mild allelic form of MPS IV (25300). For this reason no asterisk is assigned.

Danes, B. S. and Bearn, A. G.: Cellular metachromasia, a genetic marker for studying the mucopolysaccharidoses. Lancet I: 241-243, 1967.

McKusick, V. A.: Heritable Disorders of Connective Tissue. St. Louis: C. V. Mosby Co., 1972 (4th Ed.).

25240 MUCOLIPIDOSIS I (LIPOMUCOPOLYSACCHARIDOSIS)

In the terminology, classification, and numbering of this category, I have followed Spranger and Wiedemann (1970). Mucolipidosis I was formerly called lipomucopolysaccharidosis. The disorder is characterized by mild Hurler-like manifestations with moderate mental retardation, no excess mucopolysacchariduria and peculiar inclusions of the fibroblasts. Spranger and Wiedemann (1970) observed three affected sibs and parental consanguinity in one instance. They suggested that the sibs described by Pincus et al. (1967) had this disorder as did the patient reported by Sanfilippo et al. (1962). See case of Loeb et al. (1969). The fibroblasts have as striking inclusions as in mucolipidosis II (I-cell disease). However, lysosomal enzymes are normal in fibroblasts rather than low as in mucolipidosis II. Lysosomal enzymes are high in liver. This is the reason the Belgian group referred to this as GAL plus disease. The classification as a mucolipidosis is based on electron microscopy. Spranger (1972) suspects there are two forms A and B of which the second has more severe neurologic problems. Spranger (1974) found that his original case of ML I in fact had mannosidosis (24850). Indeed, Spranger (1974) knew of only three cases, two of his and one of Berard-Badier et al. (1970). (The last case we had classified as the same as the condition reported by Goldberg et al. (23325).) All three were sporadic. Features are short trunk with relatively long limbs, cherry red spot of the fundus oculi, corneal opacity, impaired hearing, muscular hypotonia and wasting, cerebellar signs, tremor, myoclonic jerks, peripheral neuropathy, vacuoles in circulating white cells and bone marrow cells, and myelin degeneration on histologic studies. The patients do not have contractures.

Berard-Badier, M., Adechy-Benkoel, L., Chamlian, A. et al.: Etude ultrastructurale duparenchyme hepatique dans les mucopolysaccharidoses. Path. Biol. (Paris) 18: 117-128, 1970.

Loeb, H., Teppel, M. and Cremer, N.: Clinical, biochemical and ultrastructural studies of an atypical form of mucopolysaccharidosis. Acta Paediat. 58: 220-228, 1969.

Pincus, J. H., Rossi, J. P. and Daroff, R. B.: Delayed development of disturbed mucopolysaccharide metabolism in a Hurler variant. Arch. Neurol. 16: 244-253, 1967.

Sanfilippo, S. J., Yunis, J. and Worthen, H. G.: An unusual storage disease resembling the Hurler-Hunter syndrome. (Abstract) Am. J. Dis. Child. 104: 553 only, 1962.

Spranger, J. W. and Wiedemann, H. R.: The genetic mucolipidoses. Diagnosis and differential diagnosis. Humangenetik 9: 113-139, 1970.

Spranger, J. W.: Kiel, Germany: personal communication, 1972.

Spranger, J. W., Wiedemann, H. R., Tolksdorf, M., Graucob, E. and Caesar, R.: Lipomucopolysaccharidose: eine neue Speicherkrankheit. Z. Kinderheilk. 103: 285-306, 1968.

Spranger, J.: Kiel, Germany, personal communication, 1974.

*25250 MUCOLIPIDOSIS II (I-CELL DISEASE)

This is a Hurler-like condition with severe clinical and radiologic features, peculiar fibroblast inclusions and no excessive mucopolysacchariduria. Congenital dislocation of the hip, thoracic deformities, hernia and hyperplastic gums are evident soon after birth. Retarded psychomotor development, clear corneas, restricted joint mobility are other features. Leroy et al. (1969) first described this condition. Both sexes have been affected, sibs were affected in two families and the parents of one of the patients of Spranger and Wiedemann (1970) were first cousins. Abnormal inclusions were found in the fibroblasts of some heterozygotes (Leroy et al., 1969). Weismann et al. (1971) concluded that the defect leads to leakage of lysosomal enzymes from the cell. Cultured fibroblasts showed low levels of four lysosomal enzymes whereas the level of these enzymes in the cultured medium was high. The designation is perhaps not the best because other disorders especially mucolipidosis I have as striking inclusions (Spranger, 1972). Hickman and Neufeld (1972) presented evidence for their hypothesis that the mutation in I-cell disease is in an enzyme which modifies several lysosomal enzymes to guarantee their recognition by cells and re-entry into cells from the intercellular space into which the enzymes have been secreted by the synthesizing cells. There is precedence for the idea that carbohydrate sidechains of glycoproteins control entry of the proteins into liner cells (Morell et al., 1971). This hypothesis would explain why multiple enzymes are high in the medium in which I-cells are grown and low in the cells themselves. It is an alternative to the 'leaky lysosome' hypothesis of Wiesmann et al. (1971). The evidence presented by Hickman and Neufeld (1972) was of several types. For example, they found that alpha-1-iduronidase produced by I-cells did not 'correct' Hurler cells whereas semipurified iduronidase from urine and medium in which normal cells have grown do correct the metabolic defect of Hurler cells. The Neufeld hypothesis is an alternative to the Novikoff hypothesis which suggests that the acid hydrolases are packaged in the lysosomes directly after synthesis in the Golgi apparatus. This may indeed be true for some lysosomal enzymes because acid phosphatase and beta-glucosidase have normal activities in I cells. Leroy et al. (1972) found no accumulation of lipid in brain and viscera and no accumulation of mucopolysaccharide in these tissues or fibroblasts. For this reason they questioned the appropriation of the designation 'mucolipidosis.'

Demars, R. I. and Leroy, J.: The remarkable cells cultured from a human with Hurler's syndrome. An approach to visual selection for in vitro genetic studies. In Vitro 2: 107, 1967.

Gilbert, E. F., Dawson, G., ZuRhein, G. M., Opitz, J. M. and Spranger, J. W.: I-cell disease, mucolipidosis II. Pathological, histochemical, ultrastructural and biochemical observations in four cases. Z. Kinderheilk. 114: 259-292, 1973.

Hanai, J., Leroy, J. and O'Brien, J. S.: Ultrastructure of cultured fibroblasts in I-cell disease. Am. J. Dis. Child. 122: 34-38, 1971.

Hickman, S. and Neufeld, E. F.: A hypothesis for I-cell disease: defective hydrolases that do not enter lysosomes. Biochem. Biophys. Res. Commun., in press, 1972.

Hickman, S. and Neufeld, E. F.: A hypotheses for I-cell disease: defective hydrolases that do not enter lysosomes. Biochem. Biophys. Res. Commun. 49: 992-999, 1972.

Leroy, J. G. and Demars, R. I.: Mutant enzymatic and cytological phenotypes in cultured human fibroblasts. Science 157: 804-806, 1967.

Leroy, J. G., Demars, R. I. and Opitz, J. M.: I-cell disease. The Clinical Delineation of Birth Defects. IV. Skeletal Dysplasias. New York: National Foundation, 1969. Pp. 174-185.

Leroy, J. G., Ho, M. W., MacBrinn, M. C., Zielke, K., Jacob, J. and O'Brien, J. S.: I-cell disease biochemical studies. Pediat. Res. 6: 752-757, 1972.

Morell, A. G., Gregoriadis, G., Scheinberg, I. H., Hickman, J. and Ashwell, G.: The role of sialic acid in determining the survival of glycoproteins in the circulation. J. Biol. Chem. 246: 1461-1467, 1971.

Spranger, J. W. and Wiedemann, H. R.: The genetic mucolipidoses. Diagnosis and differential diagnosis. Humangenetik 9: 113-139, 1970.

Spranger, J. W.: Kiel, Germany: personal communication, 1972.

Wiesmann, U. N., Rossi, E. E. and Herschkowitz, N. N.: Treatment of metachromatic leukodystrophy in fibroblasts by enzyme replacement. (Letter) New Eng. J. Med. 284: 672-673, 1971.

R
E
C
E
S
S
I
V
E

*25260 MUCOLIPIDOSIS III (PSEUDO-HURLER POLYDYSTROPHY)

Under the designation 'pseudo-polydystrophie de Hurler,' Maroteaux and Lamy (1966) described 4 cases with many of the features of the Hurler syndrome but a much slower clinical evolution and no mucopolysacchariduria. The bone marrow contained cells reminiscent of those in the Hurler syndrome but vacuoles were empty. Hypoplasia of the odontoid was noted in at least one case. The authors pointed out that this is probably the same condition as that in a patient listed among 'cases defying classification' in the report of McKusick et al. (1965). It is plausible that there should be genetic defects of mucopolysaccharide metabolism without mucopolysacchariduria and this is probably an example. It holds a relationship to mucopolysaccharidosis I comparable to the relationship of the non-keratosulfate-excreting Morquio syndrome to mucopolysaccharidosis IV. I have two brother-sister pairs among the six patients with this disorder whom I have studied in detail. Several other patients are known to me. The sibs reported by Steinbach et al. (1968) appear to have had this condition. In 1928, in Freiburg, Germany, Schinz and Furtwaengler described a sibship of 11, the offspring of a first-cousin marriage, in which a man then 29-years-old and three of his sisters were identically affected by a disorder in which a striking feature was stiff joints. Flexion contracture in the fingers and toes was combined with reduced mobility in the ankles, wrists, knees, elbows, hips, shoulders and spine. The face was red with somewhat prominent forehead, broad nose and fleshy tongue. Intelligence was normal. Umbilical hernia was present in the male, whose height was 61.4 inches. X-rays showed thick skull, short posterior cranial fossa and prominent external and internal occipital protuberance. A striking feature was extensive destruction or disturbance in the development of the carpal and tarsal bones. In 1934 Horsch described a sister from the same sibship. All features including those in the carpal and tarsal bones were identical. The brother was restudied with description of cysts in the head of the humerus and the epiphysis of the radius and digits. Langer, Kronenberg and Gorlin (1966) described a 61 year old male who appeared to have the same disorder, including changes in the joints, carpal and tarsal bones, and cornea. The urine contained no excess of acid mucopolysaccharide but did have an excess of a glycoprotein. Gorlin (1972) tells me that he is convinced of the identity of their patient to that of Schinz and Furtwaengler (1928). We have seen a patient in his late 20's with presumably the same disorder. There is more than one cause of the pseudo-Hurler polydystrophy phenotype. Of 18 patients studied by Kelly and Thomas (1974), only 12 of them met the biochemical and ultrastructural criteria for ML III. One apparently typical case proved to have a form of the Maroteaux-Lamy syndrome (25300). Others probably represent some disorder not cataloged here. It is possible that ML II (25250) and ML III represent homozygosity for genes at one and the same locus, namely one determining a 'recognition marker' for multiple lysosomal enzymes. The enzyme deficient in this disorder (and ML II) is a glycosyl transferase, presumably.

Gorlin, R. J.: Minneapolis, Minn.: personal communication, 1972.

Horsch, K.: Ueber hereditaere degenerative Osteoarthropathie. Arch. Orthop. Unfallchir. 34: 536-540, 1934.

Kelly, T. E. and Thomas, G. H.: Baltimore, personal communication, 1974.

Langer, L. O., Jr., Kronenberg, R. S. and Gorlin, R. J.: A case simulating Hurler syndrome of unusual longevity, without abnormal mucopolysacchariduria. A proposed classification of the various forms of the syndrome and similar diseases. Am. J. Med. 40: 448-457, 1966.

Maroteaux, P. and Lamy, M.: La pseudo-polydystrophie de Hurler. Presse Med. 74: 2889-2892, 1966.

McKusick, V. A., Kaplan, D., Wise, D., Hanley, W. B., Suddarth, S. B., Sevick, M. E. and Maumenee, A. E.: The genetic mucopolysaccharidoses. Medicine 44: 445-483, 1965.

Schinz, H. R. and Furtwaengler, A.: Zur Kenntnis einer hereditaeren Osteoarthropathie mit rezessivem Erbgang. Deutsch. Z. Chir. 207: 398-416, 1928.

Schmidt, R.: Eine bisher nicht beschriebene Form familiaerer Hornhautentartung in Verbindung mit Osteoarthropathie. Klin. Mbl. Augeneilk. 100: 616-620, 1938.

Steinbach, H. L., Preger, L., Williams, H. E. and Cohen, P.: The Hurler syndrome without abnormal mucopolysacchariduria. Radiology 90: 472-478, 1968.

25270 MUCOPOLYSACCHARIDOSES, UNCLASSIFIED TYPES

Not only are special studies such as those by the methods of Neufeld revealing heterogeneity within several of the six main types of mucopolysaccharidosis but also some forms remain unclassified. For example, Horton and Schimke (1970) described brother and sister, ages 13 and 11, with features like pseudo-Hurler polydystrophy (mucolipidosis III) but with mucopolysaccharides (both chondroitin sulfate B and heparitin sulfate) in the urine in amounts about 10 to 15 times the normal. Intelligence was normal. Brown and Kuwabara (1970) observed two sisters, ages 5 and 13 years, with Hurler-like facies, swollen fingers, dwarfed stature, severe progressive joint destruction and peculiar progressive peripheral annular corneal of calcification. The parents were Puerto Rican first cousins. Fibroblasts showed metachromasia and increased mucopolysaccharide. Urinary mucopolysaccharide was normal. High doses of vitamins seemed to be beneficial. Scott et al. (1973) described a male child who had mucopolysacchariduria, mental retardation, 'dysostosis multiplex' and appearance like that of a mucopolysaccharidosis. Death occurred at 47 months from pneumonia. The reticuloendothelial system remained free of mucopolysaccharide although accumulations were found in the perichondrium, coronary arteries, aorta and glomerular epithelial cells of the kidney. Lipid accumulated in peripheral neurons but not in central neurons.

Brown, S. I. and Kuwabara, T.: Peripheral corneal opacification and skeletal deformities. A newly recognized acid mucopolysaccharidosis simulating rheumatoid arthritis. Arch. Ophthal. 83: 667-677, 1970.

Horton, W. A. and Schimke, R. N.: A new mucopolysaccharidosis. J. Pediat. 77: 252-258, 1970.

Scott, C. R., Laqunoff, D. and Pritzl, P.: A mucopolysaccharide storage disease with involvement of the renal glomerular epithelium. Am. J. Med. 54: 549-556, 1973.

*25280 MUCOPOLYSACCHARIDOSIS TYPE I (HURLER SYNDROME: GARGOYLISM)

The autosomal recessive form is more frequent than type II, which is X-linked, has no clouding of the cornea and pursues a slower course. In two cases presumably of this type, Austin et al. (1964) found an increase in activity of the lysosomal enzyme arylsulphatase-B in liver, kidney and brain. Danes and Bearn (1965) found that cellular accumulation of mucopolysaccharides persists in cultured fibroblasts. Fratantoni, Hall and Neufeld (1968) showed that the accumulation results from inefficient degradation of intracellular mucopolysaccharide rather than excessive synthesis or reduced secretion. Furthermore they found that mixing of fibroblasts from Hurler and Hunter patients causes mutual correction of the intracellular accumulation of mucopolysaccharides. Medium in which cells of the other type or normal cells had been incubated was also effective in correcting the defect. Thus, isolation and identification of the corrective factor in the medium opens up possibilities of clarifying the normal mechanisms of MPS degradation, as well as therapy. Differentiation of the Sanfilippo syndrome (MPS III) from the Hurler and Hunter syndromes is also possible by this mixed culture method. Neuhauser et al. (1968) concluded that subarachnoid cysts are often responsible for the enlarged sella in the Hurler syndrome. If the mutation rates are the same and the heterozygotes for both conditions have no reproductive advantage or disadvantage, the Hunter syndrome should be one and one half times more frequent among newborns than the Hurler syndrome (McKusick, 1970). Observations probably does not agree with expectation. Improvement, clinical and chemical, with plasma infusions has been claimed (Di Ferrante et al., 1971). Results of treatment with purified preparations of Neufeld's correction factor are eagerly awaited.

Austin, J., McAfee, D., Armstrong, D., O'Rourke, M., Shearer, L. and Bachhawat, B.: Abnormal sulphatase activities in two human diseases (metachromatic leucodystrophy and gargoylism). Biochem. J. 93: 15C-17C, 1964.

Danes, B. S. and Bearn, A. G.: Hurler's syndrome: demonstration of an inherited disorder of connective tissue in cell culture. Science 149: 987-989, 1965.

Danes, B. S., Queenan, J. T., Gadow, E. C., and Cederquist, L. L.: Antenatal diagnosis of mucopolysaccharidoses. (Letter) Lancet I: 946-947, 1970.

Danes, B. S.: In-vitro confirmation of genetic compound of the Hurler and Scheie syndromes. (Letter) Lancet I: 680 only, 1974.

506

DiFerrante, N., Nichols, B. L., Donnelly, P. V., Neri, G., Hrgovcic, R. and Berglund, R. K.: Induced degradation of glycosaminoglycans in Hurler's and Hunter's syndromes by plasma infusion. Proc. Nat. Acad. Sci. 68: 303-307, 1971.

Foley, K. M., Danes, B. S. and Bearn, A. G.: White blood cell cultures in genetic studies on the human mucopolysaccharidoses. Science 164: 424-426, 1969.

Fratantoni, J. C., Hall, C. W. and Neufeld, E. F.: Hurler and Hunter syndromes: mutual correction of the defect in cultured fibroblasts. Science 162: 570-572, 1968.

Fratantoni, J. C., Hall, C. W. and Neufeld, E. F.: The defect in Hurler's and Hunter's syndromes: faulty degradation of mucopolysaccharide. Proc. Nat. Acad. Sci. 60: 699-706, 1968.

Fratantoni, J. C., Neufeld, E. F., Uhlendorf, B. W. and Jacobson, C. B.: Intrauterine diagnosis of the Hurler and Hunter syndromes. New Eng. J. Med. 280: 686-688, 1969.

Ho, M. W. and O'Brien, J. S.: Hurler's syndrome: deficiency of a specific beta galactosidase isoenzyme. Science 165: 611-613, 1969.

Leroy, J. G. and Crocker, A. C.: Studies on the genetics of the Hurler-Hunter syndrome. In, Aronson, S. M. and Volk, B. W. (eds.): Inborn Disorders of Sphingolipid Metabolism. Oxford: Pergamon Press, 1967. Pp. 455-473.

MacBrinn, M., Okada, S., Woollacott, M., Patel, V., Ho, M. W., Tappel, A. L. and O'Brien, J. S.: Beta-galactosidase deficiency in the Hurler syndrome. New Eng. J. Med. 281: 338-343, 1969.

Manley, G. and Hawksworth, J.: Diagnosis of Hurler's syndrome in the hospital laboratory and the determination of its genetic type. Arch. Dis. Child. 41: 91-96, 1966.

Matalon, R. and Dorfman, A.: Hurler's syndrome, an alpha-1-iduronidase deficiency. Biochem. Biophys. Res. Commun. 47: 959-964, 1972.

McKusick, V. A.: Heritable Disorders of Connective Tissue. St. Louis: C. V. Mosby Co., 1972 (4th. Ed.).

McKusick, V. A.: Relative frequency of the Hunter and Hurler syndromes. New Eng. J. Med. 283: 853-854, 1970.

Neufeld, E. F. and Fratantoni, J. C.: Inborn errors of mucopolysaccharide metabolism. Faulty degradative mechanisms are implicated in this group of human diseases. Science 169: 141-146, 1970.

Neuhauser, E. B. D., Griscom, N. T. and Gilles, F. H.: Arachnoid cysts in the Hurler-Hunter syndrome. Ann. Radiol. (Paris) 11: 453-469, 1968.

Schafer, I. A., Sullivan, J. C., Svejcar, J., Kofoed, J. and Robertson, W. B.: Study of the Hurler syndrome using cell culture: definition of the biochemical phenotype and the effect of ascorbic acid on the mutant cell. J. Clin. Invest. 47: 321-328, 1968.

Schafer, I. A., Sullivan, J. C., Svejcar, J., Kofoed, J. and Robertson, W. B.: Vitamin C-induced increase of dermatan sulfate in cultured Hurler's fibroblasts. Science 153: 1008-1010, 1966.

Spranger, J.: The systemic mucopolysaccharidoses. Ergeb. Inn. Med. Kinderhilk. 32: 165-265, 1972.

*25290 MUCOPOLYSACCHARIDOSIS TYPE III A (SANFILIPPO SYNDROME A)

In this variety only heparitin sulfate is excreted in the urine. The clinical features are severe mental defect with relatively mild somatic features (moderately severe claw hand and visceromegaly, little or no corneal clouding or skeletal, e.g., vertebral, change). The presenting problem may be marked overactivity, destructive tendencies and other behavioral aberrations in a child of 4 to 6. Maroteaux et al. (1966) reported a kindred in which three separate consanguineous marriages resulted in a total of four cases. The radiologic findings in the skeleton are relatively mild and consist of persistent biconvexity of the vertebral bodies, absent hydrocephalus and very thick calvarium. Two forms of Sanfilippo syndrome are identified by cocultivation experiments on fibroblasts (Kresse et al. 1971). Type A has deficiency of heparan sulfate sulfatase (Kresse and Neufeld, 1972).

Kresse, H. and Neufeld, E. F.: The Sanfilippo a corrective factor: purification and mode of action. J. Biol. Chem. 247: 2164-2170, 1972.

Kresse, H., Wiesmann, U., Cantz, M., Hall, C. W. and Neufeld, E. F.: Biochemical heterogeneity of the Sanfilippo syndrome: preliminary characterization of two deficient factors. Biochem. Biophys. Res. Commun. 42: 892, 1971.

Langer, L. O.: The radiographic manifestations of the HS-mucopolysaccharidosis of Sanfilippo, with discussion of this condition in relation to the other mucopolysaccharidoses and a classification of these fundamentally similar entities. Ann. Radiol. 7: 315-325, 1964.

Maroteaux, P., Frezal, J., Tahbaz-Zadeh and Lamy, M.: Une observation familiale d'oligophrenie polydystrophique. J. Genet. Hum. 15: 93-102, 1966.

Matalon, R. and Dorfman, A.: Sanfilippo A syndrome. Sulfamidase deficiency in cultured skin fibroblasts and liver. J. Clin. Invest. 54: 907-912, 1974.

McKusick, V. A., Kaplan, D., Wise, D., Hanley, W. B., Suddarth, S. B., Sevick, M. E. and Maumenee, A. E.: The genetic mucopolysaccharidoses. Medicine 44: 445-483, 1965.

Sanfilippo, S. J., Podosin, R., Langer, L. O. and Good, R. A.: Mental retardation associated with acid mucopolysacchariduria (heparitin sulfate type). J. Pediat. 63: 837-838, 1963.

R
E
C
E
S
S
I
V
E

Spranger, J. W., Teller, W., Kosenow, W., Murken, J. and Eckert-Huseman, E.: Die hs-mucopolysaccharidose von Sanfilippo (polydystrophe oligophrenie). Bericht Ueber 10 Patienten. Z. Kinderheilk. 101: 71-84, 1967.

Wallace, B. J., Kaplan, D., Adachi, M., Schneck, L. and Volk, B. W.: Mucopolysaccharidosis type III. Morphologic and biochemical studies of two siblings with Sanfilippo syndrome. Arch. Path. 82: 462-473, 1966.

*25292 MUCOPOLYSACCHARIDOSIS TYPE III B (SANFILIPPO SYNDROME B)

The defect in this form of Sanfilippo syndrome, which clinically is probably indistinguishable from type III A, concerns N-acetyl-alpha-D-glucosaminidase (O'Brien, 1972).

O'Brien, J. S.: Sanfilippo syndrome: profound deficiency of alpha-acetylglucosaminidase activity in organs and skin fibroblasts from type-B patients. Proc. Nat. Acad. Sci. 69: 1720-1722, 1972.

Von Figura, K. and Kresse, H.: Quantitative aspects of pinocytosis and intracellular fate of N-acetyl-alpha-D-glucosaminidase in Sanfilippo B fibroblasts. J. Clin. Invest. 53: 85-90, 1974.

Von Figura, K., Logering, M., Mersmann, G. and Kreese, H.: Sanfilippo B disease: serum assays for detection of homozygous and heterozygous individuals in three families. J. Pediat. 83: 607-611, 1973.

*25300 MUCOPOLYSACCHARIDOSIS TYPE IV (MORQUIO SYNDROME)

It seems likely that the condition described in 1929 by Morquio in Montevideo and Brailsford in Birmingham, Eng., was the entity in which we now recognize the occurrence of corneal clouding, aortic valve disease and urinary excretion of keratosulfate. Between 1929 and 1959 a miscellany of skeletal disorders was included in the Morquio category. These included various types of spondylo-epiphyseal dysplasia and multiple epiphyseal dysplasia. In the late 1950's when mucopolysacchariduria and extra-skeletal features were recognized, the eponym Morquio-Ullrich was proposed. It seems preferable, however, to retain the designation Morquio syndrome for this condition and to separate out the simulating conditions which represent entities distinct from that described by Morquio and Brailsford. This and some other forms of spondyloepiphyseal dysplasia are prone to the dangerous complications of atlantoaxial dislocation, due to hypoplasia of the odontoid (Greenberg, 1968). See 25230 for a possible allelic disorder. Gadbois et al. (1973) identified 48 cases of Morquio syndrome in the province of Quebec. They were distributed in 27 families. Although total urinary excretion of mucopolysaccharide was normal, excretion of keratan sulfate was increased two to three times over normal. Two distinct forms of keratan sulfate excreting Morquio syndrome were thought to exist in the group. Matalon et al. (1974) concluded that the enzyme deficiency involves 6-sulfatase which works on both kerstan sulfate and chondroitin sulfate.

Blaw, M. E. and Langer, L. O.: Spinal cord compression in Morquio-Brailsford's disease. J. Pediat. 74: 593-600, 1969.

Gadbois, P., Moreau, J. and Laberge, C.: La maladie de Morquio dans la province de Quebec. L'Union Medicale Du Canada. 102: 602-607, 1973.

Greenberg, A. D.: Atlantoaxial dislocations. Brain 91: 655-684, 1968.

Langer, L. O., Jr. and Carey, L. S.: The roentgenographic features of the KS mucopolysaccharidosis of Morquio (Morquio-Brailford's disease). Am. J. Roentgen. 97: 1-20, 1966.

Linker, A., Evans, L. R. and Langer, L. O.: Morquio's disease and mucopolysaccharide excretion. J. Pediat. 77: 1039-1047, 1970.

Maroteaux, P. and Lamy, M.: Opacites corneennes et troubles metaboliques dans la maladie de Morquio. Rev. Franc. Etud. Clin. Biol. 6: 481-483, 1961.

Matalon, R., Arbogast, B. and Dorfman, A.: Morquio's syndrome: a deficiency of chondroitin sulfate N-acetylhexosamine sulfate sulfatase. (Abstract) Pediat. Res. 8: 436 only, 1974.

Pedrini, V., Lennzi, L. and Zamtotti, V.: Isolation and identification of keratosulphate in urine of patients affected by Morquio-Ullrich disease. Proc. Soc. Exp. Biol. Med. 110: 847-849, 1962.

Robins, M. M., Stevens, H. F. and Linker, A.: Morquio's disease: an abnormality of mucopolysaccharide metabolism. J. Pediat. 62: 881-889, 1963.

Von Noorden, G. K., Zellweger, H. and Ponseti, I. V.: Ocular findings in Morquio-Ullrich's disease. Arch. Ophthal. 64: 585-591, 1960.

Zellweger, H., Ponseti, I. V., Pedrini, V., Stamler, F. S. and Von Noorden, G. K.: Morquio-Ullrich's disease. Report of 2 cases. J. Pediat. 59: 549-561, 1961.

25310 MUCOPOLYSACCHARIDOSIS TYPE V (SCHEIE SYNDROME, LATE HURLER SYNDROME, ETC.)

Stiff joints, clouding of the cornea most dense peripherally, survival to a late age with little if any impairment of intellect, and aortic regurgitation are features. Chondroitin sulfate B is excreted in the urine in excess. The second case of Emerit et al. (1966) was probably of this type. The parents were second-cousins. The facies and hands were characteristic and aortic regurgitation was present. The patient, a 32-year-old female, had a son with tricuspid atresia and situs inversus. The sisters, ages 47 and 55, reported by Koskenoja and Suvanto (1959) probably had this condition. The case of Poulet (1968) with two affected cousins was probably Scheie syndrome. Weismann and Neufeld (1970) found surprisingly no cross-correction of Scheie and Hurler fibroblasts, but the expected cross-correction of Scheie fibroblasts with those from Sanfilippo and Hunter patients. The possible interpretations include allelism of the two genes, either different amino acids

508 substituted at the same site in the cistron with different changes in the properties of the product protein (enzyme) as in Hb S and Hb C, or amino acids substituted at different sites in the same cistron, again with quite different effects on the properties of the product protein, as in Hb S and Hb M(Saskatoon). In the latter situation, the term heteroallele is sometimes used. It is theoretically possible that some of the phenotypically overlapping, 'new' mucopolysaccharidoses that are being described are examples of so-called compounds, comparable to the SC disease among the hemoglobinopathies. In such instances the parents would not be expected to be consanguineous. The asterisk which this entry carried in prior editions has been deleted because of the suggestion that the locus for the Scheie syndrome may be the same as that for the Hurler syndrome. My colleagues and I (1972) have suggested that the Hurler syndrome might be called MPS IH and the Scheie syndrome MPS IS. The genetic compounds which appear to exist at the MPS I locus, and must exist if the hypothesis of allelism is correct, may be called MPS IH-S.

Emerit, I., Maroteaux, P. and Vernant, P.: Deux observations de mucopolysaccharidose avec atteinte cardio-vasculaire. Arch. Franc. Pediat. 23: 1075-1087, 1966.

Koskenoja, M. and Suvanto, E.: Gargoylism: report of adult form with glaucoma in two sisters. Acta Ophthal. 37: 234-240, 1959.

McKusick, V. A., Howell, R. R., Hussels, I. E., Neufeld, E. F. and Stevenson R. E.: Allelism, nonallelism and genetic compounds among the mucopolysaccharidoses hypotheses. Lancet I: 993-996, 1972.

Poulet, J.: Mucopolysaccharidose du type Hurler I sans deterioration mentale chez un adulte et ses deux germains. Sem. Hop. Paris 44: 2545-2554, 1968.

Scheie, H. G., Hambrick, G. W., Jr. and Barness, L. A.: A newly recognized forme fruste of Hurler's disease (gargoylism). Am. J. Ophthal. 53: 753-769, 1962.

Wiesmann, U. N. and Neufeld, E. F.: Scheie and Hurler syndromes: apparent identity of the biochemical defect. Science 169: 72-74, 1970.

*25320 MUCOPOLYSACCHARIDOSIS TYPE VI (MAROTEAUX-LAMY SYNDROME)

The clinical characteristics are striking osseous and corneal changes (like those of MPS I) without intellectual impairment. Only (or predominantly) chondroitin sulfate B is excreted in the urine.

Barton, R. W. and Neufeld, E. F.: A distinct biochemical deficit in the Maroteaux-Lamy syndrome (mucopolysaccharidosis VI). J. Pediat. 80: 114-116, 1972.

DiFerrante, N., Hyman, B. H., Kish, W., Donnelly, P. V., Nichols, B. L. and Dutton, R. V.: Mucopolysaccharidosis VI (Maroteaux-Lamy disease) clinical and biochemical study of a mild variant case. Johns Hopkins Med. J. 135: 42-53, 1974.

Goldberg, M. F., Scott, C. I. and McKusick, V. A.: Hydrocephalus and papilledema in the Maroteaux-Lamy syndrome (mucopolysaccharidosis type VI). Am. J. Ophthal. 69: 969-975, 1970.

Maroteaux, P. and Lamy, M.: Hurler's disease, Morquio's disease, and related mucopolysaccharidoses. J. Pediat. 67: 312-323, 1965.

Maroteaux, P., Leveque, B., Marie, J. and Lamy, M.: Une nouvelle dysostose avec elimination urinaire de chondroitine-sulfate B. Presse Med. 71: 1849-1852, 1963.

Quigley, H. A. and Kenyon, K. R.: Ultrastructural and histochemical studies of a newly recognized form of systemic mucopolysaccharidosis (Maroteaux-Lamy syndrome, mild pehnotype). Am. J. Ophthal. 77: 809-818, 1974.

*25322 MUCOPOLYSACCHARIDOSIS VII (BETA-GLUCURONIDASE DEFICIENCY)

Sly et al. (1973) have described a single patient with skeletal changes consistent with a mucopolysaccharidosis, hepatosplenomegaly, and granular inclusions in granulocytes. Fibroblasts demonstrated deficiency of beta-glucuronidase. Both parents and several sibs of the mother showed an intermediate level of the enzyme.

Brot, F. E., Glaser, J. H., Roozen, K. J. and Sly, W. S.: In vitro corredtion of deficient human fibroblast by beta-glucuronidase from different human sources. Biochem. Biophys. Res. Commun. 57: 1-8, 1974.

Gehler, J., Cantz, M., Tolksdorf, M. and Spranger, J.: Mucopolysaccharidosis VII: beta-glucuronidase deficiency. Humangenetik 23: 149-158, 1974.

Glaser, J. H. and Sly, W. S.: Beta-glucuronidase deficiency mucopolysaccharidosis: methods for enzymatic diagnosis. J. Lab. Clin. Med. 82: 969-977, 1973.

Sly, W. S., Quinton, B. A., McAlister, W. H. and Rimoin, D. L.: Beta-glucuronidase deficiency: report of clinical, radiologic and biochemical features of a new mucopolysaccharidosis. J. Pediat. 82: 249 only, 1973.

*25325 MULIBREY NANISM

In Finland Perheentupa et al. (1973) described a new syndrome and named it mulibrey nanism for muscle, liver, brain and eye. Twenty-three patients were studied. Growth failure was evident at birth and was progressive. The characteristics were triangular face often with hydrocephaloid skull, gracility and muscular hypotonia, peculiar voice, enlarged liver, raised venous pressure due to pericardial constriction (a regular feature), and yellowish dots and pigment dispersion in the ocular fundi. Two-thirds of the patients had cutaneous naevi flammei and a third had cystic dysplasia of the tibia. The geographic accumulation of cases in a sparsely settled region of Finland, observation of three pairs of affected sibs, and parental consanguinity in three families supported recessive inheritance. It is likely that some more cases are lost through abortion or early death.

R
E
C
E
S
S
I
V
E

Perheentupa, J., Autio, S., Leisti, S., Raitta, C. and Tuuteri, L.: Mulibrey nanism, an autosomal recessive syndrome with pericardial constriction. Lancet II: 351-355, 1973.

*25330 MUSCULAR ATROPHY, INFANTILE (WERDNIG-HOFFMANN)

The age of onset is the main feature distinguishing the infantile (Werdnig-Hoffmann) and juvenile (Kugelberg-Welander) types.

Marquardt, MacLowry and Perry (1962), among others, have described the disorder in twins. Brandt (1949) reported the largest single study, involving 112 cases in 70 families. Segregation analysis yielded results consistent with autosomal recessive inheritance. Almost 6 percent of parents were consanguineous, a value 8 times that in controls. In 51 of 112, the spinal type was proved. In 2 or 3 the myopathic type was proved. In 59 the type was not determined. Werdnig-Hoffmann paralysis was present in several members of the inbred group of Scottish tinkers with familial goiter (see THYROID HORMONOGENESIS, GENETIC DEFECT IN, IV). Hogenhuis et al. (1967) reported special studies of a Chinese family in which 4 of 8 sibs succumbed to Werdnig-Hoffmann disease. Ghetti et al. (1971) claimed that in many families 'malignant' Werdnig-Hoffmann disease is found to coexist with the Werdnig-Hoffmann disease with a prolonged course, the Wohlfart-Kugelberg-Welander disease with infantile onset, and the Wohlfart-Kugelberg-Welander disease with juvenile onset. They concluded that these are one disorder.

Brandt, S.: Hereditary factors in infantile progressive muscular atrophy. Study of one-hundred and twelve cases in seventy families. Am. J. Dis. Child. 78: 226-236, 1949.

Brandt, S.: Werdnig-Hoffmann's infantile progressive muscular atrophy. Op. Ex. Domo Biol. Hered. Hum. U. Hafniensis 22: 1-328, 1950.

Gamstorp, I.: Progressive spinal muscular atrophy with onset in infancy or early childhood. Acta Paediat. Scand. 56: 408-423, 1967.

Ghetti, B., Amati, A., Turra, M. V., Pacini, A., Del Vecchio, M. and Guazzi, G. C.: Werdnig-Hoffmann-Wohlfart-Kugelberg-Welander disease: nosological unity and clinical variability in intrafamilial cases. Acta Genet. Med. Gem. 20: 43-58, 1971.

Hanhart, E.: Die infantile progressive spinale Muskelatrophie (Werdnig-Hoffmann) als einfach-rezessive, subletale Mutation auf Grund von 29 Faellen in 14 Sippen. Helv. Paediat. Acta 1: 110-133, 1945.

Hogenhuis, L. A., Spaulding, S. W. and Engel, W. K.: Neuronal RNA metabolism in infantile spinal muscular atrophy (Werdnig-Hoffmann's disease) studied by radioautography: a new technic in the investigation of neurological disease. J. Neuropath. Exp. Neurol. 26: 335-341, 1967.

Marquardt, J. E., MacLowry, J. and Perry, R. E.: Infantile progressive spinal muscular atrophy in identical Negro twins. New Eng. J. Med. 267: 386-388, 1962.

*25340 MUSCULAR ATROPHY, JUVENILE (KUGELBERG-WELANDER)

Kugelberg and Welander (1956) found 5 affected children among the 12 offspring of normal parents; two of the five were monozygotic twins. Spira (1963) described 7 affected members in two sibships of a family. In each case the affected persons were offspring of a first cousin marriage. Levy and Wittig (1962) described proximal muscular atrophy in two half-brothers, with onset at 13 and 16 years. Onset is usually between 2 and 17 years. Atrophy and weakness of proximal limb muscles, primarily in the legs, is followed by distal involvement. Usually the cases are diagnosed as limb-girdle muscular dystrophy until they are studied fully. Twitchings (fasciculations) are an important differentiating sign. Muscular biopsy and electromyography show the true nature of the process as a lower motor neuron disease. Furukawa et al. (1968) reported two families, each with affected brother and sister. The parents in one were first cousins. They pointed out that in their cases as well as those in the literature the symptoms of female patients were mild and the clinical course slow whereas male sibs were severely affected. They interpreted this as sex-influence. A dominant form represented by the mother and two children described by Ford (1961) may also exist and this may be the same as what has been termed scapuloperoneal amyotrophy (q.v.). Bundy and Filomeno (1974) described a Negro sibship in which 5 sibs out of 10 had this disorder.

Bundy, S. E. and Filomeno, A. R.: Proximal spinal muscular atrophy. In, Bergsma, D. (ed.): Clinical Delineation of Birth Defects. XVI. Urinary System and Others. Baltimore: Williams and Wilkins, 1974. Pp. 336-338.

Ford, F. R.: Diseases of the Nervous System in Infancy, Childhood and Adolescence. Springfield, Ill.: Charles C Thomas, 1961. P. 390.

Furukawa, T., Nakao, K., Sugita, H. and Tsukagoshi, H.: Kugelberg-Welander disease, with particular reference to sex-influenced manifestations. Arch. Neurol. 19: 156-162, 1968.

Furukawa, T., Tsukagoshi, H., Sugita, H., Kondo, K. and Tsubaki, T.: Clinical and genetic considerations on Kugelberg-Welander's disease. Clin. Neurol. 6: 148-155, 1966.

Hausmanowa-Petrusewicz, I., Sobkowicz, H., Zielinska, S. and Dobosz, I.: Apropos of heredofamilial juvenile muscular atrophy. Schweiz. Arch. Neurol. Psychiat. 90: 255-267, 1962.

Kugelberg, E. and Welander, L.: Heredofamilial juvenile muscular atrophy simulating muscular dystrophy. Arch. Neurol. Psychiat. 75: 500-509, 1956.

Levy, J. A. and Wittig, E. O.: Familial proximal muscular atrophy. Neuropsiquiatria 20: 233-237, 1962.

Meadows, J. C., Marsden, C. D. and Harriman, D. G. F.: Chronic spinal muscular atrophy in adults. I. The Kugelberg-Welander syndrome. J. Neurol. Sci. 9: 527-550, 1969.

Smith, J. B. and Patel, A.: The Wohlfart-Kugelberg-Welander disease. Review of the literature and report of a case. Neurology 15: 469-473, 1965.

Spira, R.: Neurogenic, familial, girdle type muscular atrophy (clinical electromyographic and pathological study). Confin. Neurol. 23: 245-255, 1963.

25350 MUSCULAR ATROPHY, PROGRESSIVE

Asano and colleagues (1960) described a form of distal muscular atrophy beginning in the first year of life. Features include impaired sensibility in the feet, dysarthria, choreic movements of arms and face, partial optic atrophy, scoliosis, incontinence, mental deficiency and increased deep tendon reflexes.

Asano, N. and colleagues: A peculiar type of progressive muscular atrophy. Jap. J. Hum. Genet. 5: 139 only, 1960.

25355 MUSCULAR ATROPHY, SPINAL, INTERMEDIATE TYPE

Fried and Emery (1971) suggested the existence of a distinct form of spinal muscular atrophy intermediate in severity between the infantile form of Werdnig-Hoffmann (SMA type I by their designation) and the juvenile form of Kugelberg and Welander (SMA III). The intermediate form, which they designate SMA II, is characterized by onset usually between 3 and 15 months and survival beyond 4 years and usually until adolescence or later. Proximal muscle weakness is the cardinal feature as in other forms of spinal muscular atrophy. They presented 14 cases of whom two were sibs. The parents were all normal and non-consanguineous. Hanson and Bundey (1974) described two brothers in a sibship of 4. SMA I (Werdnig-Hoffmann disease) and SMA III (Kugelberg-Welander disease) may be due to homozygosity of allelic genes, and SMA II could represent the genetic compound.

Fried, K. and Emery, A. E. H.: Spinal muscular atrophy type II. A separate genetic and clinical entity from type I (Werdnig-Hoffmann disease) and type III (Kugelberg-Welander disease). Clin. Genet. 2: 203-209, 1971.

Hanson, J. E. and Bundey, S. E.: Spinal muscular atrophy: an unusual variant with infantile onset and prolonged survival. In, Bergsma, D. (ed.): Clinical Delineation of Birth Defects. XVI. Urinary System and Others. Baltimore: Williams and Wilkins, 1974. Pp. 339-340.

*25360 MUSCULAR DYSTROPHY I (LIMB-GIRDLE, PELVO-FEMORAL OR LEYDEN-MOEBIUS TYPE)

R
E
C
E
S
S
I
V
E

The limb-girdle type of muscular dystrophy has its onset usually in childhood but sometimes in maturity or middle age. Involvement is first evident in either the pelvic or, less frequently, the shoulder girdle, often with asymmetry of wasting when the upper limbs are first involved. Spread from the lower to the upper limbs or vice versa occurs within twenty years. Pseudohypertrophy of the calves is uncommon but may be counterfeited by a stocky build or wasting of the vasti (Chung and Morton, 1959). The rate of progression is variable. Severe disability with inability to walk is seen within 20-30 years of onset. Contractures and facial weakness occur only late in some cases. Age at death shows a wide spread with the largest number dying in middle life.

Only 59 percent of cases of limb-girdle muscular dystrophy could, in the analysis of Chung and Morton (1959), be ascribed to autosomal recessive inheritance. The remainder were sporadic cases of unknown etiology. By an ingenious mathematical analysis Morton (1960) concluded that homozygosity at either of two loci may result in limb-girdle muscular dystrophy and that about 1.6 percent of the normal population is heterozygous for a limb-girdle muscular dystrophy gene.

Pfandler (1950) reported an extensive Swiss pedigree which was reproduced by Touraine (1955). Jackson and Carey (1961) found the same type of muscular dystrophy in the descendants of Swiss immigrants in a religious isolate (Amish) in Indiana. Cardiac involvement in brother and sister with this type was noted by Felsch et al. (1966). Moser et al. (1966) found autosomal recessive muscular dystrophy to be four times more frequent in the canton of Berne than in other countries studied. He mapped the places of origin of the parents of cases within the canton. These proved to be the same area as those from which the Amish family names are derived.

Rudman et al. (1972) concluded that patients are at least 7 times more sensitive to growth hormone than are normals.

Chung, C. S. and Morton, N. E.: Discrimination of genetic entities in muscular dystrophy. Am. J. Hum. Genet. 11: 339-359, 1959.

Felsch, G., Hoffmeyer, O. and Richter, G.: Herzbeteiligung bei dystrophia musculorum progressiva (Erb). Z. Ges. Inn. Med. 21: 73-79, 1966.

Jackson, C. E. and Carey, J. H.: Progressive muscular dystrophy: autosomal recessive type. Pediatrics 28: 77-84, 1961.

Jackson, C. E. and Strehler, D. A.: Limb-girdle muscular dystrophy: clinical manifestations and detection of preclinical disease. Pediatrics 41: 495-502, 1968.

Morton, N. E. and Chung, C. S.: Formal genetics of muscular dystrophy. Am. J. Hum. Genet. 11: 360-379, 1959.

Morton, N. E.: The mutational load due to detrimental genes in man. Am. J. Hum. Genet. 12: 348-364, 1960.

Moser, H., Wiesmann, U. N., Richterich, R. and Rossi, E.: Progressive Muskeldystrophie. VIII.
Haeufigkeit, Klinik und Genetik der Typen I und II. Schweiz. Med. Wschr. 96: 169-174, 205-211, 1966.

Pfaendler, U.: Eine einfach rezessive Form der dystrophia musculorum progressiva mit einer Sippen-stammtafel aus dem Emmental (Schweiz). Deutsch. Med. Wschr. 75: 1221-1225, 1950.

Rudman, D., Chyatte, S B., Gerron, G. G., O'Beirne, I. and Barlow, J.: Hyper-responsiveness of patients with limb-girdle dystrophy to human growth hormone. J. Clin. Endocr. 35: 256-260, 1972.

Touraine, A.: L'Heredite en Medecine. Paris: Masson, 1955. P. 710.

*25370 MUSCULAR DYSTROPHY II (RESEMBLING X-LINKED DUCHENNE MUSCULAR DYS-TROPHY)

Autosomal recessive inheritance of muscular dystrophy resembling the X-linked Duchenne type has been reported by Kloepfer and Talley (1958), Dubowitz (1960) and Skyring and McKusick (1961), among others. Onset before 5 years, confinement to wheelchair by 12 years and death usually before 20 years characterize the course. Pseudohypertrophy is present. Skyring and McKusick (1961) suggested that the signs of cardiac involvement present in the X-linked form may be lacking in the autosomal variety. In 1971, through the courtesy of Kloepfer, I had an opportunity to restudy two affected members, a brother and sister (IX,22 and IX,23 of the original pedigree), reported by Kloepfer and Talley (1958). They were then 30 and 27 years old, respectively, and had evidence of cardiac involvement with chronic congestive heart failure in the girl and arrhythmia with coronary sinus rhythm by electrocardiogram in the male. The girl had two children of ages 6 and 4 years.

Dubowitz, V.: Progressive muscular dystrophy of the Duchenne type in females and its mode of inheritance. Brain 83: 432-439, 1960.

Kloepfer, H. W. and Talley, C.: Autosomal recessive inheritance of Duchenne-type muscular dystrophy. Ann. Hum. Genet. 22: 138-143, 1958.

Skyring, A. and McKusick, V. A.: Clinical, genetic and electrocardiographic studies in childhood muscular dystrophy. Am. J. Med. Sci. 242: 534-547, 1961.

25380 MUSCULAR DYSTROPHY, CONGENITAL PROGRESSIVE, WITH MENTAL RETARDATION

Parental consanguinity was present in 6 families studied by Fukuyama et al. (1960). In two sibships multiple cases were observed.

Fukuyama, F., Kawozura, M. and Haruna, H.: A peculiar form of congenital muscular dystrophy: report of 15 cases. Pediatrica 44: 5 only, 1960.

*25390 MUSCULAR DYSTROPHY, CONGENITAL, PRODUCING ARTHROGRYPOSIS

Pearson and Fowler (1963) described non-progressive myopathy in sibs, producing the arthrogryposis syndrome (q.v.). A similar situation may have existed in the family reported by Banker et al. (1957) and possibly the same condition was reported by Lowenthal as myosclerosis (q.v.). Thus, congenital myopathy may produce in infancy the picture of arthrogryposis or that of amyotonia congenita (see MYOPATHY, CONGENITAL, BATTEN-TURNER TYPE).

Banker, B. Q., Victor, M. and Adams, R. D.: Arthrogryposis multiplex due to congenital muscular dystrophy. Brain 80: 319-334, 1957.

Pearson, C. M. and Fowler, W. G., Jr.: Hereditary non-progressive muscular dystrophy inducing arthrogryposis syndrome. Brain 86: 75-88, 1963.

25400 MUSCULAR DYSTROPHY, CONGENITAL, WITH INFANTILE CATARACT AND HYPOGO-NADISM

Bassoe (1956) described a syndrome of congenital muscular dystrophy, infantile cataract, and hypogonadism (in females ovarian agenesis, in males Klinefelter syndrome). Seven persons living in a small, isolated Norwegian village were identified.

Bassoe, H. H.: Familial congenital muscular dystrophy with gonadal dysgenesis. J. Clin. Endocr. 16: 1614-1621, 1956.

25410 MUSCULAR DYSTROPHY, CONGENITAL, WITH RAPID PROGRESSION

In addition to the slowly progressive congenital myopathy (q.v.) described by Batten and Turner, congenital muscular dystrophy producing arthrogryposis, and that associated with mental retardation, congenital and rapidly progressive muscular dystrophy was reported by De Lange (1937) in three members of each of two sibships related as second cousins. The condition described by Short (1963) and by Wharton (1965) may be the same.

De Lange, C.: Studien ueber angeborene Laehmungen bzw. angeborene Hypotonie. Acta Paediat. 20 (suppl. 3): 1-51, 1937.

Short, J. K.: Congenital muscular dystrophy. A case report with autopsy findings. Neurology 13: 526-530, 1963.

Wharton, B. A.: An unusual variety of muscular dystrophy. Lancet I: 248-249, 1965.

*25415 MUSK, INABILITY TO SMELL

Whissell-Buechy and Amoore (1973) suggested that this is an autosomal recessive trait. Musk pentadecalactone could not be smelled by about 7 percent of Caucasians, but this deficiency was not found in any Negroes. The authors stated that there were 27 then known discrete anosmias.

Whissell-Buechy, D. and Amoore, J. E.: Odour-blindness to musk: simple recessive inheritance. Nature 242: 271-273, 1973.

25420 MYASTHENIA GRAVIS

According to Celesia (1965), the disease has been limited to one generation in 18 of the 22 reported families with multiple cases. In the other four families 2 generations were affected. The familial form usually affects young children or adolescents and onset in adulthood is rare. The familial form is, furthermore, static or only slowly progressive. Walsh and Hoyt (1959) and Rothbart (1937) each reported a family with four affected brothers. Affected brother-sister pairs have been reported by Teng and Osserman (1956) and Celesia (1965) among others. Affected parent and offspring were reported by Foldes and McNall (1960), among others. Kurland and Alter (1961) reviewed the reports of familial aggregation and twin cases and concluded that 'there is as yet insufficient evidence to suggest that genetic factors are of significance in the etiology of myasthenia gravis.' Kott and Bornstein (1969) observed four affected sibs. It seems likely that a small proportion of cases are Mendelian. The characteristics are onset in the first year of life, good response to anti-cholinesterase drugs, good prognosis and absence of antimuscle antibodies in the serum. Parental consanguinity has been reported in at least two instances of multiple affected sibs. Bundy (1972) concluded that there are two forms of childhood myasthenia. A form with onset before 2 years of age and milder though persistent course may be autosomal recessive, although it is possible that the cases represent the extreme end of a multifactorial distribution. Cases with onset between ages 2 and 20 years resemble adult myasthenia, which is associated with autoimmunity and increased incidence of thyroid dysfunction.

Bundy, S.: A genetic study of infantile and juvenile myasthenia gravis. J. Neurol. Neurosurg. Psychiat. 35: 41-51, 1972.

Celesia, G. G.: Myasthenia gravis in two siblings. Arch. Neurol. 12: 206-210, 1965.

Foldes, F. F. and McNall, P. G.: Unusual familial occurrence of myasthenia gravis. J.A.M.A. 174: 418-420, 1960.

Kott, E. and Bornstein, B.: Familial early infantile myasthenia gravis with a 15-year follow-up. J. Neurol. Sci. 8: 573-578, 1969.

Kurland, L. T. and Alter, M.: Current status of the epidemiology and genetics of myasthenia gravis. Myasthenia gravis (Second International Symposium Proceedings). Viets, H. R. (ed.): Springfield, Ill.: Charles C Thomas, 1961. Pp. 307-336.

Rothbart, H. B.: Myasthenia gravis in children: its familial incidence. J.A.M.A. 108: 715-717, 1937.

Teng, P. and Osserman, K. E.: Studies in myasthenia gravis: neonatal and juvenile types. J. Mount Sinai Hosp. N.Y. 23: 711-727, 1956.

Walsh, F. B. and Hoyt, W. F.: External ophthalmoplegia as part of congenital myasthenia in siblings: myasthenia gravis in children: report of family showing congenital myasthenia. Am. J. Ophthal. 47: 28-34, 1959.

Warrier, C. B. and Pillai, T. D.: Familial myasthenia gravis. Brit. Med. J. 3: 839-840, 1967.

25430 MYASTHENIC MYOPATHY

Johns, Driefuss, Crowley and Fakadej (1966) described a sibship of 8, of whom 4 (2 males and 2 females) developed in adolescence a proximal myopathy involving the pectoral and pelvic girdles. By 10 years after onset they showed a prominent myasthenic reaction and good response to cholinesterase inhibitors. Electromyographic findings were typical on myasthenia gravis.

Johns, T. R., Dreifuss, F. E., Crowley, W. J. and Fakadej, A. V.: Familial non-progressive myasthenic myopathy. (Abstract) Neurology 16: 307 only, 1966.

25440 MYCOSIS FUNGOIDES

In brother and sister, Sandbank and Katzenellenbogen (1968) observed mycosis fungoides. Few reports of familial occurrence have appeared. Cameron (1933) reported the condition in mother and daughter.

Cameron, O. J.: Mycosis fungoides in mother and in daughter. Arch. Derm. 27: 232-236, 1933.

Sandbank, M. and Katzenellenbogen, I.: Mycosis fungoides of prolonged duration in siblings. Arch. Derm. 98: 620-627, 1968.

25450 MYELOMA, MULTIPLE

Leoncini and Korngold (1964) described multiple myeloma in two sisters and reviewed the literature on familial cases. Thomas (1964) observed myeloma in a brother and sister. Alexander and Benninghoff (1965) described 3 affected Negro sibs. Affected sibs have been reported by a number of other authors. Axelsson and Hallen (1965) found two families, one with two and one with three sibs, showing high M-component on a large population survey in Sweden. In a third family two persons with high M-component were more remotely related. These 7 were from a total group of 59 (out of 7918) found to have M-component. Their condition was considered to be a variety of essential benign monoclonal hypergammaglobulinemia. Manson (1961) reported affected sisters, one of whom also had pernicious anemia. Myeloma has also been observed in father and son (Nadeau et al., 1956). Berlin et al. (1968) described familial occurrence of M-components. Whitehouse (1971) observed affected brother and sister. One possible explanation for familial paraproteinemia would be that plasma cell clones with similar structural genes for the paraprotein synthesized by these cells proliferate in related individuals. This hypothesis predicts that paraproteins from two members of the same family would be identical. The paraproteins of a mother with multiple myeloma and a son with probably benign monoclonal gammopathy were isolated by Crant et al. (1971). Light chains were both of the lambda type but had differences on peptide map in both the common and variable regions of the proteins. These data show that the structural genes operative in paraprotein light chain production in these first-degree relatives are different. The presence of a genetic basis is suggested by the occurrence of two different monoclonal gammapathies in one patient. Humphrey (1973), for example, tells me of a patient who had an intracranial plasmacytoma which was surgically removed. Six years later she developed a plasmacytoma of one kidney. The second tumor produced a different gamma globulin from that released into the cerebrospinal fluid by the brain plasmacytoma.

Alexander, L. L. and Benninghoff, D. L.: Familial multiple myeloma. J. Nat. Med. Ass. 57: 471-475, 1965.

Axelsson, U. and Hallen, J.: Familial occurrence of pathological serum-proteins of different gamma-globulin groups. Lancet II: 369-370, 1965.

Berlin, S. O., Odeberg, H. and Weingart, L.: Familial occurrence of M-components. Acta Med. Scand. 183: 347-350, 1968.

Crant, J. A., Blumenschein, G. R. and Buckley, C. E.: Familial paraproteinemia. Arch. Intern. Med. 128: 427-431, 1971.

Goldstone, A. H., Wood, J. K and Cook, M. K.: Myeloma in mother and daughter. Acta Haemat. 49: 176-181, 1973.

Herrell, W. E., Ruff, J. D. and Bayrd, E. D.: Multiple myeloma in siblings. J.A.M.A. 167: 1485-1487, 1958.

Humphrey, R. L.: Baltimore: personal communication, 1973.

Leoncini, D. L. and Korngold, L.: Multiple myeloma in 2 sisters. An immunochemical study. Cancer 17: 733-737, 1964.

Manson, D. I.: Multiple myeloma in sisters. Scot. Med. J. 6: 188 only, 1961.

Nadeau, L. A., Magalini, S. I. and Stefanini, M.: Familial multiple myeloma. Arch. Path. 61: 101-106, 1956.

Thomas, T. F.: Multiple myeloma in siblings. New York J. Med. 64: 2096-2099, 1964.

Whitehouse, S.: Baltimore, Md.: personal communication, 1971.

R
E
C
E
S
S
I
V
E

*25460 MYELOPEROXIDASE DEFICIENCY

Lehrer and Cline (1969) found no detectable activity of the lysosomal enzyme myeloperoxidase (MPO) in neutrophils and monocytes of a patient with disseminated candidiasis. Other granule-associated enzymes were normal. Leukocytes from one of the proband's sisters also showed no MPO activity. Leukocytes from the proband's four sons showed about one-third normal levels. The proband and his relatives had not experienced frequent or unusual bacterial infections. Salmon et al. (1970) demonstrated immunologically absence of MPO protein, at least absence of cross-reacting material, in homozygotes. Eosinophilic peroxidase, which is chemically distinct from MLO was normal. The defective cellular immunity in this condition was restored to normal by transfusion of HL-A identical leukocytes from a healthy brother (Valdimarsson et al., 1972). Immune responses remained normal after 17 months. Persistence of functionally competent grafted cells was considered the likely mechanism.

Klebanoff, S. J. and Pincus, S. H.: Hydrogen peroxide utilization in myeloperoxidase-deficient leukocytes: a possible microbicidal control mechanism. J. Clin. Invest. 50: 2226-2229, 1971.

Lehrer, R. I. and Cline, M. J.: Leukocyte myeloperoxidase deficiency and disseminated candidiasis: the role of myeloperoxidase in resistance to Candida infection. J. Clin. Invest. 48: 1478-1488, 1969.

Salmon, S. E., Cline, M. J., Schultz, J. and Lehrer, R. I.: Myeloperoxidase deficiency: immunologic study of a genetic leukocyte defect. New Eng. J. Med. 282: 250-253, 1970.

Valdimarsson, H., Moss, P. D., Holt, P. J. L. and Hobbs, J. R.: Treatment of chronic mucocutaneous candidiasis with leukocytes from HL-A compatible siblings. Lancet I: 469-472, 1972.

25470 MYELOPROLIFERATIVE DISEASE

Randall, et al. (1965) observed a severe myeloproliferative disorder with features resembling chronic or subacute myeloid leukemia in 9 children related as first or second cousins. Two children recovered completely after a chronic illness of 10 to 12 years. No consistent chromosomal aberration was found. Low leukocyte alkaline phosphatase was found in all affected children and in 18 of 20 asymptomatic relatives.

Randall, D. L., Reiquam, C. W., Githens, J. H. and Robinson, A.: Familial myeloproliferative disease. A new syndrome closely simulating myelogenous leukemia in childhood. Am. J. Dis. Child. 110: 479-500, 1965.

*25480 MYOCLONIC EPILEPSY OF UNVERRICHT AND LUNDBORG

The onset, occurring between 6 and 13 years of age, is characterized by convulsions. Myoclonus begins 1 to 5 years later. The twitchings occur predominantly in the proximal muscles of the extremities and are bilaterally symmetrical, although asynchronous. At first small, they become late in the clinical course so violent that the victim is thrown to the floor. Mental deterioration and eventually dementia develop. Signs of cerebellar ataxia are present late in the course, which usually is 10 to 20 years in duration. Noad and Lance

(1960) described myoclonic epilepsy with cerebellar ataxia in several offspring of a mating of first cousins once removed.

Stevenson pointed out, in a discussion of genetic aspects of the study by Harriman and Millar (1955), that Lundborg's study is 'of considerable historic interest in human genetics.' Lundborg's data were used to test statistically the recessive hypothesis, the first such analysis in man. The statistical analysis was done first by Weinberg (1912) and later by Bernstein (1929).

Myoclonic epilepsy is a symptom of a number of the CNS disorders listed in this catalog, including amaurotic idiocy and the various degenerative disorders. In fact, myoclonus occurs with most brain diseases of children. For example, the sibs reported by Morse (1949) as myoclonic epilepsy were reported by Ford, Livingston and Pryles (1951) as 'familial degeneration of the cerebral gray matter in childhood.' In the specific entity which deserves to be called myoclonic epilepsy and which is represented by the cases of Unverricht (1891) and Lundborg (1913), intracellular LaFora bodies suggesting amyloid are found in the brain and similar inclusions in the cells of the heart and liver (Harriman and Millar, 1955). The LaFora material has the properties of an acid mucopolysaccharide. Yokoi et al. (1968) arrived at a preliminary conclusion that the LaFora body is polyglycosan in nature. They pictured the existence of an enzyme defect which leads to deposition of polyglucosans near their site of synthesis in the agranular endoplasmic reticulum. Schwarz and Yanoff (1965) described a brother and sister, offspring of a one and one half cousin marriage, with this disease. Seizures began at age 15 in the boy with slowly progressive motor and mental deterioration to death at age twenty three and one half years. The sister's seizures began at age 14 and progression to dementia and blindness occurred, with death at age 19. Intra and extracellular LaFora bodies were found in the CNS, retina, axis cylinders of spinal nerves, heart muscle, liver cells and striated muscle fibers. Diagnosis by liver biopsy or muscle biopsy was proposed. Vogel, Hafner and Diebold (1965) have suggested the existence of two recessively inherited types, both of which show LaFora bodies: (1) The Unverricht or 'classical' type has a relatively malignant course with early death. (2) The Lundborg type pursues a relatively benign course with death at a later stage. Kraus-Ruppert et al. (1970) also thought that the Lundborg and Unverricht types are distinguishable.

See also DEAF-MUTISM WITH FAMILIAL MYOCLONUS EPILEPSY. By this classification the case of Janeway et al. (1967) probably represented Unverricht's type (although the authors thought otherwise). There is also an autosomal dominant type (without LaFora bodies). Fluharty et al. (1970) described in cultured fibroblasts bodies which may be the equivalent of the LaFora body observed histologically. Sarlin et al. (1960) claimed that electroencephalographic abnormalities distinguish heterozygotes from homozygous normals.

Fluharty, A. L., Porter, M. T., Hirsh, G. A., Pevida, E. and Kihara, H.: Metachromasia in fibroblasts from a patient with LaFora's disease. (Letter) Lancet II: 109-110, 1970.

Ford, F. R., Livingston, S. and Pryles, C. V.: Familial degeneration of cerebral gray matter in childhood, with convulsions, myoclonus, spasticity, cerebellar ataxia, choreoathetosis, dementia, and death in status epilepticus: differentiation of infantile and juvenile types. J. Pediat. 39: 33-43, 1951.

Harriman, D. G. F. and Millar, J. H. D.: Progressive familial myoclonic epilepsy in 3 families: its clinical features and pathological basis. Brain 78: 325-349, 1955.

Janeway, R., Ravens, J. R., Pearce, L. A., Odor, D. L. and Suzuki, K.: Progressive myoclonus epilepsy with LaFora inclusion bodies. I. Clinical, genetic, histopathologic and biochemical aspects. Arch. Neurol. 16: 565-582, 1967.

Kraus-Ruppert, R., Ostertag, B. and Hafner, H.: A study of the late form (type Lundborg) of progressive myoclonic epilepsy. J. Neurol. Sci. 11: 1-15, 1970.

Lundborg, H. B.: Der Erbgang der progressiven Myoklonusepilepsie. (Myoklonie-Epilepsie, Unverricht's familiaere Myoklonie). Zbl. Ges Neurol. Psychiat. 9: 353-358, 1912.

Lundborg, H. B.: Die progressive Myoklonusepilepsie (Unverricht's Myoklonie). Upsala: Almqvist and Wiksell, 8: 567-570, 1903.

Lundborg, H. B.: Medizinisch-biologische Familienforschungen innerhalb eines 2232 koepfigen Bauern-geschlechtes in Schweden. Jena: Fischer, 1913.

Morse, W. I.: Hereditary myoclonus epilepsy: two cases with pathological findings. Bull. Hopkins Hosp. 84: 116-134, 1949.

Noad, K. B. and Lance, J. W.: Familial myoclonic epilepsy and its association with cerebellar disturbance. Brain 83: 618-630, 1960.

Sarlin, M. B., Kloepfer, H. W., Mickle, W. A. and Heath, R. G.: The detection of carriers in hereditary myoclonic epilepsy. Acta Genet. Med. Gem. 9: 466-471, 1960.

Schwarz, G. A. and Yanoff, M.: Lafora's disease, distinct clinico-pathologic form of Unverricht's syndrome. Arch. Neurol. 12: 172-188, 1965.

Unverricht, H.: Die Myoclonie. Berlin: Franz Deuticke, 1891.

Vogel, F., Hafner, H. and Diebold, K.: Zur Genetik der progressiven Myoklonusepilepsien (Unverricht-Lundborg). Humangenetik 1: 437-475, 1965.

Yanoff, M. and Schwartz, G. A.: Lafora's disease: a distinct genetically determined form of Unverricht's syndrome. J. Genet. Hum. 14: 235-244, 1965.

R
E
C
E
S
S
I
V
E

Yokoi, S., Austin, J., Witmer, F. and Sakai, M.: Studies in myoclonus epilepsy (Lafora body form). I. Isolation and preliminary characterization of LaFora bodies in two cases. Arch. Neurol. 19: 15-33, 1968.

25500 MYOPATHY PRODUCING CONGENITAL OPHTHALMOPLEGIA AND 'FLOPPY BABY' SYNDROME

Hurwitz et al. (1969) described affected brother and sister. They and both parents had aminoaciduria which was of uncertain relationship to the myopathy. Clinically the myopathy most resembled that described by Batten and Turner (see MYOPATHY, CONGENITAL). Ophthalmoplegia and floppiness also occur with myotubular myopathy (see MYOPATHY, CENTRONUCLEAR) but this entity was excluded by the muscle biopsy in the cases of Hurwitz et al. (1969).

Hurwitz, L. J., Carson, N. A. J., Allen, I. V. and Chopra, J. S.: Congenital ophthalmoplegia, floppy baby syndrome, myopathy and aminoaciduria. Report of a family. J. Neurol. Neurosurg. Psychiat. 32: 495-508, 1969.

*25510 MYOPATHY WITH ABNORMAL LIPID METABOLISM

Bradley et al. (1969) described the case of a 25-year-old woman, offspring of first-cousin parents, with myopathy involving the muscles of the neck and proximal limbs. Muscle biopsy showed interfibrillar and subsarcolemmal vacuoles, by histochemical study normal type-II muscle fibers with excessive neutral fat and free fatty acids in type-I fibers, and by electron microscopy degenerate mitochondria. The defect may reside in the pathway of free fatty acid oxidation. A specific lipase may be deficient. Engel et al. (1970) described identical twin sisters, aged 18 years, who from early childhood had had muscle aching with myoglobinuria, sometimes induced by exercise. Fasting or high fat, carbohydrate, isocalorie diet induced muscle aches, marked rise in the serum level of muscle enzymes, and no ketonemia or ketonuria. Since administration of medium-chain triglycerides produced the expected normal ketonemia and ketonuria, a defect in long-chain fatty acid utilization was postulated. A defect in an energy source to muscle was apparently responsible for the symptoms. Possible implication of the carnitine system was suggested by Bressler (1970). DiMauro and DiMauro (1973) studied a patient who probably had the same disorder as the twins of Engel et al. (1970) and found very low activity of muscle carnitine palmityltransferase measured by three different methods.

Bradley, W. G., Hudgson, P., Gardner-Medwin, D. and Walton, J. N.: Myopathy associated with abnormal lipid metabolism in skeletal muscle. Lancet 1: 495-498, 1969.

Bressler, R.: Carnitine and the twins. (Editorial) New Eng. J. Med. 282: 745-746, 1970.

DiMauro, S. and DiMauro, P. M. M.: Muscle carnitine palmityltransferase deficiency and myoglobinuria. Science 182: 929-930, 1973.

Engel, W. K., Vick, N. A., Glueck, C. J. and Levy, R. I.: A skeletal-muscle disorder associated with intermittent symptoms and a possible defect of lipid metabolism. New Eng. J. Med. 282: 697-704, 1970.

25513 MYOPATHY WITH CARNITINE DEFICIENCY

Engel and Angelini (1973) described a 24-year-old woman with myopathy characterized morphologically by myriads of lipid-filled vacuoles in muscle fibers and chemically by low levels of carnitine and impaired oxidation of fatty acids. Addition of carnitine increased the oxidation rate to normal levels. Carnitine stimulates oxidative catabolism of long-chain fatty acids by facilitating their transport from the cytoplasm to the intramitochondrial sites where they undergo beta oxidation. Genetic information is lacking, unless the condition reported by Engel et al. (1970) in identical twin sisters is the same.

Engel, A. G. and Angeline, C.: Carnitine deficiency of human skeletal muscle with associated lipid storage myopathy: a new syndrome. Science 179: 899-901, 1973.

Engel, A. G. and Siekert, R. G.: Lipid storage myopathy responsive to prednisone. Arch. Neurol. 27: 174-181, 1972.

Engel, W. K., Vick, N. A., Glueck, C. J. and Levy, R. I.: A skeletal-muscle disorder associated with intermittent symptoms and a possible defect of lipid metabolism. New Eng. J. Med. 282: 697-704, 1970.

*25514 MYOPATHY WITH LACTIC ACIDOSIS

Larsson et al. (1964) described 14 cases in 5 sibships. Parental consanguinity was observed. Linderholm et al. (1969) published a follow-up. The myopathy began in childhood and ran a chronic course with exacerbations and remissions, and was characterized by low physical performance. Physical exertion caused dyspnea and exhaustion, and when continued the muscles became hard and tender with cramps and sometimes weakness. Persistence in exertion led to nausea and vomiting. Lactic acidosis and sometimes myoglubinuria occurrs. Rawles and Weller (1974) described two brothers who probably had the same disorder. The first was studied at age 19 because of breathlessness on exertion and ankle edema. A high cardiac output was the only finding. The two brothers showed the additional feature of sideroblastic anemia (with sideroblasts of the congenital or ring form). Electron microscopy of muscle from one of the brothers showed paracrystalline inclusion bodies in mitochondria. The disorder was thought to be primarily cardiac until cardiac catheterization was performed. The asymptomatic father of the boys had chronic lactic acidosis.

Larsson, L. E., Linderholm, H., Muller, R., Ringqvist, T. and Sornas, R.: Hereditary metabolic myopathy with paroxysamal myoglobinuria due to abnormal glycolysis. J. Neurol. Neurosurg. Psychiat. 27: 361-380, 1964.

Linderholm, H., Muller, R., Ringqvist, T. and Sornas, R.: Hereditary abnormal muscle metabolism with hyperkinetic circulation during exercise. Acta Med. Scand. 185: 153-166, 1969.

RECESSIVE

Rawles, J. M. and Weller, R. O.: Familial association of metabolic myopathy, lactic acidosis and sideroblastic anemia. Am. J. Med. 56: 891-897, 1974.

25515 MYOPATHY WITH LYSIS OF TYPE I MYOFIBRILS

Cancilla et al. (1971) described a brother and sister with a congenital myopathy consisting of probable lysis of type I myofibrils. Finely granular material that stained intensely with the myosin ATP-ase reaction accumulated.

Cancilla, P. A., Kalyanaraman, K., Verity, M. A., Munsat, T. and Pearson, C. M.: Familial myopathy with probable lysis of myofibrils in type 1 fibers. Neurology 21: 279-285, 1971.

25520 MYOPATHY, CENTRONUCLEAR (MYOTUBULAR MYOPATHY)

Sher et al. (1967) described two Negro sisters suffering from generalized weakness and wasting. In 80 to 98 percent of muscle fibers numerous nuclei were situated centrally. Little degenerative change was evident in the muscles. The asymptomatic mother showed a mixture of small, centrally nucleated fibers and normal fibers. Clinically, the myopathy began early in life and progressed slowly, resulting in marked ptosis, generalized muscular atrophy and scoliosis. An isolated case was reported by Spiro et al. (1966) who called it myotubular myopathy. In the development of skeletal muscle a 'myotubular' stage with centrally located nuclei occurs in utero at about 10 weeks of age. Spiro et al. (1966) thought this disease may represent persistence of fetal muscle. Pearson et al. (1967) described a female patient with evidence of myopathy from birth. The mother, although clinically normal, showed minor histologic abnormalities of skeletal muscle. Bradley et al. (1970) described affected Negro brothers with weakness begun at 8 and 15 years of age and death at 34 years of age in both. Heterogeneity is suggested by the description of autosomal dominant and X-linked recessive inheritance (q.v.). Bradley et al. (1970) concluded that the disorder is a degeneration, not a maturation arrest.

Bradley, W. G., Price, D. L. and Watanabe, C. K.: Familial centronuclear myopathy. J. Neurol. Neurosurg. Psychiat. 33: 687-693, 1970.

Pearson, C. M., Coleman, R. F., Fowler, W. M., Jr., Mommaerts, W. F. H. M., Munsat, T. L. and Peter, J. B.: Skeletal muscle: basic and clinical aspects and illustrative new diseases. Ann. Intern. Med. 67: 614-650, 1967.

Sher, J. H., Rimalovski, A. B., Athanassiades, T. J. and Aronson, S. M.: Familial centronuclear myopathy: a clinical and pathological study. Neurology 17: 727-742, 1967.

Spiro, A. J., Shy, G. M. and Gonatas, N. K.: Myotubular myopathy. Arch. Neurol. 14: 1-14, 1966.

R
E
C
E
S
S
I
V
E

*25530 MYOPATHY, CONGENITAL (BATTEN-TURNER TYPE)

Batten (1910) and later Turner (1949, 1962) provided 50 years' observations on a family in which 6 sibs presented in infancy the picture of 'amyotonia congenita' and later in life a non-progressive myopathy. The parents were not related.

Batten, F. E.: The myopathies or muscular dystrophies: a critical review. Quart. J. Med. 3: 313-328, 1910.

Engel, W. K., Vick, N. A., Glueck, C. J. and Levy, R. I.: A skeletal-muscle disorder associated with intermittent symptoms and a possible defect of lipid metabolism. New Eng. J. Med. 282: 697-704,

Turner, J. W. A. and Lees, F.: Congenital myopathy — a fifty-year follow-up. Brain 85: 733-740, 1962.

Turner, J. W. A.: On myotonia congenita. Brain 72: 25-34, 1949.

25540 MYOPATHY, WITH GIANT ABNORMAL MITOCHONDRIA

Shy and Gonatas (1964) observed an 8-year-old child with hypotonia and proximal weakness. Cytochemical and electron-microscopic studies of muscle showed large bizarre mitochondria. Vascular smooth muscle, leucocytes and intramyal nerves did not show these changes. The patient's basal metabolic rate was normal. This and the morphologic findings were different from the case of Luft et al. (see HYPERMETABOLISM DUE TO DEFECT IN MITOCHONDRIA). A sister had died at 18 months of age of what was diagnosed Werdnig-Hoffmann disease. D'Agostino et al. (1968) described sisters, ages 8 and 15, with a limb-girdle type of myopathy and growth retardation. Mitochondria of excessive size and number were found. This was, then, both megaconial and pleoconial. The parents were not related (Bray, 1973).

Bray, P. F.: Salt Lake City, personal communication, Oct. 17, 1973.

D'Agostino, A. N., Ziter, F. A., Rollison, M. L. and Bray, P. F.: Familial myopathy with abnormal muscle mitochondria. Arch. Neurol. 18: 388-401, 1968.

Shy, G. M. and Gonatas, N. K.: Human myopathy with giant abnormal mitochondria. Science 145: 493-496, 1964.

Shy, G. M., Gonatas, N. K. and Perez, M.: Two childhood myopathies with abnormal mitochondria: I. Megaconial myopathy. II. Pleoconial myopathy. Brain 89: 133-158, 1966.

25550 MYOPIA, INFANTILE SEVERE

For discussion of possible recessive inheritance based on the occurrence in offspring of consanguineous matings, see Waardenburg (1963).

Waardenburg, P. J., Franceschetti, A. and Klein, D.: In, Genetics and Ophthalmology. Springfield, Ill.: Charles C Thomas, 2: 1246-1248, 1963.

25560 MYOSCLEROSIS, CONGENITAL, OF LOWENTHAL

Lowenthal (1954) described symmetrical congenital contractures of the joints in 4 sibs, offspring of normal parents. Sclerosis of both muscle and skin was thought to be present. See MUSCULAR DYSTROPHY, CONGENITAL, PRODUCING ARTHROGRYPOSIS.

Lowenthal, A.: Un groupe heredodegeneratif nouveau: les myoscleroses heredofamiliales. Acta Neurol. Belg. 54: 155-165, 1954.

*25570 MYOTONIA, GENERALIZED

Becker (1966) concluded that a recessive form of myotonia is more frequent than the dominant myotonia congenita of Thomsen. Segregation ratios and the frequency of parental consanguinity suggested recessive inheritance. The recessive form is apparently not congenital but begins usually at age 4-6 years. The involvement is more severe than in Thomsen disease. Winters (1970) described myotonia congenita in two brothers and a sister with normal parents. Harper and Johnston (1972) reported a particularly interesting family in which three children of first-cousin parents were affected.

Becker, P. E.: Generalized myotonia of recessive inheritance. Proc. Third Intern. Cong. Hum. Genet. (Chicago, Sept. 5-10, 1966).

Becker, P. E.: Zur Genetik der Myotonien. In, Kuhn, E. (Ed.): Progressive Muskeldystrophie, Myotonie, Myasthenie. Berlin: Springer-Verlag, 1966. Pp. 247-255.

Harper, P. S. and Johnston, D. M.: Recessively inherited myotonia congenita. J. Med. Genet. 9: 213-215, 1972.

Winters, J. L. and McLaughlin, L. A.: Myotonia congenita. A review of four cases. J. Bone Joint Surg. 52A: 1345-1350, 1970.

*25580 MYOTONIC MYOPATHY, DWARFISM, CHONDRODYSTROPHY, AND OCULAR AND FACIAL ABNORMALITIES

Aberfeld, Hinterbuchner and Schneider (1965) described brother and sister with an apparently progressive disorder characterized by myotonic myopathy, dystrophy of epiphyseal cartilages, joint contractures, blepharophimosis, myopia, pigeon breast. This report illustrates the confusion that can be created by multiple reports of the same family. Although not noted by Aberfeld et al. (1965) in their report which focused on neurologic aspects, the same sibs had previously been reported by Schwartz and Jampel (1962) who focused attention on the blepharophimosis. Mereu et al. (1969) described affected brother and sister with unrelated parents. Aberfeld et al. (1970) reported brother and sister. Huttenlocher et al. (1969) described affected brother and sister. They postulated a membrane defect with inability to maintain a proper gradient of sodium and potassium. Abnormally low muscle potassium was found. Procaine amide therapy helped muscle function. Beighton (1973) reported two affected offspring of a second-cousin marriage.

Aberfeld, D. C., Namba, T., Vye, M. V. and Grob, D.: Chondrodystrophic myotonia: report of two cases. Myotonic dwarfism, diffuse bone disease, and unusual ocular and facial abnormalities. Arch. Neurol. 22: 455-462, 1970.

Aberfeld, D. C., Hinterbuchner, L. P. and Schneider, M.: Myotonia, dwarfism, diffuse bone disease and unusual ocular and facial abnormalities (a new syndrome). Brain 88: 313-322, 1965.

Beighton, P.: The Schwartz syndrome in southern Africa. Clin. Genet. 4: 548-555, 1973.

Fowler, W. M., Jr., Layzer, R. B., Taylor, R. G., Eberle, E. D., Sims, G. E., Munsat, T. L., Philippart, M. and Wilson, B. W.: The Schwartz-Jampel syndrome: its clinical, physiological and histological expressions. J. Neurol. Sci. 22: 127-146, 1974.

Huttenlocher, P. R., Landwirth, J., Hanson, V., Gallagher, B. B. and Bensch, K.: Osteo-chondro-muscular dystrophy. A disorder manifested by multiple skeletal deformities, myotonia, and dystrophic changes in muscle. Pediatrics 44: 945-958, 1969.

Mereu, T. R., Porter, I. H. and Hug, G.: Myotonia, shortness of stature, and hip dysplasia. Am. J. Dis. Child. 117: 470-478, 1969.

Schwartz, O. and Jampel, R. S.: Congenital blepharophimosis associated with a unique generalized myopathy. Arch. Ophthal. 68: 52-57, 1962.

Van Huffelen, A. C., Gabreels, F. J. M., Van Luypen, J. S., Horst, V. D., Sbooff, J. L., Stadhouders, A. M. and Korten, J. J.: Chondrodystrophic myotonia. Neuropadiatrie 5: 71-90, 1974.

25590 MYXEDEMA

Hall (1965) described five families in which 14 cases of myxedema occurred in addition to the five probands. In one of these, a case of thyrotoxicosis was also observed and in each of two families a relative had non-toxic goiter. A sixth proband had a daughter with thyrotoxicosis. In the families of 32 other patients with myxedema no thyroid dysfunction was detected. Environmental factors, such as viral infection, cannot be excluded in the causation of such familial aggregation. However, the findings were considered compatible with sex-influenced recessive inheritance and also with the previous suggestion of a genetic relationship of myxedema to hyperthyroidism and to non-toxic goiter. In one family 'bilateral inheritance of thyroid disease' was demonstrated.

Hall, P. F.: Familial occurrence of myxedema. J. Med. Genet. 2: 173-180, 1965.

25595 MYXOMA, ATRIAL

Kleid et al. (1973) described left atrial myxoma in a 14-year-old boy and a right atrial myxoma in his 16-year-old brother.

Kleid, J. M., Klugman, J., Haas, J. and Battock, D.: Familial atrial myxoma. Am. J. Cardiol. 32: 361-364, 1973.

25597 MYXOMA, INTRACARDIAC

Two families with multiple affected sibs have been reported. Krause et al. (1971) treated a 34-year-old patient with a pulmonic valve complicated by bacterial endocarditis. A family history showed that a brother of the patient had died at age 25 of left atrial myxoma. Two other sibs had had rheumatic heart disease. Heydorn et al. (1973) reported the occurrence of atrial myxoma in two teen-age brothers.

Heydorn, W. H., Gomez, A. C., Kleid, J. J. and Haas, J. M.: Atrial myxoma in siblings. J. Thorac. Cardiovasc. Surg. 65: 484-486, 1973.

Krause, S., Adler, L. N., Reddy, P. S. and Magovern, G. J.: Intracardiac myxoma in siblings. Chest 60: 404-406, 1971.

*25600 NECROTIZING ENCEPHALOPATHY, INFANTILE SUBACUTE, OF LEIGH

The main pathology is gray matter degeneration with foci of necrosis and capillary proliferation in the brain stem. Feigin and Wolf (1954) observed two affected sibs from a consanguineous mating. Because of similarity to Wernicke encephalopathy, they suggested that a genetic defect in some way related to thiamine was present. Johns Hopkins' cases include K.L.M. (B5346: path 24642), who had an affected sib and is referred to by Ford (1960). Clark (1964) pictured the histopathology of this case. This may be the same condition as lactic acidosis of infancy (q.v.), which leads to necrotizing encephalopathy. This condition was first described by Leigh (1951). The main biochemical findings are high pyruvate and lactate in the blood and slightly low glucose levels in blood and CSF. Hommes et al. (1968), who studied a family with three affected sibs, concluded that gluconeogenesis is impaired. Absence of pyruvate carboxylase in the liver was demonstrated and this was suggested as the basic defect. Clayton et al. (1967) demonstrated therapeutic benefit of lipoic acid. Cooper et al. (1969, 1970) found that patients with SNE elaborate a factor found in the blood and urine which inhibits the synthesis of thiamine triphosphate (TTP) in brain tissue. The enzyme responsible for TTP synthesis is called thiamine pyrophosphate-adenosine triphosphate phosphoryl transferase. TTP is completely absent in postmortem brain. An assay for the inhibitor of TTP synthesis can be performed on urine or blood for diagnostic purposes. In the urine of heterozygotes, obligatory or presumptive, Murphy (1973) found an inhibitor of thiamine triphosphate synthesis in vitro. Pincus et al. (1969) had described the inhibitor in untreated patients. Thiamine derivatives in therapy were studied by Pincus et al. (1973). As pointed out by Gordon et al. (1974), since oxidation of pyruvate is dependent on a multi-enzyme complex, it is likely that a number of apo-enzyme and co-enzyme deficiencies can lead to this disorder.

Clark, D. B.: Infantile subacute necrotizing encephalopathy. In, Nelson, W. E. (ed.): Textbook of Pediatrics. Philadelphia: W. B. Saunders, 1964 (8th Ed.).

Clayton, B. E., Dobbs, R. H. and Patrick, A. D.: Leigh's subacute necrotizing encephalopathy: clinical and biochemical study, with special reference to therapy with lipoate. Arch. Dis. Child. 42: 467-478, 1967.

Cooper, J. R., Itokawa, Y. and Pincus, J. H.: Thiamine triphosphate deficiency in subacute necrotizing encephalomyelopathy. Science 164: 74-75, 1969.

Cooper, J. R., Pincus, J. H., Itokawa, Y. and Piros, K.: Experience with phosphoryl transferase inhibition in subacute necrotizing encephalomyelopathy. New Eng. J. Med. 283: 793-795, 1970.

David, R. B., Gomez, M. R. and Okazaki, H.: Necrotizing encephalomyelopathy (Leigh). Develop. Med. Child. Neurol. 12: 436-445, 1970.

Feigin, I. and Wolf, A.: A disease in infants resembling chronic Wernicke's encephalopathy. J. Pediat. 45: 243-263, 1954.

Ford, F. R.: A disease resembling Wernicke's encephalopathy (Feigen and Wolf). Diseases of the Nervous System in Infancy, Childhood and Adolescence. Springfield, Ill.: Charles C Thomas, 1960. (4th Ed.). Pp. 407-410.

Gordon, N., Marsden, H. B. and Lewis, D. M.: Subacute necrotising encephalomyelopathy in three siblings. Develop. Med. Child Neurol. 16: 64-78, 1974.

Hommes, F. A., Polman, H. A. and Reerink, J. D.: Leigh's encephalomyelopathy: an inborn error of gluconeogenesis. Arch. Dis. Child. 43: 423-426, 1968.

Leigh, D.: Subacute necrotizing encephalomyelopathy in an infant. J. Neurol. Neurosurg. Psychiat. 14: 216-221, 1951.

Murphy, J. V.: Subacute necrotizing encephalomyelopathy (Leigh's disease): detection of the heterozygous carrier state. Pediatrics 51: 710-715, 1973.

Pincus, J. H., Cooper, J. R., Murphy, J. V., Rabe, E. F., Lonsdale, D. and Dunn, H. G.: Thiamine derivatives in subacute necrotizing encephalomyelopathy. Pediatrics 51: 716-721, 1973.

Pincus, J. H., Itokawa, Y. and Cooper, J.R.: Enzyme-inhibiting factor in subacute necrotizing encephalomyelopathy. Neurology 19: 841-845, 1969.

Richter, R. B.: Infantile subacute necrotizing encephalopathy with predilection for the brain stem. J. Neuropath. Exp. Neurol. 16: 281-307, 1957.

*25605 NEONATAL OSSEOUS DYSPLASIA I

Radiographic studies of stillborn dwarfs are revealing multiple new forms of neonatal osseous dysplasia.

R
E
C
E
S
S
I
V
E

Thanatophoric dwarfism (27365) and achondrogenesis (20060) are examples. The terminology for these separate disorders is unsatisfactory — hence, the above system. De la Chapelle et al. (1972) described a hitherto unrecognized skeletal dysplasia in a stillborn son and daughter of consanguineous parents. The limbs were strikingly short. The fibula and ulna were almost triangular. The middle phalanges were curiously double. Both had cleft palate and patent foramen ovale and ductus Botalli. The boy but not the girl had endocrine and hematologic abnormalities. A relationship of this skeletal dysplasia to mesomelic dwarfism of the hypoplastic ulna, fibula and mandible types (24970) can be suggested. These might, for example, be allelic disorders.

De la Chapelle, A., Maroteaux, P., Havu, N. and Granroth, G.: Une rare dysplasie osseuse letale de transmission recessive autosomique. Arch. Franc. Pediat. 29: 759-770, 1972.

*25610 NEPHRONOPHTHISIS, FAMILIAL JUVENILE

Like several other Mendelizing disorders, this one was first described by Fanconi and his colleagues (1951). In the various reports anemia, polyuria, polydipsia, isosthenuria and death in uremia have been features. Hypertension and proteinuria are conspicuous in their absence. Symmetrical destruction of the kidneys involving both tubules and glomeruli (which were hyalinized) are observed. The age at death ranges from about 4 to about 15 years. Von Sydow and Ranstrom (1962) observed parental consanguinity. Mangos et al. (1964) thought decreased urine concentrating ability might be a manifestation of heterozygotes. Herdman et al. (1967) described medullary cystic disease in 7 and 5-year-old sibs and in a 7-year-old boy whose sister had died of the disease. They were impressed with the probable identity of medullary cystic disease and familial nephronophthisis. Mongeau and Worthen (1967) came to the same conclusion, as did also Strauss and Sommers (1967) who with humor commented that those who gave the name of medullary cysts of the kidney focused 'attention on the hole as the characteristic feature of the doughnut rather than on the kind of dough enclosing the hole.' Even though one form of medullary cystic disease may be the same as juvenile nephronophthisis, it is clear that a separate form of polycystic kidney, medullary type (q.v.), inherited as a dominant, also exists. The sibship reported by Meier and Hess (1965) had first cousin parents and apparently independent inheritance of two recessives, retinitis pigmentosa and nephronophthisis. Sworn and Eisinger (1972) reported 3 affected sibs in one of whom there was cystic anatomic demonstration of medullary cystic disease whereas a second was found at autopsy to have nephronophthisis. Sworn and Eisinger (1972) suggested that the morphologic findings in the kidney may be a function of age, i.e., that longer surviving patients are more likely to show the changes of medullary cystic disease.

Alexander, F. and Campbell, S.: Familial uremic medullary cystic disease. Pediatrics 45: 1024-1028, 1970.

Broberger, O., Winberg, J. and Zetterstrom, R.: Juvenile nephronophthisis. I. A genetically determined nephropathy with hypotonic polyuria and azotaemia. Acta Paediat. 49: 470-479, 1960.

Fanconi, G., Hanhart, E., Von Albertini, A., Uehlinger, E., Dolivo, G. and Prader, A.: Die familiaere juvenile Nephronophthise. (Die idiopathische Parenchymatose). Helv. Paediat. Acta 6: 1-49, 1951.

Gibson, A. A. M. and Arneil, G. C.: Nephronophthisis: report of 8 cases in Britain. Arch. Dis. Child. 47: 84-89, 1972.

Giselson, N., Heinegard, D., Holmberg, C. G., Lindberg, L. G., Lindstedt, E., Lindstedt, G. and Schersten, B.: Renal medullary cystic disease or familial juvenile nephronophthisis: a renal tubular disease. Am. J. Med. 48: 174-184, 1970.

Hackzell, G. and Lundmark, C.: Familial juvenile nephronophthisis. Acta Paediat. 47: 428-440, 1958.

Herdman, R. C., Good, R. A. and Vernier, R. L.: Medullary cystic disease in two siblings. Am. J. Med. 43: 335-344, 1967.

Mangos, J. A., Opitz, J. M., Lobeck, C. C. and Cookson, D. V.: Familial juvenile nephronophthisis. An unrecognized renal disease in the United States. Pediatrics 34: 337-345, 1964.

Meier, D. A. and Hess, J. W.: Familial nephropathy with retinitis pigmentosa: a new oculorenal syndrome in adults. Am. J. Med. 39: 58-69, 1965.

Mongeau, J. G. and Worthen, H. G.: Nephronophthisis and medullary cystic disease. Am. J. Med. 43: 345-355, 1967.

Sherman, F. E., Studnicki, F. M. and Fetterman, G. H.: Renal lesions of familial juvenile nephronophthisis examined by microdissection. Am. J. Clin. Path. 55: 391-400, 1971.

Strauss, M. B. and Sommers, S. C.: Medullary cystic disease and familial juvenile nephronophthisis. Clinical and pathological identity. New Eng. J. Med. 277: 863-864, 1967.

Sworn, M. J. and Eisinger, A. J.: Medullary cystic disease and juvenile nephronophthisis in separate members of the same family. Arch. Dis. Child. 47: 278-281, 1972.

Von Sydow, G. and Ranstrom, S.: Familial juvenile nephronophthisis. Acta Paediat. 51: 561-574, 1962.

RECESSIVE

25620 NEPHROSIS WITH DEAFNESS AND URINARY TRACT AND OTHER MALFORMATIONS

Braun and Bayer (1962) described a sibship of 12 containing 5 affected brothers. Two brothers, 5 sisters and both parents were normal. Parental consanguinity was denied. Whereas two of the affected sibs had urinary tract and digital anomalies, bifid uvula, nephrosis and deafness, one brother was deaf and had digital anomalies only, and 2 brothers had nephrosis only. The digital anomaly consisted of short and bifid distal phalanges of thumbs and big toes, for which no photographs or roentgenograms were published. Deafness was conductive, with no malformations of the middle ear bone (one of the affected sibs was autopsied). A female relative was known to be deaf. The author suggested either autosomal recessive or X-linked dominant inheritance (the mother had renal complications and hypertension during her pregnancies) of this syndrome, which was not previously described in the literature.

Braun, F. C., Jr. and Bayer, J. F.: Familial nephrosis associated with deafness and congenital urinary tract anomalies in siblings. J. Pediat. 60: 33-41, 1962.

*25630 NEPHROSIS, CONGENITAL

Whereas the usual idiopathic nephrotic syndrome of childhood almost never has its onset before the age of 18 months, congenital nephrosis shows itself in the first days or weeks of life. Furthermore, the familial occurrence including parental consanguinity is that of an autosomal recessive trait. Otherwise the clinical, chemical and pathologic features are identical with those of the idiopathic condition. A large series of cases was collected by Hallman and Hjelt (1959) in Finland and by Vernier, Brunson and Good (1957) and Worthen, Vernier and Good (1959) in Minnesota, where many persons of Finnish extraction live. The latter group was impressed with the high frequency of maternal toxemia in these cases. Giles et al. (1957) have reported two affected sibs from a first-cousin marriage and a third case, the child of cousins. Ongre (1961) described sibs with nephrosis starting in the neonatal period and with cystic-like dilation of renal tubules. It is likely that this is not congenital cystic disease but rather congenital nephrosis, as in the other series mentioned. Congenital heart disease was also present in the cases reported by Fournier et al. (1963). This disorder seems to have a relatively high frequency in Finland (Norio et al., 1964). McCrory and colleagues (1966) suggested that familial nephrosis is of two types. One simulates the sporadic form of childhood nephrosis and is separable only by the occurrence of nephrosis in more than one family member. The other, most properly called congenital, or perhaps even better neonatal, nephrosis is clearly differentiated by early age of onset, lack of responsiveness to therapy, poor prognosis and distinctive morphologic changes. Nephrosis of later onset is occasionally familial but not necessarily Mendelian (Roy and Pitcock, 1971).

Bader, P. I., Grove, J., Trygstad, C. W. and Nance, W. E.: Familial nephrotic syndrome. Am. J. Med. 56: 34-43, 1974.

Fournier, A., Paget, M., Pauli, A. and Devin, P.: Syndromes nephrotiques familiaux. Syndrome nephrotique associe a une cardiopathie congenitale chez quatre soeurs. Pediatrie 18: 677-685, 1963.

Giles, H. M., Pugh, R. C. B., Darmady, E. M., Stranack, F. and Woolf, L. I.: The nephrotic syndrome in early infancy: a report of 3 cases. Arch. Dis. Child. 32: 167-180, 1957.

Hallman, N. and Hjelt, L.: Congenital nephrotic syndrome. J. Pediat. 55: 152-162, 1959.

Hallman, N., Hjelt, L. and Ahvenainen, E. K.: Nephrotic syndrome in newborn and young infants. Ann. Paediat. Fenn. 2: 227-241, 1956.

Hallman, N., Norio, R. and Kouvalainen, K.: Main features of the congenital nephrotic syndrome. Acta Paediat. Scand. 172 (suppl.): 75-78, 1967.

McCrory, W. W., Shibuya, M. and Worthen, H. G.: Hereditary renal glomerular disease in infancy and childhood. Advances Pediat. 14: 253-280, 1966.

Norio, R.: Heredity in the congenital nephrotic syndrome. A genetic study of 57 Finnish families with a review of reported cases. Ann. Paediat. Fenn. 12 (suppl. 27): 1-94, 1966.

Norio, R., Hjelt, L. and Hallman, N.: Congenital nephrotic syndrome: an inherited disease? A preliminary report. Ann. Paediat. Fenn. 10: 223-227, 1964.

Ongre, A. A.: Nephrotic syndrome with cyst-like dilations of renal tubules: report of 2 cases in siblings in early infancy. Acta Path. Microbiol. Scand. 51: 1-8, 1961.

Roy, S. and Pitcock, J. A.: Idiopathic nephrosis in identical twins. Am. J. Dis. Child. 121: 428-430, 1971.

Vernier, R. L., Brunson, J. and Good, R. A.: Studies on familial nephrosis. I. Clinical and pathologic study of four cases in a single family. Am. J. Dis. Child. 93: 469-485, 1957.

Worthen, H. G., Vernier, R. L. and Good, R. A.: Infantile nephrosis: clinical biochemical, and morphologic studies of the syndrome. Am. J. Dis. Child. 98: 731-748, 1959.

25640 NERVOUS SYSTEM DISORDER RESEMBLING REFSUM DISEASE AND HURLER DISEASE

Shy et al. (1967) described a 21-year-old Negro girl with progressive ptosis, external ophthalmoplegia, retinitis pigmentosa, ataxia, absent deep tendon reflexes, elevated cerebrospinal fluid protein, and histologic features compatible with either Hurler syndrome (MPS I) or with Refsum disease. Neither phytanic acid nor mucopolysaccharide was found in excess in the tissues, however.

Gonatas, N. K.: A generalized disorder of nervous system, skeletal muscle and heart resembling Refsum's disease and Hurler's syndrome. II. Ultrastructure. Am. J. Med. 42: 169-178, 1967.

Shy, G. M., Silberberg, D. H., Appel, S. H., Mishkin, M. M. and Godfrey, E. H.: A generalized disorder of nervous system, skeletal muscle and heart resembling Refsum's disease and Hurler's syndrome. I. Clinical, pathologic and biochemical characteristics. Am. J. Med. 42: 163-168, 1967.

*25650 NETHERTON DISEASE

The features are 'bamboo hair' (trichorrhexis nodosa, or, because of the nodes, invaginata), congenital ichthyosiform erythroderma and atopic diathesis. It has been observed almost only in females. The parents of Wilkinson, Curtis and Hawk's patient (1964) were third cousins. They suggested that the disorder is an autosomal recessive inborn error of metabolism. Their patient also had hypogammaglobulinemia. Stankler and Cochrane (1967) described affected sisters of Italian extraction. Porter and Starke (1968) reported an affected male. Several males in the family including the proband had histologically typical X-linked ichthyosis

(left margin, vertical) R E C E S S I V E

and the relationship of these males was consistent with X-linkage. Stevanovic (1969) reported two more cases and Julius and Keeran (1971) described a fourth one. Altman and Strand (1969) suggested that the Netherton disease and ichthyosis linearis circumflexa are manifestations of the same entity. The term psoriasiform ichthyosis was proposed by them for including both diseases under the same denominator based on the report of seven cases with both disorders.

Altman, J. and Strand, J.: Netherton's syndrome and ichthyosis linearis circumflexa. Arch. Derm. 100: 550-558, 1969.

Julius, C. E. and Keeran, M.: Netherton's syndrome in a male. Arch. Derm. 104: 422-424, 1971.

Porter, P. S. and Starke, J. C.: Netherton's syndrome. Arch. Dis. Child. 43: 319-322, 1968.

Stankler, L. and Cochrane, T.: Netherton's disease in two sisters. Brit. J. Derm. 79: 187-196, 1967.

Stevanovic, D. V.: Multiple defects of the brain shaft in Netherton's disease. Brit. J. Derm. 81: 851-857, 1969.

Wilkinson, R. D., Curtis, G. H. and Hawk, W. A.: Netherton's disease: trichorrhexis invaginata (bamboo hair) congenital ichthyosiform erythroderma and the atopic diathesis. A histopathologic study. Arch. Derm. 89: 46-54, 1964.

*25660 NEUROAXONAL DYSTROPHY, INFANTILE (SEITELBERGER)

The degenerative encephalopathy described first by Seitelberger (1952) is similar to, but not identical with, Hallervorden-Spatz disease (q.v.). Visceral changes were described by Cowen and Olmstead (1963) and by Sandbank (1965). The changes in the brain are widespread focal swelling and degeneration of axons with scattered 'spheroids' (Cowen, Olmstead, 1963). Crome and Weller (1965) described a brother and sister who died at 12 and 18 months, respectively, with mental retardation, paralysis and epilepsy.

Cowen, D. and Olmstead, E. V.: Infantile neuroaxonal dystrophy. J. Neuropath. Exp. Neurol. 22: 175-236, 1963.

Crome, L. and Weller, S. D. V.: Infantile neuroaxonal dystrophy. Arch. Dis. Child. 40: 502-507, 1965.

Nakai, H., Landing, B. H. and Schubert, W. K.: Seitelberger's spastic amaurotic axonal idiocy. Report of a case in a 9-year-old boy with comment on visceral manifestation. Pediatrics 25: 441-449, 1960.

Sandbank, U.: Infantile neuroaxonal dystrophy. Arch. Neurol. 12: 155-159, 1965.

25670 NEUROBLASTOMA

Dodge and Benner (1945) reported a brother and sister with neuroblastoma of the adrenal medulla. The father and 3 of his 5 sibs in the report of Chatten and Voorhess (1967) had cafe-au-lait spots. Griffin and Bolande (1969) described two sisters with congenital disseminated neuroblastoma. In both regression of the retroperitoneal tumors to fibrocalcific residues and maturation to ganglioneuroma were observed. In one of them, metastatic nodules in the skin matured to ganglioneuromas and by progressive loss of ganglion cells came to resemble neurofibromas closely. A 15-year-old sister showed by X-ray, a small focus of adrenal calcification. These sisters were mentioned in the report of Chatten and Voorhess (1967). Wong et al. (1971) described a brother and sister in each of whom neuroblastoma was diagnosed at the age of five and one half months. The father showed increased amounts of vanillylmandelic acid in the urine. Neuroblastoma may be much more frequent than the frequency of clinical detection would suggest (Beckwith and Perrin, 1963). Helson et al. (1969) found elevated catecholamines in sibs of children with overt neuroblastomas. Hardy and Nesbit (1972) reported neuroblastoma in a brother and sister and a male first-cousin. Knudson and Strong (1972) applied to neuroblastoma Knudson's two-mutation theory of cancer and concluded that it fits. The other two conditions to which it has been applied (see 17130 and 18020) are 'dominant.' The father in the family of Wong et al. (1971) had elevated catecholamines and in the family of Zimmerman (1951) the father had a mediastinal ganglioneuroma removed at age 10 years. Wagget et al. (1973) described 2 sib pairs of which all 4 died with metastatic neuroblastoma. There was no evidence of tumor or neurofibromatosis in sibs or parents. Gerson et al. (1974) gave a follow-up on the family reported by Chatten and Voorhess (1967). The mother of four sibs with neuroblastoma had persistently elevated urinary catecholamines, but was aysmptonatic. She was subsequently found to have a posterior mediastinal mast which in retrospective review of radiographs was found to have been present and of constant size for at least 16 years.

Beckwith, J. B. and Perrin, E. V.: In situ neuroblastomas: a contribution to the natural history of neural crest tumors. Am. J. Path. 43: 1089-1104, 1963.

Chatten, J. and Voorhess, M. L.: Familial neuroblastoma. Report of a kindred with multiple disorders, including neuroblastomas in four siblings. New Eng. J. Med. 277: 1230-1236, 1967.

Dodge, H. J. and Benner, M. C.: Neuroblastoma of the adrenal medulla in siblings. Rocky Mountain Med. J. 42: 35-38, 1945.

Gerson, J. M., Chatten, J. and Eisman, S.: Familial neuroblastoma — a follow-up. (Letter) New Eng. J. Med. 290: 1487 only, 1974.

Griffin, M. E. and Bolande, R. P.: Familial neuroblastoma with regression and maturation to ganglioneurofibroma. Pediatrics 43: 377-382, 1969.

Hardy, P. C. and Nesbit, M. E., Jr.: Familial neuroblastoma: report of a kindred with a high incidence of infantile tumors. J. Pediat. 80: 74-77, 1972.

Helson, L., Blasco, P. and Murphy, M. L.: Familial neuroblastoma. (Abstract) Clin. Res. 17: 614 only, 1969.

Knudson, A. G., Jr. and Strong, L. C.: Mutation and cancer: neuroblastoma and pheochromocytoma. Am. J. Hum. Genet. 24: 514-532, 1972.

Wagget, J., Aherne, G. and Aherne, W.: Familial neuroblastoma: report of two sib pairs. Arch. Dis. Child. 48: 63-66, 1973.

Wong, K. Y., Hanenson, I. B. and Lampkin, B. C.: Familial neuroblastoma. Am. J. Dis. Child. 121: 415-416, 1971.

Zimmerman, J.: Ganglioneuroblastome als erbliche Systemerkrankung des Sympathicus. Beitr. Path. Anat. 111: 355-372, 1951.

*25673 NEURONAL CEROID-LIPOFUSCINOSIS, INFANTILE FINNISH TYPE

In a single child with unrelated parents, Hagberg et al. (1968) described an apparently new entity, characherized by mental retardation, loss of speech, minor motor seizures, regression of motor development, and ataxia. Histologically the brain showed total derangement of cortical cytoarchitecture, severe degeneration of white matter and deposits of granular material suggesting free fatty acids and unsaturated fatty acids. Biochemical studies showed a disturbance of linolenic acid metabolism. The patient of Hagberg et al. (1968) was of Finnish extraction. At least 55 cases of the same abnormality have been identified in Finland (Hagberg, 1974). Onset is at age 8 to 18 months with rapid psychomotor deterioration, ataxia and muscular hypotonia. Microcephaly and myoclonic jerks are also features. Convulsions are rare. The patient is blind by age 2-years, with optic atrophy and macular and retinal changes but no pigment aggregation. Both the ERG and the EEG undergo early extinction. The condition can be distinguished from other forms of amaurotic idiocy such as the juvenile form of Batten and Spielmeyer (20420) and the late infantile form of Jansky and Bielschowsky (20450). All of these conditions are classified as neuronal ceriod-lipofuscinoses by Zeman and Dyken (1969). Not only the clinical features (Santavuori et al., 1973) but also the morphologic findings (Haltia et al. 1973) are distinctive: severe neuronal destruction with massive accumulations of phagocytes, often binucleated, and unusually hypertrophic fibrillary astrocytes in the cerebral cortex.

Hagberg, B., Sourander, P. and Svennerholm, L.: Late infantile progressive encephalopathy with disturbed poly-unsaturated fat metabolism. Acta Paediat. Scand. 57: 495-499, 1968.

Hagberg, B.: Goteborg, personal communication, Sept. 4, 1974.

Haltia, M., Rapola, J., Santavuori, P. and Keranen, A.: Infantile type of so-called neuronal ceroid-lipofuscinosis — Part 2. Morphological and biochemical studies. J. Neuro. Sci. 18: 269-285, 1973.

Santavuori, P., Haltia, M., Rapola, J. and Raitta, C.: Infantile type of so-called neuronal ceroid-lipofuscinosis. Part I. A clinical study fo 15 patients. J. Neurol. Sci. 18: 257-267, 1973.

Zeman, W. and Dyken, P.: Neuronal ceroid-lipofuscinosis (Batten's disease). Relationship to amaurotic familial idiocy. Pediatrics 44: 570-583, 1969.

*25675 NEUROPATHY, CONGENITAL SENSORY

Murray (1973) reported 2 daughters of first cousins with a recessive form of congenital sensory neuropathy. The neuropathy affected pain, temperature and touch sensations in varying degrees on the limbs and trunk. This disorder is non-progressive and may be caused by a failure of sensory nerve formation rather than by sensory nerve degeneration. Those affected often develop painless finger and toe ulcerations which consequently lead to damage to the underlying bone. These patients may develop neuropathic joint degeneration as well. Murray compiled 33 cases of congenital sensory neuropathy from the literature, 20 of whom were from 6 families. This disorder is distinguished from hereditary sensory radicular neuropathy (16240) by the presence from infancy, non-progressive course, and recessive inheritance. It is distinguished from congenital insensitivity to pain by the involvement of all nodalities of sensation peripherally. It is distinguished from the entry no. 25680 by normal sweating.

Murray, T. J.: Congenital sensory neuropathy. Brain 96: 387-394, 1973.

*25680 NEUROPATHY, CONGENITAL SENSORY, WITH ANHIDROSIS

Pinsky and DiGeorge (1966) described three mentally retarded children, of which two were sibs, with recurrent episodes of unexplained fever, repeated traumatic and thermal injuries and self-mutilating behavior. Sweating could not be elicited by thermal, painful, emotional or chemical stimuli. Histamine evoked no axone flare. Subcutaneous administration of mecholyl or neostigmine in doses capable of producing lacrimation in normal children, failed to do so in the present patients, despite their occasional spontaneous lacrimation. One was female and two males. Swanson (1963) described the same syndrome in two male sibs. Swanson, Buchan and Alvord (1963) described the histologic findings, namely absence of Lissauer tract (thin myelinated afferent fibers) and small dorsal root axons. Since both dorsal root and sympathetic ganglia derive from the neural crest, they thought a unified anatomical basis might be provided. Dysautonomia (q.v.) has been incorrectly diagnosed in some cases. Biemond congenital and familial analgesia (q.v.) is another condition sometimes confused with dysautonomia. Wolfe and Henkin (1970) referred to the disorder in Pinsky and DiGeorge's sibs as type II familial dysautonomia. They suggested that it is the same as the disorder reported in two sibs of each of two families by Swanson (1963) and by Vassella et al. (1968).

Brown, J. W. and Podosin, R.: A syndrome of the neural crest. Arch. Neurol. 15: 294-301, 1966.

Pinsky, L. and DiGeorge, A. M.: Congenital familial sensory neuropathy with anhidrosis. J. Pediat. 68: 1-13, 1966.

Swanson, A. G.: Congenital insensitivity to pain with anhidrosis. A unique syndrome in two male siblings. Arch. Neurol. 8: 299-306, 1963.

Swanson, A. G., Buchan, G. C. and Alvord, E. D., Jr.: Absence of Lissauer's tract and small dorsal root axons in familial, congenital, universal insensitivity to pain. Trans. Am. Neurol. Assoc. 88: 99-103, 1963.

Vassella, F., Emrich, H. M., Kraus-Ruppert, R., Aufdermaur, F. and Tonz, O.: Congenital sensory neuropathy with anhidrosis. Arch. Dis. Child. 43: 124-130, 1968.

Wolfe, S. M. and Henkin, R. I.: Absence of taste in type II familial dysautonomia: unresponsiveness to methacholine despite the presence of taste buds. J. Pediat. 77: 103-108, 1970.

*25690 NEUROPATHY, PROGRESSIVE SENSORY, OF CHILDREN

Johnson and Spalding (1964) described sensory neuropathy in two boys, aged 10 years and 15 years, each of whom had consanguineous parents. The disorder began in early childhood, progressed slowly, involved all modalities of sensation with no disturbance of motor and autonomic function, and was predominantly distal with late involvement of the trunk. Loss of digits and Charcot joints at the ankles resulted. The disorder is differentiated from congenital indifference to pain by involvement of all sensory modalities, preservation of sensation including pain proximally, loss of tendon reflexes, gradual progression, and peripheral nerve degeneration. It is differentiated from hereditary sensory radicular neuropathy by its mode of inheritance (recessive, not dominant), early age of onset and ultimate involvement of the trunk. The patient reported by Ogden et al. (1959) as progressive sensory radicular neuropathy of Denny-Brown was probably this condition because symptoms began at least as early as 1 year and the parents were first cousins. Haddow et al. (1970) described a brother and sister, offspring of non-consanguineous parents (mother, Irish; father, French-Canadian), with non-progressive sensory defect leading to extensive damage to the fingers. The cases of Haddow et al. (1970) had low spinal fluid protein, suffered from unexplained chronic diarrhea in early life. They suggested that the disorder in the French-Canadian family described by Hould and Verret (1967) was the same, even though onset was not until the middle of the first decade. Ohta et al. (1973) reported further on the family described by Hould and Verret (1967). They suggested that the families of Schoene et al. (1970), Ogryzlo (1946) and Parks and Staples (1945) had the same condition. They further suggested the designation, hereditary sensory neuropathy type II, giving the number of type I to the dominant disorder (16240). They suggested that dysautonomia (22390) might be called HSN-type III (a practice which would, it seems to me, serve no useful function) and that there is yet another variety which they termed HSN-type IV and which here is called INSENSITIVITY TO PAIN WITH ANHIDROSIS (24305).

Barry, J. E., Hopkins, I. J. and Neal, B. W.: Congenital sensory neuropathy. Arch. Dis. Child. 49: 128-132, 1974.

Haddow, J. E., Shapiro, S. R. and Gall, D. G.: Congenital sensory neuropathy in siblings. Pediatrics 45: 651-655, 1970.

Hould, F. and Verret, S.: Neuropathie radiculaire hereditaire avec pertes de sensibilite: etude d'une famille Canadienne-Francaise. Laval Med. 38: 454-459, 1967.

Johnson, R. H. and Spalding, J. M. K.: Progressive sensory neuropathy in children. J. Neurol. Neurosurg. Psychiat. 27: 125-130, 1964.

Ohta, M., Ellefson, R. D., Lambert, E. H. and Dyck, P. J.: Hereditary sensory neuropathy, type II. Clinical, electrophysiologic, histologic, and biochemical studies of a Quebec kinship. Arch. Neurol. 29: 23-37, 1973.

Ogden, T. E., Robert, F. and Carmichael, E. A.: Some sensory syndromes in children: indifference to pain and sensory neuropathy. J. Neurol. Neurosurg. Psychiat. 22: 267-276, 1959.

Ogryzlo, M. A.: A familial peripheral neuropathy of unknown etiology resembling Morvan's disease. Canad. Med. Assoc. J. 54: 547-553, 1946.

Parks, H. and Staples, O. S.: Two cases of Morvan's syndrome of uncertain cause. Arch. Intern. Med. 75: 75-81, 1945.

Schoene, W. C., Asbury, A. K., Astrom, K. E. and Masters, R.: Hereditary sensory neuropathy: a clinical and ultrastructural study. J. Neurol. Sci. 11: 463-487, 1970.

25700 NEUROVISCERAL STORAGE DISEASE WITH CURVILINEAR BODIES

Duffy et al. (1968) described a single case of a 6-year-old boy with a neurovisceral storage disease with curvilinear bodies demonstrated intracellularly by electron microscopy. The diagnosis was possible in vitam by rectal or other visceral biopsy. Chemical studies showed this is not a gangliosidosis.

Duffy, P. E., Kornfeld, M. and Suzuki, K.: Neurovisceral storage disease with curvilinear bodies. J. Neuropath. Exp. Neurol. 27: 351-370, 1968.

*25705 NEUROVISCERAL STORAGE DISEASE WITH VERTICAL SUPRANUCLEAR OPHTHAL-MOPLEGIA

The distinctive features were vertical supranuclear ophthalmoplegia (VSO), foamy storage cells in the marrow ('sea-blue histiocytes') and neuronal storage with distinctive histochemical and ultrastructural appearances. Neville et al. (1973) found three pairs of affected sibs and an equal sex incidence. Two brothers were reported by Grover and Naiman (1971). In addition to VSO, neurologic manifestations include progressive dysarthria.

Grover, W. D. and Naiman, J. L.: Progressive paresis of vertical gage in lipid storage disease. Neurology 21: 896-899, 1971.

Neville, B. G. R., Lake, B. D., Stephens, R. and Sanders, M. D.: A neurovisceral storage disease with vertical supranuclear ophthalmoplegia, and its relationship to Niemann-Pick disease — a report of nine patients. Brain 96: 97-120, 1973.

R
E
C
E
S
S
I
V
E

Andrews, McClellan and Scott (1960) described two affected sibs. The parents were not known to be related. It is not entirely certain that this is an entity separate from that listed as AGRANULOCYTOSIS (20270). It is possible that some cases of neonatal neutropenia are due to fetomaternal immunization involving neutrophil-specific antigens (Lalezari and Radel, 1974).

Andrews, J. P., McClellan, J. T. and Scott, C. H.: Lethal congenital neutropenia with eosinophilia occurring in two siblings. Am. J. Med. 29: 358-362, 1960.

Lalezari, P. and Radel, E.: Neutrophil-specific antigens: immunology and clinical significance. Seminars in Hemat. 11: 281-290, 1974.

*25720 NIEMANN-PICK DISEASE (SPHINGOMYELIN LIPIDOSIS)

Lipid, mainly sphingomyelin, accumulates in reticuloendothelial and other cell types throughout the body. The accumulation in ganglion cells of the central nervous system leads to cell death. Hepatosplenomegaly, retarded physical and mental growth and severe neurologic disturbances are features. Symptoms usually develop by 6 months and death occurs by three years of age. However, recent publications (Crocker and Farber, 1958; Forsythe, McKeown and Neill, 1959) make it clear that the biological behavior can be more widely variable than the last statement might suggest and that survival to adulthood is possible if an early critical period is survived. Knudson and Kaplan (1962) emphasized the existence of different groups and suggested that three types can be distinguished: infantile cerebral, juvenile cerebral and non-cerebral types. Wiedemann and colleagues (1965) found large storage cells in the bone marrow of both clinically normal parents of a sibship with several affected children. The parents were first-cousins. About 40 percent of cases are Jewish. A possible variant studied by Crocker and Farber (1958) and by Fredrickson (1966) occurs in patients of French-Canadian extraction, coming from the vicinity of Yarmouth, Nova Scotia. The course is protracted with slow progression of neurologic abnormalities to severe disability. Jaundice is a prominent feature. Pfandler (1953) described non-Jewish Swiss brothers (out of 14 sibs) who died at ages 29 and 33 years. Terry et al. (1954) described the sporadic case of a Jewish male who died at age 51 years. It seems possible that these are instances of a separate disorder. Heterogeneity was also emphasized by Lowden et al. (1967) who described non-Jewish sibs with both clinical and chemical differences from the usual disease. In the classic infantile type Brady et al. (1966) demonstrated that the biochemical defect is a deficient activity of the enzyme which catalyzes cleavage of sphingomyelin to phosphorylcholine and ceramide. Uhlendorf et al. (1967) found that the metabolic defect persists in cell culture. Increased sphingomyelin was demonstrated in cells from bone marrow, skin and amnion. The last makes prenatal diagnosis possible. About 85 percent of patients fall into Crocker's group A, with death before age 3 years. In group B, the visceral or 'chronic' form, patients remain free of neurologic manifestations despite massive visceral involvement. In both forms a deficiency of sphingomyelinase has been demonstrated. Patients in group C have a slower progression of clinical symptoms. CNS symptoms appear between 2 and 4 years. Spasticity is striking and seizures, particularly myoclonic jerks, are common. Group D (the 'Nova Scotian type' of Crocker) also has slow progression. Neurologic abnormalities begin in early or middle childhood. The biochemical abnormalities of groups C and A are less clearly known than those of groups A and B. Five distinct forms of Niemann-Pick disease are distinguished: the classical infantile form (type A of Crocker), the visceral form (type B), the subacute or juvenile form (type C), the Nova Scotian variant (type D), and the adult form (Terry et al., 1954; Lynn and Terry, 1964). Schneider and Kennedy (1967) found that sphingomyelinase is deficient only in the infantile and visceral forms. Crocker (1961) provided the delineation of the first four types.

R
E
C
E
S
S
I
V
E

Brady, R. O.: The sphingolipidoses. New Eng. J. Med. 275: 312-318, 1966.

Brady, R. O., Kanfer, J. N., Mock, M. B. and Fredrickson, D. S.: The metabolism of sphingomyelin. II. Evidence of an enzymatic deficiency in Niemann-Pick disease. Proc. Nat. Acad. Sci. 55: 366-369, 1966.

Crocker, A. C. and Farber, S.: Niemann-Pick disease: a review of eighteen patients. Medicine 37: 1-95, 1958.

Crocker, A. C.: The cerebral defect in Tay-Sachs disease and Niemann-Pick disease. J. Neurochem. 7: 69-80, 1961.

Forsythe, W. I., McKeown, E. F. and Neill, D. W.: Three cases of Niemann-Pick's disease in children. Arch. Dis. Child. 34: 406-409, 1959.

Fredrickson, D. S. and Sloan, H. R.: Sphingomyelin lipidosis: Niemann-Pick disease. In, Stanbury, J. B., Wyngaarden, J. B. and Fredrickson, D. S. (eds.): The Metabolic Basis of Inherited Disease. New York: McGraw-Hill, 1972 (3rd Ed.). Pp. 783-807.

Kampine, J. P., Brady, R. O. and Kanfer, J. N.: Diagnosis of Gaucher's disease and Niemann-Pick disease with small samples of venous blood. Science 155: 86-88, 1967.

Knudson, A. G., Jr. and Kaplan, W. D.: Genetics of the sphingolipidoses. In, Aaronson, S. M. and Volk, B. W. (eds.): Cerebral Sphingolipidoses. A Symposium on Tay-Sachs Disease. New York: Academic Press, 1962. Pp. 395-411.

Lowden, J. A., Laramee, M. A. and Wentworth, P.: The subacute form of Niemann-Pick disease. Arch. Neurol. 17: 230-237, 1967.

Lynn, R. and Terry, R. D.: Lipid histochemistry and electron microscopy in adult Niemann-Pick disease. Am. J. Med. 37: 987-994, 1964.

Pfandler, U.: Nouvelles conceptions sur l'heredite et la pathogenie de la maladie de Niemann-Pick. Helv. Med. Acta 20: 216-241, 1953.

Philippart, M., Martin, L., Martin, J. J. and Menkes, J. H.: Niemann-Pick disease. Morphologic and biochemical studies in the visceral form with late central nervous system involvement (Crocker's group C). Arch. Neurol. 20: 227-238, 1969.

Schneider, P. B. and Kennedy, E. P.: Sphingomyelinase in normal human spleens and in spleens from subjects with Niemann-Pick disease. J. Lipid Res. 8: 202-209, 1967.

Terry, R. D., Sperry, W. M. and Brodoff, B.: Adult lipidosis resembling Niemann-Pick's disease. Am. J. Path. 30: 263-285, 1954.

Uhlendorf, B. W., Holtz, A. I., Mock, M. B. and Fredrickson, D. S.: Persistence of a metabolic defect in tissue cultures derived from patients with Niemann-Pick disease. In, Aronson, S. M. and Volk, B. W. (eds.): Inborn Disorders of Sphingolipid Metabolism. Oxford: Pergamon Press, 1967. Pp. 443-453.

Wiedemann, H. R., Gerken, H., Graucob, E. and Hansen, H. G.: Recognition of heterozygosity in sphingolipidoses. (Letter) Lancet I: 1283 only, 1965.

*25725 NIEMANN-PICK DISEASE WITHOUT SPHINGOMYELINASE DEFICIENCY

The presumption is strong that the three forms of Niemann-Pick disease (types C, D, and E) in which a deficiency of sphingomyelinase has not been demonstrated are determined by mutation at one or more loci distinct from that determining the presumably allelic types A and B.

*25727 NIGHTBLINDNESS WITH HIGH GRADE MYOPIA

Gassler's instructive pedigree of an inbred Swiss kindred (1925) with night blindness and myopia is reproduced by Francois (1961). (The term hemeralopia, which literally means 'day blindness,' is a misnomer. Nyctalopia is the proper term.) Merin et al. (1970) and Der Kaloustian and Baghdassarian (1972) reported instructive families.

Der Kaloustian, V. M. and Baghdassarian, S. A.: The autosomal recessive variety of congenital stationary night blindness with myopia. J. Med. Genet. 9: 67-69, 1972.

Francois, J.: Heredity in Ophthalmology. St. Louis: C. V. Mosby Co., 1961. P. 400, fig. 368.

Gassler, V. J.: Ueber eine bis jetzt nicht bekannte recessive Verknuopfung von hochgradiger Myopie mit angeborener Hemeralopie. Arch. Klaus Stift. Vererbungsforsch. 1: 259-272, 1925.

Merin, S., Rowe, H., Auerbach, E. and Landau, J.: Syndrome of congenital high myopia with nyctalopia. Am. J. Ophthal. 70: 541-547, 1970.

25730 NON-DISJUNCTION

The possibility of recessive genes predisposing to non-disjunction was examined by Kwiterovich et al. (1966) by determining the frequency of mongolism in an inbred Amish population and by Matsunaga (1966) and Forssman and Akesson (1966) who investigated the frequency of inbreeding among mothers of cases of mongolism. All three studies gave no suggestion of inbreeding effect — this, despite work of Gowen (1933) indicating such an effect in Drosophila melanogaster and suggestive earlier work with mongolism. Hirschhorn and Hsu (1969) described two sisters with XYY-XY-XO mosaicism whose brother had XYY-XY mosaicism. The parents were second cousins. See also SATELLITE ASSOCIATION RESULTING IN FAMILIAL CHROMOSOMAL MOSAICISM. The occurrence of multiple cases of various aneuploid states in the same sibship or kindred has been interpreted by some as indicating a familial, presumably genetic, tendency to anaphase loss or nondisjunction (e.g. Boczkowski et al., 1969). Hsu et al. (1970) described a family of Portuguese extraction in which two sisters had 45, X-46, XY-47, XYY mosaicism and a brother had 46, XY-47, XYY mosaicism. A third sister showed 5 percent aberrant cells (extra B group chromosome, extra small acrocentric, missing C group chromosome). The parents were second cousins. The authors postulated an autosomal recessive gene which predisposes the homozygote to 'mitotic instability.' Others have proposed a dominant factor for nondisjunction. See SATELLITE ASSOCIATION, etc. Beadle (1932) described in maize a recessive gene 'sticky' which predisposed to mitotic nondisjunction. Lewis and Gencarella (1952) described a similar recessive mutation in Drosophila. Distributive pairing, a phenomenon postulated but not proved for man (Grell, 1971), is a possible non-Mendelian mechanism for familial aneuploidy.

Beadle, G. W.: A gene for sticky chromosomes in Zea mays. Z. Ind. Abstam. Vererbungsl. 63: 195-217, 1932.

Boczkowski, K., Herman, E. and Jedrzejewski, M.: The presence of Turner's syndrome with 45, X karyotype in two generations. Am. J. Obstet. Gynec. 103: 597-599, 1969.

Goldstein, A., Hausknecht, R., Hsu, L. Y. F., Brendler, H. and Hirschhorn, K.: Sex chromosome mosaicism in 3 sibs. Clinical and pathologic aspects. Am. J. Obstet. Gynec. 107: 108-115, 1970.

Gowen, J. W.: Meiosis as a genetic character in Drosophila melanogaster. J. Exp. Zool. 65: 83-106, 1933.

Grell, R. F.: Distributive pairing in man? Ann. Genet. 14: 165-171, 1971.

Hsu, L. Y. F., Hirschhorn, K., Goldstein, A. and Barcinski, M. A.: Familial chromosomal mosaicism, genetic aspects. Ann. Hum. Genet. 33: 343-349, 1970.

Hirschhorn, K. and Hsu, L. Y.: Sex chromosome mosaicism in individuals with a Y chromosome. The Clinical Delineation of Birth Defects. V. Phenotypic Aspects of Chromosomal Aberrations. New York: National Foundation, 1969. Pp. 19-23.

Kwiterovich, P. O., Jr., Cross, H. E. and McKusick, V. A.: Mongolism in an inbred population. Bull. Hopkins Hosp. 119: 268-275, 1966.

Lewis, E. B. and Gencarella, W.: Claret and non-disjunction in Drosophila melanogaster. (Abstract) Genetics 37: 600-601, 1952.

Matsunaga, E.: Down's syndrome and maternal inbreeding. Acta Genet. Med. Gem. 15: 224-229, 1966.

Penrose, L. S.: Mongolism. Brit. Med. Bull. 17: 184-189, 1961.

25740 NYSTAGMUS

For evidence of autosomal recessive inheritance of an isolated variety of nystagmus, see review by Waardenburg (1962), including pedigrees (Waardenburg, 1963).

Waardenburg, P. J.: De Genetica Medica. Rome: L. Gedda (ed.) 6: 100 only, 1962.

Waardenburg, P. J., Franceschetti, A. and Klein, D.: In, Genetics and Ophthalmology. Springfield, Ill.: Charles C Thomas, 2: 1043 only, 1963.

25750 OBESITY-HYPOVENTILATION SYNDROME (PICKWICKIAN SYNDROME)

Falsetti and colleagues (1964) described affected brother and sister. The features are obesity, cyanosis, somnolence, muscular twitching and periodic breathing.

Falsetti, H. L., Hanson, J. S. and Tabakin, B. S.: Obesity-hypoventilation syndrome in siblings. Am. Rev. Resp. Dis. 90: 105-110, 1964.

*25760 OCULAR MYOPATHY WITH CURARE SENSITIVITY

In an inbred kindred of south India, Mathew et al. (1970) observed 9 persons with static ophthalmoparesis beginning in childhood. Oropharyngeal weakness was not associated but limb weakness was noted in 2. There was no response to neostigmine or echophonium, and the response to tetanic stimulation of the ulnar nerve was normal. The authors for these reasons regarded the condition as an ocular myopathy and not a form of myasthenia gravis, despite the fact that all subjects were as sensitive to tubocurarine as patients with myasthenia gravis. The pedigree is convincingly that of an autosomal recessive. Two asymptomatic presumed heterozygotes showed sensitivity to tubocurarine.

Mathew, N. T., Jacob, J. C. and Chandy, J.: Familial ocular myopathy with curare sensitivity. Arch. Neurol. 22: 68-74, 1970.

25770 OCULO-AURICULO-VERTEBRAL DYSPLASIA (OAV SYNDROME; GOLDENHAR SYNDROME)

R
E
C
E
S
S
I
V
E

The features are (1) coloboma of the eyelid and dermoid of the conjunctiva, (2) accessory auricular appendages anterior to the ear, and (3) vertebral anomalies. The zygomatic arches are hypoplastic, producing absence of the usual malar eminences, and the mandible is hypoplastic as in mandibulo-facial dysostosis (q.v.) with which the OAV syndrome is sometimes confused. Saraux, Grignon and Dhermy (1963) described 2 affected sisters born of healthy, unrelated parents. The karyotype was normal. Proto and Scullica (1966) described the condition in a father and his son and daughter. The mother was a first cousin of the father. A patient possibly with the same condition was observed by Fraser (1967) to have acro-osteolysis of the terminal phalanges. Summitt (1969) described a kindred with many affected persons in an autosomal dominant pattern including male-to-male transmission. Notable variability in the clinical picture was described. White (1969) described a girl with some of the features of Goldenhar syndrome. Krause (1970) described affected brother and sister. The proband had a hemangioma of the scalp. Saraux et al. (1963) described affected sisters.

Fraser, G. R.: Adelaide, Australia: personal communication, 1967.

Goldenhar, M.: Associations malformatives de l'oeil et de l'oreille. En particulier, le syndrome: dermoide epibulbaire-appendices auriculaires — fistula auris congenita et ses relations avec la dysostose mandibulo-faciale. J. Genet. Hum. 1: 243-282, 1952.

Gorlin, R. J. and Pindborg, J. J.: Oculoauriculovertebral dysplasia. In, Syndromes of the Head and Neck. New York: Blackiston Division, McGraw-Hill Book Co., 1964. Pp. 419-426.

Krause, U.: The syndrome of Goldenhar affecting two siblings. Acta Ophthal. 48: 494-499, 1970.

Proto, F. and Scullica, L.: Contributo allo studio della ereditarieta die dermoidi epibulbari. Acta Genet. Med. Gem. 15: 351-363, 1966.

Saraux, H., Grignon, J.-L. and Dhermy, P.: A propos d'une observation familiale de syndrome de Franceschetti-Goldenhar. Bull. Soc. Ophtal. Franc. 63: 705-707, 1963.

Summitt, R. L.: Familial goldenhar syndrome. The Clinical Delineation of Birth Defects. II. Malformation Syndromes. New York: National Foundation, 1969. Pp. 106-109.

Terhaar, B.: Oculo-auriculo-vertebral dysplasia (Goldenhar's syndrome) concordant in identical twins. Acta Genet. Med. Gem. 21: 116-124, 1972.

White, J. H.: Oculo-nasal dysplasia. J. Genet. Hum. 17: 107-114, 1969.

*25780 OCULO-CEREBRAL SYNDROME WITH HYPOPIGMENTATION

Cross, McKusick and Breen (1967) described a family in which four sibs, two male and two female, had cutaneous hypopigmentation, severe ocular anomalies, and cerebral defect manifested by spasticity, mental and physical retardation and athetoid movements.

Cross, H. E., McKusick, V. A. and Breen, W.: A new oculocerebral syndrome with hypopigmentation. J. Pediat. 70: 398-406, 1967.

Tuomaala and Haapanen (1968) described two sisters and a brother with similar anomalies of the eyes (strabismus, myopia, distichiasis), bones (short stature, brachydactyly, hypoplastic maxilla), and skin (scanty hair, hypopigmentation). The patients were mentally retarded.

Tuomaala, P. and Haapanen, E.: Three siblings with similar anomalies in the eyes, bones and skin. Acta Ophthal. 46: 365-371, 1968.

25800 ODOR, PECULIAR

A peculiar odor in association with mental retardation is a valuable clue to the presence of a metabolic defect, as witnessed by maple syrup urine disease, isovalericacidemia, phenylketonuria, Sidbury syndrome, oasthouse urine disease, methionine malabsorption.

*25810 OGUCHI DISEASE

The characteristics are congenital, static hemeralopia and diffuse yellow or gray coloration of the fundus. After 2 or 3 hours in total darkness, the normal color of the fundus returns. The condition is more frequent in Japanese. See HEMERALOPIA for a comment on the use of this term.

Caccamise, W. C.: Congenital nonprogressive night blindness. Bull. U.S. Army Med. Dept. 9: 920-928, 1949.

Franceschetti, A. and Chome-Bercioux, N.: Fundus albipunctatus cum hemeralopie (cas stationnaire depuis 49 ans). Ophthalmologica 121: 185-193, 1951.

Francois, J., Verriest, G. and De Rouck, A.: La maladie d'Oguchi. Ophthalmologica 131: 1-40, 1956.

Klien, B. A.: A case of so-called Oguchi's disease in the U.S.A. Am. J. Ophthal. 22: 953-955, 1939.

*25815 OLIGOSYNAPTIC (OR OLIGOCHIASMIC) INFERTILITY

Eight cases of infertility are known (Ferguson-Smith, 1973) in which a deficiency in synapsis during meiosis is evident by a deficiency of chiasmas in meiotic preparations from the testes. Since three of the males had first-cousin parents, the disorder is very likely to be autosomal recessive. Defective DNA repair was reported in the patient of Pearson et al. (1970), but Page (1973) could not demonstrate a defect in the patients she studied.

Ferguson-Smith, M. A.: Glasgow, personal communication, 1973.

Page, B. M.: Glasgow, personal communication, 1973.

Pearson, P. L., Ellis, J. D. and Evans, H. J.: A gross reduction in chiasma formation during meiotic prophase and a defective DNA repair mechanism associated with a case of human male infertility. Cytogenetics 9: 460-467, 1970.

25820 OLIVER SYNDROME (POSTAXIAL POLYDACTYLY AND MENTAL RETARDATION)

Oliver (1940) described two female and one male offspring of a cousin marriage with this combination.

Oliver, C. P.: Recessive polydactylism associated with mental deficiency. J. Hered. 31: 365-367, 1940.

*25830 OLIVOPONTOCEREBELLAR ATROPHY II (OPCA II, FICKLER-WINKLER TYPE)

Aside from the different mode of inheritance, OPCA II differs from OPCA I (q.v.) in a lack of involuntary movements and of sensory changes. Skre and Berg (1973) presented a family in which 4 of 11 sibs are from a consanguineous mating had both albinism and cerebellar ataxia. No sib had only one of the traits. Onset of cerebellar signs occurred at about age 50 years. The authors held the ataxia to be of the Dejerine-Thomas (1900) variety of olivopontocerebellar atrophy (Becker, 1966). An alternative possibility is pleiotropism. The exact identity of the neurologic problem in the kindred studied by Skre and Berg (1974) seems uncertain. Berg (1974) suggested it may be cerebello-parenchymal disorder II (21310).

Becker, P. E.: Typ Dejerine-Thomas der olivo-ponto-zerebellaren Atrophie. Humangenetik V-1, Pp. 250-251, 1966.

Berg, K.: Oslo, personal communication, 1974.

Dejerine, J. and Thomas, A.: L'atrophie olivo-ponto-cerebelleuse. Nouv. Iconogr. Salpetr. 13: 330-370, 1900.

Fickler, A.: Klinische und pathologisch-anatomische Beitraeg zu den Erkrankungen des Kleinhirns. Deutsch. Z. Nervenheilk. 41: 306-375, 1911.

Skre, H. and Berg, K.: Cerebellar ataxia and total albinism: a kindred suggesting pleiotropism or linkage. Clin. Genet. 5: 196-204, 1974.

Winkler, C.: A case of olivo-pontine cerebellar atrophy and our conceptions of neo- and palaio-cerebellum. Schweiz. Arch. Neurol. Psychiat. 13: 684-702, 1923.

*25840 OPHTHALMOPLEGIA TOTALIS WITH PTOSIS AND MIOSIS

For evidence supporting the existence of an autosomal recessive form, see Waardenburg (1962, 1963).

Waardenburg, P. J.: De Genetica Medica. Rome: L. Gedda (ed.) 6: 100 only, 1962.

Waardenburg, P. J., Franceschetti, A. and Klein, D.: In, Genetics and Ophthalmology. Springfield, Ill.: Charles C Thomas, 2: 78 only, 1963.

R
E
C
E
S
S
I
V
E

Many causes are recognized. Some forms are muscular whereas others are neural or nuclear. Oculopharyngeal muscular dystrophy (16430) is one form. The heterogeneity is indicated by the association with retinitis pigmentosa, heart block (16510), ataxia (16450) and other abnormalities as reviewed by Drachman (1968).

Drachman, D. A.: Ophthalmoplegia plus. The neurodegenerative disorders associated with progressive external ophthalmoplegia. Arch. Neurol. 18: 654-674, 1968.

25850 OPTIC ATROPHY, CONGENITAL OR EARLY INFANTILE

This disorder should be distinguished from congenital amaurosis (tapetoretinal dysplasia). Kjer (1959) reviewed the subject of an autosomal recessive form in connection with his study of a dominant form. Recent reports are few in number. Parental consanguinity was noted in earlier reports.

Kjer, P.: Infantile optic atrophy with dominant mode of inheritance: a clinical and genetic study of 19 Danish families. Acta Ophthal. 54 (suppl.): 1-147, 1959.

25865 OPTIC ATROPHY, NERVE DEAFNESS AND DISTAL NEUROGENIC AMYOTROPHY

In two brothers and their nephew (son of sister), Rosenberg and Chutorian (1967) found the combination of progressive polyneuropathy suggesting Charcot-Marie-Tooth disease with deafness and visual impairment due to degeneration of the acoustic and optic nerves. This syndrome was described in a Korean brother and sister by Iwashita et al. (1970) thereby excluding X-linked inheritance if the same disorder as that described by Rosenberg and Chutorian (1967) was in fact present.

Iwashita, H., Inoue, N., Araki, S. and Kuriowa, Y.: Optic atrophy, neural deafness, and distal neurogenic amyotrophy. Report of a family with two affected siblings. Arch. Neurol. 22: 357-364, 1970.

Rosenberg, R. N. and Chutorian, A.: Familial opticoacoustic nerve degeneration and polyneuropathy. Neurology 17: 827-832, 1967.

*25870 OPTICO-COCHLEO-DENTATE DEGENERATION

Muller and Zeman (1965) reported two brothers with degeneration of the optic, cochlear, dentate and medial lemniscal systems. The clinical picture could be correlated. Seven other cases are now known. Blindness with optic atrophy, deafness, little or no speech, spasticity and death before age 10 were features.

Muller, J. and Zeman, W.: Degenerescence systematisee optico-cochleo-dentelee. Acta Neuropath. 5: 26-39, 1965.

25880 ORAL SENSIBILITY, DISTURBANCE OF

Bosma (1965) has studied a condition in which because of sensory problem in the mouth the patient remains infantile in oral configuration and function. The 'labial gate' remains infantile with drooling, and nipple (suckle) feeding only is practiced, even in the adult. One expects the labial gate function to develop by age 22-24 months. Two-point discrimination is defective in the mouth. The patients appear to have facial diplegia. The smile is transverse as in dysautonomia. Often the patient stands with the head back to prevent drooling, and in some instances the salivary glands have been removed. Minor neurologic defects may be demonstrable elsewhere such as in the hands where a sensory type of incoordination is demonstrable. One 19 year old female has married. No familial cases have in fact been identified but few cases are known.

Bosma, J. F.: Bethesda, Md.: personal communication, 1965.

Bosma, J. F., Grossman, R. C. and Kavanagh, J. F.: A syndrome of impairment of oral perception. In, Bosma, J. F. (ed.): Symposium on Oral Sensation and Perception. Springfield, Ill.: Charles C Thomas, 1967. Pp. 318-335.

25885 ORAL-FACIAL-DIGITAL SYNDROME III

Sugarman et al. (1971) reported a new form of oral-facial-digital syndrome in two sisters. Features were mental retardation, eye abnormalities, lobulated hamartomatous tongue, dental abnormalities, bifid uvula, postaxial hexadactyly of hands and feet, pectus excavatum, short sternum, and kyphosis. One of the sibs showed ceaseless 'see-saw winking' of the eyes. The parents were not related.

Sugarman, G. I., Katakia, M. and Menkes, J. H.: See-saw winking in a familial oral-facial-digital syndrome. Clin. Genet. 2: 248-254, 1971.

*25887 ORNITHINEMIA

The deficiency is thought to concern ornithine ketoacid aminotransferase. Bickel et al. (1968) described 2 affected sisters with symptoms of disturbance in the brain, liver and proximal renal tubules. Shih et al. (1969) described a different type of ornithinemia in a single case. The clinical picture was different and ornithine ketoacid aminotransferase was normal. Ornithinemia presumably due to deficiency of ornithine ketoacid aminotransferase was found in 9 patients with gyrate atrophy of the choroid and retina (Simell and Takki, 1973). Ornithine levels were 10 to 20 times higher than normal in plasma, urine, spinal fluid and aqueous humor. No consistent clinical abnormality other than the ocular one was found. Hyperammonemia was now found in the fasting state or after meals or stress testing. All the patients' parents were from the same geographic area of Finland.

Bickel, H., Feist, D., Muller, H. and Quadbeck, G.: Ornithinaemie. Eine weitere Aminosaeurenstoffwechselstoerung mit Hirnschaedigung. Dtsch. Med. Wchnschr. 93: 2247-2251, 1968.

Shih, V. E., Efron, M. L. and Moser, H. W.: Hyperornithinemia, hyperammonemia, and homocitrul-

Simell, O. and Takki, K.: Raised plasma ornithine and gyrate atrophy of the choroid and retina. Lancet I: 1031-1033, 1973.

*25890 OROTICACIDURIA I

The features (Huguley et al., 1959) are megaloblastic anemia which is unresponsive to vitamin B12 and folic acid, hypochromic, microcytic circulating erythrocytes which do not change with administration of iron or pyridoxine, large amounts of orotic acid in the urine, and correction of anemia with reduction in orotic acid excretion when uridylic acid and cytidylic acid were administered. Fallon and colleagues (1964) have extensively studied the heterozygotes in the first family described (Huguley et al., 1959). A second family has been discovered in New Zealand and a third in Texas (Haggard, Lockhart, 1965). In the last patient urinary obstruction was produced by the high urinary excretion of orotic acid. Rogers et al. (1968) described another case, from North Carolina. Rogers and Porter (1968) devised a screening test which is effective in detecting either homozygotes or heterozygotes. A puzzling feature is that two enzymes are defective in this disorder: orotidine-5-prime-pyrophosphorylase and the decarboxylase for orotidine-5-prime-phosphate.

Becroft, D. M. O., Phillips, L. I. and Simmonds, A.: Hereditary orotic aciduria: long-term therapy with uridine and a trial of uracil. J. Pediat. 75: 885-891, 1969.

Fallon, H. J., Smith, L. H., Graham, J. B. and Burnett, C. H.: A genetic study of hereditary orotic aciduria. New Eng. J. Med. 270: 878-881, 1964.

Haggard, M. E. and Lockhart, L. H.: Hereditary orotic aciduria, a disorder of pyrimidine metabolism responsive to uridine therapy. (Abstract) J. Pediat. 67: 906 only, 1965.

Huguley, C. M., Jr., Bain, J. A., Rivers, S. L. and Scoggins, R. B.: Refractory megaloblastic anemia associated with excretion of orotic acid. Blood 14: 615-634, 1959.

Rogers, L. E. and Porter, F. S.: Hereditary orotic aciduria. II. A urinary screening test. Pediatrics 42: 423-428, 1968.

Rogers, L. E., Warford, L. R., Patterson, R. B. and Porter, F. S.: Hereditary orotic aciduria. I. A new case with family studies. Pediatrics 42: 415-422, 1968.

Smith, L. H., Jr.: Hereditary orotic aciduria-pyrimidine auxotrophism in man. (Editorial) Am. J. Med. 38: 1-6, 1965.

Smith, L. H., Jr., Huguley, C. M., Jr. and Bain, J. A.: Hereditary orotic aciduria. In, Stanbury, J. B., Wyngaarden, J. B. and Fredrickson, D. S. (eds.): The Metabolic Basis of Inherited Disease. New York: McGraw-Hill, 1972 (3rd Ed.). Pp. 1003-1029.

Tubergen, D. G., Krooth, R. S. and Heyn, R. M.: Hereditary orotic aciduria with normal growth and development. Am. J. Dis. Child. 118: 864-870, 1969.

*25892 OROTICACIDURIA II

This disorder differs from type I in that only one enzyme is defective: orotidine-5-prime-phosphate decarboxylase. O5P-pyrophosphorylase (also known as orotate phosphoribosyl-transferase) activity is increased. Only one case has been identified but recessive inheritance is supported by intermediate enzyme activity or urinary excretion of orotic acid in the patient's mother and brother and probably father (Fox et al., 1969).

Fox, R. M., O'Sullivan, W. J. and Firkin, B. G.: Orotic aciduria. Differing enzyme patterns. Am. J. Med. 47: 332-336, 1969.

Smith, L. H., Jr., Huguley, C. M., Jr. and Bain, J. A.: Hereditary orotic aciduria. In, Stanbury, J. B., Wyngaarden, J. B. and Fredrickson, D. S. (eds.): The Metabolic Basis of Inherited Disease. New York: McGraw-Hill, 1972 (3rd Ed.). Pp. 1003-1029.

25910 OSTEOARTHROPATHY, FAMILIAL IDIOPATHIC, OF CHILDHOOD

Currarino et al. (1961) and Chamberlain et al. (1965) reported a Negro family in which three sisters had a form of osteoarthropathy seemingly distinct from pachydermoperiostosis (q.v.). The salient features were clubbing of the fingers, eczematous skin eruption, periosteal new bone formation, and defects of the cranial bones resulting in wide fontanelles. Cremin (1970) described a case.

Chamberlain, D. S., Whitaker, J. and Silverman, F. N.: Idiopathic osteoarthropathy and cranial defects in children (familial idiopathic osteoarthropathy). Am. J. Roentgen. 93: 408-415, 1965.

Cremin, B. J.: Familial idiopathic osteoarthropathy of children: a case report and progress. Brit. J. Radiol. 43: 568-570, 1970.

Currarino, G., Tierney, R. C., Giesel, R. G. and Weihl, C.: Familial idiopathic osteoarthropathy. Am. J. Roentgen. 85: 633-644, 1961.

25920 OSTEOCHONDROSIS DEFORMANS TIBIAE, FAMILIAL INFANTILE TYPE

Osteochondrosis deformans tibiae is also called tibia vara, or Blount disease. Blount (1937) distinguished infantile and juvenile forms. Sevastikoglou and Eriksson (1967) observed four affected with the infantile form in a sibship of 6 children. Two of the affected were identical twins. See TIBIA VARA in dominant catalog.

Blount, W. P.: Tibia vara: osteochondrosis deformans tibiae. J. Bone Joint Surg. 19: 1-29, 1937.

Sevastikoglou, J. A. and Eriksson, J.: Familial infantile osteochondrosis deformans tibiae. Idiopathic tibia vara. A case report. Acta Orthop. Scand. 38: 81-87, 1967.

*25925 OSTEODYSPLASIA, FAMILIAL, ANDERSON TYPE

Anderson et al. (1972) described a unique abnormality of bone, especially of the craniofacial skeleton, in a young woman with recurrent mandibular fractures and in three of her four sibs. The sibship was the product of a consanguineous marriage of Irish descent. The designation was chosen because the calvarium, spine, clavicles, ribs, femurs and feet showed abnormalities. The mandibula was abnormally pointed with obtuse angle. The four sibs had hyperuricemia and three had diastolic hypertension. Both traits were present in the father who was otherwise unaffected.

Anderson, L. G., Cooke, A. J., Coccaro, P. J., Coro, C. J. and Bosma, J. F.: Familial osteodysplasia. J.A.M.A. 220: 1687-1693, 1972.

*25927 OSTEODYSPLASTY, PRECOCIOUS, OF DANKS, MAYNE AND KOZLOWSKI

In its skeletal changes this disorder bears some qualitative clinical similarity to osteodysplasty of Melnick and Needles. However, its mode of inheritance and early fatal outcome distinguish it. The two could be caused by allelic genes but at this writing (1972) I know of no clear example in man of allelic disorders with dominant inheritance in one and recessive inheritance in another. Danks et al. (1973) reported three cases of which two were in sibs. All three died as infants. They suffered from a generalized disturbance of modeling of the long and tubular bones and pelvis with severe hypoplasia of the bones, of the fingers and toes. Growth failure, striking susceptibility to respiratory infection and fatal outcome suggested a widespread dysfunction.

Danks, D. M., Mayne, V. and Kozlowski, K.: A precocious autosomal recessive type of osteodysplasty. The Clinical Delineation of Birth Defects. XIX. Skeletal Dysplasias (cont.). Baltimore: Williams and Wilkins, 1973.

25930 OSTEODYSTROPHY AND MENTAL RETARDATION

Ruvalcaba et al. (1971) described two brothers, born to unrelated parents, who showed mental retardation, short stature, microcephaly, peculiar facies with hooked nose and small mouth, narrow thoracic cage with pectus carinatum hypoplastic genitalia, hypoplastic 'onion skin' cutaneous lesions and skeletal deformities including short metatarsals and metacarpals and epiphysitis of the spine. Because two female maternal cousins showed some of the same features, X-linked semi-dominant inheritance was considered. One of the girls seems to have been fully affected, however. She died at age 17 years with congenital hydrocephalus and the Dandy-Walker anomaly.

Ruvalcaba, R. H., Reichert, A. and Smith, D. W.: A new familial syndrome with osseous dysplasia and mental deficiency. J. Pediat. 79: 450-455, 1971.

*25940 OSTEOGENESIS IMPERFECTA CONGENITA (VROLIK TYPE OF OSTEOGENESIS IMPERFECTA)

Smars, Beckman and Book (1961), McKusick and colleagues (1961), Awwaad and Reda (1960) and others have described families with two or more affected sibs from ostensibly normal parents. Such is probably to be expected of a dominant trait with wide expressivity and does not require a recessive explanation. Hanhart (1951), however, described a kindred with affected members in five sibships. Here incomplete dominance is not so satisfactory an explanation. In all such studies care must be taken not to confuse hypophosphatasia for osteogenesis imperfecta. Kaplan and Baldino (1953) described a kindred derived from an inbred, Arabic-speaking, polygamous sect called the Mozabites, living in southern Algeria. Nine cases occurred in four sibships among the descendants and Laplane et al. (1959) and Kaplan et al. (1958), in a follow-up of the same kindred described 19 cases. Parental consanguinity was noted by several authors, including Freund and Lehmacher (1954) and Rohwedder (1953) who described a case in which the parents were brother and sister.

Meyer (1955) reported 'atypical osteogenesis imperfecta' in several of the 11 offspring of a mentally defective woman by her own father. Manifestations were spontaneous fractures, generalized osteoporosis, and Wormian bones in the area of the lambdoidal sutures. Blue sclerae and deafness were not present. Morphologically these appear to be two forms of OI congenita, a thin boned and a broad-boned type. The latter is well illustrated by the male and female sibs reported by Remigio and Grinvalsky (1970). One had dislocated lenses, aortic coarctation, and basophilic and mucoid changes in the connective tissue of the heart valves and aorta. The other had less pronounced changes of the same nature in the aorta. Parental consanguinity was denied. The broad-boned type is also illustrated in fig. 6-3 by McKusick (1966) and the thin-bone type in fig. 6-5. The 'broad-bone' form of osteogenesis imperfecta and type IA achondrogenesis (20060) bear similarities. In the latter condition the ribs are thin and prone to fractures but the long bones of the limbs are severely shortened and bowed.

Awwaad, S. and Reda, M.: Osteogenesis imperfecta: review of literature and a report on three cases. Arch. Pediat. 77: 280-290, 1960.

Freund, R. and Lehmacher, K.: Beitrag zur Vererbung der Osteogenesis imperfecta. Geburtsh. Frauenheilk. 14: 171-177, 1954.

Goldfarb, A. A. and Ford, D., Jr.: Osteogenesis imperfecta congenita in consecutive siblings. J. Pediat. 44: 264-268, 1954.

Hanhart, E.: Ueber eine neue Form von Osteopsathyrosis congenita mit einfach-rezessivem, sowie 4 neue Sippen mit dominantem Erbgang und die Frage der Vererbung der sog. Osteogenesis imperfecta. Arch. Klaus Stift. Vererbungsforsch. 26: 426-437, 1951.

Ibsen, K. H.: Distinct varieties of osteogenesis imperfecta. Clin. Orthop. 50: 279-290, 1967.

Kaplan, M. and Baldino, C.: Dysplasie periostale paraissant familiale et transmise suivant le mode Mendelien recessif. Arch. Franc. Pediat. 10: 943-950, 1953.

Kaplan, M., Laplane, M. R., Debray, P. and Lasfargues, G.: Sur l'heredite de la dysplasie periostale complement a la communication de M. Kaplan et C. Baldino. Arch. Franc. Pediat. 15: 1097-1101, 1958.

Laplane, M. R., Lasfargues, G. and Debray, P.: Essai de classification genetique des osteogeneses imparfaites. Presse Med. 67: 893-895, 1959.

McKusick, V. A. and colleagues: Medical genetics 1960. J. Chronic Dis. 434-435, 1961. (fig 50).

McKusick, V. A.: Heritable Disorders of Connective Tissue. St. Louis: C. V. Mosby Co., 1972 (4th Ed.).

Meyer, H.: Atypical osteogenesis imperfecta: Lobstein's disease. Arch. Pediat. 72: 182-186, 1955.

Remigio, P. A. and Grinvalsky, H. T.: Osteogenesis imperfecta congenita: association with conspicuous extraskeletal connective tissue dysplasia. Am. J. Dis. Child. 119: 524-528, 1970.

Rohwedder, H. J.: Ein Beitrag zur Frage des Erbganges der Osteogenesis imperfecta Vrolik. Arch. Kinderheilk. 147: 256-262, 1953.

Schroder, G.: Eine klinisch-erbbiologische Untersuchung des Krankengutes in Westfalen. Schaetzung der Mutationsraten fuer den Regierungsbezirk Munster (Westfalen). Z. Menschl. Vererb. Konstitutionsl. 37: 632-676, 1964.

Smars, G., Beckman, L. and Book, J. A.: Osteogenesis imperfecta and blood groups. Acta Genet. Statist. Med. 11: 133-136, 1961.

Zeitoun, M. M., Ibrahim, A. H. and Kassem, A. S.: Osteogenesis imperfecta congenita in dizygotic twins. Arch. Dis. Child. 38: 289-291, 1963.

25950 OSTEOGENIC SARCOMA

Harmon and Morton (1966) reported osteogenic sarcoma in 4 sibs, with onset at 15, 20, 11 and 22 years. On the other hand, Epstein and Bixler (1970) observed osteogenic sarcoma in a father and daughter. See CHONDROSARCOMA. The demonstration of evidence of immune response (lysis of radiolabeled tumor cells by donor lymphocytes) in household contacts of patients with osteosarcoma (Levin et al., 1974) suggests that the familial aggregation may be due to a transmitted agent.

Epstein, L. I., Bixler, D. and Bennett, J. E.: An incident of familiar cancer: including 3 cases of osteogenic sarcoma. Cancer 25: 889-891, 1970.

Harmon, T. P. and Morton, K. S.: Osteogenic sarcoma in four siblings. J. Bone Joint Surg. 48B: 493-498, 1966.

Levin, A. S., Byers, V. X., Fudenberg, H. H. and Wybran, J.: Immunologic parameters for monitoring immunotherapy with tumor specific transfer factor. (Abstract) Clin. Res. 22: 570A only.

*25960 OSTEOLYSIS, HEREDITARY MULTICENTRIC

Among the offspring of double second cousins, Torg et al. (1969) described a new skeletal disorder to which they gave the above designation. In addition to collapse and resorption of the carpal and tarsal bones, there were osteoporosis, cortical thinning and increased caliber of the tubular and long bones. Clinically, the disorder was characterized by fusiform enlargement of the digits and flexion contractures of the knees, hip and elbows.

Torg, J. S., DiGeorge, A. M., Kirkpatrick, J. A., Jr. and Martinez Trujillo, M.: Hereditary multicentric osteolysis with recessive transmission: a new syndrome. J. Pediat. 75: 243-252, 1969.

25965 OSTEOMA OF MIDDLE EAR

Thomas (1964) reported bilateral osteoma of the middle ear in a 10-year-old boy and unilateral osteoma in his sister age 6 years. There was no history of deafness in other relatives.

Thomas, R.: Familial osteoma of the middle ear. J. Laryng. Otol. 78: 805-807, 1964.

*25970 OSTEOPETROSIS ('MARBLE BONES,' ALBERS-SCHONBERG DISEASE)

The features are macrocephaly, progressive deafness and blindness, hepatosplenomegaly and severe anemia beginning in early infancy or in fetal life. The condition results from defective resorption of immature bone. By X-ray the diagnosis may be made before birth of the affected fetus.

Enell and Pehrson described 2 sibs and a cousin affected with the early severe form in a highly inbred kindred. An autosomal dominant form is more benign. Osteosclerosis also occurs in pycnodysostosis, in van Buchem disease and in Engelmann disease. See HYPEROSTOSES. Similarities to the gray-lethal mutation in the mouse, which seems to be a thyrocalcitonin excess disease, has stimulated search for abnormality of this hormone in osteopetrosis and other osteosclerotic conditions. However, Walker (1973) has presented evidence that the osteopetrosis of the gray-lethal and microphthalmic mice is not primarily related to calcitonin or parathyroid hormone over-production. Temporary parabiosis with normal littermates resulted in permanent cure. He suggested that the procedure had resulted in recruitment of progenitors of competent osteolytic cells from the blood of the normal mouse. The occurrence of hypocalcemica and even tetany in cases of osteopetrosis (e.g., J.H.H. 1208323) is consistent with a thyrocalcitonin disorder. Keith (1968) presented evidence suggesting that primary retinal atrophy, not optic atrophy from nerve pressure, occurs in osteopetrosis. Moe and Skjaeveland (1969) described beneficial effects of cortisone. Brown and Dent (1971)

R
E
C
E
S
S
I
V
E

gave a good review of present theories of pathogenesis and described probable models in the mouse and rabbit. Walker (1974) showed that oseopetroasis could be induced in normal mice by intravenous injection of splenic cells into the lethally inadiated recipient from osteopetrotic sibs. This he interpreted to mean that (1) pregenitors of osteoclasts are produced exclusively by the blood forming tissues; (2) ossification centers can be seeded with osteoclastic progenitors via the blood stream because of their homing capabilities, and (3) the osteoclast is the only cell type functionally incompetent in the osteopetrotic mouse.

Brown, D. M. and Dent, P. B.: Pathogenesis of osteopetrosis: a comparison of human and animal spectra. Pediat. Res. 5: 181-191, 1971.

Enell, H. and Pehrson, M.: Studies on osteopetrosis. I. Clinical report of three cases with genetic considerations. Acta Paediat. 47: 279-287, 1958.

Hanhart, E. and Schackermann, (NI): In, Waardenburg, P. J., Franceschetti, A. and Klein, D. (eds.): Genetics and Ophthalmology. Springfield, Ill.: Charles C Thomas, 1: 336 only, 1960.

Hanhart, E.: Ueber die Genetik der einfach-rezessiven Formen der Marmorknochenkrankheit und zwei entsprechende Stammbaeume aus der Schweiz. Helv. Paediat. Acta 3: 113-125, 1948.

Keith, C. G.: Retinal atrophy in osteopetrosis. Arch. Ophthal. 79: 234-241, 1968.

Moe, P. J. and Skjaeveland, A.: Therapeutic studies in osteopetrosis: report of 4 cases. Acta Paediat. Scand. 58: 593-600, 1969.

Tips, R. L. and Lynch, H. T.: Malignant congenital osteopetrosis resulting from a consanguineous marriage. Acta Paediat. 51: 585-588, 1962.

Walker, D. G.: Osteopetrosis cured by temporary parabiosis. Science 180: 875 only, 1973.

Walker, D. G.: Spleen transplant induces osteopetrosis. In press, 1974.

*25973 OSTEOPETROSIS WITH RENAL TUBULAR ACIDOSIS

Sly et al. (1972) described three sibs ages 22, 17, and 15, born to normal unrelated parents with a form of osteopetrosis distinct from both the malignant form (25970) and the benign autosomal dominant form (16660). The disorder was manifest in the first two years because of fractures. Other features were short stature, dull mentality, dental malocclusion, and visual impairment from optic nerve compression. Mild anemia in infancy improved later and radiographic features of osteopetrosis improved some at puberty. Serum acid phosphatase was elevated and electrolyte changes suggested mild tubular acidosis. Guibaud et al. (1972) described two brothers with renal tubular acidosis and mild osteopetrosis. The unaffected parents, from North Africa, were cousins.

Guibaud, P., Larbre, F., Freycon, M. T. and Genoud, J.: Osteopetrose et acidose renale tubulaire. Deux cas de cette association dans une fratrie. Arch. Franc. Pediat. 29: 269-286, 1972.

Sly, W. S., Lang, R., Avioli, L., Haddad, J., Lubowitz, H. and McAlister, W.: Recessive osteopetrosis: new clinical phenotype. (Abstract) Am. J. Hum. Genet. 24: 34A only, 1972.

25975 OSTEOPOROSIS, JUVENILE

Idiopathic osteoporosis of childhood or adolescence without blue sclerae and other stigmata of osteogenesis imperfecta is occasionally observed and sometimes more than one sib is affected. This may be a distinct recessively inherited entity. The condition described by Chowers and colleagues (1962) may fall into this category but the presence of aminoaciduria and low serum uric acid makes a renal tubular defect of the Fanconi type likely.

Berglund, G. and Lindquist, B.: Osteopenia in adolescence. Clin. Orthop. 17: 259-264, 1960.

Chowers, I., Czaczkes, J. W., Ehrenfeld, E. N. and Landau, S.: Familial aminoaciduria in osteogenesis imperfecta. J.A.M.A. 181: 771-775, 1962.

Dent, C. E. and Friedman, M.: Idiopathic juvenile osteoporosis. Qurat. J. Med. 34: 177-210, 1965.

Jackson, W. P. U.: Osteoporosis of unknown cause in younger people. Idiopathic osteoporosis. J. Bone Joint Surg. 40B: 420-441, 1958.

*25977 OSTEOPOROSIS-PSEUDOGLIOMA SYNDROME

Bianchine et al. (1972) described three families. One of the cases had been reported by Bianchine and Murdoch (1969). This patient had had many fractures suggesting osteogenesis imperfecta. In addition, at the age of a few weeks presumed retinoblastoma was discovered in each eye. Enucleation was performed after preparatory irradiation. Histology showed pseudoglioma. Opitz (1972) observed the syndrome in two brothers and a sister who were, furthermore, mentally retarded.

Bianchine, J. W. and Murdoch, J. L.: Juvenile osteoporosis (Q) in a boy with bilaterial enucleation of the eyes for pseudoglioma. The Clinical Delineation of Birth Defects. IV. Skeletal Dysplasias. New York: National Foundation, 1969. Pp. 225-226.

Bianchine, J. W., Briard-Gullemot, M. L., Maroteaux, P., Frezal, J. and Harrison, H. E.: Generalized osteoporosis with bilateral pseudoglioma — an autosomal recessive disorder of connective tissue: report of three families — review of the literature. (Abstract) Am. J. Hum. Genet. 24: 34A only, 1972.

Opitz, J. M.: Madison, Wis.: personal communication, 1972.

*25990 OXALOSIS I (HYPEROXALURIA I; GLYCOLIC ACIDURIA)

The condition is characterized by a continuous high urinary oxalate excretion and progressive bilateral oxalate urolithiasis and nephrocalcinosis. Extra-renal deposits of oxalate occur in later stages. Death from renal failure occurs in childhood or early adult life. Williams and Smith (1968) were able to distinguish two distinct genetic disorders among cases of primary hyperoxaluria. The largest proportion had glycolic aciduria and hyperoxaluria, marked reduction in metabolism of C14-labeled glyoxylate or glycolate to carbon dioxide, increased conversion of glyoxylate to urinary glycolate and a defect of the enzyme soluble 2-oxo-glutarate: glyoxylate carboligase. Other patients with primary hyperoxaluria excreted normal amounts of glycolic acid but large amounts of l-glyceric acid, a compound not previously found in biological material. In this form the defect is thought to reside in the enzyme D-glyceric dehydrogenase (glyoxylate reductase). Presumably two separate genetic loci are involved. Klauwers et al. (1969) demonstrated that, as in cystinosis, renal transplantation is unsuccessful because the donor kidney becomes involved with functional failure. Lindenmayer (1970) reported on four cases of oxalosis in three sibships. Five of the six parents he could trace to a common ancestral couple born in the 1700's. A useful review of published cases was provided. Coltart and Hudson (1971) described a patient in whom deposition of oxalate in the conduction system caused heart block. Both soluble and mitochondrial alpha-ketoglutarate glyoxylate carboligase activity of muscle were normal in a patient with l-glycolic hyperoxaluria reported by Bourke et al. (1972). The patient may suffer from a different disorder, or the enzyme of muscle may be an isozyme of that in liver, spleen and kidney which was deficient in this patient. Boquist et al. (1973) described a patient who survived to age 46 years.

Boquist, L., Lindqvist, B., Ostberg, Y. and Steen, L.: Primary oxalosis. Am. J. Med. 54: 673-681, 1973.

Bourke, E., Frindt, G., Flynn, P. and Schreiner, G. E.: Primary hyperoxaluria with normal alpha-ketoglutarate: glyoxylate carboligase activity. Treatment with isocarboxid. Ann. Intern. Med. 76: 279-284, 1972.

Coltart, D. J. and Hudson, R. E. B.: Primary oxalosis of the heart: a cause of heart block. Brit. Heart J. 33: 315-319, 1971.

Dent, C. E. and Stamp, T. C. B.: Treatment of primary hyperoxaluria. Arch. Dis. Child. 45: 735-745, 1970.

Frederick, E. W., Rabkin, M. T., Richie, R. H., Jr. and Smith, L. H., Jr.: Studies on primary hyperoxaluria. I. In vivo demonstration of a defect in glyoxylate metabolism. New Eng. J. Med. 269: 821-829, 1963.

Hockaday, T. D. R., Clayton, J. E. and Smith, L. H., Jr.: The metabolic error in primary hyperoxaluria. Arch. Dis. Child. 40: 485-491, 1965.

Klauwers, J., Wolf, P. L. and Cohn, R.: Renal transplantation in primary oxalosis. J.A.M.A. 209: 551 only, 1969.

Koch, J., Stokstad, E. L., Williams, H. E. and Smith, L. H., Jr.: Deficiency of 2-oxo-glutarate: glyoxylate carboligase activity in primary hyperoxaluria. Proc. Nat. Acad. Sci. 57: 1123-1129, 1967.

Liban, E.: Oxalosis in a tripolitanian kinship. In, Goldschmidt, E. (ed.): Genetics of Migrant and Isolate Populations. Baltimore: Williams and Wilkins, 1963. P. 303.

Lindenmayer, J. P.: L'heredite dans l'oxalose familiale. J. Genet. Hum. 18: 31-44, 1970.

Williams, H. E. and Smith, L. H., Jr.: L-glyceric aciduria: new genetic variant of primary hyperoxaluria. New Eng. J. Med. 278: 233-239, 1968.

Williams, H. E. and Smith, L. H., Jr.: Primary hyperoxaluria. In, Stanbury, J. B., Wyngaarden, J. B. and Fredrickson, D. S. (eds.): The Metabolic Basis of Inherited Disease. New York: McGraw-Hill, 1972 (3rd Ed.). Pp. 196-219.

*26000 OXALOSIS II (HYPEROXALURIA II; GLYCERIC ACIDURIA)

See above for evidence for two separate types of hyperoxaluria which are distinct biochemically and presumably are the result of mutation at separate loci. Williams and Smith (1971) presented evidence that in this form of hyperoxaluria hydroxypyruvate, present in excess because of deficiency in the enzyme which converts it to D-glycerate, stimulates oxidation of glycolate to oxylate and decreases reduction of glyoxylate to glycolate. This is a novel explanation for the phenotypic consequences of a Garrodian inborn error of metabolism.

Williams, H. E. and Smith, L. H., Jr.: Hyperoxaluria in L-glyceric aciduria: possible pathogenetic mechanism. Science 171: 390-391, 1971.

26010 PA POLYMORPHISM OF ALPHA-2-GLOBULIN

A polymorphism of alpha-2-globulin was demonstrated by MacLaren et al. (1966) using the Ouchterlony method of immunodiffusion and antiserum produced in sheep. About 18 percent of males and young females are positive. All women in late pregnancy and women taking the contraceptive agent Enovid are positive. The designation PA was given for this reason and means 'pregnancy associated.' Cord bloods are negative. Family data best fitted the view that PA-1-positivity is an autosomal recessive trait. Thus, this system is a distinctly unusual one from several points of view. Haptoglobin and the Gc protein are also alpha-2-globulins. Dunston and Gershowitz (1973) showed that Xh (31480) and Pa 1 (26010) are identical, that X-linkage is ruled out by findings in two females, and that this is probably not a Mendelian polymorphism.

Dunstan, G. M. and Gershowitz, H.: Further studies of Xh, a serum protein antigen in man. Vox Sang. 24: 343-353, 1973.

MacLaren, J. A., Reid, D. E., Konugres, A. A. and Allen, F. H., Jr.: Pa 1, a new inherited alpha-2-globulin of human serum. Vox Sang. 11: 553-560, 1966.

Winkelman (1932) described this combination in two brothers. The early onset retinitis pigmentosa progressed to blindness. Progressive rigidity of extrapyramidal type and dysarthria were features. The pyramidal tracts were, by both clinical and pathologic evidence, unaffected, and there were no sensory changes. One brother died at age 24 years. Destruction of the pallida and reticular portions of the substantia nigra were demonstrated. X-linked inheritance is, of course, possible.

Winkelman, N. W.: Progressive pallidal degeneration. A new clinicopathologic syndrome. Arch. Neurol. Psychiat. 27: 1-21, 1932.

*26030 PALLIDO-PYRAMIDAL SYNDROME

Davison (1954) described 5 affected cases in 3 families. In one family a brother and sister with first-cousin parents were affected and in another family a brother and sister with uncle-niece parents were affected. The illness began in the second or early third decade with the picture of paralysis agitans and pyramidal tract signs. Autopsy (Davison, 1954) showed pallor of the pallidal segments, thinning of the ansa lenticularis, slight shrinkage and cellular change in the substantia nigra and early demyelination of the pyramids and crossed pyramidal tracts. One of Davison's cases had been previously reported by Ramsey Hunt (1917). Tremor and rigidity of paralysis agitans type began at age 13. Clinically, Wilson disease was considered likely for a time. The patient survived until age 65 years. The same disorder may have been described as familial progressive pallidum atrophy, in six sibs, by Lange and Poppe (1963). Lange et al. (1970) gave information on the autopsy findings.

Davison, C.: Pallido-pyramidal disease. J. Neuropath. Exp. Neurol. 13: 50-59, 1954.

Hunt, J. R.: Progressive atrophy of the globus pallidus (primary atrophy of the pallidal system). A system of the paralysis Agitans type, characterized by atrophy of the motor cells of the corpus striatum. A contribution to the functions of the corpus striatum. Brain 40: 58-148, 1917.

Jellinger, K.: Progressive Pallidumatrophie. J. Neurol. Sci. 6: 19-44, 1968.

Lange, E. and Poppe, W.: Klinischer Beitrag zum Krankheitsbild der progressiven Pallidumatrophie (van Bogaert). Psychiat. Neurol. 146: 176-192, 1963.

Lange, E., Poppe, W. and Scholtze, P.: Familial progressive pallidum atrophy. Europ. Neurol. 3: 265-267, 1970.

*26040 PANCREATIC INSUFFICIENCY AND BONE MARROW DYSFUNCTION (SHWACHMAN SYNDROME)

Shwachman et al. (1964) described a syndrome of pancreatic insufficiency (suggesting cystic fibrosis of the pancreas but with normal sweat electrolytes and no respiratory difficulties) and pancytopenia. One sibship contained two affected brothers and an affected female. The same syndrome was described by Nezelof and Watchi (1961) and more recently by other authors such as Pringle, Young and Haworth (1968). Goldstein (1968) and others before him called this condition congenital lipomatosis of the pancreas. He described one affected of a pair of fraternal twin girls. Affected sibs were referred to by Burke et al. (1967) and Pringle et al. (1968) observed associated skeletal changes of the metaphyseal dysostosis type. These are of interest because of the digestive abnormalities (not yet well characterized) and hematologic changes in cartilage-hair hypoplasia (q.v.), a form of metaphyseal dysostosis.

Bodian, M., Sheldon, W. and Lightwood, R.: Congenital hypoplasia of the exocrine pancreas. Acta Paediat. 53: 282-293, 1964.

Burke, V., Colebatch, J. H., Anderson, C. M. and Simons, M. J.: Association of pancreatic insufficiency and chronic neutropenia in childhood. Arch. Dis. Child. 42: 147-157, 1967.

Goldstein, R.: Congenital lipomatosis of the pancreas. Malabsorption, dwarfism, leukopenia with relative granulocytopenia and thrombocytopenia. Clin. Pediat. 7: 419-422, 1968.

Nezelof, C. and Watchi, M.: L'hypoplasie congenitale lipomateuse du pancreas exocrine chez l'enfant. (Deux observations et revue de la litterature). Arch. Franc. Pediat. 18: 1135-1172, 1961.

Pringle, E. M., Young, W. F. and Haworth, E. M.: Syndrome of pancreatic insufficiency, blood dyscrasia and metaphyseal dysplasia. Proc. Roy. Soc. Med. 61: 776-777, 1968.

Saint-Martin, J., Fournet, J. P., Charlas, J., Schaison, G., Nodot, A., Meyer, B. and Vialatte, J.: Insuffisance pancreatique externe avec granulopenie chronique. Arch. Franc. Pediat. 26: 861-871, 1969.

Shmerling, D. H., Prader, A., Hitzig, W. H., Giedion, A., Hadorn, B. and Kuhni, M.: The syndrome of exocrine pancreatic insufficiency, neutropenia, metaphyseal dysostosis and dwarfism. Helv. Paediat. Acta 24: 547-575, 1969.

Shwachman, H., Diamond, L. K., Oski, F. A. and Khaw, K. T.: The syndrome of pancreatic insufficiency and bone marrow dysfunction. J. Pediat. 65: 645-663, 1964.

26045 PANCREATIC INSUFFICIENCY, COMBINED EXOCRINE

Townes (1969) reported a 3-and one-half-year-old female with generalized anasarca, hypoproteinemia and congestive heart failure. A combined proteolytic and lipolytic defect was found. Activities of trypsin, chymotrypsin, carboxypeptidase and lipase were completely absent. Activation studies proved negative. Striking improvement accompanied feeding of protein hydrolysate (Townes, 1972). The child also had an imperforate anus, a point of interest because a patient with trypsinogen deficiency also had imperforate anus.

Townes, P. L.: Proteolytic and lipolytic deficiency of the exocrine pancreas. J. Pediat. 75: 221-228, 1969.

Townes, P. L.: Trypsinogen deficiency and other proteolytic deficiency diseases. The Clinical Delineation of Birth Defects. XIII. G. I. Tract Including Liver and Pancreas. Baltimore: Williams and Wilkins, 1972. Pp. 95-101.

26050 PAPILLOMA OF CHOROID PLEXUS

Komminoth et al. (1965) observed intraventricular papilloma of the choroid plexus in a 2-year-old boy and his 4-year-old sister.

Komminoth, R., Woringer, E., Baumgartner, J., Braun, J. P. and Le Maistre, D.: Papillome intraventriculaire familial. Caracteristiques angiographiques. Neurochirurgie 11: 267-272, 1965.

26053 PARANA HARD-SKIN SYNDROME

Cat et al. (1974) described a new syndrome in 8 persons in 7 Brazilian families living in a restricted area of southern Parana. Two were brothers and the parents of another were first-cousins. Beginning at the age of 2 or 3 months, the skin of the entire body become progressively thicker. All joints gradually become frozen and movement of the chest and abdomen is severely restricted. Respiratory insufficiency may lead to death. The disorder is probably distinguishable from the stiff-skin syndrome (18490) by the severe growth retardation, more malignant course, and probable mode of inheritance.

Cat, I., Rodrigues-Magdalena, N. I., Parolin-Marinoni, L., Wong, M. P., Freitas, O. T., Malfi, A., Costa, O., Esteves, L. and Giraldi, D. J.: Parana hard-skin syndrome: study of seven families. Lancet I: 215-216, 1974.

26055 PARATHYROID HORMONE, INACTIVE

Nusynowitz and Klein (1973) described a 20-year-old male college student with hypocalcemia, hyperphosphatemia, chronic tetany, and cataracts. Normal to high levels of immunoreactive parathyroid hormone were found. Renal responsiveness to exogenous PTH was demonstrated. The authors suggested that this patient suffered from a defect in conversion of proparathyroid hormone to its active form. The parents were not related and no other affected persons were found in the family (Nusynowitz, 1973).

Nusynowitz, M. L. and Klein, M. H.: Pseudoidiopathic hypoparathyroidism. Hypoparathyroidism with ineffective parathyroid hormone. Am. J. Med. 55: 677-686, 1973.

Nusynowitz, M. L.: El Paso, Texas, personal communication, Nov. 30, 1973.

26057 PELGER-HUET-LIKE ANOMALY AND EPISODIC FEVER WITH ABDOMINAL PAIN

Murros and Konttinen (1974) described a family in which four sisters suffered from recurrent attacks of abdominal pain and fever, consistent with the diagnosis of familial Mediterranean fever (24910). The four sisters had a Pelger-Huet-like abnormality of the polymorphs. Of the neutrophils 45-66 percent were unsegmented; 26-46 percent of eosinophils were unsegmented. The mother of the sisters, one of their brothers and the son of one of the sisters showed an intermediate defect (13-19 percent segmented neutrophils, normally segmented eosinophils) and no attacks. The father of the sisters and his sibs were all unavailable for study, but had no attacks. A brother and sister of the sister and the daughter of one of them had normal leukocytes and no attacks. Possibly this is a new autosomal recessive syndrome, with only expressions in the leukocytes, in heterozygotes.

Murros, J. and Konttinen, A.: Recurrent attacks of abdominal pain and fever with familial segmentation arrest of granulocytes. Blood 43: 871-874, 1974.

26060 PELIZAEUS-MERZBACHER DISEASE, INFANTILE ACUTE TYPE

Nisenbaum, Sandbank and Kohn (1965) described a family in which 6 of 7 sibs died in the first months of life. The parents, Yemenite Jews, were apparently unrelated. All six affected children were born prematurely at birth weights of 1350 to 2200 g. Complete neuropathologic study was performed in one case. Since this is clearly not the condition described by Pelizaeus and Merzbacher, the appropriateness of using this eponym can be questioned. Vomiting beginning at 1-3 weeks after birth and progressing to continuous projectile vomiting was the main feature.

Nisenbaum, C., Sandbank, U. and Kohn, R.: Pelizaeus-Merzbacher disease, 'infantile acute type.' Report of a family. Ann. Paediat. 204: 365-376, 1965.

26070 PENDRED SYNDROME (HEREDITARY GOITER AND DEAFNESS)

The thyroid is enlarged. The subjects are usually euthyroid but occasionally may be hypothyroid. Perchlorate administered after radioiodine caused discharge of iodine in the homozygotes and not in controls (Fraser, Morgans, Trotter, 1960). The deafness is perceptive in type and sometimes defective vestibular function is associated. The deafness is not caused by hypothyroidism but is rather a second expression of the same genetic defect. Batsakis and Nishiyama (1962) estimated that Pendred syndrome accounts for 1 to 10 percent of hereditary deafness. There appear to be at least two distinct varieties of Pendred syndrome, because Hollander and his colleagues (1964) found a defect involving not an inadequate iodination of tyrosine but apparently the condensation of iodotyrosines to form iodothyronines. Fraser (1965) estimated the frequency in the British Isles to be about 0.000075. Johnsen (1958) observed quasi-dominant inheritance through three generations because of marriage of affected persons. Because of the uncertainty as to whether organification defect with deafness is different from organification defect without deafness, no asterisk is used here. See THYROID HORMONOGENESIS, GENETIC DEFECT IN, IIB. Illum et al. (1972) reported 15 cases. They showed a phenomenal pedigree in which 8 proven cases and several presumed cases occurred in 3 generations of a family in a pseudo-dominant pedigree pattern. In one patient histologic examination showed a Mondini type malformation of the cochlear, i.e., only the basal cochlear turn is retained while the apical turns forms a common cavity. In 6 and perhaps 7 of the other 14 cases the same defect was demonstrated

536

by tomography of the temporal bones in the axial-pyramidal projection. The authors suggested that peroxidase deficiency may be responsible for the cochlear lesion as well as for the thyroid defect. A possible relation of progression of deafness and occurrence of trauma was noted in two patients I have seen (L. D., 1470207; W. D., 1470208). Vestibular disturbance was a striking feature in cases I saw in Glasgow with Professor J. H. Hutchinson (1969). The deafness may be present at birth or develop in early childhood. Likewise the goiter may be evident at birth or not develop until the second decade. Intelligence and growth are usually but not always normal. Thyroid carcinoma has been observed (Elman, 1958; Milutinovic et al., 1969). Deol (1973) demonstrated deafness in mice born of mothers treated with propylthiouracil durning pregnancy. Deafness was prevented by administration of thyroxine along with propythiouracil.

Batsakis, J. G. and Nishiyama, R. H.: Deafness with sporadic goiter: Pendred's syndrome. Arch. Otolaryng. 76: 401-406, 1962.

Deraemaeker, R.: Congenital deafness and goiter. Am. J. Hum. Genet. 8: 253-256, 1956.

Deol, M. S.: An experimental approach to the understanding and treatment of hereditary syndromes with congenital deafness and hypothyroidism. J. Med. Genet. 10: 235-242, 1973

Elman, D. S.: Familial association of nerve deafness with nodular goiter and thyroid carcinoma. New Eng. J. Med. 259: 219-223, 1958.

Fishman, J., Fraser, F. C., Watanabe, M., Sodhi, H. S. and Beck, J. C.: Familial nerve deafness and goitre. Canad. Med. Ass. J. 83: 889-892, 1960.

Fraser, G. R.: Association of congenital deafness with goitre (Pendred's syndrome). A study of 207 families. Ann. Hum. Genet. 28: 201-249, 1965.

Fraser, G. R., Morgans, M. E. and Trotter, W. R.: The syndrome of sporadic goitre and congenital deafness. Quart. J. Med. 29: 279-295, 1960.

Hollander, C. S., Prout, T. E., Rienhoff, M., Ruben, R. J. and Asper, S. P., Jr.: Congenital deafness and goiter. Studies of a patient with a cochlear defect and inadequate formation of iodothyronines. Am. J. Med. 37: 630-637, 1964.

Illum, P., Kiaer, H. W., Hvidberg-Hansen, J. and Sondergaard, G.: Fifteen cases of Pendred's syndrome. Arch. Otolaryng. 96: 297-304, 1972.

Johnsen, S.: Familial deafness and goitre in persons with a low level of protein-bound iodine. Acta Otolaryng. 140 (suppl.): 168-177, 1958.

Milutinovic, P. S., Stanbury, J. B., Wicken, J. V. and Wynn-Jones, E.: Thyroid function in a family with the Pendred syndrome. J. Clin. Endocr. 29: 962-969, 1969.

R
E
C
E
S
S
I
V
E

*26080 PENTOSURIA (L-XYLULOSURIA)

Subjects excrete 1-4 gms. of the pentose L-xylulose in the urine each day. It is a benign disturbance which occurs almost exclusively in Ashkenazi Jews of Polish-Russian extraction. However, Khachadurian (1962) and Politzer and Fleischmann (1962) have described it in Lebanese families. The frequency in Ashkenazim may be as high as one in each 2500 births. A loading method for demonstrating the heterozygote is available. By direct biochemical means applied to erythrocytes Wang and Van Eys (1970) demonstrated that the basic fault concerns NADP-linked xylitol dehydrogenase. Heterozygotes could be identified.

Hiatt, H. H.: Pentosuria. In, Stanbury, J. B., Wyngaarden, J. B. and Fredrickson, D. S. (eds.): The Metabolic Basis of Inherited Disease. New York: McGraw-Hill, 1972 (3rd Ed.). Pp. 119-130.

Khachadurian, A. K.: Essential pentosuria. Am. J. Hum. Genet. 14: 249-255, 1962.

Politzer, W. M. and Fleischmann, H.: L-xylulosuria in a Lebanese family. Am. J. Hum. Genet. 14: 256-260, 1962.

Roberts, P. D.: The inheritance of essential pentosuria. Brit. Med. J. 1: 1478-1479, 1960.

Wang, Y. M. and Van Eys, J.: The enzymatic defect in essential pentosuria. New Eng. J. Med. 282: 892-896, 1970.

26090 PERICARDIAL EFFUSION, CHRONIC

Genecin (1959) described young adult brothers with asymptomatic chronic pericardial effusion. In one the pericardial fluid contained abundant cholesterol crystals. The other brother also had mild polycythemia, strikingly tortuous retinal arterioles and localized areas of cutaneous flushing.

Genecin, A.: Chronic pericardial effusion in brothers, with a note on 'cholesterol pericarditis.' Am. J. Med. 26: 496-502, 1959.

*26100 PERNICIOUS ANEMIA, CONGENITAL, DUE TO DEFECT OF INTRINSIC FACTOR

Congenital PA has been described in 28 cases according to McNicholl and Egan (1968) who described affected brother and sister. The defect seems to be one of failure of intrinsic factor secretion despite normal gastric acidity and mucosal morphology. The disorder is distinct from selective B12 malabsorption and from the juvenile PA with gastric atrophy, achlorhydria, endocrine gland hypofunction, circulating antibodies and frequent return of intrinsic factor secretion with treatment with corticosteroids and thyroid hormone. It is also probably distinct from adult PA. The congenital form was manifest by megaloblastic anemia presenting at about 1 year of age and mental retardation. Katz et al. (1971) described a 13-year-old male from a consanguineous marriage with normal gastric intrinsic factor by immunoassay but none by biologic test.

Katz, M., Lee, S. K. and Cooper, B. A.: Vitamin B(12) malabsorption due to biologically inert intrinsic factor. New Eng. J. Med. 287: 425-429. 1972.

Jiji, R. M.: Juvenile pernicious anemia. New Eng. J. Med. 271: 995-1003, 1964.

McNicholl, B. and Egan, B.: Congenital pernicious anemia: effects on growth, brain, and absorption of B12. Pediatrics 42: 149-156, 1968.

*26110 PERNICIOUS ANEMIA, JUVENILE, DUE TO SELECTIVE INTESTINAL MALABSORPTION OF VITAMIN B12

Waters and Murphy (1963) reported three affected brothers. Both parents and 5 other sibs had subnormal or borderline vitamin B12 absorption. See also Lambert, Prankerd and Smellie (1961). Mollin, Baker and Doniach (1955) reported juvenile pernicious anemia in the offspring of a first-cousin marriage. The father developed classic pernicious anemia in middle age. Grasbeck (1960) described what may be a distinct condition. Whereas a defect in production of intrinsic factor was postulated by the authors cited above, Grasbeck favored a selective defect in intestinal absorption of vitamin B12 in this disorder which was uninfluenced by administration of intrinsic factor. Proteinuria and malformation of the urinary tract were also present. Imerslund and Bjornstad (1963) and Lamy et al. (1961) reported on the syndrome of chronic relapsing megaloblastic anemia and permanent proteinuria. Cases of childhood pernicious anemia have been reported in which, although the gastric mucosa was histologically normal intrinsic factor was lacking from the acid gastric juice. No antibodies to intrinsic factor or to gastric parietal cells were detected in the patient's serum. Studies in sibs, parents and grandparents showed no abnormality in the secretion of gastric acid or intrinsic factor and normal vitamin B12 absorption (McIntyre et al., 1965).

In one such family (Herbert, Streiff and Sullivan, 1964) two sibs were affected. Adult pernicious anemia shows gastric atrophy, antibodies to intrinsic factor and to parietal cells in the plasma and a relatively high frequency of associated thyroiditis and myxedema. Some juvenile cases are of this type. Other juvenile cases (described above) seem to suffer from a selective failure of intrinsic factor secretion. This may be recessive. Juvenile 'congenital' pernicious anemia was the designation suggested by Miller et al. (1966) for vitamin B12 deficiency due to congenital lack of gastric intrinsic factor without other apparent abnormality of the stomach or its secretions. Furthermore, serum antibodies to intrinsic factor and gastric parietal cells are conspicuously absent. The relation to the usual adult pernicious anemia is unclear. Mohamed et al. (1966) reported sisters with selective malabsorption of vitamin B12 with adequate gastric secretion of functionally competent intrinsic factor and hydrochloric acid. Persistent proteinuria appears to be an integral part of the syndrome (Mohamed et al., 1966). The latter authors gave a genetic analysis of published cases. In the oldest known patient, Goldberg and Fudenberg (1968) found normal amounts of biologically active intrinsic factor in the gastric juice and found neither antibodies to intrinsic factor nor inhibitors of intrinsic factor. The mechanism of defective absorption is unknown. MacKenzie et al. (1972) found no morphologic abnormality of the ileal mucosa and there seems to be no defect in ileal receptors for the complex between intrinsic factor and B12. The defect appears to be located between the attachment of B12 to the surface of the ileal cell and the binding to transcobalamin II. They studied 3 brothers. This disorder is sometimes accompanied by homocystinuria (Hollowell et al., 1969). In 1972 Grasbeck stated that 47 cases were known of which 21 have been diagnosed in Finland.

Francois, R., Revol, L., Germain, D., Bourlier, V., Karlin, Mme., Coeur, P., Pellet, H. and Manuel, Y.: Le syndrome d'Imerslund (a propos de trois cas dans une meme fratrie). Ann. Pediat. 43: 490-503, 1967.

Goldberg, L. S. and Fudenberg, H. H.: Familial selective malabsorption of vitamin B12. Re-evaluation of an in vivo intrinsic-factor inhibitor. New Eng. J. Med. 279: 405-407, 1968.

Grasbeck, R. and Kantero, I.: A case of juvenile vitamin B12 deficiency. (Abstract) Acta Paediat. 47 (suppl. 118): 140-141, 1959.

Grasbeck, R.: Familial selective vitamin B12 malabsorption. (Letter) New Eng. J. Med. 287: 358 only, 1972.

Grasbeck, R.: Familjar selektiv B12-malabsorption with proteinuri ett perniciosaliknande syndrome. Nord. Med. 63: 322-323, 1960.

Herbert, V., Streiff, R. R. and Sullivan, L. W.: Notes on vitamin B12 absorption, autoimmunity and childhood pernicious anemia, relation of intrinsic factor to blood group substance. Medicine 43: 679-687, 1964.

Hollowell, J. G., Jr., Hall, W. K., Coryell, M. E., McPherson, J., Jr. and Hahn, D. A.: Homocystinuria and organic aciduria in a patient with vitamin-B(12) deficiency. (Letter) Lancet II: 1428 only, 1969.

Imerslund, O. and Bjornstad, P.: Familial vitamin B12 malabsorption. Acta Haemat. 30: 1-7, 1963.

Lambert, H. P., Prankerd, T. A. J. and Smellie, J. M.: Pernicious anaemia in childhood. A report of two cases in one family and their relationships to the aetiology of pernicious anaemia. Quart. J. Med. 30: 71-90, 1961.

Lamy, M., Besancon, F., Loverdo, A. and Afifi, F.: Specific malabsorption of vitamin B12 and proteinuria. Megaloblastic anemia of Imerslund-Grasbeck: study of 4 cases. Arch. Franc. Pediat. 18: 1109-1120, 1961.

MacKenzie, I. L., Donaldson, R. M., Jr., Trier, J. S. and Mathan, V. I.: Ileal mucosa in familial selective vitamin B12 malabsorption. New Eng. J. Med. 286: 1021-1025, 1972.

McIntyre, O. R., Sullivan, L. W., Jeffries, G. H. and Silver, R. H.: Pernicious anemia in childhood. New Eng. J. Med. 272: 981-986, 1965.

Miller, D. R., Bloom, G. E., Streiff, R. R., Lo Buglio, A. F. and Diamond, L. K.: Juvenile 'congenital' pernicious anemia. Clinical and immunologic studies. New Eng. J. Med. 275: 978-983, 1966.

Mohamed, S. D., McKay, E. and Galloway, W. H.: Juvenile familial megaloblastic anaemia due to selective malabsorption of vitamin B(12). A family study and a review of the literature. Quart J. Med. 35: 433-453, 1966.

Mollin, D. L., Baker, S. J. and Doniach, I.: Addisonian pernicious anaemia without gastric atrophy in young man. Brit. J. Haemat. 1: 278-290, 1955.

Waters, A. H. and Murphy, M. E. B.: Familial juvenile pernicious anaemia. A study of the hereditary basis of pernicious anaemia. Brit. J. Haemat. 9: 1-12, 1963.

*26120 PEROMELIA

In a Brazilian family of Portuguese ancestry Freire-Maia, Quelce-Salgado and Koehler (1959) found an apparent recessive type of peromelia ('maimed limb'). Abnormality was confined to the upper limbs and consisted of aplasia or hypoplasia of many bones. One affected male married to the daughter of his half-sister had two affected children.

Freire-Maia, N., Quelce-Salgado, A. and Koehler, R. A.: Hereditary bone aplasias and hypoplasias of the upper extremities. Acta Genet. Statist. Med. 9: 33-40, 1959.

*26130 PEROMELIA WITH MICROGNATHISM

This syndrome is probably distinct from the Brazilian type of acheiropody (q.v.) and from simple peromelia (q.v.). In Hanhart's report of three cases, two were related and in the third the parents were consanguineous.

Hanhart, E.: Ueber die Kombination von Peromelie mit Mikrognathie, ein neues Syndrom beim Menschen, entsprechend der Akroteriasis congenita von Wriedt und Mohr beim Rindh. Arch. Klaus Stift. Vererbungsforsch. 25: 531-543, 1950.

26140 PERONEUS TERTIUS MUSCLE, ABSENCE OF

From studies in the Navajo, Spuhler (1950) concluded that absence is recessive. The muscle is a dorsiflexor of the foot. When the subject stands with the toes in sharp dorsiflexion, the tendons of the peroneus tertius become prominent over the cuboid bone just outside the most lateral tendon of the extensor digitorum longus.

Spuhler, J. N.: Genetics of three normal morphological variations: pattern of superficial veins of the anterior thorax, peroneus tertius muscle, and number of vallate papillae. Cold Spring Harbor Symposia Quant. Biol. 15: 175-188, 1950.

*26150 PEROXIDASE AND PHOSPHOLIPID DEFICIENCY IN EOSINOPHILES

In Yemenite Jews in Israel, Presentey (1969) and Presentey and Szapiro (1969) described a 'new' anomaly of eosinophiles characterized by nuclear hypersigmentation, hypogranulation and negative peroxidase and phospholipid staining. No connection between the morphologic and presumed enzymatic defect and any illness has been established. Recessive inheritance seems quite clear.

Presentey, B. Z. and Szapiro, L.: Hereditary deficiency of peroxidase and phospholipids in eosinophilic granulocytes. Acta Haemat. 41: 359-362, 1969.

Presentey, B. Z.: Morphologic observations and genetic follow-up of a familial anomaly of eosinophils. Am. J. Clin. Path. 51: 458-462, 1969.

*26155 PERSISTENT MULLERIAN DUCT SYNDROME

The typical case is that of a male with bilateral cryptorchidism and inguinal hernias but normal external genitalia. At the time of hernia repair, a uterus and fallopian tubes are found in the inguinal canal. The gonads are testes (Nilson 1939). Gruell-Gonzalez et al. (1971), Morillo-Cucci and German (1971), and Armendares et al. (1973) described affected brothers. Von Seemen (1927) observed parental consanguinity. The defect is one of male sexual differentiation, specifically failure of Mullerian duct regression in otherwise normal males.

Armendares, S., Buentello, L. and Frenk, S.: Two male sibs with uterus and fallopian tubes. A rare probably inherited disorder. Clin. Genet. 4: 291-296, 1973.

Brook, C. G. D., Wagner, H., Zachmann, M., Prader, A., Armendares, S., Frenk, S., Aleman, P., Najjar, S. S., Slim, M. S., Genton, N. and Bozic, C.: Familial occurrence of persistent mullerian structures in otherwise normal males. Brit. Med. J. 1: 771-773, 1973.

Gruell-Gonzales, J. R., Paramino-Ruibal, A. and Delgado-Morales, B.: Pseudohermafroditismo masculino con genitales interos bisexuales. Reporte de 2 hermanos. Rev. Cuba Pediat. 43: 579-586, 1971.

Morillo-Cucci, G. and German, J.: Males with a uterus and fallopian tubes, a rare disorder of sexual development. Bergsma, D.: (ed.) Clinical Delineation of Birth Defects. X. Williams and Wilkins, 1971. Pp. 229-231.

Nilson, O.: Hernia uteri inguinalis beins Manne. Acta Chir. Scand. 83: 231-249, 1939.

*26160 PHENYLKETONURIA

This cause of mental retardation is important because it is treatable by dietary means. The defect concerns phenylalanine hydroxylase. Features other than mental retardation include a 'mousey' odor, light pigmentation, peculiarities of gait, stance and sitting posture, eczema, and epilepsy (Paine, 1957). Peculiarities in the distribution of phenylketonuria have been noted. The disorder is rare in Ashkenazi Jews (Cohen et al., 1961; Centerwall and Neff, 1961). Carter and Woolf (1961) noted that of the cases seen in London and

R
E
C
E
S
S
I
V
E

presently living in southeast England, a disproportionately large number had parents and grandparents born in Ireland or west Scotland. The frequency at birth in northern Europeans may be about 1 per 10,000 (Guthrie and Susi, 1963). PKU is also rare in southern Italians. When it does occur in this group, it seems to be a different entity, namely, the form in which death occurs on low phenylalanine diet without supervision (Efron, personal communication, Nov. 2, 1965). Victor H. Auerbach (Philadelphia) also concluded there is a second variety of PKU. Evidence of heterogeneity in phenylketonuria was presented also by Woolf et al. (1968). The occurrence of mental retardation in the offspring of homozygous mothers is an example of a genetic disease based on the genotype of the mother. Kerr et al. (1968) demonstrated 'fetal PKU' by administering large amounts of phenylalanine to mother monkeys. The offspring had reduced learning ability. They pointed out that the damage is aggravated by the normal placental process which functions to maintain higher levels of amino acids in the fetus than in the mother. Huntley and Stevenson (1969) described two sisters with PKU who had in all 28 pregnancies. Sixteen ended in spontaneous first-trimester abortion. All carried to term had intrauterine growth retardation and microcephaly. Nine of the 12 term infants had cardiac malformations. Levy et al. (1970) screened the serum of 280,919 'normal' teenagers and adults whose blood had been submitted for syphilis testing. Only three adults with the biochemical findings of PKU were found. Each was mentally subnormal. Normal mentality is very rare among patients with phenylketonuria who have not received dietary therapy. Bowden and McArthur (1972) found that phenylpyruvic acid inhibits pyruvate decarboxylase in brain but not in liver. They suggested that this accounts for the defect in formation of myelin and mental retardation in this disease. Two isozymes of phenylalanine hydroxylase exist in human fetal liver (Barranger et al., 1972). The hydroxylation of phenylalanine is highly complex. At least three enzymes are known to be involved and mutation at two loci can affect at least two of these. Furthermore, multiple alleles probably exist at the locus (or loci) determining the phenylalanime hydroxylase apoenzyme. Thus, there is much opportunity for the many varieties of hyperphenylalaninemia.

Aoki, K. and Siegel, F. L.: Hyperphenylalaninemia: disaggregation of brain polyribosomes in young rats. Science 168: 129-130, 1970.

Arthur, L. J. H. and Hulme, J. D.: Intelligent, small for dates baby born to oligophrenic phenylketonuric mother after low phenylalanine diet during pregnancy. Pediatrics 46: 235-239, 1970.

Auerbach, V. H., DiGeorge, A. M. and Carpenter, G. G.: Phenylalaninemia. A study of the diversity of disorders which produce elevation of blood concentrations of phenylalanine. In, Nyhan, W. L. (ed.): Amino Acid Metabolism and Genetic Variation. New York: McGraw-Hill, 1967. Pp. 11-68.

Barranger, J. A., Geiger, P. J., Arezino, A. and Bessman, S. P.: Isozymes of phenylalanine hydroxylase. Science 175: 903-905, 1972.

Bowden, J. A. and McArthur, C. L. III: Possible biochemical model phenylketonuria. Nature 235: 230 only, 1972.

Carter, C. O. and Woolf, L. I.: The birthplaces of parents and grandparents of a series of patients with phenylketonuria in southeast England. Ann. Hum. Genet. 25: 57-64, 1961.

Centerwall, W. R. and Neff, C. A.: Phenylketonuria: a case report of children of Jewish ancestry. Arch. Paediat. 78: 379-384, 1961.

Cohen, B. E., Bodonyi, E. and Szeinberg, A.: Phenylketonuria in Jews. Lancet I: 344-345, 1961.

Cunningham, G. C., Day, R. W., Berman, J. L. and Hsia, D. Y.-Y.: Phenylalanine tolerance tests in families with phenylketonuria and hyperphenylalaninemia. Am. J. Dis. Child. 117: 626-635, 1969.

Frankenburg, W. K., Duncan, B. R., Coffelt, R. W., Koch, R., Coldwell, J. G. and Son, C. D.: Maternal phenylketonuria: implications for growth and development. J. Pediat. 73: 560-570, 1968.

Guthrie, R. and Susi, A.: A simple phenylalanine method for detecting phenylketonuria in large populations of newborn infants. Pediatrics 32: 338-343, 1963.

Howell, R. R. and Stevenson, R. E.: The offspring of phenylketonuric women. Soc Biol. 18 (suppl.): S19-S29, 1971.

Hsia, D. Y.-Y.: Phenylketonuria and its variants. Prog. Med. Genet. 7: 29-68, 1970.

Huntley, C. C. and Stevenson, R. E.: Maternal phenylketonuria. Course of two pregnancies. Obstet. Gynec. 34: 694-700, 1969.

Kerr, G. R., Chamove, A. S., Harlow, H. F. and Waisman, H. A.: 'Fetal PKU': the effect of maternal hyperphenylalaninemia during pregnancy in the rhesus monkey (Macaca mulatta). Pediatrics 42: 27-36, 1968.

Knox, W. E.: Phenylketonuria. In, Stanbury, J. B., Wyngaarden, J. B. and Fredrickson, D. S. (eds.): The Metabolic Basis of Inherited Disease. New York: McGraw-Hill, 1972 (3rd Ed.). Pp. 266-295.

Levy, H. L., Karolkewicz, V., Houghton, S. A. and MacCready, R. A.: Screening the 'normal' population in Massachusetts for phenylketonuria. New Eng. J. Med. 282: 1455-1458, 1970.

Menkes, J. H. and Aeberhard, E.: Maternal phenylketonuria. J. Pediat. 74: 924-931, 1969.

O'Flynn, M. E., Tillman, P. and Hsia, D. Y.-Y.: Hyperphenylalanemia without phenylketonuria. Am. J. Dis. Child. 113: 22-30, 1967.

Paine, R. S.: The variability in manifestations of untreated patients with phenylketonuria (phenylpyruvic aciduria). Pediatrics 20: 290-302, 1957.

Perry, T. L., Hansen, S., Tischler, B., Bunting, R. and Diamond, S.: Glutamine depletion in phenylketonuria: possible cause of the mental defect. New Eng. J. Med. 282: 761-766, 1970.

Rosenblatt, D. and Scriver, C. R.: Heterogeneity in genetic control of phenylalanine metabolism in man. Nature 218: 677-678, 1968.

Scriver, C. R.: Montreal, personal communication, 1974.

Woolf, L. I., Cranston, W. I. and Goodwin, B. L.: Genetics of phenylketonuria. I. Heterozygosity for phenylketonuria. II. Third allele at the phenylalanine hydroxylase locus in man. Nature 213: 882-885, 1967.

Woolf, L. I., Goodwin, B. L., Cranston, W. I., Wade, D. N., Woolf, F., Hudson, F. P. and McBean, M. S.: A third allele at the phenylalanine-hydroxylase locus in mild phenylketonuria (hyperphenylalaninaemia). Lancet I: 114-117, 1968.

Yu, J. S. and O'Halloran, M. T.: Atypical phenylketonuria in a family with a phenylketonuric mother. Pediatrics 46: 707-711, 1970.

*26165 PHOSPHOFRUCTOKINASE, RED CELL

Layzer and Epstein (1972) presented evidence which made it unlikely that a gene for red cell phosphofructokinase is on chromosome 21 (as had been previously suggested by Baikie et al. (1965) on the basis of apparent dosage effect).

Layzer, R. B. and Epstein, C. J.: Phosphofructokinase and chromosome 21. Am. J. Hum. Genet. 24: 533-543, 1972.

26170 PHOSPHOGLYCERATE KINASE DEFICIENCY OF ERYTHROCYTE

Kraus (1968) attributed life-long anemia in a 63-year-old Caucasian woman to deficiency of red cell phosphoglycerate kinase. No relatives were available for study, but a history of anemia in the proband's mother and two of her sibs was obtained. One would expect recessive inheritance, however. Hemolytic anemia due to deficiency of phosphoglycerate kinase appeared to be X-linked in a kindred studied by Valentine et al. and a structural locus for PGK has been confidently assigned to the long arm of the X chromosome (see 31180). Red cell PFK is composed of two nonidentical subunits, one of which is unrelated to white cell and platelet PFK, whereas fibroblast PFK is related to both (Layzar and Epstein, 1972).

Baikie, A. F., Loder, P. B., De Grouchy, G. C. and Pitt, D. B.: Phosphohexokinase activity of erythrocytes in mongolism: another possible marker for chromosome 21. Lancet I: 412-414, 1965.

Beutler, E.: Electrophoresis phosphoglycerate kinase. Biochem. Genet. 3: 189-195, 1969.

Kraus, A. P., Langston, M. F., Jr. and Lynch, B. L.: Red cell phosphoglycerate kinase deficiency. A new cause of non-spherocytic hemolytic anemia. Biochem. Biophys. Res. Commun. 30: 173-177, 1968.

26180 PIERRE ROBIN SYNDROME (GLOSSOPTOSIS, MICROGNATHIA, CLEFT PALATE)

Affected brothers were reported by Smith and Stowe (1961) and pictured by McKusick et al. (1962). (It is possible that these brothers had the Wagner syndrome: see 14320.) Sachtleben (1964) also described 2 brothers, who in addition to the usual features had bilateral syndactyly of the second and third toes and evidence of cardiac disease. The older brother had hypospadias, bipartite scrotum and mental retardation. Shah et al. (1970) observed Pierre Robin syndrome in four sibs including a set of twins. Bixler and Christian (1971) described the full Robin syndrome in two sibships related to each other as second cousins. Singh et al. (1970) reported a third pair of affected brothers. In the view of Opitz (1973), Stickler syndrome (10830) should come first to mind in cases of the Pierre Robin syndrome especially familial cases.

Bixler, D. and Christian, J. C.: Pierre Robin syndrome occurring in two unrelated sibships. The Clinical Delineation of Birth Defects. XI. Orofacial Structures. Baltimore: Williams and Wilkins, 1971. Pp. 67-71.

McKusick, V. A. and colleagues: Medical genetics 1961. J. Chronic Dis. 15: 417-572, 1962.

Opitz, J. M.: Madison, Wis., personal communication, 1973.

Russo, G., Mollica, F., Pavone, L. and Musumerci, S.: Robin's syndrome in three children of consanguineous parents. A pedigree suggesting autosomal recessive inheritance. Acta Genet. Med. Gem. 21: 349-353, 1973.

Sachtleben, P.: Zur Pathogenese und Therapie des Pierre-Robin-Syndroms. Arch. Kinderheilk. 171: 55-63, 1964.

Shah, C. V., Pruzansky, S. and Harris, W. S.: Cardiac malformations with facial clefts. Am. J. Dis. Child. 114: 238-244, 1970.

Singh, R. P., Jaco, N. T. and Vigna, V.: Pierre Robin syndrome in siblings. Am. J. Dis. Child. 120: 560-561, 1970.

Smith, J. L. and Stowe, F. R.: The Pierre Robin syndrome (glossoptosis, micrognathia, cleft palate). A review of 39 cases with emphasis on associated ocular lesions. Pediatrics 27: 128-133, 1961.

26190 PILI TORTI (TWISTED HAIR)

The shafts of the hairs are flattened at irregular intervals and twisted through 180 degrees about their axes. The hair is coarse, dry and lusterless. It breaks off leaving a stubble of variable length. In two of six families reported by Gedda and Cavalieri (1963) the parents were related and in two others of the six families two sibs were affected. Both parents were unaffected in all 6 families. The dental enamel has been hypoplastic in some of the cases. Usually the hair becomes normal at puberty. The condition was first described and named by Ronchese (1932) who observed 2 affected sisters. Appel and Messina (1942) described an affected girl of whom a brother, a sister, a paternal aunt and the paternal grandmother were also affected. A similar condition of the hair occurred in the patients with Menkes syndrome, an X-linked recessive (q.v.).

Appel, B. and Messina, S. J.: Pili torti hereditaria. New Eng. J. Med. 226: 912-915, 1942.

Gedda, L. and Cavalieri, R.: Rilievi genetici delle distrofie congenite dei capelli. Proc. Sec. Intern. Cong. Hum. Genet. (Rome, Sept. 6-12, 1961.) 2: 1070-1077, 1963.

Nichamin, S. J.: Twisted hairs (pili torti). Am. J. Dis. Child. 95: 612-615, 1958.

Ronchese, F.: Twisted hairs (pili torti). Arch. Derm. Syph. 26: 98-109, 1932.

26200 PILI TORTI AND NERVE DEAFNESS

Bjornstad (1965) first commented on this association. Among 8 cases of pili torti, five had nerve deafness. Reed (1966) observed four additional cases and Robinson and Johnston (1967) reported a case. The deafness is evident in the first year of life. The syndrome occurred in sibs among the cases of Bjornstad and Reed. Crandall et al. (1973) described three male sibs with neurosensory deafness, alopecia due to pili torti and secondary hypogonadism.

Bjornstad, R.: Pili torti and sensory-neural loss of hearing. Proc. 17th Meet. Nth. Dermat. Soc. (Copenhagen, May 27-29, 1965).

Crandall, B. F., Samec, L., Sparkes, R. S. and Wright, S. W.: A familial syndrome of deafness, alopecia, and hypogonadism. J. Pediat. 82: 461-465, 1973.

Reed, W. B.: Burbank, Calif.; personal communication, 1966.

Robinson, G. C. and Johnston, M. M.: Pili torti and sensory neural hearing loss. J. Pediat. 70: 621-623, 1967.

26220 PINEALOMA WITH HYPERPINEALISM

An increasing body of evidence suggests an endocrine function of the pineal gland and a role in regulation of hypothalamic releasing factors, particularly gonadotropins (Reiter and Fraschini, 1969). Mendenhall (1950) described a family in which 3 of 7 sibs had hirsutism, hyperpigmentation, precocious dentition, hyperglycemia and enlarged genitalia. Two of the three also had pituitary cysts. West et al. (1972) described a brother and sister with hyperinsulinemia, insulin-resistent hyperglycemia, unusual facies, enlarged and fissured tongue, advanced dentition, acanthosis nigricans, thickened nails and enlarged external genitalia. The girl died at 7-8 years from ketoacidosis and recurrent infections. Autopsy showed enlargement of the pineal gland and cystic ovaries.

Mendenhall, E. M.: Tumor of the pineal body with high insulin resistance. J. Indiana Med. Ass. 43: 32-36, 1950.

Robson, S. M. and Mendenhall, E. N.: Familial hypertrophy of pineal body, hyperplasia of adrenal cortex and diabetes mellitus: report of 3 cases. Am. J. Clin. Path. 26: 283-290, 1956.

West, R. J., Borin, H. Z., Turner, W. M. L. and Lloyd, J. K.: Familial insulin resistant diabetes mellitus. (Abstract) Arch. Dis. Child. 47: 153 only, 1972.

*26230 PINGELAPESE BLINDNESS

Brody et al. (1970) described in Pingelapese people of the eastern Caroline Islands in the Pacific, a severe ocular abnormality manifested by horizontal pendular nystagmus, photophobia, amaurosis, colorblindness and gradually developing cataract. From 4 to 10 percent of Pingelapese people are blind from infancy. Segregation analysis and equal sex distribution supported recessive inheritance. The high gene frequency was attributed to reduction in the population to about 9 surviving males by a typhoon (about 1780), combined with subsequent isolation. Whether the disorder is a form of congenital achromatopsia or a tapetoretinal degeneration with primary involvement of the cones was not clear. Carr et al. (1970) studied the same group and concluded that it is instead congenital complete achromatopsia. The impression of tapetoretinal degeneration was based, they thought, on severe myopia which was found in a majority of the affected persons. The disorder is nonprogressive. Compare retinal cone degeneration (18002).

Brody, J. A., Hussels, I., Brink, E. and Torres, J.: Hereditary blindness among Pingelapese people of eastern Caroline Islands. Lancet I: 1253-1257, 1970.

Carr, R. E., Morton, N. E. and Siegel, I. M.: Pingelap eye disease. (Letter) Lancet I: 667 only, 1970.

*26240 PITUITARY DWARFISM I (PRIMORDIAL DWARFISM, SEXUAL ATELEIOTIC DWARFISM, ISOLATED GROWTH HORMONE DEFICIENCY)

Early in this century Gilford called dwarfs with normal body proportions ateleiotic ('not arrived at perfection') and distinguished sexual and asexual types. The two types correspond to what are referred to here as pituitary dwarfism I and III. The first has an isolated deficiency of growth hormone, whereas the second has deficiency of all anterior pituitary hormones. The existence of an isolated growth hormone deficiency in recessively inherited sexual ateleiosis was demonstrated by Rimoin, Merimee and McKusick (1966). Families of this type have been reported by McKusick (1955), von Verschuer and Conradi (1938), Dzierzynski (1938) and others. Moe (1968) reported brother and sister with hypoglycemia and presumed isolated somatotropin deficiency. The father had diabetes insipidus. Illig and Prader (1972) have observed a possible distinct form of isolated growth hormone deficiency. All features are more severe than in the majority of cases and there may be an exaggerated tendency to develop antibodies which viciate therapy. The patients may be somewhat short at birth, dwarfism is more extreme than in other cases, hypoglycemia is a conspicuous feature and the puppet facies are exaggerated. It may be that the cases of the more usual HGH deficiency have some growth hormone whereas these have none.

Leisti et al. (1973) found growth hormone deficiency in a male with deletion of the short arm of chromosome

R E C E S S I V E

18. The association may be coincidence or may indicate that a locus controlling growth hormone synthesis is on the deleted segment.

Carsner, R. L. and Rennels, E. G.: Primary site of gene action in anterior pituitary dwarf mice. Science 131: 829 only, 1960.

Dzierzynski, W.: Nanosomia pituitaria hypoplastica hereditaria. Zbl. Ges. Neurol. Psychiat. 162: 411-421, 1938.

Illig, R. and Prader, A.: Zurich, Switzerland: personal communication, 1972.

Leisti, J., Leisti, S., Perheentupa, J., Savilahti, E. and Aula, P.: Absence of IgA and growth hormone deficiency associated with short arm deletion of chromosome 18. Arch. Dis. Child. 48: 320-322, 1973.

McKusick, V. A.: Primordial dwarfism and ectopia lentis. Am. J. Hum. Genet. 7: 189-198, 1955.

Moe, P. J.: Hypopituitary dwarfism. The importance of early therapy. Acta Paediat. Scand. 57: 300-304, 1968.

Rimoin, D. L., Merimee, T. J. and McKusick, V. A.: Growth-hormone deficiency in man: an isolated, recessively inherited defect. Science 152: 1635-1637, 1966.

Seip, M., Van der Hagen, C. B. and Trygstad, O.: Hereditary pituitary dwarfism with spontaneous dwarfism. Arch. Dis. Child. 43: 47-52, 1968.

Von Verschuer, O. F. and Conradi, L.: Eine Sippe mit rezessiv erblichem primordialem Zwergwuchs. Z. Menschl. Vererb. Konstitutionsl. 22: 261-267, 1938.

*26250 PITUITARY DWARFISM II (LARON TYPE)

Pertzelan et al. (1968) described a form of dwarfism in which the abnormality of pituitary hormones is limited to growth hormone, but the level of growth hormone as measured by the immuno-assay method is high rather than low. In Israel all cases (13 females, 7 males) of this type were Oriental Jews. A functionally abnormal, although immuno-reactive, growth hormone molecule was postulated. Inheritance was clearly recessive. Bailey et al. (1967) observed two sibs with severe dwarfing, retarded bone age, hypoglycemia and excessively high serum levels of growth hormone as determined by radio-immuno-assay. The parents were first-cousins. This disorder could be determined by a gene allelic to that producing lack of growth hormone. The 30-year-old man reported by Merimee et al. (1968) had raised levels of plasma HGH which was not suppressed by hyperglycemia and further augmented by insulin-induced hypoglycemia and by arginine infusion. With respect to all metabolic indices examined he showed attenuated responses to exogenous growth hormone. Similarities to isolated growth hormone deficiency cases of type I were exaggerated hypoglycemic response to exogenous insulin and insulinopenia after glucose or arginine. A 'warped' HGH molecule which saturates receptors and primary end organs unresponsiveness are two alternative explanations. The demonstration of deficient sulfation factor (somatomedin) generation (Daughaday et al., 1969) suggests that the mutation may primarily involve that substance. Laron (1974) listed a number of non-Jewish cases. Several of them were of Dutch or Arab extraction.

Bailey, J. D., Bain, H. W., Thompson, M. W., Gargliardino, J. J. and Martin, J. M.: Etiological factors in idiopathic hypopituitary dwarfism. Am. Pediat. Soc., 1967.

Daughaday, W. W., Laron, Z., Pertzelan, A. and Heins, J. N.: Defective sulfation factor generation: a possible etiological link in dwarfism. Trans. Ass. Am. Physicians 82: 129-140, 1969.

Laron, Z., Pertzelan, A. and Mannheimer, S.: Genetic pituitary dwarfism with high serum concentration of growth hormone. A new inborn error of metabolism? Israel J. Med. Sci. 2: 152-155, 1966.

Laron, Z.: The syndrome of familial dwarfism and high plasma immunoreactive human growth hormone. In, Bergsma, D. (ed.): Clinical Delineation of Birth Defects. XVI. Urinary System and Others. Baltimore: Williams and Wilkins, 1974. Pp. 231-238.

Merimee, T. J., Hall, J., Rabinowitz, D., McKusick, V. A. and Rimoin, D. L.: An unusual variety of endocrine dwarfism: subresponsiveness to growth hormone in a sexually mature dwarf. Lancet II: 191-193, 1968.

Najjar, S. S., Khachadurian, A. K., Ilbawi, M. N. and Blizzard, R. M.: Dwarfism with elevated levels of plasma growth hormone. New Eng. J. Med. 284: 809-812, 1971.

Pertzelan, A., Adam, A. and Laron, Z.: Genetic aspects of pituitary dwarfism due to absence or biological inactivity of growth hormone. Israel J. Med. Sci. 4: 895-900, 1968.

*26260 PITUITARY DWARFISM III (PANHYPOPITUITARISM)

Panhypopituitary dwarfism is not excessively rare, there probably being 7 to 10 thousand cases in the United States. The form inherited as a simple recessive probably is rare. Multiple cases in multiple sibships observed among the Hutterites, a religious isolate in the United States and Canada, indicate the recessive inheritance of panhypopituitarism. We have also observed panhypopituitarism in a 50-year-old uncle and 5-year-old niece. Furthermore, the familial cases in the inbred population of certain areas of Switzerland and of the Island of Veglia (Krk) in the Adriatic, observed by Hanhart (1925, 1953), are probably examples. This type (ateleiotic dwarfism with hypogonadism) is sometimes called Hanhart dwarfism. The nature of most panhypopituitarism as a congenital malformation with little indication of a Mendelian basis is supported by the observation by Rosenfield et al. (1967) of 16-year-old identical twins, one normal and one with panhypopituitarism. Kirchhoff (1954) described three affected sibs who may have had panhypopituitarism, the oldest being almost 18 years old. Selye (1949) pictured three brothers, ages 25, 22, and 11 with panhypopituitarism. The cases described by Schmolck (1907) may have been of the panhypopituitary type.

R
E
C
E
S
S
I
V
E

Bailey et al. (1967) reported two families with a total of 5 affected. In one the parents were first-cousins. Steiner and Boggs (1965) described brother and sister, offspring of first-cousin parents, with congenital absence of the pituitary leading to hypothyroidism, hypoadrenalism and hypogonadism. A third sib was probably also affected and died probably of hypoglycemia in the newborn period. This may be a separate entity from the other(s) discussed in this listing. The sella turcica was normal in size in the cases of Steiner and Boggs (1965). The disorder reported by Sadegi-Nejad and Senior (1974) may be the same or an allelic disorder. A male newborn infant developed hypoglycemic convulsions. Diagnostic studies showed evidence of deficiency of thyrotropin, growth hormone and prolactin. The child thrived on replacement therapy. A female sib died in the first day of life with similar clinical findings and at autopsy showed absence of the anterior pituitary and atrophic adrenal glands.

Bailey, J. D., Bain, H. W., Thompson, M. W., Gagliardino, J. J. and Martin, J. M.: Etiological factors in idiopathic hypopituitary dwarfism. Am. Pediat. Soc., 1967.

Ferrier, P. E.: Congenital absence or hypoplasia of the endocrine glands. J. Genet. Hum. 17: 325-347, 1969.

Fraser, G. R.: Studies in isolates. J. Genet. Hum. 13: 32-46, 1964.

Hanhart, E.: Die Rolle der Erbfaktoren bei den Stoerungen des Wachstums. Schweiz. Med. Wschr. 83: 198-203, 1953.

Hanhart, E.: Ueber heredodegenerativen Zwergwuchs mit dystrophia adiposogenitalis. An hand von Untersuchungen bei drei Sippen von proportionierten Zwergen. Arch. Klaus Stift. Vererbungsforsch. 1: 181-257, 1925.

Kirchhoff, H. W., Lehmann, W. and Schaefer, U.: Clinical, hereditary-biologic and constitutional studies of primordial dwarfs. Z. Kinderheilk. 75: 243-266, 1954.

Rosenfield, R. L., Root, A. W., Bongiovanni, A. M. and Eberlein, W. R.: Idiopathic anterior hypopituitarism in one of monozygotic twins. J. Pediat. 70: 115-117, 1967.

Sadeghi-Nejad, A. and Senior, B.: A familial syndrome of isolated aplasia of the anterior pituitary. Diagnostic studies and treatment in the neonatal period. J. Pediat. 84: 79-84, 1974.

Schmolck, (NI): Mehrfacher Zwergwuchs in verwandten Familien eines Hochgebirgtales. Virchow Arch. Path. Anat. 187: 105-111, 1907.

Selye, H.: Textbooks of Endocrinology. Montreal: U. Montreal, 1947. P. 268.

Steiner, M. M. and Boggs, J. D.: Absence of pituitary gland, hypothyroidism hypoadrenalism and hypogonadism in a 17-year-old dwarf. J. Clin. Endocr. 25: 1591-1598, 1965.

26270 PITUITARY DWARFISM WITH SMALL SELLA TURCICA

Ferrier and Stone (1969) described an apparently distinct form of familial pituitary insufficiency in two sisters, aged 10 and 11 years. The features were severe growth retardation from infancy, tendency to hypoglycemia, deficient production of growth hormone, TSH and ACTH, marked retardation in skeletal maturation, and very small sella turcica with abnormal morphology of the petrous bone. Ozer (1974) reported a case of pituitary dwarfism with small sella turcica. Retinitis pigmentosa was an additional feature. No other cases have, it seems, been reported (Rimoin, 1974).

Ferrier, P. E. and Stone, E. F., Jr.: Familial pituitary dwarfism associated with an abnormal sella turcica. Pediatrics 43: 858-865, 1969.

Ozer, F. L.: Pituitary dwarfism with retinitis pigmentosa and small sella turcica. In, Bergsma, D. (ed.): Clinical Delineation of Birth Defects. XVI. Urinary System and Others. Baltimore: Williams and Wilkins, 1974. P. 354 only.

Rimoin, D. L.: Torrance, Calif., personal communication, Sept. 9, 1974.

26275 PLACENTAL SULFATASE DEFICIENCY

The human placenta is rich in the enzymes 3-beta-steroid sulfatase and arylsulfatase. France and Liggins (1969) and others described deficiency of 3-beta-steroid sulfatase in the placenta. France et al. (1973) showed that arylsulfatase is also deficient in these instances. France and Downey (1974) showed that the deficiency is limited to the placenta. Multiple sibs with the defect have been observed. All those that France and Downey (1974) specifically referred to were males.

France, J. T. and Liggins, G. C.: Placental sulfatase deficiency. J. Clin. Endocr. 29: 138-141, 1969.

France, J. T., Seddons, R. J. and Liggins, G. C.: A study of a pregnancy with low estrogen production due to placental sulfatase deficiency. J. Clin. Endocr. 36: 1-9, 1973.

France, J. T. and Downey, J. A.: A study of arylsulfatase activity in children born of pregnancies affected with plancental sulfatase deficiency. Biochem. Med. 10: 167-174, 1974.

26280 PLASMA CLOT RETRACTION FACTOR, DEFICIENCY OF

Newcomb et al. (1967) described an apparently 'new' bleeding syndrome characterized by deep tissue bleeding, poor wound healing, pseudotumor formation and umbilical cord bleeding. A defect in clot retraction was correctable by a plasma protein. Family studies supported autosomal recessive inheritance.

Newcomb, T. F., Kitchens, C. S. and Berman, P. A.: A new bleeding syndrome with defective clot retraction due to deficiency of a plasma protein. Am. Soc. Hemat., Toronto, 1967.

RECESSIVE

In a case of childhood myopathy, Shy et al. (1966) found large numbers of mitochondria. The clinical features were proximal weakness and wasting, prolonged episodes of flaccid paralysis and salt-craving. Two brothers may have been affected in this sibship.

Shy, G. M., Gonatas, N. K. and Perez, M.: Two childhood myopathies with abnormal mitochondria: I. Megaconial myopathy. II. Pleoconial myopathy. Brain 89: 133-158, 1966.

26310 POLYCYSTIC KIDNEY, CATARACT AND CONGENITAL BLINDNESS

Fairley, Leighton and Kincaid-Smith (1963) observed three sibs with some type of eye defect causing blindness and some type of renal defect. One died at age 22 years of polycystic kidney, was blind from birth and showed central cataract. A second died at 18 years and had the same eye defect; atrophic kidneys with pyramidal cysts were found. The third sib had retinal dystrophy (or dysplasia) and large kidneys with medullary cysts. Pierson et al. (1963) reported two sisters who died at the ages of 10 and 15 days. Both had a complex ocular dysplasia (microcoria, hypoplastic retina, cataract, absence of ciliary body, persistence of fetal irido-corneal angle) in association with microcystic renal dysplasia. I have had a male patient (P 11614) who was blind from birth, probably as a result of retinal aplasia, and died of renal failure at age 12 years. Autopsy showed cystic disease of the kidneys.

Fairley, K. F., Leighton, P. W. and Kincaid-Smith, P.: Familial visual defects associated with polycystic kidney and medullary sponge kidney. Brit. Med. J. 1: 1060-1063, 1963.

Pierson, M., Cordier, J., Hervouet, F. and Rauber, G.: Une curieuse association malformative congenitale et familiale atteignant l'oeil et le rein. J. Genet. Hum. 12: 184-213, 1963.

*26320 POLYCYSTIC KIDNEY, INFANTILE, TYPE I

It has long been recognized that the age distribution of cases of polycystic kidneys has two peaks, one at birth and one between ages 30-60 years. Furthermore, the cases with the later peak show the familial pattern of an autosomal dominant. Three types of cystic kidneys in newborns, infants and children were distinguished by Lundin and Olow (1961). In type I the kidneys are oversized and spongy. The liver and pancreas may show fibrosis and-or cystic change. 'Potter's face' (deep-set eyes, micrognathia, large, floppy, low-set ears) is present in most or all. Lundin and Olow (1961) found 9 cases among 21 sibs. When these figures were treated by the method of Weinberg the corrected figure of 6 affected in 27 sibs was arrived at (a satisfactory agreement with the ratio expected of a recessive trait).

Type II also has large kidneys but is characterized by more abundant connective tissue than in type I. Type III has hypoplastic kidneys. In type II familial aggregation has been observed, but the evidence for recessive inheritance is not complete. Carter (1974) summarized a clinicopathologic study by Blyth and Ockenden (1969). Childhood polycystic disease fell into four classes according to age of onset, clinical course, proportion of renal tubules involved and degree of hepatic fibrosis. All four groups, termed perinatal, neonatal, infantile and juvenile, were thought to be recessive. The type was consistent within any one family. Occasionally, the 'adult' dominant form presented in childhood.

Blyth, H. M. and Ockenden, B. G.: A clinico-pathological and family study of polycystic disease of the kidneys and liver in children. (Abstract) J. Clin. Path. 22: 508 only, 1969.

Blyth, H. M. and Ockenden, B. G.: Polycystic disease of kidneys and liver presenting in childhood. J. Med. Genet. 8: 257-284, 1971.

Carter, C. O.: Polycystic disease presenting in childhood. In, Bergsma, D. (ed.): Clinical Delineation of Birth Defects. XVI. Urinary System and Others. Baltimore: Williams and Wilkins, 1974. Pp. 16-21.

Lee, K. H. and Chang, E.: Dystocia due to congenital polycystic kidneys. J. Obstet. Gynec. 77: 1115-1116, 1970.

Lundin, P. M. and Olow, I.: Polycystic kidneys in newborns, infants and children. A clinical and pathological study. Acta Paediat. 50: 185-200, 1961.

26330 POLYCYTHEMIA RUBRA VERA

Modan (1965) suggested that in only two reports of familial PRV is the diagnosis completely documented (Lawrence and Goetsch, 1950; Erf, 1956). Lawrence and Goetsch (1950) described 3 affected sibs. Two patients in the series of Erf (1956) were brothers and three others had 'a definite family history.' Levin et al. (1967) reported a curious case of two brothers with polycythemia vera and the Philadelphia chromosome. Subsequently, this was shown to be an instance of familial small Y chromosome (Levin, 1974). The precise mode of inheritance is unknown.

Erf, L. A.: Radioactive phosphorus in the treatment of primary polycythemia. Progr. Hemat. 1: 153-165, 1956.

Lawrence, J. H. and Goetsch, A. T.: Familial occurrence of polycythemia and leukemia. Calif. Med. 73: 361-364, 1950.

Levin, W. C., Houston, E. W. and Ritzman, S. E.: Polycythemia vera with Ph-1 chromosomes in two brothers. Blood 30: 503-512, 1967.

Levin, W. C.: Galveston, Texas, personal communication, Jan. 9, 1974.

Modan, B.: Polycythemia: a review of epidemiological and clinical aspects. J. Chronic Dis. 18: 605-645, 1965.

R
E
C
E
S
S
I
V
E

Auerbach, Wolff and Mettier (1958) reported three families. In one, two brothers and a sister were affected and in the second the proband and an aunt. The parents were normal. Unlike polycythemia vera, the subjects demonstrated no increase in white count, platelets or uric acid and the process was benign. Nadler and Cohn (1939) described a family in which 4 of 11 children showed polycythemia. The mother stated that these four children had red faces from the time of birth. This condition would more accurately be called benign familial erythrocytosis, since only the erythroid series is affected. See ERYTHROCYTOSIS, BENIGN FAMILIAL, in dominant catalog. Yonemitsu et al. (1973) described two affected sons of parents related as half first cousins. Both had a marked increase in erythroprotein concentration in plasma and urine. Adamson et al. (1973) studied two families with recessive erythrocytosis and found increased erythropoietin production uninfluenced by alterations in the oxygen-carrying capacity of the blood when the hematocrit was lowered by phlebotomy. Hemoglobin and red cell function and renal vasculature were normal. A genetic defect in regulation of erythropoietin production was postulated.

Adamson, J. W., Stamatoyannopoulos, G., Kontras, S., Lascari, A. and Detter, J.: Recessive familial erythrocytosis: aspects of marrow regulation in two families. Blood 41: 641-652, 1973.

Auerbach, M. L., Wolff, J. A. and Mettier, S. R.: Benign familial polycythemia in childhood: report of two cases. Pediatrics 21: 54-58, 1958.

Nadler, S. B. and Cohn, I.: Familial polycythemia. Am. J. Med. Sci. 198: 41-48, 1939.

Yonemitsu, H., Yamaguchi, K., Shigeta, H., Okuda, K. and Takaku, F.: Two cases of familial erythrocytosis with increased erythroprotein activity in plasma and urine. Blood 42: 793-797, 1973.

26350 POLYDACTYLISM

The Ellis-van Creveld, Carpenter syndrome and Lawrence-Moon-Biedl-Bardet syndromes (q.v.) are recessive disorders which have polydactylism as features. Snyder (1929) in a study of Negroes in Pamlico Co., N.C., assembled evidence interpreted as indicating a recessive form of simple polydactyly.

Snyder, L. H.: A recessive factor for polydactylism in man. Studies in human inheritance. J. Hered. 20: 73-77, 1929.

26352 POLYDACTYLY WITH NEONATAL CHONDRODYSTROPHY, TYPE I (MAJEWSKI TYPE)

Majewski et al. (1971) did much to clarify this syndrome on the basis of 4 personal cases and 32 nearly identical or similar cases from the literature. Death occurred perinatally in all. Malformations included median cleft lip, pre- and post-axial polysyndactyly, short ribs and limbs, genital abnormalities, and anomalies of epiglottis and viscera. Meckel syndrome (24900), Smity-Lemli-Opitz syndrome (27040), OFD syndrome (31120), Mohr syndrome (25210), Jeune syndrome (20850) and Ellis-van Creveld syndrome (22550) share some of these features but are distinguished with ease. Spranger et al. (1974) reported a case whose sib may have died of the same condition. Polycystic kidneys occur with this condition as well as with Meckel syndrome (24900). Spranger et al. (1974) referred to this condition as short-rib polydactyly (SRP) syndrome. The most distinctive finding in the Majewski syndrome is disproportionate shortening of the tibia. The radiologic appearance of the pelvis is normal and the metaphyseal margins of the tubular bones are regular (Spranger et al., 1974).

Majewski, F., Pfeiffer, R. A., Lenz, W., Muller, R., Feil, G. and Seiler, R.: Polysyndaktylie, verkerzte Gliedmassen, und Genitalfehlbildungen: Kennzeichen eines selbstandigen Syndrome? Z. Kinderheilk. 111: 118-138, 1971.

Spranger, J., Grimm, B., Weller, M., Weibenbacher, G., Herrmann, J., Gilbert, E. and Krepler, R.: Short rib-polydactyly (SRP) syndromes, types Majewski and Saldino-Noonan. Z. Kinderheilk. 116: 73-94, 1974.

Spranger, J., Langer, L. O., Weller, M. H. and Herrmann, J.: Short rib-polydactyly syndromes and related conditions. Birth Defects Orig. Art. Ser. 10 (9): 117-123, 1974.

26353 POLYDACTYLY WITH NEONATAL CHONDRODYSTROPHY, TYPE II (SALDINO-NOONAN TYPE)

This, like type I, is a condition lethal in the newborn period. The infant has a hydropic appearance, postaxial polydactyly, severely shortened and flipper-like limbs, and striking metaphyseal dysplasia of tubular bones. Ossification is defective in the calvaria, vertebrae, pelvis and bones of the hands and feet. As in type I, polycystic kidneys, transposition of great vessels, and atretic lesions of the gastrointestinal and genitourinary systems occur. Two patients reported by Saldino and Noonan (1972) were sibs. The disorder reported by Marec et al. (1973) in two pairs of sibs was probably this disorder. The tubular bones are short, with marked metaphyseal irregularities. The pelvis resembles that in the Ellis-van Creveld syndrome and asphyxiating thoracic dystrophy, with small ilia and osseous spurs projecting medially and laterally from the acetabular roofs.

Marec, B. L., Passarge, E., Dellenbach, P., Kerisit, J., Signargout, J., Ferrand, B. and Senecal, J.: Les formes neonatales lethales de la dysplasie chondro-ectodermique. Ann. Radiol. 16: 19-26, 1973.

Saldino, R. M. and Noonan, C. D.: Severe thoracic dystrophy with striking micromelia, abnormal osseous development, including the spine, and multiple visceral abnormalities. Am. J. Roengenol. 114: 257-263, 1972.

Spranger, J., Grimm, B., Weller, M., Weibenbacher, G., Herrmann, J., Gilbert, E. and Krepler, R.: Short rib-polydactyly (SRP) syndromes, types Majewski and Saldino-Noonan. Z. Kinderheilk. 116: 73-94, 1974.

26355 POLYNEUROPATHY, MIXED, OF EARLY ONSET

R
E
C
E
S
S
I
V
E

Mahloudji (1969) described two sisters and a brother (with first-cousin parents) who suffered from a slowly progressive mixed polyneuropathy. Onset was in the first years of life.

Mahloudji, M.: A recessively inherited mixed polyneuropathy of early onset. J. Med. Genet. 6: 411-412, 1969.

26360 POLYSACCHARIDE, STORAGE OF UNUSUAL

Craig and Uzman (1958) described two sibs affected by a metabolic disorder characterized pathologically by the storage of an unusual polysaccharide.

Craig, J. M. and Uzman, L. L.: A familial metabolic disorder with storage of an unusual polysaccharide complex. Pediatrics 22: 20-32, 1958.

26365 POPLITEAL PTERYGIUM SYNDROME

Bartsocas and Papas (1972) reported a family in which the parents were third cousins and four sibs were very severely affected. See 11950 and 17810 for dominant forms.

Bartsocas, C. S. and Papas, C. V.: Popliteal pterygium syndrome. Evidence for a severe autosomal recessive form. J. Med. Genet. 9: 222-226, 1972.

*26370 PORPHYRIA, CONGENITAL ERYTHROPOIETIC (GUNTHER DISEASE)

Forms of hereditary porphyria other than this behave as dominant traits. The congenital erythropoietic form is very rare. Drabkin (1963) reported in brief a Brazilian family in which 4 of 9 sibs were affected. Marked splenomegaly and cutaneous mutilation were features. Porphyrins are demonstrable in the erythropoietic cells, thus providing differentiation from the hepatic forms of porphyria which show porphyrins in the liver cells and not in the red blood cells. Hemolytic anemia may be helped by splenectomy. Gunther called this condition congenital haematoporphyria. Watson renamed it erythropoietic porphyria. Although recessive in cattle as well as in man, congenital erythropoietic porphyria is said to be dominant in swine and in cats (Glenn et al., 1968). Romeo and Levin (1969) concluded that the primary enzyme defect concerns uroporphyrinogen III co-synthetase.

Drabkin, D. L.: Some historical highlights in knowledge of porphyrins and porphyrias. Ann. N.Y. Acad. Sci. 104: 658-665, 1963.

Glenn, B. L., Glenn, H. G. and Omtvedt, I. T.: Congenital porphyria in the domestic cat (Felis catus): preliminary investigations on inheritance pattern. Am. J. Vet. Res. 29: 1653-1657, 1968.

Levin, E. Y. and Flyger, V.: Erythropoietic porphyria of the fox squirrel Sciurus niger. J. Clin. Invest. 52: 96-105, 1973.

Marvert, H. S. and Schmid, R.: The porphyrias. In, Stanbury, J. B., Wyngaarden, J. B. and Fredrickson, D. S. (eds.): The Metabolic Basis of Inherited Diseases. New York: McGraw-Hill, 1972 (3rd Ed.). Pp. 1087-1140.

Romeo, G. and Levin, E. Y.: Uroporphyrinogen 3 cosynthetase in human congenital erythropoietic porphyria. Proc. Nat. Acad. Sci. 63: 856-863, 1969.

Romeo, G., Glenn, B. L. and Levin, E. Y.: Uroporphyrinogen 3 cosynthetase in asymptomatic carriers of congenital erythropoietic porphyria. Biochem. Genet. 4: 719-726, 1970.

Romeo, G., Kaback, M. M. and Levin, E. Y.: Uroporphyrinogen 3 cosynthetase activity in fibroblasts from patients with congenital erythropoietic porphyria. Biochem. Genet. 4: 659-664, 1970.

Watson, C. J.: The problem of porphyria — some facts and questions. New Eng. J. Med. 263: 1205-1215, 1960.

*26380 POTASSIUM AND MAGNESIUM DEPLETION (SEE ALSO PSEUDO-ALDOSTERONISM)

Gitelman et al. (1966) reported two affected sisters who were the offspring of parents related as half-first-cousins-once-removed. They had experienced occasional mild episodes of muscle weakness and had suffered for many years from a chronic dermatitis characterized by thickening with a purple-red hue. Erythema of the skin is a feature of experimental magnesium depletion in the rat.

Earle, D. P., Sherry, S., Eichna, L. W. and Conan, N. J.: Low potassium syndrome due to defective renal tubular mechanisms for handling potassium. Am. J. Med. 11: 283-301, 1951.

France, R. and Tolleson, W. J.: Potassium depletion of undetermined origin in two brothers. Trans. Am. Clin. Climat. Ass. 69: 106-112, 1958.

Gitelman, H. J., Graham, J. B. and Welt, L. G.: A new familial disorder characterized by hypokalemia and hypomagnesemia. Trans. Ass. Am. Physicians 79: 221-235, 1966.

26390 POTASSIUM-SODIUM DISORDER OF ERYTHROCYTE

Sheep show a polymorphism of red cell potassium and sodium concentration. So-called LK sheep have low potassium and high sodium whereas HK sheep have the converse. Low potassium is dominant to high potassium. A precisely comparable situation has not been found in man. (See review by Lush, 1966.) In a child with hemolytic anemia Zarkowsky et al. (1968) found high sodium (100 meq. per liter) and low potassium (40 meq. per liter) in the red cells. Splenectomy was beneficial. Both parents were of Hungarian descent. They and a female sib had normal blood studies. In 3 males in 3 successive generations, Oski et al. (1969) found hemolytic anemia, stomatocytic red cells, and increased red cell fragility. Old cells were less dense than young cells and had a high-sodium, low-potassium content.

R
E
C
E
S
S
I
V
E

Lush, I. E.: The Biochemical Genetics of Vertebrates Except Man. Philadelphia: W. B. Saunders, 1966.

Oski, F. A., Naiman, J. L., Blum, S. F., Zarkowsky, H. S., Whaun, J., Shohet, S. B., Green, A. and Nathan, D. G.: Congenital hemolytic anemia with high-sodium, low-potassium red cells. New Eng. J. Med. 280: 909-916, 1969.

Zarkowsky, H. S., Oski, F. A., Sha'Afi, R., Shohet, S. B. and Nathan, D. G.: Congenital hemolytic anemia with high-sodium, low-potassium red cells. I. Studies of membrane permeability. New Eng. J. Med. 278: 573-581, 1968.

26400 PRADER-WILLI SYNDROME

Johnsen, Crawford and Haessler (1967) studied 7 mentally retarded cases aged 4 to 19 years. All showed poverty of fetal movements and extreme infantile hypotonia. With improvement in muscle tone, feeding difficulties abated but were replaced by uncontrollable hyperphagia. Plethoric obesity, retarded psychomotor development and diminutive hands and feet were noted. All teenagers were less than 5 feet tall. Studies showed that fat synthesis from acetate during fasting was 10 times greater in cases than unaffected sibs and hormone stimulated lipolysis was depressed. These workers suggested that the condition is comparable to the genetic obese-hyperglycemic mouse. Since during fasting substrate continues to be used for new fat and lipolysis is deficient, survival depends on a continuous supply of exogenous calories. Langdon-Down (1828-1896), who described mongolism (Down syndrome), also described this condition in 1887 (see account by Brain, 1967). The patient was a mentally subnormal girl who, when 13 years old, was 4 feet 4 inches in height, and weighed 196 lbs. At 25 years of age she weighed 210 lbs. 'Her feet and hands remained small, and contrasted remarkably with the appendages they terminated. She had no hair in the axillae, and scarcely any on the pubis. She had never menstruated, nor did she exhibit the slightest sexual instinct.' Down called the condition polysarcia. Zellweger and Schneider (1968) found one instance of affected sibs, brother and sister (Gabilan and Royer, to be published; probably the same as Gabilan, 1962) and one instance of parental consanguinity in the same report. I have observed a single case in an inbred Amish community. The fact that only one case is present speaks against recessive inheritance. However, Prader and Willi (quoted by Hoefnagel et al., 1967) favored recessive inheritance. Gabilan (1962) reported one family with affected brother and sister, as well as a second in which the parents of the proband were first cousins, but his patients were not entirely typical. The abundant fat, muscle hypotonia and small feet and hands are exactly the opposite of the sparse fat, muscle hypertrophy and large hands and feet in Seip syndrome, a recessive. Dunn (1968) found a high parental age but others have not. One of their patients had an XYY karyotype. The suggestion of a hypothalamic defect located in the ventromedial or ventrolateral nucleus is plausible, but no such lesion has been reported, nor was such found on careful search in a typical case (Warkany, 1970). Hamilton et al. (1972) showed that the hypogonadism is hypogonadotropic in type and the result of hypothalamic dysfunction. Treatment with clomiphene citrate caused rise in plasma luteinizing hormone, testosterone and urinary gonadotropin levels to normal and resulted in normal spermatogenesis and physical signs of puberty. A variant of the Prader-Willi syndrome, showing precocious puberty, was described by MacMillan et al. (1972). Jancar (1971) reported familial incidence. Hall and Smith (1972) reported two affected male maternal first-cousins. One was of normal stature and intelligence. They pointed out narrow bifrontal cranial diameter as a feature. MacMillan et al. (1972) described 2 unrelated girls with the features of this syndrome who additionally showed precocious puberty. They suggested this to be a variant and that a hypothalamic disturbance is responsible for this disorder.

RECESSIVE

Bolanos, F., Lopez-Amor, E., Vasquez, G., Lisker, R. and Morato, T.: Hypothalamic-pituitary-gonadal function in two siblings with Prader-Willi. Rev. Invest. Clin. 26: 53-62, 1974.

Brain, R. T.: In, Wolstenholme, G. E. W. and Porter, R. (eds.): Mongolism. Boston: Little Brown and Co., 1967. Pp. 1-5.

Down, J. L.: Mental Affections of Childhood and Youth. London: Churchill, 1887. P. 172.

Dunn, H. G.: The Prader-Labhart-Willi syndrome: review of the literature and report of nine cases. Acta Paediat. Scand. 186 (suppl.): 1-38, 1968.

Gabilan, J. C. and Royer, P.: Le syndrome de Prader, Labhart et Willi (etude de onze observations). Arch. Franc. Pediat., to be published.

Gabilan, J. C.: Syndrome de Prader, Labhart et Willi. J. Pediat. (Paris) 1: 179- , 1962.

Hall, B. D. and Smith, D. W.: Prader-Willi syndrome. A resume of 32 cases including an instance of affected first cousins, one of whom is of normal stature and intelligence. J. Pediat. 81: 286-293, 1972.

Hamilton, C. R., Jr., Scully, R. E. and Kliman, B.: Hypogonadotropinism in Prader-Willi syndrome. Induction of puberty and spermatogenesis by clomiphene citrate. Am. J. Med. 52: 322-329, 1972.

Hoefnagel, D., Costello, P. J. and Hatoum, K.: Prader-Willi syndrome. J. Ment. Defic. Res. 11: 1-11, 1967.

Jancar, J.: Prader-Willi syndrome (hypotonia, obesity, hypogonadism, growth and mental retardation). J. Ment. Defic. Res. 15: 20-29, 1971.

Johnsen, S., Crawford, J. D. and Haessler, H. A.: Fasting hyperlipogenesis: an inborn error of energy metabolism in Prader-Willi syndrome. Aps, 1967.

Laurance, B. M.: Hypotonia, mental retardation, obesity, and cryptorchidism associated with dwarfism and diabetes in children. Arch. Dis. Child. 42: 126-139, 1967.

MacMillan, D. R., Kim, C. B. and Weisskopf, B.: Syndrome of growth resistance, obesity, and intellectual impairment with precocious puberty. Arch. Dis. Child. 47: 119-121, 1972.

Warkany, J.: Cincinnati, Ohio: personal communication, 1970.

Zellweger, H. and Schneider, H. J.: Syndrome of hypotonia-hypomentia-hypogonadism-obesity (HHHO) or Prader-Willi syndrome. Am. J. Dis. Child. 115: 588-598, 1968.

26405 PRENATAL BOWING

Uncomplicated prenatal bowing of the long bones with dimpling has been described in sibs (Conway, 1958; Mahloudji, 1971).

Conway, T. J.: Prenatal bowing and angulation of long bones. A description of its occurrence in a brother and sister. Am. J. Dis. Child. 95: 305-308, 1958.

Mahloudji, M.: Shiraz, Iran: personal communication, 1971.

26410 PROGERIA

Precocious senility of striking degree is characteristic of this exceedingly rare disorder. Death from coronary artery disease is frequent and may occur before 10 years of age. Suggestion of recessive inheritance is provided by the report from Egypt of affected sisters, children of first-cousins (Gabr et al., 1960). Cockayne syndrome (q.v.) which resembles progeria in some respects, is clearly an autosomal recessive. Paterson (1922) recorded the cases of two affected brothers, offspring of first-cousins. Photographs were not published, however, and the diagnosis is not completely certain. The full report was simply the following: 'A boy, aged 8 years. Condition has been present since birth. The father and mother are first-cousins. There are four children in the family; the girls are unaffected, both boys are affected. The senile condition of the skin and facies should be noted. The vessels show arteriosclerosis. (There is almost complete absence of subcutaneous fat.)'

Among the 9 offspring of two sisters, Rava (1967) found 6 affected. Erecinski et al. (1961) described photographically typical progeria in 2 brothers. Debusk (1972) found information on consanguinity in 19 reported cases. In 3 the parents were related. In 20 cases in which parental age was known the mean paternal and maternal ages were 35.6 and 28.8 years, respectively, and the median ages 31 and 28 respectively. In 7 U.S. cases, the mean paternal age was 37.1. These values suggest a 'paternal age effect' as in dominant mutations. Conceivably progeria is a dominant and the rare instances of affected sibs are the result of germinal mosaicism. Ayres and Mihan (1974) suggested that a fault in vitamin E metabolism may be at the root of progeria and recommended vitamin E therapy for its anti-oxidant effect.

Ayres, S. and Mihan, R.: Progeria: a possible therapeutic approach. (Letter) J.A.M.A. 227: 1381-1382, 1974.

Debusk, F. L.: The Hutchinson-Gilford progeria syndrome. J. Pediat. 80: 697-724, 1972.

Erecinski, K., Bittel-Dobrzynska, N. and Mostowiec, S.: Zespol progerii u dwoch braci. Pol. Tyg. Lek. 16: 806-809, 1961.

Gabr, M., Hashem, N., Hashem, M., Fahmi, A. and Safouh, M.: Progeria, a pathologic study. J. Pediat. 57: 70-77, 1960.

Paterson, D.: Case of progeria. Proc. Roy. Soc. Med. 16: 42 only, 1922.

Rava, G.: Su un nucleo familiare di progeria. Minerva Med. 58: 1502-1509, 1967.

*26415 PSEUDOACHONDROPLASTIC DYSPLASIA II (FORMERLY PSEUDOACHONDROPLASTIC SPONDYLOEPIPHYSEAL DYSPLASIA)

Hall and Dorst (1969) recognized two recessive forms of pseudoachondroplastic dysplasia, designated types II and IV, types I and III being dominant. The radiologic features of II and IV are distinctive from each other and from the two dominant types.

Hall, J. G. and Dorst, J. P.: Pseudoachondroplastic SED, recessive Maroteaux-Lamy type. The Clinical Delineation of Birth Defects. IV. Skeletal Dysplasias. New York: National Foundation, 1969. Pp. 254-259.

*26416 PSEUDOACHONDROPLASTIC DYSPLASIA IV (FORMERLY PSEUDOACHONDROPLASTIC SPONDYLOEPIPHYSEAL DYSPLASIA)

Of the four types, the shortening of the limbs is most marked in this form.

McKusick, V. A.: Heritable Disorders of Connective Tissue. St. Louis: C. V. Mosby Co., 1972 (4th Ed.). Chapter 13.

26420 PSEUDOGLIOMA

Although usually inherited as an X-linked recessive, the disorder was observed in a boy and girl from a consanguineous marriage by Moutinho and Franceschetti (1954).

Moutinho, H. and Franceschetti, A.: Pseudo-gliome familial du type inflammatoire avec consanguinite des parents. J. Genet. Hum. 3: 82-85, 1954.

*26427 PSEUDOHERMAPHRODITISM, FEMALE, WITH SKELETAL ANOMALIES

In two daughters of a first-cousin marriage, Park et al. (1972) described primary amenorrhea, ambiguous external genitalia and bony abnormalities (hypoplasia and shortening of mandibular condyles, hypoplasia of maxilla, fusion of humerus and ulnar dislocation of radial heads, etc.). Karyotype was normal female. The clitoris was enlarged with marked fusion of the labioscrotal folds. The vagina was of normal size. Ovaries, tubes and uterus were normal.

R
E
C
E
S
S
I
V
E

Park, I. J., Jones, H. W., and Melhem, R. E.: Nonadrenal familial female hermaphroditism. Am. J. Obstet. Gynec. 112: 930-934, 1972.

*26428 PSEUDOHERMAPHRODITISM, MALE INTERNAL

This condition is also known as hernia uteri inguinale, male pseudohermaphroditism with Mullerian derivatives, female genital ducts in otherwise normal males, and persistent oviduct syndrome. Affected males are most often detected by the presence of an inguinal hernia containing Mullerian derivatives. The report of two affected brothers by Armendares et al. (1973) and by Morillo-Cucci and German (1971), and the parental consanguinity reported by von Seemen (1927) suggest autosomal recessive inheritance.

Armendares, S., Buentello, L. and Frenk, S.: Two male sibs with uterus and fallopian tubes: a rare, probably inherited disorder. Clin. Genet. 4: 291-296, 1973.

Morillo-Cucci, G. and German, J.: Males with a uterus and fallopian tubes, a rare disorder of sexual development. In, Bergsma, D. (ed.): Clinical Delineation of Birth Defects. X. Endocrine System. Baltimore: Williams and Wilkins, 1971. Pp. 229-231.

Von Seemen, H.: Pseudohermaphroditismus masculinus internus — Kryptorchidismus — Hernia inguinalis congenita. Bruns' Beitr. Klin. Chir. 141: 370-390, 1927.

26430 PSEUDOHERMAPHRODITISM, MALE, WITH GYNECOMASTIA

Saez et al. (1971) reported two brothers with male pseudohermaphrodism and gynecomastia in whom metabolic studies led to the conclusion that a defect in 17-ketosteroid reductase limited to the testis was the 'cause.' The parents were apparently non-consanguineous. Seven brothers and five sisters were living and apparently well. Goebelsmann et al. (1973) described this disorder in a 46-year-old phenotypic female. She was a seemingly normal girl until puberty when she developed breast, masculinized and failed to menstruate. The patient's parents were first-cousins.

Goebelsmann, U., Horton, R., Mestman, J. H., Arce, J. J., Nagata, Y., Nakamura, R. M., Thorneycroft, I. H. and Mishell, D. R., Jr.: Male pseudohermaphroditism due to testicular 17-beta-hydroxysteroid dehydrogenase deficiency. J. Clin. Endocr. Metab. 36: 867-879, 1973.

Saez, J. M., Frederich, A., De Peretti, E. and Bertrand, J.: Children with male pseudohermaphroditism: endocrine and metabolic studies. The Clinical Delineation of Birth Defects. X. The Endocrine System. Baltimore: Williams and Wilkins, 1971. Pp. 150-158.

Saez, J. M., De Peretti, E., Morera, A. M., David, M. and Bertrand, J.: Familial male pseudohermaphroditism with gynecomastia due to a testicular 17-ketosteroid reductase defect. I. Study in vivo. J. Clin. Endocr. Metab. 32: 604-610, 1971.

Saez, J. M., Morera, A. M., De Peretti, E. and Bertrand, J.: Further in vivo studies in male pseudohermaphroditism with gynecomastia due to a testicular 17-ketosteroid reductase defect (compared to a case of testicular feminization). J. Clin. Endocr. Metab. 34: 598-600, 1972.

26440 PSEUDOHYPOPARATHYROIDISM, TYPE II

Drezner et al. (1973) described a 22-month-old boy with grand-mal seizures and hypocalcemia, who showed elevated serum parathyroid hormone, increased urinary excretion of cyclic AMP and a marked rise in urinary cyclic AMP in response to exogenously administered parathyroid extract. However, neither the renal tubular handling of phosphate nor the serum calcium concentration responded appropriately to administered parathyroid hormone. They postulated a defect in the intracellular reception of the cyclic AMP message. No family data were given.

Drezner, M., Neelon, F. A. and Lebovitz, H. E.: Pseudohypoparathyroidism type II: a possible defect in the reception of the cyclic AMP signal. New Eng. J. Med. 289: 1056-1060, 1973.

26445 PSEUDOMONGOLISM

My colleagues and I have studied two Amish families with the following condition: four sibs in one family and two in the other had mental retardation, short stature and facial and other characteristics which led to the diagnosis of mongolism. Karyotype and dermatoglyphics were normal, however. Edwards (1970) described an identical situation in two brothers and suggested that Hall's case (1962) might be similar.

Edwards, J. H.: Experience (with mongolism) in Birmingham. Ann. New York Acad. Sci. 171: 304-319, 1970.

Hall, B.: Down's syndrome (mongolism) with normal chromosomes. Lancet II: 1026-1027, 1962.

26450 PSEUDOURIDINURIA AND MENTAL DEFECT

Kihara (1967) described increased urinary excretion of pseudouridine (5-ribosyluracil) in sibs institutionalized for mental deficiency.

Kihara, H.: Pseudouridinuria in mentally defective siblings. Am. J. Ment. Defic. 71: 593-596, 1967.

*26460 PSEUDOVAGINAL PERINEOSCROTAL HYPOSPADIAS (PPSH)

Simpson et al. (1971) described a family with three affected brothers whose parents were double first-cousins. Each of the affected sibs had an XY karyotype and ambiguous genitalia leading to rearing as females. No breast development or menstruation occurred at puberty, and instead typical masculation was observed. The name of the disorder stems from the finding of a blind-ending perineal opening resembling a vagina and a severely hypospadiac penis with the urethra opening onto the perineum. De Vaal (1955) reported three brothers who were thought for a time to be girls. The parents and grandparents on one side were first-cousins

R
E
C
E
S
S
I
V
E

and great-grandparents were also related. PPSH can be difficult to distinguish from the incomplete testicular feminization syndrome (ITFS) especially in the young child. The distinction is obviously important since this is a male-limited autosomal recessive with a recurrence risk of 1 in 8 whereas ITFS is probably X-linked recessive (or autosomal dominant male-limited) as is the complete syndrome. Wilson et al. (1974) chose to refer to this as type 2 familial incomplete male pseudohermaphroditism, type 1 being the Riefenstein syndrome (31230). This resembles the most severe form of type I incomplete male pseudohermaphroditism, but differs from it by the lack of breasts and by its autosomal inheritance. Dihydrotestosterone formation is defective in this condition. Testosterone and estrogen levels are normal, hence the lack of gynecomastia. Other evidence as well suggests that dihydrotestosterone is important to external virilization. In a village in the Dominican Republic, Imperato-McGinley et al. (1974) studied 12 families with 22 male pseudohermaphrodites. The affected males are born with ambiguous genitalia and masculinized at puberty without breast development. The testes are normal histologically. The patients have no Mullerian structures, complete Wolffian differentiation, small phallus, bifid scrotum, urogenital sinus with perineal hypospadias and blind vaginal pouch. At puberty, they show male habitus with excellent muscular development, voice change, enlargement of phallus and production of semen, but small prostate and scanty beard. Plasma testosterone is normal; plasma 5 alpha-dihydrotestosterone is low. An abnormally small amount of radioactive testosterone is converted to dihydrotestosterone. One woman studied showed the same biochemical defect. At critical periods in utero masculinization of the external genitalia may be dihydrotestosterone-dependent, although Wolffian differentiation is testosterone-dependent. Some of the pubertal events may be testosterone-dependent, whereas others are dependent on dihydrotestosterone. I suspect this is the same as pseudovaginal perineoscrotal hyposphadias (26460).

De Vaal, O. M.: Genital intersexuality in three brothers, connected with consanguineous marriages in the three previous generations. Acta Paediat. 44: 35-39, 1955.

Imperato-McGinley, J., Guerrero, L., Gautier, T. and Peterson, R. E.: An unusual inherited form of male psuedohermaphroditism. A model of 5 alpha-reductase deficiency in man. (Abstract) J. Clin. Invest. 53: 35A only, 1974.

Opitz, J. M., Simpson, J. L., Sarto, G. E., Summitt, R. L., New, M. and German, J.: Pseudovaginal perineoscrotal hypospadias. Clin. Genet. 3: 1-26, 1971.

Simpson, J. L., New, M., Peterson, R. E. and German, J.: Pseudovaginal perineoscrotal hypospadias (PPSH) in sibs. The Clinical Delineation of Birth Defects. X. The Endocrine System. Baltimore: Williams and Wilkins, 1971. Pp. 140-144.

Walsh, P. C., Madden, J. D., Harrod, M. J., Goldstein, J. L., MacDonald, P. C. and Wilson, J. D.: Familial incomplete male pseudohermaphroditism, type 2. Decreased dihydrotestosterone formation in pseudovaginal perineoscrotal hypospadias. In press, 1974.

Wilson, J. D., Harrod, M. J., Goldstein, J. L., Hemsell, D. L. and MacDonald, P. C.: Familial incomplete male pseudohermaphroditism type I. Evidence for androgen resistance in a family with the Reifenstein syndrome. New Eng. J. Med. 290: 1097-1103, 1974.

R
E
C
E
S
S
I
V
E

*26470 PSEUDOVITAMIN D DEFICIENCY RICKETS (VITAMIN-D-DEPENDENT RICKETS)

Dent et al. (1968) described a severely affected patient. The findings in this disorder differ from those in the X-linked vitamin D resistant rickets by the severity and the accompanying myopathy. The response to vitamin D is better in this disorder than in the X-linked condition. The severe skeletal changes suggest those of Morquio syndrome or some similar skeletal dysplasia. The beneficial effects of therapy may be overlooked. Earlier onset and depression of calcium as well as phosphorus in the blood help distinguish this disorder from the X-linked condition. Prader et al. (1961) suggested dominant inheritance but later Prader (cited by Dent et al., 1968) expressed doubts. He had a new family with first-cousin parents who were healthy with normal plasma levels of calcium and phosphorus. Dent et al. (1968) made brief mention of two other patients known to them, both with normal parents who were, however, related as first cousins. We have observed affected brother and sister. Vitamin-D-dependent rickets was the term suggested by Fraser and Salter (1958). Scriver (1970) supported autosomal recessive inheritance and suggested that the condition may be more frequent than previously realized. Hamilton et al. (1970) demonstrated defective intestinal absorption of calcium. Fraser et al. (1973) concluded that the basic defect concerns the enzyme 25-hydroxycholecalciferol-1-hydroxylase.

Fraser, D. and Salter, R. B.: The diagnosis and management of the various types of rickets. Pediat. Clin. N. Am. (May) 417-441, 1958.

Fraser, D., Kooh, S. W., Kind, H. P., Holick, M. F., Tanaka, Y. and DeLuca, H. F.: Pathogenesis of hereditary vitamin-D-dependent rickets. An inborn error of vitamin D metabolism involving defective conversion of 25-hydroxyvitamin D to 1alpha, 25-dihydroxyvitamin D. New Eng. J. Med. 289: 817-822, 1973.

Hamilton, R., Harrison, J., Fraser, D., Raddle, I., Morecki, R. and Paunier, L.: The small intestine in vitamin D dependent rickets. Pediatrics 45: 364-373, 1970.

Dent, C. E., Friedman, M. and Watson, L.: Hereditary pseudo-vitamin D deficiency rickets ('Pseudo-Mangelrachitis'). J. Bone Joint Surg. 50B: 708-719, 1968.

Prader, A., Illig, R. and Heierli, E.: Eine besondere Form der primaeren Vitamin-D-resistenten Rachitis mit Hypocalcaemie und autosomal-dominant Erbgang: die hereditaere Pseudo-Mangelrachitis. Helv. Paediat. Acta 16: 452-468, 1961.

Scriver, C. R.: Vitamin D dependency. (Editorial) Pediatrics 45: 361-363, 1970.

The features are characteristic changes in the skin of the neck, axilla and other flexural areas, in Bruch membrane resulting in angioid streaks on funduscopic examination and in arteries producing gastrointestinal and other hemorrhage, precocious calcification and occlusive vascular changes. Series ascertained because of the skin lesions show a preponderance of females, whereas series of cases of angioid streaks show a sex ratio of about 1. The possibility of an autosomal dominant form of PXE has been raised by the rather numerous families in which successive generations are affected. Wise (1966) stated that about a quarter of all families with two or more affected have cases in successive generations. This would appear to be too frequent a finding to be explicable in all instances by the phenomenon of quasi-dominance. Wise (1966) could discern no quantitative or qualitative difference between the cases in families with successive generations affected and families with unaffected but consanguineous parents.

Berlyne et al. (1961) suggested that PXE may be inherited as a partial X-linked recessive (i.e., that the gene may be on a part of the X chromosome homologous with part of the Y chromosome). If such were the case patients in any one sibship would tend always to be of the same sex. This appears not to be the case. Metachromasia of fibroblasts was reported by Cartwright et al. (1969). Pope (1974) suggests that there are two dominant and two recessive forms of PXE (see 17785). Type II recessive form is very rare, being present in 3 of 121 probands in Pope's study in the United Kingdom. It is characterized by generalized skin changes with no blood vessel or ocular manifestations.

Berlyne, G. M., Bulmer, M. G. and Platt, R.: The genetics of pseudoxanthoma elasticum. Quart. J. Med. 30: 201-212, 1961.

Cartwright, E., Danks, D. M. and Jack, I.: Metachromatic fibroblasts in pseudoxanthoma elasticum and Marfan's syndrome. (Letter) Lancet I: 533-534, 1969.

Coffman, J. D. and Sommers, S. C.: Familial pseudoxanthoma elasticum and valvular heart disease. Circulation 19: 242-250, 1959.

Goodman, R. M., Smith, E. W., Paton, D., Bergman, R. A., Siegel, C. L., Ottesen, O. E., Shelley, W. M., Pusch, A. L. and McKusick, V. A.: Pseudoxanthoma elasticum: a clinical and histopathological study. Medicine 42: 297-334, 1963.

Messis, C. P. and Budzilovich, G. N.: Pseudoxanthoma elasticum: report of an autopsied case with cerebral involvement. Neurology 20: 703-709, 1970.

Pope, F. M.: Baltimore, personal communication, 1974.

Wise, D.: In, H. Gottron and U. Schnyder (eds.): Hereditary Disorders of Connective Tissues. Vererbung von Hautkrankheiten. Berlin: Springer-Verlag, 1966. P. 471.

*26490 PTA (PLASMA THROMBOPLASTIN ANTECEDENT, FACTOR XI) DEFICIENCY

The disorder is not completely recessive because the heterozygotes have a mild but definite bleeding tendency. Almost all patients have been of Jewish extraction (Biggs and MacFarlane, 1962). Rosenthal (1964) collected 72 cases from 46 Jewish families. PTA, factor XI deficiency, analogous to that in man and cattle, has been found in a family of Springer Spaniel dogs. The defect is characterized by autosomal inheritance (determined), minor bleeding episodes, severe protracted bleeding after surgical procedures, abnormal prothrombin consumption, prolonged PTT and recalcification times and abnormal factor XI assay.

Biggs, R. and MacFarlane, R. G.: Human Blood Coagulation and Its Disorders. Oxford: Blackwell, 1962. (3rd Ed.).

Dodds, W. J. and Kull, J. E.: Canine factor XI (plasma thromboplastin antecedent) deficiency. J. Lab. Clin. Med. 78: 746-752, 1971.

Rapaport, S. I., Proctor, R. R., Patch, M. J. and Yettra, M.: The mode of inheritance of PTA deficiency: evidence for the existence of major PTA deficiency and minor PTA deficiency. Blood 18: 149-165, 1961.

Rosenthal, R. L.: Haemorrhage in PTA (factor XI) deficiency. (Abstract) Proc. 10th. Intern. Congr. Soc. Hematol., Stockholm, 1964.

Rosenthal, R. L., Dreskin, O. H. and Rosenthal, N.: Plasma thromboplastin antecedent (PTA) deficiency: clinical, coagulation, therapeutic and hereditary aspects of a new hemophilia-like disease. Blood 10: 120-131, 1955.

Vinazzer, H.: Partieller familiaerer Faktor-XI-Mangel. Blut 15: 263-267, 1967.

*26500 PTERYGIUM SYNDROME

Webbing of the neck, antecubital fossae and popliteal fossae with sternal deformity and male hypogonadism may behave sometimes as a dominant, but there appears clearly to be a recessive pterygium syndrome. I have observed a family in which each of two cousin sibships contained two cases (Norum et al. 1969). Of the 4, 3 were male and one female. Curious 'dents,' cutaneous depressions, were present on the back of the elbows and front of the knees. Matolcsy (1936) described a brother and sister with severe webbing of the neck, axillae, popliteal fossae and fingers. The boy, age 13, had cryptorchidism. The sibs reported by Srivastana (1968) as examples of arthrogryposis multiplex congenita appeared to have had this disorder. Gorlin (1974) suggests that the sibs reported by Matolcsky (1936) had this disorder, as did also case 1 in the report by Guinand-Doniol (1947). In the last case the parents were consanguineous.

Gorlin, R. J.: Minneapolis, personal communication, March 15, 1974.

R
E
C
E
S
S
I
V
E

Matolcsy, T.: Ueber die chirurgische Behandlung der angeborenen Flughaut. Langenbeck. Arch. Klin. Chir. 185: 675-681, 1936.

Srivastana, R. N.: Arthrogryposis multiplex congenita. Case report of two siblings. Clin. Pediat. 7: 691-694, 1968.

Norum, R. A., James, V. L. and Mabry, C. C.: Pterygium syndrome in three children in a recessive pedigree pattern. The Clinical Delineation of Birth Defects. II. Malformation Syndromes. New York: National Foundation, 1969. Pp. 233-235.

*26510 PULMONARY ALVEOLAR MICROLITHIASIS

The condition is characterized by multiple minute calcifications located in the alveoli and producing a typical radiographic appearance. Sibs have been affected in a number of cases. Information on consanguinity has apparently not been collected in a systematic manner; however, in several of the reported cases note was made of the fact that the parents were related. Caffrey and Altman (1965) described the disorder in premature twins who died at age 12 hours. They reviewed 66 cases in the literature of 68 cases (including theirs): 34 were familial, occurring in 13 families. A disproportionately large proportion of cases may be of Spanish extraction. In Spain Lopez-Areal et al. (1965) described 2 affected sisters in one family and a boy and his two sisters in a second family. O'Neill et al. (1967) observed three affected sibs. Affected brother and sister with first cousin parents were reported by Burguet and Reginster (1967). In Beirut Balikian et al. (1968) described the disorder in two pairs of brothers and an unrelated girl.

Balikian, J. P., Fuleihan, F. J. D. and Nucho, C. N.: Pulmonary alveolar microlithiasis. Report of five cases with special reference to roentgen manifestations. Am. J. Roentgen. 103: 509-518, 1968.

Burguet, W. and Reginster, A.: L'heredite de la microlithiase alveolaire pulmonaire. A propos d'une nouvelle observation familiale. Ann. Genet. 10: 75-81, 1967.

Caffrey, P. R. and Altman, R. S.: Pulmonary alveolar microlithiasis in premature twins. J. Pediat. 66: 758-763, 1965.

Gomez, G., Gomez, G. E., Lichlemberger, E., Santamaria, A., Carvajal, L., Jimenez-Penulea, B., Saaibi, E., Barrera, A. R., Orduz, E. and Correa-Henao, A.: Familial pulmonary alveolar microlithiasis: four cases from Colombia, S. A.: is microlithiasis also an environmental disease? Radiology 72: 550-561, 1959.

Lopez-Areal, L., Zumarraga, R., Turner, C. G., Granizo, I. F. M., Vara Cuadrado, F. and Duque Fraile, J.: Microlitiasis alveolar pulmonar familiar e infantil. (Descripcion de cinco casos in dos familias.) Rev. Clin. Esp. 97: 389-395, 1965.

O'Neill, R. P., Cohn, J. E. and Pellegrino, E. D.: Pulmonary alveolar microlithiasis — a family study. Ann. Intern. Med. 67: 957-967, 1967.

Sosman, M. C., Dodd, G. D., Jones, W. D. and Pillmore, G. U.: The familial occurrence of pulmonary alveolar microlithiasis. Am. J. Roentgen. 77: 947-1012, 1957.

Viswanathan, R.: Pulmonary alveolar microlithiasis. Thorax 17: 251-256, 1962.

26530 PULMONARY CYSTIC LYMPHANGIECTASIS (LYMPHANGIOMATOSIS)

Frank and Piper (1959) described two affected infants who were not related. One was stillborn and the other lived only about 2 hours. In one case there were similar lesions in the heart, pancreas, kidneys and mesentery. Nothing is known about possible genetic basis.

Frank, J. and Piper, P. G.: Congenital pulmonary cystic lymphangiectasis. J.A.M.A. 171: 1094-1098, 1959.

26540 PULMONARY HYPERTENSION, PRIMARY

In two sisters and a brother Coleman, Edmunds and Tregillus (1959) observed primary pulmonary hypertension and confirmed the diagnosis by post-mortem examination. All three sibs were affected in the family reported by Tsagaris and Tikoff (1968). Two were male and one female. Other reports have suggested dominant inheritance (q.v.). Hood et al. (1968) reported the condition in three sisters. Their review of the literature led them to conclude that the single generation cases tend to be predominantly in women and to have later onset than the multiple generation cases which tend to show more nearly equal sex distribution.

Coleman, P. N., Edmunds, A. W. and Tregillus, J.: Primary pulmonary hypertension in three sibs. Brit. Heart J. 21: 81-88, 1959.

Hood, W. B., Jr., Spencer, H., Lass, R. W. and Daley, R.: Primary pulmonary hypertension: familial occurrence. Brit. Heart J. 30: 336-343, 1968.

Robertson, B., Rosenhamer, G. and Lindberg, J.: Idiopathic pulmonary hypertension in two siblings. Clinical, microangiographic and histologic observations. Acta Med. Scand. 186: 569-577, 1969.

Tsagaris, T. J. and Tikoff, G.: Familial primary pulmonary hypertension. Am. Rev. Resp. Dis. 97: 127-130, 1968.

26550 PULMONIC STENOSIS

Coblentz and Mathivat (1952) described two sisters with pulmonic stenosis. Lamy, de Grouchy and Schweisguth (1957) found increased parental consanguinity in pulmonic stenosis and described one instance of two affected sibs. Consanguinity effect is to be expected of a multifactorial trait, so that this like the occurrence of affected sibs is not proof of simple recessive inheritance. David (1974) observed a family with four affected persons in three generations: grand-father, two of his daughters, and a son of one of the daughters.

Coblentz, B. and Mathivat, A.: Stenose pulmonaire congenitale chez deux soeurs. Arch. Mal. Coeur. 45: 490-495, 1952.

David, T. J.: A family with congenital pulmonary valve stenosis. Humangenetik 21: 287-288, 1974.

Lamy, M., De Grouchy, J. and Schweisguth, O.: Genetic and non-gentic factors in the etiology of congenital heart disease: a study of 1188 cases. Am. J. Hum. Genet. 9: 17-41, 1957.

26560 PULMONIC STENOSIS AND CONGENITAL NEPHROSIS

Fournier and colleagues (1963) observed a family in which 4 of 5 children had clinical and-or autopsy evidence of pulmonary stenosis and congenital nephrotic syndrome.

Fournier, A., Paget, M., Pauli, A. and Devin, P.: Syndromes nephrotiques familiaux. Syndrome nephrotique associe a une cardiopathie congenitale chez quatre soeurs. Pediatrie 18: 677-685, 1963.

*26570 PURETIC SYNDROME

Puretic and colleagues (1962) described a 'new' form of connective tissue disorder. In addition to the proband, a brother and sister were apparently affected, having died in infancy with painful flexural contractures of the elbows, shoulder joints and knees which developed at about 3 months of age. In addition to contractures, the proband showed (1) deformity of the face and skull, (2) stunted growth, (3) osteolysis of terminal phalanges, (4) multiple large subcutaneous nodes, some calcified, (5) dysseborrheic, sclerodermiform and atrophic changes of the skin, (6) recurrent suppurative infections of the skin, eyes, nose and ears. Ishikawa and Hori (1964) described a two-and-one-half-year-old Japanese infant whose sib had died at 8 months probably of the same condition. Systemic hyalinosis was suggested as a designation.

Ishikawa, H. and Hori, Y.: Systematisierte Hyalinose in Zusammenhang mit Epidermolysis bullosa polydystrophica und hyalinosis cutis et mucosae. Arch. Klin. Exp. Derm. 218: 30-51, 1964.

Puretic, S., Puretic, B., Fiser-Herman, M. and Adamcic, M.: A unique form of mesenchymal dysplasia. Brit. J. Derm. 74: 8-19, 1962.

*26580 PYCNODYSOSTOSIS (PYKNODYSOSTOSIS)

The features are deformity of the skull (including wide sutures), maxilla and phalanges (acro-osteolysis), osteosclerosis and fragility of bone. The disorder was first described and named by Maroteaux and Lamy (1962). (Andren et al. (1962) simultaneously and independently delineated this syndrome. They found 11 patients reported under various designations and added the cases of monozygotic twins.) In the past a number of these cases have probably been diagnosed as osteopetrosis (e.g., Seigman and Kilby, 1950). The patient of the latter authors was a Negro female, the offspring of first or second cousins. Kajii et al. (1966) described a Japanese case in the daughter of a first-cousin marriage. Also see CRANIOSTENOSIS. For a somewhat similar though distinct entity see ACRO-OSTEOLYSIS WITH OSTEOPOROSIS AND CHANGES IN SKULL AND MANDIBLE (dominant catalog). Sedano et al. (1968) found parental consanguinity in about 30 percent of reported cases, reflecting the rarity of the pycnodysostosis gene. Kozlowski and Yu (1972) described a child who had hematologic features, hepatosplenomegaly and anemia, like those of osteopetrosis (25970). From Portugal Almeida (1972) reported seven cases in four families of whom three had consanguineous parents.

Almeida, L. M. de: Contribution a l'etude genetique de la pycnodystostose. Ann. Genet. 15: 99-101, 1972.

Andren, L., Dymling, J. F., Hogeman, K. E. and Wendeberg, B.: Osteopetrosis acro-osteolytica. A syndrome of osteopetrosis, acro-osteolysis and open sutures of the skull. Acta Chir. Scand. 124: 496-507, 1962.

Elmore, S. M.: Pycnodysostosis: a review. J. Bone Joint Surg. 49A: 153-163, 1967.

Elmore, S. M., Nance, W. E., McGee, B. J., Engel-De Montmollin, M. and Engel, E.: Pycnodysostosis, with a familial chromosome anomaly. Am. J. Med. 40: 273-282, 1966.

Kajii, T., Homma, T. and Ohsawa, T.: Pycnodysostosis. J. Pediat. 69: 131-133, 1966.

Kozlowski, K. and Yu, J. S.: Pycnodysostosis: a variant form with visceral manifestations. Arch. Dis. Child. 47: 804-807, 1972.

Maroteaux, P. and Lamy, M.: La pycnodysostose. Presse Med. 70: 999-1002, 1962.

Nance, W. E. and Engel, E.: Autosomal deletion mapping in man. Science 155: 692-694, 1967.

Sedano, H. D., Gorlin, R. J. and Anderson, V. E.: Pycnodysostosis. Clinical and genetic considerations. Am. J. Dis. Child. 116: 70-77, 1968.

Seigman, E. L. and Kilby, W. C.: Osteopetrosis. Report of a case and review of recent literature. Am. J. Roentgen. 63: 865-874, 1950.

*26590 PYLE DISEASE (METAPHYSEAL DYSPLASIA)

Despite the bizarre roentogenographic changes, there are few clinical findings other than genu valgum. The skull is only mildly affected, thus distinguishing this disorder from the craniometaphyseal dysplasias. The femurs show an Erlenmeyer-flask conformity. The humerus is abnormally broad and 'undermodeled' in its proximal two-thirds, the radius and ulna in their distal two-thirds. Affected sibs were reported by Bakwin and Krida (1937), Daniel (1960), Pyle (1931), Feld et al. (1955) and Hermel et al. (1953), among others. Parental consanguinity was present in the cases of Daniel (1960). It is suggested by Gorlin et al. (1969) that

R
E
C
E
S
S
I
V
E

'Pyle disease' be reserved for the form of metaphyseal dysplasia with little involvement of the cranial bones. Restudy of Pyle patients showed little involvement of the skull (Silverman, 1970). See CRANIOMETA-PHYSEAL DYSPLASIA.

Bakwin, H. and Krida, A.: Familial metaphyseal dysplasia. Am. J. Dis. Child. 53: 1521-1527, 1937.

Daniel, A.: Pyle's disease. Indian J. Radiol. 14: 126-131, 1960.

Feld, H., Switzer, R. A., Dexter, M. W. and Langer, E. W.: Familial metaphyseal dysplasia. Radiology 65: 206-212, 1955.

Gorlin, R. J., Spranger, J. W. and Koszalka, M. F.: Genetic craniotubular bone dysplasias and hyperostoses. A critical analysis. The Clinical Delineation of Birth Defects. IV. Skeletal Dysplasias. New York: National Foundation, 1969. Pp. 79-95.

Hermel, M. B., Gershon-Cohen, J. and Jones, D. T.: Familial metaphyseal dysplasia. Am. J. Roentgenol. 70: 413-421, 1953.

Nema, H. V., Mathur, J. S. and Srivastava, T. P.: Craniometaphyseal dysplasia. Brit. J. Ophthal. 58: 107-109, 1974.

Pyle, E.: Case of unusual bone development. J. Bone Joint Surg. 13: 874-876, 1931.

Silverman, F. N.: Cincinnati, Ohio: personal communication, 1970.

*26595 PYLORIC ATRESIA

In two sibships, one with related parents, Bar-Maor et al. (1972) reported 5 cases of pyloric atresia. Others (e.g., Bronsther et al., 1971) have reported familial cases. The pylorus is reduced to a fibrous band or is obstructed by a diaphragm. Either may occur in the same family. Congenital pyloric atresia was observed by Tan and Murugasu (1973) in sibs, a male and a female infant. Both showed a thick membrane completely obstructing the pylorus. The parents of German and English extraction were non-consanguineous and had a third normal child.

Bar-Maor, J. A., Nissan, S. and Nevo, S.: Pyloric atresia. A hereditary congenital anomaly with autosomal recessive transmission. J. Med. Genet. 9: 7072, 1972.

Bronsther, B., Nadeau, M. R. and Abrams, M. W.: Congenital pyloric atresia: a report of three cases and review of the literature. Surgery 69: 130-136, 1971.

Tan, K. L. and Murugasu, J. J.: Congenital pyloric atresia in siblings. Arch. Surg. 106: 100-102, 1973.

26600 PYLORIC STENOSIS, INFANTILE

Mendelian inheritance of pyloric stenosis cannot be established. Carter (1961) estimated that the recurrence risk was 10 percent for males born after an affected child and 1.5 to 2 percent for females. Pyloric stenosis is an occasional feature of the Smith-Lemli-Opitz syndrome (27040).

Carter, C. O.: Genetics of infantile pyloric stenosis. The Clinical Delineation of Birth Defects. XIII. G. I. Tract Including Liver and Pancreas. Baltimore: Williams and Wilkins, 1972. Pp. 12-14.

Carter, C. O.: The inheritance of congenital pyloric stenosis. Brit. Med. Bull. 17: 251-254, 1961.

Dodge, J. A.: Infantile pyloric stenosis: a multifactorial condition. The Clinical Delineation of Birth Defects. XIII. G. I. Tract Including Liver and Pancreas. Baltimore: Williams and Wilkins, 1972. Pp. 15-21.

*26610 PYRIDOXINE DEPENDENCY WITH SEIZURES

Waldinger (1964) described three sibs of Italian ancestry in whom pyridoxine dependency was manifest at birth, by convulsions. Four previously reported sibships with more than one affected sib were referred to. Bejsovec et al. (1967) described three sibs with intrauterine convulsions. The first two (females) died in status epilepticus. The third was shown to have pyridoxine dependency. Thus, this is one form of 'convulsive disorder, familial, with prenatal or early onset' (q.v.). The disorder was first described by Hunt et al. (1954), but only recently has the defect been proposed to reside in glutamic acid decarboxylase (Scriver and Whelan, 1969; Yoshida et al., 1971).

Bejsovec, M., Kulenda, Z. and Ponca, E.: Familial intrauterine convulsions in pyridoxine dependency. Arch. Dis. Child. 42: 201-207, 1967.

Hunt, A. D., Jr., Stokes, J., Jr., McCrory, W. W. and Stroud, H. H.: Pyridoxine dependency: report of a case of intractable convulsions in an infant controlled by pyridoxine. Pediatrics 13: 140-145, 1954.

Scriver, C. R. and Hutchison, J. H.: The vitamin B6 deficiency syndrome in human infancy: biochemical and clinical observations. Pediatrics 31: 240-250, 1963.

Scriver, C. R.: Vitamin B6 deficiency and dependency in man. Am. J. Dis. Child. 113: 109-114, 1967.

Scriver, C. R. and Whelan, D. T.: Glutamic acid decarboxylase (GAD) in mammalian tissue outside the central nervous system, and its possible relevance to hereditary vitamin B6 dependency with seizures. Ann. N. Y. Acad. Sci. 166: 83-96, 1969.

Waldinger, C.: Pyridoxine deficiency and pyridoxine dependency in infants and children. Postgrad. Med. 35: 415-422, 1964.

Yoshida, T., Tada, K. and Arakuwa, T.: Vitamin B6 dependency of glutamic acid decarboxylase in the kidney from a patient with vitamin B6 dependent convulsion. Tokoku J. Exp. Med. 104: 195-198, 1971.

*26612 PYRIMIDINE 5-PRIME-NUCLEOTIDASE DEFICIENCY, HEMOLYTIC ANEMIA FROM

R E C E S S I V E

Valentine et al. (1974) showed deficiency of a pyrimidine specific 5-prime-nucleotidase in 4 subjects with hereditary hemolytic anemia. Ribosephosphate pyrophosphokinase was severely reduced, probably as an epiphenomenon resulting from inhibition of its synthesis by high concentrations of pyrimidine.

Valentine, W. N., Fink, K. F., Paglia, D. E., Harris, S. R. and Adams, W. S.: RBC pyrimidine 5(prime) nucleotidase deficiency. A new hemolytic syndrome. (Abstract) Clin. Res. 22: 563A only, 1974.

Valentine, W. N., Fink, K., Paglia, D. E., Harris, S. R. and Adams, W. S.: Hereditary homolytic anemia with human erythrocyte pyrimidine 5-prime-nucleotidase deficiency. J. Clin. Invest. 54: 866-879, 1974.

26613 PYROGLUTAMICACIDURIA

Jellum et al. (1970) discovered large amounts of pyroglutamic acid in the urine and plasma of a 19-year-old retarded male patient. The chemical search was initiated because of explained chronic metabolic acidosis. Pyroglutamic acid was isolated by gas chromatoglraphy and identified by mass spectrometry; it is ninhydrin-negative. The patient showed spastic tetraparesis and a cerebellar disorder with intention tremor and dysarthria. Deficiency of 5-oxo-prolinase in the kidney is suspected but not proved.

Jellum, E., Kluge, T., Borresen, H. C., Stokke, O. and Eldjarn, L.: Pyroglutamic acidosis — a new inborn error of metabolism. Scand. J. Clin. Invest. 26: 327-335, 1970.

*26615 PYRUVATE CARBOXYLASE DEFICIENCY

The biochemical and clinical lesions are similar to those for pyruvate decarboxylase deficiency (20880). The case reported by Tada et al. (1969) came from a family in which two sisters were presumably affected with the same physical and mental retardation. In the child investigated fully, serum alanine and pyruvate levels were elevated. Enzyme studies showed normal SGPT and liver pyruvate decarboxylase activities. However, the activity of pyruvate carboxylase (oxaloacetic decarboxylase) was deficient. Hyperalaninemia may be secondary to the increased level of pyruvate. Delvin et al. (1971) found responsiveness to thiamine administration. Thiamine pyrophosphate is the coenzyme for pyruvate dehydrogenase, a key enzyme for an alternate route of pyruvate metabolism. Pyruvate dehydrogenase activity was abnormally high in the patient's cells suggesting that thiamine restored pyruvate metabolism by facilitating an alternative mechanism for its oxidation. Delvin et al. (1972) pointed out that two forms of pyruvate carboxylase exist in liver, a high-Km and a low Km form. They reported a case with abnormality of gluconeogenesis and elevated plasma levels of pyruvate, lactate and alanine in which the low-Km enzyme was deficient. See 24540 and 25600.

Delvin, E., Scriver, C. R., Gagnan-Brunette, M. and Hazel, B.: Mechanism for thiamine responsiveness in pyruvic acidemia due to pyruvate carboxylase deficiency: a proposal. (Abstract) Proc. Canad. Fed. Biol. Sci. 14: 168 only, 1971.

Delvin, E., Neal, J. L. and Scriver, C. R.: Pyruvate carboxylase: two forms in human liver. (Abstract) Pediat. Res. 6: 392 only, 1972.

Tada, K., Yoshida, T., Konno, T., Wada, Y., Yokayama, Y. and Arakawa, T.: Hyperalaninemia with pyruvicemia. Tokoku J. Exp. Med. 97: 99-100, 1969.

*26620 PYRUVATE KINASE (PK) DEFICIENCY OF ERYTHROCYTE

The disease as described by Bowman and Procopio (1963) is much more severe than that reported by Tanaka, Valentine and Miwa (1962). Bowman and Procopio observed severe hemolytic anemia leading to death in the first years of life if not treated by transfusions and splenectomy. Tanaka, Valentine and Miwa observed a compensated hemolytic anemia in young adults who had been relatively little incapacitated. Separate alleles or even genes at different loci may be involved. Necheles et al. (1966) illustrated the variability with two unrelated patients. One had cholecystitis and cholelithiasis for which surgery was performed at age 23. He was well thereafter until age 28 when anemia developed, for which splenectomy was performed with good results. The second case was an infant who required exchange transfusion in the neonatal period because of jaundice and anemia. Results of splenectomy performed at 14 months were excellent. Further evidence of heterogeneity (possibly all allelic) in pyruvate kinase deficiency was presented by Sachs et al. (1967) and by Paglia et al. (1968), who found a PK enzyme of abnormal kinetics in patients with anemia. Leukocytes of patients with red cell PK deficiency show normal enzyme activity. The liver shows, however, deficiency of the PK isozyme which is identical to that in red cells (Bigley and Koler, 1968). Zuelzer et al. (1968) pointed out marked intrafamilial variability which studies suggested was due to heterozygosity for two distinct interacting mutants in mildly affected relatives of severely affected probands. Persons possibly heterozygous for an anomalous pyruvate kinase had anemia in the family reported by Sachs et al. (1968). The evidence of Koler et al. (1964) indicate the existence of at least two PK loci. Since PK is an essential enzyme homozygosity for the deficient state would be lethal otherwise. Although not all patients with PK deficiency responded, Blume et al. (1970) reported that intravenous administration of inosine and adenine was effective therapy, leading to decreased hemolysis.

Bigley, R. H. and Koler, R. D.: Liver pyruvate kinase (PK) isozymes in a PK-deficient patient. Ann. Hum. Genet. 31: 383-388, 1968.

Blume, K. G., Busch, D., Hoffbauer, R. W., Arnold, H. and Lohr, G. W.: The polymorphism of nucleoside effect in pyruvate kinase deficiency. Humangenetik 9: 257-259, 1970.

Boivin, P. and Galand, C.: A mutant of human red cell pyruvate kinase with high affinity for phosphoenolpyrvate. Enzyme 18: 37-47, 1974.

Bowman, H. S. and Procopio, F.: Hereditary non-spherocytic hemolytic anemia of the pyruvate-kinase deficient type. Ann. Intern. Med. 58: 567-591, 1963.

Bowman, H. S., McKusick, V. A. and Dronamraju, K. R.: Pyruvate kinase deficient hemolytic anemia in an Amish isolate. Am. J. Hum. Genet. 17: 1-8, 1965.

Keitt, A. S. and Bennett, D. C.: Pyruvate kinase deficiency and related disorders of red cell glycolysis. Am. J. Med. 41: 762-785, 1966.

Koler, R. D., Bigley, R. H., Jones, R. T., Rigas, D. A., Vanbellinghen, P. and Thompson, P.: Pyruvate kinase: molecular differences between human red cell and leukocyte enzymes. Cold Spring Harbor Symp. Quant. Biol. 24: 213-221, 1964.

Necheles, T. F., Finkel, H. E., Sheehan, R. G. and Allen, D. M.: Red cell pyruvate kinase deficiency. The effect of splenectomy. Arch. Intern. Med. 118: 75-78, 1966.

Oski, F. A. and Bowman, H.: A low k(m) phosphoenolpyruvate mutant in the amish with red cell pyruvate kinase deficiency. Brit. J. Haemat. 17: 289-297, 1969.

Paglia, D. E., Valentine, W. N., Baughan, M. A., Miller, D. R., Reed, C. F. and McIntyre, O. R.: An inherited molecular lesion of erythrocyte pyruvate kinase. Identification of a kinetically aberrant isozyme associated with premature hemolysis. J. Clin. Invest. 47: 1929-1946, 1968.

Sachs, J. R., Wicker, D. J., Gilcher, R. O., Conrad, M. E. and Cohen, R. J.: Familial hemolytic anemia resulting from an abnormal red blood cell pyruvate kinase. J. Lab. Clin. Med. 72: 359-362, 1968.

Searcy, G. P., Miller, D. R. and Tasker, J. B.: Congenital hemolytic anemia in the basenji dog due to erythrocyte pyruvate kinase deficiency. Canad. J. Comp. Med. 35: 67-70, 1971.

Tanaka, K. R., Valentine, W. N. and Miwa, S.: Pyruvate kinase (PK) deficiency hereditary nonspherocytic hemolytic anemia. Blood 19: 267-295, 1962.

Valentine, W. N. and Tanaka, K. R.: Pyruvate kinase deficiency and other enzyme-deficiency hereditary hemolytic anemias. In, Stanbury, J. B., Wyngaarden, J. B. and Fredrickson, D. S. (eds.): The Metabolic Basis of Inherited Disease. New York: McGraw-Hill, 1972 (3rd Ed.). Pp. 1338-1357.

Zuelzer, W. W., Robinson, A. R. and Hsu, T. H. J.: Erythrocyte pyruvate kinase deficiency in non-spherocytic hemolytic anemia: a system of multiple genetic markers? Blood 32: 33-48, 1968.

26630 RED HAIR

R
E
C
E
S
S
I
V
E

In Copenhagen, Hauge and Helweg-Larsen (1954) found the prevalence of 'strikingly red hair' to be 1.90 percent. Neel (1943) was of the opinion that red hair is recessive with occasional penetrance in heterozygotes and hypostasis to factors determining black or brown hair color. Reed (1952) questioned whether red hair 'segregates' when macroscopic methods for scoring subjects are used. Red hair has been present in patients with Job syndrome (q.v.). Rife (1967) concluded that the proportion of red-haired offspring in families in which one or both parents are red haired are too high to support the hypothesis that red hair is inherited as a simple recessive. The family data and gene frequency analysis suggested to him that the presence of red pigment in the hair is dominant to its absence and is hypostatic to brown or black.

Hauge, M. and Helweg-Larsen, H. F.: Studies on linkage in man: red hair versus blood groups, PTC and eye colour. Ann. Eugen. 18: 175-182, 1954.

Neel, J. V.: Concerning inheritance of red hair. J. Hered. 34: 93-96, 1943.

Reed, T. E.: Red hair colour as a genetical character. Ann. Eugen. 17: 115-139, 1952.

Rife, D. C.: The inheritance of red hair. Acta Genet. Med. Gem. 16: 342-349, 1967.

Singleton, W. R. and Ellis, B.: Inheritance of red hair for six generations. J. Hered. 55: 261-266, 1964.

*26635 RED SKIN PIGMENT ANOMALY OF NEW GUINEA

Walsh (1971) described a pigment anomaly in New Guinea natives. The skin is reddish-brown rather than black as in other natives. Melanin is present, however, and increases with age. The color of the hair varies from the usual black to almost white. Nystagmus and photophobia were variable features. An enzymatic defect in melanin formation was posited. Many pedigrees supporting recessive inheritance were presented.

Walsh, R. J.: A distinctive pigment of the skin in New Guinea natives. Ann. Hum. Genet. 34: 379-385, 1971.

26640 REESE RETINAL DYSPLASIA

This disorder consists of malformation of the retina and persistence of the primary vitreous. Absence of the definitive vitreous is not surprising since its formation is dependent on the retina. The abnormality may simulate Norrie disease (see X-linked catalog). It is the characteristic eye change in trisomy 13-15 (trisomy D-1, or the Bartholin-Patau syndrome), which is characterized by delay in the development of several proteins such as adult hemoglobin and red cell catalase (Lee et al., 1966). Multiple visceral manifestations and others such as polydactyly were known to be associated (Harris and Thomson, 1937; Reese and Blodi, 1950; Reese and Straatsma, 1958; Yudkin, 1928) long before the chromosomal basis was elucidated. Aside from the importance in the differential diagnosis of microphthalmos, anophthalmos, Norrie disease, the main reason for including mention here of Reese retinal dysplasia is that Reese and Straatsma (1958) observed two sibships with multiple affected members — 2 out of 3 in one and 3 out of 4 in a second. In reporting the case of a 10-year-old boy, Matthes and Stenzel (1968) described minor changes in the mother and two sibs. Karyotype was normal in the proband.

Harris, H. A. and Thomson, G. C.: Persistent truncus arteriosus communis with microphthalmos, orbital cyst and polydactyly. Arch. Dis. Child. 12: 59-66, 1937.

Krause, A. C.: Congenital encephalo-ophthalmic dysplasia. Arch. Ophthal. 36: 387-444, 1946.

Lee, C. S. N., Boyer, S. H., Bowen, P., Weatherall, D. J., Rosenblum, H., Clark, D. B., Duke, J. R., Liboro, C., Bias, W. B. and Borgaonkar, D. S.: The D(1) trisomy syndrome: three subjects with unequally advancing development. Bull. Johns Hopkins Hosp. 118: 374-394, 1966.

Matthes, A. and Stenzel, K.: Familiaere, encephalo-retinale Dysplasie (Krause-Reesem syndrom) mit myoklonischastatische petit mal. Z. Kinderheilk. 103: 81-89, 1968.

Reese, A. B. and Blodi, F. C.: Retinal dysplasia. Am. J. Ophthal. 33: 23-32, 1950.

Reese, A. B. and Straatsma, B. R.: Retinal dysplasia. Am. J. Ophthal. 45: 199-211, 1958.

Yudkin, A. M.: Congenital bilateral microphthalmos accompanied by other malformations of the body. Am. J. Ophthal. 11: 128-131, 1928.

*26650 REFSUM SYNDROME

Retinitis pigmentosa, chronic polyneuritis and cerebellar signs are the cardinal clinical features. Some cases have nerve deafness and most have electrocardiographic changes. Ichthyosis is present in some. Histologically interstitial hypertrophic polyneuritis and degeneration of nuclei and fiber tracts in the brain stem have been described. An instructive pedigree is that shown by Baker (1962). This condition has been shown to be a disorder of lipid metabolism. An unusual fatty acid 3, 7, 11, 15- tetramethyl-hexadecanic acid has been identified in the serum and in the lipid deposits of the liver, kidney and other organs. Klenk and Kahlke (1963) discovered the accumulation of the branched chain fatty acid, phytanic acid. Isotopic studies indicate that there is little endogenous synthesis of phytanic acid and that the metabolic defect involves degradation. In these patients exogenous phytol is readily converted to phytanic acid. Eldjarn et al. (1966) showed that with a diet free of chlorophyll and of foods which might contain phytol, phytanic acid or their precursors, phytanic acid could be reduced in the blood and clinical improvement effected. Patients and cultured fibroblasts from patients show very low oxidation of C14-labelled phytanic acid but normal oxidation of pristanic acid which is known to be the first product of phytanic acid degradation (Steinberg et al., 1967). The defect then resides in the enzyme which catalyzes the alpha-oxidative process by which phytanic acid is shortened by one carbon atom. Studies of cultured fibroblasts from patients with Refsum disease led Herndon et al. (1969) to the conclusion that the enzyme involved in alpha-hydroxylation of phytanate is deficient, while enzymes involved in later steps are normal.

Ashenhurst, E. M., Millar, J. H. D. and Milliken, T. G.: Refsum's syndrome affecting a brother and two sisters. Brit. Med. J. 2: 415-417, 1958.

Baker, A. B.: Familial primary amyloidosis with polyneuropathy. Clinical Neurology. New York: Hoeber-Harper, (2nd Ed.) 4: 2287, 1962.

Clark, D. B. and Critchley, M.: Heredopathia atactica polyneuritiformis (Refsum's syndrome). Proc. Roy. Soc. Med. 44: 689-690, 1951.

Eldjarn, L., Try, K., Stokke, O., Munthe-Kaas, A. W., Refsum, S., Steinberg, D., Avigan, J. and Mize, C. E.: Dietary effects on serum-phytanic-acid levels and on clinical manifestations in heredopathia atactica polyneuritiforms. Lancet I: 691-693, 1966.

Herndon, J. H., Jr., Steinberg, D. and Uhlendorf, B. W.: Refsum's disease: defective oxidation of phytanic acid in tissue cultures derived from homozygotes and heterozygotes. New Eng. J. Med. 281: 1034-1038, 1969.

Herndon, J. H., Jr., Steinberg, D., Uhlendorf, B. W. and Fales, H. M.: Refsum's disease: characterization of the enzyme defect in cell culture. J. Clin. Invest. 48: 1017-1032, 1969.

Kahlke, W. and Wagener, H.: Conversion of h3-phytol to phytanic acid and its incorporation into plasma lipid fractions in heredopathia atactica polyneuritiformis. Metabolism 15: 687-693, 1966.

Klenk, E. and Kahlke, W.: Ueber das Vorkommen der 3.7.11.15-tetramethyl-hexadecansaeure (Phytansaeure) in den Cholesterinestern und andern Lipoidfraktionen der Organe bei einem Krankheitsfall unbekannter Genese (Verdacht auf heredopathia atactica polyneuritiformis Refsum-syndrom). Hoppe Seyler. Z. Physiol. Chem. 333: 133-142, 1963.

Mize, C. E., Herndon, J. H., Jr., Blass, J. P., Milne, G. W. A., Follansbee, C., Laudat, P. and Steinberg, D.: Localization of the oxidative defect in phytanic acid degradation in patients with Refsum's disease. J. Clin. Invest. 48: 10331040, 1969.

Refsum, S.: Heredopathia atactica polyneuritiformis. J. Nerv. Ment. Dis. 116: 1046-1050, 1952.

Refsum, S., Salomonsen, L. and Skatvedt, M.: Heredopathia atactica polyneuritiformis in children. J. Pediat. 35: 335-343, 1949.

Richterich, R., Kahlke, W., Van Mechelen, P. and Rossi, E.: Refsum's syndrome (Heredopathia atactica polyneuritiformis): ein angeborener Defekt im lipidstoffwechsel mit Speicherung von 3,7,11,15-tetramethyl-hexadecansaure. Klin. Wschr. 41: 800-801, 1963.

Richterich, R., Van Mechelen, P. and Rossi, E.: Refsum's disease (heredopathia atactica polyneuritiformis): an inborn error of lipid metabolism with storage of 3,7,11,15-tetramethyl hexadecanoic acid. I. Report of a case. Am. J. Med. 39: 230-236, 1965.

Steinberg, D., Herndon, J. H., Jr., Uhlendorf, B. W., Mize, C. E., Avigan, J. and Milne, G. W. A.: Refsum's disease: nature of the enzyme defect. Science 156: 1740-1742, 1967.

Steinberg, D., Mize, C. E., Avigan, J., Fales, H. M., Eldjarn, L., Try, K., Stokke, O. and Refsum, S.: Studies on the metabolic error in Refsum's disease. J. Clin. Invest. 46: 313-322, 1967.

Steinberg, D., Mize, C. E., Herndon, J. H., Jr., Fales, H. M., Engel, W. K. and Vroom, F. Q.: Phytanic acid in patients with Refsum's syndrome and response to dietary treatment. Arch. Intern. Med. 125: 75-87, 1970.

Steinberg, D., Vroom, F. Q., Engel, W. K., Cammermeyer, J., Mize, C. E. and Avigan, J.: Refsum's disease — a recently characterized lipidosis involving the nervous system. Ann. Intern. Med. 66: 365-395, 1967.

26660 REGIONAL ENTERITIS

About 10 percent of persons with regional enteritis have one or more close relatives with granulomatous disease of the bowel. The familial pattern does not suggest simple Mendelian inheritance. In 5 persons of Ashkenazic Jewish origin (ancestors from area of Russia-Poland around Vilna) Sheehan et al. (1967) found red cell glucose-6-phosphate dehydrogenase deficiency associated with regional enteritis or granulomatous colitis. The affected persons were 2 males and 3 females. Regional enteritis and sarcoidosis have been observed in the same family (18100).

Sheehan, R. G., Necheles, T. F., Lindeman, R. J., Meyer, H. J. and Patterson, J. F.: Regional enteritis associated with erythrocyte G6PD-deficiency. New Eng. J. Med. 277: 1124-1126, 1967.

26670 RENAL AGENESIS, BILATERAL

There are at least two reports of the defect in sibs. On the other hand, six cases are known of twin pairs of which only one was affected (Davidson and Ross, 1954). No twins, both affected, seem to have been reported. Bilateral renal agenesis was reported in 2 male sibs by Madisson (1934). The 'Potter facies,' which are considered typical of renal agenesis, consist of wide-set eyes, 'parrot-beak' nose, receding chin and large, low-set ears deficient in cartilage (Potter, 1946). It occurs in other renal disorders which interfer with formation of amniotic fluid and in infants with normal kidneys but prolonged leakage of amniotic fluid (Bain et al., 1964). Potter syndrome is characterized by peculiarity of the facies and ears and is secondary to compression as a result of oligohydramnios whatever the cause. Deformity of the feet and hands and hypoplasia of the lungs are other features. Thus, Potter facies are not pathognomonic of — renal agenesis. Buchta et al. (1973) suggest that bilateral renal agenesis is multifactorial with a recurrence risk in sibs of about 1 percent.

Bain, A. D., Smith, I. I. and Gauld, I. K.: Newborn after prolonged leakage of liquor amnii. Brit. Med. J. 2: 598-599, 1964.

Baron, C.: Bilateral agenesis of the kidneys in two consecutive infants. Am. J. Obstet. Gynec. 67: 667-670, 1954.

Buchta, R. M., Viseskul, C., Gilbert, E. F., Sarto, G. E. and Opitz, J. M.: Familial bilateral renal agenesis and hereditary renal adysplasia. Zschr. Kinderhlk. in press, 1973.

Davidson, W. M. and Ross, G. I. M.: Bilateral absence of the kidneys and related congenital anomalies. J. Path. Bact. 68: 459-471, 1954.

Hack, M., Jaffe, J., Blankstein, J., Goodman, R. M. and Brish, M.: Familial aggregation in bilateral renal agenesis. Clin. Genet. 5: 173-177, 1974.

Madisson, H.: Ueber das Fehlen beider Nieren (Aplasia renum bilateralis). Centrabl. Path. Anat. 60: 1-8, 1934.

Potter, E. L.: Facial characteristics of infants with bilateral renal agenesis. Am. J. Obstet. Gynec. 51: 885-888, 1946.

Rizza, J. M..and Downing, S. E.: Bilateral renal agenesis in two female siblings. Am. J. Dis. Child. 121: 60-63, 1971.

Schmidt, E. C. H., Hartley, A. A. and Bower, R.: Renal aplasia in sisters. Arch. Path. 54: 403-406, 1952.

26680 RENAL AGENESIS, UNILATERAL

Gorvoy, Smulewicz and Rothfeld (1962) described affected brothers. The disorder could, as far as this information alone is concerned, be X-linked. Unilateral absence of the kidney was described in a boy and his maternal uncle by Bound (1943). Buchta et al. (1973) invented the designation hereditary renal adysplasia (combining the terms aplasia and dysplasia) for this disorder and suggested dominant, probably autosomal, inheritance. The disorder is more severe in males than in females. They raised a question of relationship between this disorder and vaginal atresia (Mayer-Rokitanski-Kuster syndrome, 27700) which they suggest may also be an autosomal dominant.

Bound, J. P.: Two cases of congenital absence of one kidney in the same family. Brit. Med. J. 2: 747 only, 1943.

Buchta, R. M., Viseskul, C., Gilbert, E. F., Sarto, G. G. and Opitz, J. M.: Familial bilateral renal agenesis and hereditary renal adysplasia. Zschr. Kinderhlk. 115: 111-129, 1973.

Gorvoy, J. D., Smulewicz, J. and Rothfeld, S. H.: Unilateral renal agenesis in two siblings. Case report. Pediatrics 29: 270-273, 1962.

*26690 RENAL DYSPLASIA AND RETINAL APLASIA

Loken and colleagues (1961) reported brother and sister with this combination. In the sister renal dysplasia was proved at autopsy. A similar syndrome is said (Waardenburg, 1963) to have been found in mice by Keeler. Senior, Friedmann and Braudo (1961) and Fairley, Leighton and Kincaid-Smith (1963) have also reported families with an oculorenal syndrome. In the former family the renal changes resembled those in

R
E
C
E
S
S
I
V
E

Fanconi familial juvenile nephronophthisis (q.v.). In the latter family the renal change was like polycystic   559
kidney. In an Amish isolate, Schimke (1969) found two cousins with vasopressin-resistant diabetes insipidus,
progressive azotemia, and retinitis pigmentosa. A more remotely related person may also have been affected.
Despite some histologic similarities to juvenile nephronophthisis and to medullary cystic disease, Schimke
concluded that the total clinicogenetic picture supported the view that this is a distinct entity. Dekaban (1969)
described two brothers with congenital retinal blindness and a developmental renal abnormality leading to
uremia. Autopsy was performed in one of the patients who died at age 10 years. The heterogeneity of the
renal-retinal syndrome is indicated by the variable age of onset of the retinal abnormality. In some families
it is congenital, whereas in others it behaves like isolated recessive retinitis pigmentosa. The heterogeneity
is further indicated by the report of other associated manifestations such as cerebellar ataxia and skeletal
abnormalities including cone epiphyses (Mainzer et al., 1970).

Bios, E. and Royer, P.: Association de nephropathie tubulo-interstitielle chronique et de degenerescence tapeto-retinienne. Etude genetique. Arch. Franc. Pediat. 27: 471-481, 1970.

Dekaban, A. S.: Familial occurrence of congenital retinal blindness and developmental retinal lesions. J. Genet. Hum. 17: 289-296, 1969.

Fairley, K. F., Leighton, P. W. and Kincaid-Smith, P.: Familial visual defects associated with polycystic kidney and medullary sponge kidney. Brit. Med. J. 1: 1060-1063, 1963.

Fontaine, J. L., Boulesteix, J., Saraux, H., Lasfargues, G., Grenet, P., Ghiem Minh Dung, N., Dhermy, P., Roy, C. and Laplane, R.: Nephropathie tubulo-interstitielle de l'enfant avec degenerescence tapeto-retinienne (syndrome de Senior). A propos d'une observation. Arch. Franc. Pediat. 27: 459-470, 1970.

Loken, A. C., Hanssen, O., Halvorsen, S. and Jolster, N. J.: Hereditary renal dysplasia and blindness. Acta Paediat. 50: 177-184, 1961.

Mainzer, F., Saldino, R. M., Ozonoff, M. B. and Minagi, H.: Familial nephropathy associated with retinitis pigmentosa, cerebellar ataxia and skeletal abnormalities. Am. J. Med. 49: 556-562, 1970.

Saraux, H., Dhermy, P., Fontaine, J. L., Boulesteix, J., Lasfargue, G., Grenet, P., N'Gheim, M. and Laplane, R.: La degenerescence retino-tubulaire de Senior et Loken. Arch. Ophthal. 30: 683-696, 1970.

Schimke, R. N.: Hereditary renal-retinal dysplasia. Ann. Intern. Med. 70: 735-744, 1969.

Senior, B., Friedmann, A. I. and Braudo, J. L.: Juvenile familial nephropathy with tapetoretinal degeneration: a new oculorenal dystrophy. Am. J. Ophthal. 52: 625-633, 1961.

Waardenburg, P. J.: Congenital and early infantile retinal dysfunction (high-graded amblyopia and amaurosis Leber). In, Genetics and Ophthalmology. Springfield, Ill.: Charles C Thomas, vol. 2, 1963. Pp. 1567-1581.

26700 RENAL HAMARTOMAS, NEPHROBLASTOMATOSIS AND FETAL GIGANTISM

Liban and Kozenitzky (1970) and Perlman et al. (1973) described, in 5 offspring of Jewish-Yemenite second-cousin parents, a disorder manifested by large birth size, bilateral renal hamartomas with or without nephroblastomatosis, hypertrophy of the islets of Langerhans and unusual facies. The longest survival was 27 days. There are some obvious similarities to the Beckwith-Wiedemann syndrome (22560).

Liban, E. and Kozenitzky, I. L.: Metanephric hamartomas and nephroblastomatosis in siblings. Cancer 25: 885-888, 1970.

Perlman, M., Goldberg, G. M., Bar-Ziv, J. and Danovitch, G.: Renal hamartomas and nephroblastomatosis with fetal gigantism: a familial syndrome. J. Pediat. 83: 414-418, 1973.

26720 RENAL TUBULAR ACIDOSIS III (DISLOCATION OR BICARBONATE WASTING)

Morris et al. (1969) observed two unrelated infant girls with a distinct form of bicarbonate wasting RTA which they referred to as dislocation type. Huth, Webster and Elkinton (1960) separated the group with onset in infancy and childhood from that with onset in later life. The former seems to be a genetic disorder transmitted as an autosomal recessive, although a predominance of males has been observed. Wilson et al. (1967) studied two families each with a case of late onset renal tubular acidosis and found elevation of serum immunoglobulins in close relatives but no other cases of renal tubular acidosis. Renal tubular acidosis becomes apparent because of (1) periodic paralysis due to hypokalemia, (2) rickets or osteomalacia, (3) kidney stones, or (4) nephrocalcinosis by abdominal X-ray.

Huth, E. J., Webster, G. D., Jr. and Elkinton, J. R.: The renal excretion of hydrogen ion in renal tubular acidosis. III. An attempt to detect latent cases in a family: comments on nosology, genetics and etiology of the primary disease. Am. J. Med. 29: 586-598, 1960.

McSherry, E., Sebastian, A. and Morris, R. C., Jr.: Renal tubular acidosis in infants: the several kinds, including bicarbonate-wasting, classic renal tubular acidosis. J. Clin. Invest. 51: 499-514, 1972.

Morris, E., Sebastian, A., Kranhold, J. and Morris, R. C.: Infantile renal tubular acidosis (RTA), a distinct type. (Abstract) Clin. Res. 17: 441 only, 1969.

Wilson, I. D., Williams, R. C., Jr. and Tobian, L., Jr.: Renal tubular acidosis: three cases with immunoglobulin abnormalities in the patients and their kindreds. Am. J. Med. 43: 356-370, 1967.

*26730 RENAL TUBULAR ACIDOSIS WITH PROGRESSIVE NERVE DEAFNESS

Konigsmark (1966) has observed a 17-year-old girl who had calculi removed from both kidneys at age 12. Studies at that time showed renal tubular acidosis and bilateral neural deafness. One brother, age 20, had similar renal disease and progressive nerve deafness. The parents and another brother were normal and the parents were unrelated. Nance (1970) has observed sibs with this combination of abnormalities. Cohen et al. (1973) described a possibly allelic form with greater severity of both the otologic and the renal defects. Shapira et al. (1974) found an inactive mutant form of red cell carbonic anhydrase B (11480) in two sisters and a first cousin once removed. All three had renal tubular acidosis and nerve deafness. The parents of both sibships were consanguineous. The mutant CA B had seven rather than eight tyrosine residues.

Cohen, T., Brand-Auraban, A., Karshai, C., Jacob, A., Gay, I., Tsitsianov, J., Shapiro, T., Jatziv, S. and Ashkenazi, A.: Familial infantile renal tubular acidosis and congenital nerve deafness: an autosomal recessive syndrome. Clin. Genet. 4: 275-278, 1973.

Konigsmark, B. W.: Baltimore, Md.: personal communication, 1966.

Nance, W. E.: Indianapolis, Ind.: personal communication, 1970.

Nance, W. E. and Sweeney, A.: Evicence for autosomal recessive inheritance of the syndrome of renal tubular acidosis with deafness. The Clinical Delineation of Birth Defects. IX. Ear. Baltimore: Williams and Wilkins, 1971. Pp. 70-72.

Nance, W. E., Sweeney, A., McLeod, A. C. and Cooper, M. C.: Hereditary deafness: a presentation of some recognized types, modes of inheritance, and aids in counseling. Sth. Med. Bull. 58: 41-57, 1970.

Shapira, E., Ben-Yoseph, Y., Eyal, G. and Russell, A.: Enzymatically inactive red cell carbonic anhydrase B in a family with renal tubular acidosis. J. Clin. Invest. 53: 59-63, 1974.

Walker, W. G.: Renal tubular acidosis and deafness. The Clinical Delineation Of Birth Defects. IX. Ear. Baltimore: Williams And Wilkins, 1971. P. 126.

26740 RENAL, GENITAL AND MIDDLE EAR ANOMALIES

In 4 female sibs Winter et al. (1968) observed renal hypoplasia or aplasia, anomalies of the internal genitalia especially vaginal atresia and in the two surviving sisters, in whom it could be investigated, anomaly of the ossicles of the middle ear. Turner (1968) described a similarly affected patient.

Turner, G.: A second family with renal, vaginal, and middle ear anomalies. J. Pediat. 76: 641 only, 1968.

Winter, J. S. D., Kohn, G., Mellman, W. J. and Wagner, S.: A familial syndrome of renal, genital, and middle ear anomalies. J. Pediat. 72: 88-93, 1968.

26745 RESPIRATORY DISTRESS SYNDROME

Karpatkin et al. (1972) observed two sibs with idiopathic respiratory distress syndrome and disseminated intravascular coagulation. A genetically determined maternal factor or homozygosity in the affected infants, a female and a male, are alternative possibilities.

Karpatkin, M., Sacker, I. and Ackerman, N.: Respiratory-distress syndrome and disseminated intravascular coagulation in two siblings. (Letter) Lancet I: 102-103, 1972.

26750 RETICULAR DYSGENESIA (CONGENITAL ALEUKIA)

In 1959 de Vaal and Seynhaeve described newborn male twins who had normal numbers of erythrocytes and platelets but no blood leukocytes at all. They died at 5 and 8 days of age of sepsis. Postmortem showed absent myeloid elements from the bone marrow and absent lymphocytes from the thymus and spleen. Seligmann et al. (1968) suggested that this may be generalized immunologic deficiency disorder. They suggested that the case of Gitlin et al. (1964) may have been the same disorder. In that case the thymus was hypoplastic without Hassal corpuscles.

De Vaal, O. M. and Seynhaeve, V.: Reticular dysgenesia. Lancet II: 1123-1125, 1959.

Gitlin, D., Vawter, G. and Craig, J. M.: Thymic alymphoplasia and congenital aleukocytosis. Pediatrics 33: 184-192, 1964.

Seligmann, M., Fudenberg, H. H. and Good, R. A.: A proposed classification of primary immunologic deficiencies. Am. J. Med. 45: 817-825, 1968.

*26770 RETICULOSIS, FAMILIAL HISTIOCYTIC (OR HEMOPHAGOCYTIC)

Anemia, granulocytopenia and thrombocytopenia are produced in part by phagocytosis of blood cells, in part by replacement of the marrow by histiocytic infiltration. Families have been reported by Marrian and Sanerkin (1963) and by Farquhar and colleagues (1952, 1958). In the latter family 4 sibs were affected. The father showed autoantibody and shortened red cell life-span. Farquhar, MacGregor and Richmond (1958) concluded that the minor changes observed in the father and one sib represented the heterozygous state. They were not concerned about the lack of changes in the mother since expression in the heterozygote is often variable. The disorder discussed by Omenn (1965) and by Miller (1966) is probably this. Omenn (1965) described an inbred American family of Irish extraction with a large number of affected persons in many related sibships. Miller (1966) described five sisters — a complete sibship, including a pair of twins — with clinical features of failure to thrive, recurrent infections, lymphadenopathy, hepatosplenomegaly, pulmonary infiltration and terminal pancytopenia and hypergammaglobulinemia. Death occurred between ages 20 months and 57 months. Autopsy showed diffuse reticulum cell infiltration of most organs including the central nervous system, obliteration of architecture of lymph glands and marked plasmacytosis.

This disorder, lymphohistiocytic infiltration (q.v.), and Letterer-Siwe disease (q.v.) are not easily distinguished and may be the same entity. The family reported by Farquhar et al. (1952, 1958) was Scottish. Another Scottish family, with 3 affected sibs, was reported by Goodall, Guthrie and Buist (1965). Bell et al. (1968) described affected brothers born 11 years apart. Meningoencephalitis during infancy was a feature in each. Hemophagocytosis in bone marrow preparations made the diagnosis. Donohue (1968) has autopsy information on 6 cases which occurred in an inbred Mennonite group in Ontario.

Barth, R. F., Khurana, S. K., Vergara, G. G., Lowman, J. T. and Beckwith, J. B.: Rapidly fatal familial histiocytosis associated with eosinophilia and primary immunological deficiency. Lancet II: 503-506, 1972.

Bell, R. J. M., Brafield, A. J. E., Barnes, N. D. and France, N. E.: Familial haemophagocytic reticulosis. Arch. Dis. Child. 43: 601-606, 1968.

Buist, N. R. M., Jones, R. N. and Cavens, T. R.: Familial haemophagocytic reticulosis in first cousins. Arch. Dis. Child. 46: 728-729, 1971.

Donohue, W. L.: Toronto, Canada: personal communication, 1968.

Farquhar, J. W. and Claireaux, A. E.: Familial haemophagocytic reticulosis. Arch. Dis. Child. 27: 519-525, 1952.

Farquhar, J. W., MacGregor, A. R. and Richmond, J.: Familial haemophagocytic reticulosis. Brit. Med. J. 2: 1561-1564, 1958.

Friedman, R. M. and Steigbigel, N. H.: Histiocytic medullary reticulosis. Am. J. Med. 38: 130-133, 1965.

Goodall, H. B., Guthrie, W. and Buist, N. R. M.: Familial haemophagocytic reticulosis. Scot. Med. J. 10: 425-438, 1965.

MacMahon, H. E., Bedizel, M. and Ellis, C. A.: Familial erythrophagocytic lymphohistiocytosis. Pediatrics 32: 868-879, 1963.

Marrian, V. J. and Sanerkin, N. G.: Familial histiocytic reticulosis (familial haemophagocytic reticulosis). J. Clin. Path. 16: 65-69, 1963.

Miller, D. R.: Familial reticuloendotheliosis: concurrence of disease in five siblings. Pediatrics 38: 986-995, 1966.

Omenn, G. S.: Familial reticuloendotheliosis with eosinophilia. New Eng. J. Med. 273: 427-432, 1965.

26775 RETINAL DETACHMENT AND OCCIPITAL ENCEPHALOCELE

In 5 of 10 sibs, Knobloch and Layer (1971) described high myopia, vitreo-retinal degeneration with retinal detachment and occipital encephalocele. The parents were unaffected and denied consanguinity.

Knobloch, W. H. and Layer, J. M.: Retinal detachment and encephalocele. J. Pediat. Ophthal. 8: 181-184, 1971.

26780 RETINAL DYSTROPHY, RETICULAR PIGMENTARY, OF POSTERIOR POLE

This condition, first described by Sjogren in 1950, is characterized by a peculiar network of black pigmented lines in the posterior pole of the retina, resembling a fishnet with its knots. In late stages the network disappears and drusen appear. Deutman and Rumke (1969) described the disorder in a Dutch brother and sister whose parents were second cousins. The parents of Sjogren's family were also related. Deafness and spherophakia in that family were probably independent recessive traits.

Deutman, A. F. and Rumke, A. M.: Reticular dystrophy of the retinal pigment epithelium. Dystrophia reticularis laminae pigmentosa retinae of H. Sjogren. Arch. Ophthal. 82: 4-9, 1969.

Sjogren, H.: Dystrophia reticularis laminae pigmentosae retinae: earlier not described hereditary eye disease. Acta Ophthal. 28: 279-295, 1950.

26790 RETINAL TELANGIECTASIA AND HYPOGAMMAGLOBULINEMIA

Frenkel and Russe (1967) described a 13 year old boy with this combination. His 10 year old sister had less extensive retinal telangiectases and impairment of delayed hypersensitivity but no deficiency of gammaglobulin.

Frenkel, M. and Russe, H. P.: Retinal telangiectasia associated with hypogammaglobulinemia. Am. J. Ophthal. 63: 215-220, 1967.

*26800 RETINITIS PIGMENTOSA

Changes which may be labelled retinitis pigmentosa (or atypical retinitis pigmentosa) are observed in a number of the other conditions listed here, e.g., abetalipoproteinemia, Alstrom syndrome, Refsum disease, Bardet-Biedl syndrome, Usher syndrome, Cockayne syndrome, pallidal degeneration. In a survey of retinitis pigmentosa in five Swiss cantons, Ammann, Klein and Boehringer (1961) found deaf-mutism associated in 16 of 118 living cases (see USHER SYNDROME). Franceschetti's striking pedigree (1953) is reproduced in Francois' book (1961). Babel (1972) suggested that heterozygotes of retinitis pigmentosa develop fundus changes typical of the homozygote after measles.

Ammann, F., Klein, D. and Boehringer, H. R.: Resultats preliminaires d'une enquete sur la frequence et la distribution geographique des degenerescences tapeto-retiniennes en Suisse (etude de cinq cantons). J. Genet. Hum. 10: 99-127, 1961.

Babel, J.: Geneva, Switzerland: cited by I. E. Hussels, 1972.

Franceschetti, A.: Degenerescence chorioretinienne familiale avec angiosclerose choroidienne, stade tardif d'une retinitis punctata albescens, constatee 54 ans auparavant. Ophthalmologia 125 (suppl. 37): 340-347, 1953.

Franceschetti, A.: Retinite pigmentaire recessive dans deux generations consecutives ('pseudo-dominance'). J. Genet. Hum. 2: 145-146, 1953.

RECESSIVE

Francois, J.: Heredity in Ophthalmology. St. Louis: C. V. Mosby Co., 1961. P. 444 fig. 391.

Kobayashi, F.: Genetic study on retinitis pigmentosa. Jap. J. Ophthal. 4: 82-91, 1960.

26805 RETINOPATHY, PIGMENTARY, AND MENTAL RETARDATION

Mirhosseini et al. (1972) described two brothers with pigmentary retinal degeneration, cataract, microcephaly, severe mental retardation, hyperextensible joints, scoliosis, and arachnodactyly. One had hypogonadism. The parents were apparently not related.

Mirhosseini, S. A., Holmes, L. B. and Walton, D. S.: Syndrome of pigmentary retinal degeneration, cataract, microcephaly, and severe mental retardation. J. Med. Genet. 9: 193-196, 1972.

*26810 RETINOSCHISIS WITH EARLY HEMERALOPIA

Favre (1958) described a brother and sister, age 16 and 15 respectively, with hemeralopia, degenerative vitreous changes, peripheral and central retinoschisis, etc. MacVicar and Wilbrandt (1970) described the disorder in two brothers whose parents were related. Night blindness had been present since childhood. Ricci (1960) added a case. This is to be distinguished from X-linked retinoschisis and from autosomal dominant hyaloideo-retinal degeneration (q.v.). It is characterized by a liquefied vitreous body with preretinal band-shaped structures (veil), macular changes in the form of retinoschisis or edema and pigmentary degeneration of the retina with hemeralopia and extinguished electroretinogram. Cataract is a complication.

Favre, M.: A propos de deux cas de degenerescence hyaloideoretinienne. Two cases of hyaloid-retinal degeneration. Ophthalmologica 135: 604-609, 1958.

MacVicar, J. E. and Wilbrandt, H. R.: Hereditary retinoschisis and early hemeralopia. A report of two cases. Arch. Ophthal. 83: 629-636, 1970.

Ricci, A.: Clinique et transmission genetique des differentes formes de degenerescences vitreo-retiniennes. Ophthalmologica 139: 338-342, 1960.

26820 RHABDOMYOLYSIS, ACUTE RECURRENT

Although the genetics remains unclear, recessive inheritance is perhaps most likely. Hed (1953) observed three affected brothers. Three other brothers and the parents were unaffected. The sister of a male patient of Bowden et al. (1956) was also affected.

Bowden, D. H., Fraser, D., Sackson, S. H. and Walker, N. F.: Acute recurrent rhabdomyolysis (paroxysmal myohaemoglobinuria). Medicine 35: 335-353, 1956.

Farmer, T. A., Hammack, W. J. and Frommeyer, W. B.: Idiopathic recurrent rhabdomyolysis associated with myoglobinuria. Report of a case. New Eng. J. Med. 264: 60-66, 1961.

Hed, R.: Myoglobinuria. Arch. Intern. Med. 92: 825-832, 1953.

Kahler, H. J.: Die Myoglobinurien. Ergebn. Inn. Med. Kinderheilk. 11: 1-103, 1959.

26827 RIBOSOMAL RNA, 5S (INCLUSION HERE JUSTIFIED BY AVAILABILITY OF DATA ON NUCLEOTIDE SEQUENCE)

Forget and Weissman (1967, 1969) sequenced 5S ribosomal RNA of human KB carcinoma cells and demonstrated two forms differing by the presence of one additional residue. The two forms have 120 and 121 nucleotides, respectively.

Forget, B. G. and Weissman, S. M.: Nucleotide sequence of KB cell 5S RNA. Science 158: 1695-1699, 1967.

Forget, B. G. and Weissman, S. M.: The nucleotide sequence of ribosomal 5S ribonucleic acid from KB cells. J. Biol. Chem. 244: 3148-3165, 1969.

*26830 ROBERTS SYNDROME (SEVERE ABSENCE DEFORMITIES OF LONG BONES OF LIMBS ASSOCIATED WITH CLEFT LIP-PALATE)

Roberts (1919) described three affected sibs and pictures were included. The parents were first-cousins of Italian extraction. The bones of the legs were almost absent and those of the arms hypoplastic. The skull looked oxycephalic with prominent eyes (as in Crouzon disease). Stroer's case (1939) may be the same entity. Again the parents were first cousins. Appelt et al. (1966) also described cases and pointed out that clitoral or penile enlargement is a feature. The SC phocomelia syndrome (q.v.) is a similar but distinct disorder. Assemany et al. (1971) described two unrelated males with phocomelia and mandibular hypoplasia. The relationship to the Roberts syndrome is unclear. Freeman et al. (1974) gave a good survey. Temtamy (1974) concluded that Roberts syndrome and the SC phocomelia syndrome (26900) are one and the same. Furthermore, we have observed recently a case of apparent Roberts syndrome in which thrombocytopenia occurred and an aunt had well-confirmed TAR syndrome (27400). Thus, the relationship of the Roberts and TAR syndromes awaits classification. Cleft palate has not been observed in the TAR syndrome, to my knowledge.

Appelt, J., Gerken, H. and Lenz, W.: Tetraphokomelie mit Lippen-Kiefer-Gaumenspalte und Klitorishypertropie — ein Syndrom. Paediat. Padol. 2: 119-124, 1966.

Assemany, S. R., Kajii, T. and Gardner, L. I.: Syndrome of phocomelia with mandibular hypoplasia. Helvet. Paediat. Acta 26: 403-409, 1971.

Freeman, M. V. R., Williams, D. W., Schimke, N. and Temtamy, S. A.: The Roberts syndrome. Clin. Genet. 5: 1-16, 1974.

R
E
C
E
S
S
I
V
E

Herrmann, J., Feingold, M., Tuffli, G. A. and Opitz, J. M.: A familial dysmorphogenetic syndrome of limb deformities, characteristic facial appearance and associated anomalies: the 'pseudothalidomide' or 'SC-syndrome.' The Clinical Delineation of Birth Defects. III. Limb Malformations. New York: National Foundation, 1969. Pp. 81-89.

Roberts, J. B.: A child with double cleft of lip and palate, protrusion of the intermaxillary portion of the upper jaw and imperfect development of the bones of the four extremities. Ann. Surg. 70: 252-254, 1919.

Stroer, W. F. H.: Ueber das Zusammentreffen von Hasenscharte mit ernsten extremitaeten Missbildungen. Erbarzt 7: 101-104, 1939.

Temtamy, S. A.: Baltimore and Cairo, personal communication, 1974.

*26840 ROTHMUND-THOMSON SYNDROME (POIKILODERMA ATROPHICANS AND CATARACT)

This is a hereditary dermatosis characterized by atrophy, pigmentation, and telangiectasia and frequently accompanied by juvenile cataract, saddle nose, congenital bone defects, disturbances of hair growth, and hypogonadism. Prognosis for survival is fairly good. Rothmund's family was further investigated by Siemens (cited by Waardenburg, 1961). It is possible that the condition described by Thomson (1936) is a different recessive disorder from that described by Rothmund. Saddle nose was not present and cataract did not occur.

Blinstrub, R. S., Lehman, R. and Steinberg, T. H.: Poikiloderma congenitale. Report of two cases. Arch. Derm. 89: 659-664, 1964.

Block, B. and Stauffer, H.: Skin diseases of endocrine system (dyshormonal dermatoses). Poikiloderma-like changes in connection with underdevelopment of the sexual glands and dystrophia adiposogenitalis. Arch. Derm. Syph. 19: 22-34, 1929.

Cole, H. N., Giffen, H. K., Simmons, J. T. and Stroud, G. M., III: Congenital cataracts in sisters with congenital ectodermal dysplasia. J.A.M.A. 129: 723-728, 1945.

Franceschetti, A.: Les dysplasies ectodermiques et les syndromes hereditaires apparentes. Dermatologica 106: 129-156, 1953.

Kraus, B. S., Gottlieb, M. A. and Meliton, H. R.: The dentition in Rothmund's syndrome. J. Am. Dent. Ass. 81: 894-915, 1970.

Rothmund, A.: Ueber Cataracten in Verbindung mit einer eigenthuemlichen Hautdegeneration. Graefe. Arch. Ophthal. 14: 159-182, 1868.

Sexton, G. B.: Thomson's syndrome (poikiloderma congenitale). Canad. Med. Ass. J. 70: 662-665, 1954.

Siemens, H. W.: In, Waardenburg, P. J., Franceschetti, A. and Klein, D. (eds.): Genetics and Ophthalmology. Springfield, Ill.: Charles C Thomas, 2: 896 only, 1963.

Taylor, W. B.: Rothmund's syndrome — Thomson's syndrome. Arch. Derm. 75: 236-244, 1957.

Thomson, M. S.: Poikiloderma congenitale. Brit. J. Derm. 48: 221-234, 1936.

26850 ROWLEY-ROSENBERG SYNDROME (GROWTH RETARDATION, PULMONARY HYPERTENSION AND AMINOACIDURIA)

Rowley and colleagues (1961) described a 'new' syndrome in three of six children. Features were growth retardation, poor muscular development, scanty adipose tissue, recurrent pulmonary infection, atelectasis, and right ventricular hypertrophy. One survivor had aminoaciduria without elevation of serum amino acids and increased plasma unesterified fatty acid concentration (Rosenberg et al., 1961). The affected sibs were two boys and a girl. The disorder is sometimes referred to as the 'Bushy syndrome,' for the surname of the affected family.

Rosenberg, L. E., Mueller, P. S. and Watkins, D. M.: A new syndrome: familial growth retardation, renal aminoaciduria and cor pulmonale. II. Investigation of renal function, amino acid metabolism, and genetic transmission. Am. J. Med. 31: 205-215, 1961.

Rowley, P. T., Mueller, P. S., Watkins, D. M. and Rosenberg, L. E.: Familial growth retardation, renal aminoaciduria and cor pulmonale. I. Description of a new syndrome, with case reports. Am. J. Med. 31: 187-204, 1961.

26860 RUBINSTEIN SYNDROME (BROAD THUMBS AND GREAT TOES, CHARACTERISTIC FACIES, MENTAL RETARDATION)

Although most of the cases have been sporadic, Johnson (1966) described affected sibs. In addition to the anomalies listed above, pulmonary stenosis, keloid formation in surgical scars, large foramen magnum, and vertebral and sternal anomalies should be mentioned. In the case reported by Jeliu and Saint-Rome (1967), the parents were second cousins. I find it difficult to accept the suggestion of multifactorial inheritance (Roy et al., 1968). I would expect a graded severity (for which there is no evidence) among cases and in close relatives, since there is no obvious mechanism for a threshold effect. The lack of much if any familial aggregation is against multifactoral inheritance just as it is against recessive inheritance. Multifactorial inheritance is unlikely in the case of such rare entities. The dermatoglyphic changes described by Giroux and Miller (1967) suggest a chromosomal abnormality. Such has not been identified but a small abnormality beyond the limits of resolution of existing methods seems the most likely cause of Rubinstein syndrome. Padfield et al. (1968) studied 17 cases and found no case among 50 sibs. The frequency of Rubinstein syndrome is about 1 per 500 institutionalized persons with mental retardation over age 5 years. Pfeiffer (1968) described the syndrome in both of monozygotic twins. Father-daughter incest produced another case

(Padfield et al., 1968). Takeuchi (1966) also observed affected sibs. Rubinstein (1969) found parental age to be about average. Der Kaloustian et al. (1972) described affected brother and sister from consanguineous parents. However, whereas the facies was characteristic, broad first digits were absent clinically and questionable radiographically. Simpson and Brissenden (1973) found two affected among 243 sibs of probands.

Coffin, G. S.: Brachydactyly, peculiar facies and mental retardation. Am. J. Dis. Child. 108: 351-359, 1964.

Der Kaloustian, V. M., Afifi, A. K., Sinno, A. A. and Mire, J.: The Rubinstein-Taybi syndrome: clinical and muscle electron microscopic study. Am. J. Dis. Child. 124: 897-902, 1972.

Giroux, J. and Miller, J. R.: Dermatoglyphics of the broad thumb and great toe syndrome. Am. J. Dis. Child. 113: 207-209, 1967.

Jeliu, G. and Saint-Rome, G.: Le syndrome de Rubinstein-Taybi. A propos d'une observation. Un. Med. Canada 96: 22-29, 1967.

Johnson, C. F.: Broad thumbs and broad great toes with facial abnormalities and mental retardation. J. Pediat. 68: 942-951, 1966.

Padfield, C. J., Partington, M. W. and Simpson, N. E.: The Rubinstein-Taybi syndrome. Arch. Dis. Child. 43: 94-101, 1968.

Pfeiffer, R. A.: Rubinstein-Taybi-syndrom bei wahrscheinlich eineiigen Zwillingen. Humangenetik 6: 84-87, 1968.

Roy, F. H., Summitt, R. L., Hiatt, R. L. and Hughes, J. G.: Ocular manifestations of the Rubinstein-Taybi syndrome. Case report and review of the literature. Arch. Ophthal. 79: 272-278, 1968.

Rubinstein, J. H. and Taybi, H.: Broad thumbs and toes and facial abnormalities. Am. J. Dis. Child. 105: 588-608, 1963.

Rubinstein, J. H.: The broad thumb syndrome — progress report 1968. The Clinical Delineation of Birth Defects. II. Malformation Syndromes. New York: National Foundation, 1969. Pp. 25-41.

Simpson, N. E. and Brissenden, J. E.: The Rubinstein-Taybi syndrome. Familial and dermatoglypic data. Am. J. Hum. Genet. 25: 225-229, 1973.

Takeuchi, M.: Rubinstein's syndrome in two siblings. Gunma J. Med. Sci. 15: 17-22, 1966.

26870 SACCHAROPINURIA

This condition was observed by Carson et al. (1968) in a 22-year-old, moderately retarded, somewhat short girl with EEG abnormalities but no history of fits. No other family members were affected. The urine contained lysine, citrulline, and histidine in addition to saccharopine. This disorder is presumably distinct from hyperlysinemia in which (in one form at least) a defect in the enzyme which converts lysine to saccharopine is present. Simell et al. (1972) described a three-and-one-half-year old girl with spastic diplegia. She had lysinuria and saccharopinuria, but plasma levels of citrulline were normal. Somatically and mentally she was normal.

Carson, N. A. J., Scally, B. G., Neill, D. W. and Carre, I. J.: Saccharopinuria: a new inborn error of lysine metabolism. Nature 218: 679 only, 1968.

Simell, O., Visakorpi, J. K. and Donner, M.: Saccharopinuria. Arch. Dis. Child. 47: 52-55, 1972.

*26880 SANDHOFF DISEASE, OR GM(2) GANGLIOSIDOSIS TYPE II

The initial description was made by Sandhoff et al. (1968). O'Brien (1971) studied two Mexican-American sisters and a boy of Anglo-Saxon extraction. All patients have been non-Jewish. However, the clinical and pathologic picture is very similar to Tay-Sachs disease. Weakness begins in the first six months of life. Startle reaction, early blindness, progressive mental and motor deterioration, doll-like face, cherry red spots and macrocephaly are all present as in Tay-Sachs disease. Death has occurred by age three. Hexosaminidases A and B are both deficient in this disorder. In the case of Krivit et al. (1972) signs of heart involvement preceded those of nervous system change. A pansystolic murmur and cardiomegaly were discovered at 3 months. Neurologic deterioration was first noted at 8 months. Coarse facies, macroglossia, megaloencephaly, minimal hepatosplenomegaly and high lumbar gibbus suggested Hurler syndrome. Srivastava and Beutler (1973) think that hexosaminidases A and B share a common subunit which is lacking in Sandhoff disease, whereas a subunit unique to hexosaminidase A is deficient in Tay-Sachs disease (27280). Spence et al. (1974) described a case of clinically, histologically and chemically typical Sandhoff disease in a Negro male. Total hexosaminidase activity in the blood was 20-24 percent of normal (compared with the usual value of less than 5 percent), whereas in the liver the level was less than 2 percent of normal. This may be an allelic variant of Sandhoff disease.

Krivit, W., Desnick, R. J., Lee, J., Moller, J., Wright, F., Sweeley, C. C., Snyder, P. D., Jr. and Sharp, H. L.: Generalized accumulation of neutral glycosphingolipids with G(m2) ganglioside accumulation in the brain. Sandhoff's disease (variant of Tay-Sachs disease). Am. J. Med. 52: 763-770, 1972.

O'Brien, J. S.: Ganglioside storage diseases. In, Harris, H. and Hirschhorn, K. (ed.): Advances in Human Genetics, (vol. 3) 1971.

Okada, S., McCrea, M. and O'Brien, J. S.: Sandhoff's disease (Gm2 gangliosidosis type 2): clinical, chemical, and enzyme studies in five patients. Pediat. Res. 6: 606-615, 1972.

Sandhoff, K., Andreae, U. and Jatzkewitz, H.: Deficient hexosaminidase activity in an exceptional case

Sandhoff, K., Harzer, K., Wassle, W. and Jatzkewitz, H.: Enzyme alterations and lipid storage in three variants of Tay-Sachs disease. J. Neurochem. 18: 2769, 1971.

Spence, M. W., Ripley, B. A., Embil, J. A. and Tibbles, A. R.: A new variant of Sandhoff's disease. Pediat. Res. 8: 628-637, 1974.

Srivastava, S. K. and Beutler, E.: Hexosaminidase-A and hexosaminidase-B: studies in Tay-Sachs' and Sandhoff's disease. Nature 241: 463 only, 1973.

Suzuki, Y., Koizumi, Y., Togari, H. and Ogawam, Y.: Sandhoff disease: diagnosis of heterozygous carriers. Clin. Chim. Acta 48: 153-158, 1973.

*26890 SARCOSINEMIA

Gerritsen and Waisman (1966) found hypersarcosinemia and sarcosinuria in brother and sister with mild mental retardation and few other abnormalities. Abnormal increases in blood and urine sarcosine occurred in 2 other sibs, the mother, a maternal aunt and the maternal grandmother (but not in the father) when sarcosine or its precursor dimethylglycine was administered. Sarcosine dehydrogenase may be defective. Scott et al. (1970) found by loading tests a decreased capacity to convert sarcosine to glycine, suggesting a deficiency of sarcosine dehydrogenase activity. The suggestion can be proven only by liver biopsy. Their patient had motor and mental retardation.

Gerritsen, T. and Waisman, H. A.: Hypersarcosinemia: an inborn error of metabolism. New Eng. J. Med. 275: 66-69, 1966.

Hagge, W., Brodehl, J. and Gellissen, K.: Hypersarcosinemia. (Abstract) Pediat. Res. 1: 409 only, 1967.

Scott, C. R., Clark, S. H., Teng, C. C. and Swedberg, K. R.: Clinical and cellular studies of sarcosinemia. J. Pediat. 77: 805-811, 1970.

Willems, C., Heusden, W. A., Hainaut, A. and Chapelle, P.: Hypersarcosinemie avec sarcosinurie — etude d'une nouvelle famille. J. Genet. Hum. 19: 101-118, 1971.

26895 SARCOTUBULAR MYOPATHY

Jerusalem et al. (1973) described this disorder in two brothers from an inbred Hutterite colony. Nonprogressive muscular weakness was present from infancy. Muscle biopsy showed selective involvement of type II fibers with changes which were vacuolar in transverse section and segmental on longitudinal section. In electron microscopy the spaces were membrane-bound. Cytochemical markers indicated that the delimiting membranes were reactive for the sarcoplasmic reticulum-associated atpase.

Jerusalem, F., Engel, A. G. and Gomez, M. R.: Sarcotubular myopathy. Neurology 23: 897-906, 1973.

*26900 SC PHOCOMELIA SYNDROME

In a family with surname beginning with S and another with surname beginning with C, Herrmann et al. (1969) described a syndrome consisting of the following features: (1) nearly symmetrical reductive malformations of the limbs resembling phocomelia; (2) flexion contractures of various joints; (3) multiple minor anomalies, including capillary hemangioma of the face, forehead and ears, hypoplastic cartilages of the ears and nose, micrognathia, scanty, silvery-blond hair, and cloudy corneas; (4) intrauterine and extrauterine growth retardation; (5) possibly mental retardation; and (6) autosomal recessive inheritance. The same syndrome was probably described by O'Brien and Mustard (1921) in 3 of 8 children of normal parents who were related as double first-cousins. Hall and Greenberg (1972) described the oldest known case (8 years old). She was mentally normal. They were impressed with hypotrichosis and midfacial hemangioma, for which reason they proposed the designation hypomelia-hypotrichosis-facial hemangioma syndrome. They emphasized a characteristic appearance of the face. Some consider this the same as Robert syndrome (26830). The usual absence of cleft palate in the SC syndrome may be a difference.

Hall, B. D. and Greenberg, M. H.: Hypomelia-hypotrichosis-facial hemangioma syndrome (pseudothalidomide, SC syndrome, SC phocomelia syndrome). Am. J. Dis. Child. 123: 602-604, 1972.

Herrmann, J., Feingold, M., Tuffli, G. A. and Opitz, J. M.: A familial dysmorphogenetic syndrome of limb deformities, characteristic facial appearance and associated anomalies: the 'pseudothalidomide' or 'SC-syndrome.' The Clinical Delineation of Birth Defects. III. Limb Malformations. New York: National Foundation, 1969. Pp. 81-89.

O'Brien, H. R. and Mustard, H. S.: An adult living case of total phocomelia. J.A.M.A. 77: 1964-1967, 1921.

26910 SCHILDER DISEASE

All cases reported as familial Schilder disease are probably in fact either Krabbe disease, sudanophilic cerebral sclerosis, or metachromatic leukencephalopathy (q.v.). If the term is to be preserved at all, its use should be confined to sudanophilic cerebral sclerosis (q.v.).

26920 SCHMIDT SYNDROME (DIABETES MELLITUS, ADDISON DISEASE, MYXEDEMA)

It is thought by many that this syndrome has an autoimmune basis. Other possible autoimmune conditions, e.g. Hashimoto struma, show familial aggregation. Whether the basis is genetic cannot be stated with certainty, and if genetic it is not certain that a single gene change is involved. Phair et al. (1965) reported brother and sister.

Carpenter, C. C. J., Solomon, N., Silverberg, S. G., Bledsoe, T., Northcutt, R. C., Klinenberg, J. R.,

Bennett, I. L. and Harvey, A. M.: Schmidt's syndrome (thyroid and adrenal insufficiency). A review of the literature and a report of fifteen new cases including ten instances of coexistent diabetes mellitus. Medicine 43: 153-180, 1964.

Phair, J. P., Bondy, P. K. and Abelson, D. M.: Diabetes mellitus, Addison's disease and myxedema report of two cases. J. Clin. Endocr. 25: 260-265, 1965.

Solomon, N., Carpenter, C. J., Bennett, I. L., Jr. and Harvey, A. M.: Schmidt's syndrome (thyroid and adrenal insufficiency) and coexistent diabetes mellitus. Diabetes 14: 300-304, 1965.

26930 SCHWARTZ-LELAK SYNDROME

Gorlin et al. (1969) suggested that the patient described by Schwartz (1960) as an example of craniometaphyseal dysplasia and that reported by Lelek (1961) as an example of Camurati-Engelmann disease suffered from a distinct disorder. Enlargement of the head and genu varum or genu valgum were main features. Long bones were widened with translucent flaring of the metaphyses. Serum alkaline phosphatase level was elevated in both cases. Both patients were males. Parents and sibs were unaffected and no mention was made of parental consanguinity.

Gorlin, R. J., Spranger, J. W. and Koszalka, M. F.: Genetic craniotubular bone dysplasias and hyperostoses: a critical analysis. The Clinical Delineation of Birth Defects. IV. Skeletal Dysplasias. New York: National Foundation, 1969. Pp. 79-95.

Lelek, I.: Camurati-Engelmann disease. Fortschr. Roentgen. 94: 702-712, 1961.

Schwartz, E.: Craniometaphyseal dysplasia. Am. J. Roentgen. 84: 461-466, 1960.

26940 SCLEROCORNEA

Sclerocornea is a congenital malformation of the cornea, such that the boundary between the cornea and the sclera is obscured. Usually the involvement is limited to the peripheral part of the cornea but it may extend to the entire cornea, so-called sclerocornea totalis. The mild form is inherited as a dominant, the severe form as a recessive. The pinnae are malformed in some cases. Bloch (1965) reviewed the familial reports. Segregation analysis showed satisfactory agreement with the recessive hypothesis. Several instances of parental consanguinity are reported. Sclerocornea is also a feature of cornea plana (q.v.).

Bloch, N.: Les differents types de sclerocornee, leurs modes d'heredite et les malformations congenitales concomitantes. J. Genet. Hum. 14: 133-172, 1965.

*26950 SCLEROSTEOSIS (CORTICAL HYPEROSTOSIS WITH SYNDACTYLY)

Sclerosteosis is a term applied by Hansen (1967) to a disorder similar to van Buchem hyperostosis corticalis generalisata (q.v.) but differing in radiologic appearance of the bone changes and in the presence of asymmetric cutaneous syndactyly of the index and middle fingers in many but not all cases. The jaw has an unusually square appearance in this condition. Affected sibs were observed by Hirsch (1929), Falconer and Ryrie (1937), Higinbotham and Alexander (1941), Kelley and Lawlah (1946), Truswell (1958) and Klintworth (1963). Parental consanguinity was observed by Falconer and Ryrie (1937) and by Truswell (1958) and the cases of Kelley and Lawlah (1946) and of Witkop (1965) were from an inbred tri-racial group of southern Maryland known as the 'We-Sorts.'

Falconer, A. W. and Ryrie, B. J.: Report on familial type of generalized osteo-sclerosis with report on pathological changes. Med. Press 195: 12-20, 1937.

Hansen, H. G.: Sklerosteose. In, Opitz, H. and Schmid, F. (eds.): Handbuch der Kinderheilkunde. Berlin: Springer, 1967. vol. VI, Pp. 351-355.

Higinbotham, N. L. and Alexander, S. F.: Osteopetrosis. Four cases in one family. Am. J. Surg. 53: 444-454, 1941.

Hirsch, I. S.: Generalized osteitis fibrosa. Radiology 13: 44-84, 1929.

Kelley, C. H. and Lawlah, J. W.: Albers-Schonberg disease. A family survey. Radiology 47: 507-513, 1946.

Klintworth, G. K.: Neurologic manifestations of osteopetrosis (Albers-Schonberg's disease). Neurology 13: 512-519, 1963.

Truswell, A. S.: Osteopetrosis with syndactyly. A morphologic variant of Albers-Schonberg's disease. J. Bone Joint Surg. 40B: 208-218, 1958.

Witkop, C. J.: Genetic disease of the oral cavity. In, Tiecke, R. W. (ed.): Oral Pathology. New York: McGraw-Hill Co., 1965.

*26960 SEA-BLUE HISTOCYTE DISEASE

This disorder is characterized by splenomegaly, mild thrombocytopenia and, in the bone marrow, numerous histocytes containing cytoplasmic granules which stain bright blue with the usual hematologic stains. The name was coined by Silverstein et al. (1970). Holland et al. (1965) suggested that the syndrome is the consequence of an inherited metabolic defect analogous to Gaucher disease and other sphingolipoidoses. Jones et al. (1970) described affected brother and sister. Parental consanguinity was possible because both parents came from the same restricted area of West Virginia. Lake et al. (1970) suggested that the 'sea-blue' designation be abandoned because the marrow contains a second variety of abnormal cell which never stains 'sea-blue' and because they had observed a 'malignant' disorder with the same type of cells and progressive neurologic disease characterized by ataxia, dementia and seizures. Heterozygotes may have some sea-blue histocytes in the bone marrow (Zlotnick, Fried, 1970). Wewalka (1970) gave a long-term follow-up on a case reported in 1950. He commented on eye changes: a white ring surrounding the macula. Berman (1972) told me of two sisters with this disorder which was at first misdiagnosed Gaucher disease. Her qualitative test for excessive mucopolysacchariduria was mildly positive in this case. Sawitsky et al. (1972) added two families. In, one, 4 brothers and a sister out of 7 sibs with normal parents were affected. The family was from Trinidad. In the second, an American black family, mother and daughter were affected. They concluded that this disorder is a lipidosis. They presented a pedigree of the family of Zlotnick and Fried (1970). The parents were first cousins in their Iranian Jewish family and showed changes consistent with carrier status. Sea-blue histiocytes have been observed in Norum disease (24590), Jacobson et al., 1972, and in neurovisceral storage disease with vertical supranuclear ophthalmoplegia (25705).

Berman, E.: Jerusalem: personal communication, 1972.

Holland, P., Hug, G. and Schubert, W. K.: Chronic reticuloendothelial cell storage disease. Am. J. Dis. Child. 110: 117-124, 1965.

Jacobson, C. D., Gjone, E, and Hovig, T.: Sea-blue histiocytes in familial lecithin cholesterol acyltransferase deficiency. Scand. J. Haemat. 9: 106-113, 1972.

Jones, B., Gilbert, E. F., Zugibe, F. T. and Thompson, H.: Sea-blue histiocyte disease in siblings. Lancet II: 73-75, 1970.

Lake, B. D., Stephens, R. and Neville, B. G. R.: Syndrome of the sea-blue histiocyte. (Letter) Lancet II: 309 only, 1970.

Sawitsky, A., Rosner, F. and Chodsky, S.: The sea-blue histiocyte syndrome, a review: genetic and biochemical studies. Sem. Hemat. 9: 285-297, 1972.

Silverstein, M. N., Ellefson, R. D. and Ahern, E. J.: The syndrome of the sea-blue histiocyte. New Eng. J. Med. 282: 1-4, 1970.

Wewalka, F. G.: Syndrome of the sea-blue histiocyte. (Letter) Lancet II: 1248 only, 1970.

Zlotnick, A. and Fried, K.: Sea-blue-histiocyte syndrome. (Letter) Lancet II: 776 only, 1970.

*26970 SEIP SYNDROME (BERARDINELLI SYNDROME, TOTAL LIPODYSTROPHY AND ACROMEGALOID GIGANTISM)

The features are generalized lipodystrophy, hyperlipemia, hepatomegaly, acanthosis nigricans, elevated basal metabolic rate and non-ketonic insulin-resistant diabetes mellitus. Studies of pituitary and adrenal function including growth hormone assays have been normal. Polycystic ovaries, muscular hypertrophy, and mental retardation have occurred in some cases. Two affected sibs have been reported in each of five families and in four other families the parents were consanguineous (Brunzell et al., 1968). Seip (1959) described affected brother and sister. Lipodystrophic muscular hypertrophy (Senior, 1961) may be the same entity. Consanguinity and multiple affected sibs are known. Substances with insulin-antagonizing and fat-mobilizing properties have been found in the urine (Hamwi et al, 1966). Leprechaunism (q.v.) has some similar features. See PRADER-WILLI SYNDROME for a condition in which abundant fat, muscle hypotonia and small hands and feet are exactly the opposite of the findings in this syndrome. See SYSTEMIC CYSTIC ANGIOMATOSIS and SEIP SYNDROME for discussion of what may be the same entity. Mabry and Hollingsworth (1971) presented evidence for abnormal pituitary function with secretion of an abnormal hormone with melanotrophic and growth hormone properties. In one case surgical hypophysectomy was followed by marked improvement. Seip (1971) published a review of published cases.

Berardinelli, W.: A undiagnosed endocrinometabolic syndrome: report of two cases. J. Clin. Endocr. 14: 193-204, 1954.

Brunzell, J. D., Shankle, S. W. and Bethune, J. E.: Congenital generalized lipodystrophy and systemic cystic angiomatosis: the simultaneous occurrence of two unusual syndromes in a single family. Ann. Intern. Med. 69: 501-516, 1968.

Hamwi, G. J., Kruger, F. A., Eymontt, M. J., Scarpelli, D. G., Gwinup, G. and Byron, R.: Lipoatrophic diabetes. Diabetes 15: 262-268, 1966.

Lawrence, R. D.: Lipodystrophy and hepatomegaly with diabetes, lipaemia, and other metabolic disturbances. A case throwing new light on the action of insulin. Lancet I: 724-731, 773-775, 1946.

Mabry, C. C. and Hollingsworth, D. R.: Generalized lipodystrophy (lipoatrophic diabetes): evidence for abnormal pituitary function. Pediat. Res. Soc., 1971.

Reed, W. B., Dexter, R., Corley, C. and Fish, C.: Congenital lipodystrophic diabetes with acanthosis nigricans. The Seip-Laurence syndrome. Arch. Derm. 91: 326-334, 1965.

Seip, M. and Trygstad, O.: Generalized lipodystrophy. Arch. Dis. Child. 38: 447-453, 1963.

Seip, M.: Generalized lipodystrophy. Ergeb. Med. Kinderheilk. 31: 59-95, 1971.

Seip, M.: Lipodystrophy and gigantism with associated endocrine manifestation. A new diencephalic syndrome? Acta Paediat. 48: 555-574, 1959.

Senior, B.: Lipodystrophic muscular hypertrophy. Arch. Dis. Child. 36: 426-431, 1961.

26980 SENILE PLAQUE FORMATION

Constantinidis and De Ajuriaguerra (1965) studied the brain from 64 elderly persons, from 30 families, with various psychiatric diagnoses, for the presence of senile plaques independent of associated cerebral lesions. Of 29 pairs of sibs, senile plaques were found in both in 22, 4 were both unaffected and 3 had one affected.

R
E
C
E
S
S
I
V
E

Although the authors postulated recessive inheritance, it should be noted that of 10 two generation observations, parent and child were affected in 3 and one generation only in 7.

Constantinidis, J. and De Ajuriaguerra, J.: L'incidence familiale des plaques seniles. Confin. Psychiat. 8: 130-137, 1965.

26985 SEX REVERSAL SYNDROME

Evidence favoring an autosomal gene contributing to testicular differentiation became available as a result of the discovery of the sex reversal mutation in the goat (Hamerton et al., 1969) and in the mouse (Cattanach et al., 1971). In these instances an autosomal mutation causes the indifferent gonad of genetic females to differentiate into a testis rather than an ovary. Over 40 men with a 46, XX karyotype have been documented (de la Chapelle, 1972). One instance of familial occurrence has been described (Kasdan et al., 1973).

Hamerton, J. L., Dickson, J. M., Pollard, C. E., Grieves, S. A. and Short, R. V.: Genetic intersexuality in goats. J. Repord. Fertil. Suppl. 7: 25-51, 1969.

Kasdan, R., Nankin, H. R., Troen, P., Wald, N., Pan, S. and Yanaihara, T.: Paternal transmission of maleness in XX human beings. New Eng. J. Med. 288: 539-545, 1973.

26990 SIALURIA

Montreuil et al. (1967) described the chemical aspects of a new form of mellituria called sialuria. A 'young patient' excreted 5.8 to 7.2 gm. of N-acetyl-neuraminic acid per day. No clinical or genetic information was provided.

Montreuil, J., Biserte, G., Strecker, G., Spik, G., Fontaine, G. and Farriaux, J.-P.: Description d'un nouveau type de meliture: la sialurie. C. R. Acad. Sci. 265: 97-99, 1967.

27000 SIDBURY SYNDROME

Sidbury, Smith and Harlan (1967) observed that three of four children of a second-cousin marriage died in the first two weeks of life with the following symptoms after the first three days: convulsions, lethargy, dehydration, moderate hepatomegaly, depressed platelets and leucocytes and an unusual urinary odor like that of sweaty feet. Postmortem examination showed mainly changes related to the hematologic findings: hypoplastic marrow, scattered hemorrhages of viscera and terminal septicemia. The unusual odor is the result of butyric and hexanoic acids. They suggest that this is an inborn error of short-chain fatty acid metabolism and more specifically that a defect in green acyl dehydrogenase may be involved. In a second family a brother and sister with unrelated parents had a similar ailment. See ISOVALERICACIDEMIA.

Sidbury, J. B., Jr., Smith, E. K. and Harlan, W.: An inborn error of short-chain fatty acid metabolism. The odor-of-sweaty-feet syndrome. J. Pediat. 70: 8-15, 1967.

27005 SILVER-RUSSELL DWARFISM

No Mendelian or chromosomal basis for this condition has been established. New dominant mutation is a possibility. The two main features are hemihypertrophy (or better, lateral asymmetry) and low birth weight dwarfism. Tanner and Ham (1969) suggested the designation of Silver dwarf be reserved for children of short stature (without microcephaly or other special features) who have low birth weight for the length of gestation, asymmetry of arms, legs, body or head and incurved 5th fingers. They suggested that the designation of Russell dwarf be reserved for the similar situation when asymmetry is lacking. Rimoin (1969) described monozygotic male twins concordant for Silver dwarfism. Fuleihan et al. (1971) observed three affected sibs among the six offspring of consanguineous Lebanese parents. Craniofacial disproportion and other minor anomalies were present. The mother was very short. Another possible familial occurence was observed by Silver (cited by Gareis et al., 1971), who found out the mother of one of his cases was only 59 inches tall and had triangular facies and incurved fifth fingers.

Fuleihan, D. S., Vazken, B. A., Der Kaloustian, M. and Najjar, S. S.: The Russell-Silver syndrome: report of three siblings. J. Pediat. 78: 654-657, 1971.

Gareis, F. J., Smith, D. W. and Summitt, R. L.: The Russell-Silver syndrome without asymmetry. J. Pediat. 79: 775-781, 1971.

Moseley, J. E., Moloshok, R. E. and Freiberger, R. H.: The Silver syndrome: congenital asymmetry, short stature and variations in sexual development. Am. J. Roentgen. 97: 74-81, 1966.

Rimoin, D. L.: The Silver syndrome in twins. The Clinical Delineation of Birth Defects. II. Malformation Syndromes. New York: National Foundation, 1969. Pp. 183-187.

Silver, H. K.: Asymmetry, short stature, and variations in sexual development: a syndrome of congenital malformations. Am. J. Dis. Child. 107: 495-515, 1964.

Tanner, J. M. and Ham, T. J.: Low birthweight dwarfism with asymmetry (Silver's syndrome): treatment with human growth hormone. Arch. Dis. Child. 44: 231-243, 1969.

27010 SITUS INVERSUS VISCERUM

Familial concentration (Leininger and Gibson, 1950) and consanguineous parents (Cockayne, 1938) have been observed.

Cockayne, E. A.: The genetics of transposition of the viscera. Quart. J. Med. 7: 479-493, 1938.

Leininger, C. R. and Gibson, S.: Transposition of viscera in siblings. J. Pediat. 37: 195-200, 1950.

*27020 SJOGREN-LARSSON SYNDROME (OLIGOPHRENIA, CONGENITAL ICHTHYOSIS, SPASTIC NEUROLOGIC DISORDER)

R
E
C
E
S
S
I
V
E

The skin changes are similar to those of congenital ichthyosiform erythroderma (q.v.), although considerable variations in severity have been described (Goldsmith et al., 1971). Link and Roldan (1958) reported cases. Blumel, Watkins and Eggers (1958) referred to the neurologic disorder as spastic quadriplegia. Sjogren and Larsson (1956, 1957) suggested that all their cases (28 in number) were derived from the same mutation, occurring about 600 years ago and that about 1.3 percent of the population of the north of Sweden is heterozygous for the gene. About half the cases have pigmentary degeneration of the retina. Lesions of the ocular fundus were discussed by Gilbert et al. (1968).

Blumel, J., Watkins, M. and Eggers, G. W. N.: Spastic quadriplegia combined with congenital ichthyosiform erythroderma and oligophrenia. Am. J. Dis. Child. 96: 724-726, 1958.

Gilbert, W. R., Jr., Smith, J. L. and Nyhan, W. L.: The Sjogren-Larsson syndrome. Arch. Ophthal. 80: 308-316, 1968.

Goldsmith, L. A., Baden, H. P. and Canty, T. G.: Sjogren-Larsson syndrome. Acta Dermatovener. 51: 374-378, 1971.

Heijer, A. and Reed, W. B.: Sjogren-Larsson syndrome: congenital ichthyosis spastic paralysis, and oligophrenia. Arch. Derm. 92: 545-552, 1965.

Link, J. K. and Roldan, E. C.: Mental deficiency, spasticity, and congenital ichthyosis. Report Of A Case. J. Pediat. 52: 712-714, 1958.

Richards, B. W.: Congenital ichthyosis, spastic diplegia and mental deficiency. (Letter) Brit. Med. J. 2: 714 only, 1960.

Selmanowitz, V. J. and Porter, M. J.: The Sjogren-Larsson syndrome. Am. J. Med. 42: 412-422, 1967.

Sjogren, T. and Larsson, T.: Oligophrenia in combination with congenital ichthyosis and spastic disorders. A clinical and genetic study. Acta Psychiat. Neurol. Scand. 32 (suppl. 113): 1-112, 1957.

Sjogren, T.: Oligophrenia combined with congenital ichthyosiform erythrodermia, spastic syndrome and macularretinal degeneration. A clinical and genetic study. Acta Genet. Statist. Med. 6: 80-91, 1956.

Zaleski, W. A.: Congenital ichthyosis, mental retardation and spasticity (Sjogren-Larsson syndrome). Canad. Med. Ass. J. 86: 951-954, 1962.

*27025 SKELETAL DYSPLASIA, SEVERE, WITH VISCERAL ANOMALIES

Saldino and Noonan (1972) described an apparently 'new' form of severe micromelic dwarfism combined with anorectal anomalies, heart malformations and pulmonary hypoplasia. The changes were different from those of thanatophoric dwarfism and asphyxiating thoracic dystrophy. Two female sibs were affected. Since this is one of the several forms leading to stillbirth or neonatal death, this might be called a form of thanatophoric dwarfism. However, the latter term should be reserved for the specific entity described elsewhere.

Saldino, R. M. and Noonan, C. D.: Severe thoracic dystrophy with striking micromelia, abnormal osseous development, including the spine, and multiple visceral anomalies. Am. J. Roentgen. 114: 257-263, 1972.

*27030 SKIN PEELING, FAMILIAL CONTINUOUS

Kurban and Azar (1969) described 3 affected males and an affected female among the 9 offspring of a first-cousin marriage. No previous instance of familial occurrence of this condition (otherwise known as deciduous skin, keratolysis exfoliativa congenita, 'skin shedding' etc.) has been described.

Kurban, A. K. and Azar, H. A.: Familial continual skin peeling. Brit. J. Derm. 81: 191-195, 1969.

27035 SKUNK N-BUTYLMERCAPTAN, INABILITY TO SMELL

This may be an autosomal recessive trait.

Patterson, P. M. and Lauder, B. A.: The incidence and probable inheritance of 'smell blindness'. J. Hered. 39: 295-297, 1948.

*27040 SMITH-LEMLI-OPITZ SYNDROME

In three unrelated males Smith, Lemli and Opitz (1964) found a strikingly similar combination of congenital anomalies: microcephaly, mental retardation, hypotonia, incomplete development of the male genitalia, short nose with anteverted nostrils, and, in two, pyloric stenosis. A deceased male sib of one of these was probably identically affected. No parental consanguinity was discovered. Pinsky and DiGeorge (1965) reported affected brother and sister. Blair and Martin (1966) also described the condition in brother and sister. The male had hypospadias. Dallaire and Fraser (1966) described affected brothers. Blepharoptosis has been a feature of many cases. Lowry, Miller and MacLean (1968) described the combination of micrognathia, polydactyly and cleft palate, resembling the syndrome known in the German literature as 'Typus Rostockiensis' or 'Ullrich-Feichtiger syndrome' but suggesting the Smith-Lemli-Opitz syndrome in respect to dermatoglyphics. Hoefnagel et al. (1969) and Fried and Fraser (1972) reported cases in adults.

Blair, H. R. and Martin, J. K.: A syndrome characterized by mental retardation, short stature, craniofacial dysplasia, and genital anomalies occurring in siblings. J. Pediat. 69: 457-459, 1966.

Cotlier, E. and Rice, P.: Cataracts in the Smith-Lemli-Opitz syndrome. Am. J. Ophthal. 72: 955-959, 1971.

Dallaire, L. and Fraser, F. C.: The syndrome of retardation with urogenital and skeletal anomalies in siblings. J. Pediat. 69: 459-460, 1966.

R
E
C
E
S
S
I
V
E

Dallaire, L.: Syndrome of retardation with urogenital and skeletal anomalies (Smith-Lemli-Opitz syndrome): clinical features and mode of inheritance. J. Med. Genet. 6: 113-120, 1969.

Deaton, J. G. and Mendoza, L. O.: Smith-Lemli-Opitz syndrome in a 23-year-old man. Arch. Intern. Med. 132: 422-426, 1973.

Fried, K. and Fraser, W. I.: Smith-Lemli-Opitz syndrome in an adult. J. Ment. Defic. Res. 16: 30-34, 1972.

Hoefnagel, D., Wurster, D., Pomeroy, J. and Benz, R.: The Smith-Lemli-Opitz syndrome in an adult. J. Ment. Defic. Res. 13: 249-257, 1969.

Kenis, H. and Hustinx, T. W.: A familial syndrome of mental retardation in association with multiple congenital anomalies resembling the syndrome of Smith-Lemli-Opitz. Maandschr. Kindergeneesk. 35: 37-48, 1967.

Lowry, R. B., Miller, J. R. and MacLean, J. R.: Micrognathia, polydactyly and cleft palate. J. Pediat. 72: 859-861, 1968.

Nevo, S., Benderly, A., Levy, J. and Katznelson, M. B.: Smith-Lemli-Opitz syndrome in an inbred family. Am. J. Dis. Child. 124: 431-435, 1972.

Pinsky, L. and DiGeorge, A. M.: A familial syndrome of facial and skeletal anomalies associated with genital abnormality in the male and normal genitals in the female. Another cause of male pseudohermaphroditism. J. Pediat. 66: 1049-1054, 1965.

Smith, D. W., Lemli, L. and Opitz, J. M.: A newly recognized syndrome of multiple congenital anomalies. J. Pediat. 64: 210-217, 1964.

Weber, J. W. and Schwartz, H.: Der typus Rostockiensis Ullrich-Feichtiger Dyskraniopygophalangie. Helv. Paediat. Acta. 15: 163-170, 1960.

*27060 SPASTIC DIPLEGIA, INFANTILE TYPE

Hanhart (1936) described 7 cases in 4 related sibships. All eight parents could be traced to a common ancestor born in the 17th century. Penrose (1963) observed the disorder with mental dificiency in two offspring of a first-cousin marriage. This is probably the same disorder as that reported by Book (1956) and Book and Sjogren (1970) as spastic oligophrenia.

Book, J. A. and Sjogren, T.: A pedigree with essential myoclonus and genetic spastic oligophrenia. Clin. Genet. 1: 95-103, 1970.

Book, J. A.: Genetical investigations in a north-swedish population. Population Structure, Spastic Oligophrenia, Deaf Mutism. Ann. Hum. Genet. 20: 239-250, 1956.

Hanhart, E.: Eine Sippe mit einfach-rezessiver Diplegia spastica infantilis (Littlescher Krankheit) aus einem schweizer Insuchtgebiet. Erbarzt 11: 165-172, 1936. (See De Genetica Medica, L. Gedda (ed.). 3: 68 only, 1963.).

Penrose, L. S.: The biology of mental defect. New York: Grune and Stratton, (3rd ed.). 1963. p. 168.

*27070 SPASTIC PARAPLEGIA AND RETINAL DEGENERATION

Louis-Bar and Pirot (1945) described two brothers with macular degeneration and spastic paraplegia referred to by the authors as 'Strumpell type.' A third brother was said to have a forme fruste of spastic paraplegia. They could find no report of similar cases. Family 1 of Ledic and Van Bogaert (1960) may be identical. We have seen a female (S.S., 1217761) with late onset spastic paraplegia and retinal degeneration more striking peripherally. A sister is identically affected, and another sister had only spastic paraplegia (Mahloudji and Chuke, 1968). Follow-up studies by Stiefel and Todorov (1974) showed that the third sister had developed the typical retinal changes and that out of the sibship of 11, two more (five in all) are affected. The affected persons are mentally dull. Onset was between ages 30 and 36 years.

Ledic, P. and Van Bogaert, L.: Cerebellar and spastic heredo-degeneration with macular degeneration. J. Genet. Hum. 9: 140-157, 1960.

Louis-Bar, D. and Pirot, G.: Sur une paraplegie spasmodique avec degenerescence maculaire chez deux freres. Opthalmologica 109: 32-43, 1945.

Mahloudji, M. and Chuke, P. O.: Familial spastic paraplegia with retinal degeneration. Johns Hopkins Med. J. 123: 142-144, 1968.

Stiefel, J. W. and Todorov, A. B.: Recessive spastic paraplegia with retinal degeneration. In, Bergsma, D. (ed.): Clinical Delineation of Birth Defects. XVI. Urinary System and Others. Baltimore: Williams and Wilkins, 1974. Pp. 343-344.

*27080 SPASTIC PARAPLEGIA, HEREDITARY

Bell and Carmichael (1939) found probable recessive inheritance in 49 of 74 pedigrees. Spastic paraplegia, like retinitis pigmentosa and optic atrophy, is a relatively non-specific manifestation. The pyramidal tracts are highly vulnerable to insult from many causes because of the long axon. The protein-synthesizing machinery is in the cell body and mitochondria are also in short supply in the axoplasm so that oxidative metabolism is limited. Interference with axoplasmic flow which occurs from the cell body to the farthest reaches of the axon can easily occur. Recessive cases were described by Freud (1893) and by Jones (1907). Four sibs (out of 8) with spastic paraparesis and mental retardation were briefly described by Allport (1971). A recessively inherited 'pure' spastic paraplegia (i.e., one unaccompanied by other features such as macular degeneration, as in 27070, or mental deterioration as in the Mast syndrome, 24890) is very rare in my experience.

Aagenaes, O.: Hereditary spastic paraplegia: a family with ten injured. Acta Psychiat. Neurol. Scand. 34: 489-494, 1959.

Allport, R. B.: Mental retardation and spastic paraparesis in four of eight siblings. (Letter) Lancet II: 1089 only, 1971.

Bell, J. and Carmichael, E. A.: On the heredity of ataxia and spastic paraplegia. In, Treasury of Human Inheritance. London: Cambridge Univ. Press, 4: (part 3) 169-172, 1939.

Freud, S.: Ueber familiaere Formen von cerebralen Diplegien. Neurol. Centralblatt (Mendel) 12: 512-515 and 542-547, 1893.

Jones, E.: Eight cases of hereditary spastic paraplegia. Rev. Neurol. Psychiat. 5: 98-106, 1907.

27090 SPASTIC PSEUDOSCLEROSIS (DISSEMINATED ENCEPHALOMYELOPATHY: CORTICOPALLIDODEGENERATION)

Davison and Rabiner (1940) described two brothers and a sister with onset in the late 20's. Autopsy was performed in one. It is not clear that a distinct entity is involved.

Davison, C. and Rabiner, A. M.: Spastic pseudosclerosis (disseminated encephalomyelopathy: corticopallidospinal degeneration): familial and non-familial incidence (clinicopathologic study). Arch. Neurol. Psychiat. 44: 578-598, 1940.

27100 SPINA BIFIDA CYSTICA

Lorber (1965) suggested recessive inheritance. However, penetrance must be greatly reduced because he estimated the risk of recurrence of spina bifida cystica, anencephaly or hydrocephalus in subsequently born offspring to be about 8 percent. Record and McKeown (1950) had estimated the risk at 4 percent. Taking spina bifida and anencephaly (q.v.), Carter and Roberts (1967) estimated the risk in England of a third child having major central nervous system malformation, two having been previously affected, to be about 1 in 10. Lorber and Levick (1967) found spina bifida occulta in 14.3 percent of 188 mothers and 26.8 percent of 179 fathers of cases, and in 5 percent of 200 controls. Spina bifida occulta was not commoner among parents with more than one affected child and in a majority of families neither parent had it. Because spina bifida and anencephaly are generally considered one entity, see ANENCEPHALY (20650).

Carter, C. O. and Roberts, J. A. F.: The risk of recurrence after two children with central-nervous-system malformations. Lancet I: 306-308, 1967.

Lorber, J. and Levick, K.: Spina bifida cystica: incidence of spina bifida occulta in parents and in controls. Arch. Dis. Child. 42: 171-173, 1967.

Lorber, J.: The family of spina bifida cystica. Pediatrics 35: 589-595, 1965.

Record, R. G. and McKeown, T.: Congenital malformation of the central nervous system. III. Risk of malformations in sibs of malformed individuals. Brit. J. Prev. Soc. Med. 4: 217-220, 1950.

27110 SPINAL EXTRADURAL CYST

Chynn (1967) described spinal extradural cyst in a Negro brother and sister, ages 12 and 10 at the time of diagnosis. Progressive weakness in the legs was the main symptom. Another sib may also have been affected. In all three sibs congenital lymphedema of the leg and double rows of eyelashes (distichiasis) were present. The syndrome of lymphedema, distichiasis and other anomalies has been observed as a dominant (q.v.). Bergland (1968) found three sibs out of 4 affected but this appears to be the same family as that described by Chynn (1967). Spinal extradural cysts are very rare. Spinal anomalies of this type were present in affected persons with lymphedema and distichiasis reported by Robinow et al. (1970) but were asymptomatic. It is likely that 'spinal extradural cyst' is not a separate genetic entity but merely part of the lymphedema-distichiasis syndrome, a dominant (15340).

Bergland, R. M.: Congenital intraspinal extradural cyst. Report of three cases in one family. J. Neurosurg. 28: 495-499, 1968.

Chynn, K.-Y.: Congenital spinal extradural cyst in two siblings. Am. J. Roentgen. 101: 204-215, 1967.

Robinow, M., Johnson, G. F. and Verhagen, A. D.: Distichiasis-lymphedema. A hereditary syndrome of multiple congenital defects. Am. J. Dis. Child. 119: 343-347, 1970.

*27120 SPINAL MUSCULAR ATROPHY, RYUKYUAN TYPE

In the Ryukyu Islands of Japan, Kondo et al. (1970) described a form of spinal muscular atrophy which may be different from any previously described. The disease began in early infancy and caused symmetric proximal muscular atrophy, more severe in the lower extremities than in the upper. Fasciculations, slight kyphoscoliosis and pes cavus were seen. The evidence of recessive inheritance is convincing. A common ancestor of all the patients was thought to be a lord who lived in northern Okinawa from 1314 to 1429. The mutation must have occurred before the 14th century. The present distribution of cases could be explained by the activities of ancestors several centuries ago. Whether this disease is separate from Kugelberg-Welander disease, a heterogeneous entity, is not certain, and it resembles limb-girdle muscular dystrophy (which is also heterogeneous).

Kondo, K., Tsubaki, T. and Sakamoto, F.: The Ryukyuan muscular atrophy. An obscure heritable neuromuscular disease found in the islands of southern Japan. J. Neurol. Sci. 11: 359-382, 1970.

In recessively inherited spinocerebellar ataxia of uncertain classification, Van Bogaert and Martin (1974) and Spoendlin (1974) described optic cochlear degeneration leading to blindness and deafness. Presumably this was not the Refsum syndrome (26650), which has simialr manifestations.

Spoendlin, H.: Optic and cochleo-vestibular degenerations in hereditary ataxias. II. Temporal bone pathology in two cases of Friedreich's ataxia with vestibulo-cochlear disorders. Brain 97: 41-48, 1974.

Van Bogaert, L. and Martin, L.: Optic and cochleo-vestibular degenerations in the hereditary ataxias. I. Clinico-pathological and genetic aspects. Brain 97: 15-40, 1974.

27130 SPLEEN, ABSENCE OF (ASPLENIA SYNDROME)

Congenital absence of the spleen is usually accompanied by complex cardiac malformations, malposition and maldevelopment of the abdominal organs, and abnormal lobation of the lungs. Heinz and Howell-Jolly bodies in the peripheral blood are hematologic signs of absent spleen. A few cases have had multiple spleens. Most cases are sporadic. However, familial incidence has been observed twice. A patient with the typical asplenia syndrome had a sib who at autopsy showed multiple accessory spleens, persistent atrioventicularis communis and partial transposition of the abdominal viscera (Polhemus and Schafer, 1952). In a second family 3 sibs had asplenia with cyanotic congenital heart disease (Ruttenberg et al., 1964).

Polhemus, D. W. and Schafer, W. B.: Congenital absence of spleen. Syndrome with atrioventricularis and situs inversus. Case reports and review of literature. Pediatrics 9: 696-708, 1952.

Ruttenberg, H. D., Neufeld, H. N., Lucas, R. V., Jr., Carey, L. S., Adams, P., Jr., Anderson, R. C. and Edwards, J. E.: Syndrome of congenital cardiac disease with asplenia. Distinction from other forms of congenital cyanotic cardiac disease. Am. J. Cardiol. 13: 387-406, 1964.

*27140 SPLENIC HYPOPLASIA

Kevy et al. (1968) described a sibship with consanguineous parents, in which one of two boys and two of three girls had splenic hypoplasia. One of the children died at 10 months of overwhelming haemophilus influenzae sepsis. The other two had repeated episodes of pneumococcal meningitis and H. influenzae sepsis. Absence of the spleen was demonstrated by radioactive scanning after injection of AU(198) colloid and chromium-tagged, heated red cells, by the presence of Howell-Jolly bodies and Heinz bodies in the peripheral blood, and by failure to synthesize antibody to sheep red blood cells injected intravenously. The situation is comparable to that in infants in whom the spleen is removed in early life.

Kevy, S. V., Tefft, M., Vawter, G. F. and Rosen, F. S.: Hereditary splenic hypoplasia. Pediatrics 42: 752-758, 1968.

27150 SPLENOPORTAL VASCULAR ANOMALIES

Barbagallo Sangiorgi, Pagliaro and La Seta (1965) described two families. In one, two of 4 brothers had splenomegaly, compensated cirrhosis and mild diabetes. Splenic venograph showed splenocaval shunt and one had chronic hyperammoniacal encephalopathy. In the second family a brother and two sisters had splenomegaly, ascites and anomalous splenoportal venous system. The father and another brother were symptom free but had splenomegaly. The vascular anomaly may have been secondary to hepatic fibrosis and the disorder may be either identical to that discussed elsewhere (see HEPATIC FIBROSIS) or non-genetic.

Barbagallo Sangiorgi, G., Pagliaro, L. and La Seta, A.: Familial occurrence of congenital splenoportal anomalies. Lancet 1: 962-963, 1965.

*27160 SPONDYLOEPIPHYSEAL DYSPLASIA TARDA

Golding (1935) and Klenerman (1961) described two sons and a daughter of a first-cousin marriage showing short stature, flat vertebrae and severe hip disease. In the proband symptoms in the back began at 15 years followed by symptoms referable to the hips. Multiple loose bodies were removed from various joints of one sib-18 from the right hip at about age 26, several from left elbow at age 28 and 30 from the left hip at age 33. The proband was about 52 years old at the time of Klenerman's report. Severe osteoarthritis of the hips was a feature. The authors suggested a relationship to Morquio-Brailsford chondro-osteodystrophy, but this seems doubtful. Martin et al. (1970) described two brothers, offspring of a second-cousin marriage, with platyspondyly, flattening of the metatarsal and metacarpal beads and symmetrical polyarticular osteoarthritis. No beta-2-globulin was demonstrated in their sera. The patients were natives of the Magdalen Islands in the Gulf of St. Lawrence and many others of that population were found to have either absence or relative deficiency of beta-2-globulin (Martin, 1970). Hence, it may represent a separate genetic trait. Carter and Sutcliffe (1970) pointed out that autosomal dominant, autosomal recessive and X-linked forms of spondyloepiphyseal dysplasia are known.

Carter, C. O. and Sutcliffe, J.: Genetic varieties of spondylo-epiphyseal dysplasia. In, Jelliffe, A. M. and Strickland, B. (eds.): Symposium Ossium. London: Livingstone, 1970.

Golding, F. C.: Chondro-osteodystrophy. Brit. J. Radiol. 8: 457-465, 1935.

Klenerman, L.: An adult case of chondro-osteodystrophy. Proc. Roy. Soc. Med. 54: 71-73, 1961.

Martin, J. R., Macewan, D. W., Blais, J. A., Metrakos, J., Gold, P., Langer, F. and Hill, R. O.: Platyspondyly, polyarticular osteoarthritis, and absent beta-2-globulin in two brothers. Arth. Rheum. 13: 53-67, 1970.

27180 SPONDYLOMETAPHYSEAL DYSPLASIA

Kozlowski et al. (1967) delineated this entity. The condition prompts medical attention because of short

R
E
C
E
S
S
I
V
E

stature, usually between ages 1 and 4 years. Shortening of the trunk is the main factor in the short stature. Unusual, perhaps unique, radiologic changes occur in the distal metaphyseal of the femur before age six. Metaphyseal changes are striking in the femoral neck and trochanteric area. Generalized platyspondyly is a striking feature. Similar cases of this condition, which is usually termed Morquio syndrome, were found in the literature. The authors suspected autosomal recessive inheritance. We have observed a type of spondylometaphyseal dysplasia that we call either the Strudwick form of SMD (from a patient's name) or SMD congenita. All six cases have been sproadic. This form may be dominant. It bears many resemblances to SED congenita (18390). Radiologically they may be indistinguishable in early life; and cleft palate, myopia and atlanto-axial instability occur in both. The X-ray changes later are characteristic in SMD congenita and consist of striking changes described as dappled metaphyses.

Kozlowski, K., Maroteaux, P. and Spranger, J. W.: La dysostose spondylo-metaphysaire. Presse Med. 75: 2769-2774, 1967.

LaQuesne, G. W. and Kozlowski, K.: Spondylometaphyseal dysplasia. Brit. J. Radiol. 46: 685-691, 1973.

Michel, J., Grenier, B., Castaing, J., Augier, J. L. and Desbuquois, G.: Deux cas familiaux de dysplasie spondylo-metaphysaire. Ann. Radiol. 13: 251-254, 1970.

Piffaretti, P. G., Delgado, H. and Nussle, D.: La dysostose spondylo-metaphysaire de Kozlowski, Maroteaux et Spranger. Ann. Radiol. 13: 405-417, 1970.

Remy, J., Nuyts, J. P., Bombart, E. and Rembert, A.: La dysostose spondylo-metaphysaire. A propos de deux observations. Ann. Radiol. 13: 419-425, 1970.

*27190 SPONGY DEGENERATION OF CENTRAL NERVOUS SYSTEM

Salient clinical features are onset in early infancy, atonia of neck muscles, hyperextension of legs and flexion of arms, blindness, severe mental defect, megalocephaly and death by 18 months on the average. Pathologic studies show spongy degeneration of the white matter. In this country the disorder has been observed in infants of Jewish extraction whose ancestors lived in Vilna (Banker et al., 1964). Spongy degeneration is a non-specific morphologic change which occurs in a number of situations. See LACTIC ACIDOSIS WITH SPONGY DEGENERATION. Spongy degeneration rather closely resembling that of Van Bogaert-Bertrand disease was observed in a case of homocystinuria (Chou and Waisman, 1965). This is also called Canavan disease. In an Iranian family with first-cousin parents, Mahloudji et al. (1970) described four affected sibs out of 9. Morphologic abnormality of the mitochondria of astrocytes was emphasized by Adornato et al. (1972).

Adornato, B. T., O'Brien, J. S., Lampert, P. W., Roe, T. F. and Neustein, H. B.: Cerebral spongy degeneration of infancy: a biochemical and ultrastructural study of affected twins. Neurology 22: 202-210, 1972.

Aduchi, M. and Aronson, S. M.: Studies on spongy degeneration of the central nervous system (van Bogaert-Bertrand type). In, Aronson, S. M. and Volk, B. W. (eds.): Inborn Disorders of Sphingolipid Metabolism. Oxford: Pergamon Press, 1967. Pp. 129-147.

Banker, B. Q., Robertson, J. T. and Victor, M.: Spongy degeneration of the central nervous system in infancy. Neurology 14: 981-1001, 1964.

Chou, S. M. and Waisman, H. A.: Spongy degeneration of the central nervous system. Case of homocystinuria. Arch. Path. 79: 357-363, 1965.

Hogan, G. R. and Richardson, E. P., Jr.: Spongy degeneration of the nervous system (Canavan's disease). Report of a case in an Irish-American family. Pediatrics 35: 284-294, 1965.

Mahloudji, M., Daneshbod, K. and Karjoo, M.: Familial spongy degeneration of the brain. Arch. Neurol. 22: 294-298, 1970.

Morcaldi, L., Salvati, G., Giordano, G. G. and Guazzi, G. C.: Congenital van bogaert-bertrand disease in a non-Jewish family. Acta Genet. Med. Gem. 18: 142-157, 1969.

Van Bogaert, L.: Familial spongy degeneration of the brain. (Complementary study of the family R). Acta Psychiat. Neurol. Scand. 39: 107-113, 1963.

ZuRhein, G. M., Eichman, P. L. and Puletti, F.: Familial idiocy with spongy degeneration of the central nervous system of van Bogaert-Bertrand type. Neurology 10: 998-1006, 1960.

27200 SUCROSURIA, HIATUS HERNIA AND MENTAL RETARDATION

Sucrosuria has been observed with mental deficiency in several cases. However, Perry et al. (1959) concluded that the association is coincidental. Furthermore, sucrosuria has not been proved to represent an inborn error. This is probably not a single gene disorder but rather a non-specific syndrome due to atonic state of severely mentally retarded children, with absorption of undigested sucrose from the atonic bowel.

Moncrieff, A. A.: Biochemistry of mental defect. Lancet II: 273-278, 1960.

Perry, T. L., Lippman, R. W., Walker, D. and Shaw, K. N. F.: Sucrosuria and mental deficiency: a coincidence. Pediatrics 24: 774-779, 1959.

Stern, J. and Sylvester, P. E.: Sucrosuria, hiatus hernia and mental retardation. Proc. London Conf. on Scientific Study of Mental Deficiency. (1960), Dagenham: May and Baker Ltd., 1962. Pp. 153-159.

Woodruff, G. G., Jr.: Sucrosuria in association with mental deficiency and hiatal hernia. J. Pediat. 52: 66-72, 1958.

The disorder seems to begin rarely in early infancy. However, the paucity of myelin in the cerebral hemispheres during the first 4-6 months of life would make histopathologic classification on the basis of myelin breakdown difficult at this stage. Progression is usually subacute in pace. Cortical blindness is often a conspicuous feature. Sibs may show great differences in the site of the lesion, age of onset and rate of progression (Meyer and Pilkington, 1936).

Greenfield, J. G.: In, Neuropathology. London: Edward Arnold Ltd., 1958. p. 460 ff.

Meyer, A. and Pilkington, F.: Some problems of pathogenesis in Schilder's disease, with description of a new familial case. J. Ment. Sci. 82: 812-826, 1936.

*27220 SULFATIDOSIS, JUVENILE, AUSTIN TYPE

At least three patients have been described (Austin, 1965; Thieffry et al., 1967). The disorder combines features of metachromatic leukodystrophy and of a mucopolysaccharidosis. Increased amounts of acid mucopolysaccharides are found in the urine and several tissues. In contrast to the classic form of metachromatic leukodystrophy arylsulfatase A, B and C are absent in the Austin type of juvenile sulfatidosis. Austin's two patients were sibs (in the M family). The gargoylism features are mild. Neurologic deterioration is rapid. Both mucopolysaccharide and sulfatide are found in the urine in excess. Cerebrospinal fluid protein is increased. Peripheral nerves show metachromatic degeneration of myelin on biopsy. Rampini et al. (1970) reported three additional cases. Murphy et al. (1971) described a case in which the mucopolysaccharides in the liver were thought to consist of both heparin sulfate and dermatan sulfate. Murphy's case also accumulated cholesterol sulfate. Mossakowski et al. (1961) observed three affected sibs, two female and one male, in a French-Canadian family.

Austin, J. H.: Metachromatic leukodystrophy. In, Carter, C. C. (ed.): Medical Aspects of Mental Retardation. Springfield, Ill.: Charles C Thomas, 1965. P. 768.

Bischel, M., Austin, J. and Kemeny, M.: Metachromatic leukodystrophy (MLD). VII. Elevated sulfate acid polysaccharide levels in urine and postmortem tissue. Arch. Neurol. 15: 13-28, 1966.

Mossakowski, M., Mathieson, G. and Cummings, J. N.: On the relationship of metachromatic leucodystrophy and amaurotic idiocy. Brain 81: 585-604, 1961.

Murphy, J. V., Wolfe, H. J., Balazs, E. A. and Moser, H. W.: A patient with deficiency of arylsulfatases A, B, C, and steroid sulfatase, associated with storage of sulfatide, cholesterol sulfate and glycosaminoglycans. In, Bernsohn, J. and Grossman, H. J. (eds.): Lipid Storage Diseases: Enzymatic Defects and Clinical Implications. New York: Academic Press, 1971. Pp. 67-110.

Rampini, S., Isler, W., Baerlocher, K., Bischoff, A., Ulrich, J. and Pluss, H. J.: Die Kombination von metachromatischer Leukodystrophie und Mukopolysaccharidose als selbstaendiges Krankheitsbild (Mukosulfatidose). Helv. Paediat. Acta 25: 436-461, 1970.

Thieffry, S., Lyon, G. and Maroteaux, P.: Encephalopathie metabolique associant une mucopolysaccharidose et une sulfatidose. Arch. Franc. Pediat. 24: 425-432, 1967.

*27230 SULFO-CYSTEINURIA (SULFITE OXIDASE DEFICIENCY)

In an infant with fatal neurologic disease and ectopia lentis, Mudd et al. (1967) found increased S-sulfite in the urine with markedly decreased inorganic sulfate excretion. A deficiency in the activity of sulfite oxidase, an enzyme which normally catalyzed conversion of sulfite to sulfate, was postulated. Sibs had died, probably of the same disorder.

Irreverre, F., Mudd, S. H., Heizer, W. D. and Laster, L.: Sulfate oxidase deficiency: studies of a patient with mental retardation, dislocated ocular lenses, and abnormal urinary excretion of S-sulfo-L-cysteine, sulfite and thiosulfate. Biochem. Med. 1: 187-199, 1967.

Mudd, S. H., Irreverre, F. and Laster, L.: Sulfite oxidase deficiency in man: demonstration of the enzymatic defect. Science 156: 1599-1602, 1967.

27235 SUMMITT SYNDROME

Summitt (1969) described two brothers with craniosynostosis and syndactyly which was severe in one and mild in the other. Both were obese. Intelligence was normal. The skull was towered as in Carpenter syndrome. The parents were first-cousins.

Summitt, R. L.: Recessive acrocephalosyndactyly with normal intelligence. The Clinical Delineation of Birth Defects. III. Limb Malformations. New York: National Foundation, 1969. Pp. 35-38.

27240 SUXAMETHONIUM SENSITIVITY (PSEUDOCHOLINESTERASE DEFICIENCY)

Homozygous persons sustained prolonged apnea after administration of the muscle relaxant suxamethonium in connection with surgical anesthesia. Pseudocholinesterase in the serum is low in its activity and is furthermore atypical in its substrate behavior. In the absence of the relaxant the homozygote is at no known disadvantage. The dibucaine number (percentage inhibition by dibucaine) identifies three genotypes. Two further alleles are a silent gene and an allele identified by fluoride inhibition. A non-allele is responsible for an electrophoretic variant. Deficiency of pseudocholinesterase is unusually frequent among Alaskan Eskimos (Gutsche et al., 1967). Heterogeneity of the 'silent' cholinesterase genes was indicated by the studies of Rubinstein et al. (1970). In an Eskimo population with a gene frequency for serum cholinesterase deficiency exceeding 10 percent, Scott et al. (1970) determined normal enzyme levels at various ages and the degree of overlap of heterozygous and homozygous classes. (No asterisk is given in this entry, because in the dominant catalog the two pseudocholinesterase loci are listed.) There is phenotypic diversity in suxamethonium sensitivity resulting from allelic series. Some of the subjects with sensitive genotypes have apnea lasting 2 or 3 hours whereas the apnea in other sensitive genotypes is considerably shorter (Lehmann and Liddle, 1972).

Goedde, H. W., Doenicke, A. and Altland, K.: Pseudocholinesterasen: Pharmakogenetik, Biochemie, Klinik. Berlin: Springer-Verlag, 1967.

Gutsche, B. B., Scott, E. M. and Wright, R. C.: Hereditary deficiency of pseudocholinesterase in Eskimos. Nature 215: 322-323, 1967.

Hodgkin, W., Giblett, E. R., Levine, H., Bauer, W. and Motulsky, A. G.: Complete pseudocholinesterase deficiency: genetic and immunologic characterization. J. Clin. Invest. 44: 486-493, 1965.

Lehmann, H. and Liddell, J.: The cholinesterase variants. In, Stanbury, J. B., Wyngaarden, J. B. and Fredrickson, D. S. (eds.): The Metabolic Basis of Inherited Disease. New York: McGraw-Hill, 1972 (3rd Ed.). Pp. 1730-1736.

Lehmann, H. and Silk, E.: Familial pseudocholinesterase deficiency. Brit. Med. J. 1: 128-129, 1961.

Rubinstein, H. M., Dietz, A. A., Hodges, L. K., Lubrano, T. and Czebotar, V.: Silent cholinesterase gene: variations in the properties of serum enzyme in apparent homozygotes. J. Clin. Invest. 49: 479-486, 1970.

Scott, E. M., Weaver, D. D. and Wright, R. C.: Discrimination of phenotypes in human serum cholinesterase deficiency. Am. J. Hum. Genet. 22: 363-369, 1970.

27250 SYSTEMIC CYSTIC ANGIOMATOSIS AND SEIP SYNDROME

In a Negro family Brunzell et al. (1968) observed a combination of congenital generalized lipodystrophy and systemic cystic angiomatosis in 5 of 12 sibs. The authors found previous reports of only 14 cases of cystic angiomatosis, none familial. Progressive incapacitating bone involvement occurred. Two had soft tissue (e.g., subcutaneous) angiomas. The lipodystrophy was accompanied by acanthosis nigricans, large hands and feet, acromegaloid facial features, lipenia, and hepatosplenomegaly and was in all ways identical to that of Seip syndrome (q.v.). Thus, one and the same gene may be responsible for the syndrome in reported cases of Seip disease and in the affected persons reported by Brunzell et al. (1968). Cystic angiomatosis may have been late in developing or overlooked in reported cases.

Brunzell, J. D., Shankle, S. W. and Bethune, J. E.: Congenital generalized lipodystrophy and systemic cystic angiomatosis: the simultaneous occurrence of two unusual syndromes in a single family. Ann. Intern. Med. 69: 501-516, 1968.

27255 TACHYCARDIA, HYPERTENSION, MICROPHTHALMOS, HYPERGLYCINURIA

Adams and Nance (1967) described a brother and sister with paroxysmal tachycardia, hypertension, syncope and seizures, associated with dominantly inherited microphthalmos, cataracts, hyperglycinuria and renal stones. A disturbance in glycine metabolism was postulated.

Adams, C. W. and Nance, W. E.: Persistent tachycardia, paroxysmal hypertension, and seizures: association with hyperglycinuria, dominantly inherited microphthalmia, and cataracts. J.A.M.A. 202: 525-530, 1967.

27260 TAPETO-RETINAL DEGENERATION WITH ATAXIA

There appear to be several types. In one variety the ataxia is of the Marie type. Although the inheritance is usually dominant, recessive pedigrees have been observed (Walsh, 1957). In a second form the ataxia is of Friedreich type (q.v.). The inheritance is recessive. Mixed or more complex types of neurologic involvement with ataxia occur in a third type. As one would expect, this is a heterogeneous category. Refsum disease and abetalipoproteinemia give this combination of findings. See also NERVOUS SYSTEM DISORDER RESEMBLING REFSUM DISEASE AND HURLER DISEASE. See OLIVOPONTOCEREBELLAR ATAXIA WITH MACULAR DYSTROPHY.

Franceschetti, A., Francois, J. and Babel, J.: Les heredo-degenerescences choroido-retiniennes (degenerescences tapeto-retiniennes). Paris: Masson, 2: 1963.

Walsh, F. B.: Clinical Neuro-Ophthalmology. Baltimore: Williams and Wilkins, 1957 (2nd Ed.). Pp. 620.

*27265 TATSUMI FACTOR DEFICIENCY

The Tatsumi clotting factor is said to be similar in its properties to Christmas factor but distinguishable from it by appropriate tests (Yoshida et al., 1960). Deficiency manifested by bleeding was observed in two consanguineous families and in both males and females. Clotting time was slightly prolonged, prothrombin consumption and thromboplastin generation were abnormal, and the bleeding time was long. Kosaki et al. (1968) suggested that Tatsumi factor is necessary for activation of Christmas factor by activated PTA.

Kosaki, G., Tanaka, K., Inoshita, K. and Nagao, M.: A role of TF (tatsumi-factor) on activation of factor IX: second report. Proc. XII Cong. Internat. Soc. Hemat. New York, 1968. P. 176.

Yoshida, K., Umegaki, K., Yoshioka, K., Fukui, H., Majima, T. and Tagawa, N.: Hemorrhagic diathesis with prolonged bleeding time, serum defect and qualitative platelet dysfunction. Proc. VIII Internat. Cong. Hemat. Tokyo: Pan Pacific Press, 1960. P. 1556.

27270 TAURODONTISM

This trait is characterized by large pulp chambers. The changes are usually most striking in the molars. Shaw (1928) claimed that the trait is inherited as an autosomal recessive but much more evidence is required. Indeed, Haunfelder (1967) presented a family suggesting dominant inheritance. Witkop and Rao (1971) found no affected parents in eight cases they investigated. Taurodontism (meaning 'bull teeth') was a frequent finding in early man and today in races such as the Eskimos who use their teeth for cutting hides. Coon (1962) suggested that the trait might have selective advantage to such groups. The genetics is likely to be polygenic. See AMELOGENESIS IMPERFECTA WITH TAURODONTISM.

Coon, C. S.: The Origin of Races. New York: Alfred A. Knoff, 1962.

Haunfelder, D.: A contribution to molars with prismatic roots (so-called taurodontism). Deutsch. Zahnaertzl. Z. 21: 419-423, 1967.

Shaw, J. C. M.: Taurodent teeth in South African races. J. Anat. 62: 476-498, 1928.

27275 TAY-SACHS DISEASE, AB VARIANT

Sandhoff et al. (1971) refer to Sandhoff disease (26880) as variant O (since both hexosaminidase A and B are missing) and classic Tay-Sachs disease as variant B (since hexosaminidase is absent but hexosaminidase B is present in increased amounts). They studied a single patient with a third form they called variant AB, because both hexosaminidase A and hexosaminidase B are increased in amounts. Because it is not certain that a locus distinct from that of Sandhoff disease and the infantile and juvenile forms of Tay-Sachs disease is involved, an asterisk is not used. Sandhoff's patient with the AB variant was studied clinically by Hugo Moser of Boston. A brother and sister were affected.

Sandhoff, K., Horzer, K., Wassle, W. and Jatzkewitz, H.: Enzyme alterations and lipid storage in three variants of Tay-Sachs disease. J. Neurochem. 18: 2469-2489, 1971.

27277 TAY-SACHS DISEASE, JUVENILE TYPE

Alternatively the gene responsible for the juvenile form may be allelic to that responsible for the classic infantile form of Tay-Sachs disease, just as allelic forms of Niemann-Pick disease, Gaucher disease and metachromatic leukodystrophy occur, with different ages of onset. Whereas classic Tay-Sachs patients with complete deficiency of hexosaminidase A die before age 5 years, patients with the partial deficiency die by age 15 years. Component A may be a group of enzymes and the partial deficiency in the juvenile form may be in fact total absence of one of these enzymes (Suzuki and Suzuki, 1970).

Suzuki, Y. and Suzuki K.: Partial deficiency of hexosaminidase component A in juvenile Gm (2)-gangliosidosis. Neurology 20: 848-851, 1970.

*27280 TAY-SACHS DISEASE: GM2-GANGLIOSIDOSIS, TYPE I

Tay-Sachs disease is characterized by the onset in infancy of developmental retardation, followed by paralysis, dementia and blindness, with death in the second or third year of life. A gray-white area around the fovea centralis, due to lipid-laden ganglion cells, leaving a central 'cherry-red' spot is a typical fundoscopic finding. Pathological verification is provided by the finding of the typically ballooned neurons in the central nervous system. The frequency of the condition is much higher in Ashkenazi Jews of Eastern European origin than in others. Parental consanguinity is frequent in non-Jewish cases, relatively infrequent in the Jewish cases — facts which also emphasize the difference in gene frequency in the two groups. The gene frequency in New York City Jews is between 0.013 and 0.016 and that in non-Jews is only about one-hundredth of this value. Fructose-1-phosphate aldolase is deficient in the serum and glutamic oxalacetic transaminase and lactic dehydrogenase are elevated. An early and persistent extension response to sound ('startle reaction') is useful for recognizing the disorder. Zeman (1966) is of the opinion that only three entities deserve being called amaurotic idiocy, namely: (1) congenital amaurotic idiocy; (2) Tay-Sachs disease; and (3) generalized gangliosidosis. In all of these excessive accumulation of gangliosides has been demonstrated by thin-layer chromatography. In the so-called juvenile and adult forms of amaurotic idiocy no abnormality of gangliosides or other lipids has been found, thus indicating the taxonomic inappropriateness of classifying these with Tay-Sachs disease. The three true gangliosidoses have onset during infancy and show striking megalencephaly. Balint et al. (1967) found that both homozygotes and heterozygotes show reduced sphingomyelin in red blood cells and found this reduction useful in carrier identification. Accumulation of a glycoprotein in red cells of patients with Tay-Sachs disease demonstrated by Balint and Kyriakides (1968) may have bearing on the nature of the primary defect. The basic enzyme defect has been shown by Okada and O'Brien (1969) to concern one component of a hexosaminidase. Total hexosaminidase activity was normal but when components A and B were separated, component A was found to be absent. Hultberg (1969) confirmed the findings of Okada and O'Brien (1969). Okada et al. (1971) compared the findings in regard to hexosaminidases A and B in the three forms of ganglioside GM(2) storage disease (Tay-Sachs disease, Sandhoff disease, and juvenile GM(2) gangliosidosis). The family was not Jewish. Kolodny (1972), who also studied the proband, states that visual function was retained and optic atrophy was not present at age 20 months. At death at 32 months, microscopic findings in the central nervous system were like those in Tay-Sachs disease. The patients showed normal results in tests which usually demonstrate the Tay-Sachs heterozygote. By study of somatic cell hybrids, Gilbert et al. (1974) showed that a locus determining hexosaminidase A is on chromosome no. 7. See 14265 for similar information concerning hexosaminidase B.

Aronson, S. M., Valsamis, M. P. and Volk, B. W.: Infantile amaurotic family idiocy: occurrence, genetic considerations and pathophysiology in the non-Jewish infant. Pediatrics 26: 229-242, 1960.

Balint, J. A. and Kyriakides, E. C.: Studies of red cell stromal proteins in Tay-Sachs disease. J. Clin. Invest. 47: 1858-1864, 1968.

Balint, J. A., Kyriakides, E. C. and Spitzer, H. L.: On the chemical changes in the red cell stroma in Tay-Sachs disease: their value as genetic tracers. In, Aronson, S. M. and Volk, B. W. (eds.): Inborn Disorders of Sphingolipid Metabolism. Oxford: Pergamon Press, 1967. Pp. 423-430.

Brady, R. O.: Cerebral lipidoses. Ann. Rev. Med. 21: 317-334, 1970.

Gilbert, F., Kucherlapati, R., Creagan, R. P., Murnane, M. J., Darlington, G. J. and Ruddle, F. H.:

R
E
C
E
S
S
I
V
E

Tay-Sachs' disease the assignment of genes for hexosaminidase A and B to chromosomes 7 and 5 in man. Proc. Nat. Acad. Sci., in press, 1974.

Hanhart, E.: Ueber 27 Sippen mit infantiler amaurotischer Idiotie (Tay-Sachs). Acta Genet. Med. Gem. 3: 331-364, 1954.

Hultberg, B.: N-acetylhexosaminidase activities in Tay-Sachs disease. (Letter) Lancet II: 1195 only, 1969.

Kolodny, E. H.: Boston, Mass.: personal communication, 1972.

O'Brien, J. S., Okada, S., Chen, A. and Fillerup, D. L.: Tay-Sachs disease: detection of heterozygotes and homozygotes by serum hexosaminidase assay. New Eng. J. Med. 283: 15-20, 1970.

O'Brien, J. S., Okada, S., Fillerup, D. L., Veath, M. L., Adornato, B., Brenner, P. H. and Leroy, J. G.: Tay-Sachs disease: prenatal diagnosis. Science 172: 61-64, 1971.

Ohman, R., Ekelund, H. and Svennerholm, L.: The diagnosis of Tay-Sachs disease. Acta Paediat. Scand. 60: 399-406, 1971.

Okada, S. and O'Brien, J. S.: Tay-sachs disease: generalized absence of a beta-d-n-acetylhexosaminidase component. Science 165: 698-700, 1969.

Okada, S., Veath, M. L., Leroy, J. and O'Brien, J. S.: Ganglioside Gm(2) storage diseases: hexosaminidase deficiencies in cultured fibroblasts. Am. J. Hum. Genet. 23: 55-61, 1971.

Schneck, L., Maisel, J. and Volk, B. W.: The startle response and serum enzyme profile in early detection of Tay-Sachs disease. J. Pediat. 65: 749-756, 1964.

Sloan, H. R. and Fredrickson, D. S.: Gm(2) gangliosidoses: Tay-Sachs disease. In, Stanbury, J. B., Wyngaarden, J. B. and Fredrickson, D. S. (eds.): The Metabolic Basis of Inherited Disease. New York: McGraw-Hill, 1972 (3rd Ed.). Pp. 615-638.

Volk, B. W.: Tay-Sachs Disease. New York: Grune and Stratton, 1964.

Zeman, W.: Indianapolis, Ind.: personal communication, 1966.

27300 TEETH, FUSED

Deppendorf (1912) described bilateral fusion of the deciduous incisors in sisters, aged 4 and 5 and one half years, and also a rarer condition, bilateral fusion of a deciduous mandibular canine with the second incisor.

Deppendorf, (NI): Beitraege zur Verschmelzung und Zwillingsbildung menschlicher Zaehne im Milch- und im bleibenden Gebiss. Deutsch. Mschr. Zahnheilk. 5: 427-432, 1912.

27310 TESTES, ABSENCE OF

Abeyaratne et al. (1969) described 16 cases of apparently complete absence of testes in phenotypic males, including one pair of affected sibs. Bobrow and Gough (1970) also described two affected brothers. This familial disorder may be unilateral in a portion of cases. Ferrier (1969) examined twins, one of whom had anorchia, and found them through blood studies to probably be monozygotic. Familial occurrence was noted by Overzier and Linden (1956).

Abeyaratne, M. R., Aherne, W. A. and Scott, J. E. S.: The vanishing testis. Lancet II: 822-824, 1969.

Bobrow, M. and Gough, M. H.: Bilateral absence of testes. (Letter) Lancet I: 366 only, 1970.

Koopman, J.: Congenital anorchia: case. Geeneesk. Gids. 8: 309-330, 1930.

Overzier, C. and Linden, H.: Echter Agonadismus (Anorchismus) bei Geschwistern. Gynaecologia 142: 215-233, 1956.

27320 TESTICULAR FEMINIZATION, INCOMPLETE TYPE

This syndrome differs from complete testicular feminization in the presence of clitoral enlargement and sometimes partial fusion of the labia at birth and virilization at puberty. The pedigree pattern is like that of an X-linked recessive in several published families, but Philip and Trolle (1965) described a family in which four sibs, the product of a consanguineous mating, and their paternal cousins were affected. Opitz et al. (1972) concluded, however, that the disorder in this family was in fact what they termed pseudovaginal perineoscrotal hypospadias (26460) which is clearly an autosomal recessive. Incomplete testicular feminization syndrome may be an X-linked recessive (or male-limited autosomal dominant) as in the 'complete' form (see 31380).

Opitz, J. M., Simpson, J. L., Sarto, G. E., Summitt, R. L., New, M. and German, J.: Pseudovaginal perineoscrotal hypospadias. Clin. Genet. 3: 1-26, 1972.

Philip, J. and Trolle, D.: Familial male hermaphroditism with delayed and partial masculinization. Am. J. Obstet. Gynec. 93: 1076-1083, 1965.

27330 TESTICULAR TUMORS

Hutter et al. (1967) reviewed the reports of testicular tumors in brothers and in twins and reported affected brothers.

Hutter, A. M., Lynch, J. J. and Shnider, B. I.: Malignant testicular tumors in brothers. A case report. J.A.M.A. 199: 1009-1010, 1967.

27340 TETRAMELIC DEFICIENCIES, ECTODERMAL DYSPLASIA, DEFORMED EARS, AND OTHER ABNORMALITIES

RECESSIVE

Freire-Maia (1970) described a Brazilian family in which a brother and sister and two deceased brothers showed severe absence deformities of all four limbs, hypotrichosis, abnormal teeth, hypoplastic nipples and areolae and deformed auricles. His consistent features included hypoplastic nails, hypogonadism, thyroid enlargement, incomplete cleft lip, mental retardation, and ECG and EEG abnormalities. Both living sibs showed an excess of tyrosine and-or tryptophane in the urine. Parental consanguinity was denied but the parents came from the same farm in one of the most inbred areas of Brazil.

Cat, I., Costa, O. and Freire-Maia, N.: Odontotrichomelic hypohidrotic dysplasia. A clinical reappraisal. Hum. Hered. 22: 91-95, 1972.

Freire-Maia, N.: A newly recognized genetic syndrome of tetramelic deficiencies, ectodermal dysplasia, deformed ears, and other abnormalities. Am. J. Hum. Genet. 22: 370-377, 1970.

27350 THALASSEMIAS

It seems justified to include thalassemia major in a catalog of rare recessive phenotypes. (No asterisk is used because it is not certain that mutation elsewhere than at the established structural loci for hemoglobin is involved.) Apparent homozygotes have been observed in the offspring of consanguineous marriages in Birmingham, England (Lloyd and Brown, 1962). The gene involved may have arisen by mutation and not been introduced by early travelers from the Mediterranean. The same argument can be proposed for the sickle homozygote (see SICKLE CELL ANEMIA). Two varieties of thalassemia have been recognized according to their behavior in the heterozygous state with alpha and beta chain mutants. Thus, beta thalassemia interacts with Hb S (a beta chain variant) to result in the clinical picture called sickle-thalassemia and alpha thalassemia interacts with Hb I in a comparable manner (Atwater and colleagues, 1960). A third variety is called delta thalassemia because the defect concerns an inability to make delta chains. The homozygote has no Hb A2 (Thompson et al., 1965). Hb Lepore (see dominant catalog) also produces a thalassemia picture. A fourth variety of thalassemia may be called beta-delta type and may like Lepore hemoglobin represent the result of fusion of the genes determining the beta and delta hemoglobin chains. (These genes by other evidence appear to be contiguous.) Comings and Motulsky (1966) showed that cis delta chains are not synthesized in this condition which is also called fetal thalassemia (because of high Hb F). In their patient with the abnormal beta-delta gene (actually perhaps a deletion) on one chromosome and the Hb B(2) gene in the other, no Hb A2 was formed. Stamatoyannopoulos (1971) postulated the existence of gamma-thalassemia (in addition to the alpha, beta, delta and betadelta forms). These mutations are tolerated by the fetus because two pairs of gamma-chain loci operate in man. Two types are envisioned, of which gamma-ala thalassemia is associated with mild anemia and gamma-gly with moderate reduction in the synthetic of Hb F. The biochemical defect in the thalassemias is in transcription; translation is normal (Kazazian, 1974). In some thalassemias globin synthesis is reduced (due either to decreased messenger RNA synthesized or transported or to increased mRNA destruction). In other thalassemias, synthesis of a specific globin chain is completely absent and no mRNA can be demonstrated, suggesting gene deletion (Kan, 1974). The phenotype in the latter situation is hydrops fetalis, a finding in homozygous alpha thalassemia such as occurs in Cantonese Chinese.

Atwater, J., Schwartz, I. R. and Tocantins, L. M.: A variety of human hemoglobin with 4 distinct electrophoretic components. Blood 15: 901-908, 1960.

Butikofer, E., Hoigne, R., Marti, H. R. and Betke, K.: Haemoglobin-h-Thalassaemie. Mitteilung eines Falles mit Familienuntersuchung. Schweiz. Med. Wschr. 90: 1215-1217, 1960.

Bannerman, R. M. and Callender, S. T.: Thalassaemia in Britain. (Letter) Brit. Med. J. 2: 1288 only, 1961.

Callender, S. T., Mallett, B. J. and Lehmann, H.: Thalassaemia in Britain. Brit. J. Haemat. 7: 1-8, 1961.

Comings, D. E. and Motulsky, A. G.: Absence of cis delta chain synthesis in delta-beta thalassemia (F-thalassemia). Blood 28: 54-69, 1966.

Dittman, W. A., Haut, A., Wintrobe, M. M. and Cartwright, G. E.: Hemoglobin H associated with an uncommon variant of thalassemia trait. Blood 16: 975-983, 1960.

Havard, C. W. H., Lehmann, H. and Scott, R. B.: Thalassaemia minor in an English woman. Brit. Med. J. 1: 304-305, 1958.

Heller, P., Yakulis, V. J., Rosenzweig, A. I., Abildgaard, C. F. and Rucknagel, D. L.: Mild homozygous beta-thalassemia: further evidence for the heterogeneity of beta-thalassemia genes. Ann. Intern. Med. 64: 52-61, 1966.

Huisman, T. H. H., Punt, K. and Schaad, J. D.: Thalassemia minor associated with hemoglobin-B2 heterozygosity: a family report. Blood 17: 747-757, 1961.

Israels, M. C. G. and Turner, R. L.: A British target-cell anaemia. Lancet II: 1363-1365, 1955.

Kan, Y. W.: San Francisco, personal communication, 1974.

Lehmann, H.: Thalassaemia in Britain. (Letter) Brit. Med. J. 2: 1288-1289, 1961.

Lloyd, J. K. and Brown, G. A.: Homozygous thalassemia in an English child. (Abstract) Proc. 10th Intern. Congr. Pediat., Lisbon, 1962. P. 23-24.

Motulsky, A. G.: Current concepts of the genetics of the thalassemias. Cold Spring Harbor Sympos. Quant. Biol. 29: 399-413, 1964.

Necheles, T. F., Allen, D. M. and Gerald, P. S.: The many forms of thalassemia: definition and classification of the thalassemia syndromes. Ann. N.Y. Acad. Sci. 165: 5-12, 1969.

Pearson, H. A. and Moore, M. M.: Human hemoglobin gene linkage: report of a family with hemoglobin

R
E
C
E
S
S
I
V
E

B(2), hemoglobin S, and beta-thalassemia, including a probable crossover between thalassemia and delta loci. Am. J. Hum. Genet. 17: 125-132, 1965.

Schwartz, E.: The silent carrier of beta thalassemia. New Eng. J. Med. 281: 1327-1333, 1969.

Stamatoyannopoulos, G.: Gamma-thalassemia. Lancet II: 192-193, 1971.

Thompson, R. B., Warrington, R., Odom, J. and Bell, W. N.: Interaction between genes for delta thalassemia and hereditary persistence of foetal hemoglobin. Acta Genet. Statist. Med. 15: 190-200, 1965.

Weatherall, D. J.: The biochemical lesion in thalassemia. Brit. J. Haemat. 15: 1-5, 1968.

Weatherall, D. J.: The Thalassaemia Syndrome. Philadelphia: F. A. Davis Co., 1965.

27360 THALIDOMIDE SUSCEPTIBILITY

Kremer and Fullerton (1961) described brother and sister who developed neuropathy at the same time interval after starting thalidomide. Genetic differences in susceptibility to the teratogenic effects of thalidomide are suspected but unproved, and nothing is known of genetic differences in the metabolism of the drug.

Kremer, M. and Fullerton, P. M.: Neuropathy after thalidomide ('Distaval'). Brit. Med. J. 2: 1498 only, 1961.

*27365 THANATOPHORIC DWARFISM

Maroteaux, Lamy and Robert (1967) gave this name to the condition in certain micromelic dwarfs who die in the first hours of life. The ribs and bones of the extremities are very short. Vertebral bodies are greatly reduced in height with wide intervertebral spaces but caudad narrowing of the spinal canal is not present. They found cases in the literature which answered this description, the earliest being one reported by Maygrier in 1898. They concluded that dominant mutation is the most likely basis but that recessive inheritance cannot be excluded. Asphyxiating thoracic dystrophy (q.v.) is to be differentiated. Maroteaux et al. (1967) referred to yet another rare type of micromelic chondrodystrophy with early death. Giedion (1968) described a Swiss case which differed from other cases in the presence of radioulnar synostosis and survival for 96 hours. In utero diagnosis was demonstrated by Keats et al. (1970). Recessive inheritance now (1971) seems quite certain. Chemke et al. (1971) described two affected offspring of first-cousin parents and quoted an observation (Harris and Patton, 1971) of two affected sibs. Langer and Gorlin (1971) reviewed the films on Chemke's cases and judged them consistent with thanatophoric dwarfism. Partington et al. (1971) described cloverleaf skull in association with a generalized skeletal dysplasia consistent with thanatophoric dwarfism. Two of their four cases were in sibs. Pena and Goodman (1973) reviewed reported cases and concluded that polygenic inheritance is most likely. They suggested an empiric recurrence risk in sibs of 2 percent. They admitted the possibility that some cases are autosomal recessive. Genetic heterogenity, with some recessive and many dominant new mutation cases, would seem a priori more likely to me. Sabry (1974) observed affected triplets whose parents were first-cousins.

Campbell, R. E.: Thanatophoric dwarfism in utero: a case report. Am. J. Roentgen. 112: 198-200, 1971.

Chemke, J., Graff, G. and Lancet, M.: Familial thanatophoric dwarfism. (Letter) Lancet I: 1358 only, 1971.

Giedion, A.: Thanatophoric dwarfism. Helv. Paediat. Acta 23: 175-183, 1968.

Harris, R. and Patton, J. T.: Achondroplasia and thanatophoric dwarfism in the newborn. Clin. Genet. 2: 61-72, 1971.

Kaufman, R. L., Rimoin, D. L., McAlister, W. H. and Kissane, J. M.: Thanatophoric dwarfism. Am. J. Dis. Child. 120: 53-57, 1970.

Keats, T. E., Riddervold, H. O. and Michaelis, L. L.: Thanatophoric dwarfism. Am. J. Roentgen. 108: 473-480, 1970.

Kozlowski, K., Prokop, E. and Zybaczynski, J.: Thanatophoric dwarfism. Brit. J. Radiol. 43: 565-568, 1970.

Langer, L. O. and Gorlin, R. J.: Minneapolis, Minn.: personal communication, 1971.

Maroteaux, P. and Lamy, M.: Le diagnostic des nanismes chondro-dystrophiques chez les nouveau-nes. Arch. Franc. Pediat. 25: 241-262, 1968.

Maroteaux, P., Lamy, M. and Robert, J.-M.: Le nanisme thanatophore. Presse Med. 75: 2519-2524, 1967.

Maygrier, C.: Foetus achondroplasique: presentation de photographies, du moulage, d'une radiographie et du squelette. Bull. Soc. Obstet. Gynec. 1: 248-255, 1898.

Partington, M. W., Gonzales-Crussi, F., Khakee, S. G. and Wollin, D. G.: Cloverleaf skull and thanatophoric dwarfism. Report of four cases, two in the same sibship. Arch. Dis. Child. 46: 656-664, 1971.

Pena, S. D. J. and Goodman, H. O.: The genetics of thanatophoric dwarfism. Pediatrics 51: 104-109, 1973.

Sabry, A.: Thanatophoric dwarfism in triplets. (Letter) Lancet II: 533 only, 1974.

27370 THIEMANN EPIPHYSEAL DISEASE

Bohme (1963) reported two male sibs with Thiemann epiphyseal disease, involving the proximal interphalangeal joints of the fingers. The metaphyses and epiphyses were broad and short. Onset was at 13 and 17 years, respectively. The parents were not related and they and other family members were not affected.

R
E
C
E
S
S
I
V
E

Boehme, A.: Kasuistischer Beitrag zur Thiemannschen Epiphysenerkrankung. Z. Ges. Inn. Med. 18: 491-495, 1963.

*27375 THREE M (3M) SYNDROME

Malvaux (1974), Miller and McKusick (1974) observed sibs with low birth weight dwarfism, narrow facies, grooved lower anterior thorax, and clinodactyly. Intelligence was normal. The brother and sister observed by McKusick and Miller were the offspring of first-cousin parents. This seems distinct from Russell-Silver dwarfism (26865).

Malvaux, P.: Louvain, personal communication, Jan. 17, 1974.

Miller, J. D. and McKusick, V. A.: To be published, 1974.

*27380 THROMBASTHENIA OF GLANZMANN AND NAEGELI

Recessive inheritance is claimed to obtain in almost all cases (Lelong, 1960; Marx and Jean, 1962). A bleeding diathesis with normal bleeding time, platelet count and coagulation time but deficient clot retraction and abnormal platelet morphology is found. There probably is more than one form of the disease. Gross et al. (1960) found that the platelets of one group have greatly reduced glyceraldehydephosphate dehydrogenase (GAPDH) and pyruvate kinase (PK) activity. The platelets show reduced adhesiveness; on blood smears there is notable absence of platelet aggregation and by electron microscopy the 'round' type of platelet predominates. Friedman et al. (1964) described the disease in a boy and girl who were double first-cousins (the mother of one was a sister of the father of the other and vice versa). No abnormality has been detected in heterozygotes. Five factors have been identified as essential to normal platelet function in hemostasis: (1) a platelet property, lacking in Glanzmann thrombasthenia, which makes platelets adhere at the site of vessel injury; (2) a collagenous and elastic fibrous substance for platelets to adhere to; (3) a plasma factor, lacking in Von Willebrand disease (a dominant, q.v.); (4) calcium; and (5) ADP which is released from damaged red cells and tissue cells. The difficult nosology of this undoubtedly heterogeneous category was discussed by Kanska et al. (1963) and by Alagille et al. (1964). An apparently unique congenital platelet disorder was described by Bowie, Thompson and Owen (1964). There is some suggestion of a dominant form (q.v.) as well as the better established recessive form (Caen et al., 1966) and this may be a heterogeneous category. Absent platelet aggregation was emphasized by Caen et al. Cronberg et al. (1967) described a kindred in which three persons in two sibships had a severe clotting defect, whereas others, including all 4 parents of the affected sibships, had a minor defect. The most impressive abnormality in vitro was complete absence of ability of the platelets to aggregate or adhere to glass. The same was observed by Zaizov et al. (1968) in brother and sister whose parents were first-cousins once removed. Papayannis and Israels (1970) concluded that the heterozygote can be identified by the clot retraction test. Some heterozygotes are mild bleeders. A classification of hereditary thrombopathies was given by Bowie and Owen (1968). They classified the disorder into three major categories: (1) thrombopathy (deficient or ineffective platelet factor 3); (2) thrombasthenia (diminished clot retraction); and (3) compound platelet defects (those associated with deficiency of either factor VIII or factor IX). The heterogeneity of thrombasthenia is coming increasingly to light as various biochemical defects are identified. Moser et al. (1968) found severe deficiency of glutathione reductase in platelets in two sibs. Karpatkin and Weiss (1972) found markedly decreased glutathione peroxidase activity of platelets in three patients. Corby et al. (1972) reported a brother and sister who had bleeding diathesis, normal platelet counts, prolonged bleeding times, deficient platelet factor 3 and absent platelet aggregation in response to ADP, collagen and epinephrine. Hathaway (1972) reviewed disorders of platelet function.

Alagille, D., Josso, F., Binet, J. L. and Blin, M. L.: La dystrophie thrombocytaire hemorragipare. Discussion nosologique. Nouv. Rev. Franc. Hemat. 4: 755-790, 1964.

Beutler, E.: Glanzmann's thrombasthenia and reduced glutathione. New Eng. J. Med. 287: 1094-1095, 1972.

Bowie, E. J. W. and Owen, C. A.: Thrombopathy. Sem. Hemat. 5: 73-82, 1968.

Bowie, E. J. W., Thompson, J. H., Jr. and Owen, C. A., Jr.: A new abnormality of platelet function. Thromb. Diath. Haemorrh. 11: 195-203, 1964.

Caen, J. P., Castaldi, P. A., Leclerc, J. C., Inceman, S., Larrieu, M. J., Probst, M. and Bernard, J.: Congenital bleeding disorders with long bleeding time and normal platelet count. I. Glanzman's thrombasthenia (report of fifteen patients). Am. J. Med. 41: 4-26, 1966.

Corby, D. G., Zirbel, C. L., Lindley, A. and Schulman, I.: Thrombasthenia. Am. J. Dis. Child. 121: 140-144, 1972.

Cronberg, S., Nilsson, I. M. and Zetterqvist, E.: Investigation of a family with members with both severe and mild degree of thrombasthenia. Acta Paediat. Scand. 56: 189-197, 1967.

Friedman, L. L., Bowie, E. J. W., Thompson, J. H., Jr., Brown, A. L., Jr. and Owen, C. A., Jr.: Familial Glanzmann's thrombasthenia. Mayo Clin. Proc. 39: 908-918, 1964.

Gross, R., Gerok, W., Lohr, G. W., Vogell, W., Waller, H. D. and Theopold, W.: Ueber die Natur der Thrombasthenie. Thrombopathie Glanzmann-Naegeli. Klin. Wschr. 38: 193-206, 1960.

Hathaway, W. E.: Bleeding disorders due to platelet dysfunction. Am. J. Dis. Child. 121: 127-134, 1972.

Kanska, B., Niewiarowski, S., Ostrowski, L., Poplawski, A. and Prokopowicz, J.: Macrothrombocytic thrombopathia. Clinical, coagulation and hereditary aspects. Thromb. Diath. Haemorrh. 10: 88-100, 1963.

Karpatkin, S. and Weiss, H. J.: Deficiency of glutathione peroxidase associated with high levels of reduced glutathione in Glanzmann's thrombasthenia. New Eng. J. Med. 287: 1062-1066, 1972.

RECESSIVE

Lelong, J. C.: La thrombopathie de Glanzmann-Naegeli. Paris: R. Foulon et Cie., 1960.

Marx, R. and Jean, G.: Studien zur Pathogenese der Thrombasthenie Glanzmann-Naegeli. Klin. Wschr. 40: 942-953, 1962.

Moser, K., Lechner, K. and Vinazzer, H.: A hitherto not described enzyme defect in thrombasthenia: glutathione reductase deficiency. Thromb. Diath. Haemorrh. 19: 46-52, 1968.

Papayannis, A. G. and Israels, M. C. G.: Glanzmann's disease and trait. (Letter) Lancet II: 44 only, 1970.

Pittman, M. A., Jr. and Graham, J. B.: Glanzmann's thrombopathy: an autosomal recessive trait in one family. Am. J. Med. Sci. 247: 293-303, 1964.

Waller, H. D. and Gross, R.: Genetische Enzymdefecte als Ursache von Thrombocytopathien. Verh. Deutsch. Ges. Inn. Med. 70: 476-494, 1964.

Zaizov, R., Cohen, I. and Matoth, Y.: Thrombasthenia: a study of two siblings. Acta Paediat. Scand. 57: 522-526, 1968.

*27390 THROMBOCYTOPENIA

Schaar (1963) described four affected brothers. No platelet-stimulating factor or anti-platelet antibody was present and there was no skeletal anomaly. Bloom et al. (1966) described a form of constitutional aplastic anemia (see ANEMIA, CONGENITAL HYPOPLASTIC) with 'amegakaryocytic thrombocytopenia present at birth or early infancy, followed later in childhood by pancytopenia.' They called it type II constitutional aplastic anemia. Maternal-fetal incompatibility of platelet antigens is a cause of neonatal thrombocytopenia in multiple sibs (Paganelli, 1969), simulating recessive inheritance. See PLATELET GROUPS in dominant catalog. These patients were chronically thrombocytopenic but responded to the transfusion of normal plasma. Autosomal recessive inheritance has been reported by Roberts and Smith (1950) and by Wilson et al. (1963).

Bloom, G. E., Warner, S., Gerald, P. S. and Diamond, L. K.: Chromosome abnormalities in constitutional aplastic anemia. New Eng. J. Med. 274: 8-14, 1966.

Paganelli, V. H.: Thrombocytopenia in newborn siblings. (Letter) J.A.M.A. 208: 1703 only, 1969.

Roberts, M. H. and Smith, M. H.: Thrombopenic purpura. Report of four cases in one family. Am. J. Dis. Child. 79: 820-825, 1950.

Schaar, F. E.: Familial idiopathic thrombocytopenic purpura. J. Pediat. 62: 546-551, 1963.

Shulman, I., Pierce, M., Lukens, A. and Currimbhoy, Z.: A factor in normal plasma required for platelet production: chronic thrombocytopenia due to its deficiency. Blood 16: 943-957, 1960.

Vildosola, J. and Emparanza, E.: Hereditary familial thrombocytopenia. (Abstract) Intern. Cong. Paediat., Lisbon, 1962. P. 36.

Wilson, S. J., Larsen, W. E., Skillman, R. S. and Walters, T. R.: Familial thrombocytopenic purpura. Blood 22: 827 only, 1963.

*27400 THROMBOCYTOPENIA — ABSENT RADIUS (TAR) SYNDROME

Shaw and Oliver (1959) described sibs with absent radii and thrombocytopenia. They suggested that this disorder is distinct from Fanconi pancytopenic syndrome (q.v.) because there was no hypoplasia of the erythron and the blood disorder was evident in the first few months of life. The rare condition had been reported in sibs by Gross, Groh and Weippl (1956). In other reported cases congenital heart disease and renal malformations were found. Thrombocytopenia usually gives rise to symptoms early in life but is transient. Thus, the process is a more benign one than is Fanconi panmyelopathy, in which leukemia is a further complication. Other differences from Fanconi disease include the absence of particular change in the thumb, of pigmentary abnormalities, and of chromosomal breaks. In a family studied in this department (Hall et al., 1969) four sisters were affected. One with tetralogy of Fallot had died. The oldest was alive at age 27 and had two normal children. The occurrence of hypoplastic radius and hypoplastic thrombocytopenia with trisomy 18 (Rabinowitz et al., 1967) is of interest although its relationship to the Mendelizing syndrome is doubtful.

Dignan, P. S. J., Mauer, A. M. and Frantz, C.: Phocomelia with congenital hypoplastic thrombocytopenia and myeloid leukemoid reactions. J. Pediat. 70: 561-573, 1967.

Gross, H., Groh, C. and Weippl, G.: Kongenitale hypoplastische Thrombopenie mit Radius-Aplasie, ein Syndrom multipler Abartungen. Neue Oest. Z. Kinderheilk. 1: 574, 1956.

Hall, J. G., Levin, J., Kuhn, J. P., Ottenheimer, E. J., Van Berkum, K. A. P. and McKusick, V. A.: Thrombocytopenia with absent radius (TAR). Medicine 48: 411-439, 1969.

Rabinowitz, J. G., Moseley, J. E., Mitty, H. A. and Hirschorn, K.: Trisomy 18, esophageal atresia, anomalies of the radius, and congenital hypoplastic thrombocytopenia. Radiology 89: 488-491, 1967.

Shaw, S. and Oliver, R. A. M.: Congenital hypoplastic thrombocytopenia with skeletal deformities in siblings. Blood 14: 374-377, 1959.

27403 THROMBOCYTOPENIA DUE TO CONGENITAL ABSENCE OF 'THROMBOPOIETIN'

Schulman et al. (1960) described an 8-year-old girl who had thrombocytopenia which responded to transfusions of blood or plasma. Deficiency of a stimulating factor which is responsible for megakaryocyte maturation and platelet production was postulated. The family history was negative. The mother's plasma induced normal platelet responses whereas the father's resulted in submaximal responses. Upshaw (1967) described a similar case.

Schulman, I., Pierce, M., Lukens, A. and Currimbhoy, Z.: Studies on thrombopoiesis. I. A factor in normal human plasma required for platelet production: chronic thrombocytopenia due to its deficiency. Blood 16: 943-957, 1960.

Upshaw, J. D.: Comment. Third Conf. Blood Platelets, 1967.

*27410 THROMBOCYTOPENIC THROMBOPATHY

Cullum, et al., (1967) described a family of Sicilian origin with a bleeding disorder characterized by thrombocytopenia, morphologically abnormal platelets, prolonged bleeding time, low platelet thromboplastic activity and normal clot retraction. Phospholipid content of platelets was increased. The authors suggested that abnormally rapid removal of the bizarre platelets may be responsible for thrombocytopenia. The morphologic abnormality of the platelet was thought to be dominant. Two members of the family were judged to be homozygotes. Their parents were first cousins. All of five children were apparent heterozygotes. None of the heterozygotes had abnormal bleeding. The same abnormality was described in a family by Kanaska et al. (1963).

Cullum, C., Cooney, D. P. and Schrier, S. L.: Familial thrombocytopenic thrombocytopathy. Brit. J. Haemat. 13: 147-159, 1967.

Kanaska, B., Niewiarowski, S. and Ostrowski, L.: Macrothrombocytic thrombopathia. Clinical, coagulation and hereditary aspects. Thromb. Diath. Haemorrh. 10: 88-100, 1963.

27420 THUMB, DISTAL HYPEREXTENSIBILITY OF

According to Glass and Kistler (1953), among whites 24.7 percent and among Negroes 35.6 percent showed the trait. Penetrance was calculated as 96.5 percent. Hyperextensible thumb was judged to be recessive, the responsible gene having a frequency of 0.496 in U.S. whites.

Glass, B. and Kistler, J. C.: Distal hyperextensibility of the thumb. Acta Genet. Statist. Med. 4: 192-206, 1953.

27423 THYMOMA, FAMILIAL

Matani and Dristsas (1973) reported a Greek sibship of three, demonstrating familial occurrence of thymoma. One of the three sibs, a 2-year-old girl, died of respiratory insufficiency resulting from a lymphocytic thymoma. Her 9-month-old brother died two years earlier of the same cause. The eldest sib, a male, and the parents were healthy. No reference was made concerning parental consanguinity. Thymomas are notably rare in persons of this young age.

Lattes, R.: Thymoma and other tumors of the thymus: an analysis of 107 cases. Cancer 15: 1224-1260, 1962.

Legg, M. A. and Brady, W. J.: Pathology and clinical behavior of thymomas: a survey of 51 cases. Cancer 18: 1131-1144, 1965.

Matani, A. and Dristsas, C.: Familial occurrence of thymoma. Arch. Path. 95: 90-91, 1973.

27425 THYROGLOBULIN SYNTHESIS (DIMINISHED OR ALTERED)

Since thyroglobulin is a large, complex protein that plays an important role in hormonogenesis, it is probable that errors in the synthesis of this protein could occur and that they would tend to cause disease. Riddick et al. (1969) has reported on three goitrous members of a sibship of four. These patients had hypothyroidism or compensated hypothyroidism, had normal or high uptake of radioiodine, and biochemical measurements on removed thyroid tissue showed absence of thyroglobulin with the appearance of abnormal light iodoproteins. Other descriptions of abnormal or altered biosynthesis of thyroglobulins are discussed by Stanbury (1972).

Riddick, F. A., Jr., Desai, K. B., Murison, P. J. and Stanbury, J. B.: Familial goiter with diminished synthesis of thyroglobulin. Z. Exp. Med. 150: 203-212, 1969.

Stanbury, J. B.: Familial goiter. In, Stanbury, J. B., Wyngaarden, J. B. and Fredrickson, D. S. (eds.): The Metabolic Basis of Inherited Disease. New York: McGraw-Hill, 1972 (3rd Ed.). Pp. 223-265.

27430 THYROID HORMONE UNRESPONSIVENESS

Among 2 of 6 children of a consanguineous marriage, Refetoff et al. (1967) observed deaf-mutism, strippled epiphyses, goiter and abnormally high PBI. They postulated end-organ unresponsiveness to thyroid hormone. Other autosomal end-organ unresponsive states behave as dominants. Exceptions to this statement include unresponsiveness to thyrotropin and adrenal unresponsiveness to ACTH. A different type of unresponsiveness to thyroid hormones, presumably genetic, was reported by Lamberg (1973), who described a 25-year-old woman who had had goiter at birth and undergone thyroidectomy twice for non-toxic goiter during childhood. Concentrations of thyroid hormones and of thyrotropin in the blood were about twice normal and responses to thyrotropin-releasing hormone were normal. The findings were considered compatible with partial resistance to thyroid hormones in peripheral tissues, including the anterior pituitary. A similar patient may have been reported by Bode et al. (1972).

Bode, H., Danon, M., Maloof, F., Weintraub, B. and Crawford, J. D.: (Abstract, p. 23) 48th Meeting of Am. Thyroid Ass., Chicago, 1972.

Lamberg, B. A.: Congenital euthyroid goiter and partial peripheral resistance to thyroid hormones. Lancet I: 854-857, 1973.

R
E
C
E
S
S
I
V
E

Refetoff, S., De Wind, L. T. and De Groot, L. J.: Familial syndrome combining deaf-mutism, stippled epiphyses, goiter and abnormally high PBI: possible target organ refractoriness to thyroid hormone. J. Clin. Endocr. 27: 279-294, 1967.

*27440 THYROID HORMONOGENESIS, GENETIC DEFECT IN, I (ACCUMULATION, TRANSPORT OR TRAPPING DEFECT)

This defect is characterized by an inability of the thyroid to maintain a concentration difference of readily exchangeable iodine between the plasma and the thyroid gland. The defect is also found in the salivary gland and gastric mucosa. It is presumed to arise either because of a deficient supply of energy for the transport system or because of abnormality of a carrier or receptor substance. Parental consanguinity was present in the case of Stanbury and Chapman (1960).

Beierwaltes, W. H.: Genetics of thyroid disease. In, Hazard, J. B. and Smith, D. E. (eds.): The Thyroid. Baltimore: Williams and Wilkins Co., 1964.

Stanbury, J. B. and Chapman, E. M.: Congenital hypothyroidism with goiter: absence of an iodide-concentrating mechanism. Lancet I: 1162-1165, 1960.

Stanbury, J. B.: Familial goiter. In, Stanbury, J. B., Wyngaarden, J. B. and Fredrickson, D. S. (eds.): The Metabolic Basis of Inherited Disease. New York: McGraw-Hill, 1972 (3rd Ed.). Pp. 223-265.

*27450 THYROID HORMONOGENESIS, GENETIC DEFECT IN, IIA (ORGANIFICATION DEFECT I)

This defect may include two distinct types. In both, the ability to iodinate tyrosyl residues with intrathyroidal iodine is impaired. A severe type may lack an iodide peroxidase. Accumulated iodide is precipitously discharged from the gland on administration of thiocyanate. Hagen et al. (1971), in a 16-year-old girl with euthyroidism, normal hearing and goiter, found deficient peroxidase activity in thyroid tissue. Enzyme activity was restored by addition of hematin, the prosthetic group of peroxidase. They concluded that the defect may concern the binding of the prosthetic group by the apoenzyme. A sister was identically affected. 50 percent of thyroidal iodine was released by perchlorate, suggesting the defect in Pendred syndrome (27460). Valenta et al. (1971) presented direct proof of a defect in thyroid peroxidase in a patient with congenital goitrous hypothyroidism.

Hagen, G. A., Niepomniszcze, H., Haibach, H., Bigazzi, M., Hati, R., Rapoport, B., Jimenez, C., Degroot, L. J. and Frawley, T. F.: Peroxidase deficiency in familial goiter with iodide organification defect. New Eng. J. Med. 285: 1394-1398, 1971.

Leszynsky, H. E.: Genetic studies in familial goitrous cretinism. (Abstract) Acta Endocr. 46: 103-110, 1964.

Parker, R. H. and Beierwaltes, W. H.: Inheritance of defective organification of iodine in familial goitrous cretinism. J. Clin. Endocr. 21: 21-30, 1961.

Stanbury, J. B.: The metabolic errors in certain types of familial goiter. Recent Prog. Hormone Res. 19: 547-577, 1963.

Valenta, L., Bode, H. H., Vickery, A. L. and Maloof, F.: Lack of thyroid peroxidase activity: a cause of congenital goitrous hypothyroidism. (Abstract) J. Clin. Invest. 50: 94A-95A, 1971.

*27460 THYROID HORMONOGENESIS, GENETIC DEFECT IN, IIB (ORGANIFICATION DEFECT II)

A milder type of organification defect is associated with congenital deafness (Pendred syndrome) and may be the result of lack of an iodinase. See PENDRED SYNDROME. Patients with the milder defect show only partial discharge of iodine when thiocyanate is given. Fraser (1967) raises the question of whether the organification defect without deafness as described by Stanbury and Hedge (1950) is different from the organification defect with deafness as described by Pendred. Fraser raises the possibility that variability in severity of one and the same defect may be involved. He supports this contention with the description of a patient with unilateral deafness whose sister, also with Pendred syndrome, had bilateral deafness. Also cases of the full syndrome and cases with near normal hearing occurred in the same family. A partial organification defect without deafness and with goiter and euthyroid state was described in 3 sibs by Furth et al. (1967).

Fraser, G. R.: Adelaide, Australia: personal communication, 1967.

Furth, E. D., Carvalho, M. and Vianna, B.: Familial goiter due to an organification defect in euthyroid siblings. J. Clin. Endocr. 27: 1137-1140, 1967.

Stanbury, J. B. and Hedge, A. N.: A study of a family of goitrous cretins. J. Clin. Endocr. 10: 1471-1484, 1950.

*27470 THYROID HORMONOGENESIS, GENETIC DEFECT IN, III (COUPLING DEFECT)

Patients with the iodotyrosyl coupling defect fail to couple enough of these residues into iodothyronine hormones. This may be the result of absence of a hypothetical 'coupling enzyme' or of a structural abnormality in thyroglobulin which makes intramolecular coupling more difficult. The defect can be detected with certainty only by showing that iodothyronines fail to appear in biopsy specimens of thyroid tissue.

Alexander, N. M. and Burrow, G. N.: Thyroxine biosynthesis in human goitrous cretinism. J. Clin. Endocr. 30: 308-315, 1970.

Morris, J. H.: Defective coupling of iodotyrosine in familial goiters: report of two patients. Arch. Intern. Med. 114: 417-423, 1964.

R E C E S S I V E

*27480 THYROID HORMONOGENESIS, GENETIC DEFECT IN, IV (DEFECT OF IODOTYROSINE DEHALOGENASE, OR DEIODINASE)

The iodotyrosine dehalogenase defect is characterized by an inability of many tissues, including the thyroid, to deiodinate MIT and DIT. As a result intravenously administered labelled DIT appears intact in the urine. This is the only thyroid defect for which the specific enzyme involved has been identified. Hutchison and McGirr (1956) studied this disorder in an inbred group of itinerant tinkers in western Scotland. Werdnig-Hoffmann paralysis occurred in the same group. Among 7 sibs from related parents, Kusakabe and Miyake (1964) found three in whom peripheral deiodination occurred but none was produced by thyroid biopsy tissue. Thus, two entities may exist in this class.

Hutchison, J. H. and McGirr, E. M.: Sporadic non-endemic goitrous cretinism. Hereditary transmission. Lancet 1: 1035-1037, 1956.

Kusakabe, T. and Miyake, T.: Thyroidal deiodination defect in three sisters with simple goiter. J. Clin. Endocr. 24: 456-459, 1964.

*27490 THYROID HORMONOGENESIS, GENETIC DEFECT IN, V (PLASMA IODOPROTEIN DEFECT)

Patients with the serum iodoprotein disorder have large amounts of an albumin-like iodoprotein in the plasma. The source of this component could be a normal but minor pathway of iodine metabolism in the thyroid which expands because of a block in the normal thyroglobulin pathway, or it may appear simply as a result of hyperplasia of the gland from some undisclosed cause, or because a structural abnormality of the cell membrane permits albumin to enter and leave the cell, being iodinated in the process. Lissitzky et al. (1967) described a 12-year-old boy with congenital goiter and hypothyroidism. The parents were second cousins. In the thyroid tissue thyroglobulin was practically absent and was replaced by iodinated albumin-like proteins. Although the sister was euthyroidal, she had goiter with high RAI uptake by the thyroid and low PBI as in her brother. Complicating interpretation is the presence of asymptomatic goiter in the mother and her sister.

Lissitzky, S., Codaccioni, J. L., Bismuth, J. and Depieds, R.: Congenital goiter with hypothyroidism and iodo-serum albumin replacing thyroglobulin. J. Clin. Endocr. 27: 185-196, 1967.

27500 THYROTOXICOSIS (GRAVES DISEASE)

R
E
C
E
S
S
I
V
E

Bartels (1941) claimed that this disorder is inherited as a simple autosomal recessive with relative sex limitation to females and a reduced penetrance (70-80 percent) in homozygotes. Martin and Fisher (1945) also postulated a recessive factor predisposing to exophthalmic goiter. In contrast, these workers (1951) could find no evidence of hereditary basis of toxic nodular goiter. Ingbar and colleagues (1956) found abnormalities of thyroid metabolism in euthyroid relatives of thyrotoxic patient. Levit in early studies in the U.S.S.R. was more inclined toward dominant inheritance (Fraser, 1967). Neither the recessive nor the dominant hypothesis has satisfactory proof. Impressively extensive involvement occurs in some families. Skillern (1972) favored polygenic inheritance for hyperthyroidism and for Hashimoto thyroiditis (14030) which may accompany it.

Bartels, E. D.: Heredity in Graves' Disease. Copenhagen: Munksgaard, 1941.

Fraser, G. R.: Adelaide, Australia: personal communication, 1967.

Ingbar, S. H., Freinkel, N., Dowling, J. T. and Kumagai, L. F.: Abnormalities of iodine metabolism in euthyroid relatives of patients with Graves' disease. (Abstract) J. Clin. Invest. 35: 714 only, 1956.

Martin, L. and Fisher, R. A.: The hereditary and familial aspects of exophthalmic goiter and nodular goitre. Quart. J. Med. 14: 207-219, 1945.

Martin, L. and Fisher, R. A.: The hereditary and familial aspects of toxic nodular goitre (secondary thyrotoxicosis). Quart. J. Med. 20: 293-297, 1951.

Skillern, P. G.: Genetics of Graves' disease. Mayo Clin. Proc. 47: 848-849, 1972.

*27510 THYROTROPIN DEFICIENCY, ISOLATED

Although more than a dozen cases of isolated thyrotropin deficiency have been reported, the first familial incidence was described by Miyai et al. (1971), who observed two sisters with cretinism. Synthetic thyrotropin-releasing hormone resulted in no rise in serum TSH levels. The parents were second cousins. A male sib, who died at age 3 years, may also have been affected. Isolated TSH deficiency has been described (Zisman et al., 1969) in patients with pseudohypoparathyroidism (Albright hereditary osteodystrophy, q.v.). Thyrotropin is more generally known as TSH (thyroid-stimulating hormone). The use of thyrotropin-releasing hormone (TRH) produced by the hypothalamus reveals the existence of isolated hypothalamic hypothyroidism indistinguishable from TSH deficiency (Pittman et al., 1971). TRH is synthesized enzymatically (Mitnick and Reichlin, 1972).

Grabow, J. D. and Chou, S. M.: Thyrotropin hormone deficiency with a peripheral neuropathy. Arch. Neurol. 19: 284-291, 1968.

Mitnick, M. and Reichlin, S.: Enzymatic synthesis of thyrotropin-releasing hormone (TRH) by hypothalamic 'TRH synthetase.' Endocrinology 91: 1145-1153, 1972.

Miyai, K., Azukizawa, M. and Kumahara, Y.: Familial isolated thyrotropin deficiency with cretinism. New Eng. J. Med. 285: 1043-1048, 1971.

O'Dell, W. D.: Isolated deficiencies of anterior pituitary hormones: symptoms and diagnosis. J.A.M.A. 197: 1006-1016, 1966.

Pittman, J. A., Jr., Haigler, E. D., Jr., Hershman, J. M. and Pittman, C. S.: Hypothalamic hypothyroidism. New Eng. J. Med. 285: 844-845, 1971.

Sawin, C. T. and McHugh, J. E.: Isolated lack of thyrotropin in man. J. Clin. Endocr. 26: 955-959, 1966.

Zisman, E., Lotz, M., Jenkins, M. E. and Bartter, F. C.: Studies in pseudohypoparathyroidism. Two new cases with a probable selective deficiency of thyrotropin. Am. J. Med. 46: 464-471, 1969.

27520 THYROTROPIN, UNRESPONSIVENESS TO

Stanbury et al. (1968) described an 8-year-old boy with congenital hypothyroidism who was the offspring of parents related as first cousins once removed. He showed high serum levels of biologically active thyrotropin but no response to thyrotropin in viro or in his thyroid tissue slices in vitro. End-organ unresponsiveness was suggested. Stanbury (1972) tells me he knows of no other case.

Stanbury, J. B.: Cambridge, Mass.: personal communication, Dec. 1972.

Stanbury, J. B., Rocmans, P., Buhler, U. K. and Ochi, Y.: Congenital hypothyroidism with impaired thyroid response to thyrotropin. New Eng. J. Med. 279: 1132-1136, 1968.

*27525 TONGUE, PIGMENTED FUNGIFORM PAPILLAE OF

Negroes in particular may show spotted pigmentation of the tip of the tongue. The melanin is located on the summit of the fungiform papillae. Davis (1968) commented on the occurrence of pigmented spots and patches of the tongue, a possibly different phenotype. Rao (1970) collected data on 132 families from West Burgal and concluded that the trait segregates, the 'normal' allele being dominant over the 'pigmented' allele, i.e., pigment spots (or patches) being a recessive trait.

Davis, T. A.: Biology in the Tropics. In, Dronamaraju, K. (ed.): Haldane and Modern Biology. Baltimore: The Johns Hopkins Press, 1968. Pp. 327-333.

Koplon, B. S. and Hurley, H. J.: Prominent pigmented papillae of the tongue. Arch. Derm. 95: 394-396, 1967.

Monash, S.: Normal pigmentation of the oral mucosa. Arch. Derm. Syph. 26: 139-147, 1932.

Rao, D. C.: Tongue pigmentation in man. Hum. Hered. 20: 8-12, 1970.

Rao, D. C., Satynarayana, M., Veerraju, P. and Rao, B. B.: Tongue pigmentation in man: ethnic studies and further pedigrees. Acta Genet. Med. Gem. 21: 221-232, 1972.

Rao, D. C.: Formal segregation analysis for tongue pigmentation in man. Hum. Hered. 23: 308-312, 1973.

27530 TRACHEOBRONCHOMEGALY

Johnston and Green (1965) presented 5 cases of which two were Negro brother and sister. Chromosome studies were normal. The parents and five other sibs appeared to be unaffected. Two sibs died in early infancy. In one mongolism was diagnosed. Although bronchopulmonary suppuration largely determines the degree of respiratory disability, infection is not responsible for the underlying lesion of the tracheobronchial tree. The characteristic bronchographic picture led several workers to call it trachiectasis with multiple diverticula. The appearance is created by enlargement of the airways and musculo-membranous tissue projecting like corrugations between the cartilaginous rings. The Negro patient reported by Aaby and Blake (1966) probably suffered from Ehlers-Danlos syndrome.

Aaby, G. V. and Blake, H. A.: Tracheobronchiomegaly. Ann. Thorac. Surg. 2: 64-70, 1966.

Johnston, R. F. and Green, R. A.: Tracheobronchiomegaly: report of five cases and demonstration of familial occurrence. Am. Rev. Resp. Dis. 91: 35-50, 1965.

*27535 TRANSCOBALAMIN II DEFICIENCY

Hakami et al. (1971) described macrocytic anemia and other manifestations of vitamin B12 deficiency in two infant sibs who had normal levels of serum B12. Deficiency in the B12 transport protein transcobalamin II was demonstrated. A partial deficiency in both parents and other hematologically normal relatives indicated autosomal recessive inheritance. Decreased intestinal absorption of B12, uncorrected by intrinsic factor, suggested that transcobalamin II is involved in B12 absorption. B12 responsive megaloblastic anemias of the pediatric age group included a form due to lack of intrinsic factor (26100) and a form due to a defect in intestinal absorption, with associated proteinuria (26110). TC II is a plasma globulin which is believed to be the primary transport protein for vitamin B12. Genetic absence leads to severe megaloblastic anemia in early infancy. Scott et al. (1972) concluded that no defect in homocysteine methyltransferase or methylmalonyl CoA mutase occurs in these patients and that TC II is normally necessary mainly for delivery of the cobalamin molecule to the hematopoietic system.

Hakami, N., Neiman, P. E., Canellos, G. P. and Lazerson, J.: Neonatal magaloblastic anemia due to inherited transcobalamin II deficiency in two siblings. New Eng. J. Med. 285: 1163-1170, 1971.

Scott, C. R., Hakami, N., Teng, C. C. and Sagerson, R. N.: Hereditary transcobalamin II deficiency: the role of transcobalamin II in vitamin B12 dependent reactions in man. J. Pediat. 81: 1106-1111, 1972.

*27537 TRICARBOXYLIC ACID CYCLE, DEFECT OF

Blass et al. (1972) studied cultured skin fibroblasts from the daughter of a couple related as second cousins once removed. An older sister had died in early childhood. The proband, aged 3 years, had severe generalized neurologic disease and persistent lactic acidosis. Radioactive citrate, palmitate and pyruvate were oxidized at a rate less than one-third of normal. Deficiency was identified in the activity of the pyruvate dehydrogenase complex although not in the thiamine-dependent first enzyme of that complex. The patient was thought to have a partial genetic defect affecting the tricarboxylic acid cycle. For discussion of the enzyme complex involved, see Reed and Cox (1970).

Blass, J. P., Schulman, J. D., Young, D. S. and Hom, E.: An inherited defect affecting the tricarboxylic acid cycle in a patient with congenital lactic acidosis. J. Clin. Invest. 51: 1845-1851, 1972.

Reed, L. J. and Cox, D. J.: Multienzyme complexes. In, Boyer, P. D.: The Enzymes. New York: Academic Press, 1970. Vol. 1, Pp. 213-240.

27540 TRICHOMEGALY (EXCESSIVE GROWTH OF EYELASHES AND BROW HAIR) WITH MENTAL RETARDATION, DWARFISM AND PIGMENTARY DEGENERATION OF RETINA

Excessive growth of eyelashes and brow hair is probably a familial trait. Oliver and McFarlane (1965) described an isolated case of a male child with low birth weight dwarfism, very long eyelashes and eyebrows, mental retardation and pigmentary degeneration of the retina. The karyotype was normal and the parents were not consanguineous. I have seen sibs with long eyelashes and mental retardation. Corby et al. (1971) reported a case of the full syndrome.

Cant, J. S.: Ectodermal dysplasia. J. Pediat. Ophthal. 4 (no. 4): 13-17, 1967.

Corby, D. G., Lowe, R. S., Jr., Haskins, R. C. and Hebertson, L. M.: Trichomegaly, pigmentary degeneration of the retina, and growth retardation. Am. J. Dis. Child. 121: 344-345, 1971.

Oliver, G. L. and McFarlane, D. C.: Congenital trichomegaly with associated pigmentary degeneration of the retina, dwarfism and mental retardation. Arch. Ophthal. 74: 169-171, 1965.

27550 TRICHORHINOPHALANGEAL SYNDROME

Giedion (1966) delineated a new syndrome consisting of thin and slowly growing hair, pear-shaped nose with high philtrum, brachyphalangy with deformation of the fingers and wedge-shaped epiphyses. Giedion's patient, a girl, had 2 supernumerary incisors. In the literature he found two previous reports each describing two affected sibs. Furthermore the parents were consanguineous in one case. One of the pairs of affected sibs was reported as pseudo-pseudohypoparathyroidism (van der Werff Ten Bosch, 1959). We have observed affected brother and sister whose parents are not related and allegedly are unaffected but the father was not available for examination (Hussels, 1971). While showing that in most instances inheritance is autosomal dominant (19035), Giedion et al. (1973) concluded that a recessive form probably exists.

Giedion, A.: Das Tricho-rhino-phalangeal syndrom. Helv. Paediat. Acta 21: 475-482, 1966.

Giedion, A.: Zapfenepiphysen. Naturgeschichte und diagnostische Bedeutung einer stoerung des enchondralen Wachstums. Ergebn. Med. Radiol. 8: 59-124, 1968.

Giedion, A., Burdea, M., Fruchter, Z., Meloni, T. and Trosc, V.: Autosomal dominant transmission of the tricho-rhino-phalangeal syndrome. Report of 4 unrelated families, review of 60 cases. Helv. Paediat. Acta 28: 249-259, 1973.

Hussels, I. E.: Trichorhinophalangeal syndrome in two sibs. The Clinical Delineation of Birth Defects. XI. Orofacial Structures. Baltimore: Williams and Wilkins, 1971. Pp. 301-303.

Van der Werff Ten Bosch, J. J.: The syndrome of brachymetacarpal dwarfism ('pseudo-pseudohypoparathyroidism') with and without gonadal dysgenesis. Lancet I: 69-71, 1959.

27555 TRICHORRHEXIS NODOSA SYNDROME

Pollitt et al. (1968) described a brother and sister with mental and physical retardation and trichorrhexis nodosa. Cystine content of the hair was about half normal (Pollitt, Stonier, 1971). This disorder bears some resemblance to that reported in the Amish and called here hair-brain syndrome (23405). Also see Netherton syndrome (25650).

Pollitt, R. J., Jenner, F. A. and Davies, M.: Sibs with mental and physical retardation and trichorrhexis nodosa with abnormal amino acid composition of the hair. Arch. Dis. Child. 43: 211-216, 1968.

Pollitt, R. J. and Stonier, P. D.: Proteins of normal hair and of cystine-deficient hair from mentally retarded siblings. Biochem. J. 122: 433-444, 1971.

27560 TRIGONOCEPHALY

Multiple affected sibs have been observed by DeMyer (1964). Agenesis of the olfactory bulbs and tracts is associated. It is an entity distinct from holoprosencephaly (q.v.) with which it, however, shares some features.

DeMyer, W.: Indianapolis, Ind.: personal communication, 1964.

27565 TRIHYDROXYCOPROSTANIC ACID IN BILE (ALLIGATOR DEFECT)

Eyssen et al. (1972) provided the first example of a possible Mendelian defect in bile acid synthesis. Normally bile acids are synthesized in the liver by hydrogenation and hydroxylation of the steroid nucleus of cholesterol, followed by oxidation of the side chain. In certain lower vertebrates, the side chain of cholesterol is oxidized but not degrated. The alligator, for example, has trihydroxycoprostanic acid as a major bile acid. Two brothers, of whom one was studied biochemically, had cholestasis and obstructive jaundice due to partial atresia of intrahepatic bile ducts. One died at 4 months, the other at 6 months. Of the bile acids in the duodenal fluid 19 percent was trihydroxycoprostanic acid. A second patient, a female, likewise had cholestatic jaundice, and trihydroxycoprostanic acid represented 45 percent of the duodenal bile acids. Hanson (1973) has a similar patient.

Eyssen, H., Parmentier, G., Compernolle, F., Boon, J. and Eggermont, E.: Trihydroxycoprostanic acid

R
E
C
E
S
S
I
V
E

in the duodenal fluid of two children with intrahepatic bile duct anomalies. Biochim. Biophys. Acta 273: 212-221, 1973.

Hanson, R.: Minneapolis: personal communication via Dr. Alan F. Hofmann, Rochester, Minn.

27570 TRIMETHYLAMINURIA (FISH-ODOR SYNDROME)

Humbert et al. (1970) described a 6 year old girl with multiple pulmonary infections beginning in the neonatal period and intermittently a fishy odor. Splenomegaly, anemia and neutropenia were also present. The urine contained increased amounts of trimethylamine. Trimethylamine (TMA) is a derivative of choline. TMA oxidase may be deficient. Defective membrane function was demonstrated in platelets, neutrophils and red cells (Humbert et al., 1971).

Humbert, J. R., Hammond, K. B., Hathaway, W. E., Marcoux, J. and O'Brien, D.: The stale-fish syndrome: a new metabolic disorder associated with trimethylaminuria. Pediat. Res. Soc., 1971.

Humbert, J. R., Hammond, K. B., Hathaway, W. E., Marcoux, J. and O'Brien, D.: Trimethylaminuria: the fish-odour syndrome. (Letter) Lancet II: 770-771, 1970.

*27580 TRIOSEPHOSPHATE ISOMERASE (TPI) DEFICIENCY

A form of non-spherocytic hemolytic anemia of Dacie's type II (in vitro autohemolysis is not corrected by added glucose) has been found to have a deficiency of red cell triosephosphate isomerase (Schneider et al., 1965). Association with recurrent infection and a progressive neurologic disorder characterized by spasticity was noted. The homozygotes show 6 percent of normal TPI activity in red cells and 20 percent in white cells. Heterozygotes show about 50 percent. From studies in the cri du chat syndrome, Sparkes et al. (1969) suggested that the TPI locus is on the short arm of chromosome 5. Others have failed to confirm this (Brock and Singer, 1970). See 19045.

Brock, D. J. H. and Singer, J. D.: Red cell triosephosphate isomerase gene. (Letter) Lancet II: 1136 only, 1970.

Peters, J., Hopkinson, D. A. and Harris, H.: Genetic and non-genetic variation of the triosephosphate isomerase isozymes in human tissues. Ann. Hum. Genet. 36: 297-312, 1973.

Rudiger, H. W., Passarge, E., Hirth, L., Goedde, H. W., Blume, K. G., Lohr, G. W., Benohr, H. C. and Waller, H. D.: Triosephosphate isomerase gene not localized on the short arm of chromosome 5 in man. (Letter) Nature 228: 1320-1321, 1970.

Schneider, A. S., Valentine, W. N., Hattori, M. and Heins, H. L., Jr.: Hereditary hemolytic anemia with triosephosphate isomerase deficiency. New Eng. J. Med. 272: 229-235, 1965.

Sparkes, R. S., Carrel, R. E. and Paglia, D. E.: Probable localization of a triosephosphate isomerase gene to the short arm of the no. 5 human chromosome. Nature 224: 367-368, 1969.

*27590 TROYER SYNDROME

In an Amish group in Ohio, Cross and McKusick (1967) observed 20 cases of spastic paraplegia with distal muscle wasting and designated it Troyer syndrome for the surname of many of the affected persons. The disorder has its onset in early childhood with dysarthria, distal muscle wasting and difficulty in learning to walk. Lower limb spasticity and contractures usually make walking impossible by the third or fourth decade. Drooling and mild cerebellar signs occur in some. All have weakness and atrophy of thenar, hypothena and dorsal interosseous muscles.

Cross, H. E. and McKusick, V. A.: The Troyer syndrome. A recessive form of spastic paraplegia with distal muscle wasting. Arch. Neurol. 16: 473-485, 1967.

*27600 TRYPSINOGEN DEFICIENCY

Failure to thrive, nutritional edema, and hypoproteinemia with normal sweat electrolytes were features of affected infants. A protein hydrolysate diet was beneficial. A male sib of Townes' first patient (1965) had died apparently of the same condition. Townes' two patients were male (1965, 1967). Morris and Fisher (1967) reported a female who also had imperforate anus. The clinical picture in enterokinase deficiency (q.v.) is closely similar but the defect is not in the synthesis of trypsinogen but in the synthesis of the enterokinase which stimulates secretion of proteolytic enzymes by the pancreas. Oral pancreatin represents a therapeutically successful form of enzyme replacement (Townes, 1972).

Morris, M. D. and Fisher, D. A.: Trypsinogen deficiency disease. Am. J. Dis. Child. 114: 203-208, 1967.

Townes, P. L.: Trypsinogen deficiency and other proteolytic deficiency diseases. The Clinical Delineation of Birth Defects. XIII. G. I. Tract Including Liver and Pancreas. Baltimore: Williams and Wilkins, 1972. Pp. 95-101.

Townes, P. L., Bryson, M. F. and Miller, G.: Further observations on trypsinogen deficiency disease: report of a case. J. Pediat. 71: 220-224, 1967.

Townes, P. L.: Trypsinogen deficiency disease. J. Pediat. 66: 275-285, 1965.

*27610 TRYPTOPHANURIA WITH DWARFISM

Tada, Ito, Wada and Arakawa (1963) described a 9 year old girl with dwarfism, mental defect, cutaneous photosensitivity and gait disturbance resembling cerebellar ataxia. The clinical features resembled Hartnup disease (q.v.) but the chemical findings were different. Tryptophane was excreted in the urine in excess without increase in indican or indole acetic acid excretion. With tryptophane loading the plasma level of tryptophane increased markedly and remained higher longer than in normals and tryptophanuria was

R
E
C
E
S
S
I
V
E

increased with relatively little increase in kynurenine excretion. The defect was thought to concern the conversion of tryptophane to kynurenine. The disorder was thought to have occurred in three children (two males and the female proband) in three sibships. All six parents were traced to a common ancestral couple. The proband showed conjunctival telangiectasia which together with ataxia creates similarities to ataxia-telangiectasia (q.v.).

Tada, K., Ito, H., Wada, Y. and Arakawa, T.: Congenital tryptophanuria with dwarfism ('H' disease-like clinical features without indicanuria and generalized aminoaciduria): a probably new inborn error of tryptophane metabolism. Tohoku J. Exp. Med. 80: 118-134, 1963.

27620 T-SUBSTANCE ANOMALY

Some of the children in whom unusual, as yet unidentified, T-substance has been found in the urine by paper chromatography have had severe mental and-or physical retardation.

Coles, H. M.: T-substance anomaly with horseshoe kidney. Proc. Roy. Soc. Med. 54: 330-331, 1961.

Coles, H. M., Priestman, A. and Wilkinson, J. H.: T-substance anomaly. An inborn error of purine metabolism. Lancet II: 1220-1223, 1960.

27630 TURCOT SYNDROME (MALIGNANT TUMORS OF THE CENTRAL NERVOUS SYSTEM ASSOCIATED WITH FAMILIAL POLYPOSIS OF THE COLON)

Turcot, Depres and St. Pierre (1959) described affected brother and sister. The parents were third cousins (personal communication from Turcot). Because of the association of colonic polyps with tumors of many types in the Gardner syndrome, it is possible that the sibs reported by Turcot and colleagues had that condition, a dominant (q.v.). The possibility is strengthened by the description by Yaffee (1964) of a case of Gardner syndrome whose 'uncle died of Turcot syndrome.' This might suggest that Turcot syndrome is merely an unusual mode of presentation of the Gardner syndrome, a dominant. The contrary view, that there exists a genuine syndrome of glioma and polyposis inherited as a recessive, is supported by the family reported by Baughman et al. (1969). A brother and two sisters had the full syndrome and another brother may have been affected. The parents were healthy and unrelated.

Baughman, F. A., Jr., List, C. F., Williams, J. R., Muldoon, J. P., Segarra, J. M. and Volkel, J. S.: The glioma-polyposis syndrome. New Eng. J. Med. 281: 1345-1346, 1969.

Turcot, J., Despres, J. P. and St. Pierre, F.: Malignant tumors of the central nervous system associated with familial polyposis of the colon: report of two cases. Dis. Colon Rectum 2: 465-468, 1959.

Yaffee, H. S.: Gastric polyposis and soft tissue tumors. A variant of Gardner's syndrome. Arch. Derm. 89: 806-808, 1964.

27640 TWINNING, DIZYGOTIC

Weinberg (1909) suggested that hereditary twinning is transmitted only through the female line, applies only to dizygotic twins, and is probably recessive. Observation of multiple births following use of pituitary gonadotropins suggests a pituitary mechanism for gene action (Milham, 1964). Wyshak and White (1965) presented evidence, based on Mormon records, which they interpreted as supporting recessive inheritance. Among the children of female DZ twins, 17.1 twins per 1000 maternities occurred as compared with 7.9 among children of male DZ twins. Female sibs of DZ twins had 17 per 1000 twins, whereas male sibs had 13.1 per 1000. Supposedly the gene is too frequent for one to expect increased consanguinity in the grandparents of dizygotic twins. Taylor (1931) reported multiple sets of dizygotic twins in four generations. In the same family mother and daughter did not menstruate until after their first pregnancies, at ages 20 and 22, respectively. The differentiation of multifactorial and monofactorial inheritance of twinning is difficult. Ethnic differences in the rate of dizygotic twinning is evidence of genetic factors. In interracial marriages the rate follows that of the mother's ethnic group. Furthermore, when the mother is a racial hybrid, the dizygotic twinning frequency is that of the race with the lower frequency, indicating the recessive nature of the genetic factors (Morton et al., 1967).

Milham, S., Jr.: Pituitary gonadotropin and dizygotic twinning. Lancet II: 566 only, 1964.

Morton, N. E., Chung, C. S. and Mi, M. P.: Genetics of interracial crosses in Hawaii. Monographs in Human Genetics, Vol. 3. Basel: S. Karger, 1967.

Taylor, C. E.: Four generations of heterosexual twins with prepartum amenorrhoea in two generations. Brit. Med. J. 2: 384 Only, 1931.

Weinberg, W.: Zur Bedeutung der Mehrlingsgeburten fur die Frage der Bestimmung des Geschlechts. Arch. Rass.-U. Ges. Biol. 6: 28-32, 1909.

Wyshak, G.: Distribution among relatives of genotypes for twinning. Biometrics 24: 179-185, 1968.

Wyshak, G. and White, C.: Genealogical study of human twinning. Am. J. Public Health 55: 1586-1593, 1965.

27650 TYROSINE METABOLISM, DELAYED MATURATION IN

Bloxam and colleagues (1960) found that 14 of 1276 infants tested had large amounts of p-hydroxyphe-nyl-pyruvic acid, p-hydroxyphenyl-lactic acid and tyrosine in the urine. The infants were on normal diet. A delay in maturation of an enzyme was postulated. A genetic basis was presumed and is indeed plausible but not proved.

Bloxam, H. R., Day, M. G., Gibbs, N. K. and Woolf, L. I.: An inborn defect in the metabolism of tyrosine in infants on a normal diet. Biochem. J. 77: 320-326, 1960.

R
E
C
E
S
S
I
V
E

Buist (1967) referred to studies of a child with tyrosinemia and tyrosine transaminase deficiency, but normal p-hydroxyphenylpyruvic acid oxidase. Phenylalanine level was normal. Hydroxyphenylpyruvic acid was elevated in the urine. Fellman et al. (1969) reported chemical studies on the same patient. Only the mitochondrial form of tyrosine aminotransferase was present in the liver. The soluble form of the enzyme was lacking. The patient had markedly elevated tyrosine blood levels and an increase in urinary p-hydroxyphenylpyruvate and p-hydroxyphenyllactate. Goldsmith et al. (1973) suggested that this child may have had the same defect as that they observed in the Richner-Hanhart syndrome (24480). A regulator gene for tyrosine transaminase is X-linked (31435).

Buist, N.: In, Nyhan, W. L. (ed.): Amino Acid Metabolism and Genetic Variation. New York: McGraw-Hill, 1967. P. 117.

Fellman, J. H., Vanbellinghen, P. J., Jones, R. T. and Koller, R. D.: Soluble and mitochondrial forms of tyrosine aminotransferase relationship to human tyrosinemia. Biochemistry 8: 615-622, 1969.

Goldsmith, L. A., Kang, E., Bienfang, D. C., Jimbow, K., Gerald, P. S. and Baden, H. P.: Tyrosinemia with plantar and palmar keratosis and keratitis. J. Pediat. 83: 798-805, 1973.

Kennaway, N. G. and Bruist, N. R. M.: Metabolic studies in a patient with hepatic cytosol tyrosine aminotransferase deficiency. Pediat. Res. 5: 287- , 1971.

*27670 TYROSINEMIA

Among the children of first-cousin parents, Lelong et al. (1963) observed two sons with cirrhosis, Fanconi syndrome and marked increase in plasma tyrosine. In the sib most extensively observed hepatosplenomegaly was discovered at 3 months of age and rickets at 18 months. Malignant changes developed in the liver and death from pulmonary metastases occurred shortly before his 5th birthday. The author suggested that the basic defect concerns an enzyme involved with tyrosine metabolism. Other cases are reported in the earlier literature. Himsworth has a similar case in his book on the liver. Gentz, Jagenburg and Zetterstrom (1965) described 7 patients in 4 families with multiple renal tubular defects like those of the de Toni-Debre-Fanconi syndrome, nodular cirrhosis of the liver and impaired tyrosine metabolism. P-hydroxyphenyllactic acid was excreted in unusually large amounts. A total lack of liver P-hydroxyphenylpyruvate oxidase activity was demonstrated. Tyrosine-alpha-ketoglutarate transaminase was normal. Scriver, Larochelle and Silverberg (1967) identified the disease in 35 French-Canadian infants of whom 16 were sibs (i.e., two or more in each of several families). Marked tyrosinemia and tyrosyluria were present. The urine contained para-hydroxy-phenylpyruvic acid (PHPPA) and lactic and acetic derivatives. Loading test with tyrosine and with PHPPA suggested deficient P-hydroxyphenylpyruvate oxidase activity, which was confirmed by assay of liver biopsy samples. In stage I infants exhibit hepatic necrosis and hypermethioninemia. In stage II nodular cirrhosis and chronic hepatic insufficiency without hypermethioninemia are found. In stage III renal tubular damage (Baber syndrome), often with hypophosphatemic rickets, appears. Low tyrosine diet arrested progression of the disease. Zetterstrom (1963) studied 7 cases coming from an isolated area of southwestern Sweden. Halvorsen et al. (1966) gave details on 6 cases from Norway. Recent evidence discussed by La Du and Gjessing (1972) is against the hypothesis that tyrosinemia is a P-hydroxyphenylpyruvic acid oxidase deficiency and they believe that further investigation is needed to explain the clinical and pathologic features of tyrosinemia.

Fritzell, S., Jagenburg, O. R. and Schnurer, L. B.: Familial cirrhosis of the liver, renal tubular defects with rickets and impaired tyrosine metabolism. Acta Paediat. 53: 18-32, 1964.

Gaull, G. E., Rassin, D. K., Sturman, J. A.: Significance of hypermethioninaemia in acute tyrosinosis. (Letter) Lancet I: 1318-1319, 1968.

Gentz, J., Jagenburg, R. and Zetterstrom, R.: Tyrosinemia. J. Pediat. 66: 670-696, 1965.

Halvorsen, S. and Gjessing, L. R.: Studies of tyrosinosis. I. Effect of low-tyrosine and low-phenylalanine diet. Brit. Med. J. 2: 1171-1173, 1964.

Halvorsen, S., Pande, H., Loken, A. C. and Gjessing, L. R.: Tyrosinosis. A Study Of 6 Cases. Arch. Dis. Child. 41: 238-249, 1966.

Kang, E. S. and Gerald, P. S.: Hereditary tyrosinemia and abnormal pyrrole metabolism. A patient with hereditary tyrosinemia is described who developed metabolic and clinical changes compatible with acute intermittent porphyria. J. Pediat. 77: 397-406, 1970.

La Du, B. N. and Gjessing, L. R.: Tyrosinosis and tyrosinemia. In, Stanbury, J. B., Wyngaarden, J. B. and Fredrickson, D. S. (eds.): The Metabolic Basis of Inherited Disease. New York: McGraw-Hill, 1972 (3rd. Ed.). Pp. 296-307.

La Du, B. N.: The enzymatic deficiency in tyrosinemia. Am. J. Dis. Child. 113: 54-57, 1967.

Laberge, C.: Hereditary tyrosinemia in a French-Canadian isolate. Am. J. Hum. Genet. 21: 36-45, 1969.

Lelong, M., Alagille, D., Gentil, C. I., Colin, J., Le Tan, V. and Gabilan, J. C.: Cirrhose congenitale et familiale avec diabete phospho-gluco-amine, rachitisme vitamin D-resistant et tyrosinurie massive. Rev. Franc. Etude. Clin. Biol. 8: 37-50, 1963.

Scriver, C. R., Larochelle, J. and Silverberg, M.: Hereditary tyrosinemia and tyrosyluria in a French-Canadian geographic isolate. Am. J. Dis. Child. 113: 41-46, 1967.

Scriver, C. R., Partington, M. W. and Sass-Kortsak, A.: Conference on hereditary tyrosinemia held at the Hospital for Sick Children. Canad. Med. Ass. J. 97: 1045-1100, 1967.

RECESSIVE

Whelan, D. T. and Zannoni, V. G.: Microassay of tyrosine-amino transferase and p-hydroxyphenyl-pyruvic acid oxidase in mammalian liver and patients with hereditary tyrosinemia. Biochem. Med. 9: 19-31, 1974.

Zetterstrom, R.: Tyrosinosis. Ann. N.Y. Acad. Sci. 111: 220-226, 1963.

27680 TYROSINOSIS

Confusion exists between the terms 'tyrosinemia' and 'tyrosinosis.' La Du (personal communication, 1966) suggests that the problem is best solved by reserving the term 'tyrosinosis' for the apparently unique condition reported by Medes (1932). The defect in her patient may have involved liver tyrosine transaminase, see 27660, not P-hydroxyphenylpyruvic acid oxidase as she postulated. The patient was a 49-year-old male Russian Jew, diagnosed as having myasthenia gravis. La Du and Gjessing (1972) have discussed the evidence supporting the localization of this defect in various steps of tyrosine metabolism. Until other patients with this disease are discovered, no definite conclusion can be reached.

La Du, B. N. and Gjessing, L. R.: Tyrosinosis and tyrosinemia. In, Stanbury, J. B., Wyngaarden, J. B. and Fredrickson, D. S. (eds.): The Metabolic Basis of Inherited Disease. New York: McGraw-Hill, 1972 (3rd. Ed.).

Medes, G.: A new error of tyrosine metabolism: tyrosinosis. The intermediary metabolism of tyrosine and phenylalanine. Biochem. J. 26: 917-940, 1932.

*27690 USHER SYNDROME (RETINITIS PIGMENTOSA AND CONGENITAL DEAFNESS)

Lang (1959) observed five affected children out of ten from a first-cousin marriage. Lindenov (1945) wrote on deaf-mutism associated with retinitis pigmentosa and feeblemindedness. Kloepfer, Laguaite and McLaurin (1966) identified 537 persons with hearing loss in a French 'Cajun' group in Louisiana. Of the 468 living persons with hearing loss at least 158 or about 30 percent were known to have retinitis pigmentosa and cataract. The first description of this syndrome was by Liebreich (1861) who commented on a relatively high frequency in Jews in Berlin. Von Graefe (1858) may have given the earliest description. Hammerschlag (1907) made a similar observation in Vienna. Hallgren (1959) found 177 affected persons in 102 families. In addition to the features noted in the title of his paper, cataract developed by age 40 in most. Mental deficiency and psychosis occurred each in about one-quarter of cases. A large majority had a disturbance of gait attributed to a lesion of the labyrinth. In Finland, Nuutila (1970) found 133 persons with retinitis pigmentosa and congenital sensory deafness, 4 with RP and progressive sensory deafness. On the basis of 133 patients in Finland, Forsius et al. (1971) concluded that there are two distinct forms of the Usher syndrome: one characterized by congenital deafness and severe retinitis pigmentosa, and a second less frequent form in which the inner ear and retina are both less severely affected. Whether these are allelic forms or not is unknown. Holland et al. (1972) found gyrate atrophy in a few heterozygotes.

De Haas, E. B. H., Van Lith, G. H. M., Rijnders, J., Rumke, A. M. L. and Volmer, C. H.: Usher's syndrome, with special reference to heterozygous manifestations. Docum. Ophthal. 28: 166-190, 1970.

Forsius, H., Erikkson, A., Nuutila, A., Vainio-Mattila, B. and Krause, U.: A genetic study of three rare retinal disorders: dystrophia retinae dysacusis syndrome, X-chromosomal retinoschisis and grouped pigments of the retina. The Clinical Delineation of Birth Defects. VIII. Eye. Baltimore: Williams and Wilkins, 1971.

Hallgren, B.: Retinitis pigmentosa combined with congenital deafness: with vestibulo-cerebellar ataxia and mental abnormality in a proportion of cases. Acta Psychiat. Neurol. Scand. 34: (suppl. 138) 9-101, 1959.

Hammerschlag, V.: Zur Kenntnis der hereditaer-degenerativen Taubstummen und ihre differential-diagnostische Bedeutung. Z. Ohrenheilk. 54: 18-36, 1907.

Holland, M. G., Cambie, E. and Kloepfer, W.: An evaluation of genetic carriers of Usher's syndrome. Am. J. Ophthal. 74: 940-947, 1972.

Kloepfer, H. W., Laguaite, J. K. and McLaurin, J. W.: The hereditary syndrome of congenital deafness and retinitis pigmentosa: (Usher's syndrome). Laryngoscope 76: 850-862, 1966.

Lang, H. A.: Retinal degeneration and nerve deafness. Brit. Med. J. 2: 1096 only, 1959.

Liebreich, R.: Abkunft aus Ehen unter Blutsverwandten als Grund von Retinitis pigmentosa. Dtsch. Klin. 13: 53, 1861.

Lindenov, H.: The Etiology of Deaf-mutism with Special Reference to Heredity. Copenhagen: E. Munksgaard, 1945.

Nuutila, A.: Dystrophia retinae pigmentosa-dysacusis syndrome (DRD): a study of the Usher or Hallgren syndrome. J. Genet. Hum. 18: 57-88, 1970.

Usher, C. H.: Bowman's lecture: on a few hereditary eye affections. Trans. Ophthal. Soc. U.K. 55: 164-245, 1935.

Von Graefe, A.: Exceptionelles Verhalten des Gesichtsfeldes bei Pigmententartung der nefzhaut. Graefes Arch. Ophthal. 4: 250-253, 1858.

Vernon, M.: Usher's syndrome-deafness and progressive blindness. Clinical cases, prevention, theory and literature survey. J. Chronic Dis. 22: 133-151, 1969.

*27700 VAGINA, ABSENCE OF (ROKITANSKY-KUSTER-HAUSER SYNDROME; UTERUS BIPARTITUS SOLIDUS RUDIMENTARIUS CUM VAGINA SOLIDA)

The features, in addition to congenital absence of the vagina, are normal female secondary sexual

R
E
C
E
S
S
I
V
E

characteristics, rudimentary uterus in the form of bilateral and non-canaliculated muscular buds, normal tubes and ovaries and normal endocrine and cytogenetic evaluations. Anger et al. (1966) reported three affected sisters. Phaneuf (1947) described the malformation in two pairs of sisters whose mothers were sisters. Las Casas dos Santos (1888) reported early familial cases. Bryan et al. (1949) mentioned that in one of their 100 cases a sister had congenital absence of the vagina and each of two had a sister with primary amenorrhea. Jones and Mermut (1972) concluded that most of the earlier reported cases except those of Anger et al. (1966) were instances of testicular feminization. They reported two affected sisters. Karyotype was normal. The abnormality in sexual development in the R-K-H syndrome is the same as that in the syndrome of Klippel-Feil deformity, conductive deafness, absent vagina (14886).

Anger, D., Hemet, J. and Ensel, J.: Forme familiale du syndrome de Rokitansky-Kuster-Hauser. Bull. Fed. Gynec. Obstet. Franc. 18: 229-234, 1966.

Bryan, A. L., Nigro, J. A. and Counseller, V. S.: One-hundred cases of congenital absence of the vagina. Surg. Gynec. Obstet. 88: 79-86, 1949.

Jones, H. W. and Mermut, S.: Familial occurrence of congenital absence of the vagina. Am. J. Obstet. Gynec. 114: 1100-1101, 1972.

Las Casas Dos Santos, (NI): Missbildungen des Uterus. Z. Geburtsh. Gynaek. 14: 140-184, 1888.

Phaneuf, L. E.: Discussion (congenital malformations of the reproductive organs). Am. J. Obstet. Gynec. 53: 48 only, 1947.

*27710 VALINEMIA

Urinary and serum valine were elevated, without elevation of leucine and isoleucine, in a child with vomiting, failure to thrive and drowsiness (Wada et al., 1963). The parents, who were not known to be related, both showed abnormally large amounts of valine in the urine. The deficient enzyme is valine transaminase. Observation of this condition and sweaty feet disease indicates that different enzymes are involved in the metabolism of valine, leucine and isoleucine. Dancis et al. (1967) presented evidence that the transamination of valine is dependent on an enzyme specific for valine. They showed further that transamination of valine is demonstrable in the normal placenta. It might be possible to make a prenatal diagnosis of valinemia by needle biopsy of the placenta, in instances of an affected previously born sib.

Dancis, J., Hutzler, J., Tada, K., Wada, Y., Morikawa, T. and Arakawa, T.: Hypervalinemia: a defect in valine transamination. Pediatrics 39: 813-817, 1967.

Tada, K., Wada, Y. and Arakawa, T.: Hypervalinemia: its metabolic lesion and therapeutic approach. Am. J. Dis. Child. 113: 64-67, 1967.

Wada, Y., Tada, K., Minagawa, A., Yoshida, T., Morikawa, T. and Okamura, T.: Idiopathic hypervalinemia. Probably a new entity of inborn error of valine metabolism. Tohoku J. Exp. Med. 81: 46-55, 1963.

*27715 VAN BOGAERT-HOZAY SYNDROME

Van Bogaert (1953) and Hozay (1953) described a form of acro-osteolysis with facial abnormalities in a brother and sister aged 27 and 28. The parents were distantly related. The fingers and toes appeared infantile. The distal end of the ulna was underdeveloped. The facies were characterized by flat nasal bridge, thickened cheeks, deformed ears, micrognathia with abnormal dental position, and absent beard. Myopia and astigmatism were present. The male was mildly retarded, the female had done well in school.

Hozay, H.: Sur une dystrophie familiale particuliere. Inhibition precoce de la croissance et osteolyse non-mutilante acrale avec dysmorphie faciale. Rev. Neurol. 89: 245- , 1953.

Van Bogaert, L.: Essai de classement et d'interpretation de quelques acro-osteolyses multilantes et non-mutilantes actuellement connues. Acta Neurol. Belg. 53: 90-115, 1953.

27720 VENTRICLE, HYPOPLASIA OF RIGHT

Hypoplasia of the right ventricle and tricuspid valve was observed in brother and sister by Davachi et al. (1967), who pointed out that at least two families with multiple affected sibs have been reported (Medd et al., 1961; Sackner et al., 1961).

Davachi, F., McLean, R. H., Moller, J. H. and Edwards, J. E.: Hypoplasia of the right ventricle and tricuspid valve in siblings. J. Pediat. 71: 869-874, 1967.

Medd, W. E., Neufeld, H. N., Weidman, W. H. and Edwards, J. E.: Isolated hypoplasia of the right ventricle and tricuspid valve in siblings. Brit. Heart J. 23: 25-30, 1961.

Sackner, M. A., Robinson, M. J., Jamison, W. L. and Lewis, D. H.: Isolated right ventricular hypoplasia with atrial septal defect or patent foramen ovale. Circulation 24: 1388-1402, 1961.

*27730 VERTEBRAL ANOMALIES

Lavy, Palmer and Merritt (1967) observed 4 of 7 offsprings of a third-cousin marriage having characteristic vertebral anomalies, including hemivertebrae and block vertebrae accompanied by deformity of the ribs. All affected children died of respiratory infection under 1 year of age. Moseley and Bonforte (1969) described the same disorder in two apparently unrelated children of non-consanguineous Puerto Rican parents. Caffey (1967) described brother and sister with short neck and trunk in contrast to extremities of normal length. Both showed 'hemivertebrae at practically all levels in the spine.' The skeletons were otherwise normal. We (Norum, 1969) have observed 4 similar cases in two related sibships in an inbred community in eastern Kentucky. Fused ribs also occurred in affected persons. See COSTOVERTEBRAL SEGMENTATION

RECESSIVE

ANOMALIES in the dominant catalog. Phenotypically the dominant and recessive forms are very similar. Eller and Morton (1970) described similar deformity of the chest and spine, with additional craniolacunia, rachischisis and urinary tract anomalies, in the offspring of a woman who admitted to a single exposure to LSD about the time of conception. Cantu et al. (1971) described five cases in an inbred kindred. Castroviejo et al. (1973) reported spondylo-thoracic dysplasia in three Spanish sisters. The sisters showed the typically short thorax, short neck with limited mobility, winged scapulae and scoliosis or kyphoscoliosis. Particularly noteworthy were the vertebral anomalies including hemivertebrae and vertibral fusions affecting the whole vertebral column. Rib abnormalities in form and number were seen. One sister showed decreased mental function and another showed incompletely formed odontoid process. Bartsocas et al. (1974) described three affected sibs (two of them identical twin sisters).

Bartsocas, C. S., Kiossoglou, K. A., Papas, C. V., Xanthou-Tsingoglou, M., Anagnostakis, D. E. and Daskalopoulou, H. D.: Costovertebral dysplasia. Birth Defects Orig. Art. Ser. 10 (9): 221-226, 1974.

Caffey, J. P.: Normal vertebral column. Pediatric X-ray Diagnosis. Chicago: Year Book Medical Publishers, 1967. Pp. 1101-1108, (5th Ed.).

Cantu, J. M., Urrusti, J., Rosales, G. and Rojas, A.: Evidence for autosomal recessive inheritance of costovertebral dysplasia. Clin. Genet., 1971.

Castroviejo, I. P., Rodrieguez-Costa, T. and Castillo, F.: Spondylo-thoracic dysplasia in three sisters. Develop. Med. Child Neurol. 15: 348-354, 1973.

Eller, J. L. and Morton, J. M.: Bizarre deformities in offspring of user of lysergic acid diethylamide. New Eng. J. Med. 283: 395-397, 1970.

Lavy, N. W., Palmer, C. G. and Merritt, A. D.: A syndrome of bizarre vertebral anomalies. J. Pediat. 69: 1121-1125, 1967.

Moseley, J. E. and Bonforte, R. J.: Spondylothoracic dysplasia — a syndrome of congenital anomalies. Am. J. Roentgen. 106: 166-169, 1969.

Norum, R. A.: Costovertebral anomalies with apparent recessive inheritance. The Clinical Delineation of Birth Defects. IV. Skeletal Dysplasias. New York: National Foundation, 1969. Pp. 326-329.

*27735 VITAMIN A METABOLIC DEFECT

McLaren and Zekian (1971) reported a case of vitamin A deficiency in a Lebanese-Arab girl, the offspring of first-cousin-once-removed parents. Night blindness, hyperkeratosis follicularis, Bitot spots of the conjunctiva and very low plasma levels of vitamin A were features. A defect in enzymatic conversion of beta-carotene to retinol in the intestine was suggested. Recessive inheritance seems likely.

McLaren, D. S. and Zekian, B.: Failure of enzymic cleavage of beta-carotene. The cause of vitamin A deficiency in a child. Am. J. Dis. Child. 121: 278-280, 1971.

*27740 VITAMIN B12 METABOLIC DEFECT

Mudd et al. (1969) described the biochemical findings in an infant boy who died at 7.5 weeks. There was a defect in the two reactions in which vitamin B12 derivatives are known to function as coenzymes: (1) methionine formation from 5-methylfolate-H(4) and homocysteine, and (2) isomerization of methylmalo-nyl-Co-A to succinyl-Co-A. The infant showed homocystinemia, cystathioninemia and cystathioninuria, decrease in blood methionine, and methylmalonic aciduria. Deficient activity was demonstrated in the two enzymes dependent on B12 derivatives as coenzymes: methylfolate-H(4) methyltransferase and methylmalo-nyl-Co-A isomerase. Since vitamin B12 was present in normal concentrations in the liver, Mudd et al. concluded that the gene-determined defect probably concerned the conversion of B12 to a coenzymatically active derivative. See the vitamin B12 responsive form of METHYLMALONIC ACIDURIA for another disorder of vitamin B12 metabolism. McCully (1969) studied the same patient as that reported by Mudd et al. (1970) and on the pathologic findings based conclusions about the genesis of atrial changes in homocystinuria and of arteriosclerosis in general. Goodman et al. (1970) reported two brothers with a milder, possibly allelic form of the disorder. The elder, a 14 year old Mexican-American, was first admitted to the hospital in an acute psychotic episode. He had an IQ of about 50, a somewhat Marfanoid habitus and mild abnormalities on neurologic examination. Ectopia lentis and chest deformity were lacking. The parents were first-cousins-once-removed.

Goodman, S. I., Moe, P. G., Hammond, K. B., Mudd, S. H. and Uhlendorf, B. W.: Homocystinuria with methylmalonic aciduria. Two cases in a sibship. Biochem. Med. 4: 500-515, 1970.

McCully, K. S.: Vascular pathology of homocysteinemia: implications for the pathogenesis of arteriosclerosis. Am. J. Path. 56: 111-128, 1969.

Mudd, S. H., Levy, H. L. and Abeles, R. H.: A derangement in B12 metabolism leading to homocystinemia, cystathioninemia and methylmalonic aciduria. Biochem. Biophys. Res. Commun. 35: 121-126, 1969.

Mudd, S. H., Levy, H. L. and Morrow, G. III: Deranged B12 metabolism: effects on sulfur amino acid metabolism. Biochem. Med. 4: 193-214, 1970.

Mudd, S. H., Uhlendorf, B. W., Hinde, K. R. and Levy, H. L.: Deranged B12 metabolism: studies of fibroblasts grown in tissue culture. Biochem. Med. 4: 215-239, 1970.

27745 VITAMIN-K DEPENDENT COAGULATION DEFECT

Prothrombin, Stuart factor, factor VII and Christmas factor all require vitamin K for their synthesis. It is theoretically possible that a genetic disorder of the metabolism of vitamin K might lead to a congenital

RECESSIVE

combined deficiency of these four clotting factors. Although combined deficiency has been reported several times, in nearly every instance the patient had access to coumarin-like drugs. A more convincing case was reported by McMillan and Roberts (1966). An infant girl had had bleeding from the first week of life. No evidence of hepatic damage or of malabsorption was found but the patient responded to the administration of vitamin K. Clotting factors were normal in both parents. The pathogenesis of the deficiency state has not been clarified further and whether the patient's defect is genetic is not known.

McMillan, C. W. and Roberts, H. R.: Congenital combined deficiency of coagulation factors II, VII, IX and X. New Eng. J. Med. 274: 1313-1315, 1966.

*27760 WEILL-MARCHESANI SYNDROME (SPHEROPHAKIA-BRACHYMORPHIA SYNDROME, CONGENITAL MESODERMAL DYSMORPHO-DYSTROPHY)

The features are ectopia lentis, short stature and brachydactyly. The lens is usually round and abnormally small, so that the spherophakia-brachymorphia syndrome is a synonym. The syndrome is apparently not completely recessive. Probert (1953) described a family in which four sibs (3 females, one male) had the full syndrome, and one of their parents and many relatives in a dominant pedigree pattern had brachymorphism. Meyer and Holstein (1941) described four affected sibs whose parents were related. Rennert (1969) described 'difficulty in extending his arms over his head' in a 9-year-old boy. The sisters reported by Feinberg (1960) clearly did not have W-M. They are the same cases as those described by Gorlin et al. (1960) as a possible new syndrome (see GORLIN SYNDROME). Gorlin et al. (1974) reported a father and two children with seemingly bona fide W-M syndrome. Since the wife was short, this may be an example of backcross mating homozygote with heterozygote.

Feinberg, S. B.: Congenital mesodermal dysmorpho-dystrophy (brachymorphic type). Radiology 74: 218-229, 1960.

Gorlin, R. J., Chaudhry, A. P. and Moss, M. L.: Craniofacial dysostosis, patent ductus arteriosus, hypertrichosis, hypoplasia of labia majora, dental and eye anomalies — a new syndrome? J. Pediat. 56: 778-785, 1960.

Gorlin, R. J., L'Heureux, R. R. and Shapiro, I.: Weill-Marchesani syndrome in two generations: genetic heterogeneity or pseudodominance? J. Pediat. Ophthal. 11: 139-144, 1974.

Kloepfer, H. W. and Rosenthal, J. W.: Possible genetic carriers in the spherophakia-brachymorphia syndrome. Am. J. Hum. Genet. 7: 398-424, 1955.

Meyer, S. J. and Holstein, T.: Spherophakia with glaucoma and brachydactyly. Am. J. Ophthal. 24: 247-257, 1941.

Probert, L. A.: Spherophakia with brachydactyly. Comparison with Marfan's syndrome. Am. J. Ophthal. 36: 1571-1574, 1953.

Rennert, O. M.: The Marchesani syndrome. A brief review. Am. J. Dis. Child. 117: 703-705, 1969.

Stadlin, W. and Klein, D.: Ectopie congenitale du cristallin avec spherophaquie et brachymorphie accompagnee de paresis du regard. (Syndrome de Marchesani). Ann. Oculist. 181: 692-701, 1948.

*27770 WERNER SYNDROME

The features are scleroderma-like skin changes, especially in the extremities, cataract, subcutaneous calcification, premature arteriosclerosis, diabetes mellitus, and a widened and prematurely aged facies. A particularly instructive pedigree was reported by McKusick et al. (1963).

Boyd, M. W. J. and Grant, A. P.: Werner's syndrome (progeria of the adult): further pathological and biochemical observations. Brit. Med. J. 2: 920-925, 1959.

Epstein, C. J., Martin, G. M., Schultz, A. L. and Motulsky, A. G.: Werner's syndrome: a review of its symptomatology, natural history, pathologic features, genetics and relationship to the natural aging process. Medicine 45: 177-222, 1966.

McKusick, V. A. and colleagues: Medical genetics 1962. J. Chronic Dis. 16: 457-634, 1963.

Motulsky, A. G., Schultz, A. and Priest, J.: Werner's syndrome: chromosomes, genes, and the ageing process. Lancet I: 160-161, 1962.

27780 WILMS TUMOR

Rather numerous instances of multiple affected sibs have been described (Fitzgerald, Hardin, 1955). Strom (1957) described a family with 5 cases in three generations. A healthy male had two affected children (out of 5) by one wife and one affected child by another wife. A sister and an aunt of his had died in infancy or early childhood of abdominal tumor. Aniridia, hemihypertrophy and other congenital anomalies have been found in some cases of Wilms tumor (Miller, Fraumeni and Manning, 1964). Jolles (1973) described Wilms tumor in a 30-month-old girl and hypernephroma in her 67-year-old paternal grandmother. Brown et al. (1972) reported the occurrence of Wilms tumor, in 4 members of 3 successive generations of a family. The affected were the proband, a girl, her mother, aunt and grandfather. The presence of Wilms tumor was histopathologically confirmed in 3 of the 4 cases. The right kidney was affected first in all. The aunt eventually developed Wilms tumor of the left kidney leading to her death at age 7. Knudson and Strong (1972) reviewed and summarized data on 58 familial cases. They concluded that bilateral tumors are more likely to be familial, that familial tumors result from two mutations, one germinal and one somatic and that sporadic tumors result from two somatic mutations. Meadows et al. (1974) described a family in which the mother had congenital hemihypertrophy and three of her children had Wilms tumor. A fourth had a urinary trait anomaly. In one of the children the Wilms tumor was bilateral and in a second it was multicentric.

Brown, W. T., Puranik, S. R., Altman, D. H. and Hardin, H. C., Jr.: Wilms' tumor in three successive generations. Surgery 72: 756-761, 1972.

Fitzgerald, W. L. and Hardin, H. C., Jr.: Bilateral Wilms' tumor in a Wilms tumor family: case report. J. Urol. 73: 468-474, 1955.

Jolles, B.: Wilms' tumor in father and son. Lancet I: 207 only, 1973.

Kaufman, R. L., Vietti, T. J. and Wabner, C. I.: Wilms' tumor in father and son. Lancet I: 43 only, 1973.

Kontras, S. B. and Newton, W. A., Jr.: Familial Wilms' tumor. In, Bergsma, D. (ed.): Clinical Delineation of Birth Defect . XVI. Urinary System and Others. Baltimore: Williams and Wilkins, 1974. Pp. 187-188.

Knudson, A. G., Jr. and Strong, L. C.: Mutation and cancer: a model for Wilms' tumor of the kidney. J. Nat. Cancer Inst. 48: 313-324, 1972.

Meadows, A. T., Lichtenfeld, J. L. and Koop, C. E.: Wilms' tumor in three children of a woman with congenital hemihypertrophy. New Eng. J. Med. 291: 23-24, 1974.

Miller, R. W., Fraumeni, J. F., Jr. and Manning, M. D.: Association of Wilms' tumor with aniridia, hemihypertrophy and other congenital malformations. New Eng. J. Med. 270: 922-927, 1964.

Strom, T.: A Wilms' tumor family. Acta Paediat. 46: 601-604, 1957.

*27790 WILSON DISEASE (HEPATOLENTICULAR DEGENERATION)

The liver and basal ganglia undergo changes which express themselves in neurologic manifestations and signs of cirrhosis. A disturbance in copper metabolism is somehow involved in the mechanism. Low ceruloplasmin is found in the serum. Shokeir and Shreffler (1969) advanced the hypothesis that ceruloplasmin functions in enzymatic transfer of copper to copper-containing enzymes such as cytochrome oxidase. Supporting the hypothesis was the finding of markedly reduced levels of activity of cytochrome oxidase in Wilson disease and moderate reductions in heterozygotes. From a study of 28 Canadian families, Cox et al. (1972) suggested that there are at least three forms of Wilson disease. In a rare 'atypical form' the heterozygotes show about 50 percent the normal level of ceruloplasmin. This gene may have been of German-Mennonite derivation. In the two typical forms heterozygotes have normal ceruloplasmin levels, although they can be identified by decreased reappearance of radioactive copper into serum and ceruloplasmin. The authors referred to the two 'typical forms' as the Slavic and the juvenile type. The Slavic type has a late age of onset and is predominantly a neurologic disease. The juvenile type which occurs in Western Europeans and several other ethnic groups has onset before age 16 years and is frequently a hepatic disease. Low levels of ceruloplasmin are normally found in the newborn (Shokeir, 1971).

R
E
C
E
S
S
I
V
E

Anderson, P. J. and Popper, H.: Changes in hepatic structure in Wilson's disease. Am. J. Path. 36: 483-497, 1960.

Bearn, A. G. and McKusick, V. A.: Azure lunulae. An unusual change in the fingernails in two patients with hepatolenticular degeneration (Wilson's disease). J.A.M.A. 166: 904-906, 1958.

Bearn, A. G.: A genetical analysis of thirty families with Wilson's disease (hepatolenticular degeneration). Ann. Hum. Genet. 24: 33-43, 1960.

Bearn, A. G.: Wilson's disease. In, Stanbury, J. B., Wyngaarden, J. B. and Fredrickson, D. S. (eds.): The Metabolic Basis of Inherited Disease. New York: McGraw-Hill, 1972 (3rd Ed.). Pp. 1033-1050.

Cox, D. W., Fraser, F. C. and Sass-Kortsak, A.: A genetic study of Wilson's disease: evidence for heterogeneity. Am. J. Hum. Genet. 24: 646-666, 1972.

Goldstein, N. P., Tauxe, W. N., McCall, J. T., Randall, R. V. and Gross, J. B.: Wilson's disease (hepatolenticular degeneration). Treatment with penicillamine and changes in hepatic trappings of radioactive copper. Arch. Neurol. 24: 391400, 1971.

Holtzman, N. A., Naughton, M. A., Iber, F. L. and Gaumnitz, B. M.: Ceruloplasmin in Wilson's disease. J. Clin. Invest. 46: 993-1002, 1967.

Levi, A. J., Sherlock, S., Scheuer, P. J. and Cumings, J. N.: Presymptomatic Wilson's disease. Lancet II: 575-579, 1967.

Shokeir, M. H. K. and Shreffler, D. C.: Cytochrome oxidase deficiency in Wilson's disease: a suggested ceruloplasmin function. Proc. Nat. Acad. Sci. 62: 867-872, 1969.

Shokeir, M. H. K.: Investigations on the nature of ceruloplasmin deficiency in the newborn. Clin. Genet. 2: 223-227, 1971.

Slovis, T. L., Dubois, R. S., Rodgerson, D. O. and Silverman, A.: The varied manifestations of Wilson's disease. J. Pediat. 78: 578-584, 1971.

Sternlieb, I. and Scheinberg, I. H.: Chronic hepatitis as a first manifestation of Wilson's disease. Ann. Intern. Med. 76: 59-64, 1972.

Strickland, G. T., Frommer, D., Leu, M. L., Pollard, R., Sherlock, S. and Cumings, J. N.: Wilson's disease in the United Kingdom and Taiwan. I. General characteristics of 142 cases and prognosis. II. A genetic analysis of 88 cases. Quart. J. Med. 42: 619-638, 1973.

Walshe, J. M. and Cumings, J. N.: Wilson's Disease. Some Current Concepts. Oxford: Blackwell, 1961. Pp. 1-292.

*27795 WINCHESTER DISEASE

In two daughters of first-cousin Puerto Rican parents, Winchester et al. (1969) described a new syndrome characterized by short stature, severe joint contractures, peripheral corneal opacities, coarsened facies, dissolution of carpal and tarsal bones and generalized osteoporosis. Changes in and about joints simulated advanced rheumatoid arthritis. Urinary mucopolysaccharide excretion was normal but cultured skin fibroblasts showed metachromasia and increased uronic acid (with intermediate levels in the parents' fibroblasts). Brown and Kuwabara (1970) described electron microscopic findings in a corneal biopsy and concluded that the findings (together with those of fibroblast study outlined above) are consistent with this being a mucopolysaccharide storage disease. Hollister et al. (1974) studied three affected persons in two sibships related as first-cousins and each apparently with consanguineous parents. On the basis of electron microscopic studies, they concluded that this is a nonlysosomal connective tissue disease.

Brown, S. I. and Kuwabara, T.: Peripheral corneal opacification and skeletal deformities: a newly recognized acid mucopolysaccharidosis simulating rheumatoid arthritis. Arch. Ophthal. 83: 667-677, 1970.

Hollister, D. W., Rimoin, D. L., Lachman, R. S. and Cohen, A. H.: The Winchester syndrome: clinical, radiographic and pathologic study. In, Rimoin, D. L. and Schimke, R. N. (eds.): Medical Genetics Today. Baltimore: Williams and Wilkins, 1973.

Hollister, D. W., Rimoin, D. L., Lachman, R. S., Cohen, A. H., Reed, W. B. and Westin, G. W.: The Winchester syndrome: a nonlysosomal connective tissue disease. J. Pediat. 84: 701-709, 1974.

Winchester, P., Grossman, H., Lim, W. N. and Danes, B. S.: A new acid mucopolysaccharidosis with skeletal deformities simulating rheumatoid arthritis. Am. J. Roentgen. 106: 121-128, 1969.

*27800 WOLMAN DISEASE

Wolman and colleagues (1961) described three sibs in whom involvement of the viscera was an important feature and death occurred at the age of about 3 months. Xanthomatous changes were observed in the liver, adrenal, spleen, lymph nodes, bone marrow, small intestine, lungs and thymus and slight change in the skin, retina and central nervous system. The adrenals were calcified. Death was thought to be due to intestinal malabsorption resulting from involvement of the gut. The parents, Persian Jews, were cousins. Lipids in the plasma were normal or moderately elevated. Several features suggested that the entity is distinct from hypercholesterolemia and the hyperlipidemias (q.v.). Three cases, the first from the U.S.A., were reported by Crocker and colleagues (1965) who gave no information on ethnicity. The relatively non-specific clinical picture includes poor weight gain, vomiting, diarrhea, increasing hepatosplenomegaly with abdominal protruberance and death in nutritional failure by 2-4 months of age. Foam cells are found in bone marrow and vacuolated lymphocytes in peripheral blood, as in Niemann-Pick disease. Diffuse punctate calcification of the adrenals is typical. Disseminated foam cell infiltration is found in many organs. Great increases in cholesterol are found in the organs. Konno et al. (1966) reported a Japanese family with three affected sibs. Spiegel-Adolf et al. (1966) reported 3 affected sibs in an American family. Patrick and Lake (1969) demonstrated deficiency of an acid lipase which apparently leads to the progressive accumulation of triglycerides and cholesterol esters in lysosomes in the tissues of affected persons. Lough et al. (1970) described an affected infant of Greek ancestry in whom calcified adrenals were demonstrated on the 5th day of life. Young and Patrick (1970) commented on the existence of cases with the same biochemical and histologic changes as in the acute infantile form but with later onset and a much less fulminant course. One of their cases was alive and well at age 8 years, showing no clinical abnormality other than moderate hepatomegaly. The same enzyme is deficient in all these cases. Hence, they suggested the term 'acid lipase deficiency' for the whole group with Wolman disease as the designation for the acute infantile form.

Crocker, A. C., Vawter, G. F., Neuhauser, E. B. D., and Rosowsky, A.: Wolman's disease: three new patients with a recently described lipidosis. Pediatrics 35: 627-640, 1965.

Kahana, D., Berant, M. and Wolman, M.: Primary familial xanthomatosis with adrenal involvement (Wolman's disease). Report of a further case with nervous system involvement and pathogenetic considerations. Pediatrics 42: 70-76, 1968.

Konno, T., Fujii, M., Watanuki, T. and Koizumi, K.: Wolman's disease: the first case in Japan. Tohoku J. Exp. Med. 90: 375-389, 1966.

Lake, B. D. and Patrick, A. D.: Wolman's disease: deficiency of 600-resistant acid esterase activity with storage of lipids in lysosomes. J. Pediat. 76: 262-266, 1970.

Lake, B. D.: Histochemical detection of the enzyme deficiency in blood films in Wolman's disease. J. Clin. Path. 24: 617-620, 1971.

Lough, J., Fawcett, J. and Wiegensberg, B.: Wolman's disease. An electron microscopic, histochemical, and biochemical study. Arch. Path. 89: 103-110, 1970.

Marshall, W. C., Ockenden, B. G., Fosbrooke, A. S. and Cumings, J. N.: Wolman's disease. A rare lipidosis with adrenal calcification. Arch. Dis. Child. 44: 331-341, 1969.

Patrick, A. D. and Lake, B. D.: Deficiency of an acid lipase in Wolman's disease. Nature 222: 1067-1068, 1969.

Spiegel-Adolf, M., Baird, H. W. and McCafferty, M.: Hematologic studies in Niemann-Pick and Wolman's disease (cytology and electrophoresis). Confin. Neurol. 28: 399-406, 1966.

Wolman, M., Sterk, V. V., Gatt, S. and Frenkel, M.: Primary family xanthomatosis with involvement and calcification of the adrenals. Report of two more cases in siblings of a previously described infant. Pediatrics 28: 742-757, 1961.

Young, E. P. and Patrick, A. D.: Deficiency of acid esterase activity in Wolman's disease. Arch. Dis. Child. 45: 664-668, 1970.

27810 WOLMAN DISEASE WITH HYPOLIPOPROTEINEMIA AND ACANTHOCYTOSIS

Eto and Kitagawa (1970) described a disorder which may be a distinct entity. Malabsorption of lipid, vomiting, growth failure, and adrenal calcification were present. Hypolipoproteinemia and acanthocytosis suggest this is an entity distinct from Wolman disease.

Eto, Y. and Kitagawa, T.: Wolman's disease with hypolipoproteinemia and acanthocytosis: clinical and biochemical observations. J. Pediat. 77: 862-867, 1970.

27820 WOOLLY HAIR, HYPOTRICHOSIS, EVERTED LOWER LIP, PSYCHOSIS, ETC.

Salamon (1963) described this syndrome as a recessive. The parents were consanguineous. Woolly hair, as an isolated trait, is a dominant (q.v.).

Salamon, T.: Ueber eine Familie mit recessiver Kraushaarigkeit, Hypotrichose und anderen Anomalien. Hautarzt 14: 540-544, 1963.

*27825 WRINKLY SKIN SYNDROME

In two and possibly three offspring of first-cousin parents, Gazit et al. (1973) described a disorder they called the wrinkly skin syndrome. It was characterized at birth by wrinkled skin of the hands and feet with an increased number of wrinkles on the palms and soles. Skeletal musculature was poorly developed and hypotonic with winging of the scapulas. The venous pattern was prominent over the anterior thorax.

Gazit, E., Goodman, R. M., Katznelson, M., Bat-Miriam, and Rotem, Y.: The wrinkly skin syndrome: a new heritable disorder of connective tissue. Clin. Genet. 4: 186-192, 1973.

*27830 XANTHINURIA

The disorder is characterized by excretion of very large amounts of xanthine in the urine and a tendency to form xanthine stones. Uric acid is strikingly diminished in serum and urine. Dickinson and Smellie (1959) described a well-studied single case, a child of unrelated, unaffected parents. Watts et al. (1964) described a 23-year-old woman in whom the disorder was suspected because of very low serum uric acid. There were no urinary calculi. Enzyme assays showed very little oxidation of both hypoxanthine and xanthine presumably due to a defect in xanthine oxidase. Affected brothers have been observed (Wyngaarden, 1966). In the eighth known patient, studied by Chalmers et al. (1969), a Negro male, crystalline deposits occurred in skeletal muscle. A myopathy with crystalline deposits was described also by Engelman et al. (1964). The defect lies in xanthine oxidase (Engelman et al., 1964; Sperling et al., 1971).

Chalmers, R. A., Johnson, M., Pallis, C. and Watts, R. W. E.: Xanthinuria with myopathy. Quart. J. Med. 38: 493-512, 1969.

Cifuentes Delatte, L. and Castro-Mendoza, H.: Xanthinuria familiar. Rev. Clin. Esp. 107: 244, 1967.

Dickinson, C. J. and Smellie, J. M.: Xanthinuria. Brit. Med. J. 2: 1217-1221, 1959.

Engelman, K., Watts, R. W. E., Klinenberg, J. R., Sjoerdsma, A. and Seegmiller, J. E.: Clinical, physiological and biochemical studies of a patient with xanthinuria and pheochromocytoma. Am. J. Med. 37: 839-861, 1964.

Sorensen, L. B., Tesar, J. T., Ellman, M. H. and Cowell, J.: A new case of xanthinuria. Am. J. Med. 53: 690-692, 1972.

Sperling, O., Liberman, U. A., Frank, M. and De Vries, A.: Xanthinuria: an additional case with demonstration of xanthine oxidase deficiency. Am. J. Clin. Path. 55: 351-354, 1971.

Watts, R. W. E., Engelman, K., Klinenberg, J. R., Seegmiller, J. E. and Sjoerdsma, A.: Enzyme defect in a case of xanthinuria. Nature 201: 395-396, 1964.

Wyngaarden, J. B.: Xanthinuria. In, Stanbury, J. B., Wyngaarden, J. B. and Fredrickson, D. S. (eds.): The Metabolic Basis of Inherited Disease. New York: McGraw-Hill, 1972 (3rd Ed.). Pp. 992-1002.

27840 XANTHISM (RUFOUS ALBINISM)

This trait occurs in Negroes and is characterized by bright copper-red coloration of the skin and hair and dilution of the color of the iris. Barnicot (1957) suggested that this is a genetic trait distinct from albinism. Pearson, Nettleship and Usher (1911-1913) are said to have cited a pedigree in which both xanthism and albinism occurred. Xanthism may be the same as type II albinism (q.v.), which in the Negro seems to answer the descriptions cited above.

Barnicot, N. A.: Human pigmentation. Man 57: 114-120, 1957.

Pearson, K., Nettleship, E. and Usher, C. H.: A Monograph on Albinism in Man. Series VI, VIII, IX, parts I, II and IV. London: Cambridge Univ. Press, 6: 1911-1913.

*27860 XANTHURENICACIDURIA

This disorder is due to a defect in kynureninase, a vitamin B6 dependent enzyme in the tryptophane catabolic pathway. Both B6-responsive and B6-nonresponsive forms are known. Tada et al, (1967) reported this disorder in a brother and sister with mental retardation. The parents were first-cousins. The patients excreted excessive amounts of xanthurenic acid, kynurenic acid, 3-hydroxykynurenine and kynurenine after tryptopham loading. This disturbance was temporarily corrected by large doses of vitamin B6. The activity

R
E
C
E
S
S
I
V
E

of kynureninase in the liver was marked reduced. The activity was appreciably restored by the addition of an excessive pyridoxal phosphate.

Tada, K., Yokoyama, Y., Nakagawa, H., Yoshida, T. and Arakawa, T.: Vitamin B6 dependent xanthurenic aciduria. Tohoku J. Exp. Med. 93: 115-124, 1967.

*27870 XERODERMA PIGMENTOSUM

Sensitivity to sunlight with the development of carcinomata at an early age is observed. Onset, with freckle-like lesions in exposed areas, usually occurs in the first years of life. The possibility of partial sex-linked recessive inheritance was suggested by Haldane but is now considered unlikely. Parental consanguinity is frequent. The sex ratio is about 1. Ruder (cited by Cockayne) observed the condition in 7 out of 13 sibs. It is not clear whether heterozygotes show changes. Increased freckling has been claimed to be such a manifestation. El-Hefnawi, Smith and Penrose (1965) presented useful pedigrees and suggested linkage with the ABO blood group locus. Cleaver (1968) showed that whereas normal skin fibroblasts can repair ultraviolet radiation damage to DNA by inserting new bases into DNA, cells from patients with xeroderma pigmentosum lack this capacity or have a much reduced capacity for repair. Goldstein and Lin (1972) showed that Xp-hamster hybrid cells had normal repair and survived ultraviolet irradiation. Cell-fusion studies indicate that complementation can take place between the fibroblasts from certain pairs of patients. The cells of each member cannot by themselves effect repair of DNA, but this can be done by the fused cells. So far four complementation groups have been found indicating that mutation at any one of at least four loci can cause defective DNA repair leading to the clinical state of xeroderma pigmentosum (Robbins et al., 1974). At least two patients with xeroderma pigmentosum and a normal in vitro DNA repair rate have been observed (Robbins et al., 1974; Cleaver, 1972). Thus, we seem justified in listing five xeroderma pigmentosum loci (27870, 27871, 27872, 27880, and 27885). The four complementation groups, called A-D, show no consistent clinical correlations (as to neurologic signs, for example) but did show correlations with DNA repair rate: group A — less than 2 percent of normal; group B — 3-to-7 percent, group C — 10-to-25 percent; group D — 25-55 percent.

Afifi, A. K., Der Kaloustian, V. M. and Mire, J. J.: Muscular abnormality in xeroderma pigmentosum. High resolution light-microscopy and electron-microscopic observations. J. Neurol. Sci. 17: 435-442, 1972.

Cleaver, J. E.: Defective repair replication of DNA in xeroderma pigmentosum. Nature 218: 652-656, 1968.

Cleaver, J. E.: Xeroderma pigmentosum: variants with normal DNA repair and normal sensitivity to ultraviolet light. J. Invest. Derm. 58: 124-128, 1972.

Cockayne, E. A.: Inherited abnormalities of the skin and its appendages. London: Oxford Univ. Press, 1933.

De Grouchy, J., De Nava, C., Feingold, J., Frezal, J. and Lamy, M.: Asynchronie chromosomique dans un cas de xeroderma pigmentosum. Ann. Genet. 10: 224-225, 1967.

El-Hefnawi, H., Smith, S. M. and Penrose, L. S.: Xeroderma pigmentosum-its inheritance and relationship to the ABO blood-group system. Ann. Hum. Genet. 28: 273-290, 1965.

Goldstein, S. and Lin, C. C.: Survival and DNA repair of somatic cell hybrids after ultraviolet irradiation. Nature N.B. 239: 142-145, 1972.

MacKlin, M. T.: Xeroderma pigmentosum: report of a case and consideration of incomplete sex linkage in inheritance of the disease. Arch. Derm. Syph. 49: 157-171, 1944.

Regan, J. D., Setlow, R. B., Kaback, M. M., Howell, R. R., Klein, E. and Burgess, G.: Xeroderma pigmentosum: a rapid sensitive method for prenatal diagnosis. Science 174: 147-150, 1971.

Robbins, J. H., Kraemer, K. H., Lutzner, M. A., Festoff, B. W. and Coon, H. G.: Xeroderma pigmentosum: an inherited disease with sun sensitivity, multiple cutaneous neoplasms, and abnormal DNA repair. Ann. Intern. Med. 80: 221-248, 1974.

*27871 XERODERMA PIGMENTOSUM II

See 27870.

*27872 XERODERMA PIGMENTOSUM III

See 27870.

27875 XERODERMA PIGMENTOSUM WITH NORMAL DNA-REPAIR RATES

As indicated in 27870, at least two patients with xeroderma pigmentosum have been found to have normal DNA-repair rates. Presumably this disorder is autosomal recessive, but the proof is not yet available.

*27880 XERODERMIC IDIOCY OF DE SANCTIS AND CACCHIONE

In addition to xeroderma pigmentosum the features are mental deficiency, dwarfism and gonadal hypoplasia. Reed, May and Nickel (1965) described the syndrome in a Caucasian brother and sister and two 'Japanese' brothers. Although these authors were of the view that this is fundamentally the same entity as xeroderma pigmentosum without associated abnormalities, it seems more likely that it is distinctive. Choreo-athetoid neurologic signs occurred in their cases. One sib developed leukemia (Reed, 1967). Yano (1950) described the autopsy findings in a Japanese case and Reed et al. (1969) reported the findings in a Japanese-American case. Cerebral and olivopontocerebellar atrophy was found. Of the 5 patients described by Reed et al. (1969), 4 had associated neurologic features (de Sanctis-Cacchione syndrome). One of the patients with the latter syndrome developed acute lymphatic leukemia at the age of 3 years. Deweerdt-Kastelein et al. (1972) found

R
E
C
E
S
S
I
V
E

complementation when cells from classic xeroderma pigmentosum were hybridized with cells from a case of the de Sanctis-Cacchione syndrome. This could be either interlocus or interallelic complementation. It is not incontrovertible evidence for separate loci for these two forms of disease. Neurologic manifestations are frequent in xeroderma pigmentosum. Thus, more than one complementation type of XP may have clinical symptoms justifying designation as the de Sanctis-Cacchione syndrome. Death of neurons may be occurring more rapidly in persons with a defect in DNA-repair than in normals (Robbins et al. 1974). Areflexia is a common finding.

Deweerdt-Kastelein, E. A., Keijzer, W. and Bootsma, D.: Genetic heterogeneity of xeroderma pigmentosum demonstrated by somatic cell hybridization. Nature (Nb) 238: 80-83, 1972.

Elsasser, G., Freusberg, O. and Theml, F.: Das Xeroderma pigmentosum und die 'xerodermische Idiotie.' Arch. Derm. 188: 651-655, 1950.

Reed, W. B.: Burbank, Calif.: personal communication, 1967.

Reed, W. B., Landing, B., Sugarman, G. I., Cleaver, J. E. and Melnyk, J.: Xeroderma pigmentosum. Clinical and laboratory investigation of its basic defect. J.A.M.A. 207: 2073-2079, 1969.

Reed, W. B., May, S. B. and Nickel, W. R.: Xeroderma pigmentosum with neurological complications. Arch. Derm. 91: 224-226, 1965.

Robbins, J. H., Kraemer, K. H., Lutzner, M. A., Festoff, B. W. and Coon, H. G.: Xeroderma pigmentosum: an inherited disease with sun sensitivity, multiple cutaneous neoplasms and abnormal DNA repair. Ann. Intern. Med. 80: 221-248, 1974.

Yano, K.: Xeroderma pigmentosum mit Storungen des Zentralnervensystems: eine histopathologische Untersuchung. Folia Psychiat. Neurol. Jap. 4: 143-151, 1950.

27890 XYLOSIDASE DEFICIENCY

Payling-Wright and Evans (1970) described a girl who had been normal until age 3 months when there was onset of seizures. At the age of nine months, she was floppy; also she made choreo-athetotic movements and appeared to lack sight or hearing. Investigations showed small head, hypsarrhythmia by EEG and dilated ventricles by air encephalography. Lymphocytes grown in short-term culture showed very low beta-xylosidase. Thus, this appears to be a lysosomal disorder. No further information is available (Evans, 1974).

Evans, P. R.: London, personal com.nunication, Apr. 22, 1974.

Payling-Wright, C. R. and Evans, P. R.: A case of beta-xylosidase deficiency. (Letter) Lancet II: 43 only, 1970.

R
E
C
E
S
S
I
V
E

X-LINKED PHENOTYPES

Fanconi, Prader, Isler, Luthy and Siebenmann (1964) suggested X-linked recessive inheritance of a syndrome of Addison disease and cerebral sclerosis. All cases have been male and in at least five instances a brother and-or a maternal uncle of the proband has been similarly affected. Hoefnagel, Van den Noort and Ingbar (1962) described the histologic findings in endocrine glands, especially the pituitary and adrenal. The locus is not closely linked to the Xg locus (Spira et al., 1971).

Aguilar, M. J., O'Brien, J. S. and Taber, P.: The syndrome of familial leukodystrophy, adrenal insufficiency and cutaneous melanosis. In, Aronson, S. M. and Volk, B. W. (eds.): Inborn disorders of Sphingolipid Metabolism. Oxford: Pergamon Press, 1967. Pp. 149-166.

Fanconi, A., Prader, A., Isler, W., Luthy, F. and Siebenmann, R. E.: Morbus Addison mit Hirnsklerose im Kindesalter. Ein hereditares Syndrom mit X-chromosomaler Vererbung? Helv. Paediat. Acta 18: 480-501, 1964.

Hoefnagel, D., Brun, A., Ingbar, S. H. and Goldman, H.: Addison's disease and diffuse cerebral sclerosis. J. Neurol. Neurosurg. Psychiatry 30: 56-60, 1967.

Hoefnagel, D., Van den Noort, S. and Ingbar, S. H.: Diffuse cerebral sclerosis with endocrine abnormalities in young males. Brain 85: 553-568, 1962.

Schaumburg, H. H., Richardson, E. P., Johnson, P. C., Cohen, R. B., Powers, J. M. and Raine, C. S.: Schilder's disease: sex-linked recessive transmission with specific adrenal changes. Arch. Neurol. 27: 458-460, 1972.

Spira, T. J., Adam, A., Goodman, R. M. and Berger, A.: Recombination between cerebral sclerosis — Addison's disease and the Xg blood-groups. (Letter) Lancet II: 820-821, 1971.

Turkington, R. W. and Stempfel, R. S., Jr.: Adrenocortical atrophy and diffuse cerebral sclerosis (Addison-Schilder's disease). J. Pediatr. 69: 406-412, 1966.

*30020 ADRENAL HYPOPLASIA

The anatomic features were both severe hypoplasia and disorganization. Death without treatment was early in life. There are probably both autosomal recessive and X-linked forms and there may be more than one of each. Weiss and Mellinger (1970) reported 3 affected brothers out of four. A different man fathered each of the three affected sons. Histologically there was lack of organization of the cortex into cords. Presence of clumps of large pale staining cells is another feature. Several other families consistent with X-linked inheritance were found (e.g., Boyd and MacDonald, 1960; Uttley, 1968; Stempfel and Engel, 1960). Brochner-Mortensen (1956) described Addison disease in two brothers and two of their maternal uncles. Three of the patients had died at ages 19, 26 and 33 years. Addison disease and cerebral sclerosis (q.v.) is a well established X-linked disorder. In brothers reported by Meakin et al. (1959), the diagnosis was made in the elder at 9 years of age and in the second at 6 years of age. Martin (1971) described a pair of brothers in whom the signs of Addison disease developed at age 5. It seems likely that Addison disease with this later onset is distinct from that due to adrenal hypoplasia as described by Weiss and Mellinger (1970) and by others.

Boyd, J. F. and MacDonald, A. M.: Adrenal cortical hypoplasia in siblings. Arch. Dis. Child. 35: 561-568, 1960.

Brochner-Mortensen, K.: Familial occurrence of Addison's disease. Acta Med. Scand. 155: 205-209, 1956.

Martin, M. M.: Familial Addison's disease. The Clinical Delineation of Birth Defects. X. The Endocrine System. Baltimore: Williams and Wilkins, 1971. Pp. 98-100.

Pakravan, P., Kenny, F. M., Depp, R. and Allen, A. C.: Familial congenital absence of adrenal glands; evaluation of glucocorticoid, mineralocorticoid, and estrogen metabolism in the perinatal period. J. Pediatr. 84: 74-78, 1974.

Stempfel, R. S., Jr. and Engel, F. L.: A congenital, familial syndrome of adrenocortical insufficiency without hypoaldosteronism. J. Pediatr. 57: 443-451, 1960.

Uttley, W. S.: Familial congenital adrenal hypoplasia. Arch. Dis. Child. 43: 724-730, 1968.

Weiss, L. and Mellinger, R. C.: Congenital adrenal hypoplasia — an X-linked disease. J. Med. Genet. 7: 27-32, 1970.

30025 ADRENAL UNRESPONSIVENESS TO ACTH

Franks and Nance (1970) suggested that one form of this phenotype may be X-linked. See 20220.

Franks, R. C. and Nance, W. E.: Hereditary adrenocortical unresponsiveness to ACTH. Pediatrics 45: 43-48, 1970.

*30030 AGAMMAGLOBULINEMIA (BRUTON TYPE)

Patients are unusually prone to bacterial infection but not to viral infection. A clinical picture resembling rheumatoid arthritis develops in many. Before antibiotics, death occurred in the first decade. In the more usual X-linked form of the disease plasma cells are lacking. A rarer form of agammaglobulinemia (Hitzig and Willi, 1961), which is inherited as an autosomal recessive (q.v.), shows marked depression of the circulating lymphocytes and lymphocytes are absent from the lymphoid tissue. The alymphocytotic type is even more virulent than the X-linked form leading to death in the first 18 months after birth, from severe thrush, chronic diarrhea, and recurrent pulmonary infections. Seligman et al. (1968) proposed a classification

X

L
I
N
K
E
D

of immunologic deficiencies which included 11 entities of which a genetic basis has been proved or suspected in all except one — DiGeorge thymic aplasia. The 10 others are Bruton sex-linked agammaglobulinemia, selective inability to produce IgA (which they state may be autosomal recessive in some cases), transient hypogammaglobulinemia of infancy, non-sex-linked immunoglobulin deficiency, agammaglobulinemia with thymoma, Wiskott-Aldrich syndrome, ataxia-telangiectasia, primary lymphopenic immunologic deficiency of the type first reported by Gitlin and Craig (1963), Swiss-type agammaglobulinemia, and autosomal recessive lymphopenia with normal immunoglobulins (Nezelof syndrome). Ament et al. (1973) pointed out that gastrointestinal infestation with Giardia lamblia is frequent in this and other forms of IDS (immunodeficiency syndrome). Geha et al. (1973) showed that males with proven X-linked agamma-globulinemias lacked bone marrow derived (B) lymphocytes from the circulating blood whereas progenitor and thymus (T) cells were normal. See 30040, 30100 and 30823 for other X-linked deficiencies of immunoglobulins.

Ament, M. E., Ochs, H. D. and Davis, S. D.: Structure and function of the gastrointestinal tract in primary immunodeficiency syndromes. A study of 39 patients. Medicine 52: 227-248, 1973.

Garvie, J. M. and Kendall, A. C.: Congenital agammaglobulinaemia. Report of two further cases. Brit. Med. J. 1: 548-550, 1961.

Geha, R. S., Rosen, F. S. and Merler, E.: Identification and characterization of subpopulations of lymphocytes in human peripheral blood after fractionation on discontinuous gradients of albumin. The cellular defect in X-linked agammaglobulinemia. J. Clin. Invest. 52: 1726-1734, 1973.

Gitlin, D. and Craig, J. M.: The thymus and other lymphoid tissues in congenital agammaglobulinemia. I. Thymic alymphoplasia and lymphocytic hypoplasia and their relation to infection. Pediatrics 32: 517-530, 1963.

Hitzig, W. H. and Willi, H.: Hereditary lymphoplasmocytic dysgenesis ('alymphocytose mit agamma-globulinamia'). Schweiz. Med. Wschr. 91: 1625-1633, 1961.

Janeway, C. A., Apt, L. and Gitlin, D.: Agammaglobulinemia. Trans. Ass. Am. Physicians 66: 200-202, 1953.

Seligman, M., Fudenberg, H. H. and Good, R. A.: A proposed classification of primary immunologic deficiencies. Am. J. Med. 45: 817-825, 1968.

*30040 AGAMMAGLOBULINEMIA, SWISS TYPE (THYMIC EPITHELIAL HYPOPLASIA)

This type of disease differs from the Bruton type by the presence of lymphocytopenia ('alymphocytosis'), earlier age of death, vulnerability to viral and fungal as well as bacterial infections, lack of delayed hypersensitivity, atrophy of the thymus, and lack of benefit by gamma globulin administration. It is usually inherited as an autosomal recessive (q.v.) but all cases in three families studied by Rosen et al. (1966) were male and one kindred (family T) had 9 affected males in 5 sibships in three generations connected through females in a typical X-linked recessive pedigree pattern. Miller and Schieken (1967) suggested that one form of thymic dysplasia is X-linked. An impressive pedigree with 6 affected males in 3 generations was published by Dooren et al. (1968), who following the recommendations of a workshop on immunological deficiency diseases in man (Sanibel Island, Fort Myers, Fla., Feb. 1-5, 1967) called the condition thymic epithelial hypoplasia. In the same workshop Rosen et al. (1968) pointed out that a difference from the autosomal recessive is less profound lymphocytopenia.

Miller, M. E. and Schieken, R. M.: Thymic dysplasia. A separable entity from 'Swiss agammaglobuline-mia.' Am. J. Med. Sci. 253: 741-750, 1967.

Rosen, F. S. and Janeway, C. A.: The gamma globulins. III. The antibody deficiency syndromes. New Eng. J. Med. 275: 709-715 and 769-775, 1966.

Rosen, F. S., Craig, J. M., Vawter, G. and Janeway, C. A.: The dysgammaglobulinemias and X-linked thymic hypoplasia. In, Good, R. A. (ed.): Immunologic Deficiency Diseases in Man. New York: National Foundation, 1968. Pp. 67-70.

Rosen, F. S., Gotoff, S. P., Craig, J. M., Ritchie, J. and Janeway, C. A.: Further observations on the Swiss type of agammaglobulinemia (alymphocytosis). The effect of syngeneic bone-marrow cells. New Eng. J. Med. 274: 18-21, 1966.

*30050 ALBINISM, OCULAR

In affected men the pupillary reflex is characteristic of albinism. The fundus is depigmented and the choroidal vessels stand out strikingly. Nystagmus, head nodding, and impaired vision also occur. Pigmentation is normal elsewhere than in the eye. In carrier females the fundus, especially in the periphery, shows a mosaic of pigmentation, as first recognized by Vogt (1942). Lyon (1962) pointed out that the fundus finding in heterozygous females supports her theory. Nystagmus is frequently an associated feature. In fact the ocular albinism has been commented on only obliquely or not at all in some reports of X-linked nystagmus in families which almost certainly had ocular albinism. Waardenburg and Van den Bosch's family was earlier reported by Engelhard as a family with hereditary nystagmus. One family studied by Fialkow et al. (1967) had been reported by Lein et al. (1956) as sex-linked nystagmus. Fundus drawings of heterozygous carriers are provided by Francois and Deweer, and by others. (See frontispiece, McKusick, 1964.) Theoretically one should be able to count the number of pigmented spots and arrive at an estimate of the number of anlage cells present at the time of Lyonization. Unfortunately most of the available drawings are probably too crude to be relied on for this use. Furthermore, the drawings suggest appreciable variation in the number and size of pigmented areas, a finding to be expected from the considerations of the Lyon hypothesis. Isolated albinism of the eye is inherited in the rabbit as an autosomal recessive (Magnussen, 1952). Fialkow et al. (1967)

Pearce et al. (1968) in an English kindred. From a Newfoundland kindred Pearce et al. (1971) presented data which reduce the estimate of the interval between Xg and ocular albinism from 17 to 15.

Engelhard, C. F.: Eine Familie mit hereditarem Nystagmus. Zbl. Ges. Neurol. Psychiat. 28: 319-338, 1915.

Fialkow, P. J., Giblett, E. R. and Motulsky, A. G.: Measurable linkage between ocular albinism and Xg. Am. J. Hum. Genet. 19: 63-69, 1967.

Francois, J. and Deweer, J. P.: Albinisme oculaire lie au sexe et alterations caracteristiques du fond d'oeil chez les femmes heterozygotes. Ophthalmologia 126: 209-221, 1953.

Gillespie, F. D.: Ocular albinism with report of a family with female carriers. Arch. Ophthalmol. 66: 774-777, 1961.

Lein, J. N., Stewart, C. T. and Moll, F. C.: Sex-linked hereditary nystagmus. Pediatrics 18: 214-217, 1956.

Lyon, M. F.: Sex chromatin and gene action in the mammalian X-chromosome. Am. J. Hum. Genet. 14: 135-148, 1962.

Magnussen, K.: Beitrag zur Genetik und Histologie eines isolierten Augenalbinismus beim Kaninchen. Z. Morph. Anthrop. 44: 127-135, 1952.

McKusick, V. A.: On the X chromosome of man. Washington: Am. Inst. Biol. Sci., 1964.

Negrelli, B. C.: L'albinisme oculaire lie au sexe dans le cadre du depistage des heterozygotes en ophtalmologie. J. Genet. Hum. 8: 108 only, 1959.

Pearce, W. G., Johnson, G. J., Gillan, J. G.: Nystagmus in a female carrier of ocular albinism. J. Med. Genet. 9: 126-128, 1972.

Pearce, W. G., Johnson, G. J. and Sanger, R.: Ocular albinism and Xg. (Letter) Lancet I: 1072 only, 1971.

Pearce, W. G., Sanger, R. and Race, R. R.: Ocular albinism and Xg. Lancet I: 1282-1283, 1968.

Vogt, A.: Die Iris: Albinismus solum bulbi. Atlas Spalt-Lampen-Mikroskopie 3: 846, 1942.

Waardenburg, P. J. and Van den Bosch, J.: X-chromosomal ocular albinism in Dutch family. Ann. Hum. Genet. 21: 101-122, 1956.

30060 ALBINISM, OCULAR (FORSIUS-ERIKSSON TYPE)

Forsius and Eriksson (1964) considered the ocular albinism they described in a family from the Aland Islands in the Sea of Bothnia to be a distinct entity. Males in 6 generations were affected. In addition to albinism of the fundus, the features were hypoplasia of the fovea, marked impairment of vision, nystagmus, myopia, astigmatism and protanomalous color blindness. Female carriers showed slight disturbances of color discrimination and electromyographically demonstrable nystagmus. Warburg (1964) described ocular albinism and protanopia in the same family. Only two of four males with ocular albinism showed dyschromatopsia. The absence of characteristic fundus pigmentary pattern in female carriers in the family of Forsius and Eriksson may be the best indication that they dealt with a distinct entity. Waardenburg et al. (1969) concluded that the disorder is entirely distinct from the X-linked ocular albinism. The pigment deficiency is not complete as in ocular albinism. They use Aland Island disease or the Forsius-Eriksson syndrome as preferable designations. Linkage studies indicate a recombination fraction of about 0.12 (confidence limits wide) with the Xg blood group locus (Race and Sanger, 1968), leading Waardenburg et al. (1969) to the suggestion that Aland Island disease and ocular albinism may be allelic, or may be pseudo-allelic, i.e., due to genes at adjacent loci. Scialfa (1967) reported a family with this disorder.

Forsius, H. and Eriksson, A. W.: Ein neues Augensyndrom mit x-chromosomaler Transmission. Eine Sippe mit Fundusalbinismus, Foveahypoplasie, Nystagmus, Myopie, Astigmatismus Und Dyschromatopsie. Klin. Monatsbl. Augenheilkd. 144: 447-457, 1964.

Race, R. R. and Sanger, R.: Blood Groups in Man. Philadelphia: F. A. Davis Co., 1968 (5th Ed.). P. 549.

Scialfa, A.: Albinisme oculaire et dyschromatopsie. Arch. Ophthalmol. 27: 483-494, 1967.

Waardenburg, P. J., Eriksson, A. W. and Forsius, H.: Aland eye disease (syndroma Forsius-Eriksson). Prog. Neuro-Ophthal. 2: 336-339, 1969.

Waardenburg, P. J.: Some notes on Aland eye disease (Forsius-Eriksson syndrome). J. Med. Genet. 7: 194-199, 1970.

Warburg, M.: Ocular albinism and protanopia in the same family. Acta Ophthalmol. 42: 444-451, 1964.

*30070 ALBINISM-DEAFNESS SYNDROME

Margolis (1962) described a 'new' X-linked syndrome — deaf-mutism and total albinism. Also from Israel, Ziprkowski and his colleagues (1962) described an X-linked syndrome consisting of deaf-mutism and partial albinism (without ocular albinism). They were reporting on the same family. The albinism is shown by the photographs to be 'partial,' as described by Ziprkowski and colleagues. Indeed, the pigmentary disorder might be called 'piebald.' Woolf (1965) observed the same phenotype in two Hopi American Indian brothers. Woolf, Dolowitz and Aldous (1965) described two Hopi brothers with congenital deafness and a remarkably similar pattern of pigmentary variegation of the piebald type. Another brother and both parents were normal and no other cases are known in southwest Indians. The deafness was subtotal nerve type. Hearing impairment in heterozygotes was demonstrated by Fried et al. (1969). Dolowitz (1966) stated that the 'Hopi children showed no marked decrease in vestibular function as judged by calorics with the Hallpike-Cawthorn test.'

Dolowitz, D. A.: Salt Lake City, Utah: personal communication, 1966.

Fried, K., Feinmesser, M. and Tsitsianov, J.: Hearing impairment in female carriers of the sex-linked syndrome of deafness with albinism. J. Med. Genet. 6: 132-134, 1969.

Margolis, E.: A new hereditary syndrome — sex-linked deaf-mutism associated with total albinism. Acta Genet. Statist. Med. 12: 12-19, 1962.

Reed, W. B., Stone, V. M., Boder, E. and Ziprkowski, L.: Pigmentary disorders in association with congenital deafness. Arch. Dermatol. 95: 176-186, 1967.

Woolf, C. M.: Albinism among Indians in Arizona and New Mexico. Am. J. Hum. Genet. 17: 23-35, 1965.

Woolf, C. M., Dolowitz, D. A. and Aldous, H. E.: Congenital deafness associated with piebaldness. Arch. Otolaryngaol. 82: 244-250, 1965.

Ziprkowski, L., Krakowski, A., Adam, A., Costeff, H. and Sade, J.: Partial albinism and deaf-mutism due to a recessive sex-linked gene. Arch. Dermatol. 86: 530-539, 1962.

*30080 ALBRIGHT HEREDITARY OSTEODYSTROPHY

This condition comprises both pseudohypoparathyroidism and pseudo-pseudohypoparathyroidism, which are probably aspects of a single entity. The facts (1) that no indubitable instance of male-to-male transmission has been observed and (2) that females are affected twice as often as males support the view that the disorder is an X-linked dominant. On the other hand, hemizygous males are not more severely affected than are heterozygous females. In fact, the tabulation of reported pedigrees (Mann, et al., 1962) shows that whereas only four of 36 female cases were of the incomplete form, six of 14 male cases failed to show full expression. This finding, contrary to that in other X-linked traits and contrary to present concepts of the X chromosome, makes it possible that this disorder is in fact a sex-influenced autosomal dominant. Type E brachydactyly (McKusick and Milch, 1964) resembles this entity in respect to short stature, the hand anomaly and round face. Mental retardation, cataract and ectopic calcification are not present. It is clearly autosomal dominant (q.v.). Male-to-male transmission was also observed in the family reported by Goeminne (1965) but the absence of ectopic calcification, mental retardation and cataract makes it virtually certain that this too was an instance of metacarpal brachydactyly and not Albright osteodystrophy. Goeminne (1970) remains of the opinion that his 'autosomal' pedigree represents PPHP. Hyperplasia of the parathyroids is the anatomic finding in these cases. Turner syndrome, a chromosomal aberration, often shows the same hand change. This Albright syndrome is not to be confused with polyostotic fibrous dysplasia (q.v.) to which Albright's name is also attached eponymously. Cases in which the picture was pseudohypoparathyroidism at one stage and later pseudo-pseudohypoparathyroidism have been reported by Palubinskas and Davis (1959) and others. Lee et al. (1968) found high parathormone and thyrocalcitonin in a mother and her affected son and daughter. The authors stated that the only other family with full expression in two generations was that of Mann et al. (1962). Whereas normal individuals show an increase in urinary excretion of cyclic AMP (which is involved in the cellular mechanisms of response to several hormones) on administration of parathormone, Chase et al. (1968) found no such response in patients with pseudohypoparathyroidism. Chase et al. (1969) found that parathyroid hormone circulates in abnormally high concentration in pseudohypoparathyroidism and secretion of the hormone responds normally to physiologic control by calcium. Unlike the normal, cyclic AMP did not increase in the urine in response to administrated parathormone. They suggested that the basic defect may be deficient amount or function of parathormone-sensitive adenyl cyclase in bone and kidney. Like others, Chase et al. (1969) found pseudopseudohypoparathyroidism and pseudohypoparathyroidism in different members of the same family, but surprising findings were that persons with pseudopseudohypoparathyroidism showed (1) abnormally high basal urinary excretion of cyclic AMP, and (2) normal increase in urinary AMP with parathormone infusion. Possibly patients change in regard to these characteristics when passing from the picture of pseudo- to pseudopseudohypoparathyroidism. Chase and Aurbach (1968) showed that parathormone and vasopressin stimulate adenyl cyclase in anatomically separate parts of the kidney, cortex and medulla, respectively. To my knowledge, the cyclic AMP system has not been examined in nephrogenic diabetes insipidus (q.v.). Intelligence is normal in some patients with pseudohypoparathyroidism. Frame et al. (1972), among others, has described renal resistance to parathormone with osteitis fibrosa produced by the secondary hyperparathyroidism. One possibility is that there are separate genetic mechanisms for renal and osseous response to parathormone and that only the former is defective in these cases. An intriguing alternative possibility is that the bones at least in a patchy distribution are responsive to parathormone because of the Lyon phenomenon.

Chase, L. R. and Aurbach, G. D.: Renal adenyl cyclase: anatomically separate sites for parathyroid hormone and vasopressin. Science 159: 545-547, 1968.

Chase, L. R., Melson, G. L. and Aurbach, G. D.: Pseudohypoparathyroidism: defective excretion of 3 (prime)-5(prime)-AMP in response to parathyroid hormone. J. Clin. Invest. 48: 1832-1844, 1969.

Frame, B., Hanson, C. A., Frost, H. M., Block, M. and Arnstein, A. R.: Renal resistance to parathyroid hormone with osteitis fibrosa: 'pseudohypoparathyroidism.' Am. J. Med. 52: 311-321, 1972.

Goeminne, L.: Albright's hereditary poly-osteochondrodystrophy (pseudo-pseudo-hypoparathyroidism with diabetes hypertension, arteritis and polyarthrosis). Acta Genet. Med. Gemellol. 14: 226-281, 1965.

Goeminne, L.: Zulte, Belgium: personal communication, 1970.

X

L
I
N
K
E
D

(Albright's hereditary osteodystrophy). A family study. Mayo Clin. Proc. 39: 81-91, 1964.

Lee, J. B., Tashjian, A. H., Jr., Streeto, J. M. and Frantz, A. G.: Familial pseudohypoparathyroidism. Role of parathyroid hormone and thyrocalcitonin. New Eng. J. Med. 279: 1179-1184, 1968.

Mann, J. B., Alterman, S. and Hill, A. G.: Albright's hereditary osteodystrophy comprising pseudohypoparathyroidism and pseudo-pseudohypoparathyroidism, with a report of two cases representing the complete syndrome occurring in successive generations. Ann. Intern. Med. 56: 315-342, 1962.

McKusick, V. A. and Milch, R. A.: The clinical behavior of genetic disease: selected aspects. Clin. Orthop. 33: 22-39, 1964.

Palubinskas, A. J. and Davies, H.: Calcification of the basal ganglia of the brain. Am. J. Roentgen. 82: 806-822, 1959.

30090 ALCOHOLISM

Cruz-Coke and Varela (1966) advanced the hypothesis that alcoholism is determined by an X-linked recessive gene. Winokur (1967) concluded from an analysis of data published by Amark (1951) that the X-linked hypothesis is untenable.

Amark, C.: A study in alcoholism. Clinical, social-psychiatric and genetic investigations. Acta Psychiatr. Neurol. Scand. 70 (Suppl.): 1-283, 1951.

Cruz-Coke, R. and Varela, A.: Inheritance of alcoholism. Its association with colour-blindness. Lancet II: 1282-1284, 1966.

Winokur, G.: X-borne recessive genes in alcoholism. (Letter) Lancet II: 466 only, 1967.

*30100 ALDRICH SYNDROME

The manifestations are eczema, thrombocytopenia, proneness to infection, and bloody diarrhea. Death occurs before age 10. Aldrich's original kindred was of Dutch extraction. Van den Bosch and Drukker (1964) described several families in the Netherlands. In 3 of 5 female carriers the platelet count was below the lower limit of normal. Several groups (Blaese et al., 1968; Cooper et al., 1968) have presented evidence that the immune defect is in the afferent limb, i.e., is one of antigen processing or recognition.

Aldrich, R. A., Steinberg, A. G. and Campbell, D. C.: Pedigree demonstrating a sex-linked recessive condition characterized by draining ears, eczematoid dermatitis and bloody diarrhea. Pediatrics 13: 133-139, 1954.

Blaese, R. M., Strober, W., Brown, R. S. and Waldmann, T. A.: The Wiskott-Aldrich syndrome. A disorder with a possible defect in antigens processing or recognition. Lancet I: 1056-1060, 1968.

Blaese, R. M., Strober, W., Levy, A. L. and Waldmann, T. A.: Hypercatabolism of IgG, IgA, IgM, and albumin in the Wiskott-Aldrich syndrome. A unique disorder of serum protein metabolism. J. Clin. Invest. 50: 2331-2338, 1971.

Cooper, M. D., Chae, H. P., Lowman, J. T., Krivit, W. and Good, R. A.: Wiskott-Aldrich syndrome. An immunologic deficiency disease involving the afferent limb Of immunity. Am. J. Med. 44: 499-513, 1968.

Gelzer, J. and Gasser, C.: Wiskott-Aldrich-syndrome. Helv. Paediat. Acta 16: 17-39, 1961.

Krivit, W. and Good, R. A.: Aldrich's syndrome (thrombocytopenia, eczema and infection in infants). Studies of the defense mechanisms. Am. J. Dis. Child. 97: 137-153, 1959.

Levin, A. S., Spitler, L. E., Stiles, D. P. and Fundenberg, H. H.: Wiskott-Aldrich syndrome, a genetically determined cellular immunologic deficiency: clinical and laboratory responses to therapy with transfer factor. Proc. Natl. Acad. Sci. 67: 821-828, 1970.

Steinberg, A. G.: Methodology in human genetics. J. Med. Educ. 34: 315-334, 1959.

Van den Bosch, J. and Drukker, J.: Het syndroom van Aldrich: een klinisch en genetisch onderzoek van enige nederlandse families. Maandschr. Kindergeneeskd. 32: 359-373, 1964.

Wolff, J. A.: Wiskott-Aldrich syndrome: clinical, immunologic, and pathologic observations. J. Pediatr. 70: 221-232, 1967.

*30110 AMELOGENESIS IMPERFECTA, HYPOMATURATION TYPE

The enamel is opaque white, soft and easily abraded but appears of normal thickness in unerupted teeth. The condition is inherited as an X-linked recessive. Witkop (1967) observed changes in the teeth of heterozygous females consistent with the Lyon hypothesis. Witkop (1967) and Sauk et al. (1972) presented evidence that the heterozygous female has vertically arranged bands of mottled enamel alternating with bands of normal appearing enamel. The findings were considered consistent with the Lyon hypothesis.

Sauk, J. J., Jr., Lyon, H. W. and Witkop, C. J., Jr.: Electron optic microanalysis of two genes products in enamel of females heterozygous for X-linked hypomaturation amelogenesis imperfecta. Am. J. Hum. Genet. 24: 267-276, 1972.

Witkop, C. J.: Hereditary defects in enamel and dentin. Acta Genet. Statist. Med. 7: 236-239, 1957.

Witkop, C. J., Jr.: Partial expression of sex-linked recessive amelogenesis imperfecta in females compatible with the Lyon hypothesis. Oral Surg. 23: 174-182, 1967.

X

L
I
N
K
E
D

*30120 AMELOGENESIS IMPERFECTA, HYPOPLASTIC TYPE (HEREDITARY ENAMEL HYPO-PLASIA)

In this condition the enamel is very hard but is abnormally thin so that the teeth appear small. The surface is rough. This type is inherited as an X-linked dominant. Possible genetic relationship, e.g. allelism, with the factor for the hypomaturation type is unknown. Therefore the two have been listed as separate loci. Rushton (1964) pointed out differences in males and females which may be based on the Lyon phenomenon. The affected males have only a very thin smooth layer of enamel which appears nearly homogeneous. The females have enamel which in parts is much thicker giving a vertically grooved appearance to the teeth. Wide variation in the involvement in females is also consistent with the Lyon hypothesis. This disorder, like hypophosphatemia, was considered to be autosomal dominant before the true inheritance was pointed out by Schulze (1952, 1957) and others. The histologic characteristic is the presence of twisted enamel rods coursing from the dentino-enamel junction to the enamel surface. Berkman and Singer (1971) presented evidence for operation of the Lyon phenomenon in heterozygous females.

Berkman, M. D. and Singer, A.: Demonstration of the Lyon hypothesis in X-linked dominant hypoplastic amelogenesis imperfecta. The Clinical Delineation of Birth Defects. XI. Orofacial Structures. Baltimore: Williams and Wilkins, 1971. Pp. 204-209.

Haldane, J. B. S.: A probable new sex-linked dominant in man. J. Hered. 28: 58-60, 1937.

Rushton, M. A.: Hereditary enamel defects. Proc. Roy. Soc. Med. 57: 53-58, 1964.

Schulze, C. and Lenz, F. R.: Uber Zahnschmelzhypoplasie von unvollstandig dominantem geschlechts-gebundenen Erbgang. Z. Menschl. Vererb. Konstitutionsl. 31: 104-114, 1952.

Schulze, C.: Erbbedingte Strukturanomalien menschlicher Zahne. Acta Genet. Statist. Med. 7: 231-235, 1957.

Shokeir, M. H. K.: Hereditary enamel hypoplasia. Clin. Genet. 2: 387-391, 1971.

Weinmann, J. P., Svoboda, J. F. and Woods, R. W.: Hereditary disturbances of enamel formation and calcification. J. Am. Dent. Assoc. 32: 397-418, 1945.

*30130 ANEMIA, HYPOCHROMIC

This condition was first described by Cooley (1945), who also first described thalassemia. He pointed out possible X-linkage in a family in which 19 males in five generations were affected, with transmission through unaffected females. Rundles and Falls reported two families, of which one was the same as that reported by Cooley.

Hypochromic anemia has, of course, other causes, notably iron deficiency. What is referred to here are the rare cases in which it is hereditary. The condition is also known as hereditary iron-loading anemia (Byrd and Cooper, 1961). The features include: (a) anemia detected first in childhood in some cases; (b) death from hemochromatosis at a relatively young age, with the number of transfusions inadequate to account for the hemochromatosis; (c) hyperferricemia; and (d) abundance of siderocytes in peripheral blood after splenectomy. Somewhat enlarged spleens and minor red cell abnormalities without anemia were observed in female carriers by Rundles and Falls (1946).

Bickers et al. (1962) described the disorder in a man whose mother, sister and five children had hematologic involvement in various degrees. Pyridoxine responsiveness was demonstrated in at least two affected members of Rundles and Falls family (Bishop and Bethel, 1959; Horrigan and Harris, 1964). Close linkage to the Xg locus was excluded by Elves, Bourne and Israels (1966). Associated hypolipidemia and hypocholesterolemia were pointed out by Spitzer, Newcomb and Noyes (1966). Two populations of cells, as to morphology, in heterozygotes were illustrated by Pinkerton (1967). Prasad et al. (1968) studied a Negro family in which both sideroblastic anemia and G6PD-deficiency were segregating. A maximum likelihood estimate of the recombination value was 0.14. In females doubly heterozygous in coupling, a correlation between small red cells and low G6PD was found. In a heterozygote Lee et al. (1968) separated two populations of red cells by centrifugation in layered gum acacia solutions of different specific gravity. The microcytes had a lower level of free protoporphyrin than did the normal cells but unimpaired capacity to convert delta-aminolevulinic acid to protoporphyrin, suggesting a defect at or before the step in which delta-aminolevulinic acid is synthesized. The enzyme defect may concern delta-aminolevulinic acid synthetase, which requires vitamin B6 as a cofactor and is the rate-limiting step in porphyrin synthesis. If so, this enzyme would appear to be determined by a structural gene on the X chromosome. Thalassemia minor is the other condition which in this country produces hereditary hypochromic anemia. Weatherall et al. (1970) were unable to demonstrate Lyonization of the Xg locus by observing two populations of cells in females heterozygous for familial sideroblastic anemia, called here X-linked hypochromic anemia. Hines (1971) observed decreased levels of pyridoxal phosphokinase in red cells and livers of patients with pyridoxine-dependent refractory sideroblastic anemia. Aoki et al. (1973) found deficiency of delta-aminolevulinic acid synthetase in the red cells of patients with sideroblastic anemia, some of whom were males with congenital anemia which in some responded to treatment with B6.

Aoki, Y., Urata, G. and Takaku, F.: Delta-aminolevulinic acid synthetase in erythroblasts of patients with primary siderblastic anemia. Acta Haematol. Jap. 36: 74-77, 1973.

Bickers, J. N., Brown, C. L. and Sprague, C. C.: Pyridoxine responsive anemia. Blood 19: 304-312, 1962.

Bishop, R. C. and Bethel, F. H.: Hereditary hypochromic anemia with transfusion hemosiderosis treated with pyridoxin. New Eng. J. Med. 261: 486-489, 1959.

Byrd, R. B. and Cooper, T.: Hereditary iron-loading anemia with secondary hemochromatosis. Ann. Intern. Med. 55: 103-123, 1961.

Cooley, T. B.: A severe type of hereditary anemia with elliptocytosis: interesting sequence of splenectomy. Am. J. Med. Sci. 209: 561-568, 1945.

Elves, M. W., Bourne, M. S. and Israels, M. C. G.: Pyridoxine-responsive anaemia determined by an X-linked gene. J. Med. Genet. 3: 1-4, 1966.

Harris, J. W. and Horrigan, D. L.: Pyridoxine-responsive anemia-prototype and variations of the theme. Vitamins Hormones 22: 721-753, 1964.

Hines, J. D.: Quantitative assessment of blood and tissue pyridoxal phosphokinase concentration in patients with vitamin B6-dependent states. J. Clin. Invest. 50: 45A only, 1971.

Horrigan, D. L. and Harris, J. W.: Pyridoxine-responsive anemia: analysis of 62 cases. Adv. Intern. Med. 12: 103-174, 1964.

Lee, G. R., MacDiarmid, W. D., Cartwright, G. E. and Wintrobe, M. M.: Hereditary, X-linked, sideroachrestic anemia. The isolation of two erythrocyte populations differing in Xg(A) blood type and porphyrin content. Blood 32: 59-70, 1968.

Pinkerton, P. H.: X-linked hypochromic anemia. (Letter) Lancet I: 1106-1107, 1967.

Prasad, A. S., Tranchida, L., Konno, E. T., Berman, L., Albert, S., Sing, C. F. and Brewer, G. J.: Hereditary sideroblastic anemia and glucose-6-phosphate dehydrogenase deficiency in a Negro family. J. Clin. Invest. 47: 1415-1424, 1968.

Rundles, R. W. and Falls, H. F.: Hereditary (sex-linked) anemia. Am. J. Med. Sci. 211: 641-658, 1946.

Spitzer, N., Newcomb, T. F. and Noyes, W. D.: Pyridoxine-responsive hypolipidemia and hypocholesterolemia in a patient with pyridoxine responsive anemia. New Eng. J. Med. 274: 772-775, 1966.

Weatherall, D. J., Pembrey, M. E., Hall, E. G., Sanger, R., Tippett, P. and Gavin, J.: Familial sideroblastic anaemia: problem of Xg and X chromosomes inactivation. Lancet II: 744-748, 1970.

*30150 ANGIOKERATOMA, DIFFUSE (FABRY DISEASE; HEREDITARY DYSTOPIC LIPIDOSIS)

Skin lesions of vascular nature are the main basis of the name. Attacks of pain in the abdomen are often misdiagnosed as appendicitis. Such pains and those elsewhere, such as in the extremities, probably have their basis in lipid changes in ganglion cells of the autonomic nervous system. Vascular lesions of lipid nature occur at other sites such as the ocular fundi and kidney. Renal failure is the usual cause of death. Heterozygous females almost never have skin lesions and survive longer despite renal involvement. Hamburger and colleagues (1964) described a familial nephropathy, manifested clinically by proteinuria and renal insufficiency. Renal biopsy showed that the epithelial cells of the glomerular tufts and to a lesser extent the tubular epithelial cells, glomerular endocapillary cells and arteriolar muscular cells were severely deformed with a large amount of cytoplasmic inclusion material. The inclusion material was thought to be lipoid in nature. The findings resemble those of angiokeratoma corporis diffusum but the absence of other signs of this disease suggested that a new entity may be involved. The mother's father died of uremia. Skin lesions are easily overlooked. It is clear, however, that they may be lacking even in patients with severe visceral manifestations (Johnston, 1967). Johnston et al. (1969) estimated the recombination fraction of angiokeratoma versus Xg to be 0.24 (95 percent probability limits, 8-49.8 percent) and of angiokeratoma versus deutan to be 0.17 (95 percent probability limits, 1-50 percent). Franceschetti et al. (1969) reexamined the family with 'cornea verticillata' reported by Gruber (1946) and showed that Fabry disease was the 'cause' of the corneal change. The extent of involvement of the cornea is about the same in males and females. Thus, carrier females can be identified. The corneal condition was formerly called also Fleischer vortex dystrophy, or whorl-like corneal dystrophy. Atabrine produces an interesting phenocopy. Kint (1970) showed that the activity of alpha-galactosidase is deficient in leukocytes of male patients with Fabry disease and that carrier females can be identified by this method. In two patients Mapes et al. (1970) demonstrated a decline in the plasma level of galactosylgalactosylglucosylceramide when normal plasma was infused to provide active enzyme (ceramide trihexosidase). The Fabry locus does 'Lyonize' (Romeo and Migeon, 1970). At a Montreal hospital in a period of a few months Clarke et al. (1971) saw two men with Fabry disease without skin lesions, suggesting that it may be a more frequent cause of proteinuria or renal failure than realized. A difference from the usual form of Fabry disease is suggested by the fact that leukocyte alpha-galactosidase deficiency was only partial rather than being complete (Kint, 1970) as in the usual cases. The relationship of the alpha-galactosidase deficiency to the primary fault, deficiency of ceramide trihexosidase, is unknown. Romeo and Migeon (1971) presented evidence for a structural change in the mutant enzyme (slower heat inactivation than in the normal and different K(m) values). Angiokeratoma occurs also with alpha-l-fucosidase deficiency (23000), an autosomal recessive (Patel et al., 1972). Localization of the alpha galactosidase locus to the X chromosome had been achieved also by cell hybridization (Grzeschik, 1972). Flynn et al. (1972) described a family without skin lesions. One affected male had severe enteropathy.

Brady, R. O., Gal, A. E., Bradley, R. M., Martensson, E., Warshaw, A. L. and Laster, L.: Enzymatic defect in Fabry's disease. Ceramidetrihexosidase deficiency. New Eng. J. Med. 276: 1163-1167, 1967.

Clarke, J. T., Knaack, J., Crawhall, J. C. and Wolfe, L. S.: Ceramide trihexosidosis (Fabry's disease) without skin lesions. New Eng. J. Med. 284: 233-235, 1971.

Flynn, D. M., Lake, B. D., Boothby, C. B. and Young, E. P.: Gut lesions in Fabry's disease without a rash. Arch. Dis. Child. 47: 26-33, 1972.

X
L
I
N
K
E
D

Franceschetti, A. T., Philippart, M. and Franceschetti, A.: A study of Fabry's disease. I. Clinical examination of a family with cornea verticillata. Dermatologica 138: 209-221, 1969.

Frost, P., Tanaka, Y. and Spaeth, G. L.: Fabry's disease — glycolipid lipidoses. Histochemical and electron microscopic studies of two cases. Am. J. Med. 40: 618-627, 1966.

Grzeschik, K. H.: Leiden, personal communication, via Dr. F. H. Ruddle, 1972.

Gruber, M.: Cornea verticillata. (Eine einfach-dominante Variante der Hornhaut des menschlichen Auges). Ophthalmologica 111: 120-129, 1946.

Gruber, M.: Cornea verticillata. II. Mitteilung. Ophthalmologica 112: 88-91, 1946.

Hamburger, J., Dormont, J., De Montera, H. and Hinglais, N.: Sur une singuliere malformation familiale de l'epithelium renal. Schweiz. Med. Wschr. 94: 871-876, 1964.

Johnston, A. W.: Fabry's disease without skin lesions. (Letter) Lancet I: 1277 only, 1967.

Johnston, A. W., Frost, P., Spaeth, G. L. and Renwick, J. H.: Linkage relationships of the angiokeratoma (Fabry) locus. Ann. Hum. Genet. 32: 369-374, 1969.

Kint, J. A.: Fabry's disease: alpha-galactosidase deficiency. Science 167: 1268-1269, 1970.

Mapes, C. A., Anderson, R. L., Sweeley, C. C., Desnick, R. J. and Krivit, W.: Enzyme replacement in Fabry's disease, an inborn error of metabolism. Science 169: 987-989, 1970.

Opitz, J. M., Stiles, F. C., Wise, D., Race, R. R., Sanger, R., Von Gemmingen, G. R., Kierland, R. R., Cross, E. G. and Degroot, W. P.: The genetics of angiokeratoma corporis diffusum (Fabry's disease) and its linkage relations with the Xg locus. Am. J. Hum. Genet. 17: 325-342, 1965.

Patel, V., Watanabe, I. and Zeman, W.: Deficiency of alpha-l-fucosidase. Science 176: 426-428, 1972.

Philippart, M., Sarlieve, L. and Manacorda, A.: Urinary glycolipids in Fabry's disease. Their examination in the detection of atypical variants and the pre-symptomatic state. Pediatrics 43: 201-206, 1969.

Rahman, A. N., Simeone, F. A., Hackel, D. B., Hall, P. W., III, Hirsch, E. Z. and Harris, J. W.: Angiokeratoma corporis diffusum universale (hereditary dystopic lipidosis). Trans. Ass. Am. Physicians 74: 366-377, 1961.

Romeo, G. and Migeon, B. R.: Genetic inactivation of the alpha-galactosidase locus in carriers of Fabry's disease. Science 170: 180-181, 1970.

Sweeley, C. C. and Klionsky, B.: Fabry's disease: classification as a sphingolipidosis and partial characterization of a novel glycolipid. J. Biol. Chem. 238: 3148-3150, 1963.

Wise, D., Wallace, H. J. and Jellinek, E. H.: Angiokeratoma corporis diffusum: a clinical study of eight affected families. Quart. J. Med. 31: 177-206, 1962.

30160 ANGIOMATOSIS, DIFFUSE CORTICO-MENINGEAL, OF DIVRY AND VAN BOGAERT

Features in addition to the cortico-meningeal angiomatosis were demyelination of the white substance of the centrum ovale with hemianopsia, and 'marbled skin' resulting from a telangiectatic network. Three affected brothers were described.

Divry, P. and Van Bogaert, L.: Une maladie familiale caracterisee par une angiomatose diffuse cortico-meningee non calcifiante et une demyelinisation progressive de la substance blanche. J. Neurol. Neurosurg. Psychiat. 9: 41-54, 1946.

30165 ANORCHIA, FAMILIAL

Hall et al. (1974) described anorchia in both of identical twins and in two brothers. In three anorchia was unilateral, in one bilateral.

Hall, J. G., Blizzard, R. and Morgan, A.: Familial anorchia. To be published, 1974.

30170 ANOSMIA

Anosmia may be an X-linked dominant trait: no male-to-male transmission has been observed, although only a few affected males have had children (Glaser, 1918). The main reason for considering anosmia separately is that it is not clear whether it is always merely part of the Kallmann syndrome (q.v.) or may be a distinct mutation. Affected males in Glaser's family in which X-linked inheritance was suggested had 'excessive sex interest.' It was a Russian Jewish family like those of Kallmann and colleagues.

The anatomic basis of anosmia is agenesis of the olfactory lobes. De Morsier collected 28 reported cases of agenesis of the olfactory lobes in which complete autopsy was performed and found that abnormalities of the sexual organs, mainly cryptorchidism and testicular atrophy, had been noted in 14. He suggested that the genital atrophy is secondary to involvement of the hypothalamus as well as the olfactory lobes.

De Morsier, G.: Etudes sur les dystrophies cranio-encephaliques. I. Agenesie des lobes olfactifs (telencephaloschizis lateral) et des commissures calleuse et anterieure (telencephaloschizis median): la dysplasie olfacto-genitale. Schweiz. Arch. Neurol. Psychiat. 74: 309-361, 1954.

Glaser, O.: Hereditary deficiencies in the sense of smell. Science 48: 647-648, 1918.

30180 ANUS, IMPERFORATE

Weinstein (1965) reported three families with multiple affected males in a pattern strongly suggesting X-linked recessive inheritance. In a later paper, Winkler and Weinstein (1970) described two families, each

X

L
I
N
K
E
D

with two sisters with imperforate anus and-or ectopic anus (rectovaginal fistula). They then proposed
autosomal recessive inheritance for some cases.

Weinstein, E. D.: Sex-linked imperforate anus. Pediatrics 35: 715-717, 1965.

Winkler, J. M. and Weinstein, E. D.: Imperforate anus and heredity. J. Pediatr. Surg. 5: 555-558, 1970.

*30190 BORJESON SYNDROME (MENTAL DEFICIENCY, EPILEPSY, ENDOCRINE DISORDERS)

Features were severe mental defect, epilepsy, hypogonadism, hypometabolism, marked obesity, swelling of subcutaneous tissue of face, narrow palpebral fissure, large but not deformed ears. Three females who might be carriers had moderate mental retardation. This is a 'new' syndrome described in a single kindred. Baar and Galindo (1965) described a single case they thought represented the same entity.

Baar, H. S. and Galindo, J.: The Borjeson-Forssman-Lehmann syndrome. J. Ment. Defic. Res. 9: 125-130, 1965.

Borjeson, M., Forssman, H. and Lehmann, O.: An X-linked, recessively inherited syndrome characterized by grave mental deficiency, epilepsy, and endocrine disorder. Acta Med. Scand. 171: 13-21, 1962.

*30200 BULLOUS DYSTROPHY, HEREDITARY MACULAR TYPE

The features are formation of bullae without evident trauma, absence of all hair, hyperpigmentation, depigmentation, acrocyanosis, dwarfism, microcephaly, mental inferiority, short tapering fingers, sometimes anomalies of the nails. Most patients die before attaining adulthood. This disorder has been recognized only in a single kindred living in the Netherlands and described in three publications as listed below.

Carol, W. L. L. and Kooij, R.: Macular type of hereditary bullous dystrophy. Maandschr. Kindergeneeskd. 6: 39-51, 1936.

Mendes da Costa, S. and Van der Valk, J. W.: Typus maculatus der bullosen hereditaren Dystophie. Arch. Dermatol. Syph. 91: 1-8, 1908.

Woerdeman, M. J.: Dystrophia bullosa hereditaria, typus maculatus. Nederl. Tijdschr. Geneeskd. 102: 111-116, 1958.

*30220 CATARACT, CONGENITAL TOTAL, WITH POSTERIOR SUTURAL OPACITIES IN HETEROZYGOTES

Walsh and Wegman (1937) described possible X-linked cataract in the 'We-Sorts,' a tri-racial group of southern Maryland. The affected males had nuclear cataracts with severe visual impairment. Heterozygous females had suture cataracts with only slight reduction in vision. Fraccaro et al. (1967) found the same type of expression in males and females. Linkage studies indicated that the Xg locus and the cataract locus may be within measurable distance. These authors pointed out that the pedigrees of Stieren (1907) and of Halbertsma (1934), which have been frequently cited as examples of X-linked cataract, are not acceptable. In Stieren's pedigree 7 of 17 affected males had congenital hydrocephalus and all affected males were born blind and died in convulsions. Thus, they may have suffered from a complex syndrome of which cataract was only one feature. Furthermore, two unaffected males had daughters who gave birth to affected sons. In Halbertsma's family, beside 10 affected males, 3 females had congenital cataract and one had senile cataract. Fraser and Friedmann (1967) observed a family with possible X-linked cataract. Krill et al. (1969) described a convincingly X-linked pedigree. Suture cataract was found as an early manifestation in hemizygous males. Cataract is a feature of nearly all cases of Lowe syndrome (q.v.). Nance et al. (1973) described a family in which affected males and carrier females had dental anomalies whereas persons without cataract did not. The affected males had microcornea, supernumerary incisors, anteverted pinnae, shortened metacarpals, and possible elevation of serum alkaline phosphatase. The carriers had posterior sutural opacities and cone-shaped teeth. Some of the features suggest the Lenz syndrome (30980).

Fraccaro, M., Morone, G., Manfredini, U. and Sanger, R.: X-linked cataract. Ann. Hum. Genet. 31: 45-50, 1967.

Fraser, G. R. and Friedmann, A. I.: The Causes of Blindness in Childhood. A Study of 776 Children with Severe Visual Handicaps. Baltimore: Johns Hopkins Press, 1967. P. 59.

Halbertsma, K. T. A.: Familiare aangeboren cataract. Nederl. Tijdschr. Geneeskd. 78: 1705-1709, 1934.

Krill, A. E., Woodbury, G. and Bowman, J. E.: X-chromosomal-linked sutural cataracts. Am. J. Ophthalmol. 68: 867-872, 1969.

Nance, W. E., Warburg, M., Bixler, D. and Helveston, E. M.: Congenital X-linked cataract, dental anomalies and brachymetacarpalia. Clinical Delineation of Birth Defects. XVI. Urinary System and Others. Baltimore: Williams and Wilkins, 1974. Pp. 285-291.

Stieren, E.: A study in atavistic descent of congenital cataract through four generations. Ophthalmol. Rec. 16: 234-238, 1907.

Walsh, F. B. and Wegman, M. E.: Pedigree of hereditary cataract, illustrating sex-limited type. Bull. Hopkins Hosp. 61: 125-135, 1937.

30230 CATARACT, CONGENITAL WITH MICROCORNEA OR SLIGHT MICROPHTHALMIA

Waardenburg (loc. cit. p. 880) observed a family with clear X-linked recessive inheritance. Witkop-Oostenrijk (1956) described a family in which X-linked dominance (possibly with lethality in the affected hemizygote) might be the genetic mechanism. Autosomal dominant and autosomal recessive forms also exist. Capella et al. (1963) also observed probable X-linked cataract. Nine men had cataract, four also had microcornea in one or both eyes and one had small phthisical eyes. It is uncertain that cataract with microcornea is an entity

610   separate from 'cataract, congenital total, with posterior sutural opacities in heterozygotes,' because some patients of Walsh and Wegman and one of Krill et al. showed microcornea.

Capella, J. A., Kaufman, H. E., Lill, F. J. and Cooper, G.: Hereditary cataracts and microphthalmia. Am. J. Ophthalmol. 56: 454-458, 1963.

Witkop-Oostenrijk, G. A.: Microphthalmus, microcornea en aangeboren cataract. Nederl. Tijdschr. Geneeskd. 100: 2910-2913, 1956.

Waardenburg, P. J., Franceschetti, A. and Klein, D.: Genetics and Ophthalmology. Springfield, Ill.: Charles C Thomas, 1: 851-888, 1961.

30240 CENTRAL INCISORS, ABSENCE OF

Huskins described an English family with affected members of at least three generations. He specifically stated that there was 'no evidence of any other defective condition being associated with this dental anomaly.' There was one affected female in the family. We know of no other report of X-linkage.

Huskins, C. L.: On the inheritance of an anomaly of human dentition. J. Hered. 21: 279-282, 1930.

*30250 CEREBELLAR ATAXIA

Shokeir (1970) described 3 kindreds with a total of 16 affected persons in an X-linked recessive pedigree pattern. One of the affected persons was a female with the XO Turner syndrome. Absence of extrapyramidal signs distinguished the disorder from that described by Malamud. The absence of kyphoscoliosis and pes cavus and preservation of posterior column function were features distinguishing the disorder from Friedreich ataxia. The disease did not seem to affect life-span and intelligence was unimpaired. Onset was in the late teens or early twenties. There was no visual difficulty except that attributable to nystagmus.

Shokeir, M. H. K.: X-linked cerebellar ataxia. Clin. Genet. 1: 225-231, 1970.

*30260 CEREBELLAR ATAXIA WITH EXTRAPYRAMIDAL INVOLVEMENT

Malamud's family had an unusual form of neurologic disease in that the clinical picture, dominated at the outset by cerebellar signs, was later characterized by extrapyramidal signs. Anatomical changes involved both the cerebellar and the extrapyramidal systems.

Malamud, N. and Cohen, P.: Unusual form of cerebellar ataxia with sex-linked inheritance. Neurology 8: 261-266, 1958.

*30270 CEREBRAL SCLEROSIS, DIFFUSE, SCHOLZ TYPE

Ford refers to this form as the subacute childhood type. It begins at age 8-10 years and is characterized by deafness, blindness, weakness and spasticity of the legs, and dementia. Survival is shorter after onset of symptoms. However, in Scholz's family, although the affected males in the youngest generation showed this picture, their maternal grandfathers, age 65 and 60, had the picture of spastic paraplegia.

Walsh (1957) described under the heading of Schilder disease, or encephalitis periaxialis diffusa, a kindred in which four males, offspring of sisters, succumbed to an illness possibly of the type shown by Scholz's youngest patients. See also Addison disease and cerebral sclerosis. Scholz (1925) used histologic techniques which would have removed metachromatic material. The cases of Scholz were restudied by Peiffer (1959) using frozen sections and striking metachromasia was demonstrated.

Becker, P. E.: Andere neurologische Erbkrankheiten. Handbuch der Inneren Medizin, Springer, Berlin-Gottingen-Heidelberg. 4. Aufl. VIII: 1003, 1953.

Peiffer, J.: Uber die metachromatischen Leukodystrophien (Typ scholz). Arch. Psychiatr. Nervenkr. 199: 386-416, 1959.

Scholz, W.: Klinische, pathologisch-anatomische und erbbiologische Untersuchungen bei familiarer, diffuser Hirnsklerose im Kindesalter. Zbl. Ges. Psychiatr. 9: 651-717, 1925.

Walsh, F. B.: Clinical Neuro-ophthalmology. Baltimore: Williams and Wilkins, 1957 (2nd ed.). P. 664 only.

*30280 CHARCOT-MARIE-TOOTH PERONEAL MUSCULAR ATROPHY

This condition is essentially a degeneration of spinal nerve roots, especially the motor roots to the distal parts of the extremities. Autosomal dominant and recessive forms also exist. Woratz (cited by Becker, 1966) studied a family in which X-linked dominant inheritance was present. A very large number of persons in 6 generations were affected. Ten affected fathers had only affected daughters (15) and only normal sons (8), whereas affected mothers (26) had affected sons (23) and affected daughters (21) as well as unaffected offspring. Males were more severely affected than females. Herringham (1889) reported a family with 20 affected males in 4 generations. Erwin (1944) observed 7 cases in 5 generations.

Allan, W.: Relation of hereditary pattern to clinical severity as illustrated by peroneal atrophy. Arch. Intern. Med. 63: 1123-1131, 1939.

Erwin, W. G.: A pedigree of sex-linked recessive peroneal atrophy. J. Hered. 35: 24-26, 1944.

Herringham, W. P.: Muscular atrophy of the peroneal type affecting many members of a family. Brain 11: 230-236, 1889.

Woratz, G.: Cited by Becker, P. E.: Humangenetik 5: 427 only, 1966.

X

L
I
N
K
E
D

In the families reported by Van Bogaert and Moreau (1939, 1941), Charcot-Marie-Tooth disease and Friedreich ataxia occurred in the same individuals in a pattern of sex-linked recessive inheritance. Possibly this is a mutation distinct from that responsible for the two disorders separately. If the genes for peroneal muscular atrophy and Friedreich ataxia are closely situated on the X chromosome, deletion is another possible explanation for the finding in this family. In Biemond's kindred some individuals had Charcot-Marie-Tooth disease (in a pedigree pattern consistent with X-linked inheritance), whereas two females of one sibship had Friedreich ataxia. In addition many members of the kindred had deaf-mutism (in a pattern consistent with autosomal recessive inheritance). Thus, three seemingly independent hereditary traits were observed in the same family. Van Bogaert's family is probably the only one in which the two neurologic diseases occurred always together in an X-linked pattern.

Biemond, A.: Neurotische Muskelatrophie und Friedreichsche Tabes in derselben Familie. Deutsch. Z. Nervenheilk. 104: 113-145, 1928.

Van Bogaert, L. and Moreau, M.: Combinaison de l'amyotrophie de Charcot-Marie-Tooth et de la maladie de Friedreich chez plusieurs membres d'une meme famille. Encephale 34: 312-320, 1939-1941.

30300 CHOROIDAL SCLEROSIS

In his atlas of the fundus oculi (1934), Wilmer showed (plate 82) the fundus of a 35-year-old affected man whose maternal grandfather was also affected. Furthermore two brothers and the maternal grandfather of the proband's maternal grandfather were also affected, i.e., the proband had inherited the disorder from his great-great-grandfather through the intermediacy of a carrier mother and great-grandmother. Follow-up by letter in 1962 provided no further information. Stankovic (1958) reported a similar family, which is of further interest because female carriers showed partial expression. A difficulty in interpretation of these reports is the uncertainty that the disorder is distinct from retinitis pigmentosa (q.v.) and perhaps choroideremia (q.v.). In retinitis pigmentosa (see Jacobson and Stephens, 1962) the fundi are sometimes reported as showing 'severe choroidal sclerosis.' Sorsby (1963) was of the opinion that the cases reported by Sorsby and Savory (1956) as X-linked choroidal sclerosis were instances of choroideremia. Krill and Archer (1971) were of the same view.

Jacobson, J. H. and Stephens, G.: Hereditary choroidoretinal degeneration. Study of a family including electroretinography and adaptometry. Arch. Ophthalmol. 67: 321-335, 1962.

Krill, A. E. and Archer, D.: Classification of the choroidal atrophies. Am. J. Ophthalmol. 72: 562-585, 1971.

Sorsby, A. and Savory, M.: Choroidal sclerosis. A possible intermediate sex-linked form. Br. J. Ophthalmol. 40: 90-95, 1956.

Sorsby, A.: Quoted by Franceschetti, A., Francois, J. and Babel, J.: Les heredo-degenerescences chorio-retiniennes (degenerescences tapeto retiniennes). Paris: Masson, 2: 1963. P. 777.

Stankovic, I.: L'angiosclerose choroidienne familiale liee au sexe. Bull. Soc. Ophthalmol. Fr. 71: 411-417, 1958.

*30310 CHOROIDEREMIA (PROGRESSIVE TAPETO-CHOROIDAL DYSTROPHY)

Affected males suffer progressive loss of vision (reduction of central vision, constriction of visual fields, night blindness) beginning at an early age, and the choroid and retina undergo complete atrophy. Heterozygous females show no visual defect but often show striking fundoscopic changes such as irregular pigmentation and atrophy around the optic disc. Fully affected females have been reported (Fraser and Friedmann, 1967; Shapira and Sitney, 1943). These raise the usual questions of X-chromosomal aberration, unfortunate Lyonization in a heterozygote, homozygosity, etc. An extensive study in Holland was conducted by Kurstjens (1965).

The term choroideremia, which is comparable to irideremia and means absence of choroid, is inappropriate, since there is no congenital absence of the choroid. The condition is an abiotrophy beginning shortly after birth and progressing gradually. Waardenburg favored an alternative designation 'tapetochoroidal dystrophy' (Pameyer, et al., 1960). Harris and Miller (1968) observed visual impairment in a heterozygote in the family reported earlier by McCulloch and McCulloch (1948). Lack of close linkage with the Xg locus was demonstrated by Bell and McCulloch (1971). Bell and McCulloch (1971) found three recombinants out of 6 in a study of linkage with Xg.

Bell, A. G. and McCulloch, J. C.: Choroideremia and the Xg locus: another look for linkage. Clin. Genet. 2: 239-241, 1971.

Fraser, G. R. and Friedmann, A. I.: The Causes of Blindness in Childhood. A Study of 776 Children with Severe Visual Handicaps. Baltimore: Johns Hopkins Press, 1967.

Harris, G. S. and Miller, J. R.: Choroideremia: visual defects in a heterozygote. Arch. Ophthalmol. 80: 423-429, 1968.

Kurstjens, J. H.: Choroideremia and gyrate atrophy of the choroid and retina. Doc. Ophthalmol. 19: 1-122, 1965.

McCulloch, C. and McCulloch, R. J. P.: A hereditary and clinical study of choroideremia. Trans. Am. Acad. Ophthalmol. Otolaryngol. 52: 160-190, 1948.

Shapira, T. M. and Sitney, J. A.: Choroideremia. Am. J. Ophthalmol. 26: 182-183, 1943.

X
L
I
N
K
E
D

Sorsby, A., Franceschetti, A., Joseph, R. and Davey, J. B.: Choroideremia. Clinical and genetic aspects. Br. J. Ophthalmol. 36: 547-581, 1952.

Pameyer, J. K., Waardenburg, P. J. and Henkes, H. E.: Choroideremia. Br. J. Ophthalmol. 44: 724-738, 1960.

*30320 CHOROIDO-RETINAL DEGENERATION WITH RETINAL REFLEX IN HETEROZYGOUS WOMEN

Falls and Cotterman (1948) described an X-linked form of choroidoretinal degeneration which is distinguished from other types by the presence in heterozygous women of a tapetal-like retinal reflex. See RETINITIS PIGMENTATION and CHOROIDORETINAL DYSTROPHY for phenotypically related entities.

Falls, H. F. and Cotterman, C. W.: Choroidoretinal degeneration. A sex-linked form in which heterozygous women exhibit a tapetal-like retinal reflex. Arch. Ophthal. 40: 685-703, 1948.

30330 CHOROIDO-RETINAL DYSTROPHY

Hoare (1965) described a chorioretinal disorder in 10 males in seven sibships which were offspring of sisters. The maternal grandfather of the affected males was probably also affected. The condition was detected in childhood. Some carrier women showed fundus abnormalities with visual impairment beginning in middle age and probably showing progression. The condition in males resembled retinitis pigmentosa in fundus picture and night blindness but differed by the absence of annular scotoma, by early involvement of central vision, and by relatively little vascular change.

Hoare, G. W.: Choroido-retinal dystrophy. Brit. J. Ophthal. 49: 449-459, 1965.

*30340 CLEFT PALATE (X-LINKED)

In a British Columbia Indian family, Lowry (1970) found 12 males with incomplete cleft of the secondary palate. In some the cleft was submucous. Palatopharyngeal incompetence was a leading feature. The pedigree pattern suggested X-linked recessive inheritance. The high sex ratio for cleft palate in British Columbia Indians could be due to the existence of an X-linked form of submucous cleft palate (Lowry and Renwick, 1969). Lowry (1974) has observed other cases born into this family but knows of no other reported kindred. Other families have, it seems, not been observed (Gorlin, 1974). The OPD syndrome (31130) is an X-linked syndrome with cleft palate as a feature.

Gorlin, R. J.: Minneapolis, personal communication, Jan. 23, 1974.

Lowry, R. B.: Vancouver, B. C., personal communication, Feb. 19, 1974.

Lowry, R. B. and Renwick, D. H.: Incidence of cleft lip and palate in British Columbia Indians. J. Med. Genet. 6: 67-69, 1969.

Lowry, R. B.: Sex linked cleft palate in a British Columbia Indian family. Pediatrics 46: 123-128, 1970.

*30360 COFFIN-LOWRY SYNDROME

The features are mental retardation with peculiar pugilistic nose, large ears, tapered fingers, drumstick terminal phalanges by X-ray, pectus carinatum. The syndrome was described in two unrelated adolescent boys by Coffin et al. (1966). The occurrence of minor manifestations in female relatives suggested a genetic basis. Procopis and Turner (1972) reported a family in which four brothers had the full syndrome and several female relatives had abnormal fingers and mild mental retardation. X linked dominant inheritance is likely. Lowry et al. (1971) described a new mental retardation syndrome with small stature retardation of bone age, hypotonia, tapering fingers, and facies characterized by hypertelorism, anteverted nares, and prominent frontal region. Arrested hydrocephalus may also be a feature. The disorder was transmitted through three generations, with no instance of male-to-male transmission.

Coffin, G. S., Siris, E. and Wegienka, L. C.: Mental retardation with osteocartilaginous anomalies. Am. J. Dis. Child. 112: 205-213, 1966.

Lowry, R. B., Miller, J. R. and Fraser, F. C.: A new dominant gene mental retardation syndrome: associated with small stature, tapering fingers, characteristic facies, and possible hydrocephalus. Am. J. Dis. Child. 121: 496-500, 1971.

Procopis, P. G. and Turner, B.: Mental retardation, abnormal fingers, and skeletal anomalies: Coffin's syndrome. Am. J. Dis. Child. 124: 258-261, 1972.

*30370 COLORBLINDNESS, BLUE-MONO-CONE-MONO-CHROMATIC TYPE

This disorder was previously interpreted as total colorblindness. Present information (Spivey, 1965) indicates that affected persons can see small blue objects on a large yellow field and vice versa. These cases have been variously called partial complete colorblindness, or incomplete achromatopsia. Blackwell and Blackwell (1961) have described achromatoptic families in which a few blue cones seemed to be present. See comments of Alpern, Falls and Lee (1960). Sloan (1964) has evidence of the presence of a few red cones in cases of otherwise complete achromatopsia. Bromley (1974) showed me a large kindred with this disorder in a typical X-linked recessive pattern.

Alpern, M., Falls, H. F. and Lee, G. B.: The enigma of typical total monochromacy. Am. J. Ophthal. 50: 996-1012, 1960.

Blackwell, H. R. and Blackwell, O. M.: Rod and cone receptor mechanisms in typical and atypical congenital achromatopsia. Vision Res. 1: 62-107, 1961.

Bromley, W.: Ellsworth, Me., personal communication, Aug. 8, 1974.

Sloan, L. L.: Baltimore, Md.: personal communication, 1964.

Sloan, L. L.: Congenital achromatopsia: a report of 19 cases. J. Opt. Soc. Am. 44: 117-128, 1954.

Spivey, B. E.: The X-linked recessive inheritance of atypical monochromatism. Arch. Ophthalmol. 74: 327-333, 1965.

*30380 COLORBLINDNESS, PARTIAL, DEUTAN SERIES

In western Europeans about 8 percent of males are colorblind. Of these about 75 percent have a defect in the deutan series and about 25 percent have a defect in the protan series. Waaler (1968) distinguished two types of normal color vision according to 'greenpoint,' i.e., the point at which the subject sees pure green, and two types according to 'bluepoint.' He presented the following genetic hypothesis: males can be of either G(1)B(1), G(1)B(2) or G(2)B(2). Females can be of six genotypes. Among 59 children of doubly heterozygous mothers one possible cross-over was found. He suggested the use of this polymorphism in linkage studies. Arias and Rodriguez (1972) concluded that the recombination fraction for the deutan and protan loci may be higher than originally thought, perhaps 0.095 combining their own data with those earlier published. It has been suggested that the colorblindness polymorphism is a heritage from frugivorous arboreal ancestors (Crossman, 1974).

Adam, A. and Fraser, G. R.: The linkage between protan and deutan loci. (Letters) Am. J. Hum. Genet. 22: 691-693, 1970.

Arias, S. and Rodriguez, A.: New families, one with two recombinants for estimation of recombination between the deutan and protan loci. Humangenetik 14: 264-268, 1972.

Arias, S. and Rodriguez, A.: An informative large pedigree with four compound hemizygotes of three combinations of deutan and protan genes. Acta Cient. Venez. 24: 44-52, 1973.

Crossman, J.: Colorblindness (concluded). (Letter) New Eng. J. Med. 290: 231 only, 1974.

Porter, I. H., Schulze, J. and McKusick, V. A.: Genetic linkage between the loci for glucose-6-phosphate dehydrogenase deficiency and colour blindness in American Negroes. Ann. Hum. Genet. 26: 107-122, 1962.

Porter, I. H., Schulze, J. and McKusick, V. A.: Linkage between glucose-6-phosphate dehydrogenase and colour-blindness. Nature 193: 506 only, 1962.

Waaler, G. H.: Heredity of two normal types of colour vision. Nature 218: 688-689, 1968.

*30390 COLORBLINDNESS, PARTIAL, PROTAN SERIES

The two-locus hypothesis for colorblindness is supported by three sets of observations.

A. The relative frequency of colorblindness in males and females is most consistent with the existence of two loci. Given a frequency of color-blind males of .08 and a total gene frequency for colorblindness also of .08, then on a one-locus hypothesis the frequecny of color-blind females should be .08 X .08, or .64 percent. On a two-locus hypothesis, with the protan and deutan series representing 25 and 75 percent, respectively, then the frequency of color-blind females should be less, assuming that doubly heterozygous females are normal:

Females color-blind for protan

Series — .02 X .02 = .04 percent

Females color-blind for deutan

Series — .06 X .06 = .36 percent.
.40 percent

(The expected frequency of doubly heterozygous females is the product of the frequencies of singly heterozygous females — (2 X .02 X .98) (2 X .06 X .94), or 0.0044.) In fact, the data on relative frequency of colorblindness in males and females collected in Norway by Waaler (1927) and in Switzerland by von Planta (1928) agree with the values predicted by a two-locus theory.

B. The two-locus theory is also supported by the fact that females who by the nature of the color vision defect in their sons are known to carry genes for both types of colorblindness usually do not show a defect in color vision. This is essentially the complementarity test of allelism. (The double heterozygotes in the pedigrees of Kondo and Brunner had normal color vision.)

Complementarity is also indicated by the findings in the families by Franceschetti and Klein (1957). It is possible, of course, that the mother in each family was a manifesting heterozygote. It is to be hoped that the presumably doubly heterozygous daughters have a large number of sons and that the color vision of these sons is tested in the future.

C. The pedigree of Vanderdonck and Verriest (1960) and that of Siniscalco et al., (1964) indicate independent assortment of deutan and protan genes among the offspring of a doubly heterozygous female.

The Nagel anomaloscope used in determination of the type of colorblindness, consists of a viewing tube with a circular bipartite field, one half illuminated with yellow and the other half with a mixture of green and red.

The yellow half is not variable except in brightness. The other half can be varied continuously from red to green. The subject's color sense is tested by having him mix colors in the variable half-field until he achieves a subjective match to the yellow field. Certain color combinations are considered normal whereas specific differences from the normal indicate the type and degree of anomalous color vision.

Ishihara plates alone are unreliable in distinguishing deutan and protan types. Although the Nagel anomaloscope is the 'last court of appeal' in making the differentiation, it is expensive, time-consuming, difficult for unsophisticated subjects, and, of course, not usable 'in the field.' Two 'book' tests, the Tokyo Medical College Test and the AO-HRR (Hardy-Rand-Rittler) pseudoisochromatic plates, especially when together, represent probably the methods which are both the easiest and the most reliable now available (Sloan, 1961).

Identification of a small proportion of deutero-heterozygotes is possible by means of the luminosity quotient, determined by a modification of the Nagel anomaloscope designed by Crone. Most cases of proto-heterozygotes can be identified as such with a high degree of certainty using this method.

It appears (Nemoto and Murao, 1961) that the order of dominance in colorblindness is normal — anomaly — anopia (Franceschetti hypothesis). Emmerson et al. (1974) excluded close linkage of the HGPRT and deutan loci.

Crone, R. A.: Spectral sensitivity in color-defective subjects and heterozygous carriers. Am. J. Ophthalmol. 48: 231-238, 1959.

Emmerson, B. T., Thompson, L., Wallace, D. C. and Spence, M. A.: Absence of measurable linkage between the loci for hypoxathine-guanine phosphoribosyltransferase and deutan color blindness. Am. J. Hum. Genet. 26: 78-82, 1974.

Franceschetti, A. and Klein, D.: Two families with parents of different types of red-green blindness. Acta Genet. Statist. Med. 7: 255-259, 1957.

Fraser, G. R.: Estimation of the recombination fraction between the protan and deutan loci. Am. J. Hum. Genet. 21: 593-599, 1969.

Kalmus, H.: Diagnosis and Genetics of Defective Colour Vision. Oxford: Pergamon Press, 1965. P. 59.

Nemoto, H. and Murao, M.: A genetic study of colorblindness. Jap. J. Hum. Genet. 6: 165-173, 1961.

Schmidt, I.: A sign of manifest heterozygosity in carriers of color deficiency. Am. J. Optom. 32: 404-408, 1955.

Siniscalco, M., Filippi, G. and Latte, B.: Recombination between protan and deutan genes: data on their relative positions in respect of the G6PD locus. Nature 204: 1062-1064, 1964.

Sloan, L. L.: Evaluation of the Tokyo Medical College color vision test. Am. J. Ophthalmol. 52: 650-659, 1961.

Thuline, H. C., Hodgkin, W. E., Fraser, G. R. and Motulsky, A. G.: Genetics of protan and deutan color-vision anomalies: an instructive family. Am. J. Hum. Genet. 21: 581-592, 1969.

Vanderdonck, R. and Verriest, G.: Femme protanomale et heterozygote mixte (genes de la protanomalie et de la deuteranopie en position de repulsion) ayant deux fils deuteranopes, un fils protanomal et deux fils normaux. Biotypologie 21: 110-120, 1960.

Von Planta, P.: Die Haufigkeit der angeborenen Farbensinnstorungen bei Knaben und Madchen und ihre Feststellung durch die ublichen klinischen Proben. Graefe Arch. Ophthalmol. 120: 253-281, 1928.

Waaler, G. H.: Uber die Erblichkeitsverhaltnisse der verschiedenen Arten von angeborener Rotgrun-blindheit. Ztsch. F. Indukt. Abstammungs- u. Vererbungsl. 45: 279-333, 1927.

*30400 COLORBLINDNESS, PARTIAL, TRITANOMALY

The defect in 'blue sense' is less severe than in tritanopia, an autosomal dominant (q.v.). This condition is considerably rarer than protan and deutan colorblindness. The frequency of tritan defects is imperfectly known because of lack of diagnostic tools and lesser practical importance in signaling and traffic control.

Kalmus, H.: Diagnosis and Genetics of Defective Colour Vision. Oxford: Pergamon Press, 1965. P. 59.

30405 CORPUS CALLOSUM, AGENESIS OF, WITH CHORIORETINAL ABNORMALITY

Flexion spasms in the infant represent the mode of clinical presentation. The chorioretinal abnormality is in the form of lacunas ('holes'). Aicardi et al. (1969) reported 15 cases, all in females. Although no familial cases have been observed, the disorder is entered here since X-linked dominance with lethality in the hemizygous male is a possibility. All cases would, on this hypothesis, be new mutations. Parental age would be of interest. Dennis and Bower (1972) also described a case in a female. In addition to infantile spasms, mental subnormality, specific chorioretinopathy, and 'split brain' they commented on the evidence of heterotopia of the brain by pneumoencephalogram, vertebral anomalies and characteristic EEG changes. They arrived at the same suggestion, that this is an X-linked dominant.

Aicardi, J., Chevrie, J. J. and Rousselie, F.: Le syndrome spasmes en flexion, agenesic calleuse, anomalies chorio-retiniennes. Arch. Franc. Pediatr. 26: 1103-1120, 1969.

Dennis, J. and Bower, B. D.: The Aicardi syndrome. Develop. Med. Child. Neurol. 14: 382-390, 1972.

30410 CORPUS CALLOSUM, PARTIAL AGENESIS OF

X
L
I
N
K
E
D

Menkes, Philippart and Clark (1964) described a family with five males (in four sibships of two generations connected through females) with partial agenesis of the corpus callosum. Clinical features included severe intellectual retardation and intractable seizures. Postmortem studies of one patient showed a combination of anatomic and chemical abnormalities. Opitz and Kaveggia (1974) described three brothers and two of their male first-cousins who were affected with mental retardation, disproportionately large head, imperforate anus and congenital hypotonia. Partial agenesis of the corpus callosium was proved in one ans suspected in a second. The authors felt that this disorder is distinct from that reported by Menkes et al. (1964).

Menkes, J. H., Philippart, M. and Clark, D. B.: Hereditary partial agenesis of corpus callosum. Arch. Neurol. 11: 198-208, 1964.

Opitz, J. M. and Kaveggia, E. G.: The FG syndrome. A X-linked recessive syndrome of multiple congenital anomalies and mental retardation. Z. Kinkerheilkd. 117: 1-18, 1974.

30420 CUTIS VERTICIS GYRATA, THYROID APLASIA AND MENTAL RETARDATION

Akesson (1965) described five males in three sibships of two generations who may have had this combination of manifestations. Only the proband was examined in full. He pointed out that although X-linked inheritance seemed likely most other cases of cutis verticis gyrata and mental retardation seem to have autosomal inheritance.

Akesson, H. O.: Cutis verticis gyrata, thyroaplasia and mental deficiency. Acta Genet. Med. Gem. 14: 200-204, 1965.

30430 CYANIDE, INABILITY TO SMELL

Initial studies (reviewed by Stern) showed male-female frequencies and family data consistent with X-linked recessive inheritance of inability to smell cyanide. Further studies seem to indicate that the situation is more complex (Kirk, 1953). The same conclusion was reached by Brown and Robinette (1967) and by Giles et al. (1968). The work of the last group of workers excludes X-linkage.

Allison, A. C.: Cyanide smelling deficiency among Africans. Man 53: 176-177, 1953.

Brown, K. S. and Robinette, R. R.: No simple pattern of inheritance in ability to smell solutions of cyanide. Nature 215: 406-408, 1967.

Brown, K. S., MacLean, C. M. and Robinette, R. R.: The distribution of the sensitivity to chemical odors in man. Hum. Biol. 40: 456-472, 1968.

Fukumoto, Y., Nakajima, H., Uetake, M., Matsuyama, A. and Yoshida, T.: Smell ability to solution of potassium cyanide and its inheritance. Jap. J. Hum. Genet. 2: 7-16, 1957.

Giles, E., Hansen, A. T., McCullough, J. M., Metzger, D. G. and Wolpoff, M. H.: Hydrogen cyanide and phenylthiocarbamide sensitivity, mid-phalangeal hair and color blindness in Yucatan, Mexico. Am. J. Phys. Anthropol. 28: 203-212, 1968.

Kirk, R. L. and Stenhouse, N. S.: Ability to smell solutions of potassium cyanide. Nature 171: 698-699, 1953.

Srivastava, R. P.: Ability to smell solutions of sodium cyanide. Eastern Anthropologist (Lucknow) 14: 189-191, 1961.

Stern, C.: In, Freeman, W. H. (ed.): Principles of Human Genetics. San Francisco: (2nd. Ed.) 1960. P. 232, Table 35.

*30440 DEAFNESS, CONDUCTIVE TYPE, WITH STAPES FIXATION

Shine and Watson (1967) described a Hawaiian-Chinese family with 9 males in two generations affected with conductive hearing loss and vestibular disturbance. At operation the footplate of the stapes was found to be fixed. When it was mobilized, profuse drainage of perilymph and cerebrospinal fluid occurred indicating abnormal patency of the cochlear aqueduct. Nance et al. (1970, 1971) have observed a similar family of European extraction, indicating that this is a bona fide syndrome.

McRae, K. N., Uchida, I. A. and Lewis, M.: Sex-linked congenital deafness. Am. J. Hum. Genet. 21: 415-419, 1969.

Nance, W. E., Setleff, R., McLeod, A. C., Sweeney, A., Cooper, M. C. and McConnell, F.: X-linked mixed deafness with congenital fixation of the stapedial footplate and perilymphatic gusher. The Clinical Delineation of Birth Defects. IX. Ear. Baltimore: Williams and Wilkins, 1971.

Nance, W. E., Sweeney, A., McLeod, A. C. and Cooper, M. C.: Hereditary deafness: a presentation of some recognized types, modes of inheritance, and aids in counseling. Sth. Med. Bull. 58: 41-57, 1970.

Shine, I. and Watson, J. R.: A new syndrome of sex-linked congenital conductive deafness. To be published, 1967.

Thorpe, P., Sellars, S. and Beighton, P.: X-linked deafness in a South African kindred. S. Afr. Med. J. 48: 587-590, 1974.

*30450 DEAFNESS, CONGENITAL, PERCEPTIVE TYPE

Probably about 1.5 percent of genetic deafness is determined by an X-borne gene. The X-linked form of congenital deafness has been described from Missouri (Dow, Poynter, 1930), Japan (Mitsuda et al., 1952), Belfast (Stevenson, cited by Deraemaeker), Belgium (Deraemaeker, 1958), Philadelphia (Sataloff et al. 1955) and Australia (Parker, 1958). Fraser (1965) found several families in England. In the family reported by Dow and Poynter four affected males married deaf-mute women who probably had the autosomal recessive form of the disease because no children were affected. The deafness is of perceptive type.

Deraemaeker, R.: Sex-linked congenital deafness. Acta Genet. Statist. Med. 8: 228-231, 1958.

Dow, G. S. and Poynter, C. I.: The Dar family. Eugen. News 15: 128-130, 1930.

Fraser, G. R.: Sex-linked recessive congenital deafness and the excess of males in profound childhood deafness. Ann. Hum. Genet. 29: 171-196, 1965.

McRae, K. N., Uchida, I. A., Lewis, M. and Denniston, C.: Sex-linked congenital deafness. Am. J. Hum. Genet. 21: 415-422, 1969.

Mitsuda, H., Inoue, S. and Kazama, Y.: Eine Familie mit rezessiv geschlechtsgebundener Taubstummheit. Jap. J. Hum. Genet. 27: 142, 1952.

Parker, N.: Congenital deafness due to a sex-linked recessive gene. Am. J. Hum. Genet. 10: 196-200, 1958.

Richards, B. W.: Sex-linked deaf-mutism. Ann. Hum. Genet. 26: 195-199, 1963.

Sataloff, J., Pastore, P. N. and Bloom, E.: Sex-linked hereditary deafness. Am. J. Hum. Genet. 7: 201-203, 1955.

30460 DEAFNESS, HIGH TONE NEURAL

Livan (1961) described an X-linked variety of nerve deafness characterized by hightone loss which may be distinct from the other forms of X-linked deafness listed here.

Livan, M.: Contribute alla conscenza della sorbita ereditarie. Arch. Ital. Otol. 72: 331-339, 1961.

*30470 DEAFNESS, PROGRESSIVE

Sufficient hearing is present at first that speech develops normally, then deteriorates.

Mohr, J. and Mageroy, K.: Sex-linked deafness of a possibly new type. Acta Genet. Statist. Med. 10: 54-62, 1960.

30475 DEXTROCARDIA WITH OTHER CARDIAC MALFORMATIONS

Soltan and Li (1974) described a family in which four males in three different sibships had dextrocardia. One had corrected transposition of great arteries, VSD and PDA. A second had corrected transposition and VSD that closed spontaneously. Third had situs inversus viscerum , VSD and pulmonic stenosis. The pedigree was strongly suggestive of X-linked recessive inheritance.

Soltan, H. C. and Li, M. D.: Hereditary dextrocardia associated with congenital heart defects: report of a pedigree. Clin. Genet. 5: 51-58, 1974.

*30480 DIABETES INSIPIDUS, NEPHROGENIC

The defect concerns the inability of the renal tubule to respond to antidiuretic hormone. A partial defect is demonstrable in females. Nakano (1969) described the disorder in four generations of a Samoan family. Ten Bensel and Peters (1970) described hydronephrosis in affected male sibs of the family reported by Cannon (1955). The pedigree they presented covering 5 generations with 12 affected males is typically of X-linkage. Cannon had claimed male-to-male transmission in 3 instances and autosomal dominant inheritance. His information must have been in error. Bode and Miettinen (1970) excluded close linkage with the Xg blood group. The same families had been investigated by Bode and Crawford (1969).

Abelson, H.: Nephrogenic diabetes insipidus. Pediatr. Res. 2: 271-282, 1968.

Bode, H. H. and Crawford, J. D.: Nephrogenic diabetes insipidus in North America — the Hopewell hypothesis. N. Engl. J. Med. 280: 750-754, 1969.

Bode, H. H. and Miettinen, O. S.: Nephrogenic diabetes insipidus: absence of close linkage with Xg. Am. J. Hum. Genet. 22: 221-227, 1970.

Cannon, J. F.: Diabetes insipidus. Clinical and experimental studies with consideration of genetic relationships. Arch. Intern. Med. 96: 215-272, 1955.

Carter, C. and Simpkiss, M.: The carrier state in nephrogenic diabetes insipidus. Lancet II: 1069-1073, 1956.

Nakano, K. K.: Familial nephrogenic diabetes insipidus. Hawaii Med. J. 28: 205-208, 1969.

Orloff, J. and Burg, M. B.: Vasopressin-resistant diabetes insipidus. In, Stanbury, J. B., Wyngaarden, J. B. and Fredrickson, D. S. (eds.): The Metabolic Basis of Inherited Diseases. New York: McGraw-Hill, 1972 (3rd Ed.). Pp. 1567-1580.

Ten Bensel, R. W. and Peters, E. R.: Progressive hydronephrosis, hydroureter, and dilatation of the bladder in siblings with congenital nephrogenic diabetes insipidus. J. Pediatr. 77: 439-443, 1970.

Uttley, W. S. and Thistlethwaite, D.: Failure to detect the carrier in congenital nephrogenic diabetes insipidus. Arch. Dis. Child. 47: 137-138, 1972.

*30490 DIABETES INSIPIDUS, NEUROHYPOPHYSEAL TYPE

In addition to the X-linked forms of diabetes insipidus, autosomal dominant forms also exist. Forssman had five families: two probably autosomal and three X-linked. Of the three X-linked families, one was of the pitressin-resistant type, whereas the other two families were susceptible. The latter two families presumably represent the neurohypophyseal type. Green et al. (1967) reported a family with diabetes insipidus in dominant pattern, either X-linked or autosomal. Autopsy in one of the affected members showed marked reduction of neurones in the supraoptic and paraventricular nuclei of the hypothalamus. Breast feeding was normal in one of these patients, despite the virtual absence of hypothalamic nuclei thought to be responsible for production of oxytocin which is considered essential for breast feeding.

Forssman, H.: On hereditary diabetes insipidus with special regard to a sex-linked form. Acta Med. Scand. 159 (Suppl.): 1945.

Forssman, H.: Two different mutations of the X-chromosome causing diabetes insipidus. Am. J. Hum. Genet. 7: 21-27, 1955.

Green, J. R., Buchan, G. C., Alvord, E. C., Jr. and Swanson, A. G.: Hereditary and idiopathic types of diabetes insipidus. Brain 90: 707-714, 1967.

*30500 DYSKERATOSIS, CONGENITA (ZINSSER-COLE-ENGMAN SYNDROME)

The features are cutaneous pigmentation, dystrophy of the nails, leukoplakia of the oral mucosa, continuous lacrimation due to atresia of the lacrimal ducts, often thrombocytopenia, anemia, and in most cases testicular atrophy. Only males are affected in a pattern consistent with X-linked recessive inheritance. Milgrom et al. (1964) described the condition in a Negro male. They pointed out that the two serious complications are anemia and cancer, which develops in the leukoplakia of the anus or mouth, or may develop in the skin. Bryan and Nixon (1965) described a pedigree with four and possibly five affected males in a relationship nicely consistent with X-linked recessive inheritance. The patients had pancytopenia which led the authors (incorrectly, I think) to the conclusion that Fanconi panmyelopathy and dyskeratosis congenita are one and the same entity. Addison and Rice (1965) described a male with seemingly typical skin and mucosal changes, as well as pancytopenia. His sister had poikiloderma and oral leukoplakia, progressing to squamous carcinoma fatal at age 24 years. Sorrow and Hitch (1963) described a female patient who had fatal cervical and vaginal squamous carcinoma. The relation of the disorder in these female patients to the condition which is clearly X-linked is not clear. Selmanowitz and van Voolen (1971) pointed out the phenotypic overlap with Fanconi anemia (22790) and raised the question 'whether Fanconi anemia and dyskeratosis congenita might be causally related. Because of the difference in inheritance (X-linked vs. autosomal) this possibility can be rejected out of hand.

Addison, M. and Rice, M. S.: The association of dyskeratosis congenita and Fanconi's anaemia. Med. J. Aust. 1: 797-799, 1965.

Bryan, H. G. and Nixon, R. K.: Dyskeratosis congenita and familial pancytopenia. J.A.M.A. 192: 203-208, 1965.

Garb, J.: Dyskeratosis congenita with pigmentation, dystrophia unguium and leukoplakia oris. Arch. Dermatol. 77: 704-712, 1958.

Milgrom, H., Stoll, H. L., Jr. and Crissey, J. T.: Dyskeratosis congenita. A case with new features. Arch. Dermatol. 89: 345-349, 1964.

Koszewski, B. J. and Hubbard, T. F.: Congenital anemia in hereditary ectodermal dysplasia. Arch. Dermatol. 74: 159-166, 1956.

Selmanowitz, V. J. and Van Voolen, G. A.: Fanconi's anemia and dyskeratosis congenita. (Letter) J.A.M.A. 216: 2015 only, 1971.

Sorrow, J. M., Jr. and Hitch, J. M.: Dyskeratosis congenita. First report of its occurrence in a female and a review of the literature. Arch. Dermatol. 88: 340-347, 1963.

Steier, W., Van Voolen, G. A. and Selmanowitz, V. J.: Dyskeratosis congenita: relationship to Fanconi's anemia. Blood 34: 510-521, 1972.

*30510 ECTODERMAL DYSPLASIA, ANHIDROTIC

The affected males show absence of teeth, hypotrichosis, and absence of sweat glands. Heterozygous women may show reduction or malformation of teeth and mild abnormalities of sweat glands and breasts. In Robert's family 1929, skin involvement in heterozygous females was patchy. Halperin and Curtis' case 1942 showed mental defect also, but this is not an invariable feature of cases, even in their family. This was the condition affecting the 'toothless men of Sind,' members of a Hindu kindred which resides in the vicinity of Hyderabad and was described by Darwin (1875) and by Thadani (1934). Darwin (1875) wrote as follows: 'I may give an analogous case, communicated to me by Mr. W. Wedderburn, of a Hindoo family in Scinde, in which ten men, in the course of four generations, were furnished, in both jaws taken together, with only four small and weak incisor teeth and with eight posterior molars. The men thus affected have very little hair on the body, and become bald early in life. They also suffer much during hot weather from excessive dryness of the skin. It is remarkable that no instance has occurred of a daughter being affected...though the daughters in the above family are never affected, they transmit the tendency to their sons: and no case has occurred of a son transmitting it to his sons. The affection thus appears only in alternate generations, or after long intervals.' Hutt (1935) called attention to Darwin's description. Singh, Jolly, and Kaur (1962) described a severe case in a 27-year-old Sikh woman in India. Two brothers had died of the disease. Whether this was a homozygous affected or a heterozygous manifesting female is uncertain, especially since no information was provided on whether the father was affected. Consanguineous matings of the types which are expected to result in homozygous affected females are frequent in some Indian groups. Other defects include saddle-nose and those involving the lacrimal glands, breasts and cornea. Most patients are short of stature and show hyperpigmentation around the eyes. Autopsy in one patient (Reed et al., 1970) showed absence of mucous glands in the pharynx, larynx, trachea, and large and small bronchi. The finding was thought to be the basis for increased susceptibility to respiratory infections observed in life. Mucous glands were also absent in the upper esophagus and hypoplastic in the colon.

Bowen, R.: Hereditary ectodermal dysplasia of the anhidrotic type. Sth. Med. J. 50: 1018-1021, 1957.

Darwin, C.: The Variation of Animals and Plants under Domestication. London: John Murray, 1875. (2nd Ed.) P. 319.

Grant, R. and Falls, H. F.: Anodontia: report of a case associated with ectodermal dysplasia of the anhidrotic type. Am. J. Orthodont. 30: 661-672, 1944.

Halperin, S. L. and Curtis, G. M.: Anhidrotic ectodermal dysplasia associated with mental deficiency. Am. J. Ment. Defic. 46: 459-463, 1942.

Hutt, F. B.: An earlier record of the toothless men of Sind. J. Hered. 26: 65-66, 1935.

Jesperson, H. G.: Hereditary ectodermal dysplasia of anhidrotic type. Acta Paediatr. 51: 712-720, 1962.

Kline, A. H., Sidbury, J. B., Jr. and Richter, C. P.: The occurrence of ectodermal dysplasia and corneal dysplasia in one family. J. Pediatr. 55: 355-366, 1959.

Malagon, V. and Taveras, J. E.: Congenital anhidrotic ectodermal and mesodermal dysplasia. Arch. Dermatol. 74: 253-258, 1956.

Passarge, E. and Fries, E.: X-chromosome inactivation in X-linked hypohidrotic ectodermal dysplasia. Nature N. B. 245: 58-59, 1973.

Reed, W. B., Lopez, D. A. and Landing, B.: Clinical spectrum of anhidrotic ectodermal dysplasia. Arch. Dermatol. 102: 134-143, 1970.

Roberts, E.: The inheritance of anhidrosis associated with anodontia. J.A.M.A. 93: 277-279, 1929.

Simpson, J. L., Allen, F. H., Jr., New, M. and German, J.: Absence of close linkage between the locus for Xg and the locus for anhidrotic ectodermal dysplasia. Vox Sang. 17: 465-467, 1969.

Singh, A., Jolly, S. S. and Kaur, S.: Hereditary ectodermal dysplasia. Br. J. Dermatol. 74: 34-37, 1962.

Thadani, K. I.: The toothless men of Sind. J. Hered. 25: 483-484, 1934.

*30520 EHLERS-DANLOS SYNDROME, TYPE V (X-LINKED E-D)

As one part of the genetic heterogeneity of this syndrome, Beighton (1968) described two families in which X-linked inheritance is probable. Close linkage with Xg blood groups and color-blindness was excluded. The clinical features included hyperextensible skin and bruising tendency. Fragility of skin was unimpressive. Di Ferrante and his colleagues (1974) presented evidence for deficient activity of lysyl oxidase in type V Ehlers-Danlos syndrome. This enzyme is responsible for oxidative deamination of lysine and hydroxylsine in collagen as a first step in cross-linking of collagen. In a boy with this form of E-D, Leachman et al. (1975) found excessive soluble collagen and low lysyl oxidase activity.

Beighton, P. H.: X-linked recessive inheritance in the Ehlers-Danlos syndrome. Brit. Med. J. 2: 409-411, 1968.

DiFerrante, N.: Houston, personal communication, 1974.

Leachman, R. D., Angelini, P., Di Ferrante, N., Donnelly, P. V., Francis, G., Almazan, A., Segni, G., Franzblau, C. and Jordan, R. E.: Lysyl oxidase deficiency in Ehlers-Danlos syndrome type V. In press, 1974.

Rowe, M. D., McGoodwin, E. B., Martin, G. R., Sussman, M. D., Grahn, D., Faris, B. and Franzblau: A sex-linked defect in the cross-linking of collagen and elastin associated with the mottled locus in mice. J. Exp. Med. 139: 180-192, 1974.

*30530 ENDOCARDIAL FIBROELASTOSIS

Endocardial fibroelastosis is a condition characterized by a widespread thickening of the mural endocardium due to proliferation of collagen and elastic fibers. The border between the overgrown endocardium and the adjacent myocardium is usually clearly defined. The left ventricle is the chamber of the heart most frequently affected. The primary type of endocardial fibroelastosis is seen primarily in infants and children. Fixler et al. (1970) described four males in three sibships, related through females, with the contracted form of endocardial fibroelastosis. The affected males died of heart failure in the first years of life. An autosomal recessive form of endocardial fibroelastosis appears to be well established and fibroelastosis is frequently found associated with malformations of the heart. Dilated and contracted forms of fibroelastosis are recognized on the basis of the state of the left ventricle at autopsy. The clinical picture of the two types differ, though it is not certain that the genetics differ. Female cases of the contracted form have been described.

Lindenbaum et al. (1973) described a case in England of two affected males in two generations of a kindred. The prepositus and a male first cousin of his mother both died in infancy of heart trouble. Autopsies on both confirmed the primary dilated type of endocardial fibroelastosis. One had no other birth defects; the other had a hypoplastic left kidney. Several other males of this kindred died before the age of two, possibly as a consequence of the respiratory complications of this condition. This pattern of inheritance along with Fixler's findings suggests X-linked transmission. Moller et al. (1966) documented an affected mother and son.

Fixler, D. E., Cole, R. B., Paul, M. H., Lev, M. and Girod, D. A.: Familial occurrence of the contracted form of endocardial fibroelastosis. Am. J. Cardiol. 26: 208-213, 1970.

Lindenbaum, R. H., Andrews, P. S. and Khan, A. S. S. I.: Two cases of endocardial fibroelastosis — possible X-linked determination. Brit. Heart J. 35: 38-39, 1973.

X

L
I
N
K
E
D

Moller, J. H., Fisch, R. O., Fromm, A. H. L. and Edwards, J. E.: Endocardial fibroelastosis occurring in a mother and son. Pediatrics 38: 918-921, 1966.

*30540 FACIOGENITAL DYSPLASIA (AARSKOG-SCOTT SYNDROME)

Aarskog (1970) has described an X-linked disorder characterized by ocular hypertelorism, antiverted nostrils, broad upper lip, and peculiar penoscrotal relations ('saddle-bag scrotum'). Affected males can reproduce. Scott (1971) emphasized the occurrence of ligamentous laxity manifest by hyperextensibility of the fingers, genu recurvatum and flat feet. Furthermore, hypermobility in the cervical spine with anomaly of the odontoid resulted in neurologic deficit. In the family he studied, 9 males in 5 sibships were affected. Sugarman et al. (1973) described a kindred with four affected males. They emphasized the occurrence of a 'peculiar curved linear dimple inferior to the lower lip.' This and other stigmata were present in an earlier female. They favored sex-influenced autosomal dominant inheritance.

Aarskog, D.: A familial syndrome of short stature associated with facial dysplasia and genital anomalies. J. Pediatr. 77: 856-861, 1970.

Berman, P., Desjardin, C. and Fraser, F. C.: Inheritance of the Aarskog syndrome. Birth Defects Orig. Art. Ser. 10 (7): 151-159, 1974.

Furukawa, C. T., Hall, B. D. and Smith, D. W.: The Aarskog syndrome. J. Pediatr. 81: 1117-1122, 1972.

Scott, C. I., Jr.: Unusual facies, joint hypermobility, genital anomaly and short stature: a new dysmorphic syndrome. The Clinical Delineation of Birth Defects. X. The Endocrine System. Baltimore: Williams and Wilkins, 1971. Pp. 240-246.

Sugarman, G. I., Rimoin, D. L. and Lachman, R. S.: The facial-digital-genital (Aarskog) syndrome. Am. J. Dis. Child. 126: 248-252, 1973.

*30550 FIBRIN-STABILIZING FACTOR (FACTOR XIII) DEFICIENCY

Fibrin-stabilizing factor (factor XIII) is a constituent of human plasma which, when activated, links adjacent molecules of fibrin to form a stable clot, characterized by insolubility in 5M urea or 1 percent monochloroacetic acid. Ratnoff and Steinberg (1968) pointed out that although in some families deficiency is unquestionably inherited as an autosomal recessive, X-linked inheritance is likely in other families. If true, the conclusion suggests that either (1) factor XIII is composed of two polypeptide chains, or (2) two or more enzymes or clotting factors are involved in fibrin-stabilization. Steinberg and Ratnoff (1970) found a highly significant difference in the frequency of parental consanguinity between families with only males affected and families with affected females. They advanced this as evidence for the existence of both X-linked and autosomal forms.

Ratnoff, O. D. and Steinberg, A. G.: Inheritance of fibrin-stabilizing-factor deficiency. Lancet I: 25-26, 1968.

Steinberg, A. G. and Ratnoff, O. D.: Inheritance of factor XIII. (Letter) Am. J. Hum. Genet. 22: 597-598, 1970.

*30560 FOCAL DERMAL HYPOPLASIA (FDH; GOLTZ SYNDROME)

FDH appears to be an X-linked dominant with lethality in males. The features include atrophy and linear pigmentation of the skin, herniation of fat through the dermal defects and multiple papillomas of the mucous membranes or skin. In addition, digital anomalies consist of syndactyly, polydactyly, camptodactyly and absence deformities. Oral anomalies, in addition to lip papillomas, include hypoplastic teeth. Ocular anomalies (coloboma of iris and choroid, strabismus, microphthalmia) have also been present in some cases. Goltz et al. (1962) noted that all five of their cases were female, that the disorder occurred only in female antecedents and other relatives and that miscarriages are frequent in these families. They had affected females in four successive generations in one family and in two generations of another. The mother of Wodniansky's female patient (1957) had skin changes and a sister had syndactyly of the 3rd and 4th fingers and toes bilaterally. Warburg (1970) observed microphthalmos with bilateral coloboma of the iris and ectopia lentis. Kistenmacher et al. (1970) described an affected male and raised the question of 'Durchbrenner' of Hadorn, i.e., the occasional survival of a lethal.

Goltz, R. W., Henderson, R. R., Hitch, J. M. and Ott, J. E.: Focal dermal hypoplasia syndrome. A review of the literature and report of two cases. Arch. Dermatol. 101: 1-11, 1970.

Goltz, R. W., Peterson, W. C., Jr., Gorlin, R. J. and Ravits, H. G.: Focal dermal hypoplasia. Arch. Dermatol. 86: 708-717, 1962.

Gorlin, R. J., Meskin, L. H., Peterson, W. C., Jr. and Goltz, R. W.: Focal dermal hypoplasia syndrome. Acta Derm. Venerol. 43: 421-440, 1963.

Holden, J. D. and Akers, W. A.: Goltz's syndrome: focal dermal hypoplasia. Am. J. Dis. Child. 114: 292-300, 1967.

Kistenmacher, M. L., Torosola, M. A., Punnett, H. H. and DiGeorge, A. M.: Focal dermal hypoplasia in a male. (Abstract) Am. J. Hum. Genet. 22: 19A only, 1970.

Warburg, M.: Focal dermal hypoplasia. Ocular and general manifestations with a survey of the literature. Acta Ophthalmol. 48: 525-536, 1970.

Wodniansky, P.: Ueber die Formen der congenitalen Poikilodermie. Arch. Klin. Exp. Dermatol. 205: 331-342, 1957.

30570 GERMINAL CELL APLASIA (SERTOLI-CELL-ONLY SYNDROME; DEL CASTILLO SYN-
DROME)

Edwards and Bannerman (1971) observed two brothers, ages 14 and 12, with gynecomastia and obesity. Their disorder might have been classified simply as adolescent or pubertal gynecomastia were it not for the existence of two maternal uncles with a history of pubertal gynecomastia and, in the one of them available for study, clinical features and testicular biopsy consistent with the Del Castillo syndrome. By the age of 26, he showed no gynecomastia. In the 14-year-old nephew the sperm count was probably low but sperm was present. The authors suggested that in this boy they had an opportunity to observe the Del Castillo syndrome at an earlier stage than had previously been possible. They suggested that, as in other similar conditions such as the testicular feminization syndrome and and Reifenstein syndrome, the inheritance is either X-linked or autosomal dominant male-limited. Several kindreds with multiple affected males are known. Goldstein (1974) suggested that this might be an instance of type I incomplete male pseudohermaphroditism (31210).

Edwards, J. A. and Bannerman, R. M.: Familial gynecomastia. The Clinical Delineation of Birth Defects. X. The Endocrine System. Baltimore: Williams and Wilkins, 1971. Pp. 193-195.

Goldstein, J. L.: Dallas, personal communication, Aug. 30, 1974.

Weyeneth, R.: Etiopathogenie et diagnostic de la sterilite masculine. Praxis 45: 21-34, 1956.

30580 GERODERMIA OSTEODYSPLASTICA

Boreux (1969) described a disorder which they concluded is inherited as an X-linked recessive with occasional manifestation in females. As the name indicates the features include changes in the skin suggesting precocious aging and osseous changes including osteoporosis and multiple lines like growth rings of a tree. Boreux suggested that the physiognomy resembles that of Walt Disney's dwarfs (from 'Snow White').

Boreux, G.: La gerodermie osteodysplasique a heredite liee au sexe, nouvelle entite clinique et genetique. J. Genet. Hum. 17: 137-178, 1969.

Brocher, J. E. W., Klein, D., Bamatter, F., Franceschetti, A. and Boreux, G.: Rontgenologische Befunde bei geroderma osteodysplastica hereditaria. Fortschr. Roentgenstr. 109: 185-198, 1968.

*30590 GLUCOSE-6-PHOSPHATE DEHYDROGENASE

Since identification of deficiency of G6PD and of its X-chromosomal determination in the 1950's and demonstration of electrophoretic variants of this enzyme in the early 1960's (Boyer et al., 1962), the genetic, clinical and biochemical significance of this polymorphism has been found to be very great. Deficiency of the red cell enzyme, in various forms, is the basis of favism, primaquine sensitivity and other drug-sensitive hemolytic anemia, anemia and jaundice in the newborn, and chronic nonspherocytic hemolytic anemia (Beutler et al., 1968). Different variants of the enzyme are found in high frequency in African, Mediterranean and Asiatic populations (Porter et al., 1964) and heterozygote advantage viz-a-viz malaria (Luzzatto et al., 1969) has been invoked to account for the high frequency of the particular alleles in particular population.

The variety of forms of the enzyme is numerous, as illustrated by the published tables of (Yoshida, Beutler and Motulsky, 1971; Beutler and Yoshida, 1973). The World Health Organization (1967) gave its attention to problems of nomenclature and standard procedures for study. The demonstrated polymorphism at this X-linked locus rivals that of the autosomal loci for the polypeptide chains of hemoglobin. As in the latter instance, single amino acid substitution has been demonstrated as the basis of the change in the G6PD molecule resulting from mutation (Yoshida et al., 1967).

Polymorphism at the G6PD locus has made it a useful X-chromosome marker, like colorblindness and the Xg blood group locus, and close linkage of the colorblindness loci, the G6PD locus and the locus for hemophilia A (Adam et al., 1966; Boyer and Graham, 1965) has been demonstrated. As a biochemical phenotype identifiable at the cellular level, G6PD variants have been useful in somatic cell genetics, permitting, for example, one of the critical proofs in man of the Lyon hypothesis (Davidson et al., 1963).

The relative stability of the X chromosome during evolution has been shown by the fact that the G6PD locus is X-borne also in a number of other species (Ohno, 1967). Gray et al. (1973) found that complete deficiency of G6PD produces not only nonspherocytic hemolytic anemia but also chronic granulomatous disease due to neutrophil dysfunction. That G6PD is X-linked in the mouse is supported by Epstein's finding (1969) that oocytes of XO females have half as much G6PD as do oocytes of XX female mice. The level of lactate dehydrogenase was the same. Epstein's conclusion was that the G6PD gene is X-linked in the mouse, that synthesis occurs in the oocyte and is dosage-dependent and that X-inactivation does not occur in oocytes.

Adam, A., Tippett, P., Gavin, J., Noades, J., Sanger, R. and Race, R. R.: The linkage relation of Xg to G6PD in Israelis: the evidence of a second series of families. Am. J. Hum. Genet. 30: 211-218, 1966.

X

L
I
N
K
E
D

Beutler, E., Mathai, C. K. and Smith, J. E.: Biochemical variants of glucose-6-phosphate dehydrogenase giving rise to congenital nonspherocytic hemolytic disease. Blood 31: 131-150, 1968.

Beutler, E. and Yoshida, A.: Human glucose-6-phosphate dehydrogenase varants: a supplementary tabulation. Ann. Hum. Genet. 37: 151-156, 1973.

Boyer, S. H. IV, and Graham, J. B.: Linkage between the X chromosome loci for glucose-6-phosphate dehydrogenase electrophoretic variation and hemophilia A. Am. J. Hum. Genet. 17: 320-324, 1965.

Boyer, S. H., IV, Porter, I. H. and Weilbaecher, R. G.: Electrophoretic heterogeneity of glucose-6-phosphate dehydrogenase and its relationship to enzyme deficiency in man. Proc. Natl. Acad. Sci. 48: 1868-1876, 1962.

Castro, G. A. M. and Snyder, L. M.: G6PD San Jose: a new variant characterized by NADPH inhibition studies. Humangenetik 21: 361-363, 1974.

Chan, T. K., Todd, D. and Lia, M. C. S.: Glucose 6-phosphate dehydrogenase: identity of erythrocyte and leukocyte enzyme with report of a new variant in Chinese. Biochem. Genet. 6: 119-124, 1972.

Davidson, R. G., Nitowsky, H. M. and Childs, B.: Demonstration of two populations of cells in the human female heterozygous for glucose-6-phosphate dehydrogenase variants. Proc. Nat. Acad. Sci. 50: 481-485, 1963.

Epstein, C. J.: Mammalian oocytes: X-chromosome activity. Science 163: 1078-1079, 1969.

Francke, U., Bakay, B., Connor, J. D., Coldwell, J. G. and Nyhan, W. L.: Linkage relationships of X-linked enzymes glucose-6-phosphate dehydrogenase and hypoxanthine guanine phosphoribosyltransferase. Am. J. Hum. Genet. 26: 512-522, 1974.

Gourdin, D., Vergnes, H., Bouloux, C., Ruffie, J. and Gherardi, M.: Polymorphism of erythrocyte G6PD in the baboon. Am. J. Phys. Anthropol. 37: 281-288, 1972.

Gray, G. R., Stamatoyannopoulos, G., Naiman, S. C., Kliman, M. R., Klebanoff, S. J., Austin, T., Yoshida, A. and Robinson, G. C. G.: Neutrophil dysfunction, chronic granulomatous disease, and non-genetic haemolytic anaemia caused by complete deficiency of glucose-6-phosphate dehydrogenase. Lancet II: 530-534, 1973.

Junien, C., Kaplan, J. C., Meienhofer, M. C., Maigret, P. and Sender, A.: G6PD Baudelocque: a new unstable variant characterized in cultured fibroblasts. Enzyme 18: 48-59, 1974.

Luzzatto, L., Usanga, E. A. and Reddy, S.: Glucose-6-phosphate dehydrogenase deficient red cells: resistance to infection by malarial parasites. Science 164: 839-842, 1969.

Nakai, T. and Yoshida, A.: G6PD heian, a glucose-6-phosphate dehydrogenase variant associated with hemolytic anemia found in Japan. Clinica Chimica Acta 51: 199-203, 1974.

Ohno, S.: Sex Chromosomes and Sex-linked Genes. Berlin, New York: Springer, 1967.

Panich, V.: G6PD Intanon. A new glucose-6-phosphate dehydrogenase variant. Humangenetik 21: 203-206, 1974.

Porter, I. H., Boyer, S. H., Watson-Williams, E. J., Adam, A., Szeinberg, A. and Siniscalco, M.: Variation of glucose-6-phosphate dehydrogenase in different populations. Lancet I: 895-899, 1964.

Ramot, B. and Brok, F.: A new glucose-6-phosphate dehydrogenase mutant (Tel-Hashomer mutant). Ann. Hum. Genet. 28: 167-172, 1964.

Smith, J. E.: Canine glucose-6-phosphate dehydrogenase (G6PD) deficiency. (Abstract) Meeting Am. Soc. Hemat., Hollywood, Fla., Dec. 3-6, 1972.

Stamatoyannopoulos, G., Voigtlander, V., Kotsakis, P. and Akrivakis, A.: Genetic diversity of the 'Mediterranean' glucose-6-phosphate dehydrogenase deficiency phenotype. J. Clin. Invest. 50: 1253-1261, 1971.

Turner, G. and Turner, B.: X-linked mental retardation. J. Med. Genet. 11: 109-113, 1974.

Wang, Y. M., Patterson, J. H. and Van Eys, J.: The potential use of xylitol in glucose-6-phosphate dehydrogenase deficiency anemia. J. Clin. Invest. 50: 1421-1428, 1971.

WHO: Nomenclature of glucose-6-phosphate dehydrogenase in man. Bull. WHO 36: 319-322, 1967. Also Canad. Med. Assoc. J. 97: 422-424, 1967.

WHO: Scientific group on the standardization of procedures for the study of glucose-6-phosphate dehydrogenase. WHO Techn. Rep. Ser. No. 366, 1967.

Yoshida, A.: A single amino acid substitution (asparagine to aspartic acid) between normal (B plus) and the common Negro variant (A plus) of human glucose-6-phosphate dehydrogenase. Proc. Natl. Acad. Sci. 57: 835-840, 1967.

Yoshida, A., Baur, E. W. and Motulsky, A. G.: A Philippino glucose-6-phosphate dehydrogenase variant (G6PD union) with enzyme deficiency and altered substrate specificity. Blood 35: 506-513, 1970.

Yoshida, A., Stamatoyannopoulos, G. and Motulsky, A. G.: Negro variant of glucose-6-phosphate dehydrogenase deficiency (A-) in man. Science 155: 97-99, 1967.

Yoshida, A., Beutler, E. and Motulsky, A. G.: Table of human glucose-6-phosphate dehydrogenase variants. Bull. WHO 45: 243-253, 1971.

*30600 GLYCOGEN STORAGE DISEASE VIII (DEFICIENCY OF PHOSPHORYLASE KINASE)

Williams and Field (1961) found low leukocyte phosphorylase activity in two affected brothers and normal activity in an unaffected brother and in the father. An intermediately low level in the mother, together with affected males, suggested X-linked inheritance. Wallis et al. (1966) restudied the family and with new methods found support for X-linkage. Huijing (1967) showed that there are two forms of the type VI (see RECESSIVE CATALOG). Both have low phosphorylase activity in the absence of adenosine monophosphate (AMP), but one (which is autosomal recessive) has normal phosphorylase kinase activity, while the other (which is X-linked recessive) has low phosphorylase kinase activity. Huijing and Fernandez (1969) studied two kindreds, one of which had 6 affected plus two possibly affected males. The other had 20 affected males, two affected females and 7 probably affected males. Since phosphorylase kinase is known to be enzymically

X
L
I
N
K
E
D

activated (Krebs et al. 1964), it is possible that it is an activating enzyme that is controlled by the X-chromosome. It may be significant, however, that phosphorylase B kinase deficiency of skeletal muscle is X-linked in mice (Lyon et al. 1967). Hug et al. (1969) studied female patients with glycogenosis due to deficiency of phosphorylase kinase. Huijing and Fernandez (1970) suggested that these patients were heterozygotes. Huijing (1970) pointed out similarities and differences of the human and murine defects. Phosphorylase kinase deficiency produces the mildest of the glycogenoses of man. Although Huijing (1970) referred to it as glycogen storage disease type VIA, it seems best for reasons stated elsewhere to give it a different number: hence VIII is used here. Hug (1974) claims that there is also an autosomal recessive form of phosphorylase kinase deficiency. Furthermore, he classifies phosphorylase kinase deficiency as type IX glycogen storage disease. (See Schimke et al., 1974.) By cloning cells of heterozygotes, Migeon and Huijing (1974) demonstrated some fibroblasts with enzymatic levels like those of affected hemizygotes. This was presented as proof of X-linkage and X inactivation of the phosphorylase kinase locus. For information on classification and morphology of the glycogenoses, see McAdams et al. (1974).

Hers, H. G.: Etudes enzymatiques sur fragments hepatiques: application a la classification des glycogenoses. Rev. Int. Hepat. 9: 35-55, 1959.

Hug, G., Schubert, W. K. and Chuck, G.: Deficient activity of dephosphophosphorylase kinase and accumulation of glycogen in the liver. J. Clin. Invest. 48: 704-715, 1969.

Hug, G.: Cincinnati, personal communication, 1974.

Huijing, F. and Fernandez, J.: Liver glycogenosis and phosphorylase kinase deficiency. (Letter) Am. J. Hum. Genet. 22: 484-485, 1970.

Huijing, F. and Fernandez, J.: X-chromosomal inheritance of liver glycogenosis with phosphorylase kinase deficiency. Am. J. Hum. Genet. 21: 275-284, 1969.

Huijing, F.: Glycogen-storage disease type VIa: low phosphorylase kinase activity caused by a low enzyme-substrate affinity. Biochim. Biophys. Acta 206: 199-201, 1970.

Huijing, F.: Phosphorylase kinase deficiency. Biochem. Genet. 4: 187-194, 1970.

Huijing, F.: Phosphorylase kinase in leucocytes of normal subjects and of patients with glycogen-storage disease. Biochim. Biophys. Acta 148: 601-603, 1967.

Krebs, E. G., Love, D. S., Bratvold, G. E., Trayser, K. A., Meyer, W. L. and Fischer, E. H.: Purification and properties of rabbit skeletal muscle phosphorylase B kinase. Biochemistry 3: 1022-1033, 1964.

Lyon, J. B., Jr., Porter, J. and Robertson, M.: Phosphorylase B kinase inheritance in mice. Science 155: 1550-1551, 1967.

McAdams, A. J., Hug, G. and Bove, K. E.: Glycogen storage disease, type I to X criteria for morphologic diagnosis. Hum. Pathol. 5: 463-487, 1974.

Migeon, B. R. and Huijing, F.: Glycogen-storage disease associated with phosphorylase kinase deficiency: evidence for X inactivitation. Am. J. Hum. Genet. 26: 360-368, 1974.

Schimke, R. N., Zakheim, R. M., Corder, R. C. and Hug, G.: Glycogen storage disease type IX: benign glycogenosis of liver and hepatic phosphorylase kinase deficiency. J. Pediat. 83: 1031-1034, 1973.

Wallis, P. G., Sidbury, J. B., Jr. and Harris, R. C.: Hepatic phosphorylase defect. Studies on peripheral blood. Am. J. Dis. Child. 111: 278-282, 1966.

Williams, H. E. and Field, J. B.: Low leukocyte phosphorylase in hepatic phosphorylase deficient glycogen storage disease. J. Clin. Invest. 40: 1841-1845, 1961.

30610 GONADAL DYSGENESIS, XY FEMALE TYPE

The patients appear to be normal females, who do not, however, develop secondary sexual characteristics at puberty, do not menstruate and have 'streak gonads.' They are chromatin negative and have a 44 + XY karyotype. Affected sisters were reported by Cohen and Shaw (1965) and twins by Frasier et al. (1964). Sternberg and Barclay (1967) observed three cases, each in a different sibship of a family, connected through normal females (proposita, maternal cousin and maternal aunt). A high incidence of neoplasia (gonadoblastomas and germinomas) in streak gonads of patients with the XY karyotype was claimed by Taylor et al. (1966). The patients are of essentially normal stature and have no somatic stigmata of Turner syndrome except, of course, the lack of secondary sexual characteristics. In this condition, as in the testicular feminization syndrome, it is unclear whether the gene which may be responsible is on the X chromosome or on an autosome and expressed only in chromosomal males. Whether the abnormal gene directly suppresses testis-determining loci on the chromosome or blocks some early stage of testicular morphogenesis is also unknown. The possibility of a chromosomal basis has not been excluded in these cases. The sisters reported by Cohen and Shaw (1965) had a marker autosome, which was present also in the mother. They referred to another instance of XY 'sisters' with an abnormal autosome. One of their 2 patients had gonadoblastoma. Two sisters reported by Fine, Mellinger and Canton (1962) were of normal stature but were chromatin negative. One of these cases and one of those reported by Baron, Rucki and Simm (1962) had gonadoblastoma. In the last family, two 'females' and a male were affected, the male showing no testes. All three sibs were sex chromatin negative. Barr et al. (1967) reported on a sibship of two genetic males. One, who had male pseudohermaphroditism, was reared as a female; he developed signs of masculinization at puberty and undescended but otherwise normal, testes and small fallopian tubes. The second genetic male (180 cm. tall) had pure gonadal dysgenesis with small uterus and streak gonads. This patient was at first thought to have the testicular feminization syndrome. A sister had a son with hypospadias (urethral orifice at the base of the penis). The sibship reported by Chemke et al. (1970) is similar to that of Barr et emphasized that the affected persons were unusually tall. See 23330 for discussion of the XX type of gonadal dysgenesis.

Barr, M. L., Carr, D. H., Plunkett, E. R., Soltan, H. C. and Wiens, R. G.: Male pseudohermaphroditism and pure gonadal dysgenesis in sisters. Am. J. Obstet. Gynecol. 99: 1047-1055, 1967.

Chemke, J., Carmichael, R., Stewart, J. M., Geer, R. H. and Robinson, A.: Familial XY gonadal dysgenesis. J. Med. Genet. 7: 105-111, 1970.

Cohen, M. M. and Shaw, M. W.: Two XY siblings with gonadal dysgenesis and a female phenotype. N. Engl. J. Med. 272: 1083-1088, 1965.

Espiner, E. A., Veale, A. M., Sands, V. E. and Fitzgerald, P. H.: Familial syndrome of streak gonads and normal male karyotype in five phenotypic females. New Eng. J. Med. 283: 6-11, 1970.

Fine, G., Mellinger, R. C. and Canton, J. N.: Gonadoblastoma occurring in a patient with familial gonadal dysgenesis. Am. J. Clin. Pathol. 38: 615-629, 1962.

Frasier, S. D., Bashore, R. A. and Mosier, H. D.: Gonadoblastoma associated with pure gonadal dysgenesis in monozygous twins. J. Pediatr. 64: 740-745, 1964.

Judd, H. L., Scully, R. E., Atkins, L., Neer, R. M. and Kliman, B.: Pure gonadal dysgenesis with progressive hirsutism. Demonstration of testosterone production by gonadal streaks. New Eng. J. Med. 282: 881-885, 1970.

Sternberg, W. H. and Barclay, D. L.: Familial XY gonadal dysgenesis. (Letter) Lancet II: 946 only, 1967.

Sternberg, W. H., Barclay, D. L. and Kloepfer, H. W.: Familial XY gonadal dysgenesis. New Eng. J. Med. 278: 695-700, 1968.

Taylor, H., Barter, R. H. and Jacobson, C. B.: Neoplasms of dysgenetic gonads. Am. J. Obstet. Gynecol. 96: 816-823, 1966.

30630 GRANULOMAS, CONGENITAL CEREBRAL

Sturgill and Brown (1966) described 4 brothers who died in the first 24 hours of life of congenital cerebral granulomas. The lesions suggested toxoplasmosis or salivary gland virus disease. However, no organisms or inclusions were demonstrated. Two sisters were healthy. Consanguinity was not commented upon.

Sturgill, B. C. and Brown, A. K.: Congenital cerebral granulomas. Report of four cases in male siblings. Pediatrics 37: 769-775, 1966.

*30640 GRANULOMATOUS DISEASE DUE TO LEUKOCYTE MALFUNCTION

Quie, White, Holmes and Good (1967) have observed a form of fatal granulomatous disease in males in an X-linked pedigree pattern. The leukocytes phagocytize staphylococci normally but are defective in their ability to digest the organism. The authors thought that the condition was X-linked. Windhorst et al. (1967) did family studies establishing X-linked recessive inheritance and demonstrating two populations of leukocytes in heterozygous females. Baehner and Nathan (1967) demonstrated a defect in a leukocyte oxidase. The intact leukocytes failed to reduce nitroblue tetrazolium or to show increased oxygen consumption during phagocytosis. Carson and colleagues (1965) reported 16 males in 8 families with a syndrome of chronic suppurative lymphadenitis, chronic dermatitis, chronic pulmonary disease and hepatosplenomegaly with subsequent fatal outcome. Hypergammaglobinemia was often present. The mother of the affected boy described by MacFarlane et al. (1967) had a chronic dermatitis of the neck (Jessner benign lymphocytic infiltration) and partial defect demonstrable in vitro qualitatively identical to that in her son. Reduced nicotinamide-adenine dinucleotide oxidase of normal human polymorphonuclear leukocytes has properties that qualify it as the enzyme responsible for the respiratory burst during phagocytosis. Baehner and Karnovsky (1968) found deficiency of the enzyme in five patients with chronic granulomatous disease. Thompson et al. (1969) found leukocyte abnormality in both parents of a patient with chronic granulomatous disease, suggesting that this was an autosomal recessive form or requiring some more complex explanation. Controversy over the inheritance, X-linked or autosomal, is illustrated by the letter of Windhorst (1969) and accompanying reply. Hohn and Lehrer (1974) found deficiency of NADPH oxidase as the presumed basic defect.

Ament, M. E. and Ochs, H. D.: Gastrointestinal manifestations of chronic granulomatous disease. New Eng. J. Med. 288: 382-387, 1973.

Baehner, R. L. and Karnovsky, M. L.: Deficiency of reduced micotinamide-adenine dinucleotide oxidase in chronic granulomatous disease. Science 162: 1277-1279, 1968.

Baehner, R. L. and Nathan, D. G.: Leukocyte oxidase: defective activity in chronic granulomatous disease. Science 155: 835-836, 1967.

Carson, M. J., Chadwick, D. L., Brubaker, C. A., Cleland, R. S. and Landing, B. H.: Thirteen boys with progressive septic granulomatosis. Pediatrics 35: 405-412, 1965.

Edwards, J. H.: Inheritance of chronic granulomatous disease. (Letter) Lancet II: 850-851, 1969.

Hohn, D. C. and Lehrer, R. I.: Identification of the defect in X-linked chronic granulomatous disease. (Abstract) Clin. Res. 22: 394A only, 1974.

Holmes, B., Page, A. R. and Good, R. A.: Studies of the metabolic activity of leukocytes from patients with a genetic abnormality of phagocytic function. J. Clin. Invest. 46: 1422-1432, 1967.

X
L
I
N
K
E
D

Kontras, S. B., Bodenbender, J. G., McClave, C. R. and Smith, J. P.: Interstitial cystitis in chronic granulomatous disease. J. Urol. 105: 575-578, 1971.

MacFarlane, P. S., Speirs, A. L. and Sommerville, R. G.: Fatal granulomatous disease of childhood and benign lymphocytic infiltration of the skin (congenital dysphagecytosis). Lancet I: 408-410, 1967.

Nathan, D. G., Baehner, R. L. and Weaver, D. K.: Failure of nitro blue tetrazolium reduction in the phagocytic vacuoles of leukocytes in chronic granulomatous disease. J. Clin. Invest. 48: 1895-1904, 1969.

Quie, P. G., White, J. G., Holmes, B. and Good, R. A.: In vitro bactericidal capacity of human polymorphonuclear leukocytes: diminished activity in chronic granulomatous disease of childhood. J. Clin. Invest. 46: 668-679, 1967.

Thompson, E. N., Chandra, R. K., Cope, W. A. and Soothill, J. F.: Leucocyte abnormality in both parents of a patient with chronic granulomatous disease. Lancet I: 799-800, 1969.

Windhorst, D. B., Holmes, B. and Good, R. A.: A newly defined X-linked trait in man with demonstration of the Lyon effect in carrier females. Lancet I: 737-739, 1967.

Windhorst, D. B.: Inheritance of chronic granulomatous disease. (Letter) Lancet 2: 543-544, 1969.

30650 GYNECOMASTIA, FAMILIAL

In some families male-to-male transmission bespeaks autosomal dominant inheritance. In the family described by Rosewater, Gwinup and Hamwi (1965), gynecomastia with hypogonadism occurred in four males of three sibships in two generations connected through females in a pattern consistent with X-linked or autosomal dominant inheritance. Their cases differ from the Reifenstein syndrome by the absence of hypospadias. However, the presence of hypogonadism places these in the category of male hypogonadism (q.v.). Also see GERMINAL CELL APLASIA. Wilson et al. (1974) suggested that this disorder is the mildest expression of what they term incomplete male pseudohermaphroditism, type I (31210). On the other hand, Gwinup (1974) rebutted by pointing out that this interpretation is made unlikely by the low levels of luteinizing hormones, by decreased Leydig cells on testicualr biopsy and by rapid masculinization when testosterone was administered. Follow-up showed maintenance of masculinization with injections of 200 mg. testosterone cypionate monthly.

Gwinup, G.: Incomplete male psuedohermaphroditism. (Letter) N. Engl. J. Med. 291: 308 only, 1974.

Rosewater, S., Gwinup, G. and Hamwi, G. J.: Familial gynecomastia. Ann. Intern. Med. 63: 377-385, 1965.

Wilson, J. D., Harrod, M. J., Goldstein, J. L., Hemsell, D. L. and MacDonald, P. C.: Familial incomplete male pseudohermaphroditism, type I. Evidence for androgen resistance and variable clinical manifestations in a family with the Reifenstein syndrome. New Eng. J. Med. 290: 1097-1103, 1974.

*30660 HEMOLYSIS OF TRYPSIN-TREATED RED CELLS

Heisto et al. (1964) found that freshly taken serum of about 12 percent of male donors and about 23 percent of female donors would hemolyze trypsin-treated red cells irrespective of the ABO or Rh groups. The male and female frequencies and family studies virtually proved X-linkage. Further investigations should be made.

Heisto, H., Harboe, M. and Godal, H. C.: Worm haemolysins active against trypsinized red cells: occurrence, inheritance and clinical significance. Proc. 10th Congr. Intern. Soc. Blood Transf. (Stockholm). Pp. 787-789, 1964.

*30670 HEMOPHILIA A (CLASSICAL HEMOPHILIA)

Classical hemophilia is the result of a hereditary defect in antihemophilic globulin (factor VIII). A partial deficiency in heterozygous carriers has been demonstrated by Rapaport et al. (1960), among several.

Alexander and Goldstein (1953) first noted low levels of factor VIII in cases of Von Willebrand disease ('vascular hemophilia'), an autosomally inherited disorder. This was confirmed by other workers including Nilsson and colleagues (1957), who studied Von Willebrand's original family in the Aland Islands. Thus, an autosomal locus seems also involved in some way in factor VIII formation. The possible allelic relationship of mild factor VIII deficiency is suggested by families such as that of Graham and colleagues (1953) and that of Bond and colleagues (1962) in which the carrier females as well as hemizygous males showed depression of factor VIII levels and sometimes clinical hemophilia, although the levels of factor VIII were not as low as in hemizygous affected males. Sutton (in Metabolic Basis of Inherited Disease, Stanbury, et al., editors, 1960) and Woolf (1962) have made the interesting suggestion that in man as in bacteria feedback repression, operating at the level of the gene or at the level of RNA, may be involved in setting the rate of protein synthesis. Specifically, if a mutation is of a type in which no protein of a particular type is formed, then no abnormality in level would be expected in heterozygotes. On the other hand, if a 'warped molecule' is synthesized as a result of the mutation, then feedback repression might occur even though the molecule was defective in the performance of its physiologic function. Sutton and Woolf suggested that the findings in the heterozygote for mild hemophilia fit the latter model, whereas those of severe hemophilia may fit the first model. The concept is compatible with the Lyon hypothesis and quite independent of it. From study of a family in which both hemophilia A and hemophilia B were segregating Woodliff and Jackson (1966) concluded that the two loci are far apart, as is also suggested by linkage studies of the individual disorders with marker traits. Splenic transplantation to dogs with hemophilia A corrects the coagulation defect (Norman et al., 1968).

Zacharski et al. (1968) showed that leukocytes (probably lymphocytes) in vitro synthesize factor VIII. As of this writing the best opinion seems to be that factor VIII like many other proteins is synthesized in the

X

L
I
N
K
E
D

liver and that its presence in the spleen is only a temporary, perhaps storage phenomenon. Rise in factor VIII level is induced, for example, by administration of epinephrine. Among 54 patients with hemophilia A, Feinstein et al. (1969) found that the plasma of 52 showed no neutralizing activity with a human antibody to factor VIII. The plasma from the other two had neutralizing activity comparable to that of normal plasma. Using neutralization of a factor-VIII inhibitor as a measure of cross-reacting material in the plasma of hemophilics, Denson (1968) found that 33 hemophilic plasmas (presumably from separate patients) showed little neutralization whereas 3 hemophilic plasmas showed about the same neutralization as normal plasma. The finding seems to indicate the presence of CRM-positive and CRM-negative forms of hemophilia. Hoyer and Breckenridge (1968) also found heterogeneity in hemophilia A. For both hemophilia A and hemophilia B two subtypes exist — one without any protein immunologically demonstrable and one with immunologically normal but hemostatically defective protein (Denson et al., 1969). In both hemophilia A and B, the CRM-positive form is the rarer. Whether hemophilia A is CRM-positive or CRM-negative may be a function of the sensitivity of the technique used to test immunologically for the presence of cross-reacting material. Stites et al. (1970) demonstrated CRM in all hemophilia A patients and in no patient with Von Willebrand disease. Linkage studies indicate that hemophilia A and B are not allelic. The independence of their loci was nicely confirmed when Robertson and Trueman (1964) found a family with both hemophilia A and hemophilia B and in it a male deficient in both factors. Early reports of hemophilia families emanated from this country beginning with a newspaper account in 1792 (McKusick, 1962) and continuing with reports by Otto in 1803 and Hay in 1813 (McKusick, 1962).

Stites et al. (1971) were able to detect factor VIII immunologically in all of 14 patients with hemophilia A they studied. Little or no factor VIII was identified in patients with Von Willebrand disease. They were using an unusually sensitive method. Zimmerman et al. (1971) found immunoreactive material in all of 22 patients with hemophilia A. Von Willebrand disease, on the other hand, appears to be true factor VIII deficiency. Hemophiliacs differ in AHF level (0-30 percent of normal). This variability may represent a series of alleles (as suggested by Haldane), environmental influence on the expression of a single allele or contribution of autosomal loci. Data of Nilsson et al. were used. The results suggested that there is little or no contribution of autosomal loci to AHF level in hemophiliacs, and little or no environmental influence. A series of alleles seemed the more likely explanation of differences in factor level. Allotype of factor VIII has been demonstrated by human but not animal antisera (Stites et al., 1971). The biologic fitness of patients with hemophilia A is on the average perhaps one-third that of patients with hemophilia B. On the other hand hemophilia A is about 5 times more frequent than hemophilia B. If no heterozygote advantage or disadvantage exists in either disorder, these two facts must indicate that the mutation rate for hemophilia A is about 15 times that for hemophilia B. A possible explanation is that the hemophilia A locus is duplicated many times and that mutation in any one of the presumably adjacent loci can result in hemophilia, whereas the hemophilia B locus is unitary. Factor VIII has a molecule weight about 15 times that of factor IX. Ratnoff and Bennett (1973) reviewed the genetics of coagulation disorders, with emphasis on CRM+ (allotypic) and CRM- (eniotypic) varieties. Direct studies of linkage between hemophilias A and B in the dog indicated that the two loci are at least 50 map units apart (Brinkhous et al. 1973).

Alexander, B. and Goldstein, R.: Dual hemostatic defect in pseudohemophilia. (Abstract) J. Clin. Invest. 32: 551 only, 1953.

Arrants, J. E., Jordan, P. H., Jr. and Newcomb, T. F.: Von Willebrand's disease: a cause for massive postoperative bleeding — report of a case. Ann. Surg. 156: 845-851, 1962.

Barrow, E. M. S. and Graham, J. B.: Factor VIII. (Letter) Lancet I: 1312-1313, 1973.

Bennett, B. and Ratnoff, O.: Deletion of the carrier state for classic hemophilia. N. Engl. J. Med. 7: 342-345, 1974.

Brinkhous, K. W., Davis, P. D., Graham, J. B. and Dodds, W. J.: Expression and linkage of genes for X-linked hemophilia A and B in the dog. Blood 41: 577-585, 1973.

Bennett, E. and Huehns, E. R.: Immunological differentiation of three types of hemophilia and identification of some female carriers. Lancet II: 956-958, 1970.

Bond, T. P., Levin, W. C., Celander, D. R. and Guest, M. M.: 'Mild hemophilia' affecting both males and females. N. Engl. J. Med. 266: 220-223, 1962.

Denson, K. W. E.: Two forms of haemophilia? (Letter) Lancet II: 222-223, 1968.

Denson, K. W. E., Biggs, R., Haddon, M. E., Borrett, R. and Cobb, K.: Two types of haemophilia (A+ and A-): a study of 48 cases. Br. J. Haematol. 17: 163-171, 1969.

Feinstein, D., Chong, M. N. Y., Kasper, C. K. and Rapaport, S. I.: Hemophilia A: polymorphism detectable by a factor VIII antibody. Science 163: 1071-1072, 1969.

Graham, J. B., McLendon, W. W. and Brinkhous, K. M.: Mild hemophilia: an allelic form of the disease. Am. J. Med. Sci. 225: 46-53, 1953.

Grozdea, J., Colombies, P., Bierme, R. and Ducos, J.: Myeloperoxidases and genetics of haemophilia A. (Letter) Lancet II: 220 only, 1969.

Hoyer, L. W. and Breckenridge, R. T.: Two forms of haemophilia? (Letter) Lancet II: 457 only, 1968.

Marchesi, S. L., Shulman, N. R. and Gralnick, H. R.: Studies on the purification and characterization of human factor VIII. J. Clin. Invest. 51: 2151-2161, 1972.

McKusick, V. A.: Hemophilia in early New England. A follow-up of four kindreds in which hemophilia occurred in pre-Revolutionary period. J. Hist. Med. 17: 342-365, 1962.

McKusick, V. A.: The earliest record of hemophilia in America? Blood 19: 243-244, 1962.

Nilsson, I. M., Blomback, M. and Ramgren, O.: Investigations on hemophilia A and B carriers. Bibl. Haematol. 26: 26-29, 1966.

Nilsson, I. M., Blomback, M. and Von Francken, I.: On an inherited autosomal hemorrhagic diathesis with antihemophilic globulin (AHG) deficiency and prolonged bleeding time. Acta Med. Scand. 159: 35-57, 1957.

Nilsson, I. M., Blomback, M., Ramgren, O. and Von Francken, I.: Haemophilia in Sweden. II. Carriers of haemophilia A and B. Acta Med. Scand. 171: 223-235, 1962.

Norman, J. C., Covelli, V. H. and Sise, H. S.: Transplantation of the spleen. (Editorial) Ann. Intern. Med. 78: 700-704, 1968.

Rapaport, S. I., Patch, M. J. and Moore, F. J.: Anti-hemophilic globulin levels in carriers of hemophilia A. J. Clin. Invest. 39: 1619-1625, 1960.

Ratnoff, O. D. and Bennett, B.: The genetics of hereditary disorders of blood coagulation. Science, 179: 1291-1298, 1973.

Roberts, D. F.: The genetic basis of variation in factor VIII levels among haemophiliacs. J. Med. Genet. 8: 136-139, 1971.

Robertson, J. H. and Trueman, R. G.: Combined hemophilia and Christmas disease. Blood 24: 281-288, 1964.

Schiffman, S. and Rapaport, S. I.: Increased factor VIII levels in suspected carriers of hemophilia A: taking contraceptives by mouth. N. Engl. J. Med. 275: 599 only, 1966.

Stites, D. P., Hershgold, E. J., Perlman, J. D. and Fudenberg, H. H.: Factor VIII detection by hemagglutination inhibition: hemophilia A and von Willebrand's disease. Science 171: 196-197, 1971.

Stites, D. P., Hershgold, E. J., Perlman, J. D. and Fudenberg, H. H.: Presence of the product of a 'silent gene' in hemophilia-A. (Abstract) Am. J. Hum. Genet. 22: 16A only, 1970.

Woodliff, H. J. and Jackson, J. M.: Combined haemophilia and Christmas disease. A genetic study of a patient and his relatives. Med. J. Aust. 53: 658-661, 1966.

Woolf, L. I.: Gene expression in heterozygotes. Nature 194: 609-610, 1962.

Zacharski, L. R., Bowie, E. J. W., Titus, J. L. and Owen, C. A., Jr.: Synthesis of antihemophilic factor (factor VIII) by leukocytes: preliminary report. Mayo Clin. Proc. 43: 617-619, 1968.

Zimmerman, T. S., Ratnoff, O. D. and Littell, A. S.: Detection of carriers of classic hemophilia using an immunologic assay for antihemophilic factor (factor VIII). J. Clin. Invest. 50: 255-258, 1971.

Zimmerman, T. S., Ratnoff, O. D. and Powell, A. E.: Immunologic differentiation of classic hemophilia (factor VIII deficiency) and von Willebrand's disease, with observations on combined deficiencies of antihemophilic factor and proaccelerin (factor V) and on an acquired circulating anticoagulant against antihemophilic factor. J. Clin. Invest. 50: 244-245, 1971.

30680 HEMOPHILIA A WITH VASCULAR ABNORMALITY

Egeberg (1965) studied a Norwegian family in which at least 7 persons had a disorder combining features of hemophilia A and of Von Willebrand disease. The affected males showed mild to moderately severe bleeding tendency and the females a less severe tendency. Factor VIII was decreased, more in males than in females. Bleeding time was prolonged and capillary fragility demonstrated in both sexes. The pedigree was compatible with X-linked transmission.

Egeberg, O.: An inherited hemorrhagic trait with characteristics resembling both mild hemophilia of type A and von Willebrand's disease. Scand. J. Clin. Lab. Invest. 17 (suppl. 84): 25-32, 1965.

*30690 HEMOPHILIA B (CHRISTMAS DISEASE)

Christmas disease is the result of a hereditary defect in factor IX (PTC: plasma thromboplastic component). Linkage studies suggest that the genes responsible for hemophilias A and B are not allelic. Blackburn and colleagues (1962) described two unrelated girls with Christmas disease (PTC deficiency) and a 'primary' vascular abnormality. In both instances all other members of the family were normal. This may be a situation comparable to the combination of AHG and vascular defects in Willebrand disease. The combination of factor IX with factor VII deficiency in an X-linked pattern of inheritance was described by several workers (e.g., Nour-Eldin and Wilkinson, 1959). However, Verstraete, Vermylen and Vandenbroucke (1962) found factor VII deficiency in all affected males of four families with Christmas disease and suggested that it is a consistent secondary phenomenon. By the latter view no separate mutation for the combined defect need be postulated. Twomey and Hougie (1967) defined a variant of hemophilia B which differs from the usual form in the presence of a prolonged prothrombin time. They presented evidence that a structurally abnormal and inactive form of factor IX, formed in these cases, acts as an inhibitor of the normal reaction between factor VII and animal brain. They called the variant hemophilia B(M), after the initial of the family surname. Only a minority of hemophilia B cases are of this type. Evidence for more than one form of hemophilia B was presented by Hougie and Twomey (1967) who found that in some families affected persons have prolonged prothrombin times thought to be due to inhibition by an abnormal and defective factor IX molecule. Heterozygous females show prolonged prothrombin times. They designated the variant hemophilia B(M). Roberts et al. (1968) also demonstrated heterogeneity in hemophilia B. About 90 percent of patients showed reduced PTC-inhibitor-neutralizing activity proportional to the reduction in PTC clotting activity. These

X

L
I
N
K
E
D

were interpreted as CRM-negative mutants. About 10 percent of patients showed fully effective PTC-inhibitor-neutralizing activity. These were interpreted as CRM-positive mutants. Lascari et al. (1969) described a daughter of an affected male who had an XX karyotype, factor IX level of 5 percent and hemarthrosis. The factor IX level in the mother was 100 percent. The girl was thought to be a manifesting heterozygote. Unfortunate Lyonization was postulated. Twomey et al. (1969) described a variant of hemophilia B in which an 'early one-stage inhibitor' believed to be an altered factor IX molecule is present. The inhibitor was found in about 14 percent of Christmas disease patients. They called this form hemophilia B(M) for the family surname which began with M. Denson et al. (1968) demonstrated what was probably the same biologically ineffective molecule by immunologic means. Unfortunate Lyonization was postulated in an affected girl probably heterozygous for the Christmas disease gene. Veltkamp et al. (1970) described a variant called hemophilia B Leyden which is characterized by disappearance of the bleeding diathesis as the patient ages. Correlated with the clinical improvement is a rise in factor IX from about 1 percent to 20 to 60 percent of normal. The Tenna kindred may have the same disorder. George et al. (1971) reported a family in which 3 of 4 members with Christmas disease developed an inhibitor to factor IX. The inhibitor was an IgG antibody directed against the activated form of factor IX (IXA). There was no immunologically detectable factor IX-like material in the affected family members without an inhibitor. This is consistent with the previous postulates that inhibitors to factor IX develop only in patients with Christmas disease who lack the factor IX antigen. The fourth member of the family, who had no factor IX antigen, was transfused several times, but failed to develop antibodies to factor IX. Inhibitors to factor IX develop infrequently compared to factor VIII. This suggested that there may be a predisposition, and studies in this family suggest a familial predisposition although others have not noted an increased familial increase. Brinkhous et al. (1973) showed that in the dog the loci for hemophelias A and B are further than 50 map units apart. The same is probably true in man because hemophilia A is close to the color-blindness loci whereas hemophilia B is far separated from these loci. Both factor IX and factor X consist of two polypeptide chains referred to as the L (light) and H (heavy) chains. Thus, two non-allelic forms of hemophilia B or factor XI deficiency may exist. The H chain bears a structural resemblance to the polypeptide chain of pancreatic trypsin. The L chain is covalently linked to the H chain by a single disulfide bond (Fujikawa et al., 1974).

Blackburn, E. K., Monaghan, J. H., Lederer, H. and MacFie, J. M.: Christmas disease associated with primary capillary abnormalities. Brit. Med. J. 1: 154-156, 1962.

Brinkhous, K. M., Davis, P. D., Graham, J. B. and Dodds, W. J.: Expression and linkage of genes for X-linked hemophilias A and B in the dog. Blood 41: 577-585, 1973.

Brown, P. E., Hougie, C. and Roberts, H. R.: The genetic heterogeneity of hemophilia B. N. Engl. J. Med. 283: 61-64, 1970.

Denson, K. W., Biggs, P. and Mannucci, P. M.: An investigation of three patients with Christmas disease due to an abnormal type of factor IX. J. Clin. Pathol. 21: 160-165, 1968.

Didisheim, P. and Vandervoort, R. L. E.: Detection of carriers for factor IX (PTC) deficiency. Blood 20: 150-155, 1962.

Fujikawa, K., Coan, M. H., Enfield, D. L., Titani, K., Ericsson, L. H. and Davie, E. W.: A comparison of bovine prothrombine, factor IX (Christmas factor), and factor X (Stuart factor). Proc. Nat. Acad. Sci., in press, 1974.

George, J. N., Miller, G. M. and Breckenridge, R. T.: Studies on Christmas disease: investigation and treatment of a familial acquired inhibitor of factor IX. Br. J. Haematol. 21: 333-342, 1971.

Hougie, C. and Twomey, J. J.: Hemophilia B(M): a new type of factor-IX deficiency. Lancet I: 698-700, 1967.

Lascari, A. D., Hoak, J. C. and Taylor, J. C.: Christmas disease in a girl. Am. J. Dis. Child. 117: 585-588, 1969.

Neal, W. R., Tayloe, D. T., Jr., Cederbaum, A. I. and Roberts, H. R.: Detection of genetic variants of haemophilia B with an immunosorbent technique. Br. J. Haematol. 25: 63-68, 1973.

Nour-Eldin, F. and Wilkinson, J. F.: Factor-VII deficiency with Christmas disease in one family. Lancet I: 1173-1176, 1959.

Roberts, H. R., Grizzle, J. E., McLester, W. D. and Penick, G. D.: Genetic variants of hemophilia B: detection by means of a specific PTC inhibitor. J. Clin. Invest. 47: 360-365, 1968.

Veltkamp, J. J., Meilof, J., Remmelts, H. G., Van der Vlerk, D. and Loeliger, E. A.: Another genetic variant of haemophilia B: haemophilia B Leyden. Scand. J. Haematol. 7: 82-90, 1970.

Verstraete, M., Vermylen, C. and Vandenbroucke, J.: Hemophilia B associated with a decreased factor VII activity. Am. J. Med. Sci. 243: 20-26, 1962.

Whittaker, D. L., Copeland, D. L. and Graham, J. B.: Linkage of color blindness with hemophilias A and B. Am. J. Hum. Genet. 14: 149-158, 1962.

30695 HERNIA, ANTERIOR DIAPHRAGMATIC

Lilly et al. (1973) described a family in which two brothers and their maternal uncle had congenital, anterior diaphragmatic hernia. Two of the three died in infancy of complications.

Lilly, J. R., Paul, M. and Rosser, S. B.: Anterior diaphragmatic hernia: familial presentation. The Clinical Delineation of Birth Defects. XVI. Urinary Systems and Others. Baltimore: Williams and Wilkins, 1974. Pp. 257-258.

*30700 HYDROCEPHALUS DUE TO CONGENITAL STENOSIS OF AQUEDUCT OF SYLVIUS (X-LINKED HYDROCEPHALUS)

The hydrocephalus may become arrested and the principal manifestations may be mental deficiency and spastic paraplegia. Hypoplasia and contracture of the thumb are characteristic (Edwards 1961) but were not present in any of the 7 affected males in the family studied by Bickers and Adams (1949) and later by Holmes and Nash (1967). See CATARACT, CONGENITAL TOTAL, for description of congenital hydrocephalus with cataract. Sajid and Copple (1968) found basilar impressions as an associated feature in two brothers and suggested its usefulness in diagnosis.

Bickers, D. S. and Adams, R. D.: Hereditary stenosis of the aqueduct of Sylvius as a cause of congenital hydrocephalus. Brain 72: 246-262, 1949.

Edwards, J. H.: The syndrome of sex-linked hydrocephalus. Arch. Dis. Child. 36: 486-493, 1961.

Edwards, J. H., Norman, R. M. and Roberts, J. M.: Sex-linked hydrocephalus. Report of a family with 15 affected members. Arch. Dis. Child. 36: 481-485, 1961.

Fanconi, G.: Zur Diagnose und Therapie hydrocephalischer und verwandter Zustande. Schweiz. Med. Wschr. 64: 214-223, 1934.

Holmes, L. B. and Nash, A.: X-linked hydrocephalus, comparison of pathology in two generations. Meeting, Am. Soc. Hum. Genet., Toronto, Dec. 13, 1967.

Holmes, L. B., Nash, A., ZuRhein, G., Levin, M. and Opitz, J. M.: X-linked aqueductal stenosis: clinical and neuropathological findings in two families. Pediatrics 51: 697-704, 1973.

Ribierre, M., Couvreur, J. and Canetti, J.: Les hydrocephalies par stenose de l'aqueduc de Sylvius dans la toxoplasmose congenitale. Arch. Franc. Pediatr. 27: 501-510, 1970.

Sajid, M. H. and Copple, P. J.: Familial aqueductal stenosis and basilar impression. Neurology 18: 260-262, 1968.

Shannon, M. W. and Nadler, H. L.: X-linked hydrocephalus. J. Med. Genet. 5: 326-328, 1968.

30710 HYPERTELORISM WITH ESOPHAGEAL ABNORMALITY AND HYPOSPADIAS (G SYNDROME)

Opitz et al. (1969) described four brothers with hypertelorism, a neuromuscular defect of the esophagus and swallowing mechanism, hoarse cry, hypospadias, cryptorchidism, bifid scrotum, and in one, imperforate anus. Two other brothers had died of aspiration. The parents were not related. The mother was thought to have minor stigmata such as hypertelorism, had difficulty swallowing fluids until age 11 months when a lingual frenulum (also present in at least one of the affected sons) was resected. Four living sisters were well except for one with Usher syndrome (congenital deafness and retinitis pigmentosa) and one with swallowing difficulties like the mother. As is his practice, Opitz (1969) designated the condition, 'G syndrome' after the family in which he observed it. Coburn (1970) described an isolated case in a male infant. Kasner et al. (1974) described a lethally affected female born into the family originally reported by Opitz' group. They suggested that this indicates autosomal dominant inheritance. Equally satisfactory is the hypothesis of unfortunate lyonization.

Coburn, T. P.: G syndrome. Am. J. Dis. Child. 120: 466 only, 1970.

Gilbert, E. F., Viseskul, C., Mossman, H. W. and Opitz, J. M.: The pathologic anatomy of the G syndrome. Z. Kinderheilk. 111: 290-298, 1972.

Kasner, J., Gilbert, E. F., Viseskul, C., Deacon, J., Herrmann, J. P. R. and Opitz, J. M.: The G syndrome — further observations. Z. Kinderheilk., in press, 1974.

Little, J. R. and Opitz, J. M.: The G syndrome. Am. J. Dis. Child. 121: 505-507, 1971.

Opitz, J. M., Frias, J. L., Gutenberger, J. E. and Pellett, J. R.: The G syndrome of multiple congenital anomalies. The Clinical Delineation of Birth Defects. II. Malformation Syndromes. New York: National Foundation, 1969. Pp. 95-101.

30720 HYPERURICEMIA, ATAXIA, DEAFNESS

Rosenberg et al. (1970) described a kindred in which five persons had hyperuricemia, renal insufficiency, ataxia and deafness. Serum urate levels were elevated in other members of the kindred who did not have renal insufficiency, indicating that the hyperuricemia was not secondary to renal disease. Red cell hypoxanthine-guanine phosphoribosyltransferase levels were normal. The pedigree was consistent with X-linked inheritance with full expression in some females, incomplete expression in others. Riccardi (1974) studied the family and concluded that autosomal dominant inheritance is likely because males seem to be no more severely affected on the average than females.

Riccardi, V. M.: Denver, personal communication, 1974.

Rosenberg, A. L., Bergstrom, L., Troost, B. T. and Bartholomew, B. A.: Hyperuricemia and neurologic deficits: a family study. New Eng. J. Med. 282: 992-997, 1970.

30730 HYPOGONADISM, MALE

Variously termed in the literature are several conditions which affect only persons with the usual male karyotype and which are familial with a pattern often suggesting X-linked inheritance. At least five distinct entities are probably involved: (1) male hypogonadism with or without gynecomastia, (2) male pseudohermaphroditism (q.v.), (3) the testicular feminization syndrome (q.v.), (4) gynecomastia (q.v.), and (5) the

Kallmann syndrome (q.v.). As seen later, there may be at least two distinct forms of the testicular feminization syndrome. Male pseudohermaphroditism is also probably a heterogeneous category. Autosomal dominant (male-limited), autosomal recessive (male-limited) or X-linked inheritance are all possible in this group of entities. When hypospadias and gynecomastia are associated with hypogonadism, the designation of Reifenstein syndrome is often attached. Gynecomastia may occur alone as a familial anomaly or be a feature of one of the other three classes. The necessity for studies, genetic and physiologic, to bring order out of this nosologic chaos is evident. Yet other forms of male hypogonadism — that associated with ichthyosis (q.v.) and that associated with ataxia (q.v.) — will be separately discussed.

Peters and colleagues (1955) described gynecomastia, inguinal testes, and slight hypogonadal traits in two half-brothers (sons of the same mother) and in a cousin, the son of the mother's sister. One affected male had intercourse and ejaculation. The family of Gilbert-Dreyfus and colleagues (1957) is yet another example: maternal uncles were affected. Reifenstein (1947) restudied the family reported by Young (1937). The anomaly is clearly identical to that in Reifenstein's family which we have also restudied. Since a separate, rather clear-cut entity seems to be represented in these cases, I proposed to refer to it as Reifenstein syndrome (q.v.).

There is likely to be heterogeneity left within the group of male hypogonadism even after the types discussed separately hereafter are removed. Some cases may be primary as indicated by high levels of urinary gonadotropins whereas others are cases of secondary hypogonadism with low gonadotropins. The cases of Sohval and Soffer and those of Reifenstein were of the primary type. Roth (1947) described four brothers of Czechoslovakian extraction, with unrelated parents, who had infantile external genitalia, hypogonadotropic hypogonadism, gynecomastia, and retinal degeneration. One was notably obese. Thus some aspects of the Biedl-Bardet syndrome were present. In the view of some, the disorder in the families reported by Gilbert-Dreyfus et al. (1957) and Reifenstein et al. (1947) are merely different degrees of severity of incomplete male pseudohermaphroditism, type I (31210).

Biben, R. L. and Gordan, G. S.: Familial hypogonadotropic eunuchoidism. J. Clin. Endocrinol. Metab. 15: 931-942, 1955.

Brimblecombe, S. L.: Bilateral cryptorchidism in three brothers. Br. Med. J. 1: 526 only, 1946.

Gilbert-Dreyfus, S., Sebaoun, C. A. Belaisch, J.: Etude d'un cas familial d'androgynoidisme avec hypospadias grave, gynecomastie et hyperoestrogenie. Ann. Endocrinol. 18: 93-101, 1957.

Hurxthal, L. M.: Sublingual use of testosterone in 7 cases of hypogonadism: report of 3 congenital eunuchoids occurring in one family. J. Clin. Endocr. 3: 551-556, 1943.

Peters, J. H., Sieber, W. K. and Davis, N.: Familial gynecomastia associated with genital abnormalities: report of a family. J. Clin. Endocrinol. Metab. 15: 182-198, 1955.

Reifenstein, E. C., Jr.: Hereditary familial hypogonadism. Proc. Am. Fed. Clin. Res. 3: 86 only, 1947. Recent Progr. Horm. Res. 3: 224-225, 1947.

Roth, A. A.: Familial eunuchoidism. The Laurence-Moon-Biedl syndrome. J. Urol. 57: 427-442, 1947.

Simpson, S. L.: Two brothers, with infantilism or eunuchoidism. Proc. R. Soc. Med. 39: 512-513, 1946.

Sohval, A. R. and Soffer, L. J.: Congenital familial testicular deficiency. Am. J. Ment. Defic. 14: 328-348, 1953.

Young, H. H.: Genital Abnormalities, Hermaphroditism and Related Adrenal Diseases. Baltimore: Williams and Wilkins, 1937. Pp. 405-409.

30740 HYPOGONADISM, MALE, AND ATAXIA

Volpe's cases had eunuchoid skeletal features and low urinary gonadotropins, and in addition there was cerebellar ataxia. Mathews (1964) described two brothers with pure cerebellar ataxia beginning at about age 20 and associated with marked hypogonadism due apparently to low gonadotropin excretion.

Mathews, W. B. and Rundle, A. T.: Familial cerebellar ataxia and hypogonadism. Brain 87: 463-468, 1964.

Volpe, R., Metzler, W. S. and Johnston, M. W.: Familial hypogonadotrophic eunuchoidism with cerebellar ataxia. J. Clin. Endocr. 23: 107-115, 1963.

30750 HYPOGONADISM, MALE, WITH MENTAL RETARDATION AND SKELETAL ANOMALIES

Sohval and Soffer (1953) described two brothers who were identically affected with mental retardation, multiple skeletal anomalies and hypogonadism. The testicular histopathology was distinctive. All the seminiferous tubules were involved by one of two distinct processes: true germinal aplasia or complete fibrosis, with no gradations between them. Both brothers had fasting hyperglycemia and glucose intolerance. Skeletal anomalies were restricted to the cervical spine and superior ribs.

Sohval, A. R. and Soffer, L. J.: Congenital familial testicular deficiency. Am. J. Ment. Defic. 14: 328-348, 1953.

*30760 HYPOMAGNESEMIC TETANY

Vainsel et al. (1970) described a 5-month-old boy who had convulsions and persistent tetany, associated with hypomagnesemia and hypocalcemia. Vitamin D therapy corrected the hypocalcemia without improving the clinical status. Autopsy showed calcinosis of the myocardium, kidneys and a cerebral artery. Two brothers of the proband had died of a clinically similar disorder and three of four surviving brothers had convulsions.

Others, e.g. Skyberg et al. (1967, 1969), have reported cases, all in males, and X-linked recessive inheritance seems likely.

Skyberg, D., Stromme, J. H., Nesbakken, R. and Harnaes, K.: Congenital primary hypomagnesemia, an inborn error of metabolism. Acta Paediatr. Scand. (suppl. 177): 26-27, 1967.

Skyberg, D., Stromme, J. H., Normann, T., Johannessen, B. K. and Seip, M.: Selective malabsorption of magnesium. An inborn error of metabolism. In, Allan, J. D. and others (eds.): Enzymopenic Anemias, Lysosomes, and Other Papers: Proc. 6th Symposium of Society for Study of Inborn Errors of Metabolism. Edinburgh and London: E. and S. Livingston, 1969.

Vainsel, M., Vandevelde, G., Smulders, J., Vosters, M., Hubain, P. and Loeb, H.: Tetany due to hypomagnesaemia with secondary hypocalcemia. Arch. Dis. Child. 45: 254-258, 1970.

*30770 HYPOPARATHYROIDISM

Penden's family showed neonatal true idiopathic hypoparathyroidism. She suggested that most familial cases of early onset are of the X-linked type. The autosomal variety has a later onset. No affected males reproduced in Penden's family and probably not in others of the X-linked type. Buchs (1957) reported three affected brothers who presented with neonatal tetany. Although maternal hyperparathyroidism with fetal parathyroid suppression was not excluded, it is unlikely because subsequent children were normal.

Buchs, S.: Familiarer Hypoparathyreoidismus. Ann. Paediatr. 188: 124-127, 1957.

Penden, V. H.: True idiopathic hypoparathyroidism as a sex-linked recessive trait. Am. J. Hum. Genet. 12: 323-337, 1960.

*30780 HYPOPHOSPHATEMIA (X-LINKED) (VITAMIN-D-RESISTANT RICKETS)

Low serum phosphorus with vitamin-D-resistant rickets behaves as a sex-linked dominant trait. Heterozygous females have on the average less pronounced depression of serum phosphate and less severe skeletal change. Affected persons show a reduction in renal phosphate Tm to about 50 percent of normal. Males and females are not significantly different in this respect. It is unsettled whether the basic defect concerns (1) renal resorption of phosphate, or (2) intestinal absorption of calcium with secondary hyperparathyroidism. Avioli et al. (1967) observed a defect in metabolism of vitamin D to a biologically active substance and suggested that this is the basic defect. Falls et al. (1968) presented data they interpreted as indicating that hyperphosphaturia is due to secondary hyperparathyroidism. See Williams' (1968) discussion of the nature of the defect. Stickler (1969) concluded that hypophosphatemia is present already in the neonatal period, that alkaline phosphatase is elevated at one month of age and that early treatment with high doses of vitamin D does not prevent growth failure. The concept of vitamin D resistance has shortcomings because the mimicry of nutritional rickets is not close. The X-linked disorder never shows myopathy, tetany or hypocalcemia. Furthermore, complete healing with vitamin D in high dosage and restoration of normal growth is difficult or impossible. Ponchon et al. (1969) concluded that the liver is the major if not the only physiologic site of hydroxylation of vitamin D3 (cholecalciferol) to its biologically active metabolite 25-hydroxycholecalciferol. The possibility of a defect in this system in hypophosphatemic rickets is being investigated. On the basis of a follow-up study McNair and Stickler (1969) questioned whether vitamin D therapy has any beneficial effect on growth. Surprisingly they further concluded that males and females are affected to an equal degree. By an oral phosphate tolerance test, Condon et al. (1970) demonstrated defective intestinal absorption of phosphate. Earp et al. (1970) found 25-HCC ineffective in five patients. Based on experience with a well-studied case, Schoen and Reynolds (1970) are of the opinion that treatment instituted the first day of life, or at least well before weight bearing, can result in normal growth. If true, this places great importance on the family history in identifying infants who need such therapy. Thomas and Fry (1970) described the development of parathyroid adenoma, hyperparathyroidism and osteitis fibrosa cystica as complications of vitamin D-resistant rickets. Negative results with 25-hydroxycholecalciferol (e.g., Cohanim et al., 1972) make it unlikely that the basic defect is in the conversion of vitamin D to the active form. Glorieux and Scriver (1972) suggested that the defect in this condition resides in the parathyroid hormone. Sensitive component of phosphate transport in kidney cells. Since calcium promotion phosphate reabsorption the authors suggest that the beneficial effect of vitamin D therapy is secondary to the effects on calcium metabolism. Glorieux et al. (1972) found restoration of growth when inorganic phosphate salt supplement and vitamin D2 were administered. They interpreted this to support their conclusion that the defect is primarily one of loss of phosphate at the level of the renal tubule. They also showed a direct correlation between the level of serum Pi (inorganic phosphate) and whole blood oxygen pressure at 50 percent oxygen saturation. They speculated that low Pi may inhibit synthesis of 2,3-diphosphoglycerate in red cells with resulting inhibition of release of oxygen to tissues. They suggested that this might be the mechanism of growth retardation. Short et al. (1973) demonstrated a defect in transport of inorganic phosphate by intestinal mucosa. Reitz and Weinstein (1973) found peripheral parathormone concentrations elevated in all subjects. Short et al. (1974) proposed an alternative hypothesis, namely, that the renal tubule is hyperresponsive to the phosphaturic effect of parathyroid hormone. Eicher (1974) has observed the homologous X-linked mutation in the mouse.

Archard, H. O. and Witkop, C. J., Jr.: Hereditary hypophosphatemia (vitamin D-resistant rickets) presenting primary dental manifestations. Oral Surg. 22: 184-193, 1966.

Avioli, L. V., Williams, T. F., Lund, J. and DeLuca, H. F.: Metabolism of vitamin D(3) — (3)H in vitamin D-resistant rickets and familial hypophosphatemia. J. Clin. Invest. 46: 1907-1915, 1967.

Blackard, W. G., Robinson, R. R. and White, J. E.: Familial hypophosphatemia: report of a case, with observations regarding pathogenesis. N. Engl. J. Med. 266: 899-905, 1962.

Burnett, C. H., Dent, C. E., Harper, C. and Warland, B. J.: Vitamin D-resistant rickets. Analysis of twenty-four pedigrees with hereditary and sporadic cases. Am. J. Med. 36: 222-232, 1964.

Cohanim, M., DeLuca, H. F. and Yendt, E. R.: Effects of prolonged treatment with 25-hydroxycholecalciferol in hypophosphatemic (vitamin D refractory) rickets and osteomalacia. Johns Hopkins Med. J. 131: 118-132, 1972.

Condon, J. R., Nassim, J. R. and Rutter, A.: Defective intestinal phosphate absorption in familial and non-familial hypophosphatemia. Br. Med. J. 3: 138-141, 1970.

Condon, J. R., Nassim, J. R. and Rutter, A.: Pathogenesis of rickets and osteomalacia in familial hypophosphataemia. Arch. Dis. Child. 46: 269-272, 1971.

Earp, H. S., Ney, R. L., Gitelman, H. J., Richman, R. and DeLuca, H. F.: Effects of 25-hydroxycholecalciferol in patients with familial hypophosphatemia and vitamin-D-resistant rickets. N. Engl. J. Med. 283: 627-630, 1970.

Eicher, E. M.: Bar Harbor, personal communication, 1974.

Falls, W. F., Jr., Carter, N. W., Rector, F. C., Jr. and Seldin, D. W.: Familial vitamin D-resistant rickets: study of six cases with evaluation of the pathogenetic role of secondary hyperparathyroidism. Ann. Intern. Med. 68: 553-560, 1968.

Glorieux, F. and Scriver, C. R.: Loss of a parathyroid hormone-sensitive component of phosphate transport in X-linked hypophosphatemia. Science 175: 997-1000, 1972.

Glorieux, F. H., Scriver, C. R., Reade, T. M., Goldman, H. and Rosenborough, A.: Use of phosphate and vitamin D to prevent dwarfism and rickets in X-linked hypophosphatemia. N. Engl. J. Med. 287: 481-487, 1972.

McNair, S. L. and Stickler, G. B.: Growth in familial hypophosphatemic vitamin-D-resistant rickets. N. Engl. J. Med. 281: 511-516, 1969.

Ponchon, G., Kennan, A. L. and DeLuca, H. F.: 'Activation' of vitamin D by the liver. J. Clin. Invest. 48: 2032-2037, 1969.

Reitz, R. E. and Weinstein, R. L.: Parathyroid hormone secretion in familial vitamin-D-resistant rickets. N. Engl. J. Med. 289: 941-945, 1973.

Schoen, E. J. and Reynolds, J. B.: Severe familial hypophosphatemic rickets. Normal growth following early treatment. Am. J. Dis. Child. 120: 58-61, 1970.

Short, E. M., Binder, J. H. and Rosenberg, L. E.: Familial hypophosphatemic rickets: defective transport of inorganic phosphate by intestinal mucosa. Science 179: 700-702, 1973.

Short, E., Sebastian, A., Spencer, M. and Morris, R. C., Jr.: Hyperresponsiveness to the phosphaturic effect of parathyroid hormone in X-linked hypophorphatemic vitamin D-resistant rickets (FHR). (Abstract) J. Clin. Invest. 53: 75A only, 1974.

Stickler, G. B.: Familial hypophosphatemic vitamin D resistant rickets. The neonatal period and infancy. Acta Paediatr. Scand. 58: 213-219, 1969.

Thomas, W. C., Jr. and Fry, R. M.: Parathyroid adenomas in chronic rickets. Am. J. Med. 49: 404-407, 1970.

Williams, T. F.: Pathogenesis of familial vitamin D-resistant rickets. (Editorial) Ann. Intern. Med. 68: 706-707, 1968.

Winters, R. W., Graham, J. B., Williams, T. F., McFalls, V. W. and Burnett, C. H.: A genetic study of familial hypophosphatemia and vitamin D resistant rickets with a review of the literature. Medicine 37: 97-142, 1958.

*30800 HYPOXANTHINE GUANINE PHOSPHORIBOSYL TRANSFERASE

Studies using human-mouse somatic cell hybrids indicate, by reasoning similar to that used for locating the thymidine kinase locus to chromosome 17, that the HGPRT locus is on the X chromosome (Nabholz et al., 1969). The features of the Lesch-Nyhan syndrome are mental retardation, spastic cerebral palsy, choreoathetosis, uric acid urinary stones and self-destructive biting of fingers and lips. A 200 fold increase in the conversion of C(14)-labelled glycine to uric acid was observed by Nyhan, Olivier and Lesch (1965). X-linkage was first suggested by Hoefnagel et al. (1965) and is supported by a rapidly accumulating number of families. Seegmiller et al. (1967) demonstrated deficiency in the enzyme hypoxanthine-guanine phosphoribosyltransferase. That the enzyme deficiency resulted in excessive purine synthesis suggests that the enzyme (or the product of its function) normally plays a controlling role in purine metabolism. Rosenbloom et al. (1967) and Migeon et al. (1968) demonstrated two populations of fibroblasts, as regards the relevant enzyme activity, in heterozygous females, thus providing support both for X-linkage and for the Lyon hypothesis. Megaloblastic anemia has been found by some (van der Zee et al., 1968). Fujimoto et al. (1968) presented evidence that the disease can be recognized in the fetus well before the 20 weeks which is considered a limit on therapeutic abortion. The method used was an autoradiographic test for HGPRT activity, applied to cells obtained by amniocentesis. Boyle et al. (1970) made the prenatal diagnosis and performed therapeutic abortion. Henderson et al. (1969) found that the locus for HGPRT is closely linked to the Xg locus. See HYPERURICEMIA, ATAXIA, DEAFNESS for a syndrome with some similarities to the Lesch-Nyhan syndrome but normal red cell HGPRT levels. McDonald and Kelley (1971) presented evidence of genetic heterogeneity in the Lesch-Nyhan syndrome. In the patient they reported, HGPRT showed altered kinetics. In mouse-man hybrid cells, when the mouse parent cell is of the type called RAG

X
L
I
N
K
E
D

which is resistant to 8-azaguanine because of a deficiency of HGPRT, the human form of HGPRT is required in order for the hybrid cells to survive in HAT selective medium. In over 100 clones of human-rag hybrid cells maintained in HAT, Ruddle (1971) saw without exception persistence of human G6PD activity. This strongly indicates either close linkage of the HGPRT and G6PD loci or a very low incidence of X-chromosome breakage and rearrangement. Emmerson et al. (1972) described a family with partial deficiency of HGPRT in which heterozygous females had an intermediate level of enzyme activity in red cells. The finding is consistent with the view that selection at the cellular level is operating against those erythropoietic cells which have a complete deficiency in females heterozygous for the Lesch-Nyhan gene. Among 425 cases of hyperuricemia with gout or uric acid stone or both, Yu et al. (1972) found 7 with partial HGPRT deficiency and 5 of these were members of one family. Mosaicism can be demonstrated by study of hair roots in women heterozygous for the Lesch-Nyhan syndrome (Silvers et al., 1972). Greene et al. (1970) concluded that the HGPRT and Xg loci 'are sufficient distance from each other on the human X chromosome that linkage cannot be detected.' Nyhan et al. (1970) observed a sibship in which both HGPRT deficiency and G6PD deficiency were segregating and found two recombinants out of four. Emmerson et al. (1974) excluded close linkage of the HGPRT and deutan loci. In five patients with gout, Kelley et al. (1967) showed a partial deficiency of hypoxanthine-guanine phosphoribosyl-transferase, the enzyme deficient in Lesch-Nyhan syndrome (an X-linked condition). All 5 were male. Two brothers in one family were 24 and 11 years old. Three brothers in a second family were 42, 49 and 55 years old. In the first family nephrolithiasis began at age 6 or 7 followed in one by gouty arthritis at age 13. In the three brothers acute gouty arthritis began between ages 20 and 31 and two had had recurrent nephrolithiasis. The two brothers of the first family had spinocerebellar derangement distinct from the neurologic disorder of the Lesch-Nyhan syndrome. The characteristics of the enzyme were the same in each family but different between families. The differences concerned relative activities for guanine and hypoxanthine and heat stability. That the HGPRT locus is X-linked in the mouse also is indicated by Epstein's finding (1972) that the activity of the enzyme at the two-cell stage in the XO product is half that in the XX. No difference is observed in late morula and blastocyst stage.

Bakay, B., Nyhan, W. L., Fawcett, N. and Kogut, M. D.: Isoenzymes of hypoxanthine-guanine-phosphoribosyl transferase in a family with partial deficiency of the enzyme. Biochem. Genet. 7: 73-86, 1972.

Benke, P. J., Hebert, A. and Herrick, N.: In vitro effects of magnesium ions on mutant cells from patients with the Lesch-Nyhan syndrome. N. Engl. J. Med. 289: 446-450, 1973.

Benke, P. J., Herrick, N. and Hebert, A.: Hypoxanthine-guanine phosphoribosyltransferase variant associated with accelerated purine synthesis. J. Clin. Invest. 52: 2234-2240, 1973.

Bland, J. H.: (General Chairman) seminars on the Lesch-Nyhan syndrome. Fed. Proc. 27: 1017-1112, 1968.

Boyle, J. A., Raivio, K. O., Astrin, K. H., Shulman, J. D., Graf, M. L., Seegmiller, J. E. and Jacobson, C. B.: Lesch-Nyhan syndrome: preventive control by prenatal diagnosis. Science 169: 688-689, 1970.

Cox, R. P., Krauss, M. R., Balis, M. E. and Dancis, J.: Evidence for transfer of enzyme product as the basis of metabolic cooperation between tissue culture fibroblasts of Lesch-Nyhan disease and normal cells. Proc. Natl. Acad. Sci. 67: 1573-1579, 1970.

Dancis, J., Yip, L. C., Cox, R. P., Piomelli, S. and Balis, M. E.: Disparate enzyme activity in erythrocytes and leukocytes: a variant of hypoxanthine phosphoribosyltransferase deficiency with an unstable enzyme. J. Clin. Invest. 52: 2068-2074, 1973.

Demars, R., Sarto, G., Felix, J. S. and Benke, P.: Lesch-Nyhan mutation: prenatal detection with amniotic fluid cells. Science 164: 1303-1305, 1969.

Emmerson, B. T., Thompson, C. J. and Wallace, D. C.: Partial deficiency hypoxanthine-guanine phosphoribosyltransferase: intermediate enzyme deficiency in heterozygote red cells. Ann. Intern. Med. 76: 285-288, 1972.

Emmerson, B. T., Thompson, L., Wallace, D. C. and Spence, M. A.: Absence of measurable linkage between the loci for hypoxathine-guanine phosphoriboxyltransferase and deutan color blindness. Am. J. Hum. Genet. 26: 78-82, 1974.

Epstein, C. J.: Expression of the mammalian X chromosome before and after fertilization. Science 175: 1467-1468, 1972.

Francke, U., Bakay, B., Connor, J. D., Coldwell, J. G. and Nyhan, W. L.: Linkage relationships of X-linked enzymes glucose-6-phosphate dehydrogenase and hypoxaminthine guanine phosphoribosyltransferase. Am. J. Hum. Genet. 26: 512-522, 1974.

Fujimoto, W. Y., Seegmiller, J. E., Uhlendorf, B. W. and Jacobson, C. B.: Biochemical diagnosis of X-linked disease in utero. (Letter) Lancet II: 511-512, 1968.

Greene, M. L.: Clinical features of patients with the 'partial' deficiency of the X-linked uricaciduria enzyme. Arch. Intern. Med. 130: 193-198, 1972.

Greene, M. L., Nyhan, W. L. and Seegmiller, J. E.: Hypoxanthine-guanine phosphoribosyltransferase deficiency and Xg blood group. Am. J. Hum. Genet. 22: 50-54, 1970.

Henderson, J. F., Kelley, W. N., Rosenbloom, F. M. and Seegmiller, J. E.: Inheritance of purine phosphoribosyltransferases in man. Am. J. Hum. Genet. 21: 61-70, 1969.

Hoefnagel, D., Andrew, E. D., Mireault, N. G. and Berndt, W. O.: Hereditary choreoathetosis, self-mutilation and hyperuricemia in young males. N. Engl. J. Med. 273: 130-135, 1965.

Kelley, W. N., Rosenbloom, F. M., Henderson, J. F. and Seegmiller, J. E.: A specific enzyme defect in gout associated with overproduction of uric acid. Proc. Natl. Acad. Sci. 57: 1735-1739, 1967.

Kelley, W. N., Green, M. L., Rosenbloom, F. M., Henderson, J. F. and Seegmiller, J. E.: Hypoxanthine-guanine phosphoribosyltransferase deficiency in gout. Ann. Intern. Med. 70: 155-206, 1969.

Kogut, M. D., Donnell, G. N., Nyhan, W. L. and Sweetman, L.: Disorder of purine metabolism due to partial deficiency of hypoxanthine-guanine phosphoribosyltransferase. Am. J. Med. 48: 148-161, 1970.

McDonald, J. A. and Kelley, W. N.: Lesch-Nyhan syndrome: absence of the mutant enzyme in erythrocytes of a heterozygote for both normal and mutant hypoxanthine-guanine phosphoribosyl transferase. Biochem. Genet. 6: 21-26, 1972.

McDonald, J. A. and Kelley, W. N.: Lesch-Nyhan syndrome: altered kinetic properties of mutant enzyme. Science 171: 689-691, 1971.

Migeon, B. R.: X-linked hypoxanthine-guanine phosphoribosyl transferase deficiency: detection of heterozygotes by selective medium. Biochem. Genet. 4: 377-383, 1970.

Migeon, B. R., Der Kaloustian, V. M., Nyhan, W. L., Young, W. J. and Childs, B.: X-linked hypoxanthine-guanine phosphoribosyl transferase deficiency: heterozygote has two clonal populations. Science 160: 425-427, 1968.

Nabholz, M., Miggiano, V. and Bodmer, W.: Genetic analysis with human-mouse somatic cell hybrids. Nature 223: 358-363, 1969.

Newcombe, D. S., Shapiro, S. L., Sheppard, G. L. and Dreifuss, F. E.: Treatment of X-linked primary hyperuricemia with allopurinol. J.A.M.A. 198: 315-317, 1966.

Nyhan, W. L., Bakay, B., Connor, J. D., Marks, J. F. and Keele, D. K.: Hemizygous expression of glucose-6-phosphate dehydrogenase in erythrocytes of heterozygotes for the Lesch-Nyhan syndrome. Proc. Natl. Acad. Sci. 65: 214-218, 1970.

Nyhan, W. L., Olivier, W. J. and Lesch, M.: A familial disorder of uric acid metabolism and central nervous system function. J. Pediatr. 67: 257-263, 1965.

Nyhan, W. L., Resek, J., Sweetman, L., Carpenter, D. G. and Carter, C. H.: Genetics of an X-linked disorder of uric acid metabolism and cerebral function. Pediatr. Res. 1: 5-13, 1967.

Race, R. R. and Sanger, R.: Blood Groups in Man. Philadelphia: F. A. Davis Co., 1968 (5th Ed.). P. 545.

Rosenbloom, F. M., Kelley, W. N., Henderson, J. F. and Seegmiller, J. E.: Lyon hypothesis and X-linked disease. (Letter) Lancet II: 305-306, 1967.

Rosenbloom, F. M., Kelley, W. N., Miller, J., Henderson, J. F. and Seegmiller, J. E.: Inherited disorder of purine metabolism. Correlation between central nervous system dysfunction and biochemical defects. J.A.M.A. 202: 175-177, 1967.

Ruddle, F. H.: Linkage studies employing mouse-man somatic cell hybrids. Fed. Proc. 30: 921-925, 1971.

Sass, J. K., Itabashi, H. H. and Dexter, R. A.: Juvenile gout with brain involvement. Arch. Neurol. 13: 639-655, 1965.

Seegmiller, J. E., Rosenbloom, F. M. and Kelley, W. N.: Enzyme defect associated with a sex-linked human neurological disorder and excessive purine synthesis. Science 155: 1682-1684, 1967.

Shapiro, S. L., Sheppard, G. L., Jr., Dreifuss, F. E. and Newcombe, D. S.: X-linked recessive inheritance of a syndrome of mental retardation with hyperuricemia. Proc. Soc. Exp. Biol. Med. 122: 609-611, 1966.

Silvers, D. N., Cox, R. P., Balis, M. E. and Dancis, J.: Detection of the heterozygote in Lesch-Nyhan disease by hair-root analysis. New Eng. J. Med. 286: 390-395, 1972.

Sperling, O., Frank, M., Ophir, R., Liberman, U. A., Adam, A. and De Vries, A.: Partial deficiency of hypoxanthine-guanine phosphoribosyltransferase associated with gout and uric acid lithiasis. Europ. J. Clin. Biol. Res. 15: 942-947, 1970.

Van der Zee, S. P. M., Schretlen, E. D. A. M. and Monnens, L. A. H.: Megaloblastic anaemia in the Lesch-Nyhan syndrome. (Letter) Lancet I: 1427 only, 1968.

Yu, T.-F., Balis, M. E., Krenitsky, T. A., Dancis, J., Silvers, D. N., Elion, G. B. and Gutman, A. B.: Rarity of X-linked partial hypoxanthine-guanine phosphoribosyltransferase deficiency in a large gouty population. Ann. Intern. Med. 76: 255-264, 1972.

*30810 ICHTHYOSIS (X-LINKED)

Czorsz (1928) described a presumed homozygous, affected female. In 1929 Orel found in the literature 10 families with the X-linked form. Turpin and his colleagues (1945) described associated changes in the fundus oculi of affected males. Kerr, Wells and Sanger (1964) presented evidence suggesting that the X-linked ichthyosis locus may be within 'mappable' distance of the Xg locus. In addition to the genetic difference between X-linked ichthyosis and ichthyosis vulgaris, clinical and histologic differences exist (Wells and Jennings, 1967). In the X-linked form onset is at birth and scalp, ears, neck and one or more flexures are involved, with more striking scaling on the abdomen than the back and extension of the scaling down the front of the leg onto the dorsum of the foot. Histologically the epidermis is atrophic in ichthyosis vulgaris and hypertrophic in the X-linked variety. Closer situation of the Xg and ichthyosis loci was indicated by studies of Adam et al. (1969) who estimated the recombination fraction as 0.105 and of Went et al. (1969)

who found a value of 0.115. Close linkage with the deutan, protan and G6PD loci was excluded (Adam et al., 1969). Went et al. (1969) found mild abnormality of the skin in about one fourth of heterozygotes. Schnyder (1970) gave a useful classification of the inherited ichthyoses. Solomon and Schoen (1971) reported a patient with XO Turner syndrome and ichthyosis which by the pedigree and by its clinical features was X-linked. Passarge et al. (1971) described an X-linked pedigree in which the clinical picture was intermediate between those of the 'classic' X-linked form and the autosomal dominant form. Possibly this is an allelic form. Sever et al. (1968) described deep corneal opacities in all of 17 affected males and in 7 of 8 heterozygous females. Eicher (1974) speculated that the scurfy (sf) mutation in the mouse may be homologous to X-linked ichthyosis of man.

Adam, A., Ziprkowski, L., Feinstein, A., Sanger, R., Tippett, P., Gavin, J. and Race, R. R.: Linkage relations of X-borne ichthyosis to the Xg blood groups and to other markers of the X in Israelis. Ann. Hum. Genet. 32: 323-332, 1969.

Cockayne, E. A.: Inherited Abnormalities of the Skin and Its Appendages. London: Oxford U. Press, 1933. P. 213.

Czorsz, B.: Mschr. Unfalheilk. Medizin. 2: 180. Also Z. Haut. Geschlechtskr. 26: 463, 1928.

Eicher, E. M.: Bar Harbor, personal communication, 1974.

Harris, H.: A pedigree of sex-linked ichthyosis vulgaris. Ann. Eugen. 14: 9 only, 1947.

Kerr, C. B. and Wells, R. S.: Sex-linked ichthyosis. Ann. Hum. Genet. 29: 33-50, 1965.

Kerr, C. B., Wells, R. S. and Sanger, R.: X-linked ichthyosis and the Xg groups. Lancet II: 1369-1370, 1964.

Orel, H.: Die vererbung der ichthyosis congenita und der ichthyosis vulgaris. Z. Kinderheilkd. 47: 312-340, 1929.

Passarge, E., Post, B. and Schopf, E.: Possible genetic heterogeneity of X-linked ichthyosis. The Clinical Delineation of Birth Defects. XII. Skin, Hair and Nails. Baltimore: Williams and Wilkins, 1971. Pp. 46-49.

Schnyder, U. W.: Inherited ichthyoses. Arch. Dermatol. 102: 240-252, 1970.

Sever, R. J., Frost, P. and Weinstein, G.: Eye changes in ichthyosis. J.A.M.A. 206: 2283-2286, 1968.

Solomon, I. L. and Schoen, E. J.: Sex-linked ichthyosis in XO gonadal dysgenesis. (Letter) Lancet I: 1304-1305, 1971.

Turpin, R., Desvignes, (NI) and Demassieux, (NI): Sem. Hop. Paris 21: 343, 1945.

Wells, R. S. and Jennings, M. C.: X-linked ichthyosis and ichthyosis vulgaris. Clinical and genetic distinctions in a second series of families. J.A.M.A. 202: 485-488, 1967.

Went, L. N., Degroot, W. P., Sanger, R., Tippett, P. and Gavin, J.: X-linked ichthyosis: linkage relationship with the Xg blood groups and other studies in a large Dutch kindred. Ann. Hum. Genet. 32: 333-346, 1969.

30820 ICHTHYOSIS AND MALE HYPOGONADISM

In the apparently unique family reported by Lynch and his colleagues five males in three generations showed both secondary hypogonadism (associated with low titers of pituitary gonadotrophic hormones) and congenital ichthyosis. This is classed as a definite X-linked recessive trait because if the syndrome were inherited as an autosomal dominant, the ichthyosis component would be expected to have been displayed by females. The authors suggested that close linkage may be responsible for the occurrence of hypogonadism with ichthyosis, a well-known X-linked trait. However, ichthyosis and hypogonadism is listed as a separate mutation since linkage can only be postulated. If indeed the two traits are due to two linked genes one can say with 95 percent confidence that the recombination value is not greater than 20 percent. The disorder was transmitted by six females in whom there was opportunity for cross-over.

Lynch, H. T., Ozer, F., McNutt, C. W., Johnson, J. E. and Jampolsky, N. A.: Secondary male hypogonadism and congenital ichthyosis. Association of two rare genetic diseases. Am. J. Hum. Genet. 12: 440-447, 1960.

30823 IMMUNODEFICIENCY WITH INCREASED IGM

In the WHO classification of immunodeficiencies, an entity termed X-linked immunodeficiency with increased IgM was listed (Fudenberg et al., 1970). Several families are known to Rosen (1973). The 'best' pedigree is that reported by Jamieson and Kerr (1962). Four affected boys in this kindred were studied by Rosen and found to fit the diagnosic criteria.

Fudenberg, H. H., et al.: Classification of the primary immunodeficiencies (WHO recommendation). N. Engl. J. Med. 283: 656-657, 1970.

Jamieson, W. M. and Kerr, M. R.: A family with several cases of hypogammaglobulinemia. Arch. Dis. Child. 37: 330-336. 1962.

Rosen, F. S.: Boston, personal communication, Aug. 23, 1973.

30825 IMMUNOGLOBULIN M, LEVEL OF

Grundbacher (1972) suggested that genes on the X chromosome determine the quantity of immunoglobulin M, because the concentration in serum is one-third higher in females than in males and intrafamilial

X
L
I
N
K
E
D

correlations are higher between sons and mothers than between sons and fathers. Even higher IgM was observed in XXX females (Rhodes et al., 1969) and XO females had levels like normal males.

Grundbacher, F. J.: Human X chromosome carries quantitative genes for immunoglobulin M. Science 176: 311-312, 1972.

Rhodes, K., Markham, R. L., Maxwell, P. M. and Monk-Jones, M. E.: Immunoglobulins and the X-chromosome. Br. Med. J. 3: 439-441, 1969.

*30830 INCONTINENTIA PIGMENTI

Incontinentia pigmenti is a disturbance of skin pigmentation inconstantly associated with a variety of malformations of the eye, teeth, skeleton, heart, etc. The pigmentary disturbance, an autochthonous tattooing, is evident at or soon after birth and may be preceded by a phase suggesting inflammation in the skin. In the fully developed disease, the skin shows swirling patterns of melanin pigmentation, especially on the trunk, suggesting the appearance of 'marble cake.' Histologically, deposits of melanin pigment are seen in the corium: the designation was based on the idea that the basal layer of the epidermis is 'incontinent' of melanin. Pedigree patterns suggest X-linked dominance with lethality in the male. The phenotype in the affected females might be consistent with random X chromosome inactivation as in the Lyon hypothesis.

The cutaneous phenotype has other interesting features, namely, that in the first months of life it has some characteristics of an inflammatory process and that the pigmentary changes have usually disappeared completely by the age of 20 years. Caffey disease (infantile hyperostosis), which is familial and possibly genetic, displays a similar behavior, with pronounced signs suggesting an inflammatory process in many bones with subsequent quiescence and in many cases disappearance of all evidence of previous disease. Kuster and Olbing (1964) reported a mentally retarded woman with incomplete dentition and a history of skin lesions at birth. She had one son and 11 daughters. Six of the girls showed incomplete dentition and incontinentia pigmenti.

Cytoplasmic (or other nonchromosomal) inheritance with lethality in the male could also account for the pedigree pattern. Features of the histologic and clinical picture have suggested viral etiology to several workers (e.g., Haber, 1952). Cytoplasmic inclusions like those of molluscum contagiosum have been identified (Thomas W. Murrell, Jr.: Richmond: personal communication).

As a third possibility, the pedigree pattern is probably consistent also with an autosome X chromosome translocation. No chromosomal abnormality was found in two cases of incontinentia pigmenti studied by Benirschke (personal communication). In the family studied, the mother and two daughters were affected; there had been one male abortion. Garrod (1906) may have described the first case, a girl with typical pigmentary changes together with mental deficiency and tetraplegia.

Carney, R. G. and Carney, R. G., Jr.: Incontinentia pigmenti. Arch. Dermatol. 102: 157-162, 1970.

Garrod, A. E.: Peculiar pigmentation of the skin in an infant. Trans. Clin. Soc. Lond. 39: 216 only, 1906.

Haber, H.: The Bloch-Sulzberger syndrome (incontinentia pigmenti). Br. J. Dermatol. 64: 129-140, 1952.

Kuster, F. and Olbing, H.: Incontinentia pigmenti. Bericht uber neun Erkrankungen in einer Familie und einem Obduktionsbefund. Ann. Paediatr. 202: 92-100, 1964.

Lenz, W.: Medizinische Genetik. Eine Einfuhrung in ihre Grundlagen und Probleme. Stuttgart: Georg Thieme Verlag, 1961. P. 89.

Pfeiffer, R. A.: Zur Frage der Vererbung der Incontinentia Pigmenti Bloch-Siemens. Z. Menschl. Vererb. Konstitutionsl. 35: 469-493, 1960.

Reed, W. B., Carter, C. and Cohen, T. M.: Incontinentia pigmenti. Dermatologica 134: 243-250, 1967.

30840 INTRAUTERINE GROWTH RETARDATION, MICROCEPHALY, AND MENTAL RETARDATION

In their report on intrauterine growth retardation, Warkany, Monroe and Sutherland (1961) described a family in which four males in three generations in a pattern consistent with X-linked recessive inheritance showed low-birth weight despite term gestation and were either stillborn or showed slow physical and mental development. Three presumed heterozygous females had low birth weight but became normal adults capable of reproduction. Microcephaly was present in the affected males and mental retardation required institutionalization. This may be the same condition as that described simply as mental retardation in this X-linked catalog.

Warkany, J., Monroe, B. B. and Sutherland, B. S.: Intrauterine growth retardation. Am. J. Dis. Child. 102: 249-279, 1961.

*30850 IRIS, HYPOPLASIA OF, WITH GLAUCOMA

Frank-Kamenetzki (1925) described this disorder in two Russian kindreds. The atrophy or hypoplasia of the iris seemed, from the findings in young family members, to be primary and glaucoma secondary. Makarow (cited by Waardenburg et al., 1961) probably described the same disorder, also in Russia. No other families are known. The similarity to Rieger anomaly (see dominant catalog) is noteworthy.

Frank-Kamenetzki, S. G.: Eine eigenartige hereditare Glaukomform mit Mangel des Irisstromas und geschlechtsgebundener Vererbung. Klin. Monatsbl. Augenheilkd. 74: 133-150, 1925.

Waardenburg, P. J., Franceschetti, A. and Klein, D.: Genetics and Ophthalmology. Springfield, Ill.: Charles C Thomas, 1961 (Vol. 1), P. 609.

McElfresh (1962) described a form of neonatal hyperbilirubinemia in six males of two generations in a pattern consistent with X-linked recessive inheritance. One affected member of the earlier generation was jaundiced with light stools for the first five months of life. He was 31 and well, with two normal children, at the time of report.

McElfresh, A. E.: Familial obstructive jaundice during infancy. (Abstract) Am. J. Dis. Child. 104: 531-532, 1962.

30870 KALLMANN SYNDROME (SECONDARY, OR HYPOGONADOTROPIC, HYPOGONADISM WITH ANOSMIA; DYSPLASIA OLFACTOGENITALIS OF DE MORSIER)

Affected males show anosmia and hypogonadism secondary to low gonadotropin production. Transmitting females have partial or complete anosmia. Gonadotropins have to our knowledge not been studied in the carrier females. Affected males at times have children. Unilateral renal agenesis has occurred in some affected males. Anosmia is due to agenesis of the olfactory lobes. Whether a mutation resulting in anosmia is separate from that for the Kallmann syndrome is discussed elsewhere. Color blindness was also segregating in Kallmann's families. However, the information was too limited to give conclusive evidence on possible X-linkage of this syndrome. Hockaday (1966) described two cases. In the second the father was found to have 'complete anosmia on testing.' Anosmia must be inquired about in cases of hypogonadism since patients rarely volunteer the information. Indeed, the patient is sometimes unaware of anosmia so that tests are necessary. Pittman (1966) found anosmia in 16 of 28 cases of hypogonadotropic hypogonadism. With treatment fertility may be restored in these cases and observations differentiating X-linked from autosomal inheritance may be forthcoming. See the autosomal recessive catalog for possible autosomal recessive inheritance of Kallmann syndrome. Bardin et al. (1969) concluded that these patients have a defect in both pituitary and Leydig cell function. They demonstrated impaired secretion of FSH and LH and Leydig cell insensitivity to gonadotropin. Sparkes et al. (1968) described hypogonadotropic hypogonadism with anosmia in two brothers and in a half-sister of theirs. The three affected sibs had the same mother who although obviously not fully affected had minor signs (late menarche and irregular menses) despite which she managed to have 9 liveborn children. The affected girl had no menses or breast development at age 18 and ovaries which were histologically exactly like those of the fetus. Anosmia was present. The authors suggested X-linked inheritance. Schroffner and Furth (1970) found failure of response to clomiphene, as measured by plasma levels of gonadotropins. The father had anosmia. The father of one of Hockaday's patients also had anosmia (1966). An affected female with two affected brothers was described by Males et al. (1973). Males et al. (1973) studied 6 unrelated subjects, 5 males and one female with Kallmann syndrome. All the males had small genitals and decreased sexual hair. Gynecomastia and eunuchoid habitus were seen in four. All six had a normal sella turcica. Testicular biopsies of the males showed decreased numbers of germ cells and a spermatogenic state at the primary spermatocyte stage. Leydig cells were not histologically identifiable. All six patients demonstrated anosmia. The affected female had 2 brothers with anosmia and hypogonadism. Urine gonadotropins were low in the two patients tested. Basal urinary 17-hydroxycorticosteroids were normal in those tested. A metyrapone test suggested low levels of ACTH in two. One male patient at operation showed agenesis of the olfactory bulbs and tracts.

The authors state that the hypogonadotropin hypogonadism with anosmia probably is the expression of a disorder of hypothalamic regulation involving the control of those releasing factors needed for effective pituitary function. Additionally, it is interesting to note that there is some evidence for a relationship between olfactory acuity (perhaps to detect pheromones) and the gonadal and adrenal system in laboratory test animals.

Henkin, R. I.: Abnormalities of taste and olfaction in patients with chromatin negative gonadal dysgenesis. J. Clin. Endocrinol. Metab. 27: 1436-1440, 1967.

Hockaday, T. D. R.: Hypogonadism and life-long anosmia. Postgrad. Med. J. 42: 572-574, 1966.

Kallmann, F. J., Schoenfeld, W. A. and Barrera, S. E.: The genetic aspects of primary eunuchoidism. Am. J. Ment. Defic. 48: 203-236, 1944.

Males, J. L., Townsend, J. L. and Schneider, R. A.: Hypogonadotropic hypogonadism with anosmia — Kallman's syndrome: a disorder of olfactory and hypothalamic function. Arch. Intern. Med. 131: 501-507, 1973.

Males, J. L., Townsend, J. L. and Schneider, R. A.: Hypogonadotropic hypogonadism with anosmia-Kallmann's syndrome. Arch. Intern. Med. 131: 501-508, 1973.

Nowakowski, H. and Lenz, W.: Genetic aspects in male hypogonadism. Recent Progr. Horm. Res. 17: 53-95, 1961.

Paulsen, C. A.: Familial hypogonadotropic hypogonadism with anosmia. Arch. Intern. Med. 121: 534-538, 1968.

Pittman, J.: Boston, Mass.: personal communication, 1966.

Schroffner, W. G. and Furth, E. D.: Hypogonadotropic hypogonadism with anosmia (Kallmann's syndrome) unresponsive to clomiphene citrate. J. Clin. Endocrinol. Metab. 31: 267-270, 1970.

Sparkes, R. S., Simpson, R. W. and Paulsen, C. A.: Familial hypogonadotropic hypogonadism with anosmia. Arch. Intern. Med. 121: 534-538, 1968.

30875 KELL 'MODIFIER'

Allen (1974) has evidence for an X-linked modifier of the expression of the Kell blood group (11090).

X

L
I
N
K
E
D

30877 KERATOSIS FOLLICULARIS, DWARFISM, CEREBRAL ATROPHY

Cantu et al. (1974) described a kindred in which three brothers and three of their maternal uncles had generalized keratosis follicularis, severe growth retardation and cerebral atrophy. Hair, eyebrows and eyelashes were almost completly absent.

Cantu, J. M., Hernandez, A., Larracilla, J., Terejo, A. and Macotela-Ruiz, E.: A new X-linked recessive disorder with dwarfism, cerebral atrophy, and generalized keratosis follicularis. J. Pediatr. 84: 564-570, 1974.

*30880 KERATOSIS FOLLICULARIS, SPINULOSA DECALVANS CUM OPHIASI

Affected men show thickening of the skin of the neck, ears, and extremities, especially the palms and soles, loss of eyebrows, eyelashes and beard, thickening of the eyelids with blepharitis and ectropion, and corneal degeneration. The term 'cum ophiasi' means 'with ophiasis,' i.e., baldness in one or more winding streaks about the head. The term comes from the Greek for snake. Decalvans refers to the loss of hair. Autosomal dominant inheritance has also been described (Thelen 1940).

In Siemens' publication pointing out X-linked inheritance, two families were described. In the one not observed personally by Siemens (described by Lameris, 1905, and by Rochat, 1906) the inheritance appeared to be X-linked recessive, whereas the other was an example of X-linked dominant (or intermediate) inheritance. The Lameris kindred was studied further by Jonkers (1950) and the pedigree was reproduced by Waardenburg, Franceschetti, and Klein (Genetics and Ophthalmology, Vol. I, 1961). Restudy indicated that the inheritance is the same as in Siemens' pedigree. Eicher (1974) speculated that the homologous mutation in the mouse may be 'sparse fur' (spf).

Eicher, E. M.: Bar Harbor, personal communication, 1974.

Jonkers, G. H.: Hyperkeratosis follicularis and cornea degeneration. Ophthalmologica 120: 365-367, 1950.

Lameris, (NI): Ichthyosis follicularia. Nederl. Tijdschr. Geneeskd. 2: 1524 only, 1905.

Rochat, (NI): La paralysie de l'oculomoteur externe d'origine auriculaire. Arch. Internat. Laryng. 21: 125-131, 1906.

Sendi, H.: Quelques cas de keratosis follicularis spinulosa decalvans (Siemens). Thesis, Geneva, 1957.

Siemens, H. W.: Ueber einen in der menschlichen Pathologie noch nicht beobachteten Vererbungsmodus: dominant geschlechtsgebundene Vererbung. Arch. Rass.-u. Ges. Biol. 17: 47-61, 1925.

30885 LARYNGEAL ABDUCTOR PARALYSIS

Plott (1964) described three brothers with permanent congenital laryngeal abductor paralysis and mental deficiency. A fourth male sib suspected of having been affected died perinatally. Dygenesis of the nucleus ambiguus was considered likely. Walters and Fitch (1973) presented a pedigree which made X-linked recessive inheritance likely. Two brothers were affected together with a first-cousin-once-removed connected through females.

Plott, D.: Congenital laryngeal-abductor paralysis due to nucleus abmiguus dysgensis in three brothers. New Eng. J. Med. 271: 593-597, 1964.

Walters, G. V. and Fitch, N.: Familial laryngeal abductor paralysis and psychomotor retardation. Clin. Genet. 4: 429-433, 1973.

30890 LEBER OPTIC ATROPHY

Part of the difficulty in studying the genetics of this disorder arises from diagnostic confusion in a disease category which is almost certainly heterogeneous. There are many peculiarities to the familial distribution of Leber optic atrophy. In Europeans 84.8 percent of cases are male but in Japanese only 59.1 percent. In Europeans the peak age of onset seems to be about age 20 years. The disorder is usually transmitted through the mother. Ninety-five percent of affected males apparently get their disease from the mother, some of whom (about a seventh) are affected whereas the remainder have affected relatives. Eighty-four percent of affected females get their disease from the mother and about half of their mothers are affected.

Recent studies raise doubts about whether males ever transmit the condition. Furthermore, the interrelationship of a genetic factor with an environmental factor (perhaps tobacco) has been raised (Wilson, 1963, 1965). The genetic component may well prove to be autosomal. Imai and Moriwaki suggest cytoplasmic inheritance. Wilson (1965) has suggested that this generalized neurologic disease results from cyanide intoxication because cyanide in the diet and in tobacco smoke is for genetic reasons not adequately detoxified to thiocyanate. Wallace (1970) presented family data which he interpreted as supporting the vertical transmission of a slow virus. Neurologic manifestations were discussed and a hitherto undescribed feature, severe and sometimes fatal encephalitis occurring most often between ages 5 and 10 years, was reported.

Bell, J.: Hereditary optic atrophy (Leber's disease). In, Treasury of Human Inheritance. London: Cambridge Univ. Press, 2: 325-423, 1933.

Erickson, R. P.: Leber's optic atrophy, a possible example of maternal inheritance. Am. J. Hum. Genet. 24: 348-349, 1972.

Imai, Y. and Moriwaki, D.: A probable case of cytoplasmic inheritance in man: a critique of Leber's disease. J. Genet. Hum. 33: 163-167, 1936.

X

L
I
N
K
E
D

Waardenburg, P. J.: Beitrag zur Vererbung der familiaren Sehnervenatrophie (Leberschen Krankheit). Klin. Monatsbl. Augenheilkd. 73: 619-652, 1924.

Wallace, D. C.: A new manifestation of Leber's disease and a new explanation for the agency responsible for its unusual pattern of inheritance. Brain 93: 121-132, 1970.

Wallace, D. C.: Leber's optic atrophy: a possible example of vertical transmission of a slow virus in man. Aust. Ann. Med. 19: 1-4, 1970.

Wilson, J.: Leber's hereditary optic atrophy: a possible defect of cyanide metabolism. Clin. Sci. 29: 505-515, 1965.

Wilson, J.: Leber's hereditary optic atrophy: some clinical and aetiological considerations. Brain 86: 347-362, 1963.

*30900 LOWE OCULOCEREBRORENAL SYNDROME

The features are hydrophthalmia, cataract, mental retardation, vitamin D resistant rickets, aminoaciduria, and reduced ammonia production by the kidney. Streiff and colleagues (1958) suggested X-linkage because all cases are male and affected brothers have been described. In one case two brothers and a cousin (the mothers were sisters) were affected. By slit lamp Richards and colleagues (1965) found lens opacities in heterozygotes. Aminoaciduria in the mother of a patient, after loading with ornithine, was reported as a heterozygote manifestation by Chutorian and Rowland (1966) and a high incidence of maternal cataract has been noted. McCance, Matheson, Gresham and Elkinton (1960) described a condition which is probably quite distinct but which may also be X-linked, their subjects having been two brothers with unrelated unaffected parents. Features were poor appetite, failure to grow, corneal opacities, partial blindness, nystagmus, mental retardation, intention tremor, hyperchloremic acidosis, very acid urine, defect in urinary production of ammonium ion, death from progressive renal failure, underdeveloped glomeruli, structural abnormalities in the brain, and absence of testes. Svorc et al. (1967) described an affected female child and referred to two others in the literature. Such cases may have a different genetic mechanism than X-linkage or may represent infelicitous Lyonization in heterozygous females. Matsuda et al. (1969) described a Japanese boy with typical clinical features of Lowe syndrome, but the metabolic acidosis was shown to be due to failure not of urinary acidification but of bicarbonate reabsorption. Matsuda et al. (1970) suggested that this is a special type of Lowe syndrome and that it may have autosomal recessive inheritance. He suggested that the cases described by Oetliker and Rossi (1969) were of this type. In Matsuda's study the father showed aminoaciduria after ornithine loading. Mild 'snowflake' lenticular opacities in carrier females were described by Martin and Carson (1967).

Acker, K. J., Roels, H., Beelaerts, W., Pasternack, A. and Valcke, R.: The histologic lesions of the kidney in the oculo-cerebro-renal syndrome of Lowe. Nephron 4: 193-214, 1967.

Auricchio, S., Frischknecht, W. and Shmerling, D.: Primare Tubulopathien. III. Ein Fall von oculo-cerebro-renalem Syndrom (Lowe-Syndrome). Helv. Paediatr. Acta 16: 647-655, 1961.

Chutorian, A. and Rowland, L. P.: Lowe's syndrome. Neurology 16: 115-122, 1966.

Harris, L. S., Gitter, K. A., Galin, M. A. and Plechaty, G. P.: Oculo-cerebro-renal syndrome. Report of a case in a baby girl. Br. J. Ophthalmol. 54: 278-280, 1970.

Lowe, C. U.: Oculo-cerebral-renal syndrome. Maandschr. Kindergeneske. 28: 77-80, 1960.

Lowe, C. U., Terrey, M. and MacLachlan, E. A.: Organic-aciduria, decreased renal ammonia production, hydrophthalmos, and mental retardation. Am. J. Dis. Child. 83: 164-184, 1952.

Matsuda, I., Sugai, M. and Kajii, T.: Ornithine loading test in Lowe's syndrome. J. Pediat. 77: 127-129, 1970.

Matsuda, I., Takeda, T., Sugai, M. and Matsuura, N.: Oculocerebrorenal syndrome. Am. J. Dis. Child. 117: 205-212, 1969.

Martin, V. A. F. and Carson, N. A. J.: Inborn metabolic disorders with associated ocular lesions in Northern Ireland. Trans. Ophthalmol. Soc. U.K. 87: 847-870, 1967.

McCance, R. A., Matheson, W. J., Gresham, G. A. and Elkinton, J. R.: The cerebro-ocular-renal dystrophies: a new variant. Arch. Dis. Child. 35: 240-249, 1960.

Oetliker, O. and Rossi, E.: The influence of extracellular fluid volume on the renal bicarbonate threshold: a study of two children with Lowe's syndrome. Pediatr. Res. 3: 140-148, 1969.

Pallisgaard, G. and Goldschmidt, E.: The oculo-cerebro-renal syndrome of Lowe in four generations of one family. Acta Paediatr. Scand. 60: 146-148, 1971.

Richards, W., Donnell, G. N., Wilson, W. A., Stowens, D. and Perry, T.: The oculo-cerebro-renal syndrome of Lowe. Am. J. Dis. Child. 109: 185-203, 1965.

Streiff, E. B., Straub, W. and Golay, L.: Les manifestations oculaires du syndrome de Lowe. Ophthalmologica 135: 632-639, 1958.

Svorc, J., Masopust, J., Komarkova, A., Macek, M. and Hyanek, J.: Oculocerebrorenal syndrome in a female child. Am. J. Dis. Child. 114: 186-190, 1967.

Wilson, W. A., Richards, W. and Donnell, G. N.: Oculo-cerebral-renal syndrome of Lowe: a review of eight cases noting the genetic inheritance. Arch. Ophthal. 70: 5-11, 1963.

X

L
I
N
K
E
D

Witzleben, C. L., Schoen, E. J., Tu, W. H. and McDonald, L. W.: Progressive morphologic renal changes in the oculo-cerebro-renal syndrome of Lowe. Am. J. Med. 44: 319-324, 1968.

*30910 MACULAR DYSTROPHY

This is dystrophy of the macular area of the fundus oculi and is not to be confused with macular (i.e., spotty) dystrophy of the skin (e.g., 30200). Halbertsma's pedigree is consistent with X-linked inheritance except for an instance of apparent father-to-son transmission in the first generation. Color blindness also was segregating in Halbertsma's family, but analysis in terms of linkage is impossible because in those males with macular dystrophy the retinal disease may have been responsible for the color blindness. Falls (1952) studied a family of X-linked macular dystrophy with affected identical male twins. A cystic maculopathy may be the only finding in X-linked retinoschisis (q.v.).

Falls, H. F.: The role of the sex chromosome in hereditary ocular pathology. Trans. Am. Ophthal. Soc. 50: 421-467, 1952.

Halbertsma, K. T. A.: Ueber einige erbliche familiare Augenerkrankungen. I. Erbliche familiare Entartung des gelben Fleckes (zusammen mit Farbenblindheit). Klin. Monatsbl. Augenheilkd. 80: 794-812, 1928.

30915 MALE PSEUDOHERMAPHRODITISM: DEFICIENCY OF TESTICULAR 17,20-DESMOLASE

This disorder seems to be X-linked. The enzyme deficient in this condition (like 17-ketosteroid reductase; see 26430) is not involved in the formation of hydrocortisone. Hence, the adrenogenital syndrome does not result. They are, however, essential enzymes in the synthesis of C-19 steroids.

Zachmann, M., Hamilton, W., Vollmin, J. A. and Prader, A.: Testicular 17, 20-desmolase deficiency causing male psuedohermaphroditism. Acta Endocrinol. (Suppl.) 155: 65-80, 1971.

Zachmann, M., Vollmin, J. A., Hamilton, W. and Prader, A.: Steroid 17, 20-desmolase deficiency: a new cause of male pseudohermaphroditism. Clin. Endocrinol. 1: 369- , 1972.

30920 MANIC-DEPRESSIVE PSYCHOSIS

Winokur and Tanna (1969) suggested X-linked dominant inheritance. The evidence is weak, at the best. Without reference to specific genetic hypothesis, Mendlewicz et al. (1972) reported that bipolar (manic-depressive) patients with a family history of similar illness responded better to lithium than those without affected relatives.

Mendlewicz, J., Fieve, R. R., Stallone, F. and Fleiss, J. L.: Genetic history as a predictor of lithium response in manic-depressive illness. (Letter) Lancet I: 599-600, 1972.

Mendlewicz, J. and Rainer, J. D.: X-linkage in manic-depressive illness. (Letter) Br. Med. J. 3: 290 only, 1973.

Winokur, G. and Tanna, V. L.: Possible role of X-linked dominant factor in manic depressive disease. Dis. Nerv. Syst. 30: 89-94, 1969.

30925 MASA SYNDROME

The acronym comes from mental retardation, aplasia, shuffling gait and adducted thumbs. Bianchine and Lewis (1974) described a Mexican-American kindred in which 6 males in 4 sibs of three generations plus a female in one of them had this combination. Other genetic explanations are possible especially sex-influenced autosomal dominance. In addition to the features covered by the acronym the patients showed small body size, exaggerated lumbar lordosis, and hyperactive deep tendon reflexes in the lower limbs.

Bianchine, J. W. and Lewis, R. C., Jr.: The MASA syndrome, a new heritable mental retardation syndrome. Clin. Genet. 5: 298-306, 1974.

*30930 MEGALOCORNEA

Affected males show large cornea as an isolated defect. Heterozygous women may show slight increase in corneal diameter (Riddell, 1941). Autosomal dominant inheritance is probably much rarer. Megalocornea occurs at times as part of the Marfan syndrome (inherited as an autosomal dominant). Two presumed homozygous females occurred in this family.

Gronholm, V.: Ueber die Vererbung der Megalokornea nebst einem Beitrag zur Frage des genetischen Zusammenhanges zwischen Megalokornea und Hydrophthalmus. Klin. Monatsbl. Augenheilkd. 67: 1-15, 1921.

Riddell, W. J. B.: Uncomplicated hereditary megalocornea. Ann. Eugen. 11: 102-107, 1941.

*30940 MENKES SYNDROME (KINKY HAIR DISEASE)

In a family of English-Irish descent living in New York, Menkes and colleagues (1962) described an X-linked recessive disorder characterized by early retardation in growth, peculiar hair and focal cerebral and cerebellar degeneration. Severe neurologic impairment began within a month or two of birth and progressed rapidly to decerebration. Five males were affected but the gene could by inference be identified in four generations. The failure to grow brought the affected infants to medical attention at the age of a few weeks and death occurred in the first or second year of life. The hair was stubby and white. Microscopically it showed twisting, varying diameter along the length of the shaft and often fractures of the shaft at regular intervals. Rather extensive biochemical investigations showed elevated plasma glutamic acid as the only consistent abnormality. The anatomic change in the central nervous system was described on the basis of two autopsies. Bray (1965) observed two brothers who died as infants with spastic dementia, seizures and defective hair. Blood and urine amino acids were normal. Whether this is the same disorder as that in Menkes' family is unclear. The condition described by Yoshida et al. (1964) may be the same. French and Sherard (1967) presented evidence that this disorder may represent an abnormality of lipid metabolism. Their 16-month-old patient showed (1) scant, whitish, lackluster, kinky hair which microscopically showed pili torti, monilethrix and trichorrhexis nodosa, (2) retarded growth, (3) micrognathia and highly arched palate, (4) decline in mental development, (5) onset of focal and generalized seizures, (6) spastic quadriparesis with clenched fists, opisthotonos and scissoring. Biochemical studies showed depressed serum tocopherol and normal amino acid content of hair serum and urine. An abnormal autofluorescence is displayed by hair and by Purkinje cells' axons. 'Kinky hair disease' has proved a designation useful in detection of new cases, since the hair change is an easily remembered feature by which physicians can be alerted to the condition (O'Brien, 1968). Changes in the metaphyses of the long bones and tortuosity of cerebral arteries have been described. Danks et al. (1971) suggested that the frequency may be 1 in 40,000 live births in Melbourne and higher than previously thought because some patients may die undiagnosed. Hypothermia and acute illness with septicemia were modes of presentation. Patchy abnormality of systemic arteries with stenosis or obliteration was observed by Danks et al. (1971). They also observed toleridine-blue-metachromasia of fibroblasts. Wesenberg et al. (1971) pointed out that the fetal hair does not show pili torti. Danks et al. (1972) presented evidence of a defect in the intestinal absorption of copper. Copper deficiency in animals leads to connective tissue changes because formation lysine-derived cross-links in elastin and collagen is interfered with, the amine oxidase responsible for the initial modification of lysine being copper-dependent. This may explain the arterial abnormalities. The striking hair changes which are the basis of one designation for the disorder are probably the result of defective formation of disulfide bones in keratin since this process is copper-dependent, and copper deficiency in sheep leads to the formation of wool with defective cross-linking. Changes in the metaphyses of the long bones resemble scurvy. Ascorbic acid oxidase is copper-dependent. The mottled series of mutations in the mouse may be homologous to Menkes syndrome (Hunt, 1974).

Billings, D. M. and Degnan, M.: Kinky hair syndrome. A new case and a review. Am. J. Dis. Child. 121: 447-449, 1971.

Bray, P. F.: Sex-linked neurodegenerative disease associated with monilethrix. Pediatrics 36: 417-420, 1965.

Bucknall, W. E., Haslam, R. H. A. and Holtzman, N. A.: Kinky hair syndrome: response to copper therapy. Pediatrics 52: 653-657, 1973.

Danks, D. M., Campbell, P. E., Stevens, B. J., Mayne, V. and Cartwright, E.: Menkes' kinky hair syndrome. An inherited defect in copper absorption with widespread effects. Pediatrics 50: 188-201, 1972.

Danks, D. M. and Cartwright, E.: Menke's kinky hair disease: further definition of the defect in copper transport. Science 179: 1140-1141, 1973.

Danks, D. M., Cartwright, E., Campbell, P. E. and Mayne, V.: Is Menkes' syndrome a heritable disorder of connective tissue? (Letter) Lancet II: 1089 only, 1971.

Danks, D. M., Stevens, B. J., Campbell, D. E., Gillespie, J. M., Walker-Smith, J., Bloomfield, J. and Turner, B.: Menkes' kinky-hair syndrome. Lancet I: 1100-1102, 1972.

French, J. H. and Sherard, E. S.: Studies of the biochemical basis of kinky hair disease. Pediatr. Res. 1: 206, 1967.

Hunt, D. M.: Primary defect in copper transport underlies mottled mutants in the mouse. Nature 249: 852-854, 1974.

Menkes, J. H., Alter, M., Steigleder, G. K., Weakley, D. R. and Sung, J. H.: A sex-linked recessive disorder with retardation of growth, peculiar hair and focal cerebral and cerebellar degeneration. Pediatrics 29: 764-779, 1962.

O'Brien, J. S.: Los Angeles, Calif.: personal communication, 1968.

Rowe, D. W., McGoodwin, E. B., Martin, G. R., Sussman, M. D., Grahn, D., Faris, B. and Franzblau, C.: A sex-linked defect in the cross-linking of collagen and elastin associated with the mottled locus in mice. J. Exp. Med. 139: 180-192, 1974.

Wesenberg, R. L., Gwinn, J. L. and Barnes, G. R., Jr.: Radiological findings in the kinky-hair syndrome. Radiology 92: 500-506, 1969.

Yoshida, T., Tada, K., Mizuno, T., Wada, Y., Akabane, J., Ogasawara, J., Minagawa, A., Morikawa, T. and Okamura, T.: A sex-linked disorder with mental and physical retardation characterized by cerebrocortical atrophy and increase of glutamic acid in the cerebrospinal fluid. Tohoku J. Med. Sci. 83: 261-269, 1964.

*30950 MENTAL DEFICIENCY (MARTIN-BELL, OR RENPENNING TYPE); X-LINKED MENTAL RETARDATION

Among the numerous types of mental deficiency an hereditary X-linked form exists. An apparently X-linked non-progressive form of mental deficiency without evident somatic malformation and without motor or sensory dysfunction was described by Martin and Bell (1943) and possibly the same mutation was described by Allan and Herndon (1944). Priest and colleagues (1961), as well as others, found more males in state institutions for mental defectives and found that affected sibs were more often male. However, males are probably more likely to be institutionalized. Furthermore, several autosomal conditions show a male preponderance which almost certainly has a basis other than X-linkage in a proportion of cases. Another kindred with convincingly X-linked mental retardation was reported by Renpenning and his colleagues (1962). Lubs (1969) found a marker X chromosome consisting of a secondary constriction near the end of the long arm giving the appearance of large satellites. The anomalous chromosome was not preferentially

Lyonized as occurs with an isochromosome X for example. The hemizygous males had mental retardation. The author thought that either the anomalous region itself or a closely linked recessive gene might account for the X-linked inheritance of mental deficiency in this family. Turner et al. (1970) emphasized the lack of physical abnormality in this disorder. Opitz (1972) suggests that this is the most frequent form of familial mental retardation in males. Among severely retarded males there is a high frequency of seizures. Performance IQ tends to be higher than verbal IQ. The intelligence of heterozygotes may be reduced as a group but this is not certain. In one relatively large kindred Fried and Sanger (1973) found evidence that 'mental retardation with or without hydrocephalus' is within measurable distance of Xg. The most likely recombination fraction was 0.11. See MASA syndrome (30925) for a mental retardation syndrome which may be X-linked. Gerrard and Renpenning (1974) gave an interesting account of the history of this disorder. Repenning was a medical student at the time of his story.

Allan, W. and Herndon, C. N.: Retinitis pigmentosa and apparently sex-linked idiocy in a single sibship. J. Hered. 35: 41-43, 1944.

Allan, W., Herndon, C. N. and Dudley, F. C.: Some examples of the inheritance of mental deficiency: apparently sex-linked idiocy and microcephaly. Am. J. Ment. Defic. 48: 325-334, 1944.

Escalante, J. A., Grunspun, H. and Frota-Pessoa, O.: Severe sex-linked mental retardation. J. Genet. Hum. 19: 137-140, 1971.

Fried, K. and Sanger, R.: Possible linkage between Xg and the locus for a gene causing mental retardation with or without hydrocephalus. J. Med. Genet. 10: 17-18, 1973.

Gerrard, J. W. and Renpenning, H. J.: Sex-linked mental retardation. (Letter) Lancet I: 1346 only, 1974.

Lehrke, R. G.: X-linked Mental Retardation and Verbal Disability. Birth Defects: Orig. Art. Ser. 10 (no. 1): 1-100, 1974.

Losowski, M. S.: Hereditary mental defect showing the pattern of sex influence. J. Ment. Defic. Res. 5: 60-62, 1961.

Lubs, H. A.: A marker X chromosome. Am. J. Hum. Genet. 21: 231-244, 1969.

Martin, J. P. and Bell, J.: A pedigree of mental defect showing sex-linkage. J. Neurol. Psychiatry 6: 154-157, 1943.

Neuhauser, G. and Zerbin-Rudin, E.: Oligophrenie mit wahrscheinlich geschlechtsgebunden-rezessiver Vererbung. Deutsch. Med. Wschr. 94: 2519-2521, 1969.

Opitz, J. M., Segal, A. T., Klove, H., Mathews, C. and Lehrke, R. L.: X-linked mental retardation. Study of a large kindred with 20 affected members. (Abstract) J. Pediatr. 67: 713-714, 1965.

Priest, J. H., Thuline, H. C., Laveck, G. D. and Jarvis, D. B.: An approach to genetic factors in mental retardation. Studies of families containing at least two siblings admitted to a state institution for the retarded. Am. J. Ment. Defic. 66: 42-50, 1961.

Renpenning, H., Gerrard, J. W., Zaleski, W. A. and Tabata, T.: Familial sex-linked mental retardation. Canad. Med. Assoc. J. 87: 954-956, 1962.

Rosanoff, A. J.: Sex-linked inheritance in mental deficiency. Am. J. Psychiatry 11: 289-297, 1931.

Snyder, R. D. and Robinson, A.: Recessive sex-linked mental retardation in the absence of other recognizable abnormalities. Report of a family. Clin. Pediatr. 8: 669-674, 1969.

Turner, G., Engisch, B., Lindsay, D. G. and Turner, B.: X-linked mental retardation without physical abnormality (Renpenning's syndrome) in sibs in an institution. J. Med. Genet. 9: 324-330, 1972.

Turner, G., Turner, B. and Collins, E.: Renpenning's syndrome — X-linked retardation. Lancet II: 365-366, 1970.

Wortis, H., Pollack, M. and Wortis, J.: Families with two or more mentally retarded or mentally disturbed siblings: the preponderance of males. Am. J. Ment. Defic. 70: 745-752, 1966.

30960 MENTAL RETARDATION AND MUSCULAR ATROPHY

Allan, Herndon and Dudley (1943-44) described a phenomenal family in which many affected males had, in addition to mental retardation, muscular weakness first noted at about six months by inability to hold up the head (giving the family's designation of 'limber-neck'). Walking was delayed or never achieved. Speech was almost unintelligible. Muscular atrophy and weakness was generalized. Contractures of the hamstring resulted in peculiar stance.

Allan, W., Herndon, C. N. and Dudley, F. C.: Some examples of the inheritance of mental deficiency: apparently sex-linked idiocy and microcephaly. Am. J. Ment. Defic. 48: 325-334, 1943-44.

*30963 METACARPAL 4-5 FUSION

Orel (1928) and Holmes et al. (1972) described fusion of the fourth and fifth metacarpals as an X-linked recessive trait. In the family of the latter study, close linkage of the locus with colorblindness could be excluded. Other reports are more consistent with autosomal dominant inheritance (e.g., Habighorst and Albers, 1965). The families of Lerch (1948) and of Habighorst and Albers (1965) suggested autosomal dominant inheritance because of affected females and male-to-male transmission.

Habighorst, L. V. and Albers, P.: Familiare synostosis metacarpi IV and V. Z. Orthop. 100: 521-525, 1965.

Holmes, L. B., Wolf, E. and Miettinen, O. S.: Metacarpal 4-5 fusion with X-linked recessive inheritance. Am. J. Hum. Genet. 24: 562-568, 1972.

Orel, H.: Kleine Beitrage zur Vererbungswissenschaft. Synostosis metacarpi quarti et quinti. Z. Anat. 14: 244-252, 1928.

30965 METHYLMANDELICACIDURIA

Two brothers were studied by Rennert et al. (1971) and two older male sibs thought to have the same condition had died before age 7 years. Symptoms began with ataxia and seizures in the second year of life. Protein restriction caused remission. Protein loading and specifically phenylalanine loading caused exacerbations.

Rennert, O., Julius, R., Aylsworth, A., Williams, C. and Greer, M.: A new disorder of phenylalanine metabolism associated with ataxia, convulsions and retardation: methylmalonic aciduria. Society of Pediat. Res. 1971.

In Stephens' cases white opacification of the cornea (possibly this should be termed sclerocornea) and blindness were present. Roberts' cases also had corneal change. Mental deficiency was present in some in Roberts' family, but intelligence was normal in at least two of six cases of microphthalmia examined. No mental defect was present except in microphthalmia cases. On the other hand, Stephens' cases were of university level of intelligence. Sjogren and Larsson (1949) described microphthalmia and oligophrenia behaving as an autosomal recessive syndrome.

30970 MICROPHTHALMIA

Anophthalmia and microphthalmia are terms used interchangeably. The family reported by Hoefnagel, Keenan, and Allen (1963) was probably one of X-linked microphthalmia. Most cases of true anophthalmos have been recessive (q.v.). Pseudoglioma, microphthalmia and Norrie disease are confused in the literature (Warburg, 1966). The affected persons in Roberts' pedigree (originally reported by Ash in 1922) were clearly instances of Norrie disease. In only about half of the cases was the eye microphthalmic or more precisely phthisical. Histologic study of the eye in one mentally retarded blind boy from this family (Whitnall and Norman, 1940) showed changes like those observed by Warburg in Norrie disease (q.v.). Stephens' patients are more difficult to evaluate, mainly because they were rather old at the time of first examination and information is limited to the facts that the eyes were small and corneas cloudy. Warburg (1966) thinks these also may have been instances of Norrie disease. Congenital cataract was also present in some of the patients in a family reported by Capella et al. (1963). Cataracts and microphthalmia was dominant (see 15685) in a second family they reported. They think this was an instance of pseudoglioma or of retinal dysplasia.

Capella, J. A., Kaufman, H. E., Lill, F. J. and Cooper, G.: Hereditary cataracts and microphthalmia. Am. J. Ophthalmol. 56: 454-458, 1963.

Hoefnagel, D., Keenan, M. E. and Allen, F. H.: Heredofamilial bilateral anophthalmia. Arch. Ophthalmol. 69: 760-764, 1963.

Roberts, J. A. F.: Sex-linked microphthalmia sometimes associated with mental defect. Br. Med. J. 2: 1213-1216, 1937. (In, Waardenburg, P. J., Franceschetti, A. and Klein, D. (eds.): Genetics and Ophthalmology. Springfield, Ill.: Charles C Thomas, 2: 768-770, 1961.

Sjogren, T. and Larsson, T.: Microphthalmos and anophthalmos with or without coincident oligophrenia. Acta Psychiat. Neurol. 56 (suppl.): 1-103, 1949.

Stephens, F. E.: A case of sex-linked microphthalmia. J. Hered. 38: 307-310, 1947.

Warburg, M.: Copenhagen, Denmark: personal communication, 1966.

Whitnall, S. E. and Norman, R. M.: Microphthalmia and visual pathways, case associated with blindness and imbecility, and sex-linked. Br. J. Ophthalmol. 24: 229-244, 1940.

*30980 MICROPHTHALMIA OR ANOPHTHALMOS, WITH ASSOCIATED ANOMALIES

The eye anomaly was unilateral in some of the affected persons in Lenz' remarkable pedigree. Narrow shoulders, double thumbs, other skeletal anomalies, and dental, urogenital and cardiovascular malformations were observed. The mother of the proband, a 13-year-old boy born blind, had a deformity of the fifth finger, suggesting mild expression. Goldberg and McKusick (1971) reported a kindred in which four males in three sibships connected through females had kyphoscoliosis, microphthalmos, mental retardation and microcephaly. The ears were simple and anteverted. There were, however, no instances of male-to-male transmission. Herrmann and Opitz (1969) described a single affected male age 11 years. Features were physical and mental retardation, hypospadias and bilateral cryptorchidism, renal dysgenesis and hydroureters, left microphthalmos, agenesis of upper lateral incisors and irregular lower incisors, long cylindrical thorax with sloping shoulders and exaggerated lumbar lordosis, and cutaneous clubbing of the right 3rd and 4th toes. The mother was short of stature and had a small head circumference. Hoefnagel et al. (1963) observed 4 affected males in 3 sibships. The pedigree with 4 affected males reported by Goldberg and McKusick (1971) is probably the same disorder. Some of the X-linked cataract families (see 30220) have shown associated dental and digital anomalies which raise the question of a relationship.

Goldberg, M. F. and McKusick, V. A.: X-linked colobomatous microphthalmos and other congenital anomalies. A disorder resembling Lenz's dysmorphogenetic syndrome. Am. J. Ophthalmol. 71: 1128-1133, 1971.

Herrmann, J. and Opitz, J. M.: The Lenz microphthalmia syndrome. The Clinical Delineation of Birth Defects. II. Malformation Syndromes. New York: National Foundation, 1969. Pp. 138-143. 1972.

X

L
I
N
K
E
D

Lenz, W.: Recessiv-geschlechtsgebundene Mikrophthalmie mit multiplen Missbildungen. Ztschr. Kinderheilk. 77: 384-390, 1955.

*30990 MUCOPOLYSACCHARIDOSIS TYPE II (HUNTER SYNDROME)

The sex-linked mucopolysaccharidosis differs from the autosomal type (MPS I) in being on the average less severe and in not showing clouding of the cornea. Features are dysostosis with dwarfism, grotesque facies, hepatosplenomegaly from mucopolysaccharide deposits, cardiovascular disorders from mucopolysaccharide deposits in the intima, mental retardation, deafness, excretion of large amounts of chondroitin sulfate B and heparitin sulfate in the urine. Danes and Bearn (1965) find that fibroblasts from patients with this disorder show metachromatic cytoplasmic inclusions and that about half the fibroblasts of heterozygotes show such inclusions. Berg et al. (1968) concluded that the Hunter locus and the Xm locus are within measurable distance of each other, the best estimate of the recombination fraction being 0.09. Two forms of MPS II are distinguishable clinically. A severe form (called MPS II A in my system) has progressive mental retardation and death before age 15 years in most cases. A mild form (called MPS II B) is compatible with survival to adulthood and reproduction is known to have occurred in one case (DiFerrante and Nichols, 1972). Erickson et al. (1972) claims that pebbly skin lesions in the scapula area occur only in the severe form. Furthermore, they can be distinguished by the serum beta-galactosidase which is elevated in the severe form and reduced in the mild form. The same corrective factor is effective in both and the disorders are presumably allelic.

Bach, G., Eisenberg, F., Jr., Cantz, M. and Neufeld, E. F.: The defect in the Hunter syndrome: deficiency of solfoiduronate sulfatase. Proc. Nat. Acad. Sci., in press, 1973.

Berg, K., Danes, B. S. and Bearn, A. G.: The linkage relation of the loci for the Xm serum system and the X-linked form of Hurler's syndrome (Hunter's syndrome). Am. J. Hum. Genet. 20: 398-401, 1968.

Booth, C. W. and Nadler, H. L.: Demonstration of the heterozygous state in Hunter's syndrome. Pediatrics 53: 396-399, 1974.

Cantz, M., Chrambach, A. and Neufeld, E. F.: Characterization of the factor deficient in the Hunter syndrome by polyacrylamide gel electrophoresis. Biochem. Biophys. Res. Commun. 39: 936-942, 1970.

Danes, B. S. and Bearn, A. G.: Hurler's syndrome: a genetic study of clones in cell culture with particular reference to the Lyon hypothesis. J. Exp. Med. 126: 509-522, 1967.

Danes, B. S. and Bearn, A. G.: Hurler's syndrome: demonstration of an inherited disorder of connective tissue in cell culture. Science 149: 987-989, 1965.

DiFerrante, N. and Nichols, B. L.: A case of the Hunter syndrome with progeny. Johns Hopkins Med. J. 130: 325-328, 1972.

Erickson, R., Sandman, R., Neufeld, E. and Epstein, C.: Biochemical differentiation of two forms of mucopolysaccharidosis II (Hunter's disease). (Abstract) Am. J. Hum. Genet. 24: 26A only, 1972.

Gerich, J. E.: Hunter's syndrome: beta-galactosidase deficiency in skin. New Eng. J. Med. 280: 799-802, 1969.

McKusick, V. A.: Heritable Disorders of Connective Tissue. St. Louis: C. V. Mosby Co., 1972 (4th Ed.).

Ockermann, P. A. and Kohlin, P.: Glycosidases in skin and plasma in Hunter's syndrome. Abnormality of a beta-galactosidase in skin. Acta Paediatr. Scand. 57: 281-284, 1968.

Van Pelt, J. F.: Gargoylism. Thesis, Nijmegen, 1960.

30995 MUSCULAR DYSTROPHY, HEMIZYGOUS LETHAL TYPE

Becker (1972) suggested that the form of muscular dystrophy limited to females as reported by Henson et al. (1967), may be X-linked dominant lethal in hemizygous males. Eight females in four sibships in two generations of the family were affected. Henson et al. (1967) favored autosomal dominant inheritance with female influence (for which reason this entity is listed as 16060 in the dominant catalog). Heyck and Lamdahn (1969) described what appears to be the same myopathy in two sisters, their mother and their grandmother. This is a slowly progressive limb-girdle form of muscular dystrophy.

Becker, P. E.: Neues zur Genetik und Klassifikation der Muskeldystrophien. Humangenetik 17: 1-22, 1972.

Henson, T. E., Muller, J. and DeMyer, W. E.: Hereditary myopathy limited to females. Arch. Neurol. 17: 238-247, 1967.

Heyck, H. and Lamdahn, G.: Die progressiv-dystrophien Myopathien. Berlin — Heidelberg — New York: Springer, 1969.

31000 MUSCULAR DYSTROPHY, MABRY TYPE

Mabry et al. (1965) described a kindred with 9 males affected by a late-onset form of muscular dystrophy. These authors thought it to be different from the types of Duchenne, Becker and Dreifuss. They suggested that it differed from the Becker type, which it resembled most closely, by earlier onset (about puberty) and some histological features.

Mabry, C. C., Roeckel, I. E., Munich, R. L. and Robertson, D.: X-linked pseudohypertrophic muscular dystrophy with a late onset and slow progression. New Eng. J. Med. 273: 1062-1070, 1965.

*31010 MUSCULAR DYSTROPHY, PROGRESSIVE, TARDIVE TYPE OF BECKER

The onset is often in the 20's and 30's and survival to a relatively advanced age is frequent. Several affected males in Becker's large kindred had produced children and the resulting pedigree pattern was consistent with X-linked inheritance. Others have described such families. Allelism with the Duchenne type is possible. Linkage studies might establish non-allelism as in the case of hemophilias A and B. There may be more than one form of X-linked late form of muscular dystrophy. Emery (1962) has restudied the family of Dreifuss and Hogan (1961) and found features different from those in the families reported by Becker. A review of reports was given by Zellweger and Hanson (1967), who also reported a family with many males affected. Emery et al. (1969) presented evidence suggesting linkage of the Becker muscular dystrophy locus and the deutan color-blindness locus. This should be checked in other families, using also G6PD as a marker. That Duchenne and Becker types are at different loci would be indicated by such a finding, since the Duchenne type is not linked to color-blindness. In further studies Emery (1974) found evidence of even closer linkage of Becker muscular dystrophy to color-blindness than previously suspected.

Becker, P. E.: Eine neue X-chromosomale Muskeldystrophie. Acta Psychiatr. Neurol. Scand. 193: 427 Only, 1955.

Becker, P. E.: Neue Ergebnisse der Genetik der Muskeldystrophien. Acta Genet. Statist. Med. 7: 303-310, 1957.

Becker, P. E.: Two new families of benign sex-linked recessive muscular dystrophy. Rev. Can. Biol. 21: 551-566, 1962.

Blyth, H. M. and Pugh, R. J.: Muscular dystrophy in childhood: the genetical aspect: a field study in the Leeds region of clinical types and their inheritance. Ann. Hum. Genet. 23: 127-163, 1959.

Dreifuss, F. E. and Hogan, G. R.: Survival in X-chromosomal muscular dystrophy. Neurology 11: 734-737, 1961.

Emery, A. E. H.: Baltimore, Md.: personal communication, 1962.

Emery, A. E. H., Clack, E. R., Simon, S. and Taylor, J. L.: Detection of carriers of benign X-linked muscular dystrophy. Br. Med. J. 4: 522-523, 1967.

Emery, A. E. H., Smith, C. A. B. and Sanger, R.: The linkage relations of the loci for benign (Becker type) X-borne muscular dystrophy, colour blindness and the Xg blood groups. Ann. Hum. Genet. 32: 261-269, 1969.

Emery, A. E. H.: Edinburgh, personal communication, 1974.

Moser, H.: Biochemische, histologische und klinische Befunde bei einer vierjahrigen Konduktorin der gutartigen X-chromosomalen Muskeldystrophie. Humangenetik 11: 328-335, 1971.

Shaw, R. F. and Dreifuss, F. E.: Mild and severe forms of X-linked muscular dystrophy. Arch. Neurol. 20: 451-460, 1969.

Zellweger, H. and Hanson, J. W.: Slowly progressive X-linked recessive muscular dystrophy (type IIIB). Report of cases and review of the literature. Arch. Intern. Med. 120: 525-535, 1967.

*31020 MUSCULAR DYSTROPHY, PSEUDOHYPERTROPHIC PROGRESSIVE, DUCHENNE TYPE

Usually the onset is before age six and the victim is chair-ridden by age 12 and dead by age 20. The myocardium is affected. An autosomal recessive form of muscular dystrophy can closely simulate the sex-linked form but the myocardium is probably not affected.

Chung, Morton, and Peters (1960), among others, have concluded that a minority of heterozygous female carriers have an increase in serum aldolase and even fewer have physical disability and creatinuria. Leyburn, Thomson and Walton (1961), on the other hand, could demonstrate no abnormality of creatine and creatinine excretion or of serum levels of aldolase and transaminases in carrier females. Serum phosphocreatine kinase (creatine phosphokinase) is elevated beyond the normal range in many female carriers, according to Schapira and colleagues (1960) and Aebi and colleagues (1961-62). Miyoshi et al. (1968) found four electrophoretically separable myoglobin subfractions in normal muscle and found in Duchenne muscular dystrophy but not other types a striking change in the quantities of the types. Decreased body potassium concentrations were reported by Blahd et al. (1967) in patients with muscular dystrophy and particularly interestingly in relatives who may have been heterozygotes. Both the Duchenne and the limb-girdle types of muscular dystrophy were represented in their series. Mental retardation of mild degree is a pleiotropic effect of the Duchenne gene, (Zellweger and Niedermeyer, 1965), although the mechanism is unknown. Roy and Dubowitz (1970) suggested that electronmicroscopy may be useful in identifying carriers. Gallup and Dubowitz (1973) reviewed evidence that muscular dystrophy is fundamentally a neural not a myal disorder. Matheson and Howland (1974) described erythrocyte deformation in patients with muscular dystrophy the proportion of distorted cells being greatest in the Duchenne type. Furthermore, carrier females showed an abnormally hight proportion of distorted cells.

Aebi, U., Richterich, R., Stillhart, H., Colombo, J. P. and Rossi, E.: Progressive muscular dystrophy. II. Biochemical identification of the carrier state in the recessive sex-linked juvenile (Duchenne) type by serum creatine-phosphokinase determinations. Enzym. Biol. Clin. 1: 61-74: Helv. Paediatr. Acta 16: 543-564, 1961-62.

Blahd, W. H., Lederer, M. and Cassen, B.: The significance of decreased body potassium concentrations in patients with muscular dystrophy and nondystrophic relatives. N. Engl. J. Med. 276: 1349-1352, 1967.

Bundey, S. E.: Extreme muscle hypertrophy in Duchenne muscular dystrophy. In, Bergsma, D. (ed.):

X

L
I
N
K
E
D

Chung, C. S., Morton, N. E. and Peters, H. A.: Serum enzymes and genetic carriers in muscular dystrophy. Am. J. Hum. Genet. 12: 52-66, 1960.

Gallup, B. and Dubowitz, V.: Failure of dystrophic neurones to support functional regeneration of normal or dystrophic muscles in culture. Nature 243: 237-239, 1973.

Gardner-Medwin, D.: Mutation rate in the Duchenne type of muscular dystrophy. J. Med. Genet. 7: 334-337, 1970.

Leyburn, P., Thomson, W. H. S. and Walton, J. N.: An investigation of the carrier state in the Duchenne type muscular dystrophy. Ann. Hum. Genet. 25: 41-49, 1961.

Matheson, D. W. and Howland, J. L.: Erythrocyte deformation in human muscular dystrophy. Science 184: 165-166, 1974.

Miyoshi, K., Saijo, K., Kuryu, Y., Oshima, Y., Nakano, M. and Kawai, H.: Myoglobin subfractions: abnormality in Duchenne type of progressive muscular dystrophy. Science 159: 736-737, 1968.

Morton, N. E. and Chung, C. S.: Formal genetics of muscular dystrophy. Am. J. Hum. Genet. 11: 360-379, 1959.

Prosser, E. J., Murphy, E. G. and Thompson, M. W.: Intelligence and the gene for Duchenne muscular dystrophy. Arch. Dis. Child. 44: 221-230, 1969.

Rosman, N. P. and Kakulas, B. A.: Mental deficiency associated with muscular dystrophy-a neurological study. Brain 89: 769-788, 1966.

Rosman, N. P.: The cerebral defect and myopathy in Duchenne muscular dystrophy. A comparative clinicopathological study. Neurology 20: 329-335, 1970.

Roy, S. and Dubowitz, V.: Carrier detection in Duchenne muscular dystrophy. A comparative study of electron microscopy, light microscopy, and serum enzymes. J. Neurol. Sci. 11: 65-79, 1970.

Schapira, F., Dreyfus, J.-C., Schapira, G. and Demos, J.: Etude de l'aldolase et de la creatine kinase du serum chez les meres de myopathies. Rev. Fr. Etud. Clin. Biol. 5: 990-994, 1960.

Skyring, A. P. and McKusick, V. A.: Clinical, genetic and electrocardiographic studies of childhood muscular dystrophy. Am. J. Med. Sci. 242: 534-547, 1961.

Zellweger, H. and Niedermeyer, E.: Central nervous system manifestations in childhood muscular dystrophy (CMD) I. Ann. Paediatr. 205: 25-42, 1965.

*31030 MUSCULAR DYSTROPHY, TARDIVE TYPE OF DREIFUSS, WITH CONTRACTURES

Dreifuss and Hogan (1961) and Emery and Dreifuss (1966) studied a Virginian kindred in which there were eight affected males in three generations in typical X-linked pedigree pattern. Onset of muscle weakness was noted around the age of four or five, first affecting the lower extremities with a tendency to walk on the toes. By the early teens waddling gait with increased lumbar lordosis was marked and weakness of the shoulder girdle musculature appeared later. Slow progression with continued gainful employment is the rule. Flexion deformities of the elbows dating from early childhood, mild pectus excavatum, signs of cardiac involvement and absence of muscle pseudohypertrophy, involvement of the forearm muscles and mental retardation distinguished the Dreifuss form from the Becker form. Pearson, Kar, Peter and Munsat (1965) found a difference of muscle LDH electrophoretic pattern in this type as compared with the Duchenne type. Becker (1972) republished illustrations of typical cases reported by Cestan and Lejonne (1902).

Becker, P. E.: Neues zur Genetik und Klassifikation der Muskeldystrophien. Humangenetik 17: 1-22, 1972.

Cestan, R. and LeJonne, N. I.: Une myopathie avec retractions familiales. Nous. Iconogr. Salpetriere 15: 38-52, 1902.

Dreifuss, F. E. and Hogan, G. R.: Survival in X-chromosomal muscular dystrophy. Neurology 11: 734-737, 1961.

Emery, A. E. H. and Dreifuss, F. E.: Unusual type of benign X-linked muscular dystrophy. J. Neurol. Neurosurg. Psychiatry 29: 338-342, 1966.

Pearson, C. M., Kar, N. C., Peter, J. B. and Munsat, T. L.: Muscle lactate dehydrogenase patterns in two types of X-linked muscular dystrophy. Am. J. Med. 39: 91-97, 1965.

Rotthauwe, H. W., and Beyer, H.: Neuer Typ einer recessiv X-chromosomal verebten Muskeldystrophie: scapulo-humero-distale Muskeldystrophie mit fruhzeitigen Kontrakuren und Herzrhythmusstorungen. Humangenetik 16: 181-200, 1972.

Thomas, P. K., Calne, D. B. and Elliott, C. F.: X-linked scapuloperoneal syndrome. J. Neurol. Neurosurg. Psychiatry 35: 208-215, 1972.

*31040 MYOPATHY, CENTRONUCLEAR (MYOTUBULAR MYOPATHY)

Van Wijngaarden et al. (1969) described this disorder in five affected males in four sibships connected through females who in two instances showed partial manifestations on muscle biopsy. The patients were born as floppy infants and had serious respiratory problems early in life, extraocular, facial and neck muscles were always affected. Bradley et al. (1970) described affected brothers. See (25520) for evidence of an autosomal

X
L
I
N
K
E
D

recessive form. X-linked inheritance is supported by the description of affected brothers by Meyers et al. (1973). Both were floppy infants and died at 7 and 18 months of age. The mother showed no abnormality or muscle biopsy or enzyme assay. One of the brothers was previously reported by Engel et al. (1968).

Bradley, W. G., Price, D. L. and Watanabe, C. K.: Familial centronuclear myopathy. J. Neurol. Neurosurg. Psychiatry 33: 687-693, 1970.

Engel, W. K., Gold, G. N. and Karpati, B.: Type I fiber hypotrophy and central nuclei. Arch. Neurol. 18: 435-444, 1968.

Meyers, K. R., Golomb, H. M. and Hansen, J. L.: Familial congential neuromuscular disease with 'myotubes.' Clin. Genet. 5: 327-337, 1974.

Van Wijngaarden, G. K., Fleury, P., Bethlem, J. and Meijer, A. E. F. H.: Familial 'myotubular' myopathy. Neurology 19: 901-908, 1969.

31045 MYOPATHY, QUADRICEPS

Espir and Matthews (1973) described two brothers with quadriceps myopathy. All three daughters of one of them had mild involvement. They found reports of no precisely similar cases. Clinically the thighs showed islands of hypertrophy in wasted quadriceps muscles. Severe aching in the thigh muscles was a feature which preceded the development of weakness by many years. Knee jerks were absent. Wasting of the hand muscles was present in one of the men. In late stages prominent areas of hypertrophy projecting from patches of atrophy gave the quadriceps a strikingly unusual appearance. Onset was in adulthood with benign course and late involvement of pelvic girdle and hand muscles.

Boddie, H. G. and Stewart-Wynne, E. G.: Quadriceps myopathy — entity or syndrome? Arch. Neurol. 31: 60-62, 1974.

Espir, M. L. E. and Matthews, W. B.: Hereditary quadriceps myopathy. J. Neurol. Neurosurg. Psychiatry 36: 1041-1045, 1973.

*31050 NIGHT BLINDNESS, CONGENITAL STATIONARY, WITH MYOPIA

Night blindness (nyctalopia) is a symptom of several chorioretinal degenerations. The distinctive feature of the mutation listed here is the stationary nature of the night blindness. There is an autosomal dominant variety reported in many families of which the most famous is that descendant from Jean Nougaret, born in Provence in 1637, and studied by Cunier (1838), Nettleship (1909, 1912) and others. (An abnormal segregation ratio with fewer affected persons than anticipated has been suggested in this family, but other large pedigrees do not show this.) The X-linked form is distinguished from the autosomal form by the association of myopia. Morton (1893) described a family with X-linked myopia and night blindness. Fraser and Friedmann (1967) described a family from the same area near Cardiff, Wales.

Myopia has not been listed as a separate X-linked mutation because it is not completely certain that it indeed occurs with this mode of inheritance and independent of night blindness or ophthalmoplegia. Worth (1906) reported four families with myopia which apparently was X-linked. At Nettleship's suggestion he looked for associated night blindness and found it in the affected members of only one of the families. In Oswald's family with myopia transmitted in a pattern otherwise consistent with X-linked inheritance apparent male-to-male transmission occurred in the first generation. Francois and de Rouck (1965) described two families with 'degenerative' myopia transmitted as an X-linked recessive. In one of the families congenital hemeralopia was associated.

Cunier, F.: Observations curieuse d'une achromatopsie hereditaire depuis 5 generations. Ann. Ocul. 1: 488-489, 1838.

Francois, J. and De Rouck, A.: Sex-linked myopic chorioretinal heredodegeneration. Am. J. Ophthalmol. 60: 670-678, 1965.

Fraser, G. R. and Friedmann, A. I.: The Causes of Blindness in Childhood. A Study of 776 Children with Severe Visual Handicaps. Baltimore: Johns Hopkins Press, 1967. P. 72.

Kleiner, W.: Uber den grossen schweizerischen Stammbaum, in dem mit Kurzsichtigkeit kombinierte Nachtblindheit sich forterbt. Arch. Rass.-u. Ges. Biol. 15: 1-17, 1923.

Morton, A. S.: Two cases of hereditary congenital night-blindness without visible fundus change. Trans. Opthalmol. Soc. U.K. 13: 147-150, 1893.

Nettleship, E.: On some hereditary diseases of the eye (Bowman lecture). Retinitis pigmentosa, night blindness with myopia, ocular albinism. Trans. Ophthalmol. Soc. U.K. 29: 57-148, 1909. A pedigree of congenital night blindness with myopia. Trans. Ophthalmol. Soc. U.K. 32: 21-45, 1912.

White, T.: Linkage and crossing-over in the human sex chromosomes. J. Genet. 40: 403-437, 1940.

Worth, C.: Hereditary influence in myopia. Trans. Ophthalmol. Soc. U.K. 26: 141-144, 1906.

*31060 NORRIE DISEASE (ATROPHIA BULBORUM HEREDITARIA: PSEUDOGLIOMA)

Warburg (1961) reported seven cases of a hereditary degenerative disease in seven generations of a Danish family. The proband was a 12-month-old boy. He was normal except for lens opacities found at initial examination at three months of age. Both irises were atrophic. The fundus was filled with a proliferating retrolental yellowish mass. At eight months of age the left eye was enucleated on suspicion of retinoblastoma. Histological examination showed a hemorrhagic necrotic mass in the posterior chamber surrounded by undifferentiated glial tissue. Histologic diagnosis was pseudotumor of the retina, retinal hyperplasia, hyperplasia of retinal, ciliary, and iris pigment epithelium, hypoplasia and necrosis of the inner layer of the

X

L
I
N
K
E
D

retina, cataract, phthisis bulbi. Six relatives had a similar ocular disease. In five of these seven cases deafness developed in later years, and in four of the seven cases the mental capacity was low. Warburg found 48 similar cases in nine families described in the literature under different categories which she believes belong to this disease.

Warburg (1963) presented two new families with 11 patients suffering from this disease. Patients examined varied from 2 months to 58 years of age. At earliest examination pseudoglioma, synechiae and atrophy of the iris were observed. Blindness was found during infants' first month of life. By eight months cataract was observed and at 10 years the eyes were atrophic with band-shaped corneal degeneration and dense cataract. By the age of 50 years the atrophy had advanced to opaque white cornea, obliterated anterior chamber, atrophic white iris, and cataractous lens. Though some afflicted had normal intelligence, many were mentally deficient. Five of nine in one family were hard of hearing and two of these five had diabetes. The mode of inheritance in both families was X-chromosomal recessive.

Whitnall and Norman (1940) reported the neuropathology of a case. The optic nerves and lateral geniculate bodies were small. Warburg, Hauge and Sanger (1965) demonstrated no linkage with the Xg blood groups. Families with Norrie disease have often been reported as pseudoglioma or as microphthalmia in the literature. The mental retardation is a deterioriation inasmuch as the affected infants seem to be normal for the first 1-2 years. In 1959 Taylor et al. reported a Greek family with this condition living in Episkopi in Cyprus. The condition was popularly known as Episkopi blindness. The published pedigree showed 16 affected males in 5 generations. All affected males were retarded. Mistakenly Duke-Elder in his system of ophthalmology classified the disorder as band-shaped keratopathy.

In the family reported by Forssman, 'pseudoglioma' was combined with mental deficiency present from infancy and apparently of progressive nature. Forssman's patients (1960) were first described by Dahlberg-Parrow (1956). Three of the blind boys were re-examined by Warburg (1966) who concluded that the histories and ocular findings were typical of Norrie disease. In the extensive pedigree from a Canadian Indian group reported by Wilson (1949), histologic changes may have been like those of Norrie disease. Zimmerman (1964) found retinal dysplasia in one of these cases.

Clarke (1898) described possible homozygous affected females. A man blind from probable bilateral 'pseudoglioma' married his first cousin. Of their six children, 2 girls and 1 boy had unilateral or bilateral 'pseudoglioma.' As discussed under MICROPHTHALMIA (q.v.), 'pseudoglioma,' microphthalmos and Norrie disease are confused in the literature.

Pseudoglioma is a non-specific term for any condition more or less mimicking retinoblastoma. Thus pseudoglioma can have as diverse causes as inflammation, hemorrhage, trauma, neoplasia or congenital malformation. Many of the causes lead only to unilateral involvement. Norrie disease is a form of bilateral and congenital pseudoglioma. It should be evident from the above discussion that pseudoglioma is merely any condition of the eye liable to be mistaken for true glioma and therefore not an acceptable diagnosis either clinically or pathologically (Duke-Elder, 1958).

Anderson, S. R. and Warburg, M.: Norrie's disease. Arch. Ophthalmol. 66: 614-618, 1961.

Clarke, E.: 'Pseudo-glioma' in both eyes. Trans. Ophthalmol. Soc. U.K. 18: 136-138, 1898.

Dahlberg-Parrow, R.: Congenital sex-linked pseudoglioma and grave mental deficiency. Acta Ophthalmol. 34: 250-254, 1956.

Duke-Elder, J. R.: Pseudoglioma in children: aspects of clinical and pathological diagnosis. Sth. Med. J. 51: 754-759, 1958.

Forssman, H.: Mental deficiency and pseudoglioma, a syndrome inherited as an X-linked recessive. Am. J. Ment. Defic. 64: 984-987, 1960.

Holmes, L. B.: Norrie's disease — an X-linked syndrome of retinal malformation, mental retardation and deafness. N. Engl. J. Med. 284: 367-368, 1971.

Nance, W. E., Hara, S., Hansen, A., Elliott, J., Lewis, M. and Chown, B.: Genetic linkage studies in a Negro kindred with Norrie's disease. Am. J. Hum. Genet. 21: 423-429, 1969.

Taylor, P. J., Coates, T. and Newhouse, M. L.: Episkopi blindness: hereditary blindness in a Greek Cypriot family. Br. J. Ophthalmol. 43: 340-344, 1959.

Warburg, M.: Copenhagen, Denmark: personal communication, 1966.

Warburg, M.: Norrie's disease (atrofia bulborum hereditaria). Acta Ophthalmol. 41: 134-146, 1963.

Warburg, M.: Norrie's disease, a congenital progressive oculo-acoustico-cerebral degeneration. Acta Ophthalmol. 89 (suppl.): 1-147, 1966.

Warburg, M., Hauge, M. and Sanger, R.: Norrie's disease and the Xg blood group system: linkage data. Acta Genet. 15: 103-115, 1965.

Whitnall, S. E. and Norman, R. M.: Microphthalmia and the visual pathways. A case associated with blindness and imbecility, and sex-linked. Br. J. Ophthalmol. 24: 229-244, 1940.

Wilson, W. M. G.: Congenital blindness (pseudoglioma) occurring as a sex-linked developmental anomaly. Canad. Med. Assoc. J. 60: 580-584, 1949.

X
LINKED

*31070 NYSTAGMUS (X-LINKED)

Nystagmus is, of course, only a symptom and has many causes. In fact it occurs as part of the symptom complex in certain other sex-linked traits (e.g., Pelizaeus-Merzbacher, spastic paraplegia, ocular albinism, etc.). What is referred to here is a hereditary form which occurs alone and of which the neuroanatomical basis is still unknown.

Autosomal dominant and recessive forms are less frequent than the X-linked form. Waardenburg (personal communication) feels there is no reason to separate an X-linked recessive from an X-linked dominant form as some have attempted. In some families the disorder is recessive in one line and dominant in another (Hemmes, 1924; Waardenburg, Franceschetti and Klein, textbook, 1961). The explanation could be that the mutation is identical but that there is a series of 'wildtype' isoalleles which have different effects on penetrance of the mutation in the heterozygous female.

Billings, M. L.: Nystagmus through four generations. J. Hered. 33: 457 only, 1942.

Cox, R. A.: Congenital head-nodding and nystagmus: report of a case. Arch. Ophthalmol. 15: 1032-1036, 1936.

Cuendet, J. F. and Della Porta, V.: Une famille de nystagmiques. Ophthalmologica 117: 199-201, 1949.

Hemmes, G. C.: Over Hereditairen Nystagmus. Thesis, Utrecht, 1924.

Rucker, C. W.: Sex-linked nystagmus associated with red-green color-blindness. Am. J. Hum. Genet. 1: 52-54, 1949.

Waardenburg, P. J.: Zum Kapitel des ausserokularen erblichen Nystagmus. Acta Genet. Statist. Med. 4: 298-312, 1953.

31080 NYSTAGMUS, MYOCLONIC

This condition may be an X-linked dominant and distinct from simple nystagmus (q.v.).

In the family described by Van Bogaert and De Savitsch (1937), ten sons of four affected men were all normal with the exception of one instance of an affected son of an affected man who was married to a relative; ten of the sons of 13 daughters of affected men were affected.

Van Bogaert, L. and De Savitsch, E.: Sur une maladie congenitale et heredofamiliale comportant un tremblement rythmique de la tete des globes oculaires et des membres superieurs. (Ses relations avec le nystagmus-myoclonie et le nystagmus congenital hereditaire.) Encephale 32: 113-139, 1937.

31090 OCCIPITAL HAIR, WHITE LOCK OF

Only a single pedigree showing X-linked inheritance is known to us, that of Karl Pearson, who stated that the pedigree was that 'of a well-known family.' The following is a quotation from Pearson (1909).

A case of some interest, the partial albinism, consisting of a white lock, appears to be inherited only through the female and to occur only in the males. II.3 (reported by IV.7), IV.7 and VI.1 had patches of white hair on the back of the head. The patch on VI.1 is about the size of a shilling, it is slightly to the right of the median plane and above the occiput: the skin from which it springs does not appear less pigmented or otherwise differentiated from the adjacent skin. Offspring of V.3 are known to exist and are said not to be affected, but details could not be ascertained.

Pearson, K., Nettleship, E. and Usher, C. H.: A Monograph on Albinism in Man. Cambridge: Drapers Company Research Memoirs, 1911-1913, 1: 255, fig. 638, plate 53.

31095 OCCIPITAL HORN SYNDROME

Rybak et al. (1974) described an unusual syndrome in an 11-year-old male and two maternal uncles. Boney 'horns', symmetrically situated on each side of the foramen magnum and pointing caudad, were demonstrable radiographically. A life-long history of frequent loose stools, obstructive uropathy requiring in one uncle ileal loop diversion, and mild mental retardation were other features.

Rybak, J. J.,,Lazoff, S. G., Parker, B. R. and Luzzatti, L.: Skeletal dysplasia, occipital horns, intestinal malabsorption, and obstructive uropathy — a new hereditary syndrome. To be published, 1974.

*31100 OPHTHALMOPLEGIA, EXTERNAL, AND MYOPIA

In the probably unique family of Salleras and Ortiz de Zarate (1950), affected men showed bilateral ptosis, complete or partial ophthalmoplegia, abnormal shape or function of the pupil, myopia, and progressive degeneration of the retina and choroid. Often there was also absence of patellar and Achilles reflexes, spina bifida, and cardiac and other congenital malformations. Some carrier women showed absent deep tendon reflexes only. Hereditary ophthalmoplegia without myopia is frequently an autosomal dominant or recessive. The pedigree was brought up to date in 1966.

Ortiz de Zarate, J. C.: Recessive sex-linked inheritance of congenital external ophthalmoplegia and myopia coincident with other dysplasias. Br. J. Ophthalmol. 50: 606-607, 1966.

Salleras, A. and Ortiz de Zarate, J. C.: Recessive sex-linked inheritance of external ophthalmoplegia and myopia coincident with other dysplasias. Brit. J. Ophthal. 34: 662-667, 1950.

31110 OPTIC ATROPHY — SPASTIC PARAPLEGIA SYNDROME

Bruyn and Went (1964) described a degenerative disorder of the central nervous system associated with optic atrophy in at least 18 members of a family. One of these was female but the diagnosis was in some doubt in this case. The neurologic disorder showed features intermediate between those of hereditary spastic paraplegia (Strumpell-Lorrain) and Hallevorden-Spatz disease. The laboratory studies (Went, 1964) showed some peculiarities, e.g., abnormal oral glucose tolerance tests and mild red cell macrocytosis, but have thus far not contributed particularly to an understanding of the disorder.

Bruyn, G. W. and Went, L. N.: A sex-linked heredo-degenerative neurological disorder, associated with Leber's optic atrophy. I. Clinical studies. J. Neurol. Sci. 1: 59-80, 1964.

Went, L. N.: A sex-linked heredo-degenerative neurological disorder associated with Leber's optic atrophy. Genetic aspects. Acta Genet. Statist. Med. 14: 220-239, 1964.

Went, L. N.: A sex-linked heredo-degenerative neurological disorder, associated with Leber's optic atrophy. II. Laboratory investigations. J. Neurol. Sci. 1: 81-87, 1964.

*31120 ORAL-FACIAL-DIGITAL (OFD) SYNDROME

Gorlin and colleagues (1961) first reported this condition in the English literature. Clefts of the jaw and tongue in the area of the lateral incisors and canines, other malformations of the face and skull, malformation of the hands, specifically syndactyly, familial trembling, and mental retardation are features. Others include small nostrils, lateral displacement of the inner canthi, lobulate tongue, peculiarly irregular and asymmetrical clefts of the palate, multiple milia on pinnae, alopecia. Abnormal frenulae in the mouth appear to lead to the clefting of jaw, tongue and upper lip. All cases (with exception mentioned below) are female. Ruess and colleagues (1962) state that the sex ratio in affected sibships differs significantly from 1:1 in the direction of 2:1 (f:m). Furthermore, an excessive number of abortions in affected sibships is reported. X-linked dominant inheritance is suggested, with the trait lethal in the hemizygous male. However, Patau and colleagues (1961) interpret this syndrome as a partial autosomal trisomy which is lethal in the male. The existence of an autosomal aberration has been claimed in several of the cases studied by this group. The possibility that the chromosomal segment inserted into a large autosome was derived from an X chromosome and that the phenotypic changes were the result of position effects was considered unlikely by Patau (personal communication). The only male reported as presumed OFD syndrome (Kushnick, Massa, Baukema, 1963) probably had Mohr syndrome (q.v.). Doege et al. (1964) reported a kindred with 15 affected females. Chromosome studies of 8 of them did not uncover any abnormality. Wahrman, Berant, Jacobs, Aviad and Ben-Hur (1966) described the condition in an XXY male. This greatly strengthens the idea that inheritance is male-lethal X-linked dominant. Incontinentia pigmenti (q.v.) may have the same inheritance. See TREMBLING CHIN in the dominant catalog for information bearing on the differential diagnosis. See MOHR SYNDROME in the recessive catalog for information bearing on the differential diagnosis. In 1960 Fuhrmann and Vogel described cleft lip-palate and syndactyly in a female infant and partial manifestation (syndactyly, finger deformity and split in tip of tongue) in the mother. The lip cleft was median. They cited other cases of this syndrome and suggested autosomal dominant inheritance. Subsequently Fuhrmann et al. (1966) concluded that this was a case of OFD syndrome and that inheritance is X-linked dominant with lethality in male. Vaillaud et al. (1968) described a remarkable pedigree in which 10 females had OFD. The grandmother and 9 of her granddaughters through three unaffected sons had OFD. The 9 affected included all daughters of the three carrier males. The authors accepted the interpretation of X-linked dominance with lethality in the hemizygous males, which has been applied to previously published pedigrees. In addition, however, to explain the findings in this specific family they postulated that the OFD gene is on a terminal segment of the X chromosome homologous with a segment of the Y chromosome and that the three carrier males had inherited a Y chromosome which in some way masked expression of the OFD gene. Gorlin (1970) suggests that the two sisters with 'severe achondroplasia' described by Wallace et al. (1970) had this condition. Certainly the appearance of the upper lip was typical of OFD in both.

Dodge, J. A. and Kernohan, D. C.: Oral-facial-digital syndrome. Arch. Dis. Child. 42: 214-219, 1967.

Doege, T. C., Campbell, M. M., Bryant, J. S. and Thuline, H. C.: Mental retardation and dermatoglyphics in a family with the oral-facial-digital syndrome. Am. J. Dis. Child. 116: 615-622, 1968.

Doege, T. C., Thuline, H. C., Priest, J. H., Norby, D. E. and Bryant, J. S.: Studies of a family with the oral-facial-digital syndrome. N. Engl. J. Med. 271: 1073-1080, 1964.

Fuhrmann, W., Stahl, A. and Schroeder, T. M.: Das oro-facio-digitale Syndrome, zugleich eine Diskussion der Erbgange mit geschlechtsbegrenztem Letaleffekt. Humangenetik 2: 133-164, 1966.

Gorlin, R. J. and Psaume, J.: Orodigitofacial dysostosis — a new syndrome. J. Pediatr. 61: 520-530, 1962.

Gorlin, R. J.: Minneapolis, Minn.: personal communication, 1970.

Gorlin, R. J., Anderson, V. E. and Scott, C. R.: Hypertrophied frenuli, oligophrenia, familial trembling and anomalies of the hand. Report of four cases in one family and a forme fruste in another. N. Engl. J. Med. 264: 486-489, 1961.

Kushnick, T., Massa, T. P. and Baukema, R.: Orofaciodigital syndrome in male: case report. J. Pediatr. 63: 1130-1134, 1963.

Patau, K., Therman, E., Inhorn, S. L., Smith, D. W. and Ruess, A. L.: Partial trisomy syndromes. II. An insertion as cause of the OFD syndrome in mother and daughter. Chromosoma 12: 573-584, 1961.

Reinwein, H., Schilli, W., Ritter, H., Brehme, H. and Wolf, V.: Untersuchungen an einer Familie mit Oral-facial-digital-syndrom. Humangenetik 2: 165-177, 1966.

Ruess, A. L., Pruzansky, S., Lis, E. F. and Patau, K.: The oral-facial-digital syndrome: a multiple congenital condition of females with associated chromosomal abnormalities. Pediatrics 29: 985-995, 1962.

Solomon, L. M., Fretzin, D. and Pruzansky, S.: Pilosebaceous dysplasia in the oral-facial-digital syndrome. Arch. Dermatol. 102: 598-602, 1970.

Vaillaud, J. C., Martin, J., Szepetowski, G. and Robert, J. M.: Le syndrome oro-facio-digital. Etude clinique et genetique a propos de 10 cas observes dans une meme famille. Rev. Pediatr. 4: 383-392, 1968.

Wahrman, J., Berant, M., Jacobs, J., Aviad, I. and Ben-Hur, N.: The oral-facial-digital syndrome: a male-lethal condition in a boy with 47-XXY chromosomes. Pediatrics 37: 812-821, 1966.

Wallace, D. C., Exton, L. A., Pritchard, D. A., Leung, Y. and Cooke, R. A.: Severe achondroplasia. Demonstration of probable heterogeneity within this clinical syndrome. J. Med. Genet. 7: 22-26, 1970.

*31125 ORNITHINE-TRANSCARBAMYLASE DEFICIENCY

Hyperammonemia due to deficiency of ornithine-transcarbamylase is listed in the recessive catalog (23720). As indicated there, there is reason to suspect that the enzyme may be encoded by an X-borne gene. Mutation in this gene may lead to partial deficiency in heterozygous females and to complete deficiency in hemizygous males (Campbell et al., 1971). Scott et al. (1972) presented two kindreds that support X-linked recessive inheritance of ornithine-transcarbamylase deficiency. Confirmation by cell culture studies is impossible because OTC activity is not present in normal fibroblasts. Short et al. (1972) studied 4 families, all consistent with X-linked inheritance.

Campbell, A. G. M., Rosenberg, L. E., Snodgrass, P. J. and Nuzum, C. T.: Lethal neonatal hyperammonaemia due to complete ornithine-transcarbamylase deficiency. (Letter) Lancet II: 217-218, 1971.

Campbell, A. G. M., Rosenberg, L. E., Snodgrass, P. J. and Nuzum, C. T.: Ornithine transcarbamylase deficiency: a cause of lethal neonatal hyperammonemia in males. N. Engl. J. Med. 288: 1-6, 1973.

Scott, C. R., Chiang Teng, C., Goodman, S. I., Greensher, A. and Mace, J. W.: X-linked transmission of ornithine-transcarbamylase deficiency. (Letter) Lancet II: 1148 only, 1972.

Short, E. M., Conn, H. O., Snodgrass, P. J. and Rosenberg, L. E.: X-linked dominant inheritance of ornithine transcarbamylase deficiency. (Abstract) Am. J. Hum. Genet. 24A only, 1972.

Short, E. M., Conn, H. O., Snodgrass, P. J., Campbell, A. G. M. and Rosenberg, L. E.: Evidence for X-linked dominant inheritance of ornithine transcarbamylase deficiency. N. Engl. J. Med. 288: 7-12, 1973.

*31130 OTO-PALATO-DIGITAL (OPD) SYNDROME

Dudding et al. (1967) described three male sibs with conduction deafness, cleft palate, characteristic facies and a generalized bone dysplasia. A broad nasal root gives the patient a pugilistic appearance. Wide-spacing of the toes creates a resemblance to the foot of a tree frog. X-linkage and autosomal inheritance could not be distinguished. Roentgenologic features were reviewed in the same patients by Langer (1967). (The male patient reported by Taybi (1962) may have had this condition). Conductive hearing loss, somewhat broad thumbs and great toes, short fingernails, fifth finger clinodactyly, dislocation of the head of the radius, pectus excavatum, mild dwarfism were also features. A secondary ossification center at the base of the second metacarpal and metatarsal is characteristic. Turner (1970) has observed affected half-brothers who had different fathers, thus supporting X-linked inheritance. Weinstein and Cohen (1966) suggested that an X-linked form of cleft palate exists. Affected males and carrier females showed hypertelorism and median frontal prominence. Four males in three sibships connected through 5 presumably heterozygous females were affected. Gorlin (1967) suggests that the condition in this family was the oto-palato-digital syndrome (31130). The Xray changes in the hands and feet were consistent (Gorlin, 1971).

Dudding, B. A., Gorlin, R. J. and Langer, L. O.: The oto-palato-digital syndrome. A new symptom-complex consisting of deafness, dwarfism, cleft palate, characteristic facies, and a generalized bone dysplasia. Am. J. Dis. Child. 113: 214221, 1967.

Gall, J. C., Jr., Stern, A. M., Poznanski, A. K., Garn, S. M., Weinstein, E. D. and Hayward, J. R.: Oto-palato-digital syndrome: comparison of clinical and radiographic manifestations in males and females. Am. J. Hum. Genet. 24: 24-36, 1972.

Gorlin, R. J.: Minneapolis, Minn.: personal communication, 1967, 1971.

Langer, L. O., Jr.: The roentgenographic features of the oto-palato-digital (OPD) syndrome. Am. J. Roentgen. 100: 63-70, 1967.

Taybi, H.: Generalized skeletal dysplasia with multiple anomalies. A note on Pyle's disease. Am. J. Roentgen. 88: 450-457, 1962.

Turner, G.: Sydney, Australia: personal communication, 1970.

Weinstein, E. D. and Cohen, M. M.: Sex-linked cleft palate. Report of a family and review of 77 kindreds. J. Med. Genet. 3: 17-22, 1966.

*31140 PAINE SYNDROME (MICROCEPHALY WITH SPASTIC DIPLEGIA)

In the French-Canadian family described by Paine (1960) the pattern of inheritance was quite consistent with X-linkage. Myoclonic fits were one feature and another was elevated level of amino acids in the spinal fluid with inversion of the usual ratio of plasma level to spinal fluid level. Autopsy in one case showed an apparent developmental malformation (hypoplasia of the cerebellum, inferior olives and pons), supporting the view that this entity is distinct from the two forms of diffuse sclerosis (q.v.) and from hydrocephalus due to stenosis of the aqueduct of Sylvius (q.v.) which is sometimes accompanied by spastic paraplegia and microcephaly after arrest of the hydrocephalus. Subsequent studies failed to substantiate the amino acid changes (Efron, 1966). Seemanova et al. (1973) reported a kindred with two affected males in each of three sibships connected through carrier females. Abdominal reflexes were absent in these cases. The level of amino acids in the cerebrospinal fluid was normal. The disorder may be the same as that reported by Paine. However, hypoplasia of the cerebellum, pons and inferior olive was not found.

Efron, M. S.: Boston, Mass.: personal communication, 1966.

Paine, R. S.: Evaluation of familial biochemically determined mental retardation in children, with special reference to aminoaciduria. New Eng. J. Med. 262: 658-665, 1960.

Paine, R. S.: Washington, D.C.: personal communication, 1963.

Seemanova, E., Lesny, I., Hyanek, J., Brachfeld, K., Rossler, M. and Proskova, M.: X-chromosomal recessive microcephaly with epilepsy, spastic tetraplegia and absent abdominal reflex. New variety of 'Paine syndrome'? Humangenetik 20: 113-117, 1973.

31145 PALLISTER W SYNDROME

Pallister et al. (1974) described two brothers with a mental retardation syndrome characterized by an unusual physiognomy (frontal prominence, anterior cowlick, hypertelorism, antimongoloid orbital slant, and broad, flat nasal bridge like that of the OPD syndrome, 31130), midline notch of upper lip and submucous cleft of the hard palate, absent upper central incisors, limited motion at the elbow due to subluxation, camptodactyly and pes cavus. In addition to the mental retardation, the patients had grand mal seizures. The mother and a sister were considered mildly affected, consistent with heterozygous manifestation of an X-linked trait.

Pallister, P. D., Herrmann, J., Spranger, J. W., Gorlin, R. J., Langer, L. O. and Opitz, J. M.: The W syndrome. Birth Defects Orig. Art. Ser. 10 (7): 51-60, 1974.

*31150 PARKINSONISM

Like some other traits listed here, Parkinsonism is only a symptom and has many causes. Cases of idiopathic paralysis agitans (that is, cases in which arteriosclerosis and encephalitis are considered unlikely causes) have been found to have family histories consistent with autosomal dominant inheritance. The Filipino kindred showing X-linked recessive inheritance (observed by McKusick and colleagues) appears to be unique. Onset of symptoms occurs at the age of about 40 years.

Johnston, A. W. and McKusick, V. A.: Sex-linked recessive inheritance in spastic paraplegia and Parkinsonism. Proc. Sec. Intern. Cong. Hum. Genet., (Rome, Sept. 6-12, 1961.) 3: 1652-1654, 1961.

*31160 PELIZAEUS-MERZBACHER DISEASE

The diffuse cerebral sclerosis group rivals the spinocerebellar degeneration group in clinical, pathologic, and genetic confusion. It is currently under intense investigation and is gradually being elucidated through biochemical characteristics. Some, e.g., Ford (1960), refer to the Pelizaeus-Merzbacher form as the chronic infantile type. It begins in infancy as early as the eighth day and usually no later than the third month and is very slowly progressive so that the victim may survive to middle age. One of Pelizaeus' patients lived to 52 years of age and in Tyler's Negro family an affected male was still living at age 51. At first, rotary movements of the head and eyes develop but curiously may later disappear. Affected children are known in these families as 'head nodders' and 'eye waggers.' Spasticity of the legs and later the arms, cerebellar ataxia, dementia, and Parkinsonian symptoms are other features developing over the first decade or two of life. Some heterozygous females show the disorder. The brain of such a female in Merzbacher's family was studied by Spielmeyer (cited by Tyler, 1958) with demonstration of changes. Sidman, Dickie and Appel (1964) described an X-linked demyelination disorder in mice which is similar to Pelizaeus-Merzbacher disease in man.

Ford, F. R.: Diseases of the Nervous System in Infancy, Childhood and Adolescence. Springfield, Ill.: Charles C Thomas, 1960 (4th Ed.). Pp. 831-833.

Gertner, M., Zalay, E. and Hirschhorn, K.: Cellular metachromasia in Pompe's disease and Pelizaeus-Merzbacher disease. Clin. Genet. 1: 28-29, 1970.

Merzbacher, L.: Gesetzmassigkeiten in der Vererbung und Verbreitung verschiedener hereditar-familiarer Erkrankungen. Arch. Rass.-u. Ges. Biol. 6: 172-198, 1909.

Nisenbaum, C., Sandbank, U. and Kohn, R.: Pelizaeus-Merzbacher disease 'infantile acute type.' Report of a family. Ann. Paediatr. 204: 365-376, 1965.

Penrose, L. S.: Biology of Mental Defect. London: Sidgwick and Jackson Ltd., (2nd Ed.) 1954.

Schneck, L., Adachi, M. and Volk, B. W.: Congenital failure of myelinization: Pelizaeus-Merzbacher disease? Neurology 21: 817-824, 1971.

Sidman, R. L., Dickie, M. M. and Appel, S. H.: Mutant mice (quaking and jimpy) with deficient myelination in the central nervous system. Science 144: 309-311, 1964.

Tyler, H. R.: Pelizaeus-Merzbacher disease: a clinical study. Arch. Neurol. Psychiatry 80: 162-169, 1958.

Zeman, W., DeMyer, W. and Falls, H. F.: Pelizaeus-Merzbacher disease. A study in nosology. J. Neuropath. Exp. Neurol. 23: 334-354, 1964.

31170 PERIODIC PARALYSIS, FAMILIAL

Khan (1935) described a large family in which 8 males were affected with familial periodic paralysis in a pattern consistent with X-linked recessive inheritance. By this hypothesis, at least 4 females were heterozygous carriers. The X-linked recessive pattern of inheritance in Khan's family was probably only fortuitous based on the disease's predilection for males. Of 627 reported cases reviewed by Sagild, 411 were men. Furthermore 99 of 109 probands were men. Among 52 cases of the disease in Denmark only 4 were female, a sex-ratio of 12:1. When affected, women show a less severe clinical picture. Some of Sagild's families, especially when only part is considered, have a pedigree pattern consistent with X-linked recessive

652   inheritance. However, numerous instances of male-to-male transmission have been observed. Sagild's conclusion was that the hypokalemic variety of familial periodic paralysis is inherited as an autosomal dominant with marked reduction in penetrance in the female. The hyperkalemic form of the disease affects males and females equally.

Khan, M. Y.: Familial periodic paralysis. Indian Med. Gaz. 70: 28-29, 1935.

Sagild, U.: Hereditary Transient Paralysis. Copenhagen, Munksgarrd, 1959.

*31180 PHOSPHOGLYCERATE KINASE (PGK)

Valentine et al. (1969) found hemolytic anemia with deficient red and white cell phosphoglycerate kinase in a large Chinese kindred. Mild hemolysis was present in presumed heterozygotes. Chen et al. (1971) described an electrophoretic variant of PGK with enzyme activity in the normal range. PGK and G6PD are probably not closely linked. From cell hybridization studies, it was concluded that the locus is on the long arm of the X chromosome (Grzeschik et al., 1972). Ricciuti and Ruddle (1973) concluded, from the study of chromosomal aberrations in cell hybridization systems, that the order on the X-chromosome is centromere — PGK — HGPRT (30800) — G6PD. The conclusion is based on his own work with the KOP 14 X translocation, and on Park Gerald's with a 19 X translocation and Bootsma's with a 3 X translocation. All have breaks involving the long arm of the X chromosome, each at a different site. From studies of X-autosome translocations it appears that the order of loci on the large arm of the X chromosome are centromere — PGK- HGPRT (30800) — G6PD (30590). In the KOP T14 X all three loci are apparently on the part of the long arm translocated to chromosome 14. In the T19 X studied by Gerald et al. (1973) the HGPRT and G6PD loci (but not PGK) are on the part of the long arm translocated to chromosome 19. In the T3 X studied by Bootsma (1972) G6PD (but not the other two) are on the part of the long arm translocated to chromosome 3. PGK is X-linked in the kangaroo also (Cooper et al., 1971). Description of various physical properties of PGK in cases of hemolytic anemia (Yoshida and Miwa, 1974) recapitulates the experience with G6PD (30590), PK (26620), etc. The conclusion was based on work with the KOP 14 X translocation.

Chen, S.-H., Malcolm, L. A., Yoshida, A. and Giblett, E. R.: Phosphoglycerate kinase: an X-linked polymorphism in man. Am. J. Hum. Genet. 23: 87-91, 1971.

Cooper, D. W., Vandeberg, J. L., Sharman, G. B. and Poole, W. E.: Phosphoglycerate kinase polymorphism in kangaroos provides further evidence for paternal inactivation. Nature N. B. 230: 155-157, 1971.

Deys, B. F., Grzeschik, K. H., Grzeschik, A., Jaffe, E. R. and Siniscalco, M.: Human phosphoglycerate kinase and inactivation of the X chromosome. Science 175: 1002-1003, 1972.

Grzeschik, K. H., Allderdice, P. W., Grzeschik, A., Opitz, J. M., Miller, O. J. and Siniscalco, M.: Cytological mapping of human X-linked genes by use of somatic cell hybrids involving an X-autosome translocation. Proc. Natl. Acad. Sci. 69: 69-73, 1972.

Huijing, F., Eicher, E. M. and Coleman, D. L.: Location of phosphorylase kinase (Phk) in the mouse X-chromosome. Biochem. Genet. 9: 193-196, 1973.

Meera Khan, P., Westerveld, A., Grzeschik, K. H., Deys, B. F., Garson, O. M. and Siniscalco, M.: X-linkage of human phosphoglycerate kinase confirmed in man-mouse and man-Chinese hamster somatic cell hybrids. Am. J. Hum. Genet. 23: 614-623, 1971.

Kozak, L. P., McLean, G. K. and Eicher, E. M.: X-linkage of phosphoglycerate kinase in the mouse. Biochem. Genet. 2: 41-47, 1974.

Ricciuti, F. C. and Ruddle, F. H.: Assignment of three gene loci (PGK, HGPRT, and G6PD) to the long arm of the human X-chromosome by somatic cell genetics. Genetics 74: 661-678, 1973.

Valentine, W. N., Hsieh, H.-S., Paglia, D. E., Anderson, H. M., Baughan, M. A., Jaffe, E. R. and Garson, O. M.: Hereditary hemolytic anemia associated with phosphoglycerate kinase deficiency in erythrocytes and leukocytes. A probable X-chromosome-linked syndrome. N. Engl. J. Med. 280: 528-534, 1969.

Yoshida, A. and Miwa, S.: Characterization of a phosphoglycerate kinase variant associated with hemolytic anemia. Am. J. Hum. Genet. 26: 378-384, 1974.

31190 PIERRE ROBIN SYNDROME WITH CONGENITAL HEART MALFORMATION AND CLUBFOOT

Gorlin et al. (1970) described a kindred in which multiple males, related through normal females had this combination. Other possible reports of the syndrome were noted, e.g., Sachtleben (1964) had two brothers with cleft palate, congenital heart disease and clubfoot. In a brief follow-up note, Gorlin et al. (1971) stated that subsequent to the time of report 'two more affected sons have been born to sisters of our proband's mother.'

Gorlin, R. J., Cervenka, J. and Pruzansky, S.: Facial clefting and its syndromes. The Clinical Delineation of Birth Defects. XI. Orofacial Structures. Baltimore: Williams and Wilkins, 1971. Pp. 3-49.

Gorlin, R. J., Cervenka, J., Anderson, R. C., Sauk, J. J. and Bevis, W. D.: Robin's syndrome. A probably X-linked recessive subvariety exhibiting persistence of left superior vena cava and atrial septal defect. Am. J. Dis. Child. 119: 176-178, 1970.

Sachtleben, P.: Zur Pathogenese und Therapie des Pierre-Robin-syndromes. Arch. Kinderheilkd. 171: 55-63, 1964.

*31200 PITUITARY DWARFISM IV (X-LINKED PANHYPOPITUITARISM)

X
L
I
N
K
E
D

Phelan et al. (1971) reported four cases in three sibships connected through females and Schimke et al. (1971)   653
described panhypopituitarism in two half-brothers with the same mother.

Phelan, P. D., Connelly, J., Martin, F. I. R. and Wettenhall, H. N. B.: X-linked recessive hypopituitarism. The Clinical Delineation of Birth Defects. X. The Endocrine System. Baltimore: Williams and Wilkins, 1971. Pp. 24-27.

Schimke, R. N., Spaulding, J. J. and Hollowell, J. G.: X-linked congenital panhypopituitarism. The Clinical Delineation of Birth Defects. X. The Endocrine System. Baltimore: Williams and Wilkins, 1971. Pp. 21-23.

31210 PSEUDOHERMAPHRODITISM, INCOMPLETE MALE, TYPE I

Goldstein and Wilson (1974) recommended the classification of male pseudohermaphroditism that is followed here. They propose that the disorders described by Lubs et al. (1959), Gilbert-Dreyfus et al. (1957), Reifenstein (Bowen et al. 1965) and Rosewater et al. (1965) may be various severities of one and the same disorder or may be allelic disorders. This conclusion was based in large part, on a family in which one or another affected member conformed to four entities (Wilson et al., 1974). The form described by Lubs is the most severe in terms of change in the external genitalia and the form described by Rosewater is the least severe. Walker et al. (1970 also described a family with wide variability in degree of severity.

Bowen, P., Lee, C. N. S., Migeon, C. J., Kaplan, N. M., Whalley, P. J., McKusick, V. A. and Reifenstein, E. C.: Hereditary male pseudohermaphroditism with hypogonadism, hypopadias and gynecomastia (Reifenstein's syndrome). Ann. Intern. Med. 62: 252-270, 1965.

Gilbert-Dreyfus, S., Sebaoun, S. A. and Belaisch, J.: Etude d'un cas familial d'androgynoidisme avec hypospadias grave, gynecomastie et hyperoestrogenie. Ann. Endocrinol. 18: 93-101, 1957.

Goldstein, J. L. and Wilson, J. D.: Hereditary disorders of sexual development in man. In, Motulsky, A. G. and Lenz, W. (ed.): Birth Defects. Amsterdam: Excepta Medica, 1974. Pp. 165-173.

Lubs, H. A., Jr., Vilar, O. and Bergenstal, D. M.: Familial male pseudohermaphroditism with labial testes and partial feminization: endocrine studies and genetic aspects. J. Clin. Endocrinol. 19: 1110-1120, 1959.

Rosewater, S., Gwinup, G. and Hamwi, G. J.: Familial gynecomastia. Ann. Intern. Med. 63: 377-385, 1965.

Walker, A. C., Stack, E. M. and Horsfall, W. A.: Familial male psuedohermaphroditism. Med. J. Aust. 1: 156-160, 1970.

Wilson, J. D., Harrod, M. J., Goldstein, J. L., Hemsell, D. L. and MacDonald, P. C.: Familial incomplete male pseudohermaphroditism, type I. Evidence for androgen resistance and variable clinical manifestations in a family with the Reifenstein syndrome. N. Engl. J. Med. 290: 1097-1103, 1974.

31215 PTERYGIUM SYNDROME (X-LINKED)

Carnevale et al. (1973) observed a family with 7 cases of pterygium syndrome in three generations and suggested X-linked dominant inheritance because father-to-son transmission did not occur and all four daughters but none of four sons of an affected male were affected. Against X-linked dominant inheritance was the fact that females were not more mildly affected than the one affected male in the pedigree.

Carnevale, A., Hernandez, A. L. and De los Cobos, L.: Sindrome de pterygium familiar con probable transmission dominante ligada al cromosoma X. Rev. Invest. Clin. 25: 237-244, 1973.

31220 RADIAL LOOP, PLAIN, ON RIGHT INDEX FINGER

Walker (1941) suggested that this pattern is sex linked. Holt (1962) could not confirm the suggestion of X-linkage.

Holt, S. B.: London, England: personal communication, 1962.

Walker, J. F.: A sex linked recessive fingerprint pattern. J. Hered. 32: 279-280, 1941.

31230 REIFENSTEIN SYNDROME

The features of this form of male pseudohermaphroditism are hypospadias, hypogonadism, gynecomastia, normal XY karyotype and a pedigree pattern consistent with X-linked recessive inheritance. Although the affected males are infertile, germ cells with mitotic (and perhaps meiotic) activity are demonstrated by testicular biopsy. No spermatozoa are found. Some of the histologic features such as Leydig cell hyperplasia and hyaline tubular ghosts resemble those of the XXY Klinefelter syndrome. However, the presence of germ cells, the hypospadias and the familial nature are distinguishing features. A defect in production of fetal androgen is thought to be responsible for the hypospadias. Some of the pathologic changes in the testis may result from high FSH secondary to androgen deficiency. Treatment with testosterone from an early age might restore fertility. Differentiation from the incomplete testicular feminization syndrome (31380) and perhaps from pseudovaginal perineoscrotal hypospadias (26460) is not always easy. Wilson et al. (1974) studied a family with 11 affected males. The phenotype in these varied from minimal changes (microphallus and bifid scrotum) in two, to almost complete male pseudohermaphrodotism. (Perineoscrotal hypospadias absent vas deferens and vaginal orifice) in one. On the basis of this and another reported pedigree they suggested that the affected members in the kindred reported by Gilbert-Dreyfus et al. (see 30730), Lubs et al. (see 31370 and 31371) and Rosewater et al. (see 30650) had the same condition as that reported by Reifenstein. Wilson et al. (1974) chose to refer to the condition as type 1 familial incomplete male pseudohermaphoditism (type 2 is autosomal recessive; 26460. From studies of blood levels of testosterone and luteinizing hormone and the rate of production of estrogen and androgen they concluded that the underlying defect is in androgen action not androgen synthesis.

X

L
I
N
K
E
D

Boczkowski, K. and Teter, J.: Familial male pseudohermaphroditism. Acta Endocrinol. 49: 497-509, 1965.

Bowen, P., Lee, C. N. S., Migeon, C. J., Kaplan, N. M., Whalley, P. J., McKusick, V. A. and Reifenstein, E. C.: Hereditary male pseudohermaphroditism with hypogonadism, hypospadias and gynecomastia (Reifenstein's syndrome). Ann. Intern. Med. 62: 252-270, 1965.

Wilson, J. D., Harrod, M. J., Goldstein, J. L., Hemsell, D. L. and MacDonald, P. C.: Familial incomplete male psuedohermpahroditism type 1. Evidence for androgen resistance and variable clinical manifestations in a family with the Reifenstein syndrome. N. Engl. J. Med. 290: 1097-1103, 1974.

31240 RENAL TUBULAR ACIDOSIS II (PROXIMAL, RATE, OR BICARBONATE WASTING TYPE)

This variety is apparently distinct from classic RTA I, which is inherited as a dominant. Most, or perhaps all, the cases have been males. Hence, X-linked recessive inheritance is possible.

Edelmann, C. M., Jr.: Bronx, N.Y.: personal communication, 1970.

Sebastian, A., McSherry, E. and Morris, R. C., Jr.: On the mechanism of renal potassium wasting in renal tubular acidosis associated with the Fanconi syndrome (type 2 RTA). J. Clin. Invest. 50: 231-243, 1971.

Soriano, J. R., Boichis, H., Stark, H. and Edelmann, C. M., Jr.: Proximal renal tubular acidosis. A defect in bicarbonate reabsorption with normal urinary acidification. Pediatr. Res. 1: 81-98, 1967.

*31250 RETICULOENDOTHELIOSIS (X-LINKED)

Falletta et al. (1970) described a Latin American family in which 17 males in two generations died under the age of 6 years, following an illness characterized by fever, pallor, jaundice, hepatosplenomegaly, and lymphadenopathy. Median age of onset was 14 months (4-62 months) and median duration of illness was 22 days (1-50 days). Histologic changes were consistent with malignant reticuloendotheliosis. All affected males were related through their mothers.

Falletta, J. M., Fernbach, D. J., Singer, D. B., Shore, N. A., Landing, B. and Heath, C. W., Jr.: An X-linked recessive 'malignant' reticuloendotheliosis. (Abstract) Society for Pediatric Research, Atlantic City, 1970.

Falletta, J. M., Fernbach, D. J., Singer, D. B., Smith, M. A., Landing, B. H., Heath, C. W., Jr., Shore, N. A. and Barrett, F. F.: A fatal X-linked recessive reticuloendothelial syndrome with hyperglobulinemia. X-linked recessive reticuloendotheliosis. J. Pediatr. 83: 549-556, 1973.

*31260 RETINITIS PIGMENTOSA (X-LINKED)

The X-linked form is also called choroidoretinal degeneration, or pigmentary retinopathy. Affected males show typical 'bone corpuscle' clumps of pigment on fundoscopic examination and progressive choroidal sclerosis leading to complete blindness. Heterozygous women may show a tapetoretinal reflex (brilliant, scintillating, golden hued, patchy appearance most striking around the macula) but no visual defect. Retinitis pigmentosa is sometimes autosomal dominant, sometimes autosomal recessive. In addition to these hereditary forms without associated manifestations, retinitis pigmentosa is one component of certain hereditary syndromes, notably the Laurence-Moon-Bardet-Biedl syndrome. Thus there may be at least seven or eight distinct genetic varieties of the phenotype. The X-linked form is one of the rarer. All families do not show the expression in female carriers described above. Thus, there seems to be a fully recessive and an intermediate X-linked form: their relation to each other is unknown. The gyrate choroidal atrophy described by Waardenburg (1932) as X-linked was found on further study to be retinitis pigmentosa (Waardenburg, Franceschetti and Klein, textbook, 1961, p. 799). As is reviewed by Jacobson and Stephens (1962), there are some phenotypic differences between families reported. The genetic significance of these differences is unknown. In the family reported by Heck (1963), heterozygous females sometimes were fully affected and sometimes showed only a blue-yellow color defect (a rare anomaly). 'Tapetal reflex' was not present, as in the heterozygotes reported by Falls and Cotterman. The degeneration of the retina was variable in type, being pigmentary degeneration, non-pigmentary degeneration and macular degeneration in different affected males. Cataract was present in two with pigmentary degeneration. The most frequent form of retinitis pigmentosa is the recessively inherited form(s), the dominant forms are next in frequency and the X-linked form is rarest, being less than 5 percent in most series. Grutzner et al. (1972) concluded that the loci for RP, for Xg blood group and for color vision are widely separated on the X chromosome.

Allan, W.: Eugenic significance of retinitis pigmentosa. Arch. Ophthalmol. 18: 938-947, 1937.

Falls, H. F.: The role of the sex chromosome in hereditary ocular pathology. Trans. Am. Ophthal. Soc. 50: 421-467, 1952.

Grutzner, P., Sanger, R. and Spivey, B. E.: Linkage studies in X-linked retinitis pigmentosa. Humangenetik 14: 155-158, 1972.

Heck, A. F.: Presumptive X-linked intermediate transmission of retinal degenerations. Variations and coincidental occurrence with ataxia in a large family. Arch. Ophthalmol. 70: 143-149, 1963.

Jacobson, J. H. and Stephens, G.: Hereditary choroidoretinal degeneration. Study of a family including electroretinography and adaptometry. Arch. Ophthalmol. 67: 321-335, 1962.

Klein, D., Franceschetti, A., Hussels, I., Race, R. R. and Sanger, R.: X-linked retinitis pigmentosa and linkage studies with the Xg blood-groups. Lancet I: 974-975, 1967.

McQuarrie, M. D.: Two pedigrees of hereditary blindness in man. J. Genet. 30: 147-153, 1935.

X

L
I
N
K
E
D

Usher, C. H.: Bowman lecture on a few hereditary eye affections. Trans. Ophthalmol. Soc. U.K. 55: 164-245, 1935.

Waardenburg, P. J.: Das menschliche Auge und seine Erbanlagean. Martinus Nijhoff, 'S-Gravenhage, 1932.

Warburg, M. and Simonsen, S. E.: Sex-linked recessive retinitis pigmentosa. A preliminary study of the carriers. Acta Ophthalmol. 46: 494-499, 1968.

*31270 RETINOSCHISIS

Retinoschisis is intraretinal splitting due to degeneration. The abnormality may not be clinically manifest until middle life. The affected males show cystic degeneration leading to split in the retina, detachment of the retina, and finally complete retinal atrophy with sclerosis of the choroid. Gieser and Falls (1961) observed a macular cyst in one eye of a possible female carrier in a kindred with nine affected males and suggested that it might represent an expression of the carrier state.

Retinoschisis is, in the opinion of Gieser and Falls (1961), the same condition as that described by Mann and MacRae (1938) as congenital vascular veil in the vitreous and also the same as the X-linked retinal detachment described by Sorsby and colleagues (1951). Retinoschisis is probably distinct from pseudoglioma, although possibly even this cannot be considered settled. So-called congenital falciform fold of the retina (ablatio falciformis retinae congenita) is probably yet another expression of the same gene as that for retinoschisis. Weve (1938) observed falciform fold and pseudoglioma in the same family. Forsius and colleagues (1963) described a family with a homozygous affected female who was the daughter of an affected male and his second cousin. All three of the homozygote's sons, by two different husbands, were affected. Yanoff et al. (1968) reported the histologic appearance in the eye of a 50-month-old boy whose brother was also affected. The splitting occurred in the sensory retina, predominantly in the nerve fiber layer. Cystic maculopathy is sometimes the only finding in these patients. The basic lesion is cystic degeneration in the deep nerve layer. Ives et al. (1970) found loose linkage with the Xg locus.

Forsius, H., Eriksson, A. and Vainio-Mattila, B.: Geschlechtsgebundene, erbliche Retinoschisis in zwei Familien in Finnland. Klin. Monatsbl. Augenheilkd. 143: 806-816, 1963.

Forsius, H., Erikkson, A., Nuutila, A., Vainio-Mattila, B. and Krause, U.: A genetic study of three rare retinal disorders: dystrophia retinae dysacusis syndrome, X-chromosomal retinoschisis and grouped pigments of the retina. The Clinical Delineation of Birth Defects. VIII. Eye. Baltimore: Williams and Wilkins, 1971.

Forsius, H., Vainio-Mattila, B. and Eriksson, A.: X-linked hereditary retinoschisis. Br. J. Ophthalmol. 46: 678-681, 1962.

Gieser, E. P. and Falls, H. F.: Hereditary retinoschisis. Am. J. Ophthalmol. 51: 1193-1200, 1961.

Ives, E. J., Ewing, C. C. and Innes, R.: X-linked juvenile retinoschisis and Xg linkage in five families. (Abstract) Am. J. Hum. Genet. 22: 17A-18A, 1970.

Kleinert, H.: Eine recessiv-geschlechtsgebundene Form der idiopathischen Netzhautspaltung bei nichtmyopen Jugendlichen. Graefe Arch. Ophthalmol. 154: 295-305, 1953.

Mann, I. and MacRae, A.: Congenital vascular veils in the vitreous. Br. J. Ophthalmol. 22: 1-10, 1938.

Manschot, W. A.: Pathology of hereditary juvenile retinoschisis. Arch. Ophthalmol. 88: 131-138, 1972.

Sorsby, A., Klein, M., Gann, J. H. and Siggins, G.: Unusual retinal detachment, possibly sex linked. Br. J. Ophthalmol. 35: 1-10, 1951.

Vainio-Mattila, B., Eriksson, A. W. and Forsius, H.: X-chromosomal recessive retinoschisis in the region of Pori. An ophthalmo-genetical analysis of 103 cases. Acta Ophthalmol. 47: 1135-1148, 1969.

Weve, H.: Ablatio falciformis congenita (retinal fold). Br. J. Ophthalmol. 22: 456-470, 1938.

Yanoff, M., Kertesz Rahn, E. and Zimmerman, L. E.: Histopathology of juvenile retinoschisis. Arch. Ophthalmol. 79: 49-53, 1968.

31280 SACRAL DEFECT WITH ANTERIOR SACRAL MENINGOCELE

Cohn and Bay-Nielsen (1969) described seven cases of anterior sacral meningocele with partial absence of the sacrum and coccyx. Symptoms included constipation and urinary incontinence. All the affected persons were female. One unaffected female appears to have transmitted the disorder. A majority of reported cases are female. The authors suggested X-linked dominant inheritance. Abortions do not seem to have been increased in the family.

Cohn, J. and Bay-Nielsen, E.: Hereditary defects of the sacrum and coccyx with anterior sacral meningocele. Acta Paediatr. Scand. 58: 268-274, 1969.

31283 SCAPULOHUMEROPERONEAL MUSCULAR ATROPHY WITH CARDIAC CONDUCTION DEFECT

5 males in 3 sibships of which the mothers were sisters were reported by Mawatori and Katayama (1973) to have a form of spinal muscular atrophy characterized by juvenile onset, scapulohumeroperoneal muscular weakness, and cardiac conduction defect. Limitation in neck flexion due to shortness (or atrophy) of posterior nuchal muscles and shortness of the Achilles tendons were early manifestations. The carrier mothers had similar but milder electrocardiographic changes. They considered this a 'new' disorder. See 31320 for discussion of other forms of X-linked spinal muscular atrophy.

Mawatori, S. and Katayama, K.: Scapulohumeral muscular atrophy with cardiomyopathy. An X-linked recessive trait. Arch. Neurol. 28: 55-59,,1973.

*31285 SCAPULOPERONEAL SYNDROME

Thomas et al. (1972) described a kindred with typical X-linked inheritance of a myopathy manifesting as muscular weakness and wasting, affecting predominantly the proximal muscles of the legs. Accompanying features were contractures of the elbows, pes cavus and in adulthood cardiomyopathy. Pseudohypotrophy was absent. Close linkage with deutan colorblindness was found. The authors pointed out similarities to the benign type of muscular dystrophy with contracture (31030) but thought that the distribution of muscular involvement distinguished the two. Rotthauwe et al. (1972) observed 17 affected males in 3 generations of a Bavarian family.

Rotthauwe, H. W., Mortier, W. and Beyer, H.: Neuer Typ einer recessiv X-chromosomal vererbten Muskeldystrophie: scapulo-humero-distale Muskeldystrophie mit fruhzeitigen Kontrakturen und Herzrhythmusstorungen. Humangenetik 16: 181-200, 1972.

Thomas, P. K., Calne, D. B. and Elliott, C. F.: X-linked scapuloperoneal syndrome. J. Neurol. Neurosurg. Psychiatry 35: 208-215, 1972.

31287 SIMPSON DYSMORPHIA SYNDROME ('BULLDOG SYNDROME')

In two males, sons of sisters, Simpson et al. (1973) observed a 'new' dysmorphism with the following features: broad stocky appearance, distinctive facies (large protruding jaw, widened nasal bridge, upturned nasal tip), enlarged tongue, and broad and short hands and fingers. Intelligence was normal. The family referred to his appearance as 'bulldog' like. In infancy hypothyroidism was suggested but excluded by laboratory tests. Close linkage with the Xg blood group locus was excluded.

Simpson, J. L., New, M., Landey, S. and German, J.: A previously unrecognized X-linked syndrome of dysmorphia. In, Clinical Delineation of Birth Defects. XVII. Malformation Syndromes (cont.). Baltimore: Williams and Wilkins, 1973.

*31290 SPASTIC PARAPLEGIA

Spastic paraplegia is an autosomal dominant in many families, an autosomal recessive in many others. The family of Johnston and McKusick (1962) showed X-linked recessive inheritance. Wolfslast's family (1943), with what he termed spastic diplegia, is another possible example. One affected male was living at age 50 and a second at age 20. Nystagmus was described in a female carrier. Professor P. E. Becker of Gottingen is of the opinion, however, that Wolfslast's family suffered from the Pelizaeus-Merzbacher syndrome, and Verschuer in his textbook states the same opinion. A more likely case of X-linked spastic paraplegia is that of Blumel et al. (1957). Early onset, slow progression, and long survival with eventual involvement of the cerebellum, cerebral cortex and optic nerves are features of the X-linked form as observed by Johnston and McKusick. Thurmon et al. (1971) has studied two kindreds rather extensively affected with probable X-linked spastic paraplegia. Ginter et al. (1974) had an opportunity to examine the central nervous system at autopsy in one patient from the Johnston-McKusick kindred. Degeneration of both corticospinal and spinocerebellar traits was found. Many but not all of the affected members showed cerebellar signs. Raggio et al. (1973) reported a kindred with 10 affected males in 7 sibships widely separated in a kindred. Nixon and Conneally (1968) described hind-leg paralysis as an X-linked trait in the Syrian hamster. This may be homologous to X-linked spastic paraplegia in man. Follow-up with autopsy information was given by Ginter et al. (1974).

Blumel, J., Evans, E. B. and Eggers, G. W. N.: Hereditary cerebral palsy. A preliminary report. J. Pediatr. 50: 454-458, 1957.

Ginter, D. N., Konigsmark, B. A. and Abbott, M. H.: X-linked spinocerebellar degeneration. In, Bergsma, D. (ed.): Clinical Delineation of Birth Defects. XVI. Urinary System and Others. Baltimore: Williams and Wilkins, 1974. Pp. 334-336.

Johnston, A. W. and McKusick, V. A.: A sex-linked recessive inheritance of spastic paraplegia. Am. J. Hum. Genet. 14: 83-94, 1962.

Nixon, C. W. and Conneally, M. E.: Hind-leg paralysis: a new sex-linked mutation in the Syrian hamster. J. Hered. 59: 276-278, 1968.

Raggio, J. F., Thurmon, T. F. and Anderson, E. E.: X-linked hereditary spastic paraplegia. J. La. State Med. Soc. 125: 4-6, 1973.

Thurmon, T. F., Walker, B. A., Scott, C. I. and Abbott, M. H.: Two kindreds with a sex-linked recessive form of spastic paraplegia. The Clinical Delineation of Birth Defects. VI. Nervous System. Baltimore: Williams and Wilkins, 1971. Pp. 219-221.

Wolfslast, W.: Eine Sippe mit recessiver geschlechtsgebundener spastischer Diplegie. Z. Menschl. Vererb. Konstitutionsl. 27: 189-198, 1943.

31300 SPATIAL VISUALIZATION, APTITUDE FOR

Stafford (1961), using the identical blocks test as a measure of spatial visualization, studied 104 fathers and mothers and their 58 teen-age sons and 70 daughters. Males showed higher average scores than females in both the paternal and offspring group. No correlation of scores existed between fathers and mothers and none between fathers and sons. The correlations between fathers and daughters, between mothers and sons and between mothers and daughters was what would be expected on the assumption that the aptitude for visualizing space is an X-linked recessive trait. Garron (1970) pointed out that if spatial and numerical abilities are determined by an X-linked recessive gene patients with Turner syndrome should show superior inheritance.

Bock, R. D. and Kolakowski, D.: Further evidence of sex-linked major gene influence on human spatial visualizing ability. Am. J. Hum. Genet. 25: 1-14, 1973.

Garron, D. C.: Sex-linked, recessive inheritance of spatial and numerical abilities, and Turner's syndrome. Psychol. Rev. 77: 147-152, 1970.

Stafford, R. E.: Sex differences in spatial visualization as evidence of sex-linked inheritance. Percept. Mot. Skills 13: 428 only, 1961.

31310 SPIEGLER-BROOKE TUMORS

The demonstration, in the same patients and same families, of cylindroma as described by Spiegler and of epithelioma adenoides cysticum as described by Brooke supports their genetic identity (Guggenheim and Schnyder, 1961). (See EPITHELIOMA, HEREDITARY BENIGN CYSTIC, in dominant catalog for further discussion of nosology.) Schmidt-Baumler (1931) raised the question of X-linked dominant inheritance. The pedigree of Blandy and colleagues (1961) showed an affected male who had all daughters affected and all sons unaffected. Up to the end of 1954, Evans found 47 reported cases, of which 30 were female. Guggenheim and Schnyder found that 132 of 212 reported cases were in females. However, against X-linkage is the fact that male-to-male transmission has been frequently observed. We have one pedigree with at least nine affected persons and at least one instance of male-to-male transmission. The disorder is probably an autosomal dominant with stronger expression in the female. Stronger expression in presumed heterozygous females than in hemizygous males is contrary to what is expected in X-linked dominant inheritance. The possibility of X-linkage in a small proportion of families is not completely excluded, however.

Blandy, J. P., Gammie, W. F. P., Stovin, P. G. I. and Swettenham, K.: Turban tumours in brother and sister. Br. J. Surg. 49: 136-140, 1961.

Chalstrey, L. J.: Turban tumors. St. Bart's Hosp. J. 59: 378-383, 1955.

Evans, C. D.: Turban tumour. Br. J. Dermatol. 66: 434-443, 1954.

Guggenheim, W. and Schnyder, U. W.: Zur Nosologie der Spiegler-Brookeschen Tumoren. Dermatologica 122: 274-278, 1961.

Regan, W. J.: Turban tumours. Proc. R. Soc. Med. 49: 337-339, 1956.

Schmidt-Baumler, H.: Familiares Cylindrome. Ein Beitrag zur Frage der geschlechtsbegrenzten Vererbung. Arch. Dermatol. Syph. 163: 114-125, 1931.

Wiedmann, A.: Weitere Beitrage zur Kenntnis der sogenannten Zylindrome der Kopfhaut. Arch. Dermatol. Syph. 159: 180-187, 1929.

*31320 SPINAL AND BULBAR MUSCULAR ATROPHY

Kennedy, Alter and Sung (1968) described 9 males in two unrelated kindreds. Onset of fasciculations followed by muscle weakness and wasting occurred at approximately 40 years of age. Bulbar signs and facial fasciculations were characteristic. Dysphagia persisted more than 10 years in one man of each family. Babinski sign was negative in all. The disorder is compatible with long life. Pyramidal, sensory and cerebellar signs were absent. Three of their patients had gynecomastia. Japanese families reported by Tsukagoshi et al. (1965) and some other isolated cases (Smith and Patel, 1965) may have had the same disorder. Infantile muscular atrophy (Werding-Hoffman disease) is an autosomal recessive. Juvenile hereditary proximal spinal muscular atrophy begins in childhood or adolescence and is slowly progressive usually without bulbar involvement. Inheritance is either autosomal recessive or autosomal dominant. The proband in Murakami's family (1957) was a 55-year-old Japanese farmer. Kurland (1957) mentioned two families seen by him in Japan. Quarfordt et al. (1970) described four brothers with adult-onset proximal spinal muscular atrophy. Type II hyperlipoproteinemia was present in all four and was absent from their one unaffected sib, a sister. Some children of affected males, too young to show the neurologic abnormality, also showed hyperlipoproteinemia. Mawatari and Katayama (1973) reported a family demonstrating juvenile onset scapulohumeroperoneal neurogenic muscular weakness and atrophy with cardiopathy. The affected were 5 Japanese males of the same generation related through the maternal line. The authors proposed X-linked recessive inheritance for this condition. The first symptom in all, shortening of the Achilles tendon at age 7 to 10, was followed by symmetrical scapulohumeroperoneal muscle weakness and limited neck flexion due to atrophy of posterior nuchal muscles. EMG testing showed neurogenic abnormalities with normal nerve conduction velocities suggesting a motor neuron problem. Only one patient showed fasciculations and all presented normal sensation, pyramidal, cerebellar and bulbar functions. Tendon reflexes were decreased. The cardiac involvement included bradycardia and ECG abnormalities with conduction defects and left axis deviation. These patients showed no symptoms of these heart problems. The maternal grandmother and two mothers (assumed carriers) of the affected males proved to have ECG abnormalities similar to, but less severe than their sons. Takahashi (1971) reported the same disorder in two brothers. The relationship of this disorder to other reported X-linked muscular atrophies is not certain.

Kennedy, W. R., Alter, M. and Sung, J. H.: Progressive proximal spinal and bulbar muscular atrophy of late onset: a sex-linked recessive trait. Neurology 18: 671-680, 1968.

Kurland, L. T.: Epidemiologic investigations of amyotrophic lateral sclerosis. III. A genetic interpretation of incidence and geographic distribution. Mayo Clin. Proc. 32: 449-462, 1957.

Lee, G. R., MacDiarmid, W. D., Cartwright, G. E. and Wintrobe, M. M.: Hereditary, X-linked, sideroachrestic anemia. The isolation of two erythrocyte populations differing in Xg(A) blood type and porphyrin content. Blood 32: 59-70, 1968.

Mawatari, S. and Katayama, K.: Scapuloperoneal muscular atrophy with cardiopathy, an X-linked recessive trait. Arch. Neurol. 28: 55-59, 1973.

Murakami, U.: Clinico-genetic study of hereditary disorders of the nervous system, especially on problems of pathogenesis. Folia Psychiat. Neurol. Jap. 1 (suppl.): 1-209, 1957.

Quarfordt, S. H., Devivo, D. C., Engel, W. K., Levy, R. I. and Fredrickson, D. S.: Familial adult-onset proximal spinal muscular atrophy. Arch. Neurol. 22: 541-549, 1970.

Smith, J. B. and Patel, A.: The Wohlfart-Kugelberg-Welander disease: review of the literature and report of a case. Neurology 15: 469-473, 1965.

Takahashi, K.: Clin. Neurol. 11: 650-658, 1971.

Takikawa, K.: A pedigree of progressive bulbar paralysis appearing in sex-linked recessive inheritance. Jap. J. Hum. Genet. 28: 116 only, 1953.

Tsukagoshi, H., Nakanishi, T., Kondo, K. and Tsubaki, T.: Hereditary, proximal, neurogenic muscular atrophy in adult. Arch. Neurol. 12: 597-603, 1965.

*31330 SPINAL ATAXIA

A kindred with X-linked inheritance of what the authors thought was probably Friedreich ataxia was reported by Turner and Roberts (1938). Onset was at about five years and the victim was bedfast by about 20 years. The first carrier female in the kindred was of English extraction. In 1910 Brandenberg described four males with Friedreich ataxia in three generations of a family, related through females in a pattern consistent with X-linkage.

Brandenberg, F.: Kasuistische Beitrage zur gleichgeschlechtlichen Vererbung. Arch. Rass.-u. Ges. Biol. 7: 290-305, 1910.

Turner, E. V. and Roberts, E.: A family with a sex-linked hereditary ataxia. J. Nerv. Ment. Dis. 87: 74-80, 1938.

*31340 SPONDYLOEPIPHYSEAL DYSPLASIA, LATE

The trunk is particularly short and the hips show degenerative disease. Changes in the spine and hips become evident between 10 and 14 years of age. In adults vertebral changes, especially in the lumbar region, are diagnostic. Ochronosis is suggested by apparent intervertebral disk calcification. In fact, the vertebral bodies are malformed and flattened and most of the dense area is part of the vertebral plate.

Barber, H. S.: An unusual form of familial osteodystrophy. Lancet I: 1220-1221: and II: 154-155, 1960.

Bannerman, R. M.: X-linked spondyloepiphyseal dysplasia tarda (SDT). The Clinical Delineation of Birth Defects. IV. Skeletal Dysplasias. New York: National Foundation, 1969. Pp. 48-51.

Bannerman, R. M., Ingall, G. B. and Mohn, J. F.: X-linked spondyloepiphyseal dysplasia tarda: clinical and linkage data. J. Med. Genet. 8: 291-301, 1971.

Hobaek, A.: Problems of Hereditary Chondrodysplasia. Oslo, Norway: Oslo U. Press, 1961.

Jacobsen, A. W.: Hereditary osteochondro-dystrophia deformans. A family with twenty members affected in five generations. J.A.M.A. 113: 121-124, 1939.

Lamy, M. and Maroteaux, P.: Les chondrodystrophies genotypiques. Paris: L'Expansion, 1960. Pp. 67ff.

Langer, L. O., Jr.: Spondyloepiphyseal dysplasia tarda. Hereditary chondrodysplasia with characteristic vertebral configuration in the adult. Radiology 82: 833-839, 1964.

Maroteaux, P., Lamy, M. and Bernard, J.: La dysplasie spondylo-epiphysaire tardive. Presse Med. 65: 1205-1208, 1957.

31350 TEETH, ABSENCE OF

Erpenstein and Pfeiffer (1967) described transmission of oligodontia or hypodontia through four generations of a family. Males had oligodontia, females had hypodontia. No male-to-male transmission was observed. However, only two affected males had children (4 unaffected sons, 1 daughter with hypodontia). X-linkage is likely. In at least 18 persons in 4 generations Dahlberg (1937) noted absence of at least six anterior teeth in both dentitions. He suggested X-linked dominant inheritance, but against this is one unaffected daughter of the one affected male with children in the kindred.

Dahlberg, A. A.: Inherited congenital absence of six incisors, deciduous and permanent. J. Dent. Res. 16: 59-62, 1937.

Erpenstein, H. and Pfeiffer, R. A.: Geschlechsgebunden-dominant erbliche Zahnunterzahl. Humangenetik 4: 280-293, 1967.

31360 TELECANTHUS WITH ASSOCIATED ABNORMALITIES

Ocular hypertelorism is often incorrectly diagnosed when a flat nasal bridge, epicanthal folds, external strabismus, widely spaced eyebrows, blepharophimosis or some combination of these is present. Telecanthus is a preferable term when increased distance separates the inner canthi. Dystopia canthorum is a synonym. Christian et al. (1969) and Opitz et al. (1969) reported, in all, four families in which telecanthus with or without hypertelorism was associated in males with hypospadias, cryptorchidism, cleft lip and palate, urinary malformations, and in some mental retardation. Female carriers have less severe telecanthus and escaped congenital malformation. Except for one alleged and unconfirmed instance in a remote branch of one of the families of Opitz et al., no male-to-male transmission was observed. Thus X-linked inheritance is possible. Michaelis and Mortier (1972) described a case. Hypospadias and hypertelorism were features of two brothers who had osteochondritis dissecans at multiple sites as described in the recessive catalog. (See HYPERTELORISM, CRYPTORCHIDISM, etc., 23970,)

Christian, J. C., Bixler, D., Blythe, S. C. and Merritt, A. D.: Familial telecanthus with associated congenital anomalies. The Clinical Delineation of Birth Defects. II. Malformation Syndromes. New York: National Foundation, 1969. Pp. 82-85.

Michaelis, E. and Mortier, W.: Association of hypertelorism and hypospadias-the BBB-syndrome. Helv. Paediat. Acta 27: 575-581, 1972.

Opitz, J. M., Summitt, R. L. and Smith, D. W.: The BBB syndrome. Familial telecanthus with associated congenital anomalies. The Clinical Delineation of Birth Defects. II. Malformation Syndromes. New York: National Foundation, 1969. Pp. 86-94.

*31370 TESTICULAR FEMINIZATION SYNDROME

This variety of sex anomaly has been of relatively long interest to geneticists largely through the publications of Pettersson and Bonnier (1937). Both the nature of the basic defect and the mode of inheritance are in question. The affected males have female external genitalia, female breast development, blind vagina, absent uterus and female adnexa, abdominal or inguinal testes, and a normal male $(2A+XY)$ karyotype. The patients often come to medical attention because of a presumed inguinal hernia. Many have absent pubic and axillary hair ('hairless pseudofemale'). The hair of the head is luxuriant, without temporal balding. The phenotype is often voluptuously feminine: Netter (1958) reported this disorder in a famous photographic model, Marshall and Harder (1958) reported affected monozygotic twins who worked as airline stewardesses, and Polaillon (1891) described prostitution in an affected person.

In one such patient studied by Wilkins (1957) the hair follicles of the axillary and pubic areas, although anatomically normal, were unresponsive to local or parenteral administration of androgens and the beard, voice, and clitoris were similarly unresponsive. Female carriers, presumed heterozygotes, may show no, or almost no, secondary sex hair but have normal menstruation, conception and pregnancies. The basic defect in cases of the hairless pseudofemale type might be end-organ unresponsiveness to androgen, a situation comparable to nephrogenic diabetes insipidus, and pseudohypoparathyroidism (inherited as an autosomal dominant). (These conditions are analogous to the situation in the Seabright Bantam Cock which has a female comb structure despite obvious demonstrations of virility.) It is likely that more than one distinct entity is included in the testicular feminization syndrome. Wilkins states: 'in about one-third of the cases of male pseudohermaphroditism 'of feminine type' sexual hair has been entirely lacking.' Miller considers 'feminizing labial testes' of the type described by Lubs, Vilar and Bergenstal (1959) to be a separate form of male pseudohermaphroditism.

The histological changes in the testis in this syndrome tend to be characteristic and not the non-specific ones of cryptorchidism. Furthermore, the degree of feminization appears to be correlated with the degree of change in the testis.

Whether the trait is X-linked or autosomal is uncertain. The evidence from linkage studies is inconclusive.

Mainly using data on the frequency of inguinal hernia in females, Jagiello and Atwell (1962) estimated the frequency of testicular feminization as being of the order of one in 65,000 males. This value implies a mutation rate of $0.5-0.4 \times 10^{-5}$ genes per generation (depending on whether the disorder is autosomal dominant or X-linked recessive).

Professor J. M. Morris, Yale University, called my attention to the following case of Gayral and colleagues (1960): a woman, who was sister, mother, and grandmother of affected males, showed asymmetry in the development of the breasts, body hair, and vulva. The right breast was smaller than the left and there was no pubic hair to the right of the mid-line. She had always had menstrual irregularity but had three children, an affected male, a carrier daughter, and a daughter who was the mother of three unaffected sons. The findings may be best explained by an X-linked recessive (or incompletely recessive) gene whose effects are to render tissues resistant to male hormone. The patchy changes in the heterozygous female suggest, furthermore, that the causative gene is X-linked with Lyonization phenomenon.

French et al. (1966) found that testosterone failed to affect the urinary excretion of nitrogen, phosphorus and citric acid when given in a dosage much greater than that which in controls decreased excretion of all three. Conversion of testosterone to estrogen does not occur, it seems. Plasma estrogen levels were those observed in the normal female. Leydig cell stimulation to estrogen production occurs probably because of failure of the feed-back repression of the pituitary which shares the unresponsiveness to testosterone. Southern et al. (1961) showed normal testosterone levels. The means for establishing X-linked inheritance included demonstration of linkage with an X chromosome marker, demonstration of Lyonization in heterozygous females and demonstration that the proportion of new mutation cases is one third rather than one-half (expected of an autosomal dominant). Possibly by artificial insemination methods, X-linked inheritance could be tested in the testicular feminization of cattle (Nes, 1966). Lyon and Hawkes (1970) described a homologous phenotype in the mouse and showed that it is genetic, the Tfm locus being situated in the middle of the X chromosome. Ohno and Lyon (1970) showed that in these mice certain enzymes of the mouse kidney, e.g., alcohol dehydrogenase, are not inducible as is usually possible. They postulated that the Tfm locus is a repressive regulatory locus controlling many testosterone inducible enzymes. In affected hemizygotes all these enzymes become non-inducible. According to their suggestion, this is a regulator mutation like the non-inducible mutation in the lac-repressor locus of E. coli as elucidated by Jacob and Monod (1963). Bardin et al. (1970) described studies of the pseudohermaphroditic rat which seems to have a disorder analogous to testicular feminization. Androgen-dependent differentiation is absent. Defective formation of dihydrotestosterone was apparently not the explanation.

Clinically cases of incomplete, or partial, testicular feminization are recognized. These differ from the classic 'complete' form in the presence of enlarged clitoris at birth and virilization at puberty. Familial occurrence has been observed. Goldstein and Wilson (1972) studied the Tfm mouse and showed that there is resistence to androgen-mediated sexual differentiation in embryos by giving dihydrotestosterone to pregnant mothers. Low serum testosterone and low production of testosterone in adult Tfm testis of the mouse was a feature different from man, but was considered by them as secondary to the defect in differentiation. They showed deficient binding of testosterone in the nuclei of the submaxillary gland of these adult Tfm animals, but again this may be the result of incomplete differentiation of an androgen-sensitive cell line. A defect in 5 alpha-reduction of testosterone to dihydrotestosterone (DTH) in TF seems unlikely because of the failure of response by patients to administered DTH and because the disorder in the mouse, which seems to be homologous, has a different defect. Shanies et al. (1972) found deficiency of the reductase in fibroblasts cultured from perineal skin of a TF patient. B. Migeon (1974) found two clones of fibroblasts in heterozygous females, one with androgen-binding and one without, thus clinching the X-linkage of this disorder. Bullock and Bardin (1972) concluded that androgen-binding proteins are absent from the cytosol of preputial gland of Tfm rats and from the kidney of Tfm mice.

Adachi, K. and Kano, M.: Adenyl cyclase in human hair follicles: its inhibition by dihydrotestosterone. Biochem. Biophys. Res. Commun. 41: 884-890, 1970.

Albright, F., Burnett, C. H., Smith, P. H. and Parson, W.: Pseudo-hypoparathyroidism, an example of 'Seabright-Bantam syndrome.' Report of 3 cases. Endocrinology 30: 922-932, 1942.

Bardin, C. W., Bullock, L., Schneider, G., Allison, J. E. and Stanley, A. J.: Pseudohermaphrodite rat: end organ insensitivity to testosterone. Science 167: 1136-1137, 1970.

Bullock, L. P. and Bardin, C. W.: Androgen receptors in testicular feminization. J. Clin. Endocrinol. Metab. 35: 935-937, 1972.

Burgermeister, J. J.: Contribution a l'etude d'un type familial d'intersexualite. J. Genet. Hum. 2: 51-82, 1953.

French, F. S., Baggett, B., Van Wyk, J. J., Talbert, L. M., Hubbard, W. R., Johnston, F. R., Weaver, R. P., Forchielli, E., Rao, G. S. and Sarda, I. R.: Testicular feminization: clinical, morphological and biochemical studies. J. Clin. Endocrinol. 25: 661-677, 1965.

French, F. S., Van Wyk, J. J., Baggett, B., Easterling, W. E., Talbert, L. M., Johnston, F. R. and Forchielli, E.: Further evidence of a target organ defect in the syndrome of testicular feminization. J. Clin. Endocrinol. Metab. 26: 493-503, 1966.

Gayral, L., Barraud, M., Carrie, J. and Candebat, L.: Pseudo-hermaphrodisme a type de 'testicule feminisant': 11 cas. Etude hormonale et etude psychologique. Toulouse Med. 61: 637-647, 1960.

Goldstein, J. L. and Wilson, J. D.: Studies on the pathogenesis of the pseudohermaphroditism in the mouse with testucular feminization. J. Clin. Invest. 51: 1647-1658, 1972.

Grumbach, M. M. and Barr, M. L.: Cytologic tests of chromosomal sex in relation to sexual anomalies in man. Recent Progr. Horm. Res. 14: 255-334, 1958.

Hauser, G. A.: Testikulare Feminisierung. In: die Intersexualitat. Overzier, C. (Ed.): Stuttgart: Georg Thieme Verlag, 1961. Pp. 261-282.

Jacob, F. and Monod, J.: General repression, allosteric inhibition, and cellular differentiation. In, Locke, M. (ed.): Cytodifferentiation and Macromolecular Synthesis. London: Academic Press, 1963. Pp. 30-64.

Jagiello, G., and Atwell, J. D.: Prevalence of testicular feminisation. Lancet I: 329 only, 1962.

Keenan, B. S., Meyer, W. .J., III, Hadjian, A. J., Jones, H. W. and Migeon, C. J.: Syndrome of androgen insensitivity in man: absence of 5-alpha-dihydrotestosterone binding protein in skin fibroblasts. J. Clin. Endocrinol. Metab. 38: 11431146, 1974.

Lubs, H. A., Jr., Vilar, O. and Bergenstal, D. M.: Familial male pseudohermaphroditism with labial testes and partial feminization: endocrine studies and genetic aspects. J. Clin. Endocrinol. Metab. 19: 1110-1120, 1959.

Lyon, M. F. and Hawkes, S. G.: X-linked gene for testicular feminization in the mouse. Nature 225: 1217-1219, 1970.

Marshall, H. K. and Harder, H. I.: Testicular feminizing syndrome in male pseudohermaphrodite: report of two cases in identical twins. Obstet. Gynec. 12: 284-293, 1958.

Mauvais-Jarvis, P., Bercovici, J. P., Crepy, O. and Gauthier, F.: Studies on testosterone metabolism in subjects with testicular feminization syndrome. J. Clin. Invest. 49: 31-40, 1970.

Migeon, B. R.: Baltimore, personal communication, July, 1974.

Miller, O. J.: Developmental sex abnormalities. In, Penrose, L. S. (ed.): Recent Advances in Human Genetics. London: J. and A. Churchill Ltd., 1961. Pp. 39-55.

X

L
I
N
K
E
D

Nes, N.: Testikulaer feminisering hos storfe. Nord. Med. 18: 19-29, 1966.

Northcutt, R. C., Island, D. P. and Liddle, G. W.: An explanation for the target organ unresponsiveness to testosterone in the testicular feminization syndrome. J. Clin. Endocrinol. Metab. 29: 422-425, 1969.

Ohno, S. and Lyon, M. F.: X-linked testicular feminization in the mouse as a non-inducible regulatory mutation of the Jacob-Monod type. Clin. Genet. 1: 121-127, 1970.

Ohno, S.: Simplicity of mammalian regulatory systems inferred by single gene determination of sex phenotypes. Nature 234: 134-137, 1971.

Pettersson, G. and Bonnier, G.: Inherited sex-mosaic in man. Hereditas 23: 49-69, 1937.

Puck, T. T., Robinson, A. and Tjio, J. H.: Familial primary amenhorrhea due to testicular feminization: a human gene affecting sex differentiation. Proc. Soc. Exp. Biol. Med. 103: 192-196, 1960.

Schreiner, W. E.: Uber eine hereditare Form von Pseudohermaphrodismus masculinus (testiculare Feminisierung). Gynaecologia 148: 355-357, 1959.

Shanies, D. D., Hirschhorn, K. and New, M. I.: Metabolism of testosterone-14C by cultured human cells. J. Clin. Invest. 51: 1459-1468, 1972.

Southern, A. L. and Saito, A.: The syndrome of testicular feminization. A report of three cases with chromatographic analysis of the urinary neutral 17-ketosteroids. Ann. Intern. Med. 55: 925-931, 1961.

Southern, A. L.: The syndrome of testicular feminization. In, Levine, R. and Luft, R. (eds.): Advances in Metabolic Diseases. New York: Academic Press, 1965. Pp. 227-256.

Stenchever, M. A., Ng, A. B. P., Jones, G. K. and Jarvis, J. A.: Testicular feminization syndrome. Chromosomal, histologic, and genetic studies in a large kindred. Obstet. Gynec. 33: 649-657, 1969.

Strickland, A. L. and French, F. S.: Absence of response to dihydrotestosterone in the syndrome of testicular feminization. J. Clin. Endocrinol. Metab. 29: 1284-1286, 1969.

Wilkins, L.: The Diagnosis and Treatment of Endocrine Disorders in Childhood and Adolescence. Springfield, Ill.: Charles C Thomas, 1957 (2nd Ed.).

31380 TESTICULAR FEMINIZATION, INCOMPLETE TYPE

This syndrome resembles the complete form in respect to female phenotype, bilateral testes and 46, XY karyotype, but differs by clitoral enlargement from birth and virilization at puberty. The labia may be partially fused. Although the degree of masculinization of the external genitalia is variable, most patients are raised as females. The testes resembles those of complete testicular feminization. In the family described by Lubs et al. (1959) some spermatogenesis was found. There is partial responsiveness to androgen (Winterborn et al. (1970). Although X-linked recessive or male-limited autosomal dominant inheritance is suggested by some pedigrees such as that of Lubs et al. (1959), an autosomal recessive form (q.v.) may exist also. However, it is difficult to distinguish the incomplete testicular feminization syndrome from pseudovaginal perineoscrotal hypospadias (26460) which is clearly autosomal recessive. Boczkowski and Teter (1965) described 3 cases among the children of two sisters.

Boczkowski, K. and Teter, J.: Familial male pseudohermaphroditism. Acta Endocrinol. 49: 497-509, 1965.

Lubs, H. A., Jr., Vilar, O. and Bergenstal, D. M.: Familial male pseudohermaphroditism with labial testes and partial feminization: endocrine studies and genetic aspects. J. Clin. Endocrinol. Metab. 19: 1110-1120, 1959.

Winterborn, M. H., France, N. E. and Raiti, S.: Incomplete testicular feminization. Arch. Dis. Child. 45: 811-812, 1970.

*31390 THROMBOCYTOPENIA

Vestermark and Vestermark (1964) found X-linked 'essential' thrombocytopenia in two generations of a family. One affected male became symptom-free spontaneously after puberty and one became symptom-free after splenectomy at the age of 18 years but died later of adrenal hemorrhage. Three other patients had, in addition to hemorrhagic diathesis, a mild tendency to infection and eczema. This condition may be distinct from Aldrich syndrome (q.v.). In addition to Aldrich syndrome and separate from it, a probable X-linked thrombocytopenia has been described by Ata, Fisher, and Holman (1965) in 9 males in 6 sibships in 4 generations of a kindred, connected by females. In addition one female was affected. She was karyologically normal and the father had no history of bleeding. Therefore, she probably represents unfortunate Lyonization. She differed from the affected males in recovering spontaneously. Canales and Mauer (1967) studied a family containing 7 thrombocytopenic males in an X-linked recessive pedigree pattern. Although no eczema or undue susceptibility to infection was noted and bleeding symptoms were mild, 5 of the 7 showed reduced or absent isohemagglutinins and increased gamma-A globulin. In the 13 affected members of the kindred reported by Chiaro et al. (1972) bleeding had its onset at about age 6 years and spontaneous remission of 'bleeding' but not of thrombocytopenia occurred in early adult life.

Ata, M., Fisher, O. D. and Holman, C. A.: Inherited thrombocytopenia. Lancet I: 119-123, 1965.

Canales, L. and Mauer, A. M.: Sex-linked hereditary thrombocytopenia as a variant of Wiskott-Aldrich syndrome. N. Engl. J. Med. 277: 899-901, 1967.

Chiaro, J. J., Dharmkrong-At, A. and Bloom, G. E.: X-linked thrombocytopenic purpura. I. Clinical and genetic studies of a kindred. Am. J. Dis. Child. 123: 565-568, 1972.

662   Vestermark, B. and Vestermark, S.: Familial sex-linked thrombocytopenia. Acta Pediat. 53: 365-370, 1964.

31400 THROMBOCYTOPENIA WITH ELEVATED SERUM IGA AND RENAL DISEASE

Gutenberger et al. (1970) described a kindred in which 10 males and two females had thrombocytopenia apparently as a result of reduced platelet production. Eight of the thrombocytopenic persons had elevated IgA levels in the serum. Renal biopsy in three thrombocytopenic brothers with hematuria showed varying degrees of glomerulonephritis. The two thrombocytopenic women were mothers of affected sons. One of these two women also had elevated IgA. The authors concluded that the disorder is X linked and probably distinct from the Wiskott-Aldrich syndrome and from 'simple' X-linked thrombocytopenia.

Gutenberger, J., Trygstad, C. W., Stiehm, E. R., Opitz, J. M., Thatcher, L. G. and Bloodworth, J. M. B., Jr.: Familial thrombocytopenia, elevated serum IgA levels and renal disease. A report of a kindred. Am. J. Med. 49: 729-741, 1970.

31410 THUMB, CONGENITAL CLASPED

In this disorder the thumb is adducted and flexed across the palm due to a defect in the extensors of the thumb. Weckesser et al. (1968) described an interesting Negro family in which 7 males in 4 sibships were affected. The pattern was entirely consistent with X-linked recessive inheritance. Findings in children and grandchildren of affected males were not described. White and Jensen (1952) observed the anomaly in mother and two children and Namba et al. (1965) described it in brother and sister. A preponderance of affected males (27 out of 42) is consistent with X-linkage, especially when the likely heterogeneity of congenital clasped thumb is taken into account. (Weckesser et al. (1968) classified their cases in 4 groups.) Clasped thumb occurs in some families with X-linked hydrocephalus due to stenosis of the aqueduct of Sylvius (q.v.).

Namba, K., Muda, Y. and Hachiguchi, T.: Congenital clasped thumb. Orthop. Surg. 16: 1031-1035, 1965.

Weckesser, E. C., Reed, J. R. and Heiple, K. G.: Congenital clasped thumb (congenital flexion-adduction deformity of the thumb). A syndrome, not a specific entity. J. Bone Joint Surg. 50A: 1417-1428, 1968.

White, J. W. and Jensen, W. E.: The infant's persistent thumb-clutched hand. J. Bone Joint Surg. 34A: 680-688, 1952.

*31420 THYROXINE-BINDING GLOBULIN (TBG) OF SERUM, VARIANTS OF

Thyroxine-binding globulin is reduced so that patients show reduced protein bound iodine (PBI) but are euthyroid. Nicoloff, Dowling and Patton (1964) observed 6 cases (3 males, 3 females) in 3 sibships of two generations of a family. No male-to-male transmission was observed. Nikolai and Seal (1966) studied two families in which X-linkage is possible. Marshall, Levy and Steinberg (1966) described an extensively studied family in which the findings were most consistent with X-linkage. Female carriers showed an intermediate level of TBG. With a mutation, presumably at the same locus, an increase in TBG can occur. Because of increase in total binding globulin protein-bound iodine is increased in four persons in three generations. The pedigree pattern was equally consistent with autosomal and X-linked dominance. Beierwaltes and Robbins (1959) found high TBG in a father and his only daughter. Both his sons had normal TBG levels. The daughter's level was not as high as the father's. Thus in this family also X-linked dominance was suggested. Jones and Seal (1967) reported a family with elevated TBG in 9 persons in 3 generations, again in a pattern suggesting X-linkage. They suggested gene duplication as the mechanism of the elevation. X-linked inheritance was strongly supported by the findings of deficiency of TBG in a patient with the XO Turner syndrome (Refetoff and Selenkow, 1968). The maternal grandfather and a half brother were also TBG-deficient and at least 3 females, including the mother, had intermediate levels. Kraemer and Wiswell (1968) presented suggestive but not conclusive evidence of autosomal transmission and some other published pedigrees are consistent with this mode. Thorson et al. (1966) presented evidence for two thyroid-binding globulins, thus creating the possibility of appreciable genetic heterogeneity in both high and low TBG. For a review, see Rivas et al. (1971). Avruskin et al. (1972) found associated retarded mental and motor development in 4 males in 3 sibships in a pattern consistent with X-linked recessive inheritance. They suggested close linkage of two separate mutant loci but an allele at the TBG locus with the neurologic features as a pleiotropic effect would seem at least equally possible.

Avruskin, T. W., Braverman, L. E. and Crigler, J. F.: Thyroxine-binding globulin deficiency and associated neurological deficit. Pediatrics 50: 638-645, 1972.

Beierwaltes, W. H. and Robbins, J.: Familial increase in thyroxine binding sites in serum alpha globulin. J. Clin. Invest. 38: 1683-1688, 1959.

Fialkow, P. J., Giblett, E. R. and Musa, B.: Increased serum thyroxine-binding globulin capacity: inheritance and linkage relationships. J. Clin. Endocrinol. Metab. 30: 66-70, 1970.

Florsheim, W. H., Dowling, J. T., Meister, L. and Bodfish, R. E.: Familial elevation of serum thyroxine-binding capacity. J. Clin. Enocrinol. Metab. 22: 735-740, 1962.

Jones, J. E. and Seal, U. S.: X-chromosome linked inheritance of elevated thyroxine-binding globulin. J. Clin. Endocrinol. Metab. 27: 1521-1528, 1967.

Kraemer, E. and Wiswell, J. G.: Familial thyroxine-binding globulin deficiency. Metabolism 17: 260-262, 1968.

Malvaux, P. and De Nayer, P.: X-chromosome linked inheritance of decreased thyroxine-binding globulin. Arch. Dis. Child. 47: 635-638, 1972.

Marshall, J. S., Levy, R. P. and Steinberg, A. G.: Human thyroxine-binding globulin deficiency. A genetic study. N. Engl. J. Med. 274: 1469-1473, 1966.

X

L
I
N
K
E
D

Nicoloff, J. T., Dowling, J. T. and Patton, D. D.: Inheritance of decreased thyroxine-binding by the thyroxine-binding globulin. J. Clin. Endocrinol. Metab.24: 294-298, 1964.

Nikolai, T. F. and Seal, U. S.: X-chromosome linked familial decrease in thyroxine-binding globulin activity. J. Clin. Endocrinol. Metab. 26: 835-841, 1966.

Nikolai, T. F. and Seal, U. S.: X-chromosome linked inheritance of thyroxine-binding globulin deficiency. J. Clin. Endocrinol. Metab. 27: 1515-1520, 1967.

Refetoff, S. and Selenkow, H. A.: Familial thyroxine-binding globulin deficiency in a patient with Turner's syndrome (XO). Genetic study of a kindred. N. Engl. J. Med. 278: 1081-1087, 1968.

Rivas, M. L., Merritt, A. D. and Oliner, L.: Genetic variants of thyroxine-binding globulin (TBG). The Clinical Delineation of Birth Defects. X. The Endocrine System. Baltimore: Williams and Wilkins, 1971. Pp. 34-41.

Thorson, S. C., Tauxe, W. N. and Taswell, H. F.: Evidence for the existence of two thyroxine-binding globulin moieties: correlation between paper and starch-gel electrophoretic patterns utilizing thyroxine-binding globulin-deficient sera. J. Clin. Endocrinol. Metab. 26: 181-188, 1966.

31430 TORTICOLLIS, KELOIDS, CRYPTORCHIDISM, AND RENAL DYSPLASIA

Goeminne (1968) described a syndrome he concluded is inherited as an X-linked trait with incomplete dominance. None of the affected males reproduced. Affected persons included (1) a male with congenital muscular torticollis, (2) a male with torticollis, cryptorchidism and varicose veins, (3) a male with torticollis, many spontaneous keloids, unilateral cryptorchidism, oligospermia, chronic pyelonephritis with unilateral renal atrophy, multiple cutaneous nevi, a basal cell epithelioma, and varicose veins, (4) a male with torticollis, keloids and cryptorchidism, (5) a female with torticollis and pigmented nevi, and (6) a female with facial asymmetry, chronic pyelonephritis and nevi. The pedigree was consistent with the postulated mode of inheritance but no affected male reproduced.

Goeminne, L.: A new probably X-linked inherited syndrome: congenital torticollis, multiple keloids, cryptorchidism and renal dysplasia. Acta Genet. Med. Gem. 17: 439-467, 1968.

*31435 TYROSINE AMINOTRANSFERASE, REGULATOR OF

From the study of rat-human cell hybrids, Croce et al. (1973) found that tyrosine aminotransferase was always inducible when the human X chromosome was absent and not inducible when it was present. The repressor was syntenic to G6PD and HGPRT but not necessarily on the long arm of the X chromosome as the latter two loci are shown to be. This is the first example of gene assignment to the X chromosome by the cell hybrid method. All other entries in this catalog have been assigned by family studies and then confirmed by cell hybrid studies.

Croce, C. M., Litwack, G. and Koprowski, H.: Human regulatory gene for inducible tyrosine aminotransferase in rat-human hybrids. Proc. Natl. Acad. Sci. 70: 1268-1272, 1973.

31440 VALVULAR HEART DISEASE, CONGENITAL

Monteleone and Fagan (1969) described 6 definite and 1 probable case of congenital heart disease in males in four sibships of three generations of a Negro kindred in a pattern suggesting X-linked recessive inheritance. Four had mitral and aortic regurgitation, of whom two also had tricuspid regurgitation. The fifth definite case had only mitral regurgitation. Histologically changes in the mitral valve of one case resembled those seen in the 'floppy valve syndrome' (Read et al., 1965) or in Marfan syndrome (which was suggested by no other feature of the cases).

Monteleone, P. L. and Fagan, L. F.: Possible X-linked congenital heart disease. Circulation 39: 611-614, 1969.

Read, R. C., Thal, A. P. and Wendt, V. E.: Symptomatic valvular myxomatous transformation (the floppy valve syndrome). A possible forme fruste of the Marfan syndrome. Circulation 32: 897-910, 1965.

*31450 VAN DEN BOSCH SYNDROME

The components of this syndrome transmitted as an X-linked recessive are (1) mental deficiency, (2) choroideremia, (3) acrokeratosis verruciformis, (4) anhidrosis, and (5) skeletal deformity. An interesting and possibly important point is that at least 3 of these five components have been described as isolated X-linked traits. The syndrome has been observed in a single kindred.

Van den Bosch, J.: A new syndrome in three generations of a Dutch family. Ophthalmologica 137: 422-423, 1959.

31460 WILDERVANCK SYNDROME (CERVICO-OCULO-ACOUSTIC SYNDROME)

The Wildervanck syndrome consists of congenital perceptive deafness, Klippel-Feil anomaly (fused cervical vertebrae), and abducens palsy with retractio bulbi (Duane syndrome). The disorder is limited, or almost completely limited, to females, raising the question of sex-linked dominance with lethality in the hemizygous male. This syndrome (at least profound childhood deafness and Klippel-Feil malformation) may be responsible for at least 1 percent of deafness among girls. The deafness is perceptive in type and has been shown by radiologic studies to be due to a bony malformation of the inner ear. Kirkham (1969) described a family which was affected through 5 generations with perceptive deafness and in which two members had Duane syndrome. See KLIPPEL-FEIL DEFORMITY, CONDUCTIVE DEAFNESS and ABSENT VAGINA (14894).

Everberg, G., Ratjen, E. and Sorensen, H.: Wildervanck's syndrome: Klippel-Feil's syndrome associated with deafness and retraction of the eyeball. Br. J. Radiol. 36: 562-567, 1963.

Fraser, W. I. and MacGillivray, R. C.: Cervico-oculo-acoustic dysplasia ('the syndrome of Wildervanck'). J. Ment. Defic. Res. 12: 322-329, 1968.

Kirkham, T. H.: Cervico-oculo-acusticus syndrome with pseudopapilloedema. Arch. Dis. Child. 44: 504-508, 1969.

Kirkham, T. H.: Duane's syndrome and familial perceptive deafness. Br. J. Ophthalmol. 53: 335-339, 1969.

McLay, K. and Maran, A. G. D.: Deafness and the Klippel-Feil syndrome. J. Laryngol. 83: 175-184, 1969.

Wildervanck, L. S.: Een cervico-oculo-acusticussyndroom. Nederl. Tijdschr. Geneeskd. 104: 2600-2605, 1960.

Wildervanck, L. S., Hoeksema, P. E. and Penning, L.: Radiological examination of the inner ear of deaf-mutes persenting the cervico-oculo-acusticus syndrome. Acta Otolaryngol. 61: 445-453, 1966.

31465 WILLVONSEDER SYNDROME

Willvonseder et al. (1973) described three brothers who had dementia, spastic dysarthria, paresis of vertical eye movements, disturbance of gait and splenomegaly. The onset was prepubertal and progression slow.

Willvonseder, R., Goldstein, N. P., McCall, J. T., Yoss, R. E. and Tauxe, W. N.: A hereditary disorder with dementia, spastic dysarthria, vertical eye movement paresis, gait disturbance, splenomegaly, and abnormal copper metabolism. Neurology 23: 1039-1049, 1973.

31467 X CHROMOSOME CONTROLLING ELEMENT

Therman et al. (1974) suggested that condensation occurs around a center (locus) on the long arm of the X-chromosome near the centromere. They based this on the observation (1) that the abnormal X-chromosomes with the assumed center in duplicate form have bipartite Barr bodies and (2) that no X short arm isochromosomes (Xpi) have been confidently identified. They suggested that Xpi is lethal because the cell has no method of dosage compensation. The existence of such a locus in man is rendered plausible by the demonstration in the mouse of a locus called Xce (X-chromosome controlling element). Grahn (1973) studied the position of the Xce locus on the mouse map. Ohno et al. (1973) and Drews et al. (1974) described an allele at the Xce locus.

Cattanach, B. M., Pollard, C. E. and Perez, J. N.: Controlling elements in the mouse X-chromosome. I. Interaction with the X-linked genes. Genet. Res. 14: 223-235, 1969.

Cattanach, B. M., Perez, J. N. and Pollard, C. E.: Controlling elements in the mouse X-chromosome. II. Location in the linkage map. Genet. Res. 15: 183-195, 1970.

Drews, U., Blecher, S. R., Owen, D. A. and Ohno, S.: Genetically directed preferential X-activation seen in mice. Cell 1: 3-8, 1974.

Grahn, D.: Mouse Newsletter, No. 48, P. 21, Feb., 1973.

Ohno, S., Christian, L., Atlardi, B. J. and Kan, J.: Modification of expression of the testicular feminization (Tfm) gene of the mouse by a 'controlling element' gene. Nature N.B. 245: 92-93, 1973.

Therman, E., Sarto, G. E. and Patau, K.: Center for Barr body condensation of the proximal part of the human Xq: a hypothesis. Chromosoma 44: 361-366, 1974.

*31470 XG BLOOD GROUP SYSTEM

The antigen called Xg(a) behaves as an X-linked dominant. It was found in 89 percent of 188 Caucasian females and in 62 percent of 154 males. The antiserum was derived from a patient with hereditary hemorrhagic telangiectasia who had received many transfusions. The antigen is well developed at birth. In the few Negroes tested the phenotype frequencies seem to be about the same as in Caucasians. 'Evidence is accumulating that homozygotes react as strongly as hemizygotes and more strongly than heterozygotes.' The efficient estimate of the frequency of the Xg(a) allele in Caucasians, making use of the data on females as well as males, is 0.651 (Sanger et al., 1962).

The Xg(a) blood group is of great use to genetics especially for study of linkage and determination where non-disjunction occurs leading to X chromosome aneuploidy. Evidence on Lyonization of the Xg locus is conflicting. Evidence for Lyonization came from a study of X-linked hypochromic anemia (q.v.) by Lee and colleagues (1968). Lawler and Sanger (1970) found that a group of females with Philadelphia-chromosome-positive myeloid leukemia cases had the frequency of Xg types expected of females. This could mean either that the Xg locus is not subject to inactivation or that all Ph-positive cells are not monoclonal. Also assumed, of course, is that the erythroid cells in the patients studied are derived from a Ph-positive cell and that no red cells derived from Ph-negative precursors persist. Data on linkage of the Xg locus with many other loci are summarized by Race and Sanger (1968). Ducos et al. (1971) studied a chimera twin pair in whom two red cell populations were easily separable because of differences in their ABO blood groups. One population was Xg(a+), the other Xg (a-). Thus the important point was established that the Xg antigen is made in the red cell precursors and not secondary acquired by red cells. Xg can, therefore, give information on Lyonization. The Xg locus cannot be on the distal third of the long arm of the X chromosome because Pearson (1973) observed a family in which the mother was Xg(a+) and had a balanced translocation of the

X
L
I
N
K
E
D

distal third of the Xq onto 3p, the karyologically normal father was Xg (a-) and an unbalanced daughter with deleted distal third of the long arm of one X chromosome (derived from the mother) was Xg (a·).

Cook, I. A., Polley, M. J. and Mollison, P. L.: A second example of anti-Xg(a). Lancet I: 857-859, 1963.

Ducos, J., Morty, Y., Sanger, R. and Race, R. R.: Xg and X chromosome inactivation. Lancet II: 219-220, 1971.

Lee, G. R., MacDiarmid, W. D., Cartwright, G. E. and Wintrobe, M. H.: Hereditary, X-linked, sideroachrestic anemia. The isolation of two erythrocyte populations differing in XgA blood type and porphyrin content. Blood 32: 59-70, 1968.

Mann, J. D., Cahan, A., Gelb, A. G., Fisher, N., Hamper, J., Tippett, P., Sanger, R. and Race, R. R.: A sex-linked blood group. Lancet I: 8-10, 1962.

Pearson, P.: Leiden: personal communication, 1973.

Race, R. R. and Sanger, R.: Blood Groups in Man. Philadelphia: F. A. Davis Co., 1968 (5th Ed.).

Sanger, R., Race, R. R., Tippett, P., Hamper, J., Gavin, J. and Cleghorn, T. E.: The X-linked blood group system Xg: more tests on unrelated people and on families. Vox Sang. 7: 571-578, 1962.

Siniscalco, M. G., Filippi, B., Latte, B., Piomelli, S., Rattazzi, M., Gavin, J., Sanger, R. and Race, R. R.: Failure to detect linkage between Xg and X-borne loci in Sardinians. Ann. Hum. Genet. 29: 231-252, 1966.

31480 XH ANTIGEN

The Xh antigen was first described by Bundschuh (1966), who suggested X-linkage because the antigen is more frequent in women (97 percent) than in men (88 percent). The antigen is demonstrated with antiserum produced by injecting rabbits with pool serum from healthy women and absorption of the immune serum with selected male sera. Genetic analysis is complicated by the fact that both genetic and non-genetic factors seem to influence the quantity of the antigen present. Dunston and Gershowitz (1973) showed that Xh (31480) and Pa 1 (26010) are identical, that X-linkage is ruled out by findings in two females, and that this is probably not a Mendelian polymorphism. See 26010 for evidence excluding X-linkage.

Dunston, G. M. and Gershowitz, H.: Further studies of Xh, a serum protein antigen in man. Vox Sang. 24: 343-353, 1973.

Kueppers, F.: Studies on the Xh antigen in human serum. Humangenetik 7: 98-103, 1969.

*31490 XM SYSTEM

Berg and Bearn (1966) discovered an X-linked serum protein type by means of heteroantiserum made specific by absorption. Since the group specific antigen appears to be located in the alpha-2-macroglobulin of serum, the name Xm was assigned to the system. The distribution of phenotypes in families and in populations was consistent with X-linkage. Berg et al. (1968) concluded that the Hunter locus and the Xm locus are within measurable distance of each other, the best estimate of the recombination fraction being 0.09. The strongest evidence of linkage was between Xm and deutan color blindness where Berg (1969) found a lod score of 2.5 at recombination fraction of 0.05 and 0.10.

Berg, K. and Bearn, A. G.: A common X-linked serum marker and its relation to other loci on the X chromosome. Trans. Assoc. Am. Physicians 79: 165-176, 1966.

Berg, K. and Bearn, A. G.: An inherited X-linked serum system in man. The Xm system. J. Exp. Med. 123: 379-397, 1966.

Berg, K., Danes, B. S. and Bearn, A. G.: The linkage relation of the loci for the Xm serum system and the X-linked form of Hurler's syndrome (Hunter's syndrome). Am. J. Hum. Genet. 20: 398-401, 1968.

Berg, K.: Mapping the X chromosome-discussion paper. Bull. Europ. Soc. Hum. Genet. 3: 29-32, 1969.

31500 ZONULAR CATARACT AND NYSTAGMUS

Falls (1952) reported a family in which this combination of traits appeared to be X-linked. He pointed out that the family was 'incompletely studied.'

Falls, H. F.: The role of the sex chromosome in hereditary ocular pathology. Trans. Am. Ophthalmol. Soc. 50: 421-467, 1952.

AUTHOR INDEX

Calvert, H. T.	20120
Camacho, A. M.	20171
Cambie, E.	27690
Cambier, J.	11820
Camejo, M. G.	21190
Cameron, A. H.	20010
Cameron, D.	23170, 23570, 24150
Cameron, J. M.	13240
Cameron, K. M.	14500
Cameron, O. J.	25440
Cameron, S. J.	19330
Camiel, M. R.	17530
Cammermeyer, J.	26650
Camp, C. D.	16950
Camp, M. B.	16240
Campailla, E.	20125
Campbell, A. G. M.	23720, 31125
Campbell, A. M. G.	12495, 14310, 16240
Campbell, B. K.	23620
Campbell, C. J.	12780
Campbell, D. C.	30100
Campbell, D. E.	30940
Campbell, M.	11520
Campbell, M. M.	31120
Campbell, P. E.	13260, 30940
Campbell, R. A.	16120, 17980, 23540, 24120
Campbell, R. E.	27365
Campbell, S.	23540, 25610
Campion, W. M.	15270
Canada, W. J.	17550
Canales, L.	31390
Canby, J. P.	23580
Cancilla, P. A.	24520, 25515
Candebat, L.	31370
Canellos, G. P.	27535
Canent, R. V.	19245
Canetti, J.	30700
Canijo, M.	10480
Canlas, Z.	21990
Cann, H. M.	23670
Cann, H. W.	17790
Cannon, F. E.	12870
Cannon, J. F.	12580, 14340, 30480
Cannon, P. J.	24120
Cant, J. S.	23020, 27540
Cantolino, S. J.	13680, 18510
Canton, J. N.	30610
Cantor, H. E.	20460
Cantu, J. M.	10320, 27730, 30877
Cantwell, A. R., Jr.	13260
Cantwell, J.	11500
Canty, T. G.	27020
Cantz, M.	25290, 25322, 30990
Capella, J. A.	15685, 30230, 30970
Caplan, D. B.	12160
Caplan, L.	10580
Caplan, R. M.	24710
Capotorti, L.	24380
Capp, G. I.	14228
Capp, G. L.	14228
Capute, A. J.	15110, 20885, 24510
Caratzali, A.	13740
Caravati, C. M.	17370
Carbonell Juanico, M.	16600
Cardinale, G. J.	25100
Caren, J.	13755, 16290

Cares, H. L.	21220
Caresano, A.	25140
Carew, J. P.	16280
Carey, J. H.	10490, 25360
Carey, L. S.	25300, 27130
Carey, M. C.	16780, 18220, 23620
Cariou, P.	16880
Carleton, R. A.	12100
Carlsen, F.	16250
Carlsen, R. B.	23000
Carlson, L. A.	14440
Carlson, W. D.	13370
Carman, C. T.	17130
Carmel, P.	23260
Carmel, R.	21170
Carmena, M.	13410
Carmichael, E. A.	24300, 25690, 27080
Carmichael, R.	30610
Carneiro, S. J.	12045
Carnes, W. H.	10420
Carnevale, A.	31215
Carney, R. G.	30830
Carney, R. G., Jr.	30830
Caro, A. J.	14310
Carol, W. L. L.	20970, 30200
Caroline, L.	24020
Carones, A. V.	23410
Carpenter, C. C. J.	26920
Carpenter, C. J.	26920
Carpenter, D. G.	30800
Carpenter, G.	20100
Carpenter, G. G.	10160, 11070, 26160
Carpenter, S.	16015, 16450, 21800
Carr, A. A.	16200
Carr, D. H.	30610
Carr, R. D.	15590, 18520
Carr, R. E.	26230
Carre, I. J.	14240, 23540, 23870, 26870
Carrea, O. T.	24170
Carrel, R. E.	19045, 27580
Carrell, R. W.	14228
Carrie, J.	31370
Carrington, C. B.	13500
Carritt, B.	14770
Carroll, F.	16350
Carroll, M.	24850
Carron, R.	20850, 24300
Carruthers, M. E.	12180
Carsner, R. L.	26240
Carson, M. J.	30640
Carson, N. A. J.	23620, 23870, 24950, 25500, 26870, 30900
Carson, P. E.	10300, 17220, 23180, 30590
Carta, S.	14228
Carter, C.	14790, 16900, 30480, 30830
Carter, C. H.	24220, 30800
Carter, C. O.	14270, 16090, 24920, 25020, 26160, 26320, 26600, 27100, 27160
Carter, D. M.	16710
Carter, H. R.	16470
Carter, N. D.	11480
Carter, N. G.	14560
Carter, N. W.	30780
Carter, S.	11508, 23730
Carter, T.	21390
Carter, T. S.	15830
Carter, W. J.	19110

Dawson, D. M. 10845, 12330, 23260
Dawson, G. 23100, 24550, 25250
Dawson, P. J. 13000, 20805
Dawson, S. P. 23040
Dawson, T. A. J. 13740
Day, E. 20805, 21910
Day, H. J. 13000
Day, M. G. 27650
Day, N. K. 21695
Day, N. K. B. 21695
Day, R. 23040
Day, R. W. 26160
Dayalan, N. 20040
Dayan, A. D. 12340, 20420
Dayhoff, M. O. 10360, 10370, 11413, 12015, 12395, 12397, 13482, 13840, 13925, 14010, 14020, 14228, 14975, 15020, 15345, 15945, 16565, 16970, 17335, 17673, 19000, 19233
Dayman, J. 23450
Da Silva Horta, J. 10480
Da Silva, L. C. 24330
Da Silva Lima, J. F. 10340
De Groot, C. J. 23730
De Jimenez, R. B. C. 10360
De Jong, B. P. 16395
De Lozzio, C. B. 22410
De Nayer, P. 31420
De Wael, J. 23180
Deacon, J. S. R. 21208, 21555
Dean, G. 17600, 17620
Deaton, J. G. 27040
Debarros, N. 24800
Debastos, O. 24170
Debray, J. 23190
Debray, P. 25940
Debre, R. 14160, 21920, 23520
Debusk, F. L. 26410
Dechaume, J. 19330
Decker, J. L. 13890
Deforest, R. E. 11390
Degenhardt, K.-H. 12260
Degnan, M. 23020, 30940
Degos, R. 13280
Degraef, P. J. 22810
Degroot, L. J. 27450
Degroot, W. P. 30150, 30810
Dehaene, P. 24900
Dehejia, H. 22275
Deicher, H. 14010, 14020
Deiss, W. P., Jr. 13110, 16660
Dejager, H. J. 14973
Dejean, C. 16350
Dejerine, J. 14590, 25830
Dejong, R. N. 12340, 14310, 16030
Dejong, W. W. 14228
Dekaban, A. 24620
Dekaban, A. S. 15620, 24950, 26690
Dekaouel, C. 17000, 17190
Dekker, G. 24500
Delamare, J. 23600
Delaney, J. R. 21060
Delaney, M. J. 14290
Delaney, R. 14710
Delaney, W. V. 14320
Delange, R. J. 14275
Delavierre, P. 15890
Delbarre, F. 10260
Delbeke, M. J. 18020
Delea, C. S. 19310

Deleon, G. A. 14590
Delgado-Morales, B. 26155
Delgado, H. 27180
Della Cella, G. 23000
Della Porta, V. 31070
Delleman, J. W. 12180
Dellenbach, P. 26353
Delree, C. 12554
Delthil, S. 16530
Deluca, H. F. 19310
Delucca, A. 10420
Delvin, E. 20375, 21990, 24540, 24860, 26615
Del Vecchio, M. 25330
Demarinis, F. 11270
Demars, R. 30800
Demars, R. I. 25250
Demarsh, Q. B. 17240
Demassieux, (NI) 30810
Demelo, J. M. 14228
Demeulenaere, L. 12070
Deminatti, M. 18160
Demis, D. J. 15480
Demos, J. 31020
Dempsey, E. F. 19170
Denaro, S. J. 16290
Denborough, M. A. 14560
Denes, G. 11410
Deneve, V. 20370
Denison, E. K. 11455
Dennehy, J. J. 10610
Dennett, X. 21420
Dennis, J. 30405
Dennis, J. P. 10080
Dennis, M. 15835
Dennis, N. R. 18990
Denniston, C. 30450
Denniston, J. C. 23790
Denny-Brown, D. 11820, 16240
Denson, K. W. 30690
Denson, K. W. E. 22750, 30670
Dent, C. E. 15650, 22780, 23450, 23620, 24150, 25975, 25990, 26470, 30780
Dent, P. B. 21450, 25970
Dent, T. E. 14560
Deodhar, S. D. 23360
Deol, M. S. 26070
Deparis, M. 23600
Depieds, R. 27490
Depp, R. 30020
Deppendorf, (NI) 27300
Der Kaloustian, M. 27005
Der Kaloustian, V. M. 10010, 22340, 24360, 24620, 25727, 26860, 27870, 30800
Deraemaeker, R. 22070, 26070, 30450
Derbes, V. 15080, 24610
Derbes, V. J. 11220, 12010, 21640, 24230, 24250
Dern, R. J. 17220, 30590
Derrick, J. R. 10500
Derry, D. M. 23060
Der Kaloustian, V. M. 21740, 22340, 22480
Desai, K. B. 27425
Desai, M. P. 14228
Desai, R. 24170
Desbuquois, B. 24750
Desbuquois, G. 21520, 27180
Deshaies, G. 12260
Deshpande, C. K. 21110
Desimone, J. 11480
Desjardin, C. 30540
Desjardins, L. 23040

Swatek, F. E. 16960
Swaye, P. 13500, 17850
Swedberg, K. R. 21950, 26890
Sweeley, C. C. 23100, 26880, 30150
Sweeney, A. 26730, 30440
Sweeney, V. P. 17600
Sweet, L. K. 21050
Sweetman, L. 24000, 30800
Sweetnam, R. 14790
Sweetnam, W. P. 24030
Sweetnan, R. 16900
Swelstad, J. 24743
Swenson, R. S. 17400
Swenson, R. T. 14228
Swettenham, K. 31310
Swieconek, J. A. 16780
Swift, M. 22765
Swift, M. R. 12390, 16090, 22765
Swift, P. N. 23690
Swinton, N. W. 17130, 17490
Swinyard, C. A. 20810
Switzer, R. A. 26590
Swoboda, H. 23900
Sworn, M. J. 25610
Sybers, H. D. 21410
Sycamore, L. K. 13240
Sydenstricker, V. P. 14228
Sylvest, B. 12420
Sylvester, P. E. 13660, 21720, 24510, 27200
Symonds, C. P. 15990, 18080
Symonds, E. M. 19230
Symons, J. S. 20850
Szabados, T. 18225
Szabo, G. 16220, 19110
Szabo, L. 21880
Szalay, G. C. 21090
Szapiro, L. 26150
Szeinberg, A. 11520, 13270, 13815, 13820, 17610, 20020, 20160, 26160, 30590
Szelenyi, J. 14228
Szelenyi, J. G. 14228
Szepetowski, G. 31120
Szijarto, L. 24620
Szily, A. von 12630
Szur, L. 14228
Szymanowska, Z. 25080
Tabakin, B. S. 25750
Tabara, K. 14228
Tabata, T. 30950
Taber, E. 14040
Taber, K. W. 20650
Taber, P. 30010
Taconis, W. K. 13450
Tada, K. 21950, 22910, 23620, 23830, 26610, 26615, 27610, 27710, 27860, 30940
Tadjoedin, M. K. 20890
Tagatz, G. 24420
Tagawa, N. 27265
Tahbaz-Zadeh 25290
Taitz, L. S. 23200, 24140
Taj-Eldin, S. 11400
Takagi, A. 15850
Takagi, T. 13482
Takahashi, H. 14228
Takahashi, K. 10540
Takahashi, Y. 22910
Takaku, F. 26340, 30130
Takeda, I. 14228
Takeda, T. 30900
Takenaka, M. 14228
Takeuchi, A. 15510
Takeuchi, M. 26860
Takeuchi, T. 13060
Takikawa, K. 31320
Takki, K. 25887
Takla, R. 24620
Talamo, R. C. 20740, 21970
Talapatra, N. C. 14228
Talbert, A. A. 11890
Talbert, L. M. 31370
Talbert, O. R. 24880
Talbert, P. C. 14500
Talbert, W. R., Jr. 13500
Talbot, N. B. 21380
Talbot, S. 11220
Talbott, J. H. 17040
Tallen, H. H. 25085
Taller, E. 23940
Talley, C. 25370
Talner, N. S. 21910
Tampas, J. P. 11400
Tamura, A. 14228
Tamura, T. 22910
Tan, B. H. 20740
Tan, K. H. 19350
Tan, K. L. 26595
Tan, Y. H. 10745, 14757, 14770
Tanaka, J. 23075
Tanaka, K. 21020, 24350, 27265
Tanaka, K. R. 18290, 26620
Tanaka, M. 21250
Tanaka, T. 23280
Tanaka, Y. 30150
Tancredi, F. 23200, 24260
Tandon, S. N. 19370
Tang, T. 21360
Tangheroni, W. 14228
Tangun, Y. 17350
Taniguchi, R. 18320
Tanna, V. L. 30920
Tannen, R. L. 19110
Tanner, J. M. 27005
Tanner, M. 10630
Tanno, K. 22910, 23830
Tantravahi, R. 17385
Tappel, A. L. 25280
Taratuto, A. 14580
Targgart, W. H. 17980
Tariverdian, G. 10270, 17220, 17240
Tariwerdian, G. 10270
Tarjan, G. 24950
Tarkoff, M. P. 20740
Tarlow, M. J. 22620
Tarm, F. 24120
Tarnoky, A. L. 10360
Tarnvik, A. 14745, 17165
Tartaglia, A. P. 10280
Tarui, S. 23280
Taschdjian, C. 24020
Tashian, R. E. 11480, 11481, 13321, 13340, 17220, 30590
Tashjian, A. H., Jr. 13110, 16230, 17140, 30080
Tasker, J. B. 26620
Tasker, W. G. 21510
Taskinen, P. J. 11960
Taswell, H. F. 18860, 31420
Tatarski, I. 14228
Tatsis, B. 14228
Tattersall, R. B. 12585, 22210

767

SUBJECT INDEX

APICAL DYSTROPHY   see COLOBOMA OF MACULA WITH TYPE B BRACHYDACTYLY (12040)
APICAL DYSTROPHY   see BRACHYDACTYLY, TYPE B (11300)
*APLASIA CUTIS CONGENITA 10760
*APLASIA CUTIS CONGENITA (CONGENITAL DEFECT OF SKIN, CONGENITAL DEFECT OF SKULL
   AND SCALP) 20770
APLASIA   see MASA SYNDROME (30925)
APLASIA CUTIS CONGENITA   see ABSENCE DEFECT OF LIMBS, SCALP AND SKULL (10030),
   EPIDERMOLYSIS BULLOSA WITH CONGENITAL LOCALIZED ABSENCE OF SKIN AND DEFOR-
   MITY OF NAILS (13200)
APOCRINE CHROMIDROSIS   see NAILBEDS, PIGMENTATION OF (16110)
APPENDICITIS, PRONENESS TO 10770
APPLE PEEL SYNDROME   see JEJUNAL ATRESIA (24360)
ARACHNODACTYLY   see CONTRACTURAL ARACHNODACTYLY (12105)
ARACHNODACTYLY   see MARFAN SYNDROME (15470), ACHARD SYNDROME (10070)
ARACHNOIDITIS   see SPINAL ARACHNOIDITIS (18295)
ARCUS CORNEAE (ARCUS SENILIS) 10780
AREFLEXIC DYSTASIA   see ROUSSY-LEVY HEREDITARY AREFLEXIC DYSTASIA (18080)
*ARGININEMIA 20780
ARGININOSUCCINIC ACID SYNTHETASE DEFICIENCY   see CITRULLINEMIA (21570)
*ARGININOSUCCINICACIDURIA 20790
ARHINENCEPHALY   see HOLOPROSENCEPHALY, FAMILIAL ALOBAR (23610)
ARM FOLDING 10785
ARMS, MALFORMATION OF 10790
ARNOLD-CHIARI MALFORMATION 20795
ARRHENOBLASTOMA — THYROID ADENOMA 10795
*ARTERIAL CALCIFICATION, GENERALIZED, OF INFANCY 20800
ARTERIAL TORTUOSITY 20805
ARTERIES, ANOMALIES OF 10800
ARTERIES, HYPOPLASIA OF   see INTERNAL CAROTID ARTERIES, HYPOPLASIA OF (24310)
ARTERIOHEPATIC DYSPLASIA 20807
ARTERIOPATHY, FAMILIAL   see SUPRAVALVULAR AORTIC STENOSIS (18550)
ARTERIOVENOUS FISTULA, PULMONARY   see TELANGIECTASIA, HEREDITARY HEMORRHAGIC
   (18730)
ARTHALGIA, PERIODIC   see BONE PAIN, PERIODIC (11227)
ARTHRITIS, SACRO-ILIAC 10810
ARTHROCHALASIS MULTIPLEX CONGENITA   see JOINT LAXITY (24380)
ARTHROGRYPOSIS MULTIPLEX CONGENITA   see NEUROPATHY, CONGENITAL, WITH ARTHRO-
   GRYPOSIS (16195)
*ARTHROGRYPOSIS MULTIPLEX CONGENITA 20810
ARTHROGRYPOSIS WITHOUT WEAKNESS 10815
*ARTHROGRYPOSIS-LIKE DISORDER 20820
ARTHROGRYPOSIS-LIKE HAND ANOMALY AND SENSORI-NEURAL DEAFNESS 10820
ARTHROGRYPOSIS   see PSEUDO-ARTHROGRYPOSIS (17730)
ARTHROGRYPOSIS MULTIPLEX CONGENITA   see MUSCULAR DYSTROPHY, CONGENITAL PRO-
   DUCING ARTHROGRYPOSIS (25390)
ARTHROGRYPOSIS-LIKE DISORDER   see PSEUDO-ARTHROGRYPOSIS (17730)
*ARTHRO-OPHTHALMOPATHY, HEREDITARY PROGRESSIVE (STICKLER SYNDROME) 10830
ARTHRO-OSTEO-ONYCHO-DYSPLASIA   see NAIL-PATELLA SYNDROME (16120)
ARTICHOKE, MODIFICATION OF TASTE BY 10833
*ARYL HYDROCARBON HYDROXYLASE (AHH) INDUCIBILITY 10834
ARYLESTERASE, SERUM 10835
ASCHER SYNDROME   see BLEPHAROCHALASIS AND 'DOUBLE LIP' (10990)
ASCITES, CHYLOUS 20830
ASCORBIC ACID, INABILITY TO SYNTHESIZE   see HYPOASCORBEMIA (24040)
ASEPTIC NECROSIS   see OSTEOCHONDRITIS DISSECANS (16580)
ASPARAGUS, URINARY EXCRETION OF ODORIFEROUS COMPONENT OF 10840
*ASPARTYLGLYCOSAMINURIA 20840
*ASPHYXIATING THORACIC DYSTROPHY OF THE NEWBORN (JEUNE SYNDROME; THORACIC-PEL-
   VIC-PHALANGEAL DYSTROPHY) 20850
*ASPLENIA WITH CARDIOVASCULAR ANOMALIES (IVEMARK SYNDROME) 20853
ASTHMA   see BRONCHOMALACIA (21145)
ASTHMA, NASAL POLYPS, ASPIRIN INTOLERANCE (ASA TRIAD) 20855
ASTHMA, SHORT STATURE AND ELEVATED IGA 20860
ASTHMA   see ATOPIC HYPERSENSITIVITY (20920)
ASTROCYTOMA   see BASAL CELL NEVUS SYNDROME (10940)
ASYMMETRY, LATERAL   see SILVER SYNDROME (18240), HEMIHYPERTROPHY (23500)
ATAXIA AND RETINITIS PIGMENTOSA   see REFSUM DISEASE (26650), NERVOUS SYSTEM DISORDER
   RESEMBLING REFSUM DISEASE AND HURLER DISEASE (25640), ABETALIPOPROTEINEMIA
   (20010)
ATAXIA WITH MYOCLONUS EPILEPSY AND PRESENILE DEMENTIA 20870
ATAXIA, HEREDITARY   see FRIEDREICH ATAXIA (13660, 22930), CEREBELLAR ATAXIA (11720, 11730,
   21290, 30250), CEREBELLO-PARENCHYMAL DISORDERS (11740, 11750, 21310-21340), OLIVOPONTO-
   CEREBELLAR ATROPHY (16440-16470, 25830)
*ATAXIA, INTERMITTENT, WITH PYRUVATE DEHYDROGENASE (DECARBOXYLASE) DEFICIENCY 20880
ATAXIA, LATE ONSET, WITH GLUCOSE INTOLERANCE (MACHADO DISEASE) 10845
ATAXIA, MENTAL RETARDATION AND CATARACT   see MARINESCO-SJOGREN SYNDROME (24880)
*ATAXIA, PERIODIC VESTIBULO-CEREBELLAR 10850
*ATAXIA, SPASTIC 10860
ATAXIA, WITH FASCICULATIONS 10870
ATAXIA-DEAFNESS-RETARDATION (ADR) SYNDROME 20885
*ATAXIA-TELANGIECTASIA 20890
ATAXIC DIPLEGIA AND DEFECTIVE CELLULAR IMMUNITY 20900
ATELEIOTIC DWARFISM   see PITUITARY DWARFISM I (26240)
ATHETOSIS   see CUTIS LAXA, CORNEAL CLOUDING, MENTAL RETARDATION (12380)

ATHETOSIS see DOUBLE ATHETOSIS (12640), HYPOXANTHINE QUANINE PHOSPHORIBOSYL TRANSFERASE DEFICIENCY (30800)
ATHROMBIA, ESSENTIAL 10875
ATHYREOTIC CRETINISM see CRETINISM, ATHYREOTIC (21870)
*ATONIC-ASTATIC SYNDROME OF FOERSTER 20910
ATOPIC DERMATITIS see DEAFNESS, NEURAL, WITH ATYPICAL ATOPIC DERMATITIS (22170)
ATOPIC DIATHESIS see NETHERTON DISEASE (25650)
ATOPIC HYPERSENSITIVITY 20920
ATOPIC HYPERSENSITIVITY see IMMUNE RESPONSE (14685)
ATP, ELEVATED, IN ERYTHROCYTES see ADENOSINE TRIPHOSPHATE, ELEVATED, OF ERYTHRO-CYTES (10290)
ATP-ASE DEFICIENCY HEMOLYTIC ANEMIA see ADENOSINE TRIPHOSPHATASE DEFICIENCY, ANEMIA DUE TO (10280)
*ATRANSFERRINEMIA 20930
ATRESIA OF ESOPHAGUS see TRACHEOESOPHAGEAL FISTULA WITH ESOPHAGEAL ATRESIA (18990), VATER ASSOCIATION (19235)
ATRESIA OF LARYNX see LARYNX, CONGENITAL PARTIAL ATRESIA OF (15030)
ATRIAL CARDIOMYOPATHY WITH HEART BLOCK 10877
ATRIAL FIBRILLATION see NODAL RHYTHM (16380)
ATRIAL MYXOMA see MYXOMA ATRIAL (25595)
*ATRIAL SEPTAL DEFECT 10880
*ATRIAL SEPTAL DEFECT WITH ATRIO-VENTRICULAR CONDUCTION DEFECTS 10890
ATRIAL SEPTAL DEFECT, PRIMUM TYPE 20940
ATRIAL SEPTAL DEFECT see ELLIS-VAN CREVELD SYNDROME (22550), HOLT-ORAM SYNDROME (14290)
*ATRICHIA WITH PAPULAR LESIONS 20950
ATRIOVENTRICULAR BLOCK see HEART BLOCK, CONGENITAL (23470), ATRIAL SEPTAL DEFECT WITH ATRIO-VENTRICULAR CONDUCTION DEFECTS (10890)
ATRIOVENTRICULAR DISSOCIATION 20960
ATROPHIA BULBORUM HEREDITARIA see NORRIE DISEASE (31060)
ATROPHIA GYRATA CHOROIDEAE ET RETINAE OF FUCHS see FUCHS ATROPHIA GYRATA CHOROIDEAE ET RETINAE (22990)
*ATROPHODERMIA VERMICULATA (FOLLICULITIS ULERYTHEMATOSA, ATROPHODERMA RETICULATA, HONEYCOMB ATROPHY, ATROPHODERMIA RETICULATA SYMMETRICA FACIEI, ETC.) 20970
ATROPHY, MUSCULAR see MUSCULAR ATROPHY (15850-15870, 25330-25350)
AUBERGER BLOOD GROUP see BLOOD GROUP-AUBERGER SYSTEM (11040)
AUDITORY CANAL, EXOSTOSES OF see EAR EXOSTOSES (12830)
*AURICULO-OSTEODYSPLASIA 10900
AUSTIN TYPE METACHROMATIC LEUKODYSTROPHY see METACHROMATIC LEUKODYSTROPHY WITH MUCOPOLYSACCHARIDURIA (24990)
AUSTRALIA ANTIGEN 20980
AUTOIMMUNE DISEASES 10910
AUTOIMMUNITY see HASHIMOTO STRUMA (14030), THYROID AUTOANTIBODIES (18850)
AXENFELD ANOMALY see RIEGER SYNDROME (18050)
BABER CONGENITAL CIRRHOSIS see CIRRHOSIS, FAMILIAL (11890, 21560), TYROSINEMIA (27670)
BAIB EXCRETION see BETA-AMINOISOBUTYRIC ACID, URINARY EXCRETION OF (21010)
BAKER CYST see POPLITEAL CYST (17575)
*BALDNESS 10920
BALLER-GEROID SYNDROME see CRANIOSYNOSTOSIS WITH RADIAL DEFECTS (21860)
BAMBOO HAIR see NETHERTON DISEASE (25650)
BAND-SHAPED KERATOPATHY see CORNEAL DYSTROPHY, BAND-SHAPED (21750)
BANKI SYNDROME 10930
*BARDET-BIEDL SYNDROME 20990
BARLOW SYNDROME see MITRAL REGURGITATION (15770)
BARTTER SYNDROME see HYPOKALEMIC ALKALOSIS (24120)
*BASAL CELL NEVUS SYNDROME (MULTIPLE BASAL CELL NEVI, ODONTOGENIC KERATOCYSTS AND SKELETAL ANOMALIES) 10940
BASAL GANGLIA, CALCIFICATION OF see CALCIFICATION OF BASAL GANGLIA, AND HYPOCAL-CEMIA (11410)
BASAN SYNDROME see ECTODERMAL DYSPLASIA, ABSENT DERMATGLYPHIC PATTERN, CHANGES IN NAILS AND SIMIAN CREASE (12920)
BASILAR IMPRESSION, PRIMARY 10950
BASILAR IMPRESSION see ACRO-OSTEOLYSIS (10240)
BASSEN-KORNZWEIG SYNDROME see ABETALIPOPROTEINEMIA (20010)
'BAT EAR' see EAR WITHOUT HELIX (12880)
BATTEN DISEASE see AMAUROTIC FAMILY IDIOCY, JUVENILE TYPE (20420)
BBB SYNDROME see TELECANTHUS WITH ASSOCIATED ABNORMALITIES (31360)
BECKER MUSCULAR DYSTROPHY see MUSCULAR DYSTROPHY, TARDIVE TYPE (31030)
BECKWITH-WIEDEMANN SYNDROME see EMG SYNDROME (22560)
BEETURIA (BETACYANINURIA) 10960
*BEHR SYNDROME (BEHR COMPLICATED FORM OF INFANTILE HEREDITARY OPTIC ATROPHY) 21000
BELL PALSY see CRANIAL NERVES, RECURRENT PARESIS (21820)
BERARDINELLI SYNDROME see SEIP SYNDROME (26970)
BEST DISEASE see MACULAR DEGENERATION, POLYMORPHIC (15370)
BETA (2A)-GLOBULIN ANOMALY see GLOBULIN ANOMALY INVOLVING BETA (2A)-GLOBULIN (13790)
BETA-AMINOISOBUTYRIC ACID (BAIB), URINARY EXCRETION OF 21010
*BETA-HYDROXYISOVALERIC ACIDURIA AND BETA-METHYLCROTONYLGLYCINURIA 21020
BETA-KETOTHIOLASE DEFICIENCY see ALPHA-METHYLACETOACETICACIDURIA (20375)
BETA-LIPOPROTEIN TYPES see LIPOPROTEIN TYPES (15200-15240)
BETA-LIPOPROTEIN, DOUBLE see LIPOPROTEIN, VARIANT OF BETA (15240)
BETA-MERCAPTOLACTATE-CYSTEINE DISULFIDURIA see MIXED DISULFIDURIA I (25205)
BETA-METHYLCROTONYLGLYCINURIA see METHYLCROTONYLGLYCINURIA (25095)

CALCITONIN 11413
CAMPOMELIC DWARFISM see BOWING, CONGENITAL OF LONG BONES WITH ASSOCIATED
SKELETAL AND OTHER DEFECTS (21135)
*CAMPTOBRACHYDACTYLY 11415
CAMPTODACTYLY WITH FIBROUS TISSUE HYPERPLASIA AND SKELETAL DYSPLASIA 21193
CAMPTODACTYLY WITH MUSCULAR HYPOPLASIA, SKELETAL DYSPLASIA AND ABNORMAL
PALMAR CREASES 21196
CAMPTODACTYLY see FIBROSCLEROSIS, MULTIFOCAL (22880), MOUTH, INABILITY TO OPEN
COMPLETELY, ETC. (15830), LICHTENSTEIN SYNDROME (24655)
CAMPTODACTYLY see ARTHROGRYPOSIS-LIKE HAND ANOMALY AND SENSORI-NEURAL DEAF-
NESS (10820)
*CAMPTODACTYLY 11420
CAMPTODACTYLY, CLEFT PALATE, CLUB FOOT 11430
CAMPTOMELIC DWARFISM see BOWING, CONGENITAL, OF LONG BONES (21130)
CAMURATI-ENGELMANN DISEASE see ENGELMANN DISEASE (13130)
CANAVAN DISEASE see SPONGY DEGENERATION OF THE CENTRAL NERVOUS SYSTEM (27190)
CANCER 11440
CANCER FAMILY SYNDROME see CANCER (11440)
CANCER OF BOWEL see SCLERO-ATROPHIC AND KERATOTIC DERMATOSIS OF LIMBS (18160)
CANCER OF THE BREAST, FAMILIAL 21200
CANCER see POLYPOSIS (17500-17540), TYLOSIS WITH ESOPHAGEAL CANCER (14850), XERODERMA
PIGMENTOSUM (19440, 27870), URETERAL CARCINOMA (19160)
CANCER OF COLON 11450
CANCER SUSCEPTIBILITY see ARYL HYDROCARBON HYDROXYLASE INDUCIBLE (10834)
CANCER, HEPATOCELLULAR 11455
CANDIDASIS, CHRONIC MUCOCUTANEOUS see LYMPHOKINE DEFICIENCY (24765), LYMPHOBLAS-
TIC TRANSFORMATION, INHIBITION OF (24743), LYMPHOBLASTIC TRANSFORMATION INTRIN-
SIC DEFECT IN (24745), MONOCYTE CHEMOTACTIC DISORDER (25225)
CANDIDIASIS, DISSEMINATED see MYELOPEROXIDASE DEFICIENCY (25460)
*CANDIDIASIS, FAMILIAL CHRONIC MUCOCUTANEOUS (FCMC) 21205
*CANINE TEETH, ABSENCE OF UPPER PERMANENT 11460
CANINE TEETH, ABSENCE OF UPPER PERMANENT see ANODONTIA, PARTIAL (10660)
CANITIES PREMATURA see BOOK SYNDROME OR PHC SYNDROME (11230), WAARDENBURG
SYNDROME (19350)
CANTHI, LATERAL DISPLACEMENT OF MEDIAL see WAARDENBURG SYNDROME (19350)
CAPDEPONT TEETH see DENTINOGENESIS IMPERFECTA (12550)
CARABELLI ANOMALY OF MAXILLARY MOLAR TEETH 11470
CARBAMYL PHOSPHATE SYNTHETASE DEFICIENCY see HYPERAMMONEMIA II (23730)
CARBOHYDRATE-INDUCIBLE (CARBOHYDRATE-EXACERABLE) HYPERLIPEMIA see HYPERLIPO-
PROTEINEMIA III AND IV (14450, 14460)
CARBONIC ANHYDRASE B see RENAL TUBULAR ACIDOSIS WITH PROGRESSIVE NERVE DEAF-
NESS (26730)
*CARBONIC ANHYDRASE, ERYTHROCYTE, ELECTROPHORETIC VARIANTS OF (CA I) 11480
*CARBONIC ANHYDRASE, ERYTHROCYTE, ELECTROPHORETIC VARIANTS OF (CA II) 11481
CARCINOID BRONCHIAL see ENDOCRINE ADENOMATOSIS, MULTIPLE (13110)
CARCINOID, INTESTINAL 11490
CARDIAC ARRHYTHMIA (EXTRASYSTOLES) 11500
*CARDIAC CONDUCTION DEFECT 11508
CARDIAC CONDUCTION SYSTEM, DEFECT IN 11510
CARDIAC CONDUCTION SYSTEM, DEFECT IN see BUNDLE BRANCH BLOCK (11390)
CARDIAC LIPIDOSIS, FAMILIAL 21208
CARDIAC MALFORMATION see COARCTATION OF AORTA (12000), ATRIAL SEPTAL DEFECT
(10880), EBSTEIN ANOMALY (22470), PULMONIC STENOSIS (26550), SUPRAVALVAR AORTIC
STENOSIS (18550)
CARDIO-AUDITORY SYNDROME OF JERVELL AND LANGE-NIELSEN see DEAFMUTISM III
CARDIO-AUDITORY SYNDROME OF SANCHEZ CASCOS 21210
CARDIOMYOPATHY, FAMILIAL IDIOPATHIC 11520
CARDIOMYOPATHY, OBSTRUCTIVE see VENTRICULAR HYPERTROPHY, HEREDITARY (19260)
CARDIOMYOPATHY see OPHTHALMOPLEGIA, PIGMENTARY DEGENERATION OF RETINA AND
CARDIOMYOPATHY (16510)
*CARNOSINEMIA 21220
CAROTENEMIA, FAMILIAL 11530
CAROTID ARTERIES, HYPOPLASIA OF see INTERNAL CAROTID ARTERIES, HYPOPLASIA OF (24310)
CAROTID BODY TUMORS see PARAGANGLIOMATA (16800)
CAROTID-CAVERNOUS FISTULA see EHLERS-DANLOS SYNDROME (13000, 22540, 30520)
CARPAL BONES, FUSION OF see MITRAL REGURGITATION (15770), SYNOSTOSES (18640), SYMPHAL-
ANGISM (18560, 18570), ELLIS-VAN CREVELD SYNDROME (22550)
CARPAL DISPLACEMENT (CARPAL BOSSING) 11540
CARPAL FUSIONS see BANKI SYNDROME (10930)
CARPAL OSTEOLYSIS see OSTEOLYSIS, HEREDITARY, OF CARPAL BONES WITH NEPHROPATHY
(16630), OSTEOARTHROPATHY OF SCHINZ AND FURTWAENGLER (25900)
CARPENTER SYNDROME see ACROCEPHALOPOLYSYNDACTYLY II (20100)
CARTILAGE-HAIR HYPOPLASIA see METAPHYSEAL CHONDRODYSPLASIA, MCKUSICK TYPE
(25025)
CARTWRIGHT BLOOD GROUP see BLOOD GROUP — CARTWRIGHT SYSTEM (11210)
*CASEIN VARIANTS 11545
CAT EYE SYNDROME (OCULAR COLOBOMA, IMPERFORATE ANUS, ETC.) 11547
*CATALASE 11550
CATALASE VARIANTS see ACATALASEMIA (20020)
CATAPLEXY see NARCOLEPSY (16140)
CATARACT, ANTERIOR POLAR see MICROPHTHALMIA-CATARACT (15685)
*CATARACT, CRYSTALLINE ACULEIFORM OR FROSTED 11570
*CATARACT, CRYSTALLINE CORALLIFORM 11580
*CATARACT, FLORIFORM 11590

CUSHING DISEASE see PHEOCHROMOCYTOMA AND AMYLOID-PRODUCING MEDULLARY THY-
ROID CARCINOMA (17140)
*CUTIS LAXA 12370
CUTIS LAXA, CORNEAL CLOUDING, MENTAL RETARDATION 12380
CUTIS LAXA see WRINKLED SKIN SYNDROME (27825)
*CUTIS LAXA 21910
CUTIS LAXA WITH BONE DYSTROPHY 21920
CUTIS VERTICIS GYRATA AND MENTAL DEFICIENCY 21930
CUTIS VERTICIS GYRATA, THYROID APLASIA AND MENTAL RETARDATION 30420
CUTIS VERTICIS see ACROMEGALOID CHANGES, CUTIS VERTICIS GYRATA AND CORNEAL
LEUKOMO (10210)
CYANIDE INTOXICATION see LEBER OPTIC ATROPHY (30890)
CYANIDE TOXICITY, QUESTION OF see LEBER OPTIC ATROPHY (30890)
CYANIDE, INABILITY TO SMELL 30430
CYANOSIS AND HEPATIC DISEASE 21940
CYANOSIS see HB M (14170), VENULAR INSUFFICIENCY, SYSTEMIC (19270), HB FREIBURG (14170)
CYCLOPIA see HOLOPROSENCEPHALY, FAMILIAL ALOBAR (23610)
CYCLOPS see HOLOPROSENCEPHALY, FAMILIAL ALOBAR (23610)
CYLINDROMATOSIS 12385
CYLINDROMA see SPIEGLER-BROOKE TUMORS (31310)
CYLINDROMATOSIS (TURBAN TUMORS) see EPITHELIOMA, HEREDITARY MULTIPLE BENIGN
CYSTIC (13270)
CYSTATHIONINE SYNTHASE DEFICIENCY see HOMOCYSTINURIA (23620)
*CYSTATHIONINURIA 21950
CYSTIC DISEASE OF KIDNEY AND-OR LIVER see ALSO POLYCYSTIC KIDNEY, INFANTILE TYPE I
(26320)
CYSTIC DISEASE OF LUNG 21960
CYSTIC DISEASE OF THE KIDNEY see POLYCYSTIC KIDNEYS (17390), TUBEROUS SCLEROSIS (19110)
CYSTIC DISEASE OF THE LUNG see FIBROCYSTIC PULMONARY DYSPLASIA (13500)
*CYSTIC FIBROSIS (MUCOVISCIDOSIS) 21970
CYSTIC KIDNEY DISEASE see NEPHRONOPHTHISIS (25610), ASPHYXIATING THORACIC DYSTRO-
PHY OF THE NEWBORN (20850)
CYSTIC LYMPHANGIOMATOSIS see PULMONARY CYSTIC LYMPHANGIECTASIS (26530)
CYSTIC MEDIAL NECROSIS OF AORTA see ERDHEIM CYSTIC MEDIAL NECROSIS OF AORTA (13290)
CYSTINOSIS, ADULT see CYSTINOSIS III (22000)
CYSTINOSIS see FANCONI SYNDROME I (22770)
*CYSTINOSIS I (EARLY ONSET NEPHROPATHIC TYPE: INFANTILE TYPE) 21980
*CYSTINOSIS II (LATE ONSET NEPHROPATHIC TYPE; JUVENILE OR ADOLESCENT TYPE) . . . 21990
*CYSTINOSIS III (BENIGN TYPE; ADULT TYPE) 22000
*CYSTINURIA I, II, III (AT LEAST 3 ALLELES AT ONE LOCUS) 22010
CYSTS OF MACULA see MACULAR DEGENERATION, POLYMORPHIC (15370)
CYSTS OF THE JAW 12390
*CYTOCHROME B(5) 12395
*CYTOCHROME C 12397
CYTOCHROME-RELATED DISEASE OF MUSCLE AND NERVOUS SYSTEM 12400
*DALMATIAN HYPOURICEMIA 22015
DANDY-WALKER ANOMALY see OSTEODYSTROPHY AND MENTAL RETARDATION (25930)
*DANDY-WALKER SYNDROME 22020
DANDY-WALKER SYNDROME see HYDROCEPHALUS (23660)
DANUBIAN ENDEMIC FAMILIAL NEPHROPATHY (DEFN; BALKAN NEPHROPATHY) 12410
*DARIER-WHITE DISEASE (KERATOSIS FOLLICULARIS) 12420
DARWINIAN POINT (OF PINNA) 12430
DARWINIAN TUBERCLE (OF PINNA) 12440
DAY-BLINDNESS see COLOR-BLINDNESS, TOTAL (21690)
DE LANGE SYNDROME see CORNELIA DE LANGE SYNDROME (21790)
DE LANGE SYNDROME see CORNELIA DE LANGE SYNDROME (21790)
DEAF-MUTISM AND FAMILIAL MYOCLONUS EPILEPSY 22030
*DEAF-MUTISM AND FUNCTIONAL HEART DISEASE (PROLONGED Q-T INTERVAL IN EKG AND
SUDDEN DEATH) 22040
*DEAF-MUTISM AND ONYCHODYSTROPHY 22050
DEAF-MUTISM AND SPLIT HANDS AND FEET 22060
*DEAF-MUTISM I (CONGENITAL DEAFNESS) 22070
*DEAFMUTISM II (CONGENITAL DEAFNESS) 22080
DEAFMUTISM WITH GROWTH HORMONE EXCESS BY RADIO-IMMUNO-ASSAY see PITUITARY
DWARFISM II (26250)
DEAF-MUTISM WITH TOTAL ALBINISM 22090
DEAF-MUTISM, SEMILETHAL 22100
DEAFNESS AND ATOPIC DERMATITIS 22110
DEAFNESS AND HIDROTIC ECTODERMAL DYSPLASIA see ECTODERMAL DYSPLASIA AND NEU-
ROSENSORY DEAFNESS (22480)
DEAFNESS, COCHLEAR, WITH MYOPIA AND INTELLECTUAL IMPAIRMENT 22120
*DEAFNESS, CONDUCTIVE, WITH MALFORMED EXTERNAL EAR 22130
DEAFNESS, CONDUCTIVE see KLIPPEL-FEIL DEFORMITY, ETC. OBLIGATE HETEROZYGOTES HAD
NORMAL URINARY CONCENTRATION. USE OF THIS PROVED ERRONEOUS IN GENETIC COUN-
SELING. (14890)
*DEAFNESS, CONDUCTIVE TYPE, WITH STAPES FIXATION 30440
*DEAFNESS, CONGENITAL, PERCEPTIVE TYPE 30450
DEAFNESS, HIGH TONE NEURAL 30460
DEAFNESS, NERVE TYPE, WITH MESENTERIC DIVERTICULA OF SMALL BOWEL AND PROGRESSIVE
NEUROPATHY 22140
DEAFNESS, NEURAL, CONGENITAL MODERATE 22150
DEAFNESS, NEURAL, EARLY ONSET 22160
DEAFNESS, NEURAL, WITH ATYPICAL ATOPIC DERMATITIS 22170
DEAFNESS, NEUROSENSORY, WITH PITUITARY DWARFISM 22175

*DYSAUTONOMIA (RILEY-DAY SYNDROME) 22390
DYSAUTONOMIA, TYPE II see NEUROPATHY, CONGENITAL SENSORY, WITH ANHIDROSIS (25680)
DYSAUTONOMIA-LIKE DISORDER 22400
DYSAUTONOMIA see NEUROPATHY, CONGENITAL SENSORY, WITH ANHIDROSIS (25680)
DYSCHONDROPLASIA see OSTEOCHONDROMATOSIS (16600)
*DYSCHONDROSTEOSIS 12730
DYSCHROMATOPSIA see COLOR BLINDNESS, PARTIAL (30380-30400)
DYSCHROMATOSIS SYMMETRICA HEREDITARIA 12740
DYSCHROMATOSIS UNIVERSALIS HEREDITARIA 12750
DYSENCEPHALIA SPLANCHNOCYSTICA see MECKEL SYNDROME (24900)
*DYSERYTHROPOIETIC ANEMIA, HEMPAS TYPE OR TYPE II 22410
*DYSERYTHROPOIETIC ANEMIA, TYPE I 22412
DYSFIBRINOGENEMIAS see FIBRINOGEN (13480)
DYSFIBRINOGENEMIA see FIBRINOGEN VARIANTS (13480)
DYSGENESIS MESODERMALIS CORNEAE ET SCLERAE 22420
DYSGENESIS MESODERMALIS see RIEGER SYNDROME (18050)
DYSKERATOSIS CONGENITA, SCOGGINS TYPE 12755
*DYSKERATOSIS, CONGENITA (ZINSSER-COLE-ENGMAN SYNDROME) 30500
*DYSKERATOSIS, HEREDITARY BENIGN INTRAEPITHELIAL 12760
DYSLEXIA, SPECIFIC ('CONGENITAL WORD-BLINDNESS') 12770
*DYSOSTEOSCLEROSIS 22430
DYSOSTOSIS, ENCHONDRAL, OF NIERHOFF-HUBNER TYPE 22440
DYSOSTOSIS, PERIPHERAL see PERIPHERAL DYSOSTOSIS (17070), ACRODYSOSTOSIS (10180)
DYSPHAGIA see ODONTOMA-DYSPHAGIA SYNDROME (16433)
DYSPLASIA EPIPHYSEALIS HEMIMELICA 12780
DYSPLASIA OF HIP see HIP, DISLOCATION OF, CONGENITAL (14270)
DYSPROTEINEMIA, FAMILIAL IDIOPATHIC see LYMPHANGIECTASIA, INTESTINAL (15280)
*DYSPROTHROMBINEMIA 12790
DYSSPONDYLY see COSTOVERTEBRAL SEGMENTATION ANOMALIES (12260), VERTEBRAL ANOM-
    ALIES (27730)
DYSSYNERGIA CEREBELLARIS MYOCLONICA see MYOCLONUS AND ATAXIA (15970)
DYSTASIA, HEREDITARY AREFLEXIC see ROUSSY-LEVY HEREDITARY AREFLEXIC DYSTASIA
    (18080)
*DYSTELEPHALANGY (KIRNER DEFORMITY) 12800
*DYSTONIA MUSCULORUM DEFORMANS 22450
DYSTONIA WITH 'RINGBINDEN' 22455
DYSTONIA, PERIODIC 22460
DYSTONIA see AMYOTROPHIC DYSTONIC PARAPLEGIA (10530)
*DYSTONIA MUSCULORUM DEFORMANS 12810
*DYSTONIA, FAMILIAL PAROXYSMAL 12820
DYSTONIC LIPIDOSIS, JUVENILE see LIPIDOSIS, JUVENILE DYSTONIC (24680)
DYSTOPIA CANTHORUM see TELECANTHUS WITH ASSOCIATED ABNORMALITIES (31360), WAAR-
    DENBURG SYNDROME (19350)
DYSTOPIC LIPIDOSIS, HEREDITARY see ANGIOKERATOMA, DIFFUSE (30150)
DYSTROPHIA MYOTONICA see MYOTONIC DYSTROPHY (16090)
DYSTROPHY OF CORNEA see CORNEAL DYSTROPHY (12150-12230, 21740-21780)
DYSTROPHY, MUSCULAR see MUSCULAR DYSTROPHY (15880-15900, 25360-25410, 31000-31030)
EAR EXOSTOSES (EXOSTOSES OF EXTERNAL AUDITORY CANAL) 12830
EAR FLARE 12840
EAR FOLDING 12850
*EAR MALFORMATION ('CUP EAR') 12860
EAR PITS 12870
EAR WAX see CERUMEN, VARIATION IN (11780)
EAR WITHOUT HELIX 12880
EAR, CHARACTERISTIC SHAPE OF see AURICULO-OSTEODYSPLASIA (10900)
EARLOBE ATTACHMENT (ATTACHED VS. UNATTACHED) 12890
EARLOBE CREASE 12895
EARS, ABILITY TO MOVE 12910
EARS, CUP-SHAPED see EAR MALFORMATION (12860)
EAR see MICROTIA WITH MEATAL ATRESIA (25180)
EAR DEFORMITY see HYPERTELORISM, MICROTIA, FACIAL CLEFTING SYNDROME (23980)
EAR PECULIARITY see FACIAL ASYMMETRY, ETC. (13390)
EAR PITS see DEAFNESS WITH EAR PITS (12510)
EAR, MALFORMATION OF see DEAFNESS, CONDUCTIVE, WITH MALFORMED EXTERNAL EAR
    (22130)
EARS, CALCIFICATION OF see DIASTROPHIC DWARFISM (22260), ALKAPTONURIA (20350), PULMO-
    NARY ARTERIAL STENOSIS ETC. (26520)
EBSTEIN ANOMALY 22470
ECHO 11 SENSITIVITY 12915
ECLAMPSIA see TOXEMIA OF PREGNANCY (18980)
ECTODERMAL DYSPLASIA AND NEURISENSORY DEAFNESS 22480
*ECTODERMAL DYSPLASIA, ANHIDROTIC 22490
ECTODERMAL DYSPLASIA, ANHYDROTIC see ANHIDROSIS (20660)
*ECTODERMAL DYSPLASIA, ANHIDROTIC 30510
ECTODERMAL DYSPLASIA, CLEFT LIP AND PALATE, HAND AND FOOT DEFORMITY AND MENTAL
    RETARDATION 22500
ECTODERMAL DYSPLASIA see DEAFNESS, ECTODERMAL DYSPLASIA, POLYDACTYLISM AND
    SYNDACTYLISM (12460), EEC SYNDROME (12990)
*ECTODERMAL DYSPLASIA, ABSENT DERMATOGLYPHIC PATTERN, CHANGES IN NAILS AND
    SIMIAN CREASE (BASAN SYNDROME) 12920
ECTODERMAL DYSPLASIA, ANHIDROTIC 12930
ECTODERMAL DYSPLASIA, ANHIDROTIC, WITH CLEFT LIP AND CLEFT PALATE . . . 12940
*ECTODERMAL DYSPLASIA, HIDROTIC 12950

FAMILIAL MEDITERRANEAN FEVER see MEDITERRANEAN FEVER, FAMILIAL (24910), PEL-
GER-HUET-LIKE ANOMALY AND EPISODIC FEVER (26057)
*FANCONI PANCYTOPENIA (CONSTITUTIONAL INFANTILE PANMYELOPATHY) 22765
FANCONI RENOTUBULAR SYNDROME 13460
FANCONI SYNDROME see BILIARY MALFORMATION WITH RENAL TUBUALR INSUFFICIENCY
(21055)
*FANCONI SYNDROME I (CHILDHOOD AND INFANTILE FORM WITHOUT CYSTINOSIS) 22770
*FANCONI SYNDROME II ('ADULT' FORM WITHOUT CYSTINOSIS) 22780
FANCONI-LIKE SYNDROME 22785
FANCONI'S NEPHRONOPHTHISIS see NEPHRONOPHTHISIS, FAMILIAL JUVENILE (25610)
*FARBER LIPOGRANULOMATOSIS 22800
FASCICULATION, MUSCULAR see ATAXIA WITH FASCICULATIONS (10870)
FASCICULATIONS, BENIGN see MYOKYMIA (16010)
FASCICULATIONS see SPINAL AND BULBAR MUSCULAR ATROPHY (31320)
FAT-INDUCED HYPERLIPEMIA see HYPERLIPOPROTEINEMIA I (23860)
FATTY METAMORPHOSIS OF VISCERA 22810
FAVISM 13470
FAVRE VITREO-RETINAL DEGENERATION see RETINOSCHISIS WITH EARLY HEMERALOPIA
(26810)
FAZIO-LONDE DISEASE see BULBAR PARALYSIS, PROGRESSIVE, OF CHILDHOOD (21150)
FDH SYNDROME see FOCAL DERMAL HYPOPLASIA (30560)
FEMALE PSEUDO-TURNER SYNDROME see PTERYGIUM COLLI SYNDROME (17810)
FEMUR-FIBULA-ULNA (FFU) SYNDROME 22820
FERTILE EUNUCH 22830
FERTILITY, DECREASED see HAIR-BRAIN SYNDROME (23405)
FETAL HEMOGLOBIN, HEREDITARY PERSISTENCE OF see HEMOGLOBIN F (14170)
FETTHALS SYNDROME see CERVICAL LIPODYSPLASIA, FAMILIAL (11785), LIPOMATOSIS, FAMIL-
IAL BENIGN CERVICAL (15180)
FEVER OF UNKNOWN ORIGIN see MEDITERRANEAN FEVER, FAMILIAL (24910), PERIODIC FEVER
(17030)
FEVER, FAMILIAL LIFELONG PERSISTENT 22840
FFU SYNDROME see FEMUR-FIBULA-ULNA SYNDROME (22820)
FG SYNDROME see CORPUS CALLOSUM, PARTIAL AGENESIS OF (30410)
FIBRIN MONOMER AGGREGATION PRODUCING CLOTTING DISTURBANCE see FIBRINOGEN
VARIANTS (13480)
*FIBRINOGEN 13480
FIBRINOGEN BALTIMORE see FIBRINOGEN, VARIANTS (13480)
FIBRINOGEN CROSS-LINKAGE DEFECT, DUE TO DEFICIENCY OF TRANSGLUTAMINASE . . . 13481
FIBRINOGEN DEFICIENCY see AFIBRINOGENEMIA, CONGENITAL (20240)
FIBRINOGEN — ALPHA POLYPEPTIDE CHAIN 13482
FIBRINOGEN — BETA POLYPEPTIDE CHAIN 13483
FIBRINOGEN — GAMMA POLYPEPTIDE CHAIN 13485
FIBRINOGENOPATHIES see FIBRINOGEN VARIANTS (13480)
FIBRINOLYTIC DEFECT 13490
*FIBRIN-STABILIZING FACTOR (FIBRINASE, OR FACTOR XIII) DEFICIENCY 22850
*FIBRIN-STABILIZING FACTOR (FACTOR XIII) DEFICIENCY 30550
*FIBROCYSTIC PULMONARY DYSPLASIA 13500
*FIBRODYSPLASIA OSSIFICANS PROGRESSIVA 13510
FIBROMATOSIS OF SMALL INTESTINE see NEUROFIBROMATOSIS (16220)
FIBROMATOSIS, CONGENITAL GENERALIZED 13520
FIBROMATOSIS, GINGIVAL 13530
*FIBROMATOSIS, GINGIVAL, WITH HYPERTRICHOSIS 13540
*FIBROMATOSIS, GINGIVAL, WITH ABNORMAL FINGERS, FINGERNAILS, NOSE AND EARS AND
SPLENOMEGALY 13550
*FIBROMATOSIS, JUVENILE 22860
FIBROMUSCULAR HYPERPLASIA OF THE RENAL ARTERIES 22870
FIBRO-OSSEOUS DYSPLASIA OF THE JAWS 13560
FIBROSCLEROSIS, MULTIFOCAL 22880
FIBROSIS OF EXTRAOCULAR MUSCLE 13570
FIBROSIS, PULMONARY see PULMONARY FIBROSIS, IDIOPATHIC (17850)
FIBROUS DYSPLASIA OF JAW see CHERUBISM (11840)
FIBROUS DYSPLASIA see POLYOSTOTIC FIBROUS DYSPLASIA (17480)
FIBULA AND ULNA DUPLICATION OF, WITH ABSENCE OF TIBIA AND RADIUS 13575
FIBULA AND ULNA, HYPOPLASIA OF see ULNA AND FIBULA, HYPOPLASIA OF (19140), NIEVER-
GELT SYNDROME (16340), MESOMELIC DWARFISM (24970)
FIBULA AND ULNA, PARTIAL ABSENCE OF see ACHONDROGENESIS II 20070), FFU SYNDROME
(22820)
FIBULA AND ULNA, TRIANGULAR see NEONATAL OSSEOUS DYSPLASIA I (25605)
FIBULA APLASIA AND COMPLEX BRACHYDACTYLY 22890
FIBULA, RECURRENT DISLOCATION OF HEAD OF 13580
FIBULA, SHORT see MENTAL RETARDATION SYNDROME (24960)
FIFTH DIGIT SYNDROME 13590
FINGER, ABSENT TERMINAL PHALANX OF FIFTH FINGERS see FIFTH FINGER SYNDROME (13590)
FINGER, RADIALLY CURVED FIFTH see CAMPTODACTYLY (11420)
*FINGERPRINTS, ABSENCE OF 13600
FINGERPRINTS see RADIAL LOOP, PLAIN, ON RIGHT INDEX FINGER (31220)
FINGERPRINTS, ABSENCE OF see ECTODERMAL DYSPLASIA, ABSENT DERMATOGLYPHIC PAT-
TERN, ETC. (12920)
FINGERS, CURVED see BRACHYDACTYLY, TYPE A2 (11260)
FINGERS, RELATIVE LENGTH OF 13610
FISH-ODOR SYNDROME see TRIMETHYLAMINURIA (27570)
FISSURED TONGUE see GEOGRAPHIC TONGUE AND FISSURED TONGUE (13740)
FISTULA AURIS CONGENITA see DEAFNESS, WITH EAR PITS (12510), BRANCHIAL CLEFT ANOMA-
LIES (11360), EARPITS (12870)

GANGLIOSIDE LIPIDOSIS see TAY-SACHS DISEASE (27280), AMAUROTIC IDIOCY, CONGENITAL
    FORM (20440)
*GANGLIOSIDOSIS, GENERALIZED GM(1), TYPE I 23050
*GANGLIOSIDOSIS, GENERALIZED GM(1), TYPE II, OR LATE INFANTILE TYPE 23060
*GANGLIOSIDOSIS, GM(2), TYPE III, OR JUVENILE TYPE 23070
 GANGLIOSIDOSIS, GM(2), TYPE I see TAY-SACHS DISEASE (27280, 27290)
 GANGLIOSIDOSIS, GM(2), TYPE II see SANDHOFF DISEASE (26880)
 GANGLIOSIDOSIS, GM(3) 23075
 GANGRENE OF SKULL, ASEPTIC see APLASIA CUTIS CONGENITA (10760)
 GARDNER SYNDROME see POLYPOSIS, INTESTINAL III (17530)
*GARGOYLISM see MUCOPOLYSACCHARIDOSIS I, II, AND III (25280, 30990, 25290)
 GASTRIC JUICE PEPTIDES 13722
 GASTRIN 13725
 GAT-TOOTHED TRAIT see DIASTEMA, DENTAL MEDIAL (12590)
 GAUCHER DISEASE 13730
*GAUCHER DISEASE TYPE I (NON-CEREBRAL, JUVENILE) 23080
 GAUCHER DISEASE TYPE II (INFANTILE, CEREBRAL) 23090
 GAUCHER DISEASE TYPE III (JUVENILE AND ADULT, CEREBRAL) 23100
 GC see GROUP-SPECIFIC COMPONENT (13920)
 GELEOPHYSIC DWARFISM 23105
 GEOGRAPHIC TONGUE AND FISSURED TONGUE 13740
 GERMINAL CELL APLASIA (SERTOLI-CELL-ONLY SYNDROME; DEL CASTILLO SYNDROME) . 30570
 GERODERMIA OSTEODYSPLASTICA 30580
*GIANT CELL HEPATITIS, NEONATAL 23110
 GIANT CELL HEPATITIS see CIRRHOSIS, FAMILIAL (11890)
 GIANT CELL HEPATITIS, NEONATAL see HEMOCHROMATOSIS, IDIOPATHIC NEONATAL (23510),
    HYPERMETHIONINURIA (23890)
*GIANT NEUTROPHILE LEUKOCYTES 13750
 GIANT PIGMENTED HAIRY NEVUS 13755
 GIGANTISM, ACROMEGALOID see SEIP SYNDROME (26970)
 GIGANTISM, CEREBRAL see CEREBRAL GIGANTISM (11760, 21380)
 GILBERT DISEASE see HYPERBILIRUBINEMIA I (14350)
 GINGIVAL FIBROMATOSIS see FIBROMATOSIS, GINGIVAL, WITH HYPERTRICHOSIS (13540)
 GINGIVAL HYPERPLASIA see RUTHERFURD SYNDROME (18090)
 GLANZMANN THROMBOPATHY see THROMBASTHENIA OF GLANZMANN AND NAEGELI (18780,
    27380)
 GLANZMANN-NAEGELI THROMBASTHENIC THROMBOPATHY see THROMBASTHENIA OF
    GLANZMANN-NAEGELI (18780, 27380)
*GLAUCOMA 13760
 GLAUCOMA WITH ELEVATED EPISCLERAL VENOUS PRESSURES 13770
*GLAUCOMA, CONGENITAL (BUPHTHALMOS) 23130
*GLAUCOMA, CONGENITAL, WITH MENTAL RETARDATION 23140
*GLAUCOMA, HEREDITARY JUVENILE 13775
*GLAUCOMA, JUVENILE 23150
 GLAUCOMA see IRIS, HYPOPLASIA OF, WITH GLAUCOMA (30850), CHONDRODYSTROPHY, JOINT
    DISLOCATION, GLAUCOMA AND MENTAL RETARDATION (21520), MICROCORNEA, GLAUCOMA
    AND ABSENT FRONTAL SINUSES (15670)
 GLIOMA OF BRAIN 13780
 GLIOMA-POLYPOSIS SYNDROME see TURCOT SYNDROME (27630)
 GLOBOID CELL SCLEROSIS see KRABBE DISEASE (24520)
 GLOBULIN ANOMALY INVOLVING BETA (2A)-GLOBULIN 13790
 GLOMUS JUGULARE TUMORS see PARAGANGLIOMATA (16800)
*GLOMUS TUMORS, MULTIPLE 13800
 GLOSSOPTYSIS see CEREBRO-COSTO-MANDIBULAR SYNDROME (21400), PIERRE ROBIN SYN-
    DROME (26180)
 GLUCOGLYCINURIA 13810
*GLUCOSE-GALACTOSE MALABSORPTION 23160
 GLUCOSEPHOSPHATE ISOMERASE (GPI) DEFICIENCY see PHOSPHOHEXOSE ISOMERASE, VARI-
    ANTS OF (17240)
 GLUCOSEPHOSPHATE ISOMERASE DEFICIENCY HEMOLYTIC ANEMIA see PHOSPHOHEXOSE
    ISOMERASE, VARIANTS OF (17240)
*GLUCOSE-6-PHOSPHATE DEHYDROGENASE 30590
 GLUCOSE-6-PHOSPHATE DEHYDROGENASE see FAVISM (13470)
 GLUCOSE-6-PHOSPHATE DEHYDROGENASE, INSTABILITY OF, IN LEUKOCYTES see CHRONIC
    GRANULOMATOUS DISEASE DUE TO LEUKOCYTE MALFUNCTION (23370, 30640)
*GLUTAMATE OXALOACETATE TRANSAMINASE, MITOCHONDRIA (GOT-2) 13815
*GLUTAMATE OXALOACETATE TRANSAMINASE, SOLUBLE (GOT-1) 13818
 GLUTAMATE-ASPARTATE TRANSPORT DEFECT 23165
*GLUTAMATE-PYRUVATE TRANSAMINASE (GPT-1) 13820
 GLUTAMATE-PYRUVATE TRANSMINASE, MITOCHONDRIAL (GPT-2) 13821
 GLUTAMICACIDEMIA see MENKES SYNDROME (30940)
*GLUTARIC ACIDEMIA 23167
*GLUTATHIONE PEROXIDASE DEFICIENCY, HEMOLYTIC ANEMIA DUE TO 23170
 GLUTATHIONE PEROXIDASE DEFICIENCY OF LEUKOCYTES see GRANULOMATOUS DISEASE DUE
    TO LEUKOCYTE MALFUNCTION (23370, 30640)
*GLUTATHIONE REDUCTASE 13830
*GLUTATHIONE REDUCTASE, HEMOLYTIC ANEMIA DUE TO DEFICIENCY OF, IN RED CELLS . 23180
*GLUTATHIONE SYNTHETASE DEFICIENCY OF ERYTHROCYTES, HEMOLYTIC ANEMIA DUE TO 23190
 GLUTEN-INDUCED ENTEROPATHY see CELIAC SPRUE (11690)
*GLYCERALDEHYDE-3-PHOSPHATE DEHYDROGENASE 13840
 GLYCERIC ACIDURIA see OXALOSIS II (26000)
 GLYCEROL KINASE 13841
*GLYCEROL-3-PHOSPHATE DEHYDROGENASE-1 13842
*GLYCEROL-3-PHOSPHATE DEHYDROGENASE-2 13843

GRUBER SYNDROME   see MECKEL SYNDROME (24900)
GUANASE 13926
*GUANYLATE KINASE 13927
GUMS, HYPERPLASIA OF   see FIBROMATOSIS, GINGIVAL (13530), RUTHERFURD SYNDROME (18090)
GYNECOMASTIA, HEREDITARY 13930
GYNECOMASTIA, HEREDITARY 23390
GYNECOMASTIA   see SPINAL AND BULBAR MUSCULAR ATROPHY (31320)
GYNECOMASTIA, FAMILIAL   see REIFENSTEIN SYNDROME (31230)
GYNECOMASTIA, FAMILIAL 30650
G6PD DEFICIENCY   see GLUCOSE-6-PHOSPHATE DEHYDROGENASE VARIANTS (30590), REGIONAL
    ENTERITIS (26660)
G6PD WORCESTER UNDER G6PD VARIANTS   see BEHR SYNDROME (21000)
*HAGEMAN FACTOR DEFICIENCY 23400
HAILEY-HAILEY DISEASE   see PEMPHIGUS, BENIGN FAMILIAL (16960)
*HAIR ALPHA-PROTEIN 13935
HAIR WHORL ('COW-LICK,' 'CROWN') 13940
HAIR, ABNORMALITY OF   see CARTILAGE-HAIR HYPOPLASIA (21230), NETHERTON DISEASE
    (25650), MENKES SYNDROME (30940), ARGINIOSUCCINICACIDURIA (20790), TRICHORRHEXIS
    NODOSA SYNDROME (27555), NONILETHRIX (15800)
HAIR, ANOMALIES OF   see MONILETHRIX (15800, 25220)
HAIR, 'BRITTLE'   see HAIR-BRAIN SYNDROME (23405)
HAIR, MIDPHALANGEAL   see MIDPHALANGEAL HAIR (15720)
*HAIR-BRAIN SYNDROME (AMISH BRITTLE HAIR SYNDROME) 23405
HAIR, RED   see RED HAIR (26630)
HAIRY EARS (HYPERTRICHOSIS PINNAE AURIS) 13950
HAIRY ELBOWS 13960
HAIR   see BLOND HAIR (21075), RED HAIR (26630)
HAIR, EARLY GRAYING OF   see GRAYING OF HAIR, EARLY (13910)
HAIR, WHITE LOCK OF OCCIPITAL   see OCCIPITAL HAIR, WHITE LOCK OF (31090)
HAIRLESSNESS   see HYPOTRICHOSIS (24190)
HALLERMANN-STREIFF SYNDROME 23410
*HALLERVORDEN AND SPATZ, SYNDROME OF 23420
HALO NEVI (LEUKODERMA ACQUISITUM CENTRIFUGUM OF SUTTON) 23430
HAMARTOMA SYNDROME   see MULTIPLE HAMARTOMA SYNDROME (15835)
HAMARTOMA SYNDROME   see MULTIPLE HAMARTOMA SYNDROME (COWDEN DISEASE) (15835)
HAMMAN-RICH SYNDROME   see PULMONARY FIBROSIS, IDIOPATHIC (17850)
HAND AND FOOT DEFORMITY WITH FLAT FACIES 13975
HAND CLASPING PATTERN 13980
HANDEDNESS 13990
HAND-FOOT-UTERUS (HFU) SYNDROME 14000
HANHART ABSENCE DEFORMITY OF LIMBS WITH MICROGNATISM   see PEROMELIA WITH
    MICROGNATHISM (26130)
HANHART DWARFISM (ATELEIOTIC DWARFISM WITH HYPOGONADISM)   see PITUITARY DWARF-
    ISM II (26250)
'HAPPY PUPPET' SYNDROME 23440
HAPSBURG JAW   see PROGNATHISM, MANDIBULAR (17670)
*HAPTOGLOBIN, ALPHA LOCUS (Hp) 14010
*HAPTOGLOBIN, BETA LOCUS (Bp) 14020
HARLEQUIN FETUS   see ICHTHYOSIS, CONGENITAL, 'HARLEQUIN FETUS' TYPE (24250)
*HARTNUP DISEASE 23450
HASHIMOTO STRUMA 14030
HAY FEVER   see ATOPIC HYPERSENSITIVITY (20920)
HEART AND HAND SYNDROME   see TABATZNIK HEART-HAND SYNDROME (18680), HOLT-ORAM
    SYNDROME (14290)
HEART AND HAND SYNDROME I   see HOLT-ORAM SYNDROME (14290)
HEART ANOMALY   see ELLIS-VAN CREVELD SYNDROME (22550), ATROPHODERMIA VER-
    MICULATA (20970)
*HEART BLOCK 14040
HEART BLOCK AND OPHTHALMOPLEGIA 23460
*HEART BLOCK, CONGENITAL 23470
HEART BLOCK   see ATRIOVENTRICULAR DISSOCATION (20960), ATRIAL SEPTAL DEFECT WITH
    ATRIO-VENTRICULAR CONDUCTION DEFECT (10890)
HEART MALFORMATION   see ATRIAL SEPTAL DEFECT (10880)
HEART, MALFORMATION OF 14050
HEART, MALFORMATION OF 23475
HEAT URTICARIA   see URTICARIA, FAMILIAL LOCALIZED HEAT (19195)
HEBERDEN NODES 14060
HEINZ BODY ANEMIA 14070
HEINZ BODY ANEMIA   see HEMOGLOBIN UBE AND HEMOGLOBIN ZURICH (14170)
HEMANGIOBLASTOMA, CEREBELLAR AND SPINAL   see VON HIPPEL-LINDAU SYNDROME (19330)
HEMANGIOMA, CAVERNOUS   see GLOMUS TUMORS, MULTIPLE (13800)
HEMANGIOMAS 14080
HEMANGIOMAS OF SMALL INTESTINE 14090
HEMANGIOMAS   see GLOMUS TUMOR, MULTIPLE (13800), BLUE RUBBER BLEB NEVUS (11220)
HEMANGIOMATA   see MACROCEPHALY (24800), KLIPPEL-TRENAUNAY-WEBER SYNDROME
    (14900), VON HIPPEL-LINDAU SYNDROME (19330), STURGE-WEBER SYNDROME (18530)
HEMANGIOMA-THROMBOCYTOPENIA SYNDROME (KASABACH-MERRITT SYNDROME) . . . 14100
HEMANGIOMATOSIS, CUTANEOUS, WITH ASSOCIATED FEATURES 23480
HEMANGIOMATOSIS, DISSEMINATED 14110
HEMATOSIDE SPHINGOLIPODYSTROPHY   see GANGLIOSIDOSIS, GM(3) (23075)
*HEMATURIA, BENIGN FAMILIAL 14120
HEMATURIA   see HYDROXYPROLINEMIA (23700)
HEMERALOPIA   see NIGHT BLINDNESS (25725), HEMERALOPIA MEANS DAY BLINDNESS BUT IS

HYPERCALCINURIA   see HYPOURICEMIA, HYPERCALCINURIA AND DECREASED BONE DENSITY (24205)
HYPERCALCIURIA 23810
HYPERCALCIURIA   see RENAL TUBULAR ACIDOSIS (17980)
HYPERCAROTINEMIA, FAMILIAL   see CAROTINEMIA, FAMILIAL (11530)
HYPERCHOLESTEROLEMIA   see HYPERLIPOPROTEINEMIAS (14430-14460, 23860)
HYPERCHYLOMICRONEMIA   see HYPERLIPOPROTEINEMIA I (23860)
HYPERCYSTINURIA, ISOLATED 23820
HYPERDIBASICAMINOACIDURIA   see DIBASICAMINOACIDURIA (12600, 22270)
HYPERELASTICA CUTIS   see EHLERS-DANLOS SYNDROME (13000, 22540, 30520), FIBRINOLYTIC DEFECT (13490)
*HYPERGLYCINEMIA, ISOLATED 23830
HYPERGLYCINEMIA   see METHYLMALONICACIDURIA (25100, 25110), GLYCINEMIA (23200)
HYPERGLYCINURIA   see GLYCINURIA WITH OR WITHOUT UROLITHIASIS (13850), TACHYCARDIA, ETC. (27255), IMINOGLYCINURIA (24260)
HYPERHEPARINEMIA 14400
HYPERHIDROSIS   see BOOK SYNDROME (11230)
HYPERHIDROSIS   see BOOK SYNDROME, OR PHC SYNDROME (11230), CHARCOT-MARIE-TOOTH DISEASE (11820, 11830), GAMSTORP-WOHLFART SYNDROME (13720)
HYPERHIDROSIS, GUSTATORY 14410
HYPERHYDROXYPROLINEMIA   see HYDROXYPROLINEMIA (23700)
HYPERKERATOSIS   see DEAFNESS, CONGENITAL WITH KERATOPACHYDERMIA AND CONSTRICTIONS OF FINGERS AND TOES (12450), KERATOSIS (14840)
HYPERKERATOSIS FOLLICULARIS ET PARAFOLLICULARIS IN CUTEM PENETRANS   see KYRLE DISEASE (14940)
HYPERKERATOSIS LENTICULARIS PERSTANS 14415
HYPERKERATOSIS PALMOPLANTARIS   see KERATOSIS PALMARIS ET PLANTARIS (14840), ALOPECIA CONGENITA WITH KERATOSIS PLANTARIS (10410)
*HYPERKERATOSIS, LOCALIZED EPIDERMOLYTIC 14420
*HYPERLIPIDEMIA, COMBINED 14425
HYPERLIPIDEMIA   see SEIP SYNDROME (26970), HYPERLIPOPROTEINEMIAS (14440-14460, 23860)
HYPERLIPIDEMIA V (FAMILIAL HYPERPREBETALIPOPROTEINEMIA, CARBOHYDRATE-INDUCIBLE HYPERLIPEMIA) 23840
HYPERLIPIDEMIA VI (FAMILIAL HYPERCHYLOMICRONEMIA WITH HYPERPREBETALIPOPROTEINEMIA, MIXED HYPERLIPEMIA, COMBINED FAT AND CARBOHYDRATE-INDUCED HYPERLIPEMIA) 23850
HYPERLIPOGENESIS   see PRADER-WILLI SYNDROME (26400)
HYPERLIPOPROTEINEMIA (TYPE II) AND DEAFNESS 14430
*HYPERLIPOPROTEINEMIA I (FAMILIAL HYPERCHYLOMICRONEMIA, IDIOPATHIC HYPERLIPEMIA OF BURGER-GRUTZ TYPE, ESSENTIAL FAMILIAL HYPERLIPEMIA) 23860
*HYPERLIPOPROTEINEMIA II (HYPERBETALIPOPROTEINEMIA, HYPER-LOW-DENSITY-LIPOPROTEINEMIA, ESSENTIAL FAMILIAL HYPERCHOLESTEROLEMIA, FAMILIAL HYPERCHOLESTEROLEMIC XANTHOMATOSIS, XANTHOMA TUBEROSUM MULTIPLEX, FAMILIAL XANTHOMA) 14440
HYPERLIPOPROTEINEMIA III (FAMILIAL HYPERBETA AND PREBETALIPOPROTEINEMIA, FAMILIAL HYPERCHOLESTEROLEMIA WITH HYPERLIPEMIA, HYPERLIPEMIA WITH FAMILIAL HYPERCHOLESTEROLEMIC XANTHOMATOSIS, CARBOHYDRATE-INDUCED HYPERLIPEMIA) . . 14450
HYPERLIPOPROTEINEMIA IV (CARBOHYDRATE INDUCED HYPERLIPEMIA) . . . 14460
*HYPERLYSINEMIA 23870
HYPERLYSINEMIA   see LYSINE INTOLERANCE (24790)
HYPERLYSINURIA WITH HYPERAMMONEMIA 23875
HYPERMETABOLISM DUE TO DEFECT IN MITOCHONDRIA 23880
HYPERMETABOLISM DUE TO DEFECT IN MITOCHONDRIA   see MYOPATHY WITH GIANT ABNORMAL MITOCHONDRIA (25540)
HYPERMETHIONINEMIA 23890
HYPERMETHIONINEMIA   see HOMOCYSTINURIA (23620)
HYPERNEPHROMA   see VON HIPPEL-LINDAU SYNDROME (19330)
HYPERNEPHROMA (ADENOCARCINOMA OF KIDNEY) 14470
*HYPEROSTOSIS CORTICALIS GENERALISATA, BENIGN FORM OF WORTH, WITH TORUS PALATINUS 14475
*HYPEROSTOSIS CORTICALIS DEFORMANS JUVENILIS (JUVENILE PAGET DISEASE, CHRONIC CONGENITAL IDIOPATHIC HYPERPHOSPHATASEMIA) 23900
*HYPEROSTOSIS CORTICALIS GENERALISATA (VAN BUCHEM DISEASE: HYPERPHOSPHATASEMIA TARDA) 23910
HYPEROSTOSIS FRONTALIS INTERNA (MORGAGNI-STEWART-MOREL SYNDROME) . . 14480
HYPEROSTOSIS GENERALISATA WITH STRIATIONS   see OSTEOPATHIA STRIATA (16650)
HYPEROXALURIA 14490
HYPEROXALURIA   see OXALOSIS I AND II (25990, 26000)
HYPERPARATHYROIDISM 14500
*HYPERPARATHYROIDISM, NEONATAL FAMILIAL PRIMARY 23920
HYPERPHOSPHATASEMIA TARDA   see HYPEROSTOSIS CORTICALIS GENERALISTA (23910)
HYPERPHOSPHATASEMIA   see HYPEROSTOSIS CORTICALIS DEFORMANS JUVENILIS (23900)
*HYPERPHOSPHATASIA WITH MENTAL RETARDATION 23930
HYPERPHOSPHATASIA, CONGENITA   see HYPEROSTOSIS CORTICALIS DEFORMANS JUVENILIS (23900)
HYPERPHOSPHATEMIA   see CALCINOSIS, TUMORAL (21190)
*HYPERPIGMENTATION OF EYELIDS 14510
HYPERPIGMENTATION OF FULDAUER AND KUIJPERS 14520
HYPERPIGMENTATION OF FULDAUER AND KUIJPERS   see NAEGELI SYNDROME (16100), INCONTINENTIA PIGMENTI (30830), ACANTHOSIS NIGRICANS (10060)
HYPERPIGMENTATION, FAMILIAL PROGRESSIVE 14525
HYPERPIPECOLATEMIA 23940
HYPERPLASIA, GINGIVAL   see FIBROMATOSIS, GINGIVAL (13530, 13540), FACIAL HYPERTRICHOSIS (13400)
*HYPERPROLINEMIA, TYPE I 23950

*HYPERPROLINEMIA, TYPE II 23951
  HYPERPYREXIA IN ANESTHESIA   see HYPERTHERMIA OF ANESTHESIA (14560), SUXAMETHONIUM
    SENSITIVITY (27240)
  HYPERPYREXIA, MALIGNANT, OF ANESTHESIA   see HYPERTHERMIA OF ANESTHESIA (14560)
  HYPER-REFLEXIA, HEREDITARY   see KOK DISEASE (14940)
  HYPERSEGMENTATION OF THE NUCLEI OF THE POLYMORPHONUCLEAR LEUKOCYTES see
    UNDRITZ ANOMALY (19150)
  HYPERSEROTONEMIA 23960
*HYPERTELORISM (GREIG SYNDROME) 14540
  HYPERTELORISM, CRYPTORCHIDISM, DIGITAL CONTRACTURES, STERNAL DEFORMITY, AND
    OSTEOCHONDRITIS DISSECANS 23970
  HYPERTELORISM, MICROTIA, FACIAL CLEFTING (HMC) SYNDROME 23980
  HYPERTELORISM   see TELECANTHUS WITH ASSOCIATED ABNORMALITIES (31360), FACIOGENI-
    TAL DYSPLASIA (30540), LISSENCEPHALY SYNDROME (24720)
  HYPERTELORISM WITH ESOPHAGEAL ABNORMALITY AND HYPOSPADIAS (G SYNDROME) . 30710
  HYPERTENSION   see FIBROMUSCULAR HYPERPLASIA OF RENAL ARTERIES (22870), PSEU-
    DO-ALDOSTERONISM (17720)
  HYPERTENSION, ESSENTIAL 14550
  HYPERTENSION, PULMONARY   see PULMONARY HYPERTENSION, PRIMARY (17860, 26540)
  HYPERTHELIA   see NIPPLES, SUPERNUMERARY (16370)
*HYPERTHERMIA OF ANESTHESIA 14560
  HYPERTHYROIDISM   see THYROTOXICOSIS (27500)
  HYPERTONIA   see KOK DISEASE (14940)
  HYPERTRICHOSIS CUBITI   see HAIRY ELBOWS (13960)
  HYPERTRICHOSIS   see FIBROMATOSIS, GINGIVAL (13530, 13540), HAIRY EARS (13950), HAIRY
    ELBOWS (13960)
*HYPERTRICHOSIS, UNIVERSALIS 14570
*HYPERTRIGLYCERIDEMIA 14575
*HYPERTROPHIA MUSCULORUM VERA 14580
*HYPERTROPHIC NEUROPATHY OF DEJERINE-SOTTAS 14590
  HYPERTROPHIC NEUROPATHY AND CATARACT 23990
  HYPERTROPHIC SUBAORTIC STENOSIS   see VENTRICULAR HYPERTROPHY, HEREDITARY (19260)
  HYPERURICEMIA, INFANTILE, WITH ABNORMAL BEHAVIOR AND NORMAL HYPOXANTHINE
    GUANINE PHOSPHORIBOSYL TRANSFERASE 24000
  HYPERURICEMIA, LIPODYSTROPHY AND NEUROLOGIC DEFECT 24010
  HYPERURICEMIA   see GOUT (13890, 30620), HYPOXANTHINE GUANINE PHOSPHORIBOSYL TRANS-
    FERASE DEFICIENCY (30800), NEPHROPATHY, FAMILIAL, WITH GOUT (16200), GLYCOGEN
    STORAGE DISEASE I (23220), FRUCTOSE INTOLERANCE, HEREDITARY (22960)
  HYPERURICEMIA, ATAXIA, DEAFNESS 30720
  HYPERVALINEMIA   see VALINEMIA (27710)
  HYPOADRENALISM   see SCHMIDT SYNDROME (26920)
*HYPOADRENOCORTICISM, FAMILIAL 24020
*HYPOADRENOCORTICISM, WITH HYPOPARATHYROIDISM AND SUPERFICIAL MONILIASIS . . 24030
  HYPOADRENOCORTICISM   see ADRENAL HYPERPLASIA, VARIOUS TYPES (20170-20210, 30020)
  HYPOALDOSTERONISM   see ALDOSTERONE SYNTHESIS, DEFECT IN (20340)
*HYPOASCORBEMIA 24040
  HYPOBETALIPOPROTEINEMIA 14595
  HYPOCALCEMIA   see DWARFISM, CORTICAL THICKENING OF TUBULAR BONES, AND TRANSIENT
    HYPOCALCEMIA (12700)
  HYPOCHOLESTEROLEMIA   see HYPOBETALIPOPROTEINEMIA (14595)
  HYPOCHONDROPLASIA 14600
  HYPOCOMPLEMENTEMIA   see COMPLEMENT COMPONENT C-PRIME-2, DEFICIENCY OF (21700)
  HYPODONTIA   see TEETH, ABSENCE OF (31350)
  HYPOFIBRINOGENEMIA 14610
*HYPOGAMMAGLOBULINEMIA 24050
  HYPOGLYCEMIA WITH ABSENT PANCREATIC ALPHA CELLS 24055
*HYPOGLYCEMIA WITH DEFICIENCY OF GLYCOGEN SYNTHETASE IN THE LIVER 24060
  HYPOGLYCEMIA, KETOTIC, OF CHILDHOOD 24065
*HYPOGLYCEMIA, LEUCINE INDUCED 24080
  HYPOGLYCEMIA, NEONATAL, SIMULATING FOETOPATHIA DIABETICA 24090
  HYPOGLYCEMIA   see EMG SYNDROME (22560), FRUCTOSE-1, 6-DIPHOSPHATASE, HEPATIC DEFI-
    CIENCY OF (22970), FRUCTOSE INTOLERANCE, HEREDITARY (22960), GALACTOSEMIA (23040),
    GLYCOGEN STORAGE DISEASE (23210-23280, 30600)
  HYPOGONADISM, MALE 30730
  HYPOGONADISM, MALE, AND ATAXIA 30740
  HYPOGONADISM, MALE, WITH MENTAL RETARDATION AND SKELETAL ANOMALIES . . . 30750
  HYPOGONADISM   see EUNUCHOIDISM, FAMILIAL HYPOGONADOTROPHIC (22720), CLEFT LIP
    AND-OR PALATE WITH MUCOUS CYSTS OF LOWER LIP (11930), HYPERTELORISM (23970),
    KALLMANN SYNDROME (24420, 24430, 30870)
  HYPOGONADISM WITH LOW-GRADE MENTAL DEFICIENCY AND MICROCEPHALY 24100
  HYPOGONADISM, MALE 24110
  HYPOKALEMIA   see PSEUDO-ALDOSTERONISM (17720), POTASSIUM AND MAGNESIUM DEPLETION
    (26380)
*HYPOKALEMIC ALKALOSIS (BARTTER SYNDROME) 24120
  HYPOKALEMIC ALKALOSIS, HYPERTENSION AND AMENORRHEA   see ADRENAL HYPERPLASIA V
    (20210)
  HYPOLIPIDEMIA   see ANALPHALIPOPROTEINEMIA (20540), ABETALIPOPROTEINEMIA (20010),
    HOOFT DISEASE (23630), ANEMIA, HYPOCHROMIC (30130)
  HYPOMAGNESEMIA, PRIMARY 24130
*HYPOMAGNESEMIC TETANY 30760
*HYPOMELANOSIS OF ITO ('INCONTINENTIA PIGMENTI ACHROMIANS') 14615
  HYPOPARATHYROIDISM 14620
*HYPOPARATHYROIDISM 24140
*HYPOPARATHYROIDISM 30770

HYPOPARATHYROIDISM   see HYPOADRENOCORTICISM, WITH HYPOPARATHYROIDISM AND SU-
PERFICIAL MONILIASIS (24030), CEREBRAL CALCIFICATION (21360)
*HYPOPHOSPHATASIA 14630
*HYPOPHOSPHATASIA (PHOSPHOETHANOLAMINURIA) 24150
*HYPOPHOSPHATEMIA (X-LINKED) (VITAMIN-D-RESISTANT RICKETS) 30780
HYPOPIGMENTATION, GENERALIZED   see OCULOCEREBRAL SYNDROME WITH HYPOPIGMENTA-
TION (25780)
HYPOPIGMENTATION   see RAINDROP HYPOPIGMENTATION (17950), DILUTION, PIGMENTARY
(12607)
HYPOPITUITARY DWARFISM   see PITUITARY DWARFISM II (26250)
HYPOPLASIA OF TEETH 14640
HYPOPLASTIC LEFT HEART SYNDROME 24155
HYPOPROCONVERTINEMIA   see FACTOR VII DEFICIENCY (22750)
HYPOPROTEINEMIA, HYPERCATABOLIC 24160
HYPOPROTEINEMIA, IDIOPATHIC   see LYMPHANGIECTASIA, INTESTINA (15280)L, ENTEROPA-
THY, PROTEIN-LOSING (22630)
*HYPOPROTHROMBINEMIA 24170
HYPOSEGMENTATION OF THE NUCLEI, OF THE POLYMORPHONUCLEAR LEUKOCYTES   see
PELGER-HUET ANOMALY (16940)
HYPOSPADIAS   see TELECANTHUS WITH ASSOCIATED ABNORMALITIES (31360), REIFENSTEIN
SYNDROME (31230), SMITH-LEMLI-OPITZ SYNDROME (27040), PSEUDOVAGINAL PERINEOSCRO-
TAL HYPOSPADIAS (26460), HYPERTELORISM SYNDROME (14540)
HYPOTENSION, ORTHOSTATIC (SHY-DRAGER SYNDROME) 14650
HYPOTHALAMIC HAMARTOMAS 24180
HYPOTHYROIDISM   see THYROID HORMONOGENESIS, DEFECT IN (27440-27490), SCHMIDT SYN-
DROME (26920), MYXEDEMA (25590), THYROID HORMONOGENESIS, GENETIC DEFECT IN, V
(27490), THYROTROPIN, UNRESPONSIVENESS TO (27520)
HYPOTONIA-HYPOMENTIA-HYPOGONADISM-OBESITY   see PRADER-WILLI SYNDROME (26400)
*HYPOTRICHOSIS WITH LIGHT-COLORED HAIR AND FACIAL MILIA 14653
*HYPOTRICHOSIS, HEREDITARY (MARIE UNNA TYPE) 14655
HYPOTRICHOSIS   see MILIA-HYPOTRICHOSIS SYNDROME (15745)
HYPOTRICHOSIS   see WOOLLY HAIR, HYPOTRICHOSIS EVERTED LOWER LIP, ETC. (27820)
*HYPOTRICHOSIS ('HAIRLESSNESS') 24190
HYPOTRICHOSIS, SYNDACTYLY AND RETINITIS PIGMENTOSA 24200
HYPOURICEMIA   see DALMATION HYPOURICEMIA (22015)
*HYPOURICEMIA, HYPERCALCINURIA, AND DECREASED BONE DENSITY 24205
*HYPOXANTHINE GUANINE PHOSPHORIBOSYL TRANSFERASE 30800
I-CELL DISEASE   see MUCOLIPIDOSIS II (25250)
ICHTHYOSIFORM ERYTHRODERMA, BULLOUS FORM   see BULLOUS ERYTHRODERMA ICH-
THYOSIFORMIS CONGENITA (BROCQ) (11380)
*ICHTHYOSIFORM ERYTHRODERMA, BROCQ CONGENITAL, NON-BULLOUS FORM 24210
ICHTHYOSIFORM ERYTHRODERMIA, CORNEAL INVOLVEMENT, DEAFNESS 24215
*ICHTHYOSIFORM ERYTHRODERMA, UNILATERAL, WITH IPSILATERAL MALFORMATIONS ESPE-
CIALLY ABSENCE DEFORMITY OF LIMBS 24220
*ICHTHYOSIS (X-LINKED) 30810
ICHTHYOSIS AND MALE HYPOGONADISM 30820
*ICHTHYOSIS CONGENITA (LAMELLAR EXFOLIATION, OR DESQUAMATION OF THE NEWBORN,
COLLODION FETUS, ETC.) 24230
ICHTHYOSIS CONGENITA AND CATARACT   see CATARACT AND CONGENITAL ICHTHYOSIS (21240)
ICHTHYOSIS CONGENITA WITH BILIARY ATRESIA 24240
ICHTHYOSIS CONGENITA, 'HARLEQUIN FETUS' TYPE 24250
ICHTHYOSIS CONGENITA   see HARLEQUIN FETUS (23440)
ICHTHYOSIS   see NEUTROPHIL CHEMOTACTIC DEFECT (16282)
*ICHTHYOSIS HYSTRIX GRAVIOR (LAMBERT TYPE ICHTHYOSIS, 'PORCUPINE MAN') 14660
*ICHTHYOSIS VULGARIS (ICHTHYOSIS SIMPLEX) 14670
ICHTHYOSIS, BULLOUS TYPE 14680
ICSH DEFICIENCY   see FERTILE EUNUCH (22830)
IHSS (IDIOPATHIC HYPERTROPHIC SUBAORTIC STENOSIS)   see VENTRICULAR HYPERTROPHY
(19260)
IMERSLUND SYNDROME   see PERNICIOUS ANEMIA, JUVENILE (26110)
IMIDAZOLE AMINOACIDURIA   see AMAUROTIC FAMILY IDIOCY, JUVENILE TYPE (20420)
*IMINOGLYCINURIA 24260
*IMMUNE DEFECT DUE TO ABSENCE OF THYMUS 24270
IMMUNE DEFECT WITH DEFICIENCY OF URIDINE MONOPHOSPHATE KINASE   see URIDINE
MONOPHOSPHATE KINASE (19173)
IMMUNE DEFECT WITH DEFICIENCY OF ADENOSINE DEAMINASE 24275
*IMMUNE DEFECT WITH LYMPHOTOXIC FACTOR 24280
IMMUNE DEFECT, CELLULAR   see CHONDROITIN-6-SULFATURIA, DEFECTIVE CELLULAR IMMU-
NITY, NEPHROTIC SYNDROME (21515)
IMMUNE DEFICIENCY DISEASE 24285
IMMUNE DEFICIENCY   see ADENOSINE DEAMINASE (10270)
*IMMUNE RESPONSE (Ir) 14685
IMMUNE RESPONSE ASSOCIATED ANTIGENS (Ia) 14686
IMMUNODEFICIENCY WITH INCREASED IGM 30823
IMMUNODEFICIENCY   see KAPPA-CHAIN DEFICIENCY (24435)
IMMUNOGLOBULIN A, LEVEL OF 14687
IMMUNOGLOBULIN A, SELECTIVE DEFICIENCY OF   see GAMMA-A-GLOBULIN, SELECTIVE DEFI-
CIENCY OF (13710)
IMMUNOGLOBULIN A, SELECTIVE DEFICIENCY OF   see GAMMA-A-GLOBULIN, SELECTIVE DEFI-
CIENCY OF (13710)
*IMMUNOGLOBULIN Am(1) 14690
*IMMUNOGLOBULIN Am(2) (IgA HEAVY CHAIN LOCUS) 14700
IMMUNOGLOBULIN E (IgE), BASIC LEVEL OF, IN SERUM 14705
*IMMUNOGLOBULIN Gm-1 (IgG HEAVY CHAIN LOCUS) 14710

JAUNDICE, NEONATAL OBSTRUCTIVE   see GIANT CELL HEPATITIS, NEONATAL (23110)
JAUNDICE   see HYPERBILIRUBINEMIA (30860)
JAUNDICE, FAMILIAL OBSTRUCTIVE, OF INFANCY 30860
JAVRE HYALOIDO-TAPETORETINAL DEGENERATION   see HYALOIDO-TAPETORETINAL DEGEN-
   ERATION OF FAVRE (23650)
JAW, CYSTS OF   see CHERUBISM (11840), BASAL CELL NEVUS SYNDROME (10940), CYSTS OF JAW
   (12390)
JAW, OSTEOMA OF   see POLYPOSIS, INTESTINAL III (17530), OSTEOMA OF MANDIBLE (16640), TORUS
   PALATINUS AND TORUS MANDIBULARIS (18970)
JAW, WINKING   see MARCUS GUNN PHENOMENON (15460)
JAW-JERKING   see EPILEPSY, PRIMARY READING (13220)
*JEJUNAL ATRESIA ('APPLE PEEL' SYNDROME) 24360
JERVELL AND LANGE-NIELSEN SYNDROME   see DEAFMUTISM AND FUNCTIONAL HEART DIS-
   EASE (22040)
JEUNE SYNDROME   see ASPHYXIATING THORACIC DYSTROPHY OF THE NEWBORN (20850)
*JOB SYNDROME 24370
JOINT CONTRACTURES WITH OTHER ABNORMALITIES 14780
JOINT CONTRACTURES   see PSEUDO-ARTHROGRYPOSIS (17720)
JOINT HYPERFLEXIBILITY   see HEMANGIOMATOSIS, CUTANEOUS, WITH ASSOCIATED FEATURES
   (23480), EHLERS-DANLOS SYNDROME (13000, 13005, 22540, 22541, 30520)
JOINT LAXITY (ARTHROCHALASIS MULTIPLEX CONGENITA) 24380
*JOINT LAXITY, FAMILIAL 14790
JORDANS ANOMALY OF LEUKOCYTES 24390
JOSEPH SYNDROME 24400
JUMPING FRENCHMAN OF MAINE (SEE ALSO HYPER-REFLEXIA, HEREDITARY) 24410
JUVENILE POLYPOSIS COLI   see POLYPOSIS COLI, JUVENILE TYPE (17490)
KALLMANN SYNDROME (HYPOGONADOTROPIC HYPOGONADISM AND ANOSMIA) 24420
KALLMANN SYNDROME (SECONDARY, OR HYPOGONADOTROPIC, HYPOGONADISM WITH ANOS-
   MIA; DYSPLASIA OLFACTOGENITALIS OF DE MORSIER) 30870
KALLMANN SYNDROME WITH FACIAL CLEFTING 24430
KAPOSI SARCOMA 14800
KAPPA-CHAIN DEFICIENCY 24435
KAPPA-CHAIN, VARIANTS OF   see IMMUNOGLOBULIN INV LOCUS (14720)
*KARTAGENER SYNDROME (DEXTROCARDIA, BRONCHIECTASIS AND SINUSITIS) 24440
KASABACH-MERRITT SYNDROME   see HEMANGIOMA-THROMBOCYTOPENIA SYNDROME (14100)
KELL BLOOD GROUP   see BLOOD GROUP KELL-CELLANO SYSTEM (11090)
KELL 'MODIFIER' 30875
KELOIDS 14810
KELOIDS   see TORTICOLLIS, KELOIDS, CRYPTORCHIDISM, AND RENAL DYSPLASIA (31430)
KENNY SYNDROME   see DWARFISM, CORTICAL THICKENING OF TUBULAR BONES, AND TRAN-
   SIENT HYPOCALCEMIA (12700)
KERATINIZED PROTEIN, POLYMORPHISM OF   see HAIR ALPHA-PROTEIN (13935)
*KERATITIS FUGAX HEREDITARIA 14820
KERATOACANTHOMA   see EPITHELIOMA, SELF-HEALING SQUAMOUS (FERGUSON-SMITH TYPE)
   (13280)
KERATOCONUS 14830
KERATOCONUS 24450
KERATOCONUS POSTICUS CIRCUMSCRIPTUS 24460
KERATOPACHYDERMIA   see DEAFNESS, CONGENITAL WITH KERATOPACHYDERMIA AND CON-
   STRICTIONS OF FINGERS AND TOES (12450)
KERATOPATHY, BAND-SHAPED   see CORNEAL DYSTROPHY, BAND-SHAPED (21750)
KERATOSES, SEBORRHEIC   see SEBORRHEIC KERATOSES (18200)
*KERATOSIS PALMARIS ET PLANTARIS FAMILIARIS (TYLOSIS) 14840
*KERATOSIS PALMARIS ET PLANTARIS WITH ESOPHAGEAL CANCER 14850
KERATOSIS PALMO-PLANTARIS PAPULOSA 14860
KERATOSIS PALMO-PLANTARIS STRIATA 14870
KERATOSIS PALMO-PLANTARIS TRANSGRADIENS OF SIEMENS   see MAL DE MELEDA (24830)
*KERATOSIS PALMO-PLANTARIS WITH CORNEAL DYSTROPHY (RICHNER-HANHART SYNDROME) 24480
*KERATOSIS PALMO-PLANTARIS WITH PERIODONTOPATHIA (PAPILLON-LEFEVRE SYNDROME) 24500
KERATOSIS   see PORKERATOSIS OF MIBELLI (17580)
KERATOSIS FOLLICULARIS   see DARIER-WHITE DISEASE (12420)
KERATOSIS FOLLICULARIS, DWARFISM, CEREBRAL ATROPHY 30877
*KERATOSIS FOLLICULARIS, SPINULOSA DECALVANS CUM OPHIASI 30880
KERATOSIS PALMARIS ET PLANTARIS   see KNUCKLE PADS LEUKONYCHIA AND SENSINEURAL
   DEAFNESS (14920)
KERATOSIS PALMO-PLANTARIS   see SCLERO-ATROPHIC AND KERATOTIC DERMATOSIS OF LIMBS
   (18160), ALOPECIA CONGENITA WITH KERATOSIS PALMO-PLANTARIS (10410)
KERATOSIS PALMO-PLANTARIS CIRCUMSCRIPTA   see RICHNER-HANHART SYNDROME (26825)
KETOACIDOSIS OF INFANCY (SUCCINYL-COA: 3-KETOACID COA-TRANSFERASE DEFICIENCY) . 24505
*KETOACIDURIA WITH MENTAL DEFICIENCY AND OTHER FEATURES (RICHARDS-RUNDLE SYN-
   DROME) 24510
KETOTHIOLASE DEFICIENCY   see ALPHA-METHYLACETOACETICACIDURIA (20375)
KEUTEL SYNDROME 24515
KIDD BLOOD GROUP   see BLOOD GROUP-KIDD SYSTEM (11100)
KIDNEY, ADENOCARCINOMA OF   see HYPERNEPHROMA (14470)
*KILLER ANTIGEN OF PUCK 14873
KINESOGENIC CHOREOATHETOSIS   see DYSTONIA, FAMILIAL PAROXYSMAL (12820)
KINKY HAIR DISEASE   see MENKES SYNDROME (30940)
KIRNER DEFORMITY   see DYSTELEPHALANGY (12800)
KLEEBLATTSCHAEDEL (CLOVERLEAF SKULL) SYNDROME 14880
KLIPPEL-FEIL DEFORMITY, CONDUCTIVE DEAFNESS, ABSENT VAGINA 14886
KLIPPEL-FEIL SYNDROME 14890
KLIPPEL-FEIL SYNDROME   see VERTEBRAL ANOMALIES (27730), WILDERVANCK SYNDROME
   (31460), CERVICAL VERTEBRAL FUSION (11810, 21430)

KLIPPEL-TRENAUNAY-WEBER SYNDROME 14900
KNEE JOINT, DISLOCATION OF   see CAMPTODACTYLY (11420)
KNIEST DISEASE   see METATROPHIC DWARFISM, TYPE II (15655)
KNUCKLE PADS 14910
*KNUCKLE PADS, LEUKONYCHIA AND SENSINEURAL DEAFNESS 14920
KOCHER-DEBRE-SEMELAIGNE SYNDROME (CHILDHOOD HYPOTHYROIDISM WITH MUSCULAR
   'HYPERTROPHY')   see CRETINISM, ATHYREOTIC (21870)
*KOILONYCHIA, HEREDITARY 14930
*KOK DISEASE 14940
KOSTMANN AGRANULOCYTOSIS   see AGRANULOCYTOSIS, INFANTILE GENETIC, OF KOSTMANN
   (20270)
*KRABBE DISEASE (GLOBOID CELL SCLEROSIS) 24520
KRAMER SYNDROME   see OCULOCEREBRAL SYNDROME WITH HYPOPIGMENTATION (25780)
KRAUSE-REESE SYNDROME   see ENCEPHALO-RETINAL DYSPLASIA (13100)
KUF DISEASE   see AMAUROTIC IDIOCY, ADULT TYPE (20430)
KUGELBERG-WELANDER DISEASE   see MUSCULAR ATROPHY, JUVENILE (15860, 25340)
KURU 24530
KUSKOKWIN DISEASE   see ARTHROGRYPOSIS-LIKE DISORDER (20820)
KYPHOSCOLIOSIS, OSTEOPENIA, CONGENITAL CONTRACTURES   see CONTRACTURAL ARACHNO-
   DACTYLY (12105)
KYPHOSCOLIOSIS   see FACIAL ABNORMALITIES ETC. (22727)
KYPHOSIS, LUMBAR   see VERTEBRAL HYPOPLASIA WITH LUMBAR KYPHOSIS (19290)
KYRLE DISEASE 14950
LABIA MINORA, INCOMPLETE ADHESION OF 14960
*LACRIMAL DUCT DEFECT 14970
LACRIMAL DUCT DEFECT   see CLEFT LIP-PALATE WITH SPLIT HAND AND FOOT (11940)
LACRIMAL DUCTS, ANOMALY OF   see ORBITAL MARGIN, HYPOPLASIA O (16560)F
*LACRIMO-AURICULO-DENTO-DIGITAL SYNDROME (LADD) 14973
LACTALBUMIN 14975
LACTASE DEFICIENCY, INTESTINAL, IN ADULT   see DISACCHARIDE INTOLERANCE III (22310)
LACTASE, DEFECT IN INTESTINAL   see DISACCHARIDE INTOLERANCE III (22310)
*LACTATE DEHYDROGENASE, LOCUS A 15000
*LACTATE DEHYDROGENASE, LOCUS B 15010
*LACTATE DEHYDROGENASE, LOCUS C (TESTICULAR VARIANT X) 15015
LACTIC ACIDOSIS, CHRONIC ADULT FORM 15017
LACTIC ACIDOSIS   see FRUCTOSE-1, 6-DIPHOSPHATASE, HEPATIC, DEFICIENCY OF, ALANINURIA,
   ETC. (20290), TRICARBOXYLIC ACID CYCLE, DEFECT OF (27535)
LACTIC ACIDOSIS   see MITOCHONDRIAL MYOPATHY WITH LACTIC ACIDOSIS (25195), NECROTIZ-
   ING ENCPEHALOPATHY, INFANTILE SUBACUTE, OF LEIGH (25600), MYOPATHY WITH LACTIC
   ACIDOSIS (25514), PYRUVATE CARBOXYLASE DEFICIENCY (26615), ATAXIA, INTERMITTENT,
   ETC. (20880)
*LACTIC ACIDOSIS, FAMILIAL INFANTILE 24540
LACTOGEN, PLACENTAL 15020
LACTOSE INTOLERANCE   see DISACCHARIDE INTOLERANCE II AND III (22300, 22310)
*LACTOSYLCERAMIDOSIS 24550
LACUNAE, SYMMETRICAL PARIETAL   see PARIETAL FORAMINA, SYMMETRICAL (16850), CRA-
   NIUM BIFIDUM OCCULTUM (12320)
LADD SYNDROME   see LACRIMO-AURICULO-DENTO-DIGITAL SYNDROME (14975)
LAFORA DISEASE   see MYOCLONIC EPILEPSY (25480)
LANDING DISEASE   see GANGLIOSIDOSIS, GENERALIZED (23050, 23060)
LANDOUZY-DEJERINE MUSCULAR DYSTROPHY   see MUSCULAR DYSTROPHY FACIO-SCAPU-
   LO-HUMERAL (15890)
LANGER-GIEDION SYNDROME 15023
LARD SYNDROME   see LACRIMO-AURICULO-DENTO-DIGITAL SYNDROME (14973)
*LARSEN SYNDROME 15025
*LARSEN SYNDROME 24560
LARYNGEAL ABDUCTOR PARALYSIS 30885
LARYNGEAL STENOSIS   see SCHINZEL SYNDROME (18145)
LARYNGEAL WEBS   see LARYNX, CONGENITAL PARTIAL ATRESIA OF (15030)
LARYNX, CONGENITAL PARTIAL ATRESIA OF 15030
LARYNX, POSTERIOR CLEFT OF   see CLEFT LARYNX, POSTERIOR (21580)
*LATERAL INCISORS, ABSENCE OF 15040
LATTICE CORNEAL DYSTROPHY   see AMYLOIDOSIS V (10512), CORNEAL DYSTROPHY, LATTICE
   TYPE (12220)
LATTICE DEGENERATION OF RETINA LEADING TO RETINAL DETACHMENT 15050
*LAURENCE-MOON SYNDROME 24580
LAWRENCE-SEIP SYNDROME   see SEIP SYNDROME (26970)
LAZY LEUKOCYTE SYNDROME 24585
LCAT DEFICIENCY   see LECITHIN: CHOLESTEROL ACETYLTRANSFERASE (LCAT) DEFICIENCY
   (24590)
LD SYSTEM   see LIPOPROTEIN TYPES — LD SYSTEM (15210)
LDH VARIANTS   see LACTIC DEHYDROGENASE VARIANTS (14990-15010)
LEBER CONGENITAL AMAUROSIS   see AMAUROSIS CONGENITA (NOT TO BE CONFUSED WITH
   LEBER OPTIC ATROPHY) (20400)
LEBER DISEASE   see LEBER OPTIC ATROPHY (30890)
LEBER OPTIC ATROPHY   see OPTIC ATROPHY — SPASTIC PARAPLEGIA SYNDROME (31110)
LEBER OPTIC ATROPHY 30890
*LECITHIN: CHOLESTEROL ACYLTRANSFERASE (LCAT) DEFICIENCY (NORUM DISEASE) . . . 24590
*LEG, ABSENCE DEFORMITY OF, WITH CONGENITAL CATARACT 24600
LEGG-CALVE-PERTHES DISEASE 15060
LEGG-PERTHES DISEASE   see EPIPHYSEAL DYSPLASIA (22695)
LEIGH ENCEPHALOMYELOPATHY   see NECROTIZING ENCEPHALOPATHY INFANTILE SUBACUTE
   (25600)
LEINER DISEASE   see COMPLEMENT COMPONENT-5, DEFICIENCY OF (12090)

MEDULLARY FIBROSARCOMA OF   see BONE DYSPLASIA WITH MEDULLARY FIBROSARCOMA
(11225)
MEDULLARY SPONGE KIDNEY   see POLYCYSTIC KIDNEYS, MEDULLARY TYPE (17400)
MEDULLARY STENOSIS OF LONG BONES   see DWARFISM, CORTICAL THICKENING OF TUBULAR
BONES, AND TRANSIENT HYPOCALCEMIA (12700)
MEDULLARY THYROID CARCINOMA   see PHEOCHROMOCYTOMA AND AMYLOID-PRODUCING
MEDULLARY THYROID CARCINOMA (17140)
MEDULLOBLASTOMA   see BASAL CELL NEVUS SYNDROME (10940)
MEGACOLON, AGANGLIONIC (HIRSCHSPRUNG DISEASE) 24920
MEGACONIAL MYOPATHY   see MYOPATHY, WITH GIANT ABNORMAL MITOCHONDRIA (25540)
MEGACYSTIS SYNDROME   see MEGADUODENUM AND-OR MEGACYSTIC (15530), MEGADUODE-
NUM AND-OR MEGACYSTIS (15530)
*MEGADUODENUM AND-OR MEGACYSTIS 15530
*MEGALENCEPHALY 15535
MEGALENCEPHALY   see MACROCEPHALY (24800)
MEGALOBLASTIC ANEMIA DUE TO DIHYDROFOLATE REDUCTASE DEFICIENCY 24925
MEGALOBLASTIC ANEMIA, THIAMINE-RESPONSIVE 24927
MEGALOBLASTIC ANEMIA   see PERNICIOUS ANEMIA, JUVENILE (26110)
MEGALOBLASTIC ANEMIA RESPONSIVE TO FOLIC ACID, ATAXIA, MENTAL RETARDATION AND
CONVULSIONS   see FOLIC ACID, TRANSPORT DEFECT OF ( )
MEGALOCORNEA 24930
*MEGALOCORNEA 30930
MEGALOCORNEA   see (24930)
MEGALODACTYLY 15550
MEGALO-URETER   see HYDRONEPHROSIS (14340)
MEIGE SYNDROME   see LYMPHEDEMA HEREDITARY II (15320)
MELANOCYTE STIMULATING HORMONE   see MELANOTROPIN (15585)
MELANOLEUKODERMA   see LEUKOMELANODERMA, ETC. (24650)
MELANOMA, MALIGNANT 15560
MELANOMA, MALIGNANT INTRAOCULAR 15570
MELANOSIS, CUTANEOUS   see ADDISON DISEASE AND CEREBRAL SCLEROSIS (30010)
MELANOSIS, NEUROCUTANEOUS 24940
*MELANOSIS, UNIVERSAL 15580
MELANOTROPIN, BETA (MELANOCYTE STIMULATING HORMONE, MSH) 15585
*MELKERSSON SYNDROME 15590
MELKERSSON SYNDROME   see FACIAL PALSY, CONGENITAL UNILATERAL (13410)
MELLITURIA   see SIALURIA (26990)
MELNICK-NEEDLES OSTEODYSTROPLASIA   see BONE DYSPLASIA OF MELNICK AND NEEDLES
MENIERE DISEASE 15600
MENINGIOMA 15610
MENINGOMYELOCELE   see CEREBELLO-PARENCHYMAL DISORDER IV (21330)
MENINGOMYELOCELE   see ARNOLD-CHIARI MALFORMATION (20795)
*MENKES SYNDROME (KINKY HAIR DISEASE) 30940
*MENSENCHYMAL DYSPLASIA OF PURETIC   see PURETIC SYNDROME (26570)
*MENTAL DEFICIENCY (MARTIN-BELL, OR RENPENNING TYPE); X-LINKED MENTAL RETARDA-
TION 30950
MENTAL RETARDATION 15620
MENTAL RETARDATION 24950
MENTAL RETARDATION SYNDROME (MIETENS-WEBER TYPE) 24960
MENTAL RETARDATION, BUENOS AIRES TYPE 24963
MENTAL RETARDATION   see LOWRY MENTAL RETARDATION SYNDROME (15245), CONVULSIVE
DISORDER WITH MENTAL RETARDATION (21720)
MENTAL RETARDATION AND MUSCULAR ATROPHY 30960
*MERCAPTOLACTATE-CYSTEINE DISULFIDURIA 24965
MESENCHYMAL DYSPLASIA OF PURETIC   see PURETIC SYNDROME (26570)
MESIODENS   see TEETH, SUPERNUMERARY (18710)
MESOECTODERMAL DYSGENESIS   see RIEGER SYNDROME (18050)
MESOECTODERMAL DYSPLASIA   see ELLIS-VAN CREVELD SYNDROME (22550)
*MESOMELIC DWARFISM OF THE HYPOPLASTIC ULNA, FIBULA AND MANDIBLE TYPE 24970
MESOMELIC DWARFISM   see ULNA AND FIBULA, HYPOPLASIA OF (19140)
*METACARPAL 4-5 FUSION 30963
METACARPALS AND METATARSALS, FUSED   see SYNDACTYLY, TYPE V (18630)
METACARPALS, SHORT   see THYROTROPIN DEFICIENCY, ISOLATED (27510), OSTEODYSTROPHY
AND MENTAL RETARDATION (25930)
METACHONDROMATOSIS 15625
METACHROMASIA OF FIBROBLASTS 15630
METACHROMATIC LEUKODYSTROPHY AND AMAUROTIC IDIOCY, COMBINED FEATURES OF . 24980
*METACHROMATIC LEUKODYSTROPHY, ADULT 25000
METACHROMATIC LEUKODYSTROPHY, LATE INFANTILE (METACHROMATIC LEUKOENCEPHA-
LOPATHY; METACHROMATIC FORM OF DIFFUSE CEREBRAL SCLEROSIS; SULFATIDE LIPIDOSIS) 25010
*METACHROMATIC LEUKODYSTROPHY, JUVENILE 25020
*METAPHYSEAL CHONDRODYSPLASIA, MURK JANSEN TYPE 15640
*METAPHYSEAL CHONDRODYSPLASIA, SCHMIDT TYPE 15650
METAPHYSEAL CHONDRODYSPLASIA WITH THYMOLYMPHOPENIA   see 'ACHONDROPLASIA'
WITH SWISS-TYPE AGAMMAGLOBULINEMIA (20090)
*METAPHYSEAL CHONDRODYSPLASIA, MCKUSICK TYPE (FORMERLY CALLED CARTILAGE-HAIR
HYPOPLASIA) 25025
METAPHYSEAL CHONDRODYSPLASIA, PENA TYPE 25030
METAPHYSEAL CHONDRODYSPLASIA, SPAHR TYPE 25040
METAPHYSEAL DYSOSTOSIS WITH DEFECT IN HAIR GROWTH   see CARTILAGE-HAIR HYPOPLA-
SIA (21230)
METAPHYSEAL DYSOSTOSIS   see IMMUNE DEFECT DUE TO ABSENCE THYMUS (24270)
METAPHYSEAL DYSPLASIA   see FRONTOMETAPHYSEAL DYSPLASIA (22940), CRANIOMETA-
PHYSEAL DYSPLASIA (12300, 21840)

MULTIPLE EXOSTOSES see EXOSTOSES, MULTIPLE (13370)
*MULTIPLE HAMARTOMA SYNDROME 15835
MULTIPLE SCLEROSIS see DISSEMINATED SCLEROSIS (12620, 22320), PELIZAEUS-MERZBACHER
    DISEASE (16950, 26060, 31160), MYELIN (A1) PROTEIN, BASIC (15943)
MULTIPLE SCLEROSIS-LIKE DISEASE (SEE ATAXIA, SPASTIC) 15840
MUSCLE CRAMPS see MYOKYMIA (16010), GLYCOGEN STORAGE DISEASE V (MCARDLE DISEASE
    (23260), CENTRAL CORE DISEASE OF MUSCLE (11700)
MUSCLE, ANOMALIES OF see POLAND SYNDROME (17380), PALMARIS LONGUS MUSCLE, ABSENCE
    OF (16760), MUSCULAR DYSTROPHY, FACIO-SCAPUTO-HUMERAL (15890), PERONEUS TERTIUS
    MUSCLE, ABSENCE OF (26140)
MUSCLE, TWITCHES see MYOKYMIA (16010)
MUSCLES, ABSENCE OF see MUSCULAR DYSTROPHY, FACIO-SCAPULO-HUMERAL (15890)
*MUSCULAR ATROPHY, ATAXIA, RETINITIS PIGMENTOSA, DIABETES INSIPIDUS 15850
*MUSCULAR ATROPHY, INFANTILE (WERDNIG-HOFFMANN) 25330
*MUSCULAR ATROPHY, JUVENILE (KUGELBERG-WELANDER SYNDROME) 15860
*MUSCULAR ATROPHY, JUVENILE (KUGELBERG-WELANDER) 25340
MUSCULAR ATROPHY, MALIGNANT NEUROGENIC 15865
MUSCULAR ATROPHY, PROGRESSIVE 15870
MUSCULAR ATROPHY, PROGRESSIVE 25350
MUSCULAR ATROPHY, PROGRESSIVE see AMYOTROPHIC LATERAL SCLEROSIS (10540, 20510)
MUSCULAR ATROPHY, PROXIMAL SPINAL, OF LATE ONSET see SPINAL AND BULBAR MUSCULAR
    ATROPHY (31320)
MUSCULAR ATROPHY, SPINAL, INTERMEDIATE TYPE 25355
*MUSCULAR DYSTROPHY I (LIMB-GIRDLE, PELVO-FEMORAL OR LEYDEN-MOEBIUS TYPE) . 25360
*MUSCULAR DYSTROPHY II (RESEMBLING X-LINKED DUCHENNE MUSCULAR DYSTROPHY) . 25370
MUSCULAR DYSTROPHY LIMITED TO FEMALES see MYOPATHY, LIMITED TO FEMALES (16060)
MUSCULAR DYSTROPHY, CONGENITAL PROGRESSIVE, WITH MENTAL RETARDATION . . . 25380
*MUSCULAR DYSTROPHY, CONGENITAL, PRODUCING ARTHROGRYPOSIS 25390
MUSCULAR DYSTROPHY, CONGENITAL, WITH INFANTILE CATARACT AND HYPOGONADISM . 25400
MUSCULAR DYSTROPHY, CONGENITAL, WITH RAPID PROGRESSION 25410
MUSCULAR DYSTROPHY, HEMIZYGOUS LETHAL TYPE 30995
MUSCULAR DYSTROPHY, MABRY TYPE 31000
*MUSCULAR DYSTROPHY, PROGRESSIVE, TARDIVE TYPE OF BECKER 31010
*MUSCULAR DYSTROPHY, PSEUDOHYPERTROPHIC PROGRESSIVE, DUCHENNE TYPE 31020
MUSCULAR DYSTROPHY, SIMULATION OF see ENGELMANN DISEASE (13130)
*MUSCULAR DYSTROPHY, TARDIVE TYPE OF DREIFUSS, WITH CONTRACTURES 31030
MUSCULAR DYSTROPHY see MUSCULAR DYSTROPHY FACIO-SCAPULO-HUMERAL (15890), MYOP-
    ATHY, LATE DISTAL HEREDITARY (16050), MYOTONIC DYSTROPHY (16090), OCULOPHARYN-
    GEAL MUSCULAR DYSTROPHY (16430), AMINOACIDURIA WITH OTHER FEATURES (20480)
MUSCULAR DYSTROPHY, BARNES TYPE 15880
*MUSCULAR DYSTROPHY, FACIO-SCAPULO-HUMERAL 15890
MUSCULAR DYSTROPHY, LIMB-GIRDLE TYPE see MYOPATHY, LIMITED TO FEMALES (16060)
*MUSCULAR DYSTROPHY, PROXIMAL 15900
MUSCULAR HYPOPLASIA, CONGENITAL UNIVERSAL, OF KRABBE 15910
MUSCULAR SHORTENING AND DYSTROPHY 15920
MUSICAL ABILITY see TUNE DEAFNESS (19120)
*MUSK, INABILITY TO SMELL 25415
MYASTHENIA GRAVIS 15930
MYASTHENIA GRAVIS 25420
MYASTHENIA GRAVIS see AUTOIMMUNE DISEASES (10910)
MYASTHENIA, FAMILIAL LIMB-GIRDLE 15940
MYASTHENIC MYOPATHY 25430
MYCOSIS FUNGOIDES 25440
MYELIN (A1) PROTEIN, BASIC 15943
MYELIN MEMBRANE ENCEPHALITOGENIC PROTEIN 15945
MYELINATED OPTIC NERVE FIBERS 15950
MYELOMA, MULTIPLE 25450
*MYELOPEROXIDASE DEFICIENCY 25460
MYELOPROLIFERATIVE DISEASE 25470
MYOCARDIOPATHY see CARDIOMYOPATHY, FAMILIAL IDIOPATHIC (11520)
*MYOCLONIC EPILEPSY, HARTUNG TYPE 15960
MYOCLONIC EPILEPSY see PHOTOMYOCLONUS, ETC. (17250)
*MYOCLONIC EPILEPSY OF UNVERRICHT AND LUNDBORG 25480
MYOCLONIC VARIANT OF CEREBRAL LIPIDOSIS see AMAUROTIC FAMILY IDIOCY, JUVENILE
    TYPE (20420)
MYOCLONUS AND ATAXIA 15970
MYOCLONUS EPILEPSY see ATAXIA WITH MYOCLONUS EPILEPSY AND PRESENILE DEMENTIA
    (20870)
MYOCLONUS, CEREBELLAR ATAXIA AND DEAFNESS 15980
*MYOCLONUS, HEREDITARY ESSENTIAL 15990
*MYOGLOBIN 16000
MYOGLOBINURIA see RHABDOMYOLYSIS, ACUTE RECURRENT (26820), GLYCOGEN STORAGE
    DISEASE V (23260), MYOPATHY WITH ABNORMAL LIPID METABOLISM
MYOKINASE see ADENYLATE KINASE (10300)
*MYOKYMIA 16010
MYOKYMIA see GAMSTORP-WOHLFART SYNDROME (13720)
MYOMATA UTERI see LEIOMYOMATA, HEREDITARY MULTIPLE, OF SKIN (15080)
MYOPATHY PRODUCING CONGENITAL OPHTHALMOPLEGIA AND 'FLOPPY BABY' SYNDROME 25500
*MYOPATHY WITH ABNORMAL LIPID METABOLISM 25510
MYOPATHY WITH CARNITINE DEFICIENCY 25513
*MYOPATHY WITH LACTIC ACIDOSIS 25514
MYOPATHY WITH LIPID STORAGE see MYOPATHY WITH CARNITINE DEFICIENCY (25513)
MYOPATHY WITH LYSIS OF TYPE I MYOFIBRILS 25515
*MYOPATHY, CENTRONUCLEAR 16015

HEREDITARY, OF CARPAL BONES WITH NEPHROPATHY (16630), ASPHYXIATING THORACIC DYSTROPHY OF THE NEWBORN (20850)
NEPHROPATHY, FAMILIAL, WITH GOUT 16200
NEPHROSIS WITH DEAFNESS AND URINARY TRACT AND OTHER MALFORMATIONS 25620
*NEPHROSIS, CONGENITAL 25630
NEPHROSIS, CONGENITAL see PULMONIC STENOSIS (26550)
NEPHROTIC SYNDROME see MICROCEPHALY, ETC. (25130)
NERVE COMPRESSION SYNDROME see NEUROPATHY, HEREDITARY, WITH LIABILITY TO PRES-SURE PALSIES (16250)
NERVOUS SYSTEM DISORDER RESEMBLING REFSUM DISEASE AND HURLER DISEASE 25640
*NETHERTON DISEASE 25650
NEURAMINICACIDURIA see SIALURIA (26990)
*NEURITIS WITH BRACHIAL PREDILECTION 16210
NEUROARTHROMYODYSPLASIA (NEURAL TYPE OF ARTHROGRYPOSIS) see ARTHROGRYPOSIS MULTIPLEX CONGENITA (20810)
*NEUROAXONAL DYSTROPHY, INFANTILE (SEITELBERGER) 25660
NEUROBLASTOMA 25670
NEUROBLASTOMA see JOINT CONTRACTURES WITH OTHER ABNORMALITIES (14780)
*NEUROFIBROMATOSIS 16220
NEUROFIBROMATOSIS see ACOUSTIC NEUROMA, BILATERAL (10100)
*NEUROMATA, MUCOSAL, WITH ENDOCRINE TUMORS 16230
*NEURONAL CEROID-LIPOFUSCINOSIS, DOMINANT OR PARRY TYPE 16235
*NEURONAL CEROID-LIPOFUSCINOSIS, INFANTILE FINNISH TYPE 25673
*NEUROPATHY, CONGENITAL SENSORY 25675
*NEUROPATHY, CONGENITAL SENSORY, WITH ANHIDROSIS 25680
*NEUROPATHY, PROGRESSIVE SENSORY, OF CHILDREN 25690
NEUROPATHY, SENSORY see DEAFNESS, NERVE TYPE, MESENTRIC DIVERTICULA, ETC. (22140)
NEUROPATHY see AMYLOIDOSIS (10480, 10490)
*NEUROPATHY, CONGENITAL, WITH ARTHROGRYPOSIS MULTIPLEX 16237
*NEUROPATHY, HEREDITARY SENSORY RADICULAR 16240
*NEUROPATHY, HEREDITARY, WITH LIABILITY TO PRESSURE PALSIES 16250
NEUROPATHY, HYPERTROPHIC OF DEJERINE-SOTTAS see HYPERTROPHIC NEUROPATHY OF DEJERINE-SOTTAS (14590)
NEUROPATHY, WITH PARAPROTEIN IN SERUM, CEREBROSPINAL FLUID AND URINE 16260
NEURO-VISCERAL LIPIDOSIS see GANGLIOSIDOSIS, GENERALIZED (23050, 23060)
NEUROVISCERAL STORAGE DISEASE WITH CURVILINEAR BODIES 25700
*NEUROVISCERAL STORAGE DISEASE WITH VERTICAL SUPRANUCLEAR OPHTHALMOPLEGIA . 25705
*NEUTROPENIA, CHRONIC FAMILIAL 16270
NEUTROPENIA, CYCLIC 16280
NEUTROPENIA see LICHTENSTEIN SYNDROME (24655)
NEUTROPENIA see AGRANULOCYTOSIS, INFANTILE GENETIC, OF KOSTMANN (20270), CHEDI-AK-HIGASHI SYNDROME (21450), FANCONI PANCYTOPENIA (22790), GLYCINEMIA (23200), LAZY LEUKOCYTE SYNDROME (24585)
NEUTROPENIA, LETHAL CONGENITAL, WITH EOSINOPHILIA 25710
NEUTROPHIL CHEMOTACTIC DEFECT 16282
NEUTROPHILIA, HEREDITARY 16283
*NEUTROPHIL-SPECIFIC ANTIGEN: NA LOCUS 16285
*NEUTROPHIL-SPECIFIC ANTIGEN: NB LOCUS 16286
*NEVI (PIGMENTED MOLES) 16290
*NEVI FLAMMEI, FAMILIAL MULTIPLE 16300
NEVI HALO see HALO NEVI (23430)
NEVI, MULTIPLE see MELANOMA, MALIGNANT (15560)
NEVI see MELANOSIS, NEUROCUTANEOUS (24940)
NEVOID BASAL CELL SYNDROME see BASAL CELL NEVUS SYNDROME (10940)
*NEVUS FLAMMEUS OF THE NAPE OF THE NECK 16310
NEVUS SEBACEUS OF JADASSOHN 16320
NEVUS SEBACEUS, LINEAR see AORTIC ARCH INTERRUPTION, FACIAL PALSY AND RETINAL DEGENERATION (10755)
NEVUS SEBACEUS, LINEAR, WITH CONVULSIONS AND MENTAL RETARDATION 16330
NIELSON SYNDROME see PTERYGIUM COLLI SYNDROME (17810)
*NIEMANN-PICK DISEASE (SPHINGOMYELIN LIPIDOSIS) 25720
*NIEMANN-PICK DISEASE WITHOUT SPHINGOMYELINASE DEFICIENCY 25725
*NIEVERGELT SYNDROME 16340
*NIGHT BLINDNESS, CONGENITAL STATIONARY (HEMERALOPIA) 16350
*NIGHT BLINDNESS, CONGENITAL STATIONARY, WITH MYOPIA 31050
NIGHTBLINDNESS see HEMERALOPIA, ESSENTIAL (23490)
*NIGHTBLINDNESS WITH HIGH GRADE MYOPIA 25727
*NIPPLES INVERTED (MAMMILLAE INVERTITA) 16360
NIPPLES, ABSENCE OF see BREASTS AND NIPPLES, ABSENCE OF (11370)
NIPPLES, SUPERNUMERARY 16370
NOACK SYNDROME see ACROCEPHALOPOLYSYNDACTYLY I (10120)
*NODAL RHYTHM 16380
NON-DISJUNCTION 25730
NON-HEME PROTEIN OF ERYTHROCYTE 16390
NONNE-MILROY DISEASE see LYMPHEDEMA (15310)
NON-SPHEROCYTIC HEMELYTIC ANEMIA see ANEMIA, NONSPHEROCYTIC HEMOLYTIC (20620)
*NOONAN SYNDROME 16395
NOONAN SYNDROME see TURNER PHENOTYPE (19130)
*NORRIE DISEASE (ATROPHIA BULBORUM HEREDITARIA: PSEUDOGLIOMA) 31060
NORUM DISEASE see LECITHIN: CHOLESTEROL ACETYLTRANSFERASE (LCAT) DEFICIENCY (24590)
NOSE, ANOMALOUS SHAPE OF ('POTATO NOSE') 16400
NOSE, ANOMALY OF see ALAR-NASAL CARTILAGES, COLOBOMA OF, WITH TELECANTHUS (20300)
NOSE, BIFID see BIFID NOSE (21040)

OPHTHALMOPLEGIA see MYOPATHY PRODUCING CONGENITAL OPHTHALMOPLEGIA AND
  'FLOPPY BABY' SYNDROME (25500), FIBROSIS OF EXTRAOCULAR MUSCLE (13570)
OPHTHALMOPLEGIA AND HEART BLOCK see HEART BLOCK AND OPHTHALMOPLEGIA (23460)
*OPHTHALMOPLEGIA, EXTERNAL, AND MYOPIA 31100
OPHTHALMOPLEGIA, FAMILIAL STATIC see PTOSIS, HEREDITARY (17830), OCULOPHARYNGEAL
  MUSCULAR DYSTROPHY (16430)
OPPENHEIM DISEASE see AMYOTONIA CONGENITA (20500)
OPSONIZATION, DEFECT IN see PHAGOCYTOSIS, PLASMA-RELATED DEFECT IN (17110)
OPTIC ATROPHY, CONGENITAL OR EARLY INFANTILE 25850
OPTIC ATROPHY, NERVE DEAFNESS AND DISTAL NEUROGENIC AMYOTROPHY 25865
OPTIC ATROPHY see LEBER OPTIC ATROPHY (30890), BEHR SYNDROME (21000)
OPTIC ATROPHY — SPASTIC PARAPLEGIA SYNDROME 31110
OPTIC ATROPHY see DEAFNESS OPTIC ATROPHY SYNDROME (12445)
OPTIC ATROPHY WITH DEMYELINATING DISEASE OF CNS 16520
OPTIC ATROPHY, CATARACT AND NEUROLOGIC DISORDER 16530
*OPTIC ATROPHY, CONGENITAL 16540
*OPTIC ATROPHY, JUVENILE 16550
*OPTICO-COCHLEO-DENTATE DEGENERATION 25870
ORAL SENSIBILITY, DISTURBANCE OF 25880
*ORAL-FACIAL-DIGITAL (OFD) SYNDROME 31120
ORAL-FACIAL-DIGITAL SYNDROME III 25885
ORBITAL MARGIN, HYPOPLASIA OF 16560
ORNITHINE TRANSCARBAMYLASE DEFICIENCY see HYPERAMMONEMIA I (23720)
ORNITHINE TRANSCARBAMYLASE DEFICIENCY see HYPERAMMONEMIA (23720)
*ORNITHINEMIA 25887
*ORNITHINE-TRANSCARBAMYLASE DEFICIENCY 31125
ORO-FACIO-DIGITAL (OFD) SYNDROME see ORAL-FACIAL-DIGITAL SYNDROME (31120)
ORO-FACIO-DIGITAL SYNDROME II see MOHR SYNDROME (25210)
OROSOMUCOID 16565
OROSOMUCOID VARIANTS see GLYCOPROTEIN VARIANTS (13860, 13870, 23290, 23300)
*OROTICACIDURIA I 25890
*OROTICACIDURIA II 25892
ORTHOSTATIC HYPOTENSION see HYPOTENSION, ORTHOSTATIC (14650)
ORTHOSTATIC SYNDROME see HYPERBRADYKININISM (14385)
OSLER-RENDU-WEBER SYNDROME see TELANGIECTASIA (18730)
OSSICLES OF MIDDLE EAR, ANOMALIES OF see RENAL, GENITAL AND MIDDLE EAR ANOMALIES
  (26740), SYMPHALANGISM (18580), DEAFNESS CONDUCTIVE, WITH MALFORMED EXTERNAL EAR
  (22130)
OSSIFIED EAR CARTILAGES 16567
*OSTEOARTHROPATHY OF FINGERS, FAMILIAL 16570
OSTEOARTHROPATHY OF SCHINZ AND FURTWAENGLER see MUCOLIPIDOSIS II (25260)
OSTEOARTHROPATHY, FAMILIAL IDIOPATHIC, OF CHILDHOOD 25910
OSTEOARTHROPATHY, PRIMARY OR IDIOPATHIC HYPERTROPHIC see PACHYDERMOPERIOSTO-
  SIS (16710)
OSTEOCHONDRITIS DISSECANS (ASEPTIC NECROSIS) 16580
OSTEOCHONDRITIS DISSECANS OF MULTIPLE SITES 16590
OSTEOCHONDRITIS DISSECANS see HYPERTELORISM, ETC. (23970)
OSTEOCHONDROMATOSIS (ENCHONDROMATOSIS, DYSCHONDROPLASIA) 16600
OSTEOCHONDROSIS DEFORMANS TIBIAE, FAMILIAL INFANTILE TYPE 25920
*OSTEODYSPLASIA, FAMILIAL, ANDERSON TYPE 25925
*OSTEODYSPLASTY OF MELNICK AND NEEDLES 16610
*OSTEODYSPLASTY, PRECOCIOUS, OF DANKS, MAYNE AND KOZLOWSKI 25927
OSTEODYSTROPHY AND MENTAL RETARDATION 25930
OSTEOECTASIA see HYPEROSTOSIS CORTICALIS DEFORMANS JUVENILIS (23900)
*OSTEOGENESIS IMPERFECTA 16620
*OSTEOGENESIS IMPERFECTA CONGENITA (VROLIK TYPE OF OSTEOGENESIS IMPERFECTA) . . 25940
OSTEOGENIC SARCOMA 25950
OSTEOLYSIS OF TERMINAL PHALANGES see PYCNODYSOSTOSIS (26580), PURETIC SYNDROME
  (26570)
OSTEOLYSIS, CARPAL AND TARSAL see WINCHESTER DISEASE (27795)
*OSTEOLYSIS, HEREDITARY MULTICENTRIC 25960
*OSTEOLYSIS, HEREDITARY, OF CARPAL BONES WITH NEPHROPATHY 16630
OSTEOMA OF MIDDLE EAR 25965
OSTEOMAS OF MANDIBLE 16640
OSTEO-ONYCHO-DYSPLASIA HEREDITARIA (ALBUMINURICA) see NAIL-PATELLA SYNDROME
  (16120)
OSTEOPATHIA STRIATA 16650
OSTEOPENIA see KYPHOSCOLIOSIS, OSTEOPENIA, CONGENITAL CONTRACTURES (14950)
*OSTEOPETROSIS ('MARBLE BONES,' OSTEOSCLEROSIS FRAGILIS GENERALISATA, ALBERS-SCHON-
  BERG DISEASE) 16660
*OSTEOPETROSIS ('MARBLE BONES,' ALBERS-SCHONBERG DISEASE) 25970
*OSTEOPETROSIS WITH RENAL TUBULAR ACIDOSIS 25973
*OSTEOPOIKILOSIS 16670
OSTEOPOROSIS see HOMOCYSTINURIA (23620), AMINOACIDURIA WITH OTHER FEATURES (20480),
  FANCONI SYNDROME I (22770)
OSTEOPOROSIS, JUVENILE 25975
*OSTEOPOROSIS-PSEUDOGLIOMA SYNDROME 25977
OSTEOSCLEROSIS see OSTEOPATHIA STRIATA (16650), DWARFISM, CORTICAL THICKENING OF
  BONE AND TRANSIENT HYPOCALCEMIA (12700)
*OTODENTAL DYSPLASIA 16675
*OTO-PALATO-DIGITAL (OPD) SYNDROME 31130
OTO-RENO-GENITAL SYNDROME see RENAL, GENITAL AND MIDDLE EAR ANOMALIES (26740)
OTOSCLEROSIS 16680
OUABAIN RESISTANCE 16685

PITUITARY DWARFISM WITH DEAFNESS see DEAFNESS NEUROSENSORY, WITH PITUITARY DWARFISM (22175)
PITUITARY DWARFISM WITH SMALL SELLA TURCICA 26270
PITUITARY GLAND, ABSENCE OF see PITUITARY DWARFISM III (26260)
*PITYRIASIS RUBRA PILARIS 17320
PIV SYNDROME see POLYDACTYLY, IMPERFORATE ANUS, VERTEBRAL ANOMALIES (17410)
PLACENTAL ALKALINE PHOSPHATASE see PHOSPHATASE, PLACENTAL ALKALINE (17180)
PLACENTAL ENZYMES 17330
PLACENTA see CIRCUMVALLATE PLACENTA SYNDROME (21555)
PLACENTAL SULFATASE DEFICIENCY 26275
PLASMA CLOT RETRACTION FACTOR, DEFICIENCY OF 26280
PLASMA THROMBOPLASTIC COMPONENT, DEFICIENCY OF see HEMOPHILIA B (30690)
PLASMINOGEN 17335
PLATELET ABNORMALITY see STORAGE POOL PLATELET DISEASE (18505)
*PLATELET GROUPS — KO SYSTEM 17350
*PLATELET GROUPS — PL(E) SYSTEM 17354
PLATELETS, DEFECTS IN see THROMBASTHENIA OF GLANZMANN AND NAEGELI (18780, 27380), SIDBURY SYNDROME (27000)
PLATELETS, DISORDERS OF see THROMBASTHENIA THROMBOCYTOPENIA, HEREDITARY (18790), THROMBOCYTOPENIA (18800, 27390, 31390), HB KOLN (14170), VON WILLEBRAND DISEASE (19340), ALDRICH SYNDROME (30100), FANCONI PANCYTOPENIA (22790)
PLATYBASIA see BASILAR IMPRESSION, PRIMARY (10950)
PLEOCONIAL MYOPATHY 26290
PNEUMOTHORAX, SPONTANEOUS 17360
POIKILODERMA CONGENITA see ROTHMUND-THOMSON SYNDROME (26840)
POIKILODERMA, HEREDITARY SCLEROSING 17370
POLAND SYNDROME (OR POLAND SYNDACTYLY) 17380
*POLIO VIRUS SUSCEPTIBILITY 17385
POLYCYSTIC KIDNEY, CATARACT AND CONGENITAL BLINDNESS see RENAL DYSPLASIA AND RETINAL APLASIA (26690)
*POLYCYSTIC KIDNEYS 17390
*POLYCYSTIC KIDNEYS, MEDULLARY TYPE 17400
POLYCYSTIC KIDNEYS see MECKEL SYNDROME (24900)
POLYCYSTIC KIDNEY see CEREBRO-HEPATO-RENAL SYNDROME (21410)
POLYCYSTIC KIDNEY, CATARACT AND CONGENITAL BLINDNESS 26310
*POLYCYSTIC KIDNEY, INFANTILE, TYPE I 26320
POLYCYSTIC LIVER see POLYCYSTIC KIDNEYS (17390, 26320)
POLYCYTHEMIA RUBRA VERA 26330
*POLYCYTHEMIA, BENIGN FAMILIAL, OF CHILDREN 26340
POLYCYTHEMIA see HEMOGLOBIN CHESAPEAKE, HEMOGLOBIN YPSI (14170)
POLYCYTHEMIA, BENIGN FAMILIAL see ERYTHROCYTOSIS, BENIGN FAMILIAL (13310)
POLYDACTYLISM 26350
POLYDACTYLY WITH NEONATAL CHONDRODYSTROPHY, TYPE I (MAJEWSKI TYPE) . 26352
POLYDACTYLY WITH NEONATAL CHONDRODYSTROPHY, TYPE II (SALDINO-NOONAN TYPE) . 26353
POLYDACTYLY, IMPERFORATE ANUS, VERTEBRAL ANOMALIES 17410
*POLYDACTYLY, POSTAXIAL (PROBABLY AT LEAST TWO TYPES) 17420
*POLYDACTYLY, POSTAXIAL, WITH MEDIAN CLEFT OF UPPER LIP 17430
POLYDACTYLY, POSTAXIAL see ELLIS-VAN CREVELD SYNDROME (22550), LAURENCE-MOON SYNDROME (24580), BIEMOND SYNDROME II (21030)
POLYDACTYLY, PREAXIAL I ('THUMB POLYDACTYLY') 17440
*POLYDACTYLY, PREAXIAL II (POLYDACTYLY OF TRIPHALANGEAL THUMB) . . . 17450
*POLYDACTYLY, PREAXIAL III ('INDEX FINGER POLYDACTYLY') 17460
*POLYDACTYLY, PREAXIAL IV (POLYSYNDACTYLY) 17470
POLYDACTYLY see ELLIS-VAN-CREVELD SYNDROME (22550), LAURENCE-MOON SYNDROME (24580), BIEMOND SYNDROME II (10970), ACROCEPHALOPOLYSYNDACTYLY (10110, 20100)
POLYDACTYLY WITHOUT THUMB see POLYDACTYLY, PREAXIAL III (17460)
POLYDACTYLY, CENTRAL see SYNDACTYLY TYPE II (SYNPOLYDACTYLY) (18600)
POLYDACTYLY, POSTAXIAL see MECKEL SYNDROME (24900)
POLYDACTYLY, PREAXIAL see TRIPHALANGEAL THUMB, OPPOSABLE (19070)
POLYDYSSPONDYLY see COSTOVERTEBRAL SEGMENTATION ANOMALIES (12260)
POLYDYSTROPHIC OLIGOPHRENIA see MUCOPOLYSACCHARIDOSIS TYPE III (25290)
POLYHYDRAMNIOS see CIRCUMVALLATE PLACENTA SYNDROME (21555)
POLYMASTIA see NIPPLES, SUPERNUMERARY (16370)
POLYNEUROPATHY, HEREDITARY see CHARCOT-MARIE-TOOTH DISEASE (11820)
POLYNEUROPATHY, MIXED, OF EARLY ONSET 26355
POLYONCOSIS, HEREDITARY CUTANEOMANDIBULAR see BASAL CELL NEVUS SYNDROME (10940)
POLYOSTOTIC FIBROUS DYSPLASIA 17480
*POLYPOSIS COLI, JUVENILE TYPE 17490
POLYPOSIS COLI see MULTIPLE HAMARTOMA SYNDROME (15835)
POLYPOSIS OF INTESTINE see TURCOT SYNDROME (27630)
POLYPOSIS, FAMILIAL, OF ENTIRE GASTROINTESTINAL TRACT 17500
*POLYPOSIS, INTESTINAL, I (FAMILIAL POLYPOSIS OF THE COLON) 17510
*POLYPOSIS, INTESTINAL, II (PEUTZ-JEGHERS SYNDROME) 17520
*POLYPOSIS, INTESTINAL, III (GARDNER SYNDROME) 17530
POLYPOSIS, INTESTINAL, IV (SCATTERED, DISCRETE POLYPS) 17540
POLYPOSIS, SKIN PIGMENTATION, ALOPECIA AND FINGERNAIL CHANGES (CRONKITE-CANADA SYNDROME) 17550
POLYSACCHARIDE, STORAGE OF UNUSUAL 26360
POLYSEROSITIS see MEDITERRANEAN FEVER, FAMILIAL (24910)
POLYSYNDACTYLY see POLYDACTYLY, PREAXIAL IV POLYSYNDACTYLY (17470)
*POLYSYNDACTYLY WITH PECULIAR SKULL SHAPE (GREIG CEPHALO-POLYSYNDACTYLY SYNDROME) 17570
POMPE DISEASE see GLYCOGEN STORAGE DISEASE II (23230)
POPLITEAL CYST (BAKER CYST) 17575

POPLITEAL PTERYGIUM SYNDROME 26365
POPLITEAL PTERYGIUM SYNDROME   see PTERYGIUM COLLI SYNDROME (17810), CLEFT LIP-PAL-
ATE, MUCOUS CYSTS OF THE LOWER LIP, POPLITEAL PTERYGIUM, ETC. (11950)
POPLITEAL WEBBING   see CLEFT LIP AND-OR PALATE WITH MUCOUS CYSTS OF THE LOWER LIP
(11930)
*POROKERATOSIS OF MIBELLI 17580
POROKERATOSIS PLANTARIS, PALMARIS ET DISSEMINATA 17585
*POROKERATOSIS, DISSEMINATED SUPERFICIAL ACTINIC (DSAP) 17590
*PORPHYRIA, CONGENITAL ERYTHROPOIETIC (GUNTHER DISEASE) 26370
PORPHYRIA   see PROTOPORPHYRIA (17700), COPROPORPHYRIA (12130)
*PORPHYRIA, ACUTE INTERMITTENT (SWEDISH TYPE OF PORPHYRIA) 17600
PORPHYRIA, HEPATIC-CUTANEOUS TYPE (PORPHYRIA CUTANEA TARDA) 17610
*PORPHYRIA, VARIEGATA (SOUTH AFRICAN TYPE OF PORPHYRIA) 17620
PORTUGUESE AMYLOIDOSIS   see AMYLOIDOSIS I (10480)
PORT-WINE STAIN   see NEVUS FLAMMEUS OF THE NAPE OF THE NECK (16310)
POSTERIOR CLEFT OF LARYNX   see CLEFT LARYNX, POSTERIOR (21580)
POSTERIOR COLUMN ATAXIA 17625
POSTERIOR POLYMORPHOUS CORNEAL DYSTROPHY OF SCHLICHTING   see CORNEAL DYSTRO-
PHY, HEREDITARY POLYMORPHOUS POSTERIOR (12200)
POSTMINIMI, PEDUNCULATED   see POLYDACTYLY, POSTAXIAL (17420)
POSTMINIMI, PEDUNCULATED   see POLYDACTYLY, POSTAXIAL (17420)
*POTASSIUM AND MAGNESIUM DEPLETION (SEE ALSO PSEUDO-ALDOSTERONISM) 26380
POTASSIUM-SODIUM DISORDER OF ERYTHROCYTE 26390
POTTER FACIES   see RENAL AGENESIS, BILATERAL (26670)
POTTER SYNDROME   see RENAL AGENESIS (26670)
PPHP   see ALBRIGHT HEREDITARY OSTEODYSTROPHY (30080)
PRADER-WILLI SYNDROME 26400
PREALBUMIN, POLYMORPHISM OF SERUM 17630
PREALBUMIN   see ANTITRYPSIN, ELECTROPHORETIC VARIANT OF SERUM (10740)
PRE-AURICULAR PITS   see BRANCHIAL CLEFT ANOMALIES, INCLUDING BRANCHIAL CYSTS
(11360), DEAFNESS WITH EAR PITS (12510), EAR PITS (12870)
*PRECOCIOUS PUBERTY 17640
PRECOCITY, SEXUAL   see PINEALOMA WITH HYPERPINEALISM (26220)
PREGNANCY-ASSOCIATED GLOBULIN   see PA POLYMORPHISM (26010)
PREKALLIKREIN DEFICIENCY   see FLETCHER FACTOR DEFICIENCY (22900)
PREMOLAR HYPODONTIA   see BOOK'S SYNDROME, OR PHC SYNDROME (11230)
PRENATAL BOWING 26405
*PRESACRAL TERATOMA 17645
PRESENILE DEMENTIA WITH SPASTIC PARALYSIS 17650
PRESENILE DEMENTIA, KRAEPELIN TYPE 17660
PRESENILE DEMENTIA   see ATAXIA WITH MYOCLONUS EPILEPSY AND PRESENILE DEMENTIA
(20870), ALZHEIMER DISEASE OF BRAIN (10430), PICK DISEASE OF BRAIN (17270)
PRESSURE PALSIES   see NEUROPATHY, HEREDITARY, WITH LIABILITY TO PRESSURE PALSIES
(16250)
PRIMORDIAL DWARFISM   see PITUITARY DWARFISM I (26240)
PROACCELERIN DEFICIENCY   see FACTOR V DEFICIENCY (22740)
PROACCELERIN EXCESS   see FACTOR V EXCESS WITH SPONTANEOUS THROMBOSIS (13440)
PROCTALGIA FUGAX   see PAIN, SUBMANDIBULAR OCULAR AND RECTAL WITH FLUSHING (16740)
PROGERIA 26410
PROGERIA-LIKE DISORDERS   see WERNER SYNDROME (27770), HALLERMANN-STREIFF SYN-
DROME (23410), MANDIBULOACRAL DYSPLASIA (24837), ABSENT EYEBROWS AND EYELASHES
WITH MENTAL RETARDATION (20013), COCKAYNE SYNDROME (21649)
*PROGNATHISM, MANDIBULAR 17670
PROGRESSIVE BULBAR ATROPHY   see AMYOTROPHIC LATERAL SCLEROSIS (10540, 20510)
PROGRESSIVE INFANTILE SPINAL MUSCULAR ATROPHY (WERDNIG-HOFFMANN)   see MUSCU-
LAR ATROPHY, INFANTILE (25330)
PROGRESSIVE SPINAL MUSCULAR ATROPHY, JUVENILE   see MUSCULAR ATROPHY, JUVENILE
(15860, 25340)
PROINSULIN 17673
PROLACTIN DEFICIENCY, ISOLATED 17675
PROLIDASE VARIANTS   see PEPTIDASE VARIANTS (16970-17020)
PROLINE RICH PROTEIN OF SALIVA   see PAROTID PROLINE RICH PROTEIN (16878)
PROLINEMIA   see HYPERPROLINEMIA TYPES I AND II (23950)
PROLINURIA   see IMINOGLYCINURIA (24260)
PRONATION-SUPINATION OF THE FOREARM, IMPAIRMENT OF 17680
PROPIONICACIDEMIA   see GLYCINEMIA (HYPERGLYCINEMIA WITH KETOACIDOSIS AND LEU-
KOPENIA (23200)
PROPIONYL COA CARBOXYLASE DEFICIENCY   see GLYCINEMIA (23200)
PROPORTIONATE DWARFISM   see PITUITARY DWARFISM I (26240)
PRO-SPCA DEFICIENCY   see FACTOR VII DEFICIENCY (22750)
PROTANOPIA   see COLOR BLINDNESS, PARTIAL (30390)
PROTEIN INTOLERANCE   see DIBASICAMINOACIDURIA (12600, 22270)
PROTEIN INTOLERANCE   see HYPERAMMONEMIA (23720, 23730)
PROTEIN, SERUM TYPES   see SERUM PROTEIN TYPES (18230)
PROTEIN-LOSING ENTEROPATHY   see LYMPHANGIECTASIA, INTESTINAL (15280)
PROTEIN-LOSING ENTERPATHY   see ENTERPATHY, PROTEIN-LOSING (22630)
PROTEINOSIS, LIPOID   see LIPOID PROTEINOSIS OF URBACH AND WIETHE (24710)
PROTEINURIA   see PERNICIOUS ANEMIA, JUVENILE (26110)
PROTEOLYTIC CAPACITY OF PLASMA 17690
PROTHROMBIN CARDEZA   see DYSPROTHROMBINEMIA (12970)
PROTHROMBIN DEFICIENCY   see HYPOPROTHROMBINEMIA (24170)
PROTHROMBIN TIME, PROLONGED   see FLOOD FACTOR DEFICIENCY (13615)
PROTHROMBIN, DEFECT OF   see DYSPROTHROMBINEMIA (12790)
*PROTOPORPHYRIA, ERYTHROPOIETIC 17700

PROXIMAL FOCAL FEMORAL DEFICIENCY (PFFD) see FEMUR-FIBULA-ULNA (FFU) SYNDROME (22820)
PRUNE BELLY SYNDROME see ABDOMINAL MUSCLES, ABSENCE OF, WITH URINARY TRACT ABNORMALITY (10010)
PRURIGO BESNIER see ATOPIC HYPERSENSITIVITY (20920)
PRURITUS, HEREDITARY LOCALIZED 17710
*PSEUDOACHONDROPLASTIC DYSPLASIA I (FORMERLY PSEUDOACHONDROPLASTIC SPONDYLO-EPIPHYSEAL DYSPLASIA) 17715
*PSEUDOACHONDROPLASTIC DYSPLASIA III (FORMERLY PSEUDOACHONDROPLASTIC SPON-DYLOEPIPHYSEAL DYSPLASIA) 17717
*PSEUDOACHONDROPLASTIC DYSPLASIA II (FORMERLY PSEUDOACHONDROPLASTIC SPONDYLO-EPIPHYSEAL DYSPLASIA) 26415
*PSEUDOACHONDROPLASTIC DYSPLASIA IV (FORMERLY PSEUDOACHONDROPLASTIC SPONDYLO-EPIPHYSEAL DYSPLASIA) 26416
PSEUDO-ACHONDROPLASTIC TYPE OF SPONDYLOEPIPHYSEAL DYSPLASIA see SPONDYLOEPI-PHYSEAL DYSPLASIA (27170)
PSEUDO-ALDOSTERONISM (LIDDLE SYNDROME) 17720
PSEUDO-ARTHROGRYPOSIS (HEREDITARY CONGENITAL RIGIDITY OF ELBOWS AND KNEES) . 17730
PSEUDOCHOLINESTERASE DEFICIENCY see SUXAMETHONIUM SENSITIVITY (27240)
*PSEUDOCHOLINESTERASE TYPES, E(1) VARIANTS 17740
*PSEUDOCHOLINESTERASE TYPES, E(2) VARIANTS 17750
PSEUDOCHOLINESTERASE TYPES see CHOLINESTERASE, REDUCTION IN RED CELL (11850)
PSEUDOCHOLINESTERASE, INCREASE IN PLASMA LEVEL OF 17760
PSEUDO-CROUZON DISEASE see CRANIAL DYSOSTOSIS WITH PRONOUNCED DIGITAL IMPRES-SIONS (12280)
PSEUDOGLAUCOMA 17770
PSEUDOGLIOMA 26420
PSEUDOGLIOMA see OSTEOPOROSIS-PSEUDOGLIOMA SYNDROME (25985)
PSEUDOGOUT see CHONDROCALCINOSIS (11860)
*PSEUDOHERMAPHRODITISM, FEMALE, WITH SKELETAL ANOMALIES 26427
PSEUDOHERMAPHRODITISM, INCOMPLETE MALE, TYPE I 31210
PSEUDOHERMAPHRODITISM, MALE see PSUEDOVAGINAL PERINESCROTAL HYPOPADIAS (26460)
*PSEUDOHERMAPHRODITISM, MALE INTERNAL 26428
PSEUDOHERMAPHRODITISM, MALE, WITH GYNECOMASTIA 26430
PSEUDOHERMAPHRODITISM, MALE see PSEUDOVAGINAL PERINEOSCROTAL HYPOSPADIAS (26460), HYPOGONADISM, MALE (24110, 30730)
PSEUDO-HURLER POLYDYSTROPHY see MUCOLIPIDOSIS III (25260)
PSEUDOHYPOPARATHYROIDISM, TYPE II 26440
PSEUDOHYPOPARATHYROIDISM AND PSEUDO-PSEUDOHYPOPARATHYROIDISM see ALBRIGHT HEREDITARY OSTEODYSTROPHY (30080)
PSEUDOHYPOPHOSPHATASIA see HYPOPHOSPHATASIA (24150)
PSEUDOMONGOLISM 26445
PSEUDOPAPILLEDEMA 17780
PSEUDOPAPILLEDEMA see MACROCEPHALY (24800)
PSEUDOSCLEROSIS, SPASTIC see SPASTIC PSEUDOSCLEROSIS (27090)
PSEUDOTUMOR CEREBRI see INTRACRANIAL HYPERTENSION, IDIOPATHIC (24320)
PSEUDOTUMOR OF ORBIT see FIBROSCLEROSIS, MULTIFOCAL (22880)
PSEUDOURIDINURIA AND MENTAL DEFECT 26450
*PSEUDOVAGINAL PERINEOSCROTAL HYPOSPADIAS (PPSH) 26460
*PSEUDOVITAMIN D DEFICIENCY RICKETS (VITAMIN-D-DEPENDENT RICKETS) 26470
*PSEUDOXANTHOMA ELASTICUM 17785
*PSEUDOXANTHOMA ELASTICUM 26480
PSORIASIFORM ICHTHYOSIS see NETHERTON DISEASE (25650)
*PSORIASIS 17790
*PTA (PLASMA THROMBOPLASTIN ANTECEDENT, FACTOR XI) DEFICIENCY 26490
PTC (PLASMA THROMBOPLASTIC COMPONENT) DEFICIENCY see HEMOPHILIA B (30690)
PTC SYNDROME see PHEOCHROMOCYTOMA AND AMYLOID-PRODUCING MEDULLARY THY-ROID CARCINOMA (17140)
PTC TASTING see PHENYLTHIOCARBAMIDE TASTING (17120)
PTERYGIA, ANTECUBITAL see WEYERS OLIGODACTYLY SYNDROME (19360)
PTERYGIUM OF CONJUNCTIVA AND CORNEA 17800
*PTERYGIUM SYNDROME 26500
PTERYGIUM SYNDROME (PTERYGIUM COLLI SYNDROME) 17810
PTERYGIUM SYNDROME (X-LINKED) 31215
PTERYGIUM, ANTECUBITAL 17820
PTERYGIUM, ANTECUBITAL see TROCHLEA OF THE HUMERUS, APLASIA OF (19100), CLEFT LIP-PALATE (11950)
PTERYGIUM, POPLITEAL see ECTODERMAL DYSPLASIA, CLEFT LIP AND PLATE, ETC. (22500)
PTERYGIUM, POPLITEAL see CLEFT LIP AND-OR PALATE WITH MUCOUS CYSTS OF LOWER LIP (11930)
PTOSIS CONGENITAL see PTOSIS, HEREDITARY (17830)
PTOSIS FAMILIAL-NON-CONGENITAL see PTOSIS, HEREDITARY (17830)
*PTOSIS, HEREDITARY 17830
PTOSIS, HEREDITARY see OCULOPHARYNGEAL MUSCULAR DYSTROPHY (16430), OPHTHALMO-PLEGIA (25840)
PTOSIS see BLEPHAROPHIMOSIS (11010), PURPURA SIMPLEX (17900), HORNER SYNDROME (14300), MYOPATHY, CENTRONUCLEAR (25520, 31040), ALACRIMIA CONGENITA (20280), VERTEBRAL FUSION, POSTERIOR LUMBOSACRAL, BLEPHAROPTOSIS (19280), FIBROSIS OF EXTRAOCULAR MUSCLE (12570), FACIOGENITAL DYSPLASIA (30540)
PUBERTY, PRECOCIOUS see PRECOCIOUS PUBERTY (17640)
*PUBIC BONE DYSPLASIA 17835
PUCK'S SURFACE ANTIGEN see KILLER ANTIGEN OF PUCK (14875)
*PULMONARY ALVEOLAR MICROLITHIASIS 26510
PULMONARY ARTERIAL STENOSES see SUPRAVALVULAR AORTIC STENOSIS (18550)

PULMONARY ARTERIOVENOUS FISTULAE   see CYANOSIS AND HEPATIC DISEASE (21940)
PULMONARY ARTERY STENOSIS   see ARTERIOHEPATIC DYSPLASIA (20870)
PULMONARY ARTERY STENOSIS   see SUPRAVALAR AORTIC STENOSIS (18550)
PULMONARY CYSTIC LYMPHANGIECTASIS (LYMPHANGIOMATOSIS)   26530
PULMONARY DISEASE, CHRONIC OBSTRUCTIVE   see EMPHYSEMA (13070)
PULMONARY DISEASE   see ANTITRYPSIN DEFICIENCY OF PLASMA (20470)
PULMONARY EDEMA OF MOUNTAINEERS   17840
PULMONARY FIBROSIS, IDIOPATHIC (SEE FIBROCYSTIC PULMONARY DYSPLASIA)   17850
PULMONARY HYPERTENSION AND GROWTH RETARDATION   see ROWLEY-ROSENBERG SYN-
   DROME (26850)
*PULMONARY HYPERTENSION, PRIMARY   17860
PULMONARY HYPERTENSION, PRIMARY   26540
PULMONARY VALVULAR DYSPLASIA   17870
PULMONARY VENOUS RETURN   see ANOMALOUS PULMONARY VENOUS RETURN (10670)
PULMONIC STENOSIS   26550
PULMONIC STENOSIS AND CONGENITAL NEPHROSIS   26560
PULMONIC STENOSIS AND VENTRICULAR SEPTAL DEFECT   see CRANIO-ACRO-FASCIAL SYN-
   DROME (12285)
PULMONIC STENOSIS   see LEOPARD SYNDROME (15110)
PULP STONES   see PULPAL DYSPLASIA (17875)
PULPAL DYSPLASIA ('PULP STONES')   17875
PUPIL, EGG-SHAPED   17880
PUPIL, SMALL   see MICROCORNEA, CONGENITAL (15660)
*PUPILLARY MEMBRANE, PERSISTENCE OF   17890
PUPILLARY PARALYSIS   see SPINOCEREBELLAR ATROPHY WITH PUPILLARY PARALYSIS (18310)
*PURETIC SYNDROME   26570
PURPURA SIMPLEX   17900
PURPURIC ERUPTION   see PIGMENTED PURPURIC ERUPTION (17290)
*PYCNODYSOSTOSIS (PYKNODYSOSTOSIS)   26580
PYCNODYSOSTOSIS OF STANESCO   see CRANIOFACIAL DYSOSTOSIS WITH DIAPHYSEAL HYPER-
   PLASIA (12290)
*PYLE DISEASE (METAPHYSEAL DYSPLASIA)   26590
*PYLORIC ATRESIA   26595
PYLORIC STENOSIS   see NEUROBLASTOMA (25670)
PYLORIC STENOSIS, INFANTILE   26600
PYLORIC STENOSIS   see SCHINZEL SYNDROME (18145)
*PYRIDOXINE DEPENDENCY WITH SEIZURES   26610
PYRIDOXINE-RESPONSIVE ANEMIA   see ANEMIA, FAMILIAL PYRIDOXINE-RESPONSIVE (20600),
   ANEMIA, HYPOCHROMIC (30130)
*PYRIMIDINE 5-PRIME-NUCLEOTIDASE DEFICIENCY, HEMOLYTIC ANEMIA FROM   26612
PYROGLUTAMICACIDURIA   26613
PYROPHOSPHATASE, ERYTHROCYTE INORGANIC   17903
*PYRUVATE CARBOXYLASE DEFICIENCY   26615
PYRUVATE DECARBOXYLASE DEFICIENCY   see ATAXIA, INTERMITTENT, WITH PYRUVATE DE-
   CARBOXYLASE DEFICIENCY (20880)
*PYRUVATE KINASE (PK) DEFICIENCY OF ERYTHROCYTE   26620
*PYRUVATE KINASE-3   17905
QT INTERVAL, PROLONGED   see VENTICULAR FIBRILLATION WITH PROLONGED Q-T INTERVAL
   (19250)
QUIVERING CHIN   see TREMBLING CHIN (19010)
RACKET NAIL ('LE POUCE EN RAQUETTE' OF DU BOIS)   see BRACHYDACTYLY TYPE D (11320)
RADIAL APLASIA   see CRANIOSYNOSTOSIS-RADIAL APLASIA SYNDROME (21860)
RADIAL ARTERIES, ANOMALY OF   see ARTERIES, ANOMALY OF (10800)
RADIAL DEFECTS (DEFICIENCY OF RADIAL RAYS AND RADIUS AND PHOCOMELIA)   17910
RADIAL HEAD, DISLOCATION OF   see OTO-PALATO-DIGITAL SYNDROME (31130), AURICU-
   LO-OSTEODYSPLASIA (10900)
RADIAL HEADS, POSTERIOR DISLOCATION OF   17920
RADIAL HEADS, POSTEROIR DISLOCATION OF   see SYNOSTOSES (18640), NAIL-PATELLA SYN-
   DROME (16120)
RADIAL LOOP, PLAIN, ON RIGHT INDEX FINGER   31220
RADIALLY CURVED FIFTH FINGER   see BRACHYDACTYLY TYPE A3 (11270)
RADICULAR NEUROPATHY, HEREDITARY SENSORY   see NEUROPATHY, HEREDITARY SENSORY
   RADICULAR (16240)
RADIOHUMERAL SYNOSTOSIS   see HUMERORADIAL SYNOSTOSIS (23640)
*RADIO-ULNAR SYNOSTOSIS   17930
RADIUS ABSENCE OF   see FIBULA AND ULNA DUPLICATION OF ETC. (13575)
RADIUS, ABSENCE OF   see THROMBOCYTOPENIA WITH ASSOCIATED MALFORMATIONS (27400),
   CRANIOSYNOSTOSIS WITH RADIAL DEFECTS (21860), ARMS MALFORMATION OF (10790)
RADIUS, APLASIA OF, WITH CLEFT LIP-PALATE   17940
RADIUS, POSTERIOR DISLOCATION OF HEAD OF   see PTERYGIUM, ANTECUBITAL (17820)
RADIUS-PLATELET HYPOPLASIA   see TAR SYNDROME (27400)
RAINDROP HYPOPIGMENTATION   17950
*RAYNAUD DISEASE ('HEREDITARY COLD FINGERS')   17960
READING EPILEPSY   see EPILEPSY, READING (13230)
RECKLINGHAUSEN DISEASE   see NEUROFIBROMATOSIS (16220)
RECTAL PAIN   see PAIN, SUBMANDIBULAR, OCULAR AND RECTAL WITH FLUSHING (16740)
RED CELL NON-HEME PROTEIN   see NON-HEME PROTEIN OF ERYTHROCYTE (16390)
*RED CELL PERMEABILITY DEFECT   17965
*RED CELL PHOSPHOLIPID DEFECT WITH HEMOLYSIS   17970
RED CELL POTASSIUM AND SODIUM   see POTASSIUM-SODIUM DISORDER OF ERYTHROCYTE
   (26390)
RED HAIR   26630
RED PALMS   see ERYTHEMA PALMARE HEREDITARIUM (13300)
*RED SKIN PIGMENT ANOMALY OF NEW GUINEA   26635

REDUCTASE, 5-ALPHA, DEFICIENCY OF   see PSUEDOVAGINAL PERINEOSCROTAL HYPOSPADIAS
(26460)
REESE RETINAL DYSPLASIA   26640
*REFSUM SYNDROME   26650
REFSUM SYNDROME   see NERVOUS SYSTEM DISORDER RESEMBLING REFSUM DISEASE AND
HURLER DISEASE (25640)
REGIONAL ENTERITIS   26660
REGULATOR FOR ESTERASE ES-2   see ESTERASE ES-2, REGULATOR FOR (13330)
REIFENSTEIN SYNDROME   see PSEUDOHERMAPHRODITISM, MALE (31210)
REIFENSTEIN SYNDROME   31230
REIS-BUCKLERS DYSTROPHY   see CORNEAL DYSTROPHY OF REIS AND BUCKLERS (12150)
RENAL AGENESIS, BILATERAL   26670
RENAL AGENESIS, UNILATERAL   26680
RENAL ARTERIES, FIBROMUSCULAR HYPERPLASIA OF   see FIBROMUSCULAR HYPERPLASIA OF
RENAL ARTERIES (22870)
RENAL DYSFUNCTION   see PERNICIOUS ANEMIA, JUVENILE (26110)
RENAL DYSPLASIA AND RETINAL APLASIA   see POLYCYSTIC KIDNEY, CATARACT AND CONGEN-
ITAL BLINDNESS (26310)
RENAL DYSPLASIA   see TORTICOLLIS, ETC. (31430)
*RENAL DYSPLASIA AND RETINAL APLASIA   26690
RENAL GLYCOSURIA   see GLYCOSURIA, RENAL (23310)
RENAL GLYCOSURIA   see DIABETES MELLITUS (12585)
RENAL HAMARTOMAS, NEPHROBLASTOMATOSIS AND FETAL GIGANTISM   26700
RENAL STONES   see GLYCINURIA (23200)
*RENAL TUBULAR ACIDOSIS I (CLASSIC, GRADIENT OR DISTAL TYPE)   17980
RENAL TUBULAR ACIDOSIS III (DISLOCATION OR BICARBONATE WASTING)   26720
*RENAL TUBULAR ACIDOSIS WITH PROGRESSIVE NERVE DEAFNESS   26730
RENAL TUBULAR ACIDOSIS   see OSTEOPETROSIS AND RENAL TUBULAR ACIDOSIS (25975)
RENAL TUBULAR ACIDOSIS II (PROXIMAL, RATE, OR BICARBONATE WASTING TYPE)   .   .   .   31240
RENAL TUBULAR DEFECTS   see POTASSIUM AND MAGNESIUM DEPLETION (26380), FANCONI
SYNDROME (22770, 22780), THE CYSTINURIAS (22010)
RENAL TUBULAR NECROSIS   see CROME SYNDROME (21890)
RENAL TUMOR   see TUBEROUS SCLEROSIS (19110)
RENAL, GENITAL AND MIDDLE EAR ANOMALIES   26740
RENDU-OSLER-WEBER HEREDITARY HEMORRHAGIC TELANGIECTASIA   see TELANGIECTASIA,
HEREDITARY HEMORRHAGIC (18730)
RENO-MAMMARY SYNDROME   see MAMMO-RENAL SYNDROME (15435)
RESPIRATORY DISTRESS SYNDROME   26745
'RESTLESS LEGS'   see ACROMELALGIA, HEREDITARY (10230)
RETICULAR DYSGENESIA (CONGENITAL ALEUKIA)   26750
*RETICULOENDOTHELIOSIS (X-LINKED)   31250
RETICULOENDOTHELIOSIS, FAMILIAL, WITH EOSINOPHILIA   see RETICULOSIS, FAMILIAL HISTI-
OCYSTIC (26770)
*RETICULOSIS, FAMILIAL HISTIOCYTIC (OR HEMOPHAGOCYTIC)   26770
RETINA, LATTICE DEGENERATION OF   see LATTICE DEGENERATION OF RETINA LEADING TO
RETINAL DETACHMENT (15050)
*RETINAL APLASIA   17990
RETINAL APLASIA   see AMAUROSIS CONGENITA OF LEBER (24000, 24010)
RETINAL APLASIA AND RENAL DYSPLASIA   see RENAL DYSPLASIA AND RETINAL APLASIA
(26690)
*RETINAL ARTERIES, TORTUOSITY OF   18000
RETINAL COLOBOMA   see AORTIC ARCH INTERRUPTION, FACIAL PALSY AND RETINAL COLO-
BOMA (10755)
*RETINAL CONE DEGENERATION   18002
*RETINAL DETACHMENT   18005
RETINAL DETACHMENT AND OCCIPITAL ENCEPHALOCELE   26775
RETINAL DETACHMENT   see RETINOSCHISIS (31270), PSEUDOGLIOMA (26420), RETINITIS PIGMEN-
TOSA (26800, 31260), LATTICE DEGENERATION OF RETINA LEADING TO RETINAL DETACHMENT
(15050), ARTHRO-OPHTHALMOPATHY, HEREDITARY PROGRESSIVE (10830), MYOPIA (16070),
EHLERS-DANLOS SYNDROME (13000, 22540, 30520)
RETINAL DYSPLASIA OF REESE   see REESE RETINAL DYSPLASIA (26640)
RETINAL DYSTROPHY, RETICULAR PIGMENTARY, OF POSTERIOR POLE   26780
RETINAL DYSTROPHY   see CHOROIDEREMIA (30310), MACULAR DYSTROPHY (30910)
RETINAL TELANGIECTASIA AND HYPOGAMMAGLOBULINEMIA   26790
*RETINITIS PIGMENTOSA   26800
*RETINITIS PIGMENTOSA (RP)   18010
*RETINITIS PIGMENTOSA (X-LINKED)   31260
RETINITIS PIGMENTOSA AND CONGENITAL DEAFNESS   see USHER SYNDROME (27690)
*RETINOBLASTOMA   18020
RETINOPATHY, PIGMENTARY, AND MENTAL RETARDATION   26805
RETINOPATHY, VASCULAR, WITH DEAFNESS, MUSCLE WEAKNESS AND MENTAL RETARDA-
TION   see COAT'S DISEASE ETC. (21635)
*RETINOSCHISIS   31270
*RETINOSCHISIS WITH EARLY HEMERALOPIA   26810
RETRACTION SYNDROME   see DUANE SYNDROME (12680)
REYE SYNDROME   see HYPERAMMONEMIA I (23720)
RHABDOMYOLYSIS, ACUTE RECURRENT   26820
RHABDOMYOMA, CARDIAC   see TUBEROUS SCLEROSIS (19110)
RHEUMATOID ARTHRITIS   18030
RHEUMATOID-ARTHRITIS-LIKE DISORDER   see WINCHESTER DISEASE (27795)
RIB GAPS WITH MICROGNATHIA AND MENTAL RETARDATION   see CEREBRO-COSTO-MANDIBU-
LAR SYNDROME (21400)
RIBBING DISEASE (HEREDITARY MULTIPLE DIAPHYSEAL SCLEROSIS)   18040
*RIBONUCLEIC ACID, 5S (5S RNA)   18042

RIBOSEPHOSPHATE PYROPHOSPHOKINASE see PHOSPHORIBOSYLPYROPHOSPHATE SYNTHE-
TASE (17245)
*RIBOSOMAL RNA 18045
RIBOSOMAL RNA, 5S (INCLUSION HERE JUSTIFIED BY AVAILABILITY OF DATA ON NUCLEOTIDE
SEQUENCE) 26827
RIBS, BIFID see BASAL CELL NEVUS SYNDROME (10940)
RICHARD-RUNDLE SYNDROME see KETOACIDURIA, ETC. (24510)
RICHNER-HANHART SYNDROME see KERATOSIS PALMO-PLANTARIS WITH CORNEAL DYSTRO-
PHY (24480)
RICKETS, VITAMIN-D-DEPENDENT see PSEUDOVITAMIN-D-DEFICIENCY RICKETS (26470)
RICKETS see HYPOPHOSPHATEMIA (30780), VITAMIN-D-RESISTANT RICKETS (19310)
RIDGES-OFF-THE-END DERMAL PATTERN see DERMAL RIDGES-OFF-THE-END (12553)
RIEDEL'S SCLEROSING THYROIDITIS see FIBROSCLEROSIS, MULTIFOCAL (22880)
*RIEGER SYNDROME (HYPODONTIA, MESOECTODERMAL DYSGENESIS OF IRIS AND CORNEA, AND
MYOTONIC DYSTROPHY) 18050
RILEY-DAY SYNDROME see DYSAUTONOMIA, FAMILIAL (22390)
*RINGED HAIR (PILI ANNULATI) 18060
*ROBERTS SYNDROME (SEVERE ABSENCE DEFORMITIES OF LONG BONES OF LIMBS ASSOCIATED
WITH CLEFT LIP-PALATE) 26830
ROBIN SYNDROME see PIERRE ROBIN SYNDROME (26180, 31190)
ROBINOW DWARFISM 18070
ROD MYOPATHY see NEMALINE MYOPATHY (16180)
ROKITANSKY-KUSTER-HAUSER SYNDROME see VAGINA, ABSENCE OF (27700)
ROMBERG SYNDROME see HEMIFACIAL ATROPHY, PROGRESSIVE (14130)
'ROOTLESS TEETH' see DENTINE DYSPLASIA (12540)
*ROTHMUND-THOMSON SYNDROME (POIKILODERMA ATROPHICANS AND CATARACT) . . . 26840
ROTOR DISEASE see HYPERBILIRUBINEMIA III (14370)
*ROUSSY-LEVY HEREDITARY AREFLEXIC DYSTASIA 18080
ROWLEY-ROSENBERG SYNDROME (GROWTH RETARDATION, PULMONARY HYPERTENSION AND
AMINOACIDURIA) 26850
RUBINSTEIN SYNDROME (BROAD THUMBS AND GREAT TOES, CHARACTERISTIC FACIES, MENTAL
RETARDATION) 26860
RUSSELL DWARFISM see SILVER-RUSSELL DWARFISM (18240)
*RUTHERFURD SYNDROME 18090
SABRE SHINS see BOWING OF LEGS, ANTERIOR, WITH DWARFISM (21130)
SACCHAROPINURIA 26870
SACK DISEASE see EHLERS-DANLOS SYNDROME — 'ARTERIAL', 'ECCHYMOTIC' OR SACK TYPE
(13005)
SACRAL ANOMALY see ANAL-SACRAL ANOMALIES (20550)
SACRAL DEFECT WITH ANTERIOR SACRAL MENINGOCELE 31280
SADDLE NOSE see DEAFNESS WITH ECTODERMAL DYSPLASIA (12520), ROTHMUND-THOMSON
SYNDROME (26840), ECTODERMAL DYSPLASIA ANHIDROTIC (30510)
SALDINO-NOONAN DWARFISM see SKELETAL DYSPLASIA, SEVERE, WITH VISCERAL ANOMALIES
(27025)
SALDINO-NOONAN SYNDROME see POLYDACTYLY WITH NEONATAL CHONDRODYSTROPHY,
SALDINO-NOONAN TYPE (26353)
SALIVARY BASIC PROTEIN see PAROTID BASIC PROTEIN (16875)
SALIVARY PROLINE-RICH PROTEIN see PAROTID PROLINE-RICH PROTEIN (16878)
*SALIVARY SUBSTANCE, CLOSTRIDUM BOTULINUM TYPE 18095
SALT CRAVING see MITOCHONDRIAL MYOPATHY WITH SALT CRAVING (25200)
SALT-LOSING SYNDROME see ADRENAL HYPERPLASIA, HYPOADRENOCORTICISM (24020), HYPO-
ALDOSTERONISM (20340)
*SANDHOFF DISEASE, OR GM(2) GANGLIOSIDOSIS TYPE II 26880
SANFILIPPO SYNDROME see MUCOPOLYSACCHARIDOSIS III (25290)
SARCOIDOSIS 18100
SARCOMA, OSTEOGENIC see OSTEOGENIC SARCOMA (25950)
SARCOMA see CHONDROSARCOMA (21530)
SARCOMA see BONE DYSPLASIA WITH MEDULLARY FIBROSARCOMS (11225)
*SARCOSINEMIA 26890
SARCOTUBULAR MYOPATHY 26895
SATELLITE ASSOCIATION RESULTING IN FAMILIAL CHROMOSOMAL MOSAICISM 18110
*SC PHOCOMELIA SYNDROME 26900
SC(1) TRAIT OF SALIVA 18120
SCALP AND SKULL, DEFECT OF see APLASIA CUTIS CONGENITA (10760)
SCALP, ABSENCE DEFORMITY OF see ABSENCE DEFECT OF LIMBS, SCALP AND SKULL (10030)
SCAPHOCEPHALY see CRANIOSTENOSIS OR CRANIOSYNOSTOSIS (12310, 21850, 21860)
SCAPULA, CONTOUR OF VERTEBRAL BORDER OF 18130
SCAPULA, HIGH see SPRENGEL DEFORMITY (18440)
SCAPULOHUMEROPERONEAL MUSCULAR ATROPHY WITH CARDIAC CONDUCTION DEFECT . 31283
SCAPULOPERONEAL AMYOTROPHY 18140
*SCAPULOPERONEAL SYNDROME 31285
SCHAMBERG DISEASE see PIGMENTED PURPURIC ERUPTION (17290)
SCHEIE SYNDROME see MUCOPOLYSACCHARIDOSIS V (25310)
SCHEUERMANN DISEASE see OSTEODYSTROPHY AND MENTAL RETARDATION
SCHILDER DISEASE 26910
SCHILDER'S DISEASE WITH ADRENAL CHANGE see ADDISON'S DISEASE AND CEREBRAL SCLE-
ROSIS (30010)
SCHIMKE SYNDROME (PTC SYNDROME) see PHEOCHROMOCYTOMA AND AMYLOID PRODUCING
MEDULLARY THYROID CARCINOMA (17140)
SCHINZEL SYNDROME 18145
SCHIZOPHRENIA 18150
SCHMIDT SYNDROME (DIABETES MELLITUS, ADDISON DISEASE, MYXEDEMA) 26920
SCHOLZ CEREBRAL SCLEROSIS see CEREBRAL SCLEROSIS, DIFFUSE, SCHOLZ TYPE (30270)
SCHWARTZ SYNDROME see MYOTONIC MYOPATHY, DWARFISM ETC. (25580)

SKULL, DEFORMITY OF see CRANIOSTENOSIS (12310, 21850), ACROCEPHALO SYNDACTYLY (10120-10160), ACROCEPHALOPOLY SYNDACTYLY (10110, 20100)
SKUNK N-BUTYLMERCAPTAN, INABILITY TO SMELL 27035
'SLIT-EYED PEOPLE' see PTOSIS, HEREDITARY (17830)
SMELL CYANIDE, INABILITY TO see CYANIDE, INABILITY TO SMELL (30430)
SMELL KETONE COMPOUNDS, ABILITY TO 18225
SMELL-BLINDNESS see ANOSMIA (30170)
*SMITH-LEMLI-OPITZ SYNDROME 27040
SMITH-OPITZ-INBORN SYNDROME see CEREBRO-HEPATO-RENAL SYNDROME (21410)
SMITH-STRANG DISEASE see METHIONINE MALABSORPTION SYNDROME (25090)
'SNOW-CAPPED' TEETH 18230
'SNUB-NOSE' DWARFISM see DWARFISM, 'SNUB-NOSED' TYPE (22360)
SODIUM AND POTASSIUM OF ERYTHROCYTE see POTASSIUM-SODIUM DISORDER OF ERYTHRO-CYTE (26390)
SOMATOMEDIN DEFECT see PITUITARY DWARFISM II (26250)
SOMATOTROPIN see GROWTH HORMONE (13925)
*SORBITOL DEHYDROGENASE VARIANTS 18250
SORSBY SYNDROME see COLOBOMA OF MACULA WITH TYPE B BRACHYDACTYLY (12040)
SOTOS SYNDROME see CEREBRAL GIGANTISM (11760, 21380)
SOUTH AFRICAN PORPHYRIA see PORPHYRIA VARIEGATA (17620)
SPASTIC ATAXIA see ATAXIA, SPASTIC (10860)
SPASTIC DIPLEGIA, INFANTILE TYPE see SJOGREN-LARSME (27020)
SPASTIC DIPLEGIA see EPILEPSY, PHOTOGENIC, SPASTIC DIPLEGIA AND MENTAL RETARDA-TION (22680), HYPOXANTHINE QUANINE PHOSPHORIBOSYL TRANSFERASE DEFICIENCY (30800), PAINE SYNDROME (31140)
*SPASTIC DIPLEGIA, INFANTILE TYPE 27060
SPASTIC OLIGOPHRENIA see SPASTIC DIPLEGIA, INFANTILE TYPE (27060)
SPASTIC PARAPEGIA see SPINAL ARACHONORDITIS (18295)
*SPASTIC PARAPLEGIA 18260
*SPASTIC PARAPLEGIA 31290
*SPASTIC PARAPLEGIA AND RETINAL DEGENERATION 27070
SPASTIC PARAPLEGIA WITH AMYOTROPHY OF HANDS 18270
SPASTIC PARAPLEGIA WITH ASSOCIATED EXTRAPYRAMIDAL SIGNS 18280
*SPASTIC PARAPLEGIA, HEREDITARY 27080
SPASTIC PARAPLEGIA see OPTIC ATROPHY — SPASTIC PARAPLEGIA SYNDROME (31110), HYDRO-CEPHALUS DUE TO CONGENITAL STENOSIS OF AQUEDUCT OF SYLVIUS (30700)
SPASTIC PARAPLEGIA, HEREDITARY see LISSENCEPHALY SYNDROME (24720), PALLIDO-PYRAMI-DAL SYNDROME (26030)
SPASTIC PSEUDOSCLEROSIS (DISSEMINATED ENCEPHALOMYELOPATHY: CORTICOPALLIDODE-GENERATION) 27090
SPATIAL VISUALIZATION, APTITUDE FOR 31300
SPATZ-HALLERVORDEN SYNDROME see HALLERVORDEN AND SPATZ, SYNDROME OF (23420)
*SPHEROCYTOSIS, HEREDITARY 18290
SPHEROPHAKIA see WEILL-MARCHESANI SYNDROME (27760)
SPHEROPHAKIA-BRACHYMORPHIA SYNDROME see WEILL-MARCHESANI SYNDROME (27760)
SPHINGOLIPODYSTROPHY, GM(3) see GANGLIOSIDOSIS, GM(3) (23075)
SPHINGOMYELIN LIPIDOSIS see NIEMANN-PICK DISEASE (25720)
SPIEGLER-BROOKE TUMORS 31310
SPIEGLER-BROOKE TUMORS see EPITHELIOMA, HEREDITARY MULTIPLE BENIGN CYSTIC (13270)
SPIELMEYER-VOGT DISEASE see AMAUROTIC FAMILY IDIOCY, JUVENILE TYPE (20420), SAND-HOFF DISEASE (26880)
SPINA BIFIDA CYSTICA 27100
*SPINAL AND BULBAR MUSCULAR ATROPHY 31320
*SPINAL ARACHNOIDITIS 18295
SPINAL ATAXIA see HYPOGONADISM MALE, WITH ATAXIA (30740)
*SPINAL ATAXIA 31330
SPINAL EXTRADURAL CYST 27110
*SPINAL MUSCULAR ATROPHY, RYUKYUAN TYPE 27120
SPINAL MUSCULAR ATROPHY see MUSCULAR ATROPHY (15850, 15860, 25330, 25340)
*SPINOCEREBELLAR ATAXIA AND PLAQUE-LIKE DEPOSITS 18300
*SPINOCEREBELLAR ATAXIA WITH RIGIDITY AND PERIPHERAL NEUROPATHY . 18305
SPINOCEREBELLAR ATAXIA WITH EXTERNAL OPHTHALMOPLEGIA AND RETINAL DEGENERA-TION see OLIVOPONTOCEREBELLAR ATROPHY III (16450)
SPINOCEREBELLAR ATAXIA see FRIEDREICH ATAXIA (13660, 22930), CEREBELLAR ATAXIA (11720, 11730, 21290, 30250, 30260)
SPINOCEREBELLAR ATAXIA WITH BLINDNESS AND DEAFNESS 27125
SPINOCEREBELLAR ATROPHY WITH PUPILLARY PARALYSIS 18310
*SPINO-PONTINE ATROPHY 18320
SPLEEN HYPOPLASIA OR ABSENCE see ASPLENIA, WITH CARDIOVASCULAR ANOMALIES (20853)
SPLEEN, ABSENCE OF (ASPLENIA SYNDROME) 27130
*SPLENIC HYPOPLASIA 27140
SPLENO-GONADAL FUSION WITH LIMB DEFECTS AND MICROGNATHIA . . . 18330
SPLENOMEGALY WITH NEUROLOGIC DISTURBANCE see WILLVONSEDER SYNDROME (31465)
SPLENOPORTAL VASCULAR ANOMALIES 27150
SPLIT HAND WITH CLEFT PALATE AND LIP see CLEFT LIP-PALATE WITH SPLIT HAND AND FOOT (11940)
SPLIT HANDS AND FEET WITH PERCEPTIVE HEARING LOSS see DEAFMUTISM AND SPLIT HANDS AND FEET (22060)
SPLIT HAND see CLEFT HAND AND ABSENT TIBIA (11910)
SPLIT LOWER LIP 18340
SPLIT-HAND AND FOOT WITH HYPODONTIA 18350
*SPLIT-HAND DEFORMITY 18360
SPLIT-HAND DEFORMITY WITH MANDIBULOFACIAL DYSOSTOSIS 18370
SPLIT-HAND DEFORMITY see CLEFT HAND AND ABSENT TIBIA (11910)

SWEAT GLAND TUMORS OF SKIN   see SYRINGOMAS, MULTIPLE (18660)
SWEATING EXCESSIVE   see HYPERHIDROSIS, GUSTATORY (14410)
SWEATY FEET DISEASE   see ISOVALERICACIDEMIA (24350), SIDBURY SYNDROME (27000)
SWEATY FEET, ODOR LIKE   see ISOVALERICACIDEMIA (24350), SIDBURY SYNDROME (27000)
SWEDISH TYPE PORPHYRIA   see PORPHYRIA, ACUTE INTERMITTENT (17600)
SWISS TYPE AGAMMAGLOBULINEMIA   see AGAMMAGLOBULINEMIA SWISS TYPE (20250, 30040)
SWYER SYNDROME   see GONADAL DYSGENESIS XY FEMALE TYPE (30610)
SYMONDS-SHAW 'FAMILIAL CLAW FOOT WITH ABSENT DEEP TENDON REFLEXES' see
   ROUSSY-LEVY HEREDITARY AREFLEXIC DYSTASIA (18080)
SYMPHALANGISM OF TOES   18560
*SYMPHALANGISM, DISTAL   18570
*SYMPHALANGISM, PROXIMAL (HEREDITARY ABSENCE OF THE PROXIMAL INTERPHALANGEAL
   JOINTS)   18580
SYMPHALANGISM   see DIASTROPHIC DWARFISM (22260)
SYMPHYSIS PUBIS, WIDE SEPARATION OF   see CLEIDOCRANIAL DYSOSTOSIS (11970)
SYNDACTYLISM   see DEAFNESS, ECTODERMAL DYSPLASIA, POLYDACTYLISM AND SYNDACTY-
   LISM (12460), LEUKONYCHIA TOTALIS (15160), ACROCEPHALOSYNDACTYLY (10120-10160), HY-
   PEROSTOSIS CORTICALIS GENERALISATA (23910)
*SYNDACTYLY, TYPE I (ZYGODACTYLY)   18590
*SYNDACTYLY, TYPE II (SYNPOLYDACTYLY)   18600
*SYNDACTYLY, TYPE III (RING AND LITTLE FINGER SYNDACTYLY)   18610
SYNDACTYLY, TYPE IV (HASS TYPE)   18620
*SYNDACTYLY, TYPE V (SYNDACTYLY WITH METACARPAL AND METATARSAL FUSION)   . . 18630
SYNDACTYLY   see ECTODERMAL DYSPLASIA, ANHIDROTIC, WITH CLEFT LIP AND CLEFT PAL-
   ATE (12940), HYPOTRICHOSIS, SYNDACTYLY AND RETINITIS PIGMENTOSA (24200), OCULODEN-
   TODIGITAL DYSPLASIA (16420), POLAND SYNDROME (17380), SCLEROSTENOSIS (26950)
SYNDESMOPLASTIC DWARFISM   see STIFF SKIN SYNDROME (18490)
SYNECHIA WITH CLEFT PALATE   see CLEFT PALATE LATERAL SYNECHIA SYNDROME (21635)
*SYNOSTOSES (TARSAL, CARPAL AND DIGITAL)   18640
SYNOSTOSES, MULTIPLE, WITH BRACHYDACTYLY   18650
*SYNOSTOSIS, CARPAL, WITH DYSPLASTIC ELBOW JOINTS AND BRACHYDACTYLY   . . . 18655
SYNOSTOSIS   see HUMERORADIAL SYNOSTOSIS (23640)
SYNPOLYDACTYLY   see SYNDACTYLY, TYPE II (18600)
SYRINGOMAS, MULTIPLE   18660
SYRINGOMYELIA, LUMBOSACRAL   18670
SYSTEMIC CYSTIC ANGIOMATOSIS AND SEIP SYNDROME   27250
SYSTOLIC CLICK SYNDROME   see METRAL REGURGITATION (15770)
TACHYCARDIA, HYPERTENSION, MICROPHTHALMOS, HYPERGLYCINURIA   27255
TALIPES EQUINOVARUS   see CLUB FOOT (11980)
TANGIER DISEASE   see ANALPHALIPOPROTEINEMIA (20540)
*T-ANTIGEN OF SV40   18680
TAPETO-CHOROIDAL DYSTROPHY   see CHOROIDEREMIA (30310)
TAPETO-RETINAL DEGENERATION WITH ATAXIA   27260
TAPETORETINAL DEGENERATION   see HYALOIDO-TAPETORETINAL DEGENERATION OF FAVRE
   (23650)
TAR SYNDROME   see THROMBOCYTOPENIA ABSENT RADIUS SYNDROME (27400)
TARGARDT MACULAR DYSTROPHY   see MACULAR DEGENERATION, JUVENILE (24820)
TARSAL BONES, FUSION OF   see SYNOSTOSES (18640)
*TARSAL FUSION   18685
*TATSUMI FACTOR DEFICIENCY   27265
TAURINURIA   see CAMPTODACTYLY (11420)
TAURODONTISM   27270
TAY-SACHS DISEASE (JUVENILE TYPE)   see GANGLIOSIDOSIS, GM(2), TYPE III, OR JUVENILE TYPE
   (23070)
TAY-SACHS DISEASE, AB VARIANT   27275
TAY-SACHS DISEASE, JUVENILE TYPE   27277
*TAY-SACHS DISEASE: GM2-GANGLIOSIDOSIS, TYPE I   27280
TAY-SACHS-LIKE DISEASE   see SANDHOFF DISEASE (26880)
TEETH PRESENT AT BIRTH (NATAL TEETH)   see PACHYONYCHIA CONGENITA (16720), ELLIS-VAN
   CREVELD SYNDROME (22550), HALLERMAN-STREIFF SYNDROME (23410)
TEETH, FUSED   27300
TEETH, GENETIC VARIATION AND DISORDER OF   18690
TEETH, MISSING   see CANINE, ABSENCE OF UPPER PERMANENT (11460), LATERAL INCISORS,
   ABSENCE OF (15040), ANODONTIA, PARTIAL (10660), WISDOM TEETH, ABSENCE OF (19410),
   CENTRAL INCISORS, ABSENCE OF (30240), RUTHERFURD SYNDROME (18090)
*TEETH, ODD SHAPES OF   18700
TEETH, PREMATURE EXFOLIATION OR LOSS OF   see ELLIS-VAN CREVELD SYNDROME (22550),
   HYPOPHOSPHATASIA (24150)
TEETH, PRESENT AT BIRTH (NATAL TEETH)   18705
TEETH, SNOW-CAPPED   see SNOW-CAPPED TEETH (18230)
TEETH, SUPERNUMERARY   18710
TEETH   see INCONTINENTIA PIGMENTI (30830), OCULODENTODIGITAL DYSPLASIA (16420)
TEETH, ABSENCE OF   31350
TEETH, HEREDITARY BROWN   see DENTINOGENESIS IMPERFECTA (12550)
TELANGIECTASES OF BRAIN   18720
*TELANGIECTASIA, HEREDITARY BENIGN   18726
*TELANGIECTASIA, HEREDITARY HEMORRHAGIC, OF RENDU, OSLER AND WEBER   18730
TELANGIECTASIA   see ATAXIA-TELANGIECTASIA (20890), TRYPTOPHANURIA WITH DWARFISM
   (27610)
TELANGIECTATIC ERYTHEMA   see BLOOM SYNDROME (21090)
TELECANTHUS   18735
TELECANTHUS   see ALAR-NASAL CARTILAGES, COLOBOMA OF, WITH TELECANTHUS (20300)
TELECANTHUS WITH ASSOCIATED ABNORMALITIES   31360
TEMPELS, DYSPLASTIC SKIN OF   see FOCAL FACIAL DERMAL DYSPLASIA (13650)

TEMPORAL-CENTRAL FOCAL EPILEPSY   see CENTRALOPATHIC EPILEPSY (11710)
*TENDO CALCANEUS, SHORT 18737
TENDON, CONGENITAL SHORT FLEXOR   see MOUTH, INABILITY TO OPEN COMPLETELY (15830)
TERATOMA, PRESACRAL   see PRESACRAL TERATOMA (17645)
TESTES, ABSENCE OF 27310
TESTES, ABSENCE OF   see LOWE OCULO-CEREBRO-RENAL SYNDROME (30900)
*TESTICULAR FEMINIZATION SYNDROME 31370
TESTICULAR FEMINIZATION, INCOMPLETE TYPE 27320
TESTICULAR FEMINIZATION, INCOMPLETE TYPE 31380
TESTICULAR TORSION 18740
TESTICULAR TUMORS 27330
TETANY   see HYPOMAGNESAMIC TETANY (30760)
TETRALOGY OF FALLOT 18750
TETRAMELIC DEFICIENCIES, ECTODERMAL DYSPLASIA, DEFORMED EARS, AND OTHER ABNOR-
MALITIES 27340
TETRAZOLIUM OXIDASE   see INDOPHENOL OXIDASE
TETRAZOLIUM OXIDASE VARIANTS   see INDOPHENOLOXIDASE A AND B (14744, 14745)
THALASSEMIA MINOR   see POLYCYTHEMIA, BENIGN FAMILIAL, OF CHILDREN (26340)
THALASSEMIAS 27350
THALIDOMIDE SUSCEPTIBILITY 27360
*THANATOPHORIC DWARFISM 27365
THANATOPHORIC DWARFISM   see SKELETAL DYSPLASIA, SEVERE, WITH VISCERAL ANOMALIES
(27025)
THIAMINE-RESPONSIVE INBORN ERROR OF METABOLISM   see MAPLE SYRUP URINE DISEASE
(24860)
THIEMANN DISEASE   see OSTEOARTHROPATHY OF FINGERS, FAMILIAL (16570)
THIEMANN EPIPHYSEAL DISEASE 27370
THOMSEN SYNDROME   see ROTHMUND-THOMSON SYNDROME (26840), MYOTONIA CONGENITA
(16080)
THORACIC DYSOSTOSIS, ISOLATED 18775
THORACIC DYSTROPHY   see ASPHYXIATING THORACIC DYSTROPHY OF THE NEWBORN (20850)
THORACIC-PELVIC-PHALANGEAL DYSTROPHY   see ASPHYXIATING THORACIC DYSTROPHY OF
THE NEWBORN (20850)
THORAX DEFORMITY AND LOW BIRTH WEIGHT DWARFISM   see THREE M'S SYNDROME (27375)
*THREE M (3M) SYNDROME 27375
*THROMBASTHENIA OF GLANZMANN AND NAEGELI 18780
*THROMBASTHENIA OF GLANZMANN AND NAEGELI 27380
*THROMBASTHENIA-THROMBOCYTOPENIA, HEREDITARY 18790
*THROMBOCYTOPENIA 18800
*THROMBOCYTOPENIA 27390
*THROMBOCYTOPENIA 31390
THROMBOCYTOPENIA, TRANSIENT NEONATAL   see PLATELET GROUP — KO SYSTEM (17350)
*THROMBOCYTOPENIA — ABSENT RADIUS (TAR) SYNDROME 27400
THROMBOCYTOPENIA DUE TO CONGENITAL ABSENCE OF 'THROMBOPOIETIN' 27403
THROMBOCYTOPENIA   see ALDRICH SYNDROME (30100), HEMANGIOMA-THROMBOCYTOPENIA
SYNDROME (14100), GLYCINEMIA (23200), CYSTATHIONINURIA (24950), HEMOGLOBIN KOLN
(14170)
THROMBOCYTOPENIA WITH ELEVATED SERUM IGA AND RENAL DISEASE 31400
THROMBOCYTOPENIA-GIANT HEMANGIOMA SYNDROME (KASSABACH-MERRITT SYNDROME) -
see HEMANGIOMA-THROMBOCYTOPENIA SYNDROME (14100)
*THROMBOCYTOPENIC THROMBOPATHY 27410
THROMBOEMBOLISM, TENDENCY TO   see ANTITHROMBIN III DEFICIENCY (20720)
THROMBOPATHY OF GLANZMANN   see THROMBASTHENIA OF GLANZMANN AND NAEGELI
(18780, 27380)
THROMBOPHILIA 18805
THROMBOPHILIA   see FIBRINOGEN VARIANTS (13480)
THROMBOTIC VASCULAR DISEASE   see HOMOCYSTINURIA (23620), FACTOR V EXCESS (13440)
THUMB ANOMALY   see HYDROCEPHALUS DUE TO CONGENITAL STENOSIS OF AQUEDUCT OF
SYLVIUS (30700)
THUMB DEFORMITY 18810
THUMB, DISTAL HYPEREXTENSIBILITY OF 27420
THUMB, STUB   see BRACHYDACTYLY, TYPE D (11310)
THUMBNAILS, ABSENT 18820
THUMB   see TRIPHALANGEAL THUMB (19050)
THUMB, CONGENITAL CLASPED 31410
THUMBS, ABNORMAL   see CLEFT LIP-PALATE WITH ABNORMAL THUMBS AND MICROCEPHALY
(21610)
THUMBS, ADDUCTED   see ADDUCTED THUMBS SYNDROME (20155), X-LINKED HYDROCEPHALUS
(30700)
THUMBS, BROAD   see OTO-PALATO-DIGITAL SYNDROME (31130), RUBINSTEIN SYNDROME (26860)
THYMIC AGENESIS   see THYMUS AND PARATHYROIDS, ABSENCE OF (18840)
THYMIC ALYMPHOPLASIA   see AGAMMAGLOBULINEMIA, SWISS OR ALYMPHOCYTOTIC TYPE
(20250)
THYMIC APLASIA   see AGAMMAGLOBULINEMIA, SWISS OR ALYMPHOCYTOTIC TYPE (20250)
THYMIC APLASIA, OR DYSPLASIA   see IMMUNE DEFECT DUE TO ABSENCE OF THYMUS (24270)
THYMIC DYSPLASIA   see 'ACHONDROPLASIA' AND SWISS-TYPE AGAMMAGLOBULINEMIA (20090)
THYMIC EPITHELIAL HYPOPLASIA   see AGAMMAGLOBULINEMIA, SWISS TYPE (30040)
*THYMIDINE KINASE 18830
THYMOMA, FAMILIAL 27423
THYMUS AND PARATHYROIDS, ABSENCE OF (DIGEORGE SYNDROME) 18840
THYMUS, ABSENCE OF   see IMMUNE DEFECT DUE TO ABSENCE OF THYMUS (24270)
THYROGLOBULIN SYNTHESIS (DIMINISHED OR ALTERED) 27425
THYROID APLASIA   see CUTIS VERTICIS GYRATA, ETC. (30420)
THYROID AUTOANTIBODIES 18850

THYROID CANCER see PHEOCHROMOCYTOMA AND AMYLOID-PRODUCING MEDULLARY THY-
    ROID CARCINOMA (17140), POLYPOSIS, INTESTINAL III (17530)
THYROID DYSFUNCTION see MYXEDEMA (25590)
THYROID DYSGENESIS see CRETINISM, ATHYREOTIC (21870)
THYROID HORMONE UNRESPONSIVENESS 27430
*THYROID HORMONOGENESIS, GENETIC DEFECT IN, I (ACCUMULATION, TRANSPORT OR TRAP-
    PING DEFECT) 27440
*THYROID HORMONOGENESIS, GENETIC DEFECT IN, IIA (ORGANIFICATION DEFECT I) . . . 27450
*THYROID HORMONOGENESIS, GENETIC DEFECT IN, IIB (ORGANIFICATION DEFECT II) . . . 27460
*THYROID HORMONOGENESIS, GENETIC DEFECT IN, III (COUPLING DEFECT) 27470
*THYROID HORMONOGENESIS, GENETIC DEFECT IN, IV (DEFECT OF IODOTYROSINE DEHALOGE-
    NASE, OR DEIODINASE) 27480
*THYROID HORMONOGENESIS, GENETIC DEFECT IN, V (PLASMA IODOPROTEIN DEFECT) . . . 27490
THYROIDITIS, RIEDEL SCLEROSING see FIBROSCLEROSIS, MULTIFOCAL (22880)
THYROIDITIS see HASHIMOTO STRUMA, THYROID AUTOANTIBODIES (18850)
THYROTOXICOSIS (GRAVES DISEASE) 27500
*THYROTROPIN DEFICIENCY, ISOLATED 27510
THYROTROPIN, UNRESPONSIVENESS TO 27520
*THYROXINE-BINDING GLOBULIN (TBG) OF SERUM, VARIANTS OF 18860
*THYROXINE-BINDING GLOBULIN (TBG) OF SERUM, VARIANTS OF 31420
TIBIA VARA (BLOUNT DISEASE, OR OSTEOCHONDROSIS DEFORMANS TIBIAE) 18870
TIBIA VARA see OSTEOCHONDROSIS DEFORMANS TIBIAE, FAMILIAL INFANTILE TYPE (25920)
TIBIA, ABSENCE OF see FIBULA AND ULNA DUPLICATION OF ETC. (13575)
TIBIA, ABSENCE OF, WITH POLYDACTYLY 18874
TIBIA, ABSENT see CLEFT HAND AND ABSENT TIBIA (11910)
TIBIA, HYPOPLASIA OF, WITH POLYDACTYLY 18877
*TIBIAL TORSION, BILATERAL MEDIAL 18880
TIC DOULOUREUX see TRIGEMINAL NEURALGIA (19040)
TIC, FACIAL see FACIAL SPASM (13430)
TOE, FIFTH ROTATED 18890
TOE, FIFTH, NUMBER OF PHALANGES IN 18900
TOE, MISSHAPEN 18910
TOES, RELATIVE LENGTH OF 1ST AND 2ND 18920
TONGUE CURLING, FOLDING, OR ROLLING 18930
TONGUE, ABSENT FUNGIFORM PALLILLAE OF see DYSAUTONOMIA (22390)
TONGUE, BIG see EMG SYNDROME (22560)
TONGUE, GEOGRAPHIC AND FISSURED see GEOGRAPHIC TONGUE AND FISSURED TONGUE
    (13740)
TONGUE, LOBATE see MOHR SYNDROME (25210)
*TONGUE, PIGMENTED FUNGIFORM PAPILLAE OF 27525
TONGUE, PROTRUDING see FACIAL ABNORMALITIES ETC. (22727)
TONGUE, SCROTAL see SCROTAL TONGUE (18190)
TOOTH ERUPTION, FAILURE OF see RUTHERFURD SYNDROME (18090)
TOOTH-AND-NAIL SYNDROME (DYSPLASIA OF NAILS WITH HYPODONTIA) 18950
TORTICOLLIS 18960
TORTICOLLIS, KELOIDS, CRYPTORCHIDISM, AND RENAL DYSPLASIA 31430
TORTION DYSTONIA see DYSTONIA MUSCULORUM DEFORMANS (12810, 22450)
TORTUOSITY OF RETINAL ARTERIES see RETINAL ARTERIES, TORTUOSITY OF (18000)
*TORUS PALATINUS AND TORUS MANDIBULARIS 18970
TOXEMIA OF PREGNANCY 18980
TOXOPACHYOSTEOSE DIAPHYSAIRE TIBIO-PERONIERE see BOWING OF LEGS, ANTERIOR, WITH
    DWARFISM (21130)
TRACHEOBRONCHOMEGALY 27530
TRACHEO-ESOPHAGEAL FISTULA see CLEFT LARYNX, POSTERIOR (21580)
TRACHEOESOPHAGEAL FISTULA 18986
TRACHEOESOPHAGEAL FISTULA WITH ESOPHAGEAL ATRESIA 18990
TRANSAMINASE see GLUTAMIC-OXALOACETIC TRANSAMINASE (13820) AND GLUTAMIC-PY-
    RUVIC TRANSAMINASE (13827)
TRANSCOBALAMIN I DEFICIENCY see B12-BINDING ALPHA GLOBULIN, DEFICIENCY OF (21170)
*TRANSCOBALAMIN II DEFICIENCY 27535
*TRANSFERRIN 19000
TRANSFERRIN DEFICIENCY see ATRANSFERRINEMIA (20930)
TRANSGLUTAMINASE, DEFICIENCY OF see FIBRINOGEN CROSS-LINKAGE DEFECT (22845)
TREACHER COLLINS SYNDROME see MANDIBULO-FACIAL DYSOSTOSIS (15440)
*TREMBLING CHIN 19010
TREMBLING, FAMILIAL see ORAL-FACIAL-DIGITAL SYNDROME (31120)
TREMOR see ANOSMIA (30170)
TREMOR OF INTENTION, ATAXIA AND LIPOFUSCINOSIS 19020
*TREMOR, HEREDITARY ESSENTIAL 19030
TRIAD SYNDROME see ABDOMINAL MUSCLES, ABSENCE OF, ETC. (10010)
*TRICARBOXYLIC ACID CYCLE, DEFECT OF 27537
TRICHO-DENTO-OSSEOUS SYNDROME see ENAMEL HYPOPLASIA WITH CURLY HAIR (13080)
TRICHOEPITHELIOMA, MULTIPLE see EPITHELIOMA, HEREDITARY MULTIPLE BENIGN CYSTIC
    (13270)
TRICHOMEGALY 19033
TRICHOMEGALY (EXCESSIVE GROWTH OF EYELASHES AND BROW HAIR) WITH MENTAL RETAR-
    DATION, DWARFISM AND PIGMENTARY DEGENERATION OF RETINA 27540
TRICHOPHYTON RUBRUM INFECTION see NEUTROPHIL CHEMOTACTIC DEFECT (16282)
*TRICHORHINOPHALANGEAL SYNDROME 19035
TRICHORHINOPHALANGEAL SYNDROME 27550
TRICHORRHEXIS INVAGINATA, OR NODOSA see NETHERTON DISEASE (25650)
TRICHORRHEXIS NODOSA SYNDROME 27555
TRICHORRHEXIS NODOSA see MENKES SYNDROME (30940), ARGININOSUCCINICACIDURIA
    (20790)